SUBJECT ENTRY SECTION

Sample Entry

D1543860

TRUTH DISCLOSURE

Ruddick, William. Hope and deception. *Bioethics.* 1999
Jul; 13(3–4): 343–357. 16 fn. BE61884.

allowing to die; autonomy; beneficence; children; *deception;
emotions; family members; futility; motivation; parents;
patients; physician patient relationship; physicians;
placebos; principle–based ethics; professional family
relationship; prognosis; *risks and benefits; terminally ill;
trust; *truth disclosure; *hope

Convinced of hope's therapeutic benefits, physicians routinely
support patients' false hopes, often with family collusion
and vague, euphemistic diagnoses and prognoses, if not
overt lies. Bioethicists charge them with paternalistic violations of Patient Autonomy. There are, I think, too many
morally significant exceptions to accept the physician's
rationales, or the bioethicist's criticisms, stated sweepingly.
Physicians need to take account of the harms caused by loss
of hopes, especially false hopes due to deception, as well as
of the harms of successfully maintained deceptive hopes.
As for autonomy, hopes—even if based on deception—can
protect and enhance autonomy, understood broadly as the
capacity to lead a chosen or embraced life. Deception
aside, patients' hopes often rest on beliefs about *possible*
rather than *probable* outcomes—beliefs themselves supported by optimism, 'denial', or self-deception. Such 'possibility–hopes' may conflict with physicians' often more
fact-sensitive 'probability hopes.' To resolve such conflicts
physicians may try to 'down-shift' patients' or parents'
hopes to lesser, more realistic hopes. Alternatively, physicians may alter or enlarge their own professional hopes to
include the 'vital hopes' that define the lives of patients or
parents, as well as 'survival hopes' needed to face and bear
the loss of loved ones, especially children. A principle of
Hope–giving might help guide such sympathetic hope-
accommodations. More generally, it would give Hope a
distinct place among Beneficence, Autonomy, and the other
moral factors already highlighted by canonical principles of
Medical Ethics. To formulate such a principle, however, we
will need a collective Project Hope to pursue deeper
philosophical and psychological studies.

BIBLIOGRAPHY
OF
BIOETHICS

BIBLIOGRAPHY
OF
BIOETHICS

Volume 26

Editors

LeRoy Walters
Tamar Joy Kahn

Associate Editors
Frances Amitay Abramson
Jeanne Ryan Furcron
Hannelore S. Ninomiya
Cecily Orr Nuckols

KENNEDY INSTITUTE OF ETHICS
GEORGETOWN UNIVERSITY
Box 571212
WASHINGTON, DC 20057-1212

Publication of the annual *Bibliography of Bioethics* is a project
of the Kennedy Institute of Ethics, Georgetown University.

ISSN 0363-0161
ISBN 1-883913-06-3

This publication was supported by funds provided under
Contract N01 LM73514 with the National Library of Medicine,
and under Grant 5 P41 HG01115-06 from the National
Human Genome Research Institute.

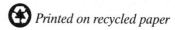 *Printed on recycled paper*

Contents

Staff ix

Editorial Advisory Board xi

Introduction 3
    The Field of Bioethics
    The Scope of the Bibliography
    Arrangement of the Bibliography
    Acknowledgments

List of Journals Cited 13

Subject Entry Section 21

    Abortion 21
        Attitudes
        Financial Support
        Foreign Countries
        Legal Aspects
        Minors
        Religious Aspects

    Advance Directives 41

    AIDS 49
        Confidentiality
        Health Personnel
        Human Experimentation
        Testing and Screening

    Allowing to Die 68
        Attitudes
        Infants
        Legal Aspects
        Religious Aspects

    Animal Experimentation 88

    Artificial Insemination 94

    Behavior Control 96

    Behavioral Genetics 98

    Behavioral Research 99
        Ethics Committees
        Foreign Countries
        Minors
        Regulation
        Research Design
        *Special Populations**

    Bioethics 103
        Codes of Ethics
        Education

    Biomedical Research 124

    Biomedical Technologies 133

    Blood Donation 137

CONTENTS

Capital Punishment 139

Cloning 139

Confidentiality 148
Legal Aspects
Mental Health

Contraception 156
Minors

Determination of Death 160
Brain Death

DNA Fingerprinting 165

Electroconvulsive Therapy 166

Embryo and Fetal Research 166

Ethicists and Ethics Committees 173

Eugenics 179

Euthanasia 184
Attitudes
Legal Aspects
Religious Aspects

Fetuses 198

Force Feeding 203

Fraud and Misconduct 203

Gene Therapy 213

Genetic Counseling 216

Genetic Intervention 220

Genetic Research 228

Genetic Screening 237

Genetic Services 256

Genome Mapping 258

Health 263

Health Care 270
Economics
Foreign Countries
Rights

Human Experimentation 303
Ethics Committees
Foreign Countries
Informed Consent
Minors
Regulation
Research Design
*Special Populations**

Immunization 353

In Vitro Fertilization 355

Informed Consent 357
Mentally Disabled
Minors

Involuntary Commitment 368
Foreign Countries
Minors

Life Extension 370

Mass Screening 370

Medical Ethics 373
Codes of Ethics
Education

Mental Health 379

Nursing Ethics 381
Education

Occupational Health 383

Organ and Tissue Donation 384

Organ and Tissue Transplantation 395

Patenting Life Forms 404

Patient Access to Records 405

Patient Care 406
Aged
Drugs
Mentally Disabled
Minors

Patients' Rights 432
Mentally Disabled

Personhood 434

Population Control 437

Prenatal Diagnosis 437

Prenatal Injuries 443

Professional Ethics 445
Codes of Ethics
Education

Professional Patient Relationship 450

Public Health 461

Recombinant DNA Research 465
Regulation

Reproduction 467

Reproductive Technologies 471

CONTENTS

Resource Allocation 481
   Biomedical Technologies

Resuscitation Orders 494

Selection for Treatment 499

Sex Determination 506

Sex Preselection 507

Sterilization 508
   Mentally Disabled

Suicide 511

Surrogate Mothers 529

Terminal Care 530
   Hospices

Torture 541

Treatment Refusal 542
   Mentally Disabled
   Minors

Truth Disclosure 549

War 552

Wrongful Life 553

Author Index 557

*The subheading *Special Populations* includes such groups as the aged, the mentally disabled, the terminally ill, prisoners, minority groups, and women.

Staff

LeRoy Walters, Ph.D.
Tamar Joy Kahn, M.L.S.
Editors

Doris M. Goldstein, M.A., M.L.S.
Director of Library and Information Services

Frances Amitay Abramson, M.A., M.S.
Jeanne Ryan Furcron, M.L.S.
Hannelore S. Ninomiya, M.A., M.L.S.
Cecily Orr Nuckols, M.L.S., M.A.
Bibliographers

Patricia C. Martin, M.A.
Data Entry Coordinator

Susan Cartier Poland, J.D.
Legal Research Associate

Laura Jane Bishop, Ph.D.
Harriet Gray, M.L.S.
Research Staff

Jonathan J. Boyles, B.A.
Legal Research Assistant

Kathleen Reynolds, MAT, M.A.
Administrative Officer

Hila Hanif
Student Assistant

Editorial Advisory Board

INTRODUCTION

INTRODUCTION

The Field of Bioethics

Bioethics can be defined as the systematic study of value questions that arise in health care delivery and in biomedicine. Specific bioethical issues that have recently received national and international attention include euthanasia, assisted suicide, new reproductive technologies, cloning, human experimentation, genetic engineering, abortion, informed consent, acquired immunodeficiency syndrome (AIDS), organ donation and transplantation, and managed care and other concerns in the allocation of health care resources.

As this list of topics suggests, the field of bioethics includes several dimensions. The first is the ethics of the professional patient relationship. Traditionally, the accent has been on the duties of health professionals—duties that, since the time of Hippocrates, have frequently been delineated in codes of professional ethics. In more recent times the rights of patients have also received considerable attention. Research ethics, the study of value problems in biomedical and behavioral research, constitutes a second dimension of bioethics. During the 20th century, as both the volume and visible achievements of such research have increased, new questions have arisen concerning the investigator-subject relationship and the potential social impact of biomedical and behavioral research and technology. In recent years a third dimension of bioethics has emerged—the quest to develop reasonable public policy guidelines for both the delivery of health care and the allocation of health care resources, as well as for the conduct of research.

No single academic discipline is adequate to discuss these various dimensions of bioethics. For this reason bioethics has been, since its inception in the late 1960s, a cross-disciplinary field. The primary participants in the interdisciplinary discussion have been physicians and other health professionals, biologists, psychologists, sociologists, lawyers, historians, and philosophical and religious ethicists.

During the past thirty years there has been a rapid growth of academic, professional, and public interest in the field of bioethics. One evidence of this interest is the establishment of numerous research institutes and teaching programs in bioethics, both in the United States and abroad. In recent years, professional societies, federal and state legislatures, and the courts have also turned increasing attention to problems in the field. In addition, during the past several years there has been a veritable explosion of literature on bioethical issues.

The literature of bioethics appears in widely scattered sources and is reported in diverse indexes which employ a bewildering variety of subject headings. This *Bibliography* is the product of a unique information retrieval system designed to identify the central issues of bioethics, to develop an indexing language appropriate to the field, and to provide comprehensive, cross-disciplinary coverage of current English-language materials on bioethical topics.

The Scope of the Bibliography

This twenty-sixth volume of the *Bibliography of Bioethics* includes materials which discuss the ethical aspects of the following major topics and subtopics:[1]

BIOETHICS, IN GENERAL
PROFESSIONAL ETHICS
    Codes of Ethics
    Medical Ethics
    Nursing Ethics
ETHICISTS AND ETHICS COMMITTEES
    Clinical Ethics Committees
    Research Ethics Committees
PROFESSIONAL PATIENT RELATIONSHIP
    Confidentiality
    Informed Consent
    Patients' Rights
    Treatment Refusal
    Truth Disclosure
HEALTH CARE AND PUBLIC HEALTH AIDS
    Care of Special Populations
    Managed Care Programs
    Resource Allocation
REPRODUCTION
    Abortion
    Contraception
    Prenatal Diagnosis
    Prenatal Injuries
    Sterilization
REPRODUCTIVE TECHNOLOGIES
    Artificial Insemination
    Cloning
    In Vitro Fertilization
    Surrogate Mothers
GENETIC INTERVENTION AND RESEARCH
    Eugenics
    Gene Therapy
    Genetic Counseling

    Genetic Research
    Genetic Screening
    Genome Mapping
    Patenting Life Forms
ORGAN AND TISSUE DONATION AND
    TRANSPLANTATION
    Fetal Tissue Donation
DEATH AND DYING
    Active Euthanasia
    Advance Directives
    Allowing to Die
    Assisted Suicide
    Determination of Death
    Resuscitation Orders
    Right to Die
    Terminal Care
MENTAL HEALTH THERAPIES
    Behavior Control
    Involuntary Commitment
    Psychoactive Drugs
HUMAN EXPERIMENTATION
    Behavioral Research
    Embryo and Fetal Research
    Research on Special Populations
ANIMAL EXPERIMENTATION
    Transgenic Animals
BIOMEDICAL RESEARCH
FRAUD AND MISCONDUCT
    Scientific Misconduct
BIOMEDICINE AND VIOLENCE
    Biological and Nuclear Warfare
    Torture.

The *Bibliography* seeks to cite all substantive English-language materials that discuss ethical aspects of the topics and subtopics listed above. It therefore incorporates a variety of media and literary forms, including journal and newspaper articles, monographs, essays in books, court decisions, bills, laws, audiovisual materials, and unpublished documents. This twenty-sixth volume of the *Bibliography* indexes documents[2] that were published since 1975, concentrating primarily on documents published in 1998 and 1999.

A cross-disciplinary monitoring system has been devised in an effort to secure documents falling within the subject-matter scope outlined above. Among the reference tools and databases the staff searches for pertinent citations are the following:

Abortion Law Reporter
AGRICOLA
AIDSLINE
All England Law Reports (subject index)
ATLA Religion Database
BioLaw
Bowker's Books in Print
Choice

Clearinghouse Review
Cumulative Index to Nursing and Allied Health
    Literature (CINAHL)
Current Contents: Clinical Medicine
Current Contents: Social and Behavioral Sciences
Current Work in the History of Medicine
Dominion Law Reports (subject index)
ERIC

---

[1] Several additional topics are closely related to the field of bioethics but have not been included in the *Bibliography*. Among these are human sexuality, ecology, and world hunger.

[2] In this Introduction the word "document" is used to refer to both print and nonprint materials.

GAO Reports, Testimony, Correspondence and Other
   Publications
Global Books in Print On Disc
GPO Access
HSTAR
Humanities Index
Index to Canadian Legal Periodical Literature
Index to Foreign Legal Periodicals
Library Journal
MEDLINE
Mental and Physical Disability Law Reporter

New Titles in Bioethics
PAIS INTERNATIONAL
PHILOSOPHER'S INDEX
POPLINE
PsycLIT
Readers' Guide to Periodical Literature
Social Sciences Index
SOCIOLOGICAL ABSTRACTS
Specialty Law Digest: Health Care Law
UMI ProQuest Digital Dissertations
WorldCat.

In addition, the *Bibliography* staff directly monitors over 150 journals and newspapers for articles and citations falling within the scope of bioethics. Please note, however, that the journal articles cited in this volume are actually drawn from 520 journals, not limited to the following directly monitored publications:

Academic Medicine
Accountability in Research
AIDS and Public Policy Journal
AIDS Policy and Law
America
American Journal of Ethics and Medicine
American Journal of Human Genetics
American Journal of Law and Medicine
American Journal of Nursing
American Journal of Psychiatry
American Journal of Public Health
Annals of Health Law
Annals of Internal Medicine
Annals of the Royal College of Physicians and Surgeons
   of Canada
Archives of Family Medicine
Archives of Internal Medicine
Assia—Jewish Medical Ethics
ATLA: Alternatives to Laboratory Animals
Bioethics
BMJ (British Medical Journal)
Brandeis Law Journal
British Journal of Nursing
Bulletin of Medical Ethics
California Law Review
Cambridge Quarterly of Healthcare Ethics
Canadian Medical Association Journal
Christian Bioethics
Christian Century
Clinical Ethics Report
Columbia Law Review
Community Genetics
Conservative Judaism
Death Studies
DePaul Journal of Health Care Law
Dolentium Hominum
Ethics
Ethics and Behavior
Ethics and Medicine: A Christian Perspective
Eubios Journal of Asian and International Bioethics
European Journal of Genetics in Society
European Journal of Health Law
Fetal Diagnosis and Therapy
First Things: A Monthly Journal of Religion and Public
   Life

Free Inquiry
Gene Therapy
Genetic Resource
Genetic Testing
Genetics in Medicine
GeneWatch
Georgetown Law Journal
Harvard Law Review
Hastings Center Report
Health Affairs
Health and Human Rights
Health Care Analysis
Health Law in Canada
Health Matrix
Health Policy
Health Progress
HEC (HealthCare Ethics Committee) Forum
Human Gene Therapy
Human Life Review
Human Reproduction
Human Reproduction and Genetic Ethics
Human Research Report
Humane Health Care International
Hypatia
International Digest of Health Legislation
International Journal of Applied Philosophy
International Journal of Bioethics
International Journal of Health Services
International Journal of Law and Psychiatry
International Journal of Technology Assessment in
   Health Care
IRB: A Review of Human Subjects Research
Issues in Law and Medicine
Issues in Science and Technology
JAMA
Joint Commission Journal on Quality Improvement
Journal of Advanced Nursing
Journal of Applied Philosophy
Journal of Business Ethics
Journal of Clinical Ethics
Journal of Contemporary Health Law and Policy
Journal of Ethics
Journal of Ethics, Law and Aging
Journal of General Internal Medicine
Journal of Genetic Counseling

Journal of Halacha and Contemporary Society
Journal of Health Politics, Policy and Law
Journal of Law and Health
Journal of Law and Medicine
Journal of Law, Medicine and Ethics
Journal of Legal Medicine
Journal of Medical Ethics
Journal of Medical Genetics
Journal of Medical Humanities
Journal of Medicine and Philosophy
Journal of Nursing Law
Journal of Palliative Care
Journal of Psychiatry and Law
Journal of Public Health Policy
Journal of Religion and Health
Journal of Religious Ethics
Journal of Social Philosophy
Journal of the American Academy of Psychiatry and the
    Law
Journal of the American Geriatrics Society
Journal of the American Medical Women's Association
Kennedy Institute of Ethics Journal
Lancet
Linacre Quarterly
Literature and Medicine
Medical Ethics and Bioethics
Medical Humanities Review
Medical Law International
Medical Law Review
Medical Trial Technique Quarterly
Medicine and Global Survival
Medicine and Law
Medicine, Conflict and Survival
Medicine, Health Care and Philosophy
Mental Retardation
Michigan Law Review
Milbank Quarterly
Minnesota Medicine
Nature
Nature Biotechnology
Nature Genetics
Nature Medicine

NCEHR (formerly NCBHR) Communiqué (National
    Council on Ethics in Human Research)
New England Journal of Medicine
New Scientist
New York Times
New York University Law Review
Newsweek
Notre Dame Journal of Law, Ethics and Public Policy
Nursing Ethics
Omega: Journal of Death and Dying
Origins
Perspectives in Biology and Medicine
Pharos
Philosophy and Public Affairs
Philosophy and Public Policy
Politics and the Life Sciences
Princeton Journal of Bioethics
Psychiatric Services
Public Affairs Quarterly
Responsive Community
Science
Science and Engineering Ethics
Science News
Science, Technology, and Human Values
The Sciences
Second Opinion
Social Justice Research
Social Philosophy and Policy
Social Science and Medicine
Social Theory and Practice
Society and Animals
Stanford Law Review
Theoretical Medicine and Bioethics
Time
Tradition
UCLA Law Review
University of Chicago Law Review
U.S. News and World Report
Virginia Law Review
Western Journal of Medicine
Women's Health Issues
Yale Law Journal.

This twenty-sixth volume of the *Bibliography* includes bibliographic data for 3,679 documents, published between 1975 and 2000. Most were published in 1998 (1,413) and 1999 (938).

All documents cited by the *Bibliography* are in the collection of the National Reference Center for Bioethics Literature (NRCBL). For information on ordering photocopies, contact the NRCBL at the Kennedy Institute of Ethics, Georgetown University, Box 571212, Washington, DC 20057-1212; telephone 202-687-3885 or 800-MED-ETHX; e-mail: medethx@georgetown.edu.

Arrangement of the Bibliography

This volume of the *Bibliography of Bioethics* is divided into four parts:

1. Introduction
2. List of Journals Cited
3. Subject Entry Section
4. Author Index.

Part 3, the Subject Entry Section, constitutes the core of the *Bibliography.*

List of Journals Cited

The second part of the *Bibliography*, the List of Journals Cited, records the title of each journal cited in the Subject Entry Section. When available, the International Standard Serial Number (ISSN) of the journal is also listed. The dual purpose of this list is to indicate precisely which journal is designated by each journal title and to obviate the need to include an ISSN number with each citation.

Subject Entry Section

The Subject Entry Section, the main part of the *Bibliography*, contains one or more entries for each of the documents processed by the bioethics information retrieval system during the preceding year. In Volume 26 of the *Bibliography*, entries for 3,679 documents have been included in the Subject Entry Section. By form, these 3,679 documents can be categorized as follows:

Journal articles	2,645
Essays in books	453
Monographs	282
Newspaper articles	198
Court decisions	34
Unpublished documents	34
Bills or laws	22
Audiovisual materials	11

The Subject Entry Section is organized under 77 major subject headings, of which 23 are further divided by subheadings. Each subheading is separated from the major subject term by a slash.

Readers of the *Bibliography* should first scan the alphabetic list of subject headings in the Table of Contents to determine where citations of interest to them are likely to be found. Only subject headings actually occurring in Volume 26 are included on this list.

The Subject Entry Section includes cross references of three types. *See* cross references lead the reader from terms that are not used as subject headings to terms that are used. *See under* cross references are generated from subheadings and guide the reader to the applicable major term in the alphabetical sequence of subject headings. *See also* cross references suggest additional subject headings where the reader may find citations of related interest.

Citation formats in the Subject Entry Section are based on the ANSI[3] standard for bibliographic references. As explained below, the citations are accompanied by indexing terms known as Keywords; in addition, 676 of the citations are accompanied by brief abstracts.

A sample subject heading and a sample entry for a journal article follow:

TRUTH DISCLOSURE

Ruddick, William. Hope and deception. *Bioethics.* 1999
Jul; 13(3–4): 343–357. 16 fn. BE61884.
allowing to die; autonomy; beneficence; children; *deception; emotions; family members; futility; motivation; parents; patients; physician patient relationship; physicians; placebos; principle–based ethics; professional family relationship; prognosis; *risks and benefits; terminally ill; trust; *truth disclosure; *hope
Convinced of hope's therapeutic benefits, physicians routinely support patients' false hopes, often with family collusion and vague, euphemistic diagnoses and prognoses, if not overt lies. Bioethicists charge them with paternalistic violations of Patient Autonomy. There are, I think, too many….

---

[3]*American National Standard for Bibliographic References,* ANSI Z39.29-1977 (New York: American National Standards Institute; 1977).

BIBLIOGRAPHY OF BIOETHICS

Eleven data elements may appear in an entry for a journal article:

1. Subject heading: **TRUTH DISCLOSURE**
2. Author(s): **Ruddick, William**
3. Title of article: Hope and deception.
4. Title of journal[4]: *Bioethics*
5. Date of publication: 1999 Jul
6. Volume and issue number: 13(3–4)
7. Pagination: 343–357
8. Number of references and/or footnotes: 16 fn.
9. Bioethics Accession Number[5]. BE61884
10. Keywords: allowing to die; autonomy, etc.
11. Abstract: Convinced of hope's. . . .

Keywords (element 10) consist of descriptors, proposed descriptors, and identifiers. Descriptors (allowing to die; etc.) are indexing terms chosen from a controlled vocabulary, the *Bioethics Thesaurus,* to represent the concepts in each document. Proposed descriptors (hope) are trial indexing terms that are being considered for possible inclusion in the *Thesaurus.* Identifiers, of which there are none in the sample entry, are proper nouns which are not part of the *Bioethics Thesaurus.* In most cases identifiers refer to a particular person, organization, legal decision, corporate body, geographic location, or time period.

Descriptor Keywords are listed first in alphabetical order in a paragraph that follows the Bioethics Accession Number. Proposed descriptors are listed next, also in alphabetical order. Identifiers are listed in alphabetical sequence following the last descriptor or proposed descriptor. Descriptors appear with every citation in the *Bibliography of Bioethics.* Proposed descriptors and identifiers are added to records as needed.

Approximately 10-20 Keywords are assigned to each document, and the general indexing policy is to employ the most specific term available. The most important concepts are designated by asterisks: *deception; etc. Keywords are included with each citation in the *Bibliography* to serve as guides to the subject content of a record.

Abstracts (element 11) appear in citations for some journal articles and all court decisions in the *Bibliography.* The abstracts in journal article citations are reprinted from journals that are major sources of information in the field of bioethics with permission from the source journals[6]. The abstracts in court decision citations were written by *Bibliography* staff, as indicated by the annotation "(KIE abstract)", to provide a brief summary of the decision.

The sample entry presented above displays the format and elements which appear in a journal article entry. Distinctive formats are used for each of the major forms of material encountered, for example, monographs, essays in monographs, and court decisions. Letters to the editor, editorials, news articles, and specific types of audiovisual materials are also identified in the bibliographic data.

Several print and nonprint forms contain data elements which do not appear in journal article entries. Among these additional elements the most important are the following: 1. Monographs: Author(s) or editor(s) of book, title of book, international standard book number (ISBN); 2. Essays in monographs (analytics): authors(s) of essay, title of essay, author(s)/editor(s) of monograph in which essay appears; 3. Court decisions: date of decision, abstract.

---

[4] International Standard Serial Numbers (ISSNs) are not included in individual entries. Instead, the ISSNs of all journals cited in the Subject Entry Section are included in the part of the *Bibliography* entitled "List of Journals Cited."

[5] The Bioethics Accession Number may be used when ordering copies of hard-to-locate documents from the National Reference Center for Bioethics Literature.

[6] *American Journal of Law and Medicine; American Journal of Public Health; Annals of Internal Medicine; Archives of Internal Medicine; Bioethics; BMJ (British Medical Journal); Cambridge Quarterly of Healthcare Ethics; Christian Bioethics; Ethics; Ethics and Behavior; Hastings Center Report; Health Care Analysis; HEC (HealthCare Ethics Committee) Forum; Human Gene Therapy; International Journal of Bioethics; JAMA; Journal of Clinical Ethics; Journal of Health Politics, Policy and Law; Journal of Law, Medicine and Ethics; Journal of Medical Ethics; Journal of Medical Humanities; Journal of Medicine and Philosophy; Kennedy Institute of Ethics Journal; Lancet; Milbank Quarterly; Nature; New England Journal of Medicine; Nursing Ethics; Philosophy and Public Affairs; Science; Social Science and Medicine; and Theoretical Medicine and Bioethics.*

Author Index

Citations in the Author Index are followed by one or more subject headings in parentheses. Readers interested in finding related citations, or in seeing the indexing Keywords, and perhaps abstracts for particular citations, can turn to an applicable subject heading in the Subject Entry Section. Citations that have no personal or corporate author are listed at the end of the Author Index under ANONYMOUS.

The *Bibliography of Bioethics* on the World Wide Web

The entries published in all of the annual volumes of the *Bibliography of Bioethics* are available as of now in the database BIOETHICSLINE®, which is updated bimonthly. BIOETHICSLINE® is produced for the U.S. National Library of Medicine (NLM), with additional support from the National Human Genome Research Institute, by the Bioethics Information Retrieval Project, part of the National Reference Center for Bioethics Literature at the Kennedy Institute of Ethics, Georgetown University. Free searching of BIOETHICSLINE® via Internet Grateful Med (IGM), an NLM World Wide Web application, is currently available at http://igm.nlm.nih.gov. Access to the database, together with an online *Searcher's Guide* and an annotated list of Keywords (see paragraph below on the *Bioethics Thesarus*), is available also through the Web gateway page of the Kennedy Institute of Ethics at http://bioethics.georgetown.edu. NLM plans to divide BIOETHICSLINE® citations between two NLM databases, MEDLINE and the LOCATOR*plus* online catalog. Information will be posted at http://bioethics.georgetown.edu when the changeover is completed.

Bioethics Thesaurus

The *Bioethics Thesaurus* is an indexing language developed by the *Bibliography* staff specifically for the cross-disciplinary field of bioethics. Keywords from the *Thesaurus,* which accompany all citations in the *Bibliography,* are used for searching the BIOETHICSLINE® database. The main part of the *Thesaurus,* an annotated alphabetic list of Keywords, is available on the World Wide Web at http://bioethics.georgetown.edu. Copies of the full *Thesaurus,* which includes several appendixes, may be purchased by contacting the Administrative Officer, *Bibliography of Bioethics,* Kennedy Institute of Ethics, Georgetown University, Box 571212, Washington, DC 20057–1212; telephone 202–687–6689 or 800–MED–ETHX; fax 202–687–6770; e–mail: medethx@georgetown.edu. Planning is underway to make the *Thesaurus* vocabulary a component of NLM's *MeSH* indexing vocabulary.

Acknowledgments

It is a pleasure to acknowledge the assistance of numerous persons who played a major role in the production of this twenty-sixth volume of the *Bibliography of Bioethics.*

The Bibliographers, Frances Amitay Abramson, Jeanne Ryan Furcron, Hannelore S. Ninomiya, and Cecily Orr Nuckols, monitored journals, indexed documents, and continued to develop the language of the Bioethics Thesaurus. Patricia C. Martin, Data Entry Coordinator, organized and supervised data entry. Susan Cartier Poland, Legal Research Associate, monitored law journals and databases, acquired legal materials and edited abstracts written for court decisions by Jonathan J. Boyle, Legal Research Assistant. Laura Jane Bishop and Harriet Gray, Research Staff, monitored the indexes listed in the Introduction and their student assistants played significant roles in securing documents. Hila Hanif assumed responsibility for the input of data. Kathleen Reynolds, Administrative Officer, provided administrative support for the project, and oversaw sales and distribution of the *Bibliography.*

The Director of Library and Information Services at the Kennedy Institute of Ethics, Doris Goldstein, provided general coordination for the project and, together with her staff, secured many of the documents which are included in the *Bibliography.* We wish to thank Librarians Martina Darragh, Lucinda Fitch Huttlinger, and Pat Milmoe McCarrick, who monitored numerous journals.

This twenty–sixth volume of the *Bibliography* has been produced with the aid of computer programs developed by Natalie A. Arluk and Karen A. Kraly, Office of Computer and Communications Systems, the National Library of Medicine.

The staff wishes to thank Stuart J. Nelson, M.D., Head of the Medical Subject Headings Section at the National Library of Medicine, who generously shared his expertise. The members of our Editorial Advisory Board contributed numerous valuable suggestions that have been incorporated into the *Bibliography.*

Funding for the costs of this twenty–sixth volume was provided through Contract N01 LM73514 with the National Library of Medicine (NLM). We wish to thank NLM for its long-term financial support, and to express our appreciation to our NLM Project Officer, Sheldon Kotzin, and to our Assistant Project Officer, Lou Knecht, for their excellent advice. We also thank Mary Smith, our Contracting Officer, and Liem T. Nguyen, Contract Specialist, for their efficiency and helpfulness. Additional funding for this volume of the *Bibliography* was provided through Grant 5 P41 HG01115-06 from the National Human Genome Research Institute (NHGRI). We thank Elizabeth Thomson, Program Director, ELSI Branch, NHGRI, for her interest and support.

Inquiries about purchasing Volumes 10-26 of the *Bibliography* should be directed to the Administrative Officer, *Bibliography of Bioethics,* Kennedy Institute of Ethics, Georgetown University, Box 571212, Washington, DC 20057-1212, telephone 202-687-6689 or 800-MED-ETHX; fax 202-687-6770, e-mail: medethx@georgetown.edu. Earlier volumes are out of print.

The bibliographic information published in volumes 1-26 of the *Bibliography of Bioethics* is also currently available as a National Library of Medicine database, BIOETHICSLINE®. For further information about free World Wide Web access to BIOETHICSLINE via Internet Grateful Med, and plans to change its future availability, contact the MEDLARS Management Section, National Library of Medicine, 8600 Rockville Pike, Bethesda, Maryland 20894; telephone 301-496-6193 or 888-FIND-NLM/888-346-3656; e-mail: mms@nlm.nih.gov; Internet (at present): http://igm.nlm.nih.gov. BIOETHICSLINE access and search aids are also available through the Web gateway of the Kennedy Institute of Ethics at http://bioethics.georgetown.edu.

The database has also been issued in CD-ROM format from two sources: BIOETHICSLINE® *Plus* is available from SilverPlatter Information, Inc., 1-800-343-0064 or www.silverplatter.com/usa, and BioethicsLine is available from OVID Technologies, Inc., 1-800-950-2035 or www.ovid.com.

* * *

The staff welcomes suggestions for the improvement of future volumes of the *Bibliography of Bioethics.* Please send all comments to:

Editors, *Bibliography of Bioethics*
Kennedy Institute of Ethics
Box 571212
Georgetown University
Washington, DC 20057-1212.

July 12, 2000

LeRoy Walters
Tamar Joy Kahn

LIST OF JOURNALS CITED

LIST OF JOURNALS CITED

A

AACN Clinical Issues in Critical Care Nursing ISSN 1046-7467

AAOHN Journal (American Association of Occupational Health Nurses) ISSN 0891-0162

ABA Journal: The Lawyer's Magazine ISSN 0747-0088

Abstract Book/Association for Health Services Research

Academic Emergency Medicine ISSN 1069-6563

Academic Medicine ISSN 1040-2446

Academic Radiology ISSN 1076-6332

Accountability in Research ISSN 0898-9621

ACOG Committee Opinions ISSN 1074-861X

Acta Anaesthesiologica Scandinavica ISSN 0001-5172

Acta Medica Portuguesa ISSN 0001-6101

Acta Obstetricia et Gynecologica Scandinavica ISSN 0001-6349

Acta Orthopaedica Scandinavica ISSN 0001-6470

Acta Psychiatrica Scandinavica ISSN 0001-690X

Acts of the Australian Parliament

Administration and Policy in Mental Health ISSN 0894-587X

Advances in Contraception ISSN 0267-4874

Advances in Medical Sociology ISSN 1057-6290

Advances in Renal Replacement Therapy ISSN 1073-4449

Ageing and Society ISSN 0144-686X

AIDS ISSN 0269-9370

AIDS and Public Policy Journal ISSN 0887-3852

AIDS Care ISSN 0954-0121

AIDS Policy and Law ISSN 0887-1493

AIPLA Quarterly Journal (American Intellectual Property Law Association) ISSN 0883-6078

Alcohol and Alcoholism ISSN 0735-0414

All England Law Reports ISSN 0002-5569

Alternative Therapies in Health and Medicine ISSN 1078-6791

Alzheimer Disease and Associated Disorders ISSN 0893-0341

America ISSN 0002-7049

American Behavioral Scientist ISSN 0002-7642

American Journal of Critical Care ISSN 1062-3264

American Journal of Health-System Pharmacy ISSN 1079-2082

American Journal of Human Genetics ISSN 0002-9297

American Journal of Kidney Diseases ISSN 0272-6386

American Journal of Law and Medicine ISSN 0098-8588

American Journal Of Managed Care ISSN 1096-1860

American Journal of Medical Genetics ISSN 0148-7299

American Journal of Medical Quality ISSN 1062-8606

American Journal of Medicine ISSN 0002-9343

American Journal of Nursing ISSN 0002-936X

American Journal of Obstetrics and Gynecology ISSN 0002-9378

American Journal of Occupational Therapy ISSN 0272-9490

American Journal of Psychiatry ISSN 0002-953X

American Journal of Psychotherapy ISSN 0002-9564

American Journal of Public Health ISSN 0090-0036

American Journal of Respiratory and Critical Care Medicine ISSN 1073-449X

American Nurses Association Center for Ethics and Human Rights Communique

American Psychologist ISSN 0003-066X

Anaesthesia and Intensive Care ISSN 0310-057X

Anesthesia and Analgesia ISSN 0003-2999

Angelicum ISSN 1123-5772

ANNA Journal (American Nephrology Nurses' Association) ISSN 8750-0779

Annals of Allergy, Asthma, and Immunology ISSN 1081-1206

Annals of Health Law ISSN 1075-2994

Annals of Internal Medicine ISSN 0003-4819

Annals of Medicine ISSN 0785-3890

Annals of Oncology ISSN 0923-7534

Annals of Periodontology ISSN 1060-0280

Annals of Pharmacotherapy ISSN 1060-0280

Annals of Saudi Medicine ISSN 0256-4947

Annals of the New York Academy of Sciences ISSN 0077-8923

Annals of the Royal Australasian College of Dental Surgeons ISSN 0158-1570

Anthropological Quarterly ISSN 0003-5491

AORN Journal (Association of Operating Room Nurses) ISSN 0001-2092

Archives of Disease in Childhood. Fetal and Neonatal Edition ISSN 1359-2998

Archives of Family Medicine ISSN 1063-3987

Archives of General Psychiatry ISSN 0003-990X

Archives of Internal Medicine ISSN 0003-9926

Archives of Neurology ISSN 0003-9942

Archives of Ophthalmology ISSN 0003-9950

Arizona Law Review ISSN 0004-153X

Artificial Organs ISSN 0160-564X

ASAIO Journal (American Society for Artificial Internal Organs) ISSN 1058-2916

Asbury Theological Journal

ATLA: Alternatives to Laboratory Animals ISSN 0261-1929

Atlantic Reporter, 2d Series

Australasian Radiology ISSN 0004-8461

Australian and New Zealand Journal of Psychiatry
    ISSN 0004-8674
Australian and New Zealand Journal of Public Health
    ISSN 1326-0200
Australian Health Review   ISSN 0156-5788
Australian Law Journal   ISSN 0004-9611

B

Berkeley Municipal Code
Bioethics   ISSN 0269-9702
Bioethics Bulletin
Bioethics Examiner
Bioethics Forum   ISSN 1065-7274
Birth   ISSN 0730-7659
BMJ (British Medical Journal)   ISSN 0959-8138
Boston University International Law Journal   ISSN
    0737-8947
British Journal of Nursing   ISSN 0966-0461
British Journal of Psychiatry   ISSN 0007-1250
British Journal of Surgery   ISSN 0007-1323
British Medical Bulletin   ISSN 0007-1420
Bulletin of Medical Ethics   ISSN 0269-1485
Bulletin of the American College of Surgeons   ISSN
    0002-8045
Bulletin of the History of Medicine   ISSN 0007-5140
Bulletin of the New York Academy of Medicine   ISSN
    0028-7091
Burns   ISSN 0305-4179
Business Ethics: A European Review   ISSN 0962-8770

C

California Law Review   ISSN 0008-1221
Cambridge Quarterly of Healthcare Ethics   ISSN
    0963-1801
Canadian Family Physician   ISSN 0008-350X
Canadian Journal of Behavioural Science   ISSN
    0008-400X
Canadian Journal of Cardiology   ISSN 0828-282X
Canadian Journal of Psychiatry   ISSN 0706-7437
Canadian Medical Association Journal   ISSN
    0008-4409
Cancer   ISSN 0008-543X
Cancer Detection and Prevention   ISSN 0361-090X
Cancer Investigation   ISSN 0735-7907
Catholic University Law Review   ISSN 0008-8390
Cellular and Molecular Biology   ISSN 0145-5680
Centennial Review   ISSN 0162-0177
Chest   ISSN 0012-3692
Child Abuse and Neglect   ISSN 0145-2134
China Journal   ISSN 0156-7365
Christian Bioethics   ISSN 1380-3603
Christian Century   ISSN 0009-5281
Christian Science Monitor   ISSN 0882-245X
Cleveland Clinic Journal of Medicine   ISSN 0891-1150
Cleveland State Law Review   ISSN 0009-8876
Clinical Genetics   ISSN 0009-9163
Clinical Neuropsychologist   ISSN 0920-1637
Clinical Obstetrics and Gynecology   ISSN 0009-9201
Clinical Otolaryngology   ISSN 0307-7772
Clinical Pediatrics   ISSN 0009-9228
Clinical Performance and Quality Health Care   ISSN
    1063-0279

Clinical Rehabilitation   ISSN 0009-9260
Clinical Transplantation   ISSN 0902-0063
Clinics in Perinatology   ISSN 0095-5108
Columbia Journal of Law and Social Problems   ISSN
    0010-1923
Columbia Law Review   ISSN 0010-1958
Community Genetics   ISSN 1422-2795
Community Mental Health Journal   ISSN 0010-3853
Connecticut Law Review   ISSN 0010-6151
Consumer Reports   ISSN 0010-7174
Cornell International Law Journal   ISSN 0010-8812
Crime and Delinquency   ISSN 0011-1287
Critical Care Clinics   ISSN 0749-0704
Critical Care Medicine   ISSN 0090-3493
Critical Care Nurse   ISSN 0279-5442
CRNA: The Clinical Forum for Nurse Anesthetists
    ISSN 1048-2687
Culture, Medicine and Psychiatry   ISSN 0165-005X
Curationis   ISSN 0379-8577
Current Opinion In Biotechnology   ISSN 0958-1669
Current Opinion in Nephrology and Hypertension
    ISSN 1062-4821
Current Opinion in Obstetrics and Gynecology   ISSN
    1040-872X
Current Opinion in Psychiatry   ISSN 0951-7367
Cutis   ISSN 0011-4162

D

Defense Council Journal   ISSN 0895-0016
Denver University Law Review   ISSN 0883-9409
Developmental Review   ISSN 0273-2297
Diabetes, Nutrition and Metabolism   ISSN 0394-3402
Diabetic Medicine   ISSN 0742-3071
Dialog: A Journal of Theology   ISSN 0012-2033
Dialysis and Transplantation   ISSN 0090-2934
Dimensions of Critical Care Nursing   ISSN 0730-4625
Dolentium Hominum: Church and Health in the World
Dominion Law Reports, 4th Series   ISSN 0012-5350
Drugs and Aging   ISSN 1170-229X
Duquesne Law Review   ISSN 0093-3058
Dynamische Psychiatrie   ISSN 0012-740X

E

East African Medical Journal   ISSN 0012-835X
Economic and Political Weekly (Bombay)   ISSN
    0012-9976
Economist   ISSN 0013-0613
Epilepsy Research   ISSN 0920-1211
Ethics and Behavior   ISSN 1050-8422
Ethics and Intellectual Disability
Ethics and Medics   ISSN 1071-3778
Ethnicity and Health   ISSN 1355-7858
European Journal of Anaesthesiology   ISSN 0265-0215
European Journal Of Clinical Pharmacology   ISSN
    0031-6970
European Journal of Genetics in Society   ISSN
    1023-9022
European Journal of Health Law   ISSN 0929-0273
European Journal of Human Genetics   ISSN
    1018-4813
European Journal of Obstetrics, Gynecology, and

Reproductive Biology ISSN 0301-2115
European Journal of Pediatrics ISSN 0340-6199

F

Family and Conciliation Courts Review ISSN 1047-5699
Family Law ISSN 0014-7281
Family Law Quarterly ISSN 0014-729X
Family Law Reports ISSN 0261-4375
Family Planning Perspectives ISSN 0014-7354
Family Systems Medicine ISSN 0736-1718
Federal Register ISSN 0097-6326
Federal Reporter, 3d Series ISSN 1048-3888
Federal Supplement ISSN 1047-7306
Federal Supplement, 2d Series ISSN 1047-7306
Feminist Studies ISSN 0046-3663
Fertility and Sterility ISSN 0015-0282
Fetal Diagnosis and Therapy ISSN 1015-3837
First Things ISSN 1047-5141
Forbes ISSN 0015-6914
Free Inquiry ISSN 0272-0701

G

General Dentistry ISSN 0363-6771
Generations (American Society on Aging) ISSN 0738-7806
GenEthics News ISSN 1354-1366
Genetic Counseling ISSN 1015-8146
Genetic Resource
GeneWATCH ISSN 0740-9737
Genome Research ISSN 1088-9051
George Mason University Civil Rights Law Journal
Georgetown Law Journal ISSN 0016-8092
Georgetown Magazine
Geriatrics ISSN 0016-867X
Good Housekeeping ISSN 0017-209X

H

Harper's Magazine ISSN 0017-789X
Harvard Human Rights Journal ISSN 1057-5057
Harvard Review of Psychiatry ISSN 1067-3229
Harvard Women's Law Journal ISSN 0270-1456
Hastings Center Report ISSN 0093-0334
Hastings Constitutional Law Quarterly ISSN 0094-5617
Hastings Law Journal ISSN 0017-8322
Hawaii Medical Journal ISSN 0017-8594
Health ISSN 0279-3547
Health Affairs ISSN 0278-2715
Health and Human Rights ISSN 1079-0969
Health and Social Work ISSN 0360-7283
Health Care Analysis ISSN 1065-3058
Health Care Ethics USA ISSN 1072-5490
Health Economics ISSN 1057-9230
Health Law News
Health Manpower Management ISSN 0955-2065
Health Policy ISSN 0168-8510
Health Policy and Planning ISSN 0268-1080
Health Progress ISSN 0882-1577
Health Psychology ISSN 0278-6133

Healthcare Alabama ISSN 1062-0257
Healthcare Forum Journal ISSN 0899-9287
HealthSpan ISSN 0883-0452
Heart and Lung ISSN 0147-9563
HEC (HealthCare Ethics Committee) Forum ISSN 0956-2737
History of Psychiatry ISSN 0957-154X
HMO Practice ISSN 0891-6624
Home Care Provider ISSN 1084-628X
Hospice Journal ISSN 0742-969X
Houston Law Review ISSN 0018-6694
Human Life Review ISSN 0097-9783
Human Reproduction ISSN 0268-1161
Human Reproduction and Genetic Ethics: An International Journal ISSN 1028-7825
Human Research Report ISSN 0885-0615
Humane Health Care International ISSN 1205-8890
Hypatia ISSN 0887-5367

I

IIC: International Review of Industrial Property and Copyright Law ISSN 0018-9855
Image: The Journal of Nursing Scholarship ISSN 0743-5150
Impact of Science on Society ISSN 0019-2872
Indian Pediatrics ISSN 0019-6061
Indiana Law Journal ISSN 0019-6665
Infants and Young Children ISSN 0896-3746
Intensive and Critical Care Nursing ISSN 0964-3397
International and Comparative Law Quarterly ISSN 0020-5893
International Digest of Health Legislation ISSN 0020-6563
International Journal of Andrology ISSN 0105-6263
International Journal of Geriatric Psychiatry ISSN 0885-6230
International Journal of Gynaecology and Obstetrics ISSN 0020-7292
International Journal of Health Care Quality Assurance ISSN 0952-6862
International Journal of Health Services ISSN 0020-7314
International Journal of Law and Psychiatry ISSN 0160-2527
International Journal of Medicine and Law
International Journal of Psychology ISSN 0020-7594
International Journal of Technology Assessment in Health Care ISSN 0266-4623
International Journal of Technology Management ISSN 0267-5730
International Journal of Trauma Nursing ISSN 1075-4210
IRB: A Review of Human Subjects Research ISSN 0193-7758
Israel Journal of Psychiatry and Related Sciences ISSN 0333-7308
Issues in Ethics (Markkula Center for Applied Ethics)
Issues in Law and Medicine ISSN 8756-8160

J

JAMA ISSN 0098-7484
Japanese Journal of Clinical Oncology ISSN 0368-2811

Jewish Medical Ethics
Joint Commission Perspectives ISSN 1044–4017
Journal of Accident and Emergency Medicine ISSN 1351–0622
Journal of Advanced Nursing ISSN 0309–2402
Journal of Applied Communication Research ISSN 0090–9882
Journal of Applied Philosophy ISSN 0264–3758
Journal of Assisted Reproduction and Genetics ISSN 1058–0468
Journal of Biolaw and Business ISSN 1095–5127
Journal of Black Studies ISSN 0021–9347
Journal of Business Ethics ISSN 0167–4544
Journal of Cellular Biochemistry. Supplement ISSN 0733–1959
Journal of Child Neurology ISSN 0883–0738
Journal of Christian Nursing ISSN 0743–2550
Journal of Clinical Ethics ISSN 1046–7890
Journal of Clinical Neuroscience ISSN 0967–5868
Journal of Clinical Nursing ISSN 0962–1067
Journal of Clinical Oncology ISSN 0732–183X
Journal of Contemporary Health Law and Policy ISSN 0882–1046
Journal of Critical Care ISSN 0883–9441
Journal of Dental Research ISSN 0022–0345
Journal of Epidemiology ISSN 0917–5040
Journal of Ethics, Law, and Aging ISSN 1076–1616
Journal of Family Practice ISSN 0094–3509
Journal of General Internal Medicine ISSN 0884–8734
Journal of Genetic Counseling ISSN 1059–7700
Journal of Gerontological Nursing ISSN 0098–9134
Journal of Head Trauma Rehabilitation ISSN 0885–9701
Journal of Health Administration Education ISSN 0735–6722
Journal of Health and Human Services Administration ISSN 0160–4198
Journal of Health Care Finance ISSN 1078–6767
Journal of Health Care for the Poor and Underserved ISSN 1049–2089
Journal of Health Economics ISSN 0167–6296
Journal of Health Politics, Policy and Law ISSN 0361–6878
Journal of Investigative Medicine ISSN 1081–5589
Journal of Law and Health ISSN 1044–6419
Journal of Law and Policy
Journal of Law and Society ISSN 0263–323X
Journal of Law, Medicine and Ethics ISSN 1073–1105
Journal of Legal Medicine ISSN 0194–7648
Journal of Long Term Home Health Care ISSN 1072–4281
Journal of Maternal–Fetal Medicine ISSN 1057–0802
Journal of Medical Ethics ISSN 0306–6800
Journal of Medical Genetics ISSN 0022–2593
Journal of Medical Humanities ISSN 1041–3545
Journal of Medicine and Philosophy ISSN 0360–5310
Journal of Moral Education ISSN 0305–7240
Journal of NIH Research ISSN 1043–609X
Journal of Nurse–Midwifery ISSN 0091–2182
Journal of Obstetric, Gynecologic and Neonatal Nursing ISSN 0884–2175
Journal of Occupational and Environmental Medicine ISSN 1076–2752

Journal of Pain and Symptom Management ISSN 0885–3924
Journal of Palliative Care ISSN 0825–8597
Journal of Public Health Medicine ISSN 0957–4832
Journal of Religion and Health ISSN 0022–4197
Journal of Religious Ethics ISSN 0384–9694
Journal of School Health ISSN 0022–4391
Journal of Social Behavior and Personality ISSN 0886–1641
Journal of Social Psychology ISSN 0022–4545
Journal of Telemedicine and Telecare ISSN 1357–633X
Journal of the American Academy of Psychiatry and the Law ISSN 1093–6793
Journal of the American Academy of Psychoanalysis ISSN 0090–3604
Journal of the American Board of Family Practice ISSN 0893–8652
Journal of the American Dental Association ISSN 0002–8177
Journal of the American Geriatrics Society ISSN 0002–8614
Journal of the American Health Information Management Association ISSN 1060–5487
Journal of the American Optometric Association ISSN 0003–0244
Journal of the American Society of Nephrology ISSN 1046–6673
Journal of the Canadian Dental Association ISSN 0709–8936
Journal of the Dental Association of South Africa ISSN 0011–8516
Journal of the National Medical Association ISSN 0027–9684
Journal of the Royal College of Physicians of London ISSN 0035–8819
Journal of the Royal Society of Medicine ISSN 0141–0768
Journal of Trauma ISSN 0022–5282
Journal of Urology ISSN 0022–5347
Journal of Women's Health ISSN 1059–7115
Judges' Journal ISSN 0047–2972

K

Kennedy Institute of Ethics Journal ISSN 1054–6863
Kentucky Law Journal ISSN 0023–026X
Kidney International ISSN 0085–2538

L

Lancet ISSN 0023–7507
Law and Inequality ISSN 0737–089X
Law and Philosophy ISSN 0167–5249
Law and Social Inquiry ISSN 0897–6546
Linacre Quarterly ISSN 0024–3639
Liver Transplantation and Surgery ISSN 1074–3022
Louisiana Law Review ISSN 0024–6859

M

Maastricht Journal of European and Comparative Law
Marquette Law Review ISSN 0025–3987

Maryland (Health–General) Code Annotated (Michie)
Maryland Journal of International Law and Trade ISSN 0884–9331
Medical Education ISSN 0308–0110
Medical Humanities Review ISSN 0892–2772
Medical Journal of Australia ISSN 0025–729X
Medical Law Review ISSN 0967–0742
Medical–Moral Newsletter ISSN 0025–7397
Medical Teacher ISSN 0142–159X
Medicine and Law ISSN 0723–1393
Medizinhistorisches Journal ISSN 0025–8431
Mental and Physical Disability Law Reporter ISSN 0883–7902
Mercer Law Review ISSN 0025–987X
Michigan Journal of Gender and Law ISSN 1095–8835
Michigan Law Review ISSN 0026–2234
Michigan Medicine ISSN 0026–2293
Milbank Quarterly ISSN 0887–378X
Minnesota Medicine ISSN 0026–556X
Missouri Medicine ISSN 0026–6620
Molecular Human Reproduction ISSN 1360–9947
Molecular Medicine Today ISSN 1357–4310
Monist ISSN 0026–9662
Mount Sinai Journal of Medicine ISSN 0027–2507

N

National Medical Journal of India ISSN 0970–258X
Nature ISSN 0028–0836
Nature Biotechnology ISSN 1087–0156
Nature Genetics ISSN 1061–4036
Nature Medicine ISSN 1078–8956
NCBHR Communiqué (National Council on Bioethics in Human Research) ISSN 1181–8778
NCCE News (Veterans Health Administration National Center for Clinical Ethics)
NCEHR Communique (National Council on Ethics in Human Research) ISSN 1181–8778
Nebraska Medical Journal ISSN 0091–6730
Nephrology, Dialysis, Transplantation ISSN 0931–0509
Neurology ISSN 0028–3878
New England Journal of Medicine ISSN 0028–4793
New Horizons ISSN 1063–7389
New Law Journal ISSN 0306–6479
New Republic ISSN 0028–6583
New Scientist ISSN 0262–4079
New York Supplement, 2d Series ISSN 1048–3624
New York Times ISSN 0362–4331
New York Times Magazine ISSN 0028–7822
New York University Review of Law and Social Change ISSN 0048–7481
New Zealand Medical Journal ISSN 0028–8446
Newsweek ISSN 0028–9604
Nordic Journal of Psychiatry ISSN 0029–1455
North Carolina Medical Journal ISSN 0029–2559
North Dakota Law Review ISSN 0029–2745
North Eastern Reporter, 2d Series ISSN 1048–3632
North Western Reporter, 2d Series ISSN 1048–3640
Northern Ireland Law Reports
Northwestern University Law Review ISSN 0029–3571
Nurse Practitioner ISSN 0361–1817
Nursing Case Management ISSN 1084–3647

Nursing Ethics ISSN 0969–7330
Nursing Standard ISSN 0029–6570
NursingConnections ISSN 0895–2809

O

Obstetrics and Gynecology Clinics of North America ISSN 0889–8545
Omega: A Journal of Death and Dying ISSN 0030–2228
Oncology Nursing Forum ISSN 0190–535X
Ontario Medical Review ISSN 0030–302X
Ophthalmology ISSN 0161–6420
Origins ISSN 0093–609X
Orthopaedic Nursing ISSN 0744–6020
Ottawa Law Review ISSN 0048–2331

P

Pacific Reporter, 2d Series ISSN 1044–9442
Palliative Medicine ISSN 0269–2163
Patient Education and Counseling ISSN 0738–3991
Pediatric Dentistry ISSN 0887–8218
Pediatric Nursing ISSN 0097–9805
Pediatric Surgery International ISSN 0179–0358
Pediatrician ISSN 0300–1245
Pediatrics ISSN 0031–4005
Perspectives in Biology and Medicine ISSN 0031–5982
PharmacoEconomics ISSN 1170–7690
Pharos ISSN 0031–7179
Philosophy and Public Policy ISSN 1067–2478
Physician Executive ISSN 0898–2759
Plastic Surgical Nursing ISSN 0741–5206
Princeton Journal of Bioethics
Professional Ethics Report ISSN 1045–8808
Professional Nurse (London) ISSN 0266–8130
Professional Psychology: Research and Practice ISSN 0735–7028
Protecting Human Subjects
Psychiatric Services ISSN 1075–2730
Psychology Today ISSN 0033–3107
Psychosomatics ISSN 0033–3182
Public Affairs Quarterly ISSN 0887–0373
Public Understanding of Science ISSN 0963–6625

Q

Quality in Health Care ISSN 0963–8172

R

Reason Papers
Reporter on Human Reproduction and the Law ISSN 8756–2057
Res Publica ISSN 1356–4765
Responsive Community ISSN 1053–0754
Revue Générale de Droit ISSN 0035–3086
Rhode Island Medicine ISSN 1061–222X

S

Saint Louis University Law Journal ISSN 0036–3030
Saint Louis University Public Law Review ISSN 0898–8404
San Diego Law Review ISSN 0036–4037

SBC Newsletter (Society for Bioethics Consultation)
Sbornik Lekarsky ISSN 0036–5327
Scandinavian Journal of Caring Sciences ISSN 0283–9318
Schweizerische Medizinische Wochenschrift ISSN 0036–7672
Science ISSN 0036–8075
Science News ISSN 0036–8423
Science, Technology, and Human Values ISSN 0162–2439
Sciences ISSN 0036–861X
Seattle University Law Review ISSN 1078–1927
Seminars in Dialysis ISSN 0894–0959
Seminars in Perioperative Nursing ISSN 1056–8670
Seton Hall Law Review ISSN 0586–5964
Social Justice Research ISSN 0885–7466
Social Philosophy and Policy ISSN 0265–0525
Social Research ISSN 0037–783X
Social Studies of Science ISSN 0306–3127
Social Work in Health Care ISSN 0098–1389
Society ISSN 0147–2011
Soundings ISSN 0038–1861
South Africa Law Reports
South African Law Journal ISSN 0038–2388
South Dakota Law Review ISSN 0038–3325
Southern California Review of Law and Women's Studies
Splice of Life
Stanford Law and Policy Review ISSN 1044–4386
Stanford Law Review ISSN 0038–9765
Stroke ISSN 0039–2499
Studies in History and Philosophy of Science ISSN 0039–3681
Suffolk University Law Review ISSN 0039–4696
Suicide and Life-Threatening Behavior ISSN 0363–0234
Supportive Care in Cancer ISSN 0941–4355

T

Theoretical Medicine and Bioethics ISSN 1386–7415
Thoracic and Cardiovascular Surgeon ISSN 0171–6425
Tikkun ISSN 0887–9982
Time ISSN 0040–781X
Today's Christian Doctor
Transplantation Proceedings ISSN 0041–1345
Trial ISSN 0041–2538

U

UCLA Law Review ISSN 0041–5650
UCLA Pacific Basin Law Journal
U.S. News and World Report ISSN 0041–5537
University of Chicago Law Review ISSN 0041–9494
University of Florida Journal of Law and Public Policy
University of Miami Law Review ISSN 0041–9818
University of Richmond Law Review ISSN 0566–2389

University of San Francisco Law Review ISSN 0042–0018
University of Tasmania Law Review ISSN 0082–2108

V

Victoria University of Wellington Law Review ISSN 0042–5117
Virginia Medical Quarterly ISSN 1052–4231

W

Wake Forest Law Review ISSN 0043–003X
Wall Street Journal ISSN 0099–9660
Washington and Lee Law Review ISSN 0043–0463
Washington Law Review ISSN 0043–0617
Washington Post ISSN 0190–8286
Washington Post Magazine ISSN 0190–8286
Washington University Law Quarterly ISSN 0043–0862
Wayne Law Review ISSN 0043–1621
West Indian Medical Journal ISSN 0043–3144
Whittier Law Review ISSN 0195–7643
Wiener Medizinische Wochenschrift ISSN 0043–5341
Wisconsin Medical Journal ISSN 0043–6542
Women and Health ISSN 0363–0242
Women and Politics ISSN 0195–7732
Women's Health Issues ISSN 1049–3867

Y

Yale Journal on Regulation ISSN 0741–9457
Yale Law Journal ISSN 0044–0094

SUBJECT ENTRY SECTION

SUBJECT ENTRY SECTION

ABORTION

See also FETUSES

Arthur, John, ed. Abortion. *In:* Arthur, John, ed. Morality and Moral Controversies. Fifth Edition. Upper Saddle River, NJ: Prentice Hall; 1999: 166–210. 9 refs. 13 fn. Includes discussion questions. ISBN 0-13-914128-6. BE60274.
  *abortion, induced; autonomy; beginning of life; cesarean section; coercion; decision making; drug abuse; *fathers; feminist ethics; fetal development; *fetuses; killing; legal aspects; *moral policy; mother fetus relationship; personhood; *pregnant women; prenatal injuries; privacy; rape; reproduction; rights; Supreme Court decisions; therapeutic abortion; treatment refusal; value of life; viability; women's rights; Roe v. Wade; United States

Beckman, Linda J.; Harvey, S. Marie, eds. The New Civil War: The Psychology, Culture, and Politics of Abortion. Washington, DC: American Psychological Association; 1998. 406 p. (Psychology of women book series). Includes references. ISBN 1-55798-517-0. BE60010.
  abortion on demand; *abortion, induced; adolescents; Asian Americans; behavioral research; blacks; counseling; decision making; domestic violence; drugs; federal government; females; government regulation; Hispanic Americans; international aspects; *knowledge, attitudes, practice; males; parental consent; *political activity; politics; pregnant women; psychological stress; psychology; psychotherapy; public policy; risks and benefits; *socioeconomic factors; statistics; Supreme Court decisions; women's health; *women's health services; *women's rights; Right to Life Movement; RU-486; *United States

Boué, A. *Primum non nocere*: prenatal diagnosis and selective abortion. *In:* Burgio, G. Roberto; Lantos, John D., eds. *Primum Non Nocere* Today. Second Edition. New York, NY: Elsevier; 1998: 49–57. ISBN 0-444-82923-7. BE60920.
  *congenital disorders; *decision making; disabled; family relationship; fetal therapy; fetuses; genetic counseling; genetic disorders; information dissemination; legal aspects; mass media; maternal health; newborns; obstetrics and gynecology; *parents; patient care team; physicians; pregnant women; *prenatal diagnosis; prognosis; quality of life; risk; *selective abortion; surgery; uncertainty; ultrasonography; France

Callum, Janet; Chalker, Rebecca; Raymond, Janice, et al. Should RU486 be legalized? *In:* Francoeur, Robert T., ed. Taking Sides: Clashing Views on Controversial Issues in Human Sexuality. Fifth Edition. Guilford, CT: Dushkin Publishing Group/Brown and Benchmark; 1996: 134–143. 9 refs. ISBN 0-697-31292-5. BE62045.
  *abortion, induced; developing countries; *drugs; government regulation; international aspects; methods; public policy; *risks and benefits; surgery; women's health; women's rights; *RU-486; United States

Chervenak, Frank A.; McCullough, Laurence B.;

Wapner, Ronald. Three ethically justified indications for selective termination in multifetal pregnancy: a practical and comprehensive management strategy. *Journal of Assisted Reproduction and Genetics.* 1995 Sep; 12(8): 531–536. 15 refs. BE60566.
  autonomy; beneficence; congenital disorders; conscience; decision making; fetuses; goals; informed consent; moral policy; morbidity; mortality; *multiple pregnancy; newborns; obstetrics and gynecology; physicians; pregnant women; prenatal diagnosis; public policy; *selective abortion; United States

Clarke, Liam. The person in abortion. *Nursing Ethics.* 1999 Jan; 6(1): 37–46. 28 refs. BE60153.
  *abortion, induced; *beginning of life; childbirth; children; emotions; *fetuses; infanticide; infants; moral development; *mother fetus relationship; *newborns; nurses; *personhood; pregnant women; speciesism; viability

Dijon, Xavier. Abortion and genetic manipulation: breaking with reasoning founded on disrespect for life and human dignity. *Medicine and Law.* 1993; 12(1–2): 85–92. 10 fn. BE60615.
  *abortion, induced; *embryo research; *embryos; humanism; legal aspects; love; moral obligations; mother fetus relationship; pregnant women; psychological stress; *value of life; women's rights; dignity

Evans, Mark I.; Johnson, Mark Paul; Quintero, Ruben A., et al. Ethical issues surrounding multifetal pregnancy reduction and selective termination. *Clinics in Perinatology.* 1996 Sep; 23(3): 437–451. 42 refs. BE60933.
  *congenital disorders; decision making; females; fetuses; *genetic disorders; males; moral obligations; *moral policy; morbidity; mortality; *multiple pregnancy; pregnant women; risks and benefits; *selective abortion; sex determination; treatment outcome; *twins

Fox-Genovese, Elizabeth. Abortion and morality revisited. *Human Life Review.* 1997 Summer; 23(3): 50–59. 9 fn. Commentary on N. Wolf, "Our bodies, our souls: rethinking pro-choice rhetoric," *New Republic*, 1995 Oct 16; 213(16): 26, 28–29, 32–35. BE61349.
  *abortion, induced; Christian ethics; fetal development; fetuses; killing; legal aspects; morality; pregnant women; quality of life; religious ethics; theology; therapeutic abortion; value of life; women's health; *women's rights; United States

Fox, Marie. A woman's right to choose? A feminist critique. *In:* Harris, John; Holm, Søren, eds. The Future of Human Reproduction: Ethics, Choice, and Regulation. New York, NY: Oxford University Press; 1998: 77–100. 95 fn. ISBN 0-19-823761-8. BE61264.
  *abortion on demand; *abortion, induced; autonomy; congenital disorders; decision making; fathers; females; feminist ethics; government regulation; international aspects; legal aspects; males; physicians; political activity; pregnant women; selective abortion; sex determination; social control; spousal consent; therapeutic abortion; women's health; *women's rights; needs; Canada; Europe; Great Britain;

BE = bioethics accession number   fn. = footnotes   refs. = references

Ireland; United States

Gans Epner, Janet E.; Jonas, Harry S.; Seckinger, Daniel L. Late-term abortion. *JAMA.* 1998 Aug 26; 280(8): 724–729. 50 refs. BE60279.
*abortion, induced; criminal law; federal government; *fetal development; fetuses; government regulation; legal aspects; legal liability; legal obligations; legislation; *methods; moral obligations; morbidity; mortality; *organizational policies; *physicians; *practice guidelines; pregnant women; *professional organizations; risks and benefits; selective abortion; state interest; statistics; Supreme Court decisions; therapeutic abortion; *viability; American College of Obstetricians and Gynecologists; American Medical Association; United States

Recent proposed federal legislation banning certain abortion procedures, particularly intact dilatation and extraction, would modify the US Criminal Code such that physicians performing these procedures would be liable for monetary and statutory damages. Clarification of medical procedures is important because some of the procedures used to induce abortion prior to viability are identical or similar to postviability procedures. This article reviews the scientific and medical information on late-term abortion and late-term abortion techniques and includes data on the prevalence of late-term abortion, abortion-related mortality and morbidity rates, and legal issues regarding fetal viability and the balance of maternal and fetal interests. According to enacted American Medical Association (AMA) policy, the use of appropriate medical terminology is critical in defining late-term abortion procedures, particularly intact dilatation and extraction, which is a variant of but distinct from dilatation and evacuation. The AMA recommends that the intact dilatation and extraction procedure not be used unless alternative procedures pose materially greater risk to the woman and that abortions not be performed in the third trimester except in cases of serious fetal anomalies incompatible with life. Major medical societies are urged to collaborate on clinical guidelines on late-term abortion techniques and circumstances that conform to standards of good medical practice. More research on the advantages and disadvantages of specific abortion procedures would help physicians make informed choices about specific abortion procedures. Expanded ongoing data surveillance systems estimating the prevalence of abortion are also needed.

Gillam, Lynn. Prenatal diagnosis and discrimination against the disabled. *Journal of Medical Ethics.* 1999 Apr; 25(2): 163–171. 34 fn. BE61921.
children; community services; *congenital disorders; *disabled; Down syndrome; fetuses; genetic disorders; genetic screening; genetic services; government financing; justice; killing; moral obligations; *moral policy; parents; personhood; pregnant women; *prenatal diagnosis; prevalence; *quality of life; *selective abortion; *social discrimination; *social impact; social worth; stigmatization; value of life; values; *wedge argument

Two versions of the argument that prenatal diagnosis discriminates against the disabled are distinguished and analysed. Both are shown to be inadequate, but some valid concerns are about the social effects of prenatal diagnosis are highlighted.

Gillam, Lynn. The 'more-abortions' objection to fetal tissue transplantation. *Journal of Medicine and Philosophy.* 1998 Aug; 23(4): 411–427. 27 refs. 14 fn. BE60631.
*aborted fetuses; *abortion, induced; *deontological ethics; double effect; *ethical analysis; *fetal tissue donation; injuries; *intention; moral complicity; *moral policy; motivation; pregnant women; social impact; utilitarianism; *wedge argument

One common objection to fetal tissue transplantation (FTT) is that, if it were to become a standard form of treatment, it would encourage or entrench the practice of abortion. This claim is at least factually plausible, although it cannot be definitively established. However, even if true, it does not constitute a compelling ethical argument against FTT. The harm allegedly brought about by FTT, when assessed by widely accepted non-consequentialist criteria, has limited moral significance. Even if FTT would cause more abortions to be performed, and abortion is taken to be a serious moral wrong, this is not sufficient in itself to make FTT wrong.

Gillon, Raanan. Eugenics, contraception, abortion and ethics. [Editorial]. *Journal of Medical Ethics.* 1998 Aug; 24(4): 219–220. 1 ref. BE61287.
coercion; *contraception; disabled; *eugenics; *genetic disorders; historical aspects; moral policy; motivation; National Socialism; philosophy; reproduction; *selective abortion; social control; social discrimination; *voluntary programs; Aristotle; Plato

Gorney, Cynthia. Articles of Faith: A Frontline History of the Abortion Wars. New York, NY: Simon and Schuster; 1998. 575 p. Bibliography: p. 528–538. ISBN 0-684-80904-4. BE60015.
abortion on demand; *abortion, induced; adults; beginning of life; fetuses; government regulation; health facilities; *historical aspects; illegal abortion; legal aspects; legal rights; legislation; maternal health; minors; *political activity; *public policy; rape; state government; Supreme Court decisions; therapeutic abortion; value of life; women's rights; Lee, Samuel; *Missouri; *Right to Life Movement; Roe v. Wade; *Twentieth Century; United States; Webster v. Reproductive Health Services; Widdicombe, Judith

Grimes, David A. A 26-year-old woman seeking an abortion. *JAMA.* 1999 Sep 22–29; 282(12): 1169–1175. 60 refs. BE62660.
*abortion, induced; attitudes; case studies; contraception; counseling; decision making; drugs; family planning; fetal development; international aspects; internship and residency; medical education; methods; physicians; pregnant women; primary health care; psychological stress; psychology; risks and benefits; statistics; United States

Grimes, David A. The continuing need for late abortions. *JAMA.* 1998 Aug 26; 280(8): 747–750. 27 refs. BE60282.
*abortion, induced; autonomy; beneficence; *decision making; federal government; *fetal development; government regulation; justice; legislation; *methods; moral policy; morbidity; mortality; *physicians; *pregnant women; prenatal diagnosis; public policy; risk; selective abortion; sex offenses; socioeconomic factors; state government; Supreme Court decisions; therapeutic abortion; *viability; women's health; United States

Hadley, Janet. Prenatal tests: blessings and burdens. In: Lee, Ellie, ed. Abortion Law and Politics Today. New York, NY: St. Martin's Press; 1998: 172–183. 27 fn. ISBN 0-312-21574-6. BE62337.
*congenital disorders; *decision making; directive counseling; *disabled; economics; *eugenics; genetic counseling; genetic disorders; genetic predisposition; genetic screening; international aspects; involuntary sterilization; late-onset disorders; parents; pregnant women; preimplantation diagnosis; *prenatal diagnosis; *public policy; rights; *selective abortion; *stigmatization; Great Britain

Hartouni, Valerie. Cultural Conceptions: On Reproductive Technologies and the Remaking of Life. Minneapolis, MN: University of Minnesota Press; 1997.

BE = bioethics accession number   fn. = footnotes   refs. = references

175 p. Bibliography: p. 157–170. ISBN 0-8166-2623-5. BE62771.

*abortion, induced; adoption; audiovisual aids; behavioral genetics; blacks; brain death; *cloning; disadvantaged; embryos; eugenics; *fetuses; genetic intervention; legal aspects; mass media; mothers; parent child relationship; personhood; political activity; posthumous reproduction; postmodernism; *pregnant women; prenatal diagnosis; prolongation of life; *reproduction; *reproductive technologies; social discrimination; *social impact; socioeconomic factors; Supreme Court decisions; *surrogate mothers; value of life; values; violence; women's rights; In re Baby M; Johnson v. Calvert; Right to Life Movement; S'Aline's Solution; The Bell Curve (Herrnstein, R.; Murray, C.); *United States

Hopkins, Patrick D., ed.; Tennessee. Supreme Court, at Knoxville. (Re)locating fetuses: technology and new body politics. *In: his* Sex/Machine: Readings in Culture, Gender, and Technology. Bloomington, IN: Indiana University Press; 1998: 171–235. 33 refs. 84 fn. ISBN 0-253-21230-8. BE62290.

*abortion, induced; alternatives; contracts; *cryopreservation; *embryo disposition; embryo transfer; *embryos; *females; feminist ethics; fetuses; human experimentation; *in vitro fertilization; infertility; intention; *legal aspects; *males; *methods; mother fetus relationship; parent child relationship; personhood; pregnant women; privacy; property rights; *reproductive technologies; *required request; *rights; *risks and benefits; social discrimination; social impact; viability; women's rights; divorce; *ectogenesis; *Davis v. Davis; Tennessee; United States

Hunt, Geoffrey. Abortion: why bioethics can have no answer -- a personal perspective. *Nursing Ethics.* 1999 Jan; 6(1): 47–57. 11 refs. BE60154.

*abortion, induced; attitudes; *beginning of life; bioethics; *dissent; embryos; ethical analysis; ethicists; fetal development; *fetuses; *moral policy; *morality; newborns; *personhood; viability; *rationality

Hunt, Jean; Joffe, Carole. Problems and prospects of contemporary abortion provision. *In:* Dan, Alice J., ed. Reframing Women's Health: Multidisciplinary Research and Practice. Thousand Oaks, CA: Sage Publications; 1994: 163–174. 13 refs. ISBN 0-8039-5860-9. BE60655.

*abortion, induced; drugs; financial support; health care reform; historical aspects; medical education; obstetrics and gynecology; physicians; political activity; violence; women's health services; women's rights; RU-486; *United States

Hunt, John. Abortion and Nazism: is there really a connection? *Linacre Quarterly.* 1996 Nov; 63(4): 53–63. 45 fn. BE59305.

abortion on demand; *abortion, induced; dehumanization; fetuses; Jews; *killing; mandatory programs; *National Socialism; personhood; political activity; public policy; *value of life; *genocide; Germany; United States

Jacoby, Kerry N. Souls, Bodies, Spirits: The Drive to Abolish Abortion Since 1973. Westport, CT: Praeger; 1998. 230 p. Bibliography: p. 205–220. ISBN 0-275-96044-7. BE60748.

*abortion, induced; fetuses; historical aspects; legal aspects; mass media; metaphor; moral policy; physicians; *political activity; politics; pregnant women; Protestants; public policy; *religion; Roman Catholics; social impact; socioeconomic factors; Supreme Court decisions; survey; values; violence; Christian Fundamentalists; Operation Rescue; *Right to Life Movement; *United States

Jeffko, Walter G. Abortion, personhood, and community. *In: his* Contemporary Ethical Issues: A Personalistic Perspective. Amherst, NY: Humanity Books; 1999:

59–84. 42 fn. ISBN 1-57392-640-X. BE62245.

*abortion, induced; *beginning of life; congenital disorders; drugs; embryos; *fetal development; *fetuses; infanticide; killing; legal aspects; methods; *moral policy; mother fetus relationship; newborns; *personhood; philosophy; population control; public policy; Roman Catholic ethics; selective abortion; sex offenses; therapeutic abortion; twinning; value of life; viability; RU-486

Kaplan, Laura. The Story of Jane: The Legendary Underground Feminist Abortion Service. Chicago, IL: University of Chicago Press; 1995. 314 p. Bibliography: p. 295–297. Originally published in 1995 by Pantheon Books, New York. ISBN 0-226-42421-9. BE60507.

counseling; *females; *historical aspects; information dissemination; *political activity; women's health services; *women's rights; *Abortion Counseling Service of Women's Liberation (Chicago); *Chicago; *Jane (Chicago); *Twentieth Century

Kittay, Eva Feder; Kittay, Leo. On the expressivity and ethics of selective abortion for disability: conversations with my son. *In:* Haber, Joram G.; Halfon, Mark S., eds. Norms and Values: Essays on the Work of Virginia Held. Lanham, MD: Rowman and Littlefield; 1998: 173–203. 19 refs. 3 fn. ISBN 0-8476-8491-1. BE62441.

abortion, induced; *congenital disorders; decision making; *disabled; Down syndrome; *family relationship; feminist ethics; love; *mentally retarded; obligations of society; *parent child relationship; pregnant women; prenatal diagnosis; *selective abortion; siblings; stigmatization; *value of life; *values; wedge argument

Larimore, Walter L.; Orr, Robert D. Medical abortion is not just a medical issue. [Editorial]. *Today's Christian Doctor.* 1997 Winter; 28(4): 4–6. 17 refs. BE60109.

*abortion, induced; drugs; killing; *morality; personhood; value of life; slavery; United States

Lavelle, Marianne. When abortions come late in pregnancy: though rare, most aren't for medical reasons. [News]. *U.S. News and World Report.* 1998 Jan 19; 124(2): 31–32. Includes inset article by E. Ackerman, "An excruciating decision over a dying fetus," p. 32. BE59168.

*abortion, induced; age factors; emotions; females; *fetal development; fetuses; government regulation; health facilities; killing; *methods; motivation; physicians; pregnant women; therapeutic abortion; time factors; United States

Lewin, Tamar. Study on late term abortion finds procedure is little used. [News]. *New York Times.* 1998 Dec 11: A12. BE60372.

*abortion, induced; drugs; *fetal development; *methods; statistics; survey; methotrexate; RU-486; *United States

Li, Hon-Lam. Abortion and degrees of personhood: understanding why the abortion problem (and the animal rights problem) are irresolvable. *Public Affairs Quarterly.* 1997 Jan; 11(1): 1–19. 26 fn. BE59161.

*abortion, induced; age factors; animal rights; *beginning of life; fetal development; *fetuses; maternal health; moral policy; morality; *personhood; *pregnant women; speciesism; therapeutic abortion; *value of life

Lundberg, George D. JAMA, abortion, and editorial responsibility. [Editorial]. *JAMA.* 1998 Aug 26; 280(8): 740. 20 refs. BE60280.

*abortion, induced; decision making; dissent; *editorial policies; fetal development; freedom; pregnant women; viability; American Medical Association; *JAMA

McCorvey, Norma. Won by Love: Norma McCorvey, Jane Roe of Roe v. Wade, Speaks Out for the Unborn

---

BE = bioethics accession number   fn. = footnotes   refs. = references

as She Shares Her New Conviction for Life. Nashville, TN: Thomas Nelson; 1997. 244 p. Written with Gary Thomas. ISBN 0-7852-7237-2. BE62775.
  *abortion, induced; Christian ethics; disadvantaged; famous persons; fetuses; legal aspects; *political activity; pregnant women; Supreme Court decisions; *value of life; *McCorvey, Norma; Operation Rescue; *Right to Life Movement; *Roe v. Wade; Texas; United States

Mullens, Anne. 7:10 am, Nov. 8, 1994. *Canadian Medical Association Journal.* 1998 Feb 24; 158(4): 528-531. BE60056.
  *abortion, induced; illegal abortion; medical education; mortality; motivation; *physicians; political activity; *violence; Canada; *Romalis, Garson

Paintin, David, ed. Ante-Natal Screening and Abortion for Fetal Abnormality. London: Birth Control Trust; 1997. 96 p. Includes references. Proceedings of a symposium held in London, 26 Sep 1996, at the Royal Society of Medicine. ISBN 0-906-233-37-2. BE59737.
  *congenital disorders; counseling; decision making; Down syndrome; economics; fetal development; methods; morality; nurse midwives; obstetrics and gynecology; parents; personhood; physicians; pregnant women; *prenatal diagnosis; preventive medicine; psychological stress; psychology; *selective abortion; needs; ultrasonography; Great Britain

Persson, Ingmar. Harming the non-conscious. *Bioethics.* 1999 Jul; 13(3-4): 294-305. 13 fn. BE61880.
  *abortion, induced; *beginning of life; brain; embryos; *fetal development; *fetal research; *fetuses; *injuries; killing; *moral policy; organ donation; personhood; prenatal injuries; quality of life; value of life; *harms; Singer, Peter
  Peter Singer has argued that nothing done to a fetus before it acquires consciousness can harm it. At the same time, he concedes that a child can be harmed by something done to it when it was a non-conscious fetus. But this implies that the non-conscious fetus can be harmed. The mistake lies in thinking that, since existence can be instrinsically bad for a being only if it is conscious, it can be harmed only if it is conscious. In fact, its being harmed only implies that it could have been conscious (and led a good life).

Porter, Elisabeth. Abortion ethics: rights and responsibilities. *Hypatia.* 1994 Summer; 9(3): 66-87. 47 refs. BE61676.
  abortion on demand; *abortion, induced; autonomy; caring; common good; communitarianism; cultural pluralism; democracy; females; *feminist ethics; fetal development; fetuses; freedom; international aspects; legal rights; males; minority groups; *moral obligations; *moral policy; *morality; mother fetus relationship; obligations to society; personhood; *pregnant women; privacy; *public policy; reproduction; *rights; self concept; socioeconomic factors; values; Western World; *women's rights; United States

Powell, Marion G. Ensuring access to abortion in an era of cutbacks. [Editorial]. *Canadian Medical Association Journal.* 1997 Jun 1; 156(11): 1545-1547. 10 refs. BE59680.
  *abortion, induced; drugs; government financing; surgery; trends; *women's health services; Canada

Reiman, Jeffrey. Abortion and the Ways We Value Human Life. Lanham, MD: Rowman and Littlefield; 1999. 127 p. 228 fn. ISBN 0-8476-9208-6. BE61274.
  *abortion, induced; adults; ancient history; children; Christian ethics; constitutional law; criminal law; double effect; fetal development; fetuses; freedom; historical aspects; human characteristics; human rights; infanticide; infants; intention; Jewish ethics; *killing; legal aspects; love;

maternal health; moral obligations; *moral policy; morality; organizational policies; personhood; *philosophy; physicians; privacy; socioeconomic factors; speciesism; Supreme Court decisions; *value of life; *values; viability; virtues; Western World; women's rights; American Medical Association; Middle Ages; Nineteenth Century; Planned Parenthood of Southeastern Pennsylvania v. Casey; Roe v. Wade; Twentieth Century; United States

Robinson, John H.; Berry, Roberta M.; McDonnell, Kevin, eds. Reproduction. *In: their* A Health Law Reader: An Interdisciplinary Approach. Durham, NC: Carolina Academic Press; 1999: 73-180. 38 fn. ISBN 0-89089-907-X. BE62292.
  *abortion, induced; attitudes; autonomy; children; cloning; *commodification; dehumanization; disabled; eugenics; family relationship; feminist ethics; fetuses; *freedom; gene therapy; *genetic intervention; genetic screening; government regulation; legal aspects; minority groups; *moral policy; morality; parent child relationship; personhood; prenatal diagnosis; *public policy; *reproduction; *reproductive technologies; rights; selective abortion; sex determination; sexuality; Supreme Court decisions; surrogate mothers; value of life; Roe v. Wade; United States

Robinson, Paul. Prenatal screening, sex selection and cloning. *In:* Kuhse, Helga; Singer, Peter, eds. A Companion to Bioethics. Malden, MA: Blackwell; 1998: 173-185. 8 refs. ISBN 0-631-19737-0. BE59493.
  autonomy; cloning; congenital disorders; costs and benefits; disabled; embryo disposition; embryos; fetuses; genetic counseling; genetic screening; killing; mass screening; moral obligations; *moral policy; pregnant women; preimplantation diagnosis; *prenatal diagnosis; psychological stress; risks and benefits; *selective abortion; sex determination; social impact; value of life

Rorty, Mary V. Feminism and elective fetal reduction. *In:* Donchin, Anne; Purdy, Laura M., eds. Embodying Bioethics: Recent Feminist Advances. Lanham, MD: Rowman and Littlefield; 1999: 159-175. 34 refs. 19 fn. ISBN 0-8476-8924-7. BE61020.
  *abortion on demand; autonomy; congenital disorders; *feminist ethics; human experimentation; informed consent; motivation; *multiple pregnancy; pregnant women; reproductive technologies; risks and benefits; *selective abortion; sex determination; twins

Runkle, Anna. In Good Conscience: A Practical, Emotional, and Spiritual Guide to Deciding Whether to Have an Abortion. San Francisco, CA: Jossey-Bass; 1998. 165 p. Bibliography: p. 159-160. ISBN 0-7879-4149-2. BE61423.
  *abortion, induced; adoption; attitudes; communication; contraception; *decision making; economics; emotions; legal aspects; methods; minors; *pregnant women; religion; values; social support; Right to Life Movement; United States

Schoen, Johanna. "A Great Thing for Poor Folks": Birth Control, Sterilization, and Abortion in Public Health and Welfare in the Twentieth Century. Ann Arbor, MI: UMI Dissertation Services; 1996. 267 p. Bibliography: p. 240-267. Dissertation, Ph.D. in History, University of North Carolina, 1995. Order No. 9631980. BE62797.
  *abortion, induced; blacks; *coercion; *contraception; eugenics; *females; government regulation; historical aspects; *indigents; *involuntary sterilization; legal aspects; males; mentally retarded; motivation; public health; *public policy; sexuality; *social control; social discrimination; state government; whites; *North Carolina; Twentieth Century; United States

Simpson, William G. A different kind of Holocaust: from

BE = bioethics accession number   fn. = footnotes   refs. = references

euthanasia to tyranny. *Linacre Quarterly*. 1997 Aug; 64(3): 87–92. BE59313.
  abortion on demand; *abortion, induced; *active euthanasia; aged; *assisted suicide; chronically ill; disabled; eugenics; historical aspects; involuntary sterilization; *killing; National Socialism; public policy; right to die; social discrimination; *social worth; terminally ill; *value of life; genocide; Darwinism; Germany; Netherlands; Twentieth Century; United States

Solinger, Rickie, ed. Abortion Wars: A Half Century of Struggle, 1950–2000. Berkeley, CA: University of California Press; 1998. 413 p. Includes references. ISBN 0–520–20952–4. BE60654.
  *abortion, induced; blacks; coercion; contraception; counseling; disabled; drug abuse; drugs; eugenics; females; fetuses; government financing; health care delivery; *historical aspects; legal aspects; morality; physicians; *political activity; politics; pregnant women; prenatal injuries; psychology; *public policy; selective abortion; social discrimination; Supreme Court decisions; violence; women's health services; *women's rights; Roe v. Wade; RU–486; *Twentieth Century; *United States

Sprague, Joey; Greer, Margaret. Standpoints and the discourse on abortion: the reproductive debate. *Women and Politics*. 1998; 19(3): 49–80. 98 refs. 1 fn. BE62437.
  abortion on demand; *abortion, induced; alternatives; autonomy; capitalism; *dissent; *feminist ethics; fetuses; legal rights; males; personhood; political activity; pregnant women; public policy; reproduction; *social dominance; socioeconomic factors; values; whites; Chodorow, Nancy; Collins, Patricia Hill; Hartsock, Nancy; O'Brien, Mary; Right to Life Movement; *United States

Sprang, M. LeRoy; Neerhof, Mark G. Rationale for banning abortions late in pregnancy. *JAMA*. 1998 Aug 26; 280(8): 744–747. 38 refs. BE60281.
  *abortion, induced; alternatives; autonomy; beneficence; federal government; *fetal development; *fetuses; *government regulation; infanticide; legislation; maternal health; *methods; moral policy; morbidity; mortality; organizational policies; pain; personhood; physicians; *pregnant women; professional organizations; public opinion; *risk; selective abortion; state government; therapeutic abortion; *viability; American College of Obstetricians and Gynecologists; American Medical Association; United States

Stetson, Dorothy McBride. Feminist perspectives on abortion and reproductive technologies. *In:* Githens, Marianne; Stetson, Dorothy McBride, eds. Abortion Politics: Public Policy in Cross–Cultural Perspective. New York, NY: Routledge; 1996: 211–223. 25 refs. 1 fn. ISBN 0–415–91225–3. BE60712.
  *abortion, induced; autonomy; contraception; females; *feminist ethics; fetuses; freedom; international aspects; legal aspects; males; pregnant women; privacy; public policy; *reproductive technologies; rights; sexuality; social dominance; *women's rights; United States

Thomson, Michael. Reproducing Narrative: Gender, Reproduction and Law. Brookfield, VT: Ashgate; 1998. 228 p. Includes references. ISBN 1–85521–929–8. BE62630.
  *abortion, induced; attitudes; contraception; employment; *females; fetuses; health hazards; historical aspects; illegal abortion; international aspects; law; *legal aspects; legislation; males; narrative ethics; occupational exposure; physicians; political activity; politics; postmodernism; pregnant women; prenatal injuries; *reproduction; reproductive technologies; *social control; social discrimination; *sociology of medicine; women's health services; Abortion Act 1967 (Great Britain); Great Britain; Human Fertilisation and Embryology Act 1990 (Great

Britain); Nineteenth Century; Twentieth Century; United States

Tollefsen, Christopher. Donagan, abortion, and civil rebellion. *Public Affairs Quarterly*. 1997 Jul; 11(3): 303–312. 10 fn. BE61732.
  *abortion, induced; fetuses; health facilities; health personnel; moral obligations; *morality; *political activity; punishment; *violence; Donagan, Alan; United States

Waldman, Steven; Ackerman, Elise; Rubin, Rita. Abortions in America: so many women have them, so few talk about them. *U.S. News and World Report*. 1998 Jan 19; 124(2): 20–22, 24–31. BE59167.
  *abortion, induced; adolescents; adoption; adults; attitudes; *communication; counseling; decision making; emotions; *females; males; *motivation; *pregnant women; *psychology; rape; sexuality; single persons; socioeconomic factors; statistics; *United States

Warren, Mary Anne. Abortion. *In:* Kuhse, Helga; Singer, Peter, eds. A Companion to Bioethics. Malden, MA: Blackwell; 1998: 127–134. 10 refs. ISBN 0–631–19737–0. BE59489.
  abortion on demand; *abortion, induced; autonomy; beginning of life; embryos; fetal development; fetuses; government regulation; *moral policy; pregnant women; public policy; value of life

Wendler, Dave. Understanding the 'conservative' view on abortion. *Bioethics*. 1999 Jan; 13(1): 32–56. 16 fn. BE60887.
  *abortion, induced; cryopreservation; *embryos; *fetal development; fetal therapy; *fetuses; genetic determinism; genetic information; in vitro fertilization; moral obligations; *moral policy; morality; *personhood; policy analysis; abortion, spontaneous; potentiality

ABORTION/ATTITUDES

Bowes, Watson; Byrne, Paul; Cavanagh, Denis, et al. True integrity for the maternal–fetal medicine physician. *Linacre Quarterly*. 1997 Aug; 64(3): 77–86. 14 refs. Response to J. Blustein and A.R. Fleischman, "The pro–life maternal–fetal medicine physician: a problem of integrity," *Hastings Center Report*, 1995 Jan–Feb; 25(1): 22–26. BE59312.
  *abortion, induced; *attitudes; *beginning of life; children; *congenital disorders; *conscience; counseling; decision making; disclosure; Down syndrome; information dissemination; medical education; *moral complicity; *moral policy; morality; *obstetrics and gynecology; *physicians; pregnant women; *prenatal diagnosis; secularism; *selective abortion; *value of life; values; *integrity

Francome, Colin. Attitudes of general practitioners in Northern Ireland toward abortion and family planning. *Family Planning Perspectives*. 1997 Sep–Oct; 29(5): 234–236. 5 fn. BE59884.
  *abortion, induced; adolescents; comparative studies; *contraception; decision making; *family planning; *family practice; females; *knowledge, attitudes, practice; married persons; *physicians; pregnant women; *Protestants; referral and consultation; *Roman Catholics; single persons; survey; *Northern Ireland

Furedi, Ann. Wrong but the right thing to do: public opinion and abortion. *In:* Lee, Ellie, ed. Abortion Law and Politics Today. New York, NY: St. Martin's Press; 1998: 159–171. 19 fn. ISBN 0–312–21574–6. BE62336.
  *abortion on demand; *abortion, induced; adolescents; adults; *congenital disorders; conscience; decision making; *fetal development; fetuses; legal aspects; mentally disabled;

morality; physically disabled; political activity; pregnant women; prenatal diagnosis; prevalence; *public opinion; public policy; rape; *selective abortion; social discrimination; socioeconomic factors; survey; *therapeutic abortion; viability; *Great Britain; Right to Life Movement

Hoedemaekers, Rogeer; ten Have, Henk. Geneticization: the Cyprus paradigm. *Journal of Medicine and Philosophy.* 1998 Jun; 23(3): 274–287. 17 refs. BE59291.
> *attitudes; carriers; *coercion; decision making; *directive counseling; economics; eugenics; *genetic counseling; *genetic screening; genetic services; genetics; *goals; health education; *health personnel; international aspects; *mass screening; parents; paternalism; *prenatal diagnosis; prevalence; preventive medicine; public health; public opinion; quality of life; *selective abortion; social control; stigmatization; *thalassemia; *Cyprus; Great Britain; Quebec

Geneticization is a broad term referring to several related processes such as a spreading tendency to use a genetic model of disease explanation, a growing influence of genetics in medical practice, and the slow changing of individual and societal attitudes towards reproduction, prevention and control of disease. These processes can be demonstrated in medical literature on preventive genetic screening and counselling programs for beta–thalassaemia in Cyprus, the United Kingdom and Canada. The preventive possibilities of the new genetic and diagnostic technologies have been quickly understood and advocated by health professionals, and their educational strategies have created a web of social control, in marked contrast to the alleged voluntary decision–making process and free choice. Genetic diagnostic technologies have led to considerable changes in control and management of beta–thalassaemia, and have generated a number of unresolved incongruities.

Klamen, Debra L.; Grossman, Linda S.; Kopacz, David R. Attitudes about abortion among second–year medical students. *Medical Teacher.* 1996 Dec; 18(4): 345–346. 5 refs. BE60697.
> *abortion, induced; *attitudes; *medical education; physicians; referral and consultation; *students; survey; Midwestern United States; University of Illinois College of Medicine

Lafayette, DeeDee; Abuelo, Dianne; Passero, Mary Ann, et al. Attitudes toward cystic fibrosis carrier and prenatal testing and utilization of carrier testing among relatives of individuals with cystic fibrosis. *Journal of Genetic Counseling.* 1999 Feb; 8(1): 17–36. 57 refs. BE61642.
> *attitudes; *carriers; *cystic fibrosis; *family members; family planning; *genetic counseling; *genetic screening; *knowledge, attitudes, practice; *prenatal diagnosis; quality of life; *selective abortion; survey; Rhode Island

Lynxwiler, John; Gay, David. The abortion attitudes of black women: 1972–1991. *Journal of Black Studies.* 1996 Nov; 27(2): 260–277. 23 refs. 2 fn. BE59448.
> *abortion, induced; age factors; *attitudes; *blacks; education; employment; *females; geographic factors; historical aspects; politics; Protestants; public opinion; public policy; religion; sexuality; single persons; *socioeconomic factors; survey; time factors; *trends; urban population; Twentieth Century; United States

McKee, Katherine; Adams, Eleanor. Nurse midwives' attitudes toward abortion performance and related procedures. *Journal of Nurse–Midwifery.* 1994 Sep–Oct; 39(5): 300–311. 25 refs. BE59185.
> *abortion, induced; *attitudes; geographic factors; *knowledge, attitudes, practice; medical education; *nurse

midwives; *nurse's role; nursing education; physicians; scarcity; stigmatization; survey; violence; American College of Nurse–Midwives; United States

Mao, Xin. Chinese geneticists approach ethics. [Letter]. *Journal of Medical Ethics.* 1998 Jan; 35(1): 83. 14 refs. BE61126.
> *attitudes; confidentiality; developing countries; *directive counseling; disclosure; eugenics; *genetic counseling; genetic disorders; genetic predisposition; genetic research; *genetic screening; genetic services; genetics; guidelines; *health personnel; international aspects; investigators; *non–Western World; *prenatal diagnosis; *selective abortion; sex determination; survey; Western World; *China

Marsiglio, William. Abortion and gender politics. *In: his* Procreative Man. New York, NY: New York University Press; 1998: 86–101, 211–213. 43 fn. ISBN 0–8147–5579–8. BE61949.
> *abortion, induced; adolescents; adults; *attitudes; autonomy; blacks; coercion; *decision making; emotions; females; legal rights; *males; married persons; parent child relationship; political activity; politics; pregnant women; sexuality; single persons; socioeconomic factors; spousal consent; spousal notification; statistics; whites; women's rights; partner notification; United States

Middleton, A.; Hewison, J.; Mueller, R.F. A pilot study of attitudes of deaf and hearing parents towards issues surrounding genetic testing for deafness. [Abstract]. *American Journal of Human Genetics.* 1997 Oct; 61(4): A190. BE59395.
> *attitudes; comparative studies; *genetic disorders; *genetic screening; *hearing disorders; *parents; *physically disabled; *prenatal diagnosis; *selective abortion; survey; Great Britain

Virgo, Katherine S.; Carr, T.R.; Hile, Allison, et al. Medical versus surgical abortion: a survey of knowledge and attitudes among abortion clinic patients. *Women's Health Issues.* 1999 May–Jun; 9(3): 143–154. 28 refs. BE62420.
> *abortion, induced; comparative studies; *drugs; *knowledge, attitudes, practice; *methods; *pregnant women; risks and benefits; socioeconomic factors; surgery; Illinois; *RU–486

ABORTION/FINANCIAL SUPPORT

Kilborn, Peter T. Definition of abortion is found to vary abroad. [News]. *New York Times.* 1999 Nov 24: A18. BE60649.
> *abortion, induced; *contraception; *developing countries; *family planning; *government financing; government regulation; *international aspects; population control; *public policy; *Bangladesh; *United States

Lewin, Tamar. A prisoner is the focus of an abortion debate. [News]. *New York Times.* 1999 Jan 10: 12. BE60124.
> *abortion, induced; coercion; *government financing; *legal aspects; municipal government; political activity; *prisoners; public opinion; Roman Catholics; Pennsylvania; *Ptaschnik, Karen

Minnesota. Supreme Court. Women of the State of Minnesota v. Gomez. *North Western Reporter, 2d Series.* 1995 Dec 15 (date of decision). 542: 17–42. BE60050.
> *abortion, induced; constitutional law; decision making; *government financing; *government regulation; indigents; *legal aspects; *legal rights; legislation; *pregnant women; privacy; sex offenses; state government; *therapeutic abortion; *Medicaid; *Minnesota; *Women v. Gomez

---

BE = bioethics accession number   fn. = footnotes   refs. = references

The Minnesota Supreme Court held unconstitutional a state law which restricted state Medicaid funding for abortions to cases where the abortion was a medical necessity, defined as a pregnancy that threatens the life of the mother in the opinion of two physicians; where the pregnancy was the product of criminal misconduct and the incident was reported to law enforcement authorities within 48 hours of the incident; or where the pregnancy was the result of incest that was reported to a valid law enforcement agency for investigation prior to the abortion procedure. The court held that Minnesota's state constitution provided broader privacy rights than the U.S. Constitution and that it protected both the right to an abortion and the right to the decision to abort. (KIE abstract)

U.S. Court of Appeals, Fifth Circuit. Hope Medical Group for Women v. Edwards. *Federal Reporter, 3d Series.* 1998 Sep 11 (date of decision). 63: 418–429. BE60052.
   *abortion, induced; death; federal government; *government financing; *government regulation; indigents; *legal aspects; legal rights; legislation; *pregnant women; sex offenses; state government; therapeutic abortion; *Hope Medical Group for Women v. Edwards; *Hyde Amendment 1994; *Louisiana; *Medicaid

The U.S. Court of Appeals for the Fifth Circuit invalidated a Louisiana law which restricted Medicaid reimbursement for abortion to instances where the pregnancy threatened the life of the mother. Although the revised 1994 Hyde Amendment permitted federal Medicaid funding for the abortion of pregnancies resulting from rape or incest, the Fifth Circuit held that the Hyde Amendment did not require states to fund these procedures. Instead, the court relied on the purposes of Medicaid to provide health–sustaining medical care and held that Louisiana's statute impermissibly restricted a women's right to abortion where medically necessary. Louisiana was enjoined from enforcing the law to the extent it restricted Medicaid reimbursement for the medically necessary abortion of pregnancies resulting from rape or incest. The court held that the state's interest in normal childbirth is not sufficient to sustain the abortion funding restriction. (KIE abstract)

U.S. District Court, D. Nebraska. Orr v. Nelson. *Federal Supplement.* 1994 Nov 4 (date of decision). 902: 1019–1022. BE59975.
   *abortion, induced; constitutional amendments; federal government; *government financing; *government regulation; indigents; *legal aspects; rape; sex offenses; *state government; therapeutic abortion; Hyde Amendment 1994; *Medicaid; *Nebraska; *Orr v. Nelson; United States

The U.S. District Court for Nebraska held invalid, under the supremacy clause of the federal Constitution, a state law which denied Medicaid reimbursement for abortion in the case of rape or incest. Since the 1994 Hyde Amendment had been revised to include federal funding for medically necessary abortion services in the case of rape or incest, the court held that a state cannot restrict Medicaid reimbursement in conflict with federal law. (KIE abstract)

ABORTION/FOREIGN COUNTRIES

Birchard, Karen. New ethical guidelines on abortion released in Ireland. [News]. *Lancet.* 1998 Dec 5; 352(9143): 1840. BE60271.
   *abortion, induced; codes of ethics; cryopreservation; embryos; *guidelines; legal aspects; misconduct; *physicians; *Ireland; *Medical Council (Ireland)

Bosch, Xavier. Spain brings forward mifepristone approval. [News]. *Lancet.* 1998 Oct 17; 352(9136): 1293. BE60269.
   *abortion, induced; *drugs; hospitals; *legal aspects; *RU–486; *Spain

Bosch, Xavier. Spain fails to extend its criteria for legal abortions. [News]. *Lancet.* 1998 Oct 3; 352(9134): 1130. BE60296.
   *abortion, induced; conscience; *government regulation; *legal aspects; physicians; standards; *Spain

Chavkin, Wendy. Unwanted pregnancy in Armenia –– the larger context. [Editorial]. *American Journal of Public Health.* 1998 May; 88(5): 732–733. 13 refs. BE60778.
   *abortion, induced; *contraception; government financing; health insurance reimbursement; *international aspects; knowledge, attitudes, practice; managed care programs; *public policy; religious hospitals; Roman Catholics; *social impact; women's health; Armenia; Eastern Europe; *United States

Ciment, James. Most deaths related to abortion occur in the developing world. [News]. *BMJ (British Medical Journal).* 1999 Jun 5; 318(7197): 1509. BE62423.
   *abortion, induced; contraception; *developing countries; illegal abortion; *international aspects; *mortality; *pregnant women; statistics; World Health Organization

Cook, Rebecca J.; Dickens, Bernard M.; Bliss, Laura E. International developments in abortion law from 1988 to 1998. *American Journal of Public Health.* 1999 Apr; 89(4): 579–586. 122 refs. BE61388.
   *abortion, induced; conscience; counseling; criminal law; developing countries; drugs; government financing; government regulation; health care delivery; health personnel; human rights; *international aspects; judicial action; *legal aspects; legislation; mandatory programs; pregnant women; rape; selective abortion; sex determination; third party consent; time factors; *trends; violence; women's health; women's rights; RU–486; United Nations

OBJECTIVES: In 2 successive decades since 1967, legal accommodation of abortion has grown in many countries. The objective of this study was to assess whether liberalizing trends have been maintained in the last decade and whether increased protection of women's human rights has influenced legal reform. METHODS: A worldwide review was conducted of legislation and judicial rulings affecting abortion, and legal reforms were measured against governmental commitments made under international human rights treaties and at United Nations conferences. RESULTS: Since 1987, 26 jurisdictions have extended grounds for lawful abortion, and 4 countries have restricted grounds. Additional limits on access to legal abortion services include restrictions on funding of services, mandatory counseling and reflection delay requirements, third–party authorizations, and blockades of abortion clinics. CONCLUSIONS: Progressive liberalization has moved abortion laws from a focus on punishment toward concern with women's health and welfare and with their human rights. However, widespread maternal mortality and morbidity show that reform must be accompanied by accessible abortion services and improved contraceptive care and information.

Cowell, Alan. Obeying pope, German bishops end role in abortion system. [News]. *New York Times.* 1998 Jan 28: A3. BE59609.
   *abortion, induced; *clergy; *counseling; health facilities; moral complicity; politics; pregnant women; *Roman Catholics; *Germany

---

BE = bioethics accession number   fn. = footnotes   refs. = references

Dolian, Gayane; Lüdicke, Frank; Katchatrian, Naira, et al. Contraception and induced abortion in Armenia: a critical need for family planning programs in Eastern Europe. *American Journal of Public Health.* 1998 May; 88(5): 803–805. 9 refs. BE60779.
*abortion, induced; age factors; *contraception; females; knowledge, attitudes, practice; methods; pregnant women; socioeconomic factors; survey; women's health; *Armenia
OBJECTIVES: The purpose of this study was to determine the number of induced abortions per woman and the reasons for selecting induced abortion among parous Armenian women. METHODS: A consecutive series of 200 women attending an abortion clinic in Yerevan, Armenia, were queried by a physician about their reproductive histories. RESULTS: Women younger than 20 years of age reported a median of 1 and women older than 40 years reported a median of 8 induced abortions in their lifetimes (overall median = 3). Lack of contraceptive information was the major reason cited for not using contraception. CONCLUSIONS: Induced abortion is the major form of birth control among parous Armenian women. Concerted public health campaigns are needed to inform women and their physicians in Armenia and other Eastern European countries about alternative contraceptive methods.

Flegel, Kenneth M. Society's interest in protection for the fetus. [Editorial]. *Canadian Medical Association Journal.* 1998 Apr 7; 158(7): 895–896. 8 refs. BE60588.
*abortion, induced; beginning of life; fetal development; *fetuses; human rights; *moral obligations; obligations of society; personhood; pregnant women; public policy; women's rights; *Canada

Forder, Caroline J. Abortion: a constitutional problem in European perspective. *Maastricht Journal of European and Comparative Law.* 1994; 1: 56–100. 186 fn. BE59705.
*abortion, induced; comparative studies; *constitutional law; counseling; criminal law; fetal development; fetuses; *government regulation; *international aspects; *legal aspects; legal liability; *legal rights; legislation; obligations of society; physicians; pregnant women; Attorney General v. X; Austria; Belgium; England; *Europe; European Commission; European Court of Human Rights; European Court of Justice; Germany; Ireland; Netherlands; Open Door Counselling v. Ireland; Pregnant Women and Family Assistance Act (Germany)

Fox, Marie. Abortion decision-making: taking men's needs seriously. *In:* Lee, Ellie, ed. Abortion Law and Politics Today. New York, NY: St. Martin's Press; 1998: 198–215. 59 fn. ISBN 0-312-21574-6. BE62339.
*abortion, induced; contraception; counseling; *decision making; *fathers; females; fetuses; judicial action; justice; *legal aspects; *legal rights; *males; married persons; maternal health; parent child relationship; physician's role; *pregnant women; public policy; *spousal consent; spousal notification; therapeutic abortion; value of life; viability; *women's rights; Abortion Act 1967 (Great Britain); C v. S.; European Court of Human Rights; *Great Britain; Paton v. British Pregnancy Advisory Service

Francome, Colin. Attitudes of general practitioners in Northern Ireland toward abortion and family planning. *Family Planning Perspectives.* 1997 Sep–Oct; 29(5): 234–236. 5 fn. BE59884.
*abortion, induced; adolescents; comparative studies; *contraception; decision making; *family planning; *family practice; females; *knowledge, attitudes, practice; married persons; *physicians; pregnant women; *Protestants; referral and consultation; *Roman Catholics; single persons; survey; *Northern Ireland

Furedi, Ann. Wrong but the right thing to do: public opinion and abortion. *In:* Lee, Ellie, ed. Abortion Law and Politics Today. New York, NY: St. Martin's Press; 1998: 159–171. 19 fn. ISBN 0-312-21574-6. BE62336.
*abortion on demand; *abortion, induced; adolescents; adults; *congenital disorders; conscience; decision making; *fetal development; fetuses; legal aspects; mentally disabled; morality; physically disabled; political activity; pregnant women; prenatal diagnosis; prevalence; *public opinion; public policy; rape; *selective abortion; social discrimination; socioeconomic factors; survey; *therapeutic abortion; viability; *Great Britain; Right to Life Movement

Gevers, Sjef. Third trimester abortion for fetal abnormality. *Bioethics.* 1999 Jul; 13(3–4): 306–313. 9 fn. BE61881.
advisory committees; *congenital disorders; decision making; *fetal development; fetuses; guidelines; *legal aspects; physicians; pregnant women; *public policy; *selective abortion; therapeutic abortion; *viability; Abortion Act 1981 (Netherlands); *Netherlands
Developments in medical technology have increased the possibility of diagnosing severe structural abnormalties in the fetus. If these occur, a woman may request termination of her pregnancy. This raises serious ethical and legal questions, in particular if the anomalies are discovered in the third trimester when the fetus is considered viable. Should doctors be allowed to act upon a request for abortion in such a situation, and, if so, which safeguards should be in place? These questions are discussed with special reference to the Netherlands where a commission established by the government recently published a report on this matter.

Githens, Marianne; Stetson, Dorothy McBride, eds. Abortion Politics: Public Policy in Cross-Cultural Perspective. New York, NY: Routledge; 1996. 234 p. Includes references. ISBN 0-415-91225-3. BE60710.
abortion on demand; *abortion, induced; comparative studies; constitutional law; contraception; criminal law; feminist ethics; fetuses; *government regulation; hospitals; *international aspects; killing; *legal aspects; legal rights; physicians; political activity; *politics; pregnant women; prenatal injuries; public opinion; *public policy; religion; reproductive technologies; rights; Roman Catholics; women's rights; wrongful life; *Canada; *Eastern Europe; European Union; France; Germany; Hungary; Ireland; *Japan; Poland; Romania; Russia; *United States; *Western Europe

Goldbeck-Wood, Sandra. Bavaria forced to lift abortion restrictions. [News]. *BMJ (British Medical Journal).* 1998 Nov 7; 317(7168): 1272. BE60929.
*abortion, induced; federal government; government regulation; *legal aspects; state government; *Bavaria; *Germany

Graham, John Remington. Natural law, our constitutions, and the unborn. *Revue Generale de Droit.* 1996; 27(1): 21–53. 110 fn. BE59409.
*abortion, induced; beginning of life; *constitutional law; contraception; *fetuses; freedom; *legal rights; *natural law; privacy; sexuality; Supreme Court decisions; value of life; *Canada; Roe v. Wade; *United States

Grossmann, Atina. The debate that will not end: the politics of abortion in Germany from Weimar to National Socialism and the postwar period. *In:* Berg, Manfred; Cocks, Geoffrey, eds. Medicine and Modernity: Public Health and Medical Care in Nineteenth- and Twentieth-Century Germany. New York, NY: Cambridge University Press; 1997: 193–211. 51 fn. ISBN 0-521-56411-5. BE59271.

BE = bioethics accession number   fn. = footnotes   refs. = references

abortion on demand; *abortion, induced; aliens; coercion; contraception; counseling; criminal law; eugenics; fetal development; government regulation; *historical aspects; illegal abortion; involuntary sterilization; *legal aspects; National Socialism; nurse midwives; physicians; politics; *public policy; rape; selective abortion; socioeconomic factors; sterilization (sexual); therapeutic abortion; war; women's rights; *East Germany; *Germany; *Twentieth Century; *West Germany; World War II

Hoedemaekers, Rogeer; ten Have, Henk.
Geneticization: the Cyprus paradigm. *Journal of Medicine and Philosophy.* 1998 Jun; 23(3): 274–287. 17 refs. BE59291.
  *attitudes; carriers; *coercion; decision making; *directive counseling; economics; eugenics; *genetic counseling; *genetic screening; genetic services; genetics; *goals; health education; *health personnel; international aspects; *mass screening; parents; paternalism; *prenatal diagnosis; prevalence; preventive medicine; public health; public opinion; quality of life; *selective abortion; social control; stigmatization; *thalassemia; *Cyprus; Great Britain; Quebec
Geneticization is a broad term referring to several related processes such as a spreading tendency to use a genetic model of disease explanation, a growing influence of genetics in medical practice, and the slow changing of individual and societal attitudes towards reproduction, prevention and control of disease. These processes can be demonstrated in medical literature on preventive genetic screening and counselling programs for beta–thalassaemia in Cyprus, the United Kingdom and Canada. The preventive possibilities of the new genetic and diagnostic technologies have been quickly understood and advocated by health professionals, and their educational strategies have created a web of social control, in marked contrast to the alleged voluntary decision–making process and free choice. Genetic diagnostic technologies have led to considerable changes in control and management of beta–thalassaemia, and have generated a number of unresolved incongruities.

Ireland. An act (No. 5 of 1995) to prescribe the conditions subject to which certain information relating to services lawfully available outside the state for termination of pregnancies and to persons who provide such services may be given to individual women or the general public, and other matters. Dated 12 May 1995. (The Regulation of Information (Services Outside the State for Termination of Pregnancies) Act, 1995). [Summary]. *International Digest of Health Legislation.* 1995. 46(4). 481–482. BE62692.
  *abortion, induced; *information dissemination; international aspects; *legal aspects; pregnant women; *Ireland

Karro, Helle. Abortion in the framework of family planning in Estonia. *Acta Obstetricia et Gynecologica Scandinavica.* 1997; 76(Suppl. 164): 46–50. 20 refs. BE59127.
  *abortion, induced; age factors; childbirth; contraception; family planning; fetal development; financial support; health education; legal aspects; minors; motivation; parental consent; statistics; therapeutic abortion; *Estonia

Kellough, Gail. Aborting Law: An Exploration of the Politics of Motherhood and Medicine. Buffalo, NY: University of Toronto Press; 1996. 340 p. Includes references. ISBN 0–8020–2971–X. BE59735.
  *abortion, induced; autonomy; caring; commodification; criminal law; deontological ethics; females; fetuses; freedom; government regulation; historical aspects; international aspects; *legal aspects; legal obligations; legal rights; males; moral policy; physicians; *political activity; *politics; pregnant women; reproduction; social dominance;

teleological ethics; therapeutic abortion; *women's rights; *Canada; Criminal Code of Canada; Ontario Coalition for Abortion Clinics; United States

Kilborn, Peter T. Definition of abortion is found to vary abroad. [News]. *New York Times.* 1999 Nov 24: A18. BE60649.
  *abortion, induced; *contraception; *developing countries; *family planning; *government financing; government regulation; *international aspects; population control; *public policy; *Bangladesh; *United States

Kligman, Gail. The Politics of Duplicity: Controlling Reproduction in Ceausescu's Romania. Berkeley, CA: University of California Press; 1998. 358 p. Bibliography: p. 331–346. ISBN 0–520–21075–1. BE60112.
  *abortion, induced; adoption; coercion; communism; contraception; deception; dehumanization; dissent; economics; females; fraud; government regulation; historical aspects; *illegal abortion; incentives; information dissemination; international aspects; legal aspects; mass media; moral complicity; morbidity; mortality; paternalism; physicians; *political systems; politics; *population control; *public policy; *reproduction; *social control; social impact; socioeconomic factors; statistics; unwanted children; women's health; *Romania; *Twentieth Century

Kulczychi, Andrzej. The Abortion Debate in the World Arena. New York, NY: Routledge; 1999. 246 p. Bibliography: p. 211–231. ISBN 0–415–92268–2. BE62140.
  *abortion, induced; comparative studies; cultural pluralism; dissent; family planning; government regulation; illegal abortion; *international aspects; physicians; political activity; *public policy; religion; Roman Catholics; statistics; women's health; women's rights; *Kenya; *Mexico; *Poland

Lee, Ellie, ed. Abortion Law and Politics Today. New York, NY: St. Martin's Press; 1998. 233 p. Includes references. ISBN 0–312–21574–6. BE62335.
  abortion on demand; *abortion, induced; autonomy; *decision making; eugenics; fathers; fetuses; genetic screening; historical aspects; illegal abortion; *international aspects; judicial action; *legal aspects; *legal rights; legislation; paternalism; physician's role; *political activity; politics; *pregnant women; prenatal diagnosis; public opinion; reproductive technologies; selective abortion; socioeconomic factors; spousal consent; spousal notification; therapeutic abortion; women's health; women's rights; Abortion Act 1967 (Great Britain); *France; *Great Britain; Human Fertilisation and Embryology Act 1990 (Great Britain); *Ireland; National Health Service; *Northern Ireland; *Poland; Twentieth Century; *United States

Lessard, Hester. The construction of health care and the ideology of the private in Canadian constitutional law. *Annals of Health Law.* 1993; 2: 121–159. 153 fn. BE59830.
  *abortion, induced; constitutional law; criminal law; economics; federal government; government regulation; *health care delivery; *historical aspects; hospitals; *legal aspects; legal rights; national health insurance; physicians; pregnant women; *private sector; *public policy; *public sector; *rights; social discrimination; therapeutic abortion; *women's rights; *Canada; Canadian Charter of Rights and Freedoms; Criminal Code of Canada; Nineteenth Century; R. v. Morgentaler; Twentieth Century

Levine, Noga Morag. Abortion in Israel: community, rights, and the context of compromise. *Law and Social Inquiry.* 1994 Spring; 19(2): 313–335. 65 fn. BE59899.
  *abortion, induced; attitudes; democracy; ethics committees; government regulation; hospitals; Jewish ethics; legal aspects; legislation; political activity; politics; pregnant women; private sector; *public policy; public sector;

BE = bioethics accession number   fn. = footnotes   refs. = references

selective abortion; socioeconomic factors; therapeutic abortion; women's health; women's rights; *Israel; Right to Life Movement; United States

Macklin, Ruth. Death and birth. *In: her* Against Relativism: Cultural Diversity and the Search for Ethical Universals in Medicine. New York, NY: Oxford University Press; 1999: 136-160. 32 fn. ISBN 0-19-511632-1. BE62782.
  *abortion, induced; autonomy; brain death; cardiac death; *cultural pluralism; *determination of death; *ethical relativism; family relationship; *females; feminist ethics; fetuses; infanticide; *international aspects; justice; morality; mortality; non-Western World; organ donation; organ transplantation; pregnant women; public policy; *selective abortion; *sex determination; *social discrimination; *social worth; value of life; values; women's rights; Cameroon; China; India; Japan; Philippines; United States

Macklin, Ruth. International feminism and reproductive rights. *In: her* Against Relativism: Cultural Diversity and the Search for Ethical Universals in Medicine. New York, NY: Oxford University Press; 1999: 161-185. 30 fn. ISBN 0-19-511632-1. BE62783.
  autonomy; *contraception; *cultural pluralism; decision making; *developing countries; *ethical relativism; females; *feminist ethics; freedom; *human rights; *international aspects; justice; legal aspects; males; methods; non-Western World; *paternalism; *political activity; postmodernism; pregnant women; public policy; *reproduction; reproductive technologies; Roman Catholic ethics; selective abortion; *sex determination; social control; social discrimination; values; Western World; *women's health; *women's rights; Brazil; China; Feminist International Network of Resistance to Reproductive and Genetic Engineering (FINRRAGE); India; International Conference on Population and Development (Cairo, 1994); Women's Global Network for Reproductive Rights

McNally, Ruth. Eugenics here and now. *In:* Glasner, Peter; Rothman, Harry, eds. Genetic Imaginations: Ethical, Legal and Social Issues in Human Genome Research. Brookfield, VT: Ashgate; 1998: 69-82. 23 refs. Based on a paper presented at a workshop hosted by the Centre for Social and Economic Research at the University of the West of England; reprinted from *The Genetic Engineer and Biotechnologist*, 1995; 15(2-3). ISBN 1-84014-356-8. BE60019.
  attitudes; congenital disorders; disabled; *eugenics; genetic counseling; *genetic disorders; genetic enhancement; genetic predisposition; genetic screening; *genetic services; genome mapping; international aspects; prenatal diagnosis; public policy; risk; *selective abortion; social impact; wrongful life; *Great Britain; National Health Service

Mao, Xin. Chinese geneticists approach ethics. [Letter]. *Journal of Medical Ethics.* 1998 Jan; 35(1): 83. 14 refs. BE61126.
  *attitudes; confidentiality; developing countries; *directive counseling; disclosure; eugenics; *genetic counseling; genetic disorders; genetic predisposition; genetic research; *genetic screening; genetic services; genetics; guidelines; *health personnel; international aspects; investigators; *non-Western World; *prenatal diagnosis; *selective abortion; sex determination; survey; Western World; *China

Mason, John Kenyon. Abortion. *In: his* Medico-Legal Aspects of Reproduction and Parenthood. Second Edition. Brookfield, VT: Ashgate; 1998: 107-141. 117 fn. ISBN 1-84104-065-8. BE61063.
  abortion on demand; *abortion, induced; adults; beginning of life; confidentiality; conscience; criminal law; decision making; embryos; fathers; fetal development; fetuses; international aspects; *legal aspects; legal liability; legal rights; mentally disabled; minors; morality; multiple

pregnancy; nurses; parental consent; personhood; physicians; *pregnant women; privacy; selective abortion; sex determination; state interest; statistics; therapeutic abortion; third party consent; value of life; viability; Abortion Act 1967 (Great Britain); Canada; Germany; *Great Britain; Human Fertilisation and Embryology Act 1990 (Great Britain); Infant Life (Preservation) Act 1929 (Great Britain); Ireland; Northern Ireland; Offences Against the Person Act 1861 (Great Britain); United States

Nolan, David. Abortion: should men have a say? *In:* Lee, Ellie, ed. Abortion Law and Politics Today. New York, NY: St. Martin's Press; 1998: 216-231. 26 fn. ISBN 0-312-21574-6. BE62340.
  *abortion, induced; coercion; contraception; *decision making; *fathers; fetuses; *legal aspects; legal obligations; *legal rights; males; maternal health; moral obligations; parent child relationship; physician's role; political activity; *pregnant women; *spousal consent; spousal notification; Supreme Court decisions; viability; *women's rights; Abortion Act 1967 (Great Britain); C v. S.; Doe v. Smith; *Great Britain; Paton v. British Pregnancy Advisory Service; Planned Parenthood of Central Missouri v. Danforth; Planned Parenthood of Southeastern Pennsylvania v. Casey; *United States

Northern Ireland. Supreme Court of Judicature, High Court of Justice, Family Division. Northern Health and Social Services Board v. F and G. *Northern Ireland Law Reports.* 1993 Oct 14 (date of decision). 1993: 268-278. BE60625.
  *abortion, induced; government regulation; international aspects; *legal aspects; *minors; pregnant women; psychological stress; therapeutic abortion; Great Britain; *Northern Health and Social Services Board v. F and G; *Northern Ireland
The Northern Ireland Supreme Court granted permission for a minor, who had been made a ward of the court upon the application of the Northern Health and Social Services Board, to have an abortion and authorized travel outside its jurisdiction for the operation. K, a 14-year-old who had been in foster care, was found to be 13 weeks pregnant and wanted an abortion. Abortion in Northern Ireland is unlawful unless "in good faith for the purpose of preserving the life or health of the woman." The court decided that abortion would be in K's best interests, after considering medical evidence that the psychological effects of continuing the pregnancy were more dangerous than those following its termination. As no doctor could be found who would perform an abortion in Northern Ireland, even one deemed lawful by its highest court, K was allowed to travel to England for the procedure. (KIE abstract)

Odlind, Viveca. Induced abortion -- a global health problem. *Acta Obstetricia et Gynecologica Scandinavica.* 1997; 76(Suppl. 164): 43-45. 11 refs. BE59126.
  *abortion, induced; contraception; developing countries; economics; family planning; health education; illegal abortion; indigents; *international aspects; legal aspects; *maternal health; morbidity; mortality; pregnant women; resource allocation; social impact; statistics; therapeutic abortion; women's health services

Payne, Doug. More British abortions for Irish women. [News]. *BMJ (British Medical Journal).* 1999 Jan 9; 318(7176): 77. BE60930.
  *abortion, induced; attitudes; *international aspects; legal aspects; pregnant women; statistics; *Great Britain; *Ireland

Poland. Law of 30 Aug 1996 amending the law on family planning, protection of human fetuses, and the conditions under which pregnancy termination is permissable, and amending other laws. (*Dziennik Ustaw*

BE = bioethics accession number   fn. = footnotes   refs. = references

Rzeczypospolitej, 4 Dec 1996, No. 139, Text No. 646, pp. 2885–2888). *International Digest of Health Legislation.* 1997; 48(2): 176–178. BE59592.
  *abortion, induced; contraception; *government regulation; health education; illegal abortion; informed consent; minors; pregnant women; prenatal injuries; selective abortion; sexuality; therapeutic abortion; third party consent; women's health services; *Poland

Schubert–Lehnhardt, Viola. Selective abortion after prenatal diagnosis. *Medicine and Law.* 1996; 15(1): 75–81. 11 fn. BE61204.
  attitudes; autonomy; *congenital disorders; *disabled; eugenics; *informal social control; mother fetus relationship; *prenatal diagnosis; quality of life; *selective abortion; *stigmatization; value of life; women's rights; *Germany

Sheiner, Eyal; Shoham–Vardi, Ilana; Weitzman, Dalia, et al. Decisions regarding pregnancy termination among Bedouin couples referred to third level ultrasound clinic. *European Journal of Obstetrics, Gynecology, and Reproductive Biology.* 1998 Feb; 76(2): 141–146. 14 refs. BE60478.
  *congenital disorders; *decision making; evaluation studies; fetal development; minority groups; parents; *pregnant women; *prenatal diagnosis; *selective abortion; ultrasonography; *Arabs; *Israel

Smit, D. Van Zyl. Reconciling the irreconcilable? Recent developments in the German law on abortion. *Medical Law Review.* 1994 Autumn; 2(3): 302–320. 107 fn. BE60604.
  *abortion, induced; constitutional law; counseling; criminal law; fetuses; government regulation; historical aspects; illegal abortion; judicial action; *legal aspects; legal liability; legal rights; physicians; pregnant women; East Germany; *Germany; Nineteenth Century; Twentieth Century; West Germany

South Africa. An act (No. 92 of 1996) to determine the circumstances in which and conditions under which the pregnancy of a woman may be terminated; and to provide for matters connected therewith. Date of assent: 12 Nov 1996. (The Choice on Termination of Pregnancy Act, 1996). (*Government Gazette*, 22 Nov 1996, Vol 377, No. 17602, pp. 1–10). [Summary]. *International Digest of Health Legislation.* 1997; 48(2): 178–181. BE59593.
  abortion on demand; *abortion, induced; counseling; fetal development; informed consent; *legal aspects; mentally disabled; minors; pregnant women; records; selective abortion; therapeutic abortion; third party consent; *South Africa

Tang, Julie. The United States' immigration laws: prospects for relief for foreign nationals seeking refuge from coercive sterilization or abortion practices in their homelands. *Saint Louis University Public Law Review.* 1996; 15(2): 371–401. 165 fn. BE59915.
  *abortion, induced; *aliens; *coercion; federal government; *human rights; *international aspects; *involuntary sterilization; judicial action; *legal aspects; *mandatory programs; political systems; *population control; *public policy; reproduction; *emigration and immigration; *China; In re Chang; U.S. Congress; *United States

Thompson, Angela. International protection of women's rights: an analysis of *Open Door Counselling Ltd. and Dublin Well Woman Centre v. Ireland. Boston University International Law Journal.* 1994; 12: 371–406. 206 fn. BE59895.
  *abortion, induced; counseling; equal protection; *human rights; *information dissemination; *international aspects;

*legal aspects; legal rights; morality; pregnant women; privacy; *women's rights; European Commission on Human Rights; European Convention on Human Rights; *European Court of Human Rights; *Ireland; *Open Door Counselling v. Ireland

Tuffs, Annette. German drug agency approves mifepristone. [News]. *BMJ (British Medical Journal).* 1999 Jul 17; 319(7203): 141. BE62513.
  *abortion, induced; *drugs; *government regulation; *Germany; *RU–486

Wheale, Peter R. Moral and legal consequences for the fetus/unborn child of medical technologies derived from human genome research. *In:* Glasner, Peter; Rothman, Harry, eds. Genetic Imaginations: Ethical, Legal and Social Issues in Human Genome Research. Brookfield, VT: Ashgate; 1998: 83–96. 35 refs. Based on a paper presented at a workshop hosted by the Centre for Social and Economic Research at the University of the West of England; reprinted from *The Genetic Engineer and Biotechnologist*, 1995; 15(2–3). ISBN 1–84014–356–8. BE60020.
  abortion, induced; *beginning of life; coercion; *congenital disorders; deontological ethics; *embryo research; *embryos; ethical analysis; fetal development; *fetuses; genetic disorders; genetic screening; genome mapping; government regulation; *legal aspects; legal liability; *moral obligations; *moral policy; negligence; *personhood; pregnant women; prenatal injuries; *public policy; *quality of life; rights; *selective abortion; social impact; treatment refusal; utilitarianism; *value of life; *wrongful life; *Great Britain

Whelan, Robert, ed. Legal Abortion Examined: 21 Years of Abortion Statistics. London: SPUC Educational Research Trust; 1992. 32 p. ISBN 0–946680–37X. BE59220.
  *abortion, induced; age factors; aliens; child abuse; childbirth; congenital disorders; fetal development; international aspects; married persons; mortality; pregnant women; private sector; selective abortion; single persons; *statistics; therapeutic abortion; Abortion Act 1967 (Great Britain); England; *Great Britain; National Health Service; Scotland; Wales

ABORTION/LEGAL ASPECTS

Alaska. Supreme Court. Valley Hospital Association, Inc. v. Mat–Su Coalition for Choice. *Pacific Reporter, 2d Series.* 1997 Nov 21 (date of decision). 948: 963–973. BE59971.
  *abortion, induced; constitutional law; government regulation; *hospitals; *institutional policies; *legal aspects; legal rights; privacy; *refusal to treat; state government; *state interest; *Alaska; *Valley Hospital Association v. Mat–Su Coalition

The Alaska Supreme Court held unconstitutional a state law that permitted hospitals to refuse to provide abortion services to the extent it applied to "quasi–public" providers and enjoined a "quasi–public" hospital from enforcing its policy not to perform abortions. The court held that the state's constitution provided a fundamental right and privilege to abortion under its privacy right, and that the law and the hospital's policy violated this right: "The reasons a doctor and patient choose a medical procedure, so long as it is legal, must not be subject to the approval of hospital's board of directors, according to their own values." The abortion right, in the opinion of the court, can only be constrained by a compelling state interest and when no less restrictive means could advance that end. The court held the hospital was a quasi–public institution and subject to the compelling state interest standard because: 1) the state

---

BE = bioethics accession number   fn. = footnotes   refs. = references

had created in it a health care monopoly by the certificate of need procedure; 2) the hospital received local, state, and federal funds; 3) the hospital received local land grants; and 4) the hospital was required to operate as a public facility. In a footnote, the court reserved the question of whether "a quasi–public hospital could have a policy based on the religious tenets of its sponsor which could be a compelling state interest." (KIE abstract)

Avallone, Fran; Focus on the Family; Family Research Council. Do parental notification laws benefit minors seeking abortions? *In:* Francoeur, Robert T., ed. Taking Sides: Clashing Views on Controversial Issues in Human Sexuality. Fifth Edition. Guilford, CT: Dushkin Publishing Group/Brown and Benchmark; 1996: 174–191. 6 refs. ISBN 0–697–31292–5. BE62047.
*abortion, induced; adolescents; alternatives; decision making; *government regulation; *legal aspects; maternal health; *minors; parental consent; *parental notification; pregnant women; risks and benefits; state government; state interest; Supreme Court decisions; United States

Benshoof, Janet; Knights of Columbus. Abortion and the "pro–life" *v.* "pro–choice" debate: should the human fetus be considered a person? *In:* Francoeur, Robert T., ed. Taking Sides: Clashing Views on Controversial Issues in Human Sexuality. Fifth Edition. Guilford, CT: Dushkin Publishing Group/Brown and Benchmark; 1996: 120–133. 9 refs. Bibliography: p. 133. ISBN 0–697–31292–5. BE62044.
*abortion, induced; *beginning of life; constitutional law; embryos; *fetuses; *legal aspects; legal liability; *legal rights; *personhood; *pregnant women; prenatal injuries; Supreme Court decisions; viability; wrongful death; Fourteenth Amendment; *Roe v. Wade; *United States; Webster v. Reproductive Health Services

Bopp, James; Cook, Curtis R.; Heilig, Steve, et al. Partial–birth abortion. [Letters and response]. *New England Journal of Medicine.* 1998 Dec 3; 339(23): 1716–1717. 10 refs. BE61713.
*abortion, induced; federal government; *fetal development; fetuses; *government regulation; killing; *legal aspects; *methods; newborns; personhood; physicians; politics; state government; terminology; viability; *United States

Bopp, James; Cook, Curtis R. Partial–birth abortion: the final frontier of abortion jurisprudence. *Issues in Law and Medicine.* 1998 Summer; 14(1): 3–57. 213 fn. BE61034.
*abortion, induced; childbirth; *constitutional law; criminal law; federal government; *fetal development; fetuses; *government regulation; infanticide; killing; *legal aspects; legal rights; maternal health; *methods; organizational policies; pain; personhood; physicians; pregnant women; professional organizations; state government; state interest; Supreme Court decisions; viability; American College of Obstetricians and Gynecologists; American Medical Association; Evans v. Kelley; *Michigan; *Partial–Birth Abortion Ban Act (1995 bill); Planned Parenthood of Southeastern Pennsylvania v. Casey; Roe v. Wade; U.S. Congress; *United States

Bostrom, Barry A. Evans v. Kelley. [Note]. *Issues in Law and Medicine.* 1998 Summer; 14(1): 103–106. BE61035.
*abortion, induced; *constitutional law; criminal law; due process; *fetal development; fetuses; *government regulation; *legal aspects; legal rights; legislation; maternal health; *methods; physicians; pregnant women; state government; *Evans v. Kelley; *Michigan

Bostrom, Barry A. Planned Parenthood of Wisconsin v.

Doyle. [Note]. *Issues in Law and Medicine.* 1998 Fall; 14(2): 209–214. BE62013.
*abortion, induced; constitutional law; *fetal development; *government regulation; *legal aspects; *methods; physicians; state government; *Planned Parenthood of Wisconsin v. Doyle; *Wisconsin

Cahill, Lisa Sowle. Catholic commitment and public responsibility. *In:* Rainey, R. Randall; Magill, Gerard, eds. Abortion and Public Policy: An Interdisciplinary Investigation within the Catholic Tradition. Omaha, NE: Creighton University Press; 1996: 131–162. 53 fn. Paper presented at a conference held at Saint Louis University, 11–13 Mar 1993. ISBN 1–881871–18–5. BE61992.
abortion on demand; *abortion, induced; autonomy; *common good; *conscience; consensus; contraception; fetal development; fetal research; fetuses; historical aspects; informed consent; *justice; law; *legal aspects; *moral policy; morality; *natural law; personhood; *politics; pregnant women; public opinion; *public policy; reproduction; *Roman Catholic ethics; sexuality; social discrimination; state government; *theology; *value of life; values; women's rights; Declaration on Abortion; Europe; United States

Cook, Rebecca J.; Dickens, Bernard M.; Bliss, Laura E. International developments in abortion law from 1988 to 1998. *American Journal of Public Health.* 1999 Apr; 89(4): 579–586. 122 refs. BE61388.
*abortion, induced; conscience; counseling; criminal law; developing countries; drugs; government financing; government regulation; health care delivery; health personnel; human rights; *international aspects; judicial action; *legal aspects; legislation; mandatory programs; pregnant women; rape; selective abortion; sex determination; third party consent; time factors; *trends; violence; women's health; women's rights; RU–486; United Nations
OBJECTIVES: In 2 successive decades since 1967, legal accommodation of abortion has grown in many countries. The objective of this study was to assess whether liberalizing trends have been maintained in the last decade and whether increased protection of women's human rights has influenced legal reform. METHODS: A worldwide review was conducted of legislation and judicial rulings affecting abortion, and legal reforms were measured against governmental commitments made under international human rights treaties and at United Nations conferences. RESULTS: Since 1987, 26 jurisdictions have extended grounds for lawful abortion, and 4 countries have restricted grounds. Additional limits on access to legal abortion services include restrictions on funding of services, mandatory counseling and reflection delay requirements, third–party authorizations, and blockades of abortion clinics. CONCLUSIONS: Progressive liberalization has moved abortion laws from a focus on punishment toward concern with women's health and welfare and with their human rights. However, widespread maternal mortality and morbidity show that reform must be accompanied by accessible abortion services and improved contraceptive care and information.

Dixon, Nicholas. The morality of anti–abortion civil disobedience. *Public Affairs Quarterly.* 1997 Jan; 11(1): 21–38. 30 fn. BE59162.
*abortion, induced; blacks; *conscience; constitutional law; *dissent; fetuses; health facilities; historical aspects; judicial action; justice; *legal aspects; legal rights; *morality; motivation; *political activity; pregnant women; public policy; punishment; value of life; slavery; Dworkin, Ronald; Fourteenth Amendment; King, Martin Luther; Nineteenth Century; *Operation Rescue; *Right to Life Movement; Roe

---

BE = bioethics accession number   fn. = footnotes   refs. = references

v. Wade; Twentieth Century; United States

Forder, Caroline J. Abortion: a constitutional problem in European perspective. *Maastricht Journal of European and Comparative Law.* 1994; 1: 56–100. 186 fn. BE59705.
  *abortion, induced; comparative studies; *constitutional law; counseling; criminal law; fetal development; fetuses; *government regulation; *international aspects; *legal aspects; legal liability; *legal rights; legislation; obligations of society; physicians; pregnant women; Attorney General v. X; Austria; Belgium; England; *Europe; European Commission; European Court of Human Rights; European Court of Justice; Germany; Ireland; Netherlands; Open Door Counselling v. Ireland; Pregnant Women and Family Assistance Act (Germany)

Fox, Marie. Abortion decision–making: taking men's needs seriously. *In:* Lee, Ellie, ed. Abortion Law and Politics Today. New York, NY: St. Martin's Press; 1998: 198–215. 59 fn. ISBN 0–312–21574–6. BE62339.
  *abortion, induced; contraception; counseling; *decision making; *fathers; females; fetuses; judicial action; justice; *legal aspects; *legal rights; *males; married persons; maternal health; parent child relationship; physician's role; *pregnant women; public policy; *spousal consent; spousal notification; therapeutic abortion; value of life; viability; *women's rights; Abortion Act 1967 (Great Britain); C v. S.; European Court of Human Rights; *Great Britain; Paton v. British Pregnancy Advisory Service

Gevers, Sjef. Third trimester abortion for fetal abnormality. *Bioethics.* 1999 Jul; 13(3–4): 306–313. 9 fn. BE61881.
  advisory committees; *congenital disorders; decision making; *fetal development; fetuses; guidelines; *legal aspects; physicians; pregnant women; *public policy; *selective abortion; therapeutic abortion; *viability; Abortion Act 1981 (Netherlands); *Netherlands
Developments in medical technology have increased the possibility of diagnosing severe structural abnormalties in the fetus. If these occur, a woman may request termination of her pregnancy. This raises serious ethical and legal questions, in particular if the anomalies are discovered in the third trimester when the fetus is considered viable. Should doctors be allowed to act upon a request for abortion in such a situation, and, if so, which safeguards should be in place? These questions are discussed with special reference to the Netherlands where a commission established by the government recently published a report on this matter.

Githens, Marianne; Stetson, Dorothy McBride, eds. Abortion Politics: Public Policy in Cross–Cultural Perspective. New York, NY: Routledge; 1996. 234 p. Includes references. ISBN 0–415–91225–3. BE60710.
  abortion on demand; *abortion, induced; comparative studies; constitutional law; contraception; criminal law; feminist ethics; fetuses; *government regulation; hospitals; *international aspects; killing; *legal aspects; legal rights; physicians; political activity; *politics; pregnant women; prenatal injuries; public opinion; *public policy; religion; reproductive technologies; rights; Roman Catholics; women's rights; wrongful life; *Canada; *Eastern Europe; European Union; France; Germany; Hungary; Ireland; *Japan; Poland; Romania; Russia; *United States; *Western Europe

Glendon, Mary Ann; Treene, Eric W. The legacy of Justice William Brennan. *Human Life Review.* 1998 Winter; 24(1): 65–76. 4 fn. BE59446.
  abortion on demand; *abortion, induced; constitutional law; fetuses; government financing; government regulation; historical aspects; *legal aspects; *legal rights; minors; parental consent; parental notification; pregnant women; privacy; state interest; *Supreme Court decisions;

therapeutic abortion; value of life; viability; Beal v. Doe; *Brennan, William; City of Akron v. Akron Center for Reproductive Health; Colautti v. Franklin; Doe v. Bolton; Eisenstadt v. Baird; Harris v. McRae; Hodgson v. Missouri; Maher v. Roe; Ohio v. Akron Center for Reproductive Health; Planned Parenthood Association of Kansas City v. Ashcroft; Poelker v. Doe; Roe v. Wade; Thornburgh v. American College of Obstetricians and Gynecologists; Twentieth Century; *United States

Graham, John Remington. Natural law, our constitutions, and the unborn. *Revue Generale de Droit.* 1996; 27(1): 21–53. 110 fn. BE59409.
  *abortion, induced; beginning of life; *constitutional law; contraception; *fetuses; freedom; *legal rights; *natural law; privacy; sexuality; Supreme Court decisions; value of life; *Canada; Roe v. Wade; *United States

Grossmann, Atina. The debate that will not end: the politics of abortion in Germany from Weimar to National Socialism and the postwar period. *In:* Berg, Manfred; Cocks, Geoffrey, eds. Medicine and Modernity: Public Health and Medical Care in Nineteenth– and Twentieth–Century Germany. New York, NY: Cambridge University Press; 1997: 193–211. 51 fn. ISBN 0–521–56411–5. BE59271.
  abortion on demand; *abortion, induced; aliens; coercion; contraception; counseling; criminal law; eugenics; fetal development; government regulation; *historical aspects; illegal abortion; involuntary sterilization; *legal aspects; National Socialism; nurse midwives; physicians; politics; *public policy; rape; selective abortion; socioeconomic factors; sterilization (sexual); therapeutic abortion; war; women's rights; *East Germany; *Germany; *Twentieth Century; *West Germany; World War II

Hanigsberg, Julia E. Homologizing pregnancy and motherhood: a consideration of abortion. *Michigan Law Review.* 1995 Nov; 94(2): 371–418. 190 fn. Paper presented at the 1995 meeting of the Law and Society Association. BE59708.
  *abortion, induced; attitudes; *autonomy; decision making; disadvantaged; drugs; *females; *feminist ethics; fetal development; fetuses; *government regulation; human body; law; legal aspects; *legal rights; mother fetus relationship; mothers; motivation; *pregnant women; prenatal injuries; privacy; reproduction; self concept; *social control; social discrimination; value of life; women's health services; *women's rights; liberalism; RU–486; United States

Holmes, Steven A. Right to abortion quietly advances in state courts. [News]. *New York Times.* 1998 Dec 6: 1, 25. BE60368.
  *abortion, induced; government financing; government regulation; indigents; *legal aspects; *legal rights; parental notification; pregnant women; *state government; trends; Medicaid; *United States

Indiana. Supreme Court. A Woman's Choice–East Side Women's Clinic v. Newman. *North Eastern Reporter, 2d Series.* 1996 Aug 7 (date of decision). 671: 104–113. Rehearing denied 30 Dec 1996. BE60047.
  *abortion, induced; *emergency care; government regulation; informed consent; *legal aspects; legislation; maternal health; mental health; *pregnant women; state government; *therapeutic abortion; *A Woman's Choice–East Side Women's Clinic v. Newman; *Indiana
Answering certified questions to a federal district court, the Indiana Supreme Court held that the state's medical emergency condition exception to the abortion informed consent rules applies when (1) compliance would pose a significant threat to the life or health of the woman in any way, and (2) when compliance would threaten to cause severe psychological harm to the woman. The

---

BE = bioethics accession number   fn. = footnotes   refs. = references

Court refused to hold that the exception would apply when compliance threatens to cause severe but temporary physical health problems for the woman. (KIE abstract)

Ireland. An act (No. 5 of 1995) to prescribe the conditions subject to which certain information relating to services lawfully available outside the state for termination of pregnancies and to persons who provide such services may be given to individual women or the general public, and other matters. Dated 12 May 1995. (The Regulation of Information (Services Outside the State for Termination of Pregnancies) Act, 1995). [Summary]. *International Digest of Health Legislation.* 1995. 46(4). 481–482. BE62692.
    *abortion, induced; *information dissemination; international aspects; *legal aspects; pregnant women; *Ireland

Janofsky, Michael. Judge backs Virginia limit on abortions. [News]. *New York Times.* 1998 Jul 2: A12. BE59616.
    *abortion, induced; fetal development; *government regulation; *legal aspects; *methods; state government; viability; *Virginia

Kellough, Gail. Aborting Law: An Exploration of the Politics of Motherhood and Medicine. Buffalo, NY: University of Toronto Press; 1996. 340 p. Includes references. ISBN 0-8020-2971-X. BE59735.
    *abortion, induced; autonomy; caring; commodification; criminal law; deontological ethics; females; fetuses; freedom; government regulation; historical aspects; international aspects; *legal aspects; legal obligations; legal rights; males; moral policy; physicians; *political activity; *politics; pregnant women; reproduction; social dominance; teleological ethics; therapeutic abortion; *women's rights; *Canada; Criminal Code of Canada; Ontario Coalition for Abortion Clinics; United States

Kocieniewski, David. Ban on a type of abortion is struck down. [News]. *New York Times.* 1998 Dec 9: B1, B4. BE60371.
    *abortion, induced; *fetal development; *government regulation; *legal aspects; *methods; state government; *New Jersey

Law, Sylvia A. Silent no more: physicians' legal and ethical obligations to patients seeking abortions. *New York University Review of Law and Social Change.* 1994-1995; 21(2): 279–321. 222 fn. BE62223.
    *abortion, induced; autonomy; conscience; *counseling; disclosure; informed consent; internship and residency; *legal aspects; legal liability; *legal obligations; medical education; medical ethics; *moral obligations; negligence; obstetrics and gynecology; organizational policies; paternalism; physician patient relationship; *physicians; *pregnant women; professional organizations; *referral and consultation; standards; Supreme Court decisions; women's health services; wrongful life; patient abandonment; American College of Obstetricians and Gynecologists; American Medical Association; *United States

Lee, Ellie, ed. Abortion Law and Politics Today. New York, NY: St. Martin's Press; 1998. 233 p. Includes references. ISBN 0-312-21574-6. BE62335.
    abortion on demand; *abortion, induced; autonomy; *decision making; eugenics; fathers; fetuses; genetic screening; historical aspects; illegal abortion; *international aspects; judicial action; *legal aspects; *legal rights; legislation; paternalism; physician's role; *political activity; politics; *pregnant women; prenatal diagnosis; public opinion; reproductive technologies; selective abortion; socioeconomic factors; spousal consent; spousal notification; therapeutic abortion; women's health; women's rights;

Abortion Act 1967 (Great Britain); *France; *Great Britain; Human Fertilisation and Embryology Act 1990 (Great Britain); *Ireland; National Health Service; *Northern Ireland; *Poland; Twentieth Century; *United States

Leibold, Peter; Gilham, Charles S. When physicians perform abortions outside the Catholic hospital. *Health Progress.* 1998 Mar-Apr; 79(2): 12–14. 14 fn. BE60591.
    *abortion, induced; conscience; employment; federal government; government financing; *institutional policies; *legal aspects; legal liability; *physicians; *religious hospitals; *Roman Catholic ethics; social discrimination; United States

Lessard, Hester. The construction of health care and the ideology of the private in Canadian constitutional law. *Annals of Health Law.* 1993; 2: 121–159. 153 fn. BE59830.
    *abortion, induced; constitutional law; criminal law; economics; federal government; government regulation; *health care delivery; *historical aspects; hospitals; *legal aspects; legal rights; national health insurance; physicians; pregnant women; *private sector; *public policy; *public sector; *rights; social discrimination; therapeutic abortion; *women's rights; *Canada; Canadian Charter of Rights and Freedoms; Criminal Code of Canada; Nineteenth Century; R. v. Morgentaler; Twentieth Century

Lewin, Tamar. A prisoner is the focus of an abortion debate. [News]. *New York Times.* 1999 Jan 10: 12. BE60124.
    *abortion, induced; coercion; *government financing; *legal aspects; municipal government; political activity; *prisoners; public opinion; Roman Catholics; Pennsylvania; *Ptaschnik, Karen

Lewin, Tamar. Wisconsin abortion clinics shut down, citing new law. [News]. *New York Times.* 1998 May 15: A27. BE59672.
    *abortion, induced; criminal law; fetal development; *government regulation; health facilities; *legal aspects; *legal liability; *methods; *physicians; refusal to treat; state government; viability; *Wisconsin

McCorvey, Norma. I Am Roe: My Life, *Roe v. Wade,* and Freedom of Choice. New York, NY: HarperPerennial; 1994. 216 p. ISBN 0-06-092638-4. BE61421.
    abortion on demand; *abortion, induced; *government regulation; *historical aspects; illegal abortion; lawyers; *legal rights; *political activity; pregnant women; state government; *Supreme Court decisions; women's rights; Right to Life Movement; *Roe v. Wade; *Roe, Jane; Texas; Twentieth Century; *United States

Mason, John Kenyon. Abortion. *In: his* Medico-Legal Aspects of Reproduction and Parenthood. Second Edition. Brookfield, VT: Ashgate; 1998: 107–141. 117 fn. ISBN 1-84104-065-8. BE61063.
    abortion on demand; *abortion, induced; adults; beginning of life; confidentiality; conscience; criminal law; decision making; embryos; fathers; fetal development; fetuses; international aspects; *legal aspects; legal liability; legal rights; mentally disabled; minors; morality; multiple pregnancy; nurses; parental consent; personhood; physicians; *pregnant women; privacy; selective abortion; sex determination; state interest; statistics; therapeutic abortion; third party consent; value of life; viability; Abortion Act 1967 (Great Britain); Canada; Germany; *Great Britain; Human Fertilisation and Embryology Act 1990 (Great Britain); Infant Life (Preservation) Act 1929 (Great Britain); Ireland; Northern Ireland; Offences Against the Person Act 1861 (Great Britain); United States

Massachusetts. Supreme Judicial Court. Planned Parenthood League of Massachusetts v. Attorney

---

BE = bioethics accession number   fn. = footnotes   refs. = references

General. *North Eastern Reporter, 2d Series.* 1997 Mar 18 (date of decision). 677: 101–114. BE60048.

*abortion, induced; constitutional law; due process; fathers; *government regulation; judicial action; *legal aspects; legal rights; *minors; mothers; *parental consent; *pregnant women; state government; state interest; *Massachusetts; *Planned Parenthood v. Attorney General

The Supreme Judicial Court of Massachusetts sustained a state statute which required pregnant unmarried minors to obtain the consent of both parents or a judge of the Superior Court in order to have an abortion. The court held that the state's interest in protecting the welfare of its minors and ensuring informed consent justified restrictions on a minor's constitutional right to choose an abortion. The court held unconstitutional, however, the law's requirement that the minor obtain the consent of both parents as an undue burden on the minor's due process rights. (KIE abstract)

Minnesota. Supreme Court. Women of the State of Minnesota v. Gomez. *North Western Reporter, 2d Series.* 1995 Dec 15 (date of decision). 542: 17–42. BE60050.

*abortion, induced; constitutional law; decision making; *government financing; *government regulation; indigents; *legal aspects; *legal rights; legislation; *pregnant women; privacy; sex offenses; state government; *therapeutic abortion; *Medicaid; *Minnesota; *Women v. Gomez

The Minnesota Supreme Court held unconstitutional a state law which restricted state Medicaid funding for abortions to cases where the abortion was a medical necessity, defined as a pregnancy that threatens the life of the mother in the opinion of two physicians; where the pregnancy was the product of criminal misconduct and the incident was reported to law enforcement authorities within 48 hours of the incident; or where the pregnancy was the result of incest that was reported to a valid law enforcement agency for investigation prior to the abortion procedure. The court held that Minnesota's state constitution provided broader privacy rights than the U.S. Constitution and that it protected both the right to an abortion and the right to the decision to abort. (KIE abstract)

Nolan, David. Abortion: should men have a say? *In:* Lee, Ellie, ed. Abortion Law and Politics Today. New York, NY: St. Martin's Press; 1998: 216–231. 26 fn. ISBN 0-312-21574-6. BE62340.

*abortion, induced; coercion; contraception; *decision making; *fathers; fetuses; *legal aspects; legal obligations; *legal rights; males; maternal health; moral obligations; parent child relationship; physician's role; political activity; *pregnant women; *spousal consent; spousal notification; Supreme Court decisions; viability; *women's rights; Abortion Act 1967 (Great Britain); C v. S.; Doe v. Smith; *Great Britain; Paton v. British Pregnancy Advisory Service; Planned Parenthood of Central Missouri v. Danforth; Planned Parenthood of Southeastern Pennsylvania v. Casey; *United States

Pear, Robert. Inquiry criticizes A.M.A. backing of abortion procedure ban. [News]. *New York Times.* 1998 Dec 4: A27. BE60375.

*abortion, induced; federal government; *fetal development; government regulation; *methods; *organizational policies; *physicians; politics; *professional organizations; *American Medical Association; United States

Poland. Law of 30 Aug 1996 amending the law on family planning, protection of human fetuses, and the conditions under which pregnancy termination is permissable, and amending other laws. (*Dziennik Ustaw Rzeczypospolitej*, 4 Dec 1996, No. 139, Text No. 646, pp. 2885–2888). *International Digest of Health Legislation.* 1997; 48(2): 176–178. BE59592.

*abortion, induced; contraception; *government regulation; health education; illegal abortion; informed consent; minors; pregnant women; prenatal injuries; selective abortion; sexuality; therapeutic abortion; third party consent; women's health services; *Poland

Robertson, John A. Abortion to obtain fetal tissue for transplant. *Suffolk University Law Review.* 1993 Winter; 27(4): 1359–1389. 75 fn. BE61595.

*aborted fetuses; *abortion, induced; advisory committees; anencephaly; attitudes; coercion; constitutional law; criminal law; *decision making; *directed donation; family members; federal government; fetal research; *fetal tissue donation; *government regulation; informed consent; killing; legal aspects; *legal rights; *moral policy; motivation; organ donation; persistent vegetative state; *pregnant women; public policy; remuneration; reproduction; sex determination; state interest; tissue transplantation; transplant recipients; *women's rights; Department of Health and Human Services; National Institutes of Health; United States

Scarnecchia, Suellyn; Field, Julie Kunce. Judging girls: decision making in parental consent to abortion cases. *Michigan Journal of Gender and Law.* 1995; 3(41): 75–123. 134 fn. BE59408.

*abortion, induced; *adolescents; *competence; counseling; *decision making; *informed consent; *judicial action; *legal aspects; legislation; *minors; *parental consent; standards; state government; Supreme Court decisions; *Michigan; United States

Smit, D. Van Zyl. Reconciling the irreconcilable? Recent developments in the German law on abortion. *Medical Law Review.* 1994 Autumn; 2(3): 302–320. 107 fn. BE60604.

*abortion, induced; constitutional law; counseling; criminal law; fetuses; government regulation; historical aspects; illegal abortion; judicial action; *legal aspects; legal liability; legal rights; physicians; pregnant women; East Germany; *Germany; Nineteenth Century; Twentieth Century; West Germany

South Africa. An act (No. 92 of 1996) to determine the circumstances in which and conditions under which the pregnancy of a woman may be terminated; and to provide for matters connected therewith. Date of assent: 12 Nov 1996. (The Choice on Termination of Pregnancy Act, 1996). (*Government Gazette*, 22 Nov 1996, Vol 377, No. 17602, pp. 1–10). [Summary]. *International Digest of Health Legislation.* 1997; 48(2): 178–181. BE59593.

abortion on demand; *abortion, induced; counseling; fetal development; informed consent; *legal aspects; mentally disabled; minors; pregnant women; records; selective abortion; therapeutic abortion; third party consent; *South Africa

Stoller, David. Prenatal genetic screening: the enigma of selective abortion. *Journal of Law and Health.* 1997–98; 12(1): 121–140. 111 fn. BE61137.

abortion, induced; congenital disorders; dehumanization; disabled; eugenics; federal government; fetuses; genetic counseling; genetic disorders; genetic enhancement; *genetic screening; genome mapping; government regulation; *legal aspects; *prenatal diagnosis; *selective abortion; sex determination; state government; state interest; stigmatization; Supreme Court decisions; viability; *United States

Thompson, Angela. International protection of women's rights: an analysis of *Open Door Counselling Ltd. and Dublin Well Woman Centre v. Ireland. Boston University International Law Journal.* 1994; 12: 371–406. 206 fn.

BE = bioethics accession number   fn. = footnotes   refs. = references

BE59895.
  *abortion, induced; counseling; equal protection; *human rights; *information dissemination; *international aspects; *legal aspects; legal rights; morality; pregnant women; privacy; *women's rights; European Commission on Human Rights; European Convention on Human Rights; *European Court of Human Rights; *Ireland; *Open Door Counselling v. Ireland

Tuffs, Annette. German drug agency approves mifepristone. [News]. *BMJ (British Medical Journal).* 1999 Jul 17; 319(7203): 141. BE62513.
  *abortion, induced; *drugs; *government regulation; *Germany; *RU–486

U.S. Court of Appeals, Fifth Circuit. Hope Medical Group for Women v. Edwards. *Federal Reporter, 3d Series.* 1998 Sep 11 (date of decision). 63: 418–429. BE60052.
  *abortion, induced; death; federal government; *government financing; *government regulation; indigents; *legal aspects; legal rights; legislation; *pregnant women; sex offenses; state government; therapeutic abortion; *Hope Medical Group for Women v. Edwards; *Hyde Amendment 1994; *Louisiana; *Medicaid

The U.S. Court of Appeals for the Fifth Circuit invalidated a Louisiana law which restricted Medicaid reimbursement for abortion to instances where the pregnancy threatened the life of the mother. Although the revised 1994 Hyde Amendment permitted federal Medicaid funding for the abortion of pregnancies resulting from rape or incest, the Fifth Circuit held that the Hyde Amendment did not require states to fund these procedures. Instead, the court relied on the purposes of Medicaid to provide health–sustaining medical care and held that Louisiana's statute impermissibly restricted a women's right to abortion where medically necessary. Louisiana was enjoined from enforcing the law to the extent it restricted Medicaid reimbursement for the medically necessary abortion of pregnancies resulting from rape or incest. The court held that the state's interest in normal childbirth is not sufficient to sustain the abortion funding restriction. (KIE abstract)

U.S. Court of Appeals, Fourth Circuit. Planned Parenthood of the Blue Ridge v. Camblos. *Federal Reporter, 3d Series.* 1997 Jun 30 (date of decision). 116: 707–721. BE61997.
  *abortion, induced; competence; constitutional law; *government regulation; *judicial action; *legal aspects; legal rights; *minors; *parental notification; pregnant women; state government; *Planned Parenthood of the Blue Ridge v. Camblos; *Virginia

The U.S. Court of Appeals for the Fourth Circuit issued a stay of the district court's injunction against enforcement of Virginia's Parental Notice Act which allows a juvenile court judge the discretion to decline authorization of an abortion without parental notice, even if the judge finds the pregnant minor to be mature and capable of informed consent for an abortion. The circuit court decided that the district court had erred in holding that the judicial bypass procedures in Virginia's parental *notice* statute must satisfy the constitutional requirements for bypass procedures in parental *consent* statutes, as interpreted by the U.S. Supreme Court. (KIE abstract)

U.S. Court of Appeals, Ninth Circuit. Wicklund v. Salvagni. *Federal Reporter, 3d Series.* 1996 Aug 16 (date of decision). 93: 567–572. BE60053.
  *abortion, induced; constitutional law; *government regulation; judicial action; *legal aspects; legal rights; *minors; *parental notification; *pregnant women; risks and

benefits; state government; *Montana; *Wicklund v. Salvagni

The U.S. Court of Appeals for the Ninth Circuit held unconstitutional a Montana parental notification law in the case of minors seeking abortion. The law provided that a physician could not perform an abortion upon a minor or an incompetent person unless the physician had given 48 hours notice to one parent or to the legal guardian of the patient. The law permitted a minor to petition a court for a waiver of the notice requirement if she was sufficiently mature to decide whether to have an abortion and if the notification of a parent or guardian was not in the best interest of the minor. The court struck down the law because it did not provide for judicial bypass where the abortion, and not just the parental notice, would be in the minor's best interest. (KIE abstract)

U.S. Court of Appeals, Sixth Circuit. Women's Medical Professional Corporation v. Voinovich. *Federal Reporter, 3d Series.* 1997 Nov 18 (date of decision). 130: 187–219. BE60054.
  *abortion, induced; constitutional law; *fetal development; fetuses; *government regulation; legislation; maternal health; *methods; *pregnant women; state government; *therapeutic abortion; viability; *Ohio; *Women's Medical Professional Corp. v. Voinovich

The U.S. Court of Appeals for the Sixth Circuit affirmed a district court ruling that held unconstitutional an Ohio abortion law which banned the dilation and extraction and dilation and evacuation procedures and restricted abortion of a viable fetus to cases where the pregnancy posed risk of death or serious injury to the pregnant woman. The law also required that a physician certify the necessity of such an abortion in writing and a second physician concur in writing after reviewing the mother's records, that the abortion be performed in a facility with a neonatal unit to care for the fetus, that the attending physician use a method of abortion offering the best ooportunity for the fetus to survive (unless the procedure poses a greater chance of death or serious risk to the health of the mother) and that a second physician be present to attend the fetus. In the event of a medical emergency, none of the requirements would apply. The court held that the statute was an undue burden on abortion because it banned the two most common methods of second trimester abortion. The court also held as unconstitutionally vague the medical emergency and medical necessity provisions of the law which required a physician to believe the abortion necessary and for that belief to be reasonable. (KIE abstract)

U.S. Court of Appeals, Tenth Circuit. Jane L. v. Bangerter. *Federal Reporter, 3d Series.* 1996 Dec 23 (date of decision). 102: 1112–1118. BE60055.
  *abortion, induced; *constitutional law; *fetal development; fetuses; *government regulation; *legal aspects; *pregnant women; selective abortion; state government; Supreme Court decisions; therapeutic abortion; *viability; *Jane L. v. Bangerter; Planned Parenthood of Southeastern Pennsylvania v. Casey; Roe v. Wade; *Utah; *Utah Abortion Act 1991

On remand from the U.S. Supreme Court, the U.S. Court of Appeal for the Tenth Circuit held unconstitutional a Utah law restricting access to abortion services after twenty weeks gestation. The law allowed abortions after twenty weeks only when necessary to save the pregnant woman's life, to prevent grave damage to the pregnant woman's health, or to prevent the birth of a child with grave defects. The court held that the restriction violated *Roe v. Wade* and its progeny in defining viability in terms of gestational weeks. Viability, the point at which

---

BE = bioethics accession number   fn. = footnotes   refs. = references

there is a reasonable likelihood of the fetus' sustained survival outside the womb, with or without artificial support, and the point also at which the state first has a compelling interest in the fetus's existence sufficient to burden a women's ability to choose whether to terminate the pregnancy, can only be determined by a physician on the particular facts of each patient. Defining viability in terms of gestational time and not in terms of gestational development could preclude access to abortion where a pregnancy has reached twenty gestational weeks, yet the fetus has not actually attained viability. Such a definition is an undue burden on a woman's right to choose to abort a nonviable fetus before the state has a compelling interest. (KIE abstract)

U.S. District Court, D. Montana, Butte Division. Wicklund v. Lambert. *Federal Supplement.* 1997 Oct 9 (date of decision). 979: 1285–1290. BE61650.
  *abortion, induced; confidentiality; equal protection; government regulation; judicial action; *legal aspects; legislation; *minors; *parental notification; state government; state interest; Supreme Court decisions; *Montana; *Wicklund v. Lambert
The U.S. District Court for the District of Montana held Montana's Parental Notice of Abortion Act constitutional on the grounds that the state law does not violate the federal equal protection clause and that the judicial bypass procedure as specified in the Act adequately protects privacy, anonymity, and confidentiality. The court recognized that Montana had a legitimate state interest in protecting the well–being of minor, pregnant females. The court determined that the Act's specific provisions, and not the general provisions of the state's Youth Court Act, applied to the parental notification bypass in cases involving a minor's abortion. (KIE abstract)

U.S. District Court, D. Nebraska. Carhart v. Stenberg. *Federal Supplement.* 1997 Aug 14 (date of decision). 972: 507–531. BE61800.
  *abortion, induced; constitutional law; due process; *fetal development; *government regulation; *legal aspects; legal rights; maternal health; *methods; physicians; pregnant women; state government; *Carhart v. Stenberg; Fourteenth Amendment; *Nebraska; United States
The U.S. District Court for the District of Nebraska issued a preliminary injunction to prevent enforcement of Nebraska's partial birth abortion law on the grounds that the law criminalized the intact dilation and extraction abortion procedure and violated the due process clause of the Fourteenth Amendment. Nebraska's ban on this particular method placed women at an appreciably greater risk of injury or death. Such a prohibition is an undue burden on a woman's right to choose an abortion and thus unconstitutional. (KIE abstract)

U.S. District Court, D. Nebraska. Orr v. Nelson. *Federal Supplement.* 1994 Nov 4 (date of decision). 902: 1019–1022. BE59975.
  *abortion, induced; constitutional amendments; federal government; *government financing; *government regulation; indigents; *legal aspects; rape; sex offenses; *state government; therapeutic abortion; Hyde Amendment 1994; *Medicaid; *Nebraska; *Orr v. Nelson; United States
The U.S. District Court for Nebraska held invalid, under the supremacy clause of the federal Constitution, a state law which denied Medicaid reimbursement for abortion in the case of rape or incest. Since the 1994 Hyde Amendment had been revised to include federal funding for medically necessary abortion services in the case of rape or incest, the court held that a state cannot restrict

Medicaid reimbursement in conflict with federal law. (KIE abstract)

U.S. District Court, E.D. Louisiana. Okpalobi v. Foster. *Federal Supplement.* 1998 Jan 7 (date of decision). 981: 977–988. BE61996.
  *abortion, induced; constitutional law; fetuses; *government regulation; health facilities; informed consent; *injuries; *legal liability; personhood; *physicians; pregnant women; prenatal injuries; state government; *torts; *Louisiana; *Okpalobi v. Foster
The U.S. District Court for the Eastern District of Louisiana granted a motion for a preliminary injunction against enforcement of a Louisiana statute which made an abortion provider liable, in tort, "for any damage occasioned or precipitated by the abortion," even when the woman had signed a consent form. The court held that the state statute was unconstitutionally vague because it failed to provide the abortion provider with a fair warning of the legal standard to be applied in determining liability. Also, the court held that the law likely violated the Fourteenth Amendment, because it ran afoul of the Supreme Court pronouncement that the word "person" does not include the unborn. Under the statute, the woman could sue for damages sustained by either her or her unborn child. (KIE abstract)

U.S. District Court, E.D. Michigan, Southern Division. Evans v. Kelley. *Federal Supplement.* 1997 Jul 31 (date of decision). 977: 1283–1320. BE61850.
  *abortion, induced; due process; *fetal development; *government regulation; *legal aspects; legal rights; maternal health; *methods; physicians; pregnant women; state government; Supreme Court decisions; *Evans v. Kelley; *Michigan; United States
The U.S. District Court for Eastern District of Michigan, Southern Division, granted an injunction against enforcement of Michigan's "Partial Birth Abortion" statute. The state law made partial birth abortion a crime except when "necessary to save the life of a pregnant woman whose life is endangered by a physical disorder, physical illness, or physical injury and no other medical procedure will accomplish that purpose." The statute is unconstitutional because it imposes an undue burden on a woman's right to seek a second trimester abortion of a previable fetus. It violated due process rights by being vague about which procedures were legal and by being overbroad in its elimination of some procedures. (KIE abstract)

U.S. District Court, W.D. Wisconsin. Karlin v. Foust. *Federal Supplement.* 1997 Oct 2 (date of decision). 975: 1177–1235. BE61734.
  *abortion, induced; constitutional law; counseling; *government regulation; informed consent; *legal aspects; legislation; physicians; pregnant women; state government; Supreme Court decisions; *Karlin v. Foust; Planned Parenthood of Southeastern Pennsylvania v. Casey; *Wisconsin
The U.S. District Court for the Western District of Wisconsin concluded that the major portion of Wisconsin's new law on abortion is constitutional in light of the Supreme Court's decision in Planned Parenthood of Southeastern Pennsylvania v. Casey. The court considered whether the three parts of the law were substantial obstacles to a woman's choice of abortion. The first part involved a 24–hour waiting period between informed consent and the procedure, which required two trips to the clinic and for some women the cost of an overnight trip. The court concluded that the effect of this part was unclear and thus did not constitute an undue burden. The second part of the law concerned informed

---

BE = bioethics accession number   fn. = footnotes   refs. = references

consent. The requirement that physicians explain that a child's father is liable for financial support was not unconstitutional, but the requirement that all pregnant women -- even those seeking abortion prior to ten to twelve weeks' gestation -- be told of the availability of services for seeing ultrasound images and hearing fetal heart tones was struck down as unconstitutional. The law's provision on performing an abortion in a medical emergency was held to depend on the physician's standard of reasonable medical care and was allowed to stand. (KIE abstract)

U.S. District Court, W.D. Wisconsin. Planned Parenthood of Wisconsin v. Doyle. *Federal Supplement, 2d Series.* 1998 Jun 15 (date of decision). 9: 1033-1046. BE61649.
   *abortion, induced; fetal development; government regulation; *legal aspects; legal liability; legislation; *methods; physicians; state government; *Planned Parenthood of Wisconsin v. Doyle; *Wisconsin

The U.S. District Court for the Western District of Wisconsin denied a motion for a preliminary injunction on Wisconsin's "partial-birth abortion" act. The court held that the act was likely to survive a vagueness challenge because its liability provisions make clear that it refers to a specific abortion procedure, intact dilation and extraction, and because its liability and culpability provisions appear to be sufficient and not unconstitutionally vague. Also, because the conventional dilation and extraction method of abortion is a safe alternative, prohibition of the intact dilation and extraction method is unlikely to constitute an undue burden on a woman's right to choose an abortion and render the statute unconstitutional. (KIE abstract)

Uddo, Basile J. The public law of abortion: a constitutional and statutory review of the present and future legal landscape. *In:* Rainey, R. Randall; Magill, Gerard, eds. Abortion and Public Policy: An Interdiscliplinary Investigation within the Catholic Tradition. Omaha, NE: Creighton University Press; 1996: 163-182. 48 fn. Paper presented at a conference held at Saint Louis University, 11-13 Mar 1993. ISBN 1-881871-18-5. BE61993.
   *abortion, induced; constitutional law; disclosure; fetuses; freedom; *government regulation; informed consent; *legal aspects; *legal rights; minors; parental consent; physicians; pregnant women; public opinion; public policy; spousal notification; *standards; state government; state interest; Supreme Court decisions; viability; Pennsylvania; *Planned Parenthood of Southeastern Pennsylvania v. Casey; Roe v. Wade; *United States

Wheale, Peter R. Moral and legal consequences for the fetus/unborn child of medical technologies derived from human genome research. *In:* Glasner, Peter; Rothman, Harry, eds. Genetic Imaginations: Ethical, Legal and Social Issues in Human Genome Research. Brookfield, VT: Ashgate; 1998: 83-96. 35 refs. Based on a paper presented at a workshop hosted by the Centre for Social and Economic Research at the University of the West of England; reprinted from *The Genetic Engineer and Biotechnologist*, 1995; 15(2-3). ISBN 1-84014-356-8. BE60020.
   abortion, induced; *beginning of life; coercion; *congenital disorders; deontological ethics; *embryo research; *embryos; ethical analysis; fetal development; *fetuses; genetic disorders; genetic screening; genome mapping; government regulation; *legal aspects; legal liability; *moral obligations; *moral policy; negligence; *personhood; pregnant women; prenatal injuries; *public policy; *quality of life; rights; *selective abortion; social impact; treatment refusal; utilitarianism; *value of life; *wrongful life; *Great Britain

Wisconsin abortion law allowed to stand. [News]. *New York Times.* 1998 May 20: A15. BE59673.
   *abortion, induced; criminal law; fetal development; *government regulation; *legal aspects; *methods; physicians; state government; viability; *Wisconsin

ABORTION/MINORS

Avallone, Fran; Focus on the Family; Family Research Council. Do parental notification laws benefit minors seeking abortions? *In:* Francoeur, Robert T., ed. Taking Sides: Clashing Views on Controversial Issues in Human Sexuality. Fifth Edition. Guilford, CT: Dushkin Publishing Group/Brown and Benchmark; 1996: 174-191. 6 refs. ISBN 0-697-31292-5. BE62047.
   *abortion, induced; adolescents; alternatives; decision making; *government regulation; *legal aspects; maternal health; *minors; parental consent; *parental notification; pregnant women; risks and benefits; state government; state interest; Supreme Court decisions; United States

Massachusetts. Supreme Judicial Court. Planned Parenthood League of Massachusetts v. Attorney General. *North Eastern Reporter, 2d Series.* 1997 Mar 18 (date of decision). 677: 101-114. BE60048.
   *abortion, induced; constitutional law; due process; fathers; *government regulation; judicial action; *legal aspects; legal rights; *minors; mothers; *parental consent; *pregnant women; state government; state interest; *Massachusetts; *Planned Parenthood v. Attorney General

The Supreme Judicial Court of Massachusetts sustained a state statute which required pregnant unmarried minors to obtain the consent of both parents or a judge of the Superior Court in order to have an abortion. The court held that the state's interest in protecting the welfare of its minors and ensuring informed consent justified restrictions on a minor's constitutional right to choose an abortion. The court held unconstitutional, however, the law's requirement that the minor obtain the consent of both parents as an undue burden on the minor's due process rights. (KIE abstract)

Northern Ireland. Supreme Court of Judicature, High Court of Justice, Family Division. Northern Health and Social Services Board v. F and G. *Northern Ireland Law Reports.* 1993 Oct 14 (date of decision). 1993: 268-278. BE60625.
   *abortion, induced; government regulation; international aspects; *legal aspects; *minors; pregnant women; psychological stress; therapeutic abortion; Great Britain; *Northern Health and Social Services Board v. F and G; *Northern Ireland

The Northern Ireland Supreme Court granted permission for a minor, who had been made a ward of the court upon the application of the Northern Health and Social Services Board, to have an abortion and authorized travel outside its jurisdiction for the operation. K, a 14-year-old who had been in foster care, was found to be 13 weeks pregnant and wanted an abortion. Abortion in Northern Ireland is unlawful unless "in good faith for the purpose of preserving the life or health of the woman." The court decided that abortion would be in K's best interests, after considering medical evidence that the psychological effects of continuing the pregnancy were more dangerous than those following its termination. As no doctor could be found who would perform an abortion in Northern Ireland, even one deemed lawful by its highest court, K was allowed to travel to England for the procedure. (KIE abstract)

Scarnecchia, Suellyn; Field, Julie Kunce. Judging girls:

BE = bioethics accession number   fn. = footnotes   refs. = references

decision making in parental consent to abortion cases. *Michigan Journal of Gender and Law.* 1995; 3(41): 75–123. 134 fn. BE59408.

*abortion, induced; *adolescents; *competence; counseling; *decision making; *informed consent; *judicial action; *legal aspects; legislation; *minors; *parental consent; standards; state government; Supreme Court decisions; *Michigan; United States

U.S. Court of Appeals, Fourth Circuit. Planned Parenthood of the Blue Ridge v. Camblos. *Federal Reporter, 3d Series.* 1997 Jun 30 (date of decision). 116: 707–721. BE61997.

*abortion, induced; competence; constitutional law; *government regulation; *judicial action; *legal aspects; legal rights; *minors; *parental notification; pregnant women; state government; *Planned Parenthood of the Blue Ridge v. Camblos; *Virginia

The U.S. Court of Appeals for the Fourth Circuit issued a stay of the district court's injunction against enforcement of Virginia's Parental Notice Act which allows a juvenile court judge the discretion to decline authorization of an abortion without parental notice, even if the judge finds the pregnant minor to be mature and capable of informed consent for an abortion. The circuit court decided that the district court had erred in holding that the judicial bypass procedures in Virginia's parental *notice* statute must satisfy the constitutional requirements for bypass procedures in parental *consent* statutes, as interpreted by the U.S. Supreme Court. (KIE abstract)

U.S. Court of Appeals, Ninth Circuit. Wicklund v. Salvagni. *Federal Reporter, 3d Series.* 1996 Aug 16 (date of decision). 93: 567–572. BE60053.

*abortion, induced; constitutional law; *government regulation; judicial action; *legal aspects; legal rights; *minors; *parental notification; *pregnant women; risks and benefits; state government; *Montana; *Wicklund v. Salvagni

The U.S. Court of Appeals for the Ninth Circuit held unconstitutional a Montana parental notification law in the case of minors seeking abortion. The law provided that a physician could not perform an abortion upon a minor or an incompetent person unless the physician had given 48 hours notice to one parent or to the legal guardian of the patient. The law permitted a minor to petition a court for a waiver of the notice requirement if she was sufficiently mature to decide whether to have an abortion and if the notification of a parent or guardian was not in the best interest of the minor. The court struck down the law because it did not provide for judicial bypass where the abortion, and not just the parental notice, would be in the minor's best interest. (KIE abstract)

U.S. District Court, D. Montana, Butte Division. Wicklund v. Lambert. *Federal Supplement.* 1997 Oct 9 (date of decision). 979: 1285–1290. BE61650.

*abortion, induced; confidentiality; equal protection; government regulation; judicial action; *legal aspects; legislation; *minors; *parental notification; state government; state interest; Supreme Court decisions; *Montana; *Wicklund v. Lambert

The U.S. District Court for the District of Montana held Montana's Parental Notice of Abortion Act constitutional on the grounds that the state law does not violate the federal equal protection clause and that the judicial bypass procedure as specified in the Act adequately protects privacy, anonymity, and confidentiality. The court recognized that Montana had a legitimate state interest in protecting the well-being

of minor, pregnant females. The court determined that the Act's specific provisions, and not the general provisions of the state's Youth Court Act, applied to the parental notification bypass in cases involving a minor's abortion. (KIE abstract)

ABORTION/RELIGIOUS ASPECTS

Anderson, J. Kerby. Abortion. *In: his* Moral Dilemmas: Biblical Perspectives on Contemporary Ethical Issues. Nashville, TN: Word Publishing; 1998: 1–15, 227–228. 17 fn. ISBN 0-8499-1446-9. BE62391.

*abortion, induced; *Christian ethics; fetuses; historical aspects; legal aspects; methods; personhood; political activity; women's rights; United States

Cahill, Lisa Sowle. Catholic commitment and public responsibility. *In:* Rainey, R. Randall; Magill, Gerard, eds. Abortion and Public Policy: An Interdisciplinary Investigation within the Catholic Tradition. Omaha, NE: Creighton University Press; 1996: 131–162. 53 fn. Paper presented at a conference held at Saint Louis University, 11–13 Mar 1993. ISBN 1-881871-18-5. BE61992.

abortion on demand; *abortion, induced; autonomy; *common good; *conscience; consensus; contraception; fetal development; fetal research; fetuses; historical aspects; informed consent; *justice; law; *legal aspects; *moral policy; morality; *natural law; personhood; *politics; pregnant women; public opinion; *public policy; reproduction; *Roman Catholic ethics; sexuality; social discrimination; state government; *theology; *value of life; values; women's rights; Declaration on Abortion; Europe; United States

Cowell, Alan. Obeying pope, German bishops end role in abortion system. [News]. *New York Times.* 1998 Jan 28: A3. BE59609.

*abortion, induced; *clergy; *counseling; health facilities; moral complicity; politics; pregnant women; *Roman Catholics; *Germany

Donovan, Patricia. Hospital mergers and reproductive health care. *Family Planning Perspectives.* 1996 Nov–Dec; 28(6): 281–284. 21 fn. BE61811.

*abortion, induced; community services; *contraception; economics; *family planning; geographic factors; government regulation; *hospitals; indigents; *institutional policies; legal aspects; political activity; prenatal diagnosis; referral and consultation; *religious hospitals; *Roman Catholic ethics; state government; trends; voluntary sterilization; *women's health services; *community hospitals; *health facility mergers; American Civil Liberties Union; Montana; New York; *United States

Episcopal Diocese of Washington, D.C. Committee on Medical Ethics (Chair: Cynthia B. Cohen). Wrestling with the Future: Our Genes and Our Choices. Harrisburg, PA: Morehouse Publishing; 1998. 132 p. Bibliography: p. 125–127. ISBN 0-8192-1762-X. BE61310.

adolescents; adults; carriers; case studies; children; chromosome abnormalities; clergy; confidentiality; congenital disorders; decision making; disclosure; employment; family members; family relationship; genetic counseling; genetic disorders; genetic information; genetic intervention; genetic predisposition; *genetic screening; health insurance; health personnel; informed consent; late-onset disorders; morality; newborns; parents; pastoral care; preimplantation diagnosis; *prenatal diagnosis; privacy; *Protestant ethics; psychological stress; reproduction; *risks and benefits; *selective abortion; sex determination; social discrimination; stigmatization; theology; uncertainty;

BE = bioethics accession number   fn. = footnotes   refs. = references

*Anglican Church; *Episcopal Church; United States

Feldman, David M. Birth Control in Jewish Law: Marital Relations, Contraception, and Abortion as Set Forth in the Classic Texts of Jewish Law. First Jason Aronson Edition. Northvale, NJ: Jason Aronson; 1998. 349 p. Includes references. ISBN 0-7657-6058-4. BE62622.
> *abortion, induced; beginning of life; Christian ethics; *contraception; drugs; embryos; females; fetuses; historical aspects; *Jewish ethics; males; *marital relationship; maternal health; methods; reproduction; *sexuality; *theology; therapeutic abortion

Hayes, Edward J.; Hayes, Paul J.; Kelly, Dorothy Ellen, et al. Principles relating to the taking of life. *In: their* Catholicism and Ethics. Norwood, MA: C.R. Publications; 1997: 121–151. Includes discussion questions and projects. References embedded in list at back of book. ISBN 0-9649087-7-8. BE61947.
> *abortion, induced; active euthanasia; advance directives; allowing to die; assisted suicide; attitudes to death; childbirth; double effect; drugs; *euthanasia; fetuses; forms; killing; methods; opioid analgesics; palliative care; pregnant women; rights; *Roman Catholic ethics; terminal care; therapeutic abortion; *value of life; abortion, spontaneous; Catholic Health Association

Hehir, J. Bryan. The Church and abortion in the 1990s: the role of institutional leadership. *In:* Rainey, R. Randall; Magill, Gerard, eds. Abortion and Public Policy: An Interdisciplinary Investigation within the Catholic Tradition. Omaha, NE: Creighton University Press; 1996: 203–228. 30 fn. Paper presented at a conference held at Saint Louis University, 11–13 Mar 1993. ISBN 1-881871-18-5. BE61994.
> abortion on demand; *abortion, induced; clergy; federal government; government financing; historical aspects; institutional policies; legal aspects; legislation; moral obligations; moral policy; politics; public opinion; *public policy; *Roman Catholic ethics; state government; theology; value of life; Hyde Amendment; National Conference of Catholic Bishops; Planned Parenthood of Southeastern Pennsylvania v. Casey; Roe v. Wade; Webster v. Reproductive Health Services

Kavanaugh, John F. Ethical commitments in health care systems. *America.* 1998 Nov 7; 179(14): 20. BE62274.
> *abortion, induced; *contraception; embryo research; euthanasia; fetal research; health care delivery; hospitals; *institutional ethics; *religious hospitals; reproduction; *Roman Catholic ethics; sterilization (sexual); *health facility mergers; Ethical and Religious Directives for Catholic Health Care Services; United States

Leibold, Peter; Gilham, Charles S. When physicians perform abortions outside the Catholic hospital. *Health Progress.* 1998 Mar–Apr; 79(2): 12–14. 14 fn. BE60591.
> *abortion, induced; conscience; employment; federal government; government financing; *institutional policies; *legal aspects; legal liability; *physicians; *religious hospitals; *Roman Catholic ethics; social discrimination; United States

O'Rourke, Kevin D. Applying the Directives: The *Ethical and Religious Directives* concerning three medical situations require some elucidation. *Health Progress.* 1998 Jul–Aug; 79(4): 64–69. 33 fn. BE61616.
> abortion, induced; *allowing to die; *artificial feeding; *contraception; double effect; drugs; fetuses; health care delivery; institutional policies; intention; methods; *persistent vegetative state; pregnant women; *rape; religious hospitals; *Roman Catholic ethics; surgery; *therapeutic abortion; withholding treatment; *ectopic pregnancy; *Ethical and Religious Directives for Catholic

Health Care Services

Powell, John. Abortion: The Silent Holocaust. Allen, TX: Tabor; 1981. 183 p. 22 refs. ISBN 0-89505-063-3. BE61375.
> aborted fetuses; abortion on demand; *abortion, induced; dehumanization; legal aspects; legislation; love; National Socialism; physicians; political activity; *Roman Catholic ethics; *value of life; Human Life Amendment; Right to Life Movement; United States

Rainey, R. Randall; Magill, Gerard, eds. Abortion and Public Policy: An Interdisciplinary Investigation within the Catholic Tradition. Omaha, NE: Creighton University Press; 1996. 254 p. Papers presented at a conference held at Saint Louis University, 11–13 Mar 1993. Includes references. ISBN 1-881871-18-5. BE61988.
> abortion on demand; *abortion, induced; beginning of life; conscience; constitutional law; cultural pluralism; embryos; fetal development; fetuses; freedom; goals; government regulation; justice; legal aspects; legal rights; maternal health; morality; natural law; personhood; politics; pregnant women; public opinion; *public policy; *Roman Catholic ethics; standards; state government; Supreme Court decisions; theology; value of life; values; women's rights; United States

Rainey, R. Randall; Magill, Gerard; O'Rourke, Kevin. Introduction: abortion, the Catholic Church, and public policy. *In:* Rainey, R. Randall; Magill, Gerard, eds. Abortion and Public Policy: An Interdisciplinary Investigation within the Catholic Tradition. Omaha, NE: Creighton University Press; 1996: 1–46. 148 fn. Paper presented at a conference held at Saint Louis University, 11–13 Mar 1993. ISBN 1-881871-18-5. BE61989.
> aborted fetuses; abortion on demand; *abortion, induced; beginning of life; constitutional law; federal government; fetal development; fetal tissue donation; fetuses; government financing; government regulation; historical aspects; human rights; killing; legal aspects; legal rights; natural law; personhood; political activity; politics; privacy; *public policy; *Roman Catholic ethics; state government; Supreme Court decisions; therapeutic abortion; *value of life; National Conference of Catholic Bishops; Nineteenth Century; Right to Life Movement; Roe v. Wade; RU-486; Twentieth Century; United States

Reitman, James S.; Calhoun, Byron C.; Hoeldtke, Nathan J. Perinatal hospice: a response to early termination for severe congenital anomalies. *In:* Demy, Timothy J.; Stewart, Gary P., eds. Genetic Engineering: A Christian Response: Crucial Considerations in Shaping Life. Grand Rapids, MI: Kregel Publications; 1999: 196–211. 63 fn. ISBN 0-8254-2357-0. BE61368.
> alternatives; autonomy; *Christian ethics; *congenital disorders; conscience; females; fetal development; fetuses; *hospices; *newborns; personhood; pregnant women; psychological stress; risks and benefits; *selective abortion; suffering; *terminal care; terminally ill; theology; viability; grief; United States

Wagner, Bertil K.J.; Christian Pharmacists Fellowship International. Pharmacists should not participate in abortion or assisted suicide. [Position paper]. *Annals of Pharmacotherapy.* 1996 Oct; 30(10): 1192–1196. 56 refs. 1 fn. BE60183.
> *abortion, induced; active euthanasia; alternatives; *assisted suicide; beneficence; *Christian ethics; *conscience; counseling; depressive disorder; *drugs; mortality; motivation; *organizational policies; palliative care; *pharmacists; pregnant women; professional ethics; psychological stress; theology; value of life; *Christian

---

BE = bioethics accession number   fn. = footnotes   refs. = references

Pharmacists Fellowship International; United States

Walter, James J. Theological parameters: Catholic doctrine on abortion in a pluralist society. *In:* Rainey, R. Randall; Magill, Gerard, eds. Abortion and Public Policy: An Interdisciplinary Investigation within the Catholic Tradition. Omaha, NE: Creighton University Press; 1996: 91–130. 101 fn. Paper presented at a conference held at Saint Louis University, 11–13 Mar 1993. ISBN 1-881871-18-5. BE61991.
*abortion, induced; anthropology; autonomy; beginning of life; *cultural pluralism; fetuses; freedom; killing; law; legal aspects; moral policy; morality; natural law; personhood; political activity; pregnant women; public policy; reproduction; *Roman Catholic ethics; sexuality; *theology; *value of life; *values; rationality; United States

Washofsky, Mark. Abortion and the halakhic conversation: a liberal perspective. *In:* Jacob, Walter; Zemer, Moshe, eds. The Fetus and Fertility in Jewish Law: Essays and Responsa. Pittsburgh, PA: Rodef Shalom Press; Freehof Institute of Progressive Halakhah; 1995: 39–89. 119 fn. ISBN 0-929699-07-6. BE61838.
*abortion, induced; childbirth; consensus; decision making; ethical analysis; fetuses; historical aspects; *Jewish ethics; personhood; pregnant women; *theology; therapeutic abortion; value of life; *Orthodox Judaism

Weber, David O. Realignments, realpolitik, religion, and reproductive health. *Healthcare Forum Journal.* 1996 May–Jun; 39(3): 76–83. BE59579.
*abortion, induced; conscience; *contraception; cultural pluralism; drug industry; economics; family planning; government financing; health facilities; *institutional policies; Jewish ethics; legal liability; managed care programs; medical devices; medical education; political activity; *Protestant ethics; *religion; *religious hospitals; reproductive technologies; *Roman Catholic ethics; statistics; trends; violence; voluntary sterilization; *women's health services; *health facility mergers; California; Ethical and Religious Directives for Catholic Health Care Services; Mormonism; Norplant; *United States; Utah

ACCESS TO HEALTH CARE *See* HEALTH CARE, RESOURCE ALLOCATION

ACQUIRED IMMUNODEFICIENCY SYNDROME
See AIDS

ADVANCE DIRECTIVES

See also TREATMENT REFUSAL

Aikman, Peter J.; Thiel, Elaine C.; Martin, Douglas K., et al. Proxy, health, and personal care preferences: implications for end-of-life care. *Cambridge Quarterly of Healthcare Ethics.* 1999 Spring; 8(2): 200–210. 31 fn. BE61236.
*advance care planning; *advance directives; *AIDS; allowing to die; *alternatives; assisted suicide; *attitudes; attitudes to death; comparative studies; *decision making; family members; family relationship; *forms; friends; *HIV seropositivity; home care; hospices; hospitals; *living wills; pain; palliative care; prolongation of life; *patients; *quality of life; survey; terminal care; third party consent; voluntary euthanasia; *values histories; Toronto

Alberta Law Reform Institute. Advance Directives and Substitute Decision-Making in Personal Healthcare: A Joint Report of the Alberta Law Reform Institute and the Health Law Institute. Edmonton, AB: The Institute;

1993 Mar. 60 p. 94 fn. Report No. 64. ISBN 0-8886-4180-X. BE60502.
*advance directives; age factors; competence; decision making; emergency care; family members; government regulation; health care; *legal aspects; legislation; model legislation; standards; *third party consent; *Alberta; Alberta Law Reform Institute; British Columbia; Canada; Manitoba; Newfoundland; Ontario; Saskatchewan

Alpers, Ann; Lo, Bernard. Avoiding family feuds: responding to surrogate demands for life-sustaining interventions. *Journal of Law, Medicine and Ethics.* 1999 Spring; 27(1): 74–80. 45 fn. BE61507.
*advance directives; *allowing to die; autonomy; *beneficence; biomedical technologies; case studies; communication; *conscience; consensus; cultural pluralism; *decision making; directive adherence; disclosure; *dissent; *family members; *family relationship; friends; *futility; intention; minority groups; moral obligations; patient care team; *physicians; *professional family relationship; prognosis; *prolongation of life; religion; resuscitation orders; risks and benefits; *suffering; *third party consent; time factors; *values; withholding treatment; integrity; *negotiation; oral directives

Awong, Linda; Miles, Al. Asking patients about revising advance directives. *American Journal of Nursing.* 1998 Apr; 98(4): 71. BE59627.
*advance directives; autonomy; critically ill; *directive adherence; health personnel; hospitals; paternalism; resuscitation orders

Berger, Jeffrey T. Culture and ethnicity in clinical care. *Archives of Internal Medicine.* 1998 Oct 26; 158(19): 2085–2090. 110 refs. BE59577.
*advance directives; *alternative therapies; American Indians; Asian Americans; *attitudes; autopsies; blacks; cancer; *cultural pluralism; family relationship; health; Hispanic Americans; knowledge, attitudes, practice; living wills; *minority groups; nutrition; *organ donation; *patient care; physicians; preventive medicine; prolongation of life; socioeconomic factors; *truth disclosure; whites; withholding treatment; United States

Blondeau, Danielle; Valois, Pierre; Keyserlingk, Edward W., et al. Comparison of patients' and health care professionals' attitudes towards advance directives. *Journal of Medical Ethics.* 1998 Oct; 24(5): 328–335. 38 fn. BE60255.
*administrators; *advance directives; *attitudes; autonomy; beneficence; comparative studies; family members; family relationship; justice; *knowledge, attitudes, practice; legal aspects; living wills; motivation; *nurses; *patients; *physicians; professional family relationship; professional patient relationship; survey; terminal care; third party consent; *Quebec
OBJECTIVES: This study was designed to identify and compare the attitudes of patients and health care professionals towards advance directives. Advance directives promote recognition of the patient's autonomy, letting the individual exercise a certain measure of control over life-sustaining care and treatment in the eventuality of becoming incompetent. DESIGN: Attitudes to advance directives were evaluated using a 44-item self-reported questionnaire. It yields an overall score as well as five factor scores: autonomy, beneficence, justice, external norms, and the affective dimension. SETTING: Health care institutions in the province of Québec, Canada. Survey sample: The sampling consisted of 921 subjects: 123 patients, 167 physicians, 340 nurses and 291 administrators of health care institutions. RESULTS: Although the general attitude of each population was favourable to the expression of autonomy, multivariate analysis of variance

---

BE = bioethics accession number   fn. = footnotes   refs. = references

(MANOVA) indicated that physicians attached less importance to this subscale than did other populations (p less than .001). Above all, they favoured legal external norms and beneficence. Physicians and administrators also attached less importance to the affective dimension than did patients and nurses. Specifically, physicians' attitudes towards advance directives were shown to be less positive than patients' attitudes. CONCLUSION: More attention should be given to the importance of adequately informing patients about advance directives because they may not represent an adequate means for patients to assert their autonomy.

Blustein, Jeffrey. Choosing for others as continuing a life story: the problem of personal identity revisited. *Journal of Law, Medicine and Ethics.* 1999 Spring; 27(1): 20–31. 37 fn. Commented on by M.G. Kuczewski, p. 32–36. BE61501.
  *advance directives; autonomy; communitarianism; competence; death; *decision making; dementia; *directive adherence; family members; friends; *moral policy; narrative ethics; patient care; persistent vegetative state; *personhood; philosophy; *self concept; standards; terminal care; *third party consent; time factors; Dresser, Rebecca; Robertson, John

Bradley, Elizabeth H.; Peiris, Vasum; Wetle, Terrie. Discussions about end-of-life care in nursing homes. *Journal of the American Geriatrics Society.* 1998 Oct; 46(10): 1235–1241. 44 refs. BE62263.
  *advance care planning; advance directives; aged; artificial feeding; *communication; competence; decision making; *family members; institutionalized persons; legislation; medical records; *nursing homes; *patient participation; *patients; *physicians; resuscitation; statistics; survey; *terminal care; third party consent; time factors; ventilators; retrospective studies; Connecticut; Patient Self-Determination Act 1990

Bradley, Elizabeth H.; Rizzo, John A. Public information and private search: evaluating the Patient Self-Determination Act. *Journal of Health Politics, Policy and Law.* 1999 Apr; 24(2): 239–273. 91 refs. BE61757.
  *advance directives; age factors; *decision making; education; empirical research; evaluation studies; females; health insurance; incentives; information dissemination; *legislation; males; *morbidity; nursing homes; patient admission; *social impact; *socioeconomic factors; statistics; personal financing; *Patient Self-Determination Act 1990; United States
Despite substantial regulatory efforts to improve consumer information regarding health and health care, little is known about the impact of such efforts on consumer behavior. This article examines the effect of federal legislation to enhance consumer information regarding the use of life-sustaining technology in end-of-life medical treatment decision making. Using a unique set of data abstracted from the medical records of six hundred elderly patients in nursing homes, the study finds a substantial impact of the law in promoting improved documentation of patient wishes for end-of-life medical care. Further, the data reveal that the effect of the law varies among identifiable subgroups. Consistent with the theory of search, the article demonstrates that the effects of regulatory efforts that promote the public provision of consumer information are greatest among individuals for whom information is most beneficial but for whom private search is costly. Implications for health policy are discussed.

Bradley, Elizabeth H.; Wetle, Terrie; Horwitz, Sarah. The Patient Self-Determination Act and advance directive completion in nursing homes. *Archives of Family Medicine.* 1998 Sep–Oct; 7(5): 417–423. 50 refs. BE61227.
  advance care planning; *advance directives; age factors; *aged; attitudes; comparative studies; competence; hospitals; information dissemination; institutionalized persons; *knowledge, attitudes, practice; *legislation; medical records; motivation; *nursing homes; patient admission; patient participation; patient transfer; *social impact; socioeconomic factors; statistics; survey; time factors; refusal to participate; *Connecticut; *Patient Self-Determination Act 1990; United States

Buss, Mary K.; Marx, Eric S.; Sulmasy, Daniel P. The preparedness of students to discuss end-of-life issues with patients. *Academic Medicine.* 1998 Apr; 73(4): 418–422. 16 refs. BE59878.
  *advance care planning; *advance directives; age factors; allowing to die; assisted suicide; communication; ethics consultation; *knowledge, attitudes, practice; *medical education; medical schools; physician patient relationship; *students; survey; *terminal care; *Georgetown University School of Medicine; Mayo Medical School

Campbell, Neil. A problem for the idea of voluntary euthanasia. *Journal of Medical Ethics.* 1999 Jun; 25(3): 242–244. BE61857.
  *advance directives; allowing to die; assisted suicide; *autonomy; *coercion; decision making; freedom; *involuntary euthanasia; *living wills; *motivation; *pain; *suffering; time factors; torture; *voluntary euthanasia
I question whether, in those cases where physician-assisted suicide is invoked to alleviate unbearable pain and suffering, there can be such a thing as voluntary euthanasia. The problem is that when a patient asks to die under such conditions there is good reason to think that the decision to die is compelled by the pain, and hence not freely chosen. Since the choice to die was not made freely it is inadvisable for physicians to act in accordance with it, for this may be contrary to the patient's genuine wishes. Thus, what were thought to be cases of voluntary euthanasia might actually be instances of involuntary euthanasia.

Canada. Alberta. Personal Directives Act [Chapter P-4.03]. Alberta, Canada: The Queen's Printer for Alberta; 1996 May 24 (date of enactment). 21 p. BE59346.
  *advance directives; competence; decision making; directive adherence; health personnel; judicial action; *legal aspects; legal liability; third party consent; *Alberta; *Personal Directives Act (AB)

Canadian Nurses Association; Canadian Home Care Association; Canadian Hospital Association; et al. Joint Statement on Advance Directives. [Policy statement]. Ottawa, ON: Issued by the Canadian Nurses Association, 50 Driveway, Ottawa, ON K2P 1E2, Canada; 1994 Sep. 4 p. Developed in collaboration with the Canadian Bar Association. Approved by the Board of Directors of the Canadian Nurses Association Sep 1994. BE62250.
  *advance directives; allowing to die; competence; decision making; family members; guidelines; health facilities; home care; informed consent; institutional policies; legal aspects; nurses; *organizational policies; palliative care; patient care; professional organizations; terminal care; third party consent; treatment refusal; withholding treatment; Canada; *Canadian Nurses Association

Capron, Alexander Morgan. Advance directives. *In:* Kuhse, Helga; Singer, Peter, eds. A Companion to Bioethics. Malden, MA: Blackwell; 1998: 261–271. 8 refs. ISBN 0-631-19737-0. BE59501.
  *advance directives; allowing to die; decision making;

BE = bioethics accession number   fn. = footnotes   refs. = references

evaluation; international aspects; legal aspects; living wills; prolongation of life; trends; United States

Castle, Nicholas G. Advance directives in nursing homes: resident and facility characteristics. *Omega: A Journal of Death and Dying.* 1996–1997; 34(4): 321–332. 31 refs. BE60059.
*advance directives; age factors; *aged; comparative studies; diagnosis; females; government financing; hospitals; indigents; institutional policies; *institutionalized persons; *knowledge, attitudes, practice; males; minority groups; *nursing homes; patient transfer; *patients; proprietary health facilities; quality of life; remuneration; resuscitation orders; socioeconomic factors; treatment refusal; Medicaid; United States

Collopy, Bart J. The moral underpinning of the proxy-provider relationship: issues of trust and distrust. *Journal of Law, Medicine and Ethics.* 1999 Spring; 27(1): 37–45. 25 fn. BE61503.
*advance directives; advisory committees; autonomy; communication; competence; conflict of interest; *consensus; *decision making; *directive adherence; *family members; *family relationship; friends; motivation; patients; physician patient relationship; physicians; *professional family relationship; *standards; terminal care; *third party consent; *trust; values; New York State Task Force on Life and the Law; President's Commission for the Study of Ethical Problems

Dietz, Sarah M.; Brakman, Sarah-Vaughan; Dresser, Rebecca, et al. The incompetent self: metamorphosis of a person? [Letters and responses]. *Hastings Center Report.* 1998 Sep–Oct; 28(5): 4–5. BE59545.
*advance directives; *allowing to die; autonomy; *competence; *decision making; living wills; personhood; prognosis; *prolongation of life; quality of life; ventilators

Douglas, Gillian. Re C (Refusal of Medical Treatment). [Comment]. *Family Law.* 1994 Mar; 24: 131–132. BE61827.
*advance directives; autonomy; *competence; critically ill; directive adherence; informed consent; institutionalized persons; *legal aspects; mental institutions; *mentally ill; schizophrenia; *surgery; *treatment refusal; *amputation; *Great Britain; *Re C (Refusal of Medical Treatment)

Duffield, Patricia. Advance directives in primary care. *American Journal of Nursing.* 1998 Apr; 98(4): 16CCC–16DDD. 4 refs. BE59649.
*advance directives; nurses; patient education; patients; *primary health care; survey

Dyer, Clare. Power of attorney change in England and Wales. [News]. *BMJ (British Medical Journal).* 1999 Jul 24; 319(7204): 211. BE62501.
*advance directives; allowing to die; competence; decision making; family members; *legal aspects; patient care; third party consent; withholding treatment; *England; *Wales

Eisemann, Martin; Richter, Jörg. Relationships between various attitudes towards self-determination in health care with special reference to an advance directive. *Journal of Medical Ethics.* 1999 Feb; 25(1): 37–41. 26 refs. BE61193.
adults; *advance directives; age factors; allowing to die; attitudes; *autonomy; critically ill; *decision making; drugs; females; intensive care units; males; pain; palliative care; patient care; *patient participation; prolongation of life; *public opinion; surgery; survey; terminal care; terminally ill; ventilators; withholding treatment; *Sweden
OBJECTIVES: The subject of patient self-determination in health care has gained broad interest because of the increasing number of incompetent

patients. In an attempt to solve the problems related to doctors' decision making in such circumstances, advance directives have been developed. The purpose of this study was to examine relationships between public attitudes towards patient autonomy and advance directives. SUBJECTS AND MAIN OUTCOME MEASURES: A stratified random sample of 600 adults in northern Sweden was surveyed by a questionnaire with a response rate of 78.2%. The subjects were asked about their wish for control of their health care, their concerns about health care, their treatment preferences in a life-threatening situation (both reversible and irreversible), and their attitudes towards the application of advance directives. RESULTS: Numerous relationships between various aspects of self-determination in health care (desire for control, fears of over-treatment, and choice of treatment level) in general and advance directives, in particular, were found. Those who wanted to have a say in their health care (about 94%) also mainly supported the use of an advance directive. CONCLUSIONS: The fact that almost 30% of the respondents were undecided concerning their personal use of advance directives points to a lack of knowledge and to the necessity of education of the public on these issues.

Fazel, Seena; Hope, Tony; Jacoby, Robin. Assessment of competence to complete advance directives: validation of a patient centred approach. *BMJ (British Medical Journal).* 1999 Feb 20; 318(7182): 493–497. 13 refs. BE61393.
*advance directives; *aged; autonomy; comparative studies; *competence; *dementia; *evaluation; evaluation studies; volunteers; Great Britain
OBJECTIVE: To develop a patient centred approach for the assessment of competence to complete advance directives ("living wills") of elderly people with cognitive impairment. DESIGN: Semistructured interviews. SETTING: Oxfordshire. SUBJECTS: 50 elderly volunteers living in the community, and 50 patients with dementia on first referral from primary care. MAIN OUTCOME MEASURES: Psychometric properties of competence assessment. RESULTS: This patient centred approach for assessing competence to complete advance directives can discriminate between elderly persons living in the community and elderly patients with dementia. The procedure has good interrater (r=0.95) and test-retest (r=0.97) reliability. Validity was examined by relating this approach with a global assessment of competence to complete an advance directive made by two of us (both specialising in old age psychiatry). The data were also used to determine the best threshold score for discriminating between those competent and those incompetent to complete an advance directive. CONCLUSION: A patient centred approach to assess competence to complete advance directives can be reliably and validly used in routine clinical practice.

Fazel, Seena; Hope, Tony; Jacoby, Robin. Dementia, intelligence, and the competence to complete advance directives. [Research letter]. *Lancet.* 1999 Jul 3; 354(9172): 48. 5 refs. BE62409.
*advance directives; *aged; *competence; *dementia; evaluation studies; *intelligence; Great Britain
At referral, a fifth of patients with dementia were competent to complete advance directives. Competence was significantly related to higher premorbid IQ estimated by the National Adult Reading Test.

Fazel, Seena; Hope, Tony; Jacoby, Robin. Ways of

BE = bioethics accession number   fn. = footnotes   refs. = references

assessing capacity to complete an advance directive should be developed. [Letter]. *BMJ (British Medical Journal)*. 1998 Apr 25; 316(7140): 1321–1322. 5 refs. BE59334.

*advance directives; *competence; comprehension; *dementia; *evaluation; recall; standards

Fellows, Lesley K. Competency and consent in dementia. *Journal of the American Geriatrics Society*. 1998 Jul; 46(7): 922–926. 20 refs. BE62261.

*advance directives; *aged; autonomy; beneficence; coercion; communication; *competence; *decision making; *dementia; family members; *informed consent; *patient care; patient participation; personhood; physicians; *risks and benefits; self concept; standards; terminal care; *third party consent; time factors; values

Fins, Joseph J. Commentary: from contract to covenant in advance care planning. *Journal of Law, Medicine and Ethics*. 1999 Spring; 27(1): 46–51. 29 fn. BE61504.

*advance care planning; *advance directives; allowing to die; artificial feeding; autonomy; case studies; clinical ethics committees; *contracts; *covenant; *decision making; dementia; *directive adherence; family members; *family relationship; friends; living wills; love; marital relationship; moral obligations; patients; physicians; prolongation of life; resuscitation; resuscitation orders; risks and benefits; terminal care; *third party consent; treatment refusal; trust; withholding treatment

Flew, Antony. Advance directives are the solution to Dr. Campbell's problem for voluntary euthanasia. *Journal of Medical Ethics*. 1999 Jun; 25(3): 245–246. BE61858.

*advance directives; allowing to die; autonomy; coercion; *involuntary euthanasia; *living wills; motivation; *pain; torture; *voluntary euthanasia; withholding treatment

Dr Neil Campbell suggests that when patients suffering extremes of protracted pain ask for help to end their lives, their requests should be discounted as made under compulsion. I contend that the doctors concerned should be referred to and then act upon advance directives made by those patients when of sound and calm mind and afflicted by no such intolerable compulsion.

Frankel, Sherman. The dementia dilemma. *Perspectives in Biology and Medicine*. 1999 Winter; 42(2): 174–178. A longer draft version of this article appears at Internet Website http://www.physics.upenn.edu/facultyinfo/frankel.html. BE62119.

*advance directives; aged; *assisted suicide; competence; *dementia; diagnosis; *directive adherence; patient advocacy; *right to die; voluntary euthanasia; Society for an Assisted Graceful Exit (SAGE); United States

Gilligan, Mary Ann; Jensen, Norman. Use of advance directives: a survey in three clinics. *Wisconsin Medical Journal*. 1995; 94(5): 239–243. 13 refs. BE61490.

adults; *advance directives; age factors; aged; cancer; chronically ill; comparative studies; females; HIV seropositivity; *knowledge, attitudes, practice; males; married persons; motivation; patients; single persons; survey; terminal care; trust; ambulatory care; refusal to participate; University of Wisconsin Hospital and Clinics; Wisconsin

Gordon, Nancy P.; Shade, Starley P. Advance directives are more likely among seniors asked about end-of-life care preferences. *Archives of Internal Medicine*. 1999 Apr 12; 159(7): 701–704. 17 refs. BE61328.

*advance care planning; *advance directives; age factors; *aged; communication; comparative studies; females; health; health maintenance organizations; health personnel; heart diseases; knowledge, attitudes, practice; males; patient participation; socioeconomic factors; statistics; survey;

terminal care; cerebrovascular disorders; California; Kaiser Permanente

OBJECTIVES: To estimate the proportion of seniors in a large health maintenance organization (HMO) who had been asked about their end-of-life care preferences (EOLCPs) by a clinician and who had completed an advance directive (AD). To examine the association of having had an EOLCP discussion and AD completion. SUBJECTS AND METHODS: A random sample of HMO members aged 65 years or older were asked to complete a mailed survey about health and health-related issues in 1996. Data provided by 5117 seniors (80% response rate) were used to estimate the prevalence of EOLCP and AD among seniors overall and in specific risk groups. Bivariate and multiple logistic regression models were used to identify predictors of AD completion, especially having been asked about EOLCP. RESULTS: One third of seniors reported having an AD on file with the HMO, but only 15% had talked with a clinician about EOLCP. Both having been asked about EOLCP and having an AD were positively associated with age, but not significantly associated with sex, race/ethnicity, marital status, or self-rated health status. Having been asked by a clinician about EOLCP was significantly associated with completion of an AD. CONCLUSION: Clinicians can play an important role in increasing AD completion rates among seniors by bringing up the subject of EOLCPs.

Haynor, Patricia M. Meeting the challenge of advance directives. *American Journal of Nursing*. 1998 Mar; 98(3): 26–33. 13 refs. BE59676.

*advance directives; allowing to die; case studies; decision making; directive adherence; family members; legislation; *nurse's role; nursing ethics; palliative care; patient care; public policy; Patient Self-Determination Act 1990; United States

Heffner, John E.; Fahy, Bonnie; Hilling, Lana, et al. Outcomes of advance directive education of pulmonary rehabilitation patients. *American Journal of Respiratory and Critical Care Medicine*. 1997 Mar; 155(3): 1055–1059. 28 refs. BE62103.

advance care planning; *advance directives; communication; control groups; evaluation studies; living wills; *patient education; patients; physicians; *rehabilitation; resuscitation; third party consent; ventilators; *lung diseases; refusal to participate; Arizona; California

Hines, Stephen C.; Glover, Jacqueline J.; Holley, Jean L., et al. Dialysis patients' preferences for family-based advance care planning. *Annals of Internal Medicine*. 1999 May 18; 130(10): 825–828. 20 refs. BE61609.

*advance care planning; *advance directives; *attitudes; *chronically ill; communication; decision making; *family members; family relationship; legal aspects; *patients; physician patient relationship; *physician's role; renal dialysis; state government; survey; *terminal care; third party consent; trust; New York; Pennsylvania; Rochester (NY); West Virginia

BACKGROUND: Most patients do not participate in advance care planning with physicians. OBJECTIVE: To examine patients' preferences for involving their physicians and families in advance care planning. DESIGN: Face-to-face interviews with randomly selected patients. SETTING: Community-based dialysis units in one rural and one urban region. PARTICIPANTS: 400 hemodialysis patients. MEASUREMENTS: Questions about whom patients involve in advance care planning, whom patients would like to include in this planning, and patients' reactions to state legislation on surrogate decision makers in end–of–life care. RESULTS: Patients more frequently discussed preferences for end–of–life care with family members than with physicians (50% compared with 6%; P less than 0.001). More patients wanted to include family members in future discussions of advance care planning than wanted to include physicians (91% compared with 36%; P less than 0.001). Patients were most comfortable with legislation that granted their family end–of–life decision–making authority in the event of their own incapacity (P less than 0.001). CONCLUSION: Most patients want to include their families more than their physicians in advance care planning.

Hoffmann, Diane E.; Zimmerman, Sheryl Itkin; Tompkins, Catherine. How close is enough? Family relationships and attitudes toward advance directives and life–sustaining treatments. *Journal of Ethics, Law, and Aging.* 1997 Spring–Summer; 3(1): 5–24. 33 fn. BE59201.
> *advance directives; age factors; *aged; *allowing to die; artificial feeding; blacks; communication; comparative studies; dementia; education; family members; *family relationship; females; geographic factors; *knowledge, attitudes, practice; lawyers; *living wills; males; motivation; persistent vegetative state; physicians; *prolongation of life; resuscitation; *social interaction; *socioeconomic factors; survey; terminally ill; third party consent; ventilators; whites; *withholding treatment; *adult offspring; Baltimore

Kapp, Marshall B. Commentary: anxieties as a legal impediment to the doctor–proxy relationship. *Journal of Law, Medicine and Ethics.* 1999 Spring; 27(1): 69–73. 31 fn. BE61506.
> administrators; *advance directives; *allowing to die; *decision making; *dissent; emotions; family members; futility; health facilities; information dissemination; institutional policies; knowledge, attitudes, practice; legal aspects; *legal liability; malpractice; motivation; *physicians; *professional family relationship; *prolongation of life; psychological stress; public policy; terminal care; *third party consent; treatment refusal; withholding treatment; risk management; United States

Kuczewski, Mark G. Commentary: narrative views of personal identity and substituted judgment in surrogate decision making. *Journal of Law, Medicine and Ethics.* 1999 Spring; 27(1): 32–36. 19 fn. Commentary on J. Blustein, p. 20–31. BE61502.
> *advance directives; allowing to die; autonomy; competence; *decision making; dementia; *directive adherence; family members; friends; legal aspects; living wills; moral policy; narrative ethics; persistent vegetative state; *personhood; philosophy; physicians; prolongation of life; *self concept; standards; terminal care; *third party consent; time factors; withholding treatment; Dresser, Rebecca; Robertson, John

Ladimer, Irving. Self–determination for life and death. *Medicine and Law.* 1996; 15(1): 83–92. BE61205.
> *advance directives; *allowing to die; autonomy; *decision making; information dissemination; legislation; living wills; *prolongation of life; state government; third party consent; treatment refusal; withholding treatment; Patient Self–Determination Act 1990; Uniform Rights of the Terminally Ill Act; United States

Larson, Edward J.; Eaton, Thomas A. The limits of advance directives: a history and assessment of the Patient Self–Determination Act. *Wake Forest Law Review.* 1997 Summer; 32(2): 249–293. 289 fn. BE60172.
> *advance directives; allowing to die; coercion; communication; comprehension; directive adherence; disadvantaged; economics; empirical research; *evaluation; goals; health care; health facilities; hospices; information dissemination; legal liability; *legislation; living wills;

minority groups; patient education; patients; physicians; policy analysis; politics; prognosis; psychological stress; *social impact; state government; terminal care; third party consent; values; withholding treatment; absence of proxy; *Patient Self–Determination Act 1990; Uniform Health–Care Decisions Act 1993; United States

Lee, Melinda A.; Smith, David M.; Fenn, Darien S., et al. Do patients' treatment decisions match advance statements of their preferences? *Journal of Clinical Ethics.* 1998 Fall; 9(3): 258–262. 10 fn. BE61334.
> *advance directives; aged; *allowing to die; artificial feeding; *attitudes; comparative studies; critically ill; *decision making; evaluation studies; males; medical records; *patients; *prolongation of life; renal dialysis; resuscitation orders; third party consent; time factors; treatment refusal; ventilators; withholding treatment; retrospective studies; Portland VA Medical Center (Portland, OR)

Leng, Ter Kah; Sy, Susanna Leong Huey. Advance medical directives in Singapore. *Medical Law Review.* 1997 Spring; 5(1): 63–101. 77 fn. Includes the full text of Singapore's Advance Medical Directive Act 1996, p. 89–101. BE60217.
> *advance directives; advisory committees; *allowing to die; autonomy; communication; comparative studies; *competence; cultural pluralism; decision making; family members; international aspects; *legal aspects; legal liability; legislation; palliative care; physicians; public participation; religious ethics; right to die; *terminally ill; treatment refusal; withholding treatment; *Advance Medical Directive Act 1996 (Singapore); Great Britain; *Singapore

McGee, Glenn. Paper shields: why advance directives still don't work. *Princeton Journal of Bioethics.* 1998 Spring; 1(1): 42–57. 7 refs. 4 fn. BE62490.
> advance care planning; *advance directives; allowing to die; alternatives; communication; competence; decision making; directive adherence; evaluation; futility; *living wills; motivation; physician patient relationship; physicians; resuscitation orders; terminally ill; third party consent; trust; values histories

Martin, Douglas K.; Thiel, Elaine C.; Singer, Peter A. A new model of advance care planning: observations from people with HIV. *Archives of Internal Medicine.* 1999 Jan 11; 159(1): 86–92. 58 refs. BE62604.
> *advance care planning; *advance directives; *AIDS; *attitudes; *attitudes to death; decision making; evaluation; *goals; *HIV seropositivity; living wills; models, theoretical; palliative care; *patient participation; patient satisfaction; *patients; survey; terminal care; terminally ill; qualitative research; Ontario

BACKGROUND: Although theoretical concepts from ethics and law have been applied, there is no conceptual model of advance care planning rooted in the perspective of individuals engaged in it. OBJECTIVE: To develop a conceptual model of advance care planning by examining the perspectives of individuals engaged in it. METHODS: In this qualitative research, we studied 140 individuals with human immunodeficiency virus (HIV) or acquired immunodeficiency syndrome who were engaged in advance care planning. Respondents' experience with and opinions about advance care planning were noted in interviews that were audiotaped, transcribed, and analyzed. RESULTS: The primary goal of advance care planning was to prepare for death, which entailed facing death, achieving a sense of control, and strengthening relationships. CONCLUSIONS: We have developed a conceptual model of advance care planning rooted in the perspectives of individuals engaged in it. The model has implications for theory, research, and practice regarding end–of–life care.

BE = bioethics accession number   fn. = footnotes   refs. = references

Maryland. Health Care Decisions Act. *Maryland (Health-General) Code Annotated (Michie).* 1993 (date approved). Sects. 5-601 to 5-618. 102-119. BE59870.
  active euthanasia; *advance directives; allowing to die; competence; emergency care; forms; *legal aspects; *living wills; patient care; resuscitation orders; third party consent; withholding treatment; *Maryland

May, Thomas. Slavery, commitment, and choice: do advance directives reflect autonomy? Response to "Advance directives and voluntary slavery" by Christopher Tollefsen (*CQ*, 1998 Fall; 7(4):405-413). *Cambridge Quarterly of Healthcare Ethics.* 1999 Summer; 8(3): 358-363. 10 fn. BE62353.
  *advance directives; *autonomy; *law; time factors; personal identity; slavery

May, William E. Making health care decisions for others. *Ethics and Medics.* 1997 Jun; 22(6): 1-3. BE61720.
  active euthanasia; adults; *advance directives; allowing to die; *decision making; *directive adherence; dissent; intention; moral obligations; *Roman Catholic ethics; *third party consent; values; withholding treatment; Ethical and Religious Directives for Catholic Health Care Services

Mezey, Mathy; Ramsey, Gloria C.; Mitty, Ethel. Making the PSDA work for the elderly. *Generations (American Society on Aging).* 1994 Winter; 18(4): 13-18. 24 refs. BE60545.
  *advance directives; *aged; clinical ethics committees; competence; economics; education; empirical research; government regulation; health personnel; *hospitals; *information dissemination; *institutional policies; knowledge, attitudes, practice; legislation; medical records; *nursing homes; statistics; oral directives; *Patient Self-Determination Act 1990; *United States

Mold, James W.; Looney, Stephen W.; Viviani, Nancy J., et al. Predicting the health-related values and preferences of geriatric patients. *Journal of Family Practice.* 1994 Nov; 39(5): 461-467. 32 refs. BE60499.
  *advance directives; *aged; *attitudes; competence; family relationship; health; patient care; *patients; persistent vegetative state; prolongation of life; *quality of life; religion; resuscitation; socioeconomic factors; survey; terminal care; *value of life; *values; ventilators; *values histories; Oklahoma Health Sciences Center Geriatric Continuity Clinic

Morrison, R. Sean; Zayas, Luis H.; Mulvihill, Michael, et al. Barriers to completion of health care proxies: an examination of ethnic differences. *Archives of Internal Medicine.* 1998 Dec 7-21; 158(22): 2493-2497. 25 refs. BE61228.
  advance care planning; *advance directives; aged; *blacks; comparative studies; family relationship; *Hispanic Americans; knowledge, attitudes, practice; minority groups; survey; terminal care; third party consent; trust; ventilators; whites; New York City
  BACKGROUND: Advance directives have not been uniformly used by different segments of the US population and studies have consistently shown a lower prevalence of advance directives among African Americans and Hispanics compared with non-Hispanic whites. OBJECTIVE: To examine barriers to completion of health care proxies for different ethnic groups. METHODS: One hundred ninety-seven subjects aged 65 years or older self-identified as African American (n = 65), Hispanic (n = 65), or non-Hispanic white (n = 67) attending a geriatrics and internal medicine outpatient clinic of a large New York City teaching hospital were administered a questionnaire. Questionnaires were developed to examine potential barriers to completion of health care proxies. Barriers were drawn from the literature and from focus groups. RESULTS: Significant predictors of proxy completion using logistic regression analysis included knowledge of health care proxies, availability of a health care agent, exposure to mechanical ventilation, age, and self-reported health status as fair to poor. Subjects who believed that a health care agent was irrelevant in the setting of involved family were significantly less likely to have completed a health care proxy. Although there were significant differences in the baseline completion rates of health care proxies for the 3 ethnic groups, ethnicity did not predict prior appointment of a health care agent in multivariate analysis. CONCLUSIONS: Differences in health care proxy completion rates across white, African American, and Hispanic elderly individuals in this New York City population seem to be related to potentially reversible barriers such as lack of knowledge and the perceived irrelevance of advance directives in the setting of involved family. Enhanced educational efforts of both health care personnel and patients could increase the rate of formal health care proxy appointment.

Newton, Michael J. Precedent autonomy: life-sustaining intervention and the demented patient. *Cambridge Quarterly of Healthcare Ethics.* 1999 Spring; 8(2): 189-199. 63 fn. BE61229.
  *advance directives; *allowing to die; *autonomy; beneficence; *competence; decision making; *dementia; directive adherence; family members; informed consent; *moral policy; personhood; *prolongation of life; *self concept; third party consent; time factors; treatment refusal; *personal identity; Ulysses contracts; Callahan, Daniel; Dresser, Rebecca; Dworkin, Ronald; Kadish, Sanford

Olick, Robert S. Deciding for Incompetent Patients: The Nature and Limits of Prospective Autonomy and Advance Directives. Ann Arbor, MI: UMI Dissertation Services; 1996. 374 p. (2 v. in 1). 436 fn. Dissertation, Ph.D. in Philosophy, Georgetown University, Dec 1996. Order No. 9720773. BE62147.
  advance care planning; *advance directives; *allowing to die; *autonomy; beneficence; case studies; clinical ethics committees; *competence; consensus; *decision making; dementia; directive adherence; ethical analysis; ethical review; ethical theory; family members; government regulation; guidelines; *intention; legal aspects; legal rights; models, theoretical; *moral policy; paternalism; persistent vegetative state; *personhood; physicians; prolongation of life; risks and benefits; standards; state government; terminally ill; *third party consent; treatment refusal; values; withholding treatment; *integrity; Cruzan v. Director, Missouri Department of Health; In re Quinlan; Patient Self-Determination Act 1990; United States

Perrin, Kathleen Ouimet. Giving voice to the wishes of elders for end-of-life care. *Journal of Gerontological Nursing.* 1997 Mar; 23(3): 18-27. 25 refs. BE60384.
  *advance care planning; *advance directives; *aged; allowing to die; communication; competence; *decision making; directive adherence; family members; informed consent; living wills; *nurse's role; patient advocacy; patient education; physician patient relationship; standards; *terminal care; third party consent; treatment refusal

Perry, Erica; Swartz, Richard; Smith-Wheelock, Linda, et al. Why is it difficult for staff to discuss advance directives with chronic dialysis patients? *Journal of the American Society of Nephrology.* 1996 Oct; 7(10): 2160-2168. 46 refs. BE62014.
  *advance directives; allied health personnel; attitudes to death; *chronically ill; *communication; comparative

---

BE = bioethics accession number   fn. = footnotes   refs. = references

studies; health facilities; *health personnel; *knowledge, attitudes, practice; nurses; patients; physicians; psychological stress; *renal dialysis; social workers; survey; questionnaires; Michigan

Post, Linda Farber; Blustein, Jeffrey; Dubler, Nancy Neveloff. The doctor–proxy relationship: an untapped resource: introduction. *Journal of Law, Medicine and Ethics.* 1999 Spring; 27(1): 5–12. 23 fn. BE61499.
  *advance care planning; *advance directives; allowing to die; alternatives; *communication; consensus; cultural pluralism; *decision making; diagnosis; disclosure; dissent; *family members; family relationship; friends; hospitals; legal aspects; living wills; mediation; medical records; models, theoretical; narrative ethics; patient care; patient education; physician patient relationship; *physicians; *professional family relationship; prognosis; prolongation of life; religion; *third party consent; trust; values; withholding treatment; values histories; United States

Powell, Tia. Extubating Mrs. K: psychological aspects of surrogate decision making. *Journal of Law, Medicine and Ethics.* 1999 Spring; 27(1): 81–86. 21 fn. BE61508.
  *advance directives; *allowing to die; caring; case studies; communication; cultural pluralism; *decision making; *dissent; *emotions; *family members; *family relationship; friends; intensive care units; justice; mediation; minority groups; physicians; *professional family relationship; *prolongation of life; psychological stress; *third party consent; treatment refusal; values; ventilators; withholding treatment; absence of proxy

Reynolds, Don F.; Garrett, Celia K. Avoiding resuscitation in non-hospital settings: *no consent* forms. *Bioethics Forum.* 1998 Spring; 14(1): 13–19. 11 refs. BE59946.
  *advance directives; autonomy; compensation; consent forms; directive adherence; *emergency care; *forms; home care; hospices; *legal aspects; *legal liability; legal rights; legislation; nursing homes; physicians; prolongation of life; resuscitation; *resuscitation orders; terminally ill; third party consent; treatment refusal; withholding treatment; Kansas; Missouri; Murphy v. Wheeler; Younts v. St. Francis Hospital and School of Nursing

Ritchie, Janet; Sklar, Ron; Steiner, Warren. Advance directives in psychiatry: resolving issues of autonomy and competence. *International Journal of Law and Psychiatry.* 1998 Summer; 21(3): 245–260. 25 refs. BE61669.
  *advance directives; *autonomy; *competence; *decision making; directive adherence; evaluation; informed consent; involuntary commitment; judicial action; lawyers; *mentally ill; *paternalism; physicians; psychiatric diagnosis; *psychiatric wills; *psychiatry; psychoactive drugs; resource allocation; standards; third party consent; treatment refusal; *Ulysses contracts; Canada

Robinson, John H.; Berry, Roberta M.; McDonnell, Kevin, eds. Death and dying. *In: their* A Health Law Reader: An Interdisciplinary Approach. Durham, NC: Carolina Academic Press; 1999: 339–426. 64 fn. ISBN 0-89089-907-X. BE62295.
  *active euthanasia; *advance directives; *allowing to die; artificial feeding; *assisted suicide; brain death; competence; decision making; determination of death; directive adherence; *disabled; economics; freedom; intention; *legal aspects; legal liability; legal rights; living wills; moral policy; physician's role; physicians; public policy; quality of life; *right to die; risks and benefits; standards; state government; state interest; third party consent; treatment refusal; value of life; withholding treatment; wrongful life; Patient Self-Determination Act 1990; *United States

Sabatino, Charles P. The legal and functional status of

the medical proxy: suggestions for statutory reform. *Journal of Law, Medicine and Ethics.* 1999 Spring; 27(1): 52–68. 92 fn. BE61505.
  *advance directives; allowing to die; autonomy; comparative studies; conflict of interest; conscience; contracts; *decision making; directive adherence; dissent; evaluation; family members; family relationship; friends; health facilities; historical aspects; institutional policies; judicial action; law; *legal aspects; *legal obligations; legislation; *living wills; model legislation; patient advocacy; patient transfer; physicians; professional family relationship; *public policy; *standards; *state government; terminal care; *third party consent; *United States

Schneiderman, Lawrence J. The family physician and end-of-life care. *Journal of Family Practice.* 1997 Sep; 45(3): 259–262. 38 refs. BE59341.
  advance care planning; *advance directives; *allowing to die; competence; economics; family practice; hospices; palliative care; physicians; resource allocation; resuscitation orders; *terminal care; withholding treatment; United States

Schonwetter, Ronald S.; Walker, Robert M.; Robinson, Bruce E. The lack of advance directives among hospice patients. *Hospice Journal.* 1995; 10(3): 1–11. 20 refs. BE59181.
  advance care planning; *advance directives; blacks; communication; comparative studies; diagnosis; home care; *hospices; medical records; patient admission; patient education; physicians; socioeconomic factors; *statistics; survey; *terminally ill; whites; prospective studies; retrospective studies; Florida

Singer, Peter A. University of Toronto Centre for Bioethics living will. *Ontario Medical Review.* 1993 Jan: 35, 37, 39–41. 5 refs. BE61589.
  *advance directives; allowing to die; decision making; forms; legal aspects; *living wills; resuscitation; third party consent; treatment refusal; Ontario; *University of Toronto Centre for Bioethics

Sosna, Dennis. Advance directives for emergency medical service workers: the struggle continues. *Bioethics Forum.* 1998 Spring; 14(1): 33–36. BE59949.
  *advance directives; *allied health personnel; directive adherence; education; *emergency care; *forms; *legal aspects; living wills; medical records; resuscitation; *resuscitation orders; *standards; withholding treatment; *Kansas; *Kansas City Area Ethics Committee Consortium; Midwest Bioethics Center

Spady, Donald W. Advance directives for severely mentally and physically handicapped adults who have never been competent. *Bioethics Bulletin.* 1996 Nov; 8(2): 10–11. BE61716.
  adults; *advance directives; allowing to die; case studies; *competence; congenital disorders; *decision making; family members; goals; health personnel; institutionalized persons; legal guardians; *mentally retarded; *physically disabled; prolongation of life; quality of life; resuscitation orders; third party consent; Canada

Stern, Kristina. Advance directives. *Medical Law Review.* 1994 Spring; 2(1): 57–76. 47 fn. BE59902.
  *advance directives; allowing to die; competence; decision making; family members; informed consent; judicial action; lawyers; *legal aspects; legal liability; physicians; pregnant women; third party consent; treatment refusal; *Great Britain; *Law Commission (Great Britain)

Szasz, Thomas. Parity for mental illness, disparity for the mental patient. *Lancet.* 1998 Oct 10; 352(9135): 1213–1215. 12 refs. BE60794.
  *advance directives; autonomy; brain pathology;

competence; dangerousness; government regulation; health insurance; involuntary commitment; *legal aspects; mental institutions; *mentally ill; *psychiatric wills; *treatment refusal; Patient Self-Determination Act 1990; United States

Teno, Joan M.; Branco, Kenneth J.; Mor, Vincent, et al. Changes in advance care planning in nursing homes before and after the Patient Self-Determination Act: report of a 10-state survey. *Journal of the American Geriatrics Society.* 1997 Aug; 45(8): 939–944. 43 refs. BE59434.
> *advance care planning; *advance directives; aged; artificial feeding; comparative studies; evaluation studies; *geographic factors; hospitals; *institutional policies; institutionalized persons; legislation; living wills; medical records; *nursing homes; patient transfer; *resuscitation orders; *social impact; statistics; survey; third party consent; *time factors; treatment refusal; withholding treatment; *Patient Self-Determination Act 1990; *United States

Tollefsen, Christopher. Advance directives and voluntary slavery: response to "Reassessing the reliability of advance directives," by Thomas May (*CQ* Vol. 6, No. 3). *Cambridge Quarterly of Healthcare Ethics.* 1998 Fall; 7(4): 405–413. 21 fn. BE59141.
> *advance directives; *autonomy; *competence; decision analysis; *decision making; *directive adherence; *evaluation; family members; informed consent; motivation; patient participation; *patients; *personhood; physicians; *self concept; third party consent; virtues; slavery

Toth, Ellen L.; Gill, Satvir; Godkin, Diane, et al. Advance directives for insulin-using diabetic patients. [Letter]. *Canadian Medical Association Journal.* 1998 May 5; 158(9): 1130–1131. 5 refs. BE60590.
> *advance directives; *diabetes; evaluation; *knowledge, attitudes, practice; *patient education; ambulatory care

Tulsky, James A.; Fischer, Gary S.; Rose, Mary R., et al. Opening the black box: how do physicians communicate about advance directives? *Annals of Internal Medicine.* 1998 Sep 15; 129(6): 441–449. 53 refs. BE59133.
> *advance care planning; *advance directives; attitudes; *communication; evaluation studies; informed consent; internal medicine; patients; physician patient relationship; *physicians; primary health care; prognosis; standards; terminology; third party consent; time factors; uncertainty; values; prospective studies; North Carolina; Pennsylvania
> BACKGROUND: The quality of communication that leads to the completion of written advance directives may influence the usefulness of these documents, but the nature of that communication remains relatively unexplored. OBJECTIVE: To describe how physicians discuss advance directives with patients. DESIGN: Prospective study. SETTING: Five outpatient primary care medicine practices in Durham, North Carolina, and Pittsburgh, Pennsylvania. PARTICIPANTS: 56 attending internists and 56 of their established patients. Eligible patients were at least 65 years of age or had a serious medical illness. MEASUREMENTS: Two raters coded transcripts of audiotaped discussions about advance directives to document how physicians introduced the topic of advance directives, discussed scenarios and treatments, provided information, elicited patient values, and identified surrogate decision makers. RESULTS: Conversations about advance directives averaged 5.6 minutes; physicians spoke for two thirds of this time. In 91% of cases, physicians discussed dire scenarios in which most patients would not want to be treated, and 48% asked patients about their preferences in reversible scenarios. Fifty-five percent of physicians discussed scenarios involving uncertainty, typically using

vague language. Patients' values were rarely explored in detail. In 88% of cases, physicians discussed surrogate decision making and documents to aid in advance care planning. CONCLUSIONS: Although they accomplished the goal of introducing patients to advance directives, discussions infrequently dealt with patients' values and attitudes toward uncertainty. Physicians may not have addressed the topic in a way that would be of substantial use in future decision making, and these discussions did not meet the standards proposed in the literature.

Veterans Affairs National Headquarters. Bioethics Committee. Surrogate-Written Advance Directives: Report. Issued by the VA National Center for Clinical Ethics, White River Junction, VT 05009; 1996 Jan. 6 p. 9 fn. BE59266.
> *advance directives; *allowing to die; *decision making; family members; federal government; institutional policies; legal guardians; patient care; patient care team; public hospitals; terminally ill; *third party consent; withholding treatment; United States; Veterans Health Administration

Walker, Leslie; Blechner, Barbara; Gruman, Cynthia, et al. Assessment of capacity to discuss advance care planning in nursing homes. [Letter]. *Journal of the American Geriatrics Society.* 1998 Aug; 46(8): 1055–1056. 11 refs. BE62262.
> administrators; *advance care planning; *advance directives; *competence; comprehension; decision making; empirical research; institutional policies; institutionalized persons; *nursing homes; *patient participation; *patients; Connecticut

Walsh, Marcia K. Difficult decisions in health care: one woman's journey. [Personal narrative]. *Bioethics Forum.* 1997 Summer; 13(2): 35–37. 13 refs. 2 fn. BE59401.
> *advance directives; *allowing to die; artificial feeding; attitudes; dementia; *patients; persistent vegetative state; *quality of life; terminally ill; *treatment refusal; withholding treatment

Wharton, Robert H.; Levine, Karen R.; Buka, Stephen, et al. Advance care planning for children with special health care needs: a survey of parental attitudes. *Pediatrics.* 1996 May; 97(5): 682–687. 38 refs. BE60404.
> *advance care planning; *advance directives; *attitudes; *children; *chronically ill; communication; comprehension; critically ill; *decision making; *disabled; knowledge, attitudes, practice; *parents; *patient care; physicians; *professional family relationship; prognosis; survey; truth disclosure; Massachusetts

Wilson, Petra. The Law Commission's report on mental incapacity: medically vulnerable adults or politically vulnerable law? *Medical Law Review.* 1996 Autumn; 4(3): 227–249. 83 refs. BE61511.
> adults; *advance directives; advisory committees; *competence; *decision making; dementia; human experimentation; informed consent; judicial action; *legal aspects; legal guardians; *mentally disabled; mentally retarded; model legislation; patient care; persistent vegetative state; public policy; standards; *third party consent; treatment refusal; *Great Britain; *Law Commission (Great Britain)

Winick, Bruce J. Advance directive instruments for those with mental illness. *University of Miami Law Review.* 1996 Oct; 51(1): 57–95. 128 fn. BE62226.
> *advance care planning; *advance directives; autonomy; coercion; *competence; constitutional law; decision making; due process; freedom; informed consent; involuntary commitment; *legal aspects; legal rights; living wills;

BE = bioethics accession number   fn. = footnotes   refs. = references

*mentally ill; patient care; *psychiatric wills; state interest; Supreme Court decisions; third party consent; treatment refusal; Cruzan v. Director, Missouri Department of Health; United States

Zelenik, Jomarie; Post, Linda Farber; Mulvihill, Michael, et al. The doctor-proxy relationship: perception and communication. *Journal of Law, Medicine and Ethics.* 1999 Spring; 27(1): 13–19. 16 fn. BE61500.
*advance care planning; *advance directives; aged; allowing to die; artificial feeding; *attitudes; *communication; comparative studies; *competence; *decision making; *family members; friends; hospitals; *knowledge, attitudes, practice; medical records; *patient care; patient care team; patient participation; *physicians; *professional family relationship; resuscitation orders; statistics; surgery; survey; *third party consent; ventilators; withholding treatment; retrospective studies; Montefiore Medical Center (Bronx, NY); New York City

Advance directive; notification; negligence; life prolongation; damages -- Allore v. Flower Hospital. *Mental and Physical Disability Law Reporter.* 1997 Sep-Oct; 21(5): 597. Synopsis of an unpublished 27 Jun 1997 opinion of the Ohio Court of Appeals; Ohio rule applies. BE59845.
*advance directives; allowing to die; *directive adherence; *hospitals; *legal liability; negligence; *physicians; *prolongation of life; withholding treatment; *Allore v. Flower Hospital; *Ohio

Some demented patients are still able to execute advance directives. [News]. *Geriatrics.* 1996 Jul; 51(7): 23. BE60535.
*advance directives; aged; *competence; comprehension; *dementia; nursing homes; values; Frances Schervier Home and Hospital (Bronx, NY)

AGED

See under
PATIENT CARE/AGED

AIDS

See also PUBLIC HEALTH

Aikman, Peter J.; Thiel, Elaine C.; Martin, Douglas K., et al. Proxy, health, and personal care preferences: implications for end-of-life care. *Cambridge Quarterly of Healthcare Ethics.* 1999 Spring; 8(2): 200–210. 31 fn. BE61236.
*advance care planning; *advance directives; *AIDS; allowing to die; *alternatives; assisted suicide; *attitudes; attitudes to death; comparative studies; *decision making; family members; family relationship; *forms; friends; *HIV seropositivity; home care; hospices; hospitals; *living wills; pain; palliative care; *patients; prolongation of life; *quality of life; survey; terminal care; third party consent; voluntary euthanasia; *values histories; Toronto

Alkas, Peri H.; Shandera, Wayne X. HIV and AIDS in Africa: African policies in response to AIDS in relation to various national legal traditions. *Journal of Legal Medicine.* 1996 Dec; 17(4): 527–546. 119 fn. BE61245.
*AIDS; AIDS serodiagnosis; aliens; blood banks; blood donation; *HIV seropositivity; *international aspects; Islamic ethics; law; *legal aspects; mandatory reporting; mandatory testing; political systems; prevalence; public policy; social discrimination; emigration and immigration; *Africa

Altman, Dennis. HIV, homophobia, and human rights. *Health and Human Rights.* 1998; 2(4): 15–22. 16 refs. BE61495.
*attitudes; developing countries; females; health education; *HIV seropositivity; *homosexuals; human rights; international aspects; *males; political activity; self induced illness; sexuality; *stigmatization; vulnerable populations; prostitution

American Hospital Association. AIDS/HIV Infection: Recommendations for Health Care Practices and Public Policy. Chicago, IL: The Association; 1992. 19 p. Approved by the Board of Trustees 1992. BE61474.
*AIDS; AIDS serodiagnosis; confidentiality; contact tracing; counseling; disclosure; duty to warn; economics; education; federal government; financial support; guidelines; health care; health personnel; *HIV seropositivity; *hospitals; iatrogenic disease; informed consent; *institutional policies; legal aspects; mandatory reporting; mandatory testing; occupational exposure; *organizational policies; patient care; patients; private sector; professional organizations; public policy; public sector; social discrimination; tuberculosis; universal precautions; *American Hospital Association; Centers for Disease Control and Prevention; United States

Beckett, Alexandra. End-of-life decisions in AIDS. *In:* Steinberg, Maurice D.; Youngner, Stuart J., eds. End-of-Life Decisions: A Psychosocial Perspective. Washington, DC: American Psychiatric Press; 1998: 179–203. 68 fn. ISBN 0-88048-756-9. BE60119.
*AIDS; alcohol abuse; *allowing to die; *assisted suicide; autonomy; case studies; competence; decision making; dementia; depressive disorder; drug abuse; drugs; futility; patient care; patients; *physicians; prognosis; psychiatric diagnosis; psychiatry; quality of life; referral and consultation; risks and benefits; *suicide; treatment refusal; withholding treatment; United States

Bolan, Robert K.; Bessesen, Mary; McCollum, Marianne, et al. AIDS exceptionalism. [Letters and response]. *Annals of Internal Medicine.* 1999 Jan 5; 130(1): 79–80. 11 refs. BE61076.
*AIDS; communicable diseases; drugs; *economics; federal government; government financing; health care; health insurance; HIV seropositivity; justice; medical education; patient care; political activity; public health; *public policy; *resource allocation; risks and benefits; *United States

Clark, Peter A. A legacy of mistrust: African-Americans, the medical profession, and AIDS. *Linacre Quarterly.* 1998 Feb; 65(1): 66–88. 62 fn. BE60454.
*AIDS; attitudes; autopsies; biomedical research; *blacks; cadavers; contraception; drugs; federal government; genetic screening; health care delivery; *historical aspects; hospitals; human experimentation; immunization; investigators; medical education; medical schools; misconduct; mortality; patient care; physicians; public health; public policy; scientific misconduct; selection for treatment; selection of subjects; sickle cell anemia; *social discrimination; sterilization (sexual); stigmatization; syphilis; *trust; withholding treatment; slavery; *Nineteenth Century; Tuskegee Syphilis Study; *Twentieth Century; *United States

Coburn, Tom; Senak, Mark S.; Stein, Robert E., et al. What can be done to curtail the AIDS epidemic? *In:* Dudley, William, ed. Epidemics: Opposing Viewpoints. San Diego, CA: Greenhaven Press; 1999: 53–85, 173. Bibliography: p. 85; discussion questions: p. 173. ISBN 1-56510-940-6. BE59824.
*AIDS; AIDS serodiagnosis; communicable diseases; confidentiality; contact tracing; drug abuse; federal government; HIV seropositivity; immunization; international aspects; legal aspects; legal rights; mandatory reporting;

BE = bioethics accession number   fn. = footnotes   refs. = references

mandatory testing; newborns; political activity; public health; *public policy; resource allocation; self induced illness; social impact; state government; stigmatization; voluntary programs; needle–exchange programs; United States

Cohen, Jon. Researchers urged not to inject virulent HIV strain into chimps. [News]. *Science.* 1999 Feb 19; 283(5405): 1090–1091. BE60846.
     *AIDS; *animal experimentation; *HIV seropositivity; immunization; investigators; *primates; research design; risks and benefits; United States

Cooper, Ellen R. Caring for children with AIDS: new challenges for medicine and society. *Pediatrician.* 1990; 17(2): 118–123. 13 refs. BE59456.
     adoption; AIDS; *children; confidentiality; disadvantaged; disclosure; family members; fetuses; *HIV seropositivity; informed consent; newborns; parental consent; patient care; *pediatrics; physicians; pregnant women; preventive medicine; research ethics committees; schools; stigmatization; therapeutic research; United States

Feldman, Eric A.; Bayer, Ronald, eds. Blood Feuds: AIDS, Blood, and the Politics of Medical Disaster. New York, NY: Oxford University Press; 1999. 375 p. 1,007 fn. ISBN 0–19–513160–6. BE60746.
     accountability; administrators; *AIDS; *blood donation; *blood transfusions; comparative studies; compensation; drug industry; economics; government regulation; *hemophilia; *HIV seropositivity; iatrogenic disease; information dissemination; *international aspects; legal aspects; legal liability; mandatory programs; metaphor; misconduct; organization and administration; political activity; politics; *public policy; self regulation; time factors; voluntary programs; Australia; Canada; Denmark; France; Germany; Italy; Japan; Red Cross; United States

Fieldston, Evan. AIDS, thalidomide and maternal–fetal rights in conflict. *Princeton Journal of Bioethics.* 1998 Spring; 1(1): 83–93. 9 refs. BE62495.
     *AIDS; autonomy; coercion; contraception; *drugs; *females; fetuses; *HIV seropositivity; iatrogenic disease; moral obligations; *patient care; preconception injuries; *pregnant women; *prenatal injuries; public health; quality of life; reproduction; selective abortion; *social control; toxicity; women's rights; *thalidomide

Freudenthal, Gad, ed. AIDS in Jewish Thought and Law. Hoboken, NJ: Ktav; 1998. 175 p. Includes references. ISBN 0–88125–610–2. BE60068.
     *AIDS; AIDS serodiagnosis; autonomy; circumcision; common good; compassion; confidentiality; drug abuse; duty to warn; health personnel; *HIV seropositivity; homosexuals; *Jewish ethics; mandatory testing; morality; natural law; occupational exposure; organizational policies; patient care; preventive medicine; privacy; public health; punishment; refusal to treat; risk; self induced illness; sexuality; suffering; *theology; condoms; needle–exchange programs; Conservative Judaism; Orthodox Judaism; Reform Judaism

Giesen, Dieter. Compensation and consent: a brief comparative examination of liability for HIV–infected blood. *In:* Bennett, Rebecca; Erin, Charles A., eds. HIV and AIDS: Testing, Screening, and Confidentiality. New York, NY: Oxford University Press; 1999: 91–106. 65 fn. ISBN 0–19–823801–0. BE62716.
     *AIDS; AIDS serodiagnosis; blood banks; *blood donation; *blood transfusions; comparative studies; compensation; disclosure; donors; *HIV seropositivity; hospitals; informed consent; international aspects; judicial action; legal aspects; *legal liability; legal rights; negligence; physicians; standards; *torts; *Germany; Great Britain; *United States

Gostin, Lawrence O.; Feldblum, Chai; Webber, David W. Disability discrimination in America: HIV/AIDS and other health conditions. *JAMA.* 1999 Feb 24; 281(8): 745–752. 78 refs. Includes a table of state legislation protecting persons with HIV infection against discrimination. BE60945.
     AIDS; AIDS serodiagnosis; carriers; dentistry; *disabled; *employment; *federal government; genetic disorders; genetic predisposition; *government regulation; health personnel; *HIV seropositivity; *judicial action; *legal aspects; *legislation; mentally disabled; morbidity; occupational exposure; physically disabled; *refusal to treat; reproduction; risk; *social discrimination; *standards; *state government; *Supreme Court decisions; *Americans with Disabilities Act 1990; *Bragdon v. Abbott; Rehabilitation Act 1973; *United States
The Americans With Disabilities Act (ADA) was widely hailed at the time of its enactment in 1990 as providing broad protection against disability discrimination, including discrimination against individuals infected with the human immunodeficiency virus (HIV). In the years since its enactment, however, courts frequently interpreted the ADA as providing far less protection than was initially anticipated. The Supreme Court's first case involving HIV and the acquired immunodeficiency syndrome, Bragdon v Abbott, addressed this trend by ruling that a woman with asymptomatic HIV infection is protected from discrimination in accessing dental services. In doing so, the Court endorsed an interpretation of the ADA that is broadly protective for individuals with disabilities. The Court also ruled that health care professionals may legally refuse to treat a patient because of concern that the patient poses a direct threat to safety only if there is an objective, scientific basis for concluding that the threat to safety is significant. In addition to the ADA, state laws frequently prohibit disability discrimination and apply to some employers and others not regulated by federal law. A state–by–state survey of those laws demonstrates that, consistent with Bragdon v Abbott, individuals with asymptomatic HIV have widespread protection on the state level.

Gostin, Lawrence O.; Webber, David W. The AIDS Litigation Project: HIV/AIDS in the courts in the 1990s, part 1. *AIDS and Public Policy Journal.* 1997 Winter; 12(4): 105–121. 23 fn. Provides an AIDS Litigation Project compilation of cases categorized under AIDS education; protection of the blood supply; public health powers and epidemiological surveillance; government restrictions of persons: criminal law; governmental regulation of products, consumer protection, and fraud; tort actions; duty to protect workers; administration of justice; and family law. BE59298.
     *AIDS; AIDS serodiagnosis; blood donation; blood transfusions; children; confidentiality; criminal law; diagnosis; disclosure; donors; drug abuse; employment; epidemiology; family members; federal government; government regulation; health education; health facilities; health personnel; hemophilia; *HIV seropositivity; injuries; *judicial action; *legal aspects; legal liability; mandatory reporting; mandatory testing; negligence; occupational exposure; parental consent; patients; prisoners; public health; public policy; schools; standards; state government; torts; voluntary programs; condoms; *United States

Gostin, Lawrence O.; Webber, David W. The AIDS Litigation Project: HIV/AIDS in the courts in the 1990s, part 2. *AIDS and Public Policy Journal.* 1998 Spring; 13(1): 3–19. 28 fn. Provides an AIDS Litigation Project compilation of cases categorized under privacy and confidentiality; the "right to know;" discrimination; insurance; the rights of vulnerable persons: disability,

---

homelessness and indigence; the rights of vulnerable persons: prisoners; and immigration and international travel. BE61342.

*AIDS; AIDS serodiagnosis; blood transfusions; community services; *confidentiality; *disclosure; *duty to warn; employment; health care; health personnel; *HIV seropositivity; iatrogenic disease; indigents; insurance; *legal aspects; legal liability; legal rights; mandatory testing; mass media; military personnel; patients; prisoners; *privacy; quarantine; refusal to treat; *social discrimination; *vulnerable populations; emigration and immigration; homeless persons; sexual partners; Americans with Disabilities Act 1990; *United States

Graham, Wendy J.; Newell, Marie-Louise. Seizing the opportunity: collaborative initiatives to reduce HIV and maternal mortality. *Lancet.* 1999 Mar 6; 353(9155): 836–839. 36 refs. BE61222.

AIDS; cesarean section; childbirth; children; contraception; costs and benefits; *developing countries; drugs; economics; females; health care delivery; health education; *HIV seropositivity; infants; *maternal health; *morbidity; *mortality; *mothers; newborns; patient care; patient education; *pregnant women; prevalence; preventive medicine; quality of health care; resource allocation; sexually transmitted diseases; social impact; *women's health; *women's health services; breast feeding; Africa; AZT; Inter-Agency Group for Safe Motherhood; UNAIDS

Green, Gill. AIDS and euthanasia. *AIDS Care.* 1995; 7(Suppl. 2): S169–S173. 6 refs. BE60344.

*active euthanasia; *AIDS; *assisted suicide; *attitudes; communication; family members; friends; health personnel; *HIV seropositivity; legal aspects; *patients; quality of life; suicide; survey; Scotland

Gruskin, Sofia; Mann, Jonathan; Tarantola, Daniel. Past, present, and future: AIDS and human rights. [Editorial]. *Health and Human Rights.* 1998; 2(4): 1–3. BE61494.

*AIDS; *HIV seropositivity; *human rights; *international aspects; public health; vulnerable populations; UNAIDS; United Nations; World Health Organization

Gruskin, Sofia. The highest priority: making use of UN conference documents to remind governments of their commitments to HIV/AIDS. *Health and Human Rights.* 1998; 3(1): 107–142. A compilation of references to HIV/AIDS in documents from United Nations global conferences, 1990–1995. BE62577.

adolescents; *AIDS; children; family planning; females; health care; *HIV seropositivity; human rights; *international aspects; obligations of society; public health; public policy; socioeconomic factors; vulnerable populations; *United Nations

Halkitis, Perry N.; Dooha, Susan M. The perceptions and experiences of managed care by HIV-positive individuals in New York City. *AIDS and Public Policy Journal.* 1998 Summer; 13(2): 75–84. 23 fn. BE61345.

*AIDS; *attitudes; communication; comparative studies; disclosure; economics; health insurance; *HIV seropositivity; homosexuals; males; *managed care programs; patient care; patient education; *patient satisfaction; *patients; physicians; primary health care; quality of health care; referral and consultation; stigmatization; survey; case managers; fee-for-service plans; personal financing; qualitative research; Gay Men's Health Crisis; Medicaid; *New York City

Heywood, Mark; Cornell, Morna. Human rights and AIDS in South Africa: from right margin to left margin. *Health and Human Rights.* 1998; 2(4): 60–82. 66 fn. BE61497.

*AIDS; AIDS serodiagnosis; confidentiality; developing countries; females; health care delivery; *HIV seropositivity; *human rights; informed consent; insurance; mandatory testing; political activity; politics; preventive medicine; prisoners; public health; *public policy; *social discrimination; *socioeconomic factors; vulnerable populations; *South Africa

Hoey, John. Human rights, ethics and the Krever inquiry. [Editorial]. *Canadian Medical Association Journal.* 1997 Nov 1; 157(9): 1231. 3 refs. BE59831.

AIDS; AIDS serodiagnosis; *blood banks; blood donation; codes of ethics; *drug industry; *duty to warn; *hepatitis; *HIV seropositivity; human rights; legal aspects; misconduct; *public health; public policy; Supreme Court decisions; Baxter Corp.; *Canada; Canadian Red Cross; *Commission of Inquiry on the Blood System in Canada

International Federation of Red Cross and Red Crescent Societies; François-Xavier Bagnoud Center for Health and Human Rights, Harvard School of Public Health. AIDS, Health and Human Rights: An Explanatory Model. Geneva: The Federation; Boston, MA: The Center; 1995. 162 p. Includes references. ISBN 92-9139-014-3. BE61599.

*AIDS; AIDS serodiagnosis; confidentiality; counseling; females; guidelines; health; health care; health promotion; *HIV seropositivity; *human rights; *international aspects; patient care; preventive medicine; prisoners; *public health; public policy; social discrimination; voluntary programs; prostitution; Convention on the Elimination of All Forms of Discrimination Against Women; Convention on the Rights of the Child; Declaration of Alma-Ata; International Covenant on Civil and Political Rights; International Covenant on Economic, Social and Cultural Rights; United Nations; Universal Declaration of Human Rights

Kaldjian, Lauris C.; Jekel, James F.; Friedland, Gerald. End-of-life decisions in HIV-positive patients: the role of spiritual beliefs. *AIDS.* 1998 Jan 1; 12(1): 103–107. 13 refs. BE60526.

*advance care planning; advance directives; assisted suicide; *attitudes to death; *decision making; disadvantaged; emotions; *HIV seropositivity; living wills; pastoral care; *patients; physician patient relationship; *religion; resuscitation; suicide; survey; *terminal care; urban population; Yale-New Haven Hospital

Khaïat, Lucette. The law and AIDS: issues and objectives (a comparative approach). *Medicine and Law.* 1993; 12(1–2): 3–10. 12 fn. BE60607.

*AIDS; AIDS serodiagnosis; coercion; confidentiality; *government regulation; health education; *HIV seropositivity; homosexuals; informed consent; *international aspects; *legal aspects; mandatory testing; physician's role; public health; risk; sexuality; *social control; social discrimination; social impact; socioeconomic factors; prostitution

Kirp, David L. Blood, sweat, and tears: the Tuskegee experiment and the era of AIDS. *Tikkun.* 1995 May–Jun; 10(3): 50–54. BE61473.

*AIDS; *attitudes; *blacks; deception; federal government; historical aspects; homosexuals; *human experimentation; investigators; morbidity; mortality; motivation; nontherapeutic research; physicians; public health; public policy; radiation; research design; research subjects; *scientific misconduct; social discrimination; syphilis; *trust; vulnerable populations; whites; withholding treatment; Centers for Disease Control and Prevention; Foster, Henry; Public Health Service; *Tuskegee Syphilis Study; Twentieth Century; United States

Laane, Henk-Maarten. Euthanasia, assisted suicide and AIDS. *AIDS Care.* 1995; 7(Suppl. 2): S163–S167. 13 refs. BE60343.

BE = bioethics accession number   fn. = footnotes   refs. = references

*AIDS; *assisted suicide; criminal law; drugs; economics; empirical research; knowledge, attitudes, practice; legal aspects; mortality; physicians; statistics; suffering; *voluntary euthanasia; *Netherlands

Layon, A. Joseph; D'Amico, Robert. Intensive care for patients with acquired immunodeficiency syndrome -- medicine versus ideology. *Critical Care Medicine.* 1990 Nov; 18(11): 1297-1299. 30 refs. BE60955.
    *AIDS; attitudes; economics; futility; HIV seropositivity; *intensive care units; patient admission; patients; prolongation of life; *resource allocation; self induced illness; social discrimination; terminally ill

Levi, Jeffrey. Can access to care for people living with HIV be expanded? *AIDS and Public Policy Journal.* 1998 Summer; 13(2): 56-74. 44 fn. BE61344.
    *AIDS; community services; drugs; federal government; *government financing; guidelines; *health care delivery; *HIV seropositivity; indigents; mortality; patient care; *public policy; quality of health care; resource allocation; standards; state government; statistics; Department of Health and Human Services; Department of Housing and Urban Development; Department of Veterans Affairs; Medicaid; Medicare; Ryan White Comprehensive AIDS Resources Emergency Act 1990; *United States

Lii, Jane H. Suit over adopted boy's H.I.V. seen as a first. [News]. *New York Times.* 1998 Feb 8: 35. BE59364.
    adolescents; *adoption; confidentiality; *disclosure; *duty to warn; *HIV seropositivity; *hospitals; *legal aspects; *legal liability; *parents; physicians; Moreau, Justin; New York; *New York Foundling Hospital

Mann, Jonathan M. AIDS and human rights: where do we go from here? *Health and Human Rights.* 1998; 3(1): 143-149. BE62578.
    *AIDS; health personnel; *HIV seropositivity; *human rights; international aspects; patient advocacy; professional role; public health; social discrimination

Martin, Douglas K.; Thiel, Elaine C.; Singer, Peter A. A new model of advance care planning: observations from people with HIV. *Archives of Internal Medicine.* 1999 Jan 11; 159(1): 86-92. 58 refs. BE62604.
    *advance care planning; *advance directives; *AIDS; *attitudes; *attitudes to death; decision making; evaluation; *goals; *HIV seropositivity; living wills; models, theoretical; palliative care; *patient participation; patient satisfaction; *patients; survey; terminal care; terminally ill; qualitative research; Ontario
    BACKGROUND: Although theoretical concepts from ethics and law have been applied, there is no conceptual model of advance care planning rooted in the perspective of individuals engaged in it. OBJECTIVE: To develop a conceptual model of advance care planning by examining the perspectives of individuals engaged in it. METHODS: In this qualitative research, we studied 140 individuals with human immunodeficiency virus (HIV) or acquired immunodeficiency syndrome who were engaged in advance care planning. Respondents' experience with and opinions about advance care planning were noted in interviews that were audiotaped, transcribed, and analyzed. RESULTS: The primary goal of advance care planning was to prepare for death, which entailed facing death, achieving a sense of control, and strengthening relationships. CONCLUSIONS: We have developed a conceptual model of advance care planning rooted in the perspectives of individuals engaged in it. The model has implications for theory, research, and practice regarding end-of-life care.

Novick, Alvin. HIV surveillance: what's hot, what's not.

AIDS and Public Policy Journal. 1998 Summer; 13(2): 51-55. 6 fn. BE61343.
    AIDS serodiagnosis; anonymous testing; confidentiality; contact tracing; *epidemiology; health care delivery; *HIV seropositivity; *mandatory reporting; mandatory testing; prevalence; public policy; research design; partner notification; Centers for Disease Control and Prevention; *United States

Oppé, Thomas E. Ethical aspects of AIDS in childhood in England. *Pediatrician.* 1990; 17(2): 115-117. 5 refs. BE59455.
    *AIDS; AIDS serodiagnosis; *children; confidentiality; disclosure; *HIV seropositivity; human experimentation; informed consent; parental consent; patient care; *pediatrics; physicians; *Great Britain

Panossian, André A.; Panossian, Vahé; Doumanian, Nancy P. Criminalization of perinatal HIV transmission. *Journal of Legal Medicine.* 1998 Jun; 19(2): 223-255. 155 fn. BE61249.
    child abuse; childbirth; *criminal law; drug abuse; females; *HIV seropositivity; infants; killing; *legal liability; males; mothers; *newborns; parent child relationship; patients; *pregnant women; *prenatal injuries; public policy; AZT; *United States

Piot, Peter; Timberlake, Susan. HIV/AIDS and human rights: continued commitment in the second decade. *Health and Human Rights.* 1998; 3(1): 1-6. BE62572.
    *AIDS; health; *HIV seropositivity; *human rights; international aspects; patient advocacy; United Nations

Qureshi, Sarah N. Global ostracism of HIV-positive aliens: international restrictions barring HIV-positive aliens. *Maryland Journal of International Law and Trade.* 1995 Spring; 19(1): 81-120. 316 fn. BE59314.
    AIDS; AIDS serodiagnosis; *aliens; *government regulation; *HIV seropositivity; *international aspects; legal aspects; mandatory testing; organizational policies; *public policy; *social discrimination; Asia; Europe; Haiti; South America; *United States; World Health Organization

Richardson, Lynda. Wave of laws aimed at people with H.I.V. [News]. *New York Times.* 1998 Sep 25: A1, B4. BE60573.
    AIDS serodiagnosis; confidentiality; contact tracing; criminal law; duty to warn; government regulation; *HIV seropositivity; *legal aspects; legal liability; legislation; *mandatory programs; mandatory reporting; mandatory testing; patients; public opinion; state government; *partner notification; sexual partners; *United States

Rojanksy, Nathan; Schenker, Joseph G. Ethical aspects of assisted reproduction in AIDS patients. *Journal of Assisted Reproduction and Genetics.* 1995 Sep; 12(8): 537-542. 48 refs. BE60567.
    *AIDS; AIDS serodiagnosis; artificial insemination; confidentiality; counseling; directive counseling; females; *HIV seropositivity; informed consent; ovum donors; physicians; privacy; refusal to treat; reproduction; *reproductive technologies; semen donors; partner notification

Schüklenk, Udo; Chokevivat, Vichai; Del Rio, Carlos, et al. AIDS: ethical issues in the developing world. *In:* Kuhse, Helga; Singer, Peter, eds. A Companion to Bioethics. Malden, MA: Blackwell; 1998: 355-365. 40 refs. ISBN 0-631-19737-0. BE59509.
    *AIDS; AIDS serodiagnosis; confidentiality; cultural pluralism; *developing countries; ethical relativism; health care; health education; human experimentation; immunization; informed consent; religion; research subjects; resource allocation; sexuality; social discrimination;

BE = bioethics accession number   fn. = footnotes   refs. = references

stigmatization; values; community consent; Africa; Asia; Latin America

Schüklenk, Udo. AIDS: individual and 'public' interests. *In:* Kuhse, Helga; Singer, Peter, eds. A Companion to Bioethics. Malden, MA: Blackwell; 1998: 343–354. 30 refs. ISBN 0-631-19737-0. BE59508.
*AIDS; AIDS serodiagnosis; confidentiality; criminal law; dangerousness; disclosure; drugs; duty to warn; friends; health personnel; *HIV seropositivity; human experimentation; iatrogenic disease; mandatory testing; moral obligations; occupational exposure; paternalism; patient care; patients; refusal to treat; terminally ill; sexual partners

Selwyn, Peter A.; Arnold, Robert. From fate to tragedy: the changing meanings of life, death, and AIDS. *Annals of Internal Medicine.* 1998 Dec 1; 129(11): 899–902. 29 refs. BE59327.
*AIDS; chronically ill; drugs; *HIV seropositivity; *palliative care; *patient care; physician patient relationship; *physician's role; psychological stress; *terminal care; terminally ill

The advent of highly active antiretroviral therapy (HAART) and quantitative viral load assays has revolutionized the care of HIV-infected patients. However, this paradigm shift has also had unexpected, sometimes adverse consequences that are not always obvious. Before antiretroviral therapy, physicians learned how to accompany patients through their illness; to bear witness to sickness and dying; and to help patients and their families with suffering, closure, and legacy. Since we have become better at treating the virus, a new temptation has emerged to dwell on quantitative aspects of HIV management and monitoring, although the skills that we learned earlier in the epidemic are no less necessary for providing good care. Our new-found therapeutic capabilities should not distract us from the sometimes more difficult and necessary task of simply "being there" for patients for whom HAART is no longer effective. The definition and practice of end-of-life care for patients with AIDS will continue to evolve as AIDS comes to resemble other chronic, treatable, but ultimately fatal illnesses, such as end-stage pulmonary disease and metastatic cancer, in which clinicians must continually readdress with their patients the balance of curative and palliative interventions as the disease process unfolds over time. The coming challenge in HIV care will be to encourage the maintenance of a "primary care" mentality–with attention to the larger psychosocial issues, end-of-life care, bereavement, and a focus on the patient as opposed to the illness–alongside our new antiretroviral paradigm. Otherwise, we run the risk of forgetting what we learned about healing, from a disease that we could not cure.

Starace, F.; Ogden, R.D. Suicidal behaviours and euthanasia. *AIDS Care.* 1997 Feb; 9(1): 106–108. Report on the XIth International Conference on AIDS, Vancouver, BC, Canada. BE62004.
*AIDS; *assisted suicide; attitudes; *HIV seropositivity; nurses; patients; physicians; statistics; *suicide; *voluntary euthanasia; British Columbia; California; Canada; Great Britain; Netherlands

Steinbrook, Robert. Caring for people with human immunodeficiency virus infection. [Editorial]. *New England Journal of Medicine.* 1998 Dec 24; 339(26): 1926–1928. 15 refs. BE60262.
adults; *AIDS; children; *disadvantaged; *drugs; *economics; federal government; *government financing; *health care delivery; *HIV seropositivity; mortality; *patient care; prevalence; *public policy; state government; statistics; Department of Veterans Affairs; Medicaid; Medicare; *United States

Stoto, Michael A.; Almario, Donna A.; McCormick, Marie C., eds.; Institute of Medicine. Committee on Perinatal Transmission of HIV; National Research Council and Institute of Medicine. Board on Children, Youth, and Families. Reducing the Odds: Preventing Perinatal Transmission of HIV in the United States. Washington, DC: National Academy Press; 1999. 397 p. Bibliography: p. 134–144. ISBN 0-309-06286-1. BE61845.
adolescents; AIDS; *AIDS serodiagnosis; children; counseling; drugs; epidemiology; evaluation; federal government; females; financial support; government financing; guidelines; health care delivery; *HIV seropositivity; human experimentation; mandatory testing; mass screening; *newborns; patient compliance; policy analysis; *pregnant women; *preventive medicine; professional organizations; public health; *public policy; state government; statistics; voluntary programs; women's health services; AZT; Public Health Service; *United States

Stringer, Jeffrey S.A.; Rouse, Dwight J.; Goldenberg, Robert L. Prophylactic cesarean delivery for the prevention of perinatal human immunodeficiency virus transmission: the case for restraint. *JAMA.* 1999 May 26; 281(20): 1946–1949. 41 refs. BE62312.
AIDS; *cesarean section; counseling; developing countries; drugs; empirical research; evaluation; *HIV seropositivity; maternal health; morbidity; mortality; *newborns; *pregnant women; *preventive medicine; research design; *risks and benefits; treatment outcome; United States

Tarantola, Daniel; Gruskin, Sofia. Children confronting HIV/AIDS: charting the confluence of rights and health. *Health and Human Rights.* 1998; 3(1): 60–86. 42 fn. BE62575.
*adolescents; age factors; *AIDS; *children; epidemiology; females; health care; *HIV seropositivity; *human rights; international aspects; males; obligations of society; sexuality; social discrimination; socioeconomic factors

Timberlake, Susan. UNAIDS: human rights, ethics, and law. *Health and Human Rights.* 1998; 3(1): 87–106. 41 fn. BE62576.
*AIDS; *HIV seropositivity; *human rights; information dissemination; *international aspects; organizational policies; social discrimination; vulnerable populations; *UNAIDS; *United Nations

University of Manchester (U.K.). Centre for Social Ethics and Policy. AIDS: Ethics, Justice and European Policy: summary of conclusions and recommendations. *In:* Bennett, Rebecca; Erin, Charles A., eds. HIV and AIDS: Testing, Screening, and Confidentiality. New York, NY: Oxford University Press; 1999: 267–270. ISBN 0-19-823801-0. BE62728.
*AIDS; AIDS serodiagnosis; confidentiality; duty to warn; *guidelines; health education; *HIV seropositivity; *international aspects; legal aspects; legal rights; mandatory testing; *moral obligations; *obligations of society; physician's role; public health; *public policy; social discrimination; voluntary programs; Europe; *European Community; European Union

Valdiserri, Ronald O.; Robinson, Carol; Lin, Lillian S., et al. Determining allocations for HIV-prevention interventions: assessing a change in federal funding policy. *AIDS and Public Policy Journal.* 1997 Winter; 12(4): 138–148. 31 fn. BE59300.
*AIDS; AIDS serodiagnosis; counseling; *federal

BE = bioethics accession number   fn. = footnotes   refs. = references

government; *government financing; *HIV seropositivity; *municipal government; *preventive medicine; public health; *public policy; *resource allocation; *state government; health planning; *HIV Prevention Community Planning; *United States

van den Boom, Frans M. AIDS, euthanasia and grief. *AIDS Care.* 1995; 7(Suppl. 2): S175–S185. 11 refs. BE60345.
*active euthanasia; *advance care planning; *AIDS; autonomy; communication; decision making; depressive disorder; emotions; *family members; patient participation; *psychological stress; statistics; suicide; terminally ill; *grief; sexual partners; *Netherlands

Waldholz, Michael. AZT price cut for Third World mothers-to-be. [News]. *Wall Street Journal.* 1998 Mar 5: B1, B12. BE59369.
*developing countries; *drug industry; *drugs; *economics; *HIV seropositivity; human experimentation; newborns; patient care; placebos; *pregnant women; research design; *AZT; *Glaxo-Wellcome

Whelan, Daniel. Human rights approaches to an expanded response to address women's vulnerability to HIV/AIDS. *Health and Human Rights.* 1998; 3(1): 20–36. 43 fn. BE62573.
adolescents; *AIDS; *females; health education; *HIV seropositivity; *human rights; international aspects; public policy; sexuality; social discrimination; socioeconomic factors; women's health; women's health services; *women's rights; United Nations

Wodak, Alex. Health, HIV infection, human rights, and injecting drug use. *Health and Human Rights.* 1998; 2(4): 24–41. 41 fn. BE61496.
developing countries; *drug abuse; government regulation; hepatitis; *HIV seropositivity; *human rights; *international aspects; *law enforcement; *public health; *public policy; social discrimination; vulnerable populations; United Nations; Universal Declaration of Human Rights; World Health Organization

Court says mother has right to stop HIV drugs for son. *AIDS Policy and Law.* 1998 Oct 2; 13(18): 1, 4–5. 1 ref. BE61300.
child abuse; *children; decision making; *drugs; *HIV seropositivity; *legal aspects; *legal rights; mothers; *parents; *risks and benefits; state interest; *treatment refusal; uncertainty; *In re Nikolas Emerson; Maine

AIDS/CONFIDENTIALITY

Baker, Debra. Positively truthful: appeal asks whether doctors have duty to disclose HIV status to patients. *ABA Journal: The Lawyer's Magazine.* 1998 Aug; 84: 38–40. BE59786.
*confidentiality; *disclosure; *HIV seropositivity; *iatrogenic disease; informed consent; *legal aspects; legal obligations; patients; *physicians; standards; *Doe v. Noe; *Illinois

Bayer, Ronald. Clinical progress and the future of HIV exceptionalism. *Archives of Internal Medicine.* 1999 May 24; 159(10): 1042–1048. 45 refs. BE61390.
*AIDS; *AIDS serodiagnosis; anonymous testing; attitudes; communicable diseases; confidentiality; drugs; federal government; government financing; government regulation; health care delivery; *HIV seropositivity; informed consent; *mandatory reporting; *mandatory testing; mass screening; *newborns; patient care; physicians; political activity; *pregnant women; public health; *public policy; state government; trends; voluntary programs; New York; *United States

In the 18 years since the first cases of the acquired immunodeficiency syndrome (AIDS) were reported by the Centers for Disease Control and Prevention (CDC), the epidemic has undergone profound transformations, and so, too, has the sociomedical context within which public health policy is fashioned and implemented. The early years of neglect and panic were also characterized by relative therapeutic impotence and deep uncertainty about the epidemiological course the new threat would take. In the United States and in other economically advanced nations, the threat of contracting the human immunodeficiency virus (HIV) has abated. The incidence of infection has declined, and the prevalence of infection has stabilized and, in some instances, begun to fall. The pattern of HIV spread, where it has continued, has been dramatically circumscribed to marginalized populations. The panic of the mid-1980s has passed, and in many nations, AIDS has lost its salience as a public issue. A sense of therapeutic impotence no longer prevails, and a new mood of triumphalism has taken hold. How have these crucial changes affected AIDS policies in America?

Bayer, Ronald. Responsibility and intimacy in the AIDS epidemic. *Responsive Community.* 1997 Fall; 7(4): 45–55. BE59719.
altruism; *disclosure; *duty to warn; *HIV seropositivity; homosexuals; *moral obligations; *patients; political activity; sexuality; trust; condoms; *partner notification; *sexual partners

Bennett, Rebecca; Erin, Charles A., eds. HIV and AIDS: Testing, Screening, and Confidentiality. New York, NY: Oxford University Press; 1999. 285 p. (Issues in biomedical ethics). Bibliography: p. 271–279. The impetus for this volume was provided by the research project "AIDS: Ethics, Justice and European Policy," supported by the Directorate General XII of the European Commission under its Biomedicine and Health Research Program (BIOMED 1). The coordinating group for this project, which ran for 3 years from Jan 1993, was centered within the Centre for Social Ethics and Policy at the University of Manchester, U.K. ISBN 0-19-823801-0. BE62712.
*AIDS; *AIDS serodiagnosis; blood donation; *confidentiality; counseling; disclosure; duty to warn; epidemiology; health care; health personnel; *HIV seropositivity; informed consent; insurance; legal aspects; legal liability; moral obligations; obligations of society; pregnant women; public health; public policy; resource allocation; risks and benefits; social discrimination; voluntary programs; right not to know; *Europe; *European Community; United States

Bosch, Xavier. Confidential Spanish registry of HIV-infected individuals. [News]. *JAMA.* 1999 Mar 17; 281(11): 977. BE60977.
AIDS; *confidentiality; *HIV seropositivity; mandatory reporting; *public policy; *registries; *Spain

Brazier, Margaret; Lobjoit, Mary. Fiduciary relationship: an ethical approach and a legal concept? *In:* Bennett, Rebecca; Erin, Charles A., eds. HIV and AIDS: Testing, Screening, and Confidentiality. New York, NY: Oxford University Press; 1999: 179–199. 63 fn. ISBN 0-19-823801-0. BE62722.
AIDS; *AIDS serodiagnosis; autonomy; blood specimen collection; *confidentiality; disclosure; duty to warn; *HIV seropositivity; iatrogenic disease; informed consent; *legal aspects; occupational exposure; paternalism; *patients; physician patient relationship; *physicians; standards; trust; Canada; *Great Britain

---

BE = bioethics accession number   fn. = footnotes   refs. = references

Colfax, Grant Nash; Bindman, Andrew B. Health benefits and risks of reporting HIV–infected individuals by name. [Comment]. *American Journal of Public Health.* 1998 Jun; 88(6): 876–879. 38 refs. BE60781.
AIDS; anonymous testing; attitudes; *confidentiality; epidemiology; *HIV seropositivity; homosexuals; *mandatory reporting; methods; *public policy; *risks and benefits; social impact; state government; voluntary programs; partner notification; United States
With more treatment options emerging for human immunodeficiency virus (HIV) infection, the policy of reporting HIV–infected individuals by name merits reevaluation. This paper reviews the benefits and risks of name reporting of persons infected with HIV. Public health departments have linked name reporting with medical referrals, risk reduction counseling, and partner notification programs. Yet some studies indicate that people are less likely to be tested for HIV infection when name reporting is implemented. Whether name reporting actually improves individual or public health, therefore justifying the increased risk of loss of confidentiality and possibly reduced testing rates, remains unknown. The lack of health outcome data on name reporting allows beliefs rather than facts to dominate debate about this policy. Before this practice is more widely adopted, a determination should be made as to whether the potential benefits of name reporting outweigh the risks.

Etzioni, Amitai. HIV testing of infants: privacy and public health. *Health Affairs.* 1998 Jul–Aug; 17(4): 170–183. 50 fn. BE61478.
*AIDS serodiagnosis; alternatives; anonymous testing; autonomy; *confidentiality; *disclosure; drugs; *HIV seropositivity; informed consent; legal aspects; mandatory testing; *mothers; *newborns; patient care; *pregnant women; privacy; *public policy; risks and benefits; social discrimination; state government; suffering; values; voluntary programs; AZT; *New York

Etzioni, Amitai. HIV testing of infants: should public health override privacy? *In: his* The Limits of Privacy. New York, NY: Basic Books; 1999: 17–42, 220–226. 88 fn. ISBN 0–465–04089–6. BE62442.
*AIDS serodiagnosis; anonymous testing; autonomy; communitarianism; confidentiality; costs and benefits; counseling; disadvantaged; *disclosure; *HIV seropositivity; informed consent; *mandatory testing; mothers; *newborns; patient care; policy analysis; pregnant women; *privacy; public health; *public policy; risks and benefits; social discrimination; *voluntary programs; New York; United States

Farsides, Calliope C.S. HIV infection and the health care worker: the case for limited disclosure. *In:* Bennett, Rebecca; Erin, Charles A., eds. HIV and AIDS: Testing, Screening, and Confidentiality. New York, NY: Oxford University Press; 1999: 166–178. 8 fn. ISBN 0–19–823801–0. BE62721.
AIDS; autonomy; beneficence; *confidentiality; *disclosure; employment; *health personnel; *HIV seropositivity; *iatrogenic disease; informed consent; interprofessional relations; moral obligations; patients; self regulation; Great Britain

Gostin, Lawrence O.; Webber, David W. The AIDS Litigation Project: HIV/AIDS in the courts in the 1990s, part 2. *AIDS and Public Policy Journal.* 1998 Spring; 13(1): 3–19. 28 fn. Provides an AIDS Litigation Project compilation of cases categorized under privacy and confidentiality; the "right to know;" discrimination; insurance; the rights of vulnerable persons: disability, homelessness and indigence; the rights of vulnerable persons: prisoners; and immigration and international travel. BE61342.
*AIDS; AIDS serodiagnosis; blood transfusions; community services; *confidentiality; *disclosure; *duty to warn; employment; health care; health personnel; *HIV seropositivity; iatrogenic disease; indigents; insurance; *legal aspects; legal liability; legal rights; mandatory testing; mass media; military personnel; patients; prisoners; *privacy; quarantine; refusal to treat; *social discrimination; *vulnerable populations; emigration and immigration; homeless persons; sexual partners; Americans with Disabilities Act 1990; *United States

Greene, Kathryn; Serovich, Julianne M. Appropriateness of disclosure of HIV testing information: the perspective of the PLWAs [people living with HIV/AIDS]. *Journal of Applied Communication Research.* 1996 Feb; 24(1): 50–65. 50 refs. 2 fn. BE60215.
*AIDS; AIDS serodiagnosis; *attitudes; *confidentiality; contact tracing; *disclosure; employment; family members; *HIV seropositivity; *patients; privacy; survey; partner notification; sexual partners; Southwestern United States

Häyry, Heta. Who should know about my HIV positivity and why? *In:* Bennett, Rebecca; Erin, Charles A., eds. HIV and AIDS: Testing, Screening, and Confidentiality. New York, NY: Oxford University Press; 1999: 240–250. 8 fn. ISBN 0–19–823801–0. BE62726.
*AIDS serodiagnosis; *confidentiality; deontological ethics; *disclosure; duty to warn; economics; *HIV seropositivity; *moral obligations; patients; privacy; public health; truth disclosure; utilitarianism; virtues; right not to know

Hayter, Mark. Confidentiality and the acquired immune deficiency syndrome (AIDS): an analysis of the legal and professional issues. *Journal of Advanced Nursing.* 1997 Jun; 25(6): 1162–1166. 33 refs. BE60540.
*AIDS; codes of ethics; *confidentiality; contact tracing; disclosure; duty to warn; health personnel; *HIV seropositivity; *legal aspects; professional ethics; partner notification; *Great Britain

Hilhorst, Medard T. Can health care workers care for their patients and be advocates of third–party interests? *In:* Bennett, Rebecca; Erin, Charles A., eds. HIV and AIDS: Testing, Screening, and Confidentiality. New York, NY: Oxford University Press; 1999: 149–165. 18 fn. ISBN 0–19–823801–0. BE62720.
AIDS serodiagnosis; *confidentiality; counseling; disclosure; *duty to warn; *health personnel; *HIV seropositivity; informed consent; *moral obligations; obligations to society; patients; physician's role; Netherlands

Kumar, Sanjay. Medical confidentiality broken to stop marriage of man infected with HIV. [News]. *Lancet.* 1998 Nov 28; 352(9142): 1764. BE60801.
blood donation; *confidentiality; *disclosure; *HIV seropositivity; *hospitals; *legal aspects; *marital relationship; *Dr. Tokugha vs. Apollo Hospital Enterprises; *India; Yepthomi, Tokugha

Mudur, Ganapati. Indian Supreme Court rules that HIV positive people inform spouses. [News]. *BMJ (British Medical Journal).* 1998 Nov 28; 317(7171): 1474. BE60953.
*AIDS; criminal law; *disclosure; *duty to warn; *HIV seropositivity; *legal aspects; *married persons; patients; *spousal notification; *India

Nakashima, Allyn K.; Horsley, Rosemarie; Frey, Robert L., et al. Effect of HIV reporting by name on use of HIV testing in publicly funded counseling and testing programs. *JAMA.* 1998 Oct 28; 280(16):

BE = bioethics accession number   fn. = footnotes   refs. = references

1421–1426. 32 refs. BE60293.
*AIDS serodiagnosis; *confidentiality; counseling; drug abuse; evaluation studies; government financing; health facilities; *HIV seropositivity; homosexuals; *mandatory reporting; public policy; *social impact; state government; statistics; retrospective studies; Louisiana; Michigan; Nebraska; Nevada; New Jersey; Tennessee
CONTEXT: Policies requiring confidential reporting by name to state health departments of persons infected with the human immunodeficiency virus (HIV) have potential to cause some of them to avoid HIV testing. OBJECTIVE: To describe trends in use of HIV testing services at publicly funded HIV counseling and testing sites before and after the implementation of HIV reporting policies. DESIGN AND SETTING: Analysis of service provision data from 6 state health departments (Louisiana, Michigan, Nebraska, Nevada, New Jersey, and Tennessee) 12 months before and 12 months after HIV reporting was introduced. MAIN OUTCOME MEASURE: Percent change in numbers of persons tested at publicly funded HIV counseling and testing sites after implementation of confidential HIV reporting by risk group. RESULTS: No significant declines in the total number of HIV tests provided at counseling and testing sites in the months immediately after implementation of HIV reporting occurred in any state, other than those expected from trends present before HIV reporting. Increases occurred in Nebraska (15.8%), Nevada (48.4%), New Jersey (21.3%), and Tennessee (62.8%). Predicted decreases occurred in Louisiana (10.5%) and Michigan (2.0%). In all areas, testing of at-risk heterosexuals increased in the year after HIV reporting was implemented (Louisiana, 10.5%; Michigan, 225.1%; Nebraska, 5.7%; Nevada, 303.3%; New Jersey, 462.9%; Tennessee, 603.8%). Declines in testing occurred among men who have sex with men in Louisiana (4.3%) and Tennessee (4.1%) after HIV reporting; testing increased for this group in Michigan (5.3%), Nebraska (19.6%), Nevada (12.5%), and New Jersey (22.4%). Among injection drug users, testing declined in Louisiana (15%), Michigan (34.3%), and New Jersey (0.6%) and increased in Nebraska (1.7%), Nevada (18.9%), and Tennessee (16.6%). CONCLUSIONS: Confidential HIV reporting by name did not appear to affect use of HIV testing in publicly funded counseling and testing programs.

Rand, Justin. AIDS and HIV: Colorado court upholds privacy rights in disclosure of test results. *Journal of Law, Medicine and Ethics.* 1998 Winter; 26(4): 353–355. 12 fn. BE61168.
*AIDS serodiagnosis; *blood specimen collection; confidentiality; criminal law; deception; *disclosure; government regulation; *HIV seropositivity; informed consent; *laboratories; *legal aspects; *legal liability; *privacy; *schools; state government; students; torts; *Cambridge College (Cambridge, MA); *Colorado; *Doe v. High-Tech Institute, Inc.

Richardson, Lynda. AIDS groups stunned by vote for partner notification. [News]. *New York Times.* 1998 Jun 20: B2. BE59366.
AIDS serodiagnosis; anonymous testing; confidentiality; *contact tracing; disclosure; *government regulation; *HIV seropositivity; *mandatory reporting; politics; registries; state government; voluntary programs; *partner notification; sexual partners; *New York

Richardson, Lynda. New Jersey's H.I.V. list: valuable, and still secret. [News]. *New York Times.* 1998 May 29: A1, B8. BE59367.
AIDS serodiagnosis; confidentiality; government regulation;

*HIV seropositivity; *mandatory reporting; *public policy; *registries; state government; *New Jersey

Roach, William H.; Aspen Health Law and Compliance Center. HIV/AIDS: mandatory reporting and confidentiality. *In: their* Medical Records and the Law. Third Edition. Gaithersburg, MD: Aspen Publishers; 1998: 213–239. 119 fn. ISBN 0-8342-1104-1. BE62749.
*AIDS; AIDS serodiagnosis; blood donation; *confidentiality; *disclosure; emergency care; government regulation; guidelines; health personnel; *HIV seropositivity; informed consent; judicial action; *legal aspects; legal liability; *mandatory reporting; medical records; spousal notification; state government; partner notification; sexual partners; *United States

Seidel, Gill. Confidentiality and HIV status in Kwazulu–Natal, South Africa: implications, resistances and challenges. *Health Policy and Planning.* 1996 Dec; 11(4): 418–427. 38 refs. BE60537.
AIDS serodiagnosis; *confidentiality; *counseling; developing countries; disadvantaged; disclosure; females; health personnel; *HIV seropositivity; males; politics; public policy; socioeconomic factors; stigmatization; sexual partners; *South Africa

Stenger, Christine E. Taking Tarasoff where no one has gone before: looking at "duty to warn" under the AIDS crisis. [Comment]. *Saint Louis University Public Law Review.* 1996; 15(2): 471–504. 235 fn. BE59921.
AIDS; blood transfusions; communicable diseases; *confidentiality; contact tracing; disclosure; *duty to warn; government regulation; *HIV seropositivity; hospitals; judicial action; *legal aspects; *legal liability; mandatory reporting; physician patient relationship; *physicians; state government; California; Reisner v. Regents of the University of California; *Tarasoff v. Regents; *United States

Vedder, Anton. HIV/AIDS and the point and scope of medical confidentiality. *In:* Bennett, Rebecca; Erin, Charles A., eds. HIV and AIDS: Testing, Screening, and Confidentiality. New York, NY: Oxford University Press; 1999: 140–148. 11 fn. ISBN 0-19-823801-0. BE62719.
*autonomy; *confidentiality; contact tracing; counseling; *disclosure; duty to warn; health personnel; *HIV seropositivity; moral obligations; patients

Partner notification for H.I.V. [Editorial]. *New York Times.* 1998 Jun 9: A20. BE59365.
AIDS serodiagnosis; confidentiality; *contact tracing; disclosure; government regulation; *HIV seropositivity; legislation; mandatory reporting; *public policy; state government; voluntary programs; *partner notification; sexual partners; *New York

AIDS/HEALTH PERSONNEL

Anderson, Donna G.; Vojir, Carol; Johnson, MeriLou. Three medical schools' responses to the HIV/AIDS epidemic and the effect on students' knowledge and attitudes. *Academic Medicine.* 1997 Feb; 72(2): 144–146. 9 refs. BE61431.
*AIDS; comparative studies; curriculum; geographic factors; *HIV seropositivity; *knowledge, attitudes, practice; *medical education; *medical schools; occupational exposure; patient care; prevalence; refusal to treat; *students; survey; Colorado; New Mexico; South Dakota; *University of Colorado School of Medicine; *University of New Mexico School of Medicine; *University of South Dakota School of Medicine

Annas, George J. Protecting patients from discrimination

BE = bioethics accession number   fn. = footnotes   refs. = references

-- the Americans with Disabilities Act and HIV infection. *New England Journal of Medicine.* 1998 Oct 22; 339(17): 1255-1259. 15 refs. BE60038.

AIDS; *dentistry; *disabled; dissent; federal government; genetic predisposition; guidelines; *health personnel; *HIV seropositivity; iatrogenic disease; *legal aspects; *legal obligations; legal rights; legislation; *occupational exposure; *patient care; professional organizations; *refusal to treat; reproduction; reproductive technologies; *risk; *social discrimination; standards; *Supreme Court decisions; universal precautions; American Dental Association; *Americans with Disabilities Act 1990; *Bragdon v. Abbott; Centers for Disease Control and Prevention; Rehabilitation Act 1973; School Board of Nassau County v. Arline; *United States

Baker, Debra. Positively truthful: appeal asks whether doctors have duty to disclose HIV status to patients. *ABA Journal: The Lawyer's Magazine.* 1998 Aug; 84: 38-40. BE59786.

*confidentiality; *disclosure; *HIV seropositivity; *iatrogenic disease; informed consent; *legal aspects; legal obligations; patients; *physicians; standards; *Doe v. Noe; *Illinois

Bosch, Xavier. Commission set up to deal with HIV infected doctors in Spain. [News]. *BMJ (British Medical Journal).* 1998 Oct 10; 317(7164): 970. BE60928.

AIDS; committee membership; counseling; *hepatitis; *HIV seropositivity; iatrogenic disease; patient care; patients; *physicians; professional organizations; risk; *self regulation; Catalonia; Official College of Physicians of Barcelona; *Spain

Brazier, Margaret; Lobjoit, Mary. Fiduciary relationship: an ethical approach and a legal concept? *In:* Bennett, Rebecca; Erin, Charles A., eds. HIV and AIDS: Testing, Screening, and Confidentiality. New York, NY: Oxford University Press; 1999: 179-199. 63 fn. ISBN 0-19-823801-0. BE62722.

AIDS; *AIDS serodiagnosis; autonomy; blood specimen collection; *confidentiality; disclosure; duty to warn; *HIV seropositivity; iatrogenic disease; informed consent; *legal aspects; occupational exposure; paternalism; *patients; physician patient relationship; *physicians; standards; trust; Canada; *Great Britain

Chavey, William E.; Cantor, Scott B.; Clover, Richard D., et al. Cost-effectiveness analysis of screening health care workers for HIV. *Journal of Family Practice.* 1994 Mar; 38(3): 249-257. 33 refs. BE59350.

*AIDS serodiagnosis; *costs and benefits; evaluation; *health personnel; *HIV seropositivity; hospitals; iatrogenic disease; risk

Chiodo, Gary T.; Tolle, Susan W. The ethical foundations of a duty to treat HIV-positive patients. *General Dentistry.* 1997 Jan-Feb; 45(1): 14, 16, 18, 20, 22. 35 refs. BE59426.

autonomy; codes of ethics; *dentistry; *health personnel; *HIV seropositivity; *legal aspects; legislation; *occupational exposure; *patient care; privacy; *professional ethics; professional organizations; *refusal to treat; risk; social discrimination; *infection control; universal precautions; *American Dental Association; *Americans with Disabilities Act 1990; United States

Farsides, Calliope C.S. HIV infection and the health care worker: the case for limited disclosure. *In:* Bennett, Rebecca; Erin, Charles A., eds. HIV and AIDS: Testing, Screening, and Confidentiality. New York, NY: Oxford University Press; 1999: 166-178. 8 fn. ISBN 0-19-823801-0. BE62721.

AIDS; autonomy; beneficence; *confidentiality; *disclosure; employment; *health personnel; *HIV seropositivity; *iatrogenic disease; informed consent; interprofessional relations; moral obligations; patients; self regulation; Great Britain

Federman, Daniel D. Protecting the future of medicine -- from themselves. [Editorial]. *Annals of Internal Medicine.* 1999 Jan 5; 130(1): 66-67. 6 refs. BE59332.

AIDS; *communicable diseases; curriculum; faculty; *hepatitis; *HIV seropositivity; *medical education; moral obligations; *occupational exposure; patient care; preventive medicine; risk; *students; *infection control; University of California, San Francisco

Fusilier, Marcelline; Manning, Michael R.; Villar, Armando J. Santini, et al. AIDS knowledge and attitudes of health-care workers in Mexico. *Journal of Social Psychology.* 1998 Apr; 138(2): 203-210. 21 refs. BE62680.

*AIDS; drug abuse; *health personnel; homosexuals; *knowledge, attitudes, practice; occupational exposure; patient care; refusal to treat; survey; *Mexico

Fusilier, Marcelline R.; Durlabhji, Subhash. Health care workers' AIDS attitudes and willingness to provide care -- India. *Journal of Health and Human Services Administration.* 1997 Fall; 20(2): 145-158. 20 refs. BE62651.

*AIDS; drug abuse; *health personnel; homosexuals; *knowledge, attitudes, practice; occupational exposure; patient care; *refusal to treat; survey; *India

Gerberding, Julie. Provider-to-patient HIV transmission: how to keep it exceedingly rare. [Editorial]. *Annals of Internal Medicine.* 1999 Jan 5; 130(1): 64-65. 19 refs. BE59331.

*HIV seropositivity; *iatrogenic disease; *occupational exposure; patients; *physicians; risk; *surgery; *infection control; France

Graham, Peter E.; Miller, Norman M.; Harel-Raviv, Mili. The law and ethics in relation to dentists treating HIV-positive patients: two recent court cases. *Journal of the Canadian Dental Association.* 1995 Jun; 61(6): 487-491. 6 refs. BE62118.

compensation; *dentistry; *disabled; *health personnel; *HIV seropositivity; *legal aspects; legal liability; legal rights; occupational exposure; referral and consultation; *refusal to treat; *social discrimination; *Canada; *Hamel v. Malaxos; *Jerome v. DeMarco; Ontario; Quebec; Quebec Charter of Rights and Freedoms

Hilhorst, Medard T. Can health care workers care for their patients and be advocates of third-party interests? *In:* Bennett, Rebecca; Erin, Charles A., eds. HIV and AIDS: Testing, Screening, and Confidentiality. New York, NY: Oxford University Press; 1999: 149-165. 18 fn. ISBN 0-19-823801-0. BE62720.

AIDS serodiagnosis; *confidentiality; counseling; disclosure; *duty to warn; *health personnel; *HIV seropositivity; informed consent; *moral obligations; obligations to society; patients; physician's role; Netherlands

Kondro, Wayne. Voluntary blood tests for Canadian doctors? [News]. *Lancet.* 1998 Oct 10; 352(9135): 1205. BE60260.

*AIDS serodiagnosis; *hepatitis; HIV seropositivity; mandatory testing; *organizational policies; *physicians; professional organizations; *voluntary programs; Ontario; *Ontario College of Physicians and Surgeons

Lot, Florence; Séguier, Jean-Christophe; Fégueux, Sophie, et al. Probable transmission of HIV from an

---

BE = bioethics accession number   fn. = footnotes   refs. = references

orthopedic surgeon to a patient in France. *Annals of Internal Medicine.* 1999 Jan 5; 130(1): 1–6. 19 refs. BE59330.

AIDS serodiagnosis; case studies; epidemiology; *HIV seropositivity; *iatrogenic disease; mandatory testing; occupational exposure; patients; *physicians; *surgery; infection control; *orthopedics; *France

BACKGROUND: Transmission of HIV from infected health care workers to patients has been documented in only one cluster involving 6 patients of a dentist in Florida. In October 1995, the French Ministry of Health offered HIV testing to patients who had been operated on by an orthopedic surgeon in whom AIDS was recently diagnosed. OBJECTIVE: To determine whether the surgeon transmitted HIV to patients during operations. DESIGN: Epidemiologic investigation. SETTING: The practice of an orthopedic surgeon in a French public hospital. PARTICIPANTS: 1 surgeon and 983 of his former patients. MEASUREMENTS: 3004 patients who had undergone invasive procedures were contacted by mail for counseling and HIV testing. One HIV-positive patient was interviewed, and DNA sequence analysis was performed to compare the genetic relation of the patient's and the surgeon's viruses. Infection-control precautions and the surgeon's practices were assessed. RESULTS: Of 983 patients in whom serologic status was ascertained, 982 were HIV negative and 1 was HIV positive. The HIV-positive patient, a woman born in 1925, tested negative for HIV before placement of a total hip prosthesis with bone graft (a prolonged operation) performed by the surgeon in 1992. She had no identified risk for HIV exposure. Molecular analysis indicated that the viral sequences obtained from the surgeon and the HIV-infected woman were closely related. Infection-control precautions were in accordance with recommendations, but blood contact between the surgeon and his patients occurred commonly during surgical procedures. CONCLUSIONS: An HIV-infected surgeon may have transmitted HIV to one of his patients during surgery.

McCarthy, Gillian M.; Koval, John J.; MacDonald, John K. Factors associated with refusal to treat HIV-infected patients: the results of a national survey of dentists in Canada. *American Journal of Public Health.* 1999 Apr; 89(4): 541–545. 34 refs. BE61387.

age factors; *attitudes; blood transfusions; *dentistry; drug abuse; education; *health personnel; hepatitis; *HIV seropositivity; homosexuals; moral obligations; motivation; occupational exposure; patients; *refusal to treat; sexually transmitted diseases; survey; *Canada

OBJECTIVES: This study investigated dentists refusal to treat patients who have HIV. METHODS: A survey was mailed to a random sample of all licensed dentists in Canada, with 3 follow-up attempts (n = 6444). Data were weighted to allow for probability of selection and nonresponse and analyzed with Pearson's chi 2 and multiple logistic regression. RESULTS: The response rate was 66%. Of the respondents, 32% had knowingly treated HIV-infected patients in the last year; 16% would refuse to treat HIV-infected patients. Respondents reported willingness to treat HIV-infected patients (81%), injection drug users (86%), hepatitis B virus-infected patients (87%), homosexual and bisexual persons (94%), individuals with sexually transmitted disease(s) (94%), and recipients of blood and blood products (97%). The best predictors of refusal to treat patients with HIV were lack of ethical responsibility (odds ratio = 9.0) and items related to fear of cross-infection or lack of knowledge of HIV. CONCLUSIONS: One in 6 dentists reported refusal to

treat HIV-infected patients, which was associated primarily with respondents' lack of belief in an ethical responsibility to treat patients with HIV and fears related to cross-infection. These results have implications for undergraduate, postgraduate, and continuing education.

Ogden, Russel. AIDS, euthanasia and nursing. *Nursing Standard.* 1996 May 29; 10(36): 49–51. 12 refs. BE60401.

*AIDS; *assisted suicide; attitudes; conscience; drugs; friends; *nurse's role; nursing ethics; physicians; suicide; terminally ill; *voluntary euthanasia; British Columbia

Puplick, Chris. Washington's teeth: patients' rights and dentists' rights -- where are we heading? *Annals of the Royal Australasian College of Dental Surgeons.* 1996 Apr; 13: 221–236. Presented at the 13th Convocation, Royal Australasian College of Dental Surgeons, Sydney, Apr 1996. BE60576.

attitudes; communicable diseases; *dentistry; disabled; government regulation; *health personnel; *HIV seropositivity; homosexuals; *legal aspects; minority groups; *refusal to treat; selection for treatment; *social discrimination; infection control; *Australia; Australian Dental Association; New South Wales Anti-Discrimination Act 1977; United States

Rosner, Fred. The imperative to heal in traditional Judaism. *Mount Sinai Journal of Medicine.* 1997 Nov; 64(6): 413–416. 19 refs. BE59342.

*AIDS; *communicable diseases; *Jewish ethics; moral obligations; occupational exposure; *patient care; patients; physician's role; *physicians; *refusal to treat; risk; value of life

Slovenko, Ralph. Informed consent: information about the physician. *Medicine and Law.* 1994; 13(5–6): 467–472. 28 fn. BE60006.

*AIDS; alcohol abuse; deception; *disclosure; iatrogenic disease; *informed consent; *internship and residency; *legal liability; malpractice; *physicians; *professional competence; psychotherapy; quality of health care; values; *physician impairment; teaching hospitals; Estate of Behringer v. Medical Center at Princeton; National Practitioner Data Bank; New Jersey; United States

Tessman, Irwin; Neiburger, Ellis J.; Greely, Henry T., et al. Bragdon v. Abbott: the Americans with Disabilities Act and HIV infection. [Letters and response]. *New England Journal of Medicine.* 1999 Apr 15; 340(15): 1212–1214. 8 refs. BE62568.

*dentistry; *disabled; genetic predisposition; *health personnel; *HIV seropositivity; *legal aspects; *occupational exposure; *patient care; *refusal to treat; risk; *social discrimination; *Supreme Court decisions; Americans with Disabilities Act 1990; *Bragdon v. Abbott

Duty to warn; negligence; AIDS/HIV; surgeon: Doe v. Noe. *Mental and Physical Disability Law Reporter.* 1998 Mar–Apr; 22(2): 250. BE61467.

*disclosure; *duty to warn; *HIV seropositivity; iatrogenic disease; informed consent; *legal aspects; *legal liability; *physicians; psychological stress; surgery; *Doe v. Noe; Faya v. Almarez; *Illinois

AIDS/HUMAN EXPERIMENTATION

Achrekar, Abinash; Gupta, Rajesh; Pichayangkura, Chart, et al. Informed consent for a clinical trial in Thailand. [Letter and responses]. *New England Journal of Medicine.* 1998 Oct 29; 339(18): 1331–1332. 3 refs. BE60149.

AIDS; audiovisual aids; *communication; *comprehension; *consent forms; control groups; *developing countries;

BE = bioethics accession number   fn. = footnotes   refs. = references

disclosure; drugs; ethical review; *HIV seropositivity; *human experimentation; *informed consent; *newborns; *placebos; *pregnant women; preventive medicine; random selection; *research design; research subjects; terminology; therapeutic research; AZT; Ministry of Public Health (Thailand); *Thailand

Altman, Lawrence K. Ethics panel urges easing of curbs on AIDS vaccine tests. [News]. *New York Times.* 1998 Jun 28: 6. BE59361.
advisory committees; AIDS; *developing countries; drugs; ethical relativism; guidelines; *HIV seropositivity; *human experimentation; *immunization; informed consent; *international aspects; placebos; research subjects; United States

Altman, Lawrence K. F.D.A. authorizes first full testing for H.I.V. vaccine. [News]. *New York Times.* 1998 Jun 4: A1, A23. BE59362.
developing countries; drug abuse; drug industry; federal government; *government regulation; *HIV seropositivity; homosexuals; *human experimentation; *immunization; international aspects; placebos; research design; risks and benefits; volunteers; *Food and Drug Administration; Thailand; *United States; Vaxgen Inc.

Annas, George J.; Grodin, Michael A. Human rights and maternal–fetal HIV transmission prevention trials in Africa. *American Journal of Public Health.* 1998 Apr; 88(4): 560–563. 17 refs. BE60130.
AIDS; comprehension; *control groups; *developing countries; disadvantaged; drugs; economics; ethical relativism; health care delivery; *HIV seropositivity; *human experimentation; *human rights; informed consent; *international aspects; justice; *moral policy; *newborns; patient care; *placebos; *pregnant women; preventive medicine; public health; *public policy; *research design; research subjects; resource allocation; socioeconomic factors; therapeutic research; Africa; AZT; Centers for Disease Control and Prevention; National Institutes of Health; Thailand; United Nations; United States; Universal Declaration of Human Rights
The human rights issues raised by the conduct of maternal–fetal human immunodeficiency virus transmission trials in Africa are not unique to either acquired immunodeficiency syndrome or Africa, but public discussion of these trials presents an opportunity for the United States and other wealthy nations to take the rights and welfare of impoverished populations seriously. The central issue at stake when developed countries perform research on subjects in developing countries is exploitation. The only way to prevent exploitation of a research population is to insist not only that informed consent be obtained but also that, should an intervention be proven beneficial, the intervention will be delivered to the impoverished population. Human rights are universal and cannot be compromised solely on the basis of beliefs or practices of any one country or group. The challenge to the developed countries is to implement programs to improve the health of the people in developing countries both by improving public health infrastructure and by delivering effective drugs and vaccines to the people.

Bayer, Ronald. The debate over maternal–fetal HIV transmission prevention trials in Africa, Asia, and the Caribbean: racist exploitation or exploitation of racism? *American Journal of Public Health.* 1998 Apr; 88(4): 567–570. 9 refs. BE60132.
AIDS; *control groups; *developing countries; disadvantaged; drugs; ethical relativism; ethical review; financial support; guidelines; *HIV seropositivity; *human experimentation; international aspects; justice; *moral policy; *newborns; patient care; *placebos; *pregnant women;

prevalence; preventive medicine; random selection; *research design; research subjects; resource allocation; risks and benefits; *social discrimination; socioeconomic factors; standards; therapeutic research; vulnerable populations; Africa; Asia; AZT; Caribbean Region; Centers for Disease Control and Prevention; Council for International Organizations of Medical Sciences; Declaration of Helsinki; Denmark; France; National Institutes of Health; South Africa; United Nations; United States

Beloqui, Jorge; Chokevivat, Vichai; Collins, Chris. HIV vaccine research and human rights: examples from three countries planning efficacy trials. *Health and Human Rights.* 1998; 3(1): 38–58. 21 fn. BE62574.
compensation; *developing countries; drug industry; economics; ethical review; health care; *HIV seropositivity; *human rights; *immunization; injuries; *international aspects; justice; preventive medicine; public policy; research design; research subjects; risks and benefits; social discrimination; stigmatization; *therapeutic research; volunteers; Brazil; Thailand

Bernstein, Nina. For subjects in Haiti study, free AIDS care has a price: a special report. *New York Times.* 1999 Jun 6: A1, A10. BE62347.
*AIDS; AIDS serodiagnosis; attitudes; conflict of interest; consent forms; counseling; deception; *developing countries; drugs; financial support; government financing; *human experimentation; immunization; incentives; indigents; informed consent; *international aspects; investigators; patient care; physicians; research design; research subjects; *standards; universities; withholding treatment; sexual partners; Cornell University; *Haiti; United States

Cohen, Jon; Ivinson, Adrian J. Clarifying AIDS vaccine trial guidelines. [Letter and response]. *Nature Medicine.* 1998 Oct; 4(10): 1091. BE61527.
AIDS; consensus; developing countries; dissent; *guidelines; *HIV seropositivity; *human experimentation; *immunization; *international aspects; *patient care; research subjects; standards

Cohen, Jon. No consensus on rules for AIDS vaccine trials. [News]. *Science.* 1998 Jul 3; 281(5373): 22–23. BE59940.
advisory committees; *AIDS; *developing countries; drugs; ethical review; HIV seropositivity; *human experimentation; *immunization; international aspects; investigators; patient care; research design; research subjects; withholding treatment; research ethics; United Nations

Collins, Harry; Pinch, Trevor. ACTing UP: AIDS cures and lay expertise. *In: their* The Golem at Large: What You Should Know About Technology. New York, NY: Cambridge University Press; 1998: 126–150. ISBN 0-521-55141-2. BE61681.
*AIDS; biomedical research; decision making; *drugs; federal government; government regulation; HIV seropositivity; *homosexuals; *human experimentation; investigator subject relationship; patient care; *patient participation; physician patient relationship; placebos; *political activity; *public participation; *research design; research subjects; technical expertise; therapeutic research; *ACT UP; Food and Drug Administration; New York City; San Francisco; United States

Crigger, Bette–Jane. The battle over babies: international research in perinatal HIV transmission. *IRB: A Review of Human Subjects Research.* 1998 Jul–Aug; 20(4): 13–15. 8 refs. BE61099.
AIDS; *control groups; *developing countries; *drugs; ethical review; guidelines; health care delivery; *HIV seropositivity; *human experimentation; international aspects; moral policy; *newborns; *placebos; *pregnant women; preventive medicine; public policy; *research

---

BE = bioethics accession number   fn. = footnotes   refs. = references

Crouch, Robert A.; Arras, John D. AZT trials and tribulations. *Hastings Center Report.* 1998 Nov–Dec; 28(6): 26–34. 32 fn. BE61283.

control groups; *developing countries; *drugs; *economics; financial support; guidelines; health care; *HIV seropositivity; *human experimentation; indigents; *international aspects; investigators; justice; moral obligations; motivation; newborns; *placebos; *pregnant women; *preventive medicine; public policy; *research design; research subjects; resource allocation; rights; *therapeutic research; Africa; *AZT; Centers for Disease Control and Prevention; Thailand; United States

del Rio, Carlos. Is ethical research feasible in developed and developing countries? *Bioethics.* 1998 Oct; 12(4): 328–330. 5 refs. Commentary on D.B. Resnik, "The ethics of HIV research in developing nations," p. 286–306. BE62281.

advisory committees; AIDS; control groups; *developing countries; drugs; economics; guidelines; health care delivery; *HIV seropositivity; *human experimentation; informed consent; *international aspects; moral policy; newborns; non–Western World; placebos; pregnant women; preventive medicine; public participation; public policy; *research design; research subjects; therapeutic research; Western World; AZT; Council for International Organizations of Medical Sciences; World Health Organization

Des Jarlais, Don C.; Vanischseni, Suphak; Marmor, Michael, et al. HIV vaccine trials. [Letters and response]. *Science.* 1998 Mar 6; 279(5356): 1433–1436. 5 refs. BE59440.

contraception; control groups; *developing countries; economics; *ethical relativism; guidelines; *HIV seropositivity; *human experimentation; immunization; international aspects; medical devices; methods; placebos; pregnant women; preventive medicine; research design; standards; therapeutic research; Africa; United States

Desvarieux, Moïse; Turner, Marie T.; Whalen, Christopher C., et al. Questions about a placebo–controlled trial of preventive therapy for tuberculosis in HIV–infected Ugandans. [Letters and responses]. *New England Journal of Medicine.* 1998 Mar 19; 338(12): 841–843. 11 refs. BE59438.

communicable diseases; control groups; *developing countries; drugs; historical aspects; *HIV seropositivity; *human experimentation; informed consent; international aspects; *placebos; preventive medicine; *random selection; research design; research ethics committees; scientific misconduct; therapeutic research; *tuberculosis; withholding treatment; Case Western Reserve University; Haiti; Tuskegee Syphilis Study; *Uganda; United States

de Zoysa, Isabelle; Elias, Christopher J.; Bentley, Margaret E. Ethical challenges in efficacy trials of vaginal microbicides for HIV prevention. *American Journal of Public Health.* 1998 Apr; 88(4): 571–575. 48 refs. BE60133.

AIDS; AIDS serodiagnosis; community services; control groups; counseling; decision making; *developing countries; *disadvantaged; *drugs; ethical review; *females; guidelines; health education; health promotion; health services research; *HIV seropositivity; *human experimentation; investigators; justice; *moral policy; *preventive medicine; public participation; *research design; research subjects; resource allocation; *risks and benefits; sexuality; *sexually transmitted diseases; women's health services; *condoms;

prostitution

This paper discusses some of the ethical challenges raised by advanced clinical trials designed to assess the safety and efficacy of vaginal microbicides in protecting women from HIV infection. The ethical principles that guide clinical research involving human subjects require that all participants in such trials be provided available measures known to reduce the risk of HIV infection. However, this will reduce the ability of the study to assess the protective effect of the test microbicide. In addition, providing extensive services to trial participants may be construed as an undue inducement if the study is being conducted among vulnerable groups such as sex workers or women from disadvantaged communities. Suggestions are provided to resolve this dilemma in the planning and implementation of HIV prevention services for trial participants.

Edi–Osagie, E.C.O.; Edi–Osagie, N.E.; Lurie, Peter, et al. Ethics and international research. [Letters and response]. *BMJ (British Medical Journal).* 1998 Feb 21; 316(7131): 625–628. 13 refs. BE59378.

*control groups; *developing countries; drugs; guidelines; *HIV seropositivity; *human experimentation; informed consent; international aspects; newborns; *placebos; *pregnant women; random selection; *research design; risks and benefits; socioeconomic factors; *Africa; AZT; Thailand; United States

Faden, Ruth; Kass, Nancy. HIV research, ethics, and the developing world. [Editorial]. *American Journal of Public Health.* 1998 Apr; 88(4): 548–550. 9 refs. BE60127.

AIDS; coercion; common good; *control groups; *developing countries; disadvantaged; disclosure; drugs; ethical relativism; ethical review; health care delivery; *HIV seropositivity; *human experimentation; *informed consent; international aspects; *moral policy; *newborns; patient care; *placebos; *pregnant women; preventive medicine; public health; *public policy; random selection; *research design; research subjects; risks and benefits; therapeutic research; retrospective studies; Africa; AZT; United States

Fairchild, Amy L.; Bayer, Ronald. Uses and abuses of Tuskegee. *Science.* 1999 May 7; 284(5416): 919–921. 23 refs. BE61403.

AIDS serodiagnosis; anonymous testing; *blacks; deception; developing countries; disclosure; *drug abuse; drugs; historical aspects; *HIV seropositivity; *human experimentation; indigents; informed consent; mandatory testing; medical devices; newborns; physicians; placebos; pregnant women; *preventive medicine; public policy; *research design; scientific misconduct; *social discrimination; syphilis; *trust; *vulnerable populations; withholding treatment; *needle–exchange programs; AZT; *Tuskegee Syphilis Study; Twentieth Century; *United States

Grady, Christine. Science in the service of healing. *Hastings Center Report.* 1998 Nov–Dec; 28(6): 34–38. 19 fn. BE61284.

control groups; *developing countries; *drugs; economics; financial support; goals; guidelines; *HIV seropositivity; *human experimentation; *international aspects; newborns; *placebos; *pregnant women; *preventive medicine; *research design; research subjects; Africa; *AZT; Thailand; United States

Hellman, Deborah. Trial and error: can good science be bad medicine? *New Republic.* 1998 Apr 27; 218(17): 14, 16–17. BE61471.

*developing countries; drugs; federal government; government financing; *HIV seropositivity; *human experimentation; international aspects; newborns; *placebos; *pregnant women; *random selection; *research design;

BE = bioethics accession number   fn. = footnotes   refs. = references

therapeutic research; Africa; Asia; AZT; Centers for Disease Control and Prevention; National Institutes of Health; United States

Hellman, Deborah. Trials on trial. *Philosophy and Public Policy.* 1998 Winter-Spring; 18(1-2): 13-18. 5 refs. BE59814.
> conflict of interest; *control groups; *developing countries; *drugs; *HIV seropositivity; *human experimentation; international aspects; investigators; physicians; *placebos; *pregnant women; public health; *research design; resource allocation; standards; therapeutic research; uncertainty; *AZT; Centers for Disease Control and Prevention; National Institutes of Health; United States

Ivinson, Adrian J. Hard-won consensus on AIDS vaccine trial guidelines. [News]. *Nature Medicine.* 1998 Aug; 4(8): 874. BE59731.
> consensus; *developing countries; dissent; drugs; economics; *guidelines; *HIV seropositivity; *human experimentation; *immunization; *international aspects; *patient care; standards; *UNAIDS; World Health Organization

Karim, Quarraisha Abdool; Karim, Salim S. Abdool; Coovadia, Hoosen M., et al. Informed consent for HIV testing in a South African hospital: is it truly informed and truly voluntary? *American Journal of Public Health.* 1998 Apr; 88(4): 637-640. 15 refs. BE60134.
> *AIDS; *AIDS serodiagnosis; coercion; control groups; *counseling; disadvantaged; evaluation studies; *health services research; *HIV seropositivity; human experimentation; *informed consent; *knowledge, attitudes, practice; newborns; *pregnant women; preventive medicine; public hospitals; quality of health care; research design; research ethics committees; research subjects; survey; therapeutic research; voluntary programs; King Edward VIII Hospital (Durban); *South Africa

OBJECTIVE: The purpose of this study was to assess informed consent to human immunodeficiency virus (HIV) testing in a perinatal HIV transmission study in a major referral hospital serving a largely Black population in South Africa. METHODS: First-time antenatal clinic attenders who were randomly selected from those enrolled in the perinatal HIV study (n = 56) answered questionnaires before and after counseling. RESULTS: Knowledge of HIV transmission and prevention, high at the outset, was little improved after counseling. The acceptance rate for HIV testing was high. Despite assurances that participation was voluntary, 88% of the women said they felt compelled to participate in the study. CONCLUSIONS: Informed consent in this setting was truly informed but not truly voluntary.

Karim, Salim S. Abdool. Placebo controls in HIV perinatal transmission trials: a South African's viewpoint. *American Journal of Public Health.* 1998 Apr; 88(4): 564-566. 10 refs. BE60131.
> AIDS; alternatives; autonomy; *control groups; *drugs; economics; ethical review; government financing; health care; *HIV seropositivity; *human experimentation; informed consent; *newborns; nutrition; patient care; *placebos; *pregnant women; *prevalence; preventive medicine; *public policy; *research design; research subjects; resource allocation; sexually transmitted diseases; therapeutic research; breast feeding; AZT; *South Africa

Kylmä, Jari; Vehviläinen-Julkunen, Katri; Lähdevirta, Juhani. Ethical considerations in a grounded theory study on the dynamics of hope in HIV-positive adults and their significant others. *Nursing Ethics.* 1999 May; 6(3): 224-239. 68 refs. BE61767.
> adults; AIDS; *behavioral research; *emotions; family

members; *HIV seropositivity; informed consent; investigator subject relationship; investigators; nurses; *nursing research; patients; research design; research subjects; selection of subjects; stigmatization; vulnerable populations; *hope; *qualitative research; research ethics; sexual partners

Lemonick, Michael D. Good news at a price : a study finds that AIDS drugs can help poor kids -- but was it ethical? *Time.* 1999 Feb 15; 153(6): 64. BE60961.
> *developing countries; drugs; *HIV seropositivity; *human experimentation; placebos; *pregnant women; research design; *therapeutic research; treatment outcome; *Africa; South Africa; Tanzania; Uganda

Levine, Carol. Placebos and HIV: lessons learned. *Hastings Center Report.* 1998 Nov-Dec; 28(6): 43-48. 10 fn. BE61286.
> *developing countries; drug industry; *drugs; economics; ethical review; goals; guidelines; *HIV seropositivity; *human experimentation; informed consent; *international aspects; newborns; *placebos; *pregnant women; *research design; risks and benefits; standards; withholding treatment; Africa; *AZT; Thailand; United States

Lie, Reidar K. Ethics of placebo-controlled trials in developing countries. *Bioethics.* 1998 Oct; 12(4): 307-311. 4 fn. Commentary on D.B. Resnik, "The ethics of HIV research in developing nations," p. 286-306. BE62278.
> AIDS; *alternatives; control groups; *developing countries; drugs; economics; *HIV seropositivity; *human experimentation; international aspects; *newborns; *placebos; *pregnant women; preventive medicine; random selection; *research design; AZT; Thailand

Lurie, Peter; Wolfe, Sidney M. Ethics of HIV trials. [Letter]. *Lancet.* 1998 Jan 17; 351(9097): 220. 5 refs. BE59384.
> *developing countries; drugs; economics; ethical relativism; *HIV seropositivity; *human experimentation; international aspects; newborns; *placebos; *pregnant women; preventive medicine; random selection; research design; time factors; AZT; Centers for Disease Control and Prevention

Lynn, Lorna A. AIDS clinical trials: is there access for all? [Editorial]. *Journal of General Internal Medicine.* 1997 Mar; 12(3): 198-199. 16 refs. BE59235.
> *AIDS; communication; *disadvantaged; drug abuse; females; health personnel; *HIV seropositivity; *human experimentation; incentives; *minority groups; *research subjects; *selection of subjects; social discrimination; United States

McIntosh, Kenneth. Short (and shorter) courses of zidovudine. [Editorial]. *New England Journal of Medicine.* 1998 Nov 12; 339(20): 1467-1468. 10 refs. BE59344.
> childbirth; developing countries; *drugs; *HIV seropositivity; *human experimentation; international aspects; *newborns; placebos; *pregnant women; preventive medicine; *therapeutic research; time factors; treatment outcome; *AZT

Maine. Supreme Judicial Court. In re Nikolas E. *Atlantic Reporter, 2d Series.* 1998 Nov 19 (date of decision). 720: 562-568. BE62344.
> *children; *HIV seropositivity; *investigational drugs; *legal aspects; minors; *mothers; parents; patient care; *risks and benefits; state interest; *therapeutic research; *treatment refusal; *In re Nikolas E.; Maine

The Supreme Judicial Court of Maine upheld a lower court decision allowing a mother who had been charged with parental neglect to retain custody of her HIV-positive four-year-old son, whose recommended, but highly aggressive and experimental antiviral drug treatment, she had delayed. Both of the child's divorced parents are HIV positive, and his older sister died at age 4 from AIDS complications after receiving the drug therapy. The court found that there was insufficient proof of likely benefit and lack of significant harm from the drug regimen. Furthermore the court was unable to determine the likely effects of treatment on the child. Consequently the court decided that the mother's decision to delay new and experimental treatment was not serious parental neglect. (KIE abstract)

Mann, Jonathan M.; Zion, Deborah; Macpherson, Cheryl Cox, et al. The ethics of AIDS vaccine trials. [Letters and response]. *Science.* 1998 May 29; 280(5368): 1327, 1329-1331. 11 refs. BE59441.
  *AIDS; codes of ethics; comprehension; *developing countries; drugs; economics; guidelines; HIV seropositivity; *human experimentation; *immunization; informed consent; international aspects; placebos; pregnant women; research design; standards; therapeutic research; vulnerable populations; Africa; Declaration of Helsinki; International Ethical Guidelines for Biomedical Research Involving Human Subjects; United States

Merson, Michael H.; Simonds, R.J.; Rogers, Martha F., et al. Ethics of placebo-controlled trials of zidovudine to prevent the perinatal transmission of HIV in the Third World. [Letters and response; editor's note]. *New England Journal of Medicine.* 1998 Mar 19; 338(12): 836-841. 25 refs. BE59387.
  conflict of interest; control groups; *developing countries; *drugs; economics; *ethical relativism; federal government; *HIV seropositivity; *human experimentation; informed consent; international aspects; investigators; justice; newborns; *placebos; *pregnant women; preventive medicine; random selection; *research design; research ethics committees; risks and benefits; scientific misconduct; standards; therapeutic research; Africa; AZT; Centers for Disease Control and Prevention; Ivory Coast; Thailand; United States; World Health Organization

Morris, Lynn; Martin, Desmond J.; Quinn, Thomas C., et al. The importance of doing HIV research in developing countries. *Nature Medicine.* 1998 Nov; 4(11): 1228-1229. 20 refs. BE62159.
  *AIDS; *biomedical research; *costs and benefits; *developing countries; drugs; economics; *HIV seropositivity; *human experimentation; newborns; patient care; pregnant women; preventive medicine; *resource allocation; *risks and benefits; sexually transmitted diseases; *Africa; AZT

Mueller, Mary-Rose. Science versus care: physicians, nurses, and the dilemma of clinical research. *In:* Elston, Mary Ann, ed. The Sociology of Medical Science and Technology. Malden, MA: Blackwell; 1997: 57-78. 39 refs. 5 fn. ISBN 0-631-20447-4. BE59725.
  *AIDS; *attitudes; confidentiality; *human experimentation; investigator subject relationship; investigators; nurse patient relationship; *nurse's role; nurses; organization and administration; patient advocacy; patients; patients' rights; *physician nurse relationship; physician patient relationship; *physician's role; physicians; primary health care; research subjects; sociology of medicine; *therapeutic research; ethnographic studies

Resnik, David B. Replies to commentaries. *Bioethics.* 1998 Oct; 12(4): 331-333. Response to commentaries by R.K. Lie, p. 307-311; by U. Schüklenk, p. 312-319; by J. Thomas, p. 320-327; and by C. Del Rio, p. 328-330 on his article, "The ethics of HIV research in developing nations," p. 286-306. BE62282.

AIDS; *developing countries; drug industry; drugs; financial support; government financing; health care delivery; *HIV seropositivity; *human experimentation; international aspects; justice; moral policy; *newborns; *placebos; *pregnant women; preventive medicine; public policy; *research design; socioeconomic factors; therapeutic research; AZT

Resnik, David B. The ethics of HIV research in developing nations. *Bioethics.* 1998 Oct; 12(4): 286-306. 62 fn. Commented on by R.K. Lie, p. 307-311; by U. Schüklenk, p. 312-319; by J. Thomas, p. 320-327; and by C. Del Rio, p. 328-330. BE62277.
  AIDS; beneficence; codes of ethics; control groups; *developing countries; drugs; *ethical relativism; *HIV seropositivity; *human experimentation; informed consent; international aspects; justice; metaethics; *moral policy; *newborns; non-Western World; *placebos; *pregnant women; preventive medicine; random selection; *research design; research subjects; socioeconomic factors; *standards; therapeutic research; utilitarianism; Africa; AZT; Centers for Disease Control and Prevention; Declaration of Helsinki; Dominican Republic; National Institutes of Health; Thailand; UNAIDS; World Health Organization
This paper discusses a dispute concerning the ethics of research on preventing the perinatal transmission of HIV in developing nations. Critics of this research argue that it is unethical because it denies a proven treatment to placebo-control groups. Since studies conducted in developed nations would not deny this treatment to subjects, the critics maintain that these experiments manifest a double standard for ethical research and that a single standard of ethics should apply to all research on human subjects. Proponents of the research, however, argue that these charges fail to understand the ethical complexities of research in developing nations, and that study designs can vary according to the social, economic, and scientific conditions of research. This essay explores some of the ethical issues raised by this controversial case in order to shed some light on the deeper, meta-ethical questions. The paper argues that standards of ethical research on human subjects are universal but not absolute: there are some general ethical principles that apply to all cases of human subjects research but the application of these principles must take into account factors inherent in particular situations.

Saegusa, Asako. Are Japanese researchers exploiting Thai HIV patients? [News]. *Nature Medicine.* 1998 May; 4(5): 540. BE59726.
  government financing; *HIV seropositivity; *human experimentation; *immunization; *international aspects; investigators; methods; *Japan; Japan Science and Technology Corporation; *Thailand

Schüklenk, Udo. Access to Experimental Drugs in Terminal Illness: Ethical Issues. New York, NY: Pharmaceutical Products Press; 1998. 228 p. Bibliography: p. 205-217. ISBN 0-7890-0563-8. BE59923.
  *AIDS; alternative therapies; altruism; *autonomy; competence; drug abuse; government regulation; health insurance reimbursement; homosexuals; *human experimentation; informed consent; *investigational drugs; *moral policy; nontherapeutic research; obligations of society; *paternalism; patient compliance; placebos; political activity; research design; risks and benefits; selection of subjects; social discrimination; socioeconomic factors; *terminally ill; *therapeutic research; vulnerable populations; withholding treatment; AZT; Food and Drug Administration; National Institutes of Health; United States

Schüklenk, Udo. Unethical perinatal HIV transmission trials establish bad precedent. *Bioethics.* 1998 Oct; 12(4):

BE = bioethics accession number   fn. = footnotes   refs. = references

312–319. 21 fn. Commentary on D.B. Resnik, "The ethics of HIV research in developing nations," p. 286–306. BE62279.

AIDS; alternative therapies; control groups; costs and benefits; *developing countries; drug industry; drugs; economics; ethical analysis; ethical review; guidelines; health care delivery; *HIV seropositivity; *human experimentation; informed consent; international aspects; *moral policy; *newborns; non-Western World; *placebos; *pregnant women; preventive medicine; *research design; research subjects; therapeutic research; Western World; Africa; Asia; AZT; Council for International Organizations of Medical Sciences; Latin America; UNAIDS

Sidley, Pat. South African research into AIDS "cure" severely criticised. [News]. *BMJ (British Medical Journal).* 1997 Mar 15; 314(7083): 771. BE60726.

administrators; *AIDS; conflict of interest; *drugs; ethical review; government financing; *human experimentation; investigators; research design; *scientific misconduct; *South Africa; University of Pretoria; *Virodene; Visser, Olga; Zuma, Nkosazana

Specter, Michael. Uganda AIDS vaccine test: urgency affects ethics rules. [News]. *New York Times.* 1998 Oct 1: A1, A6. BE60574.

*AIDS; *developing countries; drugs; economics; HIV seropositivity; *human experimentation; *immunization; informed consent; international aspects; research design; research subjects; risks and benefits; *Uganda

Stolberg, Sheryl Gay. Placebo use is suspended in overseas AIDS trials. [News]. *New York Times.* 1998 Feb 19: A16. BE59368.

*AIDS; *developing countries; *drugs; economics; federal government; *HIV seropositivity; *human experimentation; *international aspects; *placebos; *pregnant women; *public policy; *research design; *therapeutic research; *AZT; Centers for Disease Control and Prevention; United States

Susser, Mervyn. The prevention of perinatal HIV transmission in the less–developed world. [Editorial]. *American Journal of Public Health.* 1998 Apr; 88(4): 547–548. 11 refs. BE60126.

AIDS; *control groups; *costs and benefits; *developing countries; disadvantaged; *drugs; *HIV seropositivity; *human experimentation; international aspects; *newborns; *placebos; politics; *pregnant women; preventive medicine; *public policy; *research design; *risks and benefits; therapeutic research; breast feeding; AZT; Centers for Disease Control and Prevention; *France; National Institutes of Health; Thailand; *United Nations; *United States

Thomas, Joe. Ethical challenges of HIV clinical trials in developing countries. *Bioethics.* 1998 Oct; 12(4): 320–327. 25 fn. Commentary on D.B. Resnik, "The ethics of HIV research in developing nations," p. 286–306. BE62280.

AIDS; alternative therapies; autonomy; beneficence; conflict of interest; control groups; *developing countries; drug industry; drugs; economics; ethical review; guidelines; *HIV seropositivity; *human experimentation; human rights; international aspects; investigators; justice; moral policy; *newborns; non-Western World; placebos; *pregnant women; preventive medicine; public policy; *research design; research subjects; standards; therapeutic research; AZT; Council for International Organizations of Medical Sciences; Declaration of Helsinki; National Institutes of Health; United States

U.S. Department of Health and Human Services. The Conduct of Clinical Trials of Maternal–Infant Transmission of HIV Supported by the United States Department of Health and Human Services in Developing Countries: A Summary of the Needs of Developing Countries, the Scientific Applications, and the Ethical Considerations Assessed by the National Institutes of Health and the Centers for Disease Control and Prevention, 1994–1997. Downloaded from Internet Web site: http://www.nih.gov/news/mathiv/mathiv.htm and http://www.nih.gov/news/mathiv/whodoc.htm (Appendix) on 6 Dec 1997; 1997 Jul. 10 p. 1 ref. Appendix: Recommendations from the Meeting on Prevention of Mother-to-Infant Transmission of HIV by Use of Antiretrovirals, Geneva, 23–25 June 1994. BE62688.

*developing countries; drugs; economics; health care; *HIV seropositivity; *human experimentation; *international aspects; *newborns; placebos; *pregnant women; *research design; standards; therapeutic research; withholding treatment; Africa; *AZT; Centers for Disease Control and Prevention; Department of Health and Human Services; National Institutes of Health; Thailand; *United States; World Health Organization

Wilfert, Catherine M.; Ammann, Arthur; Bayer, Ronald, et al. Science, ethics, and the future of research into maternal infant transmission of HIV–1: Consensus statement. [For the Perinatal HIV Intervention Research in Developing Countries Workshop Participants]. *Lancet.* 1999 Mar 6; 353(9155): 832–835. 23 refs. BE61221.

AIDS; alternatives; childbirth; consensus; *control groups; costs and benefits; *developing countries; *drugs; *economics; *guidelines; *HIV seropositivity; *human experimentation; informed consent; international aspects; *moral policy; *mothers; *newborns; nutrition; patient care; *pregnant women; *preventive medicine; public health; quality of health care; *research design; risks and benefits; *socioeconomic factors; standards; therapeutic research; *breast feeding; *Perinatal HIV Intervention Research in Developing Countries Workshop

Zion, Deborah. Ethical considerations of clinical trials to prevent vertical transmission of HIV in developing countries. *Nature Medicine.* 1998 Jan; 4(1): 11–12. 5 refs. BE59981.

autonomy; coercion; competence; *developing countries; drugs; freedom; *HIV seropositivity; *human experimentation; informed consent; placebos; *pregnant women; *research design; research subjects; AZT

AIDS/TESTING AND SCREENING

Balano, Kirsten; Beckerman, Karen; Ng, Valerie, et al. Rapid HIV screening during labor. [Letter and response]. *JAMA.* 1998 Nov 18; 280(19): 1664. 6 refs. BE61079.

*AIDS serodiagnosis; *childbirth; drugs; *HIV seropositivity; informed consent; newborns; *pregnant women; risks and benefits; time factors; AZT

Baleta, Adele. Huge percentage of women volunteer for zidovudine project. [News]. *Lancet.* 1999 Jan 16; 353(9148): 219. BE61564.

AIDS; *AIDS serodiagnosis; counseling; *drugs; economics; *HIV seropositivity; newborns; *patient care; *pregnant women; *preventive medicine; voluntary programs; *AZT; *South Africa; Western Cape

Balter, Michael. French AIDS research pioneers to testify in trial of ministers. [News]. *Science.* 1999 Feb 12; 283(5404): 910–911. BE61715.

*AIDS; *AIDS serodiagnosis; blood donation; *blood transfusions; *criminal law; drug industry; economics; expert testimony; hemophilia; investigators; *legal aspects; legal liability; *misconduct; *politics; *France

---

BE = bioethics accession number   fn. = footnotes   refs. = references

Bayer, Ronald. Clinical progress and the future of HIV exceptionalism. *Archives of Internal Medicine.* 1999 May 24; 159(10): 1042-1048. 45 refs. BE61390.
> *AIDS; *AIDS serodiagnosis; anonymous testing; attitudes; communicable diseases; confidentiality; drugs; federal government; government financing; government regulation; health care delivery; *HIV seropositivity; informed consent; *mandatory reporting; *mandatory testing; mass screening; *newborns; patient care; physicians; political activity; *pregnant women; public health; *public policy; state government; trends; voluntary programs; New York; *United States

In the 18 years since the first cases of the acquired immunodeficiency syndrome (AIDS) were reported by the Centers for Disease Control and Prevention (CDC), the epidemic has undergone profound transformations, and so, too, has the sociomedical context within which public health policy is fashioned and implemented. The early years of neglect and panic were also characterized by relative therapeutic impotence and deep uncertainty about the epidemiological course the new threat would take. In the United States and in other economically advanced nations, the threat of contracting the human immunodeficiency virus (HIV) has abated. The incidence of infection has declined, and the prevalence of infection has stabilized and, in some instances, begun to fall. The pattern of HIV spread, where it has continued, has been dramatically circumscribed to marginalized populations. The panic of the mid-1980s has passed, and in many nations, AIDS has lost its salience as a public issue. A sense of therapeutic impotence no longer prevails, and a new mood of triumphalism has taken hold. How have these crucial changes affected AIDS policies in America?

Bennett, Rebecca; Erin, Charles A., eds. HIV and AIDS: Testing, Screening, and Confidentiality. New York, NY: Oxford University Press; 1999. 285 p. (Issues in biomedical ethics). Bibliography: p. 271-279. The impetus for this volume was provided by the research project "AIDS: Ethics, Justice and European Policy," supported by the Directorate General XII of the European Commission under its Biomedicine and Health Research Program (BIOMED 1). The coordinating group for this project, which ran for 3 years from Jan 1993, was centered within the Centre for Social Ethics and Policy at the University of Manchester, U.K. ISBN 0-19-823801-0. BE62712.
> *AIDS; *AIDS serodiagnosis; blood donation; *confidentiality; counseling; disclosure; duty to warn; epidemiology; health care; health personnel; *HIV seropositivity; informed consent; insurance; legal aspects; legal liability; moral obligations; obligations of society; pregnant women; public health; public policy; resource allocation; risks and benefits; social discrimination; voluntary programs; right not to know; *Europe; *European Community; United States

Bennett, Rebecca. Should we routinely test pregnant women for HIV? *In:* Bennett, Rebecca; Erin, Charles A., eds. HIV and AIDS: Testing, Screening, and Confidentiality. New York, NY: Oxford University Press; 1999: 228-239. 17 fn. ISBN 0-19-823801-0. BE62725.
> *AIDS serodiagnosis; epidemiology; health personnel; HIV seropositivity; informed consent; mandatory testing; mass screening; newborns; occupational exposure; *pregnant women; preventive medicine; *voluntary programs

Bindman, Andrew B.; Osmond, Dennis; Hecht, Frederick M., et al. Multistate evaluation of anonymous HIV testing and access to medical care. [For the Multistate Evaluation of Surveillance of HIV (MESH) Study Group]. *JAMA.* 1998 Oct 28; 280(16): 1416-1420. 12 refs. BE60292.
> *AIDS; *AIDS serodiagnosis; *anonymous testing; *confidentiality; evaluation studies; government financing; *HIV seropositivity; *patient care; social impact; statistics; survey; *time factors; retrospective studies; Arizona; California; Missouri; New Mexico; North Carolina; Oregon; Texas

CONTEXT: Infection with the human immunodeficiency virus (HIV) is the only infectious disease for which anonymous testing is publicly funded, an exception that has been controversial. OBJECTIVE: To assess whether anonymous HIV testing was associated with earlier HIV testing and HIV-related medical care than confidential HIV testing. DESIGN: Retrospective cohort. SETTING: Arizona, Colorado, Missouri, New Mexico, North Carolina, Oregon, and Texas. PARTICIPANTS: Probability sample of 835 new acquired immunodeficiency syndrome (AIDS) cases reported to the state health department's HIV/AIDS Reporting System from May 1995 through December 1996. All had responded to the AIDS Patient Survey; 643 had been tested confidentially for HIV, and 192 had been tested anonymously. MAIN OUTCOME MEASURES: First CD4+ cell count; number of days from HIV-positive test result to first HIV-related medical care, from first HIV-related medical care to AIDS, and from first HIV-positive test result to AIDS. RESULTS: Persons tested anonymously sought testing and medical care earlier in the course of HIV disease than did persons tested confidentially. Mean first CD4+ cell count was $0.427x$ $10(9)/L$ in persons tested anonymously vs $0.267x$ $10(9)/L$ in persons tested confidentially. Persons tested anonymously experienced an average of 918 days in HIV-related medical care before an AIDS diagnosis vs 531 days for persons tested confidentially. The mean time from learning they were HIV positive to the diagnosis of AIDS was 1246 days for persons tested anonymously vs 718 days for persons tested confidentially. After adjustment for the subject's age, sex, race/ethnicity, education, income, insurance status, HIV exposure group, whether the respondent had a regular source of care or symptoms at the time of the HIV test, and state residence, anonymous testing remained significantly associated with earlier entry into medical care (P less than .001). CONCLUSION: Anonymous testing contributes to early HIV testing and medical care.

Brazier, Margaret; Lobjoit, Mary. Fiduciary relationship: an ethical approach and a legal concept? *In:* Bennett, Rebecca; Erin, Charles A., eds. HIV and AIDS: Testing, Screening, and Confidentiality. New York, NY: Oxford University Press; 1999: 179-199. 63 fn. ISBN 0-19-823801-0. BE62722.
> AIDS; *AIDS serodiagnosis; autonomy; blood specimen collection; *confidentiality; disclosure; duty to warn; *HIV seropositivity; iatrogenic disease; informed consent; *legal aspects; occupational exposure; paternalism; *patients; physician patient relationship; *physicians; standards; trust; Canada; *Great Britain

Chavey, William E.; Cantor, Scott B.; Clover, Richard D., et al. Cost-effectiveness analysis of screening health care workers for HIV. *Journal of Family Practice.* 1994 Mar; 38(3): 249-257. 33 refs. BE59350.
> *AIDS serodiagnosis; *costs and benefits; evaluation; *health personnel; *HIV seropositivity; hospitals; iatrogenic disease; risk

Crawford, Colin; American Civil Liberties Union. Should HIV testing be required for all pregnant women?

BE = bioethics accession number   fn. = footnotes   refs. = references

In: Francoeur, Robert T., ed. Taking Sides: Clashing Views on Controversial Issues in Human Sexuality. Fifth Edition. Guilford, CT: Dushkin Publishing Group/Brown and Benchmark; 1996: 192–207. 17 refs. ISBN 0–697–31292–5. BE62048.
*AIDS serodiagnosis; counseling; drugs; guidelines; *HIV seropositivity; informed consent; legal aspects; *mandatory testing; *mass screening; *newborns; patient care; *pregnant women; preventive medicine; risks and benefits; social discrimination; *voluntary programs; AZT; Centers for Disease Control and Prevention; United States

Erin, Charles A. Is there a right to remain in ignorance of HIV status? *In:* Bennett, Rebecca; Erin, Charles A., eds. HIV and AIDS: Testing, Screening, and Confidentiality. New York, NY: Oxford University Press; 1999: 251–266. 45 fn. ISBN 0–19–823801–0. BE62727.
*AIDS serodiagnosis; autonomy; disclosure; *HIV seropositivity; *moral obligations; patients; psychological stress; *rights; risk; social discrimination; truth disclosure; harms; *right not to know

Etzioni, Amitai. HIV testing of infants: privacy and public health. *Health Affairs.* 1998 Jul–Aug; 17(4): 170–183. 50 fn. BE61478.
*AIDS serodiagnosis; alternatives; anonymous testing; autonomy; *confidentiality; *disclosure; drugs; *HIV seropositivity; informed consent; legal aspects; mandatory testing; *mothers; *newborns; patient care; *pregnant women; privacy; *public policy; risks and benefits; social discrimination; state government; suffering; values; voluntary programs; AZT; *New York

Etzioni, Amitai. HIV testing of infants: should public health override privacy? *In:* his The Limits of Privacy. New York, NY: Basic Books; 1999: 17–42, 220–226. 88 fn. ISBN 0–465–04089–6. BE62442.
*AIDS serodiagnosis; anonymous testing; autonomy; communitarianism; confidentiality; costs and benefits; counseling; disadvantaged; *disclosure; *HIV seropositivity; informed consent; *mandatory testing; mothers; *newborns; patient care; policy analysis; pregnant women; *privacy; public health; *public policy; risks and benefits; social discrimination; *voluntary programs; New York; United States

Feldman, Eric A. Testing the force: HIV and discrimination in the Australian military. *AIDS and Public Policy Journal.* 1998 Summer; 13(2): 85–90. 24 fn. BE61346.
*AIDS serodiagnosis; dangerousness; employment; *HIV seropositivity; international aspects; *legal aspects; *mandatory testing; *military personnel; public policy; *social discrimination; *Australia; Belgium; Canada; Disability Discrimination Act 1992 (Australia); United States

Felsman, Janine P. Eliminating parental consent and notification for adolescent HIV testing: a legitimate statutory response to the AIDS epidemic. [Note]. *Journal of Law and Policy.* 1996; 5(1): 339–383. 146 fn. BE59302.
*adolescents; *AIDS serodiagnosis; competence; *confidentiality; *counseling; *government regulation; *HIV seropositivity; *informed consent; *legal aspects; legal rights; *parental consent; *parental notification; parents; patient care; privacy; *public policy; social impact; state government; state interest; *voluntary programs; United States

Finn, Lisa. It's for (y)our own good: an analysis of the discourses surrounding mandatory, unblinded HIV testing of newborns. *Journal of Medical Humanities.* 1998 Summer; 19(2–3): 133–162. 63 refs. 30 fn. BE60902.
abortion, induced; AIDS; *AIDS serodiagnosis; biomedical

research; *blacks; cesarean section; children; coercion; contraception; counseling; decision making; drug abuse; drugs; females; fetuses; health care delivery; health education; Hispanic Americans; *HIV seropositivity; *indigents; *mandatory testing; mothers; *newborns; *pregnant women; prevalence; *preventive medicine; privacy; quality of health care; reproduction; rights; self induced illness; sexuality; *social discrimination; *socioeconomic factors; sterilization (sexual); *stigmatization; women's health; women's rights; AZT; United States

Fleischman, Alan R.; Post, Linda Farber; Dubler, Nancy Neveloff. Mandatory newborn screening for human immunodeficiency virus. *Bulletin of the New York Academy of Medicine.* 1994 Summer; 71(1): 4–17. 17 refs. BE61584.
*AIDS serodiagnosis; autonomy; blood specimen collection; confidentiality; constitutional law; counseling; drug abuse; equal protection; government regulation; *HIV seropositivity; informed consent; *legal aspects; legal rights; legislation; *mandatory programs; *mandatory testing; mothers; *newborns; patient care; pregnant women; privacy; public health; *public policy; *risks and benefits; social discrimination; state government; state interest; stigmatization; voluntary programs; women's rights; *New York

Frank, Stacy; Esch, Julie Funesti; Margeson, Nancy E. Mandatory HIV testing of newborns: the impact on women. *American Journal of Nursing.* 1998 Oct; 98(10): 49–51. 8 refs. BE61804.
*AIDS serodiagnosis; counseling; government regulation; *HIV seropositivity; informed consent; *mandatory testing; *mass screening; mothers; *newborns; nurses; patient care; public policy; risks and benefits; state government; *voluntary programs; New York

Gbolade, Babatunde A.; Tan, K.H.; Teo, K.P., et al. Reducing the vertical transmission of HIV. [Letters]. *BMJ (British Medical Journal).* 1998 Jun 20; 316(7148): 1899–1901. 15 refs. BE59423.
abortion, induced; *AIDS serodiagnosis; anonymous testing; attitudes; counseling; *HIV seropositivity; mass screening; obstetrics and gynecology; physicians; *pregnant women; prevalence; primary health care; public participation; *public policy; survey; voluntary programs; Department of Health (Great Britain); Great Britain; Italy; Singapore

Godfrey-Faussett, Peter; Baggaley, Rachel; Brewster, M.F. Exceptionalism in HIV. [Letters]. *BMJ (British Medical Journal).* 1998 Jun 13; 316(7147): 1826. 2 refs. BE59223.
*AIDS serodiagnosis; counseling; developing countries; *HIV seropositivity; pregnant women; preventive medicine; risks and benefits; voluntary programs; Africa; Great Britain

Greece. Circular No. 4548 of 13 Jun 1990 on indications and deontological principles in respect of laboratory tests for the detection of antibodies to the human immunodeficiency virus (HIV). [Summary]. *International Digest of Health Legislation.* 1994. 45(4). 501–502. BE62691.
*AIDS serodiagnosis; *government regulation; informed consent; mandatory programs; voluntary programs; *Greece

Häyry, Heta. Who should know about my HIV positivity and why? *In:* Bennett, Rebecca; Erin, Charles A., eds. HIV and AIDS: Testing, Screening, and Confidentiality. New York, NY: Oxford University Press; 1999: 240–250. 8 fn. ISBN 0–19–823801–0. BE62726.
*AIDS serodiagnosis; *confidentiality; deontological ethics; *disclosure; duty to warn; economics; *HIV seropositivity; *moral obligations; patients; privacy; public health; truth

---

BE = bioethics accession number   fn. = footnotes   refs. = references

disclosure; utilitarianism; virtues; right not to know

Hudson, C.N.; Sherr, Lorraine. Antenatal HIV testing in Europe. [Letter]. *Lancet.* 1997 Dec 13; 350(9093): 1783. BE59236.
     *AIDS serodiagnosis; consensus; counseling; *guidelines; *HIV seropositivity; *pregnant women; public policy; risks and benefits; voluntary programs; *Europe; European Union

Jayaraman, K.S. Indian state plans compulsory HIV testing, segregation and branding. [News]. *Nature Medicine.* 1998 Apr; 4(4): 378. BE59695.
     *AIDS serodiagnosis; females; *HIV seropositivity; *mandatory testing; *public policy; quarantine; sex offenses; state government; prostitution; *India; *Maharashtra

Karim, Quarraisha Abdool; Karim, Salim S. Abdool; Coovadia, Hoosen M., et al. Informed consent for HIV testing in a South African hospital: is it truly informed and truly voluntary? *American Journal of Public Health.* 1998 Apr; 88(4): 637–640. 15 refs. BE60134.
     *AIDS; *AIDS serodiagnosis; coercion; control groups; *counseling; disadvantaged; evaluation studies; *health services research; *HIV seropositivity; human experimentation; *informed consent; *knowledge, attitudes, practice; newborns; *pregnant women; preventive medicine; public hospitals; quality of health care; research design; research ethics committees; research subjects; survey; therapeutic research; voluntary programs; King Edward VIII Hospital (Durban); *South Africa
     OBJECTIVE: The purpose of this study was to assess informed consent to human immunodeficiency virus (HIV) testing in a perinatal HIV transmission study in a major referral hospital serving a largely Black population in South Africa. METHODS: First-time antenatal clinic attenders who were randomly selected from those enrolled in the perinatal HIV study (n = 56) answered questionnaires before and after counseling. RESULTS: Knowledge of HIV transmission and prevention, high at the outset, was little improved after counseling. The acceptance rate for HIV testing was high. Despite assurances that participation was voluntary, 88% of the women said they felt compelled to participate in the study. CONCLUSIONS: Informed consent in this setting was truly informed but not truly voluntary.

Kondro, Wayne. Voluntary blood tests for Canadian doctors? [News]. *Lancet.* 1998 Oct 10; 352(9135): 1205. BE60260.
     *AIDS serodiagnosis; *hepatitis; HIV seropositivity; mandatory testing; *organizational policies; *physicians; professional organizations; *voluntary programs; Ontario; *Ontario College of Physicians and Surgeons

Lindsay, Michael K. Routine voluntary antepartum HIV antibody counseling and testing: a sound public health prevention strategy. *Clinical Obstetrics and Gynecology.* 1996 Jun; 39(2): 305–315. 59 refs. BE62106.
     *AIDS serodiagnosis; anonymous testing; contact tracing; contraception; counseling; drugs; federal government; guidelines; *HIV seropositivity; informed consent; mandatory testing; *pregnant women; preventive medicine; risk; *voluntary programs; partner notification; AZT; Centers for Disease Control and Prevention; United States

McKenna, Juliet J. Where ignorance is not bliss: a proposal for mandatory HIV testing of pregnant women. *Stanford Law and Policy Review.* 1996 Summer; 7(2): 133–157. 163 fn. BE59211.
     *AIDS serodiagnosis; autonomy; coercion; communicable diseases; counseling; *decision making; directive counseling; disclosure; drugs; employment; federal government; fetuses;

guidelines; health insurance; *HIV seropositivity; legal aspects; *mandatory testing; mass screening; newborns; patient care; patient participation; *pregnant women; preventive medicine; risk; *risks and benefits; selective abortion; social discrimination; state government; state interest; stigmatization; treatment refusal; voluntary programs; *women's rights; AZT; Centers for Disease Control and Prevention; *United States

Madison, Melinda. Tragic life or tragic death: mandatory testing of newborns for HIV -- mothers' rights versus children's health. *Journal of Legal Medicine.* 1997 Sep; 18(3): 361–386. 230 fn. BE60084.
     *AIDS serodiagnosis; confidentiality; criminal law; disadvantaged; drugs; federal government; government regulation; *HIV seropositivity; informed consent; *legal aspects; legal liability; legal rights; *mandatory testing; mass screening; minors; *newborns; parents; *pregnant women; prenatal injuries; privacy; *risks and benefits; social discrimination; state government; state interest; voluntary programs; AZT; Ryan White Comprehensive AIDS Resources Emergency Act 1990; *United States

Manuel, Catherine. HIV screening: benefits and harms for the individual and the community. *In:* Bennett, Rebecca; Erin, Charles A., eds. HIV and AIDS: Testing, Screening, and Confidentiality. New York, NY: Oxford University Press; 1999: 61–74. 14 fn. ISBN 0-19-823801-0. BE62714.
     AIDS; *AIDS serodiagnosis; confidentiality; epidemiology; *HIV seropositivity; mandatory testing; mass screening; pregnant women; preventive medicine; psychological stress; public health; public policy; risk; *risks and benefits; stigmatization; voluntary programs

Marjan, R.S.R.; Ruminjo, J.K. Attitudes to prenatal testing and notification for HIV infection in Nairobi, Kenya. *East African Medical Journal.* 1996 Oct; 73(10): 665–669. 19 refs. BE62664.
     abortion, induced; *AIDS serodiagnosis; anonymous testing; *attitudes; confidentiality; contraception; *disclosure; hospitals; informed consent; institutional policies; knowledge, attitudes, practice; mass screening; *pregnant women; spousal notification; survey; voluntary programs; *Kenya

Nakashima, Allyn K.; Horsley, Rosemarie; Frey, Robert L., et al. Effect of HIV reporting by name on use of HIV testing in publicly funded counseling and testing programs. *JAMA.* 1998 Oct 28; 280(16): 1421–1426. 32 refs. BE60293.
     *AIDS serodiagnosis; *confidentiality; counseling; drug abuse; evaluation studies; government financing; health facilities; *HIV seropositivity; homosexuals; *mandatory reporting; public policy; *social impact; state government; statistics; retrospective studies; Louisiana; Michigan; Nebraska; Nevada; New Jersey; Tennessee
     CONTEXT: Policies requiring confidential reporting by name to state health departments of persons infected with the human immunodeficiency virus (HIV) have potential to cause some of them to avoid HIV testing. OBJECTIVE: To describe trends in use of HIV testing services at publicly funded HIV counseling and testing sites before and after the implementation of HIV reporting policies. DESIGN AND SETTING: Analysis of service provision data from 6 state health departments (Louisiana, Michigan, Nebraska, Nevada, New Jersey, and Tennessee) 12 months before and 12 months after HIV reporting was introduced. MAIN OUTCOME MEASURE: Percent change in numbers of persons tested at publicly funded HIV counseling and testing sites after implementation of confidential HIV reporting by risk group. RESULTS: No significant declines in the total number of HIV tests provided at counseling and

---

BE = bioethics accession number   fn. = footnotes   refs. = references

testing sites in the months immediately after implementation of HIV reporting occurred in any state, other than those expected from trends present before HIV reporting. Increases occurred in Nebraska (15.8%), Nevada (48.4%), New Jersey (21.3%), and Tennessee (62.8%). Predicted decreases occurred in Louisiana (10.5%) and Michigan (2.0%). In all areas, testing of at-risk heterosexuals increased in the year after HIV reporting was implemented (Louisiana, 10.5%; Michigan, 225.1%; Nebraska, 5.7%; Nevada, 303.3%; New Jersey, 462.9%; Tennessee, 603.8%). Declines in testing occurred among men who have sex with men in Louisiana (4.3%) and Tennessee (4.1%) after HIV reporting; testing increased for this group in Michigan (5.3%), Nebraska (19.6%), Nevada (12.5%), and New Jersey (22.4%). Among injection drug users, testing declined in Louisiana (15%), Michigan (34.3%), and New Jersey (0.6%) and increased in Nebraska (1.7%), Nevada (18.9%), and Tennessee (16.6%). CONCLUSIONS: Confidential HIV reporting by name did not appear to affect use of HIV testing in publicly funded counseling and testing programs.

Oldenettel, Debra; Dye, Timothy D.; Artal, Raul. Prenatal HIV screening in pregnant women: a medical-legal review. *Birth.* 1997 Sep; 24(3): 165–172. 46 refs. BE60332.
  *AIDS serodiagnosis; costs and benefits; disadvantaged; drugs; *HIV seropositivity; legal aspects; mandatory testing; methods; patient care; *pregnant women; privacy; public policy; *risks and benefits; stigmatization; voluntary programs; women's health services; AZT; United States

Olsthoorn-Heim, Els T.M. HIV testing and private insurance. *Medicine and Law.* 1993; 12(1–2): 11–14. BE60608.
  *AIDS serodiagnosis; contracts; disclosure; industry; *insurance; insurance selection bias; life insurance; mandatory testing; organizational policies; privacy; public policy; rights; risk; voluntary programs; right not to know; *Netherlands

Rand, Justin. AIDS and HIV: Colorado court upholds privacy rights in disclosure of test results. *Journal of Law, Medicine and Ethics.* 1998 Winter; 26(4): 353–355. 12 fn. BE61168.
  *AIDS serodiagnosis; *blood specimen collection; confidentiality; criminal law; deception; *disclosure; government regulation; *HIV seropositivity; informed consent; *laboratories; *legal aspects; *legal liability; *privacy; *schools; state government; students; torts; *Cambridge College (Cambridge, MA); *Colorado; *Doe v. High-Tech Institute, Inc.

Richards, Edward P. HIV testing, screening, and confidentiality: an American perspective. *In:* Bennett, Rebecca; Erin, Charles A., eds. HIV and AIDS: Testing, Screening, and Confidentiality. New York, NY: Oxford University Press; 1999: 75–90. 41 fn. ISBN 0–19–823801–0. BE62715.
  AIDS; *AIDS serodiagnosis; anonymous testing; confidentiality; contact tracing; counseling; epidemiology; *HIV seropositivity; homosexuals; informed consent; legal aspects; mandatory reporting; mass screening; military personnel; municipal government; political activity; prisoners; public health; *public policy; *state government; *United States

Sharma, Dinesh C. Indian welfare minister orders compulsory HIV testing for children in care. [News]. *Lancet.* 1999 Jan 30; 353(9150): 390. BE60982.
  *AIDS serodiagnosis; *children; *disadvantaged; *HIV seropositivity; *mandatory testing; *public policy; *India

Sherr, Lorraine. Counselling and HIV testing: ethical dilemmas. *In:* Bennett, Rebecca; Erin, Charles A., eds. HIV and AIDS: Testing, Screening, and Confidentiality. New York, NY: Oxford University Press; 1999: 39–60. 85 fn. ISBN 0–19–823801–0. BE62713.
  AIDS; *AIDS serodiagnosis; blood donation; children; competence; *counseling; decision making; health personnel; *HIV seropositivity; informed consent; newborns; patients; pregnant women; professional competence; psychology; Great Britain

Silversides, Ann. With HIV prevalence among women increasing, more provinces encourage prenatal testing. *Canadian Medical Association Journal.* 1998 Jun 2; 158(11): 1518–1519. BE62201.
  *AIDS serodiagnosis; children; counseling; drugs; guidelines; *HIV seropositivity; informed consent; organizational policies; physicians; *pregnant women; prevalence; preventive medicine; professional organizations; *public policy; *voluntary programs; Alberta; British Columbia; *Canada; Canadian Medical Association; Newfoundland; Ontario; Quebec

Simpson, Wendy M.; Johnstone, Frank D.; Goldberg, David J., et al. Antenatal HIV testing: assessment of a routine voluntary approach. *BMJ (British Medical Journal).* 1999 Jun 19; 318(7199): 1660–1661. 5 refs. BE62452.
  *AIDS serodiagnosis; evaluation studies; *HIV seropositivity; informed consent; institutional policies; *knowledge, attitudes, practice; patient satisfaction; *pregnant women; psychological stress; survey; *voluntary programs; Great Britain

Solomon, Liza; Benjamin, Georges; Fernando, M. Daniel, et al. National HIV case reporting. [Letters and response]. *New England Journal of Medicine.* 1998 Feb 26; 338(9): 626–627. 9 refs. BE59524.
  anonymous testing; confidentiality; disadvantaged; drug abuse; *epidemiology; *HIV seropositivity; *mandatory reporting; privacy; public health; *public policy; risks and benefits; Maryland; United States

Sorell, Tom; Draper, Heather. AIDS and insurance. *In:* Bennett, Rebecca; Erin, Charles A., eds. HIV and AIDS: Testing, Screening, and Confidentiality. New York, NY: Oxford University Press; 1999: 216–227. 12 fn. ISBN 0–19–823801–0. BE62724.
  *AIDS; *AIDS serodiagnosis; economics; health insurance; health personnel; *HIV seropositivity; industry; *life insurance; national health insurance; *private sector; *public sector; risk; *Great Britain

Stoto, Michael A.; Almario, Donna A.; McCormick, Marie C., eds.; Institute of Medicine. Committee on Perinatal Transmission of HIV; National Research Council and Institute of Medicine. Board on Children, Youth, and Families. Reducing the Odds: Preventing Perinatal Transmission of HIV in the United States. Washington, DC: National Academy Press; 1999. 397 p. Bibliography: p. 134–144. ISBN 0–309–06286–1. BE61845.
  adolescents; AIDS; *AIDS serodiagnosis; children; counseling; drugs; epidemiology; evaluation; federal government; females; financial support; government financing; guidelines; health care delivery; *HIV seropositivity; human experimentation; mandatory testing; mass screening; *newborns; patient compliance; policy analysis; *pregnant women; *preventive medicine; professional organizations; public health; *public policy; state government; statistics; voluntary programs; women's health services; AZT; Public Health Service; *United States

---

BE = bioethics accession number   fn. = footnotes   refs. = references

U.S. Centers for Disease Control and Prevention. HIV Counseling, Testing, and Referral: Standards and Guidelines. Washington, DC: U.S. Government Printing Office; 1994 May. 15 p. BE59420.
> *AIDS serodiagnosis; confidentiality; *counseling; disclosure; federal government; goals; *guidelines; *HIV seropositivity; patient education; preventive medicine; *public policy; records; referral and consultation; risk; *standards; *Centers for Disease Control and Prevention; United States

Wong, Jeffrey G.; Nakchbandi, Inaam A.; Longenecker, J. Craig, et al. HIV testing in pregnant women. [Letter and response]. *Annals of Internal Medicine.* 1998 Dec 15; 129(12): 1075. 4 refs. BE60226.
> *AIDS serodiagnosis; autonomy; counseling; drugs; *HIV seropositivity; *mandatory testing; newborns; patient care; *pregnant women; public policy; risks and benefits; *voluntary programs; AZT; United States

ALLOWING TO DIE

See also EUTHANASIA, RESUSCITATION ORDERS, SELECTION FOR TREATMENT, TERMINAL CARE, TREATMENT REFUSAL

Alpers, Ann; Lo, Bernard. Avoiding family feuds: responding to surrogate demands for life-sustaining interventions. *Journal of Law, Medicine and Ethics.* 1999 Spring; 27(1): 74–80. 45 fn. BE61507.
> *advance directives; *allowing to die; autonomy; *beneficence; biomedical technologies; case studies; communication; *conscience; consensus; cultural pluralism; *decision making; directive adherence; disclosure; *dissent; *family members; *family relationship; friends; *futility; intention; minority groups; moral obligations; patient care team; *physicians; *professional family relationship; prognosis; *prolongation of life; religion; resuscitation orders; risks and benefits; *suffering; *third party consent; time factors; *values; withholding treatment; integrity; *negotiation; oral directives

American Medical Association. Council on Ethical and Judicial Affairs. Medical futility in end-of-life care: report of the Council on Ethical and Judicial Affairs. *JAMA.* 1999 Mar 10; 281(10): 937–941. 38 refs. BE61243.
> *allowing to die; clinical ethics committees; *decision making; *dissent; family members; *futility; goals; *guidelines; *health facilities; *institutional policies; *organizational policies; patient advocacy; patient participation; patient transfer; patients; persistent vegetative state; physicians; prognosis; prolongation of life; public participation; resource allocation; standards; terminally ill; terminology; treatment outcome; *values; withholding treatment; *American Medical Association; United States

Use of life-sustaining or invasive interventions in patients in a persistent vegetative state or who are terminally ill may only prolong the dying process. What constitutes futile intervention remains a point of controversy in the medical literature and in clinical practice. In clinical practice, controversy arises when the patient or proxy and the physician have discrepant values or goals of care. Since definitions of futile care are value laden, universal consensus on futile care is unlikely to be achieved. Rather, the American Medical Association Council on Ethical and Judicial Affairs recommends a process-based approach to futility determinations. The process includes at least 4 steps aimed at deliberation and resolution including all involved parties, 2 steps aimed at securing alternatives in the case of irreconcilable differences, and a final step aimed at closure when all alternatives have been exhausted. The approach is placed in the context of the circumstances in which futility claims are made,

the difficulties of defining medical futility, and a discussion of how best to implement a policy on futility.

Andersen, David; Cavalier, Robert; Covey, Preston K. A Right to Die? The Dax Cowart Case. [CD-ROM computer file]. New York, NY: Routledge; 1996 Jun. 1 computer laser optical disc; sd., col.; 4 – 3/4 in. + user guide and teacher's guide.. Interactive; contains scenes of medical treatment which some may find distressing. Versions available for Windows or Macintosh (single user ISBN 0-415-91753-0, multiple user pack ISBN 0-415-91754-9); contact Routledge (e-mail: info.dax@routledge.com; http://www.routledge.com/routledge.html). BE59871.
> *allowing to die; assisted suicide; *autonomy; beneficence; *burns; case studies; coercion; decision making; dissent; moral obligations; *pain; paternalism; *patient care; patient care team; physically disabled; physician patient relationship; physicians; *prolongation of life; quality of life; rehabilitation; *right to die; *suffering; suicide; teaching methods; treatment outcome; *treatment refusal; *Cowart, Dax

Arthur, John, ed. Euthanasia. *In:* Arthur, John, ed. Morality and Moral Controversies. Fifth Edition. Upper Saddle River, NJ: Prentice Hall; 1999: 211–235. 2 refs. Includes discussion questions. ISBN 0-13-914128-6. BE60275.
> *active euthanasia; advance directives; *allowing to die; artificial feeding; assisted suicide; compassion; congenital disorders; double effect; drugs; freedom; intention; killing; legal aspects; *moral policy; newborns; pain; persistent vegetative state; physicians; quality of life; right to die; suffering; suicide; Supreme Court decisions; terminally ill; third party consent; treatment refusal; value of life; *voluntary euthanasia; withholding treatment; Cruzan v. Director, Missouri Department of Health; United States

Ashraf, Haroon. BMA address the issue of withholding and withdrawing treatment. [News]. *Lancet.* 1999 Jun 26; 353(9171): 2220. BE62580.
> *allowing to die; artificial feeding; *guidelines; *organizational policies; persistent vegetative state; physicians; professional organizations; withholding treatment; *British Medical Association; Great Britain

Baier, Kurt. Wrongful death and wrongful life. *In: his* Problems of Life and Death: A Humanist Perspective. Amherst, NY: Prometheus Books; 1997: 137–230. 74 fn. ISBN 1-57392-153-X. BE61848.
> *allowing to die; *assisted suicide; capital punishment; contraception; disabled; disclosure; ethical theory; guidelines; *humanism; intention; *killing; law; legal aspects; legal liability; moral obligations; *moral policy; *morality; negligence; organ donation; physicians; *population control; prognosis; *prolongation of life; quality of life; suffering; suicide; value of life; values; *voluntary euthanasia; wrongful death; *wrongful life; rationality

Beckel, Jean. Resolving ethical problems in long-term care. *Journal of Gerontological Nursing.* 1996 Jan; 22(1): 20–26. 11 refs. BE60191.
> administrators; *allowing to die; artificial feeding; case studies; clinical ethics committees; competence; *decision making; *dissent; ethical analysis; *family members; futility; hospitals; institutional policies; legal guardians; long-term care; *nurse's role; *nursing homes; patient advocacy; patient transfer; physician nurse relationship; *physicians; *prolongation of life; terminal care; terminally ill; third party consent; treatment refusal; withholding treatment

Beckett, Alexandra. End-of-life decisions in AIDS. *In:* Steinberg, Maurice D.; Youngner, Stuart J., eds. End-of-Life Decisions: A Psychosocial Perspective.

BE = bioethics accession number   fn. = footnotes   refs. = references

Washington, DC: American Psychiatric Press; 1998: 179–203. 68 fn. ISBN 0-88048-756-9. BE60119.

   *AIDS; alcohol abuse; *allowing to die; *assisted suicide; autonomy; case studies; competence; decision making; dementia; depressive disorder; drug abuse; drugs; futility; patient care; patients; *physicians; prognosis; psychiatric diagnosis; psychiatry; quality of life; referral and consultation; risks and benefits; *suicide; treatment refusal; withholding treatment; United States

Berghmans, Ron L.P. Ethical hazards of the substituted judgement test in decision making concerning the end of life of dementia patients. [Editorial]. *International Journal of Geriatric Psychiatry.* 1997 Mar; 12(3): 283–287. 23 refs. BE59429.

   advance directives; *aged; *allowing to die; autonomy; competence; *decision making; *dementia; family members; *patient care; personhood; physicians; prolongation of life; quality of life; risks and benefits; *third party consent; time factors; treatment refusal; value of life; oral directives; personal identity

Bernat, James L. VHA ethics rounds: [ethics committee role]. *NCCE News (Veterans Health Administration National Center for Clinical Ethics).* 1995 Spring; 3(2): 4–5. 2 fn. BE61469.

   accountability; *allowing to die; artificial feeding; case studies; *clinical ethics committees; *decision making; diagnosis; family members; legal aspects; legal guardians; persistent vegetative state; physicians; prognosis; third party consent; withholding treatment

British Columbia. Special Advisory Committee on Ethical Issues in Health Care. Euthanasia and Physician-Assisted Suicide. Victoria, BC: British Columbia Ministry of Health and Ministry Responsible for Seniors; 1994 Feb. 43 p. 52 fn. ISBN 0-7726-2137-3. BE59216.

   *active euthanasia; advance directives; advisory committees; *allowing to die; artificial feeding; *assisted suicide; autonomy; beneficence; coercion; compassion; competence; double effect; drugs; intention; justice; killing; legal aspects; *moral policy; pain; palliative care; persistent vegetative state; *physicians; public policy; quality of life; right to die; suffering; Supreme Court decisions; terminally ill; third party consent; treatment refusal; value of life; *voluntary euthanasia; vulnerable populations; wedge argument; withholding treatment; dignity; duty to die; *British Columbia; *Canada; Canadian Charter of Rights and Freedoms; Criminal Code of Canada; Law Reform Commission of Canada; Rodriguez v. British Columbia (Attorney-General); *Special Advisory Committee on Ethical Issues in Health Care (BC)

Brock, Dan W. Medical decisions at the end of life. *In:* Kuhse, Helga; Singer, Peter, eds. A Companion to Bioethics. Malden, MA: Blackwell; 1998: 231–241. 14 refs. ISBN 0-631-19737-0. BE59498.

   *allowing to die; autonomy; *decision making; *double effect; drugs; extraordinary treatment; family members; futility; informed consent; *killing; *moral policy; pain; *palliative care; paternalism; patient care; patient participation; physicians; prolongation of life; risks and benefits; terminal care; third party consent; treatment refusal; values; *withholding treatment

Brown, Norman K.; Thompson, Donovan J.; Prentice, Ross L. Nontreatment and aggressive narcotic therapy among hospitalized pancreatic cancer patients. *Journal of the American Geriatrics Society.* 1998 Jul; 46(7): 839–848. 30 refs. BE62259.

   active euthanasia; advance directives; *allowing to die; blood transfusions; *cancer; comparative studies; *decision making; drugs; evaluation studies; family members; futility; *intention; knowledge, attitudes, practice; medical records;

medical specialties; nurses; *opioid analgesics; physicians; primary health care; prognosis; religious hospitals; resuscitation orders; Roman Catholics; *sedatives; selection for treatment; statistics; surgery; *terminal care; *terminally ill; time factors; *withholding treatment; antibiotics; *coma; fluid therapy; King County (WA); Washington

Burrows, R. Removal of life support in intensive care units. *Medicine and Law.* 1994; 13(5–6): 489–500. 60 refs. BE60007.

   *allowing to die; autonomy; brain death; cardiac death; *decision making; deontological ethics; determination of death; economics; futility; informed consent; *intensive care units; legal aspects; patient admission; patient care; *physician's role; physicians; prognosis; *resource allocation; rights; *selection for treatment; third party consent; utilitarianism; withholding treatment; *South Africa

Campbell, Margaret L. Forgoing Life – Sustaining Therapy: How to Care for the Patient Who Is Near Death. Aliso Viejo, CA: AACN Critical Care; 1998. 140 p. 322 refs. ISBN 0-945812-77-9. BE60066.

   advance care planning; advance directives; *allowing to die; *artificial feeding; attitudes to death; autonomy; case studies; communication; compassion; competence; cultural pluralism; decision making; diagnosis; double effect; *drugs; family members; hospitals; informed consent; intention; legal aspects; minority groups; nurse patient relationship; nurses; *palliative care; persistent vegetative state; *practice guidelines; professional family relationship; prognosis; psychological stress; quality of life; *renal dialysis; resuscitation orders; right to die; sedatives; suffering; *terminal care; terminally ill; third party consent; treatment refusal; truth disclosure; *ventilators; *withholding treatment; analgesia; grief; United States

Cantor, Norman L. The real ethic of death and dying. [Book review essay]. *Michigan Law Review.* 1996 May; 94(6): 1718–1738. 82 fn. BE60104.

   *active euthanasia; advance directives; *allowing to die; assisted suicide; *autonomy; competence; decision making; informed consent; intention; killing; legal aspects; newborns; persistent vegetative state; personhood; physicians; prolongation of life; quality of life; right to die; risks and benefits; terminally ill; third party consent; *value of life; values; withholding treatment; *Rethinking Life and Death (Singer, P.); United States

Cavanaugh, Thomas A. Currently accepted practices that are known to lead to death, and PAS: is there an ethically relevant difference? *Cambridge Quarterly of Healthcare Ethics.* 1998 Fall; 7(4): 375–381. 8 fn. BE59138.

   *allowing to die; *assisted suicide; drugs; *ethical analysis; *intention; killing; *moral policy; pain; *palliative care; physicians; *sedatives; *terminal care; treatment refusal; withholding treatment

Charatan, Fred. AMA issues guidelines on end of life care. [News]. *BMJ (British Medical Journal).* 1999 Mar 13; 318(7185): 690. BE62571.

   advance care planning; *allowing to die; clinical ethics committees; *decision making; dissent; ethics consultation; family members; *futility; *guidelines; hospitals; institutional policies; mediation; *organizational policies; patient transfer; patients; *physicians; professional organizations; prolongation of life; terminally ill; withholding treatment; *American Medical Association; United States

Cheng, F.; Ip, Mary; Wong, K.K., et al. Critical care ethics in Hong Kong: cross-cultural conflicts as East meets West. *Journal of Medicine and Philosophy.* 1998 Dec; 23(6): 616–627. 16 refs. BE62069.

   aged; *allowing to die; autonomy; critically ill; decision making; family members; futility; *health care delivery; hospitals; *intensive care units; morbidity; non-Western

---

World; patient admission; patient discharge; physicians; prolongation of life; resource allocation; resuscitation orders; selection for treatment; values; withholding treatment; *Hong Kong

The practice of critical care medicine has long been a difficult task for most critical care physicians in the densely populated city of Hong Kong, where we face limited resources and a limited number of intensive care beds. Our triage decisions are largely based on the potential of functional reversibility of the patients. Provision of graded care beds may help to relieve some of the demands on the intensive care beds. Decisions to forego futile medical treatment are frequently physician-guided family-based decisions, which is quite contrary to the Western focus on patient autonomy. However, as people acquire knowledge about health care and they become more aware of individual rights, our critical care doctors will be able to narrow the gaps between the different concepts of medical ethics among our professionals as well as in our society. An open and caring attitude from our intensivists will be important in minimizing the cross-cultural conflict on the complex issue of medical futility.

Cohen, Lewis M. Suicide, hastening death, and psychiatry. *Archives of Internal Medicine.* 1998 Oct 12; 158(18): 1973–1976. 49 refs. BE59576.
*allowing to die; *assisted suicide; competence; drugs; historical aspects; legal aspects; palliative care; physician's role; *psychiatry; quality of life; referral and consultation; religion; renal dialysis; sedatives; *suicide; terminal care; terminally ill; treatment refusal; withholding treatment; United States

Cooper-Mahkorn, Déirdre. Guidelines on assisted deaths criticised. [News]. *BMJ (British Medical Journal).* 1998 Oct 3; 317(7163): 904. BE60851.
active euthanasia; *allowing to die; autonomy; *guidelines; newborns; physicians; politics; prematurity; professional organizations; rights; *terminal care; *terminally ill; third party consent; withholding treatment; coma; *German Medical Council; *Germany

Crelinsten, Gordon L.; Belik, Jacques; Bereza, Eugene, et al. CPR for patients in a persistent vegetative state? [Letters and response]. *Canadian Medical Association Journal.* 1998 Jul 14; 159(1): 18–19, 21. 8 refs. BE62204.
*allowing to die; *decision making; dissent; *family members; *futility; government financing; health facilities; institutional policies; *organizational policies; *persistent vegetative state; *physicians; professional organizations; *prolongation of life; refusal to treat; religious ethics; resource allocation; *resuscitation; *resuscitation orders; risks and benefits; value of life; values; withholding treatment; Canada; *Canadian Medical Association

Cusveller, Bart; Jochemsen, Henk. Life-terminating actions with severely demented patients: critical assessment of a report of the Royal Dutch Society of Medicine. *Issues in Law and Medicine.* 1996 Summer; 12(1): 31–45. 43 fn. BE61152.
*active euthanasia; advance directives; *allowing to die; artificial feeding; competence; *dementia; *double effect; *drugs; evaluation; futility; *involuntary euthanasia; *organizational policies; *palliative care; physician's role; *physicians; professional organizations; quality of life; risks and benefits; suffering; terminal care; *voluntary euthanasia; *withholding treatment; antibiotics; *Dutch Commission for the Acceptability of Life Terminating Action; *Netherlands; *Royal Dutch Medical Association

Derse, Arthur R. Making decisions about life-sustaining medical treatment in patients with dementia: the problem

of patient decision-making capacity. *Theoretical Medicine and Bioethics.* 1999 Jan; 20(1): 55–67. 42 refs. BE62124.
*aged; *allowing to die; assisted suicide; autonomy; beneficence; case studies; *compensation; comprehension; *decision making; *dementia; diagnosis; emergency care; heart diseases; human experimentation; *informed consent; patient care; patient participation; *prolongation of life; quality of life; recall; *resuscitation; standards; surgery; third party consent; *treatment refusal; truth disclosure; withholding treatment; rationality

Dietz, Sarah M.; Brakman, Sarah-Vaughan; Dresser, Rebecca, et al. The incompetent self: metamorphosis of a person? [Letters and responses]. *Hastings Center Report.* 1998 Sep–Oct; 28(5): 4–5. BE59545.
*advance directives; *allowing to die; autonomy; *competence; *decision making; living wills; personhood; prognosis; *prolongation of life; quality of life; ventilators

Eiser, Arnold R.; Seiden, Dena J. Discontinuing dialysis in persistent vegetative state: the roles of autonomy, community, and professional moral agency. *American Journal of Kidney Diseases.* 1997 Aug; 30(2): 291–296. 43 refs. BE61578.
advance directives; *allowing to die; autonomy; beneficence; clinical ethics committees; communication; consensus; *decision making; dissent; ethicists; family members; futility; *guidelines; health facilities; *institutional policies; *persistent vegetative state; physicians; *renal dialysis; resource allocation; *withholding treatment; End Stage Renal Disease Program; New York; United States

Filene, Peter G. In the Arms of Others: A Cultural History of the Right-to-Die in America. Chicago, IL: Ivan R. Dee; 1998. 282 p. 637 fn. ISBN 1-56663-188-2. BE60014.
*active euthanasia; *allowing to die; artificial feeding; *assisted suicide; attitudes; attitudes to death; autonomy; competence; congenital disorders; decision making; determination of death; ethicists; extraordinary treatment; government regulation; *historical aspects; judicial action; legal aspects; living wills; mass media; newborns; persistent vegetative state; physicians; political activity; politics; privacy; public opinion; *right to die; state government; suffering; *terminal care; terminally ill; treatment refusal; *trends; withholding treatment; Cruzan v. Director, Missouri Department of Health; Cruzan v. Harmon; In re Conroy; In re Quinlan; Netherlands; Nineteenth Century; Superintendent v. Saikewicz; *Twentieth Century; *United States

Fimbrez, Karen Jean. Life-Sustaining Treatment: The Family Decision-Making Process. Ann Arbor, MI: UMI Dissertation Services; 1995. 90 p. Bibliography: p. 87–90. Thesis, Master of Social Work, California State University, Long Beach, Jun 1995. Order No. 1362278. BE60067.
*advance care planning; advance directives; age factors; aged; *allowing to die; artificial feeding; attitudes; communication; costs and benefits; cultural pluralism; *decision making; *emotions; *family members; *family relationship; minority groups; nursing homes; patient care team; patient participation; prognosis; *prolongation of life; quality of life; religion; resuscitation; social workers; survey; *terminal care; third party consent; ventilators; withholding treatment; adult offspring; antibiotics; qualitative research; United States

Gilligan, Timothy; Raffin, Thomas A. End-of-life discussions with patients: timing and truth-telling. [Editorial]. *Chest.* 1996 Jan; 109(1): 11–12. 11 refs. BE60427.
*advance care planning; advance directives; *allowing to die; chronically ill; communication; critically ill; *decision making; *patient participation; *physician patient

---

BE = bioethics accession number   fn. = footnotes   refs. = references

relationship; *physicians; prognosis; terminally ill; *truth disclosure; ventilators

Hackler, Chris. Consensus and futility of treatment: some policy suggestions. *In:* ten Have, Henk A.M.J.; Sass, Hans–Martin, eds. Consensus Formation in Healthcare Ethics. Boston, MA: Kluwer Academic; 1998: 219–228. 13 refs. ISBN 0–7923–4944–X. BE62597.
  *allowing to die; autonomy; communication; consensus; *decision making; dissent; *family members; *futility; hospitals; infants; institutional policies; parental consent; patient care team; patient participation; *physicians; professional family relationship; prognosis; prolongation of life; resuscitation orders; risks and benefits; suffering; terminally ill; third party consent

Halevy, Amir; Brody, Baruch A. The Houston process-based approach to medical futility. *Bioethics Forum.* 1998 Summer; 14(2): 10–17. 12 refs. Includes appendix: "Guidelines on institutional policies on the determination of medically inappropriate interventions," p. 15–16. BE61580.
  *allowing to die; autonomy; *decision making; dissent; family members; *futility; *guidelines; health personnel; *hospitals; *institutional policies; patient care; patient participation; physicians; professional autonomy; *prolongation of life; values; withholding treatment; health services misuse; integrity; *Houston; Houston City-Wide Task Force on Medical Futility; Texas

Hamel, Mary Beth; Teno, Joan M.; Goldman, Lee, et al. Patient age and decisions to withhold life-sustaining treatments from seriously ill, hospitalized adults. [For the SUPPORT Investigators]. *Annals of Internal Medicine.* 1999 Jan 19; 130(2): 116–125. 47 refs. BE62556.
  *adults; *age factors; *aged; *allowing to die; attitudes; comparative studies; *decision making; dementia; evaluation studies; hospitals; medical records; patients; *physicians; *renal dialysis; resuscitation; *selection for treatment; *surgery; survey; *ventilators; *withholding treatment; seriously ill; Study to Understand Prognoses and Preferences for Outcomes and Risks of Treatments (SUPPORT); United States
BACKGROUND: Patient age may influence decisions to withhold life-sustaining treatments, independent of patients' preferences for or ability to benefit from such treatments. Controversy exists about the appropriateness of using age as a criterion for making treatment decisions. OBJECTIVE: To determine the effect of age on decisions to withhold life-sustaining therapies. DESIGN: Prospective cohort study. SETTING: Five medical centers participating in the Study to Understand Prognoses and Preferences for Outcomes and Risks of Treatments (SUPPORT). PATIENTS: 9105 hospitalized adults who had one of nine illnesses associated with an average 6-month mortality rate of 50%. MEASUREMENTS: Outcomes were the presence and timing of decisions to withhold ventilator support, surgery, and dialysis. Adjustment was made for sociodemographic characteristics, prognoses, baseline function, patients' preferences for life-extending care, and physicians' understanding of patients' preferences for life-extending care. RESULTS: The median patient age was 63 years; 44% of patients were women, and 53% survived to 180 days. In adjusted analyses, older age was associated with higher rates of withholding each of the three life-sustaining treatments studied. For ventilator support, the rate of decisions to withhold therapy increased 15% with each decade of age (hazard ratio, 1.15 [95% CI, 1.12 to 1.19]); for surgery, the increase per decade was 19% (hazard ratio, 1.19 [CI, 1.12 to 1.27]); and for dialysis, the increase per decade

was 12% (hazard ratio, 1.12 [CI, 1.06 to 1.19]). Physicians underestimated older patients' preferences for life-extending care; adjustment for this underestimation resulted in an attenuation of the association between age and decisions to withhold treatments. CONCLUSION: Even after adjustment for differences in patients' prognoses and preferences, older age was associated with higher rates of decisions to withhold ventilator support, surgery, and dialysis.

Hanson, Laura C.; Earp, Jo Anne; Garrett, Joanne, et al. Community physicians who provide terminal care. *Archives of Internal Medicine.* 1999 May 24; 159(10): 1133–1138. 25 refs. BE61392.
  advance care planning; *aged; *allowing to die; blacks; cancer; chronically ill; communication; death; *decision making; diagnosis; family members; family relationship; home care; hospices; hospitals; living wills; morbidity; palliative care; physician patient relationship; *physicians; *primary health care; professional family relationship; *prolongation of life; resuscitation; selection for treatment; survey; *terminal care; terminally ill; ventilators; whites; withholding treatment; community hospitals; *physician's practice patterns; retrospective studies; North Carolina
BACKGROUND: Most dying patients are treated by physicians in community practice, yet studies of terminal care rarely include these physicians. OBJECTIVE: To examine the frequency of life-sustaining treatment use and describe what factors influence physicians' treatment decisions in community-based practices. METHODS: Family members and treating physicians for decedents 65 years and older who died of cancer, congestive heart failure, chronic lung disease, cirrhosis, or stroke completed interviews about end-of-life care in community settings. RESULTS: Eighty percent of eligible family and 68.8% of eligible physicians participated (N = 165). Most physicians were trained in primary care and 85.4% were primary care physicians for the decedents. Physicians typically knew the decedent a year or more (68.9%), and 93.3% treated them for at least 1 month before death. In their last month of life, 2.4% of decedents received cardiopulmonary resuscitation, 5.5% received ventilatory support, and 34.1% received hospice care. Family recalled a discussion of treatment options in 78.2% of deaths. Most discussions (72.1%) took place a month or more before death. Place of death, cancer, and having a living will were independent predictors of less aggressive treatment before death. Physicians believed that advanced planning and good relationships were the major determinants of good decision making. CONCLUSIONS: Community physicians use few life-sustaining treatments for dying patients. Treatment decisions are made in the context of long-term primary care relationships, and living wills influence treatment decisions. The choice to remain in community settings with a familiar physician may influence the dying experience.

Harper, William. Judging who should live: Schneiderman and Jecker on the duty not to treat. *Journal of Medicine and Philosophy.* 1998 Oct; 23(5): 500–515. 12 refs. 1 fn. Commentary on L.J. Schneiderman and N.S. Jecker *Wrong Medicine: Doctors, Patients, and Futile Treatment*, Johns Hopkins University Press; 1995. Note: the journal issue cover shows a date of August 1998, which is incorrect. BE62115.
  *allowing to die; alternative therapies; alternatives; *autonomy; beneficence; *decision making; *futility; goals; intensive care units; medicine; moral policy; palliative care; patient care; patients; persistent vegetative state; personhood; *physicians; *prolongation of life; public

---

opinion; quality of life; resuscitation; standards; treatment outcome; value of life; *values; *withholding treatment

In this paper, I consider the thesis advanced by Lawrence J. Schneiderman and Nancy S. Jecker that physicians should be forbidden from offering futile treatments to patients. I distinguish between a version of this thesis that is trivially true and Schneiderman and Jecker's more substantive version of the thesis. I find that their positive arguments for their thesis are unsuccessful, and sometimes quite misleading. I advance an argument against their thesis, and find that, on balance, their thesis should be rejected. I briefly argue that a resolution of the debate about medical futility will require addressing deeper issues about value.

Howsepian, A.A. The 1994 Multi-Society Task Force consensus statement on the persistent vegetative state: a critical analysis. *Issues in Law and Medicine.* 1996 Summer; 12(1): 3–29. 87 fn. BE61151.
> allowing to die; anencephaly; artificial feeding; brain death; *brain pathology; consensus; decision making; *dehumanization; dementia; *diagnosis; *evaluation; family members; food; futility; pain; patient care; *persistent vegetative state; personhood; physicians; *professional organizations; prognosis; self concept; *standards; suffering; terminology; treatment outcome; *uncertainty; withholding treatment; coma; locked-in syndrome; *Multi-Society Task Force on Persistent Vegetative State

Hutcheon, R. Gordon; Mitchell, John J.; Schmerler, Susan. The Pediatric Ethics Forum: exploring the ethical dimensions of pediatric care. [Case analysis]. *HEC (HealthCare Ethics Committee) Forum.* 1998 Sep–Dec; 10(3–4): 338–349. 8 refs. BE61185.
> *adolescents; *allowing to die; bioethical issues; case studies; central nervous system diseases; *chronically ill; clinical ethics; *clinical ethics committees; continuing education; *critically ill; *decision making; *dissent; futility; health personnel; mothers; parental consent; patient care; patient care team; *pediatrics; prognosis; renal dialysis; withholding treatment; St. Joseph's Hospital and Medical Center (Paterson, NJ)

Jeffko, Walter G. Euthanasia: a reinterpretation. *In: his* Contemporary Ethical Issues: A Personalistic Perspective. Amherst, NY: Humanity Books; 1999: 85–105. 30 fn. ISBN 1-57392-640-X. BE62246.
> *active euthanasia; *allowing to die; artificial feeding; assisted suicide; competence; congenital disorders; double effect; *euthanasia; extraordinary treatment; *intention; *involuntary euthanasia; *killing; legal aspects; *moral policy; newborns; persistent vegetative state; personhood; physicians; public policy; quality of life; right to die; suffering; terminally ill; *voluntary euthanasia; wedge argument; withholding treatment; United States

Jochemsen, Henk; Keown, John. Voluntary euthanasia under control? Further empirical evidence from the Netherlands. *Journal of Medical Ethics.* 1999 Feb; 25(1): 16–21. 46 fn. BE61189.
> *active euthanasia; adults; *allowing to die; *assisted suicide; competence; decision making; depressive disorder; drugs; *empirical research; *guideline adherence; *guidelines; intention; *involuntary euthanasia; *knowledge, attitudes, practice; law enforcement; mandatory reporting; newborns; pain; palliative care; parental consent; *physicians; psychiatry; quality of life; referral and consultation; *regulation; *social control; statistics; suffering; terminal care; *voluntary euthanasia; *wedge argument; withholding treatment; *Netherlands

Nineteen ninety-six saw the publication of a major Dutch survey into euthanasia in the Netherlands. This paper outlines the main statistical findings of this survey and considers whether it shows that voluntary euthanasia

is under effective control in the Netherlands. The paper concludes that although there has been some improvement in compliance with procedural requirements, the practice of voluntary euthanasia remains beyond effective control.

Kirschbaum, Mark Stephen. Deciding to Authorize, Forego, or Withdraw Life Support: The Meaning for Parents. Ann Arbor, MI: UMI Dissertation Services; 1994. 172 p. Bibliography: p. 140–151. Dissertation, Ph.D., University of Minnesota, Jan 1994. Order No. 9415487. BE60715.
> *allowing to die; *attitudes; biomedical technologies; *children; chronically ill; critically ill; *decision making; disabled; *family relationship; infants; nurses; nursing research; parent child relationship; *parents; professional family relationship; psychological stress; quality of life; risks and benefits; suffering; survey; *values; withholding treatment; qualitative research

Koch, Kathryn A. The language of death: euthanatos et mors -- the science of uncertainty. *Critical Care Clinics.* 1996 Jan; 12(1): 1–14. 35 refs. BE59274.
> *allowing to die; assisted suicide; attitudes to death; competence; *decision making; determination of death; double effect; drugs; emotions; euthanasia; family members; futility; legal aspects; pain; palliative care; patient participation; *physicians; prognosis; *terminal care; terminally ill; third party consent; *uncertainty; withholding treatment; United States

Kuczewski, Mark G. Physician-assisted death: can philosophical bioethics aid social policy? *Cambridge Quarterly of Healthcare Ethics.* 1998 Fall; 7(4): 339–347. 19 fn. BE59135.
> *allowing to die; *assisted suicide; autonomy; bioethics; *casuistry; *communitarianism; drugs; *ethical analysis; ethical theory; *intention; killing; legal rights; *moral policy; palliative care; physicians; public policy; treatment refusal; United States

Kuhse, Helga. Critical notice: why killing is not always worse -- and is sometimes better -- than letting die. *Cambridge Quarterly of Healthcare Ethics.* 1998 Fall; 7(4): 371–374. 9 fn. Commentary on W. Nesbitt, "Is killing no worse than letting die?" *Journal of Applied Philosophy*, 1995; 12(1): 101–106. BE59137.
> *active euthanasia; *allowing to die; *intention; *killing; *moral policy; public policy

Ladimer, Irving. Self-determination for life and death. *Medicine and Law.* 1996; 15(1): 83–92. BE61205.
> *advance directives; *allowing to die; autonomy; *decision making; information dissemination; legislation; living wills; *prolongation of life; state government; third party consent; treatment refusal; withholding treatment; Patient Self-Determination Act 1990; Uniform Rights of the Terminally Ill Act; United States

Leone, Daniel A., ed. The Ethics of Euthanasia. San Diego, CA: Greenhaven Press; 1999. 88 p. (At issue: an opposing viewpoints series). Bibliography: p. 83–85. ISBN 0-7377-0004-1. BE61047.
> abortion, induced; *active euthanasia; *allowing to die; *assisted suicide; autonomy; Christian ethics; historical aspects; involuntary euthanasia; killing; legal aspects; moral policy; motivation; National Socialism; physicians; public policy; right to die; suffering; terminally ill; value of life; wedge argument; Germany; Netherlands; United States

Letvak, Richard; Pochard, Frédéric; Grassin, Marc, et al. Palliative options at the end of life. [Letters and response]. *JAMA.* 1998 Apr 8; 279(14): 1065–1067. 9 refs.

BE = bioethics accession number   fn. = footnotes   refs. = references

BE59234.
*allowing to die; artificial feeding; *assisted suicide; autonomy; beneficence; competence; conscience; cultural pluralism; double effect; *drugs; family members; food; informed consent; intention; pain; *palliative care; physicians; public policy; *sedatives; suffering; *terminal care; terminally ill; treatment refusal; *voluntary euthanasia; withholding treatment; coma; United States

McCormick, Richard A. Vive la différence! Killing and allowing to die. *America.* 1997 Dec 6; 177(18): 6-12. BE59444.
active euthanasia; *allowing to die; *assisted suicide; autonomy; ethicists; *killing; legal aspects; moral policy; physician's role; Supreme Court decisions; treatment refusal; withholding treatment; Beauchamp, Tom; Brock, Dan; Rachels, James; United States; Vacco v. Quill; Washington v. Glucksberg

McCullough, Laurence B. A transcultural, preventive ethics approach to critical-care medicine: restoring the critical care physician's power and authority. *Journal of Medicine and Philosophy.* 1998 Dec; 23(6): 628-642. 9 refs. BE62070.
*allowing to die; autonomy; beneficence; costs and benefits; *critically ill; *cultural pluralism; *decision making; family members; family relationship; futility; iatrogenic disease; institutional policies; *intensive care units; *international aspects; medical specialties; non-Western World; palliative care; *physicians; primary health care; *professional autonomy; prolongation of life; public policy; resource allocation; resuscitation; *values; withholding treatment; Confucian ethics; *preventive ethics; *China; *Hong Kong; *Japan; *Philippines; United States
This article comments on the treatment of critical-care ethics in four preceding articles about critical-care medicine and its ethical challenges in mainland China, Hong Kong, Japan, and the Philippines. These articles show how cultural values can be in both synchrony and conflict in generating these ethical challenges and in the constraints that they place on the response of critical-care ethics to them. To prevent ethical conflict in critical care the author proposes a two-step approach to the ethical justification of critical-care management: (1) the decision to resuscitate and initiate critical-care management, which is based on the obligation to prevent imminent mortality without permanent loss of consciousness; and (2) the decision to continue critical-care management, which is based on the obligation both to prevent imminent death without permanent loss of consciousness and to avoid unnecessary, significant iatrogenic costs to the patient and psychosocial costs to the family when the reduction of mortality risk is marginal. Physicians and hospitals should restore the critical-care physician's authority and power -- against prevailing cultural values, if necessary -- to control when critical-care intervention is offered, when it is recommended to continue, and when it is recommended to be discontinued and the patient allowed to die.

McDonnell, Orla. Ethical and social implications of technology in medicine: new possibilities and new dilemmas. *In:* Cleary, Anne; Treacy, Margaret P., eds. The Sociology of Health and Illness in Ireland. Dublin: University College of Dublin Press; 1997: 69-84. 13 refs. 4 fn. ISBN 1-900621-11-8. BE60509.
*allowing to die; artificial feeding; attitudes to death; autonomy; *biomedical technologies; decision making; determination of death; guidelines; infertility; killing; legal aspects; married persons; *mass media; patient advocacy; persistent vegetative state; physicians; privacy; *prolongation of life; quality of life; *reproductive technologies; *right to die; selection for treatment; self

regulation; *social impact; sociology of medicine; *values; withholding treatment; In re a Ward of Court; *Ireland

Mayo, David. Termination-of-treatment decisions: ethical underpinnings. *In:* Steinberg, Maurice D.; Youngner, Stuart J., eds. End-of-Life Decisions: A Psychosocial Perspective. Washington, DC: American Psychiatric Press; 1998: 259-281. 47 fn. ISBN 0-88048-756-9. BE60117.
advance directives; advisory committees; *allowing to die; *assisted suicide; autonomy; competence; death; *decision making; *disclosure; *double effect; drugs; historical aspects; human rights; informed consent; *intention; *killing; legal rights; palliative care; paternalism; patients; physician patient relationship; *physicians; psychiatric diagnosis; psychiatry; referral and consultation; right to die; suffering; *terminally ill; treatment refusal; values; withholding treatment; Patient Self-Determination Act 1990; President's Commission for the Study of Ethical Problems; United States

Merlino, Joseph P. The hospital ethics committee: a role for the contemporary psychoanalyst. *Journal of the American Academy of Psychoanalysis.* 1997 Summer; 25(2): 295-305. 12 refs. BE59531.
AIDS; *allowing to die; case studies; *clinical ethics committees; committee membership; *decision making; dissent; ethics consultation; *health personnel; hospitals; internship and residency; patient care team; *physician's role; physicians; *prolongation of life; *psychotherapy; terminal care

Midwest Bioethics Center. Kansas City Area Ethics Committee Consortium. Considerations regarding withholding/withdrawing life-sustaining treatment. *Bioethics Forum.* 1998 Summer; 14(2): SS1-SS8. BE61583.
advance directives; *allowing to die; autonomy; beneficence; clinical ethics committees; competence; *decision making; futility; *guidelines; health facilities; health personnel; justice; legal aspects; patients; records; resource allocation; third party consent; withholding treatment; Kansas City Area Ethics Committee Consortium; Missouri

Morrison, Mary F. Obstacles to doctor-patient communication at the end of life. *In:* Steinberg, Maurice D.; Youngner, Stuart J., eds. End-of-Life Decisions: A Psychosocial Perspective. Washington, DC: American Psychiatric Press; 1998: 109-136. 63 fn. ISBN 0-88048-756-9. BE60121.
advance directives; age factors; aged; *allowing to die; attitudes; attitudes to death; chronically ill; *communication; cultural pluralism; *decision making; diagnosis; mentally ill; minority groups; patient participation; *patients; *physician patient relationship; *physicians; primary health care; professional family relationship; prognosis; prolongation of life; *psychiatry; referral and consultation; religion; resuscitation orders; socioeconomic factors; *terminal care; *terminally ill; time factors; truth disclosure; values; withholding treatment; United States

Murphy, Donald; Buchanan, Susan Fox. Community guidelines for end-of-life care: incremental change or significant reform? *Bioethics Forum.* 1998 Summer; 14(2): 19-24. 4 refs. BE61581.
advance directives; *allowing to die; artificial feeding; congenital disorders; *decision making; dementia; dissent; ethics consultation; futility; *guidelines; *hospitals; *institutional policies; long-term care; newborns; nursing homes; palliative care; persistent vegetative state; prognosis; *public participation; *public policy; renal dialysis; resource allocation; resuscitation; *terminal care; treatment outcome; withholding treatment; *community policies; *Colorado; *Colorado Collective for Medical Decisions

Murphy, Donald J.; Barbour, Elizabeth. GUIDe

(Guidelines for the Use of Intensive Care in Denver): a community effort to define futile and inappropriate care. *New Horizons*. 1994 Aug; 2(3): 326–331. 36 refs. BE59890.

adults; *allowing to die; artificial feeding; congenital disorders; *consensus; critically ill; decision making; dementia; economics; *futility; *guidelines; health facilities; hospitals; *intensive care units; *interdisciplinary communication; legal aspects; low birth weight; newborns; palliative care; persistent vegetative state; prognosis; *program descriptions; public participation; resource allocation; resuscitation; right to die; *selection for treatment; treatment outcome; withholding treatment; *Guidelines for the Use of Intensive Care in Denver (GUIDe)

Nakata, Yoshinori; Goto, Takahisa; Morita, Shigeho. Serving the emperor without asking: critical care ethics in Japan. *Journal of Medicine and Philosophy*. 1998 Dec; 23(6): 601–615. 12 refs. BE62068.

*allowing to die; case studies; costs and benefits; *critically ill; decision making; family members; futility; *health care delivery; health insurance; hospitals; intensive care units; medical fees; moral obligations; non-Western World; patient admission; physicians; prolongation of life; resource allocation; terminally ill; *values; pragmatism; *Japan

This article is an attempt by Japanese physicians to introduce the practice patterns and moral justification of Japanese critical care to the world. Japanese health care is characterized by the fact that the fee schedule does not reward high technology medicine, such as surgery and critical care. In spite of the low reimbursement, our critical care practice pattern is characterized by continuing futile treatment for terminal patients in the intensive care unit (ICU). This apparently wasteful practice can be explained by fundamental Japanese cultural values, social factors in Japan, the availability of extensive insurance coverage, physicians' psychological factors, lack of cost-benefit considerations and the pragmatic approach the Japanese take to situations. We attempt to make some brief suggestions regarding the improvement of our critical care practices. Although we can not fully present quantitative data to support our argument, this article represents our real-world approaches to the ethical issues in the ICU in Japan.

Newton, Michael J. Precedent autonomy: life-sustaining intervention and the demented patient. *Cambridge Quarterly of Healthcare Ethics*. 1999 Spring; 8(2): 189–199. 63 fn. BE61229.

*advance directives; *allowing to die; *autonomy; beneficence; *competence; decision making; *dementia; directive adherence; family members; informed consent; *moral policy; personhood; *prolongation of life; *self concept; third party consent; time factors; treatment refusal; *personal identity; Ulysses contracts; Callahan, Daniel; Dresser, Rebecca; Dworkin, Ronald; Kadish, Sanford

Nyman, Deborah J.; Eidelman, Leonid A.; Sprung, Charles L. Euthanasia. *Critical Care Clinics*. 1996 Jan; 12(1): 85–96. 87 refs. BE59279.

*active euthanasia; *allowing to die; assisted suicide; drugs; *euthanasia; futility; guidelines; historical aspects; international aspects; involuntary euthanasia; legal aspects; moral policy; palliative care; physician's role; right to die; suffering; terminal care; trends; voluntary euthanasia; vulnerable populations; wedge argument; withholding treatment

Olick, Robert S. Deciding for Incompetent Patients: The Nature and Limits of Prospective Autonomy and Advance Directives. Ann Arbor, MI: UMI Dissertation

Services; 1996. 374 p. (2 v. in 1). 436 fn. Dissertation, Ph.D. in Philosophy, Georgetown University, Dec 1996. Order No. 9720773. BE62147.

advance care planning; *advance directives; *allowing to die; *autonomy; beneficence; case studies; clinical ethics committees; *competence; consensus; *decision making; dementia; directive adherence; ethical analysis; ethical review; ethical theory; family members; government regulation; guidelines; *intention; legal aspects; legal rights; models, theoretical; *moral policy; paternalism; persistent vegetative state; *personhood; physicians; prolongation of life; risks and benefits; standards; state government; terminally ill; *third party consent; treatment refusal; values; withholding treatment; *integrity; Cruzan v. Director, Missouri Department of Health; In re Quinlan; Patient Self-Determination Act 1990; United States

Olson, Ellen. Treatment termination in long-term care: what about the physician? What about the family? *Journal of Long Term Home Health Care*. 1997 Winter; 16(1): 14–21. 34 refs. BE62111.

advance directives; aged; *allowing to die; attitudes to death; communication; *decision making; *family members; futility; home care; hospices; *long-term care; medical education; nursing homes; *physicians; terminal care; treatment refusal; withholding treatment

O'Rourke, Kevin; Sulmasy, Daniel P.; Terry, Peter B., et al. Accuracy of substituted judgments in patients with terminal diagnoses. [Letter and response]. *Annals of Internal Medicine*. 1998 Dec 15; 129(12): 1082–1083. 4 refs. BE60077.

*allowing to die; artificial feeding; *autonomy; *decision making; *family members; *futility; patients; *persistent vegetative state; prognosis; *prolongation of life; *quality of life; risks and benefits; *third party consent; withholding treatment

Paris, John J.; Schreiber, Michael D. Physicians' refusal to provide life-prolonging medical interventions. *Clinics in Perinatology*. 1996 Sep; 23(3): 563–571. 31 refs. BE60941.

adults; *allowing to die; anencephaly; *autonomy; biomedical technologies; children; congenital disorders; *decision making; *dissent; *family members; *futility; legal aspects; moral obligations; newborns; *physicians; practice guidelines; *prolongation of life; *refusal to treat; resuscitation orders; risks and benefits; treatment outcome; values; extracorporeal membrane oxygenation; In re Baby K; United States

Pfettscher, Susan. Nephrology nurses, euthanasia, and assisted suicide. *ANNA Journal (American Nephrology Nurses' Association)*. 1996 Oct; 23(5): 524–525. 3 refs. BE62101.

*allowing to die; *assisted suicide; *attitudes; case studies; *nurses; patients; *renal dialysis; suffering; treatment refusal; voluntary euthanasia; withholding treatment

Phillips, Benjamin. The Concept of Futility in Medical Care. Ann Arbor, MI: UMI Dissertation Services; 1996 Dec. 159 p. Bibliography: p. 152–159. Dissertation, Ph.D. in Philosophy, State University of New York at Buffalo, UMI No. 9719164. BE61357.

aged; *allowing to die; autonomy; decision making; dissent; family members; *futility; human experimentation; informed consent; investigator subject relationship; killing; legal aspects; models, theoretical; *moral policy; nontherapeutic research; paternalism; patients; persistent vegetative state; physician patient relationship; physicians; placebos; prolongation of life; refusal to treat; religion; research subjects; resource allocation; rights; terminally ill; values; withholding treatment; hope; investigational therapies; In re Quinlan; In re Wanglie

---

BE = bioethics accession number   fn. = footnotes   refs. = references

Phipps, Etienne; Shelton, Wayne; Monafo, William, et al. Forgoing medical treatment in severe facial trauma. *Journal of Trauma.* 1997 Dec; 43(6): 970–974. 17 refs. BE60193.
> *allowing to die; autonomy; brain pathology; case studies; competence; *decision making; *dissent; ethicists; ethics consultation; *family members; *injuries; *patient care team; physically disabled; prognosis; *prolongation of life; *quality of life; third party consent; time factors; treatment outcome; treatment refusal; withholding treatment; *facial injuries

Potter, Robert; Emmott, Helen. Barney says "no." [Case study and study questions]. *Bioethics Forum.* 1998 Summer; 14(2): 29–30. BE61582.
> *aged; *allowing to die; communication; critically ill; *decision making; dissent; friends; goals; health personnel; *palliative care; patient care; renal dialysis; third party consent

Powell, Tia. Extubating Mrs. K: psychological aspects of surrogate decision making. *Journal of Law, Medicine and Ethics.* 1999 Spring; 27(1): 81–86. 21 fn. BE61508.
> *advance directives; *allowing to die; caring; case studies; communication; cultural pluralism; *decision making; *dissent; *emotions; *family members; *family relationship; friends; intensive care units; justice; mediation; minority groups; physicians; *professional family relationship; *prolongation of life; psychological stress; *third party consent; treatment refusal; values; ventilators; withholding treatment; absence of proxy

Preston, Thomas A. Physician involvement in life-ending practices. *Seattle University Law Review.* 1995 Spring; 18(3): 531–544. 28 fn. BE59822.
> active euthanasia; *allowing to die; *assisted suicide; attitudes to death; double effect; drugs; iatrogenic disease; intention; *killing; *knowledge, attitudes, practice; palliative care; persistent vegetative state; *physician's role; *physicians; prolongation of life; resuscitation orders; suffering; *terminal care; terminally ill; withholding treatment

Purcell, Carol. Withdrawing treatment from a critically-ill child. *Intensive and Critical Care Nursing.* 1997 Apr; 13(2): 103–107. 32 refs. BE60429.
> *allowing to die; beneficence; brain pathology; *children; *decision making; deontological ethics; disabled; futility; *intensive care units; justice; legal aspects; nurses; nursing ethics; parents; pediatrics; physicians; *prognosis; *quality of life; resource allocation; utilitarianism; ventilators; withholding treatment; Great Britain

Renal Physicians Association; American Society of Nephrology. RPA/ASN position on quality of care at the end of life. [Position paper]. *Dialysis and Transplantation.* 1997 Nov; 26(11): 776, 778–780, 782–783. 16 refs. BE60956.
> *advance care planning; advance directives; *allowing to die; assisted suicide; competence; family members; guidelines; hospices; informed consent; *kidney diseases; *organizational policies; palliative care; patient care team; *physicians; professional organizations; quality of health care; *renal dialysis; resuscitation orders; *terminal care; third party consent; treatment refusal; withholding treatment; *nephrology; *American Society of Nephrology; *Renal Physicians Association

Robb, Yvonne A. Ethical considerations relating to terminal weaning in intensive care. *Intensive and Critical Care Nursing.* 1997 Jun; 13(3): 156–162. 26 refs. BE60480.
> *allowing to die; autonomy; beneficence; case studies; decision making; disclosure; dissent; family members; futility; informed consent; intensive care units; nurses; pain; patient advocacy; persistent vegetative state; physicians; prolongation of life; quality of life; suffering; *terminal care;

> terminally ill; third party consent; treatment refusal; *ventilators; *withholding treatment

Sanders, Arthur B. Do we need a clinical decision rule for the discontinuation of cardiac arrest resuscitations? [Editorial]. *Archives of Internal Medicine.* 1999 Jan 25; 159(2): 119–121. 13 refs. BE60228.
> adults; aged; critically ill; *decision making; *futility; *hospitals; morbidity; *mortality; *patient discharge; physicians; practice guidelines; *prognosis; resource allocation; *resuscitation; *selection for treatment; time factors; *treatment outcome; *withholding treatment

Schneiderman, Lawrence J. Medical futility and aging: ethical implications. *Generations (American Society on Aging).* 1994 Winter; 18(4): 61–65. 18 refs. BE60555.
> *allowing to die; autonomy; caring; compassion; consensus; *decision making; empirical research; *futility; *goals; *medicine; moral obligations; moral policy; *patients; persistent vegetative state; *physicians; prognosis; prolongation of life; quality of life; resource allocation; resuscitation; risks and benefits; terminology; treatment outcome; truth disclosure; uncertainty; values; withholding treatment

Schneiderman, Lawrence J. The family physician and end-of-life care. *Journal of Family Practice.* 1997 Sep; 45(3): 259–262. 38 refs. BE59341.
> advance care planning; *advance directives; *allowing to die; competence; economics; family practice; hospices; palliative care; physicians; resource allocation; resuscitation orders; *terminal care; withholding treatment; United States

Scofield, Giles R. Medical futility: can we talk? *Generations (American Society on Aging).* 1994 Winter; 18(4): 66–70. 16 refs. BE60556.
> *allowing to die; autonomy; competence; *decision making; dissent; family members; *futility; informed consent; moral obligations; *patients; physician patient relationship; *physicians; resource allocation; resuscitation; rights; social dominance; terminally ill; terminology; treatment outcome; truth disclosure; uncertainty; values; withholding treatment

Shelton, Wayne. A broader look at medical futility. *Theoretical Medicine and Bioethics.* 1998 Aug; 19(4): 383–400. 18 refs. BE60160.
> *allowing to die; case studies; *common good; cultural pluralism; *decision making; democracy; *dissent; economics; family members; *freedom; *futility; goals; health care; health care delivery; justice; managed care programs; medicine; models, theoretical; obligations to society; *patient care; patients; persistent vegetative state; physicians; *prolongation of life; public policy; quality of life; resource allocation; resuscitation orders; *rights; risks and benefits; standards; statistics; technical expertise; treatment outcome; uncertainty; *values; ventilators; *withholding treatment; United States

Singer, Peter; Kuhse, Helga. More on euthanasia: a response to Pauer-Studer. *Monist.* 1993 Apr; 76(2): 158–174. 17 fn. Commentary on H. Pauer-Studer, "Peter Singer on euthanasia," p. 135–157. BE60219.
> *active euthanasia; adults; *allowing to die; death; *disabled; dissent; fetuses; infanticide; intention; *killing; *moral policy; National Socialism; *newborns; personhood; political activity; quality of life; selective abortion; suffering; *utilitarianism; value of life; withholding treatment; Austria; Germany; Singer, Peter

Singh, Meharban. Ethical considerations in pediatric intensive care unit: Indian perspective. [Editorial]. *Indian Pediatrics.* 1996 Apr; 33(4): 271–278. 16 refs. BE60186.
> *allowing to die; artificial feeding; brain death; *children; communication; costs and benefits; critically ill; death; decision making; determination of death; futility; infants;

*intensive care units; newborns; organ donation; parents; *patient care; patient care team; pediatrics; persistent vegetative state; physician patient relationship; professional family relationship; resource allocation; resuscitation; trust; withholding treatment; *India

Smith, George P. Ethical imperatives in law and medicine. Available from the author, 3600 John McCormack Rd., NE, Washington, DC 20064; 1997. 25 p. 88 fn. Derived from a lecture at the Health Center of the University of Texas, Tyler, TX, on 9 Nov 1996. BE59575.

*allowing to die; *autonomy; clinical ethics committees; communication; decision making; *futility; informed consent; legal aspects; medical ethics; moral obligations; palliative care; paternalism; persistent vegetative state; physician patient relationship; physicians; prolongation of life; quality of life; right to die; United States

Spike, Jeffrey. Brain death, pregnancy, and posthumous motherhood. [Case study]. *Journal of Clinical Ethics.* 1999 Spring; 10(1): 57-65. 9 fn. BE62707.

allowing to die; *brain death; *decision making; determination of death; dissent; ethics consultation; family members; fathers; feminist ethics; fetal development; *fetuses; health personnel; intensive care units; judicial action; moral policy; patient care; patient care team; posthumous reproduction; *pregnant women; *prolongation of life; quality of life; resource allocation; single persons; socioeconomic factors; third party consent; treatment outcome; ventilators; *withholding treatment

Spike, Jeffrey. Physicians' responsibilities in the care of suicidal patients: three case studies. *Journal of Clinical Ethics.* 1998 Fall; 9(3): 306-313. 5 fn. BE61339.

adults; advance directives; aged; *allowing to die; assisted suicide; autonomy; case studies; chronically ill; decision making; directive adherence; ethics consultation; family relationship; futility; patient care; *physician's role; physicians; *prolongation of life; resuscitation orders; right to die; *suicide; terminally ill; treatment refusal; withholding treatment

Sprung, Charles L.; Oppenheim, Arieh. End-of-life decisions in critical care medicine -- where are we headed? [Editorial]. *Critical Care Medicine.* 1998 Feb; 26(2): 200-202. 39 refs. BE62109.

*active euthanasia; *allowing to die; *assisted suicide; attitudes; autonomy; *critically ill; decision making; economics; hospitals; intensive care units; intention; international aspects; legal aspects; physician's role; physicians; right to die; suffering; terminally ill; treatment refusal; vulnerable populations; wedge argument; withholding treatment; Australia; Netherlands; United States

Steinberg, Maurice D.; Youngner, Stuart J., eds. End-of-Life Decisions: A Psychosocial Perspective. Washington, DC: American Psychiatric Press; 1998. 322 p. (Issues in psychiatry). 686 fn. ISBN 0-88048-756-9. BE60115.

adults; age factors; AIDS; *allowing to die; *assisted suicide; autonomy; children; *communication; competence; *decision making; depressive disorder; dissent; emotions; family members; family relationship; legal aspects; morality; patient care team; physician patient relationship; *physician's role; physicians; psychiatric diagnosis; *psychiatry; psychological stress; referral and consultation; *terminally ill; third party consent; treatment refusal; values; withholding treatment; rationality; United States

Swartz, Richard D.; Perry, Erica; Schneider, Carl, et al. The option to withdraw from chronic dialysis treatment. *Advances in Renal Replacement Therapy.* 1994 Oct; 1(3): 264-273. 84 refs. BE62003.

*allowing to die; autonomy; case studies; *chronically ill; communication; competence; *decision making; depressive

disorder; family members; interdisciplinary communication; legal aspects; patient care team; patients; professional patient relationship; prognosis; psychiatric diagnosis; quality of life; religious ethics; *renal dialysis; suffering; *treatment refusal

Swigart, Valerie Anne. A Study of Family Decision-Making about Life Support Using the Grounded Theory Method. Ann Arbor, MI: UMI Dissertation Services; 1994. 220 p. Bibliography: p. 212-220. Dissertation, Ph.D. in Nursing, University of Pittsburgh, 1994. BE59219.

advance directives; *allowing to die; critically ill; *decision making; *family members; *family relationship; killing; motivation; nursing research; *prolongation of life; quality of life; standards; suffering; survey; uncertainty; ventilators; withholding treatment; qualitative research

Swinburn, J.M.A.; Ali, S.M.; Banerjee, D.J., et al. Ethical dilemma: discontinuation of ventilation after brain stem death: to whom is our duty of care? *BMJ (British Medical Journal).* 1999 Jun 26; 318(7200): 1753-1754. 5 refs. BE62303.

allowing to die; brain; *brain death; case studies; determination of death; *dissent; *family members; futility; intensive care units; legal aspects; persistent vegetative state; *physicians; professional family relationship; prognosis; prolongation of life; psychological stress; resource allocation; *ventilators; *withholding treatment; Great Britain

Taylor, Carol. Medical futility and nursing. *Image: The Journal of Nursing Scholarship.* 1995 Winter; 27(4): 301-306. 37 refs. BE60687.

accountability; *allowing to die; autonomy; communication; *decision making; dissent; family members; *futility; hospitals; judicial action; lawyers; mass media; mediation; nurse patient relationship; *nurse's role; patient advocacy; patient care team; patients; physicians; professional autonomy; professional family relationship; *prolongation of life; resource allocation; values; *withholding treatment; United States

Van der Feen, Julie R.; Jellinek, Michael S. Consultation to end-of-life treatment decisions in children. *In:* Steinberg, Maurice D.; Youngner, Stuart J., eds. End-of-Life Decisions: A Psychosocial Perspective. Washington, DC: American Psychiatric Press; 1998: 137-177. 90 fn. ISBN 0-88048-756-9. BE60120.

*adolescents; age factors; *allowing to die; attitudes to death; autonomy; *children; competence; critically ill; *decision making; diagnosis; ethics consultation; family members; infants; informed consent; interprofessional relations; newborns; palliative care; parent child relationship; parental consent; *parents; patient care team; physician patient relationship; *physicians; professional family relationship; prognosis; *psychiatry; psychological stress; *referral and consultation; risks and benefits; *terminally ill; treatment refusal; trust; truth disclosure; values; withholding treatment; United States

van Walraven, Carl; Forster, Alan J.; Stiell, Ian G. Derivation of a clinical decision rule for the discontinuation of in-hospital cardiac arrest resuscitations. *Archives of Internal Medicine.* 1999 Jan 25; 159(2): 129-134. 30 refs. BE60229.

adults; age factors; aged; critically ill; *decision making; evaluation studies; *futility; *hospitals; morbidity; *mortality; *patient discharge; physicians; practice guidelines; *prognosis; resource allocation; *resuscitation; *selection for treatment; time factors; *treatment outcome; *withholding treatment; Ontario

BACKGROUND: Most patients undergoing in-hospital cardiac resuscitation will not survive to hospital discharge. OBJECTIVE: To derive a decision rule

---

BE = bioethics accession number   fn. = footnotes   refs. = references

permitting the discontinuation of futile resuscitation attempts by identifying patients with no chance of surviving to hospital discharge. PATIENTS AND METHODS: Patient, arrest, and outcome data for 1077 adult patients undergoing in-hospital cardiac resuscitation was retrieved from 2 randomized clinical trials involving 5 teaching hospitals at 2 university centers. Recursive partitioning was used to identify a decision rule using variables significantly associated with death in hospital. RESULTS: One hundred three patients (9.6%) survived to hospital discharge. Death in hospital was significantly more likely if patients were older than 75 years (P less than .001), the arrest was unwitnessed (P = .003), the resuscitation lasted longer than 10 minutes (P less than .001), and the initial cardiac rhythm was not ventricular tachycardia or fibrillation (P less than .001). All patients died if there was no pulse 10 minutes after the start of cardiopulmonary resuscitation, the initial cardiac rhythm was not ventricular tachycardia or fibrillation, and the arrest was not witnessed. As a resuscitation rule, these parameters identified all patients who survived to hospital discharge (sensitivity, 100%; 95% confidence interval, 97.1%–100%). Resuscitation could have been discontinued for 119 (12.1%) of 974 patients who did not survive, thereby avoiding 47 days of postresuscitative care. CONCLUSIONS: A practical and highly sensitive decision rule has been derived that identifies patients with no chance of surviving in-hospital cardiac arrest. Prospective validation of the rule is necessary before it can be used clinically.

Veterans Affairs National Headquarters. Bioethics Committee. Surrogate-Written Advance Directives: Report. Issued by the VA National Center for Clinical Ethics, White River Junction, VT 05009; 1996 Jan. 6 p. 9 fn. BE59266.
*advance directives; *allowing to die; *decision making; family members; federal government; institutional policies; legal guardians; patient care; patient care team; public hospitals; terminally ill; *third party consent; withholding treatment; United States; Veterans Health Administration

Walsh, Marcia K. Difficult decisions in health care: one woman's journey. [Personal narrative]. *Bioethics Forum.* 1997 Summer; 13(2): 35–37. 13 refs. 2 fn. BE59401.
*advance directives; *allowing to die; artificial feeding; attitudes; dementia; *patients; persistent vegetative state; *quality of life; terminally ill; *treatment refusal; withholding treatment

Webb, Gilbert W.; Huddleston, John F. Management of the pregnant woman who sustains severe brain damage. *Clinics in Perinatology.* 1996 Sep; 23(3): 453–464. 50 refs. BE60934.
allowing to die; autonomy; *brain pathology; economics; family members; fetal development; *fetuses; patient care; *persistent vegetative state; physicians; *pregnant women; *prolongation of life; resuscitation orders; third party consent; withholding treatment; Grady Memorial Hospital (Atlanta, GA)

Webb, Marilyn. The Good Death: The New American Search to Reshape the End of Life. New York, NY: Bantam Books; 1997. 479 p. 396 fn. Foreward by Timothy E. Quill; introduction by Joanne Lynn. ISBN 0-553-09555-2. BE60515.
advance directives; AIDS; *allowing to die; amyotrophic lateral sclerosis; artificial feeding; assisted suicide; *attitudes to death; cancer; case studies; cultural pluralism; *death; decision making; dementia; drugs; family members; family relationship; government regulation; hospices; legal aspects;

opioid analgesics; *pain; *palliative care; persistent vegetative state; physicians; psychological stress; quality of health care; regulation; right to die; standards; *terminal care; *terminally ill; treatment refusal; trends; withholding treatment; United States

Weijer, Charles; Singer, Peter A.; Dickens, Bernard M., et al. Bioethics for clinicians: 16. Dealing with demands for inappropriate treatment. *Canadian Medical Association Journal.* 1998 Oct 6; 159(7): 817–821. 39 refs. BE62360.
*allowing to die; case studies; communication; *decision making; *dissent; evidence-based medicine; *family members; *futility; legal aspects; mediation; patient care; *patients; persistent vegetative state; *physicians; *prolongation of life; *refusal to treat; resuscitation orders; standards; terminally ill; values; *withholding treatment; Canada

Weijer, Charles. Cardiopulmonary resuscitation for patients in a persistent vegetative state: futile or acceptable? [Editorial]. *Canadian Medical Association Journal.* 1998 Feb 24; 158(4): 491–493. 19 refs. BE60584.
*allowing to die; case studies; *decision making; dissent; *family members; *futility; legal aspects; organizational policies; *persistent vegetative state; *physicians; professional organizations; *prolongation of life; refusal to treat; religious ethics; *resuscitation; *resuscitation orders; risks and benefits; value of life; withholding treatment; dignity; Canada; United States

Winter, Bob; Cohen, Simon. ABC of intensive care: withdrawal of treatment. *BMJ (British Medical Journal).* 1999 Jul 31; 319(7205): 306–308. BE62455.
*allowing to die; brain death; case studies; decision making; dissent; family members; futility; *intensive care units; patients; physicians; prolongation of life; referral and consultation; treatment refusal; withholding treatment; Great Britain

Wooddell, Victor; Kaplan, Kalman J. An expanded typology of suicide, assisted suicide, and euthanasia. *Omega: A Journal of Death and Dying.* 1997–1998; 36(3): 219–226. 15 refs. BE61224.
*active euthanasia; *allowing to die; *assisted suicide; coercion; *euthanasia; health personnel; *involuntary euthanasia; legal aspects; physician patient relationship; *physician's role; *physicians; *suicide; terminology; third party consent; treatment refusal; voluntary euthanasia; United States

Woodman, Richard. BMA calls for extra safeguards for life and death decisions. [News]. *BMJ (British Medical Journal).* 1999 Jun 26; 318(7200): 1717. BE62424.
*allowing to die; *artificial feeding; *decision making; guidelines; legal aspects; physicians; professional organizations; self regulation; withholding treatment; British Medical Association; *Great Britain; Withholding or Withdrawing Life-Prolonging Medical Treatment: Guidance for Decision Making (BMA)

Youngner, Stuart J. Competence to refuse life-sustaining treatment. In: Steinberg, Maurice D.; Youngner, Stuart J., eds. End-of-Life Decisions: A Psychosocial Perspective. Washington, DC: American Psychiatric Press; 1998: 19–54. 60 fn. ISBN 0-88048-756-9. BE60122.
*allowing to die; alternatives; assisted suicide; autonomy; beneficence; communication; *competence; comprehension; *decision making; dementia; disclosure; informed consent; legal aspects; mentally ill; paternalism; *patients; physician patient relationship; *physician's role; *psychiatry; referral and consultation; risks and benefits; standards; terminally ill; *treatment refusal; values; withholding treatment; rationality; United States

---

BE = bioethics accession number   fn. = footnotes   refs. = references

Youngner, Stuart J. Medical futility. *Critical Care Clinics.* 1996 Jan; 12(1): 165–178. 31 refs. BE59285.
> *allowing to die; autonomy; communication; *decision making; disclosure; family members; *futility; goals; *hospitals; intensive care units; patient care; patients; physician patient relationship; physicians; prognosis; *prolongation of life; quality of life; resource allocation; rights; terminology; treatment outcome; trust; uncertainty; values; withholding treatment

Zawacki, Bruce E. International bioethics at the bedside. [Editorial]. *Burns.* 1997 May; 23(3): iii–iv. 6 refs. BE62457.
> *allowing to die; burns; communication; *cultural pluralism; *decision making; family members; informed consent; international aspects; *minority groups; patient care; patients; *physician patient relationship; physicians; *professional family relationship; prognosis; third party consent; truth disclosure; Canada; United States

United Kingdom Government publishes response to House of Lords report on medical ethics. [Summary of *Government Response to the Report of the Select Committee on Medical Ethics*, presented to Parliament by command of Her Majesty, May 1994]. *International Digest of Health Legislation.* 1995; 46(4): 570–572. BE62686.
> *active euthanasia; advance directives; advisory committees; *allowing to die; *assisted suicide; decision making; drugs; guidelines; legal aspects; palliative care; persistent vegetative state; *public policy; resource allocation; *terminal care; terminally ill; treatment refusal; *Great Britain; *House of Lords Select Committee on Medical Ethics

ALLOWING TO DIE/ATTITUDES

Achille, Marie A.; Ogloff, James R.P. When is a request for assisted suicide legitimate? Factors influencing public attitudes toward euthanasia. *Canadian Journal of Behavioural Science.* 1997 Jan; 29(1): 19–27. 57 refs. BE60494.
> active euthanasia; age factors; *allowing to die; competence; drugs; pain; prognosis; *public opinion; religion; right to die; socioeconomic factors; suffering; survey; *voluntary euthanasia; withholding treatment; dependency; British Columbia; *Vancouver

Cicirelli, Victor G. Elders' end-of-life decisions: implications for hospice care. *Hospice Journal.* 1997; 12(1): 57–72. 26 refs. BE59180.
> *aged; *allowing to die; *assisted suicide; *attitudes; chronically ill; comparative studies; *decision making; dementia; family members; hospices; *patient participation; physicians; *prolongation of life; *quality of life; socioeconomic factors; *suicide; survey; terminal care; terminally ill; *voluntary euthanasia; withholding treatment; Indiana

Connelly, R.J. Death with dignity: fifty years of soul-searching. *Journal of Religion and Health.* 1998 Fall; 37(3): 195–213. 58 fn. BE61218.
> *active euthanasia; advance directives; aged; *allowing to die; artificial feeding; *assisted suicide; *attitudes; consensus; depressive disorder; dissent; extraordinary treatment; health personnel; hospices; legal aspects; pain; palliative care; physicians; public opinion; public policy; *right to die; Roman Catholic ethics; Supreme Court decisions; *terminal care; *trends; ventilators; voluntary euthanasia; withholding treatment; Compassion in Dying; Cruzan v. Director, Missouri Department of Health; Death with Dignity Act (OR); Hemlock Society; In re Quinlan; *United States; Vacco v. Quill; Washington v. Glucksberg

Doukas, David J.; Gorenflo, Daniel W.; Supanich,

Barbara. Primary care physician attitudes and values toward end-of-life care and physician-assisted death. *Ethics and Behavior.* 1999; 9(3): 219–230. 12 refs. BE62083.
> *active euthanasia; advance directives; *allowing to die; *assisted suicide; *attitudes; family practice; internal medicine; *physicians; *primary health care; survey; *values; Michigan

This study explores how primary care physician attitudes toward physician-assisted death (PAD) are related to their personal values toward end-of-life care and PAD. A group of 810 Michigan family physicians, internists, and general practitioners, divided into 4 typology groups by their intention toward participating in PAD, rated their attitudes toward PAD, along with their values and preferences for their own end-of-life care. Respondents who most objected to PAD were less likely to have executed an advance directive and more likely to have values promoting continued life-sustaining treatment in their own terminal care. Furthermore, a significant number of physicians, who had strong values against their own withdrawal of treatment in terminal care, were opposed to the withdrawing or withholding of life-sustaining treatment in patient care. Considerations of personal physician values are relevant in the discussion of PAD and the withdrawal of treatment in terminal care.

Gramelspacher, Gregory P.; Zhou, Xiao-Hua; Hanna, Mark P., et al. Preferences of physicians and their patients for end-of-life care. *Journal of General Internal Medicine.* 1997 Jun; 12(6): 346–351. 33 refs. BE60248.
> advance directives; aged; *allowing to die; artificial feeding; *attitudes; chronically ill; communication; comparative studies; intensive care units; internal medicine; *patients; *physicians; primary health care; *prolongation of life; resuscitation; socioeconomic factors; survey; *terminal care; terminally ill; ventilators; withholding treatment; Indiana

Grubb, Andrew; Walsh, Pat; Lambe, Neil. Reporting on the persistent vegetative state in Europe. *Medical Law Review.* 1999 Summer; 6(2): 161–219. 270 fn. BE62172.
> advance directives; *allowing to die; artificial feeding; *attitudes; comparative studies; *decision making; diagnosis; family members; government regulation; *international aspects; judicial action; *legal aspects; legal obligations; patient care; *persistent vegetative state; *physicians; prognosis; review; survey; terminology; withholding treatment; antibiotics; *Europe; South Africa; United States

Hammerman, Cathy; Lavie, Ofer; Kornbluth, Eti, et al. Does pregnancy affect medical ethical decision making? *Journal of Medical Ethics.* 1998 Dec; 24(6): 409–413. 13 refs. BE60791.
> *allowing to die; *attitudes; comparative studies; *congenital disorders; *decision making; mother fetus relationship; *mothers; *newborns; obstetrics and gynecology; parent child relationship; physicians; *pregnant women; prolongation of life; psychological stress; religion; socioeconomic factors; survey; Israel

OBJECTIVE: We studied and compared the attitudes of pregnant women v new mothers in an attempt to confirm changing patterns of maternal response towards medical ethical decision making in critically ill or malformed neonates. DESIGN: Data were obtained by questionnaires divided into three sections: 1. sociodemographic; 2. Theoretical principles which might be utilised in the decision-making process; 3. Hypothetical case scenarios, each followed by possible treatment options. RESULTS: Pregnant women (n = 545) consistently requested less aggressive medical intervention for the hypothetical cases than did new

---

BE = bioethics accession number   fn. = footnotes   refs. = references

mothers (n = 250) [Trisomy 18: 57% v 42%; p = 0.0004; Asphyxia: 75% v 63%; p = 0.0017; Down's syndrome 81% v 62%; p = 0.0001; LBW 85% v 75%; p = 0.004]. Significant differences were also observed in the responses to the theoretical principles, with pregnant women attributing less importance to preserving life at all cost, while being more concerned with physical and emotional pain and suffering, with financial cost, and with the infant's potential for future productivity.

Hefferman, Pam; Heilig, Steve. Giving "moral distress" a voice: ethical concerns among neonatal intensive care unit personnel. *Cambridge Quarterly of Healthcare Ethics.* 1999 Spring; 8(2): 173-178. 5 fn. BE61234.
    allowing to die; *attitudes; biomedical technologies; *decision making; disabled; disclosure; futility; *intensive care units; *low birth weight; morbidity; mortality; *newborns; *nurses; parental consent; parents; patient care; physicians; practice guidelines; *prematurity; *prognosis; *prolongation of life; *psychological stress; *quality of life; *resuscitation; *selection for treatment; survey; *treatment outcome; ventilators; *viability; withholding treatment; neonatology; qualitative research; California; California Pacific Medical Center

Hermann, Robert; Méhes, Károly. Physicians' attitudes regarding Down syndrome. *Journal of Child Neurology.* 1996 Jan; 11(1): 66-69. 15 refs. BE60189.
    active euthanasia; *allowing to die; *attitudes; children; clinical ethics committees; comparative studies; congenital disorders; *decision making; *Down syndrome; education; international aspects; medical specialties; mentally retarded; *newborns; nurses; parents; *patient care; pediatrics; *physicians; *prolongation of life; quality of life; selection for treatment; *surgery; survey; *withholding treatment; neurology; Canada; *Hungary

Hoffmann, Diane E.; Zimmerman, Sheryl Itkin; Tompkins, Catherine. How close is enough? Family relationships and attitudes toward advance directives and life-sustaining treatments. *Journal of Ethics, Law, and Aging.* 1997 Spring-Summer; 3(1): 5-24. 33 fn. BE59201.
    *advance directives; age factors; *aged; *allowing to die; artificial feeding; blacks; communication; comparative studies; dementia; education; family members; *family relationship; females; geographic factors; *knowledge, attitudes, practice; lawyers; *living wills; males; motivation; persistent vegetative state; physicians; *prolongation of life; resuscitation; *social interaction; *socioeconomic factors; survey; terminally ill; third party consent; ventilators; whites; *withholding treatment; *adult offspring; Baltimore

Kunene, Sibusiso Sixtus; Zungu, Busie Maya. An investigation into the attitude of professional nurses towards euthanasia. *Curationis.* 1996 Dec; 19(4): 26-30. 8 refs. BE61435.
    *active euthanasia; adults; age factors; aged; *allowing to die; *attitudes; congenital disorders; decision making; drugs; family members; hospitals; newborns; *nurses; nursing research; prolongation of life; resuscitation orders; survey; terminal care; withholding treatment; *KwaZulu-Natal; *South Africa

Lee, Melinda A.; Smith, David M.; Fenn, Darien S., et al. Do patients' treatment decisions match advance statements of their preferences? *Journal of Clinical Ethics.* 1998 Fall; 9(3): 258-262. 10 fn. BE61334.
    *advance directives; aged; *allowing to die; artificial feeding; *attitudes; comparative studies; critically ill; *decision making; evaluation studies; males; medical records; *patients; *prolongation of life; renal dialysis; resuscitation; resuscitation orders; third party consent; time factors; treatment refusal; ventilators; withholding treatment; retrospective studies; Portland VA Medical Center

(Portland, OR)

Leggat, John E.; Swartz, Richard D.; Port, Friedrich K. Withdrawal from dialysis: a review with an emphasis on the black experience. *Advances in Renal Replacement Therapy.* 1997 Jan; 4(1): 22-29. 44 refs. BE60177.
    advance directives; age factors; aged; *allowing to die; attitudes to death; *blacks; communication; comparative studies; cultural pluralism; decision making; diabetes; family relationship; kidney diseases; *knowledge, attitudes, practice; morbidity; physician patient relationship; prolongation of life; quality of life; religion; *renal dialysis; social interaction; social worth; *socioeconomic factors; statistics; suicide; *treatment refusal; trust; *whites; *withholding treatment; United States

McHaffie, Hazel E.; Fowlie, Peter W. Life, Death and Decisions: Doctors and Nurses Reflect on Neonatal Practice. Hale, Cheshire, England: Hochland and Hochland; 1996. 294 p. 273 refs. ISBN 1-898507-55-4. BE62145.
    *allowing to die; clergy; communication; congenital disorders; *decision making; disabled; dissent; education; institutional policies; *intensive care units; interprofessional relations; *knowledge, attitudes, practice; legal aspects; *newborns; *nurses; parents; patient care; patient care team; physician nurse relationship; *physicians; practice guidelines; prematurity; professional family relationship; prognosis; *psychological stress; quality of life; referral and consultation; religion; selection for treatment; suffering; survey; terminal care; time factors; uncertainty; *withholding treatment; *neonatology; Scotland

Matzo, Marianne LaPorte. The search to end suffering: a historical perspective. *Journal of Gerontological Nursing.* 1997 Mar; 23(3): 11-17. 29 refs. BE60383.
    *active euthanasia; *allowing to die; artificial feeding; *assisted suicide; *attitudes; autonomy; historical aspects; international aspects; *nurse's role; *nurses; physicians; public policy; quality of life; religion; right to die; suffering; *suicide; terminal care; terminally ill; trends; voluntary euthanasia; withholding treatment

Meisel, Alan; Jernigan, Jan C.; Youngner, Stuart J. Prosecutors and end-of-life decision making. *Archives of Internal Medicine.* 1999 May 24; 159(10): 1089-1095. 22 refs. BE61391.
    active euthanasia; *allowing to die; artificial feeding; *assisted suicide; *attitudes; *criminal law; decision making; drugs; hospitals; killing; *knowledge, attitudes, practice; law enforcement; *lawyers; *legal liability; morality; *opioid analgesics; *palliative care; persistent vegetative state; *physicians; prolongation of life; right to die; survey; *terminal care; terminally ill; third party consent; ventilators; withholding treatment; *prosecutors; *United States
    OBJECTIVE: To examine personal beliefs and professional behavior of state criminal prosecutors toward end-of-life decisions. DESIGN: Mail survey. SETTING: District attorney offices nationwide. PARTICIPANTS: All prosecuting attorneys who are members of the National District Attorneys Association. A total of 2844 surveys were mailed with 2 follow-up mailings at 6-week intervals; 761 surveys were returned for a response rate of 26.8%. The majority of respondents were white men, Protestant, and served in rural areas. INTERVENTIONS: None. MAIN OUTCOME MEASURES: On the basis of 4 case scenarios, (1) professional behavior as determined by respondents' willingness to prosecute and what criminal charges they would seek; and (2) personal beliefs as determined by whether prosecutors believed the physicians' actions were morally wrong and whether they would want the same action taken if they were in the patient's condition. RESULTS: Most respondents

---

BE = bioethics accession number   fn. = footnotes   refs. = references

would not seek prosecution in 3 of the 4 cases. In the fourth case, involving physician-assisted suicide, only about one third of the respondents said that they definitely would prosecute. Those who would prosecute would most often seek a charge of criminal homicide. A majority of respondents believed that the physicians' actions were morally correct in each of the 4 cases and would want the same action taken if they were in the patient's position. There was a strong correlation between personal beliefs and professional behaviors. CONCLUSIONS: A large majority of responding prosecutors were unwilling to prosecute physicians in cases that clearly fall within currently accepted legal and professional boundaries. In the case of physician-assisted suicide, results reflected a surprisingly large professional unwillingness to prosecute and an even greater personal acceptance of physician-assisted suicide.

O'Rourke, Kevin. Surrogate decision making: ethical issues. *Health Care Ethics USA.* 1998 Summer; 6(3): 2-3. 6 refs. BE60820.
   allowing to die; *attitudes; consensus; *decision making; dementia; family members; futility; patients; persistent vegetative state; physicians; prognosis; *prolongation of life; terminally ill; *third party consent; values; withholding treatment

Rubenstein, Jeffrey S.; Unti, Sharon M.; Winter, Robert J. Pediatric resident attitudes about technologic support of vegetative patients and the effects of parental input -- a longitudinal study. *Pediatrics.* 1994 Jul; 94(1): 8-12. 8 refs. BE61307.
   *allowing to die; artificial feeding; *attitudes; *children; decision making; evaluation studies; *internship and residency; parents; *pediatrics; *persistent vegetative state; *physicians; prolongation of life; resuscitation; survey; *time factors; ventilators; withholding treatment; Chicago

Schlomann, Pamela; Fister, Susan. Parental perspectives related to decision-making and neonatal death. *Pediatric Nursing.* 1995 May-Jun; 21(3): 243-247, 254. 55 refs. BE59982.
   *allowing to die; *attitudes; attitudes to death; caring; communication; critically ill; death; *decision making; emotions; fathers; mothers; *newborns; nurses; parent child relationship; *parents; physicians; professional family relationship; survey; withholding treatment; grief; qualitative research

Shah, Nisha; Warner, James; Blizard, Bob, et al. National survey of UK psychiatrists' attitudes to euthanasia. [Letter]. *Lancet.* 1998 Oct 24; 352(9137): 1360. 5 refs. BE60797.
   active euthanasia; *allowing to die; *assisted suicide; *attitudes; *physicians; psychiatric diagnosis; *psychiatry; survey; *voluntary euthanasia; *Great Britain

Stevens, Christine A.; Hassan, Riaz. Nurses and the management of death, dying and euthanasia. *Medicine and Law.* 1994; 13(5-6): 541-554. 15 fn. BE60008.
   *active euthanasia; age factors; *allowing to die; autonomy; family members; females; guidelines; *knowledge, attitudes, practice; legal aspects; males; *nurses; pain; patients; public policy; quality of life; suffering; survey; terminally ill; withholding treatment; *South Australia

Sullivan, Mark; Ormel, Johan; Kempen, G.I.J.M., et al. Beliefs concerning death, dying, and hastening death among older, functionally impaired Dutch adults: a one-year longitudinal study. *Journal of the American Geriatrics Society.* 1998 Oct; 46(10): 1251-1257. 26 refs. BE62265.

*active euthanasia; age factors; *aged; *allowing to die; *assisted suicide; *attitudes; *attitudes to death; chronically ill; decision making; dementia; health; involuntary euthanasia; mental health; mentally ill; *persistent vegetative state; *physically disabled; psychological stress; religion; socioeconomic factors; suffering; survey; time factors; withholding treatment; dependency; *Netherlands

Wenger, Neil; Kagawa-Singer, Marjorie; Bito, Seiji, et al. End of life decision making model of Japanese Americans. [Abstract]. *Abstract Book/Association for Health Services Research.* 1997; 14: 256. BE60677.
   *advance care planning; *allowing to die; *Asian Americans; *attitudes; *decision making; family members; friends; physicians; survey; terminal care; Los Angeles

ALLOWING TO DIE/INFANTS

Appleyard, James. Withdrawal of treatment in children. [Letter]. *Journal of Medical Ethics.* 1998 Oct; 24(5): 350. BE60978.
   active euthanasia; *allowing to die; *decision making; drugs; futility; guidelines; *infants; *newborns; *organizational policies; parents; patient care team; *physicians; professional organizations; prognosis; *prolongation of life; risks and benefits; uncertainty; ventilators; *withholding treatment; *British Medical Association; *Great Britain; *Royal College of Paediatrics and Child Health

Burton, Laurel Arthur; Tarlos-Benka, Judy. Grief-driven ethical decision-making. *Journal of Religion and Health.* 1997 Winter; 36(4): 333-343. 10 fn. BE60600.
   *allowing to die; attitudes to death; blacks; case studies; consensus; cultural pluralism; *decision making; disadvantaged; *emotions; *family members; family relationship; females; futility; intensive care units; males; *mothers; narrative ethics; *newborns; *patient care team; persistent vegetative state; *professional family relationship; *psychological stress; quality of life; referral and consultation; religion; resuscitation orders; values; ventilators; withholding treatment; *grief

Clark, Frank I. Making sense of State v. Messenger. *Pediatrics.* 1996 Apr; 97(4): 579-583. 20 refs. BE59983.
   *allowing to die; *communication; decision making; *dissent; fathers; institutional policies; intensive care units; killing; *legal aspects; morbidity; *newborns; parental consent; *parents; physicians; prematurity; professional family relationship; prognosis; resuscitation; standards; *treatment refusal; uncertainty; ventilators; Messinger, Gregory; Michigan; *State v. Messenger

Cooper, Rebecca; Koch, Kathryn A. Neonatal and pediatric critical care: ethical decision making. *Critical Care Clinics.* 1996 Jan; 12(1): 149-164. 53 refs. BE59284.
   *allowing to die; anencephaly; autonomy; *children; competence; congenital disorders; critically ill; *decision making; emergency care; futility; government regulation; *infants; informed consent; legal aspects; minors; *newborns; organ donation; organ donors; parental consent; *parents; paternalism; *patient care; physicians; *prolongation of life; quality of life; religion; risks and benefits; standards; suffering; surgery; treatment refusal; twins; values; conjoined twins; rationality; United States

Fitzgerald, Wendy Anton. Engineering perfect offspring: devaluing children and childhood. *Hastings Constitutional Law Quarterly.* 1997 Summer; 24(4): 833-861. 183 fn. BE62163.
   adults; *allowing to die; autonomy; behavior disorders; *children; *congenital disorders; *decision making; dehumanization; *disabled; Down syndrome; *eugenics; gene therapy; genetic counseling; *genetic determinism; *genetic disorders; genetic predisposition; genetic research;

---

hyperkinesis; *legal aspects; *newborns; *normality; *parents; *personhood; physicians; prognosis; *prolongation of life; psychiatric diagnosis; *quality of life; resource allocation; social discrimination; social worth; *surgery; terminally ill; twins; *value of life; *values; *withholding treatment; *conjoined twins; dependency; seriously ill; Hensel twins; Holton twins; Lakeberg twins; Social Darwinism; United States

Fost, Norman. Decisions regarding treatment of seriously ill newborns. [Editorial]. *JAMA.* 1999 Jun 2; 281(21): 2041-2043. 18 refs. BE61905.
   adolescents; *allowing to die; attitudes; *congenital disorders; *decision making; disabled; empirical research; ethics consultation; intensive care units; *low birth weight; *newborns; nurses; parents; *patient care; physicians; prematurity; prognosis; *prolongation of life; *quality of life; resource allocation; *selection for treatment; *treatment outcome; trends; *uncertainty; withholding treatment; neonatology; United States

Gallucci, Denise. Making decisions about premature infants. *American Journal of Nursing.* 1998 Jun; 98(6): 64, 66. 10 refs. BE61802.
   *allowing to die; communication; *decision making; intensive care units; *newborns; *nurse's role; parents; *patient care; patient care team; *prematurity; selection for treatment; treatment outcome; uncertainty

Goldsmith, Jay P.; Ginsberg, Harley G.; McGettigan, Marie C. Ethical decisions in the delivery room. *Clinics in Perinatology.* 1996 Sep; 23(3): 529-550. 47 refs. BE60940.
   active euthanasia; *allowing to die; attitudes; *congenital disorders; *decision making; deontological ethics; government regulation; health personnel; intensive care units; legal aspects; *low birth weight; moral policy; *newborns; parents; *physicians; *prematurity; prenatal injuries; *resuscitation; *selection for treatment; teleological ethics; values; viability; withholding treatment; United States

Hammerman, Cathy; Lavie, Ofer; Kornbluth, Eti, et al. Does pregnancy affect medical ethical decision making? *Journal of Medical Ethics.* 1998 Dec; 24(6): 409-413. 13 refs. BE60791.
   *allowing to die; *attitudes; comparative studies; *congenital disorders; *decision making; mother fetus relationship; *mothers; *newborns; obstetrics and gynecology; parent child relationship; physicians; *pregnant women; prolongation of life; psychological stress; religion; socioeconomic factors; survey; Israel
   OBJECTIVE: We studied and compared the attitudes of pregnant women v new mothers in an attempt to confirm changing patterns of maternal response towards medical ethical decision making in critically ill or malformed neonates. DESIGN: Data were obtained by questionnaires divided into three sections: 1. sociodemographic; 2. Theoretical principles which might be utilised in the decision-making process; 3. Hypothetical case scenarios, each followed by possible treatment options. RESULTS: Pregnant women (n = 545) consistently requested less aggressive medical intervention for the hypothetical cases than did new mothers (n = 250) [Trisomy 18: 57% v 42%; p = 0.0004; Asphyxia: 75% v 63%; p = 0.0017; Down's syndrome 81% v 62%; p = 0.0001; LBW 85% v 75%; p = 0.004]. Significant differences were also observed in the responses to the theoretical principles, with pregnant women attributing less importance to preserving life at all cost, while being more concerned with physical and emotional pain and suffering, with financial cost, and with the infant's potential for future productivity.

Hefferman, Pam; Heilig, Steve. Giving "moral distress" a voice: ethical concerns among neonatal intensive care unit personnel. *Cambridge Quarterly of Healthcare Ethics.* 1999 Spring; 8(2): 173-178. 5 fn. BE61234.
   allowing to die; biomedical technologies; *decision making; disabled; disclosure; futility; *intensive care units; *low birth weight; morbidity; mortality; *newborns; *nurses; parental consent; parents; patient care; physicians; practice guidelines; *prematurity; *prognosis; *prolongation of life; *psychological stress; *quality of life; *resuscitation; *selection for treatment; survey; *treatment outcome; ventilators; *viability; withholding treatment; neonatology; qualitative research; California; California Pacific Medical Center

Hermann, Robert; Méhes, Károly. Physicians' attitudes regarding Down syndrome. *Journal of Child Neurology.* 1996 Jan; 11(1): 66-69. 15 refs. BE60189.
   active euthanasia; *allowing to die; *attitudes; children; clinical ethics committees; comparative studies; congenital disorders; *decision making; *Down syndrome; education; international aspects; medical specialties; mentally retarded; *newborns; nurses; parents; *patient care; pediatrics; *physicians; *prolongation of life; quality of life; selection for treatment; *surgery; survey; *withholding treatment; neurology; Canada; *Hungary

Howe, Edmund G. Treating infants who may die. *Journal of Clinical Ethics.* 1998 Fall; 9(3): 215-224. 25 fn. Commentary on C. Jones and J.M. Freeman, "Decision making in the nursery: an ethical dilemma," p. 314-322. BE61330.
   *allowing to die; attitudes; autonomy; case studies; coercion; communication; *critically ill; *decision making; disclosure; drug abuse; emotions; *health personnel; injuries; *newborns; *parents; paternalism; *patient care; professional family relationship; psychological stress; risks and benefits; socioeconomic factors; suffering; treatment refusal; analgesia; extracorporeal membrane oxygenation

Jain, Renu; Thomasma, David C.; Ragas, Rasa. Ethical challenges in the treatment of infants of drug-abusing mothers. *Cambridge Quarterly of Healthcare Ethics.* 1999 Spring; 8(2): 179-188. 37 fn. BE61235.
   *allowing to die; child abuse; *children; *congenital disorders; contraception; criminal law; *decision making; disabled; *drug abuse; federal government; futility; government regulation; infants; intensive care units; legal aspects; *low birth weight; mandatory programs; medical ethics; *mothers; *newborns; nursing ethics; *obligations of society; parents; paternalism; patient care; physicians; *pregnant women; *prematurity; *prenatal injuries; *prognosis; *prolongation of life; public policy; *quality of life; rehabilitation; *resuscitation; *selection for treatment; social discrimination; *social problems; standards; state government; treatment refusal; uncertainty; value of life; withholding treatment; United States

Jones, Charlotte; Freeman, John M. Decision making in the nursery: an ethical dilemma. *Journal of Clinical Ethics.* 1998 Fall; 9(3): 314-322. 2 fn. Commented on by E.G. Howe, p. 215-224. BE61340.
   *allowing to die; autonomy; brain pathology; case studies; communication; *critically ill; *decision making; disabled; disclosure; drug abuse; intensive care units; *newborns; parental consent; *parents; patient advocacy; *patient care; *physicians; prognosis; resuscitation orders; risks and benefits; socioeconomic factors; treatment outcome; uncertainty; extracorporeal membrane oxygenation

Jones, Gary E. Do the 'Baby Doe' rules discriminate against infants? *Pediatrician.* 1990; 17(2): 87-91. 13 refs. BE59452.
   adults; *allowing to die; competence; congenital disorders; decision making; disabled; family members; federal

---

BE = bioethics accession number   fn. = footnotes   refs. = references

government; *government regulation; *legal rights; *newborns; parental consent; *quality of life; social discrimination; standards; third party consent; treatment refusal; withholding treatment; *Department of Health and Human Services; *United States

Kennedy, Ian. Child: discontinuation of treatment: Re C (A Baby). [Comment]. *Medical Law Review.* 1997 Spring; 5(1): 102–104. BE59761.
    *allowing to die; *brain pathology; decision making; *legal aspects; *newborns; pain; prolongation of life; quality of life; risks and benefits; suffering; *ventilators; withholding treatment; *Great Britain; *Re C (A Baby)

Kennedy, Ian. Child: terminal illness; withdrawal of treatment -- Re C (A Minor) (Medical Treatment). [Comment]. *Medical Law Review.* 1998 Spring; 6(1): 99–103. BE62171.
    *allowing to die; decision making; dissent; futility; *infants; *legal aspects; palliative care; parents; *physically disabled; physicians; prolongation of life; religion; suffering; *terminally ill; ventilators; withholding treatment; neuromuscular diseases; *Great Britain; *Re C (A Minor) (Medical Treatment)

Kinlaw, Kathy. The changing nature of neonatal ethics in practice. *Clinics in Perinatology.* 1996 Sep; 23(3): 417–428. 20 refs. BE60931.
    *allowing to die; anencephaly; brain death; comprehension; *congenital disorders; *decision making; determination of death; disclosure; futility; government regulation; guidelines; informed consent; *intensive care units; *low birth weight; *newborns; parents; patient care; pediatrics; physicians; professional organizations; prognosis; prolongation of life; quality of life; risks and benefits; *selection for treatment; treatment outcome; uncertainty; withholding treatment; American Academy of Pediatrics; In re Baby K; United States

Kluge, Eike-Henner W. Severely disabled newborns. *In:* Kuhse, Helga; Singer, Peter, eds. A Companion to Bioethics. Malden, MA: Blackwell; 1998: 242–249. 29 refs. ISBN 0-631-19737-0. BE59499.
    *active euthanasia; *allowing to die; *congenital disorders; decision making; disabled; moral policy; *newborns; parents; prolongation of life; *quality of life; *selection for treatment; suffering

McHaffie, Hazel E.; Fowlie, Peter W. Life, Death and Decisions: Doctors and Nurses Reflect on Neonatal Practice. Hale, Cheshire, England: Hochland and Hochland; 1996. 294 p. 273 refs. ISBN 1-898507-55-4. BE62145.
    *allowing to die; clergy; communication; congenital disorders; *decision making; disabled; dissent; education; institutional policies; *intensive care units; interprofessional relations; *knowledge, attitudes, practice; legal aspects; *newborns; *nurses; parents; patient care; patient care team; physician nurse relationship; *physicians; practice guidelines; prematurity; professional family relationship; prognosis; *psychological stress; quality of life; referral and consultation; religion; selection for treatment; suffering; survey; terminal care; time factors; uncertainty; *withholding treatment; *neonatology; Scotland

Marshall, Adam. Choices for a child: an ethical and legal analysis of a failed surrogate birth contract. [Comment]. *University of Richmond Law Review.* 1996 Jan; 30(1): 275–302. 139 fn. BE59863.
    *allowing to die; beneficence; child abuse; *congenital disorders; contracts; *decision making; *dissent; Down syndrome; *legal aspects; mother fetus relationship; *newborns; parent child relationship; *parents; standards; surgery; *surrogate mothers; withholding treatment; Americans with Disabilities Act 1990; Baby Jane Doe; Child Abuse Amendments 1984; In re Baby M; In re Conroy; Johnson v. Calvert; Superintendent v. Saikewicz; *United States

Mason, John Kenyon. Defective neonates and infants. *In: his* Medico-Legal Aspects of Reproduction and Parenthood. Second Edition. Brookfield, VT: Ashgate; 1998: 281–318. 121 fn. ISBN 1-84104-065-8. BE61069.
    *allowing to die; anencephaly; artificial feeding; children; *congenital disorders; criminal law; *decision making; dissent; double effect; Down syndrome; drugs; food; *futility; infanticide; infants; international aspects; judicial action; *legal aspects; legal liability; low birth weight; mentally disabled; *newborns; organ transplantation; parental consent; *parents; personhood; physically disabled; *physicians; prematurity; prognosis; *prolongation of life; quality of life; risks and benefits; selection for treatment; *standards; suffering; surgery; treatment refusal; value of life; ventilators; *withholding treatment; Canada; *Great Britain; In re Baby K; In re Stephen Dawson; In re T (A Minor)(Wardship: Medical Treatment); Netherlands; R v. Arthur; *United States

Muraskas, Jonathan; Marshall, Patricia A.; Tomich, Paul, et al. Neonatal viability in the 1990s: held hostage by technology. *Cambridge Quarterly of Healthcare Ethics.* 1999 Spring; 8(2): 160–172. 43 refs. BE61233.
    *allowing to die; *biomedical technologies; consensus; costs and benefits; critically ill; decision analysis; *decision making; disabled; extraordinary treatment; *futility; *intensive care units; *low birth weight; morbidity; mortality; *newborns; *parents; patient admission; patient care; *physicians; practice guidelines; *prematurity; professional family relationship; *prognosis; quality of life; resource allocation; *resuscitation; resuscitation orders; *selection for treatment; standards; *treatment outcome; treatment refusal; uncertainty; ventilators; *viability; *withholding treatment; neonatology; United States

Otten, Marc. Parents refuse to allow life-saving treatment for newborn: our moral obligation. *Princeton Journal of Bioethics.* 1998 Spring; 1(1): 61–64. 2 refs. BE62492.
    *allowing to die; *congenital disorders; decision making; killing; moral obligations; *newborns; *parents; physicians; rights; selection for treatment; *treatment refusal; wedge argument; withholding treatment

Paris, John J.; Schreiber, Michael D. Parental discretion in refusal of treatment for newborns: a real but limited right. *Clinics in Perinatology.* 1996 Sep; 23(3): 573–581. 21 refs. BE60942.
    *allowing to die; *congenital disorders; *decision making; dissent; Down syndrome; legal aspects; *low birth weight; morbidity; mortality; *newborns; *parents; physicians; prognosis; resuscitation; rights; risks and benefits; selection for treatment; treatment outcome; *treatment refusal; uncertainty; values; withholding treatment; State v. Messenger; United States

Pauer-Studer, Herlinde. Peter Singer on euthanasia. *Monist.* 1993 Apr; 76(2): 135–157. 22 refs. 42 fn. BE60218.
    abortion, induced; *active euthanasia; adults; *allowing to die; congenital disorders; death; *disabled; *dissent; ethical theory; eugenics; fetuses; infanticide; involuntary euthanasia; *killing; *moral policy; National Socialism; *newborns; pain; parental consent; *personhood; political activity; *quality of life; social worth; speciesism; *utilitarianism; value of life; voluntary euthanasia; wedge argument; withholding treatment; rationality; Austria; Germany; Rachels, James; *Singer, Peter

Peabody, Joyce L.; Martin, Gilbert I. From how small is too small to how much is too much: ethical issues at the limits of neonatal viability. *Clinics in Perinatology.* 1996 Sep; 23(3): 473–489. 75 refs. BE60936.

BE = bioethics accession number   fn. = footnotes   refs. = references

*allowing to die; congenital disorders; costs and benefits; *decision making; economics; *intensive care units; *low birth weight; morbidity; *newborns; parents; patient care; physicians; prognosis; public policy; quality of life; *selection for treatment; third party consent; treatment outcome; treatment refusal; value of life; *viability; withholding treatment; Americans with Disabilities Act 1990; United States

Raffensperger, J. A philosophical approach to conjoined twins. *Pediatric Surgery International.* 1997 Apr; 12(4): 249-255. 29 refs. BE59192.
*allowing to die; attitudes; case studies; *congenital disorders; decision making; diagnosis; double effect; futility; historical aspects; intention; killing; mass media; mental health; moral policy; mortality; organ donation; parents; physicians; privacy; prognosis; *quality of life; religious ethics; risks and benefits; *selection for treatment; *surgery; *treatment outcome; *twins; withholding treatment; *conjoined twins; Lakeberg twins; United States

Robinson, John H.; Berry, Roberta M.; McDonnell, Kevin, eds. Neonates and children. *In: their* A Health Law Reader: An Interdisciplinary Approach. Durham, NC: Carolina Academic Press; 1999: 181-238. 46 fn. ISBN 0-89089-907-X. BE62293.
*allowing to die; *anencephaly; *children; Christian Scientists; *congenital disorders; cultural pluralism; *decision making; determination of death; *disabled; futility; human experimentation; informed consent; *legal aspects; legal liability; legal rights; *newborns; nontherapeutic research; *organ donation; *parents; patient care; personhood; prolongation of life; quality of life; religion; *rights; risks and benefits; social discrimination; standards; therapeutic research; third party consent; *treatment refusal; *value of life; wedge argument; withholding treatment; Americans with Disabilities Act 1990; United States

Saigal, Saroj; Stoskopf, Barbara L.; Feeny, David, et al. Differences in preferences for neonatal outcomes among health care professionals, parents, and adolescents. *JAMA.* 1999 Jun 2; 281(21): 1991-1997. 34 refs. BE62313.
*adolescents; allowing to die; *attitudes; comparative studies; control groups; *decision making; disabled; *health; intensive care units; *low birth weight; *newborns; normality; *nurses; *parents; patient satisfaction; *physicians; *prolongation of life; *quality of life; survey; *treatment outcome; *value of life; neonatology; Canada
CONTEXT: In neonatal intensive care, parents make important clinical management decisions in conjunction with health care professionals. Yet little information is available on whether preferences of health care professionals and parents for the resulting health outcomes differ. OBJECTIVE: To measure and compare preferences for selected health states from the perspectives of health care professionals (ie, neonatologists and neonatal nurses), parents of extremely low-birth-weight (ELBW) or normal birth-weight infants, and adolescents who were either ELBW or normal birth-weight infants. DESIGN: Cross-sectional cohort study. SETTING AND PARTICIPANTS: A total of 742 participants were recruited and interviewed between 1993 and 1995, including 100 neonatologists from hospitals throughout Canada; 103 neonatal nurses from 3 regional neonatal intensive care units; 264 adolescents (aged 12-16 years), including 140 who were ELBW infants and 124 sociodemographically matched term controls; and 275 parents of the recruited adolescents. MAIN OUTCOME MEASURE: Preferences (utilities) for 4 to 5 hypothetical health states of children were obtained by direct interviews using the standard gamble method. RESULTS: Overall, neonatologists and nurses had similar preferences for the

5 health states, and a similar proportion rated some health states as worse than death (59% of neonatologists and 68% of nurses; P=.20). Health care professionals rated the health states lower than did parents of ELBW and term infants (P less than .001). Overall, 64% of health care professionals and 45% of parents rated 1 or more health states to be worse than death (P less than .001). Differences in mean utility scores between health care professionals and parents and adolescent respondents were most pronounced for the 2 most severely disabled health states (P less than .001). CONCLUSIONS: When asked to rate the health-related quality of life for the hypothetical conditions of children, health care professionals tend to provide lower utility scores than do adolescents and their parents. These findings have implications for decision making in the neonatal intensive care unit.

Schlomann, Pamela; Fister, Susan. Parental perspectives related to decision-making and neonatal death. *Pediatric Nursing.* 1995 May-Jun; 21(3): 243-247, 254. 55 refs. BE59982.
*allowing to die; *attitudes; attitudes to death; caring; communication; critically ill; death; *decision making; emotions; fathers; mothers; *newborns; nurses; parent child relationship; *parents; physicians; professional family relationship; survey; withholding treatment; grief; qualitative research

Sexson, William R.; Overall, Stephen W. Ethical decision making in perinatal asphyxia. *Clinics in Perinatology.* 1996 Sep; 23(3): 509-518. 9 refs. BE60938.
*allowing to die; brain pathology; communication; *congenital disorders; *decision making; futility; government regulation; morbidity; mortality; *newborns; palliative care; *parents; *physicians; professional family relationship; prognosis; prolongation of life; risks and benefits; treatment outcome; uncertainty; *values; withholding treatment; United States

Singer, Peter; Kuhse, Helga. More on euthanasia: a response to Pauer-Studer. *Monist.* 1993 Apr; 76(2): 158-174. 17 fn. Commentary on H. Pauer-Studer, "Peter Singer on euthanasia," p. 135-157. BE60219.
*active euthanasia; adults; *allowing to die; death; *disabled; dissent; fetuses; infanticide; intention; *killing; *moral policy; National Socialism; *newborns; personhood; political activity; quality of life; selective abortion; suffering; *utilitarianism; value of life; withholding treatment; Austria; Germany; Singer, Peter

Smith, Stacey. Parents refuse to allow life-saving treatment for newborn: the right to choose. *Princeton Journal of Bioethics.* 1998 Spring; 1(1): 58-60. 4 refs. BE62491.
*allowing to die; case studies; *congenital disorders; decision making; *newborns; *parents; physicians; prognosis; risks and benefits; standards; state interest; surgery; *treatment refusal; withholding treatment

Stevenson, David K.; Goldworth, Amnon. Commentary: neonatal viability in the 1990s: held hostage by technology. *Cambridge Quarterly of Healthcare Ethics.* 1999 Spring; 8(2): 170-172. BE61253.
advance care planning; *allowing to die; biomedical technologies; childbirth; *decision making; intensive care units; *low birth weight; *newborns; *parents; *physicians; *prematurity; prognosis; quality of life; *resuscitation; *selection for treatment; suffering; *treatment outcome; treatment refusal; uncertainty; *viability; *withholding treatment

Way, Ruth L. Seriously ill, extremely low birthweight

BE = bioethics accession number   fn. = footnotes   refs. = references

infants: ethical dilemmas of treatment. *New Zealand Medical Journal.* 1996 Oct 25; 109(1032): 391–393. 31 refs. BE60087.
*allowing to die; beneficence; clinical ethics committees; critically ill; *decision making; financial support; iatrogenic disease; intensive care units; *low birth weight; *newborns; palliative care; parental consent; parents; physicians; *prematurity; prognosis; *prolongation of life; quality of life; resource allocation; risks and benefits; treatment outcome; uncertainty; value of life; withholding treatment

Yu, Victor Y.H. Ethical decision–making in newborn infants. *Acta Medica Portuguesa.* 1997 Feb–Mar; 10(2–3): 197–204. 116 refs. BE61552.
*allowing to die; clinical ethics committees; congenital disorders; *decision making; institutional policies; *intensive care units; international aspects; low birth weight; mortality; *newborns; palliative care; parental consent; patient care; patient care team; physicians; prematurity; prognosis; quality of life; resuscitation; selection for treatment; standards; treatment outcome; uncertainty; *withholding treatment; neonatology; Australia; Monash Medical Center (Melbourne, VIC)

ALLOWING TO DIE/LEGAL ASPECTS

Annas, George J. The "right to die" in America: sloganeering from Quinlan and Cruzan to Quill and Kevorkian. *Duquesne Law Review.* 1996 Summer; 34(4): 875–897. 37 fn. BE62533.
*allowing to die; anencephaly; artificial feeding; *assisted suicide; brain death; competence; congenital disorders; *decision making; determination of death; Down syndrome; family members; futility; informed consent; *legal aspects; *legal rights; newborns; paternalism; patients; persistent vegetative state; physicians; resuscitation orders; *right to die; risks and benefits; social discrimination; standards; state government; terminally ill; third party consent; treatment refusal; ventilators; withholding treatment; Cruzan v. Director, Missouri Department of Health; In re Quinlan; *United States

Bostrom, Barry A. In the matter of the guardianship and protective placement of Edna M.F. [Note]. *Issues in Law and Medicine.* 1998 Fall; 14(2): 205–207. BE62012.
advance directives; aged; *allowing to die; artificial feeding; communication; competence; *dementia; *legal aspects; legal guardians; persistent vegetative state; quality of life; risks and benefits; third party consent; withholding treatment; oral directives; *In re Guardianship and Protective Placement of Edna M.F.; *Wisconsin

Bragg, Rick. A family shooting and a twist like no other. [News]. *New York Times.* 1999 May 19: A1, A16. BE61009.
*allowing to die; criminal law; *family members; *killing; *legal aspects; *legal liability; withholding treatment; *Egan, Shirley; *Florida; *Smith, Georgette

Bragg, Rick. Woman avoids murder charge over daughter. [News]. *New York Times.* 1999 May 26: A26. BE62346.
*allowing to die; *family members; hospitals; *killing; *legal liability; ventilators; withholding treatment; *Egan, Shirley; *Florida; *Smith, Georgette

Bridgeman, Jo. Declared innocent? *Medical Law Review.* 1995 Summer; 3(2): 117–141. 92 fn. BE59256.
abortion, induced; adults; *allowing to die; artificial feeding; competence; conscience; contraception; *criminal law; *decision making; *judicial action; *legal aspects; *legal liability; mentally retarded; minors; nurses; parental consent; persistent vegetative state; physicians; sterilization (sexual); withholding treatment; *Airedale NHS Trust v. Bland; Gillick v. West Norfolk and Wisbech AHA; *Great Britain;

Re S.G. (Adult Mental Patient: Abortion)

Brown, Lowell C.; Paine, Shirley J. Thunder from California: the *Thor* decision and the ever–expanding right to die. *HealthSpan.* 1993 Oct; 10(9): 13–17. 56 fn. BE61559.
*allowing to die; *artificial feeding; autonomy; competence; food; force feeding; *legal aspects; legal liability; legal obligations; *legal rights; paralysis; patients; *physically disabled; physicians; *prisoners; quality of life; *right to die; state interest; suicide; surgery; *treatment refusal; value of life; withholding treatment; quadriplegia; *California; California Medical Association; *Thor v. Superior Court (Andrews)

Clark, Frank I. Making sense of State v. Messenger. *Pediatrics.* 1996 Apr; 97(4): 579–583. 20 refs. BE59983.
*allowing to die; *communication; decision making; *dissent; fathers; institutional policies; intensive care units; killing; *legal aspects; morbidity; *newborns; parental consent; *parents; physicians; prematurity; professional family relationship; prognosis; resuscitation; standards; *treatment refusal; uncertainty; ventilators; Messinger, Gregory; Michigan; *State v. Messenger

Doyle, Kathy; Carroll, Alex. The slippery slope [comparison of treatment withdrawal in English and Irish law]. *New Law Journal.* 1996 May 24; 146(6745): 759–761. BE61588.
*allowing to die; *artificial feeding; *brain pathology; comparative studies; constitutional law; decision making; diagnosis; family members; guidelines; judicial action; *legal aspects; nurses; organizational policies; *persistent vegetative state; physicians; professional organizations; right to die; state interest; third party consent; treatment refusal; value of life; *withholding treatment; *Airedale NHS Trust v. Bland; British Medical Association; General Medical Council (Great Britain); *Great Britain; *In re a Ward of Court; *Ireland; Irish Medical Council; United Kingdom Central Council for Nursing, Midwifery and Health Visiting

Ferguson, P.R. Causing death or allowing to die? A rejoinder to Randall's comments. [Letter]. *Journal of Medical Ethics.* 1998 Aug; 24(4): 281–282. 3 refs. BE61702.
*active euthanasia; *allowing to die; artificial feeding; criminal law; *intention; *legal aspects; moral obligations; *persistent vegetative state; *physicians; terminally ill; withholding treatment; Airedale NHS Trust v. Bland; Great Britain; R v. Cox

Frolik, Lawrence A., ed. Health care decision making. *In: his* Aging and the Law: An Interdisciplinary Reader. Philadelphia, PA: Temple University Press; 1999: 295–394. 14 refs. 296 fn. ISBN 1-56639-653-0. BE61059.
advance care planning; advance directives; *aged; *allowing to die; *assisted suicide; attitudes; *autonomy; chronically ill; clinical ethics; coercion; communication; *competence; critically ill; cultural pluralism; *decision making; disclosure; family members; hospitals; *informed consent; judicial action; *legal aspects; mentally disabled; minority groups; nursing homes; patient advocacy; *patient care; patient care team; patients; persistent vegetative state; physicians; prolongation of life; resource allocation; resuscitation; *right to die; standards; suffering; *terminal care; terminally ill; *third party consent; treatment refusal; truth disclosure; voluntary euthanasia; wedge argument; withholding treatment; In re Fiori; In re Milton; Medicaid; Medicare; Pocono Medical Center v. Harley; Study to Understand Prognoses and Preferences for Outcomes and Risks of Treatments (SUPPORT); Uniform Health Care Decisions Act 1993; *United States

Goff, Robert. A matter of life and death. *Medical Law Review.* 1995 Spring; 3(1): 1–21. 19 fn. Text of the Cassel

---

Lecture at the University of Stockholm, 4 June 1993. BE59255.

*active euthanasia; advisory committees; *allowing to die; artificial feeding; assisted suicide; competence; criminal law; decision making; drugs; guidelines; hospices; international aspects; involuntary euthanasia; killing; *legal aspects; *legal liability; pain; palliative care; persistent vegetative state; *physicians; public opinion; public policy; right to die; suffering; *terminal care; treatment refusal; *voluntary euthanasia; wedge argument; withholding treatment; *Airedale NHS Trust v. Bland; *Great Britain; House of Lords Select Committee on Medical Ethics; Netherlands; *R v. Cox; Sweden

Grubb, Andrew. Incompetent patient in PVS: views of relatives and "best interests": Re G. [Comment]. *Medical Law Review.* 1995 Spring; 3(1): 80-84. BE59253.

*allowing to die; artificial feeding; *decision making; dissent; family members; futility; judicial action; *legal aspects; *persistent vegetative state; physicians; *risks and benefits; third party consent; *withholding treatment; Airedale NHS Trust v. Bland; *Great Britain; *Re G

Grubb, Andrew. Incompetent patient (PVS): withdrawal of feeding (Scotland) -- Law Hospital N.H.S. Trust v. The Lord Advocate. [Comment]. *Medical Law Review.* 1996 Autumn; 4(3): 300-311. BE61514.

*allowing to die; *artificial feeding; decision making; *legal aspects; *persistent vegetative state; risks and benefits; standards; *withholding treatment; Great Britain; *Law Hospital NHS Trust v. The Lord Advocate; *Scotland

Grubb, Andrew; Walsh, Pat; Lambe, Neil. Reporting on the persistent vegetative state in Europe. *Medical Law Review.* 1999 Summer; 6(2): 161-219. 270 fn. BE62172.

advance directives; *allowing to die; artificial feeding; *attitudes; comparative studies; *decision making; diagnosis; family members; government regulation; *international aspects; judicial action; *legal aspects; legal obligations; patient care; *persistent vegetative state; *physicians; prognosis; review; survey; terminology; withholding treatment; antibiotics; *Europe; South Africa; United States

Kapp, Marshall B. Commentary: anxieties as a legal impediment to the doctor-proxy relationship. *Journal of Law, Medicine and Ethics.* 1999 Spring; 27(1): 69-73. 31 fn. BE61506.

administrators; *advance directives; *allowing to die; *decision making; *dissent; emotions; family members; futility; health facilities; information dissemination; institutional policies; knowledge, attitudes, practice; legal aspects; *legal liability; malpractice; motivation; *physicians; *professional family relationship; *prolongation of life; psychological stress; public policy; terminal care; *third party consent; treatment refusal; withholding treatment; risk management; United States

Kennedy, Ian. Child: discontinuation of treatment: Re C (A Baby). [Comment]. *Medical Law Review.* 1997 Spring; 5(1): 102-104. BE59761.

*allowing to die; *brain pathology; decision making; *legal aspects; *newborns; pain; prolongation of life; quality of life; risks and benefits; suffering; *ventilators; withholding treatment; *Great Britain; *Re C (A Baby)

Kennedy, Ian. Child: terminal illness; withdrawal of treatment -- Re C (A Minor) (Medical Treatment). [Comment]. *Medical Law Review.* 1998 Spring; 6(1): 99-103. BE62171.

*allowing to die; decision making; dissent; futility; *infants; *legal aspects; palliative care; parents; *physically disabled; physicians; prolongation of life; religion; suffering; *terminally ill; ventilators; withholding treatment; neuromuscular diseases; *Great Britain; *Re C (A Minor) (Medical Treatment)

Leng, Ter Kah; Sy, Susanna Leong Huey. Advance medical directives in Singapore. *Medical Law Review.* 1997 Spring; 5(1): 63-101. 77 fn. Includes the full text of Singapore's Advance Medical Directive Act 1996, p. 89-101. BE60217.

*advance directives; advisory committees; *allowing to die; autonomy; communication; comparative studies; *competence; cultural pluralism; decision making; family members; international aspects; *legal aspects; legal liability; legislation; palliative care; physicians; public participation; religious ethics; right to die; *terminally ill; treatment refusal; withholding treatment; *Advance Medical Directive Act 1996 (Singapore); Great Britain; *Singapore

Levi, Joel. Refusal of life-sustaining treatment recognized by court of law. *Medicine and Law.* 1993; 12(1-2): 191-192. BE60621.

*allowing to die; amyotrophic lateral sclerosis; decision making; Jewish ethics; *legal aspects; physicians; *right to die; terminally ill; *treatment refusal; ventilators; withholding treatment; *Israel

Linder, Douglas O. The other right-to-life debate: when does Fourteenth Amendment "life" end? *Arizona Law Review.* 1995; 37(4): 1183-1207. 138 fn. BE62218.

*allowing to die; artificial feeding; bioethical issues; *brain death; brain pathology; coercion; constitutional law; *determination of death; due process; federal government; government financing; *legal aspects; legal rights; *persistent vegetative state; *personhood; *prolongation of life; *public policy; resource allocation; self concept; state government; Supreme Court decisions; *value of life; vulnerable populations; wedge argument; *withholding treatment; *Fourteenth Amendment; *United States

Luttrell, Steven. Withdrawing or withholding life prolonging treatment: a new BMA report fills an ethical vacuum. [Editorial]. *BMJ (British Medical Journal).* 1999 Jun 26; 318(7200): 1709-1710. 4 refs. BE62366.

*allowing to die; artificial feeding; decision making; *guidelines; *legal aspects; *organizational policies; persistent vegetative state; physicians; professional organizations; quality of life; risks and benefits; *withholding treatment; *British Medical Association; *Great Britain

Masters, Brooke A. Family's life-and-death battle plays out in court. [News]. *Washington Post.* 1998 Sep 9: A1, A14. BE60325.

*allowing to die; *artificial feeding; *decision making; *dissent; *family members; *legal aspects; persistent vegetative state; prolongation of life; Roman Catholic ethics; *withholding treatment; *Finn, Hugh; *Finn, Michele; Virginia

Meisel, Alan. Legal aspects of end-of-life decision making. *In:* Steinberg, Maurice D.; Youngner, Stuart J., eds. End-of-Life Decisions: A Psychosocial Perspective. Washington, DC: American Psychiatric Press; 1998: 235-257. 45 fn. ISBN 0-88048-756-9. BE60118.

adults; advance directives; *allowing to die; assisted suicide; autonomy; blood transfusions; *competence; consensus; *decision making; double effect; drugs; family members; informed consent; intention; Jehovah's Witnesses; judicial action; *legal aspects; legal rights; legislation; living wills; palliative care; physically disabled; physicians; privacy; religion; *right to die; standards; state government; state interest; Supreme Court decisions; terminally ill; third party consent; treatment refusal; *withholding treatment; oral directives; *United States; Vacco v. Quill; Washington v. Glucksberg

New York State Task Force on Life and the Law. When Death Is Sought: Assisted Suicide and Euthanasia in the Medical Context; Supplement to Report. New

---

BE = bioethics accession number   fn. = footnotes   refs. = references

York, NY: The Task Force; 1997 Apr. 18 p. 70 fn. ISBN 1-881268-02-0. BE62735.

    *active euthanasia; advisory committees; *allowing to die; *assisted suicide; competence; double effect; due process; equal protection; government regulation; *guidelines; judicial action; *legal aspects; legal rights; opioid analgesics; pain; *palliative care; physicians; *public policy; right to die; risks and benefits; state government; suffering; terminally ill; treatment refusal; vulnerable populations; withholding treatment; *New York; *New York State Task Force on Life and the Law; United States; *Vacco v. Quill; Washington; *Washington v. Glucksberg

New York. Supreme Court, Queens County. In re Christopher. *New York Supplement, 2d Series.* 1998 May 21 (date of decision). 675: 807–810. BE62438.

    advance directives; aged; *allowing to die; *artificial feeding; dementia; *family members; hospitals; quality of life; *right to die; terminally ill; third party consent; treatment refusal; withholding treatment; oral directives; *In re Christopher; New York

The New York Supreme Court, Queens County, denied a hospital's application to perform a percutaneous endoscopic gastrostomy procedure, the surgical insertion of a feeding tube into the stomach and intestines, on a seventy-nine-year-old incompetent woman suffering from Alzheimer's disease. The patient's son refused to consent to the procedure, citing his mother's statement ten years previously that she did not wish to end up like Sunny Von Bulow. This statement satisfied the statutory clear and convincing evidence standard in evaluating an incompetent's wishes when deciding whether to refuse treatment. (KIE abstract)

Orentlicher, David. The Supreme Court and terminal sedation: rejecting assisted suicide, embracing euthanasia. *Hastings Constitutional Law Quarterly.* 1997 Summer; 24(4): 947–968. 100 fn. BE62166.

    *allowing to die; *artificial feeding; *assisted suicide; competence; double effect; drugs; *euthanasia; government regulation; *intention; involuntary euthanasia; *legal aspects; moral policy; pain; *palliative care; *physicians; right to die; *sedatives; suffering; *Supreme Court decisions; terminally ill; vulnerable populations; wedge argument; *withholding treatment; *United States; *Vacco v. Quill; *Washington v. Glucksberg

Peters, Ellen Ash. The care and treatment of the terminally ill: questions raised by *McConnell v. Beverly Enterprises-Connecticut, Inc.. Connecticut Law Review.* 1989 Spring; 21(3): 543–550. 11 fn. BE62126.

    *allowing to die; *artificial feeding; autonomy; conflict of interest; *decision making; *dissent; employment; *family members; financial support; *hospitals; lawyers; *legal guardians; nurses; nursing homes; patient care; *patients; *persistent vegetative state; physicians; professional family relationship; prolongation of life; psychological stress; *state interest; terminally ill; *third party consent; treatment refusal; *withholding treatment; Connecticut; *McConnell v. Beverly Enterprises

Peters, Philip G. When physicians balk at futile care: implications of the disability rights laws. *Northwestern University Law Review.* 1997 Spring; 91(3): 798–864. 266 fn. BE59810.

    adults; AIDS; *allowing to die; *decision making; *disabled; dissent; family members; federal government; *futility; *legal aspects; minors; patient transfer; persistent vegetative state; physician's role; *physicians; prolongation of life; *quality of life; resource allocation; selection for treatment; *social discrimination; *withholding treatment; Americans with Disabilities Act 1990; Rehabilitation Act 1973; *United States

Plachta, Michael. The right to die in Canadian legislation, case law and legal doctrine. *Medicine and Law.* 1994; 13(7–8): 639–680. 188 fn. BE59968.

    advance directives; *allowing to die; amyotrophic lateral sclerosis; assisted suicide; autonomy; competence; constitutional law; criminal law; family members; informed consent; *legal aspects; legal liability; *legal rights; legislation; living wills; minors; parents; physicians; public policy; *right to die; risks and benefits; standards; state interest; terminally ill; third party consent; treatment refusal; ventilators; withholding treatment; *Canada; Canadian Charter of Rights and Freedoms; Criminal Code of Canada; Law Reform Commission of Canada; Nancy B. v. Hotel-Dieu de Quebec; Rodriguez v. British Columbia (Attorney-General)

Robertson, Donald. The withdrawal of medical treatment from patients: fundamental legal issues. *Australian Law Journal.* 1996 Sep; 70(9): 723–746. 146 fn. BE62161.

    *allowing to die; assisted suicide; autonomy; Christian ethics; competence; conscience; decision making; double effect; *euthanasia; informed consent; intention; international aspects; involuntary euthanasia; judicial action; *legal aspects; patient care; quality of life; right to die; terminal care; third party consent; value of life; voluntary euthanasia; withholding treatment; *Australia; *Great Britain; *United States

Robinson, John H.; Berry, Roberta M.; McDonnell, Kevin, eds. Death and dying. *In: their* A Health Law Reader: An Interdisciplinary Approach. Durham, NC: Carolina Academic Press; 1999: 339–426. 64 fn. ISBN 0-89089-907-X. BE62295.

    *active euthanasia; *advance directives; *allowing to die; artificial feeding; *assisted suicide; brain death; competence; decision making; determination of death; directive adherence; *disabled; economics; freedom; intention; *legal aspects; legal liability; legal rights; living wills; moral policy; physician's role; physicians; public policy; quality of life; *right to die; risks and benefits; standards; state government; state interest; third party consent; treatment refusal; value of life; withholding treatment; wrongful life; Patient Self-Determination Act 1990; *United States

Robinson, John H.; Berry, Roberta M.; McDonnell, Kevin, eds. Neonates and children. *In: their* A Health Law Reader: An Interdisciplinary Approach. Durham, NC: Carolina Academic Press; 1999: 181–238. 46 fn. ISBN 0-89089-907-X. BE62293.

    *allowing to die; *anencephaly; *children; Christian Scientists; *congenital disorders; cultural pluralism; *decision making; determination of death; *disabled; futility; human experimentation; informed consent; *legal aspects; legal liability; legal rights; *newborns; nontherapeutic research; *organ donation; *parents; patient care; personhood; prolongation of life; quality of life; religion; *rights; risks and benefits; social discrimination; standards; therapeutic research; third party consent; *treatment refusal; *value of life; wedge argument; withholding treatment; Americans with Disabilities Act 1990; United States

Scherer, Jennifer M.; Simon, Rita J. Euthanasia and the Right to Die: A Comparative View. Lanham, MD: Rowman and Littlefield; 1999. 151 p. 270 fn. Includes tables of "Status of Right-to-Die Legislation in the U.S., by State, July 1997," and "Social Indicators, Euthanasia and Right-to-Die Regulations, Twenty Countries." ISBN 0-8476-9167-5. BE61316.

    *active euthanasia; advance directives; *allowing to die; *assisted suicide; attitudes to death; autonomy; beneficence; coercion; comparative studies; compassion; *cultural pluralism; disabled; economics; eugenics; goals; health care delivery; historical aspects; *international aspects; involuntary euthanasia; knowledge, attitudes, practice; *legal aspects; medicine; National Socialism; pain; palliative care;

    BE = bioethics accession number   fn. = footnotes   refs. = references

persistent vegetative state; physicians; political activity; *public opinion; *public policy; quality of life; religious ethics; *right to die; standards; *state government; suffering; suicide; terminal care; terminally ill; treatment refusal; value of life; *voluntary euthanasia; wedge argument; withholding treatment; Australia; Canada; China; Colombia; France; Germany; Great Britain; India; Iran; Israel; Japan; Netherlands; South Africa; Spain; Switzerland; United States

Shapiro, Robyn S. In re Edna MF: case law confusion in surrogate decision making. *Theoretical Medicine and Bioethics.* 1999 Jan; 20(1): 45–54. 22 refs. 3 fn. BE62123.
advance directives; *allowing to die; artificial feeding; competence; constitutional law; *decision making; *dementia; equal protection; freedom; judicial action; *legal aspects; legal guardians; legal rights; persistent vegetative state; *risks and benefits; terminally ill; *third party consent; withholding treatment; Fourteenth Amendment; *In re Guardianship and Protective Placement of Edna M.; *Wisconsin

Shiner, Keith. Medical futility: a futile concept? [Note]. *Washington and Lee Law Review.* 1996; 53(2): 803–848. 261 fn. BE59720.
*allowing to die; anencephaly; autonomy; brain death; competence; consensus; *decision making; dissent; family members; *futility; hospitals; *legal aspects; medical ethics; patient transfer; persistent vegetative state; *physician patient relationship; physician's role; *physicians; *prolongation of life; *refusal to treat; resource allocation; resuscitation; rights; state interest; treatment outcome; value of life; *withholding treatment; duty to die; In re Baby K; In re Wanglie; United States

Smith, George P. Death. *In: his* Family Values and the New Society: Dilemmas of the 21st Century. Westport, CT: Praeger; 1998: 217–246. 192 fn. ISBN 0-275-96221-0. BE62298.
*active euthanasia; *allowing to die; artificial feeding; *assisted suicide; attitudes to death; beneficence; double effect; extraordinary treatment; futility; government regulation; *legal aspects; legal liability; moral policy; physicians; quality of life; *right to die; Roman Catholic ethics; standards; state government; terminal care; terminology; treatment refusal; *withholding treatment; *United States

Stell, Lance K. Stopping treatment on grounds of futility: a role for institutional policy. *Saint Louis University Public Law Review.* 1992; 11(2): 481–497. 46 fn. BE62224.
advance directives; *allowing to die; clinical ethics committees; *decision making; dissent; family members; *futility; guidelines; *hospitals; informed consent; *institutional policies; *legal aspects; legal rights; patients; physicians; *prolongation of life; refusal to treat; right to die; terminally ill; third party consent; treatment refusal; *withholding treatment; In re Wanglie; United States

Stewart, J.A.D. Best interests and persistent vegetative state. [Letter]. *Journal of Medical Ethics.* 1998 Oct; 24(5): 350. 1 ref. BE61704.
*allowing to die; *decision making; family members; futility; *legal aspects; *persistent vegetative state; physicians; *standards; withholding treatment; England

Advance directive; notification; negligence; life prolongation; damages -- Allore v. Flower Hospital. *Mental and Physical Disability Law Reporter.* 1997 Sep–Oct; 21(5): 597. Synopsis of an unpublished 27 Jun 1997 opinion of the Ohio Court of Appeals; Ohio rule applies. BE59845.
*advance directives; allowing to die; *directive adherence; *hospitals; *legal liability; negligence; *physicians; *prolongation of life; withholding treatment; *Allore v. Flower Hospital; *Ohio

ALLOWING TO DIE/RELIGIOUS ASPECTS

Cohen, Lynne. Jewish and secular medical ethics share themes but diverge on issues such as heroic measures. *Canadian Medical Association Journal.* 1997 Nov 15; 157(10): 1415–1416. BE59683.
active euthanasia; *allowing to die; autonomy; bioethical issues; *euthanasia; *Jewish ethics; medical ethics; physicians; prolongation of life; secularism; treatment refusal; *value of life; withholding treatment; Rosner, Fred

Conner, Paul. Euthanasia -- why not? *Rhode Island Medicine.* 1993 Dec; 76(12): 595–599. Commentary on D.W. Brock, "Euthanasia," p. 585–589. Reprinted from *Providence*, 1993; 1: 241. BE59413.
advance directives; *allowing to die; artificial feeding; assisted suicide; attitudes; economics; *euthanasia; extraordinary treatment; *killing; persistent vegetative state; right to die; *Roman Catholic ethics; suffering; treatment refusal; *value of life; withholding treatment; United States

Cutter, William. Rabbi Judah's handmaid: narrative influence on life's important decisions. *In:* Jacob, Walter; Zemer, Moshe, eds. Death and Euthanasia in Jewish Law: Essays and Responsa. Pittsburgh, PA: Freehof Institute of Progressive Halakhah; Rodef Shalom Press; 1995: 61–87. 36 fn. ISBN 0-929699-06-8. BE60073.
*allowing to die; attitudes to death; *Jewish ethics; *narrative ethics; prolongation of life; suffering; value of life; *Reform Judaism

Jacob, Walter; Zemer, Moshe, eds. Death and Euthanasia in Jewish Law: Essays and Responsa. Pittsburgh, PA: Freehof Institute of Progressive Halakhah: Rodef Shalom Press; 1995. 204 p. (Studies in progressive halakha; v. 4). 202 fn. ISBN 0-929699-06-8. BE60069.
active euthanasia; advance directives; aged; *allowing to die; artificial feeding; assisted suicide; brain death; cardiac death; cesarean section; covenant; determination of death; drugs; *euthanasia; human experimentation; *Jewish ethics; killing; narrative ethics; nontherapeutic research; palliative care; persistent vegetative state; pregnant women; prognosis; prolongation of life; quality of life; resuscitation orders; risks and benefits; scarcity; selection for treatment; suffering; suicide; surgery; terminally ill; *theology; therapeutic research; treatment refusal; truth disclosure; value of life; ventilators; withholding treatment; Orthodox Judaism; *Reform Judaism

Jacob, Walter. End-stage euthanasia: some other considerations. *In:* Jacob, Walter; Zemer, Moshe, eds. Death and Euthanasia in Jewish Law: Essays and Responsa. Pittsburgh, PA: Freehof Institute of Progressive Halakhah; Rodef Shalom Press; 1995: 89–103. 32 fn. ISBN 0-929699-06-8. BE60074.
active euthanasia; *allowing to die; attitudes to death; historical aspects; *Jewish ethics; physician's role; *quality of life; resource allocation; suffering; *terminally ill; theology; value of life; withholding treatment; *Reform Judaism

Kopfensteiner, Thomas R. Death with dignity: a Roman Catholic perspective. *Linacre Quarterly.* 1996 Nov; 63(4): 64–75. 23 fn. BE59306.
*allowing to die; artificial feeding; *attitudes to death; biomedical technologies; caring; compassion; double effect; drugs; extraordinary treatment; metaphor; pain; palliative care; persistent vegetative state; physician patient relationship; *Roman Catholic ethics; suffering; *terminal care; terminally ill; theology; treatment refusal; truth disclosure; value of life; withholding treatment; analgesia; dignity; patient abandonment

---

BE = bioethics accession number   fn. = footnotes   refs. = references

Kravitz, Leonard. Euthanasia. *In:* Jacob, Walter; Zemer, Moshe, eds. Death and Euthanasia in Jewish Law: Essays and Responsa. Pittsburgh, PA: Freehof Institute of Progressive Halakhah; Rodef Shalom Press; 1995: 11–25. 26 fn. ISBN 0-929699-06-8. BE60071.
　　*active euthanasia; advance directives; *allowing to die; *euthanasia; historical aspects; intention; *Jewish ethics; killing; pain; suffering; terminally ill; theology; withholding treatment; *Reform Judaism

MacFarquhar, Neil. In Islam, brain death ends life support. *New York Times.* 1999 Feb 6: A6. BE60972.
　　*allowing to die; *brain death; *determination of death; famous persons; *Islamic ethics; terminally ill; ventilators; King Hussein

Nairn, Thomas A. Reclaiming our moral tradition: Catholic teaching calls us to accept the limits of medical technology. *Health Progress.* 1997 Nov–Dec; 78(6): 36–39, 42. 22 fn. BE61613.
　　*allowing to die; assisted suicide; autonomy; biomedical technologies; decision making; *extraordinary treatment; futility; prolongation of life; risks and benefits; *Roman Catholic ethics; suffering; terminal care; value of life; voluntary euthanasia; withholding treatment; United States

O'Rourke, Kevin D. Applying the Directives: The *Ethical and Religious Directives* concerning three medical situations require some elucidation. *Health Progress.* 1998 Jul–Aug; 79(4): 64–69. 33 fn. BE61616.
　　abortion, induced; *allowing to die; *artificial feeding; *contraception; double effect; drugs; fetuses; health care delivery; institutional policies; intention; methods; *persistent vegetative state; pregnant women; *rape; religious hospitals; *Roman Catholic ethics; surgery; *therapeutic abortion; withholding treatment; *ectopic pregnancy; *Ethical and Religious Directives for Catholic Health Care Services

Orr, Robert D.; Genesen, Leigh B. Medicine, ethics and religion: rational or irrational? *Journal of Medical Ethics.* 1998 Dec; 24(6): 385–387. 10 fn. Commentary on J. Savulescu, p. 382–384. BE60787.
　　cultural pluralism; decision making; futility; justice; *patient care; physicians; *prolongation of life; refusal to treat; *religion; resource allocation; social discrimination; suffering; values; atheists; rationality
Savulescu maintains that our paper, which encourages clinicians to honour requests for "inappropriate treatment" is prejudicial to his atheistic beliefs, and therefore wrong. In this paper we clarify and expand on our ideas, and respond to his assertion that medicine, ethics and atheism are objective, rational and true, while religion is irrational and false.

Paris, John J. Hugh Finn's "right to die." *America.* 1998 Oct 31; 179(13): 13–15. BE62273.
　　*allowing to die; *artificial feeding; dissent; family members; killing; legal aspects; *persistent vegetative state; prolongation of life; right to die; *Roman Catholic ethics; withholding treatment; *Finn, Hugh; Virginia

Rayner, John D. A matter of life and death. *In: his* Jewish Religious Law: A Progressive Perspective. New York, NY: Berghahn Books; 1998: 130–137. ISBN 1-57181-976-2. BE62136.
　　*allowing to die; brain death; cardiac death; *determination of death; double effect; drugs; *Jewish ethics; pain; persistent vegetative state; prolongation of life; terminally ill; value of life; withholding treatment; Orthodox Judaism; *Reform Judaism

Rayner, John D. Euthanasia. *In: his* Jewish Religious

Law: A Progressive Perspective. New York, NY: Berghahn Books; 1998: 138–143. ISBN 1-57181-976-2. BE62137.
　　*active euthanasia; *allowing to die; artificial feeding; double effect; drugs; *Jewish ethics; legal aspects; prolongation of life; suffering; suicide; terminally ill; withholding treatment; Orthodox Judaism; *Reform Judaism

Savulescu, Julian. Two worlds apart: religion and ethics. *Journal of Medical Ethics.* 1998 Dec; 24(6): 382–384. 5 fn. Commentary on R.D. Orr and L.B. Genesen, "Requests for "inappropriate" treatment based on religious beliefs," *JME* 1997 Jun; 23(3): 142–147. BE60786.
　　allowing to die; Christian ethics; cultural pluralism; decision making; futility; justice; *patient care; physicians; *prolongation of life; refusal to treat; *religion; resource allocation; social discrimination; *values; atheists
In a recent article entitled, Requests "for inappropriate" treatment based on religious beliefs, Orr and Genesen claim that futile treatment should be provided to patients who request it if their request is based on a religious belief. I claim that this implies that we should also accede to requests for harmful or cost-ineffective treatments based on religious beliefs. This special treatment of religious requests is an example of special pleading on the part of theists and morally objectionable discrimination against atheists. It also provides an excellent illustration of how different the practices of religion and ethics are.

Staitman, Mark N. Withdrawing or withholding nutrition, hydration or oxygen from patients. *In:* Jacob, Walter; Zemer, Moshe, eds. Death and Euthanasia in Jewish Law: Essays and Responsa. Pittsburgh, PA: Freehof Institute of Progressive Halakhah: Rodef Shalom Press; 1995: 1–10. 12 fn. ISBN 0-929699-06-8. BE60070.
　　*allowing to die; *artificial feeding; autonomy; covenant; *Jewish ethics; *persistent vegetative state; resuscitation orders; theology; value of life; *ventilators; *withholding treatment; *Reform Judaism

ANIMAL EXPERIMENTATION

Abrams, Judith Z.; Abrams, Steven A. The use of animals in medical research -- the health of the fetus and the newborn: a liberal halakhic perspective. *In:* Jacob, Walter; Zemer, Moshe, eds. The Fetus and Fertility in Jewish Law: Essays and Responsa. Pittsburgh, PA: Rodef Shalom Press; Freehof Institute of Progressive Halakhah; 1995: 119–130. 16 fn. ISBN 0-929699-07-6. BE61840.
　　animal care committees; *animal experimentation; animal rights; biomedical research; drugs; fetal research; fetal therapy; government regulation; *Jewish ethics; newborns; pain; speciesism; suffering; surgery; transgenic animals; Reform Judaism; United States

Anderson, Warwick P.; Perry, Michael A. Australian animal ethics committees: we have come a long way. *Cambridge Quarterly of Healthcare Ethics.* 1999 Winter; 8(1): 80–86. 1 ref. BE61146.
　　*animal care committees; *animal experimentation; animal rights; animal testing alternatives; committee membership; government regulation; guidelines; interdisciplinary communication; investigators; organization and administration; political activity; public participation; *Australia; Australian Code of Practice for the Care and Use of Animals for Scientific Purposes

Arluke, Arnold. Moral elevation in medical research. *Advances in Medical Sociology.* 1990; 1: 189–204. 22 refs.

BE = bioethics accession number　　　　fn. = footnotes　　　refs. = references

BE61626.
*animal experimentation; attitudes; emotions; investigator subject relationship; investigators; killing; social interaction; domestic animals

Arluke, Arnold; Groves, Julian. Pushing the boundaries: scientists in the public arena. *In:* Hart, Lynette A., ed. Responsible Conduct with Animals in Research. New York, NY: Oxford University Press; 1998: 145–164. 25 refs. 5 fn. ISBN 0-19-510512-5. BE62234.
*animal experimentation; animal rights; *attitudes; deception; *investigators; *political activity; public opinion; risks and benefits; survey; violence; People for the Ethical Treatment of Animals; United States

Bagla, Pallava. Animal experimentation: strict rules rile Indian scientists. [News]. *Science.* 1998 Sep 18; 281(5384): 1777–1778. BE59942.
animal care committees; *animal experimentation; *attitudes; *government regulation; guidelines; *investigators; professional organizations; research institutes; self regulation; voluntary programs; *India; National Science Academy (India)

Bagla, Pallava. Animal research: 50 monkeys taken from Indian lab. [News]. *Science.* 1999 Aug 13; 285(5430): 997. BE62569.
*animal experimentation; government regulation; laboratories; *political activity; *primates; research institutes; scientific misconduct; *India; *National Center for Laboratory Animal Sciences (Hyderabad)

Bagla, Pallava. India backs off on central control. [News]. *Science.* 1998 Dec 11; 282(5396): 1967. BE60303.
animal care committees; *animal experimentation; committee membership; government regulation; public policy; research institutes; *self regulation; universities; *India

Bagla, Pallava. New Indian rules disrupt research. [News]. *Science.* 1999 Jul 9; 285(5425): 180–181. BE62435.
*animal experimentation; *government regulation; *India

Balls, Michael. Reducing animal testing: tests matter more than what is tested. [Editorial]. *ATLA: Alternatives to Laboratory Animals.* 1997 Nov–Dec; 25(6): 613–617. 3 fn. BE59195.
*animal experimentation; drugs; *government regulation; politics; primates; statistics; toxicity; cosmetics; *Great Britain

Balls, Michael. The precautionary principle should be used with caution -- and should be applied to animal experimentation and genetic manipulation, not merely to protection of the environment. [Editorial]. *ATLA: Alternatives to Laboratory Animals.* 1999 Jan–Feb; 27(1): 1–5. 12 refs. BE62543.
*animal experimentation; animal organs; cloning; *ecology; evaluation; federal government; *genetic intervention; genome mapping; government regulation; health hazards; organ transplantation; politics; *public policy; research design; risks and benefits; standards; toxicity; transgenic animals; prudence; Great Britain; United States

Balls, Michael. The Three Rs concept of alternatives to animal experimentation. *In:* van Zutphen, L.F.M.; Balls, M., eds. Animal Alternatives, Welfare and Ethics. New York, NY: Elsevier; 1997: 27–41. 29 refs. ISBN 0-444-82424-3. BE61683.
*animal experimentation; *animal testing alternatives; historical aspects; international aspects; Great Britain; Twentieth Century; Universities Federation for Animal Welfare

Basu, Sandip K.; Rath, Satyajit. Animal experimentation rules in India. [Letter]. *Science.* 1998 Oct 16; 282(5388): 415. BE61090.
animal care committees; *animal experimentation; *attitudes; *government regulation; *investigators; *India

Beauchamp, Tom L. Hume on the nonhuman animal. *Journal of Medicine and Philosophy.* 1999 Aug; 24(4): 322–335. 28 refs. 12 fn. BE62611.
*animal rights; emotions; historical aspects; human characteristics; intelligence; moral policy; philosophy; *speciesism; rationality; *Hume, David

Hume wrote about fundamental similarities and dissimilarities between human and nonhuman animals. His work was centered on the cognitive and emotional lives of animals, rather than their moral or legal standing, but his theories have implications for issues of moral standing. The historical background of these controversies reaches to ancient philosophy and to several prominent figures in early modern philosophy. Hume develops several of the themes in this literature. His underlying method is analogical argument and his conclusions are generally favorable regarding the abilities in animals. Hume does not attribute a moral sense or capacity of judgment to animals, but he does suggest that their actions exhibit moral qualities, such as other-regarding instincts. Hume allows in-kind differences in both demonstrative reason and moral judgment, but in the domains of both causal reason and moral agency he believes there are differences of degree rather than of kind. Hume's most significant philosophical contribution was to move as far as anyone before him to a naturalistic explanation of human and nonhuman minds that invited psychological and epistemological examination of minds by using the identical methods and categories for man and beast.

Boisvert, D.P.J. Editorial policies and animal welfare. *In:* van Zutphen, L.F.M.; Balls, M., eds. Animal Alternatives, Welfare and Ethics. New York, NY: Elsevier; 1997: 399–404. 9 refs. ISBN 0-444-82424-3. BE61695.
*animal experimentation; *editorial policies; ethical review; international aspects; pain; research design; *standards; survey; analgesia

Boyd, Kenneth. Bringing both sides together. *Cambridge Quarterly of Healthcare Ethics.* 1999 Winter; 8(1): 43–45. 2 fn. BE61140.
animal care committees; *animal experimentation; biomedical research; consensus; dissent; ethical review; goals; investigators; *political activity; suffering; transgenic animals; *Boyd Group (Great Britain); Great Britain

Brennan, Andrew. Ethics, codes and animal research. *In:* van Zutphen, L.F.M.; Balls, M., eds. Animal Alternatives, Welfare and Ethics. New York, NY: Elsevier; 1997: 43–54. 20 refs. ISBN 0-444-82424-3. BE61684.
advisory committees; animal care committees; *animal experimentation; animal rights; animal testing alternatives; biomedical research; committee membership; government regulation; guidelines; intention; international aspects; investigators; *moral policy; pain; *regulation; risks and benefits; self regulation; sociobiology; *speciesism; *standards; suffering; teleological ethics; trust; universities; *Australia

Broadhead, Caren. Challenging the regulatory authorities to justify their requirements. *ATLA: Alternatives to Laboratory Animals.* 1998 Jan–Feb; 26(1): 69–70. 3 refs. BE59789.

BE = bioethics accession number   fn. = footnotes   refs. = references

*animal experimentation; *government regulation; toxicity; *domestic animals; Animals (Scientific Procedures) Act 1986; *Great Britain

Broadhead, Caren. The ethical review process. [Meeting report]. *ATLA: Alternatives to Laboratory Animals.* 1998 Jan–Feb; 26(1): 71–72. Report of a workshop held in London on 22 Oct 1997. BE59790.
animal care committees; *animal experimentation; *ethical review; government regulation; institutional policies; research institutes; universities; Great Britain

Choi, Hae Won. Koreans honor dead lab animals (who knows -- they may return). [News]. *Wall Street Journal.* 1998 Nov 10: B1. BE59320.
*animal experimentation; animal rights; *attitudes; attitudes to death; Buddhist ethics; investigators; *Korea

Cohen, Jon. Researchers urged not to inject virulent HIV strain into chimps. [News]. *Science.* 1999 Feb 19; 283(5405): 1090–1091. BE60846.
*AIDS; *animal experimentation; *HIV seropositivity; immunization; investigators; *primates; research design; risks and benefits; United States

Conn, P. Michael; Parker, James. Animal rights: reaching the public. [Editorial]. *Science.* 1998 Nov 20; 282(5393): 1417. 1 ref. BE60301.
*animal experimentation; *animal rights; information dissemination; *investigators; *political activity; risks and benefits; United States

Dalton, Rex. Salk Institute investigated after claims of inhumane research. [News]. *Nature.* 1998 Aug 20; 394(6695): 709. BE61108.
administrators; animal care committees; *animal experimentation; employment; federal government; *government regulation; interprofessional relations; investigators; research institutes; *scientific misconduct; self regulation; whistleblowing; Department of Agriculture; National Institutes of Health; Office for Protection from Research Risks; *Salk Institute; Sylvina, Teresa; United States

Daube, Jasper R. Searching for cures: the necessity of animal research. [Editorial]. *Minnesota Medicine.* 1997 Sep; 80(9): 27–29. 4 refs. BE59933.
*animal experimentation; biomedical research; education; information dissemination; political activity; United States

de Cock Buning, Tjard. Training members of ethics committees. *In:* van Zutphen, L.F.M.; Balls, M., eds. Animal Alternatives, Welfare and Ethics. New York, NY: Elsevier; 1997: 379–383. 4 refs. ISBN 0-444-82424-3. BE61692.
*animal care committees; animal experimentation; *committee membership; *education

DeGrazia, David. The ethics of animal research: what are the prospects for agreement? *Cambridge Quarterly of Healthcare Ethics.* 1999 Winter; 8(1): 23–34. 33 fn. BE61138.
anesthesia; *animal experimentation; *animal rights; animal testing alternatives; biomedical research; *consensus; *dissent; goals; health; industry; investigators; killing; moral obligations; *moral policy; pain; *political activity; primates; quality of life; regulation; risks and benefits; *speciesism; standards; suffering; United States

Dewsbury, Donald A. Is the fox guarding the henhouse? A historical study of the dual role of the Committee on Animal Research and Ethics. *In:* Hart, Lynette A., ed. Responsible Conduct with Animals in Research.

New York, NY: Oxford University Press; 1998: 18–29. 30 refs. 1 fn. ISBN 0-19-510512-5. BE62230.
*animal care committees; *animal experimentation; committee membership; conflict of interest; guidelines; investigators; organization and administration; professional organizations; psychology; American Psychological Association; *Committee on Animal Research and Ethics (American Psychological Association); Psychologists for the Ethical Treatment of Animals

Donnellan, Craig, ed. Animal experiments. *In:* Donnellan, Craig, ed. Do Animals Have Rights? Cambridge, England: Independence Educational Publishers; 1995: 1–21. ISBN 1-872995-50-0. BE59560.
*animal experimentation; *animal rights; *animal testing alternatives; biomedical research; drugs; government regulation; pain; *risks and benefits; speciesism; suffering; surgery; toxicity; Animals (Scientific Procedures) Act 1986; Great Britain

Fano, Alix. Lethal Laws: Animal Testing, Human Health and Environmental Policy. New York, NY: Zed Books; 1997. 242 p. 843 fn. ISBN 1-85649-498-5. BE60745.
*animal experimentation; animal testing alternatives; cancer; ecology; economics; federal government; government regulation; *health hazards; industry; international aspects; political activity; public policy; research design; risk; *toxicity; United States

Festing, M.F.W.; van Zutphen, L.F.M. Guidelines for reviewing manuscripts on studies involving live animals: synopsis of the workshop. *In:* van Zutphen, L.F.M.; Balls, M., eds. Animal Alternatives, Welfare and Ethics. New York, NY: Elsevier; 1997: 405–410. 4 refs. ISBN 0-444-82424-3. BE61696.
*animal experimentation; animal testing alternatives; *editorial policies; ethical review; euthanasia; *guidelines; pain; research design; standards; suffering; toxicity

Fox, Michael W. Concepts in Ethology: Animal Behavior and Bioethics. Second Edition. Malabar, FL: Krieger; 1998. 163 p. Bibliography: p. 153–160. ISBN 1-57524-044-0. BE61046.
*animal experimentation; animal rights; *behavioral research; bioethics; comparative studies; ecology; human characteristics

Frey, R.G. Medicine, animal experimentation, and the moral problem of unfortunate humans. *In:* Paul, Ellen Frankel; Miller, Fred D.; Paul, Jeffrey, eds. Scientific Innovation, Philosophy, and Public Policy. New York, NY: Cambridge University Press; 1996: 181–211. 56 fn. ISBN 0-521-58994-0. BE62746.
*animal experimentation; animal organs; biomedical research; disabled; health; killing; *moral policy; organ donation; organ transplantation; pain; patents; primates; property rights; public policy; quality of life; risks and benefits; scarcity; *speciesism; suffering; transgenic animals; *value of life; values

Galloway, John. Dogged by controversy [review of *The Brown Dog Affair*, by Peter Mason; and of *Lethal Laws: Animal Testing, Human Health, and Environmental Policy*, by Alix Fano]. [Book review essay]. *Nature.* 1998 Aug 13; 394(6694): 635–636. BE59159.
*animal experimentation; *animal rights; ecology; government regulation; health; historical aspects; legal aspects; *political activity; *Great Britain; *Lethal Laws: Animal Testing, Human Health, and Environmental Policy (Fano, A.); *The Brown Dog Affair (Mason, P.); Twentieth Century

Gallup, Gordon G.; Eddy, Timothy J. Animal facilities survey. *American Psychologist.* 1990 Mar; 45(3): 400–401.

BE = bioethics accession number   fn. = footnotes   refs. = references

BE60202.
  *animal experimentation; behavioral research; *psychology; standards; statistics; survey; *universities; *United States

Garattini, Silvio. Alternatives to animal experiments: expectations and limitations. *In:* van Zutphen, L.F.M.; Balls, M., eds. Animal Alternatives, Welfare and Ethics. New York, NY: Elsevier; 1997: 55–66. 47 refs. ISBN 0–444–82424–3. BE61685.
  *animal experimentation; *animal testing alternatives; drugs; research design

Garner, Robert. Animal research and pluralist politics: the British and American experience. *In:* van Zutphen, L.F.M.; Balls, M., eds. Animal Alternatives, Welfare and Ethics. New York, NY: Elsevier; 1997: 67–79. 16 refs. ISBN 0–444–82424–3. BE61686.
  *animal experimentation; cultural pluralism; government regulation; *international aspects; legislation; *political activity; political systems; *politics; *public policy; Animal Welfare Act; *Great Britain; *United States

Gluck, John P. Change during a life in animal research: the loss and regaining of ambivalence. *In:* Hart, Lynette A., ed. Responsible Conduct with Animals in Research. New York, NY: Oxford University Press; 1998: 30–48. 26 refs. ISBN 0–19–510512–5. BE62231.
  *animal experimentation; *attitudes; behavioral research; *education; emotions; *investigators; killing; laboratories; primates; suffering; universities; animal behavior

Gordon, Meg. Space monkeys 'were put at risk.' [News]. *New Scientist.* 1997 May 3; 154(2080): 6. BE60456.
  *animal experimentation; death; federal government; international aspects; primates; public policy; research design; aerospace medicine; *National Aeronautics and Space Administration; Russia; United States

Gruber, Franz P.; Kolar, Roman. Animal test advisory commissions: ethics committees in Germany. *In:* van Zutphen, L.F.M.; Balls, M., eds. Animal Alternatives, Welfare and Ethics. New York, NY: Elsevier; 1997: 373–376. ISBN 0–444–82424–3. BE61691.
  *animal care committees; animal experimentation; committee membership; ethical relativism; evaluation; statistics; *Germany

Guither, Harold D. The debate over animals in research, testing, and teaching. *In: his* Animal Rights: History and Scope of a Radical Social Movement. Carbondale, IL: Southern Illinois University Press; 1998: 73–85, 240–241. 50 fn. ISBN 0–8093–2199–8. BE62098.
  animal care committees; *animal experimentation; *animal rights; *animal testing alternatives; biology; biomedical research; education; federal government; government regulation; human animals; investigators; medical education; organizational policies; pain; peer review; political activity; professional organizations; research design; risks and benefits; suffering; toxicity; secondary schools; veterinary medicine; Animal Welfare Act; United States

Hagelin, Joakim; Carlsson, Hans–Erik; Hau, Jann. The use of animals in biomedical research. [Letter]. *Nursing Ethics.* 1999 Mar; 6(2): 173. BE61937.
  age factors; *animal experimentation; *attitudes; females; males; nurses; *nursing education; *students; survey; Sweden; *Uppsala University

Hart, Lynette A. Responsible animal care and use: moving toward a less–troubled middle ground. *In:* Hart, Lynette A., ed. Responsible Conduct with Animals in Research. New York, NY: Oxford University Press; 1998: 3–17. 47 refs. ISBN 0–19–510512–5. BE62229.

  animal care committees; *animal experimentation; animal testing alternatives; government regulation; guidelines; *international aspects; investigators; laboratories; organizational policies; professional organizations; *regulation; self regulation; universities; Australia; European Community; Great Britain; New Zealand; United States

Hart, Lynette A., ed. Responsible Conduct with Animals in Research. New York, NY: Oxford University Press; 1998. 193 p. 506 refs. 7 fn. ISBN 0–19–510512–5. BE62228.
  animal care committees; *animal experimentation; animal rights; animal testing alternatives; attitudes; behavioral research; ecology; emotions; international aspects; investigators; organizational policies; pain; political activity; professional organizations; regulation; suffering; animal behavior; United States

Herzog, Harold A. Understanding animal activism. *In:* Hart, Lynette A., ed. Responsible Conduct with Animals in Research. New York, NY: Oxford University Press; 1998: 165–183. 50 refs. ISBN 0–19–510512–5. BE62235.
  *animal experimentation; *animal rights; *attitudes; deontological ethics; moral obligations; *political activity; psychology; speciesism; utilitarianism

Hill, Richard N.; Stokes, William S. Validation and regulatory acceptance of alternatives. *Cambridge Quarterly of Healthcare Ethics.* 1999 Winter; 8(1): 73–79. 16 refs. BE61145.
  *animal experimentation; *animal testing alternatives; evaluation; federal government; *government regulation; information dissemination; peer review; *Interagency Coordinating Committee on the Validation of Alternative Methods (ICCVAM); United States

Hill, Ruaraidh; Stanisstreet, Martin; Boyes, Edward, et al. Animal experimentation needs dissection. [Letter]. *Nature.* 1998 Jan 8; 391(6663): 117. BE59186.
  *animal experimentation; attitudes; pain; public opinion; students; *transgenic animals; universities

Hoge, Warren. British researchers on animal rights death list. [News]. *New York Times.* 1999 Jan 10: 10. BE60225.
  *animal experimentation; *animal rights; food; investigators; killing; *political activity; prisoners; public policy; treatment refusal; *violence; Blakemore, Colin; *Great Britain; Horne, Barry

Jayaraman, K.S. Row in India over rules on animal experiments. [News]. *Nature.* 1998 Sep 10; 395(6698): 108. BE59155.
  *animal experimentation; *dissent; *government regulation; guidelines; investigators; professional organizations; research institutes; Council of Medical Research (India); *India; National Academy of Sciences (India)

Johnson, N.E.; Rusche, B. Ethics committees: how do they contribute to the Three Rs? Synopsis of the workshop. *In:* van Zutphen, L.F.M.; Balls, M., eds. Animal Alternatives, Welfare and Ethics. New York, NY: Elsevier; 1997: 391–395. ISBN 0–444–82424–3. BE61694.
  *animal care committees; *animal experimentation; committee membership; ethical review; *evaluation; *international aspects; pain; suffering

Kaiser, Jocelyn. Activists ransack Minnesota labs. [News]. *Science.* 1999 Apr 16; 284(5413): 410–411. BE62160.
  *animal experimentation; animal rights; laboratories; *political activity; *violence; *Animal Liberation Front; *University of Minnesota

---

Koenig, Robert. European researchers grapple with animal rights. [News]. *Science.* 1999 Jun 4; 284(5420): 1604–1606. Includes inset articles by R. Koenig, "Doing research under seige," p. 1605, and "Getting a measure of the problem," p. 1606. BE62272.
*animal experimentation; animal rights; animal testing alternatives; constitutional amendments; government regulation; international aspects; *investigators; *political activity; politics; primates; public opinion; statistics; *violence; *Germany; *Great Britain

Lamberg, Lynne. Researchers urged to tell public how animal studies benefit human health. [News]. *JAMA.* 1999 Aug 18; 282(7): 619–621. BE62654.
*animal experimentation; attitudes; *information dissemination; *investigators; mass media; *political activity; public opinion; *risks and benefits; United States

Langley, Gill. Animal tests and alternatives: an animal protection viewpoint. *In:* van Zutphen, L.F.M.; Balls, M., eds. Animal Alternatives, Welfare and Ethics. New York, NY: Elsevier; 1997: 347–354. 12 refs. ISBN 0-444-82424-3. BE61687.
*animal experimentation; *animal rights; animal testing alternatives; attitudes; government regulation; *political activity; *toxicity; *rodents; Great Britain

Lasley, Elizabeth Norton. Research lab to surrender chimps. [News]. *Science.* 1999 Sep 10; 285(5434): 1649–1650. BE62570.
*animal experimentation; federal government; government financing; government regulation; laboratories; political activity; *primates; research institutes; scientific misconduct; *Coulston Foundation; Department of Agriculture; National Institutes of Health; United States

Malakoff, David. Alternatives to animals urged for producing antibodies. [News]. *Science.* 1999 Apr 9; 284(5412): 230. 1 ref. BE61968.
*animal experimentation; animal rights; *animal testing alternatives; federal government; government regulation; international aspects; political activity; rodents; Germany; Great Britain; *National Academy of Sciences; *National Institutes of Health; Netherlands; Switzerland; United States

Malakoff, David. Groups sue to tighten oversight of rodents. [News]. *Science.* 1999 Feb 5; 283(5403): 767, 769. 1 ref. BE61111.
*animal experimentation; animal rights; animal testing alternatives; economics; federal government; *government regulation, investigators; *legal aspects; political activity; *rodents; Animal Welfare Act; Department of Agriculture; *United States

Medical Research Council (Great Britain). Responsibility in the Use of Animals in Medical Research: Guidance Issued by the Medical Research Council. [Pamphlet]. London: The Council; 1993 Jul. 13 p. (MRC ethics series). 10 refs. BE59217.
*animal experimentation; ethical review; *guidelines; investigators; legal aspects; regulation; research design; *standards; suffering; Great Britain; *Medical Research Council (Great Britain)

Mepham, T. Ben; Combes, Robert D.; Balls, Michael, et al. The Use of Transgenic Animals in the European Union: The Report and Recommendations of ECVAM [European Centre for the Validation of Alternative Methods] Workshop 28. *ATLA: Alternatives to Laboratory Animals.* 1998 Jan–Feb; 26(1): 21–43. 81 refs. Report on ECVAM workshop 28 held in Southwell, Nottinghamshire, England, 7–11 Apr 1997. BE59892.
*animal experimentation; animal organs; animal testing alternatives; biomedical research; *guidelines; *international aspects; methods; public opinion; regulation; risks and benefits; toxicity; *transgenic animals; agriculture; *Europe; *European Union

Minnesota Medical Association. Use and care of animals in research and teaching: MMA policy statement. *Minnesota Medicine.* 1997 Sep; 80(9): 28. Developed by the MMA Committee on Ethics and Medical-Legal Affairs and adopted by the Board of Trustees in May 1997. BE59969.
*animal experimentation; guidelines; *organizational policies; physicians; professional organizations; *Minnesota Medical Association

Motluk, Alison. Young people question vivisection. [News]. *New Scientist.* 1998 Jun 6; 158(2137): 23. BE59717.
adolescents; adults; *age factors; *animal experimentation; political activity; *public opinion; risks and benefits; *Great Britain

Munro, Lyle. From vilification to accommodation: making a common cause movement. *Cambridge Quarterly of Healthcare Ethics.* 1999 Winter; 8(1): 46–57. 50 fn. BE61142.
*animal experimentation; animal rights; animal testing alternatives; biomedical research; common good; *consensus; ecology; industry; investigators; motivation; *political activity; toxicity; Spira, Henry; United States

Nowak, Rachel. Almost human. [News]. *New Scientist.* 1999 Feb 13; 161(2173): 20–21. BE61795.
*animal experimentation; *animal rights; *human characteristics; *legal rights; personhood; *primates; speciesism; suffering; value of life; Great Ape Project; *New Zealand

Office for Protection from Research Risks Review Panel. Report to the Advisory Committee to the Director, NIH. The Panel [online]. Downloaded from Internet Web site: http://www.nih.gov/grants/oprr/references/060399b. html on 7 Jun 1999; 1999 Jun 3. 16 p. BE60825.
advisory committees; *animal experimentation; conflict of interest; ethical review; evaluation; *federal government; financial support; government financing; *government regulation; *human experimentation; *organization and administration; private sector; multicenter studies; *Department of Health and Human Services; *National Institutes of Health; *Office for Protection from Research Risks; *United States

Orlans, F. Barbara. Ethical evaluation of animal research protocols: how it can be enhanced. *In:* van Zutphen, L.F.M.; Balls, M., eds. Animal Alternatives, Welfare and Ethics. New York, NY: Elsevier; 1997: 385–390. 6 refs. ISBN 0-444-82424-3. BE61693.
*animal care committees; *animal experimentation; committee membership; *ethical review; evaluation; guidelines; *international aspects; pain; research design; risks and benefits; suffering

Orlans, F. Barbara. History and ethical regulation of animal experimentation: an international perspective. *In:* Kuhse, Helga; Singer, Peter, eds. A Companion to Bioethics. Malden, MA: Blackwell; 1998: 399–410. 13 refs. ISBN 0-631-19737-0. BE59513.
animal care committees; *animal experimentation; animal rights; animal testing alternatives; attitudes; *government regulation; historical aspects; *international aspects; investigators; pain; primates; professional competence; research institutes; risks and benefits; *standards; statistics; suffering; trends

---

BE = bioethics accession number   fn. = footnotes   refs. = references

Petrinovich, Lewis. Morality and animal research: research is...; setting research and educational policy. *In: his* Darwinian Dominion: Animal Welfare and Human Interests. Cambridge, MA: MIT Press; 1999: 239–337. Bibliography: p. 395–417. ISBN 0–262–16178–8. BE59742.
    animal care committees; *animal experimentation; animal rights; animal testing alternatives; behavioral research; biomedical research; cancer; drugs; education; ethical review; government regulation; guidelines; historical aspects; immunization; international aspects; investigational drugs; moral policy; pain; peer review; political activity; primates; professional organizations; psychology; public opinion; risks and benefits; speciesism; suffering; toxicity; value of life; cosmetics; Europe; Great Britain; United States

Reichhardt, Tony. Europe will fly animals on space station. [News]. *Nature.* 1999 Apr 22; 398(6729): 642. BE62073.
    *animal experimentation; international aspects; *aerospace medicine; rodents; *Europe; European Space Agency; International Space Station

Rollin, Bernard E. The moral status of animals and their use as experimental subjects. *In:* Kuhse, Helga; Singer, Peter, eds. A Companion to Bioethics. Malden, MA: Blackwell; 1998: 411–422. 23 refs. ISBN 0–631–19737–0. BE59514.
    *animal experimentation; *animal rights; animal testing alternatives; attitudes; behavioral research; government regulation; investigators; *moral policy; pain; risks and benefits; *speciesism; suffering; agriculture; rationality

Rollin, Bernard E. The Unheeded Cry: Animal Consciousness, Animal Pain, and Science. Expanded Edition. Ames, IA: Iowa State University Press; 1998. 330 p. Bibliography: p. 309–321. ISBN 0–8138–2576–8. BE60717.
    anesthesia; *animal experimentation; animal rights; behavioral research; government regulation; international aspects; *moral policy; *pain; philosophy; psychological stress; psychology; *science; *self concept; *speciesism; suffering; Australia; Canada; Europe; Great Britain; United States

Rose, Margaret. Animal ethics committees: do we need to re-examine their purpose? *In:* van Zutphen, L.F.M.; Balls, M., eds. Animal Alternatives, Welfare and Ethics. New York, NY: Elsevier; 1997: 361–366. 8 refs. ISBN 0–444–82424–3. BE61689.
    *animal care committees; *animal experimentation; committee membership; ethical review; international aspects; legislation; public policy; *Australia; New South Wales

Rowan, Andrew N. Scientists and animal research: Dr. Jekyll or Mr. Hyde? *Social Research.* 1995 Fall; 62(3): 787–800. 27 refs. BE59856.
    *animal experimentation; animal rights; *attitudes; biomedical research; historical aspects; *investigators; killing; literature; mass media; *public opinion; science; speciesism; Great Britain; Nineteenth Century; Twentieth Century; United States

Rowan, Andrew N. The search for animal well-being. *In:* Hart, Lynette A., ed. Responsible Conduct with Animals in Research. New York, NY: Oxford University Press; 1998: 119–131. 37 refs. ISBN 0–19–510512–5. BE62233.
    *animal experimentation; behavioral research; *pain; psychological stress; *suffering; surgery; animal behavior

Ryder, Richard D. Painism: some moral rules for the civilized experimenter. *Cambridge Quarterly of Healthcare Ethics.* 1999 Winter; 8(1): 35–42. 14 fn.

BE61139.
    *animal experimentation; animal rights; ethical analysis; goals; intention; *investigators; *moral policy; *pain; rights; self regulation; *speciesism; suffering; utilitarianism

Schiermeier, Quirin. Animal rights activists turn the screw. [News]. *Nature.* 1998 Dec 10; 396(6711): 505. BE60299.
    *animal experimentation; *animal rights; attitudes; investigators; *political activity; professional organizations; *violence; Animal Liberation Front; *Germany; *Great Britain

Shapiro, Kenneth Joel. Animal Models of Human Psychology: Critique of Science, Ethics, and Policy. Seattle, WA: Hogrefe and Huber; 1998. 328 p. Bibliography: p. 293–320. ISBN 0–88937–189–X. BE60750.
    *animal experimentation; animal rights; attitudes; behavior disorders; *behavioral research; food; investigators; political activity; *psychology; research design; risks and benefits; speciesism; suffering; utilitarianism; anorexia nervosa; bulimia

Silverman, Jerald. The use of animals in biomedical research and teaching: searching for a common goal. *Cambridge Quarterly of Healthcare Ethics.* 1999 Winter; 8(1): 64–72. 10 fn. BE61144.
    *animal experimentation; animal testing alternatives; attitudes; biomedical research; consensus; *education; financial support; goals; *investigators; *political activity; schools; speciesism; students; universities; domestic animals; rodents; veterinary medicine; United States

Singer, Peter. Ethics into Action: Henry Spira and the Animal Rights Movement. Lanham, MD: Rowman and Littlefield; 1998. 222 p. Includes references. ISBN 0–8476–9073–3. BE59739.
    *animal experimentation; *animal rights; animal testing alternatives; financial support; industry; *political activity; public policy; suffering; cosmetics; *Spira, Henry; United States

Singer, Peter. Henry Spira's search for common ground on animal testing. *Cambridge Quarterly of Healthcare Ethics.* 1999 Winter; 8(1): 9–22. 42 fn. An edited extract from P. Singer's *Ethics into Action: Henry Spira and the Animal Rights Movement,* Lanham, MD: Rowman and Littlefield; 1998. BE61141.
    *animal experimentation; *animal rights; *animal testing alternatives; consensus; drug industry; government regulation; historical aspects; *industry; mass media; pain; *political activity; research design; self regulation; suffering; toxicity; cosmetics; Europe; Great Britain; *Spira, Henry; Twentieth Century; United States

Singer, Peter. Living and dying. [Interview]. *Psychology Today.* 1999 Jan–Feb; 32(1): 56–59, 78–79. BE61518.
    *active euthanasia; allowing to die; *animal experimentation; brain death; *disabled; *ethicists; human experimentation; killing; morality; National Socialism; newborns; persistent vegetative state; primates; quality of life; speciesism; suffering; utilitarianism; value of life; *Singer, Peter

Trull, Frankie L.; Rich, Barbara A. More regulation of rodents. [Editorial]. *Science.* 1999 May 28; 284(5419): 1463. BE61571.
    *animal experimentation; economics; federal government; government financing; *government regulation; legal aspects; public policy; transgenic animals; *rodents; Animal Welfare Act; *Department of Agriculture; *United States

Turner, J.Z. I don't want to see the pictures: science writing and the visibility of animal experiments. *Public*

BE = bioethics accession number   fn. = footnotes   refs. = references

Understanding of Science. 1998 Jan; 7(1): 27–40. 95 fn. BE60904.
>*animal experimentation; animal organs; attitudes; cloning; comparative studies; *editorial policies; empirical research; *information dissemination; investigators; literature; organ transplantation; science; photography; *Economist; *Nature; *New Scientist; *Science; *Times Higher Education Supplement

Vandenbergh, John G. Animal welfare issues in animal behavior research. *In:* Hart, Lynette A., ed. Responsible Conduct with Animals in Research. New York, NY: Oxford University Press; 1998: 67–76. 23 refs. ISBN 0-19-510512-5. BE62232.
>animal care committees; *animal experimentation; behavioral research; federal government; government regulation; guidelines; standards; *animal behavior; Animal Welfare Act 1966; Guide for the Care and Use of Laboratory Animals (National Research Council); United States

van der Valk, Jan; Dewhurst, David; Hughes, Ian, et al. Alternatives to the Use of Animals in Higher Education: The Report and Recommendations of ECVAM (European Centre for the Validation of Alternate Methods) Workshop 33. *ATLA: Alternatives to Laboratory Animals.* 1999 Jan–Feb; 27(1): 39–52. 25 refs. BE62536.
>*animal experimentation; *animal testing alternatives; *education; evaluation; international aspects; public policy; teaching methods; Europe; European Community

van Zutphen, L.F.M.; Balls, M., eds. Animal Alternatives, Welfare and Ethics. New York, NY: Elsevier; 1997. 1,260 p. (Developments in animal and veterinary sciences; 27). Includes references.
Proceedings of the 2nd World Congress on Alternatives and Animal Use in the Life Sciences, held in Utrecht, the Netherlands, 20–24 Oct 1996. ISBN 0-444-82424-3. BE61682.
>animal care committees; *animal experimentation; animal organs; animal rights; *animal testing alternatives; audiovisual aids; computers; data banks; drugs; editorial policies; education; *international aspects; medical devices; moral policy; organ transplantation; pain; political activity; politics; public policy; regulation; risks and benefits; speciesism; standards; suffering; toxicity; transgenic animals; Australia; Europe; Germany; Great Britain; Japan; New Zealand; United States

Wadman, Meredith. Financial doubts over future of chimp lab. [News]. *Nature.* 1999 Apr 22; 398(6729): 644. BE62074.
>AIDS; *animal experimentation; federal government; financial support; government financing; HIV seropositivity; laboratories; misconduct; political activity; *primates; private sector; *research institutes; Animal Welfare Act; *Coulston Foundation; National Institutes of Health; United States

Wuensch, Karl L.; Poteat, G. Michael. Evaluating the morality of animal research: effects of ethical ideology, gender, and purpose. *Journal of Social Behavior and Personality.* 1998 Mar; 13(1): 139–150. 22 fn. BE62427.
>*animal experimentation; *attitudes; biomedical research; ethical relativism; females; males; motivation; *students; survey; universities; values; agriculture; cosmetics; veterinary medicine; United States

Yates, R. Animal ethics committees and the implementation of the Three Rs. *In:* van Zutphen, L.F.M.; Balls, M., eds. Animal Alternatives, Welfare and Ethics. New York, NY: Elsevier; 1997: 367–371. 2 refs. ISBN 0-444-82424-3. BE61690.
>*animal care committees; *animal experimentation;

committee membership; organization and administration; *Flinders University of South Australia; *South Australia

Zurlo, Joanne; Goldberg, Alan M. The role of an academic center in promoting common goals. *Cambridge Quarterly of Healthcare Ethics.* 1999 Winter; 8(1): 58–63. 8 refs. BE61143.
>*animal experimentation; *animal testing alternatives; consensus; federal government; industry; political activity; *research institutes; universities; *Center for Alternatives to Animal Testing (CAAT); Office for Protection from Research Risks; Spira, Henry; United States

The great divide? [Editorial]. *New Scientist.* 1999 Feb 13; 161(2173): 3. BE61794.
>*animal rights; *human characteristics; legal rights; personhood; *primates; speciesism; New Zealand

Unneccessary Fuss. [Videorecording].Available from People for the Ethical Treatment of Animals (PETA), P.O. Box 42516, Washington, DC 20015-0516, (202) 726-0156, (301) 770-7444.; 1985. Videocassette; 26 min.; sd.; color; VHS. Filmed by researchers at the University of Pennsylvania Head Injury Clinic and removed from the laboratories by members of the Animal Liberation Front. Narrated by Ingrid Newkirk of People for the Ethical Treatment of Animals. BE62195.
>*animal experimentation; attitudes; *brain; federal government; government financing; *injuries; investigators; *pain; *primates; research design; research institutes; *scientific misconduct; *suffering; Department of Health and Human Services; United States; *University of Pennsylvania

ANIMAL ORGANS *See* ORGAN AND TISSUE TRANSPLANTATION, ORGAN AND TISSUE DONATION

ANIMALS, TRANSGENIC *See* GENETIC INTERVENTION, PATENTING LIFE FORMS, RECOMBINANT DNA RESEARCH

ARTIFICIAL INSEMINATION

See also REPRODUCTIVE TECHNOLOGIES

Baetens, P.; Ponjaert-Kristoffersen, I.; Devroey, P., et al. Artificial insemination by donor: an alternative for single women. *Human Reproduction.* 1995 Jun; 10(6): 1537–1542. 17 refs. BE60412.
>*artificial insemination; *counseling; *females; health facilities; institutional policies; mothers; motivation; parent child relationship; program descriptions; refusal to treat; *selection for treatment; semen donors; *single persons; socioeconomic factors; Belgium; Free University of Brussels

Critser, John K. Current status of semen banking in the USA. [Article and discussion]. *Human Reproduction.* 1998 May; 13(Suppl. 2): 55–69. 14 refs. BE61481.
>age factors; artificial insemination; federal government; government regulation; guidelines; mass screening; private sector; professional organizations; registries; semen donors; sexually transmitted diseases; *sperm; standards; survey; *tissue banks; treatment outcome; American Association of Tissue Banks; American Survey for Reproductive Medicine; *United States

Grubb, Andrew. Infertility treatment: posthumous use of sperm -- R. v. Human Fertilisation and Embryology Authority, ex parte D.B. [Comment]. *Medical Law Review.* 1996 Autumn; 4(3): 329–335. BE61517.
>*artificial insemination; *cryopreservation; death; informed

consent; international aspects; *legal aspects; males; married persons; *posthumous reproduction; *sperm; coma; Belgium; *Great Britain; *R v. Human Fertilisation and Embryology Authority (ex parte Blood)

Hopkins, Patrick D., ed. (Mis?)conceptions: morality and gender politics in reproductive technology. *In: his* Sex/Machine: Readings in Culture, Gender, and Technology. Bloomington, IN: Indiana University Press; 1998: 95–170. 227 fn. ISBN 0–253–21230–8. BE62289.
abortion, induced; *artificial insemination; attitudes; children; developing countries; eugenics; family relationship; *fathers; *females; feminist ethics; genetic disorders; informed consent; international aspects; legal aspects; *males; methods; moral obligations; motivation; *parent child relationship; population control; pregnant women; public policy; remuneration; rights; *risks and benefits; selective abortion; *semen donors; *sex determination; *sex preselection; sexuality; single persons; social discrimination; social impact; socioeconomic factors; spousal notification; *surrogate mothers; wedge argument; women's rights; harms; United States

Horn, David. Unnatural acts: procreation and the genealogy of artifice. *In:* Terry, Jennifer; Calvert, Melodie, eds. Processed Lives: Gender and Technology in Everyday Life. New York, NY: Routledge; 1997: 145–154. 31 refs. 10 fn. ISBN 0–415–14932–0. BE61945.
*artificial insemination; *attitudes; confidentiality; *deception; disclosure; *eugenics; fathers; *historical aspects; international aspects; *males; married persons; parent child relationship; physicians; reproductive technologies; *semen donors; *sexuality; *nature; Europe; Hurd, Addison Davis; Nineteenth Century; Pancoast, William; Twentieth Century; United States

Loff, Bebe; Cordner, Stephen. Confusion over use of cadaver gametes for assisted fertilisation. [News]. *Lancet.* 1998 Aug 1; 352(9125): 382. BE59638.
*artificial insemination; *cadavers; *legal aspects; *married persons; *posthumous reproduction; *semen donors; *Victoria

Lui, S.C.; Weaver, S.M.; Robinson, J., et al. A survey of semen donor attitudes. *Human Reproduction.* 1995 Jan; 10(1): 234–238. 25 refs. BE60557.
altruism; *artificial insemination; *attitudes; confidentiality; disclosure; *motivation; parent child relationship; remuneration; *semen donors; survey; *Great Britain

Mason, John Kenyon. The infertile man. *In: his* Medico–Legal Aspects of Reproduction and Parenthood. Second Edition. Brookfield, VT: Ashgate; 1998: 207–226. 59 fn. ISBN 1–84104–065–8. BE61066.
age factors; *artificial insemination; children; confidentiality; cryopreservation; disclosure; fathers; females; genetic information; government regulation; homosexuals; *infertility; informed consent; *legal aspects; *males; married persons; parent child relationship; posthumous reproduction; public policy; registries; selection for treatment; semen donors; single persons; sperm; spousal consent; coma; *Great Britain; *Human Fertilisation and Embryology Act 1990; Human Fertilisation and Embryology Authority; *R v. Human Fertilisation and Embryology Authority (ex parte Blood)

Murphy, Julien S. Should lesbians count as infertile couples? Antilesbian discrimination in assisted reproduction. *In:* Donchin, Anne; Purdy, Laura M., eds. Embodying Bioethics: Recent Feminist Advances. Lanham, MD: Rowman and Littlefield; 1999: 103–120. 24 refs. 10 fn. ISBN 0–8476–8924–7. BE61017.
*artificial insemination; *diagnosis; *females; *feminist ethics; health insurance reimbursement; *homosexuals; *infertility; legal rights; marital relationship; parent child relationship; physicians; refusal to treat; reproductive technologies; *selection for treatment; *social discrimination; United States

Nachtigall, Robert D.; Tschann, Jeanne M.; Quiroga, Seline Szkupinski, et al. Stigma, disclosure, and family functioning among parents of children conceived through donor insemination. *Fertility and Sterility.* 1997 Jul; 68(1): 83–89. 22 refs. BE60333.
*artificial insemination; attitudes; children; confidentiality; *disclosure; evaluation studies; *fathers; females; males; *mothers; *parent child relationship; semen donors; socioeconomic factors; *stigmatization; California

Pennings, Guido. The internal coherence of donor insemination practice: attracting the right type of donor without paying. *Human Reproduction.* 1997 Sep; 12(9): 1842–1844. 7 refs. BE59182.
*altruism; *artificial insemination; confidentiality; economics; gifts; guidelines; incentives; informed consent; motivation; parent child relationship; *public policy; *remuneration; risks and benefits; *semen donors; Great Britain; *Human Fertilisation and Embryology Authority

Shenfield, Françoise. Recruitment and counselling of sperm donors: ethical problems. *Human Reproduction.* 1998 May; 13(Suppl. 2): 70–75. 29 refs. BE61482.
advertising; altruism; attitudes; coercion; confidentiality; *counseling; fathers; guidelines; informed consent; international aspects; motivation; remuneration; *semen donors; sperm; *tissue donation; France; Great Britain

Sootak, Jaan; Kurm, Margus. A wish to have a baby and the dignity of the child and embryo: about the law on artificial insemination and embryo protection of the Republic of Estonia. *European Journal of Health Law.* 1998 Jun; 5(2): 191–201. 7 fn. BE60900.
abortion, induced; *artificial insemination; children; disclosure; embryo disposition; embryo research; embryo transfer; embryos; females; fetal development; *government regulation; in vitro fertilization; informed consent; *legal aspects; *legislation; married persons; ovum donors; parent child relationship; reproductive technologies; semen donors; single persons; *Artificial Insemination and Embryo Protection Act (Estonia); *Estonia

Steinbock, Bonnie. Sperm as property. *In:* Harris, John; Holm, Søren, eds. The Future of Human Reproduction: Ethics, Choice, and Regulation. New York, NY: Oxford University Press; 1998: 150–161. 39 fn. ISBN 0–19–823761–8. BE61267.
*artificial insemination; autonomy; body parts and fluids; commodification; cryopreservation; decision making; dissent; *legal aspects; moral policy; *posthumous reproduction; *property rights; public policy; remuneration; reproduction; reproductive technologies; semen donors; *sperm; suicide; tissue banks; California; *Hecht v. Superior Court (Kane)

White, Caroline. Banking on interest: "Test Tube Dads" (*Inside Story*, BBC1, 25 August 1998). [Medicine and the media]. *BMJ (British Medical Journal).* 1998 Aug 29; 317(7158): 607. BE59157.
*artificial insemination; attitudes; children; confidentiality; emotions; eugenics; fathers; mass media; mothers; motivation; parent child relationship; *semen donors; *sperm; *tissue banks

ASSISTED SUICIDE *See* SUICIDE

BE = bioethics accession number   fn. = footnotes   refs. = references

ATTITUDES
See under
ABORTION/ATTITUDES
ALLOWING TO DIE/ATTITUDES
EUTHANASIA/ATTITUDES

BEHAVIOR CONTROL

Allen, Keith D.; Hodges, Eric D.; Knudsen, Sharon K. Comparing four methods to inform parents about child behavior management: how to inform for consent. *Pediatric Dentistry.* 1995 May–Jun; 17(3): 180–186. 20 refs. BE62416.
*attitudes; audiovisual aids; *behavior control; *communication; comparative studies; consent forms; *dentistry; *disclosure; informed consent; *methods; *minors; *parental consent; *parents; patient compliance; pediatrics; Nebraska; University of Nebraska Pediatric Dental Clinic

Baker, Tina; Cooper, Colleen. What happens next? [Case study and commentaries]. *Hastings Center Report.* 1999 Mar–Apr; 29(2): 24–25. BE61657.
administrators; *aged; allied health personnel; *behavior control; behavior disorders; brain pathology; case studies; death; government regulation; health personnel; institutional policies; *nursing homes; *patient care; *physical restraint; cerebrovascular disorders

Byk, Christian. International Association for Law, Ethics and Science organizes third international meeting (Paris, 23–24 Sep 1994). *International Digest of Health Legislation.* 1995; 46(4): 572–574. BE62687.
aborted fetuses; *behavior control; *behavioral research; *brain; brain pathology; fetal research; fetal tissue donation; human experimentation; informed consent; international aspects; legal aspects; *mentally ill; professional organizations; psychiatry; *psychoactive drugs; *neurosciences; International Association for Law, Ethics and Science

Cohen, Elias S.; Kruschwitz, Ann L. Restraint reduction: lessons from the asylum. *Journal of Ethics, Law, and Aging.* 1997 Spring–Summer; 3(1): 25–43. 72 fn. BE59202.
*aged; *behavior control; decision making; *dementia; education; federal government; government regulation; health personnel; historical aspects; *institutional policies; international aspects; legal aspects; *mental institutions; *mentally disabled; moral obligations; *nursing homes; patient advocacy; *patient care; *physical restraint; psychoactive drugs; quality of health care; state government; Eighteenth Century; Europe; Great Britain; Medicaid; Medicare; Nineteenth Century; Twentieth Century; *United States; Youngberg v. Romeo

Constantino, Rose E.; Boneysteele, Ginger; Gesmond, Sharyn A., et al. Restraining an aggressive suicidal, paraplegic patient: a look at the ethical and legal issues. *Dimensions of Critical Care Nursing.* 1997 May–Jun; 16(3): 144–151. 12 refs. BE59177.
aggression; *behavior control; beneficence; case studies; decision making; freedom; hospitals; informed consent; *injuries; *intensive care units; legal liability; *nurses; nursing ethics; paralysis; *patient care; patient care team; *physical restraint; professional family relationship; referral and consultation; suicide; *violence

DeSantis, Joe; Engberg, Sandra; Rogers, Joan. Geropsychiatric restraint use. *Journal of the American Geriatrics Society.* 1997 Dec; 45(12): 1515–1518. 25 refs. BE59692.
age factors; *aged; *behavior control; *behavior disorders; comparative studies; *dementia; hospitals; injuries; mental institutions; mentally ill; motivation; nurses; *patient care; *physical restraint; prospective studies

Elliott, Carl. The tyranny of happiness: ethics and cosmetic psychopharmacology. *In:* Parens, Erik, ed. Enhancing Human Traits: Ethical and Social Implications. Washington, DC: Georgetown University Press; 1998: 177–188. 11 fn. ISBN 0–87840–703–0. BE59752.
*behavior control; depressive disorder; *emotions; enhancement technologies; literature; *mental health; normality; psychiatry; *psychoactive drugs; psychological stress; *quality of life; *self concept; uncertainty; value of life; *values; Western World; authenticity; Listening to Prozac (Kramer, P.); Percy, Walker; Prozac; Twentieth Century; United States

Fairman, Julie; Happ, Mary Beth. For their own good? A historical examination of restraint use. *HEC (HealthCare Ethics Committee) Forum.* 1998 Sep–Dec; 10(3–4): 290–299. 36 refs. BE61180.
aged; attitudes; *behavior control; biomedical technologies; government regulation; historical aspects; hospitals; *nurses; nursing education; *patient care; *physical restraint; risks and benefits; United States

Fleetwood, Janet. Editor's introduction [to a set of nine articles on the use of restraints in healthcare]. *HEC (HealthCare Ethics Committee) Forum.* 1998 Sep–Dec; 10(3–4): 231–234. BE61216.
aged; *behavior control; case studies; children; hospitals; intensive care units; legal aspects; mentally ill; motivation; nursing homes; pain; patient care; patient compliance; *physical restraint; psychological stress; treatment refusal; ventilators

Frank, Martina W.; Bauer, Heidi M.; Arican, Nadir, et al. Virginity examinations in Turkey: role of forensic physicians in controlling female sexuality. *JAMA.* 1999 Aug 4; 282(5): 485–490. 30 refs. BE62565.
adults; *behavior control; coercion; *females; *forensic medicine; *human rights; *knowledge, attitudes, practice; law enforcement; medical ethics; minors; obstetrics and gynecology; organizational policies; *physician's role; *physicians; professional organizations; psychological stress; public policy; risks and benefits; sex offenses; *sexuality; social control; *social discrimination; survey; *women's rights; *Turkey; Turkish Medical Association
CONTEXT: Although the Turkish Medical Association has deemed "virginity examinations" a form of gender–based violence, women in Turkey are often subjected to such examinations by forensic physicians for both legal and social reasons. Little is known about these physicians' role and attitudes in this practice. OBJECTIVES: To assess forensic physicians' experiences and attitudes regarding virginity examinations in Turkey and suggest potential solutions to the problems identified. DESIGN: Cross–sectional self–administered survey. SETTING: Surveys were completed during the Forensic Science Congress held in Kusadasi in April 1998 as well as in urban academic and medical practice settings between April and October 1998. PARTICIPANTS: Of 158 physicians who practice, are formally trained in, or are in training for forensic medicine, 118 completed the survey (response rate, 74.7%). MAIN OUTCOME MEASURES: Frequency and circumstances of conducting virginity examinations, opinions regarding beneficial and adverse consequences of these examinations, and recommendations for changing the practice, as measured by a 100–item questionnaire. RESULTS: Overall, survey respondents reported conducting 5901 examinations in the previous 12 months; 4045 were conducted because

---

BE = bioethics accession number   fn. = footnotes   refs. = references

of alleged sexual assault and 1856 for social reasons. Although 68% of forensic physicians indicated that they believed virginity examinations are inappropriate in the absence of an allegation of sexual assault, 45% had conducted examinations for social reasons. The majority of the respondents (93%) agreed that the examinations are psychologically traumatic for the patient. In addition, more than half (58%) reported that at least 50% of patients undergo examinations against their will. CONCLUSIONS: Nearly half of forensic physicians in Turkey conduct virginity examinations for social reasons despite beliefs that such examinations are inappropriate, traumatic to the patient, and often performed against the patient's will. Physicians' participation in such practices is inconsistent with principles of bioethics and international human rights.

Goldberg, Susan L. Legal aspects of restraint use in hospitals and nursing homes. *HEC (HealthCare Ethics Committee) Forum.* 1998 Sep–Dec; 10(3–4): 276–289. 30 refs. BE61179.
    *behavior control; drugs; federal government; *government regulation; *hospitals; informed consent; legal liability; medical devices; *nursing homes; *patient care; patients' rights; *physical restraint; self regulation; standards; state government; treatment refusal; Joint Commission on Accreditation of Healthcare Organizations; Medicaid; Medicare; Nursing Home Reform Act 1987; United States

Goldman, Marina. Physical restraints. [Bibliography]. *HEC (HealthCare Ethics Committee) Forum.* 1998 Sep–Dec; 10(3–4): 323–337. BE61184.
    aged; alternatives; behavior control; family members; hospitals; mentally ill; nurses; nursing homes; *physical restraint

Holland, Anthony J.; Wong, Josephine. Genetically determined obesity in Prader–Willi syndrome: the ethics and legality of treatment. *Journal of Medical Ethics.* 1999 Jun; 25(3): 230–236. 19 fn. BE61855.
    adults; *autonomy; *behavior control; *behavior disorders; behavioral genetics; *beneficence; coercion; *competence; comprehension; *decision making; family members; *food; *genetic determinism; *genetic disorders; informed consent; *legal aspects; legal rights; mentally disabled; moral policy; morbidity; mortality; patient care; patient education; patient participation; physicians; risk; anorexia nervosa; *eating disorders; *obesity; *Great Britain; Mental Health Act 1983 (Great Britain)
A central characteristic of people with Prader–Willi Syndrome (PWS) is an apparent insatiable appetite leading to severe overeating and the potential for marked obesity and associated serious health problems and premature death. This behaviour may be due to the effects of the genetic defect resulting from the chromosome 15 abnormalities associated with the syndrome. We examine the ethical and legal dilemmas that can arise in the care of people with PWS. A tension exists between a genetic deterministic perspective and that of individual choice. We conclude that the determination of the capacity of a person with PWS to make decisions about his/her eating behaviour and to control that behaviour is of particular importance in resolving this dilemma. If the person is found to lack capacity, the common law principles of acting in a person's "best interests" using the "least restrictive alternative" may be helpful. Allowing serious weight gain in the absence of careful consideration of these issues is an abdication of responsibility.

Joint Commission on Accreditation of Healthcare Organizations. Standards for restraint and seclusion. *Joint Commission Perspectives.* 1996 Jan–Feb; 16(1): RS1–RS8. 2 fn. BE60382.
    *behavior control; *health facilities; institutional policies; patient care; patients' rights; *physical restraint; *standards; time factors; *Joint Commission on Accreditation of Healthcare Organizations; United States

Joy, Mark; Hemmings, Gwynneth; Al–Adwani, Andrew, et al. Parity of mental illness, disparity for the mental patient. [Letters and response]. *Lancet.* 1999 Jan 2; 353(9146): 73–74. 8 refs. BE61620.
    advance directives; *behavior control; coercion; competence; dangerousness; involuntary commitment; law enforcement; *mental health; *mentally ill; physicians; prisoners; psychiatric diagnosis; psychiatric wills; psychiatry; schizophrenia; stigmatization; suicide

Lamdan, Ruth M.; Ahmed, Ziauddin; Lee, Jean. General anesthesia: an extreme form of chemical and physical restraint. [Case analysis]. *HEC (HealthCare Ethics Committee) Forum.* 1998 Sep–Dec; 10(3–4): 317–322. BE61183.
    *anesthesia; *behavior control; case studies; competence; *critically ill; *mentally disabled; patient compliance; *physical restraint; *psychoactive drugs; renal dialysis; treatment refusal

Miles, Steven H. Restraints: controlling a symptom or a symptom of control. *HEC (HealthCare Ethics Committee) Forum.* 1998 Sep–Dec; 10(3–4): 235–243. 18 refs. Paper presented at the 1990 Annual Meeting Convention of the American Geriatrics Society. BE61176.
    *aged; *behavior control; consent forms; dehumanization; informed consent; injuries; institutional policies; legal aspects; *nursing homes; patient care; *physical restraint; risks and benefits; United States

Molnar, Beth E. Juveniles and psychiatric institutionalization: toward better due process and treatment review in the United States. *Health and Human Rights.* 1997; 2(2): 99–116. 46 fn. BE62089.
    *behavior control; behavior disorders; child abuse; *due process; health insurance reimbursement; homosexuals; *human rights; international aspects; *involuntary commitment; *legal aspects; mental institutions; *minors; misconduct; operant conditioning; parents; physical restraint; proprietary health facilities; voluntary admission; *Convention on the Rights of the Child; United Nations; *United States

O'Connor, Bonnie B. Culture and the use of patient restraints. *HEC (HealthCare Ethics Committee) Forum.* 1998 Sep–Dec; 10(3–4): 263–275. 35 refs. BE61177.
    aged; alternatives; attitudes; *behavior control; comparative studies; cultural pluralism; economics; health personnel; historical aspects; hospitals; *international aspects; legal aspects; legal liability; nursing homes; *patient care; *physical restraint; professional patient relationship; risk; risks and benefits; standards; *values; *Great Britain; *United States

Pelin, Serap Sahinoglu. The question of virginity testing in Turkey. *Bioethics.* 1999 Jul; 13(3–4): 256–261. 10 fn. BE61876.
    *behavior control; coercion; *females; feminist ethics; forensic medicine; human rights; legal aspects; moral obligations; patient care; physician patient relationship; *physician's role; *sexuality; *single persons; *social control; stigmatization; *Turkey
Pre-marital sex for a woman is regarded as wrong in my country. As a result, it is socially forbidden for a woman to engage in this act. In order to present a woman as a virgin on her marriage day, she is subjected to

---

BE = bioethics accession number   fn. = footnotes   refs. = references

pressure, and put under control both by her family and societal norms. However, a man is free and never made to suffer any of the above. A woman found to be a virgin on her first night of marriage is seen as a normal person while one suspected to have lost her virginity is made to undergo a series of medical examinations to bring clarity to her situation.

Rose, Steven P.R. Neurogenetic determinism and the new euphenics. *BMJ (British Medical Journal).* 1998 Dec 19–26; 317(7174): 1707–1708. 5 refs. BE60839.
aggression; *behavior control; behavior disorders; *behavioral genetics; brain pathology; drug industry; *genetic determinism; genetic predisposition; hyperkinesis; *psychoactive drugs; social problems; trends

Royal College of Psychiatrists. Consent of Non–Volitional Patients and *De Facto* Detention of Informal Patients. Issued by the Royal College of Psychiatrists, 17 Belgrave Sq., London SW1X 8PG, England; 1989 Oct. 23 p. 18 refs. Council Report CR6. Appendixes include "Legal minors" by J. Hendriks, "Assent to operation by medical staff where patient unable to give consent" by Frenchay Health Authority, "Exercising restraint" by B. Pitt, and "Sterilisation of a mentally incapable woman" by D. Brahams. BE60353.
*behavior control; coercion; *competence; consent forms; decision making; dementia; *informed consent; institutionalized persons; legal aspects; *mentally disabled; mentally retarded; minors; organizational policies; *patient care; *physical restraint; professional organizations; sterilization (sexual); third party consent; *Great Britain; *Royal College of Psychiatrists; Scotland

Royal College of Psychiatrists. Guidelines to Good Practice in the Use of Behavioral Treatments. Issued by the Royal College of Psychiatrists, 17 Belgrave Sq., London SW1X 8PG, England; 1989 Oct. 26 p. 5 refs. Council Report CR9; approved Oct 1989. BE60354.
aged; *behavior control; children; dementia; forensic psychiatry; informed consent; *mentally disabled; mentally retarded; *operant conditioning; organizational policies; physical restraint; physicians; *practice guidelines; professional organizations; psychiatry; psychotherapy; sexuality; Great Britain; *Royal College of Psychiatrists

Slomka, Jacquelyn; Agich, George J.; Stagno, Susan J., et al. Physical restraint elimination in the acute care setting: ethical considerations. *HEC (HealthCare Ethics Committee) Forum.* 1998 Sep–Dec; 10(3–4): 244–262. 35 refs. BE61178.
aged; autonomy; *behavior control; cultural pluralism; dangerousness; economics; family members; health care reform; health personnel; *hospitals; injuries; institutional policies; institutionalized persons; intention; international aspects; *mentally ill; paternalism; *patient care; patients; *physical restraint; physicians; psychiatry; psychological stress; risk; technical expertise; treatment refusal; values; United States

Vaught, Wayne; Lamdan, Ruth M. An ethics committee explores restraint use and practices. *HEC (HealthCare Ethics Committee) Forum.* 1998 Sep–Dec; 10(3–4): 306–316. 2 refs. BE61182.
aged; *behavior control; case studies; clinical ethics committees; competence; emergency care; *hospitals; informed consent; injuries; institutional policies; intensive care units; mentally ill; *patient care; *physical restraint; Allegheny University Hospital (Philadelphia)

Watts, Jonathan. Patients not to be tied up in Japanese sanatoriums. [News]. *Lancet.* 1999 Jul 24; 354(9175): 316. BE62528.

aged; *behavior control; dementia; government regulation; *guidelines; *institutionalized persons; *mental institutions; *mentally ill; *physical restraint; public hospitals; *public policy; residential facilities; *Japan

White, D.M.D.; Hillam, Jonathan; Harper, Max, et al. Suspension of nurse who gave drug on consultant's instructions. [Letters]. *BMJ (British Medical Journal).* 1997 Jan 25; 314(7076): 299–301. 8 refs. BE59380.
*administrators; aged; *behavior control; behavior disorders; coercion; dangerousness; *deception; *misconduct; *nurse's role; *nurses; patient care; *patient care team; peer review; physician nurse relationship; *physicians; psychiatry; *psychoactive drugs; *punishment; treatment refusal; *Great Britain; Mental Health Act 1983 (Great Britain); National Health Service

Witte, Kim. The manipulative nature of health communication research: ethical issues and guidelines. *American Behavioral Scientist.* 1994 Nov; 38(2): 285–293. 26 refs. BE61210.
*behavior control; common good; *communication; decision making; goals; guidelines; *health education; health hazards; *health promotion; informal social control; information dissemination; preventive medicine; public participation; risk; standards

BEHAVIORAL GENETICS

Beckwith, Jon. The responsibility of scientists in the genetics and race controversies. *In:* Smith, Edward; Sapp, Walter, eds. Plain Talk about the the Human Genome Project: A Tuskegee University Conference on Its Promise and Perils ... and Matters of Race. Tuskegee, AL: Tuskegee University Press; 1997: 83–94. 57 refs. ISBN 1–891196–01–4. BE61737.
advisory committees; *behavioral genetics; *blacks; eugenics; females; genetic determinism; genetic predisposition; genetic research; genome mapping; intelligence; *investigators; males; *moral obligations; science; *social discrimination; social impact; values; whites; Human Genome Project; NCHGR Program on Ethical, Legal, and Social Implications (ELSI); United States

Billauer, Barbara Pfeffer. On Judaism and genes: a response to Paul Root Wolpe. *Kennedy Institute of Ethics Journal.* 1999 Jun; 9(2): 159–165. 4 refs. 6 fn. Commentary on P.R. Wolpe, "If I am only my genes, what am I? Genetic essentialism and a Jewish response," *KIE Journal*, 1997 Sep; 7(3): 213–230. BE62383.
behavioral genetics; *genetic determinism; genetic identity; genetic intervention; human body; *Jewish ethics; personhood; religion; science; social sciences
The following comments on Paul Root Wolpe's article "If I Am Only My Genes, What Am I? Genetic Essentialism and a Jewish Response" address (1) his presentation of the relationship between science and culture or religion as unimodal; (2) his misconception of the Jewish view of the physical corpus; and (3) his essential question of genetic determinism by examining the traditional Jewish view of the spiritual aspects of the human.

Charles, J. Daryl. Blame it on the beta–boosters: genetics, self–determination, and moral accountability. *In:* Demy, Timothy J.; Stewart, Gary P., eds. Genetic Engineering: A Christian Response: Crucial Considerations in Shaping Life. Grand Rapids, MI: Kregel Publications; 1999: 240–258. 63 fn. ISBN 0–8254–2357–0. BE61369.
*accountability; autonomy; *behavioral genetics; *Christian ethics; coercion; conscience; freedom; *genetic determinism; *genetic predisposition; justice; law enforcement; natural law; preventive medicine; *violence; rationality; United

---

BE = bioethics accession number   fn. = footnotes   refs. = references

States

Duster, Troy. Molecular halos and behavioral glows. *In:* Smith, Edward; Sapp, Walter, eds. Plain Talk about the Human Genome Project: A Tuskegee University Conference on Its Promise and Perils ... and Matters of Race. Tuskegee, AL: Tuskegee University Press; 1997: 215–222. 4 refs. ISBN 1-891196-01-4. BE61750.
   *behavioral genetics; behavioral research; *blacks; genetic predisposition; genome mapping; law enforcement; minority groups; population genetics; risks and benefits; science; social discrimination; social sciences

Friedland, Steven I. The criminal law implications of the Human Genome Project: reimagining a genetically oriented criminal justice system. *Kentucky Law Journal.* 1997–1998; 86(2): 303–366. 276 fn. BE62429.
   *behavioral genetics; *criminal law; dangerousness; eugenics; gene therapy; *genetic determinism; genetic predisposition; genetic screening; *genetics; genome mapping; law enforcement; legal liability; normality; prisoners; public policy; science; social discrimination; social impact; social problems; violence; United States

Newson, Ainsley; Williamson, Robert. Should we undertake genetic research on intelligence? *Bioethics.* 1999 Jul; 13(3–4): 327–342. 36 fn. BE61883.
   *behavioral genetics; eugenics; family relationship; genes; *genetic enhancement; genetic information; *genetic research; genetic screening; *intelligence; resource allocation; risks and benefits; social discrimination; social impact; values
Although the concept of intelligence is difficult to define, research has provided evidence for a significant genetic component. Attempts are now being made to use molecular genetic approaches to identify genes contributing to intelligence, and to determine the ways in which they interact with environmental variables. This research is then likely to determine the developmental pathways of intelligence, in an effort to understand mental handicap and learning disorders and develop new treatment strategies. This paper reviews research on the genetic basis of intelligence, and discusses the ethical concerns, including the role of genetic information, the value we place on intelligence and the allocation of resources. It will be argued that the objections raised are problematic, and that because of the value of this knowledge and the prospect of improving lives, this research is morally required. We will then provide a brief analysis of the issues raised by enhancement of intelligence using genetic technology, and will argue that there is no intrinsic difference between this and other means of optimising intelligence.

Nygaard, Richard Lowell. The ten commandments of behavioral genetic data and criminology. *Judges' Journal.* 1997 Summer; 36(3): 59–64, 94–96. 22 fn. BE59807.
   accountability; autonomy; *behavior disorders; *behavioral genetics; *criminal law; expert testimony; genetic information; genetic predisposition; genetic research; *guidelines; interdisciplinary communication; *law enforcement; operant conditioning; prisoners; punishment; socioeconomic factors; standards; ELSI-funded publication; United States

Rose, Steven P.R. Neurogenetic determinism and the new euphenics. *BMJ (British Medical Journal).* 1998 Dec 19–26; 317(7174): 1707–1708. 5 refs. BE60839.
   aggression; *behavior control; behavior disorders; *behavioral genetics; brain pathology; drug industry; *genetic determinism; genetic predisposition; hyperkinesis; *psychoactive drugs; social problems; trends

Shickle, Darren. Do 'all men desire to know'? A right of society to choose not to know about the genetics of personality traits. *In:* Chadwick, Ruth; Levitt, Mairi; Shickle, Darren, eds. The Right to Know and the Right Not to Know. Brookfield, VT: Ashgate; 1997: 69–77. 22 refs. ISBN 1-85972-424-8. BE62190.
   autonomy; *behavioral genetics; common good; decision making; genetic enhancement; genetic predisposition; *genetic research; government financing; government regulation; investigators; normality; *public participation; recombinant DNA research; *science; self regulation; *social control; right not to know

Wolpe, Paul Root. Reply to Barbara Pfeffer Billauer's "On Judaism and genes." *Kennedy Institute of Ethics Journal.* 1999 Jun; 9(2): 167–174. 4 refs. 4 fn. BE62384.
   behavioral genetics; *genetic determinism; genetic identity; human body; *Jewish ethics; religion; science; social sciences
The response of Barbara Pfeffer Billauer to my article "If I Am Only My Genes, What Am I? Genetic Essentialism and a Jewish Response" highlights the conflict between a sociological understanding of religion and the resistance to such analysis from within a faith tradition. Ms. Billauer makes three main points; the first strangely credits to me, and then attacks, an argument the article takes great pains to refute, but does so to emphasize the faith's prescient guidance in matters scientific. The second attempts to rebut my critical analysis of the tensions inhernet in Jewish views of the body with an insistence that Judaism so perfectly balances the relation between the sacred and profane that there is not now, and never was, the slightest tension between corporeality and divinity in the Jewish corpus. The third uses my article as vehicle for her to expound on an interesting but tangential formulation of three Jewish terms. In all, the need to defend her interpretation of Judaism's solutions to the problems the article raises results in un-self-critical and ahistorical theorizing, making the utility of her arguments in a discussion of the sociology of religion unsatisfactory.

Zweig, Franklin M.; Walsh, Joseph T.; Freeman, Daniel M. Adjudicating neurogenetics at the crossroads: privacy, adoption, and the death sentence. *Judges' Journal.* 1997 Summer; 36(3): 52–55, 57–58, 90–93. 14 fn. BE59806.
   *adoption; *behavior disorders; *behavioral genetics; capital punishment; case studies; *confidentiality; *criminal law; federal government; *genetic information; *genetic predisposition; *genetic screening; government regulation; killing; *law enforcement; legislation; mandatory testing; parents; prisoners; *privacy; public policy; records; social discrimination; state government; *violence; Colorado; Connecticut; *United States

BEHAVIORAL RESEARCH

See also BIOMEDICAL RESEARCH, HUMAN EXPERIMENTATION

Chastain, Garvin; Landrum, R. Eric, eds. Protecting Human Subjects: Departmental Subject Pools and Institutional Review Boards. Washington, DC: American Psychological Association; 1999. 228 p. Includes references. ISBN 1-55798-575-8. BE62730.
   attitudes; *behavioral research; evaluation; evaluation studies; faculty; informed consent; investigators; misconduct; *organization and administration; program descriptions; *psychology; research design; *research ethics committees; *research subjects; *selection of subjects; sexuality; *students; survey; *universities; volunteers; vulnerable populations; United States

---

BE = bioethics accession number   fn. = footnotes   refs. = references

Fox, Michael W. Concepts in Ethology: Animal Behavior and Bioethics. Second Edition. Malabar, FL: Krieger; 1998. 163 p. Bibliography: p. 153–160. ISBN 1-57524-044-0. BE61046.
> *animal experimentation; animal rights; *behavioral research; bioethics; comparative studies; ecology; human characteristics

Herrera, C.D. Research ethics at the empirical side: Research Ethics: A Psychological Approach, edited by Barbara Stanley, Joan Sieber, and Gary Melton; Illusions of Reality: A History of Deception in Social Psychology, by James Korn. [Book review essay]. *Theoretical Medicine and Bioethics.* 1999 April; 20(2): 191–200. 18 fn. BE62225.
> attitudes; *behavioral research; *deception; disclosure; *empirical research; informed consent; investigators; professional ethics; *psychology; research design; research subjects; risks and benefits; debriefing; *Illusions of Reality: A History of Deception in Social Psychology (Korn, J.); *Research Ethics: A Psychological Approach (Stanley, B.; Sieber, J.; Melton, G., eds.)

Kaiser, Jocelyn, ed. Ethics of studying cybernauts. [News]. *Science.* 1999 Jun 25; 284(5423): 2051. BE62388.
> *behavioral research; *computer communication networks; federal government; guidelines; human experimentation; professional organizations; American Association for the Advancement of Science; *Internet; Office for Protection from Research Risks; United States

Karli, Pierre. Conceptual and ethical problems raised by the study of brain-behavior relationships underlying aggression. *In:* Feshbach, Seymour; Zagrodzka, Jolanta, eds. Aggression: Biological, Developmental, and Social Perspectives. New York, NY: Plenum Press; 1997: 3–14. 24 refs. BE60022.
> *aggression; behavioral genetics; *behavioral research; *brain; brain pathology; electrical stimulation of the brain; *neurology

Korn, James H. Illusions of Reality: A History of Deception in Social Psychology. Albany, NY: State University of New York Press; 1997. 204 p. Bibliography: p. 185–199. ISBN 0-7914-3308-0. BE61313.
> *behavioral research; *deception; empirical research; *historical aspects; informed consent; investigators; military personnel; professional ethics; psychological stress; *psychology; research design; statistics; trends; Festinger, Leon; Lewin, Kurt; Milgram, Stanley; *Twentieth Century; United States

Shapiro, Kenneth Joel. Animal Models of Human Psychology: Critique of Science, Ethics, and Policy. Seattle, WA: Hogrefe and Huber; 1998. 328 p. Bibliography: p. 293–320. ISBN 0-88937-189-X. BE60750.
> *animal experimentation; animal rights; attitudes; behavior disorders; *behavioral research; food; investigators; political activity; *psychology; research design; risks and benefits; speciesism; suffering; utilitarianism; anorexia nervosa; bulimia

Trickett, Edison J. Toward a framework for defining and resolving ethical issues in the protection of communities involved in primary prevention projects. *Ethics and Behavior.* 1998; 8(4): 321–337. 34 refs. BE60164.
> adolescents; *alcohol abuse; aliens; anthropology; behavior disorders; *behavioral research; children; cultural pluralism; disadvantaged; *drug abuse; ecology; education; health education; *health promotion; health services research; informed consent; injuries; investigator subject relationship; *mental health; mentally ill; metaphor; minority groups;

patient education; *preventive medicine; professional ethics; psychology; public health; sexually transmitted diseases; social dominance; *social problems; trust; values; *community medicine; *intervention studies

Ethical issues flow from and are embedded in contexts of practice. *Contexts of practice* refer to the diverse social settings where interventions occur. Primary prevention activities require new professional roles in these diverse social settings. These new roles engage the professional in new activities, which in turn allow new ethical issues to arise. This article takes an ecological perspective on ethical issues arising from the enactment of new preventive roles intended to affect groups or communities. Within this perspective, the concepts of context and culture take on special conceptual significance. Four ecological assumptions about preventive interventions intended to affect groups or communities are offered as a means of framing ethical issues in such interventions. Finally, several approaches to developing ecological knowledge about the contexts of practice are presented as ways of furthering our ability to conceptualize and cope with ethical issues in preventive interventions intended to affect groups or communities.

Wadeley, Alison. Ethics in Psychological Research and Practice. Leicester, England: British Psychological Association; 1991. 41 p. 29 refs. Open learning unit: models and methods in psychology. ISBN 1-85433-045-4. BE59462.
> animal experimentation; animal testing alternatives; *behavioral research; *education; evaluation; guidelines; operant conditioning; *professional ethics; *psychology; teaching methods; British Psychological Society; Great Britain

Wilkie, Patricia. Ethical issues in qualitative research in palliative care. *Palliative Medicine.* 1997 Jul; 11(4): 321–324. 9 refs. Paper delivered at the Qualitative Research Workshop organized jointly by the Institute of Cancer Research and Marie Curie Cancer Care, held 11 Sep 1996 at the Royal Marsden Hospital, England. BE60044.
> *behavioral research; codes of ethics; confidentiality; deception; disclosure; emotions; informed consent; motivation; *palliative care; patients; psychology; research design; research subjects; risks and benefits; *qualitative research; Declaration of Helsinki

BEHAVIORAL RESEARCH/ETHICS COMMITTEES

Chapman, Simon. When outcomes threaten incomes: a case study of the obstruction of research to reduce teenage smoking. *Health Policy.* 1997 Jan; 39(1): 55–68. 54 refs. BE59796.
> *adolescents; advertising; *behavioral research; deception; economics; *ethical review; evidence-based medicine; *health promotion; *health services research; industry; *law enforcement; mass media; *public health; public policy; research design; *research ethics committees; risks and benefits; *smoking; state government; intervention studies; Australia; *New South Wales

Chastain, Garvin; Landrum, R. Eric, eds. Protecting Human Subjects: Departmental Subject Pools and Institutional Review Boards. Washington, DC: American Psychological Association; 1999. 228 p. Includes references. ISBN 1-55798-575-8. BE62730.
> attitudes; *behavioral research; evaluation; evaluation studies; faculty; informed consent; investigators; misconduct; *organization and administration; program descriptions;

BE = bioethics accession number   fn. = footnotes   refs. = references

*psychology; research design; *research ethics committees; *research subjects; *selection of subjects; sexuality; *students; survey; *universities; volunteers; vulnerable populations; United States

BEHAVIORAL RESEARCH/FOREIGN COUNTRIES

Spurgeon, David. Canadian research councils publish joint code on ethics. [News]. *Nature.* 1998 Oct 1; 395(6701): 420. BE60808.
  advisory committees; *behavioral research; *guidelines; *human experimentation; interdisciplinary communication; *regulation; research ethics committees; *Canada; *Code of Conduct for Research involving Humans; *Medical Research Council of Canada; *Natural Sciences and Engineering Research Council (Canada); *Social Sciences and Humanities Research Council (Canada)

BEHAVIORAL RESEARCH/MINORS

Barr, Bernadine Courtright. Spare Children, 1900–1945: Inmates of Orphanages as Subjects of Research in Medicine and in the Social Sciences in America. Ann Arbor, MI: University Microfilms International; 1992. 341 p. Bibliography: p. 325–341. Dissertation, Ph.D. in Education, Stanford University, Jun 1992. Order No. 9302170. BE59732.
  attitudes; *behavioral research; *children; disadvantaged; emotions; epidemiology; historical aspects; *human experimentation; *infants; *institutionalized persons; intelligence; investigators; mentally retarded; normality; parent child relationship; physicians; psychology; *residential facilities; risks and benefits; selection of subjects; socioeconomic factors; diphtheria; Twentieth Century; United States

Fisher, Celia B.; Hoagwood, Kimberly; Jensen, Peter S. Casebook on ethical issues in research with children and adolescents with mental disorders. *In:* Hoagwood, Kimberly; Jensen, Peter S.; Fisher, Celia B., eds. Ethical Issues in Mental Health Research with Children and Adolescents. Mahwah, NJ: Lawrence Erlbaum Associates; 1996: 135–266. 188 refs. ISBN 0–8058–1953–3. BE62642.
  *adolescents; aggression; AIDS; alcohol abuse; *behavior disorders; *behavioral research; *case studies; child abuse; *children; competence; confidentiality; control groups; deception; drug abuse; empirical research; forensic psychiatry; genetic screening; HIV seropositivity; homosexuals; *human experimentation; incentives; infants; informed consent; *mentally ill; mentally retarded; minority groups; parent child relationship; parental consent; parents; placebos; privacy; psychoactive drugs; random selection; research design; research subjects; risks and benefits; selection of subjects; suicide; violence; war; withholding treatment; foster care

Hibbs, Euthymia D.; Krener, Penelope. Ethical issues in psychosocial treatment research with children and adolescents. *In:* Hoagwood, Kimberly; Jensen, Peter S.; Fisher, Celia B., eds. Ethical Issues in Mental Health Research with Children and Adolescents. Mahwah, NJ: Lawrence Erlbaum Associates; 1996: 59–71. 28 refs. ISBN 0–8058–1953–3. BE62638.
  *adolescents; audiovisual aids; *behavioral research; *children; confidentiality; control groups; disclosure; *health services research; incentives; informed consent; investigators; *mentally ill; parental consent; parents; placebos; professional competence; psychotherapy; research design; selection of subjects

Putnam, Frank W.; Liss, Marsha B.; Landsverk, John.

Ethical issues in maltreatment research with children and adolescents. *In:* Hoagwood, Kimberly; Jensen, Peter S.; Fisher, Celia B., eds. Ethical Issues in Mental Health Research with Children and Adolescents. Mahwah, NJ: Lawrence Erlbaum Associates; 1996: 113–132. 41 refs. ISBN 0–8058–1953–3. BE62641.
  *adolescents; behavior disorders; *behavioral research; *child abuse; *children; confidentiality; disclosure; empirical research; family members; informed consent; investigators; legal guardians; mandatory reporting; mentally ill; parent child relationship; parental consent; parents; patient advocacy; psychological stress; sex offenses; stigmatization; third party consent; foster care; multicenter studies; United States

BEHAVIORAL RESEARCH/REGULATION

Leigh, Wilhelmina A. Participant protection with the use of records: ethical issues and recommendations. *Ethics and Behavior.* 1998; 8(4): 305–319. 25 refs. BE60163.
  alcohol abuse; behavioral research; computer communication networks; *confidentiality; consent forms; data banks; *disclosure; *drug abuse; epidemiology; federal government; *government regulation; guidelines; health facilities; *health services research; informed consent; injuries; legal liability; *mentally ill; organizational policies; patient care; program descriptions; *records; *research subjects; time factors; recontact; Department of Health and Human Services; *Substance Abuse and Mental Health Services Administration; *United States
This article explores the ethical concerns and protections that may be required when individually identifiable data originally collected solely for clinical or administrative purposes are used in research or evaluation. It asks the following broad question with respect to the interim policy developed by the Substance Abuse and Mental Health Services Administration (SAMHSA) to protect the rights and welfare of participants in its programs: For those programs and projects not classified as research, are the protections and system for review adequate? Background information on SAMHSA's interim policy is provided, along with issues and questions related to the use of clinical and administrative records in research and evaluation. The article concludes with recommendations for modifying the existing participant protection guidelines, based on the preceding discussion of issues and questions.

Sewell, Dorita. Introduction [to a set of articles by T.F. McGovern, W.A. Leigh, E.J. Trickett, and J. de Jong and N. Reatig; and a report on the Annapolis Participant Protection Conference held by the Substance Abuse and Mental Health Services Administration (SAMHSA)]. *Ethics and Behavior.* 1998; 8(4): 285–291. 5 refs. BE60161.
  *behavioral research; confidentiality; *drug abuse; ethical review; federal government; *government regulation; guidelines; *health services research; legal aspects; *mentally ill; preventive medicine; research subjects; standards; vulnerable populations; *Substance Abuse and Mental Health Services Administration; United States

Spurgeon, David. Canadian research councils publish joint code on ethics. [News]. *Nature.* 1998 Oct 1; 395(6701): 420. BE60808.
  advisory committees; *behavioral research; *guidelines; *human experimentation; interdisciplinary communication; *regulation; research ethics committees; *Canada; *Code of Conduct for Research involving Humans; *Medical Research Council of Canada; *Natural Sciences and Engineering Research Council (Canada); *Social Sciences and Humanities Research Council (Canada)

BE = bioethics accession number   fn. = footnotes   refs. = references

BEHAVIORAL RESEARCH/RESEARCH DESIGN

Bower, Bruce. Psychology's tangled web: deceptive methods may backfire on behavioral researchers. *Science News.* 1998 Jun 20; 153(25): 394–395. BE59816.
> *behavioral research; *deception; empirical research; investigators; *psychology; research design; research subjects; trust; universities; volunteers

Häggman–Laitila, Arja. The authenticity and ethics of phenomenological research: how to overcome the researcher's own views. *Nursing Ethics.* 1999 Jan; 6(1): 12–22. 37 refs. BE60151.
> attitudes; *behavioral research; *communication; comprehension; *health; *investigator subject relationship; *investigators; nursing ethics; *nursing research; professional ethics; psychology; *research design; research subjects; *qualitative research

BEHAVIORAL RESEARCH/SPECIAL POPULATIONS

Byk, Christian. International Association for Law, Ethics and Science organizes third international meeting (Paris, 23–24 Sep 1994). *International Digest of Health Legislation.* 1995; 46(4): 572–574. BE62687.
> aborted fetuses; *behavior control; *behavioral research; *brain; brain pathology; fetal research; fetal tissue donation; human experimentation; informed consent; international aspects; legal aspects; *mentally ill; professional organizations; psychiatry; *psychoactive drugs; *neurosciences; International Association for Law, Ethics and Science

Downs, Murna. The emergence of the person in dementia research. *Ageing and Society.* 1997 Sep; 17(5): 597–607. 56 refs. BE59196.
> aged; autonomy; *behavioral research; communication; competence; *dementia; diagnosis; empirical research; family members; health services research; informed consent; *patient care; *patient participation; personhood; *research design; rights; risks and benefits; self concept; truth disclosure; support groups; United States

Fisher, Celia B.; Hoagwood, Kimberly; Jensen, Peter S. Casebook on ethical issues in research with children and adolescents with mental disorders. *In:* Hoagwood, Kimberly; Jensen, Peter S.; Fisher, Celia B., eds. Ethical Issues in Mental Health Research with Children and Adolescents. Mahwah, NJ: Lawrence Erlbaum Associates; 1996: 135–266. 188 refs. ISBN 0-8058-1953-3. BE62642.
> *adolescents; aggression; AIDS; alcohol abuse; *behavior disorders; *behavioral research; *case studies; child abuse; *children; competence; confidentiality; control groups; deception; drug abuse; empirical research; forensic psychiatry; genetic screening; HIV seropositivity; homosexuals; *human experimentation; incentives; infants; informed consent; *mentally ill; mentally retarded; minority groups; parent child relationship; parental consent; parents; placebos; privacy; psychoactive drugs; random selection; research design; research subjects; risks and benefits; selection of subjects; suicide; violence; war; withholding treatment; foster care

Hibbs, Euthymia D.; Krener, Penelope. Ethical issues in psychosocial treatment research with children and adolescents. *In:* Hoagwood, Kimberly; Jensen, Peter S.; Fisher, Celia B., eds. Ethical Issues in Mental Health Research with Children and Adolescents. Mahwah, NJ: Lawrence Erlbaum Associates; 1996: 59–71. 28 refs. ISBN 0-8058-1953-3. BE62638.
> *adolescents; audiovisual aids; *behavioral research; *children; confidentiality; control groups; disclosure; *health services research; incentives; informed consent; investigators; *mentally ill; parental consent; parents; placebos; professional competence; psychotherapy; research design; selection of subjects

James, Trudi; Platzer, Hazel. Ethical considerations in qualitative research with vulnerable groups: exploring lesbians' and gay men's experiences of health care -- a personal perspective. *Nursing Ethics.* 1999 Jan; 6(1): 73–81. 15 refs. BE60155.
> *behavioral research; emotions; females; *homosexuals; human rights; investigator subject relationship; investigators; males; nursing ethics; *nursing research; postmodernism; professional ethics; professional patient relationship; psychological stress; *stigmatization; vulnerable populations; *qualitative research

Kottow, Michael H.; Hammerman, Cathy; Kornbluth, Eti. Decision making in the critically ill neonate. [Letter and response]. *Journal of Medical Ethics.* 1998 Aug; 24(4): 280–281. 4 refs. BE61134.
> allowing to die; *behavioral research; *congenital disorders; critically ill; cultural pluralism; *decision making; newborns; nontherapeutic research; patient care; *pregnant women; prolongation of life; psychological stress; research design; research ethics committees; *survey

Kylmä, Jari; Vehviläinen–Julkunen, Katri; Lähdevirta, Juhani. Ethical considerations in a grounded theory study on the dynamics of hope in HIV–positive adults and their significant others. *Nursing Ethics.* 1999 May; 6(3): 224–239. 68 refs. BE61767.
> adults; AIDS; *behavioral research; *emotions; family members; *HIV seropositivity; informed consent; investigator subject relationship; investigators; nurses; *nursing research; patients; research design; research subjects; selection of subjects; stigmatization; vulnerable populations; *hope; *qualitative research; research ethics; sexual partners

McGovern, Thomas F. Vulnerability: reflection on its ethical implications for the protection of participants in SAMHSA programs. *Ethics and Behavior.* 1998; 8(4): 293–304. 18 refs. BE60162.
> alcohol abuse; autonomy; *behavioral research; beneficence; common good; confidentiality; *drug abuse; federal government; government regulation; *guidelines; *health services research; institutional ethics; justice; *mentally ill; preventive medicine; privacy; public participation; research ethics committees; research subjects; resource allocation; *stigmatization; *vulnerable populations; dignity; *Substance Abuse and Mental Health Services Administration; United States

The vulnerability of participants in Substance Abuse and Mental Health Services Administration (SAMHSA) programs is a consequence of the illnesses that they are experiencing; ethical guarantees must be in place that ensure the dignity of the persons involved in such programs. Dignity is more than an individual concern; it has individual, institutional, and societal dimensions. An ethical framework is proposed that involves the interrelated vulnerabilities and needs of individuals and communities and our societal response to them. Among the issues given particular attention are individual and community stigmatization, target population involvement in program planning, balance with regard to confidentiality and privacy, the place of proportionality grounded in a rich sense of community as a guiding ethical prinicple, and guidelines for SAMHSA programs.

Martin, Richard J.; Gwyther, Lisa P.; Whitehouse,

Peter J. Special care unit research: ethical issues. *Alzheimer Disease and Associated Disorders.* 1994; 8(Suppl. 1): S360–S367. 40 refs. BE61577.

> advance directives; attitudes; *behavioral research; coercion; competence; *dementia; health personnel; *health services research; human experimentation; informed consent; institutionalized persons; *long-term care; *nursing homes; patients; research design; research subjects; risks and benefits; third party consent; United States

Putnam, Frank W.; Liss, Marsha B.; Landsverk, John. Ethical issues in maltreatment research with children and adolescents. *In:* Hoagwood, Kimberly; Jensen, Peter S.; Fisher, Celia B., eds. Ethical Issues in Mental Health Research with Children and Adolescents. Mahwah, NJ: Lawrence Erlbaum Associates; 1996: 113–132. 41 refs. ISBN 0-8058-1953-3. BE62641.

> *adolescents; behavior disorders; *behavioral research; *child abuse; *children; confidentiality; disclosure; empirical research; family members; informed consent; investigators; legal guardians; mandatory reporting; mentally ill; parent child relationship; parental consent; parents; patient advocacy; psychological stress; sex offenses; stigmatization; third party consent; foster care; multicenter studies; United States

Sewell, Dorita. Introduction [to a set of articles by T.F. McGovern, W.A. Leigh, E.J. Trickett, and J. de Jong and N. Reatig; and a report on the Annapolis Participant Protection Conference held by the Substance Abuse and Mental Health Services Administration (SAMHSA)]. *Ethics and Behavior.* 1998; 8(4): 285–291. 5 refs. BE60161.

> *behavioral research; confidentiality; *drug abuse; ethical review; federal government; *government regulation; guidelines; *health services research; legal aspects; *mentally ill; preventive medicine; research subjects; standards; vulnerable populations; *Substance Abuse and Mental Health Services Administration; United States

BIOETHICS

See also MEDICAL ETHICS, NURSING ETHICS, PROFESSIONAL ETHICS

Andre, Judith; Fleck, Leonard; Tomlinson, Tom. Improving our aim. [Bioethics and the press]. *Journal of Medicine and Philosophy.* 1999 Apr; 24(2): 130–147. 29 refs. 5 fn. BE61438.

> assisted suicide; *bioethical issues; *bioethics; cloning; communication; democracy; disclosure; education; empirical research; *ethicist's role; *ethicists; guidelines; *interprofessional relations; *journalism; justice; knowledge, attitudes, practice; *mass media; public policy; religion; *technical expertise; uncertainty

Bioethicists appearing in the media have been accused of "shooting from the hip" (Rachels, 1991). The criticism is sometimes justified. We identify some reasons our interactions with the press can have bad results and suggest remedies. In particular we describe a target (fostering better public dialogue), obstacles to hitting the target (such as intrinsic and accidental defects in our knowledge) and suggest some practical ways to surmont those obstacles (including seeking out ways to write or speak at length, rather than in sound bites). We make use of our own research into the way journalists quote bioethicists. We end by suggesting that the profession as a whole look into this question more fully.

Annas, George J. Some Choice: Law, Medicine, and the Market. New York, NY: Oxford University Press; 1998. 303 p. 506 fn. ISBN 0-19-511832-4. BE60651.

> AIDS; allowing to die; assisted suicide; *bioethical issues; cancer; childbirth; cloning; confidentiality; disclosure; DNA data banks; drug abuse; *economics; famous persons; federal government; females; fetuses; *freedom; genetic information; genetic screening; *government regulation; guidelines; health; health care delivery; health care reform; human experimentation; human rights; informed consent; international aspects; *legal aspects; managed care programs; metaphor; paternalism; patient care; physicians; prenatal injuries; privacy; professional organizations; prognosis; *public policy; resource allocation; scientific misconduct; self regulation; smoking; state government; tuberculosis; marijuana; *United States

Arras, John D. A case approach. *In:* Kuhse, Helga; Singer, Peter, eds. A Companion to Bioethics. Malden, MA: Blackwell; 1998: 106–114. 23 refs. ISBN 0-631-19737-0. BE59487.

> bioethics; case studies; *casuistry; consensus; cultural pluralism; *ethical analysis; methods; moral policy; principle-based ethics

Aulisio, Mark P. The foundations of bioethics: contingency and relevance. *Journal of Medicine and Philosophy.* 1998 Aug; 23(4): 428–438. 11 refs. 2 fn. BE60632.

> *bioethics; *cultural pluralism; ethical analysis; ethicists; informed consent; personhood; *postmodernism; secularism; values; *Engelhardt, H. Tristram

In this essay, I proceed by, first, laying out H. Tristram Engelhardt's argument for the principle of permission as the proper foundation for a secular bioethic. After considering how a number of commentators have tried to undermine this argument, I show why it is immune to some of these advances. I then offer my own critique of Engelhardt's project. This critique is two pronged. First, I argue that Engelhardt is unable to establish his own foundation for a secular bioethic. This inability leaves him with only contingent points of departure for a secular bioethic, some of the more salient of which he has ignored. Second, I argue that even if Engelhardt's project succeeds, it is in danger of being irrelevant in a practical sense because it ignores important contextual dimensions of the peculiar enterprise we call bioethics. Ultimately, the proper foundations for a relevant secular bioethic. I argue, must appeal to certain contingent features of the context that gives rise to the need for it.

Baker, Robert. A theory of international bioethics: multiculturalism, postmodernism, and the bankruptcy of fundamentalism. *Kennedy Institute of Ethics Journal.* 1998 Sep; 8(3): 201–231. 33 refs. 9 fn. BE60166.

> *accountability; advisory committees; animal experimentation; anthropology; autonomy; *bioethics; codes of ethics; communitarianism; compensation; consensus; *cultural pluralism; dehumanization; *ethical analysis; *ethical relativism; *ethical theory; eugenics; evaluation; *guidelines; historical aspects; *human experimentation; *human rights; informed consent; *international aspects; investigators; *misconduct; models, theoretical; *morality; *National Socialism; philosophy; physicians; *postmodernism; principle-based ethics; privacy; public policy; *radiation; research subjects; *retrospective moral judgment; *scientific misconduct; standards; terminology; *values; *culpability; slavery; *Advisory Committee on Human Radiation Experiments; Cold War; *Germany; Macklin, Ruth; Nuremberg Code; Nuremberg Trials; Twentieth Century; United States

The first of two articles analyzing the justifiability of international bioethical codes and of cross-cultural moral judgments reviews "moral fundamentalism," the theory that cross-cultural moral judgments and international bioethical codes are justified by certain "basic" or "fundamental" moral priniciples that are universally

---

accepted in all cultures and eras. Initially propounded by the judges at the 1947 Nuremberg Tribunal, moral fundamentalism has become the received justification of international bioethics, and of cross-temporal and cross-cultural moral judgments. Yet today we are said to live in a multicultural and postmodern world. This article assesses the challenges that multiculturalism and postmodernism pose to fundamentalism and concludes that these challenges render the position philosophically untenable, thereby undermining the received conception of the foundations of international bioethics. The second article, which follows, offers an alternative model -- a model of negotiated moral order -- as a viable justification for international bioethics and for transcultural and transtemporal moral judgments.

Baker, Robert. A theory of international bioethics: the negotiable and the non-negotiable. *Kennedy Institute of Ethics Journal.* 1998 Sep; 8(3): 233-273. 50 refs. 12 fn. BE60167.
> *bioethics; circumcision; clinical ethics; codes of ethics; competence; *contracts; covenant; *cultural pluralism; developing countries; drugs; *ethical relativism; *ethical theory; federal government; females; *guidelines; HIV seropositivity; *human experimentation; *human rights; informed consent; *international aspects; investigator subject relationship; investigators; legal rights; medical schools; models, theoretical; *morality; National Socialism; philosophy; physicians; placebos; *postmodernism; pregnant women; privacy; professional ethics; professional organizations; regulation; research subjects; retrospective moral judgment; scientific misconduct; *standards; therapeutic research; third party consent; values; culpability; slavery; Council for International Organizations of Medical Sciences; Declaration of Helsinki; European Convention on Human Rights and Biomedicine; Germany; Harvard Medical School; Nuremberg Code; Nuremberg Trials; United States; World Medical Association

The preceding article in this issue of the *Kennedy Institute of Ethics Journal* presents the argument that "moral fundamentalism," the position that international bioethics rests on "basic" or "fundamental" moral prinicples that are universally accepted in all eras and cultures, collapses under a variety of multicultural and postmodern critiques. The present article looks to the contractarian tradition of Hobbes and Locke -- as reinterpreted by David Gauthier, Robert Nozick, and John Rawls -- for an alternative justification for international bioethics. Drawing on the central themes of this tradition, it is argued that international bioethics can be rationally reconstructed as a negotiated moral order that respects culturally and individually defined areas of nonnegotiability. Further, the theory of a negotiated moral order is consistent with traditional ideals about human rights, is flexible enough to absorb the genuine insights of multiculturalism and postmodernism, and yet is strong enough to justify transcultural and transtemporal moral judgments, including the condemnation of the Nazi doctors at Nuremberg. This theory also is consistent with the history of the ethics of human subjects experimentation and offers insights into current controversies such as the controversy over changing the consent rule for experiments in emergency medicine and the controversy over exempting certain clinical trials of inexpensive treatments for preventing the perinatal transmission of AIDS from the ethical standards of the sponsoring country.

Baker, Robert. Negotiating international bioethics: a response to Tom Beauchamp and Ruth Macklin. *Kennedy Institute of Ethics Journal.* 1998 Dec; 8(4): 423-453. 33

refs. 10 fn. BE62377.
> accountability; advisory committees; beneficence; *bioethics; circumcision; contracts; *cultural pluralism; *ethical analysis; *ethical relativism; *ethical theory; females; historical aspects; *human experimentation; *human rights; *international aspects; investigators; *morality; National Socialism; nontherapeutic research; philosophy; physicians; *postmodernism; *principle-based ethics; *radiation; research subjects; *retrospective moral judgment; scientific misconduct; sexuality; social discrimination; stigmatization; values; women's rights; *culpability; *Advisory Committee on Human Radiation Experiments; Asia; Europe; Germany; Twentieth Century; United States

Can the bioethical theories that have served American bioethics so well, serve international bioethics as well? In two papers in the previous issue of the *Kennedy Institute of Ethics Journal*, I contend that the form of principlist fundamentalism endorsed by American bioethicists like Tom Beauchamp and Ruth Macklin will not play on an international stage. Deploying techniques of postmodern scholarship, I argue that principlist fundamentalism justifies neither the condemnation of the Nazi doctors at Nuremberg, nor, as the *Report of the Advisory Committee on the Human Radiation Experiments* (ACHRE) demonstrates, condemnation of Cold War radiation researchers. Principlist fundamentalism thus appears to be philosophy bankrupt. In this issue of the *Journal*, Beauchamp and Macklin reject this claim, arguing that I have misread the ACHRE report and misunderstood Nazism. They also argue that the form of post-postmodern negotiated human rights theory that I proffer is adequate only insofar as it is itself really fundamentalist; insofar as I take postmodernism seriously, however, I mire international bioethics in relativism. In this response, I reaffirm my anti-fundamentalism, provide further evidence in support of my reading of the ACHRE report, and defend my post-postmodern version of rights theory. I also develop criteria for a minimally adequate theoretical framework for international bioethics.

Beauchamp, Tom L.; Walters, LeRoy, eds. Contemporary Issues in Bioethics. Fifth Edition. Belmont, CA: Wadsworth; 1999. 786 p. Includes references. ISBN 0-534-50476-0. BE60065.
> abortion, induced; active euthanasia; advance directives; AIDS; allowing to die; animal experimentation; assisted suicide; autonomy; beneficence; *bioethical issues; *bioethics; cloning; codes of ethics; confidentiality; developing countries; *ethical analysis; ethical theory; ethics; eugenics; genetic intervention; genome mapping; health care; health care delivery; HIV seropositivity; human experimentation; infertility; informed consent; international aspects; justice; managed care programs; *moral policy; mother fetus relationship; patients' rights; professional ethics; professional patient relationship; public policy; reproductive technologies; resource allocation; review; right to die; rights; scientific misconduct; treatment refusal; truth disclosure; vulnerable populations

Beauchamp, Tom L. The mettle of moral fundamentalism: a reply to Robert Baker. *Kennedy Institute of Ethics Journal.* 1998 Dec.; 8(4): 389-401. 7 refs. 2 fn. BE62375.
> accountability; advisory committees; *bioethics; contracts; *cultural pluralism; *ethical analysis; *ethical relativism; *ethical theory; historical aspects; *human experimentation; *human rights; informed consent; *international aspects; investigators; *morality; National Socialism; nontherapeutic research; philosophy; physicians; *principle-based ethics; public policy; *radiation; research subjects; *retrospective moral judgment; scientific misconduct; standards; values; culpability; *Advisory Committee on Human Radiation Experiments; Germany; Twentieth Century; United States

This article is a reply to Robert Baker's attempt to rebut

BE = bioethics accession number   fn. = footnotes   refs. = references

moral fundamentalism, while grounding international bioethics in a form of contractarianism. Baker is mistaken in several of his interpretations of the alleged moral fundamentalism and findings of the Advisory Committee on Human Radiation Experiments. He also misunderstands moral fundamentalism generally and wrongly categorizes it as morally bankrupt. His negotiated contract model is, in the final analysis, itself a form of the moral fundamentalism he declares bankrupt.

Belgium. Agreement on cooperation establishing a Consultative Committee on Bioethics, done at Brussels on 15 Jan 1993 between the State, the Flemish Community, the French Community, the German–Speaking Community, and the Joint Inter–Community Commission. (*Moniteur Belge*, 12 May 1993, No. 93, p. 10824–10828). [Summary]. *International Digest of Health Legislation.* 1994. 45(1). 47–48. BE62690.
  *advisory committees; *bioethical issues; committee membership; cultural pluralism; information dissemination; public policy; *Belgium; *Consultative Committee on Bioethics (Belgium)

Berglund, Catherine Anne. Bioethics: a balancing of concerns in context. *Australian Health Review.* 1997; 20(1): 43–52. 19 refs. BE60683.
  autonomy; beneficence; *bioethical issues; *bioethics; human experimentation; informed consent; justice; legal aspects; patient care; principle–based ethics; Australia

Berglund, Catherine Anne. Ethics for Health Care. New York, NY: Oxford University Press; 1998. 228 p. Bibliography: p. 211–224. Appendixes include medical and nursing codes of ethics from Australia and New Zealand. ISBN 0–19–554172–3. BE60704.
  abortion, induced; active euthanasia; assisted suicide; autonomy; beginning of life; *bioethical issues; biomedical research; caring; case studies; codes of ethics; competence; confidentiality; critically ill; drugs; economics; education; ethical theory; genome mapping; guidelines; health care; health care delivery; *health personnel; human experimentation; informed consent; institutional ethics; justice; patient care team; personhood; privacy; *professional ethics; professional organizations; professional patient relationship; public participation; quality of life; religious ethics; research ethics committees; risks and benefits; standards; trust; Australia; Australian Medical Association; Australian Nursing Council; National Health and Medical Research Council (Australia); New Zealand Medical Association

Bin Saeed, Khalid Saad. How physician executives and clinicians perceive ethical issues in Saudi Arabian hospitals. *Journal of Medical Ethics.* 1999 Feb; 25(1): 51–56. 12 refs. BE61196.
  *administrators; allowing to die; *attitudes; *bioethical issues; codes of ethics; comparative studies; confidentiality; conflict of interest; continuing education; cultural pluralism; deontological ethics; ethics committees; gifts; *hospitals; *institutional ethics; institutional policies; interprofessional relations; medical education; *medical ethics; misconduct; patient advocacy; patient care; patients' rights; physician patient relationship; *physicians; professional autonomy; prolongation of life; regulation; resource allocation; social discrimination; socioeconomic factors; survey; terminally ill; utilitarianism; values; withholding treatment; *Saudi Arabia
  OBJECTIVES: To compare the perceptions of physician executives and clinicians regarding ethical issues in Saudi Arabian hospitals and the attributes that might lead to the existence of these ethical issues. DESIGN: Self-completion questionnaire administered from February to July 1997. SETTING: Different health regions in the Kingdom of Saudi Arabia. PARTICIPANTS: Random sample of 457 physicians (317 clinicians and 140 physician executives) from several hospitals in various regions across the kingdom. RESULTS: There were statistically significant differences in the perceptions of physician executives and clinicians regarding the existence of various ethical issues in their hospitals. The vast majority of physician executives did not perceive that seven of the eight issues addressed by the study were ethical concerns in their hospitals. However, the majority of the clinicians perceived that six of the same eight issues were ethical considerations in their hospitals. Statistically significant differences in the perceptions of physician executives and clinicians were observed in only three out of eight attributes that might possibly lead to the existence of ethical issues. The most significant attribute that was perceived to result in ethical issues was that of hospitals having a multinational staff. CONCLUSION: The study calls for the formulation of a code of ethics that will address specifically the physicians who work in the kingdom of Saudi Arabia. As a more immediate initiative, it is recommended that seminars and workshops be conducted to provide physicians with an opportunity to discuss the ethical dilemmas they face in their medical practice.

Birmingham, Karen. UK leads on science and technology bioethics. [News]. *Nature Medicine.* 1998 Jun; 4(6): 651–652. BE59729.
  accountability; *bioethical issues; DNA data banks; *DNA fingerprinting; embryo research; forensic medicine; gene therapy; *genetic intervention; government regulation; *international aspects; law enforcement; prisoners; *public policy; *regulation; reproductive technologies; science; *Great Britain; United States

Bleich, J. David. Bioethical Dilemmas: A Jewish Perspective. Hoboken, NJ: Ktav; 1998. 375 p. 438 fn. ISBN 0–88125–473–8. BE60915.
  active euthanasia; AIDS; AIDS serodiagnosis; allowing to die; artificial feeding; artificial insemination; autonomy; *bioethical issues; confidentiality; deception; diagnosis; duty to warn; embryo disposition; embryo transfer; fathers; homosexuals; in vitro fertilization; *Jewish ethics; killing; multiple pregnancy; newborns; palliative care; parent child relationship; physician patient relationship; physicians; privacy; prognosis; prolongation of life; psychological stress; reproduction; reproductive technologies; risk; selective abortion; sperm; suffering; surrogate mothers; terminally ill; *theology; tissue banks; trust; truth disclosure; value of life; ventilators; withholding treatment; conjoined twins; Orthodox Judaism

Boyle, Joseph. An absolute rule approach. *In:* Kuhse, Helga; Singer, Peter, eds. A Companion to Bioethics. Malden, MA: Blackwell; 1998: 72–79. 8 refs. ISBN 0–631–19737–0. BE59483.
  bioethics; casuistry; *deontological ethics; ethical theory; methods; natural law; Roman Catholic ethics; teleological ethics

Brody, Baruch. Religion and bioethics. *In:* Kuhse, Helga; Singer, Peter, eds. A Companion to Bioethics. Malden, MA: Blackwell; 1998: 41–48. 15 refs. ISBN 0–631–19737–0. BE59480.
  *bioethics; conscience; covenant; *cultural pluralism; double effect; ethical analysis; public policy; *religious ethics; secularism

Burgio, G. Roberto; Lantos, John D., eds. *Primum Non Nocere* Today. Second Edition. New York, NY: Elsevier; 1998. 171 p. (International congress series; no.

BE = bioethics accession number   fn. = footnotes   refs. = references

1171). Includes references. New edition of the proceedings of the international Symposium on Pediatric Bioethics, held in Pavia, Italy, 26–28 May 1994. ISBN 0–444–82923–7. BE60917.

active euthanasia; adolescents; allowing to die; anthropology; *beneficence; *bioethical issues; *bioethics; biomedical technologies; bone marrow; cancer; children; cord blood; decision making; directed donation; disease; drugs; ethical theory; evidence–based medicine; fetal research; fetal therapy; gene therapy; genetic predisposition; genetic screening; historical aspects; human experimentation; immunization; informed consent; international aspects; medical education; minors; moral policy; newborns; organ donation; palliative care; parental consent; *patient care; *pediatrics; practice guidelines; prenatal diagnosis; quality of life; risks and benefits; selective abortion; stem cells; tissue donation; ear diseases

Byk, Christian. International colloquy, "From Ethics to Law, from Law to Ethics" (Lausanne, 17–18 Oct 1996). [Meeting report]. *International Digest of Health Legislation.* 1997; 48(2): 252–254. BE59601.

*bioethics; ethics committees; government regulation; human rights; *international aspects; *law; values; *Europe

Callahan, Daniel. Calling scientific ideology to account. *Society.* 1996 May–Jun; 33(4): 14–19. BE60064.

*accountability; *bioethics; biomedical research; biomedical technologies; ecology; economics; humanism; interdisciplinary communication; *religion; *science; secularism; *social dominance; social impact; *values; nature

Callahan, Daniel. The Hastings Center and the early years of bioethics. *Kennedy Institute of Ethics Journal.* 1999 Mar; 9(1): 53–71. 10 refs. BE62329.

*bioethics; education; ethical theory; ethicists; financial support; *historical aspects; *interdisciplinary communication; medicine; philosophy; public policy; *research institutes; science; secularism; social sciences; theology; *Callahan, Daniel; *Hastings Center; Twentieth Century; United States

The Hastings Center was founded in 1969 to study ethical problems in medicine and biology. The Center arose from a confluence of three social currents: the increased public scrutiny of medicine and its practices, the concern about the moral problems being generated by technological developments, and the desire of one its founders (Callahan) to make use of his philosophical training in a more applied way. The early years of the Center were devoted to raising money, developing an early agenda of issues, and identifying a cadre of people around the country interested in the issues. Various stresses and strains in the Center and the field are identified, and some final reflections are offered on the nature and value of the contributions made by bioethics as an academic field.

Callari Galli, M. Viewing bioethics from an anthropological viewpoint. *In:* Burgio, G. Roberto; Lantos, John D., eds. *Primum Non Nocere* Today. Second Edition. New York, NY: Elsevier; 1998: 23–26. 11 refs. ISBN 0–444–82923–7. BE60919.

*anthropology; *bioethical issues; *bioethics; biomedical technologies; *cultural pluralism; ethical relativism; interdisciplinary communication; morality; social impact; *values

Campbell, Alastair V. Presidential address: Global bioethics -- dream or nightmare? *Bioethics.* 1999 Jul; 13(3–4): 183–190. Address to the Fourth World Congress of Bioethics sponsored jointly by the International Association of Bioethics and the Asian Bioethics Association. BE61867.

*bioethics; biomedical technologies; capitalism; communication; cultural pluralism; *economics; ethical theory; *international aspects; justice; methods; social control; social dominance; *values; Western World; rationality

Caplan, Arthur. Bioethics: *The Birth of Bioethics* by Albert R. Jonsen. [Book review essay]. *JAMA.* 1999 Mar 3; 281(9): 849–850. BE60267.

advisory committees; bioethical issues; *bioethics; ethicists; *historical aspects; interdisciplinary communication; *The Birth of Bioethics (Jonsen, A.R.); *Twentieth Century; United States

Caplan, Arthur. Due Consideration: Controversy in the Age of Medical Miracles. New York, NY: Wiley; 1998. 282 p. 1998 ISBN 0–471–18344–X. BE60174.

abortion, induced; AIDS; AIDS serodiagnosis; allowing to die; animal experimentation; animal organs; assisted suicide; *bioethical issues; biomedical research; biomedical technologies; bone marrow; breast cancer; cloning; communicable diseases; determination of death; DNA fingerprinting; fetal development; fetal therapy; fetal tissue donation; fraud; genetic enhancement; genetic screening; health; health care; HIV seropositivity; human experimentation; managed care programs; mandatory testing; normality; organ transplantation; patents; posthumous reproduction; reproduction; reproductive technologies; resource allocation; scientific misconduct; smoking; tissue transplantation; war

Carlberg, Axel. The Moral Rubicon: A Study of the Principles of Sanctity of Life and Quality of Life in Bioethics. Lund, Sweden: Lund University Press; 1998. 208 p. (Lund studies in ethics and theology; 5). Bibliography: p. 197–206. ISBN 91–7966–521–7. BE62729.

abortion, induced; active euthanasia; allowing to die; autonomy; *bioethics; Christian ethics; cultural pluralism; decision making; ethical theory; fetuses; historical aspects; Jewish ethics; killing; medicine; moral obligations; moral policy; newborns; personhood; philosophy; *quality of life; secularism; speciesism; standards; utilitarianism; *value of life; values; Engelhardt, H. Tristram; Kekes, John; Kuhse, Helga; Singer, Peter

Carnevale, Franco A. The utility of futility: the construction of bioethical problems. *Nursing Ethics.* 1998 Nov; 5(6): 509–517. 29 refs. BE60885.

age factors; allowing to die; bioethical issues; *bioethics; communication; dissent; *futility; literature; patient discharge; philosophy; quality of life; *resuscitation; sociology of medicine; terminology; treatment outcome; trends; values; withholding treatment

Carse, Alisa L. Facing up to moral perils: the virtues of care in bioethics. *In:* Gordon, Suzanne; Benner, Patricia; Noddings, Nel, eds. Caregiving: Readings in Knowledge, Practice, Ethics, and Politics. Philadelphia, PA: University of Pennsylvania Press; 1996: 83–110. 81 refs. 9 fn. ISBN 0–8122–1582–6. BE62131.

autonomy; beneficence; *bioethics; *caring; communication; compassion; comprehension; decision making; education; emotions; empathy; *ethical analysis; *ethical theory; females; health personnel; informed consent; *justice; males; methods; *moral development; moral obligations; morality; *narrative ethics; nurse's role; paternalism; personhood; physician's role; principle–based ethics; professional ethics; professional patient relationship; *rights; social dominance; social interaction; suffering; trust; *virtues; vulnerable populations; dependency; Aristotle

Casarett, David J.; Daskal, Frona; Lantos, John. Experts in ethics? The authority of the clinical ethicist. *Hastings Center Report.* 1998 Nov–Dec; 28(6): 6–11. 19

fn. BE61278.

> *clinical ethics; *communication; *consensus; cultural pluralism; *decision making; dissent; *ethical analysis; ethical theory; *ethicist's role; *ethicists; *ethics consultation; goals; mediation; methods; principle-based ethics; technical expertise; values; Habermas, Jürgen

Mediator? Moral Expert? Or both? "Discourse Ethics" suggests that consensus provides the foundation for defensible moral norms. Thus in building consensus on a moral problem, an ethicist is not just negotiating a compromise but is contributing to the construction of moral rules and principles that have a genuine claim on us. In this way, not only does expertise on a variety of moral positions facilitate mediation, but mediation opens the way to a kind of moral expertise.

Chambers, Tod. Retrodiction and the histories of bioethics. *Medical Humanities Review.* 1998 Spring; 12(1): 9–22. 57 fn. BE62222.

> *bioethics; casuistry; communitarianism; cultural pluralism; decision making; *ethical theory; ethicists; *historical aspects; medical ethics; methods; narrative ethics; physicians; politics; postmodernism; secularism; socioeconomic factors; virtues; liberalism; The Abuse of Casuistry (Jonsen, A.; Toulmin, S.); The Ends of Human Life: Medical Ethics in a Liberal Polity (Emanuel, E.J.); The Foundations of Bioethics (Engelhardt, H.T.); The Virtues in Medical Practice (Pellegrino, E.D.; Thomasma, D.C.); United States

Chambers, Tod. The Fiction of Bioethics: Cases as Literary Text. New York, NY: Routledge; 1999. 207 p. (Reflective bioethics). Bibliography: p. 179–192. ISBN 0–415–91989–4. BE62754.

> audiovisual aids; bioethical issues; *bioethics; *case studies; ethical analysis; ethical theory; ethicist's role; ethics consultation; feminist ethics; *literature; methods; *narrative ethics; Cowart, Dax

Childress, James F. A principle-based approach. *In:* Kuhse, Helga; Singer, Peter, eds. A Companion to Bioethics. Malden, MA: Blackwell; 1998: 61–71. 25 refs. ISBN 0–631–19737–0. BE59482.

> bioethics; caring; casuistry; deontological ethics; ethical theory; methods; moral obligations; *moral policy; *principle-based ethics; utilitarianism; virtues

Connor, Susan Scholle; Fuenzalida-Puelma, Hernán L., eds. Bioethics: Issues and Perspectives. Washington, DC: Pan American Health Organization; 1990. 239 p. (Scientific publication; no. 527) Includes references. Published also as a special issue of the *Bulletin of the Pan American Health Organization*, 1990; 24(4). Appendixes include international codes of ethics, international research codes of ethics, patients' bills of rights, and various statements on human rights. Published also in Spanish as *Bioetica: Temas y Perspectivas*, 1990. ISBN 92–75–11527–3. BE60705.

> AIDS; allowing to die; autonomy; beneficence; *bioethical issues; *bioethics; biomedical technologies; clinical ethics; clinical ethics committees; codes of ethics; coercion; confidentiality; cultural pluralism; democracy; determination of death; developing countries; duty to warn; economics; education; ethical theory; health care delivery; hospitals; human experimentation; human rights; informed consent; *international aspects; justice; medical ethics; nursing ethics; organ donation; organ donors; organ transplantation; patients; philosophy; physician patient relationship; physicians; prolongation of life; religious ethics; reproduction; reproductive technologies; required request; resource allocation; selection for treatment; terminal care; virtues; integrity; Argentina; Brazil; Canada; Caribbean Region; Chile; Colombia; Latin America; Mexico; Peru; Spain; United States

Cook-Deegan, Robert Mullan. Finding a voice for bioethics in public policy: federal initiatives in the United States, 1974–1991. *In:* ten Have, Henk A.M.J.; Sass, Hans-Martin, eds. Consensus Formation in Healthcare Ethics. Boston, MA: Kluwer Academic; 1998: 107–140. 69 refs. 7 fn. ISBN 0–7923–4944–X. BE62591.

> *advisory committees; *bioethical issues; bioethics; committee membership; consensus; decision making; evaluation; *federal government; genome mapping; goals; *historical aspects; organization and administration; politics; *public policy; Biomedical Ethics Advisory Committee; Ethics Advisory Board; Human Fetal Tissue Transplantation Research Panel; Institute of Medicine; National Commission for the Protection of Human Subjects; NIH-DOE Working Group on Ethical, Legal, and Social Implications (ELSI); Office of Technology Assessment; President's Commission for the Study of Ethical Problems; *Twentieth Century; U.S. Congress; *United States

Coward, Harold; Ratanakul, Pinit, eds. A Cross-Cultural Dialogue on Health Care Ethics. Waterloo, ON: Wilfrid Laurier University Press; 1999. 274 p. Includes references. This book is the result of the work of a Canada-Thailand interdisciplinary research team of the Centre for Studies in Religion and Society at the University of Victoria in Canada. ISBN 0–88920–325–3. BE62785.

> alternative therapies; American Indians; attitudes to death; autonomy; *bioethical issues; Buddhist ethics; *cultural pluralism; *decision making; disease; ecology; family relationship; *health; *health care; *health care delivery; informed consent; international aspects; minority groups; minors; patient participation; physician patient relationship; public participation; *public policy; religion; risks and benefits; standards; terminal care; treatment refusal; *values; Confucian ethics; Taoist ethics; Canada; China; Thailand

Crosthwaite, Jan. Gender and bioethics. *In:* Kuhse, Helga; Singer, Peter, eds. A Companion to Bioethics. Malden, MA: Blackwell; 1998: 32–40. 26 refs. ISBN 0–631–19737–0. BE59479.

> *bioethics; caring; ethical theory; *females; *feminist ethics; health care; human experimentation; justice; males; patient care; social control; social discrimination; social dominance; women's health

Darragh, Martina. BIOETHICSLINE on the World Wide Web. [News]. *Kennedy Institute of Ethics Journal.* 1998 Dec; 8(4): 467–468. BE62379.

> *bioethics; *computer communication networks; *data banks; literature; *BIOETHICSLINE; *Internet; National Library of Medicine; National Reference Center for Bioethics Literature

Davis, Dena S.; Forster, Heidi P. Legal trends in bioethics. *Journal of Clinical Ethics.* 1998 Fall; 9(3): 323–332. 29 fn. BE61341.

> abortion, induced; advisory committees; AIDS serodiagnosis; assisted suicide; *bioethical issues; confidentiality; disabled; due process; electroconvulsive therapy; employment; fetal development; genetic disorders; genetic information; health personnel; HIV seropositivity; human experimentation; *legal aspects; legal liability; managed care programs; mentally ill; patient care; physician patient relationship; physicians; privacy; refusal to treat; reproduction; reproductive technologies; selective abortion; torts; marijuana; Americans with Disabilities Act 1990; Medicare; National Bioethics Advisory Commission; *United States

de Castro, Leonardo D. Is there an Asian bioethics? *Bioethics.* 1999 Jul; 13(3–4): 227–235. 15 fn. BE61872.

> autonomy; *bioethics; cultural pluralism; *ethical relativism; international aspects; non-Western World; values; Western World; *Asia

---

BE = bioethics accession number   fn. = footnotes   refs. = references

Is there an Asian bioethics? Some people might consider it blasphemous even to ask this question. But this paper asks it not so much to seek an answer as to clarify what it could actually mean. The idea is to sort out the presuppositions and possible implications of asserting the existence of an Asian bioethics. In the end, this paper makes the following points: (1) In the attempt to assert an Asian identity, one must be careful not to commit the mistake of universalizing (among Asians) a single Asian perspective; and (2) In the face of pluralism and multi–culturalism, there is some room for a kind of universalist ethics that is founded on a collage of culturally inspired perspectives rather than on a single standard of morality.

den Hartogh, Govert. The slippery slope argument. *In:* Kuhse, Helga; Singer, Peter, eds. A Companion to Bioethics. Malden, MA: Blackwell; 1998: 280–290. 6 refs. ISBN 0–631–19737–0. BE59503.
bioethical issues; bioethics; moral policy; philosophy; *wedge argument

DesAutels, Peggy. Religious women, medical settings, and moral risk. *In:* Walker, Margaret Urban, ed. Mother Time: Women, Aging, and Ethics. Lanham, MD: Rowman and Littlefield; 1999: 175–187. 23 refs. 5 fn. ISBN 0–8476–9260–4. BE61899.
adults; age factors; aged; alternative therapies; attitudes; *bioethical issues; bioethics; Christian Scientists; clergy; clinical ethics committees; decision making; ethicists; *females; *feminist ethics; health; hospitals; palliative care; *paternalism; patient care; patient participation; *physician patient relationship; *religion; religious hospitals; Roman Catholics; *secularism; sociology of medicine; stigmatization; suffering; treatment refusal; *values; faith healing

de Wachter, Maurice A.M. Sociology and bioethics in the U.S.A. [Book review essay]. *Hastings Center Report.* 1998 Sep–Oct; 28(5): 40–42. BE59553.
autonomy; *bioethics; ethicists; ethics committees; interdisciplinary communication; *social sciences; *Bioethics and Society: Constructing the Ethical Enterprise (DeVries, R.; Subedi, J., eds.); Europe; United States

Dickenson, Donna L. Cross–cultural issues in European bioethics. *Bioethics.* 1999 Jul; 13(3–4): 249–255. 19 fn. BE61875.
autonomy; *bioethics; competence; *cultural pluralism; deontological ethics; ethical theory; informed consent; *international aspects; medical ethics; models, theoretical; paternalism; patient compliance; patients' rights; physicians; professional autonomy; treatment refusal; *Europe
European biomedical ethics is often contrasted to American autonomy–based approaches, and both are usually distinguished as 'Western'. But at least three 'different voices' within European bioethics can be identified: the deontological codes of southern Europe (and Ireland), in which the patient has a positive duty to maximise his or her own health and to follow the doctor's instructions, whilst the physician is constrained more by professional norms than by patient rights; the liberal, rights–based models of Western Europe, in which the patient retains the negative right to override medical opinion, even if his or her mental capacity is in doubt; the social welfarist models of the Nordic countries, which concentrate on positive rights and entitlements to universal healthcare provision and entrust dispute resolution to non–elected administrative officials.

Dickson, David. Wellcome Trust funds new "Medicine in Society" program. [News]. *Nature Medicine.* 1998 May;

4(5): 542. BE59840.
*bioethics; biomedical research; biomedical technologies; *financial support; international aspects; public participation; public policy; *science; *social impact; *Great Britain; National Human Genome Research Institute; NHGRI Program on Ethical, Legal, and Social Implications (ELSI); United States; *Wellcome Trust

Diniz, Debora; Guilhem, Dirce Bellezi; Garrafa, Volnei. Biothics in Brazil. *Bioethics.* 1999 Jul; 13(3–4): 244–248. 7 fn. BE61874.
*bioethics; education; historical aspects; international aspects; literature; principle–based ethics; professional organizations; research ethics committees; *Brazil
In this article the authors briefly sketch the nature of Brazilian bioethics. Bioethics emerged in Brazil later than in other Western countries and the 1990's were the most important period for the spread of the discipline in the country. It is in this period that some structural elements of bioethics were established, such as research groups, regulation of Local Research Ethics Committees (Comitês Locais de Ética em Pesquisa -- CEP), the creation of the National Commission of Ethics in Research with Human Beings (Comissão Nacional de Ética em Pesquisa com Seres Humanos -- CONEP) and the Brazilian Bioethics Society (Sociedade Brasileira de Bioética -- SBB). With regard to theoretical work, Brazilian bioethics is clearly an importer of theories from countries central to the studies of bioethics, or, in other words, countries where biothics first emerged and was established. The most commonly used theory among Brazilian researchers is principalism.

Donchin, Anne; Purdy, Laura M., eds. Embodying Bioethics: Recent Feminist Advances. Lanham, MD: Rowman and Littlefield; 1999. 286 p. Includes references. ISBN 0–8476–8924–7. BE61012.
autonomy; *bioethical issues; *bioethics; caring; developing countries; disabled; disadvantaged; drug abuse; drugs; ethical analysis; ethical theory; ethicists; eugenics; *females; *feminist ethics; genetic counseling; genetic disorders; goals; health care; human experimentation; infertility; international aspects; justice; minority groups; moral obligations; physicians; pregnant women; prenatal injuries; public policy; reproduction; reproductive technologies; selective abortion; social control; social discrimination; socioeconomic factors; values; women's health; women's rights; menopause; Australia; Canada; China; Ukraine; United States

Dorff, Elliot N. Matters of Life and Death: A Jewish Approach to Modern Medical Ethics. Philadelphia, PA: Jewish Publication Society; 1998. 456 p. Bibliography: p. 424–442. ISBN 0–8276–0647–8. BE59663.
abortion, induced; active euthanasia; advance directives; allowing to die; artificial feeding; artificial insemination; assisted suicide; autopsies; *bioethical issues; bioethics; cloning; contraception; cosmetic surgery; disabled; embryo disposition; embryo transfer; gamete intrafallopian transfer; gene therapy; genetic counseling; genetic screening; health; health care; homosexuals; hospices; in vitro fertilization; infertility; *Jewish ethics; multiple pregnancy; obligations of society; organ donation; ovum donors; persistent vegetative state; physician's role; quality of life; reproduction; reproductive technologies; resource allocation; selection for treatment; semen donors; sterilization (sexual); suicide; surrogate mothers; terminal care; *theology; value of life; *Conservative Judaism

Dorff, Elliot N. The Jewish Tradition: Religious Beliefs and Health Care Decisions. [Booklet]. Chicago, IL: Park Ridge Center for the Study of Health, Faith, and Ethics; 1996. 23 p. (Religious beliefs and health care decisions series). 53 refs. 44 fn. BE62179.
abortion, induced; active euthanasia; advance directives;

allowing to die; animal experimentation; animal organs; artificial feeding; autonomy; autopsies; *bioethical issues; cadavers; congenital disorders; conscience; contraception; determination of death; disclosure; gene therapy; genetic screening; health; health care; human experimentation; informed consent; *Jewish ethics; marital relationship; mental health; organ donation; organ transplantation; ovum donors; palliative care; patient care; physician patient relationship; physician's role; prenatal diagnosis; reproductive technologies; semen donors; sex determination; sexuality; suicide; surrogate mothers; *theology; third party consent; truth disclosure; value of life; voluntary sterilization; withholding treatment; Conservative Judaism; Orthodox Judaism; Reform Judaism

Dósa, Agnes. Bioethics and health law in Hungary. *Saint Louis University Public Law Review.* 1996; 15(2): 403–409. 40 fn. BE59916.
    *bioethical issues; coercion; decision making; economics; *health care; informed consent; involuntary commitment; *legal aspects; minors; organ donation; paternalism; patient access to records; patients' rights; physician patient relationship; presumed consent; public health; truth disclosure; *Hungary

Drane, James F. Decisionmaking and consensus formation in clinical ethics. *In:* ten Have, Henk A.M.J.; Sass, Hans-Martin, eds. Consensus Formation in Healthcare Ethics. Boston, MA: Kluwer Academic; 1998: 143–157. 13 refs. 7 fn. ISBN 0-7923-4944-X. BE62592.
    bioethics; casuistry; *clinical ethics; *consensus; cultural pluralism; *decision making; ethical analysis; ethical relativism; *international aspects; medical ethics; methods; patient care; Europe; Latin America; North America

Drutchas, Geoffrey G. Is Life Sacred? Cleveland, OH: Pilgrim Press; 1998. 209 p. Includes references. ISBN 0-8298-1275-X. BE61353.
    abortion, induced; active euthanasia; allowing to die; attitudes to death; bioethical issues; capital punishment; *Christian ethics; fetuses; historical aspects; humanism; infanticide; killing; natural law; prolongation of life; Protestant ethics; Roman Catholic ethics; secularism; suicide; *theology; *value of life; wedge argument

Dubler, Nancy Neveloff. Current ethical issues in aging: introduction. *Generations (American Society on Aging).* 1994 Winter; 18(4): 5–8. BE60543.
    advance directives; aged; autonomy; *bioethical issues; *bioethics; caring; clinical ethics; common good; communication; decision making; dissent; ethics consultation; family members; health care delivery; health facilities; health personnel; home care; justice; legal aspects; long-term care; mediation; minority groups; patient care; patients' rights; religion; socioeconomic factors; terminal care; *trends; values; United States

DuBose, Edwin R., ed. The Jehovah's Witness Tradition: Religious Beliefs and Health Care Decisions. [Booklet]. Chicago, IL: Park Ridge Center for the Study of Health, Faith, and Ethics; 1995. 10 p. (Religious beliefs and health care decisions series). 55 refs. 8 fn. BE62180.
    abortion, induced; active euthanasia; advance directives; alcohol abuse; allowing to die; assisted suicide; attitudes to death; autonomy; autopsies; *bioethical issues; *blood transfusions; confidentiality; contraception; drug abuse; electroconvulsive therapy; family relationship; genetic research; health; health care; informed consent; *Jehovah's Witnesses; mental health; mentally ill; organ transplantation; patient care; psychoactive drugs; psychotherapy; reproductive technologies; sexuality; suicide; theology; third party consent; treatment refusal; truth disclosure; voluntary sterilization

DuBose, Edwin R., ed. The Seventh-Day Adventist Tradition: Religious Beliefs and Health Care Decisions. [Booklet]. Chicago, IL: Park Ridge Center for the Study of Health, Faith, and Ethics; 1996. 7 p. (Religious beliefs and health care decisions series). 12 refs. BE62181.
    abortion, induced; active euthanasia; advance directives; AIDS; alcohol abuse; allowing to die; assisted suicide; autonomy; *bioethical issues; blood transfusions; confidentiality; contraception; drug abuse; drugs; gene therapy; genetic intervention; genetic research; genetic screening; health; health care; hypnosis; informed consent; organ donation; organ transplantation; palliative care; patient care; *Protestant ethics; quality of life; reproduction; reproductive technologies; sexuality; suffering; terminal care; theology; third party consent; truth disclosure; value of life; *Adventists; RU-486

Elliott, Carl. A Philosophical Disease: Bioethics, Culture and Identity. New York, NY: Routledge; 1999. 188 p. (Reflective bioethics). 246 fn. ISBN 0-415-91940-1. BE62623.
    bioethical issues; *bioethics; biomedical technologies; case studies; casuistry; clinical ethics; competence; conflict of interest; conscience; cultural pluralism; depressive disorder; enhancement technologies; ethical analysis; ethical theory; ethicists; ethics consultation; goals; health; hearing disorders; hospitals; human experimentation; intersexuality; law; literature; managed care programs; medicine; mental health; methods; morality; narrative ethics; normality; patient care; personhood; *philosophy; physically disabled; physician patient relationship; postmodernism; psychiatric diagnosis; psychiatry; psychotherapy; remuneration; sociology of medicine; trends; values; pragmatism; Percy, Walker; Prozac; United States; Wittgenstein, Ludwig

Elshtain, Jean Bethke; Cloyd, J. Timothy, eds. Politics and the Human Body: Assault on Dignity. Nashville, TN: Vanderbilt University Press; 1995. 323 p. 366 fn. ISBN 0-8265-1259-3. BE61045.
    allowing to die; attitudes to death; autonomy; *bioethical issues; bioethics; body parts and fluids; cadavers; chronically ill; commodification; compassion; contracts; dehumanization; democracy; DNA fingerprinting; education; eugenics; females; feminist ethics; freedom; futility; gene therapy; genome mapping; *human body; human rights; incentives; intensive care units; international aspects; legal aspects; males; organ donation; pain; personhood; politics; property rights; remuneration; reproductive technologies; schools; self concept; social control; social dominance; *suffering; surrogate mothers; terminal care; torture; *slavery

Emanuel, Ezekiel J. The blossoming of bioethics at NIH. *Kennedy Institute of Ethics Journal.* 1998 Dec; 8(4): 455–466. 3 refs. 2 fn. BE62378.
    advisory committees; bioethical issues; *bioethics; clinical ethics; education; ethicists; ethics consultation; faculty; federal government; goals; government financing; historical aspects; human experimentation; *organization and administration; *program descriptions; public policy; research ethics committees; *research institutes; teaching methods; National Human Genome Research Institute; *National Institutes of Health; NHGRI Program on Ethical, Legal, and Social Implications (ELSI); Twentieth Century; United States

The establishment of the Department of Clinical Bioethics at the Warren G. Magnuson Clinical Center of the National Institutes of Health (NIH) has coincided with a burgeoning of interest and activity related to bioethical issues at NIH. The department has precipitated a reexamination and revitalization of existing bioethics activities in the Clinical Center and has launched new programs especially in the areas of education and research. In addition, the department contributes to the work of others throughout NIH who address bioethical issues.

Engelhardt, H. Tristram. Critical care: why there is no global bioethics. *Journal of Medicine and Philosophy.* 1998 Dec; 23(6): 643–651. 4 refs. 1 fn. BE62071.

autonomy; *bioethics; critically ill; *cultural pluralism; decision making; developing countries; economics; *ethical relativism; *health care delivery; informed consent; *international aspects; justice; morality; non–Western World; public policy; quality of health care; resource allocation; secularism; standards; third party consent; *values; Western World; egalitarianism; United States

The high technology and the costs involved in critical care disclose the implausibility of applying the American standard version of bioethics in the developing world. The American standard version of bioethics was framed during the rapid secularization of the American culture, the emergence of a new image for the medical profession, the development of high technology medicine, an ever greater demand in resources, and a shift of focus from families and communities to individuals. This all brought with it a particular ideology of health care which promised Americans (1) the best of care, (2) equal care, and (3) physician/patient choice, without (4) runaway costs. This essay argues that this moral project is impossible in practice. This impossibility is especially salient in developing countries. In addition to the fact that it is financially impossible to provide all in the developing world with the standard of care accepted by law, policy, and convention in developed countries, different moral perspectives with different orderings of values will seem more or less plausible in different cultures. Indeed, such an approach would be harmful. A concrete bioethics applicable across the world does not appear possible.

European Federation of Scientific Networks. European Scientific Co-operation Network: "Medicine and Human Rights". The Human Rights, Ethical and Moral Dimensions of Health Care. Strasbourg, France: Council of Europe Publishing; 1998 Mar. 485 p. "One hundred and twenty cases examined from the standpoint of legal norms, international and European ethics, and the Catholic, Protestant, Jewish, Muslim, Buddhist and agnostic moralties, presented as an aid to decision-making and teaching." ISBN 92-871-3055-8. BE60570.

abortion, induced; active euthanasia; AIDS; allowing to die; *bioethical issues; bioethics; blood transfusions; *case studies; circumcision; coercion; confidentiality; ecology; genetic intervention; guidelines; human experimentation; *human rights; informed consent; *international aspects; killing; legal aspects; medical education; misconduct; nursing ethics; organ donation; physicians; psychiatry; *religious ethics; reproductive technologies; secularism; sterilization (sexual); torture; transsexualism; treatment refusal; value of life; vulnerable populations; Council of Europe; *Europe

European Parliament. Scientific and Technological Options Assessment (STOA) Programme Contractor. Bioethics in Europe. Final Report, July 1992. Luxembourg: European Parliament, Directorate General for Research; 1992 Sep 8. 257 p. Includes references. Pub. No. PE 158.453. BE62499.

advisory committees; attitudes; *bioethical issues; bioethics; biological warfare; *biomedical technologies; *comparative studies; *ecology; embryo research; fetal research; fetal tissue donation; food; gene therapy; *genetic intervention; genetic screening; genome mapping; germ cells; government regulation; hormones; in vitro fertilization; *international aspects; patents; preimplantation diagnosis; prenatal diagnosis; professional organizations; public opinion; *public policy; recombinant DNA research; reproductive technologies; risks and benefits; *social impact; technology assessment; transgenic animals; transgenic organisms;

agriculture; *biotechnology; *Denmark; *Europe; European Community; *European Parliament; *France; *Germany; *Great Britain; *Greece; *Italy; *Spain

Evans, Martyn. Bioethics and the newspapers. *Journal of Medicine and Philosophy.* 1999 Apr; 24(2): 164–180. 14 refs. 9 fn. BE61440.

*bioethical issues; *bioethics; brain death; communication; confidentiality; determination of death; disclosure; ethical analysis; ethicists; goals; interprofessional relations; *journalism; *mass media; narrative ethics; philosophy; values

Many bioethics questions are resistant to journalistic exploration on account of their inherently philosophical dimensions. Such dimensions are ill-suited to what we may term the internal goods (in MacIntyre's sense) of the newspapers and mass media generally, which constrain newspaper coverage to an abbreviated form of narrative that, whilst not in itself objectionable, is nonetheless inimical to the conduct of philosophical reflection. The internal goods of academic bioethics, by contrast, include attention to philosophical questions inherent in bioethical issues and value-enquiry. The danger for bioethics is that its agenda for reflective enquiry will, if dictated by this abbreviated narrative, be distorted in terms of both range and priorities, to the inevitable neglect of questions having a philosophical dimension to them. This danger can be avoided by a constructive partnership between the media and academic bioethics. The success of this partnership relies on four suggested provisos, for the meeting of which both journalists and academics bear responsibility.

Evans, Martyn. The utility of the body. *In:* ten Have, Henk A.M.J.; Welie, Jos V.M., eds. Ownership of the Human Body: Philosophical Considerations on the Use of the Human Body and Its Parts in Healthcare. Boston, MA: Kluwer Academic; 1998: 207–226. 9 refs. 12 fn. ISBN 0-7923-5150-9. BE61324.

aborted fetuses; altruism; autopsies; *bioethical issues; blood donation; cadavers; common good; family members; *human body; mandatory programs; *moral policy; *property rights; public policy; remuneration; risks and benefits; third party consent; tissue transplantation; *utilitarianism; voluntary programs

Fagot-Largeault, Anne. Ownership of the human body: judicial and legislative responses in France. *In:* ten Have, Henk A.M.J.; Welie, Jos V.M., eds. Ownership of the Human Body: Philosophical Considerations on the Use of the Human Body and Its Parts in Healthcare. Boston, MA: Kluwer Academic; 1998: 115–140. 39 refs. 2 fn. ISBN 0-7923-5150-9. BE61321.

abortion, induced; advisory committees; *bioethical issues; blood donation; *body parts and fluids; commodification; contraception; government regulation; historical aspects; *human body; human experimentation; human rights; informed consent; *legal aspects; nontherapeutic research; obligations to society; organ donation; presumed consent; privacy; *property rights; remuneration; sexuality; therapeutic research; women's rights; national ethics committees; *France; National Ethics Advisory Committee (France)

Fielding, Helen A. Body measures: phenomenological considerations of corporeal ethics. *Journal of Medicine and Philosophy.* 1998 Oct; 23(5): 533–545. 11 refs. 3 fn. Note: the journal issue cover shows a date of August 1998, which is incorrect. BE62117.

audiovisual aids; *bioethics; body parts and fluids; commodification; *human body; mass media; motivation; *organ donation; philosophy; *remuneration; *phenomenology; Dekalog 10: Thou Shall Not Covet Thy

Neighbour's Goods; Heidegger, Martin; Kieślowski, Krzysztof; Merleau-Ponty, Maurice

The development of bioethics primarily at the cognitive level further perpetuates the tendency to construe all aspects of our lives, including our bodies, as technical systems. For example, if we consider the moral issue of organ sales without taking our embodiment into account, there appear to be no sound arguments for opposing such sales. However, it is important to consider the aspects of the phenomenal body that challenge rational deliberation by exploring an embodied approach to the ethical dilemma produced by a proposed kidney exchange as presented in Krzysztof Kieślowski's *Dekalog* films. What is sought is a description of a body-measure that would serve as a critique of strictly cognitive bioethical deliberations.

Fins, Joseph J.; Miller, Franklin G.; Bacchetta, Matthew D. Clinical pragmatism: bridging theory and practice. *Kennedy Institute of Ethics Journal.* 1998 Mar; 8(1): 37-42. 11 refs. 1 fn. Commentary on L.A. Jansen, p. 23-36. BE59353.
    bioethics; *clinical ethics; consensus; *ethical analysis; ethical theory; *methods; principle-based ethics; *pragmatism; Dewey, John
This response to Lynn Jansen's critique of clinical pragmatism concentrates on two themes: (1) contrasting approaches to moral epistemology and (2) the connection between theory and practice in clinical ethics. Particular attention is paid to the status of principles and the role of consensus, with some closing speculations on how Dewey might view the current state of bioethics.

Flynn, Eileen P. Issues in Medical Ethics. Kansas City, MO: Sheed and Ward; 1997. 384 p. Bibliography: p. 376-380 ISBN 1-55612-917-3. BE61354.
    abortion, induced; adults; advance directives; AIDS; allowing to die; artificial feeding; autonomy; *bioethical issues; case studies; children; common good; congenital disorders; decision making; economics; ethical analysis; fetal research; fetal tissue donation; futility; genetic intervention; health care delivery; HIV seropositivity; human experimentation; informed consent; legal aspects; managed care programs; moral policy; newborns; organ donation; organ transplantation; paternalism; physicians; religious ethics; reproductive technologies; terminal care; voluntary euthanasia; withholding treatment; United States

Forster, Heidi P. Legal trends in bioethics. *Journal of Clinical Ethics.* 1998 Winter; 9(4): 421-430. 27 fn. BE60492.
    abortion, induced; AIDS serodiagnosis; allowing to die; *bioethical issues; body parts and fluids; brain death; cadavers; cloning; embryo disposition; eugenics; government regulation; HIV seropositivity; human experimentation; international aspects; *legal aspects; managed care programs; minors; negligence; organ donation; organ transplantation; prisoners; prolongation of life; psychoactive drugs; reproductive technologies; resource allocation; right to die; voluntary euthanasia; wrongful life; marijuana; *United States

Forster, Heidi P. Legal trends in bioethics. *Journal of Clinical Ethics.* 1999 Spring; 10(1): 66-75. 28 fn. BE62708.
    abortion, induced; active euthanasia; AIDS; allowing to die; assisted suicide; *bioethical issues; children; circumcision; cloning; drug industry; drugs; duty to warn; economics; embryo research; federal government; females; fetal development; government regulation; guidelines; HIV seropositivity; human experimentation; informed consent; international aspects; *legal aspects; legal liability; managed care programs; mentally disabled; organ donation; palliative care; patient transfer; physicians; psychiatry; refusal to treat;

state government; stem cells; surrogate mothers; withholding treatment; marijuana; Canada; Finn, Hugh; Germany; Great Britain; Kevorkian, Jack; Senegal; *United States; Youk, Thomas

Fox, Jeffrey L. U.S. Bioethics Commission meets, outlines agenda. [News]. *Nature Biotechnology.* 1996 Nov; 14(11): 1533. BE61419.
    *advisory committees; *bioethical issues; federal government; genetic information; genetic screening; government regulation; human experimentation; privacy; *public policy; research ethics committees; *National Bioethics Advisory Commission; Office for Protection from Research Risks; *United States

Freedman, Benjamin. Duty and Healing: Foundations of a Jewish Bioethic. New York, NY: Routledge; 1999. 344 p. (Reflective bioethics). 413 fn. With an introduction by Charles Weijer. ISBN 0-415-92180-5. BE61646.
    aged; allowing to die; artificial feeding; autonomy; *bioethical issues; *bioethics; case studies; coercion; *competence; cosmetic surgery; *decision making; drugs; ethical analysis; *ethicist's role; *ethics consultation; *family members; *family relationship; health; hospitals; human experimentation; *informed consent; *Jewish ethics; mentally ill; methods; *moral obligations; occupational exposure; palliative care; paralysis; parent child relationship; *patient care; physician's role; prolongation of life; quality of life; *rights; risks and benefits; secularism; suffering; terminal care; theology; third party consent; treatment refusal; truth disclosure; uncertainty; value of life; unproven therapies

Gastmans, Chris. The significance of the Convention on Human Rights and Biomedicine of the Council of Europe for healthcare ethics committees. *HEC (HealthCare Ethics Committee) Forum.* 1998 Sep-Dec; 10(3-4): 350-358. 8 refs. BE61186.
    advisory committees; *bioethical issues; clinical ethics committees; *ethics committees; guidelines; health care; *human rights; international aspects; public participation; national ethics committees; Council of Europe; *Europe; *European Convention on Human Rights and Biomedicine

Gatter, Robert. Communicative ethics for bioethics. *Bioethics Examiner.* 1997 Fall; 1(3): 4-5. 6 fn. BE59793.
    *bioethics; casuistry; *communication; consensus; cultural pluralism; *methods; principle-based ethics; *communicative ethics

Gbadegesin, Segun. Bioethics and cultural diversity. *In:* Kuhse, Helga; Singer, Peter, eds. A Companion to Bioethics. Malden, MA: Blackwell; 1998: 24-31. 14 refs. ISBN 0-631-19737-0. BE59478.
    *bioethics; *cultural pluralism; *ethical relativism; *international aspects; *non-Western World; *values; *Western World; Africa

General Conference of Seventh-Day Adventists. Christian View of Human Life Committee. The Seventh-Day Adventist Church Focuses on Ethical Issues. Washington, DC: General Conference of Seventh-Day Adventists; 1996 Jul. 39 p. 6 fn. Includes the following statements: Considerations on Assisted Human Reproduction (July 26, 1994); Seventh-Day Adventist Guidelines on Abortion (October 12, 1992); Recommendations: Use of Mifepristone (RU-486) (July 26, 1994); Seventh-Day Adventist Statement of Consensus on Care for the Dying (October 9, 1992); Christian Principles of Genetic Interventions (June 13, 1995); Birth Control: A Seventh-Day Adventist Statement of Consensus (June 1996 -- draft, approval pending). BE60859.
    abortion, induced; allowing to die; autonomy; *bioethical

---

BE = bioethics accession number   fn. = footnotes   refs. = references

issues; biological warfare; confidentiality; conscience; contraception; gene therapy; genetic intervention; genetic screening; parent child relationship; pregnant women; *Protestant ethics; reproductive technologies; suffering; terminal care; theology; value of life; *Adventists; RU–486

Goldstein, Doris Mueller, comp. Bibliography of resources by and about André Hellegers. *Kennedy Institute of Ethics Journal.* 1999 Mar; 9(1): 89–107. BE62331.
    *bioethical issues; biomedical research; ethicists; fetal development; fetuses; pregnant women; *Hellegers, André

Goodman, Kenneth W. Philosophy as news: bioethics, journalism and public policy. *Journal of Medicine and Philosophy.* 1999 Apr; 24(2): 181–200. 25 refs. 4 fn. BE61441.
    *bioethical issues; *bioethics; communication; decision making; democracy; education; *ethicist's role; *ethicists; evaluation; *goals; information dissemination; *interprofessional relations; *journalism; *mass media; moral obligations; obligations to society; philosophy; professional competence; *public policy; *standards; *technical expertise; values
News media accounts of issues in bioethics gain significance to the extent that the media influence public policy and inform personal decision making. The increasingly frequent appearance of bioethics in the news thus imposes responsibilities on journalists and their sources. These responsibilities are identified and discussed, as is (i) the concept of "news-worthiness" as applied to bioethics, (ii) the variable quality of bioethics reportage and (iii) journalists' reliance on ethicists to pass judgment. Because of the potential social and other benefits of high quality reporting on ethical issues, it is argued that journalists and their bioethics sources should explore and accommodate more productive relationships. An optimal journalism–ethics relationship will be one characterized by "para-ethics," in which journalistic constraints are noted but also in which issues and arguments are presented without oversimplification and credible disagreement is given appropriate attention.

Grisez, Germain. About health care issues. *In: his* The Way of the Lord Jesus. Volume 3: Difficult Moral Questions. Chicago, IL: Franciscan Herald Press; 1997: 203–419. 144 fn. Title supplied. ISBN 0-8199-0981-5. BE60741.
    aborted fetuses; abortion, induced; active euthanasia; allowing to die; artificial feeding; *bioethical issues; confidentiality; conscience; contraception; cosmetic surgery; deception; disclosure; employment; family members; fetal research; genetic counseling; health; HIV seropositivity; infertility; informed consent; intention; living wills; maternal health; mentally retarded; nurses; organ transplantation; patient care; persistent vegetative state; pharmacists; physicians; placebos; prolongation of life; referral and consultation; religious hospitals; remuneration; reproductive technologies; *Roman Catholic ethics; selective abortion; spousal consent; sterilization (sexual); suicide; treatment refusal; truth disclosure; twins; conjoined twins

Gudorf, Christine E. Gender and culture in the globalization of bioethics. *Saint Louis University Public Law Review.* 1996; 15(2): 331–351. 122 fn. BE59913.
    autonomy; beneficence; *bioethics; children; *circumcision; *coercion; *common good; contraception; *cultural pluralism; developing countries; ecology; *females; *feminist ethics; human rights; injuries; *international aspects; involuntary sterilization; justice; males; non–Western World; obligations to society; physicians; *population control; public policy; religion; reproduction; risks and benefits; sexuality; social control; Western World; *women's health

Hare, R.M. A utilitarian approach. *In:* Kuhse, Helga; Singer, Peter, eds. A Companion to Bioethics. Malden, MA: Blackwell; 1998: 80–85. 11 refs. ISBN 0-631-19737-0. BE59484.
    bioethics; methods; teleological ethics; *utilitarianism

Harris–Abbott, Deborah, ed. The Latter-Day Saints Tradition: Religious Beliefs and Health Care Decisions. [Booklet]. Chicago, IL: Park Ridge Center for the Study of Health, Faith, and Ethics; 1995. 19 p. (Religious beliefs and health care decisions series). 24 refs. BE62182.
    abortion, induced; active euthanasia; advance directives; allowing to die; assisted suicide; attitudes to death; autonomy; autopsies; *bioethical issues; congenital disorders; conscience; contraception; decision making; drug abuse; family members; fetal tissue donation; gene therapy; genetic research; health; health care; human body; informed consent; marital relationship; mental health; organ donation; organ transplantation; pastoral care; patient care; physician patient relationship; *Protestant ethics; psychotherapy; reproduction; reproductive technologies; selective abortion; sex determination; sex preselection; sexuality; suicide; surrogate mothers; *theology; third party consent; treatment refusal; voluntary sterilization; *Mormonism

Hayes, Edward J.; Hayes, Paul J.; Kelly, Dorothy Ellen, et al. Principles relating to the preservation of life. *In: their* Catholicism and Ethics. Norwood, MA: C.R. Publications; 1997: 153–175. Includes discussion questions and projects. References embedded in list at back of book. ISBN 0-9649087-7-8. BE61948.
    aborted fetuses; *alcohol abuse; allowing to die; artificial feeding; *bioethical issues; circumcision; *cosmetic surgery; fetal tissue donation; *human body; *hypnosis; institutional policies; males; *organ donation; *organ transplantation; persistent vegetative state; religious hospitals; *Roman Catholic ethics; sterilization (sexual); *surgery; *terminally ill; *tissue donation; *tissue transplantation; *value of life; withholding treatment

Hernández–Arriaga, Jorge; Navarrete de Olivares, Victoria; Iserson, Kenneth V. The development of bioethics in Mexico. *Cambridge Quarterly of Healthcare Ethics.* 1999 Summer; 8(3): 382–385. 12 refs. BE62480.
    advisory committees; animal experimentation; *bioethics; education; ethical review; human experimentation; medical education; medical ethics; public policy; research institutes; publishing; *Mexico; National Bioethics Commission (Mexico)

Hoffmaster, Barry. Part II, conclusion. *In:* Coward, Harold; Ratanakul, Pinit, eds. A Cross–Cultural Dialogue on Health Care Ethics. Waterloo, ON: Wilfrid Laurier University Press; 1999: 146–153. 13 refs. ISBN 0-88920-325-3. BE62791.
    autonomy; *bioethical issues; competence; *cultural pluralism; decision making; disclosure; family members; health care delivery; health personnel; patient care; physician patient relationship; public policy; truth disclosure; North America

Hoffmaster, Barry. Secular health care ethics. *In:* Coward, Harold; Ratanakul, Pinit, eds. A Cross–Cultural Dialogue on Health Care Ethics. Waterloo, ON: Wilfrid Laurier University Press; 1999: 139–145. 12 refs. ISBN 0-88920-325-3. BE62790.
    autonomy; *bioethical issues; competence; *decision making; family members; feminist ethics; health care; law; paternalism; patients; philosophy; physician patient relationship; physicians; secularism; theology; third party consent; values

Holmes, Helen Bequaert. Closing the gaps: an imperative for feminist bioethics. *In:* Donchin, Anne; Purdy, Laura

---

BE = bioethics accession number   fn. = footnotes   refs. = references

M., eds. Embodying Bioethics: Recent Feminist Advances. Lanham, MD: Rowman and Littlefield; 1999: 45-63. 50 refs. 16 fn. ISBN 0-8476-8924-7. BE61014.
    autonomy; bioethical issues; *bioethics; clinical ethics committees; conflict of interest; *disadvantaged; employment; ethicist's role; ethicists; ethics consultation; *evaluation; females; *feminist ethics; *health care; health personnel; interprofessional relations; *justice; managed care programs; medicine; minority groups; physicians; social dominance; social impact; *socioeconomic factors; *values; United States

Hope, Tony. Empirical medical ethics. [Editorial]. *Journal of Medical Ethics.* 1999 Jun; 25(3): 219-220. 4 refs. BE61853.
    advance directives; behavior disorders; *bioethical issues; *bioethics; competence; confidentiality; *empirical research; ethical theory; informed consent; interdisciplinary communication; medical ethics; *methods; narrative ethics; quality adjusted life years; research ethics committees; treatment refusal

Hoyle, Russ. US national bioethics commission: politics as usual? *Nature Biotechnology.* 1996 Aug; 14(8): 927. BE61399.
    *advisory committees; *bioethical issues; federal government; genetic research; genetic screening; genome mapping; historical aspects; human experimentation; international aspects; politics; *public policy; *National Bioethics Advisory Commission; NCHGR Program on Ethical, Legal, and Social Implications (ELSI); *United States

Hui, Edwin. Chinese health care ethics. *In:* Coward, Harold; Ratanakul, Pinit, eds. A Cross-Cultural Dialogue on Health Care Ethics. Waterloo, ON: Wilfrid Laurier University Press; 1999: 128-138. 10 refs. 40 fn. ISBN 0-88920-325-3. BE62789.
    abortion, induced; attitudes to death; autonomy; *bioethical issues; decision making; family relationship; futility; informed consent; males; parent child relationship; personhood; physician patient relationship; prolongation of life; religious ethics; reproductive technologies; suffering; third party consent; *Confucian ethics; *Taoist ethics; *China

Idziak, Janine M. Ethical Dilemmas in Allied Health. Dubuque, IA: Simon and Kolz; 2000. 288 p. Includes references. ISBN 0-9659350-3-5. BE61835.
    aborted fetuses; abortion, induced; active euthanasia; advance directives; AIDS; *allied health personnel; allowing to die; artificial feeding; assisted suicide; *bioethical issues; case studies; clinical ethics committees; confidentiality; congenital disorders; conscience; cultural pluralism; decision making; employment; ethical theory; health care; human experimentation; informed consent; moral policy; newborns; organ donation; palliative care; persistent vegetative state; prenatal diagnosis; *professional ethics; reproductive technologies; resource allocation; resuscitation orders; selective abortion; third party consent; truth disclosure; withholding treatment; United States

Jacob, Walter; Zemer, Moshe, eds. The Fetus and Fertility in Jewish Law: Essays and Responsa. Pittsburgh, PA: Rodef Shalom Press; Freehof Institute of Progressive Halakhah; 1995. 224 p. (Studies in Progressive Halakhah; v. 5). Includes references. ISBN 0-929699-07-6. BE61836.
    aborted fetuses; abortion, induced; animal experimentation; *bioethical issues; contraception; fetal research; *Jewish ethics; reproduction; reproductive technologies; sex preselection; *theology; Orthodox Judaism; Reform Judaism

Jansen, Lynn A. Assessing clinical pragmatism. *Kennedy Institute of Ethics Journal.* 1998 Mar; 8(1): 23-36. 14 refs.

9 fn. Commentary on J.J. Fins, M.D. Bacchetta, F.G. Miller, "Clinical pragmatism: a method of moral problem solving," *KIEJ* 1997 Jun; 7(2):129-145; commented on by J.J. Fins, F.G. Miller, and M.D. Bacchetta, p. 37-42. BE59352.
    bioethics; case studies; *clinical ethics; communication; consensus; decision making; dissent; *ethical analysis; ethical theory; evaluation; family members; futility; *methods; patient participation; physician patient relationship; physicians; principle-based ethics; prolongation of life; resuscitation orders; *pragmatism; Dewey, John
"Clinical pragmatism" is an important new method of moral problem-solving in clinical practice. This method draws on the pragmatic philosophy of John Dewey and recommends an experimental approach to solving moral problems in clinical practice. Although the method may shed some light on how clinicians and their patients ought to interact when moral problems are at hand, it nonetheless is deficient in a number of respects. Clinical pragmatism fails to explain adequately how moral poblems can be solved experimentally, it underestimates the relevance and importance of judgment in clinical ethics, and it presents a questionable account of the role that moral principles should play in moral problem solving.

Joint Commission on Accreditation of Healthcare Organizations. Ethical Issues and Patient Rights: Across the Continuum of Care. Oakbrook Terrace, IL: The Commission; 1998. 156 p. Includes references. ISBN 0-86688-591-9. BE62778.
    advance directives; allowing to die; bioethics; case studies; *clinical ethics; clinical ethics committees; competence; decision making; education; ethical analysis; ethical theory; ethics consultation; forms; guidelines; health care; health care delivery; *health facilities; home care; *institutional ethics; *institutional policies; organization and administration; patient care; *patients' rights; professional organizations; resuscitation orders; standards; terminal care; terminology; third party consent; values; withholding treatment; Joint Commission on Accreditation of Healthcare Organizations

Jonsen, Albert R. The birth of bioethics: the origins and evolution of a demi-discipline. *Medical Humanities Review.* 1997 Spring; 11(1): 9-21. 17 fn. Paper originally presented as the Annual Faculty Oration at the Society for Health and Human Values annual meeting in Cleveland, OH, 10 Oct 1996. BE59964.
    aborted fetuses; advisory committees; *bioethical issues; *bioethics; biomedical research; biomedical technologies; fetal research; government financing; *historical aspects; human experimentation; medical ethics; philosophy; physicians; public participation; public policy; Roman Catholic ethics; scientific misconduct; theology; National Commission for the Protection of Human Subjects; Twentieth Century; *United States

Kahn, Jeffrey. Bioethics and tobacco. *Bioethics Examiner.* 1997 Fall; 1(3): 1, 7. BE59792.
    *bioethics; economics; federal government; government regulation; industry; international aspects; *public health; *public policy; *smoking; United States

Kaiser, Jocelyn, ed. Weighing in on bioethics. [News]. *Science.* 1999 Apr 23; 284(5414): 551. BE61798.
    *bioethics; *computer communication networks; *information dissemination; *Bioethics Internet Project; *Internet; *University of Pennsylvania Center for Bioethics

Kennedy Institute of Ethics (Georgetown University). Bioethics Information Retrieval Project. Bioethics Thesaurus. 1999 Edition. Washington, DC: The Institute;

BE = bioethics accession number   fn. = footnotes   refs. = references

1999. 92 p. Also available at Web address http://bioethics.Georgetown.edu. BE61355.
*bioethical issues; *bioethics; data banks; *terminology; *BIOETHICSLINE

Kerin, Jacinta. Double standards: principled or arbitrary? [Editorial]. *Bioethics.* 1998 Oct; 12(4): iii–vii. 8 fn. BE62275.
*bioethical issues; circumcision; cosmetic surgery; *cultural pluralism; developing countries; *ethical relativism; ethics; females; HIV seropositivity; human experimentation; human rights; *international aspects; non–Western World; research design; standards; Western World

Koch, Tom. The Limits of Principle: Deciding Who Lives and What Dies. Westport, CT: Praeger; 1998. 176 p. Bibliography: p. 159–168. ISBN 0–275–96407–8. BE60113.
allowing to die; amyotrophic lateral sclerosis; *anencephaly; animal rights; *bioethical issues; bioethics; biomedical technologies; consensus; cultural pluralism; *decision making; disabled; Down syndrome; ethical analysis; eugenics; guidelines; historical aspects; intelligence; international aspects; legal aspects; methods; moral policy; newborns; organ donation; *organ transplantation; patient compliance; personhood; prognosis; prolongation of life; *quality of life; renal dialysis; *resource allocation; rights; scarcity; *selection for treatment; selective abortion; social worth; speciesism; transplant recipients; treatment outcome; *value of life; values

Kopelman, Loretta M. Bioethics and humanities: what makes us one field? *Journal of Medicine and Philosophy.* 1998 Aug; 23(4): 356–368. 15 refs. 5 fn. Presidential address to the 8 November 1997 joint meeting of the American Association for Bioethics, the Society for Bioethics Consultation, and the Society for Health and Human Values. BE60628.
bioethical issues; *bioethics; education; ethicist's role; *humanities; *interdisciplinary communication; *methods; teaching methods

Bioethics and humanities (inclusive of medical ethics, health care ethics, environmental ethics, research ethics, philosophy and medicine, literature and medicine, and so on) seems like one field; yet colleagues come from different academic disciplines with distinct languages, methods, traditions, core curriculum and competency examinations. The author marks six related "framework" features that unite and make it one distinct field. It is a commitment to (1) work systematically on some of the momentous and well–defined sets of problems about the human condition that drive our field (such as death and dying, disability, confidentiality, professionalism, informed consent, abortion, euthanasia, assisted suicide, personhood, health–care resource allocation and environmental ethics, as well as the impact of new technologies, including genetic and reproductive); (2) use interdisciplinary approaches to unravel them; (3) employ cases and practical reasoning to understand problems and solve answers; (4) apply teaching methods and goals associated with John Dewey to make students better problem–solvers; (5) find morally justifiable solutions to the problems driving our field; and (6) seek interdisciplinary and collaborative scholarship, service or teaching.

Kopelman, Loretta M.; McCullough, Laurence B. Hume, bioethics, and philosophy of medicine. [Introduction to a set of articles by T.L. Beauchamp, R.G. Frey, L.R. Churchill, K.F. Schaffner, L.B. McCullough, and L.M. Kopelman]. *Journal of Medicine and Philosophy.* 1999 Aug; 24(4): 315–321. 14 refs. BE62610.
animal rights; bioethical issues; bioethics; health; health care; historical aspects; humanities; justice; managed care programs; medical ethics; medicine; *philosophy; suicide; Eighteenth Century; *Hume, David

Krakauer, Eric L. Prescriptions: autonomy, humanism and the purpose of health technology. *Theoretical Medicine and Bioethics.* 1998 Dec; 19(6): 525–545. 27 refs. 11 fn. BE61154.
*autonomy; bioethics; *biomedical technologies; goals; health; *humanism; iatrogenic disease; medicine; moral obligations; personhood; *philosophy; suffering; rationality; Derrida, Jacques; Heidegger, Martin; Illich, Ivan; Kant, Immanuel

Kuczewski, Mark. Casuistry and principlism: the convergence of method in biomedical ethics. *Theoretical Medicine and Bioethics.* 1998 Dec; 19(6): 509–524. 40 fn. BE61153.
*bioethics; case studies; *casuistry; ethical analysis; *ethical theory; medical ethics; *methods; moral policy; *principle–based ethics; virtues

Kuczewski, Mark G.; Pinkus, Rosa Lynn B. An Ethics Casebook for Hospitals: Practical Approaches to Everyday Cases. Washington, DC: Georgetown University Press; 1999. 219 p. Bibliography: p. 203–212. ISBN 0–87840–723–5. BE62774.
advance directives; aged; allowing to die; artificial feeding; autonomy; *bioethical issues; *case studies; *clinical ethics; clinical ethics committees; communication; competence; confidentiality; continuing education; decision making; duty to warn; ethicists; family members; *hospitals; informed consent; institutional ethics; interprofessional relations; managed care programs; occupational medicine; physician patient relationship; pregnant women; professional family relationship; rehabilitation; resuscitation orders; social discrimination; teaching methods; third party consent; truth disclosure; withholding treatment; *community hospitals; United States

Kuhse, Helga; Singer, Peter, eds. A Companion to Bioethics. Malden, MA: Blackwell; 1998. 512 p. (Blackwell companions to philosophy). 961 refs. ISBN 0–631–19737–0. BE59476.
abortion, induced; active euthanasia; advance directives; AIDS; allowing to die; animal experimentation; assisted suicide; *bioethical issues; *bioethics; clinical ethics committees; confidentiality; cultural pluralism; determination of death; education; embryo research; ethical theory; ethicists; feminist ethics; genetic intervention; genome mapping; health care; human experimentation; informed consent; international aspects; killing; *methods; mother fetus relationship; organ donation; organ transplantation; personhood; population control; prenatal diagnosis; prenatal injuries; quality of life; religious ethics; reproductive technologies; resource allocation; rights; selection for treatment; suicide; treatment refusal; truth disclosure; virtues; wedge argument

Leonir, Noëlle. French, European, and international legislation on bioethics. *Suffolk University Law Review.* 1993 Winter; 27(4): 1249–1270. 6 fn. BE60700.
active euthanasia; advisory committees; *bioethical issues; body parts and fluids; cadavers; embryo research; epidemiology; gene therapy; genetic intervention; genetic screening; health care delivery; human experimentation; human rights; *international aspects; *legal aspects; legal rights; organ donation; organ donors; preimplantation diagnosis; prenatal diagnosis; reproductive technologies; Council of Europe; *Europe; European Union; *France; International Bioethics Committee (Unesco)

Levine, Carol, ed. Taking Sides: Clashing Views on Controversial Bioethical Issues. Eighth Edition.

BE = bioethics accession number   fn. = footnotes   refs. = references

Guilford, CT: Dushkin Publishing Group; 1999. 355 p. Includes references. ISBN 0-07-303190-9. BE62773.
abortion, induced; advance directives; aged; allowing to die; animal experimentation; assisted suicide; *bioethical issues; blood transfusions; body parts and fluids; cloning; developing countries; family members; family relationship; fetal development; futility; genetic screening; government regulation; health insurance; hearing disorders; HIV seropositivity; human experimentation; informed consent; managed care programs; mandatory reporting; medical devices; minors; *moral policy; parents; physically disabled; physician patient relationship; placebos; pregnant women; prenatal injuries; prolongation of life; public policy; religion; remuneration; resource allocation; treatment refusal; truth disclosure; voluntary euthanasia; withholding treatment; cochlear implants

Little, Margaret Olivia. Let me count the ways: feminism illuminating bioethics. [Book review essay]. *Medical Humanities Review.* 1997 Spring; 11(1): 76-81. BE59967.
abortion, induced; adoption; bioethical issues; *bioethics; drug abuse; employment; ethical theory; females; *feminist ethics; fetuses; HIV seropositivity; human experimentation; justice; males; parent child relationship; pregnant women; prenatal injuries; public policy; *reproduction; *reproductive technologies; rights; selection of subjects; social discrimination; *Feminism and Bioethics: Beyond Reproduction (Wolf, S.M., ed.); *Reproduction, Ethics, and the Law (Callahan, J.C., ed.)

Loewy, Erich H. Curiosity, imagination, compassion, science and ethics: do curiosity and imagination serve a central function? *Health Care Analysis.* 1998 Dec; 6(4): 286-294. 9 fn. BE60686.
capitalism; commodification; communism; compassion; cultural pluralism; democracy; *emotions; *ethics; health care; *human characteristics; libertarianism; obligations of society; science; self concept; virtues; *rationality
Curiosity and imagination have been neglected in epistemology. This paper argues that the role of curiosity and imagination is central to the way we think, regardless of whether it is thinking about problems of ethics or problems of science. In our ever more materialistic society, curiosity and reason are either discouraged or narrowly channeled. I shall argue that the role of curiosity and imagination for both science and ethics is so important that nurturing them can be seen as an ethical obligation and suppressing them as ethically problematic.

Lustig, B. Andrew. Concepts and methods in recent bioethics: critical responses. [Introduction to articles by R.M. Veatch, B.C. White and J. Zimbelman, W. Harper, P. McGrath, and H. Fielding]. *Journal of Medicine and Philosophy.* 1998 Oct; 23(5): 445-455. 27 refs. 4 fn. Note: the journal issue cover shows a date of August 1998, which is incorrect. BE62112.
allowing to die; *bioethical issues; *bioethics; clinical ethics; commodification; directed donation; ethical theory; futility; human body; informed consent; justice; methods; organ donation; philosophy; physician patient relationship; postmodernism; principle-based ethics; remuneration; social discrimination; standards; values; phenomenology

McCullough, Laurence B.; Reich, Warren Thomas. Laying medicine open: innovative interaction between medicine and the humanities. [Introduction to articles by L.B. McCullough, W.T. Reich, D. Callahan, and E.D. Pellegrino, and to a bibliography of resources prepared by and about A.E. Hellegers compiled by D.M. Goldstein]. *Kennedy Institute of Ethics Journal.* 1999 Mar; 9(1): 1-5. 7 refs. BE62326.
*bioethics; ethicists; *historical aspects; humanities; interdisciplinary communication; medical ethics; medicine; research institutes; values; Hellegers, André; United States

McCullough, Laurence B. Laying medicine open: understanding major turning points in the history of medical ethics. *Kennedy Institute of Ethics Journal.* 1999 Mar; 9(1): 7-23. 15 refs. BE62327.
*accountability; *bioethics; conflict of interest; economics; entrepreneurship; *evidence-based medicine; *historical aspects; incentives; institutional ethics; managed care programs; *medical ethics; *medicine; moral obligations; physician patient relationship; *physicians; professional competence; quality of health care; resource allocation; virtues; Eighteenth Century; Gregory, John; Scotland; Twentieth Century; United States
At different times during its history medicine has been laid open to accountability for its scientific and moral quality. This phenonmenon of laying medicine open has sometimes resulted in major turning points in the history of medical ethics. In this paper, I examine two examples of when the laying open of medicine has generated such turning points: eighteenth-century British medicine and late twentieth-century American medicine. In the eighteenth century, the Scottish physician-philosopher, John Gregory (1724-1773), concerned with the unscientific, entrepreneurial, self-interested nature of then current medical practice, laid medicine open to accountability using the tools of ethics and philosophy of medicine. In the process, Gregory wrote the first professional ethics of medicine in the English-language literature, based on the physician's fiduciary responsibility to the patient. In the late twentieth century, the managed practice of medicine has laid medicine open to accountability for its scientific quality and economic cost. This current laying open of medicine creates the challenge of developing medical ethics and bioethics for population-based medical science and practice.

Macer, Darryl R.J. Bioethics Is Love of Life: An Alternative Textbook. Christchurch, NZ: Eubios Ethics Institute; 1998. 158 p. Bibliography: p. 150-156. ISBN 0-908897-13-8. BE62142.
altruism; autonomy; beneficence; *bioethics; conscience; cultural pluralism; ecology; ethical theory; freedom; genetic intervention; international aspects; justice; *love; personhood; quality of life; religious ethics; sexuality; social interaction; speciesism; value of life; virtues; environmental ethics

McGee, Glenn. Breaking bioethics: an introduction and mission. *Cambridge Quarterly of Healthcare Ethics.* 1998 Fall; 7(4): 414-416. BE59158.
advisory committees; *bioethical issues; *bioethics; communication; education; *ethicist's role; genes; mass media; patents; public participation; public policy; time factors; *trends; United States

McGee, Glenn, ed. Pragmatic Bioethics. Nashville, TN: Vanderbilt University Press; 1999. 302 p. (Vanderbilt library of American philosophy). Bibliography: p. 289-293. ISBN 0-8265-1321-2. BE60659.
allowing to die; assisted suicide; attitudes to death; autonomy; *bioethical issues; *bioethics; casuistry; clinical ethics; clinical ethics committees; communication; competence; consensus; covenant; decision making; determination of death; ethicists; eugenics; family members; genetic enhancement; genetic information; genetics; health care delivery; health care reform; managed care programs; medical ethics; medicine; mentally ill; methods; models, theoretical; paternalism; patient participation; personhood; philosophy; physician patient relationship; physicians; professional family relationship; psychoactive drugs; resource allocation; suicide; terminal care; terminally ill; treatment refusal; voluntary euthanasia; *pragmatism

McGee, Glenn. Pragmatic method and bioethics. *In:*

BE = bioethics accession number   fn. = footnotes   refs. = references

McGee, Glenn, ed. Pragmatic Bioethics. Nashville, TN: Vanderbilt University Press; 1999: 18–29, 258–260. 44 fn. ISBN 0–8265–1321–2. BE60661.
    *bioethics; biology; decision making; education; ethical analysis; ethical theory; health; human characteristics; *methods; models, theoretical; narrative ethics; *philosophy; science; *pragmatism; Dewey, John

McGrath, Pam. Autonomy, discourse, and power: a postmodern reflection on principlism and bioethics. *Journal of Medicine and Philosophy.* 1998 Oct; 23(5): 516–532. 75 refs. 2 fn. Note: the journal issue cover shows a date of August 1998, which is incorrect. BE62116.
    alternatives; *autonomy; *bioethics; biomedical technologies; Buddhist ethics; decision making; ethicists; *home care; *hospices; hospitals; philosophy; physicians; *postmodernism; *principle–based ethics; *social discrimination; *sociology of medicine; *terminal care; terminally ill; empowerment; Foucault, Michel; Karuna Hospice Service (Brisbane, QLD)
In recent years there has been an increasing critique of the philosophy based reasoning in bioethics which is known as principlism. This article seeks to make a postmodern contribution to this emerging debate by using notions of power and discourse to highlight the limits and superficiality of this abstract, rationalistic mode of reflection. The focus of the discussion will be on the principle of autonomy. Recent doctoral research on a hospice organization (Karuna Hospice Service) will be used to contextualize the debate to end–of–life ethical dilemmas. The conclusion will be reached that the discursive richness of this organization's notion of autonomy or choice, which incorporates a holistic respect for the individual and the active creation of alternatives, can provide important insights to our understanding of autonomy in bioethics. The concern is raised that if autonomy is reified as a principle outside of the context of discourse, it may only complement the hegemonic power of biomedicine.

Macklin, Ruth. A defense of fundamental principles and human rights: a reply to Robert Baker. *Kennedy Institute of Ethics Journal.* 1998 Dec; 8(4): 403–422. 15 refs. 6 fn. BE62376.
    accountability; advisory committees; autonomy; beneficence; *bioethics; circumcision; coercion; communitarianism; *cultural pluralism; dissent; *ethical analysis; *ethical relativism; *ethical theory; females; historical aspects; *human experimentation; *human rights; informed consent; *international aspects; investigators; *misconduct; *morality; *National Socialism; *non–Western World; nontherapeutic research; physicians; *postmodernism; principle–based ethics; *radiation; research subjects; *retrospective moral judgment; *scientific misconduct; values; *Western World; women's rights; *culpability; *Advisory Committee on Human Radiation Experiments; Asia; Germany; Twentieth Century; United States
This article seeks to rebut Robert Baker's contention that attempts to ground international bioethics in fundamental principles cannot withstand the challenges posed by multiculturalism and postmodernism. First, several corrections are provided of Baker's account of the conclusions reached by the Advisory Committee on Human Radiation Experiments. Second, a rebuttal is offered to Baker's claim that an unbridgeable moral gap exists between Western individualism and non–Western communalism. In conclusion, this article argues that Baker's "nonnegotiable primary goods" cannot do the work of "classical human rights" and that the latter framework is preferable from both a practical and a theoretical standpoint.

Macklin, Ruth. Against Relativism: Cultural Diversity and the Search for Ethical Universals in Medicine. New York, NY: Oxford University Press; 1999. 290 p. 307 fn. ISBN 0–19–511632–1. BE62780.
    anthropology; autonomy; beneficence; *bioethical issues; circumcision; confidentiality; contraception; *cultural pluralism; determination of death; *developing countries; *ethical relativism; females; feminist ethics; health; historical aspects; human experimentation; *human rights; informed consent; *international aspects; justice; morality; *non–Western World; organ donation; philosophy; physician patient relationship; religious ethics; reproduction; selective abortion; sex determination; truth disclosure; values; *Western World; women's health; women's rights

Mahowald, Mary B. Collaboration and casuistry. *In:* McGee, Glenn, ed. Pragmatic Bioethics. Nashville, TN: Vanderbilt University Press; 1999: 73–83, 265–266. 24 fn. ISBN 0–8265–1321–2. BE60664.
    autonomy; *casuistry; *clinical ethics; decision making; ethics consultation; *interprofessional relations; investigators; *medicine; methods; paternalism; *philosophy; physician patient relationship; physicians; uncertainty; *pragmatism; *Pierce, Charles

Maloney, Dennis M. New federal commission proposed on bioethics. *Human Research Report.* 1998 Mar; 13(3): 6. BE59955.
    *advisory committees; *bioethical issues; cloning; federal government; government regulation; legislation; organization and administration; public participation; public policy; science; *Commission to Promote a National Dialogue on Bioethics; National Bioethics Advisory Commission; *United States

Manning, Rita C. A care approach. *In:* Kuhse, Helga; Singer, Peter, eds. A Companion to Bioethics. Malden, MA: Blackwell; 1998: 98–105. 13 refs. ISBN 0–631–19737–0. BE59486.
    autonomy; bioethical issues; bioethics; *caring; empathy; *ethical theory; health personnel; justice; methods; moral development; patients' rights; professional patient relationship; self concept; social interaction; terminal care

May, William E. Bioethics and human life. *In:* Forte, David F., ed. Natural Law and Contemporary Public Policy. Washington, DC: Georgetown University Press; 1998: 41–54. 19 fn. ISBN 0–87840–692–1. BE59724.
    autonomy; *bioethics; *decision making; freedom; human body; moral obligations; *moral policy; *natural law; personhood; public policy; *value of life; Golden Rule

Moreno, Jonathan D. Bioethics is a naturalism. *In:* McGee, Glenn, ed. Pragmatic Bioethics. Nashville, TN: Vanderbilt University Press; 1999: 5–17, 257–258. 17 fn. ISBN 0–8265–1321–2. BE60660.
    *bioethics; consensus; cultural pluralism; decision making; ethical analysis; ethical theory; ethicist's role; ethics; *methods; *philosophy; public policy; science; values; knowledge; *pragmatism; Dewey, John; United States

Morreim, E. Haavi. Bioethics and the press. *Journal of Medicine and Philosophy.* 1999 Apr; 24(2): 103–107. 12 refs. BE61436.
    *bioethical issues; *bioethics; communication; ethicist's role; interprofessional relations; *journalism; *mass media; whistleblowing; United States

Murray, Thomas H. What do we mean by "narrative ethics"? *Medical Humanities Review.* 1997 Fall; 11(2): 44–57. 33 refs. This article is a revised version of a chapter in Hilde Lindemann Nelson, ed., *Stories and Their Limits: Approaches to Narrative Bioethics,* 1997; New York: Routledge. BE59706.

BE = bioethics accession number   fn. = footnotes   refs. = references

bioethics; casuistry; cultural pluralism; ethical theory; *ethics; literature; metaphor; methods; moral development; *morality; *narrative ethics; philosophy; principle-based ethics

Nelson, Hilde Lindemann. *Feminist Approaches to Bioethics: Theoretical Reflections and Practical Applications*, by Rosemarie Tong. [Book review essay]. *Hypatia.* 1998 Fall; 13(4): 112-116. 13 refs. BE61679.
    *bioethical issues; *bioethics; *feminist ethics; *Feminist Approaches to Bioethics (Tong, R.)

Nelson, James Lindemann. Bioethics as several kinds of writing. *Journal of Medicine and Philosophy.* 1999 Apr; 24(2): 148-163. 21 refs. 9 fn. BE61439.
    *bioethical issues; *bioethics; communication; education; ethical theory; *ethicist's role; *ethicists; interprofessional relations; *journalism; literature; *mass media; technical expertise; publishing
Three different models are described of the relationship of bioethics to the press. The first two are familiar: bioethicists often are interviewed by journalists seeking background and short quotes to insert in a story; alternately, bioethicists sometimes themselves act as journalists of a sort, writing op-eds, articles or even longer works designed for wide readership. These models share the notion that bioethicists can provide information and ideas that increase the quality of people's thinking on moral matters. They share also a common difficulty: do the constraints the media impose on bioethical discourse keep bioethicists from deepening public reflection, and if not, how can those constraints be most effectively kept from distorting what bioethicists wish to say? The third model reverses--in part--the presupposition that bioethics bestows moral sophistication on a public naive about ethical issues, holding rather that matters run both ways; bioethicists stand to learn a great deal from their interactions with various publics and the media that serve them. On this view, the constraints imposed by media conventions constitute opportunities for new and potentially important forms of bioethical writing. Various concerns generated by the first two models are surveyed. It is concluded that while none of the difficulties constitute knock-down arguments against these forms of collaborating with the press, the worries are problematic enough to provide some support for considering the less familiar third approach. Further reason for taking the third model seriously draws on moral theoretic considerations.

Nicholas, Barbara. Strategies for effective transformation. *In:* Donchin, Anne; Purdy, Laura M., eds. Embodying Bioethics: Recent Feminist Advances. Lanham, MD: Rowman and Littlefield; 1999: 239-252. 37 refs. 10 fn. ISBN 0-8476-8924-7. BE61024.
    *bioethics; ethical relativism; ethical theory; *ethicist's role; *females; *feminist ethics; goals; health facilities; interdisciplinary communication; interprofessional relations; postmodernism; *social dominance

Nordio, S. Beneficence, virtues and ethical committees in pediatrics: epistemology, bioethics and medical pedagogy in pediatrics. *In:* Burgio, G. Roberto; Lantos, John D., eds. *Primum Non Nocere* Today. Second Edition. New York, NY: Elsevier; 1998: 147-158. 53 refs. ISBN 0-444-82923-7. BE60925.
    adolescents; age factors; autonomy; beneficence; *bioethics; children; clinical ethics committees; cultural pluralism; disclosure; ethical theory; informed consent; *medical education; *medical ethics; newborns; parental consent; paternalism; patient care; *pediatrics; philosophy; physician

patient relationship; physicians; principle-based ethics; research ethics committees; teleological ethics; trends; virtues

Oakley, Justin. A virtue ethics approach. *In:* Kuhse, Helga; Singer, Peter, eds. A Companion to bioethics. Malden, MA: Blackwell; 1998: 86-97. 38 refs. ISBN 0-631-19737-0. BE59485.
    bioethical issues; bioethics; *ethical theory; methods; *virtues

O'Neill, Terry. Biomedical Ethics. [Juvenile literature]. San Diego, CA: Greenhaven Press; 1999. 144 p. (Opposing viewpoints digests). Bibliography: p. 131-140. Includes study questions. ISBN 1-56510-874-4. BE61051.
    animal experimentation; *bioethical issues; body parts and fluids; cloning; gene therapy; genetic screening; government regulation; human experimentation; organ donation; privacy; remuneration; social discrimination

O'Rourke, Kevin D.; Boyle, Philip. Medical Ethics: Sources of Catholic Teachings. Third Edition. Washington, DC: Georgetown University Press; 1999. 442 p. Includes references. ISBN 0-87840-722-7. BE61314.
    abortion, induced; advance directives; aged; AIDS; allowing to die; artificial feeding; assisted suicide; *bioethical issues; brain death; cloning; confidentiality; conscience; contraception; determination of death; disabled; double effect; embryo research; euthanasia; genetic screening; health care; homosexuals; human experimentation; informed consent; marital relationship; medical ethics; national health insurance; nurses; organ donation; organ transplantation; pain; physicians; psychotherapy; rape; religious hospitals; reproductive technologies; *Roman Catholic ethics; sterilization (sexual); suffering; terminal care; *theology; third party consent; truth disclosure; value of life; Instruction on Respect for Human Life

Palmer, Michael. Moral Problems in Medicine: A Practical Coursebook. Buffalo, NY: University of Toronto Press; 1999. 190 p. Includes references. ISBN 0-8020-8257-2. BE61315.
    abortion, induced; active euthanasia; allowing to die; animal experimentation; behavior control; *bioethical issues; case studies; confidentiality; deontological ethics; *ethical theory; eugenics; freedom; genetic intervention; human experimentation; informed consent; involuntary sterilization; justice; libertarianism; mentally retarded; metaethics; motivation; paternalism; selective abortion; teleological ethics; therapeutic abortion; truth disclosure; utilitarianism; value of life; egoism

Peerenboom, Ellen. Germany funds two new bioethics programs. [News]. *Nature Medicine.* 1998 Mar; 4(3): 261. BE59839.
    *bioethics; *financial support; government financing; interdisciplinary communication; *research institutes; Bundesministerium für Bildung, Wissenschaft, Forschung und Technologie; Deutsche Forschungsgemeinschaft; *Germany

Pellegrino, Edmund D. The origins and evolution of bioethics: some personal reflections. *Kennedy Institute of Ethics Journal.* 1999 Mar; 9(1): 73-88. 32 refs. BE62330.
    *bioethics; curriculum; ethicists; ethics; *historical aspects; humanities; *interdisciplinary communication; medical education; medical schools; medicine; philosophy; physicians; religion; research institutes; values; Institute on Human Values in Medicine; Twentieth Century; United States
Bioethics was officially baptized in 1972, but its birth took place a decade or so before that date. Since its

---

BE = bioethics accession number   fn. = footnotes   refs. = references

birth, what is known today as bioethics has undergone a complex conceptual metamorphosis. This essay loosely divides that metamorphosis into three stages: an educational, an ethical, and a global stage. In the educational era, bioethics focused on a perceived "dehumanization" of medicine by the rising power of science and technology. Remedies were sought by introducing humanities, ethics, and human "values" into the medical curriculum. Ethics was one among the humanistic disciplines, but not the dominant one. In the second era, ethics assumed a dominant role as ever more complex dilemmas emerged from the rapid pace of biological research. As such dilemmas were applied to medical practice, the need for a more rigorous and more formal analysis of their moral status was clear. Philosophically-trained ethicists had an obvious role. They began to teach, write, and profoundly influence medical education and practice. In the third -- and present -- period, the breadth of problems has become so broad that ethicists must, themselves, draw on disciplines well beyond their expertise -- e.g., law, religion, anthropology, economics, political science, psychology, and the like. The era of bioethics as a global enterprise is upon us. The original hope for humanizing medicine has not been overtly successful; however, much has been accomplished of value to patients, the profession, and society. Medical morality has been transformed into a formal, systematic study of a whole range of issues of the greatest significance to humanity. Now the major challenge is one of identity, or inter-relationships and connections between the theoretical and the practical. Bioethics has outgrown its beginnings.

Pellegrino, Edmund D. What the philosophy of medicine is. *Theoretical Medicine and Bioethics.* 1998 Aug; 19(4): 315-336. 103 refs. BE60156.
  bioethics; interdisciplinary communication; *medicine; *models, theoretical; *philosophy

Poland, Susan Cartier. Bioethics commissions: town meetings with a "blue, blue ribbon". [Bibliography]. *Kennedy Institute of Ethics Journal.* 1998 Mar; 8(1): 91-109. Also available, as Scope Note 34, from the National Reference Center for Bioethics Literature, Kennedy Institute of Ethics, Georgetown University; Box 571212, Washington, DC 20057-1212, (202) 687-6738 or (800) MED-ETHX. BE59357.
  *advisory committees; *bioethical issues; *international aspects; public policy; United States

Potter, Van Rensselaer. Bioethics, biology, *and* the biosphere: fragmented ethics and "bridge bioethics". *Hastings Center Report.* 1999 Jan-Feb; 29(1): 38-40. 17 fn. BE61636.
  bioethical issues; *bioethics; capitalism; common good; democracy; developing countries; *ecology; health; human rights; humanities; interdisciplinary communication; international aspects; justice; medical ethics; obligations to society; population control; property rights; science; social problems; socioeconomic factors; *nature

Rachels, James. Ethical theory and bioethics. *In:* Kuhse, Helga; Singer, Peter, eds. A Companion to Bioethics. Malden, MA: Blackwell; 1998: 15-23. 10 refs. ISBN 0-631-19737-0. BE59477.
  *bioethics; case studies; ethical relativism; *ethical theory; *methods; moral policy; principle-based ethics

Rae, Scott B.; Cox, Paul M. Bioethics: A Christian Approach in a Pluralistic Age. Grand Rapids, MI: W.B.

Eerdmans; 1999. 326 p. (Critical issues in bioethics). 503 fn. ISBN 0-8028-4595-9. BE61422.
  abortion, induced; active euthanasia; allowing to die; assisted suicide; attitudes to death; autonomy; *bioethical issues; *bioethics; biomedical technologies; case studies; *Christian ethics; common good; confidentiality; cultural pluralism; *decision making; embryo research; embryos; ethical theory; fetal research; fetuses; genetic intervention; health care delivery; informed consent; Jewish ethics; justice; managed care programs; moral policy; personhood; physician patient relationship; physicians; postmodernism; Protestant ethics; reproductive technologies; Roman Catholic ethics; secularism; terminal care; terminally ill; theology; value of life; United States

Randall, Vernellia R. Slavery, segregation and racism: trusting the health care system ain't always easy! An African American perspective on bioethics. *Saint Louis University Public Law Review.* 1996; 15(2): 191-235. 264 fn. BE59908.
  abortion, induced; *bioethical issues; *bioethics; *blacks; contraception; *cultural pluralism; eugenics; family planning; females; genetic screening; *health care; *health care delivery; health hazards; historical aspects; human experimentation; indigents; involuntary sterilization; males; managed care programs; mass screening; morbidity; mortality; occupational exposure; organ donation; organ transplantation; prisoners; quality of health care; reproductive technologies; resource allocation; scientific misconduct; selection for treatment; sickle cell anemia; *social discrimination; stigmatization; *trust; values; violence; genocide; slavery; Nineteenth Century; Twentieth Century; *United States

Ratanakul, Pinit. Buddhist health care ethics. *In:* Coward, Harold; Ratanakul, Pinit, eds. A Cross-Cultural Dialogue on Health Care Ethics. Waterloo, ON: Wilfrid Laurier University Press; 1999: 119-127. 7 fn. ISBN 0-88920-325-3. BE62788.
  active euthanasia; allowing to die; attitudes to death; autonomy; *bioethical issues; *Buddhist ethics; compassion; health care delivery; justice; killing; pain; personhood; physician patient relationship; resource allocation; suffering; terminal care; value of life

Reich, Warren Thomas. Experiential ethics as a foundation for dialogue between health communication and health-care ethics. *Journal of Applied Communication Research.* 1988 Spring; 16(1): 16-28. 27 refs. BE59802.
  autonomy; *bioethics; biomedical research; *communication; ethical theory; literature; medicine; mentally retarded; *methods; models, theoretical; *narrative ethics; physician patient relationship; principle-based ethics; values; *communicative ethics; Arrowsmith (Lewis, S.)

Reich, Warren Thomas. The "wider view": André Helleger's passionate, integrating intellect and the creation of bioethics. *Kennedy Institute of Ethics Journal.* 1999 Mar; 9(1): 25-51. 14 refs. 5 fn. BE62328.
  advisory committees; *bioethics; compassion; contraception; disadvantaged; disease; ethicists; family members; fetal research; health; *historical aspects; *interdisciplinary communication; medicine; physicians; research institutes; Roman Catholic ethics; value of life; *values; war; *Hellegers, André; *Kennedy Institute of Ethics; Twentieth Century

This article provides an account of how André Hellegers, founder and first Director of the Kennedy Institute of Ethics at Georgetown University, laid medicine open to bioethics. Helleger's approach to bioethics, as to morality generally and also to medicine and biomedical science, involved taking the "wider view" -- a value-filled vision that integrated and gave meaning to what otherwise was disparate, precarious, and conflicting. This article shows how Helleger's wider

---

BE = bioethics accession number   fn. = footnotes   refs. = references

view of bioethics was shaped by events in his own life, his resultant sense of the precariousness of life and health, his commitment to religious inclusiveness, his research in fetal medicine, his clinical experience in obstetrics, his role in the struggle to change the teaching of the Roman Catholic Church on fertility control, and his developing concepts of health and disease. Hellegers was committed to and worked toward bioethics as a self-consciously interdisciplinary field in which the contributing disciplines adapt to each other -- rather than sustain themselves as autonomous disciplines -- to create a dynamic and complex intellectual, clinical, and social activity.

Roberts, Laura Weiss; Battaglia, John; Smithpeter, Margaret, et al. An office on Main Street: health care dilemmas in small communities. *Hastings Center Report.* 1999 Jul–Aug; 29(4): 28–37. 35 fn. Includes inset article, "The problems of rural care: four new studies," p. 30–31. BE62467.
   *clinical ethics; community services; confidentiality; conflict of interest; cultural pluralism; *geographic factors; health; *health care delivery; mental health; *patient care; physician patient relationship; physicians; psychological stress; resource allocation; scarcity; social interaction; *socioeconomic factors; values; *rural population; United States

Robinson, John H.; Berry, Roberta M.; McDonnell, Kevin, eds. Bioethics. *In: their* A Health Law Reader: An Interdisciplinary Approach. Durham, NC: Carolina Academic Press; 1999: 5–72. 18 fn. ISBN 0–89089–907–X. BE62291.
   *bioethics; caring; *casuistry; Christian ethics; cultural pluralism; deontological ethics; ethical analysis; *ethical theory; feminist ethics; medical ethics; methods; morality; postmodernism; *principle-based ethics; utilitarianism; *virtues

Rosen, Elisabeth. Bioethics committees as consensus shapers. *Bulletin of Medical Ethics.* 1999 Feb; No. 145: 13–18. 18 refs. BE61891.
   *advisory committees; *bioethical issues; cloning; comparative studies; consensus; cultural pluralism; enhancement technologies; evaluation; genetic intervention; interdisciplinary communication; international aspects; organization and administration; patents; *public policy; trust; values; Europe; *European Group on Ethics in Science and New Technologies; *National Bioethics Advisory Commission; United States

Rosenfeld, Albert. The journalist's role in bioethics. *Journal of Medicine and Philosophy.* 1999 Apr; 24(2): 108–129. 102 refs. 4 fn. BE61437.
   *bioethical issues; *bioethics; ethicists; historical aspects; interprofessional relations; *journalism; *mass media; professional role; science; scientific misconduct; trends; whistleblowing; Twentieth Century; United States
In the late 1950s and early 1960s, emerging advances in the biomedical sciences raised insufficiently noticed ethical issues, prompting science reporters to serve as a sort of Early Warning System. As awareness of bioethical issues increased rapidly everywhere, and bioethics itself arrived as a recognized discipline, the need for this early-warning press role has clearly diminished. A secondary but important role for the science journalist is that of investigative reporter/whistleblower, as in the Tuskegee syphilis trials and the government's secret plutonium experiments. Because the general public gets most of its information from the popular media, ways are suggested for journalists and bioethicists to work together.

Ross, Saul; Malloy, David Cruise. Biomedical Ethics: Concepts and Cases for Health Care Professionals. Buffalo, NY: Thompson Educational Publishing; 1999. 192 p. Bibliography: p. 186–189 ISBN 1–55077–090–X. BE62148.
   *bioethical issues; *bioethics; *case studies; decision making; deontological ethics; ethical analysis; *ethical theory; medical education; *medical ethics; moral development; moral policy; physician patient relationship; teleological ethics

Rudin, Edward. A critique from the siding: response to "Paradigms for clinical ethics consultation practice" by Mark D. Fox, Glenn McGee, and Arthur L. Caplan (*CQ*, 1998 Summer; 7(3): 308–314). *Cambridge Quarterly of Healthcare Ethics.* 1999 Summer; 8(3): 351–357. 3 refs. BE62352.
   *clinical ethics; *ethicist's role; *ethicists; *ethics consultation; health personnel; hospitals; interprofessional relations; lawyers; mental health; models, theoretical; patient care team; *referral and consultation; technical expertise; preventive ethics

Sakai, Akio. Consensus formation in bioethical decisionmaking in Japan: present contexts and future perspectives. *In:* ten Have, Henk A.M.J.; Sass, Hans–Martin, eds. Consensus Formation in Healthcare Ethics. Boston, MA: Kluwer Academic; 1998: 93–105. 34 refs. 1 fn. ISBN 0–7923–4944–X. BE62590.
   *attitudes; *bioethical issues; *biomedical technologies; *brain death; cadavers; *consensus; decision making; *determination of death; empirical research; ethics committees; medical schools; organ donation; physicians; professional organizations; *public opinion; public policy; religion; values; *Japan

Sakamoto, Hyakudai. Towards a new "global bioethics". *Bioethics.* 1999 Jul; 13(3–4): 191–197. Address to the Fourth World Congress of Bioethics sponsored jointly by the International Association of Bioethics and the Asian Bioethics Association. BE61868.
   autonomy; *bioethics; biomedical technologies; *cultural pluralism; ecology; genetic intervention; goals; *human rights; *international aspects; non-Western World; obligations to society; personhood; *values; *Western World; nature; *Asia

Sass, Hans–Martin. Action driven consensus formation. *In:* ten Have, Henk A.M.J.; Sass, Hans-Martin, eds. Consensus Formation in Healthcare Ethics. Boston, MA: Kluwer Academic; 1998: 159–173. 20 refs. ISBN 0–7923–4944–X. BE62593.
   abortion, induced; autonomy; beginning of life; bioethical issues; *bioethics; brain death; *conscience; *consensus; cultural pluralism; *decision making; democracy; determination of death; *dissent; *ethical analysis; ethical theory; ethics; interdisciplinary communication; interprofessional relations; models, theoretical; professional patient relationship; public participation; public policy; risk; technical expertise; technology assessment; trust; values; negotiation

Sherwin, Susan. Foundations, frameworks, lenses: the role of theories in bioethics. *Bioethics.* 1999 Jul; 13(3–4): 198–205. 2 refs. BE61869.
   *bioethics; ethical analysis; *ethical theory; ethics; *metaphor; methods; moral policy
I explore the implications of the foundation metaphor for understanding the role of moral theories in ethics and bioethics and argue that its disadvantages outweigh its advantages. I then consider two other metaphors that might be used instead, those of frameworks and lenses. I propose that the metaphor of lenses is most promising

---

BE = bioethics accession number   fn. = footnotes   refs. = references

in providing methodological guidance for drawing on moral theories when deliberating about bioethical problems.

Siddiqui, Ataullah. Ethics in Islam: key concepts and contemporary challenges. *Journal of Moral Education.* 1997 Dec; 26(4): 423–431. 13 fn. BE59962.
*bioethics; codes of ethics; cultural pluralism; historical aspects; interdisciplinary communication; international aspects; *Islamic ethics; medical ethics; minority groups; morality; property rights; terminology; Europe; Middle East

Silverman, William A. Where's the Evidence? Controversies in Modern Medicine. New York, NY: Oxford University Press; 1998. 259 p. Bibliography: p. 225–247. A collection of essays and responses originally published in the journal *Paediatric and Perinatal Epidemiology* between 1987 and 1997. ISBN 0-19-262934-4. BE59723.
active euthanasia; allowing to die; autonomy; *bioethical issues; biomedical technologies; conflict of interest; congenital disorders; control groups; *decision making; drug industry; *evidence-based medicine; futility; hearts; historical aspects; *human experimentation; informed consent; investigators; low birth weight; *newborns; organ transplantation; pain; parents; *patient care; physicians; *prematurity; prolongation of life; quality of life; *random selection; refusal to treat; *research design; research ethics committees; resource allocation; selection for treatment; social dominance; socioeconomic factors; therapeutic research; treatment outcome; withholding treatment; *neonatology; Great Britain; United States

Silvers, Anita. On not iterating women's disability: a crossover perspective on genetic dilemmas. *In:* Donchin, Anne; Purdy, Laura M., eds. Embodying Bioethics: Recent Feminist Advances. Lanham, MD: Rowman and Littlefield; 1999: 177–202. 65 fn. ISBN 0-8476-8924-7. BE61021.
*autonomy; *bioethics; children; directive counseling; *disabled/disadvantaged; *females; *feminist ethics; *genetic counseling; *hearing disorders; models, theoretical; parent child relationship; parents; *physically disabled; quality of life; social discrimination; social interaction; suffering; *values; Americans with Disabilities Act 1990; United States

Smith, Alexander McCall. Beyond autonomy. *Journal of Contemporary Health Law and Policy.* 1997 Fall; 14(1): 23–39. 43 fn. BE60878.
abortion, induced; allowing to die; assisted suicide; *autonomy; *bioethical issues; cultural pluralism; *decision making; disclosure; ethical relativism; human experimentation; informed consent; *legal aspects; legal rights; mentally ill; minors; moral policy; parents; pregnant women; reproductive technologies; right to die; state interest; sterilization (sexual); surrogate mothers; third party consent; treatment refusal; *values; voluntary euthanasia; Canada; *Great Britain; *United States

Smith, George P. Bioethics and the Administration of Justice. Available from the author, Catholic University of America School of Law, 3600 John McCormack Rd., NE, Washington, DC 20064; 1998. 32 p. BE62198.
bioethical issues; *bioethics; biomedical technologies; cloning; democracy; ethicists; *expert testimony; government regulation; *judicial action; law; mass media; morality; public policy; religion; science; technical expertise; United States

Spicker, Stuart F. Introduction: bioethic(s): one or many? *Journal of Medicine and Philosophy.* 1998 Aug; 23(4): 347–355. 14 refs. 1 fn. BE60627.
*bioethics; consensus; *cultural pluralism; ethical relativism; fetal tissue donation; humanities; interdisciplinary

communication; managed care programs; medical ethics; medicine; philosophy; postmodernism

Steinberg, Avraham. Medical–halachic decisions of Rabbi Shlomo Zalman Auerbach (1910–1995). *Jewish Medical Ethics.* 1997 Jan; 3(1): 30–43. 256 fn. BE59247.
allowing to die; anencephaly; artificial feeding; artificial insemination; autopsies; *bioethical issues; brain death; cadavers; cardiac death; circumcision; confidentiality; congenital disorders; contraception; determination of death; disabled; duty to warn; genetic intervention; informed consent; *Jewish ethics; males; medical education; multiple pregnancy; newborns; organ donation; organ donors; persistent vegetative state; prenatal diagnosis; resource allocation; resuscitation; selective abortion; sex preselection; strikes; suffering; surgery; surrogate mothers; terminally ill; theology; treatment refusal; ventilators; withholding treatment; intubation; *Auerbach, Shlomo Zalman

Steinberg, Avraham. The foundations and the development of modern medical ethics. *Journal of Assisted Reproduction and Genetics.* 1995 Sep; 12(8): 473–476. 13 refs. BE60558.
autonomy; *bioethical issues; *bioethics; biomedical technologies; cultural pluralism; international aspects; medical ethics; physician patient relationship; principle-based ethics; public policy; trends; values; Western World

Steinfels, Peter; Callahan, Daniel. A longtime leader in biomedical ethics reflects on his field's explosive growth, the backlash against it and 'false hopes' in America's health care quest. [Interview]. *New York Times.* 1998 May 2: A11. BE59569.
bioethical issues; *bioethics; economics; ethicists; ethics; health care; resource allocation; *Callahan, Daniel

Strong, Carson. Is there no common morality? [Book review essay]. *Medical Humanities Review.* 1997 Spring; 11(1): 39–45. 7 fn. BE59965.
bioethical issues; *bioethics; casuistry; *cultural pluralism; *ethical theory; freedom; libertarianism; *moral policy; morality; principle-based ethics; public policy; secularism; *The Foundations of Bioethics (Engelhardt, H.T.)

Tangwa, Godfrey B. Globalisation or Westernisation? Ethical concerns in the whole bio-business. *Bioethics.* 1999 Jul; 13(3–4): 218–226. 4 refs. BE61871.
*bioethics; biomedical technologies; *cultural pluralism; ecology; *international aspects; morality; non-Western World; religion; *social dominance; values; *Western World; nature; Africa

Increasing awareness of the importance of the biodiversity of the whole global biosphere has led to further awareness that the problems which arise in connection with preservation and exploitation of our planet's biodiversity are best tackled from a global perspective. The 'Biodiversity Convention' and the 'Human Genome Project' are some of the concrete attempts at such globalisation. But, while these efforts are certainly very good at the intentional level and on paper, there is, at the practical level of implementation, the danger that globalisation may simply translate into westernisation, given the Western world's dominance and will to dominate the rest of the globe. How is 'global bioethics' to be possible in a world inhabited by different cultural groups whose material situation, powers, ideas, experiences and attitudes differ rather markedly and who are not, in any case, equally represented in globalisation efforts and fora? One index of the pertinence of this question is that talk about biodiversity, biotechnology, biotrade etc. is being increasingly matched by talk about biopiracy, biorade, biocolonialism etc. In this paper, I

BE = bioethics accession number   fn. = footnotes   refs. = references

attempt to explore and develop these very general concerns.

ten Have, Henk A.M.J.; Sass, Hans–Martin, eds.
Consensus Formation in Healthcare Ethics. Boston, MA: Kluwer Academic; 1998. 256 p. (Philosophy and medicine; 58). 329 refs. 49 fn. ISBN 0–7923–4944–X. BE62584.
advisory committees; allowing to die; attitudes; *bioethical issues; *bioethics; biomedical technologies; brain death; clinical ethics; clinical ethics committees; communication; conscience; *consensus; *cultural pluralism; *decision making; determination of death; dissent; family members; federal government; futility; genetic counseling; government regulation; health care; health care delivery; historical aspects; international aspects; mental health; methods; models, theoretical; moral policy; patient care; physician's role; postmodernism; psychiatric diagnosis; psychiatry; public opinion; public policy; reproductive technologies; resource allocation; terminal care; third party consent; values; Europe; Japan; United States

ten Have, Henk A.M.J.; Welie, Jos V.M., eds.
Ownership of the Human Body: Philosophical Considerations on the Use of the Human Body and Its Parts in Healthcare. Boston, MA: Kluwer Academic; 1998. 235 p. (Philosophy and medicine; v. 59). 284 refs. 45 fn. ISBN 0–7923–5150. BE61317.
altruism; autonomy; autopsies; *bioethical issues; biomedical research; blood donation; *body parts and fluids; cadavers; commodification; common good; deontological ethics; ethical theory; historical aspects; *human body; human experimentation; legal aspects; libertarianism; mandatory programs; *moral policy; organ donation; philosophy; postmodernism; *property rights; public policy; religion; remuneration; rights; Roman Catholic ethics; *tissue donation; utilitarianism; voluntary programs; Denmark; Europe; France; Germany; Netherlands

Thomasma, David C. Bioethics and international human rights. *Journal of Law, Medicine and Ethics.* 1997 Winter; 25(4): 295–306. 81 fn. BE62675.
abortion, induced; autonomy; *bioethical issues; *bioethics; capital punishment; common good; communication; communitarianism; contraception; *cultural pluralism; economics; embryo research; *ethical relativism; *human rights; informed consent; *international aspects; non–Western World; organ donation; postmodernism; prisoners; religion; remuneration; reproductive technologies; social interaction; *values; Western World; women's rights; China; India; Middle East; Pakistan; United States

Thomasma, David C. Toward a 21st century bioethic. *Alternative Therapies in Health and Medicine.* 1995 Mar; 1(1): 74–75. 8 refs. BE62005.
*alternative therapies; bioethical issues; *bioethics; biomedical technologies; *cultural pluralism; ecology; international aspects; medicine; *non–Western World; professional patient relationship; trends; *Western World; United States

Tichtchenko, Pavel. New bioethics association is founded for the post–socialist countries. [News]. *Bulletin of Medical Ethics.* 1999 Apr; No. 147: 6. BE61822.
*bioethics; *ethicists; international aspects; *professional organizations; *Central and East European Association of Bioethics; *Eastern Europe; Europe

Tong, Rosemarie. The way of feminist bioethics. [Book review essay]. *Medical Humanities Review.* 1997 Spring; 11(1): 72–75. BE59966.
abortion on demand; abortion, induced; *bioethics; decision making; females; *feminist ethics; fetuses; moral obligations; pregnant women; *reproduction; reproductive technologies; *rights; risks and benefits; selective abortion; surrogate

mothers; utilitarianism; *Reproducing Persons: Issues in Feminist Bioethics (Purdy, L.M.)

Unesco. International Bioethics Committee.
Proceedings of the Fourth Session, October 1996. Volume I. Paris: The Committee; 1998. 164 p. Includes references. BE61056.
advisory committees; AIDS; autonomy; beneficence; *bioethical issues; committee membership; drugs; ecology; economics; food; *genetic intervention; *genetic research; *genome mapping; government regulation; *guidelines; *human experimentation; *human rights; *international aspects; investigators; justice; moral obligations; random selection; recombinant DNA research; regulation; remuneration; research subjects; risks and benefits; selection of subjects; standards; transgenic organisms; vulnerable populations; women's health; agriculture; *transgenic plants; Declaration of Helsinki; *International Bioethics Committee (Unesco); Unesco; United Nations; *Universal Declaration on the Human Genome and Human Rights (Unesco)

Unesco. International Bioethics Committee.
Proceedings of the Fourth Session, October 1996. Volume II. Paris: The Committee; 1998. 94 p. Includes references. Papers in English and in French. BE61057.
adults; advisory committees; autonomy; *bioethical issues; children; females; food; guidelines; *human experimentation; *human rights; immunization; informed consent; *international aspects; nontherapeutic research; privacy; random selection; regulation; research ethics committees; research subjects; therapeutic research; transgenic organisms; women's health; women's rights; agriculture; *transgenic plants; Argentina; Belmont Report; China; Colombia; Great Britain; International Bioethics Committee (Unesco); National Commission for the Protection of Human Subjects; Sweden; Tunisia; Unesco; United States

United Nations. Economic and Social Council. Commission on Human Rights. Human Rights and Scientific and Technological Developments –– Human Rights and Bioethics. Report of the Secretary–General. New York, NY: United Nations; 1994 Nov 15. 34 p. 10 fn. E/CN.4/1995/74. BE60624.
abortion, induced; *bioethical issues; biomedical research; confidentiality; developing countries; embryo research; family planning; genetic intervention; genetic research; *government regulation; health care delivery; human experimentation; *human rights; informed consent; *international aspects; legal aspects; medical records; organ donation; organ transplantation; physician patient relationship; *public policy; reproductive technologies; resource allocation; treatment refusal; vulnerable populations; United Nations

van der Burg, Wibren. Law and bioethics. *In:* Kuhse, Helga; Singer, Peter, eds. A Companion to Bioethics. Malden, MA: Blackwell; 1998: 49–57. 25 refs. ISBN 0–631–19737–0. BE59481.
bioethical issues; *bioethics; cultural pluralism; *interdisciplinary communication; *law; models, theoretical; *morality; paternalism; *public policy; liberalism

van Hooft, Stan. The meanings of suffering. *Hastings Center Report.* 1998 Sep–Oct; 28(5): 13–19. 14 fn. BE59548.
attitudes; Christian ethics; compassion; historical aspects; humanism; philosophy; postmodernism; secularism; *suffering; values
Western thinkers have usually falsified our experience of suffering in trying to make sense of it. In a postmodern age, their accounts seem implausible. We need a way of making sense of suffering while admitting its horror.

Veatch, Robert M. Ethical consensus formation in clinical

---

cases. *In:* ten Have, Henk A.M.J.; Sass, Hans–Martin, eds. Consensus Formation in Healthcare Ethics. Boston, MA: Kluwer Academic; 1998: 17–34. 25 refs. ISBN 0–7923–4944–X. BE62585.

   autonomy; *clinical ethics; *clinical ethics committees; competence; *consensus; contracts; covenant; cultural pluralism; *decision making; ethical theory; family members; health facilities; informed consent; legal guardians; moral policy; patient advocacy; *patient care; *patient care team; patient participation; *patients; peer review; *physicians; religious ethics; secularism; third party consent; values; absence of proxy

Veatch, Robert M. The foundations of bioethics. *Bioethics.* 1999 Jul; 13(3–4): 206–217. 20 fn. BE61870.

   *bioethics; codes of ethics; consensus; ethical relativism; *ethical theory; medical ethics; moral obligations; *morality; physicians; principle–based ethics; professional organizations; public participation; standards; values; virtues

Vorspan, Albert; Saperstein, David. Bioethics: thinking the unthinkable. *In: their* Jewish Dimensions of Social Justice: Tough Moral Choices of Our Time. New York, NY: UAHC Press; 1998: 47–73. ISBN 0–8074–0650–3. BE62633.

   advance directives; allowing to die; artificial feeding; assisted suicide; *bioethical issues; brain death; breast cancer; cardiac death; cloning; determination of death; fetal tissue donation; gene therapy; genetic disorders; genetic information; genetic intervention; genetic predisposition; genetic screening; germ cells; *Jewish ethics; organ donation; organ donors; organizational policies; persistent vegetative state; physicians; privacy; prognosis; public policy; scarcity; selection for treatment; social discrimination; terminally ill; third party consent; treatment refusal; value of life; voluntary euthanasia; withholding treatment; dignity; Orthodox Judaism; Reform Judaism; United States

Vorspan, Albert; Saperstein, David. Life and death issues: policy on the edge. *In: their* Jewish Dimensions of Social Justice: Tough Moral Choices of Our Time. New York, NY: UAHC Press; 1998: 11–46. ISBN 0–8074–0650–3. BE62632.

   abortion, induced; AIDS; alcohol abuse; *bioethical issues; capital punishment; compassion; conscience; drug abuse; *Jewish ethics; minors; organizational policies; pregnant women; selective abortion; smoking; social problems; therapeutic abortion; value of life; violence; Reform Judaism; United States

Walters, LeRoy; Kahn, Tamar Joy, eds. Bibliography of Bioethics, Volume 24. Washington, DC: Georgetown University, Kennedy Institute of Ethics; 1998. 766 p. ISBN 1–883913–04–7. BE60513.

   *bioethical issues; *bioethics

Walters, LeRoy; Kahn, Tamar Joy, eds. Bibliography of Bioethics, Volume 25. Washington, DC: Georgetown University, Kennedy Institute of Ethics; 1999. 752 p. ISBN 1–883913–0505. BE61425.

   *bioethical issues; *bioethics

Watson, Sidney Dean. In search of the story: physicians and charity care. *Saint Louis University Public Law Review.* 1996; 15(2): 353–369. 92 fn. BE59914.

   *altruism; *bioethical issues; *bioethics; caring; case studies; economics; emergency care; ethicists; *health care delivery; hospitals; *indigents; literature; medical education; medical ethics; methods; minority groups; *moral obligations; *narrative ethics; obligations of society; *patient care; patient compliance; patient transfer; physician patient relationship; *physicians; *refusal to treat; remuneration; social problems; *socioeconomic factors; Medicaid; United States

Welie, Jos V.M. In the Face of Suffering: The Philosophical–Anthropological Foundations of Clinical Ethics. Omaha, NE: Creighton University Press; 1998. 304 p. Bibliography: p. 279–293. ISBN 1–881871–26–6. BE62440.

   anthropology; *autonomy; *beneficence; bioethics; caring; *clinical ethics; *compassion; cultural pluralism; *decision making; empathy; *ethical theory; freedom; human characteristics; paternalism; patients; personhood; *philosophy; *physician patient relationship; physicians; self concept; suffering; treatment refusal; trust; authenticity; patient abandonment; sick role; *sympathy; von Gebsattel, Viktor

Werner, D. Leonard. Guest editorial: imperialism, research ethics and global health. [Letter]. *Journal of Medical Ethics.* 1999 Feb; 25(1): 62. 1 ref. BE61705.

   *bioethics; *cultural pluralism; data banks; ethical relativism; *international aspects; literature; *non–Western World; terminology; *values; *Western World; research ethics; MEDLINE

Whitehouse, Peter J. Bioethics, biology, *and* the biosphere: the ecomedical disconnection syndrome. *Hastings Center Report.* 1999 Jan–Feb; 29(1): 41–44. 15 fn. BE61637.

   *bioethics; biomedical technologies; *common good; democracy; *ecology; education; evolution; future generations; genetics; goals; health care; health hazards; *interdisciplinary communication; medical ethics; medicine; moral development; public health; public participation; religion; science; social problems; values; nature

Wildes, Kevin W. Libertarianism and ownership of the human body. *In:* ten Have, Henk A.M.J.; Welie, Jos V.M., eds. Ownership of the Human Body: Philosophical Considerations on the Use of the Human Body and Its Parts in Healthcare. Boston, MA: Kluwer Academic; 1998: 143–157. 26 refs. 2 fn. ISBN 0–7923–5150–9. BE61322.

   *bioethics; body parts and fluids; casuistry; cultural pluralism; decision making; ethical theory; *human body; informed consent; *libertarianism; *morality; organ donation; postmodernism; principle–based ethics; *property rights; remuneration; Roman Catholic ethics; secularism; values

Wolf, Susan M. Bioethics and law symposium: deconstructing traditional paradigms in bioethics: race, gender, class, and culture. Foreword: bioethics -- from mirror to window. *Saint Louis University Public Law Review.* 1996; 15(2): 183–189. 23 fn. Introduction to a set of articles by V.R. Randall, A. Jurevic, C.L. Barrow and K.A. Easley, J. Barrow, J. Downie and S. Sherwin, C.E. Gudorf, S.D. Watson, J. Tang, A. Dósa, E.S. Monahan, and H.M. Mannan. BE59907.

   *bioethics; *cultural pluralism; ethicist's role; evaluation; feminist ethics; international aspects; methods; minority groups; socioeconomic factors; *trends; United States

Wolf, Susan M. Erasing difference: race, ethnicity, and gender in bioethics. *In:* Donchin, Anne; Purdy, Laura M., eds. Embodying Bioethics: Recent Feminist Advances. Lanham, MD: Rowman and Littlefield; 1999: 65–81. 90 refs. 3 fn. ISBN 0–8476–8924–7. BE61015.

   *bioethics; cultural pluralism; *disadvantaged; empirical research; *ethical analysis; ethical theory; eugenics; *evaluation; *females; *feminist ethics; human experimentation; justice; *minority groups; misconduct; quality of health care; *social discrimination; *socioeconomic factors; United States

---

BE = bioethics accession number   fn. = footnotes   refs. = references

Wolf, Susan M. Shifting paradigms in bioethics and health law: the rise of a new pragmatism. *American Journal of Law and Medicine.* 1994; 20(4): 395–415. 130 fn. BE62535.
   bioethical issues; *bioethics; clinical ethics; cultural pluralism; decision making; empirical research; ethical theory; feminist ethics; health care; interdisciplinary communication; *law; *methods; minority groups; patient care; principle-based ethics; socioeconomic factors; *trends; *pragmatism

Wulff, Henrik R. Contemporary trends in healthcare ethics. *In:* ten Have, Henk A.M.J.; Sass, Hans–Martin, eds. Consensus Formation in Healthcare Ethics. Boston, MA: Kluwer Academic; 1998: 63–72. 6 refs. ISBN 0-7923-4944-X. BE62588.
   autonomy; bioethical issues; *bioethics; clinical ethics; comparative studies; *consensus; *cultural pluralism; decision making; deontological ethics; dissent; health care delivery; *international aspects; justice; moral obligations; physician patient relationship; principle-based ethics; public policy; rights; teleological ethics; trends; *values; *Europe; *United States

Zuckerman, Connie. Clinical ethics in geriatric care settings. *Generations (American Society on Aging).* 1994 Winter; 18(4): 9–12. 11 refs. BE60544.
   *aged; autonomy; chronically ill; *clinical ethics; clinical ethics committees; *decision making; family members; home care; interdisciplinary communication; long–term care; mediation; nursing homes; *patient care; patient care team

Zwart, Hub. Moral deliberation and moral warfare: consensus formation in a pluralistic society. *In:* ten Have, Henk A.M.J.; Sass, Hans–Martin, eds. Consensus Formation in Healthcare Ethics. Boston, MA: Kluwer Academic; 1998: 73–91. 14 refs. ISBN 0-7923-4944-X. BE62589.
   autonomy; *bioethics; communication; *consensus; *cultural pluralism; *decision making; *dissent; historical aspects; morality; postmodernism; values; negotiation

Educational resources: finding bioethics journal literature. *NCCE News (Veterans Health Administration National Center for Clinical Ethics).* 1994 Fall; 2(4): 8. BE59851.
   *bioethics; *data banks; *information dissemination; *literature; *BIOETHICSLINE; MEDLINE

European Group on Ethics in Science and New Technologies. [News]. *Journal of Medical Ethics.* 1998 Aug; 24(4): 247. BE61302.
   *advisory committees; *bioethical issues; biomedical technologies; genetic intervention; *international aspects; *European Commission; *European Group on Ethics in Science and New Technologies; Group of Advisers on the Ethical Implications of Biotechnology (European Commission)

Organisation of African Unity adopts resolution on bioethics. [Text of resolution]. *International Digest of Health Legislation.* 1997; 48(2): 239–240. Adopted by the Assembly of Heads of State and Government of the OAU at its Thirty–Second Ordinary Session in Yaoundé, Cameroon, 8–10 Jul 1996. BE59599.
   *bioethical issues; common good; embryo research; genetic materials; health care; human experimentation; *human rights; informed consent; *international aspects; organ donation; organ transplantation; *organizational policies; prisoners; torture; *Africa; *Organization of African Unity

WHO steps closer to its responsibilities. [Editorial]. *Nature.* 1999 Mar 18; 398(6724): 175. BE61960.
   *bioethical issues; *biomedical research; cloning; genetic research; *guidelines; *international aspects; *World Health Organization

BIOETHICS/CODES OF ETHICS

American Medical Association. Council on Ethical and Judicial Affairs. Code of Medical Ethics: Current Opinions with Annotations, 1998–1999 Edition. Chicago, IL: American Medical Association; 1998. 228 p. ISBN 0-89970-960-5. BE61043.
   abortion, induced; active euthanasia; advance directives; advertising; AIDS serodiagnosis; allowing to die; attitudes; *bioethical issues; biomedical technologies; capital punishment; clinical ethics committees; *codes of ethics; confidentiality; conflict of interest; cord blood; domestic violence; economics; fetal research; futility; gene therapy; genetic counseling; genetic screening; ghost surgery; gifts; health care; HIV seropositivity; human experimentation; interprofessional relations; *medical ethics; medical etiquette; medical records; misconduct; organ donation; *organizational policies; patents; physician patient relationship; *physicians; professional organizations; referral and consultation; remuneration; reproductive technologies; resource allocation; resuscitation orders; social discrimination; sports medicine; physician impairment; *American Medical Association

BIOETHICS/EDUCATION

Crausman, Robert S.; Armstrong, John D. Ethically based medical decision making in the intensive care unit: residency teaching strategies. *Critical Care Clinics.* 1996 Jan; 12(1): 71–84. 54 refs. BE59278.
   *bioethics; *clinical ethics; communication; curriculum; decision making; dissent; ethicists; faculty; family members; *intensive care units; interdisciplinary communication; *internship and residency; *medical education; *medical ethics; patient care; patient care team; physician patient relationship; *physicians; teaching methods; uncertainty; values

Higgs, Roger. Do studies of the nature of cases mislead about the reality of cases? A response to Pattison *et al. Journal of Medical Ethics.* 1999 Feb; 25(1): 47–50. 13 refs. BE61195.
   authorship; *bioethics; *case studies; *clinical ethics; dehumanization; *education; emotions; evaluation; literature; *medical ethics; *teaching methods; values
This article questions whether many are misled by current case studies. Three broad types of style of case study are described. A stark style, based on medical case studies, a fictionalised style in reaction, and a personal statement made in discussion groups by an original protagonist. Only the second type fits Pattison's category. Language remains an important issue, but to be examined as the case is lived in discussion rather than as a potentially reductionist study of the case as text.

Meyer, G. Rex, ed. Bioethics in Education. Münster, Germany: Lit; 1991. 190 p. (Erziehungswissenschaften; Bd. 27). Includes references. ISBN 3-88660-795-X. BE62146.
   bioethical issues; *bioethics; *biology; biomedical technologies; *curriculum; developing countries; *education; ethics; genetic intervention; goals; international aspects; Islamic ethics; medical education; medical ethics; physician patient relationship; science; students; teaching methods; values; secondary schools; Egypt

Myser, Catherine. How bioethics is being taught: a critical review. *In:* Kuhse, Helga; Singer, Peter, eds. A Companion to Bioethics. Malden, MA: Blackwell; 1998: 484–500. 89 refs. ISBN 0-631-19737-0. BE59521.

---

*bioethics; consensus; cultural pluralism; *curriculum; developing countries; education; evaluation; goals; *international aspects; *medical education; review; teaching methods

Newell, Christopher. The ethics of narrative ethics: some teaching reflections. *Health Care Analysis.* 1998 Jun; 6(2): 171–174. 7 refs. BE59885.
> attitudes; *bioethics; *case studies; disabled; *medical education; *narrative ethics; pastoral care; patient participation; *teaching methods; Australia

Narrative is reemerging as a teaching tool. Narrative ethics is being seen as a rich endeavour both for clinical practice and academic teaching and research. Narrative helps put ethics into context. However, the use of narrative increasingly raises issues in teaching and research: for instance, how do we do justice to the people and narratives we utilise, and what does our practice reveal about our ethics? In this article examples are drawn from clinical practice, teaching and case notes to draw out some lessons to help further critical understanding.

Pattison, Stephen; Dickenson, Donna; Parker, Michael, et al. Do case studies mislead about the nature of reality? *Journal of Medical Ethics.* 1999 Feb; 25(1): 42–46. 14 refs. BE61194.
> authorship; *bioethics; *case studies; *clinical ethics; *education; *evaluation; literature; narrative ethics; postmodernism; *teaching methods; values

This paper attempts a partial, critical look at the construction and use of case studies in ethics education. It argues that the authors and users of case studies are often insufficiently aware of the literary nature of these artefacts: this may lead to some confusion between fiction and reality. Issues of the nature of the genre, the fictional, story-constructing aspect of case studies, the nature of authorship, and the purposes and uses of case studies as "texts" are outlined and discussed. The paper concludes with some critical questions that can be applied to the construction and use of case studies in the light of the foregoing analysis.

Peters, Malte; Ono, Yumiko; Shimizu, Koji, et al. Selected bioethical issues in Japanese and German textbooks of biology for lower secondary schools. *Journal of Moral Education.* 1997 Dec; 26(4): 473–489. 32 refs. BE59963.
> *bioethical issues; *biology; comparative studies; *ecology; *education; goals; *international aspects; literature; teaching methods; values; *secondary schools; *Germany; *Japan

Reiter-Theil, Stella. The voice of the patient: experiences with the patients' medical ethics forum. *Bulletin of Medical Ethics.* 1998 Feb; No. 135: 18–21. 6 refs. BE61888.
> *bioethical issues; bioethics; *communication; *education; family members; *health personnel; medical education; patient education; *patient participation; students; *Germany; *Patientenforum Medizinische Ethik (Germany)

BIOLOGICAL WARFARE *See* WAR

BIOMEDICAL RESEARCH

See also BEHAVIORAL RESEARCH, EMBRYO AND FETAL RESEARCH, GENETIC RESEARCH, HUMAN EXPERIMENTATION

Abbott, Alison. German scientists may escape fraud trial.

[News]. *Nature.* 1998 Oct 8; 395(6702): 532–533. Includes inset article by A. Abbott, "Task force set up to determine the damage," p. 533. BE59642.
> biomedical research; *fraud; investigators; *legal aspects; *scientific misconduct; universities; *Brach, Marion; *Germany; *Herrmann, Friedhelm; University of Ulm

Abbott, Alison. Science comes to terms with the lessons of fraud. [News]. *Nature.* 1999 Mar 4; 398(6722): 13–17. Includes inset articles, "Japanese scandals raise public distrust," by A. Saegusa, p. 14; "Editors debate whether to blow the whistle on suspect papers," p. 15; and "US stalks on new definitions of misconduct," by R. Dalton, p. 16. BE61866.
> attitudes; biomedical research; due process; editorial policies; federal government; *fraud; government regulation; guidelines; *international aspects; interprofessional relations; investigators; public policy; research institutes; *science; *scientific misconduct; *self regulation; social dominance; time factors; universities; whistleblowing; retraction of publication; Europe; Germany; Japan; United States

Alper, Joseph. A man in a hurry: stem cells. [Profile of Michael West]. *Science.* 1999 Mar 5; 283(5407): 1434–1435. BE61401.
> *biomedical research; cloning; embryo research; genetic intervention; *genetic research; hybrids; industry; investigators; life extension; *stem cells; Advanced Cell Technology Inc.; *West, Michael

Altman, Ellen; Hernon, Peter, eds. Research Misconduct: Issues, Implications, and Strategies. Greenwich, CT: Ablex; 1997. 206 p. (Contemporary studies in information management, policy, and services). Bibliography: p. 187–194. ISBN 1-56750-341-1. BE62439.
> attitudes; authorship; biomedical research; codes of ethics; conflict of interest; editorial policies; faculty; humanities; international aspects; investigators; journalism; professional organizations; regulation; science; *scientific misconduct; social sciences; students; survey; universities; publishing; retraction of publication; United States

Altman, Lawrence K. British cast spotlight on misconduct in scientific research. [News]. *New York Times.* 1998 Jun 9: F3. BE59608.
> *biomedical research; community services; editorial policies; fraud; health services research; *international aspects; interprofessional relations; investigators; physically disabled; *scientific misconduct; self regulation; BMJ (British Medical Journal); Great Britain; United States; Williams, Mark H.

Angelides, Kimon; Pianelli, James V. It will take more than notebooks to stop fraud. [Letter]. *Nature.* 1998 Dec 3; 396(6710): 404. BE61089.
> *accountability; *biomedical research; *records; *research institutes; *scientific misconduct; self regulation; standards

Annas, George J. Burden of proof: judging science and protecting public health in (and out of) the courtroom. *American Journal of Public Health.* 1999 Apr; 89(4): 490–493. 4 refs. BE61385.
> compensation; cosmetic surgery; economics; *epidemiology; expert testimony; federal government; *females; government regulation; *industry; *injuries; judicial action; *legal liability; literature; *medical devices; public health; review committees; science; *standards; technical expertise; torts; women's health; *breast implants; *Dow Corning; United States

Bayer, Ronald. Science, justice, and breast implants. [Editorial]. *American Journal of Public Health.* 1999 Apr; 89(4): 483. 5 refs. BE61383.
> compensation; cosmetic surgery; *epidemiology; *females;

BE = bioethics accession number   fn. = footnotes   refs. = references

*industry; injuries; judicial action; justice; *legal liability; *medical devices; science; *uncertainty; women's health; *breast implants; United States

Biagioli, Mario. Publication and promotion: long live the deans! *Lancet.* 1998 Sep 12; 352(9131): 899–900. 1 ref. BE60145.
*accountability; *authorship; *biomedical research; fraud; *investigators; *scientific misconduct; universities

Blank, Robert H. Brain Policy: How the New Neuroscience Will Change Our Lives and Our Politics. Washington, DC: Georgetown University Press; 1999. 199 p. Bibliography: p.179–191. ISBN 0-87840-712-X. BE62619.
aggression; autonomy; behavioral genetics; *biomedical research; *biomedical technologies; *brain; brain death; *brain pathology; central nervous system diseases; competence; decision making; electrical stimulation of the brain; enhancement technologies; eugenics; fetal tissue donation; gene therapy; genetic intervention; genetic research; health hazards; informed consent; legal aspects; mentally ill; patient care; pregnant women; prenatal injuries; psychoactive drugs; psychosurgery; public participation; public policy; recall; resource allocation; risks and benefits; self concept; sexuality; social impact; stigmatization; technology assessment; therapeutic research; tissue transplantation; treatment refusal; violence; *neurosciences; United States

Blumenthal, David. Ethics issues in academic–industry relationships in the life sciences: the continuing debate. *Academic Medicine.* 1996 Dec; 71(12): 1291–1296. 15 refs. BE61378.
*biomedical research; *conflict of interest; decision making; disclosure; faculty; *financial support; human experimentation; *industry; information dissemination; *investigators; regulation; risks and benefits; *universities

Bonetta, Laura. Inquiry into clinical trial scandal at Canadian research hospital. [News]. *Nature Medicine.* 1998 Oct; 4(10): 1095. BE61528.
administrators; *biomedical research; conflict of interest; disclosure; *drug industry; drugs; *financial support; *hospitals; *human experimentation; *institutional policies; *investigators; misconduct; regulation; thalassemia; toxicity; *Apotex; *Canada; *deferiprone; *Hospital for Sick Children (Toronto); *Olivieri, Nancy

Breimer, Lars; Brown, Laura; Skinner, Andrew, et al. Fraud. [Letters]. *BMJ (British Medical Journal).* 1998 Dec 5; 317(7172): 1590–1591. 9 refs. BE61135.
authorship; biomedical research; drug industry; economics; *fraud; guidelines; human experimentation; investigators; *regulation; *scientific misconduct; Great Britain

Burton, Thomas M. A prostate researcher tested firm's product -- and sat on its board. [News]. *Wall Street Journal.* 1998 Mar 19: A1, A8. BE59671.
*biomedical research; *conflict of interest; disclosure; *drug industry; drugs; editorial policies; *financial support; fraud; investigators; medical devices; *misconduct; *physicians; *remuneration; surgery; *therapeutic research; *Oesterling, Joseph; University of Michigan

Butler, Declan. Fraud squad files report to prosecutor in INSERM case. [News]. *Nature.* 1998 Jul 23; 394(6691): 308. BE59936.
biomedical research; fraud; industry; *investigators; legal aspects; patents; *research institutes; *scientific misconduct; universities; whistleblowing; *Bihain, Bernard; *France; Genset; *INSERM; University of Rennes

Cahill, Lisa Sowle. The new biotech world order.

[Symposium: human primordial stem cells]. *Hastings Center Report.* 1999 Mar–Apr; 29(2): 45–48. 9 fn. BE61666.
advisory committees; autonomy; *biomedical research; biomedical technologies; commodification; *common good; economics; *embryo research; ethics committees; federal government; financial support; freedom; *genetic research; genetic services; government financing; human rights; *industry; informed consent; *international aspects; *justice; organizational policies; *regulation; resource allocation; *stem cells; values; Geron Corp.; Geron Ethics Advisory Board; United States

Callahan, Daniel. Calling scientific ideology to account. *Society.* 1996 May–Jun; 33(4): 14–19. BE60064.
*accountability; *bioethics; biomedical research; biomedical technologies; ecology; economics; humanism; interdisciplinary communication; *religion; *science; secularism; *social dominance; social impact; *values; nature

Campbell, Courtney S. Religion and the body in medical research. *Kennedy Institute of Ethics Journal.* 1998 Sep; 8(3): 275–305. 36 refs. 2 fn. BE60168.
advisory committees; altruism; American Indians; attitudes; *autopsies; *biomedical research; *body parts and fluids; *cadavers; commodification; *common good; confidentiality; cultural pluralism; fetal tissue donation; genetic information; *genetic research; genome mapping; *gifts; *human body; informed consent; investigators; Islamic ethics; Jewish ethics; medical education; metaphor; moral obligations; *nontherapeutic research; *organ donation; organ transplantation; property rights; Protestant ethics; *religious ethics; remuneration; Roman Catholic ethics; science; self concept; *theology; *tissue banks; *tissue donation; transplant recipients; values; National Bioethics Advisory Commission

Religious discussion of human organs and tissues has concentrated largely on donation for therapeutic purposes. The retrieval and use of human tissue samples in diagnostic, research, and education contexts have, by contrast, received very little direct theological attention. Initially undertaken at the behest of the National Bioethics Advisory Commission, this essay seeks to explore the theological and religious questions embedded in nontherapeutic use of human tissue. It finds that the "donation paradigm" typically invoked in religious discourse to justify uses of the body for therapeutic reasons is inadequate in the context of nontherapeutic research, while the "resource paradigm" implicit in scientific discourse presumes a reductionist account of the body that runs contrary to important religious values about embodiment. The essay proposes a "contribution paradigm" that provides a religious perspective within which research on human tissue can be both justified and limited.

Chalmers, Iain. Publication and promotion: the public interest. *Lancet.* 1998 Sep 12; 352(9131): 893–894. 2 refs. BE60139.
*authorship; *biomedical research; data banks; editorial policies; human experimentation; literature; research design; statistics; trends; *multicenter studies

Clarke, Adele E. Disciplining Reproduction: Modernity, American Life Sciences, and "the Problems of Sex." Berkeley, CA: University of California Press; 1998. 421 p. Bibliography: p. 333–410. ISBN 0-520-20720-3. BE60503.
animal experimentation; *biology; *biomedical research; *contraception; eugenics; family planning; federal government; females; *financial support; genetics; government financing; historical aspects; infertility; interdisciplinary communication; investigators; males; medicine; morality; political activity; population control;

---

private sector; *reproduction; reproductive technologies; *sexuality; *social control; social dominance; *sociology of medicine; universities; women's health; women's rights; agriculture; Ford Foundation; National Research Council; Rockefeller Foundation; *Twentieth Century; *United States

Concar, David. Their learned friends: was a scientific society really a front for one of the world's biggest tobacco firms? [News]. *New Scientist.* 1998 May 16; 158(2134): 5. BE59205.
*biomedical research; *conflict of interest; editorial policies; *financial support; health hazards; *industry; international aspects; *investigators; professional organizations; research institutes; scientific misconduct; *smoking; Great Britain; Indoor Air International; *Philip Morris; United States

Cowen, Robert C. Academics face abuse of rules designed to protect research. *Christian Science Monitor.* 1998 Mar 25: 13. BE59606.
*biomedical research; conflict of interest; drug industry; *due process; *financial support; information dissemination; interprofessional relations; *investigators; political activity; science; *scientific misconduct; self regulation; universities; *whistleblowing; United States

Dalton, Rex. Arizona professor files lawsuit after being fired for misconduct. [News]. *Nature.* 1998 Aug 27; 394(6696): 817. BE60633.
biomedical research; fraud; investigators; *scientific misconduct; self regulation; universities; Arizona; *Kay, Marguerite; University of Arizona

Dalton, Rex. Federal panel endorses Baylor fraud claim. [News]. *Nature.* 1999 Feb 18; 397(6720): 549. BE60636.
biomedical research; federal government; *fraud; government regulation; legal aspects; *scientific misconduct; self regulation; universities; *Angelides, Kimon; Baylor College of Medicine; United States

David, Edward E. Non-starters and no brainers: an outside perspective. *Accountability in Research.* 1997; 5(4): 255–263. Paper presented at the symposium, "Ethical Issues in Research Relationships between Universities and Industry," held in Baltimore, MD, 3–4 Nov 1995. BE60423.
*biomedical research; *conflict of interest; disclosure; financial support; guidelines; *industry; investigators; peer review; property rights; *scientific misconduct; *universities; National Academy of Sciences; National Institutes of Health; National Science Foundation; United States

Davidoff, Frank. Publication and promotion: intelligence work. *Lancet.* 1998 Sep 12; 352(9131): 895–896. 2 refs. BE60141.
*authorship; *biomedical research; disclosure; *editorial policies; investigators

Davies, Huw T.O.; Rennie, Drummond. Independence, governance, and trust: redefining the relationship between JAMA and the AMA. [Editorial]. *JAMA.* 1999 Jun 23–30; 281(24): 2344–2346. 24 refs. BE62152.
*accountability; advertising; *biomedical research; conflict of interest; disclosure; *editorial policies; *freedom; investigators; *journalism; *peer review; physicians; professional autonomy; *professional organizations; property rights; science; *standards; *trust; *American Medical Association; *JAMA; United States

Dekkers, Wim J.M.; ten Have, Henk A.M.J. Biomedical research with human body "parts". *In:* ten Have, Henk A.M.J.; Welie, Jos V.M., eds. Ownership of the Human Body: Philosophical Considerations on the Use of the Human Body and Its Parts in Health Care.

Boston, MA: Kluwer Academic; 1998: 49–63. 20 refs. 1 fn. Translated from the Dutch. ISBN 0–7923–5150–9. BE61319.
*biomedical research; *body parts and fluids; donors; ethical review; fetal tissue donation; genetic materials; human body; human experimentation; informed consent; *organ donation; property rights; remuneration; *tissue donation; cell lines

Djerassi, Carl. Who will mentor the mentors? *Nature.* 1999 Jan 28; 397(6717): 291. BE60959.
authorship; biomedical research; communication; *faculty; institutional policies; *interprofessional relations; *misconduct; *science; self regulation; *students; *universities; research ethics

Durán, Deborah Guadalupe. Lack of Hispanics' involvement in research -- is it Hispanics or scientists? *Community Genetics.* 1998; 1(3): 183–189. 22 refs. BE62368.
*attitudes; behavioral research; *biomedical research; cultural pluralism; *genetic research; health; *Hispanic Americans; *investigators; population genetics; *science; selection of subjects; socioeconomic factors; trust; United States

Dworkin, Gerald; Kennedy, Ian. Human tissue: rights in the body and its parts. *Medical Law Review.* 1993 Autumn; 1(3): 291–319. 78 fn. BE59900.
*biomedical research; *body parts and fluids; cadavers; embryos; genetic intervention; government regulation; *human body; informed consent; investigators; judicial action; *legal aspects; *legal rights; *organ donation; organ donors; patents; patients; *property rights; public policy; remuneration; third party consent; *tissue donation; Europe; *Great Britain; Moore v. Regents of the University of California; United States

Egilman, David; Wallace, Wes; Hom, Candace. Corporate corruption of medical literature: asbestos studies concealed by W.R. Grace & Co. *Accountability in Research.* 1998 Jan; 6(1–2): 127–147. 76 refs. BE61547.
animal experimentation; biomedical research; cancer; compensation; contracts; *deception; *disclosure; economics; employment; *epidemiology; federal government; financial support; government regulation; *health hazards; *industry; information dissemination; injuries; institutional ethics; insurance; investigators; legal liability; *morbidity; mortality; *occupational exposure; *scientific misconduct; *lung diseases; Montana; National Institutes of Occupational Safety and Health; United States; *W.R. Grace & Co.

Farthing, Michael J.G. Fraud in medicine: coping with fraud. *Lancet.* 1998 Dec 19–26; 352 (Suppl. 4): 11. 5 refs. BE60146.
authorship; *biomedical research; *editorial policies; fraud; international aspects; investigators; *regulation; *scientific misconduct; BMJ (British Medical Journal); *Committee on Publication Ethics (Great Britain); General Medical Council (Great Britain); *Great Britain; JAMA

Fox, Daniel M. Comment: epidemiology and the new political economy of medicine. *American Journal of Public Health.* 1999 Apr; 89(4): 493–496. 19 refs. BE61386.
*accountability; contracts; cosmetic surgery; *economics; *epidemiology; *females; *industry; informed consent; injuries; managed care programs; *medical devices; patient care; physician patient relationship; *physicians; *risk; standards; *breast implants; Dow Corning; United States

Frankel, Mark S. Perception, reality, and the political context of conflict of interest in university–industry relationships. *Academic Medicine.* 1996 Dec; 71(12):

1297–1304. 44 refs. BE61379.
  *biomedical research; *conflict of interest; disclosure; economics; empirical research; entrepreneurship; federal government; *financial support; government financing; government regulation; guidelines; *industry; information dissemination; investigators; politics; *public policy; risks and benefits; *science; *universities; values; technology transfer; National Institutes of Health; Public Health Service; *United States

Gifford, Fred. Teaching scientific integrity. *Centennial Review.* 1994 Spring; 38(2): 297–314. 6 fn. BE59404.
  *biomedical research; conflict of interest; curriculum; deception; *education; federal government; fraud; government regulation; interprofessional relations; *investigators; motivation; negligence; *professional ethics; science; *scientific misconduct; self regulation; *students; teaching methods; truth disclosure; *universities; Michigan State University; National Institutes of Health; United States

Gold, Richard. Owning our bodies: an examination of property law and biotechnology. *San Diego Law Review.* 1995; 32(4): 1167–1247. 320 fn. BE59853.
  *biomedical research; *body parts and fluids; commodification; *economics; health; *human body; informed consent; *legal aspects; patents; patients; politics; *property rights; recombinant DNA research; religion; Supreme Court decisions; *tissue donation; transgenic organisms; *values; cell lines; Diamond v. Chakrabarty; Moore v. Regents of the University of California; United States

Gottlieb, Scott. NCI defends research involving minority groups. [News]. *Nature Medicine.* 1999 Mar; 5(3): 254. BE62541.
  behavioral research; *biomedical research; *cancer; evaluation; *federal government; *government financing; *human experimentation; indigents; *minority groups; organizational policies; preventive medicine; research institutes; resource allocation; *socioeconomic factors; Institute of Medicine; *National Cancer Institute; *The Unequal Burden of Cancer (Institute of Medicine); *United States

Greenfield, Barak; Kaufman, Jeffrey L.; Hueston, William J., et al. Authors vs contributors: accuracy, accountability, and responsibility. [Letters and response]. *JAMA.* 1998 Feb 4; 279(5): 356–357. 6 refs. BE59225.
  *accountability; *authorship; *biomedical research; *scientific misconduct

Gross, Cary P.; Anderson, Gerard F.; Powe, Neil R. The relation between funding by the National Institutes of Health and the burden of disease. *New England Journal of Medicine.* 1999 Jun 17; 340(24): 1881–1887. 34 refs. BE62032.
  age factors; AIDS; *biomedical research; breast cancer; comparative studies; decision making; dementia; depressive disorder; diabetes; diagnosis; disabled; *disease; federal government; financial support; *government financing; heart diseases; industry; morbidity; mortality; patient advocacy; political activity; prevalence; *resource allocation; schizophrenia; statistics; trends; values; *disability adjusted life years; *National Institutes of Health; *United States
BACKGROUND: The Institute of Medicine has proposed that the amount of disease-specific research funding provided by the National Institutes of Health (NIH) be systematically and consistently compared with the burden of disease for society. METHODS: We performed a cross-sectional study comparing estimates of disease-specific funding in 1996 with data on six measures of the burden of disease. The measures were total mortality, years of life lost, and number of hospital days in 1994 and incidence, prevalence, and

disability-adjusted life-years (one disability-adjusted life-year is defined as the loss of one year of healthy life to disease) in 1990. With the use of these measures as explanatory variables in a regression analysis, predicted funding was calculated and compared with actual funding. RESULTS: There was no relation between the amount of NIH funding and the incidence, prevalence, or number of hospital days attributed to each condition or disease ($P=0.82$, $P=0.23$, and $P=0.21$, respectively). The numbers of deaths ($r=0.40$, $P=0.03$) and years of life lost ($r=0.42$, $P=0.02$) were weakly associated with funding, whereas the number of disability-adjusted life-years was strongly predictive of funding ($r=0.62$, P less than 0.001). When the latter three measures were used to predict expected funding, the conclusions about the appropriateness of funding for some diseases varied according to the measure used. However, the acquired immunodeficiency syndrome, breast cancer, diabetes mellitus, and dementia all received relatively generous funding, regardless of which measure was used as the basis for calculating support. Research on chronic obstructive pulmonary disease, perinatal conditions, and peptic ulcer was relatively underfunded. CONCLUSIONS: The amount of NIH funding for research on a disease is associated with the burden of the disease; however, different measures of the burden of disease may yield different conclusions about the appropriateness of disease-specific funding levels.

Guenin, Louis M. The logical geography of concepts and shared responsibilities concerning research misconduct. *Academic Medicine.* 1996 Jun; 71(6): 595–603. 14 refs. BE61427.
  *accountability; biomedical research; codes of ethics; due process; *federal government; government financing; *government regulation; industry; investigators; professional ethics; professional organizations; punishment; science; *scientific misconduct; *self regulation; standards; state interest; *universities; Office of Research Integrity; *United States

Guston, David H. The demise of the social contract for science: misconduct in science and the nonmodern world. *Centennial Review.* 1994 Spring; 38(2): 215–248. 80 refs. 45 fn. BE59402.
  biomedical research; economics; federal government; government financing; *government regulation; investigators; *politics; *science; *scientific misconduct; *self regulation; universities; whistleblowing; *National Institutes of Health; *Office of Scientific Integrity; *U.S. Congress; *United States

Haber, Edgar. Industry and the university. *Nature Biotechnology.* 1996 Apr; 14(4): 441–442. 6 refs. BE61965.
  *biomedical research; *drug industry; evaluation; *financial support; freedom; *industry; information dissemination; international aspects; investigators; patents; property rights; *risks and benefits; statistics; *trends; *universities; United States

Hamajima, Nobuyuki; Tajima, Kazuo. Patients' views on reference to clinical data. *Journal of Epidemiology.* 1997 Mar; 7(1): 17–19. 10 refs. BE60190.
  age factors; *attitudes; cancer; epidemiology; females; *health services research; *hospitals; males; *medical records; *patients; *privacy; quality of health care; survey; Aichi Cancer Center Hospital; *Japan

Harper, William. The role of futility judgments in improperly limiting the scope of clinical research. *Journal of Medical Ethics.* 1998 Oct; 24(5): 308–313. 53

---

fn. BE60251.
*biomedical research; costs and benefits; critically ill; decision making; disclosure; *futility; hospitals; *investigators; *mortality; patient discharge; *patient participation; physicians; quality of life; *research design; resuscitation; statistics; *therapeutic research; *time factors; *treatment outcome; value of life; *values; withholding treatment

In medical research, the gathering and presenting of data can be limited in accordance with the futility judgments of the researchers. In that case, research results falling below the threshold of what the researchers deem beneficial would not be reported in detail. As a result, the reported information would tend to be useful only to those who share the valuational assumptions of the researchers. Should this practice become entrenched, it would reduce public confidence in the medical establishment, aggravate factionalism within the research community, and unduly influence treatment decisions. I suggest alternative frameworks for measuring survival outcomes.

Holm, Søren; Rossel, Peter. Ethical aspects of the use of 'sensitive information' in health care research. *In:* Bennett, Rebecca; Erin, Charles A., eds. HIV and AIDS: Testing, Screening, and Confidentiality. New York, NY: Oxford University Press; 1999: 200–215. 12 fn. ISBN 0–19–823801–0. BE62723.
*confidentiality; *epidemiology; HIV seropositivity; medical records; privacy; property rights; *registries; harms; integrity; Denmark

Hope, Tony. Medical research needs lay involvement. [Editorial]. *Journal of Medical Ethics.* 1998 Oct; 24(5): 291–292. 7 refs. BE60249.
*biomedical research; costs and benefits; decision making; *futility; hospitals; *investigators; mortality; patient discharge; *patient participation; *public participation; quality of life; *research design; resource allocation; resuscitation; *therapeutic research; time factors; *treatment outcome; *values; Great Britain

Horton, Richard. Publication and promotion: a fair reward. *Lancet.* 1998 Sep 12; 352(9131): 892. 2 refs. BE60137.
*authorship; biomedical research; editorial policies

Horton, Richard. Scientific misconduct: exaggerated fear but still real and requiring a proportionate response. *Lancet.* 1999 Jul 3; 354(9172): 7–8. 15 refs. BE62408.
attitudes; biomedical research; *due process; editorial policies; government regulation; international aspects; investigators; physician patient relationship; professional autonomy; *regulation; review committees; *scientific misconduct; trust; Europe; Scandinavia; United States

Hsu, John; Trevett, Kenneth P.; Campbell, Eric G., et al. Corporate gifts to academic researchers. [Letters and responses]. *JAMA.* 1998 Sep 9; 280(10): 883–884. 4 refs. BE61077.
*biomedical research; conflict of interest; contracts; *faculty; *financial support; *gifts; *industry; institutional policies; *investigators; property rights; *universities; *United States

International Committee of Medical Journal Editors. Statement on project-specific industry support for research. [Editorial]. *Canadian Medical Association Journal.* 1998 Mar 10; 158(5): 615–616. Statement adopted 7 May 1997. BE60586.
*biomedical research; *conflict of interest; disclosure; *editorial policies; *financial support; *industry; *investigators; *International Committee of Medical Journal Editors

Jones, Anne Hudson. Publication and promotion: is the system really broken? *Lancet.* 1998 Sep 12; 352(9131): 894–895. 10 refs. BE60140.
*authorship; *biomedical research; editorial policies; guidelines; international aspects; International Committee of Medical Journal Editors

Kaiser, Jocelyn. Baylor saga comes to an end. [News]. *Science.* 1999 Feb 19; 283(5405): 1091. BE60951.
biomedical research; federal government; *fraud; *government regulation; investigators; *legal aspects; legal liability; medical schools; *scientific misconduct; self regulation; universities; *Angelides, Kimon; Association of American Medical Colleges; *Baylor College of Medicine; *Department of Health and Human Services; Office of Research Integrity; *United States

Kaiser, Jocelyn. ORI report tracks gun-shy feds. [News]. *Science.* 1999 May 7; 284(5416): 901. BE61772.
biomedical research; faculty; federal government; *government regulation; punishment; *scientific misconduct; *self regulation; statistics; *universities; whistleblowing; *Office of Research Integrity; Public Health Service; *United States

Kaiser, Jocelyn. Tulane inquiry clears lead researcher. [News]. *Science.* 1999 Jun 18; 284(5422): 1905. BE61774.
biomedical research; *fraud; investigators; *scientific misconduct; universities; *Arnold, Steven; *McLachlan, John; *Tulane University Medical Center

Kern, David G.; Kern, Robin K.; Durand, Kate T.H., et al. Secrecy in science: the flock worker's lung investigation. [Letter and response]. *Annals of Internal Medicine.* 1999 Apr 6; 130(7): 616. 6 refs. BE62562.
biomedical research; confidentiality; contracts; *disclosure; editorial policies; employment; *epidemiology; *health hazards; hospitals; *industry; investigators; *occupational exposure; physicians; toxicity; universities; *lung diseases

Kevles, Daniel J. Star chambers will result in injustice. [Letter]. *Nature.* 1998 Sep 24; 395(6700): 317. BE61109.
*biomedical research; due process; federal government; fraud; *government regulation; *investigators; *legal rights; *scientific misconduct; Baltimore, David; *Imanishi-Kari, Thereza; *Office of Research Integrity; *United States

Kevles, Daniel J. The Baltimore Case: A Trial of Politics, Science, and Character. New York, NY: Norton; 1998. 509 p. 1,054 fn. ISBN 0–393–04103–4. BE60016.
*biomedical research; *due process; famous persons; federal government; *fraud; government regulation; historical aspects; interprofessional relations; *investigators; *politics; science; *scientific misconduct; universities; whistleblowing; *Baltimore, David; Cell; *Dingell, John; Feder, Ned; Hadley, Suzanne; *Imanishi-Kari, Thereza; Massachusetts Institute of Technology; National Institutes of Health; *O'Toole, Margot; Office of Research Integrity; Office of Scientific Integrity; Rockefeller University; Stewart, Walter; Twentieth Century; U.S. Congress; *United States

Kirsch, Michael; Rothschild, Bruce M.; Ridzon, Renée, et al. Patient consent for publication. [Letters and responses]. *JAMA.* 1997 Dec 24–31; 278(24): 2139–2141. 9 refs. BE60135.
authorship; autonomy; *confidentiality; *disclosure; *editorial policies; *epidemiology; guidelines; health services research; human experimentation; *information dissemination; *informed consent; justice; obligations to society; patient participation; *patients; *privacy; professional organizations; public health; *research subjects; International Committee of Medical Journal Editors

Knowles, Lori P. Property, progeny, and patents.

BE = bioethics accession number   fn. = footnotes   refs. = references

[Symposium: human primordial stem cells]. *Hastings Center Report.* 1999 Mar–Apr; 29(2): 38–40. 2 refs. BE61663.
> aborted fetuses; advisory committees; altruism; beginning of life; *biomedical research; body parts and fluids; cryopreservation; decision making; donors; economics; embryo disposition; *embryo research; embryos; fetal tissue donation; guidelines; *industry; informed consent; institutional ethics; investigators; justice; legal aspects; organizational policies; *patents; personhood; *property rights; regulation; risks and benefits; *stem cells; tissue donation; embryo donation; Geron Corp.; Geron Ethics Advisory Board; United States

Kodish, Eric; Murray, Thomas; Whitehouse, Peter. Conflict of interest in university–industry research relationships: realities, politics, and values. *Academic Medicine.* 1996 Dec; 71(12): 1287–1290. 7 refs. BE61377.
> *biomedical research; *conflict of interest; faculty; *financial support; *industry; information dissemination; institutional policies; *investigators; public policy; *science; self regulation; trust; *universities; values; research ethics

Koepp, Robert; Miles, Stephen H.; Qizilbash, Nawab, et al. Meta–analysis of tacrine for Alzheimer disease: the influence of industry sponsors. [Letter and response]. *JAMA.* 1999 Jun 23–30; 281(24): 2287–2288. 7 refs. BE62210.
> *biomedical research; *conflict of interest; *dementia; *drug industry; *drugs; *financial support; human experimentation; *investigators; patient care; *research design; *therapeutic research; treatment outcome; *metaanalysis; Great Britain; *tacrine; United States

Kondro, Wayne. Canadian panel calls for review of drug–trial confidentiality agreements. [News]. *Lancet.* 1998 Dec 19–26; 352(9145): 1996. BE60958.
> *biomedical research; confidentiality; *conflict of interest; *contracts; *disclosure; *drug industry; *drugs; *financial support; *hospitals; *human experimentation; *investigators; thalassemia; toxicity; *Apotex; *Canada; *deferiprone; *Hospital for Sick Children (Toronto); *Olivieri, Nancy

Larkin, Marilynn. Whose article is it anyway? *Lancet.* 1999 Jul 10; 354(9173): 136. BE62411.
> *authorship; *biomedical research; conflict of interest; deception; disclosure; *drug industry; *editorial policies; *financial support; information dissemination; investigators; peer review; *scientific misconduct

Loehle, Craig. Untainted by money. *New Scientist.* 1997 Aug 16; 155(2095): 44. BE59714.
> *biomedical research; conflict of interest; drug industry; drugs; *financial support; human experimentation; incentives; investigators; *patents; peer review

Luna, Florencia. Corruption and research. *Bioethics.* 1999 Jul; 13(3–4): 262–271. 19 fn. BE61877.
> *biomedical research; developing countries; ethical relativism; *human experimentation; incentives; *international aspects; investigators; legal aspects; *misconduct; politics; regulation; remuneration; research design; research ethics committees; *scientific misconduct; selection of subjects; socioeconomic factors; bribes; *multicenter studies

Last year there was a heated debate regarding clinical trials with AZT carried out in developing countries. AIDS vaccine trials also posed various dilemmas and ethical problems. In this paper I will consider the possibility of corruption in bioethics, and international multi–centre research will be taken as an example. International clinical trials will be seen from another perspective. I will try to show that the possibility of systemic corruption should be considered when designing an international multi–centre research trial which may involve countries in very different situations regarding corruption. I will analyze three different approaches to this problem and suggest some strategies regarding their capacity to exclude the possibility of corruption.

Lundberg, George D. Publication and promotion: writing is all. *Lancet.* 1998 Sep 12; 352(9131): 898. 5 refs. BE60144.
> *authorship; *biomedical research; *editorial policies; guidelines; *international aspects; International Committee of Medical Journal Editors; JAMA

Macklin, Ruth. Ethics, epidemiology, and law: the case of silicone breast implants. *American Journal of Public Health.* 1999 Apr; 89(4): 487–489. 10 refs. BE61384.
> biomedical research; compensation; cosmetic surgery; *epidemiology; expert testimony; *females; *industry; *injuries; justice; *legal liability; literature; *medical devices; review committees; risk; science; technical expertise; *uncertainty; *breast implants; United States

Marshall, Eliot. Investigations on trial in a Texas court. [News]. *Science.* 1999 Feb 12; 283(5404): 913–914. BE61131.
> biomedical research; due process; federal government; fraud; government regulation; investigators; *legal aspects; *scientific misconduct; self regulation; universities; *Angelides, Kimon; Baylor College of Medicine; Department of Health and Human Services; Office of Research Integrity; Texas; United States

Martensen, Robert. If only it were so: medical physics, U.S. human radiation experiments, and the *Final Report* of the President's Advisory Committee (ACHRE). *Medical Humanities Review.* 1997 Fall; 11(2): 21–36. 26 fn. Commented on by R. Faden and Dan Guttman, p. 37–43. BE59808.
> *advisory committees; *biomedical research; cancer; conflict of interest; disclosure; drug industry; entrepreneurship; ethical analysis; ethical review; ethicist's role; *evaluation; *federal government; *financial support; government financing; government regulation; guidelines; *historical aspects; *human experimentation; informed consent; investigators; justice; motivation; physicians; policy analysis; politics; *public policy; *radiation; research subjects; resource allocation; science; *scientific misconduct; standards; trust; universities; *Advisory Committee on Human Radiation Experiments; Department of Energy; *Twentieth Century; *United States; University of California, Berkeley

Meguid, Michael M. Editors' responsibility in defeating fraud. [Letter]. *Nature.* 1999 May 6; 399(6731): 13. BE62566.
> biomedical research; *disclosure; *editorial policies; fraud; moral obligations; organizational policies; *scientific misconduct; Nutrition

Miller, Linda J.; Bloom, Floyd E. Publishing controversial research. [Editorial]. *Science.* 1998 Nov 6; 282(5391): 1045. BE59537.
> *biomedical research; *editorial policies; *embryo research; federal government; financial support; government regulation; guidelines; *information dissemination; international aspects; peer review; private sector; public policy; *stem cells; cell lines; *Science; United States

Morris, Lynn; Martin, Desmond J.; Quinn, Thomas C., et al. The importance of doing HIV research in developing countries. *Nature Medicine.* 1998 Nov; 4(11): 1228–1229. 20 refs. BE62159.
> *AIDS; *biomedical research; *costs and benefits;

BE = bioethics accession number   fn. = footnotes   refs. = references

*developing countries; drugs; economics; *HIV seropositivity; *human experimentation; newborns; patient care; pregnant women; preventive medicine; *resource allocation; *risks and benefits; sexually transmitted diseases; *Africa; AZT

Nadis, Steve. US concern grows over secrecy clauses. [News]. *Nature.* 1999 Apr 1; 398(6726): 359. BE60845.
*biomedical research; confidentiality; *contracts; *disclosure; employment; faculty; *financial support; *industry; *information dissemination; institutional policies; *investigators; occupational exposure; *universities; whistleblowing; lung diseases; Brown University School of Medicine; *Kern, David; United States

Nathan, D.G.; Weatherall, D.J. Academia and industry: lessons from the unfortunate events in Toronto. *Lancet.* 1999 Mar 6; 353(9155): 771–772. 9 refs. BE61219.
*administrators; *biomedical research; *conflict of interest; developing countries; *disclosure; *drug industry; *drugs; *financial support; *hospitals; *human experimentation; *information dissemination; institutional policies; *investigators; minors; regulation; review committees; *thalassemia; therapeutic research; *toxicity; *universities; whistleblowing; *Apotex; *Canada; *deferiprone; *Hospital for Sick Children (Toronto); *Olivieri, Nancy; University of Toronto

Nelkin, Dorothy; Andrews, Lori. Homo economicus: commercialization of body tissue in the age of biotechnology. *Hastings Center Report.* 1998 Sep–Oct; 28(5): 30–39. 64 fn. BE59552.
advertising; *biomedical research; blood donation; *body parts and fluids; cadavers; *commodification; conflict of interest; *cord blood; dehumanization; DNA data banks; DNA sequences; *economics; embryos; entrepreneurship; eugenics; financial support; gene therapy; genes; genetic diversity; *genetic materials; *genetic research; historical aspects; *human body; incentives; *industry; informed consent; international aspects; investigators; minority groups; misconduct; organ donation; *patents; physicians; population genetics; *property rights; public policy; social discrimination; stem cells; *tissue banks; *tissue donation; trends; trust; universities; vulnerable populations; cell lines; Human Genome Diversity Project; Moore v. Regents of the University of California; United States
The human body is becoming hot property, a resource to be "mined," "harvested," patented, and traded commercially for profit as well as scientific and therapeutic advances. Under the new entrepreneurial approach to the body old tensions take on new dimensions -- about consent, the fair distribution of tissues and products developed from them, the individual and cultural values represented by the body, and public policy governing the use of organs and tissues.

Nelkin, Dorothy. Publication and promotion: the performance of science. *Lancet.* 1998 Sep 12; 352(9131): 893. BE60138.
*authorship; *biomedical research; *economics; *editorial policies; entrepreneurship; *investigators

Northridge, Mary. Annotation: new rules for authorship in the Journal: your contributions are recognized -- and published! [Editorial]. *American Journal of Public Health.* 1998 May; 88(5): 733–734. 13 refs. BE60180.
*authorship; biomedical research; *editorial policies; guidelines; *American Journal of Public Health

Nylenna, Magne; Andersen, Daniel; Dahlquist, Gisela, et al.; National Committees on Scientific Dishonesty in the Nordic Countries. Handling of scientific dishonesty in the Nordic countries. *Lancet.* 1999 Jul 3; 354(9172): 57–61. 23 refs. BE62410.

authorship; biomedical research; committee membership; comparative studies; drug industry; international aspects; investigators; misconduct; peer review; public policy; *regulation; *review committees; *scientific misconduct; statistics; publishing; *Denmark; *Finland; *Norway; *Scandinavia; *Sweden
Despite a widely recognised need, most countries still have no coherent system to deal with scientific misconduct. Committees have been established by the national medical research councils in Denmark (1992), Norway (1994), and Sweden (1997), and by the Ministry of Education in Finland (1994), to deal with scientific misconduct -- i.e., to initiate preventive measures, to investigate alleged cases, or both. Each committee includes both scientifically and legally qualified members. The employing institutions are responsible for possible sanctions or punishments. So far, 47 cases have been accepted for investigation, the majority (25) being Danish. Disputed authorship was the most frequent reason for investigation. Junior researchers made complaints in only three of the investigated cases. Investigations have been completed in 37 cases; in nine cases, dishonesty was revealed -- two of them were related to the same researchers. Cooperation between the four Nordic committees has shown close agreement on specific issues and cases, despite minor differences in definitions, organisation, and procedures.

Paneth, Nigel. Separating authorship responsibility and authorship credit: a proposal for biomedical journals. *American Journal of Public Health.* 1998 May; 88(5): 824–826. 6 refs. BE60181.
*authorship; biomedical research; *editorial policies; forms; guidelines

Pownall, Mark. Falsifying data is main problem in US research fraud review. [News]. *BMJ (British Medical Journal).* 1999 May 1; 318(7192): 1164. BE62422.
biomedical research; faculty; federal government; fraud; government financing; government regulation; *investigators; *scientific misconduct; statistics; whistleblowing; Office of Research Integrity; Public Health Service; Scientific Misconduct Investigations 1993–1997 (ORI); United States

Pritchard, Michael S. Conflicts of interest: conceptual and normative issues. *Academic Medicine.* 1996 Dec; 71(12): 1305–1313. 13 refs. BE61380.
*biomedical research; *conflict of interest; disclosure; federal government; *financial support; government financing; government regulation; guidelines; *industry; institutional ethics; investigators; lawyers; professional ethics; professional role; *public policy; self regulation; terminology; trust; *universities; business ethics; National Science Foundation; Public Health Service; United States

Resnik, David. Social epistemology and the ethics of research. *Studies in History and Philosophy of Science.* 1996 Dec; 27(4): 565–586. 39 fn. BE60462.
authorship; biomedical research; codes of ethics; deception; fraud; freedom; goals; information dissemination; interprofessional relations; investigators; moral obligations; moral policy; *philosophy; *professional ethics; *science; scientific misconduct; standards; values; knowledge; *research ethics

Resnik, David B. The Ethics of Science: An Introduction. New York, NY: Routledge; 1998. 221 p. (Philosophical issues in science). Bibliography: 206–216. ISBN 0-415-16698-5. BE61844.
animal experimentation; authorship; *biomedical research; case studies; conflict of interest; ecology; economics; education; ethical theory; expert testimony; faculty; fraud;

BE = bioethics accession number   fn. = footnotes   refs. = references

goals; government financing; human experimentation; industry; information dissemination; interprofessional relations; *investigators; mass media; obligations to society; patents; peer review; *professional ethics; property rights; *science; *scientific misconduct; self regulation; standards; students; values; whistleblowing; publishing; *research ethics

Rule, James T.; Shamoo, Adil E. Ethical issues in research relationships between universities and industry. *Accountability in Research.* 1997; 5(4): 239–249. 21 refs. Paper presented at the symposium, "Ethical Issues in Research Relationships between Universities and Industry," held in Baltimore, MD, 3–4 Nov 1995. BE60421.
*biomedical research; *conflict of interest; disclosure; faculty; *financial support; guidelines; *industry; investigators; property rights; risks and benefits; scientific misconduct; students; *universities; United States

Saegusa, Asako. Private deal puts Japanese researcher in hot water. [News]. *Nature.* 1998 Nov 19; 396(6708): 205. BE59643.
*biomedical research; *conflict of interest; *drug industry; *financial support; *investigators; legal aspects; *scientific misconduct; *universities; *Hidaka, Hiroyoshi; *Japan; Nagoya University; *Otsuka Pharmaceutical Co.

Schmitt, Roland W. Conflict or synergy: university–industry research relations. *Accountability in Research.* 1997; 5(4): 251–254. Paper presented at the symposium, "Ethical Issues in Research Relationships between Universities and Industry," held in Baltimore, MD, 3–4 Nov 1995. BE60422.
*biomedical research; *conflict of interest; financial support; *industry; investigators; risks and benefits; *universities

Shanner, Laura. Abortion, Chernobyl, and unanswered genetic questions. *In:* Donchin, Anne; Purdy, Laura M., eds. Embodying Bioethics: Recent Feminist Advances. Lanham, MD: Rowman and Littlefield; 1999: 85–102. 18 refs. 1 fn. ISBN 0-8476-8924-7. BE61016.
childbirth; *decision making; *epidemiology; females; feminist ethics; fetuses; *genetic disorders; genetic screening; *health hazards; international aspects; methods; morbidity; nuclear energy; politics; pregnant women; prenatal diagnosis; psychological stress; public health; *radiation; *reproduction; research design; selective abortion; *social impact; socioeconomic factors; *uncertainty; *Chernobyl; Europe; Ukraine

Sherwood, Thomas; Peters, Keith. Publication and promotion: the value of discrimination. *Lancet.* 1998 Sep 12; 352(9131): 896–897. 7 refs. BE60142.
*authorship; *biomedical research; *editorial policies; investigators

Shuchman, Miriam. Independent review adds to controversy at Sick Kids. *Canadian Medical Association Journal.* 1999 Feb 9; 160(3): 386–388. BE62307.
administrators; *biomedical research; *conflict of interest; contracts; *disclosure; *drug industry; *drugs; *financial support; *hospitals; *human experimentation; institutional policies; *investigators; legal liability; minors; misconduct; review committees; thalassemia; therapeutic research; *toxicity; whistleblowing; *Apotex; *Canada; *deferiprone; *Hospital for Sick Children (Toronto); Naimark, Arnold; *Olivieri, Nancy

Silberner, Joanne. Federal science policy: changing battle lines, new fronts. *Hastings Center Report.* 1999 Jul–Aug; 29(4): 6. BE62462.
advisory committees; *biomedical research; embryo research; *federal government; government financing; government regulation; information dissemination;

psychoactive drugs; *public policy; *science; stem cells; marijuana; National Bioethics Advisory Commission; National Institutes of Health; U.S. Congress; *United States

Silversides, Ann. Private sector becoming the key to research funding in Canada. *Canadian Medical Association Journal.* 1998 Aug 25; 159(4): 397–398. BE61128.
*biomedical research; conflict of interest; *drug industry; editorial policies; *financial support; human experimentation; investigators; patents; *private sector; public policy; public sector; statistics; universities; *Canada

Skolnick, Andrew A. Drug firm suit fails to halt publication of Canadian Health Technology Report. [News]. *JAMA.* 1998 Aug 26; 280(8): 683–684. BE59690.
*biomedical research; *drug industry; *drugs; economics; *legal aspects; *technology assessment; *Bristol–Myers Squibb Canada; Canada; *Canadian Coordinating Office of Health Technology Assessment

Sly, R. Michael. Ethical scientific writing and responsible medical practice. *Annals of Allergy, Asthma, and Immunology.* 1997 Dec; 79(6): 489–494. 42 refs. Presented as the Bela Schick Lecture at the annual meeting of the American College of Allergy, Asthma, and Immunology, 11 Nov 1997. BE59528.
authorship; *biomedical research; conflict of interest; continuing education; drug industry; editorial policies; guidelines; investigators; medical education; peer review; physicians; professional competence; property rights; *scientific misconduct; plagiarism

Spurgeon, David. Canadian case questions funding. [News]. *BMJ (British Medical Journal).* 1999 Jan 9; 318(7176): 77. BE60842.
*biomedical research; confidentiality; conflict of interest; contracts; disclosure; *drug industry; *drugs; *financial support; *hospitals; *human experimentation; institutional policies; *investigators; legal aspects; regulation; therapeutic research; *toxicity; *whistleblowing; *Apotex; *Canada; deferiprone; *Hospital for Sick Children (Toronto); Medical Research Council of Canada; *Olivieri, Nancy

Spurgeon, David. Canadian whistleblower row prompts broader code of conduct. [News]. *Nature.* 1998 Dec 24–31; 396(6713): 715. BE59536.
*biomedical research; conflict of interest; disclosure; *drug industry; *drugs; *financial support; guidelines; *human experimentation; *investigators; toxicity; whistleblowing; Apotex; *Canada; Hospital for Sick Children (Toronto); *Medical Research Council of Canada; *Olivieri, Nancy

Stolberg, Sheryl Gay. New rules will force doctors to disclose ties to drug industry. [News]. *New York Times.* 1998 Feb 3: A12. BE59669.
*biomedical research; *conflict of interest; *disclosure; *drug industry; *drugs; federal government; financial support; *government regulation; *incentives; *investigators; *mandatory reporting; medical devices; *physicians; *therapeutic research; *Food and Drug Administration; United States

Svatos, Michele. Biotechnology and the utilitarian argument for patents. *In:* Paul, Ellen Frankel; Miller, Fred D.; Paul, Jeffrey, eds. Scientific Innovation, Philosophy, and Public Policy. New York, NY: Cambridge University Press; 1996: 113–144. 84 fn. ISBN 0-521-58994-0. BE62745.
alternatives; *biomedical research; *biomedical technologies; developing countries; drugs; *economics; genetic intervention; government financing; incentives; industry; information dissemination; international aspects; investigators; legal aspects; *patents; property rights; *public

---

policy; recombinant DNA research; resource allocation; *risks and benefits; social impact; transgenic organisms; universities; *utilitarianism; *agriculture; *biotechnology; *United States

Tarnow, Eugene. When extra authors get in on the act. [Letter]. *Nature.* 1999 Apr 22; 398(6729): 657. 2 refs. BE61792.
  attitudes; *authorship; biomedical research; *faculty; interprofessional relations; *investigators; science; *scientific misconduct; standards; Europe; United States

Topol, Eric J. Publication and promotion: drafter and draftees. *Lancet.* 1998 Sep 12; 352(9131): 897–898. 6 refs. BE60143.
  *authorship; biomedical research; disclosure; *editorial policies; human experimentation; investigators; multicenter studies

Tuffs, Annette. Max–Planck Society investigates misconduct. [News]. *BMJ (British Medical Journal).* 1999 Jul 31; 319(7205): 274. BE62527.
  growth disorders; hormones; industry; investigators; legal aspects; patents; property rights; research institutes; *scientific misconduct; universities; Genentech; Germany; Max Planck Society; Nature; *Seeburg, Peter; University of California

Varmus, Harold. Evaluating the burden of disease and spending the research dollars of the National Institutes of Health. [Editorial]. *New England Journal of Medicine.* 1999 Jun 17; 340(24): 1914–1915. 9 refs. BE62033.
  *biomedical research; decision making; *disease; federal government; financial support; *government financing; industry; political activity; public participation; *resource allocation; trends; *disability adjusted life years; *National Institutes of Health; *United States

Wadman, Meredith. Dilemma for journals over tobacco cash. [News]. *Nature.* 1998 Aug 13; 394(6694): 609. BE59187.
  biomedical research; cancer; *conflict of interest; *editorial policies; *financial support; *health hazards; *industry; *investigators; scientific misconduct; *smoking; Environmental Protection Agency; JAMA; Journal of the National Cancer Institute; Lancet; Pediatrics; *Tobacco Institute; United States

Wadman, Meredith. NIH 'should help sharing of research tools.' [News]. *Nature.* 1998 Jun 11; 393(6685): 505. BE59385.
  advisory committees; *biomedical research; biomedical technologies; *federal government; government financing; guidelines; *industry; *information dissemination; investigators; patents; *property rights; *public policy; *universities; technology transfer; *National Institutes of Health; *United States

Weed, Douglas L. Preventing scientific misconduct. *American Journal of Public Health.* 1998 Jan; 88(1): 125–129. 50 refs. BE62601.
  biomedical research; due process; education; empirical research; *investigators; motivation; *professional ethics; regulation; science; *scientific misconduct; statistics; terminology; virtues; whistleblowing

Wenger, Neil S.; Korenman, Stanley G.; Berk, Richard, et al. The ethics of scientific research: an analysis of focus groups of scientists and institutional representatives. *Journal of Investigative Medicine.* 1997 Aug; 45(6): 371–380. 20 refs. BE60389.
  accountability; *administrators; *attitudes; authorship; biomedical research; comparative studies; conflict of interest; education; financial support; fraud; information

dissemination; interprofessional relations; *investigators; *professional ethics; punishment; *science; *scientific misconduct; self regulation; survey; universities; values; whistleblowing; *research ethics; United States

Wolpert, Lewis. Is science dangerous? *Nature.* 1999 Mar 25; 398(6725): 281–282. 4 refs. BE61395.
  behavioral genetics; cloning; conflict of interest; decision making; disclosure; employment; eugenics; food; *genetic intervention; *genetic research; *investigators; moral obligations; obligations to society; prenatal diagnosis; public participation; *risks and benefits; *science; transgenic organisms; whistleblowing; research ethics; transgenic plants

Wright, David E. The federal research misconduct regulations as viewed from the research universities. *Centennial Review.* 1994 Spring; 38(2): 249–272. 57 fn. BE59403.
  biomedical research; case studies; due process; federal government; *government regulation; investigators; science; *scientific misconduct; *universities; Department of Health and Human Services; Office of Research Integrity; *United States

Yank, Veronica; Rennie, Drummond. Disclosure of researcher contributions: a study of original research articles in *The Lancet. Annals of Internal Medicine.* 1999 Apr 20; 130(8): 661–670. 23 refs. BE61601.
  *authorship; *biomedical research; *disclosure; *editorial policies; evaluation studies; guideline adherence; *guidelines; investigators; BMJ (British Medical Journal); International Committee of Medical Journal Editors; *Lancet
  BACKGROUND: Authorship disputes and abuses have increased in recent years. In response to a proposal that researcher contributions be specified for readers, The Lancet began disclosing such contributions at the end of original articles. OBJECTIVE: To analyze the descriptions researchers use for their contributions and to determine how the order of names on the byline corresponds to these contributions, whether persons listed on the byline fulfill a lenient version of the criteria for authorship specified by the International Committee of Medical Journal Editors (the Vancouver Group), and whether the contributions of persons listed as contributors overlap with the contributions of those who are acknowledged. DESIGN: Descriptive study. MEASUREMENTS: A taxonomy of researchers' contributions was developed and applied to researchers' self-reported contributions to original research articles published in The Lancet from July to December 1997. RESULTS: Contributors lists occupied little page space (mean, 2.5 cm of column length). Placement on the byline did not indicate the specific category of task performed, although the first-contributor position corresponded to a significantly greater number of contributions (mean numbers of contributions: first-contributor position, 3.23; second-contributor position, 2.51; third-contributor position, 2.20; and fourth-contributor position, 2.51) (P less than 0.01). Forty-four percent of contributors on the byline did not fulfill a lenient version of the Vancouver Group's criteria for authorship. Sixty percent of the most common categories of activities described on contributors lists overlapped with those on acknowledgements lists. CONCLUSIONS: Publication of lists that specify contributions to research articles is feasible and seems to impart important information. The criteria for authorship outlined by the Vancouver Group do not seem to be congruent with the self-identified contributions of researchers.

Ziman, John M. Why must scientists become more

---

ethically sensitive than they used to be? *Science*. 1998 Dec 4; 282(5395): 1813–1814. 1 fn. BE59556.
  biomedical research; financial support; *industry; *investigators; *professional ethics; *science; *universities

A duty to publish. [Editorial]. *Nature Medicine*. 1998 Oct; 4(10): 1089. BE61526.
  administrators; *biomedical research; conflict of interest; contracts; *drug industry; drugs; *financial support; hospitals; human experimentation; *information dissemination; *institutional policies; investigators; misconduct; toxicity; universities; publication bias; *publishing; Apotex; Boots Pharmaceuticals, Ltd.; deferiprone; *Dong, Betty; Hospital for Sick Children (Toronto); *Olivieri, Nancy; Synthroid; University of California, San Francisco

NIH peer review: time for some changes. [Editorial]. *Nature Biotechnology*. 1998 May; 16(5): 395. BE62362.
  *biomedical research; *conflict of interest; federal government; financial support; *government financing; guidelines; industry; *investigators; *peer review; *National Institutes of Health; United States

Policy on papers' contributors. [Editorial]. *Nature*. 1999 Jun 3; 399(6735): 393. BE61762.
  *authorship; biomedical research; *editorial policies; *science; *scientific misconduct; *Nature

State funding and data disclosure. [Editorial]. *Lancet*. 1999 Mar 27; 353(9158): 1027. BE61565.
  *biomedical research; *disclosure; ecology; epidemiology; federal government; government financing; *government regulation; industry; information dissemination; investigators; *legislation; property rights; public policy; records; *science; universities; *publishing; *Freedom of Information Act; *United States

Surviving misconduct is one thing, accountability is another. [Editorial]. *Nature*. 1998 Oct 22; 395(6704): 727. BE59585.
  *accountability; *biomedical research; government financing; international aspects; investigators; records; *research institutes; *scientific misconduct; *self regulation; Europe

Taking stock of scientific fraud. [Editorial]. *Nature Biotechnology*. 1998 May; 16(5): 395. BE62318.
  *biomedical research; *conflict of interest; *drug industry; *economics; *fraud; *investigators; medical schools; universities; United States

The Farmington Consensus. *Alcohol and Alcoholism*. 1998 Jan–Feb; 33(1): 6–8. BE60681.
  advertising; alcohol abuse; *authorship; *biomedical research; conflict of interest; disclosure; drug abuse; *editorial policies; financial support; industry; investigators; *peer review; scientific misconduct

Where next on misconduct? [Editorial]. *Nature*. 1999 Mar 4; 398(6722): 1. BE60983.
  biomedical research; investigators; regulation; *scientific misconduct; whistleblowing; United States

WHO steps closer to its responsibilities. [Editorial]. *Nature*. 1999 Mar 18; 398(6724): 175. BE61960.
  *bioethical issues; *biomedical research; cloning; genetic research; *guidelines; *international aspects; *World Health Organization

BIOMEDICAL TECHNOLOGIES

See also HEALTH CARE, ORGAN AND TISSUE TRANSPLANTATION, REPRODUCTIVE

TECHNOLOGIES
See also under
RESOURCE ALLOCATION/BIOMEDICAL TECHNOLOGIES

Annas, George J. Burden of proof: judging science and protecting public health in (and out of) the courtroom. *American Journal of Public Health*. 1999 Apr; 89(4): 490–493. 4 refs. BE61385.
  compensation; cosmetic surgery; economics; *epidemiology; expert testimony; federal government; *females; government regulation; *industry; *injuries; judicial action; *legal liability; literature; *medical devices; public health; review committees; science; *standards; technical expertise; torts; women's health; *breast implants; *Dow Corning; United States

Arnow, Kathryn Smul. Medical technology transfer and physician–patient conversation. *International Journal of Technology Management*. 1996; 11(1–2): 70–88. 48 fn. BE59407.
  *alternatives; autonomy; beneficence; *biomedical technologies; caring; *chronically ill; *communication; compassion; comprehension; *decision making; diagnosis; *disclosure; drugs; *emotions; *empathy; informed consent; malpractice; *medical devices; metaphor; narrative ethics; *patient care; *patient compliance; *patient participation; patients; *physician patient relationship; physicians; prognosis; psychological stress; psychology; quality of life; *rehabilitation; *risks and benefits; self induced illness; *smoking; suffering; technical expertise; therapeutic research; treatment outcome; *trust; truth disclosure; *uncertainty; empowerment; *lung diseases; sick role; *technology transfer

Barnett, Michael L. The assessment of new biotechnologies: would the world be different if Napoleon had received recombinant growth hormone? [Editorial]. *Journal of Dental Research*. 1995 Dec; 74(12): 1820–1821. 6 refs. BE60592.
  *biomedical technologies; dentistry; genetic intervention; growth disorders; hormones; psychoactive drugs; risks and benefits; technology assessment; treatment outcome

Bayer, Ronald. Science, justice, and breast implants. [Editorial]. *American Journal of Public Health*. 1999 Apr; 89(4): 483. 5 refs. BE61383.
  compensation; cosmetic surgery; *epidemiology; *females; *industry; injuries; judicial action; justice; *legal liability; *medical devices; science; *uncertainty; women's health; *breast implants; United States

Blank, Robert H. Brain Policy: How the New Neuroscience Will Change Our Lives and Our Politics. Washington, DC: Georgetown University Press; 1999. 199 p. Bibliography: p.179–191. ISBN 0-87840-712-X. BE62619.
  aggression; autonomy; behavioral genetics; *biomedical research; *biomedical technologies; *brain; brain death; *brain pathology; central nervous system diseases; competence; decision making; electrical stimulation of the brain; enhancement technologies; eugenics; fetal tissue donation; gene therapy; genetic intervention; genetic research; health hazards; informed consent; legal aspects; mentally ill; patient care; pregnant women; prenatal injuries; psychoactive drugs; psychosurgery; public participation; public policy; recall; resource allocation; risks and benefits; self concept; sexuality; social impact; stigmatization; technology assessment; therapeutic research; tissue transplantation; treatment refusal; violence; *neurosciences; United States

Bordo, Susan. *Braveheart*, *Babe*, and the contemporary body. *In:* Parens, Erik, ed. Enhancing Human Traits:

BE = bioethics accession number   fn. = footnotes   refs. = references

Ethical and Social Implications. Washington, DC: Georgetown University Press; 1998: 189–221. 16 fn. ISBN 0-87840-703-0. BE59753.

advertising; age factors; autonomy; biomedical technologies; capitalism; coercion; communication; *cosmetic surgery; *enhancement technologies; females; *feminist ethics; freedom; *health; *human body; males; *mass media; *normality; pain; physician's role; *self concept; *values; beauty; empowerment; *self care; United States

Brock, Dan W. Enhancements of human function: some distinctions for policymakers. In: Parens, Erik, ed. Enhancing Human Traits: Ethical and Social Implications. Washington, DC: Georgetown University Press; 1998: 48–69. 14 fn. ISBN 0-87840-703-0. BE59745.

autonomy; *biomedical technologies; coercion; cosmetic surgery; disabled; disease; education; *enhancement technologies; freedom; genetic enhancement; government regulation; growth disorders; health; health care; health insurance reimbursement; hormones; immunization; incentives; justice; mandatory programs; moral policy; *normality; parents; paternalism; psychoactive drugs; *public policy; resource allocation; risks and benefits; sports medicine; stigmatization; uncertainty; voluntary programs

Clark, Reese H. The safe introduction of new technologies into neonatal medicine. Clinics in Perinatology. 1996 Sep; 23(3): 519–527. 28 refs. BE60939.

*biomedical technologies; *evaluation; health personnel; *human experimentation; mortality; *newborns; *patient care; research design; *risks and benefits; technical expertise; *technology assessment; *therapeutic research; treatment outcome; ventilators; extracorporeal membrane oxygenation; multicenter studies

Cole-Turner, Ronald. Do means matter? In: Parens, Erik, ed. Enhancing Human Traits: Ethical and Social Implications. Washington, DC: Georgetown University Press; 1998: 151–161. 4 fn. ISBN 0-87840-703-0. BE59750.

*biomedical technologies; *enhancement technologies; genetic enhancement; *goals; justice; moral policy; psychoactive drugs; self concept; *values

Dresser, Rebecca. Science in the courtroom: a new approach. Hastings Center Report. 1999 May–Jun; 29(3): 26–27. 4 refs. BE61410.

biomedical research; *biomedical technologies; cosmetic surgery; decision making; epidemiology; *evaluation; *expert testimony; federal government; females; industry; injuries; *investigators; lawyers; *legal aspects; legal liability; medical devices; research design; review committees; *risk; *science; technical expertise; uncertainty; *breast implants; judges; United States

European Parliament. Scientific and Technological Options Assessment (STOA) Programme Contractor. Bioethics in Europe. Final Report, July 1992. Luxembourg: European Parliament, Directorate General for Research; 1992 Sep 8. 257 p. Includes references. Pub. No. PE 158.453. BE62499.

advisory committees; attitudes; *bioethical issues; bioethics; biological warfare; *biomedical technologies; *comparative studies; *ecology; embryo research; fetal research; fetal tissue donation; food; gene therapy; *genetic intervention; genetic screening; genome mapping; germ cells; government regulation; hormones; in vitro fertilization; *international aspects; patents; preimplantation diagnosis; prenatal diagnosis; professional organizations; public opinion; *public policy; recombinant DNA research; reproductive technologies; risks and benefits; *social impact; technology assessment; transgenic animals; transgenic organisms; agriculture; *biotechnology; *Denmark; *Europe; European Community; *European Parliament; *France; *Germany;

*Great Britain; *Greece; *Italy; *Spain

Fisher, Elliott S.; Welch, H. Gilbert. Avoiding the unintended consequences of growth in medical care: how might more be worse? JAMA. 1999 Feb 3; 281(5): 446–453. 75 refs. BE60239.

*biomedical technologies; chronically ill; decision making; *diagnosis; disease; drugs; economics; *health care; health care delivery; health services research; iatrogenic disease; mass screening; *medicine; morbidity; mortality; *patient care; prevalence; resource allocation; *risks and benefits; stigmatization; surgery; *technology assessment; treatment outcome; trends; uncertainty; *health services misuse

The United States has experienced dramatic growth in both the technical capabilities and share of resources devoted to medical care. While the benefits of more medical care are widely recognized, the possibility that harm may result from growth has received little attention. Because harm from more medical care is unexpected, findings of harm are discounted or ignored. We suggest that such findings may indicate a more general problem and deserve serious consideration. First, we delineate 2 levels of decision making where more medical care may be introduced: (1) decisions about whether or not to use a discrete diagnostic or therapeutic intervention and (2) decisions about whether to add system capacity, e.g., the decision to purchase another scanner or employ another physician. Second, we explore how more medical care at either level may lead to harm. More diagnosis creates the potential for labeling and detection of pseudodisease -- disease that would never become apparent to patients during their lifetime without testing. More treatment may lead to tampering, interventions to correct random rather than systematic variation, and lower treatment thresholds, where the risks outweigh the potential benefits. Because there are more diagnoses to treat and more treatments to provide, physicians may be more likely to make mistakes and to be distracted from the issues of greatest concern to their patients. Finally, we turn to the fundamental challenge -- reducing the risk of harm from more medical care. We identify 4 ways in which inadequate information and improper reasoning may allow harmful practices to be adopted -- a constrained model of disease, excessive extrapolation, a missing level of analysis, and the assumption that more is better.

Fisher, Ian. Families providing complex medical care, tubes and all. New York Times. 1998 Jun 7: 1, 30. BE60473.

adults; aged; *biomedical technologies; children; *chronically ill; economics; *family members; *home care; managed care programs; psychological stress; risks and benefits; technical expertise; Family and Medical Leave Act; United States

Fox, Daniel M. Comment: epidemiology and the new political economy of medicine. American Journal of Public Health. 1999 Apr; 89(4): 493–496. 19 refs. BE61386.

*accountability; contracts; cosmetic surgery; *economics; *epidemiology; *females; *industry; informed consent; injuries; managed care programs; *medical devices; patient care; physician patient relationship; *physicians; *risk; standards; *breast implants; Dow Corning; United States

Frankford, David M. The treatment/enhancement distinction as an armament in the policy wars. In: Parens, Erik, ed. Enhancing Human Traits: Ethical and Social Implications. Washington, DC: Georgetown University Press; 1998: 70–94. 87 fn. ISBN 0-87840-703-0. BE59746.

BE = bioethics accession number   fn. = footnotes   refs. = references

*biomedical technologies; contracts; *enhancement technologies; evaluation; health care; *health insurance reimbursement; human experimentation; medicine; moral policy; normality; patient care; policy analysis; *public policy; resource allocation; technology assessment; terminology; therapeutic research; utilitarianism; values; *investigational therapies; United States

Garcia, Sandra Anderson. Sociocultural and legal implications of creating and sustaining life through biomedical technology. *Journal of Legal Medicine.* 1996 Dec; 17(4): 469–525. 220 fn. BE61244.
abortion, induced; allowing to die; bioethics; biomedical research; *biomedical technologies; cultural pluralism; decision making; determination of death; disadvantaged; fetal research; futility; genetic counseling; *genetic intervention; genetic screening; genome mapping; intensive care units; international aspects; investigators; justice; law; legal aspects; minority groups; misconduct; newborns; physicians; political activity; prolongation of life; public policy; religion; reproduction; *reproductive technologies; resource allocation; rights; science; selection for treatment; socioeconomic factors; withholding treatment; United States

Haiken, Elizabeth. Venus Envy: A History of Cosmetic Surgery. Baltimore, MD: Johns Hopkins University Press; 1997. 370 p. 461 fn. ISBN 0–8018–5763–5. BE62626.
aged; attitudes; blacks; *cosmetic surgery; famous persons; females; *historical aspects; males; mass media; medical devices; medical specialties; minority groups; motivation; physicians; professional organizations; public opinion; risks and benefits; self concept; socioeconomic factors; stigmatization; artificial implants; beauty; mammaplasty; *Twentieth Century; United States

Hanson, Mark J. The idea of progress and the goals of medicine. *In:* Hanson, Mark J.; Callahan, Daniel, eds. The Goals of Medicine: The Forgotten Issue in Health Care Reform. Washington, DC: Georgetown University Press; 1999: 137–151. 38 fn. ISBN 0–87840–707–3. BE60522.
bioethics; *biomedical technologies; economics; *goals; *medicine; religious ethics; risks and benefits; trends; values

Jacobson, Nora. The socially constructed breast: breast implants and the medical construction of need. *American Journal of Public Health.* 1998 Aug; 88(8): 1254–1261. 81 fn. BE60376.
attitudes; autonomy; breast cancer; *cosmetic surgery; federal government; *females; government regulation; *historical aspects; human experimentation; mass media; *medical devices; physicians; politics; preventive medicine; psychology; public health; rehabilitation; risks and benefits; *sociology of medicine; surgery; *values; women's health; *breast implants; *needs; Food and Drug Administration; Nineteenth Century; *Twentieth Century; United States
When silicone gel breast implants became the subject of a public health controversy in the early 1990s, the most pressing concern was safety. This paper looks at another, less publicized issue: the need for implants. Using a symbolic interactionist approach, the author explores the social construction of the need for implants by tracing the history of the 3 surgical procedures for which implants were used. Stakeholders in this history constructed need as legitimized individual desire, the form of which shifted with changes in the technological and social context.

Juengst, Eric T. What does *enhancement* mean? *In:* Parens, Erik, ed. Enhancing Human Traits: Ethical and Social Implications. Washington, DC: Georgetown University Press; 1998: 29–47. 27 fn. ISBN 0–87840–703–0. BE59744.

*biomedical technologies; disease; *enhancement technologies; genetic enhancement; *goals; *health; *health care; justice; *medicine; *moral policy; *normality; patient care; preventive medicine; psychoactive drugs; public policy; risks and benefits; self concept; terminology; *values; NHGRI–funded publication

Kin, Curtis A. Coming soon to the "genetic supermarket" near you. [Note]. *Stanford Law Review.* 1996 Jul; 48(6): 1573–1604. 159 fn. BE62176.
biomedical technologies; children; drugs; *enhancement technologies; federal government; gene therapy; *genetic enhancement; *government regulation; *growth disorders; *hormones; industry; legal aspects; *normality; recombinant DNA research; risks and benefits; *biotechnology; Food and Drug Administration; *United States

Kolata, Gina. Where marketing and medicine meet. [News]. *New York Times.* 1998 Feb 10: A14. BE59363.
advertising; *conflict of interest; financial support; *gifts; heart diseases; *industry; *medical devices; medical specialties; *physicians; surgery; *cardiology

Krakauer, Eric L. Prescriptions: autonomy, humanism and the purpose of health technology. *Theoretical Medicine and Bioethics.* 1998 Dec; 19(6): 525–545. 27 refs. 11 fn. BE61154.
*autonomy; bioethics; *biomedical technologies; goals; health; *humanism; iatrogenic disease; medicine; moral obligations; personhood; *philosophy; suffering; rationality; Derrida, Jacques; Heidegger, Martin; Illich, Ivan; Kant, Immanuel

Little, Margaret Olivia. Cosmetic surgery, suspect norms, and the ethics of complicity. *In:* Parens, Erik, ed. Enhancing Human Traits: Ethical and Social Implications. Washington, DC: Georgetown University Press; 1998: 162–176. 8 fn. ISBN 0–87840–703–0. BE59751.
advertising; blacks; *cosmetic surgery; enhancement technologies; females; goals; health care; informed consent; justice; *medicine; *moral complicity; *moral policy; motivation; normality; *physicians; social discrimination; suffering; values; beauty

Loff, Bebe; Cordner, Stephen. Aboriginal people trade land claim for dialysis. [News]. *Lancet.* 1998 Oct 31; 352(9138): 1451. BE59640.
*health care delivery; *minority groups; public policy; *renal dialysis; Australia; *Northern Territory

McDonnell, Orla. Ethical and social implications of technology in medicine: new possibilities and new dilemmas. *In:* Cleary, Anne; Treacy, Margaret P., eds. The Sociology of Health and Illness in Ireland. Dublin: University College of Dublin Press; 1997: 69–84. 13 refs. 4 fn. ISBN 1–900621–11–8. BE60509.
*allowing to die; artificial feeding; attitudes to death; autonomy; *biomedical technologies; decision making; determination of death; guidelines; infertility; killing; legal aspects; married persons; *mass media; patient advocacy; persistent vegetative state; physicians; privacy; *prolongation of life; quality of life; *reproductive technologies; *right to die; selection for treatment; self regulation; *social impact; sociology of medicine; *values; withholding treatment; In re a Ward of Court; *Ireland

MacKay, Karen; Moss, Alvin H. To dialyze or not to dialyze: an ethical and evidence-based approach to the patient with acute renal failure in the intensive care unit. *Advances in Renal Replacement Therapy.* 1997 Jul; 4(3): 288–296. 41 refs. BE62516.
case studies; critically ill; *decision making; evidence-based medicine; family members; *intensive care units; *kidney

diseases; mortality; patient care; patients; physicians; *prognosis; quality of life; *renal dialysis; *selection for treatment; time factors; *treatment outcome; withholding treatment

McKenny, Gerald P. Enhancements and the ethical significance of vulnerability. *In:* Parens, Erik, ed. Enhancing Human Traits: Ethical and Social Implications. Washington, DC: Georgetown University Press; 1998: 222–237. 15 fn. ISBN 0-87840-703-0. BE59754.
*biomedical technologies; *enhancement technologies; goals; *health; *human body; medicine; moral obligations; moral policy; normality; *philosophy; postmodernism; self concept; values; virtues; Aristotle; Levinas, Emmanuel; Stoicism

Macklin, Ruth. Ethics, epidemiology, and law: the case of silicone breast implants. *American Journal of Public Health.* 1999 Apr; 89(4): 487–489. 10 refs. BE61384.
biomedical research; compensation; cosmetic surgery; *epidemiology; expert testimony; *females; *industry; *injuries; justice; *legal liability; literature; *medical devices; review committees; risk; science; technical expertise; *uncertainty; *breast implants; United States

Maguire, G.Q.; McGee, Ellen M. Implantable brain chips? Time for debate. *Hastings Center Report.* 1999 Jan–Feb; 29(1): 7–13. 35 fn. BE61630.
autonomy; behavior control; *biomedical technologies; *brain; computer communication networks; *computers; *enhancement technologies; human body; human characteristics; intelligence; justice; *medical devices; mentally disabled; normality; patient care; personhood; physically disabled; recall; rehabilitation; *risks and benefits; self concept; social control; social impact; socioeconomic factors; cognitive enhancement; cybernetics
We have long used mechanical devices to compensate for physical disability. Soon, however, it may be possible to augment mental capacity –– to add memory or upgrade processing power. We should ponder the enormous moral implications of the machine-assisted mind now, before it is accomplished.

Merrill, Sonya. Genetic screening: suffering and sovereignty. *In:* Demy, Timothy J.; Stewart, Gary P., eds. Genetic Engineering: A Christian Response: Crucial Considerations in Shaping Life. Grand Rapids, MI: Kregel Publications; 1999: 304–313. 7 fn. ISBN 0-8254-2357-0. BE61373.
*biomedical technologies; *Christian ethics; compassion; gene therapy; genetic disorders; genetic predisposition; *genetic screening; genome mapping; *goals; intention; mandatory testing; moral obligations; moral policy; motivation; newborns; pain; prenatal diagnosis; preventive medicine; selective abortion; *suffering; *theology

Muraskas, Jonathan; Marshall, Patricia A.; Tomich, Paul, et al. Neonatal viability in the 1990s: held hostage by technology. *Cambridge Quarterly of Healthcare Ethics.* 1999 Spring; 8(2): 160–172. 43 refs. BE61233.
*allowing to die; *biomedical technologies; consensus; costs and benefits; critically ill; decision analysis; *decision making; disabled; extraordinary treatment; *futility; *intensive care units; *low birth weight; morbidity; mortality; *newborns; *parents; patient admission; patient care; *physicians; practice guidelines; *prematurity; professional family relationship; *prognosis; quality of life; resource allocation; *resuscitation; resuscitation orders; *selection for treatment; standards; *treatment outcome; treatment refusal; uncertainty; ventilators; *viability; *withholding treatment; neonatology; United States

Nelson, Robert M. Ethics in the intensive care unit:

creating an ethical environment. *Critical Care Clinics.* 1997 Jul; 13(3): 691–701. 28 refs. BE61557.
adults; advance directives; allowing to die; attitudes; attitudes to death; *communication; compassion; covenant; *critically ill; *decision making; dissent; informed consent; *institutional ethics; *intensive care units; interprofessional relations; newborns; nurses; parental consent; parents; *patient advocacy; *patient care; *patient care team; patient participation; pediatrics; *physician nurse relationship; physician patient relationship; physicians; professional autonomy; professional competence; professional family relationship; psychological stress; suffering; third party consent; trust; values; withholding treatment

Parens, Erik, ed. Enhancing Human Traits: Ethical and Social Implications. Washington, DC: Georgetown University Press; 1998. 258 p. (Hastings Center studies in ethics). 316 fn. ISBN 0-87840-703-0. BE59743.
advertising; age factors; autonomy; behavior control; *biomedical technologies; blacks; cosmetic surgery; disabled; disease; *enhancement technologies; females; feminist ethics; genetic enhancement; goals; growth disorders; *health; *health care; health insurance reimbursement; hormones; human body; immunization; justice; literature; mass media; medicine; mental health; moral complicity; *moral policy; *normality; patient care; physicians; preventive medicine; psychoactive drugs; psychological stress; public policy; quality of life; resource allocation; review; self concept; social control; suffering; uncertainty; values; beauty; Hastings Center; Project on the Prospect of Technologies Aimed at the Enhancement of Human Capabilities and Traits; United States

Pierce, Jessica; Kerby, Christina. The global ethics of latex gloves: reflections on natural resource use in healthcare. *Cambridge Quarterly of Healthcare Ethics.* 1999 Winter; 8(1): 98–107. 29 fn. BE60531.
*ecology; economics; health hazards; *hospitals; institutional ethics; international aspects; *medical devices; social impact; United States

Ramsey, Scott D.; Hillman, Alan L.; Pauly, Mark V. The effects of health insurance on access to new medical technologies. *International Journal of Technology Assessment in Health Care.* 1997 Spring; 13(2): 357–367. 26 refs. BE61147.
*biomedical technologies; bone marrow; comparative studies; *economics; *health insurance; health maintenance organizations; health services research; heart diseases; kidney diseases; leukemia; *managed care programs; patient care; selection for treatment; statistics; tissue transplantation; angioplasty; *fee-for-service plans; proprietary organizations; *utilization review; Blue Cross-Blue Shield; California; Medicaid; Medicare

Richards, Bill. How a corporate feud doomed human trials of promising therapy. [News]. *Wall Street Journal.* 1999 Aug 6: A1, A6. BE62400.
*biomedical technologies; *bone marrow; *cancer; *economics; federal government; government financing; human experimentation; *industry; legal aspects; leukemia; methods; *patents; terminally ill; *therapeutic research; *tissue transplantation; *Baxter International Inc.; *Cell Pro Inc.; National Institutes of Health; United States

Sakai, Akio. Consensus formation in bioethical decisionmaking in Japan: present contexts and future perspectives. *In:* ten Have, Henk A.M.J.; Sass, Hans-Martin, eds. Consensus Formation in Healthcare Ethics. Boston, MA: Kluwer Academic; 1998: 93–105. 34 refs. 1 fn. ISBN 0-7923-4944-X. BE62590.
*attitudes; *bioethical issues; *biomedical technologies; *brain death; cadavers; *consensus; decision making; *determination of death; empirical research; ethics committees; medical schools; organ donation; physicians;

---

professional organizations; *public opinion; public policy; religion; values; *Japan

Sass, Hans–Martin. Moral aspects of risk and innovation. *Artificial Organs.* 1997 Nov; 21(11): 1217–1221. 16 refs. BE60079.
    artificial organs; autonomy; beneficence; *biomedical technologies; cultural pluralism; education; government regulation; health hazards; human experimentation; informed consent; medical devices; *moral policy; paternalism; patient care; politics; *regulation; research design; *risk; risks and benefits; *technology assessment; *uncertainty; *values

Silvers, Anita. A fatal attraction to normalizing: treating disabilities as deviations from "species-typical" functioning. *In:* Parens, Erik, ed. Enhancing Human Traits: Ethical and Social Implications. Washington, DC: Georgetown University Press; 1998: 95–123. 43 fn. ISBN 0–87840–703–0. BE59747.
    *biomedical technologies; community services; cosmetic surgery; costs and benefits; *disabled; disease; *enhancement technologies; genetic predisposition; *health; *health care; hearing disorders; *justice; medicine; *normality; obligations of society; *physically disabled; public policy; *quality of life; *resource allocation; Daniels, Norman

Skolnick, Andrew A. Drug firm suit fails to halt publication of Canadian Health Technology Report. [News]. *JAMA.* 1998 Aug 26; 280(8): 683–684. BE59690.
    *biomedical research; *drug industry; *drugs; economics; *legal aspects; *technology assessment; *Bristol-Myers Squibb Canada; Canada; *Canadian Coordinating Office of Health Technology Assessment

Smith, George P. Pathways to immortality in the new millenium: human responsibility, theological direction, or legal mandate. *Saint Louis University Public Law Review.* 1996; 15(2): 447–469. 133 fn. BE59920.
    assisted suicide; *biomedical technologies; cloning; *cryopreservation; decision making; determination of death; eugenics; freedom; *genetic intervention; genetic research; historical aspects; killing; *legal aspects; *life extension; religion; reproduction; reproductive technologies; right to die; risks and benefits; science; terminally ill; California; Donaldson v. Van de Kamp

Svatos, Michele. Biotechnology and the utilitarian argument for patents. *In:* Paul, Ellen Frankel; Miller, Fred D.; Paul, Jeffrey, eds. Scientific Innovation, Philosophy, and Public Policy. New York, NY: Cambridge University Press; 1996: 113–144. 84 fn. ISBN 0–521–58994–0. BE62745.
    alternatives; *biomedical research; *biomedical technologies; developing countries; drugs; *economics; genetic intervention; government financing; incentives; industry; information dissemination; international aspects; investigators; legal aspects; *patents; property rights; *public policy; recombinant DNA research; resource allocation; *risks and benefits; social impact; transgenic organisms; universities; *utilitarianism; *agriculture; *biotechnology; *United States

Thomasma, David C. Toward a 21st century bioethic. *Alternative Therapies in Health and Medicine.* 1995 Mar; 1(1): 74–75. 8 refs. BE62005.
    *alternative therapies; bioethical issues; *bioethics; biomedical technologies; *cultural pluralism; ecology; international aspects; medicine; *non-Western World; professional patient relationship; trends; *Western World; United States

Winkler, Mary G. Devices and desires of our own hearts. *In:* Parens, Erik, ed. Enhancing Human Traits: Ethical and Social Implications. Washington, DC: Georgetown University Press; 1998: 238–250. 18 fn. ISBN 0–87840–703–0. BE59755.
    *advertising; autonomy; *biomedical technologies; cosmetic surgery; *enhancement technologies; historical aspects; *human body; literature; *self concept; *social control; social impact; Brave New World (Huxley, A.)

BLOOD DONATION

See also ORGAN AND TISSUE DONATION

Annas, George J. Waste and longing –– the legal status of placental-blood banking. *New England Journal of Medicine.* 1999 May 13; 340(19): 1521–1524. 26 fn. BE62030.
    advertising; biomedical research; *blood banks; *blood donation; commodification; confidentiality; conflict of interest; *cord blood; directed donation; economics; fetal tissue donation; genetic information; genetic screening; hospitals; human experimentation; industry; *legal aspects; mothers; *newborns; organ donation; parental consent; physicians; privacy; property rights; public policy; *stem cells; tissue transplantation; unrelated donors; United States

Burgio, G. Roberto; Locatelli, F.; Nespoli, L. Hematopoietic stem cell transplantation in pediatric practice: a bioethical reassessment. *In:* Burgio, G. Roberto; Lantos, John D., eds. *Primum Non Nocere* Today. Second Edition. New York, NY: Elsevier; 1998: 85–99. 64 refs. ISBN 0–444–82923–7. BE60921.
    beneficence; *blood donation; *bone marrow; *children; *cord blood; donors; economics; family members; informed consent; intention; justice; moral policy; *newborns; parents; pediatrics; pregnant women; private sector; reproduction; resource allocation; *risks and benefits; siblings; *stem cells; *tissue banks; *tissue donation; tissue transplantation; placentas; unrelated donors

Cash, John; Boyd, Kenneth. Blood transfusion: Bayer's initiative. *Lancet.* 1999 Feb 27; 353(9154): 691–692. 7 refs. BE61198.
    *advisory committees; bioethical issues; *blood banks; blood donation; *blood transfusions; commodification; *communicable diseases; conflict of interest; donors; *drug industry; *ethics committees; *financial support; gifts; information dissemination; international aspects; organizational policies; *private sector; public policy; remuneration; *risk; self regulation; *Bayer Advisory Coucil on Bioethics; Bayer Foundation; *Bayer Inc.; *Canada

Caulfield, Timothy; Dossetor, John; Boshkov, Lynn, et al. Notifying patients exposed to blood products associated with Creutzfeldt–Jakob disease: integrating science, legal duties and ethical mandates. *Canadian Medical Association Journal.* 1997 Nov 15; 157(10): 1389–1392. 41 refs. BE59682.
    autonomy; beneficence; *blood transfusions; brain pathology; central nervous system diseases; *disclosure; *duty to warn; health personnel; hemophilia; iatrogenic disease; *information dissemination; informed consent; *legal obligations; *moral obligations; *moral policy; patients; *public policy; resource allocation; *risk; risks and benefits; *truth disclosure; *Creutzfeldt-Jakob syndrome; recontact; Canada

Eckholm, Erik. Hoping to control spread of AIDS, China bans the sale of blood. [News]. *New York Times.* 1998 Oct 1: A7. BE60366.
    AIDS; blood banks; *blood donation; *donors; *government regulation; *remuneration; scarcity; *China

Feldman, Eric A.; Bayer, Ronald, eds. Blood Feuds:

AIDS, Blood, and the Politics of Medical Disaster. New York, NY: Oxford University Press; 1999. 375 p. 1,007 fn. ISBN 0-19-513160-6. BE60746.
> accountability; administrators; *AIDS; *blood donation; *blood transfusions; comparative studies; compensation; drug industry; economics; government regulation; *hemophilia; *HIV seropositivity; iatrogenic disease; information dissemination; *international aspects; legal aspects; legal liability; mandatory programs; metaphor; misconduct; organization and administration; political activity; politics; *public policy; self regulation; time factors; voluntary programs; Australia; Canada; Denmark; France; Germany; Italy; Japan; Red Cross; United States

Giesen, Dieter. Compensation and consent: a brief comparative examination of liability for HIV-infected blood. *In:* Bennett, Rebecca; Erin, Charles A., eds. HIV and AIDS: Testing, Screening, and Confidentiality. New York, NY: Oxford University Press; 1999: 91-106. 65 fn. ISBN 0-19-823801-0. BE62716.
> *AIDS; AIDS serodiagnosis; blood banks; *blood donation; *blood transfusions; comparative studies; compensation; disclosure; donors; *HIV seropositivity; hospitals; informed consent; international aspects; judicial action; legal aspects; *legal liability; legal rights; negligence; physicians; standards; *torts; *Germany; Great Britain; *United States

Hass, Janis. Storage of cord blood attracts private-sector interest. *Canadian Medical Association Journal.* 1999 Feb 23; 160(4): 551-552. BE62308.
> *blood banks; blood donation; *cord blood; cryopreservation; economics; industry; newborns; *private sector; standards; *stem cells; time factors; *Canada

Jayaraman, K.S. Ban on sale may cause Indian blood shortage. [News]. *Nature Medicine.* 1998 Feb; 4(2): 139. BE60441.
> *blood donation; donors; government regulation; incentives; legislation; *public policy; *remuneration; *scarcity; social impact; voluntary programs; *India

Keown, John. A reply to McLachlan. *Journal of Medical Ethics.* 1998 Aug; 24(4): 255-256. 3 refs. Commentary on H.V. McLachlan, p. 252-254. BE61303.
> *altruism; *blood donation; common good; *motivation; *public policy; *voluntary programs

In an earlier article in this journal, I advanced five ethical arguments in favour of a voluntary, unpaid system of blood donation. In his reply to my article, Hugh McLachlan criticised one of those arguments, namely, the argument that an unpaid system promotes altruism and social solidarity. In this reply to Dr. McLachlan, I maintain that his criticism is misguided, and that he appears unclear not only about my own argument, but also about his own.

King, Susan M.; Watson, Heather; Heurter, Helen, et al. Notifying patients exposed to blood products associated with Creutzfeldt-Jakob disease: theoretical risk for real people. *Canadian Medical Association Journal.* 1998 Oct 6; 159(7): 771-774. 23 refs. BE62357.
> adolescents; *attitudes; *blood transfusions; central nervous system diseases; children; communication; *disclosure; duty to warn; iatrogenic disease; parental notification; *parents; *patients; psychological stress; *risk; risks and benefits; survey; *truth disclosure; *Creutzfeldt-Jakob syndrome; recontact; Canada; Hospital for Sick Children (Toronto); Ontario

Larke, Bryce. The quandary of Creutzfeldt-Jakob disease. [Editorial]. *Canadian Medical Association Journal.* 1998 Oct 6; 159(7): 789-792. 22 refs. BE62359.
> attitudes; blood donation; *blood transfusions; brain pathology; central nervous system diseases; *disclosure; *duty to warn; iatrogenic disease; industry; patients; physicians; public policy; *risk; risks and benefits; *truth disclosure; uncertainty; *Creutzfeldt-Jakob syndrome; recontact; Canada

McLachlan, Hugh V. The unpaid donation of blood and altruism: a comment on Keown. *Journal of Medical Ethics.* 1998 Aug; 24(4): 252-254. 7 fn. Commentary on J. Keown, "The gift of blood in Europe: an ethical defence of EC directive 89/381," *JME* 1997 Apr; 23(2): 96-100. Commented on by J. Keown, p. 255-256. BE61291.
> *altruism; *blood donation; common good; *motivation; *public policy; remuneration; risks and benefits; *voluntary programs

In line with article 3.4 of EC directive 89/381, Keown has presented an ethical case in support of the policy of voluntary, unpaid donation of blood. Although no doubt is cast on the desirability of the policy, that part of Keown's argument which pertains to the suggested laudability of altruism and of its encouragment by social policy is examined and shown to be dubious.

Peerenboom, Ellen. Germany still pays donors. [News]. *Nature Medicine.* 1998 Feb; 4(2): 139. BE60442.
> *blood donation; donors; international aspects; public policy; *remuneration; Europe; *Germany

Rajagopalan, M.; Pulimood, R. Attitudes of medical and nursing students towards blood donation. *National Medical Journal of India.* 1998 Jan-Feb; 11(1): 12-13. 14 refs. BE61488.
> *attitudes; *blood donation; knowledge, attitudes, practice; medical education; nursing education; *students; survey; *India

Sibbald, Barbara. Blood recipients and CJD: to notify or not to notify, that is the question. *Canadian Medical Association Journal.* 1998 Oct 6; 159(7): 829-831. BE62361.
> *attitudes; blood donation; *blood transfusions; central nervous system diseases; *disclosure; *duty to warn; iatrogenic disease; parents; *patients; public policy; *risk; risks and benefits; *truth disclosure; *Creutzfeldt-Jakob syndrome; recontact; Canada

Starr, Douglas. Blood: An Epic History of Medicine and Commerce. New York, NY: Alfred A. Knopf; 1998. 441 p. 355 fn. ISBN 0-679-41875-X. BE62629.
> AIDS; biomedical research; *blood banks; *blood donation; *blood transfusions; body parts and fluids; cadavers; commodification; developing countries; donors; drug industry; economics; gifts; hemophilia; hepatitis; *historical aspects; HIV seropositivity; homosexuals; *international aspects; misconduct; negligence; remuneration; social discrimination; sociology of medicine; war; Europe; Japan; Red Cross; United States; USSR

Zwart, Hub A.E. Why should remunerated blood donation be unethical? Ethical reflections on current blood donation policies and their philosophical origins. *In:* ten Have, Henk A.M.J.; Welie, Jos V.M., eds. Ownership of the Human Body: Philosophical Considerations on the Use of the Human Body and Its Parts in Healthcare. Boston, MA: Kluwer Academic; 1998: 39-48. 13 refs. ISBN 0-7923-5150-9. BE61318.
> *altruism; *blood donation; body parts and fluids; commodification; common good; gifts; human body; *moral policy; motivation; personhood; philosophy; property rights; public policy; *remuneration; risks and benefits; voluntary programs; liberalism

---

BE = bioethics accession number   fn. = footnotes   refs. = references

BRAIN DEATH
See under
    DETERMINATION OF DEATH/BRAIN
    DEATH

CAPITAL PUNISHMENT

Beck, James C. Psychiatry and the death penalty. *Harvard Review of Psychiatry.* 1996 Nov–Dec; 4(4): 225–229. 27 refs. BE61477.
    *capital punishment; competence; dangerousness; due process; evaluation; *forensic psychiatry; informed consent; justice; *legal aspects; medical ethics; patient care; *physician's role; prisoners; psychoactive drugs; Supreme Court decisions; *United States

Becker, Carl. Money talks, money kills -- the economics of transplantation in Japan and China. *Bioethics.* 1999 Jul; 13(3–4): 236–243. 33 fn. BE61873.
    allowing to die; *brain death; *capital punishment; *determination of death; directed donation; *economics; hospitals; institutional policies; *legal aspects; *motivation; non–Western World; *organ donation; *organ transplantation; *prisoners; *public policy; *China; *Japan
    Japan and China have long resisted the Western trend of organ transplantation from brain–dead patients, based on a 'Confucian' respect for integrity of ancestors' bodies. While their general publics continue to harbor grave doubts about such practices, their medical and political elites are hastening towards the road of organ–harvesting and organ–marketing, largely for economic reasons. This report illustrates the ways that economics is motivating brain–death legislation in Japan and criminal executions in China.

Caelleigh, Addeane S. The guillotine. *Academic Medicine.* 1997 Mar; 72(3): 166. BE59893.
    *capital punishment; *historical aspects; *methods; physician's role; Eighteenth Century; Europe; France

Halpern, Abraham L.; Freedman, Alfred M.; Schoenholtz, Jack C., et al. Ethics in forensic psychiatry. [Letter and response]. *American Journal of Psychiatry.* 1998 Apr; 155(4): 575–577. 13 refs. BE60179.
    *capital punishment; codes of ethics; *competence; conflict of interest; *expert testimony; *forensic psychiatry; law enforcement; *medical ethics; organizational policies; patient care; physician patient relationship; *physician's role; physicians; professional organizations; psychiatric diagnosis; psychiatry; American Academy of Psychiatry and the Law; American Medical Association; American Psychiatric Association

Josefson, Deborah. U.S. doctors want no part in executions. [News]. *BMJ (British Medical Journal).* 1998 Sep 12; 317(7160): 702. BE59894.
    *capital punishment; *legal aspects; *organizational policies; patient care; *physician's role; physicians; political activity; prisoners; professional organizations; state government; American College of Physicians; American Medical Association; California; United States

Palmer, Louis J. Organ Transplants from Executed Prisoners: An Argument for the Creation of Death Sentence Organ Removal Statutes. Jefferson, NC: McFarland; 1999. 156 p. 429 fn. ISBN 0–7864–0673–9. BE61943.
    anesthesia; body parts and fluids; brain death; cadavers; *capital punishment; constitutional amendments; *constitutional law; due process; equal protection; federal government; *legal aspects; *mandatory programs; methods; *model legislation; *organ donation; *prisoners; property

rights; public policy; punishment; remuneration; scarcity; state government; voluntary programs; China; Great Britain; Uniform Anatomical Gift Act; *United States

Schoenholtz, Jack C.; Freedman, Alfred M.; Halpern, Abraham L. The "legal" abuse of physicians in deaths in the United States: the erosion of ethics and morality in medicine. *Wayne Law Review.* 1996 Spring; 42(3): 1505–1601. 306 fn. BE62178.
    active euthanasia; allowing to die; *assisted suicide; *capital punishment; competence; economics; forensic medicine; forensic psychiatry; health care delivery; *killing; *legal aspects; medical ethics; moral obligations; organizational policies; patient care; *physicians; prisoners; professional organizations; psychiatric diagnosis; psychiatry; quality of life; wedge argument; American Medical Association; American Psychiatric Association; United States

An organ donation offer on death row is refused. [News]. *New York Times.* 1998 Sep 9: A23. BE61118.
    *capital punishment; *organ donation; *prisoners; public policy; state government; *Nobles, Jonathan; *Texas

CIVIL COMMITMENT *See* INVOLUNTARY COMMITMENT

CLINICAL ETHICISTS *See* ETHICISTS AND ETHICS COMMITTEES

CLINICAL ETHICS *See* BIOETHICS, ETHICISTS AND ETHICS COMMITTEES, MEDICAL ETHICS, NURSING ETHICS, PROFESSIONAL ETHICS

CLINICAL ETHICS COMMITTEES *See* ETHICISTS AND ETHICS COMMITTEES

CLINICAL RESEARCH *See* HUMAN EXPERIMENTATION

CLONING

See also REPRODUCTIVE TECHNOLOGIES, GENETIC INTERVENTION

Admiraal, Pieter; Ardila, Ruben; Berlin, Isaiah, et al.; Humanist Laureates of the International Academy of Humanism. Declaration in defense of cloning and the integrity of scientific research. *Free Inquiry.* 1997 Summer; 17(3): 11–12. BE60205.
    *cloning; freedom; humanism; religion; risks and benefits; science; International Academy of Humanism

Aldhous, Peter. The fears of a clone. *New Scientist.* 1998 Feb 21; 157(2122): 8. BE61644.
    *cloning; government regulation; reproductive technologies; United States

Alvarez, Lizette. Senate, 54–42, rejects Republican bill to ban human cloning. [News]. *New York Times.* 1998 Feb 12: A10. BE59470.
    attitudes; *cloning; embryo research; federal government; *government regulation; investigators; politics; nuclear transplantation; *U.S. Congress; *United States

Amer, Mona S. Breaking the mold: human embryo cloning and its implications for a right to individuality. [Comment]. *UCLA Law Review.* 1996 Jun; 43(5):

BE = bioethics accession number   fn. = footnotes   refs. = references

1659–1688. 158 fn. BE59212.
> body parts and fluids; children; *cloning; *cryopreservation; *embryos; genetic identity; genetic information; *genetic materials; in vitro fertilization; *legal aspects; *legal rights; parents; personhood; *property rights; reproduction; *siblings; twins; cell lines; *embryo splitting; Moore v. Regents of the University of California; United States

Anderson, J. Kerby. The ethics of genetic engineering and artificial reproduction. *In:* Demy, Timothy J.; Stewart, Gary P., eds. Genetic Engineering: A Christian Response: Crucial Considerations in Shaping Life. Grand Rapids, MI: Kregel Publications; 1999: 140–152. 20 fn. ISBN 0–8254–2357–0. BE61365.
> age factors; artificial insemination; *Christian ethics; *cloning; cryopreservation; embryo disposition; embryo research; embryo transfer; embryos; gamete intrafallopian transfer; gene therapy; in vitro fertilization; legal aspects; marital relationship; ovum donors; *parent child relationship; patents; pregnant women; *recombinant DNA research; *reproductive technologies; semen donors; sex preselection; social impact; surrogate mothers; theology; transgenic organisms; value of life; United States

Annas, George J. The prospect of human cloning: an opportunity for national and international cooperation in bioethics. *In:* Humber, James M.; Almeder, Robert F., eds. Human Cloning. Totowa, NJ: Humana Press; 1998: 51–63. 6 refs. ISBN 0–89603–565–4. BE59465.
> advisory committees; attitudes; *cloning; dehumanization; federal government; *government regulation; human experimentation; international aspects; *public policy; reproduction; reproductive technologies; risks and benefits; values; personal identity; United States

Ayd, Frank J. Human cloning and the rights of human beings. *Medical–Moral Newsletter.* 1998 May–Jun; 35(5–6): 17–23. BE61463.
> beginning of life; *cloning; *embryo research; embryos; genetic identity; government regulation; human rights; parent child relationship; personhood; public policy; risks and benefits; sexuality; value of life; nuclear transplantation; United States

Baker, Michael. Korean report sparks anger and inquiry. [News]. *Science.* 1999 Jan 1; 283(5398): 16–17. BE61091.
> attitudes; *cloning; embryo research; government regulation; investigators; reproductive technologies; *Korea

Baker, Michael. Report casts doubt on Korean experiment. [News]. *Science.* 1999 Jan 29; 283(5402): 617, 619. BE61092.
> *cloning; embryo research; ethical review; government regulation; human experimentation; investigators; methods; *Korea; Korean Medical Association

Balls, Michael. The production of genetically modified animals and humans: an inescapable moral challenge to scientists and laypeople alike. [Editorial]. *ATLA: Alternatives to Laboratory Animals.* 1998 Jan–Feb; 26(1): 1–2. 5 refs. BE59788.
> *cloning; government regulation; hybrids; primates; risks and benefits; *transgenic animals

Bard, Jennifer S. When a woman doesn't need a man: legal issues regarding cloning as an infertility treatment. *Journal of Biolaw and Business.* 1998 Spring; 1(3): 56–58. 21 fn. BE62093.
> *cloning; cryopreservation; embryos; *legal aspects; marital relationship; multiple pregnancy; parent child relationship; regulation; *reproductive technologies; risks and benefits; single persons

Berg, Paul; Singer, Maxine. Regulating human cloning.

[Editorial]. *Science.* 1998 Oct 16; 282(5388): 413. BE59645.
> *cloning; government regulation; guidelines; international aspects; recombinant DNA research; *regulation; risks and benefits; self regulation

Bilger, Burkhard. Cell block: moral relativism and news of practical benefits are nudging human cloning toward public acceptance, even as the first laws are written to ban it. *Sciences.* 1997 Sep–Oct; 37(5): 17–19. BE61521.
> advisory committees; animal experimentation; animal organs; *cloning; federal government; genetic intervention; government regulation; human experimentation; organ donation; public policy; risks and benefits; state government; transgenic animals; agriculture; transgenic plants; National Bioethics Advisory Commission; United States

Bohlin, Raymond G. The possibilities and ethics of human cloning. *In:* Demy, Timothy J.; Stewart, Gary P., eds. Genetic Engineering: A Christian Response: Crucial Considerations in Shaping Life. Grand Rapids, MI: Kregel Publications; 1999: 260–277. 51 fn. ISBN 0–8254–2357–0. BE61370.
> adults; advisory committees; animal experimentation; attitudes; Christian ethics; *cloning; cryopreservation; embryo research; embryos; human experimentation; investigators; literature; mass media; methods; organ donation; public policy; reproductive technologies; *risks and benefits; *twinning; nuclear transplantation; In His Image (Rorvik, D.); Jurassic Park (Crichton, M.); National Bioethics Advisory Commission; The Boys from Brazil (Levin, I.); United States

Bonnicksen, Andrea L. Procreation by cloning: crafting anticipatory guidelines. *Journal of Law, Medicine and Ethics.* 1997 Winter; 25(4): 273–282. 64 fn. BE62672.
> advisory committees; children; *cloning; *commodification; dehumanization; donors; embryo disposition; *embryo research; embryos; federal government; fetal research; *government regulation; guidelines; international aspects; *methods; multiple pregnancy; ovum donors; *public policy; reproductive technologies; *risks and benefits; semen donors; state government; *twinning; *embryo splitting; *nuclear transplantation; Canada; Europe; *United States

Bosch, Xavier. Spanish watchdog sees way ahead for stem–cell research. [News]. *Nature.* 1999 Apr 22; 398(6729): 645. BE61759.
> advisory committees; alternatives; *cloning; embryo research; government regulation; *stem cells; National Commission on Assisted Reproduction (Spain); *Spain

Brock, Dan W. Cloning human beings: an assessment of the ethical issues pro and con. *In:* Nussbaum, Martha C.; Sunstein, Cass R., eds. Clones and Clones: Facts and Fantasies About Human Cloning. New York, NY: Norton; 1998: 141–164. 34 refs. This essay is a shorter version of a paper prepared for the National Bioethics Advisory Commission. ISBN 0–393–04648–6. BE60359.
> *cloning; commodification; dehumanization; freedom; genetic determinism; genetic identity; genetic intervention; *moral policy; motivation; public policy; reproduction; reproductive technologies; *rights; *risks and benefits

Brower, Vicki. Experts criticize NBAC cloning report's defensive posture. [News]. *Nature Biotechnology.* 1997 Aug; 15(8): 705. BE62040.
> advisory committees; attitudes; *cloning; embryo research; ethicists; government regulation; guidelines; investigators; *public policy; *National Bioethics Advisory Commission; United States

Bruce, Donald M. Cloning -- a step too far? An article on the ethical aspects of cloning in animals and humans.

BE = bioethics accession number   fn. = footnotes   refs. = references

Human Reproduction and Genetic Ethics: An International Journal. 1998; 4(2): 34–38. BE61455.
  animal experimentation; animal rights; body parts and fluids; Christian ethics; *cloning; commodification; embryo research; genetic diversity; genetic intervention; moral policy; public policy; reproductive technologies; risks and benefits; transgenic animals; agriculture; dignity; Church of Scotland

Burley, Justine; Harris, John. Human cloning and child welfare. *Journal of Medical Ethics.* 1999 Apr; 25(2): 108–113. 18 fn. BE61912.
  *autonomy; children; *cloning; *freedom; government regulation; injuries; *moral policy; parents; *public policy; reproduction; reproductive technologies; social discrimination; stigmatization; harms
In this paper we discuss an objection to human cloning which appeals to the welfare of the child. This objection varies according to the sort of harm it is expected the clone will suffer. The three formulations of it that we will consider are: 1. Clones will be harmed by the fearful or prejudicial attitudes people may have about or towards them (H1); 2. Clones will be harmed by the demands and expectations of parents or genotype donors (H2); 3. Clones will be harmed by their own awareness of their origins, for example the knowledge that the genetic donor is a stranger (H3). We will show why these three versions of the child welfare objection do not necessarily supply compelling reasons to ban human reproductive cloning. The claim that we will develop and defend in the course of our discussion is that even if it is the case that a cloned child will suffer harms of the type H1–H3, it is none the less permissible to conceive by cloning so long as these cloning–induced welfare deficits are not such as to blight the existence of the resultant child, whoever this may be.

Campbell, Courtney S.; Woolfrey, Joan. Norms and narratives: religious reflections on the human cloning controversy. *Journal of Biolaw and Business.* 1998 Spring; 1(3): 8–20. 47 fn. BE62092.
  accountability; advisory committees; American Indians; blacks; Buddhist ethics; Christian ethics; *cloning; cultural pluralism; Eastern Orthodox ethics; education; embryo research; Hindu ethics; Islamic ethics; Jewish ethics; justice; metaphor; moral obligations; parent child relationship; Protestant ethics; public policy; *religion; *religious ethics; reproduction; reproductive technologies; risks and benefits; Roman Catholic ethics; science; theology; therapeutic research; value of life; values; National Bioethics Advisory Commission; United States

Campbell, Keith. Look on the bright side of cloning. *Nature Medicine.* 1998 May; 4(5): 557–558. 13 refs. BE59841.
  animal experimentation; animal organs; *cloning; fetal tissue donation; methods; risks and benefits; tissue transplantation; transgenic animals; nuclear transplantation

Caplan, Arthur L. Why the rush to ban cloning? *New York Times.* 1998 Jan 28: A25. BE59564.
  *cloning; embryo research; federal government; *government regulation; politics; state government; Food and Drug Administration; *United States

Cohen, Jonathan R. In God's garden: creation and cloning in Jewish thought. *Hastings Center Report.* 1999 Jul–Aug; 29(4): 7–12. 19 fn. An earlier version of this article appeared in *Journal of Progressive Judaism*, 1998 May; 10: 46–62. BE62463.
  *cloning; genetic intervention; *Jewish ethics; life extension; morality; motivation; reproduction; theology; value of life
The possibility of cloning–human beings challenges

Western beliefs about creation and our relationship to God. If we understand God as the Creator and creation as a completed act, cloning will be a transgression. If, however, we understand God as the Power of Creation and creation as a transformative process, we may find a role for human participation, sharing that power as beings created in the image of God.

Dawkins, Richard. Thinking clearly about clones: how dogma and ignorance get in the way. *Free Inquiry.* 1997 Summer; 17(3): 13–14. Adapted from materials published in *The Independent* and the London *Evening Standard.* BE60206.
  clergy; *cloning; mass media; *religion; technical expertise; twins

de Pomerai, David. Dolly mixtures: retrospect and prospects for animal and human cloning. *Human Reproduction and Genetic Ethics: An International Journal.* 1998; 4(2): 39–48. 50 refs. BE61456.
  animal experimentation; Christian ethics; *cloning; embryo research; ethical theory; government regulation; methods; moral policy; parent child relationship; public policy; reproductive technologies; risks and benefits; tissue donation; dignity; nuclear transplantation

Eisenberg, Leon. Would cloned humans really be like sheep? *New England Journal of Medicine.* 1999 Feb 11; 340(6): 471–475. 30 fn. BE60993.
  biology; brain; *cloning; evolution; fetal development; future generations; *genetic determinism; *genetic diversity; human experimentation; infants; reproductive technologies; *social impact; nuclear transplantation

Elshtain, Jean Bethke. The hard questions: our bodies, our clones. *New Republic.* 1997 Aug 4; 217(5): 25. BE60455.
  *cloning; reproductive technologies; self concept; values

Elshtain, Jean Bethke. To clone or not to clone. *In:* Nussbaum, Martha C.; Sunstein, Cass R., eds. Clones and Clones: Facts and Fantasies About Human Cloning. New York, NY: Norton; 1998: 181–189. This article appeared, in slightly different form, in the *New Republic*, 1997 Aug 4. ISBN 0–393–0468–6. BE60360.
  *cloning; dehumanization; genetic identity; motivation; reproductive technologies; risks and benefits

Epstein, Richard A. A rush to caution: cloning human beings. *In:* Nussbaum, Martha C.; Sunstein, Cass R. eds. Clones and Clones: Facts and Fantasies About Human Cloning. New York, NY: Norton; 1998: 262–279. 19 fn. ISBN 0–393–04648–6. BE60365.
  advisory committees; *cloning; freedom; genetic diversity; *government regulation; *public policy; reproductive technologies; risks and benefits; social impact; uncertainty; National Bioethics Advisory Commission

Firn, David. Roslin Institute upset by human cloning suggestions. [News]. *Nature Medicine.* 1999 Mar; 5(3): 253. BE62540.
  animal experimentation; *cloning; economics; embryo research; industry; investigators; private sector; public sector; *research institutes; stem cells; Great Britain; *Roslin Institute (Scotland)

Fishman, Rachelle H.B. Israeli cloning ban endorsed by scientists. [News]. *Lancet.* 1999 Jan 16; 353(9148): 218. BE61107.
  advisory committees; *cloning; embryo research; gene therapy; germ cells; *government regulation; human experimentation; *Israel

---

BE = bioethics accession number   fn. = footnotes   refs. = references

Fox, Jeffrey L. US bioethicists say continue human cloning moratorium. [News]. *Nature Biotechnology.* 1997 Jul; 15(7): 609. BE62018.

advisory committees; *cloning; embryo research; federal government; government regulation; private sector; *public policy; public sector; reproductive technologies; *National Bioethics Advisory Commission; United States

Galton, D.J.; Doyal, L. "Goodbye Dolly?" The ethics of human cloning. [Letter]. *Journal of Medical Ethics.* 1998 Aug; 24(4): 279. 4 refs. BE62063.

*cloning; embryo research; genetic disorders; reproductive technologies; *risks and benefits

Galton, D.J.; Kay, A.; Cavanna, J.S. Human cloning: safety is the issue. [Letter]. *Nature Medicine.* 1998 Jun; 4(6): 644. 5 refs. BE59728.

*cloning; public policy; reproductive technologies; *risk; nuclear transplantation

Glannon, Walter. The ethics of human cloning. *Public Affairs Quarterly.* 1998 Jul; 12(3): 287–305. 31 refs. 24 fn. BE61225.

autonomy; beneficence; children; *cloning; embryos; eugenics; genetic disorders; genetic diversity; genetic enhancement; genetic identity; *moral policy; motivation; organ donation; parents; reproductive technologies; risks and benefits; tissue donation; wedge argument; personal identity

Golub, Edward S. Finding a vocabulary for the extrascientific significance of technology. *Nature Biotechnology.* 1997 May; 15(5): 394. BE62015.

*cloning; confidentiality; genetic determinism; genetic information; *genetic intervention; investigators; public opinion; risks and benefits; *social impact; technology assessment

Gould, Stephen Jay. Individuality: cloning and the discomfiting cases of Siamese twins. *Sciences.* 1997 Sep–Oct; 37(5): 14–16. BE61520.

*cloning; evolution; normality; *personhood; *twins; *conjoined twins

Hadfield, Peter. Cloning's maverick goes east. [News]. *New Scientist.* 1998 Dec 12; 160(2164): 26. *cloning BE61545.

embryo research; government regulation; international aspects; investigators; laboratories; reproductive technologies; *Japan; *Seed, Richard; United States

Haglund, Keith. Research coalition promises no human cloning by members. [News]. *Journal of NIH Research.* 1997 Nov; 9(11): 20–21. BE59758.

*cloning; embryo research; genetic research; government regulation; investigators; legislation; *organizational policies; professional organizations; voluntary programs; *Federation of American Societies for Experimental Biology; United States

Hartouni, Valerie. Cultural Conceptions: On Reproductive Technologies and the Remaking of Life. Minneapolis, MN: University of Minnesota Press; 1997. 175 p. Bibliography: p. 157–170. ISBN 0-8166-2623-5. BE62771.

*abortion, induced; adoption; audiovisual aids; behavioral genetics; blacks; brain death; *cloning; disadvantaged; embryos; eugenics; *fetuses; genetic intervention; legal aspects; mass media; mothers; parent child relationship; personhood; political activity; posthumous reproduction; postmodernism; *pregnant women; prenatal diagnosis; prolongation of life; *reproduction; *reproductive technologies; social discrimination; *social impact; socioeconomic factors; Supreme Court decisions; *surrogate mothers; value of life; values; violence; women's rights; In

re Baby M; Johnson v. Calvert; Right to Life Movement; S'Aline's Solution; The Bell Curve (Herrnstein, R.; Murray, C.); *United States

Heller, Jan C. Religiously based objections to human cloning: are they sustainable? *In:* Humber, James M.; Almeder, Robert F.,eds. Human Cloning. Totowa, NJ: Humana Press; 1998: 153–176. 21 fn. ISBN 0-89603-565-4. BE59468.

*Christian ethics; *cloning; cultural pluralism; family relationship; religious ethics; reproduction; secularism; *theology; dignity; personal identity; National Bioethics Advisory Commission; United States

Holden, Constance, ed. Clone rangers. [News]. *Science.* 1999 Jun 25; 284(5423): 2083. BE62389.

*cloning; industry; *Clonaid

Hoyle, Russ. Clinton's cloning ban may threaten genetic research. *Nature Biotechnology.* 1997 Jul; 15(7): 600. BE62017.

advisory committees; *cloning; embryo research; federal government; genetic research; *government regulation; legislation; politics; *public policy; reproductive technologies; National Bioethics Advisory Commission; *United States

Hull, Richard T. No fear: how a humanist faces science's new creation. *Free Inquiry.* 1997 Summer; 17(3): 18–20. BE60208.

*cloning; freedom; humanism; regulation; religion; science; tissue donation

Human Genetics Advisory Commission (Great Britain). Cloning Issues in Reproduction, Science and Medicine. [Consultation paper]. London: The Commission [online]. Internet Web site: http://www.dti.gov.uk/hgac/papers/papers—c.htm [1998 December 7]; 1998 Jan. 23 p. 14 refs. HGAC papers. BE59316.

advisory committees; *cloning; embryo research; genetic identity; government regulation; human experimentation; legal aspects; methods; motivation; public participation; public policy; reproductive technologies; risks and benefits; stem cells; therapeutic research; embryo splitting; nuclear transplantation; Great Britain; Human Fertilisation and Embryology Authority

Human Genetics Advisory Commission (Great Britain); Great Britain. Human Fertilisation and Embryology Authority. Cloning Issues in Reproduction, Science and Medicine. [Report]. London: The Commission [online]. Web site: http://www.dti.gov.uk/hgac/papers/papers—d.htm [1998 December 9]; 1998 Dec. 39 p. 20 refs. HGAC papers. BE59317.

advisory committees; *attitudes; *cloning; confidentiality; embryo research; genetic identity; *government regulation; informed consent; international aspects; legislation; methods; motivation; public opinion; public participation; *public policy; reproductive technologies; risks and benefits; survey; therapeutic research; tissue transplantation; cell lines; nuclear transplantation; *Great Britain; Human Fertilisation and Embryology Act 1990; *Human Fertilisation and Embryology Authority; *Human Genetics Advisory Commission (Great Britain)

Humber, James M.; Almeder, Robert F., eds. Human Cloning. Totowa, NJ: Humana Press; 1998. 214 p. (Biomedical ethics reviews). 40 refs. 282 fn. ISBN 0-89603-565-4. BE59463.

Christian ethics; *cloning; ethical analysis; genetic identity; goals; government regulation; historical aspects; literature;

BE = bioethics accession number   fn. = footnotes   refs. = references

moral policy; motivation; public policy; review; risks and benefits; theology; trends

Iozzio, M.J. Science, ethics, and cloning technologies. *Linacre Quarterly.* 1997 Nov; 64(4): 46–52. 6 fn. BE61789.
> *cloning; embryo research; embryos; mass media; personhood; reproductive technologies; risks and benefits; *Roman Catholic ethics; social control; value of life

Kass, Leon R.; Wilson, James Q. The Ethics of Human Cloning. Washington, DC: AEI Press; 1998. 101 p. 4 fn. ISBN 0-8447-4050-0. BE59866.
> advisory committees; animal experimentation; autonomy; *cloning; commodification; dehumanization; embryo research; ethicists; eugenics; family relationship; genetic identity; government regulation; infertility; married persons; *moral policy; mothers; parent child relationship; *public policy; reproduction; reproductive technologies; rights; *risks and benefits; sexuality; social impact; utilitarianism; values; wedge argument; nuclear transplantation; National Bioethics Advisory Commission; United States

Kaye, Howard L. Anxiety and genetic manipulation: a sociological view. *Perspectives in Biology and Medicine.* 1998 Summer; 41(4): 483–490. 27 refs. BE61110.
> attitudes; autonomy; bioethics; *cloning; *dehumanization; emotions; eugenics; family relationship; future generations; *genetic determinism; genetic identity; *genetic intervention; interdisciplinary communication; *morality; *psychological stress; *public opinion; reproductive technologies; science; self concept; *social impact; social sciences; value of life; *values; dignity; sociology

Kelly, Robert. On human cloning. *Nature Biotechnology.* 1998 Sep; 16(9): 798. BE62025.
> *cloning; goals; human characteristics; personhood; reproductive technologies

King, David. Led by the nose. *GenEthics News.* 1997 Jan–Mar; No. 16: 7. BE60103.
> *cloning; dehumanization; motivation; reproduction; reproductive technologies; risks and benefits; science; social control; social dominance; transgenic animals; agriculture

Kitcher, Philip. Whose self is it, anyway? *Sciences.* 1997 Sep–Oct; 37(5): 58–62. BE61522.
> autonomy; *cloning; genetic information; moral policy; motivation; parent child relationship; personhood; public policy; reproductive technologies; resource allocation

Klugman, Craig M.; Murray, Thomas H. Cloning, historical ethics, and NBAC. *In:* Humber, James M.; Almeder, Robert F.,eds. Human Cloning. Totowa, NJ: Humana Press; 1998: 1–50. 99 fn. ISBN 0-89603-565-4. BE59464.
> advisory committees; animal experimentation; *attitudes; children; *cloning; commodification; dehumanization; embryos; ethicists; eugenics; family relationship; freedom; genetic diversity; genetic intervention; government regulation; guidelines; *historical aspects; human body; human experimentation; international aspects; investigators; legal aspects; *literature; mass media; metaphor; methods; moral policy; morality; personhood; philosophy; public policy; reproduction; reproductive technologies; *risks and benefits; social impact; terminology; theology; *trends; value of life; embryo splitting; nuclear transplantation; Cloning Human Beings (NBAC); National Bioethics Advisory Commission; Nineteenth Century; Twentieth Century; United States

Koch, Tom; Rowell, Mary. Humanness, personhood, and a lamb named Dolly: response to "Cloning: technology, policy, and ethics" (*CQ* Vol. 7, No. 2). *Cambridge Quarterly of Healthcare Ethics.* 1999 Spring; 8(2):

241–245. 13 refs. BE61240.
> attitudes; *cloning; decision analysis; health personnel; human characteristics; *personhood; social interaction; *standards

Kolata, Gina. In big advance in cloning, biologists create 50 mice. [News]. *New York Times.* 1998 Jul 23: A1, A20. BE62648.
> animal experimentation; *cloning; *rodents

Kolata, Gina. In the game of cloning, women hold all the cards. [News]. *New York Times.* 1998 Feb 22: 6. BE59566.
> *cloning; commodification; *females; ovum donors

Kondro, Wayne. Canadian government will revisit human-cloning legislation. [News]. *Lancet.* 1999 May 8; 353(9164): 1599. BE62288.
> animal experimentation; *cloning; *government regulation; industry; legislation; reproductive technologies; transgenic animals; *Canada

Krauthammer, Charles. Of headless mice...and men: the ultimate cloning horror: human organ farms. *Time.* 1998 Jan 19; 151(2): 76. BE59164.
> animal experimentation; body parts and fluids; *cloning; investigators; motivation; *organ donation; personhood; *headless organisms; Seed, Richard

Lampman, Jane. Cloning's double trouble. [News]. *Christian Science Monitor.* 1998 Aug 13: B1, B3–B4. BE59215.
> *cloning; morality; regulation; religious ethics; social impact

Lindsay, Ronald A. Taboos without a clue: sizing up religious objections to cloning. *Free Inquiry.* 1997 Summer; 17(3): 15–17. BE60207.
> *cloning; morality; *religion; reproduction; risks and benefits; secularism; sexuality; tissue donation; dignity

Lipschutz, Joshua H. To clone or not to clone -- a Jewish perspective. *Journal of Medical Ethics.* 1999 Apr; 25(2): 105–107. 13 refs. BE61911.
> brain; *cloning; genetic identity; *Jewish ethics; reproductive technologies; personal identity
> Many new reproductive methods such as artificial insemination, in vitro fertilisation, freezing of human embryos, and surrogate motherhood were at first widely condemned but are now seen in Western society as not just ethically and morally acceptable, but beneficial in that they allow otherwise infertile couples to have children. The idea of human cloning was also quickly condemned but debate is now emerging. This article examines cloning from a Jewish perspective and finds evidence to support the view that there is nothing inherently wrong with the idea of human cloning. A hypothesis is also advanced suggesting that even if a body was cloned, the brain, which is the essence of humanity, would remain unique. This author suggests that the debate should be changed from "Is cloning wrong?" to "When is cloning wrong?".

Loder, Natasha. Allow cloning in embryo research, says UK report. [News]. *Nature.* 1998 Dec 10; 396(6711): 503. BE59540.
> advisory committees; *cloning; *embryo research; *government regulation; public participation; *public policy; stem cells; *Great Britain; Human Fertilisation and Embryology Authority; Human Genetics Advisory Commission (Great Britain)

McCarthy, David. Persons and their copies. *Journal of*

BE = bioethics accession number   fn. = footnotes   refs. = references

Medical Ethics. 1999 Apr; 25(2): 98-104. 8 fn. BE61910.
  *autonomy; *cloning; ethical theory; genetic determinism; genetic identity; genetic information; injuries; *moral policy; personhood; reproductive technologies; harms; Kant, Immanuel

Is cloning human beings morally wrong? The basis for the one serious objection to cloning is that, because of what a clone is, clones would have much worse lives than non-clones. I sketch a fragment of moral theory to make sense of the objection. I then outline several ways in which it might be claimed that, because of what a clone is, clones would have much worse lives than non-clones. In particular, I look at various ideas connected with autonomy. I conclude that there is no basis to the claim that, because of what a clone is, clones would have much worse lives than non-clones. I therefore reject the claim that cloning human beings is morally wrong.

McMahan, Jeff. Cloning, killing, and identity. *Journal of Medical Ethics.* 1999 Apr; 25(2): 77-86. 8 fn. BE61907.
  *beginning of life; brain; *cloning; embryos; fetal development; fetuses; *killing; *moral policy; organ donation; *personhood; philosophy; self concept; tissue donation; twinning; twins; conjoined twins; nuclear transplantation; personal identity

One potentially valuable use of cloning is to provide a source of tissues or organs for transplantation. The most important objection to this use of cloning is that a human clone would be the sort of entity that it would be seriously wrong to kill. I argue that entities of the sort that you and I essentially are do not begin to exist until around the seventh month of fetal gestation. Therefore to kill a clone prior to that would not be to kill someone like you or me but would be only to prevent one of us from existing. And even after one of us begins to exist, the objections to killing it remain comparatively weak until its psychological capacities reach a certain level of maturation. These claims support the permissibility of killing a clone during the early stages of its development in order to use its organs for transplantation.

Madigan, Timothy J. Cloning and human dignity. [Editorial]. *Free Inquiry.* 1998 Spring; 18(2): 57-58. BE60447.
  *cloning; reproductive technologies; dignity

Malinowski, Michael J. Regulation of genetic modification of organisms: science or emotion? *Journal of Biolaw and Business.* 1998 Spring; 1(3): 3-7. 49 fn. BE62091.
  advisory committees; *cloning; drugs; federal government; food; *government regulation; human experimentation; international aspects; *public policy; *recombinant DNA research; *regulation; reproductive technologies; risks and benefits; *transgenic organisms; agriculture; Department of Agriculture; Environmental Protection Agency; European Union; Food and Drug Administration; National Bioethics Advisory Commission; *United States

Marlin, George J. Eugenics and cloning. *In: his* The Politician's Guide to Assisted Suicide, Cloning, and Other Current Controversies. Washington, DC: Morley Books; 1998: 125-168, 212-216. 146 fn. ISBN 0-9660597-1-9. BE62396.
  body parts and fluids; *cloning; commodification; determination of death; *eugenics; historical aspects; involuntary sterilization; killing; *legal aspects; National Socialism; organ donation; parent child relationship; personhood; reproduction; reproductive technologies; social discrimination; social worth; socioeconomic factors; Germany; United States

Matthews, Hugh. British public opposes human cloning. [News]. *BMJ (British Medical Journal).* 1998 Dec 12; 317(7173): 1613. BE61093.
  *cloning; embryo research; *public opinion; reproductive technologies; *Great Britain

Mayor, Susan. UK authorities recommend human cloning for therapeutic research. [News]. *BMJ (British Medical Journal).* 1998 Dec 12; 317(7173): 1613. BE61301.
  advisory committees; *cloning; *embryo research; *government regulation; *public policy; reproductive technologies; therapeutic research; nuclear transplantation; *Great Britain; Human Fertilisation and Embryology Authority; Human Genetics Advisory Commission (Great Britain)

Meade, Harry M. Dairy gene. *Sciences.* 1997 Sep-Oct; 37(5): 20-25. BE61519.
  *cloning; drug industry; drugs; *economics; *methods; *risks and benefits; *transgenic animals

Meilaender, Gilbert. Begetting and cloning. *First Things.* 1997 Jun-Jul; No. 74: 41-43. Remarks presented to the National Bioethics Advisory Commission on 13 Mar 1997. BE60102.
  *cloning; love; motivation; *Protestant ethics; reproduction; reproductive technologies; research embryo creation; sexuality; theology

Michael, Adam. Europe/Japan face up to legal hurdles to cloning. [News]. *Nature Biotechnology.* 1997 Jul; 15(7): 609-610. BE62019.
  advisory committees; *cloning; embryo research; *government regulation; *international aspects; legislation; reproductive technologies; *Europe; Group of Advisers on the Ethical Implications of Biotechnology (European Commission); *Japan

Moraczewski, Albert S. Cloning testimony. *Ethics and Medics.* 1997 May; 22(5): 3-4. Modified text of testimony delivered before the National Bioethics Advisory Commission on 13 Mar 1997. BE60410.
  *cloning; risks and benefits; *Roman Catholic ethics; dignity

Murphy, Timothy F. Entitlement to cloning: response to "Cloning and infertilty" by Carson Strong (*CQ*, 1998 Summer; 7(3): 279-293). *Cambridge Quarterly of Healthcare Ethics.* 1999 Summer; 8(3): 364-368. 15 refs. BE62354.
  children; *cloning; females; *homosexuals; *infertility; injuries; males; methods; parent child relationship; reproduction; reproductive technologies; rights; *selection for treatment; harms; nuclear transplantation

Nader, Claire; Newman, Stuart A. Human cloning. [Letter]. *Science.* 1998 Dec 4; 282(5395): 1824-1825. 4 refs. BE60089.
  advisory committees; *cloning; decision making; government regulation; guidelines; public participation; recombinant DNA research; *regulation; self regulation; National Bioethics Advisory Commission; United States

Nash, J. Madeleine. Cloning's Kevorkian. [News]. *Time.* 1998 Jan 19; 151(2): 58. BE59163.
  *cloning; investigators; reproductive technologies; *Seed, Richard

Nash, J. Madeleine. The case for cloning. [News]. *Time.* 1998 Feb 9; 151(5): 81. BE59165.
  *cloning; genetic disorders; genetic enhancement; government regulation; *risks and benefits; tissue donation; United States

---

BE = bioethics accession number   fn. = footnotes   refs. = references

National Bioethics Advisory Commission. Cloning Human Beings: Report and Recommendations of the National Bioethics Advisory Commission. Executive Summary. Rockville, MD: The Commission; 1997 Jun. 5 p. BE61050.

advisory committees; biomedical research; *cloning; embryo research; embryo transfer; family relationship; federal government; freedom; government financing; government regulation; human experimentation; industry; methods; *moral policy; *organizational policies; private sector; *public policy; public sector; reproductive technologies; *risks and benefits; self regulation; values; *nuclear transplantation; *National Bioethics Advisory Commission; *United States

National Bioethics Advisory Commission. Cloning Human Beings: Report and Recommendations of the National Bioethics Advisory Commission. Volumme II: Commission Papers. Rockville, MD: The Commission; 1997 Jun. 289 p. Includes references. Papers by S.H. Orkin, J. Rossant, E. Eiseman, C.S. Campbell, D.W. Brock, L.B. Andrews, B.M. Knoppers, and R.M. Cook-Deegan. BE61049.

advisory committees; animal experimentation; autonomy; biomedical research; children; *cloning; constitutional law; cultural pluralism; embryo research; embryo transfer; federal government; freedom; genetic identity; government regulation; human experimentation; industry; international aspects; legal aspects; methods; moral policy; organizational policies; parent child relationship; private sector; professional organizations; public policy; public sector; religious ethics; reproduction; reproductive technologies; research embryo creation; *risks and benefits; self regulation; social impact; state government; terminology; theology; twinning; values; *nuclear transplantation; National Bioethics Advisory Commission; *United States

Newman, Stuart A. Cloning our way to "the next level." *Nature Biotechnology.* 1997 Jun; 15(6): 488. 7 refs. BE62016.

attitudes; *cloning; reproductive technologies; *risks and benefits; social impact

Newman, Stuart A. Human cloning and the law. *Journal of Biolaw and Business.* 1998 Spring; 1(3): 59-62. 22 fn. BE62094.

advisory committees; *cloning; embryo research; federal government; genetic identity; germ cells; government financing; *government regulation; *legal aspects; public policy; reproductive technologies; Europe; National Bioethics Advisory Commission; United States

Norris, Patrick. Sheep cloning: what next? *Health Care Ethics USA.* 1997 Spring; 5(2): 6-7. 3 refs. BE61724.

animal experimentation; *cloning; reproductive technologies; risks and benefits

Nussbaum, Martha C.; Sunstein, Cass R., eds. Clones and Clones: Facts and Fantasies about Human Cloning. New York, NY: Norton; 1998. 351 p. Includes references. ISBN 0-393-04648-6. BE60358.

advisory committees; *cloning; eugenics; females; government regulation; homosexuals; legal aspects; literature; males; methods; moral policy; motivation; public policy; religious ethics; reproduction; risks and benefits; social control; social impact; twins; values; National Bioethics Advisory Commission

Orr, Robert D. The temptation of human cloning. *Today's Christian Doctor.* 1997 Fall; 28(3): 4-7. BE60420.

*Christian ethics; *cloning; morality

Pardo, Antonio. Human cloning. *Dolentium Hominum: Church and Health in the World.* 1997; 36(12th Yr., No.

3): 28-31. 19 fn. BE60597.

animal experimentation; *cloning; deontological ethics; embryo research; public policy; reproductive technologies; risks and benefits; transgenic animals; Europe; United States

Parker, Lisa S. Reproduction: *Who's Afraid of Human Cloning?* by Gregory E. Pence. [Book review essay]. *JAMA.* 1998 Nov 25; 280(20): 1798-1799. BE59603.

advisory committees; autonomy; *cloning; emotions; females; philosophy; *public policy; religion; reproductive technologies; risks and benefits; values; National Bioethics Advisory Commission; *Who's Afraid of Human Cloning? (Pence, G.E.)

Pence, Gregory E.; Smolkin, Mitchell T.; Effros, Richard M., et al. Human cloning. [Letters and responses]. *New England Journal of Medicine.* 1998 Nov 19; 339(21): 1558-1559. 7 refs. BE61712.

*cloning; dehumanization; federal government; freedom; genetic enhancement; government regulation; investigators; legal aspects; *public policy; reproduction; reproductive technologies; *risks and benefits; social control; twins; *United States

Posner, Eric A.; Posner, Richard A. The demand for human cloning. *In:* Nussbaum, Martha C.; Sunstein, Cass R., eds. Clones and Clones: Facts and Fantasies About Human Cloning. New York, NY: Norton; 1998: 233-261. 33 fn. ISBN 0-393-04648-6. BE60364.

*cloning; eugenics; evolution; females; future generations; genetic diversity; government regulation; infertility; males; marital relationship; married persons; models, theoretical; *motivation; parent child relationship; public policy; *reproduction; reproductive technologies; risks and benefits; single persons; *social impact; socioeconomic factors

Rae, Scott B. Ethical issues and concerns about human cloning. *In:* Demy, Timothy J.; Stewart, Gary P., eds. Genetic Engineering: A Christian Response: Crucial Considerations in Shaping Life. Grand Rapids, MI: Kregel Publications; 1999: 278-292. 16 fn. ISBN 0-8254-2357-0. BE61371.

adults; bone marrow; Christian ethics; *cloning; commodification; criminal law; embryo disposition; *embryo research; *embryo transfer; *embryos; family members; genetic diversity; genetic identity; in vitro fertilization; industry; intention; international aspects; personhood; preimplantation diagnosis; reproduction; tissue donation; *twinning; personal identity; Ayala, Anissa; Ayala, Marissa; Europe

Ramsay, Sarah. Call to strengthen UK ban on human clones. [News]. *Lancet.* 1998 Dec 12; 352(9144): 1917. BE61104.

advisory committees; *cloning; embryo research; *government regulation; *public policy; reproductive technologies; nuclear transplantation; *Great Britain; Human Fertilisation and Embryology Authority; Human Genetics Advisory Commission (Great Britain)

Roberts, Melinda A. Child versus Childmaker: Future Persons and Present Duties in Ethics and the Law. Lanham, MD: Rowman and Littlefield; 1998. 235 p. (Studies in social, political, and legal philosophy). Bibliography: p. 221-226. ISBN 0-8476-8901-8. BE59868.

children; *cloning; congenital disorders; constitutional law; embryos; freedom; *future generations; injuries; justice; legal aspects; *moral obligations; negligence; philosophy; privacy; quality of life; *reproduction; reproductive technologies; suffering; *teleological ethics; torts; value of life; *wrongful life; Broome, John; Fourteenth Amendment; United States

Robertson, Stephen. The ethics of human cloning.

BE = bioethics accession number   fn. = footnotes   refs. = references

[Letter]. *Journal of Medical Ethics.* 1998 Aug; 24(4): 282. 1 ref. BE62064.
　　autonomy; *cloning; deontological ethics; embryo research; eugenics; intention; preimplantation diagnosis; prenatal diagnosis; reproduction; reproductive technologies; risks and benefits; twinning

Roscam Abbing, Henriette D.C. New developments in international health law. *European Journal of Health Law.* 1998 Jun; 5(2): 155–169. Includes text of the Universal Declaration on the Human Genome and Human Rights, p. 163–167. BE60901.
　　animal organs; *cloning; communicable diseases; genetic intervention; *genetic research; *genome mapping; *guidelines; *human rights; *international aspects; *regulation; risks and benefits; *tissue transplantation; Council of Europe; *Europe; European Union; Unesco; *Universal Declaration on the Human Genome and Human Rights; World Health Organization

Rushbrooke, Rupert. Knowing me isn't knowing you. *Splice of Life.* 1998 Mar–Apr; 4(4): 6–7. BE59857.
　　adoption; children; *cloning; deception; family relationship; *self concept

Saegusa, Asako. Japan to ban human cloning. [News]. *Nature Medicine.* 1998 Sep; 4(9): 993. BE62174.
　　advisory committees; animal experimentation; *cloning; ethical review; *government regulation; guidelines; human experimentation; research institutes; universities; Council for Science and Technology (Japan); *Japan; Science Council (Japan)

Saegusa, Asako. South Korean researchers under fire for claims of human cloning. [News]. *Nature.* 1998 Dec 24–31; 396(6713): 713. BE59587.
　　attitudes; *cloning; embryo research; government regulation; investigators; methods; reproductive technologies; *Korea

Savulescu, Julian. Should doctors intentionally do less than the best? *Journal of Medical Ethics.* 1999 Apr; 25(2): 121–126. 11 fn. BE61914.
　　artificial insemination; *autonomy; *beneficence; *cloning; *congenital disorders; conscience; *decision making; disabled; *embryo transfer; eugenics; freedom; *genetic disorders; *goals; in vitro fertilization; *medicine; mentally retarded; *moral complicity; *moral obligations; moral policy; *motivation; parent child relationship; *parents; *patients; *physicians; *preimplantation diagnosis; *quality of life; refusal to treat; *reproduction; *reproductive technologies; rights; selection for treatment; sex preselection; suffering; *values; rationality
The papers of Burley and Harris, and Draper and Chadwick, in this issue, raise a problem: what should doctors do when patients request an option which is not the best available? This commentary argues that doctors have a duty to offer that option which will result in the individual affected by that choice enjoying the highest level of wellbeing. Doctors can deviate from this duty and submaximise -- bring about an outcome that is less than the best -- only if there are good reasons to do so. The desire to have a child which is genetically related provides little, if any, reason to submaximise. The implication for cloning, preimplantation diagnosis and embryo transfer is that doctors should only produce a clone or transfer embryos expected to enjoy a level of wellbeing which is less than that enjoyed by other children the couple could have, if there is a good reason to employ that technology. This paper sketches what might constitute a good reason to submaximise.

Savulescu, Julian. Should we clone human beings? Cloning as a source of tissue for transplantation. *Journal of Medical Ethics.* 1999 Apr; 25(2): 87–95. 45 fn. BE61908.
　　aborted fetuses; abortion, induced; autonomy; beginning of life; beneficence; bone marrow; *cloning; embryo research; fetal tissue donation; killing; *moral obligations; *moral policy; *motivation; organ transplantation; personhood; reproductive technologies; risks and benefits; stem cells; tissue banks; tissue transplantation; nuclear transplantation
The most publicly justifiable application of human cloning, if there is one at all, is to provide self-compatible cells or tissues for medical use, especially transplantation. Some have argued that this raises no new ethical issues above those raised by any form of embryo experimentation. I argue that this research is less morally problematic than other embryo research. Indeed, it is not merely morally permissible but morally required that we employ cloning to produce embryos or fetuses for the sake of providing cells, tissues or even organs for therapy, followed by abortion of the embryo or fetus.

Shapiro, David. Think before you squawk. *New Scientist.* 1997 Aug 2; 155(2093): 47. BE60457.
　　*advisory committees; *cloning; evaluation; government regulation; *international aspects; politics; public policy; France; Germany; Great Britain; United States

Solter, Davor. Dolly *is* a clone -- and no longer alone. [News]. *Nature.* 1998 Jul 23; 394(6691): 315–316. 12 refs. BE59937.
　　animal experimentation; *cloning; genetic research; methods; reproductive technologies; risks and benefits; stem cells; nuclear transplantation; rodents

Sunstein, Cass R. The Constitution and the clone. *In:* Nussbaum, Martha C.; Sunstein, Cass R., eds. Clones and Clones: Facts and Fantasies About Human Cloning. New York, NY: Norton; 1998: 207–220. ISBN 0–393–04648–6. BE60362.
　　*cloning; constitutional law; *government regulation; *legal aspects; *legal rights; privacy; reproduction; *state interest; Supreme Court decisions; United States

Tattam, Amanda. Australia considers human cloning for therapeutic purposes. [News]. *Lancet.* 1999 Mar 27; 353(9158): 1076. BE61984.
　　biomedical research; *cloning; embryo research; germ cells; *organizational policies; professional organizations; public policy; regulation; stem cells; *Australia; *Australian Academy of Science

Tiefel, Hans O. Human cloning in ethical perspectives. *In:* Humber, James M.; Almeder, Robert F.,eds. Human Cloning. Totowa, NJ: Humana Press; 1998: 177–207. 17 refs. 34 fn. ISBN 0–89603–565–4. BE59469.
　　attitudes; children; *cloning; communitarianism; personhood; reproduction; reproductive technologies; rights; risks and benefits; liberalism; United States

Tooley, Michael. The moral status of the cloning of humans. *In:* Humber, James M.;Almeder, Robert F.,eds. Human Cloning. Totowa, NJ: Humana Press; 1998: 65–101. 17 refs. 15 fn. ISBN 0–89603–565–4. BE59466.
　　abortion, induced; autonomy; behavioral genetics; brain; *cloning; *ethical analysis; eugenics; genetic determinism; *genetic identity; *goals; homosexuals; infertility; killing; methods; *moral policy; *motivation; organ donation; personhood; philosophy; reproductive technologies; rights; *risks and benefits; suffering; tissue donation; twins

Tracy, David. Human cloning and the public realm: a defense of intuitions of the good. *In:* Nussbaum, Martha C.; Sunstein, Cass R., eds. Clones and Clones: Facts and Fantasies About Human Cloning. New York, NY:

BE = bioethics accession number　　　　fn. = footnotes　　　refs. = references

Norton; 1998: 190–203. ISBN 0–393–0468–6. BE60361.
*cloning; commodification; consensus; cultural pluralism; human rights; international aspects; morality; religion; religious ethics; *values

Tribe, Laurence. On not banning cloning for the wrong reasons. *In:* Nussbaum, Martha C.; Sunstein, Cass R., eds. Clones and Clones: Facts and Fantasies About Human Cloning. New York, NY: Norton; 1998: 221–232. 13 fn. ISBN 0–393–04648–6. BE60363.
biomedical technologies; *cloning; dehumanization; genetic intervention; *government regulation; privacy; *public policy; reproduction; reproductive technologies; single persons; social control; stigmatization; values

U.S. Congress. House. Committee on Commerce. Subcommittee on Health and Environment. Cloning: Legal, Medical, Ethical, and Social Issues. Hearing, 12 Feb 1998. Washington, DC: U.S. Government Printing Office; 1998. 141 p. Serial No. 105–70. ISBN 0–16–056510–3. BE62739.
advisory committees; *cloning; embryo research; embryos; federal government; *government regulation; moral policy; *public policy; religious ethics; reproductive technologies; research embryo creation; *risks and benefits; stem cells; nuclear transplantation; National Bioethics Advisory Commission; *United States

Vial Correa, Juan de Dios; Sgreccia, Elio; Pontifical Academy for Life. Reflections on cloning. [English translation]. *Origins.* 1998 May 21; 28(1): 14–16. Translation of the Pontifical Academy for Life's Statement on cloning issues 25 Jun 1997 in Italian in *L'Osservatore Romano.* BE59813.
biomedical research; *cloning; embryo research; family relationship; freedom; reproductive technologies; *Roman Catholic ethics; *Pontifical Academy for Life

Wadman, Meredith. Cloned mice fail to rekindle ethics debate. [News]. *Nature.* 1998 Jul 30; 394(6692): 408–409. Includes inset article by A. Saegusa, "Japanese fear that new publicity rules could hinder their ressearch," p. 408. BE59938.
advisory committees; *cloning; federal government; *government regulation; industry; legislation; public policy; reproductive technologies; Japan; rodents; U.S. Congress; *United States

Wadman, Meredith. Cloning without human clones. [News]. *Wall Street Journal.* 1998 Jan 20: A18. BE59570.
*cloning; embryo research; federal government; genetic research; government financing; *government regulation; reproductive technologies; state government; *United States

Watts, Jonathan; Morris, Kelly. Human cloning trial met with outrage and scepticism. [News]. *Lancet.* 1999 Jan 2; 353(9146): 43. BE61083.
attitudes; *cloning; embryo research; human experimentation; investigators; methods; nuclear transplantation; Korea

Watts, Jonathan. Japan dashes Seed's plans for clone clinic. [News]. *Lancet.* 1998 Dec 12; 352(9144): 1917. BE61105.
*cloning; government regulation; *health facilities; human experimentation; international aspects; investigators; private sector; reproductive technologies; *Japan; *Seed, Richard

Watts, Jonathan. Japan proposes ban on human cloning. [News]. *Lancet.* 1998 Aug 8; 352(9126): 465. BE61304.
advisory committees; *cloning; embryo research; *government regulation; *Japan; Science Council (Japan)

Williamson, Robert. Human reproductive cloning is unethical because it undermines autonomy: commentary on Savulescu. *Journal of Medical Ethics.* 1999 Apr; 25(2): 96–97. 4 refs. BE61909.
autonomy; behavioral genetics; *cloning; genetic diversity; genetic identity; moral policy; motivation; reproductive technologies; stem cells; tissue donation

Wilmut, Ian. Dolly's false legacy. *Time.* 1999 Jan 11; 153(1): 74, 76–77. BE60316.
adults; children; *cloning; family relationship; famous persons; parents; regulation; risks and benefits; treatment outcome

Young, Frank E. Worldviews in conflict: human cloning and embryo manipulation. *In:* Demy, Timothy J.; Stewart, Gary P., eds. Genetic Engineering: A Christian Response: Crucial Considerations in Shaping Life. Grand Rapids, MI: Kregel Publications; 1999: 70–86. 41 fn. ISBN 0–8254–2357–0. BE61361.
American Indians; beginning of life; blacks; Buddhist ethics; *Christian ethics; *cloning; decision making; Eastern Orthodox ethics; *embryo research; ethical relativism; eugenics; fetal development; government regulation; Hindu ethics; hybrids; interdisciplinary communication; investigators; Jewish ethics; killing; personhood; Protestant ethics; public participation; *public policy; quality of life; *religious ethics; resource allocation; Roman Catholic ethics; secularism; self regulation; *social impact; theology; value of life; nuclear transplantation; Evangelical Christians; United States

Zaner, Richard M. Surprise! You're just like me! Reflections on cloning, eugenics, and other utopias. *In:* Humber, James M.; Almeder, Robert F.,eds. Human Cloning. Totowa, NJ: Humana Press; 1998: 103–151. 113 fn. ISBN 0–89603–565–4. BE59467.
attitudes; biomedical research; biomedical technologies; *cloning; eugenics; genetic identity; genetic intervention; genetic research; genome mapping; government regulation; mass media; medicine; personhood; privacy; reproductive technologies; *risks and benefits; science; social impact; wedge argument

Adult cloning marches on. [Editorial]. *Nature.* 1998 Jul 23; 394(6691): 303. BE59935.
*cloning; federal government; government regulation; industry; methods; private sector; reproductive technologies; United States

Australian call for repeal of restrictive cloning laws. [News]. *Nature.* 1999 Apr 15; 398(6728): 552. BE61731.
*cloning; embryo research; *government regulation; state government; *Australia

Churches condemn plan to clone humans. [News]. *Christian Science Monitor.* 1998 Jan 13: 13. BE59561.
*cloning; Protestant ethics; *religion; Anglican Church; Great Britain; Methodist Church; Seed, Richard; United States

Cloning a human cell. [Editorial]. *New York Times.* 1998 Dec 18: A34. BE60644.
*cloning; reproductive technologies; Korea

First principles in cloning. [Editorial]. *Lancet.* 1999 Jan 9; 353(9147): 81. BE61106.
*cloning; embryo research; human rights; international aspects; investigators; reproductive technologies; Korea

Hello, Dolly. [Editorial]. *Economist.* 1997 Mar 1: 17–18. BE60349.
*cloning; eugenics; *risks and benefits; twins

BE = bioethics accession number   fn. = footnotes   refs. = references

Japan bans human cloning. [News]. *Nature Biotechnology.* 1998 Sep; 16(9): 803. BE62043.
   advisory committees; *cloning; embryo research; *government regulation; guidelines; legal aspects; *Japan; Science Council (Japan)

CODES OF ETHICS
See under
   BIOETHICS/CODES OF ETHICS
   MEDICAL ETHICS/CODES OF ETHICS
   PROFESSIONAL ETHICS/CODES OF ETHICS

CONFIDENTIALITY

See also PATIENT ACCESS TO RECORDS
See also under
   AIDS/CONFIDENTIALITY

Allen, Arthur. Exposed: why doctor-patient confidentiality isn't what it used to be. *Washington Post Magazine.* 1998 Feb 8: 11–15, 27–32. BE59371.
   computer communication networks; *confidentiality; *disclosure; employment; genetic information; genetic screening; health insurance; insurance selection bias; law enforcement; legal aspects; managed care programs; *medical records; privacy; psychotherapy; United States

American Association of Occupational Health Nurses; American College of Occupational and Environmental Medicine. AAOHN and ACOEM consensus statement for confidentiality of employee health information. *AAOHN Journal (American Association of Occupational Health Nurses).* 1997 Nov; 45(11): 613. Approved by the Board of Directors of both organizations on 4 May 1997. BE59926.
   *confidentiality; disclosure; employment; informed consent; law enforcement; legal aspects; *medical records; *nurses; *occupational medicine; *organizational policies; *physicians; professional organizations; public health; *American Association of Occupational Health Nurses; *American College of Occupational and Environmental Medicine; United States

American College of Healthcare Executives. Health information confidentiality: ethical policy statement, November 1997. *Journal of the American Health Information Management Association.* 1998 Mar; 69(3): 27. Originated Feb 1994; revised Nov 1997; approved by the Board of Governors 2 Nov 1997. BE60432.
   *administrators; computers; *confidentiality; *guidelines; health care; health facilities; institutional policies; legal aspects; *medical records; *organizational policies; patient access to records; professional organizations; *American College of Healthcare Executives; United States

Boetzkes, Elisabeth. Genetic knowledge and third-party interests. *Cambridge Quarterly of Healthcare Ethics.* 1999 Summer; 8(3): 386–392. 12 fn. BE62481.
   carriers; children; communitarianism; *confidentiality; decision making; *disclosure; *family members; females; genetic disorders; *genetic information; genetic predisposition; *genetic screening; health personnel; informed consent; moral obligations; professional patient relationship; reproduction; standards; values; *harms; *negotiation

Butler, Dennis J.; Edwards, Ann; Tzelepis, Angela, et al. Informed consent for videotaping. [Letter and response]. *Academic Medicine.* 1996 Dec; 71(12): 1276–1277. 1 ref. BE61376.
   *audiovisual aids; *confidentiality; disclosure; *informed consent; internship and residency; *medical education; physician patient relationship; privacy; teaching methods; *video recording

Clayton, Paul D. Improving the privacy and security of electronic health information. *Academic Medicine.* 1997 Jun; 72(6): 522–523. BE61433.
   advisory committees; *computer communication networks; *computers; *confidentiality; federal government; government regulation; information dissemination; institutional policies; *medical records; organizational policies; privacy; *public policy; standards; *computer security; Department of Health and Human Services; Health Insurance Portability and Accountability Act 1996; National Research Council; *United States

Denley, Ian; Smith, Simon Weston; Gardner, Martin, et al. Privacy in clinical information systems in secondary care. [Article and commentaries]. *BMJ (British Medical Journal).* 1999 May 15; 318(7194): 1328–1331. 5 refs. BE62518.
   computer communication networks; *computers; *confidentiality; guidelines; health services research; *hospitals; *institutional policies; *medical records; patient care; patient care team; privacy; professional patient relationship; *computer security; *Great Britain; *National Health Service

Doyal, Len. Human need and the right of patients to privacy. *Journal of Contemporary Health Law and Policy.* 1997 Fall; 14(1): 1–21. 55 fn. BE60877.
   abortion, induced; allowing to die; *autonomy; common good; *confidentiality; disclosure; domestic violence; ethical analysis; freedom; health; human rights; injuries; legal aspects; moral obligations; *moral policy; paternalism; physicians; *privacy; professional patient relationship; regulation; right to die; *rights; truth disclosure; utilitarianism; *needs; General Medical Council (Great Britain); *Great Britain; *United States

Etzioni, Amitai. Medical records: big brother versus big bucks. *In: his* The Limits of Privacy. New York, NY: Basic Books; 1999: 139–182, 248–258. 139 fn. ISBN 0–465–04089–6. BE62443.
   biomedical research; common good; *communitarianism; computers; *confidentiality; consent forms; data banks; *disclosure; employment; government regulation; health facilities; health insurance; health services research; informed consent; institutional policies; law enforcement; *medical records; methods; policy analysis; presumed consent; *privacy; private sector; public health; public policy; risks and benefits; self regulation; computer security; United States

Etzioni, Amitai. Medical records: enhancing privacy, preserving the common good. *Hastings Center Report.* 1999 Mar–Apr; 29(2): 14–23. 53 fn. BE61656.
   advertising; coercion; *common good; communitarianism; computer communication networks; computers; *confidentiality; consent forms; *data banks; *disclosure; employment; epidemiology; fraud; genetic information; health insurance; health services research; industry; informed consent; law enforcement; libertarianism; life insurance; managed care programs; mass media; *medical records; mental health; methods; misconduct; organization and administration; patient access to records; patient care team; presumed consent; *privacy; public opinion; public policy; quality of health care; records; remuneration; *trends; computer security; patient identifiers; quality assurance; utilization review; *United States
Personal medical information is now bought and sold on the open market. Companies use it to make hiring and firing decisions and to identify customers for new products. The justification for providing such access to medical information is that doing so benefits the public by securing public safety, controlling costs, and

---

supporting medical research. And individuals have supposedly consented to it. But we can achieve the common goods while better protecting privacy by making institutional changes in the way information is maintained and protected.

Flegel, Kenneth M.; Lant, Mary. Sound privacy for patients. [Editorial]. *Canadian Medical Association Journal.* 1998 Mar 10; 158(5): 613–614. 7 refs. BE60031.
   *communication; *confidentiality; *hospitals; patient care; physicians; *privacy

Freudenheim, Milt. Medicine at the click of a mouse: on-line health files are convenient; are they private? [News]. *New York Times.* 1998 Aug 12: Business 1,8. BE61117.
   attitudes; communication; *computer communication networks; *confidentiality; health care delivery; health facilities; hospitals; informed consent; *medical records; patients; physicians; privacy; risks and benefits; computer security; Internet

Gillon, Raanan. Confidentiality. *In:* Kuhse, Helga; Singer, Peter, eds. A Companion to Bioethics. Malden, MA: Blackwell; 1998: 425–431. 15 refs. ISBN 0–631–19737–0. BE59515.
   autonomy; beneficence; *confidentiality; disclosure; duty to warn; medical ethics; moral obligations; moral policy; patient care; physician patient relationship; privacy; risks and benefits; trust

Goldworth, Amnon. Informed consent in the genetic age. *Cambridge Quarterly of Healthcare Ethics.* 1999 Summer; 8(3): 393–400. 15 fn. BE62482.
   *autonomy; breast cancer; *cancer; *confidentiality; cultural pluralism; *disclosure; family members; genetic counseling; *genetic information; genetic predisposition; *genetic screening; *informed consent; physician patient relationship; risk; risks and benefits; standards; trust

Goodman, Kenneth W. A DiMaggio rule on medical privacy. *New York Times.* 1998 Dec 30: A17. BE60969.
   *confidentiality; *disclosure; famous persons; *health; mass media; physicians; privacy

Goodman, Kenneth W. Critical care computing: outcomes, confidentiality, and appropriate use. *Critical Care Clinics.* 1996 Jan; 12(1): 109–122. 36 refs. BE59281.
   allowing to die; *computer communication networks; *computers; *confidentiality; *critically ill; data banks; decision analysis; *decision making; disclosure; epidemiology; evaluation; *futility; health services research; HIV seropositivity; informed consent; intensive care units; medical records; *patient care; physicians; privacy; *prognosis; research subjects; resource allocation; *statistics; *treatment outcome; truth disclosure; *uncertainty; withholding treatment; severity of illness index

Gostin, Lawrence O.; Hadley, Jack. Health services research: public benefits, personal privacy, and proprietary interests. [Editorial]. *Annals of Internal Medicine.* 1998 Nov 15; 129(10): 833–835. 15 refs. BE59325.
   computer communication networks; *confidentiality; data banks; disclosure; economics; federal government; government regulation; *health services research; industry; informed consent; managed care programs; medical records; *privacy; private sector; standards; Health Insurance Portability and Accountability Act 1996; United States

Healy, Bernadine. Hippocrates vs. Big Brother. *New York Times.* 1998 Jul 24: A25. BE61116.
   biomedical research; *computer communication networks; *confidentiality; data banks; epidemiology; federal government; health care delivery; informed consent; legislation; *medical records; physician patient relationship; privacy; *public policy; Health Insurance Portability and Accountability Act 1996; *United States

Holm, Søren; Rossel, Peter. Ethical aspects of the use of 'sensitive information' in health care research. *In:* Bennett, Rebecca; Erin, Charles A., eds. HIV and AIDS: Testing, Screening, and Confidentiality. New York, NY: Oxford University Press; 1999: 200–215. 12 fn. ISBN 0–19–823801–0. BE62723.
   *confidentiality; *epidemiology; HIV seropositivity; medical records; privacy; property rights; *registries; harms; integrity; Denmark

Kirsch, Michael; Rothschild, Bruce M.; Ridzon, Renée, et al. Patient consent for publication. [Letters and responses]. *JAMA.* 1997 Dec 24–31; 278(24): 2139–2141. 9 refs. BE60135.
   authorship; autonomy; *confidentiality; *disclosure; *editorial policies; *epidemiology; guidelines; health services research; human experimentation; *information dissemination; *informed consent; justice; obligations to society; patient participation; *patients; *privacy; professional organizations; public health; *research subjects; International Committee of Medical Journal Editors

Lasby, Clarence G. Eisenhower's Heart Attack: How Ike Beat Heart Disease and Held on to the Presidency. Lawrence, KS: University Press of Kansas; 1997. 384 p. Bibliography: p. 369–376. ISBN 0–7006–0822–2. BE60508.
   *confidentiality; *deception; disclosure; *famous persons; *health; *heart diseases; historical aspects; mass media; patient care; physicians; *politics; professional competence; *Eisenhower, Dwight; *Twentieth Century; United States

Mathews, Steve. Protection of personal data -- the European view. *Journal of the American Health Information Management Association.* 1998 Mar; 69(3): 42–44. 3 fn. BE60434.
   computer communication networks; computers; *confidentiality; international aspects; legal aspects; *medical records; patient access to records; patients; *public policy; standards; computer security; *Europe; European Union; European Union Directive on the Protection of Personal Data; United States

Mitka, Mike. Do-it-yourself report on patient privacy. [News]. *JAMA.* 1998 Dec 9; 280(22): 1897. BE59691.
   accountability; *confidentiality; disclosure; government regulation; health facilities; health services research; informed consent; institutional policies; law enforcement; *managed care programs; medical records; organizational policies; physicians; privacy; professional organizations; self regulation; standards; American Medical Association; Joint Commission on Accreditation of Healthcare Organizations; National Committee for Quality Assurance; United States

Mlinek, Edward J.; Pierce, Jessica. Confidentiality and privacy breaches in a university hospital emergency department. *Academic Emergency Medicine.* 1997 Dec; 4(12): 1142–1146. 12 refs. BE59125.
   *confidentiality; *disclosure; *emergency care; guideline adherence; guidelines; *hospitals; *knowledge, attitudes, practice; *patient care team; *privacy; statistics; survey; prospective studies; University of Nebraska Medical Center

Pouloudi, Athanasia. Conflicting concerns over the privacy of electronic medical records in the NHSnet. *Business Ethics: A European Review.* 1997 Apr; 6(2): 94–101. 35 refs. BE59794.
   *computer communication networks; *confidentiality; data banks; decision making; disclosure; health care delivery;

BE = bioethics accession number   fn. = footnotes   refs. = references

*medical records; organization and administration; patient participation; physicians; privacy; professional organizations; computer security; British Medical Association; *Great Britain; *National Health Service; *NHSnet

Rabinowitz, Jonathan. A method for preserving confidentiality when linking computerized registries. [Letter]. *American Journal of Public Health.* 1998 May; 88(5): 836. BE60780.
*computers; *confidentiality; *epidemiology; methods; morbidity; *registries; *computer security

Rayner, John D. Medical confidentiality. *In: his* Jewish Religious Law: A Progressive Perspective. New York, NY: Berghahn Books; 1998: 116–123. ISBN 1–57181–976–2. BE62134.
codes of ethics; *confidentiality; conscience; *disclosure; duty to warn; *Jewish ethics; medical ethics; physicians; *Reform Judaism

Regan, Priscilla M. Genetic testing and workplace surveillance: implications for privacy. *In:* Lyon, David; Zureik, Elia, eds. Computers, Surveillance, and Privacy. Minneapolis, MN: University of Minnesota Press; 1996: 21–46. 54 refs. 10 fn. ISBN 0–8166–2653–7. BE62133.
computer communication networks; *confidentiality; *employment; evaluation; genetic information; genetic predisposition; *genetic screening; insurance; legal aspects; *privacy; public opinion; *public policy; records; *values; United States

Roberts, John; Decter, Sheila R.; Nagel, Denise, et al. Confidentiality and electronic medical records. [Letter and response]. *Annals of Internal Medicine.* 1998 Mar 15; 128(6): 510–511. 1 ref. BE59377.
*computer communication networks; *confidentiality; informed consent; institutional policies; *medical records; patients; *computer security; *Internet; World Wide Web Electronic Medical Record System (W3–EMRS)

Rylance, George. Privacy, dignity, and confidentiality: interview study with structured questionnaire. *BMJ (British Medical Journal).* 1999 Jan 30; 318(7179): 301. 4 refs. BE60580.
*children; *confidentiality; disclosure; *hospitals; institutional policies; knowledge, attitudes, practice; *parents; *patient care; *privacy; survey; dignity; questionnaires; Great Britain

Schick, Ida Critelli. Protecting patients' privacy. *Health Progress.* 1998 May–Jun; 79(3): 26–31. 12 refs. Includes inset article, "Developing a culture of patient privacy," p. 29–30, 31. BE61615.
computer communication networks; *confidentiality; disclosure; health care delivery; *health facilities; health personnel; information dissemination; institutional ethics; *medical records; patient access to records; patients' rights; *privacy; computer security; Franciscan Health System of the Ohio Valley–Cincinnati; United States

Schrock, Charles R.; Botkin, Jeffrey R.; McMahon, William M., et al. Permission and confidentiality in publishing pedigrees. [Letter and response]. *JAMA.* 1998 Dec 2; 280(21): 1826–1827. 3 refs. BE61242.
*confidentiality; *editorial policies; *family members; *genetic information; *genetic research; guidelines; *informed consent; investigator subject relationship; *patients; research subjects; medical illustration; *pedigree studies; publishing; International Committee of Medical Journal Editors

Sommerville, Ann; English, Veronica. Genetic privacy: orthodoxy or oxymoron? *Journal of Medical Ethics.* 1999 Apr; 25(2): 144–150. 14 refs. BE61918.
*autonomy; *beneficence; *communitarianism; *confidentiality; decision making; directive counseling; *disclosure; *duty to warn; *family members; freedom; genetic counseling; genetic disorders; *genetic information; *genetic screening; informed consent; married persons; *moral obligations; *moral policy; paternalism; *patients; physician patient relationship; *physicians; *privacy; prognosis; reproduction; rights; risk; risks and benefits; teleological ethics; treatment refusal; truth disclosure; values; harms; *right not to know

In this paper we question whether the concept of "genetic privacy" is a contradiction in terms. And, if so, whether the implications of such a conclusion, inevitably impact on how society comes to perceive privacy and responsibility generally. Current law and ethical discourse place a high value on self–determination and the rights of individuals. In the medical sphere, the recognition of patient "rights" has resulted in health professionals being given clear duties of candour and frankness. Dilemmas arise, however, when patients decline to know relevant information or, knowing it, refuse to share it with others who may also need to know. This paper considers the notions of interconnectedness and responsibility to others which are brought to the fore in the genetic sphere and which challenge the primacy afforded to personal autonomy. It also explores the extent to which an individual's perceived moral obligations can or should be enforced.

Stolberg, Sheryl Gay. Health identifier for all Americans runs into hurdles: privacy debate heats up. [News]. *New York Times.* 1998 Jul 20: A1, A11. BE61115.
*computer communication networks; *confidentiality; data banks; federal government; government regulation; health care delivery; legislation; *medical records; privacy; *public policy; Health Insurance Portability and Accountability Act 1996; *United States

Van Haeringen, Alison R.; Dadds, Mark; Armstrong, Kenneth L. The child abuse lottery –– will the doctor suspect and report? Physician attitudes towards and reporting of suspected child abuse and neglect. *Child Abuse and Neglect.* 1998 Mar; 22(3): 159–169. 22 refs. BE61809.
*child abuse; comparative studies; confidentiality; decision making; diagnosis; injuries; *knowledge, attitudes, practice; legal aspects; *mandatory reporting; parents; pediatrics; *physicians; survey; Australia; *Queensland

van Veenendaal, E. Child abuse: does disclosing the fact have implications for medical secrecy? *Medicine and Law.* 1993; 12(1–2): 25–28. BE60609.
*child abuse; *confidentiality; *disclosure; duty to warn; health facilities; law enforcement; legal obligations; legal rights; mandatory reporting; parents; physicians; *public policy; *Netherlands

Wachbroit, Robert. Rethinking medical confidentiality: the impact of genetics. *Suffolk University Law Review.* 1993 Winter; 27(4): 1391–1410. 23 fn. BE61596.
autonomy; *confidentiality; *disclosure; *duty to warn; *family members; *genetic counseling; genetic disorders; *genetic information; genetic predisposition; genetic screening; health personnel; injuries; moral obligations; *patients; *privacy; professional patient relationship; public health; *standards; trust; NCHGR–funded publication; right not to know

Weiss, J.O.; Kozma, C.; Lapham, E.V. Whom would you trust with your genetic information? [Abstract]. *American Journal of Human Genetics.* 1997 Oct; 61(4): A24. BE59390.

*attitudes; clergy; *confidentiality; *disclosure; employment; *family members; genetic disorders; *genetic information; genetic predisposition; genetic research; *genetic screening; insurance; *patients; survey; District of Columbia

Wilkie, Tom. Genetics and insurance in Britain: why more than just the Atlantic divides the English-speaking nations. *Nature Genetics.* 1998 Oct; 20(2): 119–121. 7 refs. BE61622.
advisory committees; aged; *confidentiality; *disclosure; genetic disorders; *genetic information; *genetic screening; industry; insurance; international aspects; *life insurance; long-term care; national health insurance; *public policy; *Association of British Insurers; *Great Britain; *Human Genetics Advisory Commission (Great Britain); United States

Privacy matters. [Editorial]. *Nature Genetics.* 1998 Jul; 19(3): 207–208. 3 refs. BE61710.
*confidentiality; disclosure; *editorial policies; family members; *genetic information; *genetic research; genetic screening; guideline adherence; guidelines; *informed consent; investigators; privacy; *research subjects; *pedigree studies; publishing; International Committee of Medical Journal Editors; National Institutes of Health; Office for Protection from Research Risks

CONFIDENTIALITY/LEGAL ASPECTS

American College of Obstetricians and Gynecologists. Committee on Health Care for Underserved Women. Mandatory reporting of domestic violence. ACOG Committee Opinion No. 200. *ACOG Committee Opinions.* 1998 Mar; No. 200: 3 p. 13 refs. BE61299.
autonomy; community services; *confidentiality; *domestic violence; *females; *government regulation; law enforcement; legal obligations; *mandatory reporting; obstetrics and gynecology; *organizational policies; patient care; physician patient relationship; *physicians; professional organizations; referral and consultation; risks and benefits; state government; trust; support groups; *American College of Obstetricians and Gynecologists; *United States

Andrews, Lori B. Genetic privacy: from the laboratory to the legislature. *Genome Research.* 1995 Oct; 5(3): 209–213. 17 refs. BE60876.
*confidentiality; disclosure; employment; *genetic information; genetic research; *genetic screening; health insurance; informed consent; *legal aspects; privacy; public policy; self concept; social discrimination; stigmatization; ELSI-funded publication; right not to know; United States

Anfang, Stuart A.; Appelbaum, Paul S. Twenty years after *Tarasoff*: reviewing the duty to protect. *Harvard Review of Psychiatry.* 1996 Jul–Aug; 4(2): 67–76. 104 refs. BE61476.
*alcohol abuse; *confidentiality; *dangerousness; *duty to warn; *health personnel; HIV seropositivity; law enforcement; *legal aspects; legal liability; legal obligations; *mandatory reporting; *mentally ill; physicians; professional patient relationship; *psychiatry; psychology; *psychotherapy; social impact; state government; traffic accidents; violence; automobile driving; *Tarasoff v. Regents of the University of California; *United States

Appelbaum, Paul S. Child abuse reporting laws: time for reform? *Psychiatric Services.* 1999 Jan; 50(1): 27–29. 15 refs. BE62075.
*child abuse; confidentiality; disclosure; *guideline adherence; *health personnel; legal aspects; *legal obligations; legislation; *mandatory reporting; psychology; *psychotherapy; Netherlands; United States

Appelbaum, Paul S. Jaffee v. Redmond:

psychotherapist–patient privilege in the federal courts. *Psychiatric Services.* 1996 Oct; 47(10): 1033–1034, 1052. 9 refs. BE61532.
*confidentiality; disclosure; federal government; law enforcement; *legal aspects; *privileged communication; *psychotherapy; Supreme Court decisions; *Jaffee v. Redmond; United States

Ault, Alicia. Drug industry hopes to moderate genetic privacy laws. [News]. *Nature Medicine.* 1998 Jan; 4(1): 6. BE59979.
*confidentiality; *drug industry; *genetic information; *genetic research; *government regulation; informed consent; privacy; professional organizations; property rights; state government; Pharmaceutical Research and Manufacturers of America (PhRMA)

Beran, Roy Gary. Professional privilege, driving and epilepsy, the doctor's responsibility. *Epilepsy Research.* 1997 Mar; 26(3): 415–421. 35 refs. BE60185.
*attitudes; *confidentiality; *epilepsy; legal liability; *legal obligations; *mandatory reporting; moral obligations; obligations to society; patient compliance; physician patient relationship; *physicians; *privileged communication; *risk; survey; *traffic accidents; *automobile driving; Australia

Birchard, Karen. Irish doctors concerned by information access. [News]. *Lancet.* 1998 Oct 24; 352(9137): 1368. BE60823.
attitudes; children; *confidentiality; disclosure; *government regulation; HIV seropositivity; legal liability; legal rights; legislation; *medical records; parents; *patient access to records; physician patient relationship; physicians; sexual partners; Freedom of Information Act (Ireland); *Ireland

Brown, Barry. Genetic testing, access to genetic data and discrimination: conceptual legislative models. *Suffolk University Law Review.* 1993 Winter; 27(4): 1573–1592. 79 fn. BE60739.
*confidentiality; disclosure; employment; genetic counseling; genetic disorders; genetic research; *genetic screening; informed consent; insurance; *legal aspects; mandatory programs; *model legislation; newborns; parental consent; parents; *social discrimination; voluntary programs; United States

Budai, Pamela. Mandatory reporting of child abuse: is it in the best interests of the child? *Australian and New Zealand Journal of Psychiatry.* 1996 Dec; 30(6): 794–804. 62 refs. BE60682.
alternatives; attitudes; *child abuse; *confidentiality; decision making; disclosure; domestic violence; duty to warn; empirical research; forensic psychiatry; *health personnel; informed consent; international aspects; knowledge, attitudes, practice; legal aspects; *legal obligations; *mandatory reporting; medical ethics; medical specialties; moral obligations; parents; *physicians; professional patient relationship; *psychiatry; *psychotherapy; risks and benefits; sex offenses; social impact; trust; *Australia; New Zealand; United States

Callens, Stefaan H. The automatic processing of medical data in Belgium: is the individual protected? *Medicine and Law.* 1993; 12(1–2): 55–59. 9 fn. BE60613.
*computer communication networks; *confidentiality; disclosure; *government regulation; information dissemination; informed consent; legal aspects; legal rights; legislation; *medical records; patients; physicians; privacy; *Belgium

DeCew, Judith Wagner. In Pursuit of Privacy: Law, Ethics, and the Rise of Technology. Ithaca, NY: Cornell University Press; 1997. 199 p. Bibliography: p. 189–191. ISBN 0-8014-8411-1. BE62620.

BE = bioethics accession number   fn. = footnotes   refs. = references

abortion, induced; autonomy; computers; constitutional law; drug abuse; employment; feminist ethics; fetuses; freedom; historical aspects; homosexuals; law; *legal aspects; legal rights; mass screening; philosophy; pregnant women; *privacy; *public policy; reproduction; *rights; sexuality; Supreme Court decisions; torts; values; Roe v. Wade; *United States

Dyer, Clare. Sale of prescription data breaches confidentiality. [News]. *BMJ (British Medical Journal).* 1999 Jun 5; 318(7197): 1505. BE62521.
  biomedical research; *confidentiality; *data banks; drug industry; *drugs; *legal aspects; *medical records; *Great Britain

Felsman, Janine P. Eliminating parental consent and notification for adolescent HIV testing: a legitimate statutory response to the AIDS epidemic. [Note]. *Journal of Law and Policy.* 1996; 5(1): 339–383. 146 fn. BE59302.
  *adolescents; *AIDS serodiagnosis; competence; *confidentiality; *counseling; *government regulation; *HIV seropositivity; *informed consent; *legal aspects; legal rights; *parental consent; *parental notification; parents; patient care; privacy; *public policy; social impact; state government; state interest; *voluntary programs; United States

Ferris, Lorraine E.; Barkun, Harvey; Carlisle, John, et al. Defining the physician's duty to warn: consensus statement of Ontario's Medical Expert Panel on Duty to Inform. *Canadian Medical Association Journal.* 1998 Jun 2; 158(11): 1473–1479. 42 refs. BE61127.
  advisory committees; *confidentiality; consensus; *dangerousness; *disclosure; *duty to warn; *legal aspects; *legal liability; *legal obligations; *mandatory reporting; mentally ill; negligence; physician patient relationship; *physicians; professional organizations; psychiatric diagnosis; psychiatry; *psychotherapy; risk; *standards; *violence; Canada; Canadian Medical Protective Association; *College of Physicians and Surgeons of Ontario; *Ontario; Ontario College of Family Physicians; Ontario Medical Association; *Ontario's Medical Expert Panel on Duty to Inform; Royal College of Physicians and Surgeons of Canada; Tarasoff v. Regents of the University of California; United States

Geltman, Paul L.; Meyers, Alan F. Immigration reporting laws: ethical dilemmas in pediatric practice. *American Journal of Public Health.* 1998 Jun; 88(6): 967–968. 16 refs. BE60782.
  *aliens; *attitudes; *child abuse; children; *confidentiality; *legal aspects; *mandatory reporting; *pediatrics; *physicians; state government; survey; *emigration and immigration; Massachusetts

Grabois, Ellen W. The liability of psychotherapists for breach of confidentiality. *Journal of Law and Health.* 1997–98; 12(1): 39–84. 327 fn. BE61136.
  codes of ethics; compensation; *confidentiality; contracts; disclosure; expert testimony; health personnel; injuries; *legal aspects; *legal liability; legal obligations; malpractice; medical ethics; privacy; privileged communication; professional ethics; professional patient relationship; psychiatry; psychology; *psychotherapy; public policy; torts; trust; *United States

Grubb, Andrew. PVS patient: disclosure after death: Re C (Adult Patient: Restriction of Publicity After Death). [Comment]. *Medical Law Review.* 1997 Spring; 5(1): 108–110. BE59763.
  allowing to die; artificial feeding; *confidentiality; *death; *disclosure; family members; *freedom; health personnel; *legal aspects; *mass media; organizational policies; patients; *persistent vegetative state; physicians; professional organizations; *withholding treatment; General Medical

Council (Great Britain); *Great Britain; *Re C (Adult Patient: Restriction of Publicity After Death)

Hayter, Mark. Confidentiality and the acquired immune deficiency syndrome (AIDS): an analysis of the legal and professional issues. *Journal of Advanced Nursing.* 1997 Jun; 25(6): 1162–1166. 33 refs. BE60540.
  *AIDS; codes of ethics; *confidentiality; contact tracing; disclosure; duty to warn; health personnel; *HIV seropositivity; *legal aspects; professional ethics; partner notification; *Great Britain

Hodge, James G. Privacy and antidiscrimination issues: genetics legislation in the United States. *Community Genetics.* 1998; 1(3): 169–174. 70 refs. BE62287.
  carriers; *confidentiality; disclosure; employment; *genetic information; genetic predisposition; *genetic screening; *government regulation; insurance; *legislation; medical records; *privacy; *social discrimination; *state government; *United States

Kennedy, Ian. Physicians' duty of confidentiality : Saur v. Probes. [Comment]. *Medical Law Review.* 1993 Summer; 1(2): 254–256. BE59252.
  *confidentiality; *disclosure; *legal aspects; legal liability; mentally ill; negligence; *physicians; *privileged communication; *psychiatry; Great Britain; Michigan; *Saur v. Probes; W v. Egdell

Kumar, Sanjay. Medical confidentiality broken to stop marriage of man infected with HIV. [News]. *Lancet.* 1998 Nov 28; 352(9142): 1764. BE60801.
  blood donation; *confidentiality; *disclosure; *HIV seropositivity; *hospitals; *legal aspects; *marital relationship; *Dr. Tokugha vs. Apollo Hospital Enterprises; *India; Yepthomi, Tokugha

Loftus, Elizabeth F.; Paddock, John R.; Guernsey, Thomas F. Patient–psychotherapist privilege: access to clinical records in the tangled web of repressed memory litigation. *University of Richmond Law Review.* 1996 Jan; 30(1): 109–154. 205 fn. BE59859.
  *confidentiality; constitutional law; disclosure; expert testimony; family members; health personnel; *legal aspects; legal liability; legal rights; malpractice; medical records; methods; patients; privacy; *privileged communication; *psychotherapy; *recall; sex offenses; time factors; *United States

McGleenan, Tony. Rights to know and not to know: is there a need for a genetic privacy law? *In:* Chadwick, Ruth; Levitt, Mairi; Shickle, Darren, eds. The Right to Know and the Right Not to Know. Brookfield, VT: Ashgate; 1997: 43–54. 19 refs. 9 fn. ISBN 1-85972-424-8. BE62188.
  common good; *confidentiality; constitutional law; *disclosure; DNA data banks; *genetic information; genetic research; *genetic screening; informed consent; law enforcement; *legal aspects; *legal rights; legislation; *model legislation; moral policy; *privacy; *public policy; social discrimination; Supreme Court decisions; tissue donation; torts; truth disclosure; right not to know; *Genetic Privacy Act (1995 bill); United States

McNiel, Dale E.; Binder, Renée L.; Fulton, Forrest M. Management of threats of violence under California's duty-to-protect statute. *American Journal of Psychiatry.* 1998 Aug; 155(8): 1097–1101. 28 refs. BE61226.
  blacks; *confidentiality; *dangerousness; *duty to warn; family members; *health personnel; institutionalized persons; involuntary commitment; *knowledge, attitudes, practice; law enforcement; *legal obligations; males; *mandatory reporting; mental institutions; mentally ill; *psychotherapy; public hospitals; socioeconomic factors; state government;

BE = bioethics accession number   fn. = footnotes   refs. = references

survey; *violence; California; *San Francisco

Maloney, Dennis M. Researchers and the privacy act: Fisher v. National Institutes of Health (Part I). *Human Research Report.* 1998 Sep; 13(9): 4–5. BE61728.
  biomedical research; *confidentiality; data banks; disclosure; *federal government; *investigators; *legal aspects; privacy; records; *scientific misconduct; *Fisher v. National Institutes of Health; *Fisher, Bernard; National Surgical Adjuvant Breast and Bowel Project; *Privacy Act 1974; United States

Michalowski, Sabine. Medical confidentiality and medical privilege -- a comparison of French and German law. *European Journal of Health Law.* 1998 Jun; 5(2): 89–116. 116 fn. BE60899.
  comparative studies; *confidentiality; constitutional law; criminal law; disclosure; expert testimony; informed consent; *international aspects; *legal aspects; legal obligations; legal rights; patients; physicians; prisoners; privacy; *privileged communication; *France; *Germany

Michel, Lee. Consent: Ohio appellate court affirms confidentiality claim. *Journal of Law, Medicine and Ethics.* 1998 Winter; 26(4): 355–356. BE61169.
  *confidentiality; *disclosure; *hospitals; lawyers; *legal liability; *records; *torts; *Biddle v. Warren General Hospital; *Ohio

Montgomery, Jonathan. Confidentiality in the modernised NHS: the challenge of data protection. *Bulletin of Medical Ethics.* 1999 Mar; No. 146: 18–21. 8 fn. Includes excerpts from the British Data Protection Act 1998. BE61821.
  *confidentiality; health care delivery; health facilities; health personnel; *legal aspects; legislation; *medical records; public policy; *Data Protection Act 1998 (Great Britain); *Great Britain; *National Health Service

Nease, Donald E.; Doukas, David J. Research privacy or freedom of information? [News]. *Hastings Center Report.* 1999 May-Jun; 29(3): 47. BE61415.
  biomedical research; *confidentiality; disclosure; federal government; freedom; government financing; *government regulation; *human experimentation; *information dissemination; informed consent; legislation; *research subjects; Freedom of Information Act; *United States

Pear, Robert. Future bleak for bill to keep health records confidential. [News]. *New York Times.* 1999 Jun 21: A12. BE62348.
  *confidentiality; disclosure; federal government; government financing; health care delivery; law enforcement; *legislation; *medical records; privacy; United States

Rand, Justin. AIDS and HIV: Colorado court upholds privacy rights in disclosure of test results. *Journal of Law, Medicine and Ethics.* 1998 Winter; 26(4): 353–355. 12 fn. BE61168.
  *AIDS serodiagnosis; *blood specimen collection; confidentiality; criminal law; deception; *disclosure; government regulation; *HIV seropositivity; informed consent; *laboratories; *legal aspects; *legal liability; *privacy; *schools; state government; students; torts; *Cambridge College (Cambridge, MA); *Colorado; *Doe v. High-Tech Institute, Inc.

Reilly, Philip R. Public policy and legal issues raised by advances in genetic screening and testing. *Suffolk University Law Review.* 1993 Winter; 27(4): 1327–1357. 54 fn. BE60737.
  adoption; carriers; children; *confidentiality; *disclosure; duty to warn; economics; employment; family members; genetic disorders; *genetic information; *genetic screening;

government regulation; health care delivery; health insurance reimbursement; industry; insurance selection bias; *legal aspects; life insurance; parent child relationship; pregnant women; prenatal diagnosis; *public policy; social discrimination; state government; twins; United States

Roach, William H.; Aspen Health Law and Compliance Center. Access to medical record information. *In: their* Medical Records and the Law. Third Edition. Gaithersburg, MD: Aspen Publishers; 1998: 87–139. 291 fn. ISBN 0-8342-1104-1. BE62748.
  alcohol abuse; *confidentiality; disclosure; drug abuse; epidemiology; federal government; genetic information; government regulation; health facilities; health personnel; *legal aspects; legislation; *medical records; mentally ill; minors; patient access to records; peer review; *property rights; remuneration; state government; quality assurance; utilization review; *United States

Roach, William H.; Aspen Health Law and Compliance Center. HIV/AIDS: mandatory reporting and confidentiality. *In: their* Medical Records and the Law. Third Edition. Gaithersburg, MD: Aspen Publishers; 1998: 213–239. 119 fn. ISBN 0-8342-1104-1. BE62749.
  *AIDS; AIDS serodiagnosis; blood donation; *confidentiality; *disclosure; emergency care; government regulation; guidelines; health personnel; *HIV seropositivity; informed consent; judicial action; *legal aspects; legal liability; *mandatory reporting; medical records; spousal notification; state government; partner notification; sexual partners; *United States

Robinson, John H.; Berry, Roberta M.; McDonnell, Kevin, eds. Issues in adult health care. *In: their* A Health Law Reader: An Interdisciplinary Approach. Durham, NC: Carolina Academic Press; 1999: 239–337. 17 fn. ISBN 0-89089-907-X. BE62294.
  adults; altruism; autonomy; cadavers; commodification; competence; computers; *confidentiality; conflict of interest; data banks; decision making; *disclosure; duty to warn; genetic information; health care delivery; human experimentation; *informed consent; justice; *legal aspects; legal liability; medical records; mentally ill; negligence; *organ donation; organ donors; *organ transplantation; patient care; physician patient relationship; physicians; *privacy; psychotherapy; public health; public policy; quality of health care; remuneration; resource allocation; risks and benefits; social dominance; torts; Tarasoff v. Regents of the University of California; Uniform Anatomical Gift Act; United States

Roche, Patricia; Glantz, Leonard H.; Annas, George J. The Genetic Privacy Act: a proposal for national legislation. *In:* Smith, Edward; Sapp, Walter, eds. Plain Talk about the Human Genome Project: A Tuskegee University Conference on Its Promise and Perils ... and Matters of Race. Tuskegee, AL: Tuskegee University Press; 1997: 187–196. 28 fn. ISBN 1-891196-01-4. BE61746.
  competence; *confidentiality; disclosure; *DNA data banks; federal government; *genetic information; *genetic screening; genome mapping; *government regulation; guidelines; informed consent; *legislation; minors; pregnant women; preimplantation diagnosis; prenatal diagnosis; *privacy; risks and benefits; third party consent; tissue banks; DNA analysis; *Genetic Confidentiality and Nondiscrimination Act (1996 bill); *Genetic Privacy Act (1995 bill); United States

Rothstein, Mark A. Preventing the discovery of plaintiff genetic profiles by defendants seeking to limit damages in personal injury litigation. *Indiana Law Journal.* 1996 Fall; 71(4): 877–910. 218 fn. BE62666.
  compensation; *confidentiality; *disclosure; economics;

BE = bioethics accession number   fn. = footnotes   refs. = references

*genetic information; genetic predisposition; genetic screening; late-onset disorders; *legal aspects; legal liability; mandatory testing; medical records; *torts; *life expectancy; United States

Royal College of Psychiatrists. Position Statement on Confidentiality. Issued by the Royal College of Psychiatrists, 17 Belgrave Sq., London SW1X 8PG, England; 1989 Oct. 21 p. Council Report CR7; approved Oct 1989. BE60355.
adults; children; competence; *confidentiality; disclosure; education; family members; *forensic psychiatry; guidelines; health personnel; human experimentation; interdisciplinary communication; *legal aspects; medical records; mentally disabled; *organizational policies; patient access to records; patient care team; physicians; privacy; professional organizations; property rights; *psychiatry; Data Protection Act 1984 (Great Britain); Department of Health (Great Britain); Department of Health and Social Security (Great Britain); General Medical Council (Great Britain); *Great Britain; *Royal College of Psychiatrists

Rubinstein, Helena Gail. If I am only for myself, what am I? A communitarian look at the privacy stalemate. *American Journal of Law and Medicine.* 1999; 25(2-3): 203-231. 214 fn. BE62507.
autonomy; biomedical research; *common good; *communitarianism; computers; *confidentiality; *disclosure; *federal government; *government regulation; guidelines; health care delivery; health insurance; health services research; industry; informed consent; *legal aspects; legal rights; legislation; *medical records; obligations to society; *privacy; *public policy; rights; risks and benefits; state government; trust; Department of Health and Human Services; U.S. Congress; *United States

Spielberg, Alissa R. On call and online: sociohistorical, legal, and ethical implications of e-mail for the patient-physician relationship. *JAMA.* 1998 Oct 21; 280(15): 1353-1359. 48 refs. BE60289.
*communication; *computer communication networks; *confidentiality; disclosure; government regulation; historical aspects; informed consent; *legal aspects; *medical records; patient care; *physician patient relationship; *physicians; privacy; referral and consultation; risks and benefits; sociology of medicine; *standards; state government; trends; computer security; *physician's practice patterns; American Medical Association; American Medical Informatics Association; Internet; United States

Increased use of e-mail by physicians, patients, and other health care organizations and staff has the potential to reshape the current boundaries of relationships in medical practice. By comparing reception of e-mail technology in medical practice with its historical analogue, reception of the telephone, this article suggests that new expectations, practice standards, and potential liabilities emerge with the introduction of this new communication technology. Physicians using e-mail should be aware of these considerations and construct their e-mail communications accordingly, recognizing that e-mail may be included in the patient's medical record. Likewise, physicians should discuss the ramifications of communicating electronically with patients and obtain documented informed consent before using e-mail. Physicians must keep patient information confidential, which will require taking precautions (including encryption to prevent interception) to preserve patient information, trust, and the integrity of the patient-physician relationship.

Spielberg, Alissa R. Online without a net: physician-patient communication by electronic mail. *American Journal of Law and Medicine.* 1999; 25(2-3): 267-295. 228 fn. BE62509.

*communication; *computer communication networks; *confidentiality; constitutional law; diagnosis; disclosure; federal government; health care delivery; health insurance reimbursement; informed consent; *legal aspects; legal liability; legal rights; malpractice; *medical records; *methods; *patient care; *physician patient relationship; *privacy; psychotherapy; public health; risks and benefits; standards; state government; Supreme Court decisions; *telemedicine; Internet; *United States

Starr, Paul. Health and the right to privacy. *American Journal of Law and Medicine.* 1999; 25(2-3): 193-201. 17 fn. First Annual Justice Louis Brandeis Lecture delivered at the 21st Annual Meeting of the Massachusetts Health Data Consortium, Boston, MA, 16 April 1999. BE62506.
advertising; biomedical research; computers; *confidentiality; *disclosure; federal government; *government regulation; health care delivery; health insurance; informed consent; law enforcement; legal rights; mass media; *medical records; misconduct; *privacy; public health; public policy; *United States

Stenger, Christine E. Taking Tarasoff where no one has gone before: looking at "duty to warn" under the AIDS crisis. [Comment]. *Saint Louis University Public Law Review.* 1996; 15(2): 471-504. 235 fn. BE59921.
AIDS; blood transfusions; communicable diseases; *confidentiality; contact tracing; disclosure; *duty to warn; government regulation; *HIV seropositivity; hospitals; judicial action; *legal aspects; *legal liability; mandatory reporting; physician patient relationship; *physicians; state government; California; Reisner v. Regents of the University of California; *Tarasoff v. Regents; *United States

Stepanuk, Natalie Anne. Genetic information and third party access to information: New Jersey's pioneering legislation as a model for federal privacy protection of genetic information. [Comment]. *Catholic University Law Review.* 1998 Spring; 47(3): 1105-1144. 239 fn. BE62036.
*confidentiality; *disclosure; duty to warn; employment; family members; federal government; genetic disorders; *genetic information; genetic predisposition; genetic research; *genetic screening; *government regulation; health insurance; *legal aspects; legislation; medical records; physician patient relationship; *privacy; *property rights; *social discrimination; state government; *Genetic Privacy Act 1996 (NJ); *New Jersey

Studdert, David M. Direct contracts, data sharing and employee risk selection: new stakes for patient privacy in tomorrow's health insurance markets. *American Journal of Law and Medicine.* 1999; 25(2-3): 233-265. 242 fn. BE62508.
compensation; computers; *confidentiality; conflict of interest; *contracts; disabled; *disclosure; economics; *employment; federal government; government regulation; health care delivery; *health insurance; *incentives; insurance selection bias; *legal aspects; legislation; *managed care programs; occupational medicine; *organization and administration; patient care; *physicians; *privacy; risk; social discrimination; state government; Americans with Disabilities Act 1990; *United States

Troy, Edwin S. Flores. The Genetic Privacy Act: an analysis of privacy and research concerns. *Journal of Law, Medicine and Ethics.* 1997 Winter; 25(4): 256-272. 150 fn. BE62671.
*confidentiality; consent forms; *disclosure; DNA data banks; eugenics; federal government; genes; genetic disorders; *genetic information; genetic materials; genetic predisposition; genetic research; *genetic screening; *government regulation; guidelines; informed consent; insurance; law enforcement; *legal aspects; legal liability; *legislation; physicians; preventive medicine; *privacy; risks

---

BE = bioethics accession number   fn. = footnotes   refs. = references

and benefits; social discrimination; state government; terminology; tissue banks; trends; *Genetic Privacy Act; *United States

U.S. Congress. House. A bill to establish federal penalties for prohibited uses and disclosures of individually identifiable health information, to establish a right in an individual to inspect and copy their own health information, and for other purposes [Consumer Health and Research technology (CHART) Protection Act]. H.R. 3900, 105th Cong., 2d Sess. Introduced by Christopher Shays.; 1998 May 19. 48 p. Referred to the Committee on Commerce, and in addition to the Committees on Ways and Means and on Government Reform and Oversight. BE62444.
    biomedical research; computers; *confidentiality; criminal law; *disclosure; epidemiology; federal government; government regulation; informed consent; law enforcement; *legal aspects; legislation; *medical records; *patient access to records; state government; *Consumer Health and Research Technology (CHART) Protection Act (1998 bill); *United States

Waller, Adele A.; Alcantara, Oscar L. Ownership of health information in the information age. *Journal of the American Health Information Management Association.* 1998 Mar; 69(3): 28–40. 36 fn. Includes a continuing education quiz, p. 39–40. BE60433.
    *computer communication networks; confidentiality; contracts; *data banks; disclosure; genetic information; health care delivery; health personnel; hospitals; *legal aspects; *medical records; *patient access to records; patients; *property rights; United States

Zweig, Franklin M.; Walsh, Joseph T.; Freeman, Daniel M. Adjudicating neurogenetics at the crossroads: privacy, adoption, and the death sentence. *Judges' Journal.* 1997 Summer; 36(3): 52–55, 57–58, 90–93. 14 fn. BE59806.
    *adoption; *behavior disorders; *behavioral genetics; capital punishment; case studies; *confidentiality; *criminal law; federal government; *genetic information; *genetic predisposition; *genetic screening; government regulation; killing; *law enforcement; legislation; mandatory testing; parents; prisoners; *privacy; public policy; records; social discrimination; state government; *violence; Colorado; Connecticut; *United States

Physician–patient privilege; depression; alcoholism: McCormick v. England. *Mental and Physical Disability Law Reporter.* 1998 Mar–Apr; 22(2): 235–236. BE61466.
    alcohol abuse; *confidentiality; depressive disorder; disclosure; *legal aspects; *legal liability; physician patient relationship; *physicians; *privileged communication; *McCormick v. England; *South Carolina

CONFIDENTIALITY/MENTAL HEALTH

American Psychiatric Association. Committee on Confidentiality; American Psychiatric Association. Council on Psychiatry and Law. American Psychiatric Association resource document on preserving patient confidentiality in the era of information technology. *Journal of the American Academy of Psychiatry and the Law.* 1997; 25(4): 551–559. This document updates the APA's 1987 "Guidelines on Confidentiality." It does not represent official policy of the APA. BE59151.
    biomedical research; *computer communication networks; *confidentiality; data banks; fraud; *guidelines; health care delivery; informed consent; law enforcement; legal aspects; *medical records; organizational policies; patient access to records; physicians; professional organizations; *psychiatry;

psychotherapy; standards; *computer security; *American Psychiatric Association; United States

Anfang, Stuart A.; Appelbaum, Paul S. Twenty years after *Tarasoff*: reviewing the duty to protect. *Harvard Review of Psychiatry.* 1996 Jul–Aug; 4(2): 67–76. 104 refs. BE61476.
    *alcohol abuse; *confidentiality; *dangerousness; *duty to warn; *health personnel; HIV seropositivity; law enforcement; *legal aspects; legal liability; legal obligations; *mandatory reporting; *mentally ill; physicians; professional patient relationship; *psychiatry; psychology; *psychotherapy; social impact; state government; traffic accidents; violence; automobile driving; *Tarasoff v. Regents of the University of California; *United States

Appelbaum, Paul S. Child abuse reporting laws: time for reform? *Psychiatric Services.* 1999 Jan; 50(1): 27–29. 15 refs. BE62075.
    *child abuse; confidentiality; disclosure; *guideline adherence; *health personnel; legal aspects; *legal obligations; legislation; *mandatory reporting; psychology; *psychotherapy; Netherlands; United States

Appelbaum, Paul S. Jaffee v. Redmond: psychotherapist–patient privilege in the federal courts. *Psychiatric Services.* 1996 Oct; 47(10): 1033–1034, 1052. 9 refs. BE61532.
    *confidentiality; disclosure; federal government; law enforcement; *legal aspects; *privileged communication; *psychotherapy; Supreme Court decisions; *Jaffee v. Redmond; United States

Budai, Pamela. Mandatory reporting of child abuse: is it in the best interests of the child? *Australian and New Zealand Journal of Psychiatry.* 1996 Dec; 30(6): 794–804. 62 refs. BE60682.
    alternatives; attitudes; *child abuse; *confidentiality; decision making; disclosure; domestic violence; duty to warn; empirical research; forensic psychiatry; *health personnel; informed consent; international aspects; knowledge, attitudes, practice; legal aspects; *legal obligations; *mandatory reporting; medical ethics; medical specialties; moral obligations; parents; *physicians; professional patient relationship; *psychiatry; *psychotherapy; risks and benefits; sex offenses; social impact; trust; *Australia; New Zealand; United States

Ferriman, Annabel. Trial by video: *Someone to watch over me*, ITV, 12 January. *BMJ (British Medical Journal).* 1999 Jan 23; 318(7178): 269. BE60347.
    attitudes; *behavior disorders; *child abuse; children; *confidentiality; *deception; diagnosis; *forensic medicine; health personnel; hospitals; *mass media; *parents; risks and benefits; *covert monitoring; *Munchausen syndrome by proxy; *video recording; Great Britain

Ferris, Lorraine E.; Barkun, Harvey; Carlisle, John, et al. Defining the physician's duty to warn: consensus statement of Ontario's Medical Expert Panel on Duty to Inform. *Canadian Medical Association Journal.* 1998 Jun 2; 158(11): 1473–1479. 42 refs. BE61127.
    advisory committees; *confidentiality; consensus; *dangerousness; *disclosure; *duty to warn; *legal aspects; *legal liability; *legal obligations; *mandatory reporting; mentally ill; negligence; physician patient relationship; *physicians; professional organizations; psychiatric diagnosis; psychiatry; *psychotherapy; risk; *standards; *violence; Canada; Canadian Medical Protective Association; *College of Physicians and Surgeons of Ontario; *Ontario; Ontario College of Family Physicians; Ontario Medical Association; *Ontario's Medical Expert Panel on Duty to Inform; Royal College of Physicians and Surgeons of Canada; Tarasoff v. Regents of the University of California; United States

---

BE = bioethics accession number   fn. = footnotes   refs. = references

Grabois, Ellen W. The liability of psychotherapists for breach of confidentiality. *Journal of Law and Health.* 1997–98; 12(1): 39–84. 327 fn. BE61136.
codes of ethics; compensation; *confidentiality; contracts; disclosure; expert testimony; health personnel; injuries; *legal aspects; *legal liability; legal obligations; malpractice; medical ethics; privacy; privileged communication; professional ethics; professional patient relationship; psychiatry; psychology; *psychotherapy; public policy; torts; trust; *United States

Kennedy, Ian. Physicians' duty of confidentiality : Saur v. Probes. [Comment]. *Medical Law Review.* 1993 Summer; 1(2): 254–256. BE59252.
*confidentiality; *disclosure; *legal aspects; legal liability; mentally ill; negligence; *physicians; *privileged communication; *psychiatry; Great Britain; Michigan; *Saur v. Probes; W v. Egdell

Leigh, Wilhelmina A. Participant protection with the use of records: ethical issues and recommendations. *Ethics and Behavior.* 1998; 8(4): 305–319. 25 refs. BE60163.
alcohol abuse; behavioral research; computer communication networks; *confidentiality; consent forms; data banks; *disclosure; *drug abuse; epidemiology; federal government; *government regulation; guidelines; health facilities; *health services research; informed consent; injuries; legal liability; *mentally ill; organizational policies; patient care; program descriptions; *records; *research subjects; time factors; recontact; Department of Health and Human Services; *Substance Abuse and Mental Health Services Administration; *United States
This article explores the ethical concerns and protections that may be required when individually identifiable data originally collected solely for clinical or administrative purposes are used in research or evaluation. It asks the following broad question with respect to the interim policy developed by the Substance Abuse and Mental Health Services Administration (SAMHSA) to protect the rights and welfare of participants in its programs: For those programs and projects not classified as research, are the protections and system for review adequate? Background information on SAMHSA's interim policy is provided, along with issues and questions related to the use of clinical and administrative records in research and evaluation. The article concludes with recommendations for modifying the existing participant protection guidelines, based on the preceding discussion of issues and questions.

Loftus, Elizabeth F.; Paddock, John R.; Guernsey, Thomas F. Patient–psychotherapist privilege: access to clinical records in the tangled web of repressed memory litigation. *University of Richmond Law Review.* 1996 Jan; 30(1): 109–154. 205 fn. BE59859.
*confidentiality; constitutional law; disclosure; expert testimony; family members; health personnel; *legal aspects; legal liability; legal rights; malpractice; medical records; methods; patients; privacy; *privileged communication; *psychotherapy; *recall; sex offenses; time factors; *United States

Lynn, David J.; Vaillant, George E. Anonymity, neutrality, and confidentiality in the actual methods of Sigmund Freud: a review of 43 cases, 1907–1939. *American Journal of Psychiatry.* 1998 Feb; 155(2): 163–171. 59 refs. BE59677.
*confidentiality; directive counseling; disclosure; evaluation studies; family members; famous persons; *historical aspects; interprofessional relations; mentally ill; *methods; patients; physician patient relationship; physicians; psychiatry; *psychotherapy; social interaction; Austria; *Freud, Sigmund; Twentieth Century

McNiel, Dale E.; Binder, Renée L.; Fulton, Forrest M. Management of threats of violence under California's duty-to-protect statute. *American Journal of Psychiatry.* 1998 Aug; 155(8): 1097–1101. 28 refs. BE61226.
blacks; *confidentiality; *dangerousness; *duty to warn; family members; *health personnel; institutionalized persons; involuntary commitment; *knowledge, attitudes, practice; law enforcement; *legal obligations; males; *mandatory reporting; mental institutions; mentally ill; *psychotherapy; public hospitals; socioeconomic factors; state government; survey; *violence; California; *San Francisco

Miles, Steven H. A challenge to licensing boards: the stigma of mental illness. *JAMA.* 1998 Sep 9; 280(10): 865. 5 refs. BE60283.
*confidentiality; *depressive disorder; disclosure; interprofessional relations; medical records; organizational policies; *physicians; professional competence; professional organizations; *psychiatry; self regulation; *stigmatization; *licensing boards; *physician impairment; American Psychiatric Association; Minnesota

Perkins, David V.; Hudson, Brenda L.; Gray, Diana M., et al. Decisions and justifications by community mental health providers about hypothetical ethical dilemmas. *Psychiatric Services.* 1998 Oct; 49(10): 1317–1322. 23 refs. BE61448.
administrators; age factors; *community services; comparative studies; *confidentiality; *decision making; disclosure; education; *geographic factors; gifts; *health personnel; *mentally ill; nurses; *professional ethics; *professional patient relationship; psychology; *social interaction; social workers; survey; *case managers; *mental health services; rural population; urban population; Midwestern United States

Royal College of Psychiatrists. Position Statement on Confidentiality. Issued by the Royal College of Psychiatrists, 17 Belgrave Sq., London SW1X 8PG, England; 1989 Oct. 21 p. Council Report CR7; approved Oct 1989. BE60355.
adults; children; competence; *confidentiality; disclosure; education; family members; *forensic psychiatry; guidelines; health personnel; human experimentation; interdisciplinary communication; *legal aspects; medical records; mentally disabled; *organizational policies; patient access to records; patient care team; physicians; privacy; professional organizations; property rights; *psychiatry; Data Protection Act 1984 (Great Britain); Department of Health (Great Britain); Department of Health and Social Security (Great Britain); General Medical Council (Great Britain); *Great Britain; *Royal College of Psychiatrists

Slovenko, Ralph. Psychotherapy and Confidentiality: Testimonial Privileged Communication, Breach of Confidentiality, and Reporting Duties. Springfield, IL: Charles C. Thomas; 1998. 640 p. Includes references and Table of Cases. ISBN 0–398–06827–5. BE62399.
accountability; *confidentiality; criminal law; dangerousness; *disclosure; *duty to warn; famous persons; *forensic psychiatry; group therapy; health insurance; health personnel; *legal aspects; mandatory reporting; marital relationship; medical records; minors; parent child relationship; physician patient relationship; prisoners; *privileged communication; *psychiatry; *psychotherapy; sex offenses; stigmatization; terminology; torts; publishing; Tarasoff v. Regents of the University of California; United States

CONTRACEPTION

See also POPULATION CONTROL, STERILIZATION

Appleby, Brenda Margaret. Responsible Parenthood: Decriminalizing Contraception in Canada. Toronto, ON: University of Toronto Press; 1999. 301 p. Bibliography: p. 269-281. ISBN 0-8020-8189-4. BE62618.
  abortion, induced; common good; conscience; *contraception; criminal law; cultural pluralism; developing countries; *family planning; family relationship; government regulation; *historical aspects; information dissemination; *legal aspects; *legislation; married persons; medical devices; methods; *moral obligations; *morality; organizational policies; *parents; patient advocacy; physicians; *political activity; *politics; population control; professional organizations; *Protestant ethics; public opinion; *public policy; *Roman Catholic ethics; women's health; *Canada; Canadian Bar Association; Canadian Catholic Conference; Canadian Council of Churches; Canadian Medical Association; Criminal Code of Canada; Family Planning Federation of Canada; Food and Drugs Act (Canada); *Twentieth Century

Benagiano, G.; Cottingham, J. Contraceptive methods: potential for abuse. *International Journal of Gynaecology and Obstetrics.* 1997 Jan; 56(1): 39-46. 23 fn. BE60688.
  coercion; *contraception; developing countries; disclosure; family planning; females; guidelines; hormones; human experimentation; human rights; informed consent; *international aspects; medical devices; methods; population control; professional organizations; regulation; risks and benefits; sterilization (sexual); women's health

Benagiano, G. Reproductive health as an essential human right. *Advances in Contraception.* 1996 Dec; 12(4): 243-250. 20 refs. BE60732.
  children; developing countries; education; *family planning; human rights; *international aspects; maternal health; *reproduction; *women's health; *women's rights

Brown, Harold O.J.; Budziszewski, J.; Chaput, Charles J., et al. Contraception: a symposium. *First Things.* 1998 Dec; No. 88: 17-29. BE61938.
  abortion, induced; *contraception; females; Jewish ethics; males; marital relationship; morality; natural law; population control; Protestant ethics; reproductive technologies; *Roman Catholic ethics; sexuality; *Humanae Vitae

Chavkin, Wendy. Unwanted pregnancy in Armenia -- the larger context. [Editorial]. *American Journal of Public Health.* 1998 May; 88(5): 732-733. 13 refs. BE60778.
  *abortion, induced; *contraception; government financing; health insurance reimbursement; *international aspects; knowledge, attitudes, practice; managed care programs; *public policy; religious hospitals; Roman Catholics; *social impact; women's health; Armenia; Eastern Europe; *United States

Clarke, Adele E. Disciplining Reproduction: Modernity, American Life Sciences, and "the Problems of Sex." Berkeley, CA: University of California Press; 1998. 421 p. Bibliography: p. 333-410. ISBN 0-520-20720-3. BE60503.
  animal experimentation; *biology; *biomedical research; *contraception; eugenics; family planning; federal government; females; *financial support; genetics; government financing; historical aspects; infertility; interdisciplinary communication; investigators; males; medicine; morality; political activity; population control; private sector; *reproduction; reproductive technologies; *sexuality; *social control; social dominance; *sociology of medicine; universities; women's health; women's rights; agriculture; Ford Foundation; National Research Council; Rockefeller Foundation; *Twentieth Century; *United States

Dolian, Gayane; Lüdicke, Frank; Katchatrian, Naira, et al. Contraception and induced abortion in Armenia: a critical need for family planning programs in Eastern Europe. *American Journal of Public Health.* 1998 May; 88(5): 803-805. 9 refs. BE60779.
  *abortion, induced; age factors; *contraception; females; knowledge, attitudes, practice; methods; pregnant women; socioeconomic factors; survey; women's health; *Armenia
  OBJECTIVES: The purpose of this study was to determine the number of induced abortions per woman and the reasons for selecting induced abortion among parous Armenian women. METHODS: A consecutive series of 200 women attending an abortion clinic in Yerevan, Armenia, were queried by a physician about their reproductive histories. RESULTS: Women younger than 20 years of age reported a median of 1 and women older than 40 years reported a median of 8 induced abortions in their lifetimes (overall median = 3). Lack of contraceptive information was the major reason cited for not using contraception.
  CONCLUSIONS: Induced abortion is the major form of birth control among parous Armenian women. Concerted public health campaigns are needed to inform women and their physicians in Armenia and other Eastern European countries about alternative contraceptive methods.

Donovan, Patricia. Hospital mergers and reproductive health care. *Family Planning Perspectives.* 1996 Nov-Dec; 28(6): 281-284. 21 fn. BE61811.
  *abortion, induced; community services; *contraception; economics; *family planning; geographic factors; government regulation; *hospitals; indigents; *institutional policies; legal aspects; political activity; prenatal diagnosis; referral and consultation; *religious hospitals; *Roman Catholic ethics; state government; trends; voluntary sterilization; women's health services; *community hospitals; *health facility mergers; American Civil Liberties Union; Montana; New York; *United States

Feldman, David M. Birth Control in Jewish Law: Marital Relations, Contraception, and Abortion as Set Forth in the Classic Texts of Jewish Law. First Jason Aronson Edition. Northvale, NJ: Jason Aronson; 1998. 349 p. Includes references. ISBN 0-7657-6058-4. BE62622.
  *abortion, induced; beginning of life; Christian ethics; *contraception; drugs; embryos; females; fetuses; historical aspects; *Jewish ethics; males; *marital relationship; maternal health; methods; reproduction; *sexuality; *theology; therapeutic abortion

Foster, Peggy; Hudson, Stephanie. From compliance to concordance: a challenge for contraceptive prescribers. *Health Care Analysis.* 1998 Jun; 6(2): 123-130. 24 refs. BE59976.
  alternatives; attitudes; autonomy; blacks; *contraception; disadvantaged; drugs; family planning; *females; *hormones; informed consent; methods; models, theoretical; *patient compliance; *patient participation; physician patient relationship; risks and benefits; stigmatization; Great Britain
  In 1997 the Royal Pharmaceutical Society of Great Britain published a report entitled From Compliance to Concordance: Achieving Shared Goals in Medicine Taking. This article applies this new model -- of doctors and patients working together towards a shared goal -- to the prescribing of hormonal forms of contraception. It begins by critically evaluating the current dominant model of contraceptive prescribing. It claims that this model tends to stereotype all women, but particularly young, poor and black women, as unreliable and ill-informed contraceptors who need to be advised and even controlled by much more knowledgeable and socially responsible family planning experts. The article then suggests how a much more egalitarian model of contraceptive prescribing might be put into practice,

---

whilst acknowledging the existence of many serious obstacles to such a radical shift within family planning services. In conclusion, the article suggests that until contraceptive prescribers begin to take women's experiences of, and concerns about, hormonal contraceptives seriously they will fail to develop a potentially much more effective and liberating model of family planning.

Francome, Colin. Attitudes of general practitioners in Northern Ireland toward abortion and family planning. *Family Planning Perspectives.* 1997 Sep–Oct; 29(5): 234–236. 5 fn. BE59884.
    *abortion, induced; adolescents; comparative studies; *contraception; decision making; *family planning; *family practice; females; *knowledge, attitudes, practice; married persons; *physicians; pregnant women; *Protestants; referral and consultation; *Roman Catholics; single persons; survey; *Northern Ireland

Gillon, Raanan. Eugenics, contraception, abortion and ethics. [Editorial]. *Journal of Medical Ethics.* 1998 Aug; 24(4): 219–220. 1 ref. BE61287.
    coercion; *contraception; disabled; *eugenics; *genetic disorders; historical aspects; moral policy; motivation; National Socialism; philosophy; reproduction; *selective abortion; social control; social discrimination; *voluntary programs; Aristotle; Plato

Gold, Rachel Benson; Richards, Cory L. Managed care and unintended pregnancy. *Women's Health Issues.* 1998 May–Jun; 8(3): 134–147. 18 refs. BE60444.
    confidentiality; *contraception; *family planning; federal government; *females; government financing; government regulation; *health insurance reimbursement; health maintenance organizations; *managed care programs; obstetrics and gynecology; primary health care; *public policy; state government; *women's health services; Medicaid; United States

Goldberg, Carey. Insurance for Viagra spurs coverage for birth control. [News]. *New York Times.* 1999 Jun 30: A1, A16. BE62445.
    *contraception; *drugs; *females; *government regulation; *health insurance reimbursement; *hormones; justice; *males; politics; state government; women's rights; United States; *Viagra

Gonen, Julianna S. Managed care and unintended pregnancy: testing the limits of prevention. *Women's Health Issues.* 1999 Mar–Apr; 9(2, Suppl.): 26S–35S. 24 refs. BE61969.
    *adolescents; adults; confidentiality; *contraception; costs and benefits; *family planning; federal government; government financing; health insurance; *health insurance reimbursement; health maintenance organizations; *managed care programs; methods; organizational policies; parental consent; parental notification; *public policy; *quality of health care; religious hospitals; Roman Catholics; state government; statistics; *women's health services; Medicaid; United States

Hardon, Anita; Hayes, Elizabeth, eds. Reproductive Rights in Practice: A Feminist Report on Quality of Care. New York, NY: Zed Books; 1997. 235 p. Bibliography: p. 223–228. ISBN 1–85649–452–7. BE61834.
    abortion, induced; adolescents; comparative studies; *contraception; counseling; developing countries; economics; *family planning; family practice; females; guidelines; health care delivery; incentives; information dissemination; *international aspects; knowledge, attitudes, practice; males; methods; paternalism; physicians; population control; *public policy; *quality of health care; statistics;

*women's health; *women's health services; women's rights; Bangladesh; Bolivia; Finland; Kenya; Mexico; Netherlands; Nigeria; Thailand

Hayes, Edward J.; Hayes, Paul J.; Kelly, Dorothy Ellen, et al. Principles relating to the origin of life. *In: their* Catholicism and Ethics. Norwood, MA: C.R. Publications; 1997: 79–119. Includes discussion questions and projects. References embedded in list at back of book. ISBN 0–9649087–7–8. BE61946.
    abortion, induced; artificial insemination; clergy; cloning; *contraception; double effect; family planning; health personnel; historical aspects; in vitro fertilization; infertility; marital relationship; methods; prenatal diagnosis; reproduction; *reproductive technologies; *Roman Catholic ethics; sexuality; surrogate mothers; value of life

Kavanaugh, John F. Ethical commitments in health care systems. *America.* 1998 Nov 7; 179(14): 20. BE62274.
    *abortion, induced; *contraception; embryo research; euthanasia; fetal research; health care delivery; hospitals; *institutional ethics; *religious hospitals; reproduction; *Roman Catholic ethics; sterilization (sexual); *health facility mergers; Ethical and Religious Directives for Catholic Health Care Services; United States

Kilborn, Peter T. Definition of abortion is found to vary abroad. [News]. *New York Times.* 1999 Nov 24: A18. BE60649.
    *abortion, induced; *contraception; *developing countries; *family planning; *government financing; government regulation; *international aspects; population control; *public policy; *Bangladesh; *United States

Kilborn, Peter T. Pressure growing to cover the cost of birth control. [News]. *New York Times.* 1998 Aug 2: 1, 30. BE60967.
    *contraception; drugs; employment; federal government; government regulation; *health insurance reimbursement; males; patient advocacy; *political activity; private sector; Roman Catholic ethics; sexuality; state government; Right to Life Movement; *United States

King, Ralph T. The pill U.S. drug companies dare not market. [News]. *Wall Street Journal.* 1998 Jun 26: B1, B6. BE59621.
    abortion, induced; *contraception; *drug industry; *drugs; economics; federal government; females; legal liability; political activity; public policy; *postcoital contraceptives; Food and Drug Administration; Great Britain; *United States

Kumar, Sanjay. Research into anti-fertility vaccine continues despite protests. [News]. *Lancet.* 1998 Nov 7; 352(9139): 1528. BE60305.
    *contraception; developing countries; *females; *human experimentation; immunization; international aspects; political activity; *risks and benefits; scientific misconduct; women's health; India

Macklin, Ruth. International feminism and reproductive rights. *In: her* Against Relativism: Cultural Diversity and the Search for Ethical Universals in Medicine. New York, NY: Oxford University Press; 1999: 161–185. 30 fn. ISBN 0–19–511632–1. BE62783.
    autonomy; *contraception; *cultural pluralism; decision making; *developing countries; *ethical relativism; females; *feminist ethics; freedom; *human rights; *international aspects; justice; legal aspects; males; methods; non-Western World; *paternalism; *political activity; postmodernism; pregnant women; public policy; *reproduction; reproductive technologies; Roman Catholic ethics; selective abortion; *sex determination; social control; social discrimination; values; Western World; *women's health; *women's rights; Brazil;

BE = bioethics accession number   fn. = footnotes   refs. = references

China; Feminist International Network of Resistance to Reproductive and Genetic Engineering (FINRRAGE); India; International Conference on Population and Development (Cairo, 1994); Women's Global Network for Reproductive Rights

Maher, Daniel P. The moral triangle. *Ethics and Medics.* 1997 May; 22(5): 1–2. BE60409.
*contraception; cultural pluralism; *institutional ethics; institutional policies; physician patient relationship; *religious hospitals; *Roman Catholic ethics; sterilization (sexual)

Mason, John Kenyon. Contraception. *In: his* Medico–Legal Aspects of Reproduction and Parenthood. Second Edition. Brookfield, VT: Ashgate; 1998: 41–65. 85 fn. ISBN 1–84104–065–8. BE61061.
adults; *contraception; drug industry; family planning; hormones; informed consent; *legal aspects; legal liability; marital relationship; medical devices; mentally retarded; *methods; minors; negligence; parental consent; parental notification; physicians; risks and benefits; Roman Catholic ethics; Abortion Act 1967 (Great Britain); Gillick v. West Norfolk and Wisbech AHA; *Great Britain; Offences Against the Person Act 1861 (Great Britain); Re R (A Minor)(Wardship: Medical Treatment)

Mirsky, Judith; Radlett, Marty, eds.; Panos Institute. Private Decisions, Public Debate: Women, Reproduction and Population. London: Panos Publications; 1994. 185 p. Includes references. Journalists' case studies from India, Tanzania, South Korea, Burkina Faso, Philippines, Brazil, Ghana, Ethiopia, Thailand, Pakistan, Chile, and Egypt. ISBN 1–870670–34–5. BE59736.
abortion, induced; cesarean section; childbirth; circumcision; *contraception; *developing countries; education; employment; *family planning; *females; HIV seropositivity; illegal abortion; infertility; *international aspects; males; nurse midwives; politics; population control; reproduction; Roman Catholics; sex determination; sexually transmitted diseases; social discrimination; socioeconomic factors; sterilization (sexual); *women's health; women's health services; *women's rights; *Brazil; *Burkina Faso; *Chile; *Egypt; *Ethiopia; *Ghana; *India; *Korea; *Pakistan; *Philippines; *Tanzania; *Thailand

Mudur, Ganapati. Indian women's groups question contraceptive vaccine research. [News]. *BMJ (British Medical Journal).* 1998 Nov 14; 317(7169): 1340. BE60855.
*contraception; developing countries; *females; *human experimentation; immunization; *political activity; risks and benefits; *India

O'Rourke, Kevin D. Applying the Directives: The *Ethical and Religious Directives* concerning three medical situations require some elucidation. *Health Progress.* 1998 Jul–Aug; 79(4): 64–69. 33 fn. BE61616.
abortion, induced; *allowing to die; *artificial feeding; *contraception; double effect; drugs; fetuses; health care delivery; institutional policies; intention; methods; *persistent vegetative state; pregnant women; *rape; religious hospitals; *Roman Catholic ethics; surgery; *therapeutic abortion; withholding treatment; *ectopic pregnancy; *Ethical and Religious Directives for Catholic Health Care Services

Schoen, Johanna. "A Great Thing for Poor Folks": Birth Control, Sterilization, and Abortion in Public Health and Welfare in the Twentieth Century. Ann Arbor, MI: UMI Dissertation Services; 1996. 267 p. Bibliography: p. 240–267. Dissertation, Ph.D. in History, University of North Carolina, 1995. Order No. 9631980. BE62797.
*abortion, induced; blacks; *coercion; *contraception; eugenics; *females; government regulation; historical

aspects; *indigents; *involuntary sterilization; legal aspects; males; mentally retarded; motivation; public health; *public policy; sexuality; *social control; social discrimination; state government; whites; *North Carolina; Twentieth Century; United States

Watkins, Elizabeth Siegel. On the Pill: A Social History of Oral Contraceptives, 1950–1970. Baltimore, MD: Johns Hopkins University Press; 1998. 183 p. 480 fn. ISBN 0–8018–5876–3. BE60017.
advertising; attitudes; biomedical research; *contraception; drug industry; *drugs; family planning; federal government; *females; financial support; government regulation; *historical aspects; *hormones; information dissemination; informed consent; mass media; morality; patients; physician patient relationship; physicians; political activity; population control; risks and benefits; Roman Catholic ethics; sexuality; *social impact; socioeconomic factors; women's health; women's rights; Food and Drug Administration; *Twentieth Century; *United States

Watts, Jonathan. When impotence leads contraception. [News]. *Lancet.* 1999 Mar 6; 353(9155): 819. BE61038.
*contraception; *drugs; *females; *government regulation; *hormones; *males; mass media; political activity; public policy; sexuality; social discrimination; *impotence; *Japan; *Viagra

Weber, David O. Realignments, realpolitik, religion, and reproductive health. *Healthcare Forum Journal.* 1996 May–Jun; 39(3): 76–83. BE59579.
*abortion, induced; conscience; *contraception; cultural pluralism; drug industry; economics; family planning; government financing; health facilities; *institutional policies; Jewish ethics; legal liability; managed care programs; medical devices; medical education; political activity; *Protestant ethics; *religion; *religious hospitals; reproductive technologies; *Roman Catholic ethics; statistics; trends; violence; voluntary sterilization; *women's health services; *health facility mergers; California; Ethical and Religious Directives for Catholic Health Care Services; Mormonism; Norplant; *United States; Utah

Paying for family planning. [Editorial]. *Lancet.* 1998 Sep 12; 352(9131): 831. BE60792.
abortion, induced; *contraception; developing countries; *family planning; federal government; females; *government financing; *health insurance reimbursement; international aspects; legislation; political activity; politics; *public policy; women's health services; *United States

World Medical Association adopts statements, etc., on miscellaneous matters. [Texts of statements and declarations]. *International Digest of Health Legislation.* 1997; 48(1): 92–97. Statements and declarations adopted by the 48th General Assembly of the World Medical Association, held in Somerset West, Republic of South Africa, Oct 1996; including the Declaration of Helsinki as amended Oct 1996. BE59591.
*bioethical issues; biomedical research; *contraception; *domestic violence; *drugs; *family planning; *guidelines; *human experimentation; informed consent; *international aspects; medical education; nontherapeutic research; *organizational policies; *patient care; *physicians; *professional competence; professional organizations; public policy; quality of health care; research ethics committees; self regulation; therapeutic research; third party consent; women's rights; *antibiotics; *Declaration of Helsinki; *World Medical Association

CONTRACEPTION/MINORS

Gonen, Julianna S. Managed care and unintended pregnancy: testing the limits of prevention. *Women's*

BE = bioethics accession number   fn. = footnotes   refs. = references

Health Issues. 1999 Mar–Apr; 9(2, Suppl.): 26S–35S. 24 refs. BE61969.

> *adolescents; adults; confidentiality; *contraception; costs and benefits; *family planning; federal government; government financing; health insurance; *health insurance reimbursement; health maintenance organizations; *managed care programs; methods; organizational policies; parental consent; parental notification; *public policy; *quality of health care; religious hospitals; Roman Catholics; state government; statistics; *women's health services; Medicaid; United States

Martin, Jeanett. Contraception and the under-16s: the legal issues. *Nursing Standard.* 1996 Jun 12; 10(38): 46–48. 17 refs. BE60402.

> competence; confidentiality; *contraception; females; informed consent; *legal aspects; mentally retarded; *minors; parental consent; *Great Britain

COST OF HEALTH CARE *See* HEALTH CARE/ECONOMICS

DANGEROUSNESS *See* CONFIDENTIALITY/MENTAL HEALTH

DEATH *See* DETERMINATION OF DEATH

DEATH WITH DIGNITY *See* ALLOWING TO DIE, EUTHANASIA, SUICIDE, TERMINAL CARE

DELIVERY OF HEALTH CARE *See* HEALTH CARE

DETERMINATION OF DEATH

Benjamin, Martin. Pragmatism and the determination of death. *In:* McGee, Glenn, ed. Pragmatic Bioethics. Nashville, TN: Vanderbilt University Press; 1999: 181–193, 280–281. 14 fn. ISBN 0-8265-1321-2. BE60671.

> advisory committees; *anencephaly; brain death; *determination of death; legal aspects; organ donation; *persistent vegetative state; *personhood; philosophy; standards; values; withholding treatment; pragmatism; Harvard Committee on Brain Death; Uniform Determination of Death Act

Brock, Dan W. The role of the public in public policy on the definition of death. *In:* Youngner, Stuart J., Arnold, Robert M.; Schapiro, Renie, eds. The Definition of Death: Contemporary Controversies. Baltimore, MD: Johns Hopkins University Press; 1999: 293–307. 7 refs. ISBN 0-8018-5985-9. BE60772.

> *attitudes to death; brain; brain death; cardiac death; *decision making; *determination of death; family members; organ donation; personhood; *public participation; *public policy; resuscitation; standards; time factors; United States

Burt, Robert A. Where do we go from here? *In:* Youngner, Stuart J.; Arnold, Robert M.; Schapiro, Renie, eds. The Definition of Death: Contemporary Controversies. Baltimore, MD: Johns Hopkins University Press; 1999: 332–339. ISBN 0-8018-5985-9. BE60775.

> brain death; cardiac death; *cultural pluralism; decision making; dementia; *determination of death; legal aspects; organ donation; personhood; prolongation of life; psychology; resource allocation; *standards; suffering; treatment refusal; values; withholding treatment

Capron, Alexander Morgan. The bifurcated legal

standard for determining death: does it work? *In:* Youngner, Stuart J.; Arnold, Robert M.; Schapiro, Renie, eds. The Definition of Death: Contemporary Controversies. Baltimore, MD: Johns Hopkins University Press; 1999: 117–136. 32 fn. ISBN 0-8018-5985-9. BE60762.

> allowing to die; alternatives; *brain death; *cardiac death; *determination of death; diagnosis; *legal aspects; legislation; methods; organ donation; public policy; *standards; withholding treatment; National Conference of Commissioners on Uniform State Laws; Uniform Anatomical Gift Act; *Uniform Determination of Death Act; *United States

Charo, R. Alta. Dusk, dawn, and defining death: legal classifications and biological categories. *In:* Youngner, Stuart J., Arnold, Robert M., Schapiro, Renie, eds. The Definition of Death: Contemporary Controversies. Baltimore, MD: Johns Hopkins University Press; 1999: 277–292. 24 fn. ISBN 0-8018-5985-9. BE60771.

> *determination of death; females; fetuses; genetic determinism; *legal aspects; males; minority groups; parent child relationship; persistent vegetative state; personhood; *public policy; standards; United States

Engelhardt, H. Tristram. Redefining death: the mirage of consensus. *In:* Youngner, Stuart J.; Arnold, Robert M.; Schapiro, Renie, eds. The Definition of Death: Contemporary Controversies. Baltimore, MD: Johns Hopkins University Press; 1999: 319–331. 1 ref. ISBN 0-8018-5985-9. BE60774.

> attitudes to death; biomedical technologies; brain death; cardiac death; *consensus; *cultural pluralism; decision making; *determination of death; *dissent; methods; organ donation; *public policy; religion; secularism; standards; values; withholding treatment

Engelhart, Karlheinz; King, T.T.; Bakran, A., et al. Organ donation and permanent vegetative state. [Letters and response]. *Lancet.* 1998 Jan 17; 351(9097): 211–213. 4 refs. BE59303.

> allowing to die; artificial feeding; *determination of death; drugs; involuntary euthanasia; *killing; National Socialism; *organ donation; *persistent vegetative state; withholding treatment; Great Britain

France. Decree No. 96-1041 of 2 Dec 1996 on the determination of death prior to the removal of organs, tissues, and cells for therapeutic or scientific purposes, and amending the Public Health Code (Second Part): decrees made after consulting the *Conseil d'Etat). (Journal officiel de la Republique fran3aise, Lois et Decrets,* 4 Dec 1996, No. 282, p. 17615). *International Digest of Health Legislation.* 1997; 48(2): 197–198. 1 fn. BE59595.

> brain death; *cadavers; *determination of death; *legal aspects; *organ donation; *France

Gavin, William J. On "tame" and "untamed" death: Jamesian reflections. *In:* McGee, Glenn, ed. Pragmatic Bioethics. Nashville, TN: Vanderbilt Univesity Press; 1999: 97–112, 269–271. 56 fn. ISBN 0-8265-1321-2. BE60666.

> *attitudes to death; cultural pluralism; *death; *determination of death; emotions; historical aspects; narrative ethics; philosophy; psychology; public policy; *terminal care; *terminally ill; dignity; pragmatism; James, William

Lachs, John. The element of choice in criteria of death. *In: his* The Relevance of Philosophy to Life. Nashville, TN: Vanderbilt University Press; 1995: 209–227. 2 fn. ISBN 0-8265-1262-3. BE60867.

BE = bioethics accession number   fn. = footnotes   refs. = references

advisory committees; attitudes to death; autonomy; *brain death; cultural pluralism; death; decision making; *determination of death; personhood; public policy; standards; *values; withholding treatment; President's Commission for the Study of Ethical Problems

Lynn, Joanne; Cranford, Ronald. The persisting perplexities in the determination of death. *In:* Youngner, Stuart J.; Arnold, Robert M.; Schapiro, Renie, eds. The Definition of Death: Contemporary Controversies. Baltimore, MD: Johns Hopkins University Press; 1999: 101–114. 25 refs. ISBN 0–8018–5985–9. BE60761.
   brain death; brain pathology; cardiac death; *determination of death; organ donation; public policy; resuscitation; *standards; time factors; uncertainty

Macklin, Ruth. Death and birth. *In: her* Against Relativism: Cultural Diversity and the Search for Ethical Universals in Medicine. New York, NY: Oxford University Press; 1999: 136–160. 32 fn. ISBN 0–19–511632–1. BE62782.
   *abortion, induced; autonomy; brain death; cardiac death; *cultural pluralism; *determination of death; *ethical relativism; family relationship; *females; feminist ethics; fetuses; infanticide; *international aspects; justice; morality; mortality; non–Western World; organ donation; organ transplantation; pregnant women; public policy; *selective abortion; *sex determination; *social discrimination; *social worth; value of life; values; women's rights; Cameroon; China; India; Japan; Philippines; United States

Menikoff, Jerry. Doubts about death: the silence of the Institute of Medicine. *Journal of Law, Medicine and Ethics.* 1998 Summer; 26(2): 157–165. 63 fn. Commented on by J.T. Potts et al., p. 166–168. BE62678.
   advisory committees; brain death; *cadavers; *cardiac death; *determination of death; disclosure; *evaluation; *guidelines; informed consent; model legislation; *organ donation; organizational policies; policy analysis; *standards; *time factors; ventilators; *Institute of Medicine; Uniform Determination of Death Act; *United States

Miles, Steven. Death in a technological and pluralistic culture. *In:* Youngner, Stuart J.; Arnold, Robert M.; Schapiro, Renie, eds. The Definition of Death: Contemporary Controversies. Baltimore, MD: Johns Hopkins University Press; 1999: 311–318. 11 refs. ISBN 0–8018–5985–9. BE60773.
   brain; brain death; cardiac death; consensus; *cultural pluralism; decision making; dementia; *determination of death; organ donation; persistent vegetative state; *public policy; resuscitation; standards; withholding treatment; United States

Potts, John T.; Herdman, Roger C.; Beauchamp, Thomas L., et al. Commentary: clear thinking and open discussion guide IOM's report on organ donation. *Journal of Law, Medicine and Ethics.* 1998 Summer; 26(2): 166–168. 10 fn. Commentary on J. Menikoff, p. 157–168. BE62679.
   advisory committees; brain death; *cadavers; *cardiac death; *determination of death; disclosure; *guidelines; informed consent; institutional policies; *organ donation; policy analysis; public policy; standards; *time factors; *Institute of Medicine; *United States

Rayner, John D. A matter of life and death. *In: his* Jewish Religious Law: A Progressive Perspective. New York, NY: Berghahn Books; 1998: 130–137. ISBN 1–57181–976–2. BE62136.
   *allowing to die; brain death; cardiac death; *determination of death; double effect; drugs; *Jewish ethics; pain; persistent vegetative state; prolongation of life; terminally ill; value of life; withholding treatment; Orthodox Judaism; *Reform

Judaism

Veatch, Robert M. The conscience clause: how much individual choice in defining death can our society tolerate? *In:* Youngner, Stuart J.; Arnold, Robert M.; Schapiro, Renie, eds. The Definition of Death: Contemporary Controversies. Baltimore, MD: Johns Hopkins University Press; 1999: 137–160. 34 fn. ISBN 0–8018–5985–9. BE60763.
   advance directives; autonomy; brain; *brain death; *cardiac death; *conscience; constitutional law; *cultural pluralism; *decision making; *determination of death; dissent; family members; health insurance; health personnel; legal aspects; life insurance; married persons; moral policy; organ donation; physicians; politics; *public policy; religion; social impact; *standards; state government; terminally ill; third party consent; values; withholding treatment; New Jersey; United States

Youngner, Stuart J.; Arnold, Robert M.; Schapiro, Renie, eds. The Definition of Death: Contemporary Controversies. Baltimore, MD: Johns Hopkins University Press; 1999. 436 refs. 111 fn. ISBN 0–8018–5985–9. BE60755.
   anencephaly; attitudes to death; brain; *brain death; cardiac death; conscience; cultural pluralism; decision making; *determination of death; dissent; international aspects; Jewish ethics; legal aspects; methods; organ donation; organ transplantation; organizational policies; persistent vegetative state; personhood; physicians; professional organizations; Protestant ethics; public opinion; public participation; public policy; resuscitation; review; *standards; withholding treatment; Denmark; Germany; Japan; United States

Zemer, Moshe. Determining death in Jewish law. *In:* Jacob, Walter; Zemer, Moshe, eds. Death and Euthanasia in Jewish Law: Essays and Responsa. Pittsburgh, PA: Freehof Institute of Progressive Halakhah; Rodef Shalom Press; 1995: 105–119. 28 fn. ISBN 0–929699–06–8. BE60075.
   brain death; cardiac death; *determination of death; dissent; *Jewish ethics; organ donation; organ transplantation; Orthodox Judaism; Reform Judaism

DETERMINATION OF DEATH/BRAIN DEATH

Akabayashi, Akira. Transplantation from a brain dead donor in Japan. [News]. *Hastings Center Report.* 1999 May–Jun; 29(3): 48. BE61416.
   *brain death; determination of death; donor cards; family members; *legal aspects; legislation; *organ donation; organ transplantation; third party consent; *Japan

Asian Society of Transplantation. Declaration of Seoul on brain death. *International Digest of Health Legislation.* 1997; 48(2): 229. Adopted by the Society at its 4th Congress on 28 Aug 1995. BE59596.
   *brain death; *determination of death; *guidelines; international aspects; *legal aspects; organ donation; professional organizations; public policy; *Asia; *Asian Society of Transplantation; *Declaration of Seoul

Becker, Carl. Money talks, money kills -- the economics of transplantation in Japan and China. *Bioethics.* 1999 Jul; 13(3–4): 236–243. 33 fn. BE61873.
   allowing to die; *brain death; *capital punishment; *determination of death; directed donation; *economics; hospitals; institutional policies; *legal aspects; *motivation; non–Western World; *organ donation; *organ transplantation; *prisoners; *public policy; *China; *Japan
   Japan and China have long resisted the Western trend of organ transplantation from brain–dead patients, based on a 'Confucian' respect for integrity of ancestors'

BE = bioethics accession number   fn. = footnotes   refs. = references

bodies. While their general publics continue to harbor grave doubts about such practices, their medical and political elites are hastening towards the road of organ-harvesting and organ-marketing, largely for economic reasons. This report illustrates the ways that economics is motivating brain-death legislation in Japan and criminal executions in China.

Bernat, James L. Refinements in the definition and criterion of death. *In:* Youngner, Stuart J.; Arnold, Robert M.; Schapiro, Renie, eds. The Definition of Death: Contemporary Controversies. Baltimore, MD: Johns Hopkins University Press; 1999: 83–92. 21 fn. ISBN 0-8018-5985-9. BE60759.
> allowing to die; alternatives; brain; *brain death; cardiac death; *determination of death; moral policy; persistent vegetative state; personhood; *standards; ventilators; withholding treatment; President's Commission for the Study of Ethical Problems; United States

Bleich, J. David; Caplan, Arthur L.; Murray, Joseph E., et al. Defining the limits of organ and tissue research and transplantation. [Proceedings of the International Symposium on Law and Science at the Crossroads: Biomedical Technology, Ethics, Public Policy, and the Law; panel discussion]. *Suffolk University Law Review.* 1993 Winter; 27(4): 1457–1476. Moderator: Raja B. Khauli. BE60701.
> aborted fetuses; autonomy; body parts and fluids; *brain death; cadavers; cardiac death; *determination of death; *fetal tissue donation; *organ donation; organ donors; presumed consent; public policy; remuneration; values

Bleich, J. David. Moral debate and semantic sleight of hand. *Suffolk University Law Review.* 1993 Winter; 27(4): 1173–1193. 44 fn. BE60698.
> *aborted fetuses; abortion, induced; beginning of life; *brain death; cultural pluralism; decision making; democracy; *determination of death; fetal research; *fetal tissue donation; fetuses; government financing; legal aspects; legal rights; moral policy; newborns; prolongation of life; public policy; quality of life; religion; religious ethics; standards; state interest; theology; value of life; *values; withholding treatment

Brazil. Federal Medical Council. Federal Medical Council (CFM) of Brazil adopts resolutions on criteria for death and on medically assisted procreation. [Texts of Resolution CFM No. 1346/91, adopted 8 Aug 1991; and Resolution CFM No. 1358/92, adopted 11 Nov 1992]. *International Digest of Health Legislation.* 1994; 45(1): 100–102. BE62685.
> *brain death; confidentiality; cryopreservation; *determination of death; government regulation; *guidelines; health facilities; *legal aspects; multiple pregnancy; ovum donors; preimplantation diagnosis; records; *reproductive technologies; research embryo creation; selective abortion; sex preselection; standards; surrogate mothers; *Brazil; *Federal Medical Council (Brazil)

Brody, Baruch A. How much of the brain must be dead? *In:* Youngner, Stuart J.; Arnold, Robert M.; Schapiro, Renie, eds. The Definition of Death: Contemporary Controversies. Baltimore, MD: Johns Hopkins University Press; 1999: 71–82. 11 refs. ISBN 0-8018-5985-9. BE60758.
> allowing to die; anencephaly; *brain; *brain death; cardiac death; *determination of death; methods; moral policy; organ donation; organizational policies; personhood; professional organizations; *standards; ventilators; withholding treatment; American Medical Association

Campbell, Courtney S. Fundamentals of life and death:

Christian fundamentalism and medical science. *In:* Youngner, Stuart J.; Arnold, Robert M.; Schapiro, Renie, eds. The Definition of Death: Contemporary Controversies. Baltimore, MD: Johns Hopkins University Press; 1999: 194–209. 30 refs. ISBN 0-8018-5985-9. BE60766.
> allowing to die; *attitudes to death; autonomy; brain; *brain death; *determination of death; medicine; organ donation; personhood; *Protestant ethics; public policy; science; secularism; standards; theology; withholding treatment; coma; *Christian Fundamentalists

Capron, Alexander Morgan. The bifurcated legal standard for determining death: does it work? *In:* Youngner, Stuart J.; Arnold, Robert M.; Schapiro, Renie, eds. The Definition of Death: Contemporary Controversies. Baltimore, MD: Johns Hopkins University Press; 1999: 117–136. 32 fn. ISBN 0-8018-5985-9. BE60762.
> allowing to die; alternatives; *brain death; *cardiac death; *determination of death; diagnosis; *legal aspects; legislation; methods; organ donation; public policy; *standards; withholding treatment; National Conference of Commissioners on Uniform State Laws; Uniform Anatomical Gift Act; *Uniform Determination of Death Act; *United States

Cranford, Ronald E. Discontinuation of ventilation after brain stem death: policy should be balanced with concern for the family. *BMJ (British Medical Journal).* 1999 Jun 26; 318(7200): 1754–1755. 1 ref. BE62304.
> *brain death; *communication; *determination of death; *family members; health personnel; hospitals; institutional policies; professional family relationship; psychological stress

DeGrazia, David. Biology, consciousness, and the definition of death. *Philosophy and Public Policy.* 1998 Winter–Spring; 18(1–2): 18–22. 10 refs. BE59815.
> *brain death; *determination of death; organ donation; persistent vegetative state; personhood; prolongation of life; standards

DuBois, James M. Recent attacks on brain death: do they merit a reconsideration of our current policies? *Health Care Ethics USA.* 1998 Summer; 6(3): 4–5. 11 fn. BE60821.
> anencephaly; *brain death; *determination of death; fetuses; organ donation; personhood; quality of life; Roman Catholic ethics; standards

Fost, Norman. The unimportance of death. *In:* Youngner, Stuart J.; Arnold, Robert M.; Schapiro, Renie, eds. The Definition of Death: Contemporary Controversies. Baltimore, MD: Johns Hopkins University Press; 1999: 161–178. 39 fn. ISBN 0-8018-5985-9. BE60764.
> advisory committees; allowing to die; anencephaly; body parts and fluids; brain; *brain death; cardiac death; *determination of death; *legal aspects; legislation; *organ donation; persistent vegetative state; presumed consent; prolongation of life; *public policy; required request; standards; terminally ill; utilitarianism; withholding treatment; coma; health services misuse; Harvard Committee on Brain Death; United States

Jennett, Bryan. Discontinuation of ventilation after brain stem death: brain stem death defines death in law. *BMJ (British Medical Journal).* 1999 Jun 26; 318(7200): 1755. 5 refs. BE62305.
> *brain death; decision making; *determination of death; diagnosis; family members; *legal aspects; persistent vegetative state; physicians; third party consent; ventilators; withholding treatment; *Great Britain

---

BE = bioethics accession number   fn. = footnotes   refs. = references

Jones, D. Gareth. The problematic symmetry between brain birth and brain death. *Journal of Medical Ethics.* 1998 Aug; 24(4): 237–242. 37 refs. BE61288.
*beginning of life; *brain; *brain death; determination of death; *embryos; *fetal development; *fetuses; moral policy; *personhood; standards; terminology

The possible symmetry between the concepts of brain death and brain birth (life) is explored. Since the symmetry argument has tended to overlook the most appropriate definition of brain death, the fundamental concepts of whole brain death and higher brain death are assessed. In this way, a context is provided for a discussion of brain birth. Different writers have placed brain birth at numerous points: 25–40 days, eight weeks, 22–24 weeks, and 32–36 weeks gestation. For others, the concept itself is open to question. Apart from this, it needs to be asked whether a unitary concept is an oversimplification. The merits of defining two stages of brain birth, to parallel the two definitions of brain death, are discussed. An attempt is then made to map these various stages of brain birth and brain death onto a developmental continuum. Although the results hold biological interest, their ethical significance is less evident. Development and degeneration are not interchangeable, and definitions of death apply specifically to those who are dying, not those who are developing. I conclude that while a dual concept of brain death has proved helpful, a dual concept of brain birth still has problems, and the underlying concept of brain birth itself continues to be elusive.

Lachs, John. The element of choice in criteria of death. *In: his* The Relevance of Philosophy to Life. Nashville, TN: Vanderbilt University Press; 1995: 209–227. 2 fn. ISBN 0-8265-1262-3. BE60867.
advisory committees; attitudes to death; autonomy; *brain death; cultural pluralism; death; decision making; *determination of death; personhood; public policy; standards; *values; withholding treatment; President's Commission for the Study of Ethical Problems

Lamb, David. Organ transplants, death, and policies for procurement. *Monist.* 1993 Apr; 76(2): 203–221. 27 refs. BE60221.
altruism; body parts and fluids; *brain death; cadavers; coercion; commodification; cultural pluralism; *determination of death; family members; gifts; human body; intensive care units; international aspects; mentally disabled; minors; moral obligations; *organ donation; *organ donors; organ transplantation; patient transfer; presumed consent; religious ethics; remuneration; required request; resource allocation; risks and benefits; selection for treatment; standards; terminally ill; transplant recipients; ventilators; refusal to donate; Europe; Great Britain; Japan; United States

Linder, Douglas O. The other right-to-life debate: when does Fourteenth Amendment "life" end? *Arizona Law Review.* 1995; 37(4): 1183–1207. 138 fn. BE62218.
*allowing to die; artificial feeding; bioethical issues; *brain death; brain pathology; coercion; constitutional law; *determination of death; due process; federal government; government financing; *legal aspects; legal rights; *persistent vegetative state; *personhood; *prolongation of life; *public policy; resource allocation; self concept; state government; Supreme Court decisions; *value of life; vulnerable populations; wedge argument; *withholding treatment; *Fourteenth Amendment; *United States

Lizza, John B.; Truog, Robert D.; Robertson, John A., et al. Death: merely biological? [Letters and response]. *Hastings Center Report.* 1999 Jan-Feb; 29(1): 4–5. BE61627.

allowing to die; brain; *brain death; cardiac death; *determination of death; killing; organ donation; personhood; standards

Lock, Margaret. The problem of brain death: Japanese disputes about bodies and modernity. *In:* Youngner, Stuart J., Arnold, Robert M., Schapiro, Renie, eds. The Definition of Death: Contemporary Controversies. Baltimore, MD: Johns Hopkins University Press; 1999: 239–256. 35 fn. ISBN 0-8018-5985-9. BE60769.
advisory committees; *attitudes to death; *brain death; Buddhist ethics; cardiac death; consensus; *determination of death; diagnosis; *dissent; family members; gifts; international aspects; legal aspects; mass media; non-Western World; *organ donation; organ transplantation; organizational policies; persistent vegetative state; physicians; professional organizations; public opinion; *public policy; secularism; values; Western World; Confucian ethics; Brain Death Advisory Council (Japan); *Japan; Japan Society for Transplantation; Patients' Rights Committee (Japan); Special Cabinet Committee on Brain Death and Organ Transplants (Japan)

MacFarquhar, Neil. In Islam, brain death ends life support. *New York Times.* 1999 Feb 6: A6. BE60972.
*allowing to die; *brain death; *determination of death; famous persons; *Islamic ethics; terminally ill; ventilators; King Hussein

McMahan, Jeff. Brain death, cortical death and persistent vegetative state. *In:* Kuhse, Helga; Singer, Peter, eds. A Companion to Bioethics. Malden, MA: Blackwell; 1998: 250–260. 15 refs. ISBN 0-631-19737-0. BE59500.
*brain; *brain death; *brain pathology; dementia; *determination of death; organ donation; *persistent vegetative state; *personhood; philosophy; self concept; uncertainty; withholding treatment; conjoined twins; locked-in syndrome

Pallis, Chris. On the brainstem criterion of death. *In:* Youngner, Stuart J.; Arnold, Robert M.; Schapiro, Renie, eds. The Definition of Death: Contemporary Controversies Baltimore, MD: Johns Hopkins University Press; 1999: 93–100. 20 refs. ISBN 0-8018-5985-9. BE60760.
*brain; *brain death; *determination of death; organ donation; persistent vegetative state; *standards; withholding treatment

Pernick, Martin S. Brain death in a cultural context: the reconstruction of death, 1967–1981. *In:* Youngner, Stuart J.; Arnold, Robert M.; Schapiro, Renie, eds. The Definition of Death: Contemporary Controversies. Baltimore, MD: Johns Hopkins University Press; 1999: 3–33. 90 fn. ISBN 0-8018-5985-9. BE60756.
advisory committees; attitudes to death; autonomy; blacks; brain; *brain death; decision making; *determination of death; historical aspects; legal aspects; mass media; organ donation; organizational policies; patients; physicians; professional organizations; public opinion; public policy; resuscitation; standards; American Medical Association; Harvard Committee on Brain Death; President's Commission for the Study of Ethical Problems; Twentieth Century; United States

Plum, Fred. Clinical standards and technological confirmatory tests in diagnosing brain death. *In:* Youngner, Stuart J.; Arnold, Robert M.; Schapiro, Renie, eds. The Definition of Death: Contemporary Controversies. Baltimore, MD: Johns Hopkins University Press; 1999: 34–65. 65 refs. ISBN 0-8018-5985-6. BE60757.
advisory committees; allowing to die; brain; *brain death; brain pathology; children; *determination of death;

diagnosis; methods; mortality; organ donation; persistent vegetative state; *practice guidelines; *standards; withholding treatment; coma; locked-in syndrome; Great Britain; New York State Guidelines for Determination of Death; President's Commission for the Study of Ethical Problems; Uniform Determination of Death Act; United States

Rix, Bo Andreassen. Brain death, ethics, and politics in Denmark. *In:* Youngner, Stuart J.; Arnold, Robert M.; Schapiro, Renie, eds. The Definition of Death: Contemporary Controversies. Baltimore, MD: Johns Hopkins University Press; 1999: 227-238. 5 refs. ISBN 0-8018-5985-9. BE60768.
   advisory committees; attitudes to death; *brain death; *cardiac death; committee membership; decision making; *determination of death; diagnosis; information dissemination; mass media; organ donation; persistent vegetative state; physicians; public opinion; public participation; *public policy; *standards; Danish Council of Ethics; *Denmark

Rosner, Fred. The definition of death in Jewish law. *In:* Youngner, Stuart J.; Arnold, Robert M.; Schapiro, Renie, eds. The Definition of Death: Contemporary Controversies. Baltimore, MD: Johns Hopkins University Press; 1999: 210-221. 19 refs. ISBN 0-8018-5985-9. BE60767.
   attitudes to death; brain; *brain death; cardiac death; *determination of death; *Jewish ethics; personhood; secularism; *standards; theology; value of life

Sakai, Akio. Consensus formation in bioethical decisionmaking in Japan: present contexts and future perspectives. *In:* ten Have, Henk A.M.J.; Sass, Hans-Martin, eds. Consensus Formation in Healthcare Ethics. Boston, MA: Kluwer Academic; 1998: 93-105. 34 refs. 1 fn. ISBN 0-7923-4944-X. BE62590.
   *attitudes; *bioethical issues; *biomedical technologies; *brain death; cadavers; *consensus; decision making; *determination of death; empirical research; ethics committees; medical schools; organ donation; physicians; professional organizations; *public opinion; public policy; religion; values; *Japan

Schöne-Seifert, Bettina. Defining death in Germany: brain death and its discontents. *In:* Youngner, Stuart J.; Arnold, Robert M.; Schapiro, Renie eds. The Definition of Death: Contemporary Controversies. Baltimore, MD: Johns Hopkins University Press; 1999: 257-271. 41 refs. ISBN 0-8018-5985-9. BE60770.
   *attitudes to death; bioethics; *brain death; cardiac death; *determination of death; dissent; hearts; kidneys; legal aspects; organ donation; persistent vegetative state; physicians; practice guidelines; professional organizations; *public policy; religion; standards; third party consent; German Medical Association; German Scientific Societies; German Surgical Society; *Germany

Seifert, Josef. Is 'brain death' actually death? *Monist.* 1993 Apr; 76(2): 175-202. 18 refs. 19 fn. BE60220.
   anencephaly; brain; *brain death; cardiac death; *death; *determination of death; fetal development; human body; organ donation; personhood; *philosophy; standards; tissue transplantation; uncertainty

Shewmon, D. Alan. "Brainstem death," "brain death" and death: a critical re-evaluation of the purported equivalence. *Issues in Law and Medicine.* 1998 Fall; 14(2): 125-145. 52 fn. BE62009.
   *brain; *brain death; brain pathology; cardiac death; death; *determination of death; dissent; evaluation; informed consent; legal aspects; organ donation; prolongation of life; *standards; value of life; withholding treatment; Great

Britain; United States

Shewmon, D. Alan. Recovery from "brain death": a neurologist's apologia. *Linacre Quarterly.* 1997 Feb; 64(1): 30-96. 268 refs. 9 fn. BE59309.
   adults; anencephaly; artificial feeding; *brain; *brain death; *brain pathology; cadavers; *cardiac death; childbirth; children; consensus; dementia; *determination of death; *dissent; historical aspects; infants; killing; legal aspects; organ donation; organizational policies; pain; *persistent vegetative state; *personhood; *philosophy; physicians; pregnant women; professional organizations; Roman Catholic ethics; standards; suffering; *uncertainty; utilitarianism; withholding treatment; Guillain-Barre syndrome; locked-in syndrome; neurology; American Academy of Neurology; American Medical Association; Aristotle; President's Commission for the Study of Ethical Problems; Thomas Aquinas; Twentieth Century

Siminoff, Laura A.; Bloch, Alexia. American attitudes and beliefs about brain death: the empirical literature. *In:* Youngner, Stuart J.; Arnold, Robert M.; Schapiro, Renie, eds. The Definition of Death: Contemporary Controversies. Baltimore, MD: Johns Hopkins University Press; 1999: 183-193. 37 refs. ISBN 0-8018-5985-9. BE60765.
   *attitudes to death; *brain death; cardiac death; cultural pluralism; *determination of death; donor cards; *empirical research; family members; international aspects; *knowledge, attitudes, practice; minority groups; nurses; *organ donation; physicians; presumed consent; *public opinion; *standards; Japan; *United States

Swinburn, J.M.A.; Ali, S.M.; Banerjee, D.J., et al. Ethical dilemma: discontinuation of ventilation after brain stem death: to whom is our duty of care? *BMJ (British Medical Journal).* 1999 Jun 26; 318(7200): 1753-1754. 5 refs. BE62303.
   allowing to die; brain; *brain death; case studies; determination of death; *dissent; *family members; futility; intensive care units; legal aspects; persistent vegetative state; *physicians; professional family relationship; prognosis; prolongation of life; psychological stress; resource allocation; *ventilators; *withholding treatment; Great Britain

Veatch, Robert M. The conscience clause: how much individual choice in defining death can our society tolerate? *In:* Youngner, Stuart J.; Arnold, Robert M.; Schapiro, Renie, eds. The Definition of Death: Contemporary Controversies. Baltimore, MD: Johns Hopkins University Press; 1999: 137-160. 34 fn. ISBN 0-8018-5985-9. BE60763.
   advance directives; autonomy; brain; *brain death; *cardiac death; *conscience; constitutional law; *cultural pluralism; *decision making; *determination of death; dissent; family members; health insurance; health personnel; legal aspects; life insurance; married persons; moral policy; organ donation; physicians; politics; *public policy; religion; social impact; *standards; state government; terminally ill; third party consent; values; withholding treatment; New Jersey; United States

Watts, Jonathan. Concept of brain death to be accepted in South Korea. [News]. *Lancet.* 1998 Dec 19-26; 352(9145): 1996. BE60272.
   *brain death; cadavers; *determination of death; family members; *legal aspects; *organ donation; third party consent; *Korea

Watts, Jonathan. Japan does its first official heart and liver transplantations. [News]. *Lancet.* 1999 Mar 6; 353(9155): 821. BE61039.
   *brain death; cadavers; *determination of death; donor

BE = bioethics accession number   fn. = footnotes   refs. = references

cards; hearts; kidneys; legal aspects; livers; mass media; organ donation; *organ transplantation; public opinion; corneas; *Japan; Organ and Transplant Law 1997 (Japan)

WuDunn, Sheryl. Death taboo weakening, Japan sees 1st transplant. [News]. *New York Times.* 1999 Mar 1: A8. BE60973.
advance directives; *brain death; cardiac death; *determination of death; hearts; *legal aspects; *organ donation; *organ transplantation; *Japan

Youngner, Stuart J.; Arnold, Robert M.; Schapiro, Renie, eds. The Definition of Death: Contemporary Controversies. Baltimore, MD: Johns Hopkins University Press; 1999. 436 refs. 111 fn. ISBN 0–8018–5985–9. BE60755.
anencephaly; attitudes to death; brain; *brain death; cardiac death; conscience; cultural pluralism; decision making; *determination of death; dissent; international aspects; Jewish ethics; legal aspects; methods; organ donation; organ transplantation; organizational policies; persistent vegetative state; personhood; physicians; professional organizations; Protestant ethics; public opinion; public participation; public policy; resuscitation; review; *standards; withholding treatment; Denmark; Germany; Japan; United States

DISCLOSURE *See* CONFIDENTIALITY, INFORMED CONSENT, PATIENT ACCESS TO RECORDS, TRUTH DISCLOSURE

DISTRIBUTIVE JUSTICE *See* RESOURCE ALLOCATION

DNA FINGERPRINTING

See also GENETIC SCREENING

Birmingham, Karen. UK leads on science and technology bioethics. [News]. *Nature Medicine.* 1998 Jun; 4(6): 651–652. BE59729.
accountability; *bioethical issues; DNA data banks; *DNA fingerprinting; embryo research; forensic medicine; gene therapy; *genetic intervention; government regulation; *international aspects; law enforcement; prisoners; *public policy; *regulation; reproductive technologies; science; *Great Britain; United States

Burk, Dan L.; Hess, Jennifer A. Genetic privacy: constitutional considerations in forensic DNA testing. *George Mason University Civil Rights Law Journal.* 1994 Winter; 5(1): 1–53. 337 refs. BE59651.
autonomy; blood specimen collection; constitutional law; *DNA data banks; *DNA fingerprinting; genetic information; law enforcement; *legal aspects; legal rights; legislation; prisoners; *privacy; tissue banks; DNA Identification Act 1994; Fifth Amendment; First Amendment; Fourteenth Amendment; Fourth Amendment; *United States

Clark, William R. The ethics of molecular medicine. *In: his:* The New Healers: The Promise and Problems of Molecular Medicine in the Twenty–First Century. New York, NY: Oxford University Press; 1997: 207–231, 236. 8 refs. ISBN 0–19–511730–1. BE60572.
confidentiality; containment; disclosure; DNA data banks; *DNA fingerprinting; donors; employment; ethical review; forensic medicine; future generations; *gene therapy; genetic counseling; genetic disorders; genetic enhancement; *genetic information; genetic materials; genetic predisposition; *genetic screening; genome mapping; germ cells; government regulation; guidelines; *health insurance; informed consent; insurance selection bias; late-onset

disorders; legislation; methods; preimplantation diagnosis; privacy; public policy; recombinant DNA research; *risks and benefits; social discrimination; NIH/DOE Working Group on Ethical, Legal, and Social Issues (ELSI); United States

Goldberg, Carey. DNA databanks giving police a powerful weapon, and critics. [News]. *New York Times.* 1998 Feb 19: A1, A12. BE59565.
blood specimen collection; costs and benefits; criminal law; *DNA data banks; *DNA fingerprinting; federal government; *law enforcement; *prisoners; privacy; standards; state government; *United States

Greenberg, Daniel S. DNA in the mortuary. *Washington Post.* 1999 Jan 1: A25. BE60110.
*cadavers; *death; *DNA fingerprinting; economics; genetic screening; *industry; informed consent; United States

Hoyle, Russ. Forensics: the FBI's national DNA database. *Nature Biotechnology.* 1998 Nov; 16(11): 987. BE62363.
confidentiality; criminal law; *DNA data banks; *DNA fingerprinting; federal government; genetic information; *law enforcement; minors; *prisoners; state government; violence; *Federal Bureau of Investigation; *United States

Kluger, Jeffrey. DNA detectives. *Time.* 1999 Jan 11; 153(1): 62–63. BE60311.
constitutional law; DNA data banks; *DNA fingerprinting; *law enforcement; legal rights; mass screening; Great Britain; United States

Lambert, Bruce. Giuliani backs DNA testing of newborns for identification. [News]. *New York Times.* 1998 Dec 17: B4. BE61122.
DNA data banks; *DNA fingerprinting; genetic information; law enforcement; legal aspects; municipal government; *newborns; prisoners; privacy; public policy; New York City

Lehrman, Sally. Prisoner's DNA database ruled unlawful. [News]. *Nature.* 1998 Aug 27; 394(6696): 818. BE61566.
blood specimen collection; constitutional law; *DNA data banks; *DNA fingerprinting; genetic research; law enforcement; *legal aspects; legal rights; mandatory programs; *prisoners; privacy; state interest; *tissue banks; Fourth Amendment; *Massachusetts

Pérez–Peña, Richard; Blair, Jayson. Albany plan widely expands sampling of criminals DNA. [News]. *New York Times.* 1999 Aug 7: A1, B4. BE62350.
*DNA data banks; *DNA fingerprinting; *law enforcement; *prisoners; public policy; state government; *New York; United States

Rohde, David. Quietly, DNA testing transforms sleuth's job –– but practice alarms civil libertarians. *New York Times.* 1999 Mar 9: B1, B5. BE61275.
DNA data banks; *DNA fingerprinting; genetic information; indigents; *law enforcement; *legal aspects; minority groups; privacy; social discrimination; social impact; *New York City; United States

Banking Our Genes: DNA Data on the Information Highway. [Videorecording].Boston, MA: Fanlight Productions; 1995. 1 videocassette; 33 min.; sd.; color; VHS. Producers: Dan Small and Jean E. McEwen. Produced under a grant from the Human Genome Project, U.S. Department of Energy, Ethical, Legal and Social Implications Program, Copyright by the Eunice Kennedy Shriver Center, Waltham, MA. ISBN 1–57295–155–9. Order No. CS–155. BE62711.
computer communication networks; confidentiality; disclosure; *DNA data banks; *DNA fingerprinting;

---

*forensic medicine; genetic disorders; *genetic information; genetic materials; genetic predisposition; *genetic screening; insurance; military personnel; *privacy; social discrimination; state government; *tissue banks; ELSI-funded publication; United States

DNA testing proposals. [Editorial]. *New York Times.* 1998 Dec 17: A32. BE61121.
DNA data banks; *DNA fingerprinting; genetic information; *law enforcement; legal aspects; newborns; *prisoners; privacy; New York City

Florida tries DNA sampling to protect children. [News]. *New York Times.* 1999 Jan 27: A14. BE61123.
blood specimen collection; children; *DNA fingerprinting; forensic medicine; hospitals; law enforcement; *newborns; public policy; state government; voluntary programs; *Florida

DRUGS
See under
PATIENT CARE/DRUGS

DURABLE POWERS OF ATTORNEY *See*
ADVANCE DIRECTIVES

ECONOMICS
See under
HEALTH CARE/ECONOMICS

EDUCATION
See under
BIOETHICS/EDUCATION
MEDICAL ETHICS/EDUCATION
NURSING ETHICS/EDUCATION
PROFESSIONAL ETHICS/EDUCATION

ELECTROCONVULSIVE THERAPY

Berkeley (CA). Use of electric shock treatment prohibited. *Berkeley Municipal Code.* 1982 Dec 30 (date effective). Sect. 12.26.010 to 12.26.050. 2 p. BE59345.
*electroconvulsive therapy; *government regulation; municipal government; *Berkeley (CA); California

Boronow, John; Stoline, Anne; Sharfstein, Steven S. Refusal of ECT by a patient with recurrent depression, psychosis, and catatonia. *American Journal of Psychiatry.* 1997 Sep; 154(9): 1285–1291. 19 refs. BE60201.
beneficence; case studies; chronically ill; communication; competence; *decision making; *depressive disorder; economics; *electroconvulsive therapy; *family members; family relationship; food; government financing; hospitals; institutionalized persons; judicial action; justice; *mentally ill; paternalism; *patient care; patient care team; professional family relationship; professional patient relationship; psychiatric diagnosis; *psychoactive drugs; *schizophrenia; *treatment refusal; *catatonia; Medicare; United States

EMBRYO AND FETAL RESEARCH

See also FETUSES

Abbott, Alison. 'Don't try to change embryo research law.' [News]. *Nature.* 1999 Mar 25; 398(6725): 275. BE61962.
aborted fetuses; cloning; *embryo research; financial support; germ cells; human rights; *legal aspects; ovum; *stem cells; Deutsche Forschungsgemeinschaft; Embryo

Protection Act 1990 (Germany); *Germany

American Society for Reproductive Medicine. Ethics Committee. Informed consent and the use of gametes and embryos for research. *Fertility and Sterility.* 1997 Nov; 68(5): 780–781. 1 ref. BE62008.
disclosure; *donors; embryo disposition; *embryo research; *embryos; *germ cells; *informed consent; investigators; *ovum donors; patients; reproductive technologies; *research embryo creation; research ethics committees; *semen donors; *tissue donation; viability; American Society for Reproductive Medicine

Andrews, Lori; Elster, Nanette. International regulation of human embryo research: embryo research in the US. *Human Reproduction.* 1998 Jan; 13(1): 1–4. 13 refs. BE62220.
cloning; cryopreservation; donors; *embryo research; embryo transfer; embryos; *federal government; gene therapy; goals; government financing; *government regulation; in vitro fertilization; nontherapeutic research; preimplantation diagnosis; remuneration; *state government; therapeutic research; cell lines; embryo donation; embryo splitting; *United States

Australia. Victoria. The Infertility Treatment Act 1995. No. 63 of 1995. Date of assent: 27 Jun 1995. [Summary]. *International Digest of Health Legislation.* 1997; 48(1): 24–33. BE59589.
advisory committees; artificial insemination; counseling; donors; embryo disposition; *embryo research; embryo transfer; genetic intervention; *government regulation; in vitro fertilization; informed consent; *legal aspects; posthumous reproduction; records; *reproductive technologies; sex preselection; spousal consent; surrogate mothers; terminology; Australia; *Infertility Treatment Act 1995 (Victoria); Infertility Treatment Authority (Victoria); Standing Review and Advisory Committee on Infertility (Victoria); *Victoria

Ayd, Frank J. Human cloning and the rights of human beings. *Medical–Moral Newsletter.* 1998 May–Jun; 35(5–6): 17–23. BE61463.
beginning of life; *cloning; *embryo research; embryos; genetic identity; government regulation; human rights; parent child relationship; personhood; public policy; risks and benefits; sexuality; value of life; nuclear transplantation; United States

Bagness, Carmel. Genetics, the Fetus and Our Future. Hale, Cheshire, England: Hochland and Hochland; 1998. 105 p. Includes references. ISBN 1–898507–65–1. BE59721.
aborted fetuses; cadavers; confidentiality; criminal law; disabled; embryo disposition; *embryo research; *embryos; eugenics; fetuses; gene therapy; genetic disorders; genetic enhancement; *genetic intervention; genetic materials; genome mapping; germ cells; legal aspects; moral obligations; multiple pregnancy; ovum donors; patents; personhood; preimplantation diagnosis; property rights; recombinant DNA research; regulation; remuneration; *reproductive technologies; research embryo creation; *risks and benefits; selective abortion; semen donors; social discrimination; social impact; torts; Great Britain; Human Genome Project

Baird, Patricia. Human embryo research in Canada: legal and policy aspects. *Human Reproduction.* 1997 Nov; 12(11): 2343–2345. 4 refs. BE62209.
advisory committees; *embryo research; embryos; fetal development; guidelines; in vitro fertilization; legal aspects; peer review; *public policy; regulation; research embryo creation; research ethics committees; self regulation; voluntary programs; *Canada; *Medical Research Council of Canada; *Royal Commission on New Reproductive

Technologies (Canada)

Billings, Paul R.; Newman, Stuart A. Crossing the germline. *GeneWATCH.* 1999 Jan; 11(5–6): 1, 3–4. BE62370.

dissent; eugenics; federal government; *fetal research; fetal therapy; future generations; *gene therapy; genetic disorders; genetic intervention; *germ cells; government regulation; *risks and benefits; thalassemia; adenosine deaminase deficiency; Anderson, W. French; Council for Responsible Genetics; Recombinant DNA Advisory Committee; United States

Billings, Paul R.; Schneider, Holm; Coutelle, Charles. In utero gene therapy: the case against [and] the case for. *Nature Medicine.* 1999 Mar; 5(3): 255–257. 7 refs. BE62542.

advisory committees; animal experimentation; federal government; *fetal research; *fetal therapy; *gene therapy; genetic disorders; germ cells; government regulation; human experimentation; *risks and benefits; treatment outcome; Recombinant DNA Advisory Committee; United States

Biven, Miranda. Administrative developments: NIH backs federal funding for stem cell research. *Journal of Law, Medicine and Ethics.* 1999 Spring; 27(1): 95–99. 30 fn. BE61510.

aborted fetuses; cloning; *embryo research; *federal government; fetal tissue donation; *government financing; *government regulation; guidelines; legal aspects; politics; private sector; *stem cells; Department of Health and Human Services; *National Institutes of Health; U.S. Congress; *United States

Bonnicksen, Andrea L. Procreation by cloning: crafting anticipatory guidelines. *Journal of Law, Medicine and Ethics.* 1997 Winter; 25(4): 273–282. 64 fn. BE62672.

advisory committees; children; *cloning; commodification; dehumanization; donors; embryo disposition; *embryo research; embryos; federal government; fetal research; *government regulation; guidelines; international aspects; *methods; multiple pregnancy; ovum donors; *public policy; reproductive technologies; *risks and benefits; semen donors; state government; *twinning; *embryo splitting; *nuclear transplantation; Canada; Europe; *United States

Butler, Declan. Breakthrough stirs US embryo debate ... while Europe contemplates funding ban. [News]. *Nature.* 1998 Nov 12; 396(6707): 104–105. Includes inset articles, "Company seeks strict controls on access," by D. Butler, and "Swiss to vote on ban on *in vitro* fertilization," by U. Bahnsen. BE59586.

*embryo research; federal government; *financial support; government financing; *government regulation; industry; *international aspects; patents; private sector; regulation; reproductive technologies; *stem cells; *Europe; *European Parliament; Geron; National Institutes of Health; Switzerland; *United States

Butler, Declan. Pressure grows for relaxation of French embryo research laws. [News]. *Nature.* 1998 Oct 8; 395(6702): 532–533. BE59584.

advisory committees; embryo disposition; *embryo research; *government regulation; in vitro fertilization; investigators; parental consent; research embryo creation; *France; National Academy of Medicine (France); National Ethics Advisory Committee (France)

Byk, Christian. Reply to Lebech or the ontological humility of the lawyer faced with philosophical consistency. *Journal of Medical Ethics.* 1998 Oct; 24(5): 348–349. 1 refs. BE60259.

cryopreservation; embryo disposition; *embryo research; embryos; *fetal research; *guidelines; in vitro fertilization;

international aspects; nontherapeutic research; pregnant women; *regulation; therapeutic research; Council of Europe; Europe; *European Convention on Human Rights and Biomedicine

Replying to the criticisms of Lebech, the author tries, regarding the issue of embryo research, to draw a line between what could be an international legal approach and what is a philosophical ontological quest. It is then up to the reader to decide if, and how far, these two different approaches can be complementary.

Cahill, Lisa Sowle. The new biotech world order. [Symposium: human primordial stem cells]. *Hastings Center Report.* 1999 Mar–Apr; 29(2): 45–48. 9 fn. BE61666.

advisory committees; autonomy; *biomedical research; biomedical technologies; commodification; *common good; economics; *embryo research; ethics committees; federal government; financial support; freedom; *genetic research; genetic services; government financing; human rights; *industry; informed consent; *international aspects; *justice; organizational policies; *regulation; resource allocation; *stem cells; values; Geron Corp.; Geron Ethics Advisory Board; United States

Canada. Health Canada. Discussion Group on Embryo Research. Research on Human Embryos in Canada. Final Report of the Discussion Group on Embryo Research. Ottawa, ON: Health Canada; 1995 Nov 15. 33 p. 32 fn. BE59458.

advisory committees; children; cloning; cultural pluralism; donors; embryo disposition; *embryo research; embryos; females; fetal development; genetic screening; germ cells; *government regulation; *guidelines; hybrids; incentives; industry; informed consent; moral obligations; moral policy; ovum donors; peer review; *preimplantation diagnosis; *public policy; remuneration; *reproductive technologies; research embryo creation; risk; risks and benefits; time factors; transgenic organisms; viability; women's health; *Canada; *Discussion Group on Embryo Research (Canada)

Capron, Alexander Morgan. Good intentions. *Hastings Center Report.* 1999 Mar–Apr; 29(2): 26–27. BE61658.

aborted fetuses; cloning; embryo disposition; *embryo research; *federal government; *fetal research; fetal tissue donation; financial support; *government financing; *government regulation; guidelines; in vitro fertilization; industry; informed consent; intention; legal aspects; *research embryo creation; *stem cells; National Institutes of Health; U.S. Congress; *United States

Couzin, Jennifer. RAC confronts in utero gene therapy proposals. [News]. *Science.* 1998 Oct 2; 282(5386): 27. BE62617.

advisory committees; federal government; *fetal research; *fetal therapy; future generations; *gene therapy; *public policy; risks and benefits; thalassemia; immunologic deficiency syndromes; National Institutes of Health; *Recombinant DNA Advisory Committee; *United States

Cutrer, William; Glahn, Sandra. Dealing with genetic reality: theological and clinical perspectives. *In:* Demy, Timothy J.; Stewart, Gary P., eds. Genetic Engineering: A Christian Response: Crucial Considerations in Shaping Life. Grand Rapids, MI: Kregel Publications; 1999: 154–169. 11 fn. ISBN 0-8254-2357-0. BE61366.

autonomy; beginning of life; beneficence; *Christian ethics; cloning; decision making; deontological ethics; *embryo research; embryos; ethical analysis; gene therapy; genetic disorders; genetic enhancement; genetic information; *genetic research; intention; justice; killing; moral complicity; moral policy; personhood; preimplantation diagnosis; *reproductive technologies; *risks and benefits; value of life; virtues; Human Embryo Research Panel; United States

---

BE = bioethics accession number   fn. = footnotes   refs. = references

Dijon, Xavier. Abortion and genetic manipulation: breaking with reasoning founded on disrespect for life and human dignity. *Medicine and Law.* 1993; 12(1–2): 85–92. 10 fn. BE60615.

> *abortion, induced; *embryo research; *embryos; humanism; legal aspects; love; moral obligations; mother fetus relationship; pregnant women; psychological stress; *value of life; women's rights; dignity

Doerflinger, Richard M. The ethics of funding embryonic stem cell research: a Catholic viewpoint. *Kennedy Institute of Ethics Journal.* 1999 Jun; 9(2): 137–150. 27 refs. 7 fn. BE62381.

> aborted fetuses; alternatives; beginning of life; cultural pluralism; *embryo research; *embryos; federal government; fetal tissue donation; *government financing; legal aspects; *moral complicity; moral obligations; *moral policy; personhood; *public policy; research embryo creation; *Roman Catholic ethics; *stem cells; *value of life; *United States

Stem cell research that requires the destruction of human embryos is incompatible with Catholic moral principles, and with any ethic that gives serious weight to the moral status of the human embryo. Moreover, because there are promising and morally acceptable alternative approaches to the repair and regeneration of human tissues, and because treatments that rely on destruction of human embryos would be morally offensive to many patients, embryonic stem cell research may play a far less significant role in medical progress than proponents believe.

Dunstan, G.R. Pre-embryo research. *Journal of Assisted Reproduction and Genetics.* 1995 Sep; 12(8): 517–523. 30 fn. BE60564.

> aborted fetuses; abortion, induced; cadavers; *embryo research; *embryos; fetal tissue donation; gene therapy; international aspects; moral policy; ovum donors; preimplantation diagnosis; public policy; regulation; religious ethics; remuneration; research embryo creation; *risks and benefits; Roman Catholic ethics; tissue transplantation; value of life; Great Britain

Easterbrook, Gregg. Medical evolution: will *Homo sapiens* become obsolete? *New Republic.* 1999 Mar 1; 220(9): 20–25. BE62097.

> aborted fetuses; beginning of life; cloning; cord blood; *embryo research; embryos; federal government; fetal research; financial support; gene therapy; genetic intervention; germ cells; government financing; government regulation; industry; private sector; risks and benefits; *stem cells; United States

Fletcher, John C.; Richter, Gerd. Ethical issues of perinatal human gene therapy. *Journal of Maternal–Fetal Medicine.* 1996 Sep–Oct; 5(5): 232–244. 93 refs. BE60136.

> advisory committees; age factors; beneficence; *children; disclosure; embryo research; ethical review; federal government; *fetal research; *fetal therapy; *gene therapy; genetic disorders; genetic enhancement; germ cells; government regulation; growth disorders; historical aspects; hormones; *human experimentation; *infants; informed consent; justice; parents; pregnant women; prenatal diagnosis; privacy; research ethics committees; resource allocation; *risks and benefits; scientific misconduct; selection of subjects; selective abortion; stem cells; thalassemia; adenosine deaminase deficiency; immunologic deficiency syndromes; Germany; National Institutes of Health; Recombinant DNA Advisory Committee; United States

Fox, Jeffrey L. Future tense for in utero gene therapy. [News]. *Nature Biotechnology.* 1998 Nov; 16(11): 1002–1003. BE62320.

> advisory committees; ethical review; federal government; *fetal research; *fetal therapy; *gene therapy; genetic disorders; public policy; risks and benefits; Food and Drug Administration; National Institutes of Health; Recombinant DNA Advisory Committee; United States

Gates, Elena. Two challenges for research ethics: innovative treatment and fetal therapy. *Women's Health Issues.* 1999 Jul–Aug; 9(4): 208–210. 14 refs. BE61974.

> coercion; *fetal research; *fetal therapy; fetuses; *human experimentation; informed consent; nontherapeutic research; obstetrics and gynecology; organizational policies; patient care; physicians; *pregnant women; professional organizations; research subjects; *risks and benefits; *surgery; therapeutic research; treatment refusal; *investigational therapies; American College of Obstetricians and Gynecologists

Gavaghan, Helen. Embryo research tests NIH's mettle. [News]. *Nature Medicine.* 1995 Jan; 1(1): 5–6. BE59766.

> advisory committees; comparative studies; *embryo research; embryo transfer; federal government; fetal development; government financing; government regulation; guidelines; in vitro fertilization; international aspects; ovum donors; *public policy; research embryo creation; time factors; Human Embryo Research Panel; National Institutes of Health; *United States

Gearhart, John. New potential for human embryonic stem cells. *Science.* 1998 Nov 6; 282(5391): 1061–1062. 27 fn. BE59539.

> *embryo research; federal government; financial support; government financing; government regulation; methods; private sector; risks and benefits; *stem cells; cell lines; United States

Gemelli, Agostino. Against experimentation on human embryos. *European Journal of Genetics in Society.* 1997; 3(1): 13–15. BE61452.

> beginning of life; embryo disposition; *embryo research; fetal development; reproductive technologies; research embryo creation; value of life

Great Britain. Human Fertilisation and Embryology Authority. Sixth Annual Report [1995–1996]. London: The Authority; 1997. 45 p. Includes references. "This report covers the year beginning 1 Nov 1995 with a foreward look for the year beginning 1 Nov 1996." BE60714.

> age factors; artificial insemination; cloning; cryopreservation; *embryo research; embryos; genetic screening; *government regulation; guidelines; *health facilities; HIV seropositivity; *in vitro fertilization; information dissemination; informed consent; posthumous reproduction; preimplantation diagnosis; remuneration; *reproductive technologies; semen donors; sperm; *standards; statistics; *Great Britain; Human Fertilisation and Embryology Act 1990; *Human Fertilisation and Embryology Authority

Hicks, Stephen C. The regulation of fetal tissue transplantation: different legislative models for different purposes. *Suffolk University Law Review.* 1993 Winter; 27(4): 1613–1629. 46 fn. BE61598.

> *aborted fetuses; abortion, induced; criminal law; directed donation; embryo disposition; embryo research; embryos; federal government; *fetal research; *fetal tissue donation; government financing; *government regulation; informed consent; *model legislation; nontherapeutic research; organ donation; organ transplantation; remuneration; research ethics committees; state government; therapeutic research; tissue donation; tissue transplantation; abortion, spontaneous; NIH Revitalization Act 1993; Uniform Anatomical Gift Act; *United States

---

BE = bioethics accession number   fn. = footnotes   refs. = references

Klotzko, Arlene Judith. Immortal longings. *New Scientist.* 1998 Dec 5; 160(2163): 49. BE61544.
  *embryo research; government financing; government regulation; industry; *life extension; *stem cells; United States

Knowles, Lori P. Property, progeny, and patents. [Symposium: human primordial stem cells]. *Hastings Center Report.* 1999 Mar–Apr; 29(2): 38–40. 2 refs. BE61663.
  aborted fetuses; advisory committees; altruism; beginning of life; *biomedical research; body parts and fluids; cryopreservation; decision making; donors; economics; embryo disposition; *embryo research; embryos; fetal tissue donation; guidelines; *industry; informed consent; institutional ethics; investigators; justice; legal aspects; organizational policies; *patents; personhood; *property rights; regulation; risks and benefits; *stem cells; tissue donation; embryo donation; Geron Corp.; Geron Ethics Advisory Board; United States

Kolata, Gina. When a cell does an embryo's work, a debate is born. *New York Times.* 1999 Feb 9: F2. BE60646.
  *beginning of life; *embryo research; *embryos; *stem cells

Kolehmainen, Sophia. CRG brings ethics into NIH prenatal gene therapy debate. *GeneWATCH.* 1999 Feb; 12(1): 15–16. BE62372.
  dissent; eugenics; federal government; *fetal research; *gene therapy; genetic intervention; *germ cells; government regulation; risks and benefits; Council for Responsible Genetics; Recombinant DNA Advisory Committee; United States

Lafferty, Kevin J.; Furer, Julie J. Legal and medical implications of fetal tissue transplantation. *Suffolk University Law Review.* 1993 Winter; 27(4): 1237–1248. 59 fn. BE61594.
  aborted fetuses; diabetes; federal government; *fetal research; *fetal tissue donation; *government financing; *government regulation; *legal aspects; methods; private sector; *public policy; state government; *tissue transplantation; pancreases; United States

Lanza, Robert P.; Arrow, Kenneth J.; Axelrod, Julius, et al. Science over politics. [Letter]. *Science.* 1999 Mar 19; 283(5409): 1849–1850. Additional signers: David Baltimore, Baruj Benacerraf, Konrad E. Bloch, Nicolaas Bloembergen, Herbert C. Brown, Michael S. Brown, Jose B. Cibelli, Stanley Cohen, Leon N. Cooper, E. J. Corey, Reneto Dulbecco, Edmond H. Fischer, Val L. Fitch, Jerome I. Friedman, Milton Friedman, Robert F. Furchgott, Murray Gell-Mann, Donald A. Glaser, Sheldon Lee Glashow, Walter Gilbert, Joseph L. Goldstein, Stephen Jay Gould, Roger Guillemin, Herbert A. Hauptman, Dudley Herschbach, Roald Hoffman, and 43 others. BE61170.
  biomedical research; *embryo research; federal government; *government financing; government regulation; guidelines; politics; *public policy; *risks and benefits; *stem cells; Department of Health and Human Services; National Institutes of Health; U.S. Congress; *United States

Lebacqz, Karen. Research with human embryonic stem cells: ethical considerations. [Symposium: human primordial stem cells]. *Hastings Center Report.* 1999 Mar–Apr; 29(2): 31–36. 26 fn. Board members: Karen Lebacqz (Chair), Michael M. Mendiola, Ted Peters, Ernlé W.D. Young, and Laurie Zoloth-Dorfman. BE61661.
  aborted fetuses; advisory committees; animal experimentation; beginning of life; biomedical research; cloning; consent forms; cultural pluralism; decision making; disclosure; donors; economics; *embryo research; embryos; ethical review; fetal tissue donation; financial support; germ cells; *guidelines; human experimentation; hybrids; in vitro fertilization; *industry; informed consent; moral obligations; nontherapeutic research; *organizational policies; patents; personhood; private sector; property rights; research ethics committees; risks and benefits; *stem cells; value of life; embryo donation; *Geron Corp.; *Geron Ethics Advisory Board

Lebacqz, Karen; Tauer, Carol; McGee, Glenn, et al. Stem cells. [Letter and responses]. *Hastings Center Report.* 1999 Jul–Aug; 29(4): 4–5. BE62460.
  advisory committees; *embryo research; *ethical review; fetal development; industry; private sector; research ethics committees; *stem cells; Geron Corp.; Geron Ethics Advisory Board

Lebech, Mette Maria. Comment on a proposed draft protocol for the European Convention on Biomedicine relating to research on the human embryo and fetus. *Journal of Medical Ethics.* 1998 Oct; 24(5): 345–347. 3 fn. BE60258.
  cryopreservation; embryo disposition; *embryo research; embryos; *fetal research; gene therapy; *guidelines; in vitro fertilization; international aspects; nontherapeutic research; pregnant women; regulation; research embryo creation; therapeutic research; Council of Europe; Europe; *European Convention on Human Rights and Biomedicine
Judge Christian Byk renders service to the Steering Committee on Bioethics of the Council of Europe (CDBI) by proposing a draft of the protocol destined to fill in a gap in international law on the status of the human embryo. This proposal, printed in a previous issue of the Journal of Medical Ethics deserves nevertheless to be questioned on important points. Is Christian Byk proposing to legalise research on human embryos not only in vitro but also in utero?

Lemonick, Michael D. The biological mother lode. [News]. *Time.* 1998 Nov 16; 152(20): 96–97. BE60907.
  aborted fetuses; *embryo research; embryos; federal government; financial support; government regulation; industry; risks and benefits; *stem cells; United States

Loder, Natasha. Allow cloning in embryo research, says UK report. [News]. *Nature.* 1998 Dec 10; 396(6711): 503. BE59540.
  advisory committees; *cloning; *embryo research; *government regulation; public participation; *public policy; stem cells; *Great Britain; Human Fertilisation and Embryology Authority; Human Genetics Advisory Commission (Great Britain)

McGee, Glenn; Caplan, Arthur. The ethics and politics of small sacrifices in stem cell research. *Kennedy Institute of Ethics Journal.* 1999 June; 9(2): 151–158. 9 refs. BE62382.
  aborted fetuses; beginning of life; common good; compassion; cryopreservation; *embryo research; *embryos; federal government; fetal tissue donation; government financing; moral complicity; *moral policy; politics; *public policy; risks and benefits; *stem cells; value of life; United States
Pluripotent human stem cell research may offer new treatments for hundreds of diseases, but opponents of this research argue that such therapy comes attached to a Faustian bargain: cures at the cost of the destruction of many frozen embryos. The National Bioethics Advisory Commission (NBAC), government officials, and many scholars of bioethics, including, in these pages, John Robertson, have not offered an adequate response to ethical objections to stem cell research. Instead of examining the ethical issues involved in sacrificing

---

BE = bioethics accession number   fn. = footnotes   refs. = references

human embryos for the goal of curing fatal and disabling diseases, they seek to either dismiss the moral concerns of those with objections or to find an "accomodation" with those opposed to stem cell research. An ethical argument can be made that it is justifiable to modify or destroy certain human embryos in the pursuit of cures for dread and lethal diseases. Until this argument is made, the case for stem cell research will rest on political foundations rather than on the ethical foundations that the funding of stem cell research requires.

McGee, Glenn; Caplan, Arthur L. What's in the dish? [Symposium: human primordial stem cells]. *Hastings Center Report.* 1999 Mar–Apr; 29(2): 36–38. BE61662.
   aborted fetuses; advisory committees; beginning of life; *embryo research; *embryos; ethical review; fetal development; fetal tissue donation; fetuses; financial support; germ cells; guidelines; *industry; *moral obligations; organizational policies; personhood; private sector; risks and benefits; *stem cells; viability; Geron Corp.; Geron Ethics Advisory Board

Marshall, Eliot. A versatile cell line raises scientific hopes, legal questions. [News]. *Science.* 1998 Nov 6; 282(5391): 1014–1015. BE59538.
   *embryo research; federal government; financial support; germ cells; government financing; government regulation; industry; methods; private sector; risks and benefits; *stem cells; *cell lines; Geron; National Institutes of Health; United States

Marshall, Eliot. Britain urged to expand embryo studies. [News]. *Science.* 1998 Dec 18; 282(5397): 2167–2168. BE59542.
   advisory committees; cloning; *embryo research; government regulation; *public policy; *stem cells; *Great Britain; Human Fertilisation and Embryology Authority; Human Genetics Advisory Commission (Great Britain)

Marshall, Eliot. Ethicists back stem cell research, White House treads cautiously. [News]. *Science.* 1999 Jul 23; 285(5427): 502. BE62522.
   advisory committees; *embryo research; federal government; government financing; guidelines; politics; private sector; *public policy; *stem cells; National Bioethics Advisory Commission; *United States

Marshall, Eliot. Ruling may free NIH to fund stem cell studies. [News]. *Science.* 1999 Jan 22; 283(5401): 465, 467. BE60639.
   advisory committees; *embryo research; federal government; *government financing; *government regulation; legal aspects; *stem cells; Department of Health and Human Services; National Bioethics Advisory Commission; *National Institutes of Health; *United States

Marshall, Eliot. Stem cell research: NIH plans ethics review of proposals. [News]. *Science.* 1999 Apr 16; 284(5413): 413, 415. BE61770.
   aborted fetuses; advisory committees; *embryo research; federal government; fetal research; fetal tissue donation; *government financing; *government regulation; guidelines; *stem cells; *National Institutes of Health; *United States

Marshall, Eliot. Use of stem cells still legally murky, but hearing offers hope. [News]. *Science.* 1998 Dec 11; 282(5396): 1962–1963. BE59541.
   *embryo research; federal government; financial support; *government financing; *government regulation; private sector; *stem cells; *United States

Marwick, Charles. Funding stem cell research. [News]. *JAMA.* 1999 Feb 24; 281(8): 692–693. BE62609.

advisory committees; *embryo research; *federal government; *government financing; legal aspects; politics; *public policy; *stem cells; National Bioethics Advisory Commission; *National Institutes of Health; *United States

Mason, John Kenyon. Fetal experimentation. *In: his* Medico–Legal Aspects of Reproduction and Parenthood. Second Edition. Brookfield, VT: Ashgate; 1998: 187–206. 62 fn. ISBN 1-84104-065-8. BE61065.
   *aborted fetuses; advisory committees; anencephaly; brain; determination of death; *fetal research; *fetal tissue donation; *fetuses; incentives; informed consent; *legal aspects; moral policy; newborns; nontherapeutic research; organ donation; pregnant women; prolongation of life; public policy; research ethics committees; risk; therapeutic research; tissue transplantation; viability; ovaries; Abortion Act 1967 (Great Britain); British Medical Association; *Great Britain; Human Fertilisation and Embryology Act 1990; Human Tissue Act 1961 (Great Britain); Infant Life (Preservation) Act 1929 (Great Britain); Offences Against the Person Act 1861 (Great Britain); Peel Committee Report; Polkinghorne Report

Mayor, Susan. UK authorities recommend human cloning for therapeutic research. [News]. *BMJ (British Medical Journal).* 1998 Dec 12; 317(7173): 1613. BE61301.
   advisory committees; *cloning; *embryo research; *government regulation; *public policy; reproductive technologies; therapeutic research; nuclear transplantation; *Great Britain; Human Fertilisation and Embryology Authority; Human Genetics Advisory Commission (Great Britain)

Merchant, Jennifer. Confronting the consequences of medical technology: policy frontiers in the United States and France. *In:* Githens, Marianne; Stetson, Dorothy McBride, eds. Abortion Politics: Public Policy in Cross–Cultural Perspective. New York, NY: Routledge; 1996: 189–209. 32 fn. ISBN 0-415-91225-3. BE60711.
   abortion, induced; advisory committees; comparative studies; cryopreservation; embryo disposition; *embryo research; eugenics; federal government; feminist ethics; *fetal research; fetuses; government financing; in vitro fertilization; infertility; international aspects; *legal aspects; legal liability; personhood; physicians; pregnant women; prenatal diagnosis; prenatal injuries; *public policy; *reproductive technologies; selective abortion; surrogate mothers; *women's rights; wrongful life; *France; *United States

Miller, Linda J.; Bloom, Floyd E. Publishing controversial research. [Editorial]. *Science.* 1998 Nov 6; 282(5391): 1045. BE59537.
   *biomedical research; *editorial policies; *embryo research; federal government; financial support; government regulation; guidelines; *information dissemination; international aspects; peer review; private sector; public policy; *stem cells; cell lines; *Science; United States

Mulkay, Michael. Galileo and the embryos: religion and science in parliamentary debate over research on human embryos. *Social Studies of Science.* 1995 Aug; 25(3): 499–532. 84 fn. BE60106.
   beginning of life; *Christian ethics; clergy; common good; *embryo research; embryos; expert testimony; government regulation; historical aspects; interprofessional relations; investigators; moral policy; political activity; *politics; preimplantation diagnosis; Protestant ethics; *public policy; *religion; *risks and benefits; Roman Catholic ethics; *science; *values; rationality; Anglican Church; *Great Britain; *House of Lords; Warnock Committee

Okarma, Thomas B. Human primordial stem cells. [Symposium introduction]. *Hastings Center Report.* 1999

Mar–Apr; 29(2): 30. Introduction to a set of articles by the Geron Ethics Advisory Board (Karen Lebacqz, Chair); Glenn McGee and Arthur L. Caplan; Lori P. Knowles; Gladys B. White; Carol A. Tauer; and Lisa S. Cahill. BE61660.
  aborted fetuses; advisory committees; biomedical research; *embryo research; fetal tissue donation; financial support; government financing; *industry; *stem cells; Geron Corp.; Geron Ethics Advisory Board; United States

Parens, Erik. Researchers close in on primordial stem cells. [News]. *Hastings Center Report.* 1999 Jan–Feb; 29(1): 51–52. BE61639.
  aborted fetuses; *embryo research; embryos; fetal tissue donation; financial support; gene therapy; hybrids; industry; methods; *stem cells; nuclear transplantation; United States

Persson, Ingmar. Harming the non-conscious. *Bioethics.* 1999 Jul; 13(3–4): 294–305. 13 fn. BE61880.
  *abortion, induced; *beginning of life; brain; embryos; *fetal development; *fetal research; *fetuses; *injuries; *killing; *moral policy; organ donation; personhood; prenatal injuries; quality of life; value of life; *harms; Singer, Peter
  Peter Singer has argued that nothing done to a fetus before it acquires consciousness can harm it. At the same time, he concedes that a child can be harmed by something done to it when it was a non-conscious fetus. But this implies that the non-conscious fetus can be harmed. The mistake lies in thinking that, since existence can be instrinsically bad for a being only if it is conscious, it can be harmed only if it is conscious. In fact, its being harmed only implies that it could have been conscious (and led a good life).

Rae, Scott B. Ethical issues and concerns about human cloning. *In:* Demy, Timothy J.; Stewart, Gary P., eds. Genetic Engineering: A Christian Response: Crucial Considerations in Shaping Life. Grand Rapids, MI: Kregel Publications; 1999: 278–292. 16 fn. ISBN 0-8254-2357-0. BE61371.
  adults; bone marrow; Christian ethics; *cloning; commodification; criminal law; embryo disposition; *embryo research; *embryo transfer; *embryos; family members; genetic diversity; genetic identity; in vitro fertilization; industry; intention; international aspects; personhood; preimplantation diagnosis; reproduction; tissue donation; *twinning; personal identity; Ayala, Anissa; Ayala, Marissa; Europe

Robertson, John A. Ethics and policy in embryonic stem cell research. *Kennedy Institute of Ethics Journal.* 1999 June; 9(2): 109–136. 33 refs. 12 fn. BE62380.
  aborted fetuses; accountability; advisory committees; beginning of life; commodification; deontological ethics; embryo disposition; *embryo research; embryos; federal government; fetal tissue donation; financial support; *government financing; government regulation; guidelines; in vitro fertilization; international aspects; legal aspects; *moral complicity; moral obligations; *moral policy; ovum donors; private sector; *public policy; *research embryo creation; risks and benefits; *stem cells; teleological ethics; value of life; wedge argument; Great Britain; Human Embryo Research Panel; National Bioethics Advisory Commission; *United States
  Embryonic stem cells, which have the potential to save many lives, must be recovered from aborted fetuses or live embyros. Although tissue from aborted fetuses can be used without moral complicity in the underlying abortion, obtaining stem cells from embryos necessarily kills them, thus raising difficult questions about the use of embryonic human material to save others. This article draws on previous controversies over embryo research and distinctions between intrinsic and symbolic moral status to analyze these issues. It argues that stem

cell research with spare embryos produced during infertility treatment, or even embryos created specifically for research or therapeutic purposes, is ethically acceptable and should receive federal funding.

Rovner, Julie. Politicians squabble over stem-cell research. [News]. *Lancet.* 1999 Jun 5; 353(9168): 1948. BE62579.
  advisory committees; *embryo research; federal government; *government financing; *government regulation; *politics; public policy; *stem cells; Department of Health and Human Services; National Bioethics Advisory Commission; U.S. Congress; *United States

Serour, Gamal I. Reproductive choice: a Muslim perspective. *In:* Harris, John; Holm, Søren, eds. The Future of Human Reproduction: Ethics, Choice, and Regulation. New York, NY: Oxford University Press; 1998: 191–202. 37 fn. ISBN 0-19-823761-8. BE61270.
  aborted fetuses; abortion, induced; age factors; contraception; *embryo research; females; *fetal research; fetal tissue donation; gene therapy; genetic counseling; genetic enhancement; *Islamic ethics; multiple pregnancy; *reproduction; *reproductive technologies; research embryo creation; selection for treatment; sex determination; sex preselection; *theology

Silberner, Joanne. Turning pages, if not heads. *Hastings Center Report.* 1999 Mar–Apr; 29(2): 6. BE61654.
  advisory committees; bioethical issues; economics; *embryo research; federal government; *government financing; government regulation; health care; human experimentation; mentally ill; political activity; *politics; *public policy; stem cells; *National Bioethics Advisory Commission; National Institutes of Health; U.S. Congress; *United States; Varmus, Harold

Summer, David. Maryland court rules on embryo standing. [News]. *Journal of Law, Medicine and Ethics.* 1995 Spring; 23(1): 108. BE62534.
  advisory committees; Down syndrome; *embryo research; *embryos; federal government; fetal research; *government financing; *legal aspects; personhood; Department of Health and Human Services; *Doe v. Shalala; Human Embryo Research Panel; *United States

Tauer, Carol A. Private ethics boards and public debate. [Symposium: human primordial stem cells]. *Hastings Center Report.* 1999 Mar–Apr; 29(2): 43–45. 3 refs. BE61665.
  advisory committees; decision making; donors; *embryo research; *ethical review; federal government; fetal development; government financing; government regulation; guidelines; *industry; informed consent; moral obligations; *private sector; public participation; *public sector; research embryo creation; research ethics committees; *stem cells; Geron Corp.; Geron Ethics Advisory Board; Human Embryo Research Panel; National Institutes of Health; United States

U.S. Congress. Senate. Committee on Appropriations. Subcommitte on Departments of Labor, Health and Human Services, and Education, and Related Agencies. Stem Cell Research. Special Hearings, 2 Dec 1998, 12 Jan 1999, 26 Jan 1999. Washington, DC: U.S. Government Printing Office; 1999. 148 p. S.Hrg. 105-939. Available via the World Wide Web at http://www.access.gpo.gov/congress/senate. ISBN 0-16-058361-6. BE61995.
  aborted fetuses; abortion, induced; central nervous system diseases; cloning; diabetes; embryo disposition; *embryo research; embryos; federal government; *fetal research; financial support; *government financing; government regulation; in vitro fertilization; industry; legal aspects; moral

---

BE = bioethics accession number   fn. = footnotes   refs. = references

policy; patents; private sector; *public policy; research embryo creation; risks and benefits; *stem cells; tissue transplantation; Department of Health and Human Services; Human Embryo Research Panel; National Bioethics Advisory Commission; National Institutes of Health; Right to Life Movement; United States

Wade, Nicholas. Advisory panel votes for use of embryonic cells in research. [News]. *New York Times.* 1999 Jun 29: A15. BE62549.
> aborted fetuses; advisory committees; *embryo research; federal government; fetal tissue donation; financial support; government financing; government regulation; private sector; *public policy; *stem cells; National Bioethics Advisory Commission; U.S. Congress; *United States

Wade, Nicholas. Clinton asks study of bid to form part-human, part-cow cells. [News]. *New York Times.* 1998 Nov 15: 31. BE59321.
> advisory committees; *embryo research; *federal government; government financing; government regulation; *hybrids; politics; *public policy; research embryo creation; *stem cells; National Bioethics Advisory Commission; United States

Wade, Nicholas. Embryo cell research: a clash of values. *New York Times.* 1999 Jul 2: A13. BE62548.
> aborted fetuses; advisory committees; beginning of life; *embryo research; embryos; fetal tissue donation; government financing; moral obligations; morality; public policy; religious ethics; *stem cells; National Bioethics Advisory Commission; United States

Wade, Nicholas. Government says ban on human embryo research does not apply to cells. [News]. *New York Times.* 1999 Jan 20: A29. BE60125.
> aborted fetuses; *embryo research; federal government; government financing; *government regulation; research embryo creation; *stem cells; abortion, spontaneous; Department of Health and Human Services; *United States

Wade, Nicholas. No research on cloning of embryos, Geron says. [News]. *New York Times.* 1999 Jun 15: A21. BE62550.
> cloning; *embryo research; hybrids; *industry; methods; *stem cells; Advanced Cell Technology; *Geron Corp.; United States

Wade, Nicholas. Primordial cells fuel debate on ethics. [News]. *New York Times.* 1998 Nov 10: F1, F2. BE60641.
> aborted fetuses; *embryo research; *embryos; federal government; fetal tissue donation; financial support; government financing; government regulation; private sector; *stem cells; National Bioethics Advisory Commission; United States

Wade, Nicholas. Recommendation is near on embryo cell research: ethics panel expected to urge end to ban. [News]. *New York Times.* 1999 May 24: A18. BE62547.
> advisory committees; *embryo research; federal government; government financing; government regulation; *public policy; *stem cells; *National Bioethics Advisory Commission; U.S. Congress; *United States

Wade, Nicholas. Researchers claim embryonic cell mix of human and cow. [News]. *New York Times.* 1998 Nov 12: A1, A26. BE62599.
> autoexperimentation; cloning; *embryo research; embryos; *hybrids; industry; investigators; research embryo creation; *stem cells; Advanced Cell Technology; Cibelli, Jose

Wadman, Meredith. Congress may block stem-cell research. [News]. *Nature.* 1999 Feb 25; 397(6721): 639. BE60637.
> *embryo research; federal government; *government financing; *government regulation; politics; *stem cells; Department of Health and Human Services; National Institutes of Health; *U.S. Congress; *United States

Wadman, Meredith. Embryonic stem-cell research exempt from ban, NIH is told. [News]. *Nature.* 1999 Jan 21; 397(6716): 185-186. BE60634.
> *embryo research; federal government; *government financing; *government regulation; legal aspects; politics; *stem cells; *Department of Health and Human Services; *National Institutes of Health; U.S. Congress; *United States

Wadman, Meredith. Ethicists urge funding for extraction of embryo cells. [News]. *Nature.* 1999 May 27; 399(6734): 292. BE61761.
> aborted fetuses; advisory committees; *embryo research; *federal government; fetal tissue donation; *government financing; *government regulation; public opinion; research embryo creation; risks and benefits; *stem cells; *National Bioethics Advisory Commission; National Institutes of Health; *United States

Wadman, Meredith. Gene therapy pushes on, despite doubts. [News]. *Nature.* 1999 Jan 14; 397(6715): 94. BE60396.
> animal experimentation; federal government; *fetal research; *fetal therapy; *gene therapy; guidelines; human experimentation; *public policy; *risks and benefits; Council for Responsible Genetics; Food and Drug Administration; National Institutes of Health; NIH Guidelines; *United States

Wadman, Meredith. NIH stem-cell guidelines face stormy ride. [News]. *Nature.* 1999 Apr 15; 398(6728): 551. BE61709.
> advisory committees; alternatives; *embryo research; federal government; *government financing; *government regulation; guidelines; political activity; public policy; *stem cells; *National Institutes of Health; *United States

Warnock, Mary. Experimentation on human embryos and fetuses. *In:* Kuhse, Helga; Singer, Peter, eds. A Companion to Bioethics. Malden, MA: Blackwell; 1998: 390-396. 5 refs. ISBN 0-631-19737-0. BE59512.
> beginning of life; *embryo research; embryo transfer; embryos; fetal development; *fetal research; in vitro fertilization; moral policy; public policy; risks and benefits; utilitarianism; value of life; wedge argument; ectogenesis; Great Britain

Weiss, Rick. Federal embryo research is backed: ethicists see benefits overriding qualms. [News]. *Washington Post.* 1999 May 23: A1, A16. BE61700.
> advisory committees; *embryo research; embryos; *federal government; *government financing; *government regulation; guidelines; in vitro fertilization; public opinion; *public policy; risks and benefits; *stem cells; tissue donation; *National Bioethics Advisory Commission; National Institutes of Health; *United States

Wheale, Peter R. Moral and legal consequences for the fetus/unborn child of medical technologies derived from human genome research. *In:* Glasner, Peter; Rothman, Harry, eds. Genetic Imaginations: Ethical, Legal and Social Issues in Human Genome Research. Brookfield, VT: Ashgate; 1998: 83-96. 35 refs. Based on a paper presented at a workshop hosted by the Centre for Social and Economic Research at the University of the West of England; reprinted from *The Genetic Engineer and Biotechnologist,* 1995; 15(2-3). ISBN 1-84014-356-8. BE60020.
> abortion, induced; *beginning of life; coercion; *congenital disorders; deontological ethics; *embryo research; *embryos;

BE = bioethics accession number   fn. = footnotes   refs. = references

ethical analysis; fetal development; *fetuses; genetic disorders; genetic screening; genome mapping; government regulation; *legal aspects; legal liability; *moral obligations; *moral policy; negligence; *personhood; pregnant women; prenatal injuries; *public policy; *quality of life; rights; *selective abortion; social impact; treatment refusal; utilitarianism; *value of life; *wrongful life; *Great Britain

White, Gladys B. Foresight, insight, oversight. [Symposium: human primordial stem cells]. *Hastings Center Report.* 1999 Mar–Apr; 29(2): 41–42. 4 refs. BE61664.
advisory committees; biomedical research; conflict of interest; *embryo research; embryos; *ethical review; federal government; financial support; government financing; government regulation; guidelines; *industry; moral obligations; *private sector; public policy; *public sector; regulation; research ethics committees; *stem cells; Geron Corp.; Geron Ethics Advisory Board; Human Embryo Research Panel; National Institutes of Health; United States

Young, Frank E. Worldviews in conflict: human cloning and embryo manipulation. *In:* Demy, Timothy J.; Stewart, Gary P., eds. Genetic Engineering: A Christian Response: Crucial Considerations in Shaping Life. Grand Rapids, MI: Kregel Publications; 1999: 70–86. 41 fn. ISBN 0-8254-2357-0. BE61361.
American Indians; beginning of life; blacks; Buddhist ethics; *Christian ethics; *cloning; decision making; Eastern Orthodox ethics; *embryo research; ethical relativism; eugenics; fetal development; government regulation; Hindu ethics; hybrids; interdisciplinary communication; investigators; Jewish ethics; killing; personhood; Protestant ethics; public participation; *public policy; quality of life; *religious ethics; resource allocation; Roman Catholic ethics; secularism; self regulation; *social impact; theology; value of life; nuclear transplantation; Evangelical Christians; United States

Time to lift embryo research ban. [Editorial]. *Nature.* 1998 Nov 12; 396(6707): 97. BE59343.
*embryo research; federal government; *government regulation; industry; *stem cells; *United States

Towards the acceptance of embryo stem-cell therapies. [Editorial]. *Nature.* 1999 Jan 28; 397(6717): 279. BE60635.
cloning; *embryo research; federal government; government financing; government regulation; *stem cells; National Institutes of Health; *United States

EMBRYOS *See* EMBRYO AND FETAL RESEARCH, FETUSES

EPIDEMIOLOGY *See* BIOMEDICAL RESEARCH

ETHICISTS AND ETHICS COMMITTEES

Agich, George J. From Pittsburgh to Cleveland: NHBD [non–heart–beating donor] controversies and bioethics. *Cambridge Quarterly of Healthcare Ethics.* 1999 Summer; 8(3): 269–274. 12 fn. BE62470.
advance directives; allowing to die; autonomy; bioethical issues; *cadavers; *cardiac death; determination of death; donor cards; *ethicist's role; family members; hospitals; informed consent; *institutional policies; interdisciplinary communication; killing; *mass media; *organ donation; patients; third party consent; trust; withholding treatment; *Cleveland Clinic Foundation; 60 Minutes (CBS News television program)

Andre, Judith; Fleck, Leonard; Tomlinson, Tom.

Improving our aim. [Bioethics and the press]. *Journal of Medicine and Philosophy.* 1999 Apr; 24(2): 130–147. 29 refs. 5 fn. BE61438.
assisted suicide; *bioethical issues; *bioethics; cloning; communication; democracy; disclosure; education; empirical research; *ethicist's role; *ethicists; guidelines; *interprofessional relations; *journalism; justice; knowledge, attitudes, practice; *mass media; public policy; religion; *technical expertise; uncertainty
Bioethicists appearing in the media have been accused of "shooting from the hip" (Rachels, 1991). The criticism is sometimes justified. We identify some reasons our interactions with the press can have bad results and suggest remedies. In particular we describe a target (fostering better public dialogue), obstacles to hitting the target (such as intrinsic and accidental defects in our knowledge) and suggest some practical ways to surmount those obstacles (including seeking out ways to write or speak at length, rather than in sound bites). We make use of our own research into the way journalists quote bioethicists. We end by suggesting that the profession as a whole look into this question more fully.

Aulisio, Mark P.; Arnold, Robert M.; Youngner, Stuart J. An ongoing conversation: the Task Force report and bioethics consultation. [Introduction to a set of articles by E.D. Pellegrino, E.G. Howe, J.W. Ross, R. Pentz, A.H. Moss, and the authors]. *Journal of Clinical Ethics.* 1999 Spring; 10(1): 3–4. List of members of the SHHV–SBC Task Force on Standards for Bioethics Consultation, p. 4. BE62709.
bioethics; *clinical ethics committees; consensus; *ethicists; *ethics consultation; guidelines; organizational policies; *professional competence; professional organizations; self regulation; *standards; American Society for Bioethics and Humanities; Core Competencies for Health Care Ethics Consultation (SHHV–SBC Task Force); Society for Bioethics Consultation; Society for Health and Human Values; United States

Aulisio, Mark P.; Arnold, Robert M.; Youngner, Stuart J. Moving the conversation forward. *Journal of Clinical Ethics.* 1999 Spring; 10(1): 49–56. 8 fn. BE62706.
bioethics; clinical ethics; *clinical ethics committees; conflict of interest; consensus; decision making; education; *ethicist's role; *ethicists; *ethics consultation; *evaluation; geographic factors; guidelines; hospitals; institutional ethics; *professional competence; professional organizations; professional patient relationship; religion; social dominance; *standards; technical expertise; trust; values; preventive ethics; *Core Competencies for Health Care Ethics Consultation (SHHV–SBC Task Force)

Bartels, Dianne; Youngner, Stuart; Levine, June. HealthCare Ethics Forum '94: ethics committees: living up to your potential. *AACN Clinical Issues in Critical Care Nursing.* 1994 Aug; 5(3): 313–323. BE60676.
*clinical ethics committees; committee membership; education; ethicists; ethics consultation; *evaluation; goals; hospitals; institutional policies; *organization and administration; patient education; patient participation

Batzel, Alice M. The HIM professional's role on the ethics committee. *Journal of the American Health Information Management Association.* 1996 Nov–Dec; 67(10): 58–60. BE60431.
*allied health personnel; *clinical ethics committees; *committee membership; hospitals; *medical records; patient advocacy

Belgium. Agreement on cooperation establishing a Consultative Committee on Bioethics, done at Brussels on 15 Jan 1993 between the State, the Flemish

---

BE = bioethics accession number   fn. = footnotes   refs. = references

Community, the French Community, the German–Speaking Community, and the Joint Inter–Community Commission. (*Moniteur Belge*, 12 May 1993, No. 93, p. 10824–10828). [Summary]. *International Digest of Health Legislation*. 1994. 45(1). 47–48. BE62690.
    *advisory committees; *bioethical issues; committee membership; cultural pluralism; information dissemination; public policy; *Belgium; *Consultative Committee on Bioethics (Belgium)

Bernat, James L. VHA ethics rounds: [ethics committee role]. *NCCE News (Veterans Health Administration National Center for Clinical Ethics)*. 1995 Spring; 3(2): 4–5. 2 fn. BE61469.
    accountability; *allowing to die; artificial feeding; case studies; *clinical ethics committees; *decision making; diagnosis; family members; legal aspects; legal guardians; persistent vegetative state; physicians; prognosis; third party consent; withholding treatment

Bottum, J. Debriefing the philosophers. *First Things*. 1997 Jun–Jul; No. 74: 26–30. BE60101.
    *assisted suicide; attitudes; coercion; disadvantaged; *ethicists; indigents; *philosophy; physicians; professional competence; public policy; regulation; *right to die; social impact; *Supreme Court decisions; value of life; wedge argument; liberalism; Dworkin, Ronald; Nagel, Thomas; Nozick, Robert; Rawls, John; Scanlon, Thomas; Thomson, Judith Jarvis; United States; Vacco v. Quill; Washington v. Glucksberg

Bourke, Brian. Decisions, decisions. *Healthcare Alabama*. 1997 Mar; 10(1): 12–15, 20. BE61812.
    allowing to die; *clinical ethics committees; decision making; *hospitals; organization and administration; standards; treatment refusal; withholding treatment; Alabama; Joint Commission on Accreditation of Healthcare Organizations

Brower, Vicki. Bioethics commission "constituted for consensus." [News]. *Nature Biotechnology*. 1996 Sep; 14(9): 1069. BE61418.
    *advisory committees; bioethical issues; committee membership; consensus; genetic information; genetic screening; human experimentation; patents; public policy; *National Bioethics Advisory Commission; *United States

Cartwright, Will. The pig, the transplant surgeon and the Nuffield Council. *Medical Law Review*. 1996 Autumn; 4(3): 250–269. 39 fn. BE61512.
    *advisory committees; animal experimentation; *animal organs; *animal rights; consensus; decision making; food; government regulation; human characteristics; human experimentation; *moral policy; morality; organ donation; *organ transplantation; pain; philosophy; primates; risk; risks and benefits; self concept; *speciesism; transgenic animals; values; domestic animals; *swine; Advisory Committee on Xenotransplantation (Great Britain); Great Britain; *Institute of Medical Ethics (Great Britain); *Nuffield Council on Bioethics

Casarett, David J.; Daskal, Frona; Lantos, John. Experts in ethics? The authority of the clinical ethicist. *Hastings Center Report*. 1998 Nov–Dec; 28(6): 6–11. 19 fn. BE61278.
    *clinical ethics; *communication; *consensus; cultural pluralism; *decision making; dissent; *ethical analysis; ethical theory; *ethicist's role; *ethicists; *ethics consultation; goals; mediation; methods; principle–based ethics; technical expertise; values; Habermas, Jürgen
Mediator? Moral Expert? Or both? "Discourse Ethics" suggests that consensus provides the foundation for defensible moral norms. Thus in building consensus on a moral problem, an ethicist is not just negotiating a

compromise but is contributing to the construction of moral rules and principles that have a genuine claim on us. In this way, not only does expertise on a variety of moral positions facilitate mediation, but mediation opens the way to a kind of moral expertise.

Cash, John; Boyd, Kenneth. Blood transfusion: Bayer's initiative. *Lancet*. 1999 Feb 27; 353(9154): 691–692. 7 refs. BE61198.
    *advisory committees; bioethical issues; *blood banks; blood donation; *blood transfusions; commodification; *communicable diseases; conflict of interest; donors; *drug industry; *ethics committees; *financial support; gifts; information dissemination; international aspects; organizational policies; *private sector; public policy; remuneration; *risk; self regulation; *Bayer Advisory Coucil on Bioethics; Bayer Foundation; *Bayer Inc.; *Canada

Charo, R. Alta. Update on the National Bioethics Advisory Commission. *Protecting Human Subjects*. 1997 Fall: 10–11. BE60060.
    *advisory committees; cloning; genetic information; human experimentation; public policy; *National Bioethics Advisory Commission; United States

Cook–Deegan, Robert Mullan. Finding a voice for bioethics in public policy: federal initiatives in the United States, 1974–1991. *In:* ten Have, Henk A.M.J.; Sass, Hans–Martin, eds. Consensus Formation in Healthcare Ethics. Boston, MA: Kluwer Academic; 1998: 107–140. 69 refs. 7 fn. ISBN 0–7923–4944–X. BE62591.
    *advisory committees; *bioethical issues; bioethics; committee membership; consensus; decision making; evaluation; *federal government; genome mapping; goals; *historical aspects; organization and administration; politics; *public policy; Biomedical Ethics Advisory Committee; Ethics Advisory Board; Human Fetal Tissue Transplantation Research Panel; Institute of Medicine; National Commission for the Protection of Human Subjects; NIH–DOE Working Group on Ethical, Legal, and Social Implications (ELSI); Office of Technology Assessment; President's Commission for the Study of Ethical Problems; *Twentieth Century; U.S. Congress; *United States

Durnan, Richard J.; Lomax, Karen J. Ethics consultation: the need for continuing education and outcome evaluation, not credentialing. [Article and commentary]. *NCCE News (Veterans Health Administration National Center for Clinical Ethics)*. 1995 Spring; 3(2): 1–2, 5, 9, 11. 6 refs. BE61468.
    clinical ethics committees; committee membership; *continuing education; ethicist's role; *ethicists; *ethics consultation; evaluation; physicians; *professional competence; *standards; United States

Elliott, Carl. Bioethics as commodity: does the exchange of money alter the nature of an ethics consultation? *Bioethics Examiner*. 1997 Fall; 1(3): 1–2. BE59791.
    commodification; *conflict of interest; *ethicists; *ethics consultation; hospitals; *remuneration; trust

European Commission. Group of Advisers to the European Commission on the Ethical Implications of Biotechnology. Luxembourg: Office for Official Publications of the European Communities; 1996. 24 p. Includes summaries of GAEIB opinions on (1) bovine somatotrophin or BST; (2) manufacture of human blood and human plasma products; (3) legal protection of biological inventions; (4) gene therapy; (5) labelling of food derived from modern biotechnology; (6) prenatal diagnosis; and (7) the genetic modification of animals. ISBN 98–827–7350–7. BE59459.
    *advisory committees; bioethical issues; biomedical

BE = bioethics accession number   fn. = footnotes   refs. = references

technologies; committee membership; food; gene therapy; *genetic intervention; germ cells; human rights; *international aspects; *organization and administration; patents; prenatal diagnosis; regulation; science; transgenic animals; *Europe; *European Commission; *Group of Advisers on the Ethical Implications of Biotechnology (European Commission)

Faden, Ruth; Guttman, Dan. In response: speaking truth to historiography. *Medical Humanities Review.* 1997 Fall; 11(2): 37–43. 6 fn. Commentary on R. Martensen, p. 21–36. BE59809.
  *advisory committees; biomedical research; entrepreneurship; ethical analysis; *evaluation; *federal government; financial support; government financing; government regulation; guidelines; *historical aspects; *human experimentation; informed consent; investigators; motivation; nontherapeutic research; physicians; politics; public participation; *public policy; *radiation; research subjects; *scientific misconduct; universities; *Advisory Committee on Human Radiation Experiments; Twentieth Century; *United States; University of California, Berkeley

Finder, Stuart G.; Fox, Mark D.; Frist, William H., et al. The ethicist's role on the transplant team: a study of heart, lung, and liver transplantation programs in the United States. *Clinical Transplantation.* 1993 Dec; 7(6): 559–564. 22 refs. BE60203.
  clinical ethics; *decision making; education; *ethicist's role; *ethics consultation; hearts; hospitals; institutional policies; livers; organ donation; *organ transplantation; *patient care team; program descriptions; resource allocation; review committees; selection for treatment; self concept; statistics; survey; transplant recipients; lungs; *United States; Vanderbilt University Medical Center

Fox, Jeffrey L. U.S. Bioethics Commission meets, outlines agenda. [News]. *Nature Biotechnology.* 1996 Nov; 14(11): 1533. BE61419.
  *advisory committees; *bioethical issues; federal government; genetic information; genetic screening; government regulation; human experimentation; privacy; *public policy; research ethics committees; *National Bioethics Advisory Commission; Office for Protection from Research Risks; *United States

Freedman, Benjamin. Duty and Healing: Foundations of a Jewish Bioethic. New York, NY: Routledge; 1999. 344 p. (Reflective bioethics). 413 fn. With an introduction by Charles Weijer. ISBN 0-415-92180-5. BE61646.
  aged; allowing to die; artificial feeding; autonomy; *bioethical issues; *bioethics; case studies; coercion; *competence; cosmetic surgery; *decision making; drugs; ethical analysis; *ethicist's role; *ethics consultation; *family members; *family relationship; health; hospitals; human experimentation; *informed consent; *Jewish ethics; mentally ill; methods; *moral obligations; occupational exposure; palliative care; paralysis; parent child relationship; *patient care; physician's role; prolongation of life; quality of life; *rights; risks and benefits; secularism; suffering; terminal care; theology; third party consent; treatment refusal; truth disclosure; uncertainty; value of life; unproven therapies

Freiberg, Nancy. The ethos of ethics [Edmund D. Pellegrino]. *Georgetown Magazine.* 1996 Fall; 28(2-3-4): 14–18. BE59952.
  *ethicists; faculty; medical ethics; *physicians; Roman Catholic ethics; universities; *Pellegrino, Edmund

Gastmans, Chris. The significance of the Convention on Human Rights and Biomedicine of the Council of Europe for healthcare ethics committees. *HEC (HealthCare Ethics Committee) Forum.* 1998 Sep-Dec; 10(3-4): 350–358. 8 refs. BE61186.

advisory committees; *bioethical issues; clinical ethics committees; *ethics committees; guidelines; health care; *human rights; international aspects; public participation; national ethics committees; Council of Europe; *Europe; *European Convention on Human Rights and Biomedicine

Gibson, Joan McIver. Mediation for ethics committees: a promising process. *Generations (American Society on Aging).* 1994 Winter; 18(4): 58–60. 9 fn. BE60554.
  *clinical ethics committees; ethicist's role; *ethics consultation; goals; *mediation

Golway, Terry. Life in the 90's. [Peter Singer]. *America.* 1998 Sep 12; 179(6): 4. ethicists BE61537.
  active euthanasia; animal rights; attitudes; bioethics; disabled; dissent; faculty; infanticide; newborns; speciesism; universities; *value of life; *Princeton University; *Singer, Peter

Goodman, Kenneth W. Philosophy as news: bioethics, journalism and public policy. *Journal of Medicine and Philosophy.* 1999 Apr; 24(2): 181–200. 25 refs. 4 fn. BE61441.
  *bioethical issues; *bioethics; communication; decision making; democracy; education; *ethicist's role; *ethicists; evaluation; *goals; information dissemination; *interprofessional relations; *journalism; *mass media; moral obligations; obligations to society; philosophy; professional competence; *public policy; *standards; *technical expertise; values

News media accounts of issues in bioethics gain significance to the extent that the media influence public policy and inform personal decision making. The increasingly frequent appearance of bioethics in the news thus imposes responsibilities on journalists and their sources. These responsibilities are identified and discussed, as is (i) the concept of "news-worthiness" as applied to bioethics, (ii) the variable quality of bioethics reportage and (iii) journalists' reliance on ethicists to pass judgment. Because of the potential social and other benefits of high quality reporting on ethical issues, it is argued that journalists and their bioethics sources should explore and accommodate more productive relationships. An optimal journalism-ethics relationship will be one characterized by "para-ethics," in which journalistic constraints are noted but also in which issues and arguments are presented without oversimplification and credible disagreement is given appropriate attention.

Howe, Edmund G. Ethics consultants: could they do better? *Journal of Clinical Ethics.* 1999 Spring; 10(1): 13–25. 23 fn. BE62702.
  case studies; *clinical ethics committees; communication; *conflict of interest; consensus; deception; decision making; dissent; emotions; *ethicist's role; *ethicists; *ethics consultation; evaluation; guidelines; interprofessional relations; patient advocacy; patient care team; professional competence; *professional family relationship; *professional patient relationship; psychology; social dominance; standards; *trust; Core Competencies for Health Care Ethics Consultation (SHHV-SBC Task Force)

Hoyle, Russ. US national bioethics commission: politics as usual? *Nature Biotechnology.* 1996 Aug; 14(8): 927. BE61399.
  *advisory committees; *bioethical issues; federal government; genetic research; genetic screening; genome mapping; historical aspects; human experimentation; international aspects; politics; *public policy; *National Bioethics Advisory Commission; NCHGR Program on Ethical, Legal, and Social Implications (ELSI); *United States

Hutcheon, R. Gordon; Mitchell, John J.; Schmerler,

BE = bioethics accession number   fn. = footnotes   refs. = references

Susan. The Pediatric Ethics Forum: exploring the ethical dimensions of pediatric care. [Case analysis]. *HEC (HealthCare Ethics Committee) Forum.* 1998 Sep–Dec; 10(3–4): 338–349. 8 refs. BE61185.

*adolescents; *allowing to die; bioethical issues; case studies; central nervous system diseases; *chronically ill; clinical ethics; *clinical ethics committees; continuing education; *critically ill; *decision making; *dissent; futility; health personnel; mothers; parental consent; patient care; patient care team; *pediatrics; prognosis; renal dialysis; withholding treatment; St. Joseph's Hospital and Medical Center (Paterson, NJ)

Kantor, Jay E. Ethics consultations in psychiatric private practice. *SBC Newsletter (Society for Bioethics Consultation).* 1996 Spring: 10–12. 4 fn. Reprinted from the *Bulletin of the New York State Psychiatric Association.* BE60417.

*clinical ethics committees; competence; ethicists; *ethics consultation; health facilities; informed consent; patient care; professional competence; *psychiatry; psychotherapy

Kelly, David F.; Hoyt, John W. Ethics consultation. *Critical Care Clinics.* 1996 Jan; 12(1): 49–70. 62 refs. BE59277.

administrators; allowing to die; clergy; *clinical ethics committees; *committee membership; communication; critically ill; decision making; dissent; education; ethicists; *ethics consultation; evaluation; family members; forms; futility; *hospitals; institutional policies; intensive care units; interprofessional relations; lawyers; nurses; *organization and administration; patient advocacy; patient care; physicians; program descriptions; religious hospitals; Roman Catholics; social workers; standards; statistics; withholding treatment; St. Francis Medical Center (Pittsburgh, PA); United States

La Puma, John. Satisfying managed care patients through ethics consultation. *SBC Newsletter (Society for Bioethics Consultation).* 1996 Spring: 12–13. Reprinted from *Managed Care,* 1995 Oct; 4(10): 53–54. BE60418.

attitudes; *ethics consultation; goals; *managed care programs; patient advocacy; patient care; *patient satisfaction; patients; physicians; resource allocation

Lagnado, Lucette. Their role growing, Catholic hospitals juggle doctrine and medicine. *Wall Street Journal.* 1999 Feb 4: A1, A8. BE61011.

abortion, induced; contraception; *ethicist's role; *ethics consultation; *health care delivery; *hospitals; *institutional policies; political activity; program descriptions; referral and consultation; *religious hospitals; *Roman Catholic ethics; sterilization (sexual); therapeutic abortion; ambulatory care; *health facility mergers; Daughters of Charity National Health System; Florida; New York; Niagara Falls Memorial Hospital; Tennessee

Lederberg, Marguerite S. Making a situational diagnosis: psychiatrists at the interface of psychiatry and ethics in the consultation–liaison setting. *Psychosomatics.* 1997 Jul–Aug; 38(4): 327–338. 40 refs. BE62080.

case studies; clinical ethics; competence; decision making; *ethicists; *ethics consultation; family relationship; guidelines; interprofessional relations; legal aspects; medical education; *physicians; psychiatric diagnosis; *psychiatry; referral and consultation; resuscitation orders; terminally ill

Levine, Richard S. Avoiding conflicts of interest in surrogate decision making: why ethics committees should assign surrogacy to a separate committee. *Journal of Clinical Ethics.* 1998 Fall; 9(3): 273–290. 87 fn. BE61336.

accountability; administrators; advance directives; allowing to die; *clinical ethics committees; committee membership;

competence; *conflict of interest; *decision making; due process; education; *ethics consultation; *guidelines; health personnel; hospitals; institutional policies; managed care programs; mediation; models, theoretical; *organization and administration; *patient advocacy; resource allocation; *standards; terminal care; third party consent; withholding treatment

Lowy, Cathy. What is 'ethics'? [Comment]. *Australian and New Zealand Journal of Psychiatry.* 1997 Feb; 31(1): 83–84. Commentary on R. Pargiter and S. Bloch, "The ethics committee of a psychiatric college: its procedures and themes," p. 76–82. BE60278.

economics; *ethics committees; forensic psychiatry; *medical ethics; organization and administration; *physicians; *professional organizations; *psychiatry; Australia; New Zealand; *Royal Australian and New Zealand College of Psychiatrists

McGee, Glenn. Breaking bioethics: an introduction and mission. *Cambridge Quarterly of Healthcare Ethics.* 1998 Fall; 7(4): 414–416. BE59158.

advisory committees; *bioethical issues; *bioethics; communication; education; *ethicist's role; genes; mass media; patents; public participation; public policy; time factors; *trends; United States

Maloney, Dennis M. New federal commission proposed on bioethics. *Human Research Report.* 1998 Mar; 13(3): 6. BE59955.

*advisory committees; *bioethical issues; cloning; federal government; government regulation; legislation; organization and administration; public participation; public policy; science; *Commission to Promote a National Dialogue on Bioethics; National Bioethics Advisory Commission; *United States

Martensen, Robert. If only it were so: medical physics, U.S. human radiation experiments, and the *Final Report* of the President's Advisory Committee (ACHRE). *Medical Humanities Review.* 1997 Fall; 11(2): 21–36. 26 fn. Commented on by R. Faden and Dan Guttman, p. 37–43. BE59808.

*advisory committees; *biomedical research; cancer; conflict of interest; disclosure; drug industry; entrepreneurship; ethical analysis; ethical review; ethicist's role; *evaluation; *federal government; *financial support; government financing; government regulation; guidelines; *historical aspects; *human experimentation; informed consent; investigators; justice; motivation; physicians; policy analysis; politics; *public policy; *radiation; research subjects; resource allocation; science; *scientific misconduct; standards; trust; universities; *Advisory Committee on Human Radiation Experiments; Department of Energy; *Twentieth Century; *United States; University of California, Berkeley

Merlino, Joseph P. The hospital ethics committee: a role for the contemporary psychoanalyst. *Journal of the American Academy of Psychoanalysis.* 1997 Summer; 25(2): 295–305. 12 refs. BE59531.

AIDS; *allowing to die; case studies; *clinical ethics committees; committee membership; *decision making; dissent; ethics consultation; *health personnel; hospitals; internship and residency; patient care team; *physician's role; physicians; *prolongation of life; *psychotherapy; terminal care

Mishkin, Douglas B. Proffering bioethicists as experts. *Judges' Journal.* 1997 Summer; 36(3): 50–51, 88–89. 7 fn. BE59805.

bioethical issues; bioethics; *ethicist's role; *ethicists; *expert testimony; judicial action; legal aspects; *professional competence; standards; technical expertise; ELSI-funded publication; United States

---

BE = bioethics accession number   fn. = footnotes   refs. = references

Moreno, Jonathan D. Ethics committees and ethics consultants. *In:* Kuhse, Helga; Singer, Peter, eds. A Companion to Bioethics. Malden, MA: Blackwell; 1998: 475–484. 20 refs. ISBN 0–631–19737–0. BE59520.
  bioethics; *clinical ethics committees; ethicist's role; *ethicists; *ethics consultation; historical aspects; Twentieth Century; United States

Moss, Alvin H. The application of the Task Force report in rural and frontier settings. *Journal of Clinical Ethics.* 1999 Spring; 10(1): 42–48. 11 fn. BE62705.
  bioethics; *clinical ethics committees; education; *ethicists; *ethics consultation; *geographic factors; guidelines; health facilities; hospitals; institutional policies; *professional competence; regional ethics committees; socioeconomic factors; *standards; *rural population; Core Competencies for Health Care Ethics Consultation (SHHV–SBC Task Force); Northwestern United States; *United States; West Virginia

Nasar, Sylvia. Princeton's new philosopher draws a stir. [News]. *New York Times.* 1999 Apr 10: 1, B11. BE62699.
  attitudes; bioethical issues; *ethicists; universities; *Princeton University; *Singer, Peter

Nelson, James Lindemann. Bioethics as several kinds of writing. *Journal of Medicine and Philosophy.* 1999 Apr; 24(2): 148–163. 21 refs. 9 fn. BE61439.
  *bioethical issues; *bioethics; communication; education; ethical theory; *ethicist's role; *ethicists; interprofessional relations; *journalism; literature; *mass media; technical expertise; publishing
  Three different models are described of the relationship of bioethics to the press. The first two are familiar: bioethicists often are interviewed by journalists seeking background and short quotes to insert in a story; alternately, bioethicists sometimes themselves act as journalists of a sort, writing op–eds, articles or even longer works designed for wide readership. These models share the notion that bioethicists can provide information and ideas that increase the quality of people's thinking on moral matters. They share also a common difficulty: do the constraints the media impose on bioethical discourse keep bioethicists from deepening public reflection, and if not, how can those constraints be most effectively kept from distorting what bioethicists wish to say? The third model reverses–-in part–-the presupposition that bioethics bestows moral
  sophistication on a public naive about ethical issues, holding rather that matters run both ways; bioethicists stand to learn a great deal from their interactions with various publics and the media that serve them. On this view, the constraints imposed by media conventions constitute opportunities for new and potentially important forms of bioethical writing. Various concerns generated by the first two models are surveyed. It is concluded that while none of the difficulties constitute knock–down arguments against these forms of collaborating with the press, the worries are problematic enough to provide some support for considering the less familiar third approach. Further reason for taking the third model seriously draws on moral theoretic considerations.

Nicholas, Barbara. Strategies for effective transformation. *In:* Donchin, Anne; Purdy, Laura M., eds. Embodying Bioethics: Recent Feminist Advances. Lanham, MD: Rowman and Littlefield; 1999: 239–252. 37 refs. 10 fn. ISBN 0–8476–8924–7. BE61024.
  *bioethics; ethical relativism; ethical theory; *ethicist's role; *females; *feminist ethics; goals; health facilities; interdisciplinary communication; interprofessional relations;

postmodernism; *social dominance

Pargiter, Russell; Bloch, Sidney. The ethics committee of a psychiatric college: its procedures and themes. *Australian and New Zealand Journal of Psychiatry.* 1997 Feb; 31(1): 76–82. 18 refs. Commented on by C. Lowy, p. 83–84. BE60277.
  codes of ethics; economics; *ethics committees; forensic psychiatry; guidelines; medical education; *medical ethics; organization and administration; *physicians; *professional organizations; *psychiatry; self regulation; Australia; New Zealand; *Royal Australian and New Zealand College of Psychiatrists

Parker, Kelly A. The bioethics committee: a consensus–recommendation model. *In:* McGee, Glenn, ed. Pragamatic Bioethics. Nashville, TN: Vanderbilt University Press; 1999: 60–70, 264–265. 10 fn. ISBN 0–8265–1321–2. BE60663.
  accountability; *clinical ethics committees; committee membership; conscience; *consensus; decision making; health facilities; health personnel; institutional policies; interprofessional relations; mediation; medicine; loyalty; pragmatism

Pellegrino, Edmund D. Clinical ethics consultations: some reflections on the report of the SHHV–SBC. *Journal of Clinical Ethics.* 1999 Spring; 10(1): 5–12. 4 refs. BE62701.
  accountability; bioethics; clinical ethics; *clinical ethics committees; conflict of interest; conscience; consensus; cultural pluralism; dissent; *ethicist's role; *ethicists; *ethics consultation; *evaluation; goals; guidelines; health personnel; hospitals; institutional ethics; law; moral obligations; patient advocacy; *professional competence; professional ethics; professional organizations; psychology; religion; *standards; virtues; *Core Competencies for Health Care Ethics Consultation (SHHV–SBC Task Force)

Pentz, Rebecca D. Beyond case consultation: an expanded model for organizational ethics. *Journal of Clinical Ethics.* 1999 Spring; 10(1): 34–41. 31 fn. BE62704.
  administrators; bioethics; bone marrow; clinical ethics; *clinical ethics committees; committee membership; conflict of interest; decision making; dissent; donors; *ethicists; *ethics consultation; evaluation; futility; hospitals; *institutional ethics; institutional policies; *models, theoretical; patient advocacy; physicians; professional competence; resource allocation; standards; tissue donation; withholding treatment; business ethics; preventive ethics; Core Competencies for Health Care Ethics Consultation (SHHV–SBC Task Force); *M.D. Anderson Cancer Center

Phillips, Donald F. New report rejects accrediting of those who provide ethics consultation services. [News]. *JAMA.* 1999 Jun 2; 281(21): 1976. BE61953.
  *clinical ethics committees; *ethicists; *ethics consultation; guidelines; organizational policies; *professional competence; professional organizations; self regulation; *standards; technical expertise; Society for Bioethics Consultation; Society for Health and Human Values; United States

Pinkus, Rosa Lynn. Editorial comment on 'the ethicist's role.' *Clinical Transplantation.* 1993 Dec; 7(6): 565–566. 4 refs. BE60204.
  clinical ethics; decision making; *ethicist's role; ethics consultation; *organ transplantation; patient care team; technical expertise; United States

Poland, Susan Cartier. Bioethics commissions: town meetings with a "blue, blue ribbon". [Bibliography]. *Kennedy Institute of Ethics Journal.* 1998 Mar; 8(1): 91–109. Also available, as Scope Note 34, from the

National Reference Center for Bioethics Literature, Kennedy Institute of Ethics, Georgetown University; Box 571212, Washington, DC 20057-1212, (202) 687-6738 or (800) MED-ETHX. BE59357.
*advisory committees; *bioethical issues; *international aspects; public policy; United States

Powell, Tia. Consultation-liaison psychiatry and clinical ethics: representative cases. *Psychosomatics.* 1997 Jul-Aug; 38(4): 321-326. 8 refs. BE62079.
case studies; *clinical ethics; decision making; *ethicists; *ethics consultation; family members; living wills; *physicians; *psychiatry; resuscitation orders; suicide; terminally ill; therapeutic research

Rosen, Elisabeth. Bioethics committees as consensus shapers. *Bulletin of Medical Ethics.* 1999 Feb; No. 145: 13-18. 18 refs. BE61891.
*advisory committees; *bioethical issues; cloning; comparative studies; consensus; cultural pluralism; enhancement technologies; evaluation; genetic intervention; interdisciplinary communication; international aspects; organization and administration; patents; *public policy; trust; values; Europe; *European Group on Ethics in Science and New Technologies; *National Bioethics Advisory Commission; United States

Ross, Judith Wilson. The Task Force report: comprehensible forest or unknown beetles? *Journal of Clinical Ethics.* 1999 Spring; 10(1): 26-33. 3 fn. BE62703.
bioethics; *clinical ethics committees; conflict of interest; consensus; ethicist's role; *ethicists; *ethics consultation; *evaluation; goals; guidelines; mandatory programs; *professional competence; professional organizations; self regulation; *standards; technical expertise; uncertainty; voluntary programs; *Core Competencies for Health Care Ethics Consultation (SHHV-SBC Task Force)

Rudin, Edward. A critique from the siding: response to "Paradigms for clinical ethics consultation practice" by Mark D. Fox, Glenn McGee, and Arthur L. Caplan (*CQ*, 1998 Summer; 7(3): 308-314). *Cambridge Quarterly of Healthcare Ethics.* 1999 Summer; 8(3): 351-357. 3 refs. BE62352.
*clinical ethics; *ethicist's role; *ethicists; *ethics consultation; health personnel; hospitals; interprofessional relations; lawyers; mental health; models, theoretical; patient care team; *referral and consultation; technical expertise; preventive ethics

Schyve, Paul. Critiques and new directions [bioethics services]. *SBC Newsletter (Society for Bioethics Consultation).* 1996 Spring: 4-8. Reprinted from *Bioethics Matters: A Newsletter for Friends of the Clinical Center for Biomedical Ethics* at the University of Virginia at Charlottesville. BE60415.
*accountability; clinical ethics committees; codes of ethics; conflict of interest; disclosure; economics; ethicists; *ethics consultation; guidelines; health facilities; *hospitals; incentives; *institutional ethics; managed care programs; organization and administration; patient admission; patient participation; patient transfer; patients' rights; professional competence; *standards; *business ethics; *Joint Commission on Accreditation of Healthcare Organizations

Secundy, Marian Gray. Ethical literacy and cultural competence. *In:* McGee, Glenn, ed. Pragmatic Bioethics. Nashville, TN: Vanderbilt University Press; 1999: 246-253, 288. 18 fn. ISBN 0-8265-1321-2. BE60675.
clinical ethics; conflict of interest; cultural pluralism; economics; *ethicist's role; *ethicists; ethics consultation; health facilities; interdisciplinary communication; *professional competence; standards; technical expertise; United States

Seligman, Dan. Talking back to the ethicists. *Forbes.* 1997 May 5; 159(9): 198-199. BE59406.
bioethical issues; *ethicists; industry; technical expertise; business ethics

Sexson, William R.; Thigpen, Janet. Organization and function of a hospital ethics committee. *Clinics in Perinatology.* 1996 Sep; 23(3): 429-436. 3 refs. BE60932.
*clinical ethics committees; committee membership; communication; education; ethical review; ethics consultation; health personnel; *hospitals; institutional ethics; institutional policies; *organization and administration; patient education; patients' rights; standards; Grady Memorial Hospital (Atlanta, GA); Joint Commission on Accreditation of Healthcare Organizations

Shapiro, David. Think before you squawk. *New Scientist.* 1997 Aug 2; 155(2093): 47. BE60457.
*advisory committees; *cloning; evaluation; government regulation; *international aspects; politics; public policy; France; Germany; Great Britain; United States

Silberner, Joanne. Turning pages, if not heads. *Hastings Center Report.* 1999 Mar-Apr; 29(2): 6. BE61654.
advisory committees; bioethical issues; economics; *embryo research; federal government; *government financing; government regulation; health care; human experimentation; mentally ill; political activity; *politics; *public policy; stem cells; *National Bioethics Advisory Commission; National Institutes of Health; U.S. Congress; *United States; Varmus, Harold

Simon, Alfred. Establishing clinical [healthcare] ethics committees in Germany. [Letter]. *HEC (HealthCare Ethics Committee) Forum.* 1998 Sep-Dec; 10(3-4): 359-360. BE61003.
*clinical ethics committees; hospitals; Akademie für Ethik in der Medizin; Christian Association of Hospitals; *Germany

Singer, Peter. Living and dying. [Interview]. *Psychology Today.* 1999 Jan-Feb; 32(1): 56-59, 78-79. BE61518.
*active euthanasia; allowing to die; *animal experimentation; brain death; *disabled; *ethicists; human experimentation; killing; morality; National Socialism; newborns; persistent vegetative state; primates; quality of life; speciesism; suffering; utilitarianism; value of life; *Singer, Peter

Spencer, Edward M. Ethical conundrums: "Are ethics programs obsolete?" *SBC Newsletter (Society for Bioethics Consultation).* 1996 Spring: 8-9. Reprinted from *Bioethics Matters: A Newsletter for Friends of the Clinical Center for Biomedical Ethics* at the University of Virginia at Charlottesville. BE60416.
*clinical ethics committees; codes of ethics; committee membership; economics; ethics consultation; goals; health facilities; institutional ethics; organization and administration; standards; business ethics; Joint Commission on Accreditation of Healthcare Organizations

Spicker, Stuart F. The process of coherence formation in healthcare ethics committees: the consensus process, social authority and ethical judgments. *In:* ten Have, Henk A.M.J.; Sass, Hans-Martin, eds. Consensus Formation in Healthcare Ethics. Boston, MA: Kluwer Academic; 1998: 35-44. 15 refs. 2 fn. ISBN 0-7923-4944-X. BE62586.
*clinical ethics committees; *consensus; *decision making; dissent; ethics consultation; goals; hospitals; mediation; patient care

Steinberg, Maurice D. Psychiatry and bioethics: an exploration of the relationship. *Psychosomatics.* 1997

BE = bioethics accession number   fn. = footnotes   refs. = references

Jul–Aug; 38(4): 313–320. 48 refs. BE62078.
  bioethical issues; bioethics; clinical ethics; clinical ethics
  committees; communication; competence; decision making;
  emotions; *ethicists; *ethics consultation; informed consent;
  mediation; patient advocacy; *physician's role; *physicians;
  *psychiatry; referral and consultation; terminal care;
  treatment refusal; withholding treatment

Tichtchenko, Pavel. New bioethics association is founded
  for the post-socialist countries. [News]. *Bulletin of
  Medical Ethics.* 1999 Apr; No. 147: 6. BE61822.
  *bioethics; *ethicists; international aspects; *professional
  organizations; *Central and East European Association of
  Bioethics; *Eastern Europe; Europe

**U.S. Congress. House. Committee on Government
Reform and Oversight. Subcommittee on Human
Resources.** Institutional Review Boards: A System in
Jeopardy. Hearing, 11 Jun 1998. Washington, DC: U.S.
Government Printing Office; 1999. 179 p. Serial No.
105-166. ISBN 0-16-058021-8. BE62631.
  accountability; advisory committees; children; committee
  membership; competence; conflict of interest; continuing
  education; drug industry; *ethical review; *evaluation;
  federal government; financial support; government
  financing; government regulation; *human experimentation;
  industry; informed consent; investigational drugs;
  investigators; medical devices; mentally disabled; patient
  advocacy; placebos; public participation; *public policy;
  research design; *research ethics committees; research
  subjects; risks and benefits; selection of subjects; technical
  expertise; universities; vulnerable populations; multicenter
  studies; Department of Health and Human Services; Food
  and Drug Administration; National Bioethics Advisory
  Commission; National Institutes of Health; Office for
  Protection from Research Risks; *United States

Unesco. International Bioethics Committee. First
Session. [Report of the first session of the International
Bioethics Committee, Paris, 15–16 Sep 1993]. Paris:
International Bioethics Committee; 1994 Feb 1. 10 p.
plus annexes (90 p.). SHS-93/CONF.015/4. Original in
French. BE59221.
  *advisory committees; bioethical issues; committee
  membership; *ethics committees; gene therapy; genetic
  information; genetic research; genetic screening;
  *international aspects; organization and administration;
  population genetics; *International Bioethics Committee
  (Unesco); *Unesco

Uzych, Leo. Bioethics and NBAC. [Letter]. *Nature
Biotechnology.* 1996 Sep; 14(9): 1057. BE61417.
  *advisory committees; bioethical issues; consensus; politics;
  *public policy; *National Bioethics Advisory Commission;
  *United States

Veatch, Robert M. Ethical consensus formation in clinical
cases. *In:* ten Have, Henk A.M.J.; Sass, Hans–Martin,
eds. Consensus Formation in Healthcare Ethics. Boston,
MA: Kluwer Academic; 1998: 17–34. 25 refs. ISBN
0-7923-4944-X. BE62585.
  autonomy; *clinical ethics; *clinical ethics committees;
  competence; *consensus; contracts; covenant; cultural
  pluralism; *decision making; ethical theory; family members;
  health facilities; informed consent; legal guardians; moral
  policy; patient advocacy; *patient care; *patient care team;
  patient participation; *patients; peer review; *physicians;
  religious ethics; secularism; third party consent; values;
  absence of proxy

Weber, Leonard J. Taking on organizational ethics.
Health Progress. 1997 May–Jun; 78(3): 20–23, 32.
BE59684.
  administrators; case studies; *clinical ethics committees;

committee membership; economics; employment; ethicists;
ethics consultation; *health facilities; *institutional ethics;
institutional policies; organization and administration; patient
care; professional competence; resource allocation; business
ethics

Weijer, Charles. Duty and healing: the lifework of
Benjamin Freedman. [Editorial]. *Canadian Medical
Association Journal.* 1997 Jun 1; 156(11): 1553-1555. 12
refs. BE59679.
  bioethical issues; ethicists; Canada; *Freedman, Benjamin

Wolpe, Paul Root. The freelance bioethicist, chapter one.
[Irony]. *Cambridge Quarterly of Healthcare Ethics.* 1999
Winter; 8(1): 118–119. BE60542.
  communication; *ethicists; professional patient relationship

Yoder, Scot D. Experts in ethics? The nature of ethical
expertise. *Hastings Center Report.* 1998 Nov–Dec; 28(6):
11–19. 35 fn. BE61279.
  clinical ethics; decision making; dissent; education; *ethicists;
  ethics; ethics consultation; evaluation; goals; professional
  competence; public policy; *technical expertise
Critics of clinical ethicists sometimes claim that if there
were expertise in ethics, then there would have to be
objective moral knowledge. They also assume that there
would be only one kind of ethics expertise, and that it
would be a kind of professional specialization. All three
assumptions are mistaken.

Youngner, Stuart J. Consultation–liaison psychiatry and
clinical ethics: historical parallels and diversions.
Psychosomatics. 1997 Jul–Aug; 38(4): 309–312. 8 refs.
BE62077.
  attitudes; *clinical ethics; *ethicist's role; *ethicists; *ethics
  committees; hospitals; *physician's role; *psychiatry;
  psychotherapy; referral and consultation

EC ethics group established. [News]. *Nature Biotechnology.*
1998 Feb; 16(2): 121. BE62042.
  *advisory committees; *genetic intervention; *international
  aspects; organization and administration; *Europe;
  *European Commission; *European Group on Ethics,
  Science and Biotechnology; Group of Advisers on the
  Ethical Implications of Biotechnology (European
  Commission)

European Group on Ethics in Science and New
Technologies. [News]. *Journal of Medical Ethics.* 1998
Aug; 24(4): 247. BE61302.
  *advisory committees; *bioethical issues; biomedical
  technologies; genetic intervention; *international aspects;
  *European Commission; *European Group on Ethics in
  Science and New Technologies; Group of Advisers on the
  Ethical Implications of Biotechnology (European
  Commission)

ETHICS COMMITTEES See ETHICISTS AND
ETHICS COMMITTEES
See under
  BEHAVIORAL RESEARCH/ETHICS
    COMMITTEES
  HUMAN EXPERIMENTATION/ETHICS
    COMMITTEES

EUGENICS

See also GENETIC INTERVENTION

Agar, Nicholas. Liberal eugenics. *Public Affairs Quarterly.*
1998 Apr; 12(2): 137–155. 31 fn. BE62387.
  children; *eugenics; *freedom; *future generations; *genetic

---

BE = bioethics accession number   fn. = footnotes   refs. = references

enhancement; *genetic intervention; goals; human rights; intelligence; justice; *parents; *quality of life; regulation; reproduction; risks and benefits; values; liberalism

Alderson, Priscilla. Childhood, genetics, ethics and the social context. *In:* Clarke, Angus, ed. The Genetic Testing of Children. Washington, DC: BIOS Scientific Publishers; 1998: 223–235. 60 refs. ISBN 1-85996-146-0. BE62764.

adolescents; *attitudes; behavioral genetics; *children; congenital disorders; directive counseling; *disabled; empirical research; ethicists; *eugenics; genetic counseling; genetic determinism; genetic disorders; genetic screening; *genetics; goals; health personnel; obligations of society; prenatal diagnosis; selective abortion; social control; social problems; *social worth; socioeconomic factors; stigmatization; value of life; Great Britain

American Society of Human Genetics. Board of Directors. Eugenics and the misuse of genetic information to restrict reproductive freedom: ASHG statement. *American Journal of Human Genetics.* 1999 Feb; 64(2): 335–338. 16 refs. BE62217.

coercion; disabled; *eugenics; *freedom; genetic disorders; *genetic information; genetic screening; health personnel; historical aspects; incentives; *international aspects; investigators; involuntary sterilization; mentally retarded; National Socialism; *organizational policies; prenatal diagnosis; professional organizations; public policy; *reproduction; terminology; voluntary programs; *American Society of Human Genetics; China; Europe; Germany; Japan; United States

Appleyard, Bryan. Brave New Worlds: Staying Human in the Genetic Future. New York, NY: Viking; 1998. 198 p. Bibliography: p. 183–186. ISBN 0-670-86989-9. BE60356.

*attitudes; behavioral genetics; biology; cloning; dehumanization; ecology; *eugenics; evolution; freedom; gene therapy; genetic counseling; genetic determinism; genetic disorders; *genetic intervention; genetic predisposition; genetic research; genetic screening; *genetics; genome mapping; historical aspects; humanism; investigators; life extension; minority groups; morality; National Socialism; normality; politics; preimplantation diagnosis; prenatal diagnosis; preventive medicine; public opinion; public policy; *recombinant DNA research; reproduction; *risks and benefits; *science; selective abortion; self regulation; social control; social discrimination; *social impact; transgenic organisms; value of life; *values; nature; Asilomar Conference

Barondess, Jeremiah A. Care of the medical ethos: reflections on Social Darwinism, racial hygiene, and the Holocaust. *Annals of Internal Medicine.* 1998 Dec 1; 129(11): 891–898. 34 refs. BE59326.

dehumanization; disabled; disadvantaged; *eugenics; evolution; genetics; health care delivery; *historical aspects; human experimentation; international aspects; investigators; involuntary euthanasia; involuntary sterilization; justice; killing; *medical ethics; *medicine; minority groups; *misconduct; *moral complicity; *National Socialism; physician's role; *physicians; prisoners; psychiatry; public health; public policy; science; suffering; values; Darwinism; *Germany; *Twentieth Century; United States

Berger, Joseph. Yale gene pool seen as route to better baby. *New York Times.* 1999 Jan 10: 19. BE60023.

*advertising; *eugenics; intelligence; *ovum donors; parents; remuneration; students; universities; United States; *Yale University

Bock, Gisela. Sterilization and "medical" massacres in National Socialist Germany: ethics, politics, and the law. *In:* Berg, Manfred; Cocks, Geoffrey, eds. Medicine and

Modernity: Public Health and Medical Care in Nineteenth- and Twentieth-Century Germany. New York, NY: Cambridge University Press; 1997: 149–172. 85 fn. ISBN 0-521-56411-5. BE59269.

aliens; chronically ill; *dehumanization; *disabled; *eugenics; genetic disorders; *historical aspects; *involuntary euthanasia; *involuntary sterilization; Jews; *killing; mentally disabled; minority groups; *National Socialism; *physicians; *psychiatry; public health; *public policy; selective abortion; social control; social discrimination; *social worth; socioeconomic factors; *sociology of medicine; genocide; *Germany; *Twentieth Century

Coghlan, Andy. Perfect People's Republic. [News]. *New Scientist.* 1998 Oct 24; 160(2157): 18. BE61540.

*attitudes; carriers; common good; cultural pluralism; disabled; empirical research; employment; *eugenics; genetic screening; *health personnel; international aspects; late-onset disorders; mandatory testing; non-Western World; population control; public policy; reproduction; selective abortion; social discrimination; Western World; *China

DauBach, Penelope P. Homegrown Eugenics: Socioeconomic Differentials in Utilization of Prenatal Testing. Ann Arbor, MI: University Microfilms International; 1997. 299 p. Bibliography: p. 269–299. Dissertation, Ph.D. in Anthropology, University of Kansas, 1997. UMI No. 9811292. BE60012.

children; comparative studies; congenital disorders; costs and benefits; *decision making; *eugenics; females; genetic counseling; government financing; health insurance; indigents; *knowledge, attitudes, practice; minority groups; motivation; *pregnant women; *prenatal diagnosis; selective abortion; *socioeconomic factors; survey; whites; Medicaid; United States

Dickson, David. Congress grabs eugenics common ground. [News]. *Nature.* 1998 Aug 20; 394(6695): 711. Report of a workshop held during the 18th International Congress on Genetics in Beijing, 10–15 Oct 1998. BE60393.

*eugenics; genetic counseling; genetic disorders; genetic screening; informed consent; *international aspects; involuntary sterilization; legislation; *public policy; terminology; *China; *International Congress on Genetics; Law on Maternal and Infant Health Care (China)

Dickson, David. Survey: some countries side with China on genetic issues. [News]. *Nature Medicine.* 1998 Oct; 4(10): 1096. BE61538.

*attitudes; *cultural pluralism; developing countries; empirical research; *eugenics; genetic screening; genetic services; goals; government regulation; *health personnel; *international aspects; non-Western World; prenatal diagnosis; Western World; *China

Dikötter, Frank. Imperfect Conceptions: Medical Knowledge, Birth Defects and Eugenics in China. New York, NY: Columbia University Press; 1998. 226 p. Bibliography: p. 187–216. ISBN 0-231-11370-6. BE60707.

active euthanasia; *congenital disorders; *disabled; emotions; *eugenics; family relationship; genetic disorders; government regulation; *historical aspects; involuntary sterilization; medicine; political systems; pregnant women; *public policy; *reproduction; sexuality; *social control; value of life; values; *China; Eighteenth Century; Nineteenth Century; Seventeenth Century; Sixteenth Century; Twentieth Century

Dubow, Saul. Scientific Racism in Modern South Africa. New York, NY: Cambridge University Press; 1995. 320 p. Bibliography: p. 292–314. ISBN 0-521-47907-X.

BE60013.
*blacks; *eugenics; *historical aspects; paternalism; politics; Protestants; *social discrimination; social dominance; whites; *Nineteenth Century; Social Darwinism; *South Africa; *Twentieth Century

Dunne, Cara; Warren, Catherine. Lethal autonomy: the malfunction of the informed consent mechanism within the context of prenatal diagnosis of genetic variants. *Issues in Law and Medicine.* 1998 Fall; 14(2): 165-202. 75 fn. BE62011.
*autonomy; cancer; directive counseling; disclosure; Down syndrome; *eugenics; *genetic counseling; genetic disorders; genetic screening; genome mapping; health personnel; historical aspects; *informed consent; killing; legal liability; mentally retarded; minority groups; National Socialism; physician's role; *prenatal diagnosis; quality of life; selective abortion; social discrimination; sterilization (sexual); wrongful life; Germany; Human Genome Project; Twentieth Century; United States

Fitzgerald, Wendy Anton. Engineering perfect offspring: devaluing children and childhood. *Hastings Constitutional Law Quarterly.* 1997 Summer; 24(4): 833-861. 183 fn. BE62163.
adults; *allowing to die; autonomy; behavior disorders; *children; *congenital disorders; *decision making; dehumanization; *disabled; Down syndrome; *eugenics; gene therapy; genetic counseling; *genetic determinism; *genetic disorders; genetic predisposition; genetic research; hyperkinesis; *legal aspects; *newborns; *normality; *parents; *personhood; physicians; prognosis; *prolongation of life; psychiatric diagnosis; *quality of life; resource allocation; social discrimination; social worth; *surgery; terminally ill; twins; *value of life; *values; *withholding treatment; *conjoined twins; dependency; seriously ill; Hensel twins; Holton twins; Lakeberg twins; Social Darwinism; United States

Galton, David J. Greek theories on eugenics. *Journal of Medical Ethics.* 1998 Aug; 24(4): 263-267. 21 refs. BE61293.
*ancient history; carriers; children; disabled; *eugenics; females; *historical aspects; involuntary sterilization; legal aspects; males; mandatory programs; marital relationship; obligations to society; philosophy; population control; *reproduction; *social control; social discrimination; socioeconomic factors; *Aristotle; Athens; Europe; Galton, Francis; Great Britain; Greece; Nineteenth Century; *Plato; Twentieth Century; United States
With the recent developments in the Human Genome Mapping Project and the new technologies that are developing from it there is a renewal of concern about eugenic applications. Francis Galton (b1822, d1911), who developed the subject of eugenics, suggested that the ancient Greeks had contributed very little to social theories of eugenics. In fact the Greeks had a profound interest in methods of supplying their city states with the finest possible progeny. This paper therefore reviews the works of Plato (The Republic and Politics) and Aristotle (The Politics and The Athenian Constitution) which have a direct bearing on eugenic techniques and relates them to methods used in the present century.

Garver, Kenneth L.; Santorum, Rick. Eugenics and Catholic medicine. *Ethics and Medics.* 1998 Jul; 23(7): 1-2. BE60818.
aged; congenital disorders; economics; *eugenics; genetics; health maintenance organizations; *historical aspects; involuntary sterilization; mentally disabled; newborns; prenatal diagnosis; *public policy; *Roman Catholic ethics; selective abortion; utilitarianism; withholding treatment; Nineteenth Century; Twentieth Century; *United States

Gillon, Raanan. Eugenics, contraception, abortion and ethics. [Editorial]. *Journal of Medical Ethics.* 1998 Aug; 24(4): 219-220. 1 ref. BE61287.
coercion; *contraception; disabled; *eugenics; *genetic disorders; historical aspects; moral policy; motivation; National Socialism; philosophy; reproduction; *selective abortion; social control; social discrimination; *voluntary programs; Aristotle; Plato

Glover, Jonathan. Eugenics: some lessons from the Nazi experience. *In:* Harris, John; Holm, Søren, eds. The Future of Human Reproduction: Ethics, Choice, and Regulation. New York, NY: Oxford University Press; 1998: 55-65. 15 fn. ISBN 0-19-823761-8. BE61262.
bioethics; dehumanization; disabled; disease; *eugenics; historical aspects; international aspects; involuntary sterilization; Jews; *killing; metaphor; minority groups; *National Socialism; reproduction; social discrimination; wedge argument; *Germany; *Social Darwinism; Twentieth Century

Gray, Paul. Cursed by eugenics. *Time.* 1999 Jan 11; 153(1): 84-85. BE60317.
*eugenics; historical aspects; institutionalized persons; involuntary commitment; mentally disabled; minority groups; National Socialism; physically disabled; public policy; Supreme Court decisions; genocide; Germany; Great Britain; Twentieth Century; United States

Hadley, Janet. Prenatal tests: blessings and burdens. *In:* Lee, Ellie, ed. Abortion Law and Politics Today. New York, NY: St. Martin's Press; 1998: 172-183. 27 fn. ISBN 0-312-21574-6. BE62337.
*congenital disorders; *decision making; directive counseling; *disabled; economics; *eugenics; genetic counseling; genetic disorders; genetic predisposition; genetic screening; international aspects; involuntary sterilization; late-onset disorders; parents; pregnant women; preimplantation diagnosis; *prenatal diagnosis; *public policy; rights; *selective abortion; *stigmatization; Great Britain

Hasian, Marouf Arif. The Uses of "Necessity" in Anglo-American Discourse: An Ideographic Analysis of the Eugenics Movement, 1900-1940. Ann Arbor, MI: UMI Dissertation Services; 1993. 447 p. Bibliography: p. 408-443. Dissertation, Ph.D., University of Georgia, 1993. Order No. 9416261 BE60747.
behavioral genetics; blacks; comparative studies; contraception; education; *eugenics; females; genetic disorders; genetic screening; genome mapping; *historical aspects; indigents; involuntary sterilization; legal aspects; legislation; mass media; mothers; obligations to society; politics; reproduction; rights; Roman Catholics; social control; social discrimination; social problems; socialism; socioeconomic factors; state interest; *terminology; women's rights; *Great Britain; Human Genome Project; Nineteenth Century; *Twentieth Century; *United States

Hodges, Jeffrey Alan. Euthenics, Eugenics and Compulsory Sterilization in Michigan: 1897-1960. Ann Arbor, MI: UMI Dissertation Services; 1995. 181 p. Bibliography: p. 176-181. Thesis, Master of Arts in History, Michigan State University, 1995. UMI No. 1378034. BE60650.
behavior control; blacks; *eugenics; females; *historical aspects; institutionalized persons; *involuntary sterilization; legislation; males; mentally ill; mentally retarded; National Socialism; prisoners; *public policy; sex offenses; social problems; socioeconomic factors; state government; whites; *Michigan; *Twentieth Century; United States

Horn, David. Unnatural acts: procreation and the genealogy of artifice. *In:* Terry, Jennifer; Calvert,

---

BE = bioethics accession number   fn. = footnotes   refs. = references

Melodie, eds. Processed Lives: Gender and Technology in Everyday Life. New York, NY: Routledge; 1997: 145-154. 31 refs. 10 fn. ISBN 0-415-14932-0. BE61945.
*artificial insemination; *attitudes; confidentiality; *deception; disclosure; *eugenics; fathers; *historical aspects; international aspects; *males; married persons; parent child relationship; physicians; reproductive technologies; *semen donors; *sexuality; *nature; Europe; Hurd, Addison Davis; Nineteenth Century; Pancoast, William; Twentieth Century; United States

Johnson, Linda. Expanding eugenics or improving health care in China: commentary on the Provisions of the Standing Committee of the Gansu People's Congress concerning the prohibition of reproduction by intellectually impaired persons. *Journal of Law and Society.* 1997 Jun; 24(2): 199-234. 126 fn. BE62168.
abortion, induced; coercion; *eugenics; females; *intelligence; *involuntary sterilization; *legal aspects; legislation; *mandatory programs; married persons; *mentally retarded; normality; population control; pregnant women; *public policy; reproduction; *China; *Gansu Province; Law on Maternal and Infant Health Care 1994 (China)

King, David. The persistence of eugenics. *GenEthics News.* 1998 Feb-Mar; No. 22: 6-8. 4 refs. BE61094.
*attitudes; behavioral genetics; *directive counseling; *eugenics; *genetic counseling; genetic determinism; genetic screening; *genetics; *health personnel; historical aspects; informal social control; international aspects; investigators; parents; prenatal diagnosis; reproduction; selective abortion; social control; Twentieth Century

King, David S. Preimplantation genetic diagnosis and the 'new' eugenics. *Journal of Medical Ethics.* 1999 Apr; 25(2): 176-182. 33 refs. BE61923.
carriers; coercion; congenital disorders; decision making; directive counseling; disabled; embryo disposition; embryo transfer; embryos; *eugenics; gene pool; genetic counseling; genetic disorders; genetic predisposition; *genetic screening; goals; government regulation; health personnel; in vitro fertilization; informal social control; international aspects; knowledge, attitudes, practice; *moral policy; normality; parent child relationship; parents; physicians; *preimplantation diagnosis; prenatal diagnosis; public policy; selective abortion; social discrimination; *social impact; socioeconomic factors; trends
Preimplantation genetic diagnosis (PID) is often seen as an improvement upon prenatal testing. I argue that PID may exacerbate the eugenic features of prenatal testing and make possible an expanded form of free-market eugenics. The current practice of prenatal testing is eugenic in that its aim is to reduce the numbers of people with genetic disorders. Due to social pressures and eugenic attitudes held by clinical geneticists in most countries, it results in eugenic outcomes even though no state coercion is involved. I argue that technological advances may soon make PID widely accessible. Because abortion is not involved, and multiple embryos are available, PID is radically more effective as a tool of genetic selection. It will also make possible selection on the basis of non-pathological characteristics, leading, potentially, to a full-blown free-market eugenics. For these reasons, I argue that PID should be strictly regulated.

Larson, Edward J. Confronting scientific authority with religious values: eugenics in American history. *In:* Demy, Timothy J.; Stewart, Gary P., eds. Genetic Engineering: A Christian Response: Crucial Considerations in Shaping Life. Grand Rapids, MI: Kregel Publications; 1999: 104-124. 80 fn. ISBN 0-8254-2357-0. BE61363.
clergy; contraception; disadvantaged; *eugenics; gene

therapy; genetic determinism; genetic information; genetic screening; genome mapping; *historical aspects; human rights; institutionalized persons; *involuntary sterilization; justice; *legislation; mass media; *mentally ill; *mentally retarded; organizational policies; patient discharge; physicians; *political activity; *politics; prisoners; privacy; *religion; Roman Catholic ethics; *Roman Catholics; sex offenses; state government; Supreme Court decisions; value of life; *Alabama; *Buck v. Bell; *Christian Fundamentalists; *Louisiana; Medical Association of Alabama; Twentieth Century; United States

McNally, Ruth. Eugenics here and now. *In:* Glasner, Peter; Rothman, Harry, eds. Genetic Imaginations: Ethical, Legal and Social Issues in Human Genome Research. Brookfield, VT: Ashgate; 1998: 69-82. 23 refs. Based on a paper presented at a workshop hosted by the Centre for Social and Economic Research at the University of the West of England; reprinted from *The Genetic Engineer and Biotechnologist*, 1995; 15(2-3). ISBN 1-84014-356-8. BE60019.
attitudes; congenital disorders; disabled; *eugenics; genetic counseling; *genetic disorders; genetic enhancement; genetic predisposition; genetic screening; *genetic services; genome mapping; international aspects; prenatal diagnosis; public policy; risk; *selective abortion; social impact; wrongful life; *Great Britain; National Health Service

Mao, Xin. Ethics and genetics in China: an inside story. [Letter]. *Nature Genetics.* 1997 Sep; 17(1): 20. 5 refs. BE60439.
*attitudes; cultural pluralism; ethical relativism; *eugenics; *genetic counseling; *genetic research; *genetics; health personnel; historical aspects; international aspects; investigators; paternalism; politics; values; *China

Marlin, George J. Eugenics and cloning. *In: his* The Politician's Guide to Assisted Suicide, Cloning, and Other Current Controversies. Washington, DC: Morley Books; 1998: 125-168, 212-216. 146 fn. ISBN 0-9660597-1-9. BE62396.
body parts and fluids; *cloning; commodification; determination of death; *eugenics; historical aspects; involuntary sterilization; killing; *legal aspects; National Socialism; organ donation; parent child relationship; personhood; reproduction; reproductive technologies; social discrimination; social worth; socioeconomic factors; Germany; United States

Morton, Newton E. Hippocratic or hypocritic: birth pangs of an ethical code. [Letter]. *Nature Genetics.* 1998 Jan; 18(1): 18. 9 refs. BE59693.
coercion; directive counseling; disadvantaged; *eugenics; genetic counseling; genetics; international aspects; involuntary sterilization; minority groups; *public policy; social discrimination; *China

Normile, Dennis. Geneticists debate eugenics and China's infant health law. [News]. *Science.* 1998 Aug 21; 281(5380): 1118-1119. 1 fn. Report on the 18th International Congress of Genetics, held 10-15 Aug 1998 in Beijing. BE59891.
congenital disorders; contraception; *eugenics; gene pool; genetic counseling; genetic disorders; informed consent; involuntary sterilization; law enforcement; *legislation; married persons; *public policy; reproduction; selective abortion; *China; Law on Maternal and Infant Health Care (China)

Palmer, Eileen Alexa. Genetic Choice, Disability, and Regret. Ann Arbor, MI: UMI Dissertation Services; 1997. 159 p. Bibliography: p. 146-159. Dissertation, Ph.D. in philosophy, University of Wisconsin-Madison, 1997 May. UMI No. 9711004. BE61843.

BE = bioethics accession number   fn. = footnotes   refs. = references

children; congenital disorders; decision making; *disabled; *ethical analysis; *eugenics; *future generations; genetic disorders; genetic intervention; hearing disorders; intention; *moral obligations; *moral policy; *parents; philosophy; *quality of life; *reproduction; reproductive technologies; rights; teleological ethics; theology; time factors; value of life; harms; Adams, Robert; Heyd, David; Parfit, Derek; Woodward, James

Paul, Diane B. The Politics of Heredity: Essays on Eugenics, Biomedicine, and the Nature-Nurture Debate. Albany, NY: State University of New York Press; 1998. 219 p. (SUNY series, philosophy and biology). Bibliography: p. 187-208. ISBN 0-7914-3822-8. BE59218.
autonomy; behavioral genetics; carriers; coercion; communism; *eugenics; genetic counseling; genetic disorders; genetic screening; genetics; historical aspects; intelligence; international aspects; investigators; mass screening; mentally retarded; metaphor; newborns; phenylketonuria; politics; public policy; reproduction; review; science; selective abortion; social control; socialism; sterilization (sexual); nature; Twentieth Century; United States

Rifkin, Jeremy. Who will decide between defect and perfect? *Washington Post.* 1998 Apr 19: C4. BE59370.
*eugenics; future generations; genetic disorders; *genetic enhancement; *genetic intervention; *germ cells; normality

Rosenthal, Elisabeth. Scientists debate China's law on sterilizing the carriers of genetic defects. [News]. *New York Times.* 1998 Aug 16: 14. BE59567.
attitudes; *eugenics; genetic counseling; *genetic disorders; informed consent; *international aspects; investigators; *involuntary sterilization; legislation; *public policy; sterilization (sexual); *China; International Congress on Genetics; Law on Maternal and Infant Health Care (China)

Saatkamp, Herman J. Genetics and pragmatism. *In:* McGee, Glenn, ed. Pragmatic Bioethics. Nashville, TN: Vanderbilt University Press; 1999: 152-167, 278-279. 8 fn. ISBN 0-8265-1321-2. BE60669.
autonomy; behavioral genetics; decision making; education; *eugenics; freedom; future generations; genetic counseling; genetic determinism; genetic disorders; genetic enhancement; genetic information; *genetic intervention; genetic research; genetic screening; *genetics; genome mapping; moral obligations; parents; philosophy; preimplantation diagnosis; prenatal diagnosis; social control; teleological ethics; *pragmatism

Schmacke, Norbert. Overdramatization of the burdens on health and social services: a continuing debate in the history of German medicine. *International Journal of Health Services.* 1997; 27(3): 559-574. 40 refs. This article is a revised and extended version of a lecture given on 24 Mar 1988, in the context of an exhibition on the government-planned and executed elimination of "lives unworthy of living" in National Socialism. Translated by Sean Mullan and Jutta Rateike-Fear. BE60082.
advisory committees; *aged; AIDS; attitudes; *chronically ill; dementia; *disabled; *economics; *eugenics; euthanasia; *health care delivery; health care reform; health insurance; *historical aspects; homosexuals; killing; *National Socialism; patient care; physicians; political systems; psychiatry; social worth; socioeconomic factors; sociology of medicine; *stigmatization; terminal care; *trends; *Germany; *Twentieth Century; United States

Selden, Steven. Inheriting Shame: The Story of Eugenics and Racism in America. New York, NY: Teachers College Press; 1999. 177 p. (Advances in contemporary educational thought series). Bibliography: p. 159-167.

ISBN 0-8077-3812-3. BE62776.
attitudes; behavioral genetics; biology; blacks; disadvantaged; *education; *eugenics; genetic determinism; *historical aspects; intelligence; international aspects; involuntary sterilization; legal aspects; literature; mentally retarded; minority groups; public policy; schools; *social discrimination; universities; XYY karyotype; secondary schools; American Eugenics Society; Buck v. Bell; *Twentieth Century; *United States

Shattuck, Roger. Knowledge exploding: science and technology. *In: his* Forbidden Knowledge: From Prometheus to Pornography. San Diego, CA: Harcourt Brace; 1996: 173-225. 12 fn. ISBN 0-15-600551-4. BE61060.
behavioral genetics; case studies; *eugenics; evolution; expert testimony; freedom; gene therapy; *genetic intervention; *genetic research; genetic screening; *genome mapping; germ cells; government regulation; historical aspects; international aspects; investigators; involuntary sterilization; legal aspects; mentally retarded; National Socialism; nuclear warfare; prenatal diagnosis; recombinant DNA research; *risks and benefits; *science; self regulation; social impact; Supreme Court decisions; wrongful life; *knowledge; Asilomar Conference; Buck v. Bell; Manhattan Project; Twentieth Century

Telling, Douglas Cushman. Science in Politics: Eugenics, Sterilization, and Genetic Screening. Ann Arbor, MI: UMI Dissertation Services; 1988. 264 p. Bibliography: p. 251-264. Dissertation, Ph.D. in Political Science, University of Massachusetts, 1988. Order No. 8906337. BE61053.
bioethical issues; carriers; coercion; employment; *eugenics; fetuses; *genetic screening; government regulation; health hazards; historical aspects; industry; involuntary sterilization; legal aspects; legal liability; newborns; normality; *politics; prenatal diagnosis; *public policy; reproduction; reproductive technologies; science; selective abortion; *social control; social discrimination; socioeconomic factors; state government; *sterilization (sexual); trends; wrongful life; Galton, Francis; Muller, Hermann; Osborn, Frederick; Sanger, Margaret; Twentieth Century; *United States

Thomson, Mathew. Sterilization, segregation and community care: ideology and solutions to the problem of mental deficiency in inter-war Britain. *History of Psychiatry.* 1992 Dec; 3(12): 473-498. 119 fn. BE61498.
attitudes; deinstitutionalized persons; *eugenics; family relationship; females; *historical aspects; indigents; involuntary sterilization; males; mental institutions; *mentally retarded; motivation; paternalism; physicians; political systems; psychiatry; public policy; residential facilities; sexuality; *social control; social discrimination; social problems; social workers; socioeconomic factors; sociology of medicine; *voluntary sterilization; *Great Britain; *Nineteenth Century; *Twentieth Century

Thomson, Mathew. The Problem of Mental Deficiency: Eugenics, Democracy, and Social Policy in Britain c. 1870-1959. New York, NY: Oxford University Press; 1998. 351 p. Bibliography: p. 307-342. ISBN 0-19-820692-5. BE60511.
attitudes; community services; democracy; *eugenics; females; *historical aspects; legal aspects; males; mental institutions; *mentally retarded; organization and administration; physicians; politics; psychiatry; *public policy; social discrimination; socioeconomic factors; *sterilization (sexual); Board of Control (Great Britain); *Great Britain; Mental Deficiency Act 1913 (Great Britain); *Nineteenth Century; Royal Commission on Care and Control of the Feeble-Minded; *Twentieth Century

Tsuchiya, Takashi. Eugenic sterilizations in Japan and recent demands for an apology: a report. *Ethics and*

Intellectual Disability. 1997 Fall; 3(1): 1–4. BE59951.
    compensation; *disabled; *eugenics; females; historical
    aspects; *involuntary sterilization; *legal aspects;
    *mandatory programs; *mentally disabled; physically
    disabled; political activity; public policy; voluntary
    sterilization; *Eugenic Protection Law (Japan); *Japan;
    Twentieth Century

Wiesing, Urban. Individual rights and genetics: the
historical perspective. A comment on Ruth Chadwick's
paper. *In:* Chadwick, Ruth; Levitt, Mairi; Shickle,
Darren, eds. The Right to Know and the Right Not
to Know. Brookfield, VT: Ashgate; 1997: 23–27. 9 refs.
ISBN 1-85972-424-8. BE62185.
    autonomy; *ethical analysis; *ethical theory; *eugenics;
    *genetic information; genetic screening; *genetics; goals;
    *historical aspects; *human rights; medicine; National
    Socialism; patient advocacy; philosophy; physician patient
    relationship; politics; public policy; rights; truth disclosure;
    right not to know; Germany

Wikler, Daniel. Can we learn from eugenics? *Journal of
Medical Ethics.* 1999 Apr; 25(2): 183–194. 40 refs.
BE61924.
    attitudes; behavioral genetics; coercion; common good;
    cultural pluralism; directive counseling; disabled; *eugenics;
    future generations; genetic counseling; genetic determinism;
    genetic intervention; genetic screening; genetics; goals;
    health personnel; historical aspects; indigents; international
    aspects; involuntary sterilization; justice; mandatory
    programs; minority groups; moral obligations; *moral policy;
    National Socialism; public health; public policy;
    reproduction; review; rights; social discrimination; social
    problems; socioeconomic factors; values; voluntary
    programs; Germany; Great Britain; Nineteenth Century;
    Scandinavia; Twentieth Century; United States
Eugenics casts a long shadow over contemporary
genetics. Any measure, whether in clinical genetics or
biotechnology, which is suspected of eugenic intent is
likely to be opposed on that ground. Yet there is little
consensus on what this word signifies, and often only
a remote connection to the very complex set of social
movements which took that name. After a brief historical
summary of eugenics, this essay attempts to locate any
wrongs inherent in eugenic doctrines. Four candidates
are examined and rejected. The moral challenge posed
by eugenics for genetics in our own time, I argue, is
to achieve social justice.

Wright, Robert. Who gets the good genes? *Time.* 1999
Jan 11; 153(1): 67. BE60313.
    decision making; *eugenics; *genetic enhancement; genetic
    intervention; government regulation; parents;
    preimplantation diagnosis; prenatal diagnosis; selective
    abortion; socioeconomic factors; Brave New World (Huxley,
    A.)

China's 'eugenics' law still disturbing despite relabelling.
[Editorial]. *Nature.* 1998 Aug 20; 394(6695): 707.
BE61088.
    coercion; directive counseling; *eugenics; genetic
    counseling; genetic disorders; genetic screening; government
    regulation; human rights; involuntary sterilization;
    *legislation; minority groups; paternalism; prenatal diagnosis;
    *public policy; reproduction; selective abortion; *China;
    Law on Maternal and Infant Health Care 1995 (China);
    Universal Declaration of Human Rights

Cultural reaction. [Editorial]. *New Scientist.* 1998 Oct 24;
160(2157): 3. BE61539.
    attitudes; common good; cultural pluralism; *eugenics;
    health personnel; human rights; international aspects;
    non-Western World; prenatal diagnosis; Western World;
    *China

The Lynchburg Story: Eugenic Sterilization in America.
[Videorecording].New York, NY: Filmakers Library;
1994. 1 videocassette; 55 min.; sd.; color; VHS.
Director: Stephen Trombley; producer: Bruce Eadie. A
Worldview Pictures Production. Certificate of Merit,
San Francisco International Film Festival, 1994.
BE59872.
    adolescents; attitudes; children; *disabled; *eugenics;
    females; *historical aspects; *indigents; institutionalized
    persons; investigators; *involuntary sterilization; legal
    aspects; males; mass media; *mentally retarded; National
    Socialism; nurses; physically disabled; physicians; public
    hospitals; public opinion; *public policy; state government;
    Supreme Court decisions; *whites; Buck v. Bell; Germany;
    Laughlin, Harry; *Lynchburg Colony for the Epileptic and
    Feebleminded; Priddy, Albert; *Twentieth Century; *United
    States; Virginia

What price perfection? [Editorial]. *New Scientist.* 1997 Feb
22; 153(2070): 3. BE59711.
    *eugenics; genetic predisposition; genetic research; *genetic
    screening; homosexuals; *prenatal diagnosis; selective
    abortion

EUTHANASIA

See also ALLOWING TO DIE, SUICIDE

Anderson, Jeremy. A prayer from the dying: [an
advertisement sponsored by the Voluntary Euthanasia
Society of New South Wales]. *BMJ (British Medical
Journal).* 1999 Apr 17; 318(7190): 1084. BE62468.
    *advertising; *mass media; organizational policies; political
    activity; public opinion; *right to die; *terminally ill;
    *voluntary euthanasia; Australia; *Burns, June; *Voluntary
    Euthanasia Society (New South Wales)

Arthur, John, ed. Euthanasia. *In:* Arthur, John, ed.
Morality and Moral Controversies. Fifth Edition. Upper
Saddle River, NJ: Prentice Hall; 1999: 211–235. 2 refs.
Includes discussion questions. ISBN 0-13-914128-6.
BE60275.
    *active euthanasia; advance directives; *allowing to die;
    artificial feeding; assisted suicide; compassion; congenital
    disorders; double effect; drugs; freedom; intention; killing;
    legal aspects; *moral policy; newborns; pain; persistent
    vegetative state; physicians; quality of life; right to die;
    suffering; suicide; Supreme Court decisions; terminally ill;
    third party consent; treatment refusal; value of life;
    *voluntary euthanasia; withholding treatment; Cruzan v.
    Director, Missouri Department of Health; United States

Baier, Kurt. Wrongful death and wrongful life. *In: his*
Problems of Life and Death: A Humanist Perspective.
Amherst, NY: Prometheus Books; 1997: 137–230. 74 fn.
ISBN 1-57392-153-X. BE61848.
    *allowing to die; *assisted suicide; capital punishment;
    contraception; disabled; disclosure; ethical theory;
    guidelines; *humanism; intention; *killing; law; legal aspects;
    legal liability; moral obligations; *moral policy; *morality;
    negligence; organ donation; physicians; *population control;
    prognosis; *prolongation of life; quality of life; suffering;
    suicide; value of life; values; *voluntary euthanasia; wrongful
    death; *wrongful life; rationality

Begley, Anne Marie; Farsides, Bobby. Response to the
National Council for Hospice and Specialist Palliative
Care Services -- voluntary euthanasia: the Council's
view, by Ann Marie Begley, with reply by Bobby
Farsides on behalf of the National Council for Hospice
and Specialist Palliative Care Services. *Nursing Ethics.*
1999 Mar; 6(2): 157–161. 11 refs. BE61935.
    autonomy; double effect; drugs; health personnel; hospices;

BE = bioethics accession number   fn. = footnotes   refs. = references

*organizational policies; pain; *palliative care; paternalism; public policy; right to die; *terminal care; terminally ill; values; *voluntary euthanasia; wedge argument; analgesia; Great Britain; *National Council for Hospice and Specialist Palliative Care Services (Great Britain)

Bock, Gisela. Sterilization and "medical" massacres in National Socialist Germany: ethics, politics, and the law. *In:* Berg, Manfred; Cocks, Geoffrey, eds. Medicine and Modernity: Public Health and Medical Care in Nineteenth- and Twentieth-Century Germany. New York, NY: Cambridge University Press; 1997: 149–172. 85 fn. ISBN 0-521-56411-5. BE59269.
    aliens; chronically ill; *dehumanization; *disabled; *eugenics; genetic disorders; *historical aspects; *involuntary euthanasia; *involuntary sterilization; Jews; *killing; mentally disabled; minority groups; *National Socialism; *physicians; *psychiatry; public health; *public policy; selective abortion; social control; social discrimination; *social worth; socioeconomic factors; *sociology of medicine; genocide; *Germany; *Twentieth Century

British Columbia. Special Advisory Committee on Ethical Issues in Health Care. Euthanasia and Physician-Assisted Suicide. Victoria, BC: British Columbia Ministry of Health and Ministry Responsible for Seniors; 1994 Feb. 43 p. 52 fn. ISBN 0-7726-2137-3. BE59216.
    *active euthanasia; advance directives; advisory committees; *allowing to die; artificial feeding; *assisted suicide; autonomy; beneficence; coercion; compassion; competence; double effect; drugs; intention; justice; killing; legal aspects; *moral policy; pain; palliative care; persistent vegetative state; *physicians; public policy; quality of life; right to die; suffering; Supreme Court decisions; terminally ill; third party consent; treatment refusal; value of life; *voluntary euthanasia; vulnerable populations; wedge argument; withholding treatment; dignity; duty to die; *British Columbia; *Canada; Canadian Charter of Rights and Freedoms; Criminal Code of Canada; Law Reform Commission of Canada; Rodriguez v. British Columbia (Attorney-General); *Special Advisory Committee on Ethical Issues in Health Care (BC)

Brock, Dan W. Euthanasia. *Rhode Island Medicine.* 1993 Dec; 76(12): 585–589. 9 refs. Commented on by M.W. Hamolsky, p. 590–591; J.C. Nelson, p. 592–594; P. Conner, p. 595–599; J. Rosenberg, p. 600; J.T. McIlwain, p. 602; and J.D. Burke, p. 603–604. BE59410.
    *active euthanasia; allowing to die; assisted suicide; autonomy; beneficence; competence; economics; intention; killing; medical ethics; *moral policy; motivation; palliative care; *physician's role; physicians; *public policy; right to die; social impact; suffering; third party consent; *voluntary euthanasia; wedge argument; withholding treatment; United States

Campbell, Neil. A problem for the idea of voluntary euthanasia. *Journal of Medical Ethics.* 1999 Jun; 25(3): 242–244. BE61857.
    *advance directives; allowing to die; assisted suicide; *autonomy; *coercion; decision making; freedom; *involuntary euthanasia; *living wills; *motivation; *pain; *suffering; time factors; torture; *voluntary euthanasia
I question whether, in those cases where physician-assisted suicide is invoked to alleviate unbearable pain and suffering, there can be such a thing as voluntary euthanasia. The problem is that when a patient asks to die under such conditions there is good reason to think that the decision to die is compelled by the pain, and hence not freely chosen. Since the choice to die was not made freely it is inadvisable for physicians to act in accordance with it, for this may be contrary to the patient's genuine wishes. Thus, what were thought

to be cases of voluntary euthanasia might actually be instances of involuntary euthanasia.

Cantor, Norman L. The real ethic of death and dying. [Book review essay]. *Michigan Law Review.* 1996 May; 94(6): 1718–1738. 82 fn. BE60104.
    *active euthanasia; advance directives; *allowing to die; assisted suicide; *autonomy; competence; decision making; informed consent; intention; killing; legal aspects; newborns; persistent vegetative state; personhood; physicians; prolongation of life; quality of life; right to die; risks and benefits; terminally ill; third party consent; *value of life; values; withholding treatment; *Rethinking Life and Death (Singer, P.); United States

CBS Video. 60 Minutes: Death by Doctor. [Videorecording]. Produced by 60 Minutes, 524 West 57th St., New York, NY 10019; 1998. 1 videocassette; 14 min.; sd.; color; VHS. Television program broadcast 22 Nov 1998. Narrated by Mike Wallace; produced by Robert G. Anderson. To order transcript: 1-800-777-TEXT; to order a videotape: 1-800-848-3256. BE62752.
    *active euthanasia; amyotrophic lateral sclerosis; assisted suicide; criminal law; ethicists; family members; informed consent; legal aspects; *mass media; methods; motivation; paralysis; physician's role; *physicians; records; suffering; *voluntary euthanasia; *Kevorkian, Jack; Michigan; *Youk, Thomas; *60 Minutes (CBS News television program)

Cohen, Adam. Showdown for Doctor Death. *Time.* 1998 Dec 7; 152(23): 46–47. BE60960.
    *active euthanasia; assisted suicide; criminal law; killing; *legal liability; mass media; *physicians; *Kevorkian, Jack; United States; *Youk, Thomas; *60 Minutes

Colebunders, Robert; Schrooten, W.; Singer, Peter A., et al. Euthanasia and end-of-life care. [Letter and response]. *JAMA.* 1999 Apr 28; 281(16): 1488. 2 refs. BE62564.
    *active euthanasia; *attitudes; HIV seropositivity; legal aspects; pain; *patients; quality of life; *terminal care; *terminally ill; *voluntary euthanasia; Belgium; Ontario

Conner, Paul. Is there a secular answer to euthanasia, American style? *Angelicum.* 1996; 73: 381–400. 24 fn. BE60098.
    *active euthanasia; allowing to die; *assisted suicide; attitudes; autonomy; compassion; criminal law; ethicists; intention; killing; moral policy; *morality; motivation; palliative care; physicians; public policy; quality of life; Roman Catholic ethics; suffering; terminally ill; *voluntary euthanasia; withholding treatment; Brock, Dan; Kevorkian, Jack; United States

Cuperus-Bosma, Jacqueline M.; van der Wal, Gerrit; Looman, Caspar W.N., et al. Assessment of physician-assisted death by members of the public prosecution in the Netherlands. *Journal of Medical Ethics.* 1999 Feb; 25(1): 8–15. 7 fn. BE61188.
    *active euthanasia; advance directives; *assisted suicide; cancer; case studies; *decision making; drugs; evaluation studies; family members; guideline adherence; guidelines; involuntary euthanasia; knowledge, attitudes, practice; *law enforcement; lawyers; legal liability; mandatory reporting; pain; *physicians; prognosis; referral and consultation; standards; suffering; *survey; terminally ill; third party consent; voluntary euthanasia; dignity; life expectancy; *prosecutors; *Netherlands
OBJECTIVES: To identify the factors that influence the assessment of reported cases of physician-assisted death by members of the public prosecution. DESIGN/SETTING: At the beginning of 1996, during verbal interviews, 12 short case-descriptions were

---

BE = bioethics accession number   fn. = footnotes   refs. = references

presented to a representative group of 47 members of the public prosecution in the Netherlands. RESULTS: Assessment varied considerably between respondents. Some respondents made more "lenient" assessments than others. Characteristics of the respondents, such as function, personal–life philosophy and age, were not related to the assessment. Case characteristics, i.e. the presence of an explicit request, life expectancy and the type of suffering, strongly influenced the assessment. Of these characteristics, the presence or absence of an explicit request was the most important determinant of the decision whether or not to hold an inquest. CONCLUSIONS: Although the presence of an explicit request, life expectancy and the type of suffering each influenced the assessment, each individual assessment was dependent on the assessor. The resulting danger of legal inequality and legal uncertainty, particularly in complicated cases, should be kept to a minimum by the introduction of some form of protocol and consultation in doubtful or boundary cases. The notification procedure already promotes a certain degree of uniformity in the prosecution policy.

Cusveller, Bart; Jochemsen, Henk. Life–terminating actions with severely demented patients: critical assessment of a report of the Royal Dutch Society of Medicine. *Issues in Law and Medicine.* 1996 Summer; 12(1): 31–45. 43 fn. BE61152.
> *active euthanasia; advance directives; *allowing to die; artificial feeding; competence; *dementia; *double effect; *drugs; evaluation; futility; *involuntary euthanasia; *organizational policies; *palliative care; physician's role; *physicians; professional organizations; quality of life; risks and benefits; suffering; terminal care; *voluntary euthanasia; *withholding treatment; antibiotics; *Dutch Commission for the Acceptability of Life Terminating Action; *Netherlands; *Royal Dutch Medical Association

de Bousingen, Denis Durand. Euthanasia and pain relief discussed in Europe. [News]. *Lancet.* 1998 Oct 3; 352(9134): 1129. BE60453.
> assisted suicide; euthanasia; health care delivery; hospices; information dissemination; organizational policies; pain; *palliative care; physicians; professional organizations; *public policy; *terminal care; Austria; Council of Europe; *Europe; France; Germany

Dixon, Nicholas. On the difference between physician–assisted suicide and active euthanasia. *Hastings Center Report.* 1998 Sep–Oct; 28(5): 25–29. 12 fn. BE59551.
> *active euthanasia; *assisted suicide; coercion; *killing; *moral policy; *physician's role; *public policy; socioeconomic factors; *voluntary euthanasia; wedge argument; United States

Those who defend physician–assisted suicide often seek to distinguish it from active euthanasia, but in fact, the two acts face the same objections. Both can lead to abuse, both implicate the physician in the death of a patient, and both violate whatever objections there are to killing. Their moral similarity derives from the similar roles of the physician.

Downie, Jocelyn; Sherwin, Susan. A feminist exploration of issues around assisted death. *Saint Louis University Public Law Review.* 1996; 15(2): 303–330. 78 fn. BE59912.
> abortion, induced; *active euthanasia; allowing to die; *assisted suicide; *autonomy; coercion; competence; decision making; *females; *feminist ethics; guidelines; home care; involuntary euthanasia; killing; *legal aspects; palliative care; *public policy; right to die; *social discrimination; *social impact; terminal care; treatment refusal; *voluntary euthanasia; wedge argument; Canada; United States

Dunphy, Kilian. Death on request: euthanasia revisited. [Editorial]. *British Journal of Nursing.* 1995 Apr 13–26; 4(7): 365–366. 8 refs. BE60426.
> *active euthanasia; autonomy; palliative care; public policy; quality of life; voluntary euthanasia; wedge argument

Dworkin, Gerald; Frey, R.G.; Bok, Sissela. Euthanasia and Physician–Assisted Suicide: For and Against. New York, NY: Cambridge University Press; 1998. 139 p. Includes references. ISBN 0–521–58789–1. BE60708.
> *active euthanasia; allowing to die; artificial feeding; *assisted suicide; autonomy; Christian ethics; double effect; intention; *killing; legal rights; medical ethics; medicine; *moral policy; natural law; palliative care; physician patient relationship; *physician's role; *physicians; *public policy; quality of life; risks and benefits; suffering; terminal care; terminally ill; treatment refusal; *voluntary euthanasia; *wedge argument; withholding treatment; United States

Englert, Y. From medically assisted procreation to euthanasia: a modern way to deal with ethical dilemmas in modern medicine. *European Journal of Genetics in Society.* 1997; 3(2): 22–26. 3 refs. BE61454.
> assisted suicide; beginning of life; bioethics; embryo research; embryos; legal aspects; moral obligations; palliative care; personhood; physicians; *reproductive technologies; Roman Catholic ethics; suffering; terminal care; value of life; *voluntary euthanasia; wedge argument; Netherlands

Filene, Peter G. In the Arms of Others: A Cultural History of the Right–to–Die in America. Chicago, IL: Ivan R. Dee; 1998. 282 p. 637 fn. ISBN 1–56663–188–2. BE60014.
> *active euthanasia; *allowing to die; artificial feeding; *assisted suicide; attitudes; attitudes to death; autonomy; competence; congenital disorders; decision making; determination of death; ethicists; extraordinary treatment; government regulation; *historical aspects; judicial action; legal aspects; living wills; mass media; newborns; persistent vegetative state; physicians; political activity; politics; privacy; public opinion; *right to die; state government; suffering; *terminal care; terminally ill; treatment refusal; *trends; withholding treatment; Cruzan v. Director, Missouri Department of Health; Cruzan v. Harmon; In re Conroy; In re Quinlan; Netherlands; Nineteenth Century; Superintendent v. Saikewicz; *Twentieth Century; *United States

Flew, Antony. Advance directives are the solution to Dr. Campbell's problem for voluntary euthanasia. *Journal of Medical Ethics.* 1999 Jun; 25(3): 245–246. BE61858.
> *advance directives; allowing to die; autonomy; coercion; *involuntary euthanasia; *living wills; motivation; *pain; torture; *voluntary euthanasia; withholding treatment

Dr Neil Campbell suggests that when patients suffering extremes of protracted pain ask for help to end their lives, their requests should be discounted as made under compulsion. I contend that the doctors concerned should be referred to and then act upon advance directives made by those patients when of sound and calm mind and afflicted by no such intolerable compulsion.

Gillon, Raanan. Euthanasia in the Netherlands –– down the slippery slope? [Editorial]. *Journal of Medical Ethics.* 1999 Feb; 25(1): 3–4. 3 refs. BE61187.
> *active euthanasia; adults; allowing to die; *assisted suicide; autonomy; coercion; decision making; drugs; *empirical research; *guideline adherence; guidelines; infants; intention; *involuntary euthanasia; legal liability; palliative care; *physicians; *public policy; referral and consultation; right to die; statistics; suffering; treatment refusal; *voluntary euthanasia; *wedge argument; withholding treatment; *Netherlands

---

BE = bioethics accession number   fn. = footnotes   refs. = references

Glick, Shimon M. Euthanasia: an unbiased decision? *American Journal of Medicine.* 1997 Mar; 102(3): 294–296. 21 refs. BE62007.
  *active euthanasia; aged; *assisted suicide; autonomy; chronically ill; coercion; communication; conflict of interest; guideline adherence; involuntary euthanasia; managed care programs; patient advocacy; patients; physician patient relationship; physicians; suffering; suicide; terminally ill; trust; vulnerable populations; wedge argument; *duty to die

Hamolsky, Milton W. Some reflections on Brock's "Euthanasia." *Rhode Island Medicine.* 1993 Dec; 76(12): 590–591. Commentary on D.W. Brock, "Euthanasia," p. 585–589. BE59411.
  abortion, induced; *active euthanasia; allowing to die; assisted suicide; autonomy; medical ethics; moral policy; physician's role; voluntary euthanasia; wedge argument; withholding treatment

Hendin, Herbert. Seduced by Death: Doctors, Patients, and Assisted Suicide. Revised and Updated. New York, NY: W.W. Norton; 1998. 304 p. 359 fn. ISBN 0–393–31791–9. BE59170.
  *active euthanasia; allowing to die; *assisted suicide; attitudes to death; autonomy; chronically ill; coercion; competence; *decision making; depressive disorder; futility; guidelines; intention; involuntary euthanasia; judicial action; legal aspects; legal liability; mass media; palliative care; physician patient relationship; *physician's role; *physicians; political activity; politics; professional organizations; psychiatry; psychological stress; *public policy; referral and consultation; right to die; self regulation; statistics; suffering; suicide; Supreme Court decisions; terminally ill; treatment refusal; voluntary euthanasia; wedge argument; withholding treatment; Chabot, Boudewijn; Cohen, Herbert; Compassion in Dying; Dutch Voluntary Euthanasia Society; Hemlock Society; Kevorkian, Jack; Mulder-Meiss, Wine; *Netherlands; Quill, Timothy; Remmelink Commission; Royal Dutch Medical Association; *United States

Hendlin, Herbert. Physician–assisted suicide: what next? *Responsive Community.* 1997 Fall; 7(4): 21–34. BE59718.
  *active euthanasia; *assisted suicide; autonomy; coercion; competence; depressive disorder; drugs; government regulation; guideline adherence; guidelines; involuntary euthanasia; motivation; pain; palliative care; physicians; public policy; quality of health care; right to die; suffering; suicide; *terminal care; terminally ill; treatment refusal; *voluntary euthanasia; vulnerable populations; wedge argument; Netherlands; United States

Hester, D. Micah. Significance at the end of life. *In:* McGee, Glenn, ed. Pragmatic Bioethics. Nashville, TN: Vanderbilt University Press; 1999: 113–128, 271–274. 31 fn. ISBN 0–8265–1321–2. BE60667.
  *assisted suicide; attitudes to death; autonomy; family members; friends; health personnel; killing; *moral obligations; right to die; rights; suicide; terminal care; *terminally ill; *voluntary euthanasia; dignity; James, William

Huser, Frank A. Palliative Care and Euthanasia. Edinburgh: Campion Press; 1995. 69 p. 61 refs. Papers presented at a symposium entitled, "Palliative Care and Euthanasia," held in London, Fall 1993. ISBN 1–873732–16–3. BE60506.
  allowing to die; artificial feeding; cancer; caring; competence; criminal law; ethics; guidelines; hospices; informed consent; killing; legal aspects; nurses; *palliative care; persistent vegetative state; philosophy; politics; principle-based ethics; *public policy; quality of life; resource allocation; suffering; *terminal care; terminally ill; treatment refusal; *voluntary euthanasia; withholding treatment; *Great Britain; *Netherlands

James, Caryn. '60 Minutes,' Kevorkian and a death for the cameras. *New York Times.* 1998 Nov 23: A12. BE60369.
  *active euthanasia; *mass media; physicians; *voluntary euthanasia; *Kevorkian, Jack; United States; *Youk, Thomas; *60 Minutes (CBS News television program)

Jeffko, Walter G. Euthanasia: a reinterpretation. *In: his* Contemporary Ethical Issues: A Personalistic Perspective. Amherst, NY: Humanity Books; 1999: 85–105. 30 fn. ISBN 1–57392–640–X. BE62246.
  *active euthanasia; *allowing to die; artificial feeding; assisted suicide; competence; congenital disorders; double effect; *euthanasia; extraordinary treatment; *intention; *involuntary euthanasia; *killing; legal aspects; *moral policy; newborns; persistent vegetative state; personhood; physicians; public policy; quality of life; right to die; suffering; terminally ill; *voluntary euthanasia; wedge argument; withholding treatment; United States

Jochemsen, Henk; Keown, John. Voluntary euthanasia under control? Further empirical evidence from the Netherlands. *Journal of Medical Ethics.* 1999 Feb; 25(1): 16–21. 46 fn. BE61189.
  *active euthanasia; adults; *allowing to die; *assisted suicide; competence; decision making; depressive disorder; drugs; *empirical research; *guideline adherence; *guidelines; intention; *involuntary euthanasia; *knowledge, attitudes, practice; law enforcement; mandatory reporting; newborns; pain; palliative care; parental consent; *physicians; psychiatry; quality of life; referral and consultation; *regulation; *social control; statistics; suffering; terminal care; *voluntary euthanasia; *wedge argument; withholding treatment; *Netherlands
Nineteen ninety-six saw the publication of a major Dutch survey into euthanasia in the Netherlands. This paper outlines the main statistical findings of this survey and considers whether it shows that voluntary euthanasia is under effective control in the Netherlands. The paper concludes that although there has been some improvement in compliance with procedural requirements, the practice of voluntary euthanasia remains beyond effective control.

Kater, Michael H. The Sewering scandal of 1993 and the German medical establishment. *In:* Berg, Manfred; Cocks, Geoffrey, eds. Medicine and Modernity: Public Health and Medical Care in Nineteenth- and Twentieth-Century Germany. New York, NY: Cambridge University Press; 1997: 213–234. 109 fn. ISBN 0–521–56411–5. BE59272.
  historical aspects; *international aspects; *involuntary euthanasia; killing; mass media; medical education; medical ethics; mentally disabled; *misconduct; moral complicity; *National Socialism; organizational policies; *physicians; *professional organizations; self regulation; *sociology of medicine; American Medical Association; *German Chamber of Physicians; *Germany; *Sewering, Hans-Joachim; Twentieth Century; Vilmar, Karsten; *World Medical Association

Kissane, David W.; Street, Annette; Nitschke, Philip. Seven deaths in Darwin: case studies under the Rights of the Terminally Ill Act, Northern Territory, Australia. *Lancet.* 1998 Oct 3; 352(9134): 1097–1102. 19 refs. BE60438.
  assisted suicide; *cancer; *case studies; competence; *decision making; *depressive disorder; diagnosis; *evaluation; family relationship; *gatekeeping; *guideline adherence; guidelines; legislation; palliative care; *patients; *physician's role; *physicians; *prognosis; *psychiatric diagnosis; *psychiatry; *referral and consultation; right to die; social interaction; suffering; suicide; terminally ill; treatment refusal; *uncertainty; *voluntary euthanasia;

BE = bioethics accession number   fn. = footnotes   refs. = references

qualitative research; Australia; *Nitschke, Philip; *Northern Territory; *Rights of the Terminally Ill Act (NT)

BACKGROUND: During the 9 months between July, 1996, and March, 1997, the provision of euthanasia for the terminally ill was legal in the Northern Territory of Australia. Seven patients made formal use of the Rights of the Terminally Ill (ROTI) Act; four died under the Act. We report their clinical details and the decision-making process required by the Act. METHODS: We taped in-depth interviews with the general practitioner who provided euthanasia. Further information was available from public texts created by patients, the media, and the coroner. FINDINGS: All seven patients had cancer, most at advanced stages. Three were socially isolated. Symptoms of depression were common. Having met criteria of the Act, some patients deferred their decision for a time before proceeding with euthanasia. Medical opinions about the terminal nature of illness differed. INTERPRETATION: Provision of opinions about the terminal nature of illness and the mental health of the patient, as required by the ROTI Act, created problematic gatekeeping roles for the doctors involved.

Kitchener, Betty; Jorm, Anthony F. Conditions required for a law on active voluntary euthanasia: a survey of nurses' opinions in the Australian Capital Territory. *Journal of Medical Ethics.* 1999 Feb; 25(1): 25-30. 27 refs. BE61191.

advance directives; age factors; AIDS; *assisted suicide; *attitudes; cancer; case studies; competence; counseling; dementia; depressive disorder; drugs; family members; government regulation; *guidelines; informed consent; legal aspects; legislation; *nurses; pain; palliative care; paralysis; physicians; public opinion; *public policy; quality of life; referral and consultation; statistics; suffering; survey; terminally ill; *voluntary euthanasia; Australia; *Australian Capital Territory

OBJECTIVES: To ascertain which conditions nurses believe should be in a law allowing active voluntary euthanasia (AVE). DESIGN: Survey questionnaire posted to registered nurses (RNs). SETTING: Australian Capital Territory (ACT) at the end of 1996, when active voluntary euthanasia was legal in the Northern Territory. SURVEY SAMPLE: A random sample of 2,000 RNs, representing 54 per cent of the RN population in the ACT. MAIN MEASURES: Two methods were used to look at nurses' opinions. The first involved four vignettes which varied in terms of critical characteristics of each patient who was requesting help to die. The respondents were asked if the law should be changed to allow any of these requests. There was also a checklist of conditions, most of which have commonly been included in Australian proposed laws on AVE. The respondents chose those which they believed should apply in a law on AVE. RESULTS: The response rate was 61%. Support for a change in the law to allow AVE was 38% for a young man with AIDS, 39% for an elderly man with early stage Alzheimer's disease, 44% for a young woman who had become quadriplegic and 71% for a middle-aged woman with metastases from breast cancer. The conditions most strongly supported in any future AVE law were: "second doctor's opinion," "cooling off period," "unbearable protracted suffering," "patient fully informed about illness and treatment" and "terminally ill." There was only minority support for "not suffering from treatable depression," "administer the fatal dose themselves" and "over a certain age." CONCLUSION: Given the lack of support for some conditions included in proposed AVE laws, there needs to be further debate about the conditions required in any future AVE bills.

Kluge, Eike-Henner W. Severely disabled newborns. *In:* Kuhse, Helga; Singer, Peter, eds. A Companion to Bioethics. Malden, MA: Blackwell; 1998: 242-249. 29 refs. ISBN 0-631-19737-0. BE59499.

*active euthanasia; *allowing to die; *congenital disorders; decision making; disabled; moral policy; *newborns; parents; prolongation of life; *quality of life; *selection for treatment; suffering

Koch, Tom; Heilig, Steve. On the subject(s) of Jack Kevorkian, M.D.: a retrospective analysis. [Article and commentary]. *Cambridge Quarterly of Healthcare Ethics.* 1998 Fall; 7(4): 436-442. 7 fn. BE59147.

amyotrophic lateral sclerosis; *assisted suicide; autonomy; autopsies; cancer; central nervous system diseases; *chronically ill; depressive disorder; *diagnosis; family members; *motivation; pain; palliative care; *patients; physicians; prognosis; quality of life; treatment refusal; *voluntary euthanasia; dependency; multiple sclerosis; *Kevorkian, Jack

Kuhse, Helga. Critical notice: why killing is not always worse -- and is sometimes better -- than letting die. *Cambridge Quarterly of Healthcare Ethics.* 1998 Fall; 7(4): 371-374. 9 fn. Commentary on W. Nesbitt, "Is killing no worse than letting die?" *Journal of Applied Philosophy,* 1995; 12(1): 101-106. BE59137.

*active euthanasia; *allowing to die; *intention; *killing; *moral policy; public policy

Kuhse, Helga; Singer, Peter. Still no academic freedom in Germany. [Editorial]. *Bioethics.* 1999 Apr; 13(2): iii-vi. 7 fn. BE61156.

active euthanasia; allowing to die; assisted suicide; disabled; *euthanasia; *faculty; *freedom; *political activity; right to die; students; *universities; *Germany; *Hoerster, Norbert

Laane, Henk-Maarten. Euthanasia, assisted suicide and AIDS. *AIDS Care.* 1995; 7(Suppl. 2): S163-S167. 13 refs. BE60343.

*AIDS; *assisted suicide; criminal law; drugs; economics; empirical research; knowledge, attitudes, practice; legal aspects; mortality; physicians; statistics; suffering; *voluntary euthanasia; *Netherlands

Lachs, John. Active euthanasia. *In: his* The Relevance of Philosophy to Life. Nashville, TN: Vanderbilt University Press; 1995: 181-187. 1 fn. ISBN 0-8265-1262-3. BE60863.

*active euthanasia; adults; allowing to die; *anencephaly; *brain pathology; decision making; emotions; family members; health personnel; moral policy; newborns; *persistent vegetative state; *personhood; prolongation of life; public policy; quality of life; suffering

Lachs, John. When abstract moralizing runs amok. *In: his* The Relevance of Philosophy to Life. Nashville, TN: Vanderbilt University Press; 1995: 188-194. 7 fn. ISBN 0-8265-1262-3. BE60864.

*active euthanasia; *assisted suicide; *autonomy; drugs; moral policy; physicians; public policy; quality of life; *right to die; rights; suffering; voluntary euthanasia; wedge argument; *Callahan, Daniel

Leone, Daniel A., ed. The Ethics of Euthanasia. San Diego, CA: Greenhaven Press; 1999. 88 p. (At issue: an opposing viewpoints series). Bibliography: p. 83-85. ISBN 0-7377-0004-1. BE61047.

abortion, induced; *active euthanasia; *allowing to die; *assisted suicide; autonomy; Christian ethics; historical aspects; involuntary euthanasia; killing; legal aspects; moral policy; motivation; National Socialism; physicians; public policy; right to die; suffering; terminally ill; value of life; wedge argument; Germany; Netherlands; United States

---

BE = bioethics accession number   fn. = footnotes   refs. = references

Letvak, Richard; Pochard, Frédéric; Grassin, Marc, et al. Palliative options at the end of life. [Letters and response]. *JAMA*. 1998 Apr 8; 279(14): 1065–1067. 9 refs. BE59234.
 *allowing to die; artificial feeding; *assisted suicide; autonomy; beneficence; competence; conscience; cultural pluralism; double effect; *drugs; family members; food; informed consent; intention; pain; *palliative care; physicians; public policy; *sedatives; suffering; *terminal care; terminally ill; treatment refusal; *voluntary euthanasia; withholding treatment; coma; United States

Lindsay, Ronald Alan. Self-Determination, Suicide and Euthanasia: The Implications of Autonomy for the Morality and Legality of Assisted Suicide and Voluntary Active Euthanasia. Ann Arbor, MI: UMI Dissertation Services; 1996. 592 p. Bibliography: p. 572–592. Dissertation, Ph.D. in Philosophy, Georgetown University, August 1996. UMI No. 9713205. BE61112.
 active euthanasia; *assisted suicide; *autonomy; beneficence; coercion; competence; government regulation; guidelines; involuntary euthanasia; legal aspects; medical fees; model legislation; *moral policy; palliative care; paternalism; philosophy; physically disabled; physician patient relationship; physician's role; physicians; *public policy; *right to die; suffering; suicide; terminally ill; treatment refusal; trust; value of life; *voluntary euthanasia; vulnerable populations; wedge argument; Engelhardt, H. Tristram; Feinberg, Joel; Rachels, James

Loff, Bebe; Cordner, Stephen. Australian doctor reveals details of assisted suicides. [News]. *Lancet*. 1998 Dec 5; 352(9143): 1838. BE60824.
 assisted suicide; legal aspects; patients; *physicians; records; *voluntary euthanasia; *video recording; *Australia; *Nitschke, Philip

McIlwain, James T. Comments on "Euthanasia." *Rhode Island Medicine*. 1993 Dec; 76(12): 602. Commentary on D.W. Brock, "Euthanasia," p. 585–589. BE59415.
 *assisted suicide; attitudes to death; autonomy; *euthanasia; medical ethics; physician's role; *public policy; value of life; values; voluntary euthanasia; wedge argument; United States

McKhann, Charles F. A Time to Die: The Place for Physician Assistance. New Haven, CT: Yale University Press; 1999. 268 p. 240 fn. ISBN 0-300-07631-2. BE62341.
 *active euthanasia; advance directives; allowing to die; *assisted suicide; autonomy; chronically ill; competence; dementia; depressive disorder; double effect; economics; family members; guidelines; hospices; killing; legal aspects; medical ethics; organizational policies; palliative care; physician's role; *physicians; professional organizations; public opinion; *public policy; religious ethics; suffering; suicide; terminal care; terminally ill; treatment refusal; *voluntary euthanasia; wedge argument; rationality; Netherlands; *United States

Maltsberger, John T.; American Association of Suicidology. Committee on Physician–Assisted Death. Report of the Committee on Physician–Assisted Suicide and Euthanasia. *Suicide and Life–Threatening Behavior*. 1996; 26(Suppl.): 1–19. 36 fn. BE61572.
 *active euthanasia; aged; allowing to die; *assisted suicide; attitudes; autonomy; chronically ill; depressive disorder; disadvantaged; double effect; drugs; economics; females; intention; involuntary euthanasia; managed care programs; nurses; *organizational policies; pain; *palliative care; physician patient relationship; *physicians; public policy; right to die; suffering; *suicide; terminal care; terminally ill; voluntary euthanasia; withholding treatment; duty to die; *American Association of Suicidology; Netherlands; United States

Matthews, Hugh. Better palliative care could cut euthanasia. [News]. *BMJ (British Medical Journal)*. 1998 Dec 12; 317(7173): 1613. BE60733.
 *active euthanasia; attitudes; guidelines; involuntary euthanasia; killing; *palliative care; physicians; quality of health care; suffering; *terminal care; *Netherlands

Miller, Bradley W. A time to kill: Ronald Dworkin and the ethics of euthanasia. *Res Publica*. 1996; 2(1): 31–61. 105 fn. BE59210.
 abortion, induced; advance directives; *assisted suicide; *autonomy; competence; intention; involuntary euthanasia; justice; killing; law; mentally disabled; moral policy; morality; *natural law; persistent vegetative state; personhood; physicians; *public policy; quality of life; state interest; utilitarianism; *value of life; *voluntary euthanasia; wedge argument; dignity; *Dworkin, Ronald

Morgan, John, ed. An Easeful Death? Perspectives on Death, Dying and Euthanasia. Sydney, NSW, Australia: Federation Press; 1996. 218 p. 276 fn. ISBN 1-86287-222-8. BE62373.
 *active euthanasia; allowing to die; assisted suicide; *attitudes to death; autonomy; biomedical technologies; caring; determination of death; emotions; historical aspects; hospices; involuntary euthanasia; killing; legal aspects; legislation; nurses; palliative care; physicians; prolongation of life; quality of life; resource allocation; right to die; suffering; suicide; *terminal care; terminally ill; value of life; *values; voluntary euthanasia; withholding treatment; *Australia; Netherlands; Northern Territory; South Australia; Victoria

Morrison, R. Sean; Meier, Diane E. Physician–assisted dying: fashioning public policy with an absence of data. *Generations (American Society on Aging)*. 1994 Winter; 18(4): 48–53. 21 refs. BE60552.
 *assisted suicide; autonomy; *empirical research; hospices; international aspects; involuntary euthanasia; knowledge, attitudes, practice; legal aspects; motivation; pain; palliative care; physicians; public opinion; *public policy; risks and benefits; suffering; terminally ill; *voluntary euthanasia; wedge argument; Netherlands; *United States

Nelson, Janet Cooper. Mistaking the periphery for the center: a response to "Euthanasia" by Dan W. Brock. *Rhode Island Medicine*. 1993 Dec; 76(12): 592–594. 3 refs. Commentary on D.W. Brock, "Euthanasia," p. 585–589. BE59412.
 *active euthanasia; assisted suicide; attitudes; autonomy; *decision making; freedom; government regulation; medical ethics; patient participation; physician's role; physicians; *public participation; public policy; right to die; state interest; terminal care; values; United States

Nyman, Deborah J.; Eidelman, Leonid A.; Sprung, Charles L. Euthanasia. *Critical Care Clinics*. 1996 Jan; 12(1): 85–96. 87 refs. BE59279.
 *active euthanasia; *allowing to die; assisted suicide; drugs; *euthanasia; futility; guidelines; historical aspects; international aspects; involuntary euthanasia; legal aspects; moral policy; palliative care; physician's role; right to die; suffering; terminal care; trends; voluntary euthanasia; vulnerable populations; wedge argument; withholding treatment

Ogden, Russel. AIDS, euthanasia and nursing. *Nursing Standard*. 1996 May 29; 10(36): 49–51. 12 refs. BE60401.
 *AIDS; *assisted suicide; attitudes; conscience; drugs; friends; *nurse's role; nursing ethics; physicians; suicide; terminally ill; *voluntary euthanasia; British Columbia

Onwuteaka–Philipsen, Bregje D.; Muller, Martien T.; van der Wal, Gerrit. Euthanatics: implementation of a protocol to standardise euthanatics among pharmacists and GPs. *Patient Education and Counseling.* 1997 Jun; 31(2): 131–137. 9 refs. BE59389.

*active euthanasia; *assisted suicide; *drugs; knowledge, attitudes, practice; *methods; *pharmacists; *physicians; *practice guidelines; *standards; survey; *Netherlands

Pauer–Studer, Herlinde. Peter Singer on euthanasia. *Monist.* 1993 Apr; 76(2): 135–157. 22 refs. 42 fn. BE60218.

abortion, induced; *active euthanasia; adults; *allowing to die; congenital disorders; death; *disabled; *dissent; ethical theory; eugenics; fetuses; infanticide; involuntary euthanasia; *killing; *moral policy; National Socialism; *newborns; pain; parental consent; *personhood; political activity; *quality of life; social worth; speciesism; *utilitarianism; value of life; voluntary euthanasia; wedge argument; withholding treatment; rationality; Austria; Germany; Rachels, James; *Singer, Peter

Reiling, Jennifer, ed. *JAMA* 100 years ago: euphoria vs. euthanasia. [Reprint]. *JAMA.* 1999 Mar 24–31; 281(12): 1068f. BE60957.

attitudes; drugs; editorial policies; *euthanasia; *historical aspects; intention; pain; physicians; suffering; terminal care; Great Britain; JAMA; Lancet; *Nineteenth Century

Reinders, Hans S. Euthanasia and justice: response to "Euthanasia and health reform in Canada" by Michael Stingl (*CQ* Vol. 7, No. 4). *Cambridge Quarterly of Healthcare Ethics.* 1999 Spring; 8(2): 238–240. BE61239.

aged; autonomy; coercion; health care delivery; *health care reform; justice; motivation; primary health care; public policy; *quality of health care; quality of life; right to die; suffering; terminal care; values; *voluntary euthanasia; Canada; Netherlands

Ryan, Christopher James. Pulling up the runaway: the effect of new evidence on euthanasia's slippery slope. *Journal of Medical Ethics.* 1998 Oct; 24(5): 341–344. 29 refs. BE60257.

*assisted suicide; empirical research; *involuntary euthanasia; legal aspects; physician patient relationship; physicians; *public policy; *social impact; statistics; *voluntary euthanasia; *wedge argument; *Australia; *Netherlands; Remmelink Commission

The slippery slope argument has been the mainstay of many of those opposed to the legalisation of physician–assisted suicide and euthanasia. In this paper I re–examine the slippery slope in the light of two recent studies that examined the prevalence of medical decisions concerning the end of life in the Netherlands and in Australia. I argue that these two studies have robbed the slippery slope of the source of its power -- its intuitive obviousness. Finally I propose that, contrary to the warnings of the slippery slope, the available evidence suggests that the legalisation of physician–assisted suicide might actually decrease the prevalence of non–voluntary and involuntary euthanasia.

Scherer, Jennifer M.; Simon, Rita J. Euthanasia and the Right to Die: A Comparative View. Lanham, MD: Rowman and Littlefield; 1999. 151 p. 270 fn. Includes tables of "Status of Right–to–Die Legislation in the U.S., by State, July 1997," and "Social Indicators, Euthanasia and Right–to–Die Regulations, Twenty Countries." ISBN 0–8476–9167–5. BE61316.

*active euthanasia; advance directives; *allowing to die; *assisted suicide; attitudes to death; autonomy; beneficence; coercion; comparative studies; compassion; *cultural pluralism; disabled; economics; eugenics; goals; health care delivery; historical aspects; *international aspects; involuntary euthanasia; knowledge, attitudes, practice; *legal aspects; medicine; National Socialism; pain; palliative care; persistent vegetative state; physicians; political activity;

*public opinion; *public policy; quality of life; religious ethics; *right to die; standards; *state government; suffering; suicide; terminal care; terminally ill; treatment refusal; value of life; *voluntary euthanasia; wedge argument; withholding treatment; Australia; Canada; China; Colombia; France; Germany; Great Britain; India; Iran; Israel; Japan; Netherlands; South Africa; Spain; Switzerland; United States

Simpson, William G. A different kind of Holocaust: from euthanasia to tyranny. *Linacre Quarterly.* 1997 Aug; 64(3): 87–92. BE59313.

abortion on demand; *abortion, induced; *active euthanasia; aged; *assisted suicide; chronically ill; disabled; eugenics; historical aspects; involuntary sterilization; *killing; National Socialism; public policy; right to die; social discrimination; *social worth; terminally ill; *value of life; genocide; Darwinism; Germany; Netherlands; Twentieth Century; United States

Singer, Peter. Living and dying. [Interview]. *Psychology Today.* 1999 Jan–Feb; 32(1): 56–59, 78–79. BE61518.

*active euthanasia; allowing to die; *animal experimentation; brain death; *disabled; *ethicists; human experimentation; killing; morality; National Socialism; newborns; persistent vegetative state; primates; quality of life; speciesism; suffering; utilitarianism; value of life; *Singer, Peter

Singer, Peter; Kuhse, Helga. More on euthanasia: a response to Pauer–Studer. *Monist.* 1993 Apr; 76(2): 158–174. 17 fn. Commentary on H. Pauer–Studer, "Peter Singer on euthanasia," p. 135–157. BE60219.

*active euthanasia; adults; *allowing to die; death; *disabled; dissent; fetuses; infanticide; intention; *killing; *moral policy; National Socialism; *newborns; personhood; political activity; quality of life; selective abortion; suffering; *utilitarianism; value of life; withholding treatment; Austria; Germany; Singer, Peter

Smith, Wesley J. Forced Exit: The Slippery Slope from Assisted Suicide to Legalized Murder. New York, NY: Times Books; 1997. 291 p. 657 fn. ISBN 0–8129–2790–7. BE59666.

allowing to die; artificial feeding; *assisted suicide; coercion; compassion; disabled; economics; *euthanasia; guideline adherence; guidelines; hospices; *involuntary euthanasia; killing; legal aspects; managed care programs; pain; palliative care; *public policy; quality of life; resource allocation; right to die; terminal care; value of life; values; vulnerable populations; wedge argument; withholding treatment; Netherlands; United States

Somerville, Margaret A. Euthanasia in the media: jounalists' values, media ethics and "public square" messages. *Humane Health Care International.* 1997 Spring; 13(1): 17–20. 17 fn. BE59958.

*active euthanasia; *assisted suicide; attitudes to death; autonomy; chronically ill; compassion; disabled; journalism; *mass media; professional ethics; right to die; suffering; terminally ill; *values; Australia; Canada; Netherlands; United States

Sprung, Charles L.; Oppenheim, Arieh. End–of–life decisions in critical care medicine -- where are we headed? [Editorial]. *Critical Care Medicine.* 1998 Feb; 26(2): 200–202. 39 refs. BE62109.

*active euthanasia; *allowing to die; *assisted suicide; attitudes; autonomy; *critically ill; decision making; economics; hospitals; intensive care units; intention; international aspects; legal aspects; physician's role; physicians; right to die; suffering; terminally ill; treatment refusal; vulnerable populations; wedge argument; withholding treatment; Australia; Netherlands; United States

Starace, F.; Ogden, R.D. Suicidal behaviours and euthanasia. *AIDS Care.* 1997 Feb; 9(1): 106–108. Report

---

on the XIth International Conference on AIDS, Vancouver, BC, Canada. BE62004.
*AIDS; *assisted suicide; attitudes; *HIV seropositivity; nurses; patients; physicians; statistics; *suicide; *voluntary euthanasia; British Columbia; California; Canada; Great Britain; Netherlands

Steinfels, Peter. Beliefs: wide-ranging, tough questions have been provoked by the broadcast of Kevorkian's video. *New York Times.* 1998 Nov 28: B7. BE60575.
*active euthanasia; assisted suicide; killing; *mass media; physicians; public policy; social impact; *voluntary euthanasia; *Kevorkian, Jack; United States; *Youk, Thomas; *60 Minutes (CBS News television program)

Stingl, Michael; Burgess, Michael M.; Hubert, John, et al. Euthanasia and health reform in Canada. [Article and commentaries]. *Cambridge Quarterly of Healthcare Ethics.* 1998 Fall; 7(4): 348–370. 46 fn. BE59136.
*active euthanasia; aged; caring; chronically ill; community services; competence; economics; goals; *health care delivery; *health care reform; home care; involuntary euthanasia; *justice; obligations of society; organization and administration; palliative care; primary health care; *public policy; *quality of health care; quality of life; socioeconomic factors; suffering; *terminal care; terminally ill; *voluntary euthanasia; *Canada; Netherlands

Stoffell, Brian. Voluntary euthanasia, suicide and physician-assisted suicide. *In:* Kuhse, Helga; Singer, Peter, eds. A Companion to Bioethics. Malden, MA: Blackwell; 1998: 272–279. 14 refs. ISBN 0-631-19737-0. BE59502.
*assisted suicide; autonomy; cultural pluralism; historical aspects; justice; killing; *moral policy; morality; physicians; *public policy; right to die; suffering; *suicide; *voluntary euthanasia; rationality

ten Have, Henk A.M.J.; Welie, Jos V.M. Euthanasia in the Netherlands. *Critical Care Clinics.* 1996 Jan; 12(1): 97–108. 27 refs. BE59280.
*active euthanasia; allowing to die; assisted suicide; competence; decision making; drugs; empirical research; futility; government regulation; guidelines; intention; involuntary euthanasia; knowledge, attitudes, practice; legal aspects; legal liability; moral policy; pain; palliative care; *physicians; psychological stress; statistics; suffering; terminally ill; treatment refusal; *trends; voluntary euthanasia; withholding treatment; *Netherlands; Remmelink Commission

Thomasma, David C.; Kimbrough-Kushner, Thomasine; Kimsma, Gerrit K., et al, eds. Asking to Die: Inside the Dutch Debate About Euthanasia. Boston, MA: Kluwer Academic; 1998. 584 p. Includes reference. ISBN 0-7923-5185-1. BE61054.
accountability; *active euthanasia; advisory committees; allowing to die; alternatives; *assisted suicide; case studies; Christian ethics; competence; continuing education; criminal law; disclosure; double effect; drugs; empirical research; ethical analysis; guidelines; hospices; hospitals; informed consent; institutional policies; international aspects; involuntary euthanasia; judicial action; killing; legal aspects; legislation; mandatory reporting; *moral policy; motivation; organizational policies; palliative care; patients; physicians; professional organizations; psychiatry; public opinion; *public policy; referral and consultation; review; *standards; suffering; *voluntary euthanasia; wedge argument; dignity; Free University of Amsterdam Academic Hospital; Medical Center of Alkmaar (Netherlands); *Netherlands; Remmelink Commission; Royal Dutch Medical Association; United States

Thomasma, David C. Assessing the arguments for and against euthanasia and assisted suicide: part two.

Cambridge Quarterly of Healthcare Ethics. 1998 Fall; 7(4): 388–401. 37 fn. BE59140.
*active euthanasia; advance directives; aged; allowing to die; *assisted suicide; autonomy; compassion; economics; ethical analysis; eugenics; *intention; killing; mentally disabled; moral obligations; *moral policy; *motivation; National Socialism; physician's role; public policy; quality of life; right to die; social worth; suffering; values; *voluntary euthanasia; withholding treatment; Germany; Kevorkian, Jack; United States

Tonelli, Mark R.; Lynn, Joanne; Orentlicher, David. Terminal sedation. [Letters and response]. *New England Journal of Medicine.* 1998 Apr 23; 338(17): 1230–1231. 5 refs. BE59238.
*active euthanasia; artificial feeding; assisted suicide; double effect; *drugs; *intention; pain; physicians; *sedatives; suffering; *terminal care; *terminally ill; time factors; withholding treatment; coma

van de Scheur, Ada; van der Arend, Arie. The role of nurses in euthanasia: a Dutch study. *Nursing Ethics.* 1998 Nov; 5(6): 497–508. 19 refs. BE60811.
communication; conscience; decision making; hospitals; knowledge, attitudes, practice; legal aspects; nurse patient relationship; *nurse's role; *nurses; physicians; professional family relationship; survey; *voluntary euthanasia; qualitative research; *Netherlands

van Delden, Johannes J.M. Slippery slopes in flat countries -- a response. *Journal of Medical Ethics.* 1999 Feb; 25(1): 22–24. 8 refs. BE61190.
*active euthanasia; assisted suicide; *autonomy; *empirical research; guideline adherence; guidelines; *involuntary euthanasia; law enforcement; legal liability; legal obligations; mandatory reporting; moral policy; pain; palliative care; physicians; public policy; regulation; right to die; social control; suffering; trends; *voluntary euthanasia; *wedge argument; *Netherlands
In response to the paper by Keown and Jochemsen in which the latest empirical data concerning euthanasia and other end-of-life decisions in the Netherlands is discussed, this paper discusses three points. The use of euthanasia in cases in which palliative care was a viable alternative may be taken as proof of a slippery slope. However, it could also be interpreted as an indication of a shift towards more autonomy-based end-of-life decisions. The cases of non-voluntary euthanasia are a serious problem in the Netherlands and they are only rarely justifiable. However, they do not prove the existence of a slippery slope. Persuading the physician to bring euthanasia cases to the knowledge of the authorities is a problem of any euthanasia policy. The Dutch notification procedure has recently been changed to reduce the underreporting of cases. However, many questions remain.

van den Boom, Frans M. AIDS, euthanasia and grief. *AIDS Care.* 1995; 7(Suppl. 2): S175–S185. 11 refs. BE60345.
*active euthanasia; *advance care planning; *AIDS; autonomy; communication; decision making; depressive disorder; emotions; *family members; patient participation; *psychological stress; statistics; suicide; terminally ill; *grief; sexual partners; *Netherlands

Vander Veer, Joseph B. Euthanasia and Law in the Netherlands, by John Griffiths, et al. [Book review essay]. *JAMA.* 1999 Feb 10; 281(6): 568–569. 3 refs. BE60413.
allowing to die; assisted suicide; attitudes; *euthanasia; guideline adherence; guidelines; historical aspects; legal aspects; physicians; professional organizations; public policy; terminal care; *voluntary euthanasia; wedge argument;

*Euthanasia and Law in the Netherlands (Griffiths, J.; Bood, A.; Weyers, H.); *Netherlands; Royal Dutch Medical Association; Twentieth Century

Vlaardingerbroek, W.F.C., comp.; Netherlands. Ministry of Health, Welfare and Sport. Documentation and Library Department. Euthanasia and Physician–Assisted Suicide in the Netherlands: Bibliography 1984–1995. Rijswijk, Netherlands: Ministry of Health, Welfare and Sport; 1995 Feb. 20 p. BE59475.
*active euthanasia; *assisted suicide; physicians; *Netherlands; Remmelink Commission

Volkenandt, Matthias. Supportive care and euthanasia –– an ethical dilemma? *Supportive Care in Cancer.* 1998 Mar; 6(2): 114–119. 15 refs. Presented at the 9th International Symposium on Supportive Care in Cancer, held in St. Gallen, Switzerland, 26 Feb–1 Mar 1997. BE61573.
*active euthanasia; allowing to die; *assisted suicide; autonomy; beneficence; *cancer; double effect; drugs; economics; intention; involuntary euthanasia; *moral obligations; moral policy; pain; *palliative care; *physician patient relationship; *physicians; resource allocation; social impact; suffering; *terminal care; *terminally ill; trust; voluntary euthanasia; wedge argument; withholding treatment; United States

Widdershoven, Guy A.M. Euthanasia in the Netherlands: some first experiences of evaluation committees. [News]. *Hastings Center Report.* 1999 Jul–Aug; 29(4): 47–48. BE62486.
*active euthanasia; disclosure; *evaluation; *guideline adherence; guidelines; legal aspects; mandatory reporting; palliative care; physicians; *public policy; referral and consultation; *review committees; voluntary euthanasia; *Netherlands

Wooddell, Victor; Kaplan, Kalman J. An expanded typology of suicide, assisted suicide, and euthanasia. *Omega: A Journal of Death and Dying.* 1997–1998; 36(3): 219–226. 15 refs. BE61224.
*active euthanasia; *allowing to die; *assisted suicide; coercion; *euthanasia; health personnel; *involuntary euthanasia; legal aspects; physician patient relationship; *physician's role; *physicians; *suicide; terminology; third party consent; treatment refusal; voluntary euthanasia; United States

Zalcberg, John R.; Buchanan, John D. Clinical issues in euthanasia. [Editorial]. *Medical Journal of Australia.* 1997 Feb 3; 166(3): 150–152. 16 refs. BE60195.
allowing to die; cancer; communication; depressive disorder; family members; palliative care; physicians; professional competence; public policy; suffering; *terminal care; terminally ill; *voluntary euthanasia; vulnerable populations; withholding treatment; Australia

Euthanasia study challenged. *American Nurses Association Center for Ethics and Human Rights Communique.* 1996 Spring; 5(1): 6. *nurses BE60406.
*active euthanasia; *assisted suicide; intensive care units; palliative care; *research design; terminal care

The euthanasia war: last rights –– human beings do not start their own life; do they have the right to invite a doctor to end it? The pros and cons of doctor–assisted suicide. *Economist.* 1997 Jun 21; 343(8022): 21–24. BE60898.
*active euthanasia; allowing to die; *assisted suicide; chronically ill; double effect; futility; international aspects; involuntary euthanasia; legal aspects; pain; palliative care; physicians; regulation; *right to die; suicide; terminally ill; *voluntary euthanasia; vulnerable populations; wedge argument; withholding treatment; Australia; Colombia;

Netherlands; United States

United Kingdom Government publishes response to House of Lords report on medical ethics. [Summary of *Government Response to the Report of the Select Committee on Medical Ethics,* presented to Parliament by command of Her Majesty, May 1994]. *International Digest of Health Legislation.* 1995; 46(4): 570–572. BE62686.
*active euthanasia; advance directives; advisory committees; *allowing to die; *assisted suicide; decision making; drugs; guidelines; legal aspects; palliative care; persistent vegetative state; *public policy; resource allocation; *terminal care; terminally ill; treatment refusal; *Great Britain; *House of Lords Select Committee on Medical Ethics

EUTHANASIA/ATTITUDES

Achille, Marie A.; Ogloff, James R.P. When is a request for assisted suicide legitimate? Factors influencing public attitudes toward euthanasia. *Canadian Journal of Behavioural Science.* 1997 Jan; 29(1): 19–27. 57 refs. BE60494.
active euthanasia; age factors; *allowing to die; competence; drugs; pain; prognosis; *public opinion; religion; right to die; socioeconomic factors; suffering; survey; *voluntary euthanasia; withholding treatment; dependency; British Columbia; *Vancouver

CBS Video. 60 Minutes: Choosing Life (A.L.S.). [Videorecording]. Produced by 60 Minutes, 524 West 57th St., New York, NY 10019; 1999. 1 videocassette; 14 min.; sd.; color; VHS.. Television program broadcast 28 Feb 1999. Narrated by Mike Wallace; produced by Robert G. Anderson. To order a transcript: 1–800–777–TEXT; to order a videotape: 1–800–848–3256. BE62753.
*amyotrophic lateral sclerosis; assisted suicide; *attitudes; biomedical technologies; case studies; decision making; hospices; palliative care; paralysis; *patients; quality of life; suicide; terminal care; *voluntary euthanasia; Youk, Thomas

Cicirelli, Victor G. Elders' end–of–life decisions: implications for hospice care. *Hospice Journal.* 1997; 12(1): 57–72. 26 refs. BE59180.
*aged; *allowing to die; *assisted suicide; *attitudes; chronically ill; comparative studies; *decision making; dementia; family members; hospices; *patient participation; physicians; *prolongation of life; *quality of life; socioeconomic factors; *suicide; survey; terminal care; terminally ill; *voluntary euthanasia; withholding treatment; Indiana

Connelly, R.J. Death with dignity: fifty years of soul–searching. *Journal of Religion and Health.* 1998 Fall; 37(3): 195–213. 58 fn. BE61218.
*active euthanasia; advance directives; aged; *allowing to die; artificial feeding; *assisted suicide; *attitudes; consensus; depressive disorder; dissent; extraordinary treatment; health personnel; hospices; legal aspects; pain; palliative care; physicians; public opinion; public policy; *right to die; Roman Catholic ethics; Supreme Court decisions; *terminal care; *trends; ventilators; voluntary euthanasia; withholding treatment; Compassion in Dying; Cruzan v. Director, Missouri Department of Health; Death with Dignity Act (OR); Hemlock Society; In re Quinlan; *United States; Vacco v. Quill; Washington v. Glucksberg

Dickinson, George E.; Lancaster, Carol J.; Sumner, Edward D., et al. Attitudes toward assisted suicide and euthanasia among physicians in South Carolina and Washington. *Omega: A Journal of Death and Dying.* 1997–1998; 36(3): 201–218. 17 refs. BE61223.

BE = bioethics accession number   fn. = footnotes   refs. = references

*active euthanasia; *assisted suicide; *attitudes; clinical ethics committees; comparative studies; competence; decision making; family members; guidelines; medical specialties; morality; pain; physician patient relationship; *physicians; public opinion; public policy; quality of life; referral and consultation; right to die; survey; terminally ill; *voluntary euthanasia; *South Carolina; United States; *Washington

Doukas, David J.; Gorenflo, Daniel W.; Supanich, Barbara. Primary care physician attitudes and values toward end-of-life care and physician-assisted death. *Ethics and Behavior.* 1999; 9(3): 219-230. 12 refs. BE62083.

*active euthanasia; advance directives; *allowing to die; *assisted suicide; *attitudes; family practice; internal medicine; *physicians; *primary health care; survey; *values; Michigan

This study explores how primary care physician attitudes toward physician-assisted death (PAD) are related to their personal values toward end-of-life care and PAD. A group of 810 Michigan family physicians, internists, and general practitioners, divided into 4 typology groups by their intention toward participating in PAD, rated their attitudes toward PAD, along with their values and preferences for their own end-of-life care. Respondents who most objected to PAD were less likely to have executed an advance directive and more likely to have values promoting continued life-sustaining treatment in their own terminal care. Furthermore, a significant number of physicians, who had strong values against their own withdrawal of treatment in terminal care, were opposed to the withdrawing or withholding of life-sustaining treatment in patient care. Considerations of personal physician values are relevant in the discussion of PAD and the withdrawal of treatment in terminal care.

Green, Gill. AIDS and euthanasia. *AIDS Care.* 1995; 7(Suppl. 2): S169-S173. 6 refs. BE60344.

*active euthanasia; *AIDS; *assisted suicide; *attitudes; communication; family members; friends; health personnel; *HIV seropositivity; legal aspects; *patients; quality of life; suicide; survey; Scotland

Haverkate, Ilinka; van der Wal, Gerrit; van der Maas, Paul J., et al. Guidelines on euthanasia and pain alleviation: compliance and opinions of physicians. *Health Policy.* 1998 Apr; 44(1): 45-55. 13 refs. BE59927.

*active euthanasia; administrators; *assisted suicide; double effect; family practice; *guideline adherence; *guidelines; hospitals; *institutional policies; *knowledge, attitudes, practice; medical specialties; nursing homes; *palliative care; *physicians; referral and consultation; suffering; survey; *Netherlands

Hu, Peicheng. The acceptability of active euthanasia in China. *Medicine and Law.* 1993; 12(1-2): 47-53. 5 refs. BE60612.

*active euthanasia; *attitudes; attitudes to death; case studies; decision making; family members; females; health personnel; legal aspects; males; patients; physicians; *public opinion; resource allocation; *social impact; socioeconomic factors; suffering; survey; terminally ill; value of life; Confucian ethics; *China

Humphry, Derek; Clement, Mary. Freedom to Die: People, Politics, and the Right-to-Die Movement. New York, NY: St. Martin's Press; 1998. 388 p. 523 fn. Appendixes include "A twentieth-century chronology of voluntary euthanasia and physician-assisted suicide," "Laws on physician-assisted suicide in the United States," and "The Oregon Death with Dignity Act." ISBN

0-312-19415-3. BE62300.

advance directives; AIDS; allowing to die; *assisted suicide; *attitudes; biomedical technologies; federal government; government regulation; historical aspects; international aspects; *legal aspects; palliative care; patient advocacy; patients' rights; physician patient relationship; physicians; political activity; politics; public opinion; *public policy; religion; resource allocation; *right to die; rights; state government; terminal care; *trends; *voluntary euthanasia; Australia; Hemlock Society; In re Quinlan; Kevorkian, Jack; Netherlands; Oregon; Quill, Timothy; Twentieth Century; *United States

Jacobson, Jay A. Preaching to the choir: new voices in the end of life discussion. [Editorial]. *Journal of Clinical Oncology.* 1997 Feb; 15(2): 413-415. 5 refs. BE59533.

*active euthanasia; allowing to die; *assisted suicide; *attitudes; cancer; empirical research; food; patients; physicians; public opinion; terminally ill; treatment refusal; trends; voluntary euthanasia; oncology; United States

Kunene, Sibusiso Sixtus; Zungu, Busie Maya. An investigation into the attitude of professional nurses towards euthanasia. *Curationis.* 1996 Dec; 19(4): 26-30. 8 refs. BE61435.

*active euthanasia; adults; age factors; aged; *allowing to die; *attitudes; congenital disorders; decision making; drugs; family members; hospitals; newborns; *nurses; nursing research; prolongation of life; resuscitation orders; survey; terminal care; withholding treatment; *KwaZulu-Natal; *South Africa

Matzo, Marianne LaPorte. The search to end suffering: a historical perspective. *Journal of Gerontological Nursing.* 1997 Mar; 23(3): 11-17. 29 refs. BE60383.

*active euthanasia; *allowing to die; artificial feeding; *assisted suicide; *attitudes; autonomy; historical aspects; international aspects; *nurse's role; *nurses; physicians; public policy; quality of life; religion; right to die; suffering; *suicide; terminal care; terminally ill; trends; voluntary euthanasia; withholding treatment

Reiling, Jennifer, ed. JAMA 100 years ago: the right to die. [Reprint]. *JAMA.* 1999 Sep 22-29; 282(12): 1112*b*. BE62668.

*assisted suicide; *attitudes; *historical aspects; *physicians; *right to die; *voluntary euthanasia; *Nineteenth Century

Shah, Nisha; Warner, James; Blizard, Bob, et al. National survey of UK psychiatrists' attitudes to euthanasia. [Letter]. *Lancet.* 1998 Oct 24; 352(9137): 1360. 5 refs. BE60797.

active euthanasia; *allowing to die; *assisted suicide; *attitudes; *physicians; psychiatric diagnosis; *psychiatry; survey; *voluntary euthanasia; *Great Britain

Stevens, Christine A.; Hassan, Riaz. Nurses and the management of death, dying and euthanasia. *Medicine and Law.* 1994; 13(5-6): 541-554. 15 fn. BE60008.

*active euthanasia; age factors; *allowing to die; autonomy; family members; females; guidelines; *knowledge, attitudes, practice; legal aspects; males; *nurses; pain; patients; public policy; quality of life; suffering; survey; terminally ill; withholding treatment; *South Australia

Stolberg, Sheryl Gay. Assisted suicides are rare, survey of doctors finds. [News]. *New York Times.* 1998 Apr 23: A1, A21. BE60323.

*active euthanasia; *assisted suicide; double effect; drugs; *knowledge, attitudes, practice; legal aspects; motivation; *physicians; suffering; terminally ill; United States

Sullivan, Mark; Ormel, Johan; Kempen, G.I.J.M., et al. Beliefs concerning death, dying, and hastening death

---

BE = bioethics accession number   fn. = footnotes   refs. = references

among older, functionally impaired Dutch adults: a one-year longitudinal study. *Journal of the American Geriatrics Society.* 1998 Oct; 46(10): 1251–1257. 26 refs. BE62265.
    *active euthanasia; age factors; *aged; *allowing to die; *assisted suicide; *attitudes; *attitudes to death; chronically ill; decision making; dementia; health; involuntary euthanasia; mental health; mentally ill; *persistent vegetative state; *physically disabled; psychological stress; religion; socioeconomic factors; suffering; survey; time factors; withholding treatment; dependency; *Netherlands

Webb, Cynthia M.; Sheckard, Denise; Wilder, Pauline, et al. Over the past year, how many patients have asked you to inject drugs to intentionally end their lives? Have you ever injected drugs to intentionally end a patient's life? [Letters]. *Journal of Gerontological Nursing.* 1997 Mar; 23(3): 57–59. 6 refs. BE60414.
    assisted suicide; cancer; *knowledge, attitudes, practice; motivation; *nurses; pain; palliative care; patients; resuscitation orders; survey; terminal care; *voluntary euthanasia; United States

Wehrwein, Peter. US physicians confused about end-of-life care. [News]. *Lancet.* 1998 Aug 15; 352(9127): 549. BE59656.
    *active euthanasia; allowing to die; *assisted suicide; cancer; empirical research; *euthanasia; guideline adherence; *knowledge, attitudes, practice; *physicians; *terminally ill; withholding treatment; United States

Yuan, Zong F.; Baume, Peter. Attitudes of Sydney Chinese to voluntary euthanasia. [Letter]. *Australian and New Zealand Journal of Public Health.* 1997 Feb; 21(1): 106–107. BE60577.
    advance directives; age factors; allowing to die; *attitudes; education; *minority groups; morbidity; right to die; survey; *voluntary euthanasia; *Australia

EUTHANASIA/LEGAL ASPECTS

Australia. Euthanasia Laws Act 1997. *Acts of the Australian Parliament.* 1997 Mar 27 (date effective). 7 p. Nov 17, 1997, passed by the Senate and the House of Representatives, assented to by the Governor-General, 27 Mar 1997. BE59924.
    *active euthanasia; allowing to die; *assisted suicide; federal government; intention; killing; *legal aspects; *legislation; palliative care; state government; suicide; third party consent; withholding treatment; *Australia; *Euthanasia Laws Act 1997 (Australia); Rights of the Terminally Ill Act 1995 (Northern Territory)

Belluck, Pam. Dr. Kevorkian is a murderer, the jury finds. [News]. *New York Times.* 1999 Mar 27: A1, A9. BE60912.
    amyotrophic lateral sclerosis; assisted suicide; criminal law; *killing; *legal liability; *physicians; suffering; *voluntary euthanasia; *Kevorkian, Jack; Michigan; *Youk, Thomas

Belluck, Pam. For Kevorkian, a fifth but very different, trial. [News]. *New York Times.* 1999 Mar 20: A1, A11. BE60910.
    amyotrophic lateral sclerosis; assisted suicide; criminal law; *killing; *legal liability; mass media; *physicians; public opinion; suffering; *voluntary euthanasia; *Kevorkian, Jack; Michigan; *Youk, Thomas

Belluck, Pam. Kevorkian seen as 'distraction' on suicide aid. [News]. *New York Times.* 1999 Mar 30: A1, A17. BE60911.
    *active euthanasia; *assisted suicide; chronically ill; *legal aspects; legal liability; palliative care; *physicians; public opinion; public policy; right to die; terminally ill; wedge

argument: *Kevorkian, Jack; United States; Youk, Thomas

Chesterman, Simon. Last rights: euthanasia, the sanctity of life, and the law in the Netherlands and the Northern Territory of Australia. *International and Comparative Law Quarterly.* 1998 Apr; 47(2): 362–393. 201 fn. BE61460.
    *active euthanasia; adults; allowing to die; *assisted suicide; attitudes; autonomy; comparative studies; depressive disorder; double effect; drugs; government regulation; guidelines; intention; international aspects; involuntary euthanasia; judicial action; killing; *legal aspects; legal liability; legislation; moral policy; newborns; pain; palliative care; physicians; political activity; public policy; statistics; suffering; terminally ill; *value of life; *voluntary euthanasia; *wedge argument; Australia; Euthanasia Laws Act 1997 (Australia); *Netherlands; Nitschke, Philip; *Northern Territory; Rights of the Terminally Ill Act 1995 (NT)

Dyer, Clare. British GP cleared of murder charge. [News]. *BMJ (British Medical Journal).* 1999 May 15; 318(7194): 1306. BE62563.
    *active euthanasia; double effect; drugs; killing; *legal liability; *physicians; terminally ill; *Great Britain; *Moor, David

Ferguson, P.R. Causing death or allowing to die? A rejoinder to Randall's comments. [Letter]. *Journal of Medical Ethics.* 1998 Aug; 24(4): 281–282. 3 refs. BE61702.
    *active euthanasia; *allowing to die; artificial feeding; criminal law; *intention; *legal aspects; moral obligations; *persistent vegetative state; *physicians; terminally ill; withholding treatment; Airedale NHS Trust v. Bland; Great Britain; R v. Cox

Goff, Robert. A matter of life and death. *Medical Law Review.* 1995 Spring; 3(1): 1–21. 19 fn. Text of the Cassel Lecture at the University of Stockholm, 4 June 1993. BE59255.
    *active euthanasia; advisory committees; *allowing to die; artificial feeding; assisted suicide; competence; criminal law; decision making; drugs; guidelines; hospices; international aspects; involuntary euthanasia; killing; *legal aspects; *legal liability; pain; palliative care; persistent vegetative state; *physicians; public opinion; public policy; right to die; suffering; *terminal care; treatment refusal; *voluntary euthanasia; wedge argument; withholding treatment; *Airedale NHS Trust v. Bland; *Great Britain; House of Lords Select Committee on Medical Ethics; Netherlands; *R v. Cox; Sweden

Griffiths, John; Bood, Alex; Weyers, Heleen. Euthanasia and Law in the Netherlands. Amsterdam: Amsterdam University Press; 1998. 382 p. Bibliography: p. 353–375. ISBN 90–5356–275–3. BE61941.
    *active euthanasia; adults; advance directives; aged; allowing to die; assisted suicide; common good; congenital disorders; criminal law; *decision making; double effect; empirical research; futility; guidelines; health care delivery; health facilities; historical aspects; intention; involuntary euthanasia; judicial action; killing; *legal aspects; legislation; mandatory reporting; mentally disabled; *moral policy; newborns; pain; palliative care; persistent vegetative state; physicians; public opinion; *public policy; *regulation; review; right to die; socioeconomic factors; statistics; suffering; terminal care; treatment refusal; trends; voluntary euthanasia; wedge argument; analgesia; *Netherlands; Royal Dutch Medical Association; Twentieth Century

Griffiths, Pauline. Physician-assisted suicide and voluntary euthanasia: is it time the UK law caught up? *Nursing Ethics.* 1999 Mar; 6(2): 107–117. 35 refs. BE61930.
    allowing to die; *assisted suicide; congenital disorders;

BE = bioethics accession number   fn. = footnotes   refs. = references

criminal law; double effect; guidelines; international aspects; involuntary euthanasia; killing; knowledge, attitudes, practice; *legal aspects; *legal liability; newborns; *nurses; opioid analgesics; pain; palliative care; *physicians; public policy; *right to die; treatment refusal; *voluntary euthanasia; wedge argument; withholding treatment; Australia; *Great Britain; Netherlands; Suicide Act 1961 (Great Britain); United States

Grubb, Andrew. Attempted murder of terminally ill patient: R. v. Cox. [Comment]. *Medical Law Review.* 1993 Summer; 1(2): 232–234. BE60602.
　　*active euthanasia; double effect; drugs; intention; *killing; *legal aspects; *legal liability; pain; *physicians; *terminally ill; *Great Britain; *R. v. Cox

Humphry, Derek; Clement, Mary. Freedom to Die: People, Politics, and the Right-to-Die Movement. New York, NY: St. Martin's Press; 1998. 388 p. 523 fn. Appendixes include "A twentieth-century chronology of voluntary euthanasia and physician-assisted suicide," "Laws on physician-assisted suicide in the United States," and "The Oregon Death with Dignity Act." ISBN 0-312-19415-3. BE62300.
　　advance directives; AIDS; allowing to die; *assisted suicide; *attitudes; biomedical technologies; federal government; government regulation; historical aspects; international aspects; *legal aspects; palliative care; patient advocacy; patients' rights; physician patient relationship; physicians; political activity; politics; public opinion; *public policy; religion; resource allocation; *right to die; rights; state government; terminal care; *trends; *voluntary euthanasia; Australia; Hemlock Society; In re Quinlan; Kevorkian, Jack; Netherlands; Oregon; Quill, Timothy; Twentieth Century; *United States

Johnson, Dirk. Kevorkian faces a murder charge in death of man. [News]. *New York Times.* 1998 Nov 26: A1, A18. BE60370.
　　*active euthanasia; assisted suicide; *killing; *legal liability; mass media; physicians; right to die; *voluntary euthanasia; *Kevorkian, Jack; *Michigan; *Youk, Thomas

Johnson, Dirk. Kevorkian sentenced to 10 to 25 years in prison. [News]. *New York Times.* 1999 Apr 14: A1, A23. BE60914.
　　amyotrophic lateral sclerosis; assisted suicide; criminal law; *killing; *legal liability; *physicians; punishment; *voluntary euthanasia; *Kevorkian, Jack; Michigan; *Youk, Thomas

Marlin, George J. Assisted suicide and euthanasia. *In: his* The Politician's Guide to Assisted Suicide, Cloning, and Other Current Controversies. Washington, DC: Morley Books; 1998: 63–124, 205–211. 172 fn. ISBN 0-9660597-1-9. BE62395.
　　*active euthanasia; allowing to die; artificial feeding; *assisted suicide; Christian ethics; government regulation; historical aspects; human rights; killing; *legal aspects; legal rights; National Socialism; physician's role; physicians; politics; public policy; right to die; social impact; social worth; Supreme Court decisions; wedge argument; Germany; Kevorkian, Jack; Netherlands; United States

Monahan, Emmy S. An analysis of the mandatory notification procedure pertaining to termination of life in the Netherlands and recent developments. *Saint Louis University Public Law Review.* 1996; 15(2): 411–422. 77 fn. BE59917.
　　*active euthanasia; adults; *assisted suicide; competence; criminal law; depressive disorder; guidelines; *legal aspects; legal liability; *mandatory reporting; mentally ill; newborns; nurses; physician patient relationship; physicians; psychiatry; public policy; referral and consultation; suffering; *Netherlands

New York State Task Force on Life and the Law. When Death Is Sought: Assisted Suicide and Euthanasia in the Medical Context; Supplement to Report. New York, NY: The Task Force; 1997 Apr. 18 p. 70 fn. ISBN 1-881268-02-0. BE62735.
　　*active euthanasia; advisory committees; *allowing to die; *assisted suicide; competence; double effect; due process; equal protection; government regulation; *guidelines; judicial action; *legal aspects; legal rights; opioid analgesics; pain; *palliative care; physicians; *public policy; right to die; risks and benefits; state government; suffering; terminally ill; treatment refusal; vulnerable populations; withholding treatment; *New York; *New York State Task Force on Life and the Law; United States; *Vacco v. Quill; Washington; *Washington v. Glucksberg

Orentlicher, David. The Supreme Court and terminal sedation: rejecting assisted suicide, embracing euthanasia. *Hastings Constitutional Law Quarterly.* 1997 Summer; 24(4): 947–968. 100 fn. BE62166.
　　*allowing to die; *artificial feeding; *assisted suicide; competence; double effect; drugs; *euthanasia; government regulation; *intention; involuntary euthanasia; *legal aspects; moral policy; pain; *palliative care; *physicians; right to die; *sedatives; suffering; *Supreme Court decisions; terminally ill; vulnerable populations; wedge argument; *withholding treatment; *United States; *Vacco v. Quill; *Washington v. Glucksberg

Robb, Nancy. The Morrison ruling: the case may be closed but the issues it raised are not. *Canadian Medical Association Journal.* 1998 Apr 21; 158(8): 1071–1072. BE60589.
　　*active euthanasia; compassion; criminal law; *killing; *legal liability; *physicians; terminal care; *terminally ill; *Morrison, Nancy; *Nova Scotia

Robertson, Donald. The withdrawal of medical treatment from patients: fundamental legal issues. *Australian Law Journal.* 1996 Sep; 70(9): 723–746. 146 fn. BE62161.
　　*allowing to die; assisted suicide; autonomy; Christian ethics; competence; conscience; decision making; double effect; *euthanasia; informed consent; intention; international aspects; involuntary euthanasia; judicial action; *legal aspects; patient care; quality of life; right to die; terminal care; third party consent; value of life; voluntary euthanasia; withholding treatment; *Australia; *Great Britain; *United States

Robinson, John H.; Berry, Roberta M.; McDonnell, Kevin, eds. Death and dying. *In: their* A Health Law Reader: An Interdisciplinary Approach. Durham, NC: Carolina Academic Press; 1999: 339–426. 64 fn. ISBN 0-89089-907-X. BE62295.
　　*active euthanasia; *advance directives; *allowing to die; artificial feeding; *assisted suicide; brain death; competence; decision making; determination of death; directive adherence; *disabled; economics; freedom; intention; *legal aspects; legal liability; legal rights; living wills; moral policy; physician's role; physicians; public policy; quality of life; *right to die; risks and benefits; standards; state government; state interest; third party consent; treatment refusal; value of life; withholding treatment; wrongful life; Patient Self-Determination Act 1990; *United States

Scherer, Jennifer M.; Simon, Rita J. Euthanasia and the Right to Die: A Comparative View. Lanham, MD: Rowman and Littlefield; 1999. 151 p. 270 fn. Includes tables of "Status of Right-to-Die Legislation in the U.S., by State, July 1997," and "Social Indicators, Euthanasia and Right-to-Die Regulations, Twenty Countries." ISBN 0-8476-9167-5. BE61316.
　　*active euthanasia; advance directives; *allowing to die; *assisted suicide; attitudes to death; autonomy; beneficence;

BE = bioethics accession number   fn. = footnotes   refs. = references

coercion; comparative studies; compassion; *cultural pluralism; disabled; economics; eugenics; goals; health care delivery; historical aspects; *international aspects; involuntary euthanasia; knowledge, attitudes, practice; *legal aspects; medicine; National Socialism; pain; palliative care; persistent vegetative state; physicians; political activity; *public opinion; *public policy; quality of life; religious ethics; *right to die; standards; *state government; suffering; suicide; terminal care; terminally ill; treatment refusal; value of life; *voluntary euthanasia; wedge argument; withholding treatment; Australia; Canada; China; Colombia; France; Germany; Great Britain; India; Iran; Israel; Japan; Netherlands; South Africa; Spain; Switzerland; United States

Smith, George P. Death. *In: his* Family Values and the New Society: Dilemmas of the 21st Century. Westport, CT: Praeger; 1998: 217–246. 192 fn. ISBN 0-275-96221-0. BE62298.
*active euthanasia; *allowing to die; artificial feeding; *assisted suicide; attitudes to death; beneficence; double effect; extraordinary treatment; futility; government regulation; *legal aspects; legal liability; moral policy; physicians; quality of life; *right to die; Roman Catholic ethics; standards; state government; terminal care; terminology; treatment refusal; *withholding treatment; *United States

Underwood, James L. The Supreme Court's assisted suicide opinions in international perspective: avoiding a bureaucracy of death. *North Dakota Law Review.* 1997; 73(4): 641–684. 296 fn. BE62434.
*active euthanasia; allowing to die; *assisted suicide; autonomy; depressive disorder; due process; equal protection; freedom; government regulation; guideline adherence; guidelines; historical aspects; *international aspects; *legal aspects; legal liability; legal rights; mentally ill; pain; physically disabled; physicians; privacy; *right to die; state government; suffering; Supreme Court decisions; terminally ill; value of life; vulnerable populations; *Australia; *Canada; Chabot, Boudewijn; *Colombia; *Netherlands; Northern Territory; Rodriguez v. British Columbia (Attorney-General); *United States; Vacco v. Quill; Washington v. Glucksberg

Wise, Jacqui. Australian euthanasia law throws up many difficulties. [News]. *BMJ (British Medical Journal).* 1998 Oct 10; 317(7164): 969. BE60852.
cancer; *depressive disorder; diagnosis; dissent; *legal aspects; palliative care; physicians; *prognosis; psychiatric diagnosis; *terminally ill; *voluntary euthanasia; Australia; *Northern Territory; *Rights of the Terminally Ill Act (NT)

Dr. Kevorkian's luck runs out. [Editorial]. *New York Times.* 1999 Mar 27: A16. BE60913.
amyotrophic lateral sclerosis; assisted suicide; criminal law; *killing; *legal liability; *physicians; suffering; *voluntary euthanasia; *Kevorkian, Jack; Michigan; *Youk, Thomas

Jail time for Dr. Kevorkian. [Editorial]. *New York Times.* 1999 Apr 15: A30. BE61008.
*active euthanasia; amyotrophic lateral sclerosis; assisted suicide; killing; *legal liability; physicians; punishment; suffering; voluntary euthanasia; *Kevorkian, Jack; Michigan; *Youk, Thomas

EUTHANASIA/RELIGIOUS ASPECTS

Anderson, J. Kerby. Euthanasia. *In: his* Moral Dilemmas: Biblical Perspectives on Contemporary Ethical Issues. Nashville, TN: Word Publishing; 1998: 17–31, 228–229. 14 fn. ISBN 0-8499-1446-9. BE62392.
active euthanasia; advance directives; allowing to die; assisted suicide; *Christian ethics; *euthanasia; historical aspects; involuntary euthanasia; terminal care; value of life; voluntary euthanasia; withholding treatment; Netherlands;

United States

Burke, J. Daniel. A comment on Dan Brock's essay, "Euthanasia." *Rhode Island Medicine.* 1993 Dec; 76(12): 603–604. Commentary on D.W. Brock, "Euthanasia," p. 585–589. BE59416.
*Christian ethics; killing; moral policy; public policy; quality of life; suffering; theology; *voluntary euthanasia

Cohen, Lynne. Jewish and secular medical ethics share themes but diverge on issues such as heroic measures. *Canadian Medical Association Journal.* 1997 Nov 15; 157(10): 1415–1416. BE59683.
active euthanasia; *allowing to die; autonomy; bioethical issues; *euthanasia; *Jewish ethics; medical ethics; physicians; prolongation of life; secularism; treatment refusal; *value of life; withholding treatment; Rosner, Fred

Coleman, Gerald. Basic issues in the debate over dying. *Origins.* 1998 Mar 19; 27(39): 663–668. 56 fn. Address delivered to the annual Archbishop John R. Quinn Colloquim on Catholic Social Teaching, University of San Francisco, 28 Feb 1998. BE59812.
*active euthanasia; allowing to die; artificial feeding; *assisted suicide; autonomy; extraordinary treatment; killing; persistent vegetative state; quality of life; right to die; *Roman Catholic ethics; suffering; terminal care; value of life; United States

Conner, Paul. Euthanasia -- why not? *Rhode Island Medicine.* 1993 Dec; 76(12): 595–599. Commentary on D.W. Brock, "Euthanasia," p. 585–589. Reprinted from *Providence,* 1993; 1: 241. BE59413.
advance directives; *allowing to die; artificial feeding; assisted suicide; attitudes; economics; *euthanasia; extraordinary treatment; *killing; persistent vegetative state; right to die; *Roman Catholic ethics; suffering; treatment refusal; *value of life; withholding treatment; United States

Demy, Timothy J.; Stewart, Gary P. Suicide: A Christian Response: Crucial Considerations for Choosing Life. Grand Rapids, MI: Kregel Publications; 1998. 490 p. Includes references. Foreword by Carl F.H. Henry. ISBN 0-8254-2355-4. BE61352.
*active euthanasia; adolescents; advance directives; allowing to die; *assisted suicide; autonomy; beneficence; cancer; *Christian ethics; disabled; killing; legal aspects; morality; pain; palliative care; paternalism; physicians; Protestant ethics; public policy; quality of life; right to die; social discrimination; suffering; *suicide; terminally ill; *theology; treatment refusal; value of life; *voluntary euthanasia; wedge argument; withholding treatment; *Evangelical Christians; United States

Engelhardt, H. Tristram. Physician-assisted death: doctrinal develoment vs. Christian tradition. [Introduction to five articles]. *Christian Bioethics.* 1998 Aug; 4(2): 115–121. 7 refs. 3 fn. Introduction to a set of articles by D.C. Thomasma, H.T. Engelhardt, A. Young, C. Kaczor, and W.E. Stempsey. BE61157.
*active euthanasia; *assisted suicide; attitudes to death; *Christian ethics; Eastern Orthodox ethics; historical aspects; intention; killing; physicians; Roman Catholic ethics; suicide; theology; *voluntary euthanasia

Physician-assisted suicide offers a moral and theological Rorschach test. Foundational commitments regarding morality and theology are disclosed by how the issue is perceived and by what moral problems it is seen to present. One of the cardinal differences disclosed is that between Western and Orthodox Christian approaches to theology in general, and the theology of dying and suicide in particular. Confrontation with the issue of suicide is likely to bring further doctrinal development

---

BE = bioethics accession number   fn. = footnotes   refs. = references

in many of the Western Christian religions, so as to be able to accept physician-assisted suicide and euthanasia.

Engelhardt, H. Tristram. Physician-assisted suicide reconsidered: dying as a Christian in a post-Christian age. *Christian Bioethics.* 1998 Aug; 4(2): 143–167. 41 refs. 31 fn. Commented on by C. Kaczor, p. 183–201. BE61159.
> *active euthanasia; *assisted suicide; attitudes to death; autonomy; *Christian ethics; Eastern Orthodox ethics; freedom; legal aspects; morality; physicians; *postmodernism; right to die; *secularism; suffering; suicide; *theology; trends; *values; *voluntary euthanasia; dignity; United States

The traditional Christian focus concerning dying is on repentance, not dignity. The goal of a traditional Christian death is not a pleasing, final chapter to life, but union with God: holiness. The pursuit of holiness requires putting on Christ and accepting His cross. In contrast, post-traditional Christian and secular concerns with self-determination, control, dignity, and self-esteem make physician-assisted suicide and voluntary active euthanasia plausible moral choices. Such is not the case within the context of the traditional Christian experience of God, which throughout its 2000 years has sternly condemned suicide and assisted suicide. The wrongness of such actions cannot adequately be appreciated outside the experience of that Christian life. Traditional Christian appreciations of death involve an epistemology and metaphysics of values in discordance with those of secular morality. This difference in the appreciation of the meaning of dying and death, as well as in the appreciation of the moral significance of suicide, discloses a new battle in the culture wars separating traditional Christian morality from that of the surrounding society.

Hayes, Edward J.; Hayes, Paul J.; Kelly, Dorothy Ellen, et al. Principles relating to the taking of life. *In: their* Catholicism and Ethics. Norwood, MA: C.R. Publications; 1997: 121–151. Includes discussion questions and projects. References embedded in list at back of book. ISBN 0-9649087-7-8. BE61947.
> *abortion, induced; active euthanasia; advance directives; allowing to die; assisted suicide; attitudes to death; childbirth; double effect; drugs; *euthanasia; fetuses; forms; killing; methods; opioid analgesics; palliative care; pregnant women; rights; *Roman Catholic ethics; terminal care; therapeutic abortion; *value of life; abortion, spontaneous; Catholic Health Association

Jacob, Walter; Zemer, Moshe, eds. Death and Euthanasia in Jewish Law: Essays and Responsa. Pittsburgh, PA: Freehof Institute of Progressive Halakhah: Rodef Shalom Press; 1995. 204 p. (Studies in progressive halakha; v. 4). 202 fn. ISBN 0-929699-06-8. BE60069.
> active euthanasia; advance directives; aged; *allowing to die; artificial feeding; assisted suicide; brain death; cardiac death; cesarean section; covenant; determination of death; drugs; *euthanasia; human experimentation; *Jewish ethics; killing; narrative ethics; nontherapeutic research; palliative care; persistent vegetative state; pregnant women; prognosis; prolongation of life; quality of life; resuscitation orders; risks and benefits; scarcity; selection for treatment; suffering; suicide; surgery; terminally ill; *theology; therapeutic research; treatment refusal; truth disclosure; value of life; ventilators; withholding treatment; Orthodox Judaism; *Reform Judaism

Knobel, Peter. Suicide, assisted suicide, active euthanasia: a *Halakhic* inquiry. *In:* Jacob, Walter; Zemer, Moshe, eds. Death and Euthanasia in Jewish Law: Essays and

Responsa. Pittsburgh, PA: Freehof Institute of Progressive Halakhah; Rodef Shalom Press; 1995: 27–59. 68 fn. ISBN 0-929699-06-8. BE60072.
> advance directives; *assisted suicide; autonomy; compassion; competence; *covenant; decision making; guidelines; informed consent; *Jewish ethics; justice; killing; methods; pain; quality of life; suffering; *suicide; terminally ill; theology; value of life; virtues; *voluntary euthanasia; dignity; *Reform Judaism

Kravitz, Leonard. Euthanasia. *In:* Jacob, Walter; Zemer, Moshe, eds. Death and Euthanasia in Jewish Law: Essays and Responsa. Pittsburgh, PA: Freehof Institute of Progressive Halakhah; Rodef Shalom Press; 1995: 11–25. 26 fn. ISBN 0-929699-06-8. BE60071.
> *active euthanasia; advance directives; *allowing to die; *euthanasia; historical aspects; intention; *Jewish ethics; killing; pain; suffering; terminally ill; theology; withholding treatment; *Reform Judaism

Manning, Michael. Euthanasia and Physician-Assisted Suicide: Killing or Caring? New York, NY: Paulist Press; 1998. 120 p. Bibliography: p.108–120. ISBN 0-8091-3804-2. BE61048.
> *active euthanasia; allowing to die; artificial feeding; *assisted suicide; autonomy; common good; compassion; double effect; drugs; historical aspects; involuntary euthanasia; *killing; legal aspects; medical ethics; National Socialism; physician patient relationship; physicians; right to die; *Roman Catholic ethics; socioeconomic factors; theology; trust; wedge argument; withholding treatment; Germany; Netherlands; United States

Rayner, John D. Euthanasia. *In: his* Jewish Religious Law: A Progressive Perspective. New York, NY: Berghahn Books; 1998: 138–143. ISBN 1-57181-976-2. BE62137.
> *active euthanasia; *allowing to die; artificial feeding; double effect; drugs; *Jewish ethics; legal aspects; prolongation of life; suffering; suicide; terminally ill; withholding treatment; Orthodox Judaism; *Reform Judaism

Rosenberg, James. The voice of God. *Rhode Island Medicine.* 1993 Dec; 76(12): 600. Commentary on D.W. Brock, "Euthanasia," p. 585–589. BE59414.
> *active euthanasia; allowing to die; amyotrophic lateral sclerosis; autonomy; *Jewish ethics; killing; paralysis; physicians; *public policy; right to die; *voluntary euthanasia

Thomasma, David C. Assisted death and martyrdom. *Christian Bioethics.* 1998 Aug; 4(2): 122–142. 53 refs. 15 fn. Commented on by C. Kaczor, p. 183–201. BE61158.
> *active euthanasia; *assisted suicide; attitudes to death; capital punishment; *historical aspects; *intention; *killing; love; *Roman Catholic ethics; theology; value of life; violence; *voluntary euthanasia; war; Jesus

Against the backdrop of ancient, mediaeval and modern Catholic teaching prohibiting killing (the rule against killing), the question of assisted suicide and euthanasia is examined. In the past the Church has modified its initial repugnance for killing by developing specific guidelines for permitting killing under strict conditions. This took place with respect to capital punishment and a just war, for example. One wonders why in the least objectionable instance, when a person is already dying, suffering, and repeatedly requesting assistance in dying, there is still such widespread condemnation of assisted suicide and euthanasia. In a *Gedankexperiment*, I suggest that certain stories of martyrdom in the history of the Christian Church shed some light on the role of taking one's life, or putting one's life in danger out of love. I further suggest that requesting assisted suicide and/or

---

BE = bioethics accession number   fn. = footnotes   refs. = references

euthanasia from the motive of love of one's family or care givers might possibly qualify as one instance of justifiable euthanasia, although I acknowledge that the Church will not be making changes in its stance any time soon.

FAMILY PLANNING *See* CONTRACEPTION, POPULATION CONTROL

FETUSES

See also ABORTION, EMBRYO AND FETAL RESEARCH, PRENATAL INJURIES

Arthur, John, ed. Abortion. *In:* Arthur, John, ed. Morality and Moral Controversies. Fifth Edition. Upper Saddle River, NJ: Prentice Hall; 1999: 166–210. 9 refs. 13 fn. Includes discussion questions. ISBN 0-13-914128-6. BE60274.
> *abortion, induced; autonomy; beginning of life; cesarean section; coercion; decision making; drug abuse; *fathers; feminist ethics; fetal development; *fetuses; killing; legal aspects; *moral policy; mother fetus relationship; personhood; *pregnant women; prenatal injuries; privacy; rape; reproduction; rights; Supreme Court decisions; therapeutic abortion; treatment refusal; value of life; viability; women's rights; Roe v. Wade; United States

Beller, Fritz K.; Zlatnik, Gail P. The beginning of human life. *Journal of Assisted Reproduction and Genetics.* 1995 Sep; 12(8): 477–483. 31 fn. BE60559.
> abortion, induced; *beginning of life; brain; contraception; *embryos; fetal development; *fetuses; legal aspects; personhood; pregnant women; viability

Benedict, James. The use of fetal tissue: a cautious approval. *Christian Century.* 1998 Feb 18; 115(5): 164–165. BE60446.
> *aborted fetuses; *Christian ethics; *fetal tissue donation; risks and benefits

Benshoof, Janet; Knights of Columbus. Abortion and the "pro-life" *v.* "pro-choice" debate: should the human fetus be considered a person? *In:* Francoeur, Robert T., ed. Taking Sides: Clashing Views on Controversial Issues in Human Sexuality. Fifth Edition. Guilford, CT: Dushkin Publishing Group/Brown and Benchmark; 1996: 120–133. 9 refs. Bibliography: p. 133. ISBN 0-697-31292-5. BE62044.
> *abortion, induced; *beginning of life; constitutional law; embryos; *fetuses; *legal aspects; legal liability; *legal rights; *personhood; *pregnant women; prenatal injuries; Supreme Court decisions; viability; wrongful death; Fourteenth Amendment; *Roe v. Wade; *United States; Webster v. Reproductive Health Services

Bleich, J. David; Caplan, Arthur L.; Murray, Joseph E., et al. Defining the limits of organ and tissue research and transplantation. [Proceedings of the International Symposium on Law and Science at the Crossroads: Biomedical Technology, Ethics, Public Policy, and the Law; panel discussion]. *Suffolk University Law Review.* 1993 Winter; 27(4): 1457–1476. Moderator: Raja B. Khauli. BE60701.
> aborted fetuses; autonomy; body parts and fluids; *brain death; cadavers; cardiac death; *determination of death; *fetal tissue donation; *organ donation; organ donors; presumed consent; public policy; remuneration; values

Bleich, J. David. Moral debate and semantic sleight of hand. *Suffolk University Law Review.* 1993 Winter; 27(4):

1173–1193. 44 fn. BE60698.
> *aborted fetuses; abortion, induced; beginning of life; *brain death; cultural pluralism; decision making; democracy; *determination of death; fetal research; *fetal tissue donation; fetuses; government financing; legal aspects; legal rights; moral policy; newborns; prolongation of life; public policy; quality of life; religion; religious ethics; standards; state interest; theology; value of life; *values; withholding treatment

Bridgeman, Jo. Medical treatment: the mother's rights. *Family Law.* 1993 Sep; 23: 534–535. BE61825.
> *cesarean section; competence; *fetuses; judicial action; *legal aspects; legal rights; *pregnant women; *treatment refusal; *Great Britain; *Re S (An Adult: Surgical Treatment)

Casper, Monica J. Working on and around human fetuses: the contested domain of fetal surgery. *In:* Berg, Marc; Mol, Annemarie, eds. Differences in Medicine: Unraveling Practices, Techniques, and Bodies. Durham, NC: Duke University Press; 1998: 28–52. 23 fn. ISBN 0-8223-2174-2. BE62132.
> conflict of interest; *congenital disorders; decision making; *dissent; fetal research; *fetal therapy; *fetuses; *goals; hospitals; human experimentation; *interdisciplinary communication; *interprofessional relations; investigators; maternal health; *medical specialties; morbidity; mortality; mother fetus relationship; newborns; nurses; *obstetrics and gynecology; patient advocacy; *patient care team; pediatrics; physician patient relationship; *physicians; *pregnant women; prenatal diagnosis; psychological stress; *risks and benefits; selection for treatment; social dominance; *social workers; *sociology of medicine; *surgery; technical expertise; therapeutic research; treatment outcome; negotiation; neonatology; perinatology

Clarke, Liam. The person in abortion. *Nursing Ethics.* 1999 Jan; 6(1): 37–46. 28 refs. BE60153.
> *abortion, induced; *beginning of life; childbirth; children; emotions; *fetuses; infanticide; infants; moral development; *mother fetus relationship; *newborns; nurses; *personhood; pregnant women; speciesism; viability

Derbyshire, Stuart W.G. Locating the beginnings of pain. *Bioethics.* 1999 Jan; 13(1): 1–31. 100 fn. BE60886.
> abortion, induced; anesthesia; *brain; drugs; *fetal development; fetal therapy; *fetuses; newborns; *pain; physicians; practice guidelines; professional organizations; self concept; surgery; analgesia; Great Britain; *Royal College of Obstetricians and Gynaecologists (Great Britain)

Doyle, John P. Reflections on persons in petri dishes. *Linacre Quarterly.* 1997 Nov; 64(4): 62–76. 26 fn. BE61791.
> cloning; embryo disposition; embryo research; *embryos; human characteristics; in vitro fertilization; intelligence; morality; natural law; parent child relationship; *personhood; reproduction; self concept

Erin, Charles A. Some comments on the ethics of consent to the use of ovarian tissue from aborted fetuses and dead women. *In:* Harris, John; Holm, Søren, eds. The Future of Human Reproduction: Ethics, Choice, and Regulation. New York, NY: Oxford University Press; 1998: 162–175. 33 fn. ISBN 0-19-823761-8. BE61268.
> *aborted fetuses; advance directives; autonomy; *cadavers; decision making; disclosure; dissent; family members; *fetal tissue donation; germ cells; *informed consent; legal aspects; *ovum donors; parental consent; posthumous reproduction; presumed consent; third party consent; *tissue donation; *ovaries; Great Britain; Human Tissue Act 1961 (Great Britain)

Forster, Heidi P.; Robertson, John. Frozen embryo

BE = bioethics accession number   fn. = footnotes   refs. = references

disposition. [Letter and response]. *Hastings Center Report.* 1999 Mar–Apr; 29(2): 4–5. BE61652.
    contracts; *cryopreservation; *decision making; *dissent; *embryo disposition; embryo research; embryo transfer; *embryos; *in vitro fertilization; informed consent; *legal aspects; married persons; ovum donors; property rights; semen donors; divorce; Kass v. Kass; New York

Gillam, Lynn. The 'more–abortions' objection to fetal tissue transplantation. *Journal of Medicine and Philosophy.* 1998 Aug; 23(4): 411–427. 27 refs. 14 fn. BE60631.
    *aborted fetuses; *abortion, induced; *deontological ethics; double effect; *ethical analysis; *fetal tissue donation; injuries; *intention; moral complicity; *moral policy; motivation; pregnant women; social impact; utilitarianism; *wedge argument

One common objection to fetal tissue transplantation (FTT) is that, if it were to become a standard form of treatment, it would encourage or entrench the practice of abortion. This claim is at least factually plausible, although it cannot be definitively established. However, even if true, it does not constitute a compelling ethical argument against FTT. The harm allegedly brought about by FTT, when assessed by widely accepted non–consequentialist criteria, has limited moral significance. Even if FTT would cause more abortions to be performed, and abortion is taken to be a serious moral wrong, this is not sufficient in itself to make FTT wrong.

Golden, Frederic. The ice babies: long–lost frozen embryos are popping up all over. [News]. *Time.* 1998 Mar 2; 151(8): 65. BE59166.
    *cryopreservation; *embryo transfer; *embryos; in vitro fertilization; *time factors; United States

Grubb, Andrew. Frozen embryos: rights of inheritance: In Re the Estate of the Late K. [Comment]. *Medical Law Review.* 1997 Spring; 5(1): 121–124. BE59764.
    childbirth; *cryopreservation; embryo transfer; *embryos; fathers; fetuses; in vitro fertilization; *legal aspects; *legal rights; newborns; parent child relationship; personhood; *posthumous reproduction; property rights; *Australia; Great Britain; *In re Estate of the Late K; *Tasmania

Grubb, Andrew. Use of fetal eggs and infertility treatment: Human Fertilisation and Embryology Act 1990, section 3A. [Comment]. *Medical Law Review.* 1995 Summer; 3(2): 203–204. BE59254.
    aborted fetuses; criminal law; embryo transfer; embryos; *fetal tissue donation; germ cells; *government regulation; in vitro fertilization; *legislation; *ovum; *reproductive technologies; *Great Britain; *Human Fertilisation and Embryology Act 1990

Hartouni, Valerie. Cultural Conceptions: On Reproductive Technologies and the Remaking of Life. Minneapolis, MN: University of Minnesota Press; 1997. 175 p. Bibliography: p. 157–170. ISBN 0–8166–2623–5. BE62771.
    *abortion, induced; adoption; audiovisual aids; behavioral genetics; blacks; brain death; *cloning; disadvantaged; embryos; eugenics; *fetuses; genetic intervention; legal aspects; mass media; mothers; parent child relationship; personhood; political activity; posthumous reproduction; postmodernism; *pregnant women; prenatal diagnosis; prolongation of life; *reproduction; *reproductive technologies; social discrimination; *social impact; socioeconomic factors; Supreme Court decisions; *surrogate mothers; value of life; values; violence; women's rights; In re Baby M; Johnson v. Calvert; Right to Life Movement; S'Aline's Solution; The Bell Curve (Herrnstein, R.; Murray, C.); *United States

Hicks, Stephen C. The regulation of fetal tissue transplantation: different legislative models for different purposes. *Suffolk University Law Review.* 1993 Winter; 27(4): 1613–1629. 46 fn. BE61598.
    *aborted fetuses; abortion, induced; criminal law; directed donation; embryo disposition; embryo research; embryos; federal government; *fetal research; *fetal tissue donation; government financing; *government regulation; informed consent; *model legislation; nontherapeutic research; organ donation; organ transplantation; remuneration; research ethics committees; state government; therapeutic research; tissue donation; tissue transplantation; abortion, spontaneous; NIH Revitalization Act 1993; Uniform Anatomical Gift Act; *United States

Hopkins, Patrick D., ed.; Tennessee. Supreme Court, at Knoxville. (Re)locating fetuses: technology and new body politics. *In: his* Sex/Machine: Readings in Culture, Gender, and Technology. Bloomington, IN: Indiana University Press; 1998: 171–235. 33 refs. 84 fn. ISBN 0–253–21230–8. BE62290.
    *abortion, induced; alternatives; contracts; *cryopreservation; *embryo disposition; embryo transfer; *embryos; *females; feminist ethics; fetuses; human experimentation; *in vitro fertilization; infertility; intention; *legal aspects; *males; *methods; mother fetus relationship; parent child relationship; personhood; pregnant women; privacy; property rights; *reproductive technologies; *required request; *rights; *risks and benefits; social discrimination; social impact; viability; women's rights; divorce; *ectogenesis; *Davis v. Davis; Tennessee; United States

Hunt, Geoffrey. Abortion: why bioethics can have no answer –– a personal perspective. *Nursing Ethics.* 1999 Jan; 6(1): 47–57. 11 refs. BE60154.
    *abortion, induced; attitudes; *beginning of life; bioethics; *dissent; embryos; ethical analysis; ethicists; fetal development; *fetuses; *moral policy; *morality; newborns; *personhood; viability; *rationality

Illinois. Appellate Court, First District, Fifth Division. In re Brown. *North Eastern Reporter, 2d Series.* 1997 Dec 31 (date of decision). 689: 397–406. BE60046.
    autonomy; *blood transfusions; coercion; *fetuses; *Jehovah's Witnesses; *legal aspects; legal guardians; legal rights; *pregnant women; religion; state interest; third party consent; *treatment refusal; value of life; viability; *Illinois; *In re Brown

The Appellate Court of Illinois, First District, held that a competent pregnant woman's right to refuse medical treatment overrides the state's substantial interest in the welfare of a viable fetus. Darlene Brown entered a hospital for a cystoscopy and removal of a urethral mass. She lost 1,500 cubic centimeters of blood and refused blood transfusions because of her beliefs as a Jehovah's Witness. In her physician's opinion, Brown's chances of survival, as well as those of the fetus, were only 5%. The trial court appointed a guardian *ad litem* pursuant to the state's request to protect the interest of the fetus. The guardian ordered Brown to undergo transfusions and she gave birth to a healthy child. The court here held that the trial court abused its discretion in appointing the guardian and forcing Brown to undergo treatment, reasoning that the state's interest in preserving the life of the mother and of the fetus cannot override a pregnant woman's competent refusal of recommended invasive medical procedures. (KIE abstract)

Jeffko, Walter G. Abortion, personhood, and community. *In: his* Contemporary Ethical Issues: A Personalistic Perspective. Amherst, NY: Humanity Books; 1999: 59–84. 42 fn. ISBN 1–57392–640–X. BE62245.

---

*abortion, induced; *beginning of life; congenital disorders; drugs; embryos; *fetal development; *fetuses; infanticide; killing; legal aspects; methods; *moral policy; mother fetus relationship; newborns; *personhood; philosophy; population control; public policy; Roman Catholic ethics; selective abortion; sex offenses; therapeutic abortion; twinning; value of life; viability; RU-486

Jones, D. Gareth. The problematic symmetry between brain birth and brain death. *Journal of Medical Ethics.* 1998 Aug; 24(4): 237-242. 37 refs. BE61288.
> *beginning of life; *brain; *brain death; determination of death; *embryos; *fetal development; *fetuses; moral policy; *personhood; standards; terminology

The possible symmetry between the concepts of brain death and brain birth (life) is explored. Since the symmetry argument has tended to overlook the most appropriate definition of brain death, the fundamental concepts of whole brain death and higher brain death are assessed. In this way, a context is provided for a discussion of brain birth. Different writers have placed brain birth at numerous points: 25-40 days, eight weeks, 22-24 weeks, and 32-36 weeks gestation. For others, the concept itself is open to question. Apart from this, it needs to be asked whether a unitary concept is an oversimplification. The merits of defining two stages of brain birth, to parallel the two definitions of brain death, are discussed. An attempt is then made to map these various stages of brain birth and brain death onto a developmental continuum. Although the results hold biological interest, their ethical significance is less evident. Development and degeneration are not interchangeable, and definitions of death apply specifically to those who are dying, not those who are developing. I conclude that while a dual concept of brain death has proved helpful, a dual concept of brain birth still has problems, and the underlying concept of brain birth itself continues to be elusive.

Jonsson, Lena. The Swedish transplantation law. *International Digest of Health Legislation.* 1997; 48(2): 237-239. BE59598.
> aborted fetuses; abortion, induced; autonomy; beneficence; cadavers; decision making; family members; *fetal tissue donation; informed consent; *legal aspects; *organ donation; organ donors; presumed consent; third party consent; tissue donation; *Sweden

Kischer, C. Ward. The big lie in human embryology: the case of the preembryo. *Linacre Quarterly.* 1997 Nov; 64(4): 53-61. 20 fn. BE61790.
> advisory committees; embryo research; *embryos; fetal development; moral obligations; *personhood; *terminology; twinning; American Fertility Society; Grobstein, Clifford; Human Embryo Research Panel; Warnock Committee

Klen, Rudolf. Aborted embryos -- law and ethics. *Bulletin of Medical Ethics.* 1998 Feb; No. 135: 22-23. BE61889.
> *aborted fetuses; abortion, induced; confidentiality; decision making; *embryo disposition; embryo research; fetal research; *fetal tissue donation; government regulation; informed consent; international aspects; pregnant women; tissue banks; tissue transplantation; Czech Republic

Lafferty, Kevin J.; Furer, Julie J. Legal and medical implications of fetal tissue transplantation. *Suffolk University Law Review.* 1993 Winter; 27(4): 1237-1248. 59 fn. BE61594.
> aborted fetuses; diabetes; federal government; *fetal research; *fetal tissue donation; *government financing; *government regulation; *legal aspects; methods; private sector; *public policy; state government; *tissue transplantation; pancreases; United States

Lebech, Anne Mette Maria. Principles, compromise and human embryos in Europe. *Bulletin of Medical Ethics.* 1997 Aug; No. 130: 18-21. 14 refs. Paper presented at a Biolaw in Europe Project meeting, held in Sheffield, U.K., Apr 1997. BE61718.
> beginning of life; embryo research; *embryos; international aspects; legal aspects; personhood; *value of life; Council of Europe; *Europe; France

Li, Hon-Lam. Abortion and degrees of personhood: understanding why the abortion problem (and the animal rights problem) are irresolvable. *Public Affairs Quarterly.* 1997 Jan; 11(1): 1-19. 26 fn. BE59161.
> *abortion, induced; age factors; animal rights; *beginning of life; fetal development; *fetuses; maternal health; moral policy; morality; *personhood; *pregnant women; speciesism; therapeutic abortion; *value of life

Markens, Susan; Browner, C.H.; Press, Nancy. Feeding the fetus: on interrogating the notion of maternal-fetal conflict. *Feminist Studies.* 1997 Summer; 23(2): 351-372. 46 fn. BE59795.
> attitudes; behavior control; feminist ethics; *fetuses; food; health education; health maintenance organizations; informal social control; *mother fetus relationship; motivation; *nutrition; *patient compliance; *pregnant women; prenatal injuries; smoking; socioeconomic factors; survey; life style; *self care; California

Mason, John Kenyon. Protection of the fetus. *In: his* Medico-Legal Aspects of Reproduction and Parenthood. Second Edition. Brookfield, VT: Ashgate; 1998: 143-186. 179 fn. ISBN 1-84104-065-8. BE61064.
> *aborted fetuses; abortion, induced; alcohol abuse; allowing to die; autonomy; beginning of life; brain death; cesarean section; coercion; compensation; competence; congenital disorders; criminal law; drug abuse; fetal development; *fetal therapy; *fetuses; genetic counseling; genetic disorders; infanticide; international aspects; *legal aspects; *legal liability; *legal rights; mentally ill; methods; negligence; personhood; physicians; *pregnant women; prenatal diagnosis; *prenatal injuries; prolongation of life; public policy; selective abortion; terminally ill; torts; treatment refusal; value of life; *ventilators; viability; *wrongful death; *wrongful life; Abortion Act 1967 (Great Britain); Congenital Disabilities (Civil Liability) Act 1976 (Great Britain); *Great Britain; Infant Life (Preservation) Act 1929 (Great Britain); Scotland; United States

Massachusetts. Trial Court, Probate and Family Department, Suffolk County. AZ v. BZ. Unpublished redacted copy; 1996. 31 p. Permanent restraining order injunction and findings of fact and conclusions of law on request for restraining order. BE60049.
> consent forms; *contracts; *cryopreservation; decision making; *embryo disposition; embryo transfer; *embryos; *in vitro fertilization; informed consent; *legal aspects; *legal rights; *marital relationship; ovum donors; personhood; privacy; property rights; reproduction; semen donors; time factors; unwanted children; *divorce; *AZ v. BZ; Davis v. Davis; Kass v. Kass; *Massachusetts; New York; Tennessee

The Massachusetts Trial Court, Probate and Family Department, for Suffolk County resolved the issue of disposition of cryopreserved embryos prior to entry of a divorce judgment. The court decided in favor of the husband AZ who sought to avoid parenthood, provided that the wife BZ has a reasonable possibility of achieving parenthood through other means. Because BZ had lost both fallopian tubes in ectopic pregnancies, she and her husband AZ conceived twin daughters through in vitro fertilization (IVF) and froze the remaining seven pre-embryos in two vials. Unknown to her husband, BZ underwent an unsuccessful embryo transfer using the embryos from one vial in the month before AZ and BZ separated. Four cryopreserved embryos remained in the last vial. The judge held that a "special status" category best recognizes the dual characteristics of pre-embryos as property and as persons. Discussing the issue of procreational autonomy, the judge found that IVF differs from natural reproduction and has none of the concerns about a woman's bodily integrity. Because the disposition agreement signed by both AZ and BZ at the time of ovum harvest is seven years old and subject to an unforeseeable change of circumstances, the court balanced the interests of the gamete providers and those of a subsequent child. (KIE abstract)

Morgan, G.L. Is there a right to fetal tissue transplantation? *University of Tasmania Law Review.* 1991; 10(2): 129–156. 152 fn. BE62177.
  aborted fetuses; autonomy; disclosure; *fetal tissue donation; government financing; government regulation; health care; *human experimentation; informed consent; investigator subject relationship; investigators; legal aspects; *legal obligations; legal rights; moral obligations; morbidity; mortality; *obligations of society; paternalism; patients; pregnant women; research subjects; *rights; risks and benefits; therapeutic research; *tissue transplantation; Parkinson disease; *Australia

Morgan, Lynn M. Fetal relationality in feminist philosophy: an anthropological critique. *Hypatia.* 1996 Summer; 11(3): 47–70. 78 refs. 13 fn. BE61458.
  abortion, induced; anthropology; beginning of life; embryos; *feminist ethics; fetal development; *fetuses; infanticide; *mother fetus relationship; mothers; newborns; non-Western World; *personhood; philosophy; pregnant women; social interaction; value of life; Western World; relational ethics

Mori, Maurizio. On the concept of pre-embryo: the basis for a new "Copernican revolution" in the current view about human reproduction. *In:* Harris, John; Holm, Søren, eds. The Future of Human Reproduction: Ethics, Choice, and Regulation. New York, NY: Oxford University Press; 1998: 38–54. 15 fn. ISBN 0-19-823761-8. BE61261.
  abortion, induced; *beginning of life; biology; contraception; *embryos; *personhood; terminology; twinning; value of life

Neerhof, Mark G.; MacGregor, Scott N.; Kilner, John F. Congenital diaphragmatic hernia: in utero therapy and ethical considerations. *Clinics in Perinatology.* 1996 Sep; 23(3): 465–472. 20 refs. BE60935.
  congenital disorders; decision making; *fetal therapy; fetuses; methods; pregnant women; prenatal diagnosis; prognosis; risks and benefits; *surgery; therapeutic research; treatment outcome

New York. Supreme Court, Appellate Division, Second Department. Kass v. Kass. *New York Supplement, 2d Series.* 1997 Sep 8 (date of decision). 663: 581–602. BE60051.
  *contracts; *cryopreservation; decision making; dissent; *embryo disposition; embryo research; embryo transfer; *embryos; *in vitro fertilization; informed consent; *legal aspects; legal rights; *marital relationship; ovum donors; personhood; property rights; reproduction; semen donors; *divorce; *Kass v. Kass; New York
The New York Supreme Court, Appellate Division, enforced an informed consent agreement between husband and wife concerning disposition of cryopreserved embryos, following in vitro fertilization (IVF), for use in scientific research. Maureen and Steven Kass had provided for the use of their frozen pre-zygotes in an IVF consent form, and later affirmed that use in an uncontested divorce agreement. Maureen Kass then

changed her mind and sought legal possession and custody of the five pre-embryos for transfer into herself. The trial court had granted her exclusive control based on the determination that a husband's procreative rights in IVF were no greater than those in vivo. The appellate court, however, reversed the trial court and upheld the agreement because the couple's original mutual intent on disposition in the event of a contingency was clear and unequivocal. (KIE abstract)

Persson, Ingmar. Harming the non-conscious. *Bioethics.* 1999 Jul; 13(3–4): 294–305. 13 fn. BE61880.
  *abortion, induced; *beginning of life; brain; embryos; *fetal development; *fetal research; *fetuses; *injuries; killing; *moral policy; organ donation; personhood; prenatal injuries; quality of life; value of life; *harms; Singer, Peter
Peter Singer has argued that nothing done to a fetus before it acquires consciousness can harm it. At the same time, he concedes that a child can be harmed by something done to it when it was a non-conscious fetus. But this implies that the non-conscious fetus can be harmed. The mistake lies in thinking that, since existence can be instrinsically bad for a being only if it is conscious, it can be harmed only if it is conscious. In fact, its being harmed only implies that it could have been conscious (and led a good life).

Resnik, David B. The commodification of human reproductive materials. *Journal of Medical Ethics.* 1998 Dec; 24(6): 388–393. 21 refs. BE60788.
  autonomy; *body parts and fluids; *commodification; *embryos; *genes; *genetic materials; *germ cells; human body; moral policy; ovum donors; patents; personhood; property rights; regulation; *remuneration; reproductive technologies; semen donors; tissue donation; transgenic organisms
This essay develops a framework for thinking about the moral basis for the commodification of human reproductive materials. It argues that selling and buying gametes and genes is morally acceptable although there should not be a market for zygotes, embryos, or genomes. Also a market in gametes and genes should be regulated in order to address concerns about the adverse social consequences of commodification.

Resnik, Robert. Cancer during pregnancy. [Editorial]. *New England Journal of Medicine.* 1999 Jul 8; 341(2): 120–121. 12 refs. BE62034.
  *cancer; drugs; fetal development; *fetuses; *patient care; *pregnant women; radiology; risks and benefits; surgery; time factors; treatment outcome

Richardson, Michael K.; Reiss, Michael J. What does the human embryo look like, and does it matter? *Lancet.* 1999 Jul 17; 354(9174): 246–248. 25 refs. BE62520.
  abortion, induced; embryo research; *embryos; emotions; *fetal development; *human characteristics; personhood; speciesism; value of life

Robertson, John A. Abortion to obtain fetal tissue for transplant. *Suffolk University Law Review.* 1993 Winter; 27(4): 1359–1389. 75 fn. BE61595.
  *aborted fetuses; *abortion, induced; advisory committees; anencephaly; attitudes; coercion; constitutional law; criminal law; *decision making; *directed donation; family members; federal government; fetal research; *fetal tissue donation; *government regulation; informed consent; killing; legal aspects; *legal rights; *moral policy; motivation; organ donation; persistent vegetative state; *pregnant women; public policy; remuneration; reproduction; sex determination; state interest; tissue transplantation; transplant recipients; *women's rights; Department of Health and Human Services; National Institutes of Health; United States

---

BE = bioethics accession number   fn. = footnotes   refs. = references

Rowan, Cathy. Court-ordered caesareans -- choice or control? *Nursing Ethics.* 1998 Nov; 5(6): 542-544. 10 refs. BE60815.
> *cesarean section; *coercion; competence; *fetuses; *judicial action; *legal aspects; nurse midwives; *pregnant women; *treatment refusal; *Great Britain

Scholl, Ann. Legally protecting fetuses: a study of the legal protections afforded organically united individuals. *Public Affairs Quarterly.* 1997 Apr; 11(2): 141-161. 17 refs. 26 fn. BE61896.
> abortion on demand; cesarean section; coercion; *fetuses; legal obligations; *legal rights; mother fetus relationship; *personhood; *pregnant women; therapeutic abortion; treatment refusal; twins; *women's rights; conjoined twins; Warren, Mary Anne

Sly, William S. When does human life begin? Does science provide the answer? *In:* Rainey, R. Randall; Magill, Gerard, eds. Abortion and Public Policy: An Interdisciplinary Investigation within the Catholic Tradition. Omaha, NE: Creighton University Press; 1996: 62-71. 23 fn. Paper presented at a conference held at Saint Louis University, 11-13 Mar 1993. ISBN 1-881871-18-5. BE61990.
> abortion, induced; *beginning of life; cryopreservation; embryo disposition; *embryos; *fetal development; legal aspects; *personhood; preimplantation diagnosis; public policy; *Roman Catholic ethics; science; United States

Spike, Jeffrey. Brain death, pregnancy, and posthumous motherhood. [Case study]. *Journal of Clinical Ethics.* 1999 Spring; 10(1): 57-65. 9 fn. BE62707.
> allowing to die; *brain death; *decision making; determination of death; dissent; ethics consultation; family members; fathers; feminist ethics; fetal development; *fetuses; health personnel; intensive care units; judicial action; moral policy; patient care; patient care team; posthumous reproduction; *pregnant women; *prolongation of life; quality of life; resource allocation; single persons; socioeconomic factors; third party consent; treatment outcome; ventilators; *withholding treatment

Steinbock, Bonnie. Mother-fetus conflict. *In:* Kuhse, Helga; Singer, Peter, eds. A Companion to Bioethics. Malden, MA: Blackwell; 1998: 135-146. 36 refs. ISBN 0-631-19737-0. BE59490.
> abortion, induced; alcohol abuse; *cesarean section; children; coercion; decision making; drug abuse; fetal development; fetal therapy; *fetuses; legal aspects; *moral obligations; moral policy; *mother fetus relationship; pain; physicians; *pregnant women; *prenatal injuries; public policy; surgery; *treatment refusal

Vial Correa, Juan de Dios; Sgreccia, Elio, eds.; Pontificia Academia pro Vita. Identity and Statute [Status] of [the] Human Embryo: Proceedings of [the] Third Assembly of the Pontifical Academy for Life (Vatican City, February 14-16, 1997). Vatican City: Libreria Editrice Vaticana; 1998. 458 p. ISBN 88-209-2470-6. BE60114.
> abortion, induced; advisory committees; anthropology; *beginning of life; biology; embryo research; *embryos; fetal development; fetuses; historical aspects; human characteristics; human rights; international aspects; legal aspects; moral policy; morality; *personhood; philosophy; preimplantation diagnosis; prenatal diagnosis; public policy; reproductive technologies; *Roman Catholic ethics; *theology; *value of life; abortion, spontaneous; personal identity; United Nations; Universal Declaration of Human Rights

Wadman, Meredith. NIH launches discussion of in utero gene therapy ... and seeks to repair 'flaw' in review process. [News]. *Nature.* 1998 Oct 1; 395(6701): 420. BE60261.
> advisory committees; federal government; *fetal therapy; *gene therapy; government regulation; human experimentation; newborns; pregnant women; *risks and benefits; thalassemia; immunologic deficiency syndromes; Anderson, W. French; *National Institutes of Health; *Recombinant DNA Advisory Committee; United States

Webb, Gilbert W.; Huddleston, John F. Management of the pregnant woman who sustains severe brain damage. *Clinics in Perinatology.* 1996 Sep; 23(3): 453-464. 50 refs. BE60934.
> allowing to die; autonomy; *brain pathology; economics; family members; fetal development; *fetuses; patient care; *persistent vegetative state; physicians; *pregnant women; *prolongation of life; resuscitation orders; third party consent; withholding treatment; Grady Memorial Hospital (Atlanta, GA)

Wendler, Dave. Understanding the 'conservative' view on abortion. *Bioethics.* 1999 Jan; 13(1): 32-56. 16 fn. BE60887.
> *abortion, induced; cryopreservation; *embryos; *fetal development; fetal therapy; *fetuses; genetic determinism; genetic information; in vitro fertilization; moral obligations; *moral policy; morality; *personhood; policy analysis; abortion, spontaneous; potentiality

Wheale, Peter R. Moral and legal consequences for the fetus/unborn child of medical technologies derived from human genome research. *In:* Glasner, Peter; Rothman, Harry, eds. Genetic Imaginations: Ethical, Legal and Social Issues in Human Genome Research. Brookfield, VT: Ashgate; 1998: 83-96. 35 refs. Based on a paper presented at a workshop hosted by the Centre for Social and Economic Research at the University of the West of England; reprinted from *The Genetic Engineer and Biotechnologist*, 1995; 15(2-3). ISBN 1-84014-356-8. BE60020.
> abortion, induced; *beginning of life; coercion; *congenital disorders; deontological ethics; *embryo research; *embryos; ethical analysis; fetal development; *fetuses; genetic disorders; genetic screening; genome mapping; government regulation; *legal aspects; legal liability; *moral obligations; *moral policy; negligence; *personhood; pregnant women; prenatal injuries; *public policy; *quality of life; rights; *selective abortion; social impact; treatment refusal; utilitarianism; *value of life; *wrongful life; *Great Britain

Clinic plans to destroy unclaimed embryos. [News]. *New York Times.* 1999 Jul 13: F14. BE62546.
> *cryopreservation; *embryo disposition; *embryos; *health facilities; *in vitro fertilization; institutional policies; *Arizona Institute of Reproductive Medicine; United States

Court rules that fetuses are not "persons" entitled to be counted in the census: John Desmond Slattery v. William J. Clinton and William M. Daley, et al. (U.S. District Court, Southern District of New York, 1997). [News]. *Reporter on Human Reproduction and the Law.* 1997 Nov-Dec; No. 11-12: 62-63. BE60062.
> federal government; *fetuses; *legal aspects; *personhood; statistics; *Slattery v. Clinton and Daley; *United States

Judge orders divorcing couple's frozen embryos destroyed. [News]. *New York Times.* 1998 Sep 29: B6. BE60968.
> advance directives; contracts; cryopreservation; decision making; *dissent; *embryo disposition; *embryos; *in vitro fertilization; *legal aspects; married persons; *divorce; *New Jersey

No ABA embryo policy. [News]. *Washington Post.* 1998 Feb 3: A5. BE59675.

BE = bioethics accession number   fn. = footnotes   refs. = references

*cryopreservation; dissent; *embryo disposition; embryo transfer; *embryos; *in vitro fertilization; lawyers; *legal aspects; *organizational policies; professional organizations; property rights; divorce; *American Bar Association; United States

FINANCIAL SUPPORT See BIOMEDICAL
RESEARCH, HEALTH CARE/ECONOMICS
See under
ABORTION/FINANCIAL SUPPORT

FORCE FEEDING

Grubb, Andrew. Treatment without consent (anorexia nervosa): adult -- Riverside Mental Health Trust v. Fox. [Comment]. *Medical Law Review.* 1994 Spring; 2(1): 95–99. BE59904.
artificial feeding; *behavior disorders; females; *food; *force feeding; judicial action; *legal aspects; mentally ill; *treatment refusal; *anorexia nervosa; *Great Britain; *Riverside Mental Health NHS Trust v. Fox

Kennedy, Ian. Treatment without consent (adult): force feeding of detainee -- Department of Immigration v. Mok and Another. [Comment]. *Medical Law Review.* 1994 Spring; 2(1): 102–105. BE59905.
adults; *aliens; emergency care; *force feeding; law enforcement; *legal aspects; *prisoners; *treatment refusal; emigration and immigration; *Australia; *Department of Immigration v. Mok

Oliver, Jo. Anorexia and the refusal of medical treatment. *Victoria University of Wellington Law Review.* 1997 Dec; 27(4): 621–647. 105 fn. BE61524.
artificial feeding; autonomy; behavior disorders; *competence; females; food; *force feeding; *legal aspects; mentally ill; mothers; paternalism; *treatment refusal; *anorexia nervosa; *New Zealand; *Re CMC

FOREIGN COUNTRIES
See under
ABORTION/FOREIGN COUNTRIES
BEHAVIORAL RESEARCH/FOREIGN
COUNTRIES
HEALTH CARE/FOREIGN COUNTRIES
HUMAN EXPERIMENTATION/FOREIGN
COUNTRIES
INVOLUNTARY COMMITMENT/FOREIGN
COUNTRIES

FRAUD AND MISCONDUCT

Abbott, Alison. German scientists may escape fraud trial. [News]. *Nature.* 1998 Oct 8; 395(6702): 532–533. Includes inset article by A. Abbott, "Task force set up to determine the damage," p. 533. BE59642.
biomedical research; *fraud; investigators; *legal aspects; *scientific misconduct; universities; *Brach, Marion; *Germany; *Herrmann, Friedhelm; University of Ulm

Abbott, Alison. Science comes to terms with the lessons of fraud. [News]. *Nature.* 1999 Mar 4; 398(6722): 13–17. Includes inset articles, "Japanese scandals raise public distrust," by A. Saegusa, p. 14; "Editors debate whether to blow the whistle on suspect papers," p. 15; and "US stalks on new definitions of misconduct," by R. Dalton, p. 16. BE61866.
attitudes; biomedical research; due process; editorial policies; federal government; *fraud; government regulation; guidelines; *international aspects; interprofessional relations;

investigators; public policy; research institutes; *science; *scientific misconduct; *self regulation; social dominance; time factors; universities; whistleblowing; retraction of publication; Europe; Germany; Japan; United States

Altman, Ellen; Hernon, Peter, eds. Research Misconduct: Issues, Implications, and Strategies. Greenwich, CT: Ablex; 1997. 206 p. (Contemporary studies in information management, policy, and services). Bibliography: p. 187–194. ISBN 1–56750–341–1. BE62439.
attitudes; authorship; biomedical research; codes of ethics; conflict of interest; editorial policies; faculty; humanities; international aspects; investigators; journalism; professional organizations; regulation; science; *scientific misconduct; social sciences; students; survey; universities; publishing; retraction of publication; United States

Altman, Lawrence K. British cast spotlight on misconduct in scientific research. [News]. *New York Times.* 1998 Jun 9: F3. BE59608.
*biomedical research; community services; editorial policies; fraud; health services research; *international aspects; interprofessional relations; investigators; physically disabled; *scientific misconduct; self regulation; BMJ (British Medical Journal); Great Britain; United States; Williams, Mark H.

Angelides, Kimon; Pianelli, James V. It will take more than notebooks to stop fraud. [Letter]. *Nature.* 1998 Dec 3; 396(6710): 404. BE61089.
*accountability; *biomedical research; *records; *research institutes; *scientific misconduct; self regulation; standards

Annas, George J.; Grodin, Michael A. Reflections on the fiftieth anniversary of the Doctors' Trial. *Health and Human Rights.* 1996; 2(1): 7–21. 29 fn. BE62085.
force feeding; guidelines; *historical aspects; *human experimentation; *human rights; informed consent; *international aspects; *misconduct; *National Socialism; organizational policies; *physician's role; *physicians; prisoners; professional organizations; registries; self regulation; torture; British Medical Association; Germany; *Nuremberg Code; *Nuremberg Trials; Twentieth Century; World Medical Association

Baker, Robert. A theory of international bioethics: multiculturalism, postmodernism, and the bankruptcy of fundamentalism. *Kennedy Institute of Ethics Journal.* 1998 Sep; 8(3): 201–231. 33 refs. 9 fn. BE60166.
*accountability; advisory committees; animal experimentation; anthropology; autonomy; *bioethics; codes of ethics; communitarianism; compensation; consensus; *cultural pluralism; dehumanization; *ethical analysis; *ethical relativism; *ethical theory; eugenics; evaluation; *guidelines; historical aspects; *human experimentation; *human rights; informed consent; *international aspects; investigators; *misconduct; models, theoretical; *morality; *National Socialism; philosophy; physicians; *postmodernism; principle-based ethics; privacy; public policy; *radiation; research subjects; *retrospective moral judgment; *scientific misconduct; standards; terminology; *values; *culpability; slavery; *Advisory Committee on Human Radiation Experiments; Cold War; *Germany; Macklin, Ruth; Nuremberg Code; Nuremberg Trials; Twentieth Century; United States
The first of two articles analyzing the justifiability of international bioethical codes and of cross-cultural moral judgments reviews "moral fundamentalism," the theory that cross-cultural moral judgments and international bioethical codes are justified by certain "basic" or "fundamental" moral priniciples that are universally accepted in all cultures and eras. Initially propounded by the judges at the 1947 Nuremberg Tribunal, moral fundamentalism has become the received justification of international bioethics, and of cross-temporal and

---

BE = bioethics accession number   fn. = footnotes   refs. = references

cross–cultural moral judgments. Yet today we are said to live in a multicultural and postmodern world. This article assesses the challenges that multiculturalism and postmodernism pose to fundamentalism and concludes that these challenges render the position philosophically untenable, thereby undermining the received conception of the foundations of international bioethics. The second article, which follows, offers an alternative model –– a model of negotiated moral order –– as a viable justification for international bioethics and for transcultural and transtemporal moral judgments.

Balter, Michael. French AIDS research pioneers to testify in trial of ministers. [News]. *Science.* 1999 Feb 12; 283(5404): 910–911. BE61715.
    *AIDS; *AIDS serodiagnosis; blood donation; *blood transfusions; *criminal law; drug industry; economics; expert testimony; hemophilia; investigators; *legal aspects; legal liability; *misconduct; *politics; *France

Barondess, Jeremiah A. Care of the medical ethos: reflections on Social Darwinism, racial hygiene, and the Holocaust. *Annals of Internal Medicine.* 1998 Dec 1; 129(11): 891–898. 34 refs. BE59326.
    dehumanization; disabled; disadvantaged; *eugenics; evolution; genetics; health care delivery; *historical aspects; human experimentation; international aspects; investigators; involuntary euthanasia; involuntary sterilization; justice; killing; *medical ethics; *medicine; minority groups; *misconduct; *moral complicity; *National Socialism; physician's role; *physicians; prisoners; psychiatry; public health; public policy; science; suffering; values; Darwinism; *Germany; *Twentieth Century; United States

Bell, Elmerine Allen Whitfield. Testimony of Elmerine Allen Whitfield Bell [concerning human experimentation with plutonium]. *Accountability in Research.* 1998 Jan; 6(1–2): 167–181. Testimony delivered 18 Jan 1994 to the Subcommittee on Energy and Power of the Committee on Energy and Commerce, U.S. House of Representatives. BE61549.
    blacks; compensation; death; deception; disabled; disclosure; family members; federal government; *historical aspects; *human experimentation; indigents; information dissemination; informed consent; injuries; investigators; medical records; *nontherapeutic research; patients; physicians; public policy; *radiation; research subjects; *scientific misconduct; *Allen, Elmer; Department of Energy; *Twentieth Century; United States; *University of California, San Francisco

Biagioli, Mario. Publication and promotion: long live the deans! *Lancet.* 1998 Sep 12; 352(9131): 899–900. 1 ref. BE60145.
    *accountability; *authorship; *biomedical research; fraud; *investigators; *scientific misconduct; universities

Blumenthal, Ralph; Miller, Judith. Japanese germ–war atrocities: a half–century of stonewalling the world. *New York Times.* 1999 Mar 4: A12. BE60974.
    *biological warfare; dehumanization; disclosure; federal government; historical aspects; *human experimentation; investigators; military personnel; *misconduct; moral complicity; *prisoners; *public policy; records; *scientific misconduct; torture; China; *Japan; Twentieth Century; United States; *World War II

Boettcher, Brian. Fatal episodes in medical history. [Personal view]. *BMJ (British Medical Journal).* 1998 Dec 5; 317(7172): 1603. BE60265.
    alternative therapies; legal liability; medical education; mental institutions; mentally ill; *misconduct; mortality; *patient care; peer review; *physicians; *professional competence; psychiatry; regulation; social impact; standards;

*whistleblowing; deep sleep therapy; Australia; Chelmsford Private Hospital (Sydney); Royal Commission into Deep Sleep (Australia)

Breimer, Lars; Brown, Laura; Skinner, Andrew, et al. Fraud. [Letters]. *BMJ (British Medical Journal).* 1998 Dec 5; 317(7172): 1590–1591. 9 refs. BE61135.
    authorship; biomedical research; drug industry; economics; *fraud; guidelines; human experimentation; investigators; *regulation; *scientific misconduct; Great Britain

Briant, Robin H.; St. George, Ian M.; White, Gillian. Sexual activity between doctors and patients. [Letter and response]. *New Zealand Medical Journal.* 1996 Apr 12; 109(1019): 127–128. 9 refs. BE60086.
    attitudes; evaluation; family practice; *misconduct; morality; organizational policies; *physician patient relationship; *physicians; *sex offenses; standards; survey; Medical Council of New Zealand; *New Zealand

Burton, Thomas M. A prostate researcher tested firm's product –– and sat on its board. [News]. *Wall Street Journal.* 1998 Mar 19: A1, A8. BE59671.
    *biomedical research; *conflict of interest; disclosure; *drug industry; drugs; editorial policies; *financial support; fraud; investigators; medical devices; *misconduct; *physicians; *remuneration; surgery; *therapeutic research; *Oesterling, Joseph; University of Michigan

Butler, Declan. Fraud squad files report to prosecutor in INSERM case. [News]. *Nature.* 1998 Jul 23; 394(6691): 308. BE59936.
    biomedical research; fraud; industry; *investigators; legal aspects; patents; *research institutes; *scientific misconduct; universities; whistleblowing; *Bihain, Bernard; *France; Genset; *INSERM; University of Rennes

Charatan, Fred. Brazil challenges doctors accused of torture. [News]. *BMJ (British Medical Journal).* 1999 Mar 20; 318(7186): 757. BE62511.
    human rights; military personnel; *misconduct; *physicians; prisoners; professional organizations; self regulation; *torture; *Brazil

Cocks, Geoffrey. The old as new: the Nuremberg Doctors' Trial and medicine in modern Germany. *In:* Berg, Manfred; Cocks, Geoffrey, eds. Medicine and Modernity: Public Health and Medical Care in Nineteenth– and Twentieth–Century Germany. New York, NY: Cambridge University Press; 1997: 173–191. 71 fn. ISBN 0–521–56411–5. BE59270.
    aliens; disabled; eugenics; guidelines; *historical aspects; *human experimentation; investigators; Jews; killing; *misconduct; moral complicity; *National Socialism; nontherapeutic research; *physicians; politics; prisoners; public health; public policy; *scientific misconduct; social control; social discrimination; social dominance; *sociology of medicine; war; Declaration of Helsinki; *Germany; Nuremberg Code; *Nuremberg Trials; *Twentieth Century; World Medical Association; World War II

Cocks, Geoffrey. The old as new: the Nuremberg Doctors' Trial and medicine in modern Germany. *In: his* Treating Mind and Body: Essays in the History of Science, Professions, and Society Under Extreme Conditions. New Brunswick, NJ: Transaction Publishers; 1998: 193–213. 71 fn. ISBN 1–56000–310–3. BE62049.
    aliens; disabled; eugenics; guidelines; *historical aspects; *human experimentation; investigators; Jews; killing; *misconduct; moral complicity; *National Socialism; nontherapeutic research; *physicians; politics; prisoners; public health; public policy; *scientific misconduct; social control; social discrimination; social dominance; *sociology of medicine; war; *Germany; Guidelines for Novel

---

BE = bioethics accession number   fn. = footnotes   refs. = references

Treatment and for the Undertaking of Experiments on Humans 1931 (Germany); Nuremberg Trials; *Twentieth Century; World War II

Coghlan, Andy. Named and shamed: genetic engineers who flouted the rules are brought to book. [News]. *New Scientist.* 1998 Apr 4; 158(2128): 4. BE59716.
   disclosure; *ecology; *genetic intervention; *government regulation; *industry; investigators; research institutes; *scientific misconduct; transgenic organisms; *agriculture; *transgenic plants; Advisory Committee on Releases to the Environment (Great Britain); *Great Britain

Cohen, Jon. Research shutdown roils Los Angeles VA. [News]. *Science.* 1999 Apr 2; 284(5411): 18–19, 21. BE60847.
   administrators; animal experimentation; *federal government; *government regulation; *human experimentation; public hospitals; research ethics committees; *scientific misconduct; Department of Veterans Affairs; Los Angeles; Office for Protection from Research Risks; United States; *West Los Angeles Veterans Affairs Medical Center

Cowen, Robert C. Academics face abuse of rules designed to protect research. *Christian Science Monitor.* 1998 Mar 25: 13. BE59606.
   *biomedical research; conflict of interest; drug industry; *due process; *financial support; information dissemination; interprofessional relations; *investigators; political activity; science; *scientific misconduct; self regulation; universities; *whistleblowing; United States

Dalton, Rex. Arizona professor files lawsuit after being fired for misconduct. [News]. *Nature.* 1998 Aug 27; 394(6696): 817. BE60633.
   biomedical research; fraud; investigators; *scientific misconduct; self regulation; universities; Arizona; *Kay, Marguerite; University of Arizona

Dalton, Rex. Federal panel endorses Baylor fraud claim. [News]. *Nature.* 1999 Feb 18; 397(6720): 549. BE60636.
   biomedical research; federal government; *fraud; government regulation; legal aspects; *scientific misconduct; self regulation; universities; *Angelides, Kimon; Baylor College of Medicine; United States

Dalton, Rex. Salk Institute investigated after claims of inhumane research. [News]. *Nature.* 1998 Aug 20; 394(6695): 709. BE61108.
   administrators; animal care committees; *animal experimentation; employment; federal government; *government regulation; interprofessional relations; investigators; research institutes; *scientific misconduct; self regulation; whistleblowing; Department of Agriculture; National Institutes of Health; Office for Protection from Research Risks; *Salk Institute; Sylvina, Teresa; United States

David, Edward E. Non–starters and no brainers: an outside perspective. *Accountability in Research.* 1997; 5(4): 255–263. Paper presented at the symposium, "Ethical Issues in Research Relationships between Universities and Industry," held in Baltimore, MD, 3–4 Nov 1995. BE60423.
   *biomedical research; *conflict of interest; disclosure; financial support; guidelines; *industry; investigators; peer review; property rights; *scientific misconduct; *universities; National Academy of Sciences; National Institutes of Health; National Science Foundation; United States

Djerassi, Carl. Who will mentor the mentors? *Nature.* 1999 Jan 28; 397(6717): 291. BE60959.
   authorship; biomedical research; communication; *faculty;

Dwyer, James; Shih, Anthony. The ethics of tailoring the patient's chart. *Psychiatric Services.* 1998 Oct; 49(10): 1309–1312. 16 refs. BE61447.
   beneficence; case studies; dangerousness; *deception; depressive disorder; health insurance reimbursement; involuntary commitment; legal liability; malpractice; managed care programs; *medical records; *mentally ill; *moral policy; *motivation; patient care; *physicians; *psychiatry; referral and consultation; resource allocation; schizophrenia; suicide; trust

Dyer, Owen. GP found guilty of forging trial consent forms. [News]. *BMJ (British Medical Journal).* 1998 Nov 28; 317(7171): 1475. BE60954.
   *consent forms; *fraud; *human experimentation; *informed consent; *physicians; punishment; *scientific misconduct; *Bochsler, James; *General Medical Council (Great Britain); *Great Britain

Egilman, David; Wallace, Wes; Stubbs, Cassandra, et al. A little too much of the Buchenwald touch? Military radiation research at the University of Cincinnati, 1960–1972. *Accountability in Research.* 1998 Jan; 6(1–2): 63–102. 83 refs. BE61535.
   adults; advisory committees; bone marrow; cancer; children; compensation; competence; conflict of interest; consent forms; death; deception; disadvantaged; disclosure; editorial policies; federal government; government financing; guideline adherence; guidelines; *historical aspects; hospitals; *human experimentation; informed consent; injuries; investigators; military personnel; mortality; *nontherapeutic research; nuclear warfare; *patients; physicians; professional organizations; public policy; *radiation; research design; research ethics committees; research subjects; review committees; risk; *scientific misconduct; selection of subjects; self regulation; therapeutic research; tissue transplantation; universities; withholding treatment; Advisory Committee on Human Radiation Experiments; American College of Radiology; Atomic Energy Commission; *Department of Defense; Ohio; *Saenger, Eugene; *Twentieth Century; *United States; *University of Cincinnati

Egilman, David; Wallace, Wes; Hom, Candace. Corporate corruption of medical literature: asbestos studies concealed by W.R. Grace & Co. *Accountability in Research.* 1998 Jan; 6(1–2): 127–147. 76 refs. BE61547.
   animal experimentation; biomedical research; cancer; compensation; contracts; *deception; *disclosure; economics; employment; *epidemiology; federal government; financial support; government regulation; *health hazards; *industry; information dissemination; injuries; institutional ethics; insurance; investigators; legal liability; *morbidity; mortality; *occupational exposure; *scientific misconduct; *lung diseases; Montana; National Institutes of Occupational Safety and Health; United States; *W.R. Grace & Co.

Egilman, David; Wallace, Wes; Stubbs, Cassandra, et al. Ethical aerobics: ACHRE's flight from responsibility. *Accountability in Research.* 1998 Jan; 6(1–2): 15–61. 94 refs. BE61534.
   advisory committees; cancer; children; codes of ethics; committee membership; *compensation; *conflict of interest; consensus; disclosure; ethical relativism; *evaluation; *federal government; *historical aspects; *human experimentation; *informed consent; *injuries; international aspects; investigators; legal aspects; medical ethics; military personnel; morbidity; mortality; National Socialism; *nontherapeutic research; patient care; patients; physicians; politics; prisoners; professional organizations; *public policy; *radiation; research subjects; retrospective moral judgment;

*risk; *scientific misconduct; *standards; volunteers; culpability; recontact; *Advisory Committee on Human Radiation Experiments; American Medical Association; Cold War; Declaration of Helsinki; Faden, Ruth; Feinberg, Kenneth; Katz, Jay; Nuremberg Code; *Twentieth Century; *United States; World Medical Association

Eichenwald, Kurt; Kolata, Gina. A doctor's drug studies turn into fraud. [Research for hire: second of two articles]. *New York Times.* 1999 May 17: A1, A16. BE61175.
biomedical research; coercion; *conflict of interest; *drug industry; *drugs; economics; *entrepreneurship; federal government; financial support; *fraud; government regulation; *human experimentation; *incentives; investigators; managed care programs; misconduct; patient care; *physicians; *remuneration; research subjects; *scientific misconduct; *selection of subjects; trends; *private practice; California; *Fiddes, Robert; Food and Drug Administration; Southern California Research Institute; United States

Eichenwald, Kurt; Kolata, Gina. Drug trials hide conflicts for doctors. [Research for hire: first of two articles]. *New York Times.* 1999 May 16: 1, 34. BE61174.
authorship; biomedical research; coercion; *conflict of interest; contracts; disclosure; *drug industry; *drugs; economics; *entrepreneurship; *human experimentation; *incentives; investigators; misconduct; nurses; *physicians; professional competence; *remuneration; research ethics committees; *selection of subjects; trends; universities; *private practice; United States

Enbom, John A.; Thomas, Claire D. Evaluation of sexual misconduct complaints: the Oregon Board of Medical Examiners, 1991 to 1995. [Article and discussion]. *American Journal of Obstetrics and Gynecology.* 1997 Jun; 176(6): 1340–1348. 22 refs. BE59373.
age factors; comparative studies; emergency care; family practice; females; government regulation; internal medicine; males; medical specialties; *misconduct; obstetrics and gynecology; *physician patient relationship; *physicians; psychiatry; punishment; radiology; *sex offenses; *sexuality; sports medicine; state government; statistics; surgery; survey; *Oregon; *Oregon Board of Medical Examiners

Faden, Ruth; Guttman, Dan. In response: speaking truth to historiography. *Medical Humanities Review.* 1997 Fall; 11(2): 37–43. 6 fn. Commentary on R. Martensen, p. 21–36. BE59809.
*advisory committees; biomedical research; entrepreneurship; ethical analysis; *evaluation; *federal government; financial support; government financing; government regulation; guidelines; *historical aspects; *human experimentation; informed consent; investigators; motivation; nontherapeutic research; physicians; politics; public participation; *public policy; *radiation; research subjects; *scientific misconduct; universities; *Advisory Committee on Human Radiation Experiments; Twentieth Century; *United States; University of California, Berkeley

Faraone, Stephen V.; Gottesman, Irving I.; Tsuang, Ming T. Fifty years of the Nuremberg Code: a time for retrospection and introspection. [Editorial]. *American Journal of Medical Genetics.* 1997 Jul 25; 74(4): 345–347. 16 refs. Includes text of the Nuremberg Code. BE59128.
codes of ethics; eugenics; *genetic research; *genetics; genome mapping; historical aspects; *human experimentation; *investigators; involuntary euthanasia; involuntary sterilization; medical ethics; *misconduct; National Socialism; *physicians; *psychiatry; Germany; Nuremberg Code; Twentieth Century

Farthing, Michael J.G. Fraud in medicine: coping with fraud. *Lancet.* 1998 Dec 19–26; 352 (Suppl. 4): 11. 5 refs.

BE60146.
authorship; *biomedical research; *editorial policies; fraud; international aspects; investigators; *regulation; *scientific misconduct; BMJ (British Medical Journal); *Committee on Publication Ethics (Great Britain); General Medical Council (Great Britain); *Great Britain; JAMA

Gabbard, Glen O. Lessons to be learned from the study of sexual boundary violations. *American Journal of Psychotherapy.* 1996 Summer; 50(3): 311–322. 17 refs. BE62054.
health personnel; intention; love; *misconduct; privacy; *professional patient relationship; *psychotherapy; referral and consultation; self regulation; *sex offenses; sexuality

Gaudiani, Vincent A. It's the patient. [Editorial]. *Pharos.* 1996 Fall; 59(4): 33. BE59699.
biomedical research; health care delivery; historical aspects; international aspects; managed care programs; *misconduct; National Socialism; *physician patient relationship; *physicians; *scientific misconduct; *trends; Germany; Twentieth Century; United States

Gifford, Fred. Teaching scientific integrity. *Centennial Review.* 1994 Spring; 38(2): 297–314. 6 fn. BE59404.
*biomedical research; conflict of interest; curriculum; deception; *education; federal government; fraud; government regulation; interprofessional relations; *investigators; motivation; negligence; *professional ethics; science; *scientific misconduct; self regulation; *students; teaching methods; truth disclosure; *universities; Michigan State University; National Institutes of Health; United States

Grady, Denise. Fraud found in analyzing breast cancer. [News]. *New York Times.* 1999 Feb 6: A13. BE61124.
*breast cancer; federal government; *fraud; *government regulation; *human experimentation; medical records; nurses; *scientific misconduct; National Cancer Institute; *National Surgical Adjuvant Breast and Bowel Project; Office of Research Integrity; Philpot, Thomas; tamoxifen

Greenfield, Barak; Kaufman, Jeffrey L.; Hueston, William J., et al. Authors vs contributors: accuracy, accountability, and responsibility. [Letters and response]. *JAMA.* 1998 Feb 4; 279(5): 356–357. 6 refs. BE59225.
*accountability; *authorship; *biomedical research; *scientific misconduct

Guenin, Louis M. The logical geography of concepts and shared responsibilities concerning research misconduct. *Academic Medicine.* 1996 Jun; 71(6): 595–603. 14 refs. BE61427.
*accountability; biomedical research; codes of ethics; due process; *federal government; government financing; *government regulation; industry; investigators; professional ethics; professional organizations; punishment; science; *scientific misconduct; *self regulation; standards; state interest; *universities; Office of Research Integrity; *United States

Guston, David H. The demise of the social contract for science: misconduct in science and the nonmodern world. *Centennial Review.* 1994 Spring; 38(2): 215–248. 80 refs. 45 fn. BE59402.
biomedical research; economics; federal government; government financing; *government regulation; investigators; *politics; *science; *scientific misconduct; *self regulation; universities; whistleblowing; *National Institutes of Health; *Office of Scientific Integrity; *U.S. Congress; *United States

Hammerschmidt, Dale E. "There is no substantive due process right to conduct human-subject research": the saga of the Minnesota Gamma Hydroxybutyrate Study.

IRB: A Review of Human Subjects Research. 1997 May–Aug; 19(3–4): 13–15. 2 fn. BE60214.
    drug abuse; *due process; *ethical review; *human experimentation; informed consent; investigational drugs; *investigators; judicial action; *legal aspects; legal liability; legal rights; punishment; *research ethics committees; research subjects; *scientific misconduct; universities; University of Minnesota

Hannibal, Kari; Lawrence, Robert S. The health professional as human rights promoter: ten years of Physicians for Human Rights (USA). *Health and Human Rights.* 1996; 2(1): 111–127. 9 fn. BE62087.
    dissent; education; health; *human rights; information dissemination; *international aspects; killing; *misconduct; *physicians; *political activity; prisoners; professional organizations; torture; war; *Physicians for Human Rights; United States

Hilts, Philip J. Duke's plan ends the ban on research. [News]. *New York Times.* 1999 May 15: A10. BE61699.
    federal government; *government regulation; *human experimentation; organization and administration; research ethics committees; *scientific misconduct; self regulation; *universities; *Duke University Medical Center; *Office for Protection from Research Risks; United States

Hilts, Philip J.; Stolberg, Sheryl Gay. Ethics lapses at Duke halt dozens of human experiments. [News]. *New York Times.* 1999 May 13: A26. BE61698.
    disclosure; federal government; *government regulation; *human experimentation; informed consent; injuries; nontherapeutic research; organization and administration; research ethics committees; research subjects; *scientific misconduct; universities; volunteers; *Duke University Medical Center; *Office for Protection from Research Risks; United States

Hilts, Philip J. Psychiatric unit's ethics faulted. [News]. *New York Times.* 1998 May 28: A26. BE59614.
    federal government; *government regulation; *human experimentation; informed consent; *mentally ill; psychoactive drugs; research institutes; schizophrenia; *scientific misconduct; *withholding treatment; *Office for Protection from Research Risks; *University of Maryland at Baltimore

Hilts, Philip J. V.A. hospital is told to halt all research. [News]. *New York Times.* 1999 Mar 25: A25. BE60872.
    administrators; animal experimentation; *federal government; *government regulation; *human experimentation; informed consent; *mentally ill; psychoactive drugs; *public hospitals; research ethics committees; *scientific misconduct; withholding treatment; Department of Veterans Affairs; Los Angeles; Office for Protection from Research Risks; United States; *West Los Angeles Veterans Affairs Medical Center

Horton, Richard. Scientific misconduct: exaggerated fear but still real and requiring a proportionate response. *Lancet.* 1999 Jul 3; 354(9172): 7–8. 15 refs. BE62408.
    attitudes; biomedical research; due process; editorial policies; government regulation; international aspects; investigators; physician patient relationship; professional autonomy; *regulation; review committees; *scientific misconduct; trust; Europe; Scandinavia; United States

Kaiser, Jocelyn. Baylor saga comes to an end. [News]. *Science.* 1999 Feb 19; 283(5405): 1091. BE60951.
    biomedical research; federal government; *fraud; *government regulation; investigators; *legal aspects; legal liability; medical schools; *scientific misconduct; self regulation; universities; *Angelides, Kimon; Association of American Medical Colleges; *Baylor College of Medicine; *Department of Health and Human Services; Office of

Research Integrity; *United States

Kaiser, Jocelyn. ORI report tracks gun-shy feds. [News]. *Science.* 1999 May 7; 284(5416): 901. BE61772.
    biomedical research; faculty; federal government; *government regulation; punishment; *scientific misconduct; *self regulation; statistics; *universities; whistleblowing; *Office of Research Integrity; Public Health Service; *United States

Kaiser, Jocelyn. Tulane inquiry clears lead researcher. [News]. *Science.* 1999 Jun 18; 284(5422): 1905. BE61774.
    biomedical research; *fraud; investigators; *scientific misconduct; universities; *Arnold, Steven; *McLachlan, John; *Tulane University Medical Center

Kakkar, Supriya. Unauthorized embryo transfer at the University of California, Irvine Center for Reproductive Health. [Note]. *Hastings Constitutional Law Quarterly.* 1997 Summer; 24(4): 1015–1033. 168 fn. BE62167.
    children; constitutional law; contracts; cryopreservation; embryo disposition; *embryo transfer; embryos; genetic materials; health facilities; in vitro fertilization; industry; *legal aspects; *misconduct; *parent child relationship; physicians; privacy; property rights; *reproductive technologies; standards; *United States; *University of California, Irvine Center for Reproductive Health

Kalb, Paul E. Health care fraud and abuse. *JAMA.* 1999 Sep 22–29; 282(12): 1163–1168. 63 refs. BE62659.
    conflict of interest; *economics; federal government; *fraud; government financing; *government regulation; *health insurance reimbursement; health personnel; *law enforcement; legal liability; legislation; *physician self-referral; *remuneration; state government; whistleblowing; Ethics in Patient Referral Act 1998; False Claims Act; *United States

In recent years, health care fraud and abuse have become major issues, in part because of the rising cost of health care, industry consolidation, the emergence of private "whistle-blowers," and a change in the concept of fraud to include an emerging concern about quality of care. The 3 types of conduct that are generally prohibited by health care fraud laws are false claims, kickbacks, and self-referrals. False claims are subject to several criminal, civil, and administrative prohibitions, notably the federal civil False Claims Act. Kickbacks, or inducements with the intent to influence the purchase or sale of health care–related goods or services, are prohibited under the federal Anti-Kickback statute as well as by state laws. Finally, self-referrals -- the referral of patients to an entity with which the referring physician has a financial relationship -- are outlawed by the Ethics in Patient Referral Act as well as numerous state statutes. Consequences of violations of these laws can include, in addition to imprisonment and fines, civil monetary penalties, loss of licensure, loss of staff privileges, and exclusion from participation in federal health care programs. Federal criminal and civil statutes are enforced by the US Department of Justice; administrative actions are pursued by the Department of Health and Human Services' Office of Inspector General; and all state actions are pursued by the individual states. In addition, private whistle-blowers may, acting in the name of the United States, file suit against an entity under the False Claims Act. Enforcement of health care fraud and abuse laws has become increasingly commonplace and now affects many mainstream providers. This trend is likely to continue.

Kater, Michael H. The Sewering scandal of 1993 and the German medical establishment. *In:* Berg, Manfred;

BE = bioethics accession number   fn. = footnotes   refs. = references

Cocks, Geoffrey, eds. Medicine and Modernity: Public Health and Medical Care in Nineteenth- and Twentieth-Century Germany. New York, NY: Cambridge University Press; 1997: 213–234. 109 fn. ISBN 0–521–56411–5. BE59272.
    historical aspects; *international aspects; *involuntary euthanasia; killing; mass media; medical education; medical ethics; mentally disabled; *misconduct; moral complicity; *National Socialism; organizational policies; *physicians; *professional organizations; self regulation; *sociology of medicine; American Medical Association; *German Chamber of Physicians; *Germany; *Sewering, Hans-Joachim; Twentieth Century; Vilmar, Karsten; *World Medical Association

Kenyon, Georgina. Australian army infected troops and internees in Second World War. [News]. BMJ (British Medical Journal). 1999 May 8; 318(7193): 1233. BE62517.
    communicable diseases; drugs; *historical aspects; *human experimentation; Jews; military personnel; *nontherapeutic research; prisoners; *public policy; *scientific misconduct; malaria; *Australia; Twentieth Century; World War II

Kevles, Daniel J. Star chambers will result in injustice. [Letter]. Nature. 1998 Sep 24; 395(6700): 317. BE61109.
    *biomedical research; due process; federal government; fraud; *government regulation; *investigators; *legal rights; *scientific misconduct; Baltimore, David; *Imanishi-Kari, Thereza; *Office of Research Integrity; *United States

Kevles, Daniel J. The Baltimore Case: A Trial of Politics, Science, and Character. New York, NY: Norton; 1998. 509 p. 1,054 fn. ISBN 0–393–04103–4. BE60016.
    *biomedical research; *due process; famous persons; federal government; *fraud; government regulation; historical aspects; interprofessional relations; *investigators; *politics; science; *scientific misconduct; universities; whistleblowing; *Baltimore, David; Cell; *Dingell, John; Feder, Ned; Hadley, Suzanne; *Imanishi-Kari, Thereza; Massachusetts Institute of Technology; National Institutes of Health; *O'Toole, Margot; Office of Research Integrity; Office of Scientific Integrity; Rockefeller University; Stewart, Walter; Twentieth Century; U.S. Congress; *United States

Kirp, David L. Blood, sweat, and tears: the Tuskegee experiment and the era of AIDS. Tikkun. 1995 May–Jun; 10(3): 50–54. BE61473.
    *AIDS; *attitudes; *blacks; deception; federal government; historical aspects; homosexuals; *human experimentation; investigators; morbidity; mortality; motivation; nontherapeutic research; physicians; public health; public policy; radiation; research design; research subjects; *scientific misconduct; social discrimination; syphilis; *trust; vulnerable populations; whites; withholding treatment; Centers for Disease Control and Prevention; Foster, Henry; Public Health Service; *Tuskegee Syphilis Study; Twentieth Century; United States

Kissell, Judith Lee. Complicity in thought and language: toleration of wrong. Journal of Medical Humanities. 1999 Spring; 20(1): 49–60. 20 refs. 14 fn. BE61729.
    *accountability; bioethical issues; biomedical research; communication; famous persons; historical aspects; *misconduct; *moral complicity; moral development; *moral obligations; National Socialism; obligations to society; social discrimination; slavery; Germany; Pius XII, Pope; United States; Wythe, George

Lagnado, Lucette. Transplant patients ply an illicit market for vital medicines. [News]. Wall Street Journal. 1999 Jun 21: 1, A8. BE62450.
    *drugs; *economics; health insurance reimbursement; health personnel; hospitals; institutional policies; legal aspects; *misconduct; motivation; *organ transplantation; *patient care; patients; *transplant recipients; Medicaid; Medicare;

United States

Larkin, Marilynn. Whose article is it anyway? Lancet. 1999 Jul 10; 354(9173): 136. BE62411.
    *authorship; *biomedical research; conflict of interest; deception; disclosure; *drug industry; *editorial policies; *financial support; information dissemination; investigators; peer review; *scientific misconduct

Loff, Bebe; Cordner, Stephen. Learning a culture of respect for human rights. [Commentary]. Lancet. 1998 Dec 5; 352(9143): 1800. 3 refs. BE60803.
    disadvantaged; forensic medicine; *health care delivery; *human rights; *minority groups; *misconduct; *physicians; *prisoners; *social discrimination; torture; *aborigines; *Australia; *South Africa

Loff, Bebe; Cordner, Stephen. World War II malaria trials revisited. [News]. Lancet. 1999 May 8; 353(9164): 1597. BE62529.
    communicable diseases; drugs; *historical aspects; *human experimentation; Jews; military personnel; *nontherapeutic research; prisoners; *public policy; *scientific misconduct; malaria; *Australia; Twentieth Century; World War II

Luna, Florencia. Corruption and research. Bioethics. 1999 Jul; 13(3–4): 262–271. 19 fn. BE61877.
    *biomedical research; developing countries; ethical relativism; *human experimentation; incentives; *international aspects; investigators; legal aspects; *misconduct; politics; regulation; remuneration; research design; research ethics committees; *scientific misconduct; selection of subjects; socioeconomic factors; bribes; *multicenter studies
    Last year there was a heated debate regarding clinical trials with AZT carried out in developing countries. AIDS vaccine trials also posed various dilemmas and ethical problems. In this paper I will consider the possibility of corruption in bioethics, and international multi-centre research will be taken as an example. International clinical trials will be seen from another perspective. I will try to show that the possibility of systemic corruption should be considered when designing an international multi-centre research trial which may involve countries in very different situations regarding corruption. I will analyze three different approaches to this problem and suggest some strategies regarding their capacity to exclude the possibility of corruption.

McCaffery, Margo; Ferrell, Betty Rolling. Pain and placebos: ethical and professional issues. [Editorial]. Orthopaedic Nursing. 1997 Sep–Oct; 16(5): 8–11. 22 refs. Commentary on J. Brown et al., "Placebos and the need for good communication," ON 1997 Apr–May; 16(3): 61–65. BE60263.
    *attitudes; *deception; guideline adherence; health facilities; institutional policies; knowledge, attitudes, practice; misconduct; motivation; *nurses; *organizational policies; *pain; patient advocacy; *patient care; *placebos; practice guidelines; *professional organizations; risks and benefits; trust; analgesia

Macklin, Ruth. A defense of fundamental principles and human rights: a reply to Robert Baker. Kennedy Institute of Ethics Journal. 1998 Dec; 8(4): 403–422. 15 refs. 6 fn. BE62376.
    accountability; advisory committees; autonomy; beneficence; *bioethics; circumcision; coercion; communitarianism; *cultural pluralism; dissent; *ethical analysis; *ethical relativism; *ethical theory; females; historical aspects; *human experimentation; *human rights; informed consent; *international aspects; investigators; *misconduct; *morality; *National Socialism; *non-Western World; nontherapeutic

research; physicians; *postmodernism; principle-based ethics; *radiation; research subjects; *retrospective moral judgment; *scientific misconduct; values; *Western World; women's rights; *culpability; *Advisory Committee on Human Radiation Experiments; Asia; Germany; Twentieth Century; United States

This article seeks to rebut Robert Baker's contention that attempts to ground international bioethics in fundamental principles cannot withstand the challenges posed by multiculturalism and postmodernism. First, several corrections are provided of Baker's account of the conclusions reached by the Advisory Committee on Human Radiation Experiments. Second, a rebuttal is offered to Baker's claim that an unbridgeable moral gap exists between Western individualism and non–Western communalism. In conclusion, this article argues that Baker's "nonnegotiable primary goods" cannot do the work of "classical human rights" and that the latter framework is preferable from both a practical and a theoretical standpoint.

Maloney, Dennis M. Researchers and the privacy act: Fisher v. National Institutes of Health (Part I). *Human Research Report.* 1998 Sep; 13(9): 4–5. BE61728.
   biomedical research; *confidentiality; data banks; disclosure; *federal government; *investigators; *legal aspects; privacy; records; *scientific misconduct; *Fisher v. National Institutes of Health; *Fisher, Bernard; National Surgical Adjuvant Breast and Bowel Project; *Privacy Act 1974; United States

Marshall, Eliot. Investigations on trial in a Texas court. [News]. *Science.* 1999 Feb 12; 283(5404): 913–914. BE61131.
   biomedical research; due process; federal government; fraud; government regulation; investigators; *legal aspects; *scientific misconduct; self regulation; universities; *Angelides, Kimon; Baylor College of Medicine; Department of Health and Human Services; Office of Research Integrity; Texas; United States

Marshall, Eliot. Shutdown of research at Duke sends a message. [News]. *Science.* 1999 May 21; 284(5418): 1246. BE61773.
   administrators; federal government; government financing; *government regulation; hospitals; *human experimentation; research ethics committees; *scientific misconduct; universities; *Duke University Medical Center; *Office for Protection from Research Risks; United States

Martensen, Robert. If only it were so: medical physics, U.S. human radiation experiments, and the *Final Report* of the President's Advisory Committee (ACHRE). *Medical Humanities Review.* 1997 Fall; 11(2): 21–36. 26 fn. Commented on by R. Faden and Dan Guttman, p. 37–43. BE59808.
   *advisory committees; *biomedical research; cancer; conflict of interest; disclosure; drug industry; entrepreneurship; ethical analysis; ethical review; ethicist's role; *evaluation; *federal government; *financial support; government financing; government regulation; guidelines; *historical aspects; *human experimentation; informed consent; investigators; justice; motivation; physicians; policy analysis; politics; *public policy; *radiation; research subjects; resource allocation; science; *scientific misconduct; standards; trust; universities; *Advisory Committee on Human Radiation Experiments; Department of Energy; *Twentieth Century; *United States; University of California, Berkeley

Meguid, Michael M. Editors' responsibility in defeating fraud. [Letter]. *Nature.* 1999 May 6; 399(6731): 13. BE62566.
   biomedical research; *disclosure; *editorial policies; fraud;

moral obligations; organizational policies; *scientific misconduct; Nutrition

Nylenna, Magne; Andersen, Daniel; Dahlquist, Gisela, et al.; National Committees on Scientific Dishonesty in the Nordic Countries. Handling of scientific dishonesty in the Nordic countries. *Lancet.* 1999 Jul 3; 354(9172): 57–61. 23 refs. BE62410.
   authorship; biomedical research; committee membership; comparative studies; drug industry; international aspects; investigators; misconduct; peer review; public policy; *regulation; *review committees; *scientific misconduct; statistics; publishing; *Denmark; *Finland; *Norway; *Scandinavia; *Sweden

Despite a widely recognised need, most countries still have no coherent system to deal with scientific misconduct. Committees have been established by the national medical research councils in Denmark (1992), Norway (1994), and Sweden (1997), and by the Ministry of Education in Finland (1994), to deal with scientific misconduct -- i.e., to initiate preventive measures, to investigate alleged cases, or both. Each committee includes both scientifically and legally qualified members. The employing institutions are responsible for possible sanctions or punishments. So far, 47 cases have been accepted for investigation, the majority (25) being Danish. Disputed authorship was the most frequent reason for investigation. Junior researchers made complaints in only three of the investigated cases. Investigations have been completed in 37 cases; in nine cases, dishonesty was revealed -- two of them were related to the same researchers. Cooperation between the four Nordic committees has shown close agreement on specific issues and cases, despite minor differences in definitions, organisation, and procedures.

O'Rourke, Dennis. Half Life: A Parable for the Nuclear Age. [Videorecording]. Available from Direct Cinema Ltd., P.O. Box 69799, Los Angeles, CA, 90069, (213)396–4774; 1986. Videocassette; 86 min.; sd., color; VHS. ISBN 1-55974-135-X. Written, directed, and produced by Dennis O'Rourke. BE62227.
   cancer; deception; developing countries; federal government; genetic disorders; health hazards; *human experimentation; injuries; *morbidity; *nontherapeutic research; *nuclear warfare; *public policy; *radiation; *scientific misconduct; Atomic Energy Commission; Department of Energy; *Micronesia; *United States

Panush, Richard S. Upon finding a Nazi anatomy atlas: the lessons of Nazi medicine. *Pharos.* 1996 Fall; 59(4): 18–22. 26 refs. BE59697.
   active euthanasia; assisted suicide; biomedical research; capital punishment; dehumanization; economics; eugenics; health care delivery; *historical aspects; human experimentation; *international aspects; involuntary sterilization; *killing; literature; medical education; medical ethics; minority groups; *misconduct; moral complicity; *National Socialism; physician patient relationship; *physicians; prisoners; *scientific misconduct; social discrimination; torture; *trends; *values; genocide; medical illustration; Austria; *Germany; *Pernkopf Anatomy (Pernkopf, E.); *Twentieth Century; United States

Perry, Clifton; Kuruc, Joan Wallman. Psychotherapists' sexual relationships with their patients. *Annals of Health Law.* 1993; 2: 35–54. 126 fn. BE59827.
   compensation; criminal law; *health personnel; *legal aspects; legal liability; legislation; malpractice; mentally ill; *misconduct; *professional patient relationship; psychological stress; *psychotherapy; sex offenses; *sexuality; state government; torts; *United States

---

BE = bioethics accession number   fn. = footnotes   refs. = references

Pownall, Mark. Falsifying data is main problem in US research fraud review. [News]. *BMJ (British Medical Journal)*. 1999 May 1; 318(7192): 1164. BE62422.
   biomedical research; faculty; federal government; fraud; government financing; government regulation; *investigators; *scientific misconduct; statistics; whistleblowing; Office of Research Integrity; Public Health Service; Scientific Misconduct Investigations 1993–1997 (ORI); United States

Ramsay, Sarah. UK "Bristol case" inquiry formally opened. [News]. *Lancet.* 1999 Mar 20; 353(9157): 987. BE61957.
   children; heart diseases; hospitals; *misconduct; morbidity; mortality; patient care; *pediatrics; *physicians; *professional competence; quality of health care; self regulation; *surgery; technical expertise; Bristol; General Medical Council (Great Britain); *Great Britain; National Health Service

Resnik, David B. The Ethics of Science: An Introduction. New York, NY: Routledge; 1998. 221 p. (Philosophical issues in science). Bibliography: 206–216. ISBN 0–415–16698–5. BE61844.
   animal experimentation; authorship; *biomedical research; case studies; conflict of interest; ecology; economics; education; ethical theory; expert testimony; faculty; fraud; goals; government financing; human experimentation; industry; information dissemination; interprofessional relations; *investigators; mass media; obligations to society; patents; peer review; *professional ethics; property rights; *science; *scientific misconduct; self regulation; standards; students; values; whistleblowing; publishing; *research ethics

Richards, Karlotta A.; Noblin, Charles D. Sanctions for ethics violations: does licensure of socioeconomic status matter? *Ethics and Behavior.* 1999; 9(2): 119–126. 10 refs. BE61784.
   *attitudes; comparative studies; education; evaluation studies; *government regulation; guidelines; *health personnel; *misconduct; *patients; professional organizations; *professional patient relationship; *psychology; psychotherapy; *punishment; *sex offenses; *sexuality; *socioeconomic factors; state government; American Psychological Association; Mississippi
Although sexual relationships between therapists and their clients are unethical, such beahviors still occur. This study investigated whether psychologists with applied versus nonapplied training differed in the severity of sanctions advocated for psychologists charged with sexual ethical violations toward high- or low–socioeconomic status victims. Licensed and Nonlicensed psychologists (N=48) viewed a 15–min videotape simulating the adjudication process about an alleged sexual involvement between client and psychologist, then prescribed either: Dismissal of Charges, Educative Advisory, Educative Warning, Reprimand, Censure, Stipulated Resignation, Permitted Resignation, or Expulsion. The alleged victim was described as a college professor of home economics or a hairdresser. Licensed psychologists chose more severe sanctions ("Stipulated or Permitted Resignation") than did Nonlicensed psychologists ("Censure").
Socioeconomic status made no significant difference in sanctions. Apparently, applied therapy training results in more severe judgements toward those who violate American Psychological Association ethical guidelines than other types of psychology training.

Riggs, Garrett. What should we do about Eduard Pernkopf's atlas? *Academic Medicine.* 1998 Apr; 73(4): 380–386. 43 refs. BE59877.
   biomedical research; *cadavers; historical aspects; killing;

*literature; medical education; *medicine; *misconduct; moral complicity; *National Socialism; *physicians; prisoners; wedge argument; *medical illustration; Austria; *Pernkopf Anatomy (Pernkopf, E.); *Pernkopf, Eduard; Twentieth Century

Roberts, E. Francine. Academic misconduct in schools of nursing. *NursingConnections.* 1997 Fall; 10(3): 28–36. 24 refs. BE59191.
   attitudes; faculty; institutional policies; *misconduct; moral development; nurses; *nursing education; *nursing ethics; schools; *students; teaching methods

Saegusa, Asako. Private deal puts Japanese researcher in hot water. [News]. *Nature.* 1998 Nov 19; 396(6708): 205. BE59643.
   *biomedical research; *conflict of interest; *drug industry; *financial support; *investigators; legal aspects; *scientific misconduct; *universities; *Hidaka, Hiroyoshi; *Japan; Nagoya University; *Otsuka Pharmaceutical Co.

Sage, William M. Fraud and abuse law. [Editorial]. *JAMA.* 1999 Sep 22–29; 282(12): 1179–1181. 9 refs. BE62661.
   *economics; federal government; *fraud; government financing; *government regulation; health insurance reimbursement; health personnel; law enforcement; managed care programs; physician self-referral; remuneration; whistleblowing; Medicare; *United States

Scott, P. Anne. Professional ethics: are we on the wrong track? *Nursing Ethics.* 1998 Nov; 5(6): 477–485. 16 refs. BE60809.
   accountability; alternatives; autonomy; behavior control; behavior disorders; case studies; codes of ethics; deception; decision making; interprofessional relations; *misconduct; *nurse's role; *nurses; *nursing ethics; patient care team; physicians; principle–based ethics; psychoactive drugs; *punishment; regulation; standards; treatment refusal; *Great Britain; United Kingdom Central Council for Nursing, Midwifery and Health Visiting

Shamoo, Adil E.; Quist, Norman; Howe, Edmund G. Attempts at suppressing data. [Article and responses]. *Professional Ethics Report.* 1997 Winter; 10(1): 3–6. 5 refs. BE59206.
   accountability; biomedical research; confidentiality; *editorial policies; human experimentation; informed consent; investigators; legal liability; mentally ill; peer review; placebos; psychoactive drugs; records; schizophrenia; *scientific misconduct; *whistleblowing; withholding treatment; *Journal of Clinical Ethics

Sharkey, Joe. Bedlam: Greed, Profiteering, and Fraud in a Mental Health System Gone Crazy. New York, NY: St. Martin's Press; 1994. 294 p. ISBN 0–312–10421–9. BE62500.
   adolescents; adults; advertising; alcohol abuse; behavior disorders; children; coercion; drug abuse; *fraud; *health insurance reimbursement; involuntary commitment; legal aspects; mental health; *mental institutions; *misconduct; patient admission; *proprietary health facilities; psychiatric diagnosis; *referral and consultation; voluntary admission; *mental health services; National Medical Enterprises; Texas; *United States

Sidley, Pat. Doctors contributed to poor health of black South Africans. [News]. *BMJ (British Medical Journal).* 1998 Nov 7; 317(7168): 1269. BE62645.
   biological warfare; *blacks; *health care delivery; *misconduct; moral complicity; nurses; *physicians; prisoners; professional organizations; public policy; *social discrimination; torture; *South Africa

Sidley, Pat. South African research into AIDS "cure"

severely criticised. [News]. *BMJ (British Medical Journal).* 1997 Mar 15; 314(7083): 771. BE60726.

administrators; *AIDS; conflict of interest; *drugs; ethical review; government financing; *human experimentation; investigators; research design; *scientific misconduct; *South Africa; University of Pretoria; *Virodene; Visser, Olga; Zuma, Nkosazana

Skolnick, Andrew A. Critics denounce staffing jails and prisons with physicians convicted of misconduct. [News]. *JAMA.* 1998 Oct 28; 280(16): 1391–1392. BE60291.

*criminal law; *legal liability; *misconduct; patient care; *physicians; *prisoners; *professional competence; psychiatry; *quality of health care; *regulation; sex offenses; *licensing boards; *physician impairment; National Commission on Correctional Health Care; United States

Skolnick, Andrew A. Prison deaths spotlight how boards handle impaired, disciplined physicians. [News]. *JAMA.* 1998 Oct 28; 280(16): 1387–1390. Includes inset article, "Only the tip of the iceberg," by A.A. Skolnick, p. 1388–1389. BE60290.

*criminal law; fraud; *legal liability; *malpractice; mentally ill; *misconduct; negligence; patient care; *physicians; *prisoners; *professional competence; *quality of health care; *regulation; rehabilitation; *sex offenses; withholding treatment; *wrongful death; *licensing boards; *physician impairment; Correctional Medical Services; Mauney, Walter; United States; Williams, Gail

Sly, R. Michael. Ethical scientific writing and responsible medical practice. *Annals of Allergy, Asthma, and Immunology.* 1997 Dec; 79(6): 489–494. 42 refs. Presented as the Bela Schick Lecture at the annual meeting of the American College of Allergy, Asthma, and Immunology, 11 Nov 1997. BE59528.

authorship; *biomedical research; conflict of interest; continuing education; drug industry; editorial policies; guidelines; investigators; medical education; peer review; physicians; professional competence; property rights; *scientific misconduct; plagiarism

Tanaka, Yuki. Japanese biological warfare plans and experiments on POWs. *In: his* Hidden Horrors: Japanese War Crimes in World War II. Boulder, CO: Westview Press; 1996: 135–165, 238–242. 72 fn. ISBN 0–8133–2718–0. BE60510.

*biological warfare; communicable diseases; *dehumanization; *historical aspects; *human experimentation; international aspects; *investigators; killing; military personnel; misconduct; National Socialism; nutrition; *physicians; *prisoners; psychology; public policy; *scientific misconduct; China; *Japan; Manchuria; Rabaul; *Twentieth Century; World War II

Tarnow, Eugene. When extra authors get in on the act. [Letter]. *Nature.* 1999 Apr 22; 398(6729): 657. 2 refs. BE61792.

attitudes; *authorship; biomedical research; *faculty; interprofessional relations; *investigators; science; *scientific misconduct; standards; Europe; United States

Thomasma, David C.; Micetich, Kenneth C.; Brems, John, et al. The ethics of competition in liver transplantation. *Cambridge Quarterly of Healthcare Ethics.* 1999 Summer; 8(3): 321–329. 28 fn. BE62475.

beneficence; economics; federal government; *geographic factors; *government regulation; guidelines; hospitals; institutional policies; *justice; *livers; *misconduct; organ donation; organ donors; *organ transplantation; physicians; prisoners; public policy; *resource allocation; scarcity; *selection for treatment; standards; technical expertise; time factors; *transplant recipients; needs; *waiting lists;

Department of Health and Human Services; United Network for Organ Sharing; *United States

Thorns, Andrew; Lloyd, Geoffrey; Szmukler, George, et al. Certifying fitness for corporal punishment: ethical debate. [Case study, commentaries, and response]. *BMJ (British Medical Journal).* 1998 Oct 3; 317(7163): 939–941. 5 refs. BE60829.

conscience; cultural pluralism; *deception; health; human rights; international aspects; law; medical ethics; *misconduct; *physician's role; *prisoners; *punishment; torture; truth disclosure; values; Africa

Tuffs, Annette. Max–Planck Society investigates misconduct. [News]. *BMJ (British Medical Journal).* 1999 Jul 31; 319(7205): 274. BE62527.

growth disorders; hormones; industry; investigators; legal aspects; patents; property rights; research institutes; *scientific misconduct; universities; Genentech; Germany; Max Planck Society; Nature; *Seeburg, Peter; University of California

Wadman, Meredith. Dilemma for journals over tobacco cash. [News]. *Nature.* 1998 Aug 13; 394(6694): 609. BE59187.

biomedical research; cancer; *conflict of interest; *editorial policies; *financial support; *health hazards; *industry; *investigators; scientific misconduct; *smoking; Environmental Protection Agency; JAMA; Journal of the National Cancer Institute; Lancet; Pediatrics; *Tobacco Institute; United States

Wadman, Meredith. NIH ethics office clamps down on Duke...as basic scientists feel the pinch in LA. [News]. *Nature.* 1999 May 20; 399(6733): 190. BE61760.

advisory committees; ethical review; federal government; government financing; *government regulation; hospitals; *human experimentation; investigators; organization and administration; research ethics committees; *scientific misconduct; universities; Department of Veterans Affairs; *Duke University Medical Center; National Bioethics Advisory Commission; National Institutes of Health; *Office for Protection from Research Risks; *United States; *West Los Angeles Veterans Affairs Medical Center

Wang, Justin. Scientific misconduct: Chinese journals pledge crackdown. [News]. *Science.* 1999 Mar 5; 283(5407): 1427. BE61797.

codes of ethics; *editorial policies; investigators; professional organizations; punishment; science; *scientific misconduct; *self regulation; *China; China Association for Science and Technology

Weed, Douglas L. Preventing scientific misconduct. *American Journal of Public Health.* 1998 Jan; 88(1): 125–129. 50 refs. BE62601.

biomedical research; due process; education; empirical research; *investigators; motivation; *professional ethics; regulation; science; *scientific misconduct; statistics; terminology; virtues; whistleblowing

Weindling, Paul. Human experiments in Nazi Germany: reflections on Ernst Klee's book "Auschwitz, die NS–Medizin und ihre Opfer" (1997) and film "Arzte ohne Gewissen" (1996). *Medizinhistorisches Journal.* 1998; 33(2): 161–178. 45 refs. 6 fn. BE61443.

dentistry; eugenics; health personnel; *historical aspects; *human experimentation; investigators; involuntary euthanasia; literature; mass media; *National Socialism; physicians; public policy; *scientific misconduct; motion pictures; *Germany; *Klee, Ernst; Nuremberg Trials; Twentieth Century

Wells, Barron; Spinks, Nelda. The context of ethics in

BE = bioethics accession number   fn. = footnotes   refs. = references

the health care industry. *Health Manpower Management.* 1996; 22(1): 21–29. 8 refs. BE59338.
   *administrators; *advertising; aged; disabled; drug industry; drugs; economics; *employment; females; *health care delivery; *health facilities; *institutional ethics; medical fees; minority groups; *misconduct; social discrimination; standards; *business ethics; quality assurance; United States

Welsh, James; van Es, Adriaan. Health and human rights: an international minefield. *Lancet.* 1998 Dec 19–26; 352 (Suppl. 4): 14. 5 refs. BE60807.
   capital punishment; circumcision; females; *human rights; *international aspects; *misconduct; *physicians; political activity; public health; *torture; war

Welsh, James. Truth and reconciliation ... and justice. *Lancet.* 1998 Dec 5; 352(9143): 1852–1853. 5 refs. BE60806.
   accountability; blacks; *human rights; justice; *misconduct; *physicians; prisoners; social discrimination; *torture; *Chile; *South Africa

Wenger, Neil S.; Korenman, Stanley G.; Berk, Richard, et al. The ethics of scientific research: an analysis of focus groups of scientists and institutional representatives. *Journal of Investigative Medicine.* 1997 Aug; 45(6): 371–380. 20 refs. BE60389.
   accountability; *administrators; *attitudes; authorship; biomedical research; comparative studies; conflict of interest; education; financial support; fraud; information dissemination; interprofessional relations; *investigators; *professional ethics; punishment; *science; *scientific misconduct; self regulation; survey; universities; values; whistleblowing; *research ethics; United States

West, Doe. Radiation experiments on children at the Fernald and Wrentham schools: lessons for protocols in human subject research. *Accountability in Research.* 1998 Jan; 6(1–2): 103–125. 43 refs. BE61536.
   advisory committees; *children; competence; deception; disclosure; federal government; government financing; guideline adherence; guidelines; *historical aspects; *human experimentation; incentives; informed consent; injuries; *institutionalized persons; investigators; legal guardians; mass media; *mental institutions; *mentally retarded; *nontherapeutic research; nutrition; parental consent; physicians; public hospitals; public policy; *radiation; records; regulation; *residential facilities; retrospective moral judgment; *scientific misconduct; selection of subjects; state government; stigmatization; students; therapeutic research; third party consent; universities; Advisory Committee on Human Radiation Experiments; *Fernald State School (MA); Harvard University; *Massachusetts; Massachusetts Institute of Technology; *Task Force to Review Human Subject Research (MA); *Twentieth Century; United States; *Wrentham State School (MA)

Weyers, Wolfgang. Death of Medicine in Nazi Germany: Dermatology and Dermatopathology under the Swastika. Philadelphia, PA; Lanham, MD: Ardor Scribendi; Madison Books; 1998. 442 p. Edited by A. Bernard Ackerman. Bibliography: p. 397–413. ISBN 1-56833-122-3. BE59740.
   employment; eugenics; faculty; *historical aspects; *Jews; killing; medical education; medical specialties; *medicine; *misconduct; moral complicity; *National Socialism; *physicians; public policy; *social discrimination; universities; *dermatology; *Germany; *Twentieth Century

White, D.M.D.; Hillam, Jonathan; Harper, Max, et al. Suspension of nurse who gave drug on consultant's instructions. [Letters]. *BMJ (British Medical Journal).* 1997 Jan 25; 314(7076): 299–301. 8 refs. BE59380.
   *administrators; aged; *behavior control; behavior disorders; coercion; dangerousness; *deception; *misconduct; *nurse's role; *nurses; patient care; *patient care team; peer review; physician nurse relationship; *physicians; psychiatry; *psychoactive drugs; *punishment; treatment refusal; *Great Britain; Mental Health Act 1983 (Great Britain); National Health Service

Wincze, John P.; Richards, Jeff; Parsons, John, et al. A comparative survey of therapist sexual misconduct between an American state and an Australian state. *Professional Psychology: Research and Practice.* 1996 Jun; 27(3): 289–294. 25 refs. BE60223.
   comparative studies; disclosure; drug abuse; employment; females; fraud; health insurance reimbursement; *health personnel; international aspects; *knowledge, attitudes, practice; males; *misconduct; patients; *physicians; *professional patient relationship; *psychiatry; *psychology; *psychotherapy; *sexuality; social workers; statistics; survey; Australia; *Rhode Island; United States; *Western Australia

Wright, David E. The federal research misconduct regulations as viewed from the research universities. *Centennial Review.* 1994 Spring; 38(2): 249–272. 57 fn. BE59403.
   biomedical research; case studies; due process; federal government; *government regulation; investigators; science; *scientific misconduct; *universities; Department of Health and Human Services; Office of Research Integrity; *United States

Yankauer, Alfred. The neglected lesson of the Tuskegee study. [Letter]. *American Journal of Public Health.* 1998 Sep; 88(9): 1406. 8 refs. BE62555.
   *blacks; editorial policies; *human experimentation; informed consent; *scientific misconduct; *social discrimination; syphilis; withholding treatment; Public Health Service; *Tuskegee Syphilis Study; United States

Zelas, Karen. Sex and the doctor–patient relationship. *New Zealand Medical Journal.* 1997 Feb 28; 110(1038): 60–62. 16 refs. BE60088.
   beneficence; continuing education; geographic factors; *misconduct; moral obligations; patients; *physician patient relationship; physicians; *sex offenses; *sexuality; social dominance; trust; dependency; physician impairment; New Zealand

A suitable case for treatment. [Editorial]. *Nature.* 1999 May 20; 399(6733): 183. BE61758.
   government financing; *government regulation; *human experimentation; research ethics committees; *scientific misconduct; universities; *Duke University Medical Center; *Office for Protection from Research Risks; United States

Miss Evers' Boys. [Videorecording; "based on the true story of the infamous Tuskegee Experiment"].New York, NY: HBO Home Video; 1997. 1 videocassette; 118 min.; sd.; color; VHS. HBO in association with Anasazi Productions; a Joseph Sargent film. BE62194.
   *blacks; deception; federal government; government financing; *historical aspects; human experimentation; indigents; informed consent; investigators; *nontherapeutic research; nurses; physicians; public policy; research subjects; *scientific misconduct; *social discrimination; *syphilis; therapeutic research; *withholding treatment; Alabama; Evers, Eunice; *Public Health Service; *Tuskegee Syphilis Study; *Twentieth Century; *United States

Policy on papers' contributors. [Editorial]. *Nature.* 1999 Jun 3; 399(6735): 393. BE61762.
   *authorship; biomedical research; *editorial policies; *science; *scientific misconduct; *Nature

Surviving misconduct is one thing, accountability is another.

[Editorial]. *Nature*. 1998 Oct 22; 395(6704): 727.
BE59585.
  *accountability; *biomedical research; government
  financing; international aspects; investigators; records;
  *research institutes; *scientific misconduct; *self regulation;
  Europe

Taking stock of scientific fraud. [Editorial]. *Nature
Biotechnology*. 1998 May; 16(5): 395. BE62318.
  *biomedical research; *conflict of interest; *drug industry;
  *economics; *fraud; *investigators; medical schools;
  universities; United States

The perils of paediatric research. [Editorial]. *Lancet*. 1999
Feb 27; 353(9154): 685. BE61029.
  alternatives; comparative studies; control groups; ethical
  review; *human experimentation; intensive care units;
  investigators; methods; morbidity; mortality; *newborns;
  *parental consent; physicians; prematurity; research design;
  research ethics committees; *scientific misconduct;
  *therapeutic research; treatment outcome; *ventilators;
  *respiratory distress syndrome; *Great Britain; *North
  Staffordshire Hospital Trust; *Southall, David

Unneccessary Fuss. [Videorecording].Available from
People for the Ethical Treatment of Animals (PETA),
P.O. Box 42516, Washington, DC 20015-0516, (202)
726-0156, (301) 770-7444.; 1985. Videocassette; 26 min.;
sd.; color; VHS. Filmed by researchers at the University
of Pennsylvania Head Injury Clinic and removed from
the laboratories by members of the Animal Liberation
Front. Narrated by Ingrid Newkirk of People for the
Ethical Treatment of Animals. BE62195.
  *animal experimentation; attitudes; *brain; federal
  government; government financing; *injuries; investigators;
  *pain; *primates; research design; research institutes;
  *scientific misconduct; *suffering; Department of Health and
  Human Services; United States; *University of Pennsylvania

When mental patients are at risk. [Editorial]. *New York
Times*. 1999 Mar 31: A24. BE60909.
  *federal government; *government regulation; *human
  experimentation; *mentally ill; psychoactive drugs; public
  hospitals; schizophrenia; *scientific misconduct; withholding
  treatment; Department of Veterans Affairs; Los Angeles;
  United States; West Los Angeles Veterans Affairs Medical
  Center

Where next on misconduct? [Editorial]. *Nature*. 1999 Mar
4; 398(6722): 1. BE60983.
  biomedical research; investigators; regulation; *scientific
  misconduct; whistleblowing; United States

GENE THERAPY

See also GENETIC INTERVENTION,
    RECOMBINANT DNA RESEARCH, GENETIC
    SERVICES

**Baram, Michael; Proctor, Susan; Andalman, Robert,
et al.** Human gene therapy research: technological
temptations and social control. *Genetic Resource*. 1993;
7(2): 10-15. 45 fn. BE60209.
  eugenics; federal government; *gene therapy; genetic
  disorders; genetic enhancement; germ cells; government
  regulation; human experimentation; methods; risks and
  benefits; social control; Food and Drug Administration;
  National Institutes of Health; United States

Billings, Paul R.; Newman, Stuart A. Crossing the
germline. *GeneWATCH*. 1999 Jan; 11(5-6): 1, 3-4.
BE62370.
  dissent; eugenics; federal government; *fetal research; fetal

therapy; future generations; *gene therapy; genetic
disorders; genetic intervention; *germ cells; government
regulation; *risks and benefits; thalassemia; adenosine
deaminase deficiency; Anderson, W. French; Council for
Responsible Genetics; Recombinant DNA Advisory
Committee; United States

Billings, Paul R.; Schneider, Holm; Coutelle, Charles.
In utero gene therapy: the case against [and] the case
for. *Nature Medicine*. 1999 Mar; 5(3): 255-257. 7 refs.
BE62542.
  advisory committees; animal experimentation; federal
  government; *fetal research; *fetal therapy; *gene therapy;
  genetic disorders; germ cells; government regulation; human
  experimentation; *risks and benefits; treatment outcome;
  Recombinant DNA Advisory Committee; United States

**Candotti, Fabio; Notarangelo, Luigi D.; Ugazio,
Alberto G.** Gene therapy: current status, perspectives
and problematic issues. *In:* Burgio, G. Roberto; Lantos,
John D., eds. *Primum Non Nocere* Today. Second
Edition. New York, NY: Elsevier; 1998: 133-145. 43
refs. ISBN 0-444-82923-7. BE60924.
  AIDS; animal experimentation; cancer; *gene therapy;
  genetic disorders; human experimentation; international
  aspects; methods; nontherapeutic research; stem cells;
  therapeutic research; *treatment outcome

Chadwick, Ruth. Gene therapy. *In:* Kuhse, Helga; Singer,
Peter, eds. A Companion to Bioethics. Malden, MA:
Blackwell; 1998: 189-197. 16 refs. ISBN 0-631-19737-0.
BE59494.
  autonomy; eugenics; future generations; gene pool; *gene
  therapy; genetic enhancement; germ cells; human
  experimentation; moral obligations; *moral policy; public
  health; public policy; resource allocation; risks and benefits;
  wrongful life; personal identity

Clark, William R. The ethics of molecular medicine. *In:
his*: The New Healers: The Promise and Problems of
Molecular Medicine in the Twenty-First Century. New
York, NY: Oxford University Press; 1997: 207-231, 236.
8 refs. ISBN 0-19-511730-1. BE60572.
  confidentiality; containment; disclosure; DNA data banks;
  *DNA fingerprinting; donors; employment; ethical review;
  forensic medicine; future generations; *gene therapy; genetic
  counseling; genetic disorders; genetic enhancement; *genetic
  information; genetic materials; genetic predisposition;
  *genetic screening; genome mapping; germ cells;
  government regulation; guidelines; *health insurance;
  informed consent; insurance selection bias; late-onset
  disorders; legislation; methods; preimplantation diagnosis;
  privacy; public policy; recombinant DNA research; *risks
  and benefits; social discrimination; NIH/DOE Working
  Group on Ethical, Legal, and Social Issues (ELSI); United
  States

Cohen-Haguenauer, Odile. Gene therapy: regulatory
issues and international approaches to regulation. *Current
Opinion In Biotechnology*. 1997 Jun; 8(3): 361-369. 24 refs.
BE59148.
  advisory committees; financial support; *gene therapy;
  *government regulation; guidelines; human experimentation;
  industry; *international aspects; investigators; private sector;
  public sector; recombinant DNA research; *regulation;
  research ethics committees; risks and benefits; toxicity;
  transgenic organisms; Austria; Belgium; European Medicines
  Evaluation Agency; European Union; Food and Drug
  Administration; France; Gene Therapy Advisory Committee
  (Great Britain); Germany; Great Britain; Italy; Japan;
  National Institutes of Health; Netherlands; Recombinant
  DNA Advisory Committee; Spain; Sweden; Switzerland;
  United States

Couzin, Jennifer. RAC confronts in utero gene therapy

proposals. [News]. *Science.* 1998 Oct 2; 282(5386): 27. BE62617.
> advisory committees; federal government; *fetal research; *fetal therapy; future generations; *gene therapy; *public policy; risks and benefits; thalassemia; immunologic deficiency syndromes; National Institutes of Health; *Recombinant DNA Advisory Committee; *United States

Eisenberg, Vered H.; Schenker, Joseph G. Genetic engineering: moral aspects and control of practice. *Journal of Assisted Reproduction and Genetics.* 1997 Jul; 14(6): 297–316. 98 refs. BE62404.
> AIDS; cancer; Christian ethics; cloning; eugenics; *gene therapy; genetic enhancement; *genetic intervention; germ cells; government regulation; human experimentation; informed consent; international aspects; Islamic ethics; Jewish ethics; resource allocation; risks and benefits

Engelhardt, H. Tristram. Germ–line genetic engineering and moral diversity: moral controversies in a post–Christian world. *In:* Paul, Ellen Frankel; Miller, Fred D.; Paul, Jeffrey, eds. Scientific Innovation, Philosophy, and Public Policy. New York, NY: Cambridge University Press; 1996: 47–62. 23 fn. ISBN 0–521–58994–0. BE62743.
> beneficence; *cultural pluralism; *gene therapy; genetic enhancement; *genetic intervention; *germ cells; goals; health; *human characteristics; medicine; *moral policy; morality; philosophy; public policy; *secularism; theology; values

Fiddler, Morris; Pergament, Eugene. Germline gene therapy: its time is near. *Molecular Human Reproduction.* 1996 Feb; 2(2): 75–76. 9 refs. BE62212.
> common good; eugenics; future generations; *gene therapy; genetic enhancement; *germ cells; resource allocation; risks and benefits; wedge argument

Fletcher, John C.; Richter, Gerd. Ethical issues of perinatal human gene therapy. *Journal of Maternal–Fetal Medicine.* 1996 Sep–Oct; 5(5): 232–244. 93 refs. BE60136.
> advisory committees; age factors; beneficence; *children; disclosure; embryo research; ethical review; federal government; *fetal research; *fetal therapy; *gene therapy; genetic disorders; genetic enhancement; germ cells; government regulation; growth disorders; historical aspects; hormones; *human experimentation; *infants; informed consent; justice; parents; pregnant women; prenatal diagnosis; privacy; research ethics committees; resource allocation; *risks and benefits; scientific misconduct; selection of subjects; selective abortion; stem cells; thalassemia; adenosine deaminase deficiency; immunologic deficiency syndromes; Germany; National Institutes of Health; Recombinant DNA Advisory Committee; United States

Fox, Jeffrey L. Future tense for in utero gene therapy. [News]. *Nature Biotechnology.* 1998 Nov; 16(11): 1002–1003. BE62320.
> advisory committees; ethical review; federal government; *fetal research; *fetal therapy; *gene therapy; genetic disorders; public policy; risks and benefits; Food and Drug Administration; National Institutes of Health; Recombinant DNA Advisory Committee; United States

Fox, Jeffrey L. Gene therapy experts ponder readiness for enhancements. [News]. *Nature Biotechnology.* 1997 Nov; 15(12): 1236–1237. BE62041.
> advisory committees; attitudes; federal government; *gene therapy; *genetic enhancement; human experimentation; investigators; *public policy; National Institutes of Health; United States

Fox, Jeffrey L. Germline gene therapy contemplated.

[News]. *Nature Biotechnology.* 1998 May; 16(5): 407. BE62319.
> federal government; *gene therapy; *germ cells; government regulation; *human experimentation; United States

Hannay, Timo. Japan on verge of first gene therapy trial. [News]. *Nature Medicine.* 1995 Jan; 1(1): 9. BE59767.
> advisory committees; *gene therapy; genetic disorders; *government regulation; *human experimentation; international aspects; universities; adenosine deaminase deficiency; *Japan; Ministry of Education, Science and Culture (Japan); Ministry of Health and Welfare (Japan); United States

Hollinger, Dennis P. A theology of healing and genetic engineering. *In:* Demy, Timothy J.; Stewart, Gary P., eds. Genetic Engineering: A Christian Response: Crucial Considerations in Shaping Life. Grand Rapids, MI: Kregel Publications; 1999: 294–303. 11 fn. ISBN 0–8254–2357–0. BE61372.
> *Christian ethics; dehumanization; economics; eugenics; *gene therapy; *genetic disorders; genetic enhancement; *genetic intervention; *intention; *moral policy; *motivation; religion; social discrimination; theology; value of life; dignity; empowerment; *faith healing

Holtug, Nils. Does justice require genetic enhancements? *Journal of Medical Ethics.* 1999 Apr; 25(2): 137–143. 15 fn. BE61917.
> *compensation; cosmetic surgery; disabled; disease; enhancement technologies; *gene therapy; *genetic disorders; *genetic enhancement; *goals; government financing; growth disorders; health; health care; hormones; *justice; *medicine; *moral policy; normality; patient care; preventive medicine; psychological stress; public policy; resource allocation; social discrimination

It is argued that justice in some cases provides a pro tanto reason genetically to enhance victims of the genetic lottery. Various arguments -- both to the effect that justice provides no such reason and to the effect that while there may be such reasons, they are overridden by certain moral constraints -- are considered and rejected. Finally, it is argued that justice provides stronger reasons to perform more traditional medical tasks (treatments), and that therefore genetic enhancements should not play an important role in a public health care system.

Jaroff, Leon. Fixing the genes. *Time.* 1999 Jan 11; 153(1): 68–70, 73. BE60314.
> disease; fetal therapy; *gene therapy; genetic disorders; government regulation; human experimentation; methods; patient care; preventive medicine; public opinion; United States

Jaroff, Leon. Success stories: the verdict on the pioneering children of gene therapy -- so far, so good. *Time.* 1999 Jan 11; 153(1): 72–73. BE60315.
> *children; drugs; *gene therapy; human experimentation; methods; patient care; treatment outcome; *immunologic deficiency syndromes; Anderson, W. French; Blaese, R. Michael; Cutshall, Cindy; DeSilva, Ashanthi; National Institutes of Health; United States

Kaplan, Starr (Esther) Rose. Germ–line genetic engineering revisited. *Pharos.* 1997 Fall; 60(4): 21–25. 14 refs. BE60443.
> beneficence; common good; embryos; eugenics; fetal therapy; gene pool; *gene therapy; genetic disorders; *genetic enhancement; *germ cells; justice; nontherapeutic research; normality; regulation; resource allocation; risks and benefits; social problems; therapeutic research

Kolata, Gina. Scientists brace for changes in path of human evolution. [News]. *New York Times*. 1998 Mar 21: A1, A12. BE59619.

> attitudes; *evolution; future generations; *gene therapy; genetic disorders; genetic enhancement; *germ cells; investigators; life extension

Kolehmainen, Sophia. CRG brings ethics into NIH prenatal gene therapy debate. *GeneWATCH*. 1999 Feb; 12(1): 15–16. BE62372.

> dissent; eugenics; federal government; *fetal research; *gene therapy; genetic intervention; *germ cells; government regulation; risks and benefits; Council for Responsible Genetics; Recombinant DNA Advisory Committee; United States

Lagay, Faith L. Science, rhetoric, and public discourse in genetic research. *Cambridge Quarterly of Healthcare Ethics*. 1999 Spring; 8(2): 226–237. 33 fn. BE61238.

> alcohol abuse; bioethical issues; *consensus; *cultural pluralism; *decision making; *democracy; emotions; gene therapy; genetic disorders; *genetic enhancement; *genetic intervention; genetic predisposition; *genetic research; justice; models, theoretical; moral policy; normality; obligations of society; philosophy; postmodernism; public participation; *public policy; values; virtues; needs; rationality; *rhetoric

Lehrman, Sally. Virus treatment questioned after gene therapy death. [News]. *Nature*. 1999 Oct 7; 401(6753): 517–518. BE62683.

> advisory committees; *death; federal government; *gene therapy; government regulation; *human experimentation; livers; *research subjects; risks and benefits; toxicity; Food and Drug Administration; *Gelsinger, Jesse; National Institutes of Health; Recombinant DNA Advisory Committee; United States; *University of Pennsylvania

Lupton, M.L. Behaviour modification by genetic intervention -- the law's response. *Medicine and Law*. 1994; 13(5–6): 417–431. 47 fn. BE60004.

> advisory committees; behavioral genetics; dementia; depressive disorder; developing countries; eugenics; *gene therapy; genetic disorders; genetic enhancement; genetic predisposition; genetic research; genome mapping; germ cells; *government regulation; *guidelines; human rights; informed consent; *international aspects; *mentally disabled; mentally ill; methods; *regulation; resource allocation; Australia; Canada; Clothier Committee; Council of Ethics (Denmark); Council of Europe; Denmark; Europe; France; Great Britain; Human Genome Project; Medical Research Council (South Africa); National Ethics Advisory Committee (France); National Health and Medical Research Council (Australia); South Africa

McDonough, Paul G. The ethics of somatic and germline gene therapy. *Annals of the New York Academy of Sciences*. 1997 Jun 17; 816: 378–382. 9 refs. BE59425.

> advisory committees; federal government; *gene therapy; genetic disorders; germ cells; government regulation; human experimentation; risks and benefits; Food and Drug Administration; National Institutes of Health; Recombinant DNA Advisory Committee; United States

Mitchell, Peter. Alleged unlicensed gene-therapy trial comes to light. [News]. *Lancet*. 1999 Jul 17; 354(9174): 225. BE62662.

> advisory committees; cancer; death; *gene therapy; *government regulation; guideline adherence; *human experimentation; *international aspects; investigators; research subjects; scientific misconduct; *Denmark; Department of Health (Great Britain); *Gene Therapy Advisory Committee (Great Britain); *Great Britain; *Habib, Nagy; *Hammersmith Hospital (London); *Lindkear, Sheen

Pentz, Rebecca D. Genetic counseling: guidance for chilling choices. *In:* Demy, Timothy J.; Stewart, Gary P., eds. Genetic Engineering: A Christian Response: Crucial Considerations in Shaping Life. Grand Rapids, MI: Kregel Publications; 1999: 188–195. 3 fn. ISBN 0-8254-2357-0. BE61367.

> breast cancer; *Christian ethics; chromosome abnormalities; costs and benefits; decision making; directive counseling; disabled; employment; family members; *gene therapy; *genetic counseling; *genetic enhancement; genetic information; *genetic screening; germ cells; health personnel; insurance; pastoral care; patients; prenatal diagnosis; prolongation of life; quality of life; *risks and benefits; social discrimination; theology; values

Rehmann-Sutter, Christoph. Liberating gene therapy. [Book review essay]. *Hastings Center Report*. 1999 May–Jun; 29(3): 43. BE61414.

> cloning; *gene therapy; genetic enhancement; genetic intervention; *germ cells; *goals; normality; risks and benefits; self concept; nature; *The Ethics of Human Gene Therapy (Walters, L.; Palmer, J.G.)

Resnik, David B.; Steinkraus, Holly B.; Langer, Pamela J. Human Germline Gene Therapy: Scientific, Moral and Political Issues. Austin, TX: R.G. Landes; 1999. 189 p. (Medical intelligence unit; 9). Includes references. ISBN 1-57059-586-0. BE61052.

> alternatives; artificial insemination; autonomy; beneficence; children; confidentiality; embryo transfer; eugenics; future generations; gene pool; *gene therapy; genetic determinism; genetic disorders; genetic diversity; genetic enhancement; *genetic intervention; genetic screening; *germ cells; government regulation; human characteristics; human rights; in vitro fertilization; injuries; justice; legal rights; methods; moral obligations; *moral policy; natural law; parents; patents; preimplantation diagnosis; prenatal diagnosis; preventive medicine; privacy; *public policy; risk; *risks and benefits; selection for treatment; selective abortion; social discrimination; *social impact; socioeconomic factors; utilitarianism

Richter, Gerd; Bacchetta, Matthew D. Interventions in the human genome: some moral and ethical considerations. *Journal of Medicine and Philosophy*. 1998 Jun; 23(3): 303–317. 35 refs. BE59294.

> autonomy; children; costs and benefits; disclosure; embryo research; *ethical analysis; eugenics; future generations; *gene therapy; *genetic enhancement; *genetic intervention; *germ cells; human experimentation; informed consent; intention; international aspects; justice; *methods; *moral policy; parental consent; preimplantation diagnosis; preventive medicine; public policy; regulation; risk; *risks and benefits; stem cells; Germany

In the debate regarding the different possibilities for gene therapy, it is presupposed that the manipulations are limited to the nuclear genome (nDNA). Given recent advances in genetics, mitochondrial genome (mtDNA) and diseases must be considered as well. In this paper, we propose a three dimensional framework for the ethical debate of gene therapy where we add the genomic type (nDNA vs. mtDNA) as a third dimension to be considered beside the paradigmatic dimensions of target cell (somatic vs. germ–line) and purpose (therapeutic vs. enhancement). Somatic gene therapy can be viewed today as generally accepted, and we review the contemporary arguments surrounding it on the basis of bioethical–pragmatic, socio–political and deontological classifications. Many of the supposed ethical questions of somatic gene therapy today are not new; they are well–known issues of research ethics. We also critically summarize the different international perspectives and the German ethical discussion regarding manipulations of germ–line cells.

BE = bioethics accession number   fn. = footnotes   refs. = references

Saegusa, Asako; Nathan, Richard. Japan renews gene therapy efforts ... and plans transgenic medicine guidelines. [News]. *Nature Medicine.* 1998 Nov; 4(11): 1213. BE62158.
> cancer; *drugs; *gene therapy; government regulation; guidelines; *human experimentation; industry; recombinant DNA research; *transgenic animals; universities; *Japan; Ministry of Health and Welfare (Japan); National Institute of Health Sciences (Japan); Tokyo University

Szebik, Imre. Altering the mitochondrial genome: is it just a technical issue? Response to "Germ line therapy to cure mitochondrial disease: protocol and ethics of in vitro ovum nuclear transplantation" by Donald S. Rubenstein, David C. Thomasma, Eric A. Schon, and Michael J. Zinaman (*CQ*, 1995 Summer; 4(3): 316–339). *Cambridge Quarterly of Healthcare Ethics.* 1999 Summer; 8(3): 369–374. 22 fn. BE62355.
> future generations; *gene therapy; genetic disorders; genetic identity; *germ cells; *ovum; *risks and benefits; therapeutic research; nuclear transplantation

Taylor, Robert. Superhumans. *New Scientist.* 1998 Oct 3; 160(2154): 24–29. 4 refs. BE61940.
> cloning; DNA sequences; *gene therapy; genetic disorders; genetic enhancement; *genetic intervention; *germ cells; government regulation; hybrids; intelligence; methods; *risks and benefits; stem cells; transgenic animals; United States

U.S. National Institutes of Health. Recombinant DNA research: actions under the guidelines; notice. *Federal Register.* 1995 Apr 27; 60(81): 20726–20737. BE59544.
> *advisory committees; confidentiality; containment; *ethical review; federal government; *gene therapy; *government regulation; guidelines; *human experimentation; informed consent; organization and administration; *recombinant DNA research; *Food and Drug Administration; *National Institutes of Health; *NIH Guidelines; Office of Recombinant DNA Activities; Points to Consider: Transfer of Recombinant DNA into Human Subjects; *Recombinant DNA Advisory Committee; *United States

Wadman, Meredith. Gene therapy pushes on, despite doubts. [News]. *Nature.* 1999 Jan 14; 397(6715): 94. BE60396.
> animal experimentation; federal government; *fetal research; *fetal therapy; *gene therapy; guidelines; human experimentation; *public policy; *risks and benefits; Council for Responsible Genetics; Food and Drug Administration; National Institutes of Health; NIH Guidelines; *United States

Wadman, Meredith. NIH launches discussion of in utero gene therapy ... and seeks to repair 'flaw' in review process. [News]. *Nature.* 1998 Oct 1; 395(6701): 420. BE60261.
> advisory committees; federal government; *fetal therapy; *gene therapy; government regulation; human experimentation; newborns; pregnant women; *risks and benefits; thalassemia; immunologic deficiency syndromes; Anderson, W. French; *National Institutes of Health; *Recombinant DNA Advisory Committee; United States

Watt, Helen. Germ-line therapy for mitochondrial disease: some ethical objections. *Cambridge Quarterly of Healthcare Ethics.* 1999 Winter; 8(1): 88–96. 39 fn. Response to D.S. Rubenstein, D.C. Thomasma, E.A. Schon, and M.J. Zinaman, "Germ-line therapy to cure mitochondrial disease: protocol and ethics of *in vitro* ovum nuclear transplantation, *CQ*, 1995 Summer; 4(3): 316–339. BE60530.
> beginning of life; embryo disposition; embryo transfer; embryos; future generations; *gene therapy; *genetic disorders; *germ cells; in vitro fertilization; *methods; moral

obligations; moral policy; *ovum; ovum donors; parent child relationship; preconception injuries; preimplantation diagnosis; *risks and benefits; semen donors; therapeutic research; *value of life; wrongful life; *nuclear transplantation

Winerup, Michael. Fighting for Jacob [experimental gene therapy for Canavan disease]. *New York Times Magazine.* 1998 Dec 6: 56–63, 78, 80, 82, 112. BE60648.
> brain; children; congenital disorders; disabled; ethical review; federal government; *gene therapy; *genetic disorders; genetic research; government regulation; *human experimentation; *infants; investigators; marital relationship; *parents; psychological stress; review committees; *surgery; terminally ill; *therapeutic research; treatment outcome; expedited review; *Canavan disease; Karlin, Lindsay; National Institutes of Health; Seashore, Margretta; *Sontag, Jacob; Sontag, Jordanna; Sontag, Richard; United States; Yale University; Yale–New Haven Hospital

Gene therapy and the germline. [Editorial]. *Nature Medicine.* 1999 Mar; 5(3): 245. BE62537.
> federal government; fetal research; fetal therapy; *gene therapy; *germ cells; government regulation; human experimentation; risks and benefits; Food and Drug Administration; United States

GENETIC COUNSELING

See also GENETIC INTERVENTION, GENETIC SCREENING, PRENATAL DIAGNOSIS, GENETIC SERVICES

Allert, Gebhard; Sponholz, Gerlinde; Baitsch, Helmut, et al. Consensus formation in genetic counseling: a complex process. *In:* ten Have, Henk A.M.J.; Sass, Hans–Martin, eds. Consensus Formation in Healthcare Ethics. Boston, MA: Kluwer Academic; 1998: 193–207. 17 refs. ISBN 0-7923-4944-X. BE62595.
> case studies; *communication; comprehension; *consensus; dissent; family members; family relationship; *genetic counseling; genetic disorders; genetic screening; prenatal diagnosis; professional patient relationship; Germany

Anderson, Gwen. Nondirectiveness in prenatal genetics: patients read between the lines. *Nursing Ethics.* 1999 Mar; 6(2): 126–136. 33 refs. BE61932.
> age factors; *attitudes; communication; congenital disorders; costs and benefits; decision making; *directive counseling; disclosure; fathers; females; *genetic counseling; genetic information; *genetic screening; genetic services; health personnel; males; marital relationship; married persons; moral obligations; narrative ethics; nurses; nursing research; *patients; *pregnant women; *prenatal diagnosis; professional patient relationship; quality of life; selective abortion; suffering; uncertainty; *values; qualitative research; right not to know

Bernard, Lynn E.; McGillivray, Barbara; Van Allen, Margot I., et al. Duty to re-contact: a study of families at risk for Fragile X. *Journal of Genetic Counseling.* 1999 Feb; 8(1): 3–15. 11 refs. BE61641.
> *attitudes; carriers; *chromosome abnormalities; disclosure; *family members; *genetic counseling; genetic predisposition; *genetic screening; mentally retarded; motivation; *patients; prevalence; risks and benefits; survey; *recontact; British Columbia; Fragile X syndrome

British Medical Association. Human Genetics: Choice and Responsibility. New York, NY: Oxford University Press; 1998. 236 p. 227 fn. Appendixes provide names and addresses of regional genetics centers in the United Kingdom and of concerned organizations in the UK and

---

BE = bioethics accession number   fn. = footnotes   refs. = references

elsewhere. ISBN 0-19-288055-1. BE61351.
 adolescents; adults; advisory committees; carriers; children; cloning; competence; confidentiality; decision making; disabled; disclosure; employment; eugenics; family members; gene therapy; *genetic counseling; genetic disorders; genetic information; genetic predisposition; genetic research; *genetic screening; *genetic services; *genetics; government financing; guidelines; health personnel; informed consent; insurance; late-onset disorders; mass screening; moral obligations; *organizational policies; parents; patients; physicians; prenatal diagnosis; primary health care; professional ethics; professional organizations; registries; regulation; risks and benefits; terminology; incidental findings; paternity; *British Medical Association; Great Britain; National Health Service

Burgess, Michael M.; Laberge, Claude M.; Knoppers, Bartha Maria. Bioethics for clinicians: 14. Ethics and genetics in medicine. *Canadian Medical Association Journal.* 1998 May 19; 158(10): 1309-1313. 42 refs. BE59832.
 confidentiality; duty to warn; family members; *genetic counseling; *genetic information; *genetic predisposition; *genetic screening; guidelines; health personnel; informed consent; insurance; knowledge, attitudes, practice; late-onset disorders; legal aspects; physicians; prenatal diagnosis; psychological stress; risk; social discrimination; Canada

Chadwick, Ruth. Dimensions of quality in genetic services -- an ethical comment. *European Journal of Human Genetics.* 1997; 5(Suppl. 2): 22-24. 7 refs. BE62208.
 autonomy; costs and benefits; *evaluation; *genetic counseling; genetic disorders; genetic information; genetic screening; *genetic services; goals; international aspects; justice; patient satisfaction; prenatal diagnosis; public health; quality of health care; resource allocation; social discrimination; stigmatization; right not to know; Europe

Clarke, Angus. Genetic screening and counselling. *In:* Kuhse, Helga; Singer, Peter, eds. A Companion to Bioethics. Malden, MA: Blackwell; 1998: 215-228. 42 refs. ISBN 0-631-19737-0. BE59497.
 adults; autonomy; carriers; children; confidentiality; disclosure; family members; *genetic counseling; genetic disorders; genetic information; genetic predisposition; *genetic screening; goals; informed consent; late-onset disorders; mass screening; newborns; parental consent; prenatal diagnosis; psychological stress; public health; risks and benefits; social discrimination

Deftos, L.J. Genomic torts: the law of the future -- the duty of physicians to disclose the presence of a genetic disease to the relatives of their patients with the disease. *University of San Francisco Law Review.* 1997 Fall; 32(1): 105-137. 256 fn. BE59864.
 confidentiality; *disclosure; *duty to warn; *family members; *genetic counseling; *genetic disorders; *genetic information; *genetic predisposition; genetic screening; genome mapping; informed consent; *legal aspects; *legal liability; legal obligations; physician patient relationship; *physicians; state government; *torts; wrongful life; *United States

Dunne, Cara; Warren, Catherine. Lethal autonomy: the malfunction of the informed consent mechanism within the context of prenatal diagnosis of genetic variants. *Issues in Law and Medicine.* 1998 Fall; 14(2): 165-202. 75 fn. BE62011.
 *autonomy; cancer; directive counseling; disclosure; Down syndrome; *eugenics; *genetic counseling; genetic disorders; genetic screening; genome mapping; health personnel; historical aspects; *informed consent; killing; legal liability; mentally retarded; minority groups; National Socialism; physician's role; *prenatal diagnosis; quality of life; selective abortion; social discrimination; sterilization (sexual);

wrongful life; Germany; Human Genome Project; Twentieth Century; United States

Fitzpatrick, J.; Hahn, C.; Costa, T., et al. The duty to recontact: attitudes of genetics service providers. [Abstract]. *American Journal of Human Genetics.* 1997 Oct; 61(4): A57. BE59392.
 *attitudes; *genetic counseling; genetic research; *genetic services; *health personnel; legal obligations; moral obligations; physicians; standards; survey; *recontact; Canada; United States

Gillon, Raanan. 'Wrongful life' claims. [Editorial]. *Journal of Medical Ethics.* 1998 Dec; 24(6): 363-364. 1 ref. BE60784.
 abortion, induced; children; contraception; *disabled; *genetic counseling; health personnel; *legal liability; *negligence; wedge argument; *wrongful life

Headings, V.E. Revisiting foundations of autonomy and beneficence in genetic counseling. *Genetic Counseling.* 1997; 8(4): 291-294. 8 refs. BE60685.
 *autonomy; *beneficence; *genetic counseling; health personnel; professional patient relationship

Hodge, Susan E. Paternalistic and protective? [Letter]. *Journal of Genetic Counseling.* 1995 Dec; 4(4): 351-352. 1 ref. BE60452.
 autonomy; confidentiality; *directive counseling; disclosure; family members; *genetic counseling; *genetic screening; *Huntington disease; informed consent; paternalism; *twins

Hoedemaekers, Rogeer; ten Have, Henk. Geneticization: the Cyprus paradigm. *Journal of Medicine and Philosophy.* 1998 Jun; 23(3): 274-287. 17 refs. BE59291.
 *attitudes; carriers; *coercion; decision making; *directive counseling; economics; eugenics; *genetic counseling; *genetic screening; genetic services; genetics; *goals; health education; *health personnel; international aspects; *mass screening; parents; paternalism; *prenatal diagnosis; prevalence; preventive medicine; public health; public opinion; quality of life; *selective abortion; social control; stigmatization; *thalassemia; *Cyprus; Great Britain; Quebec
Geneticization is a broad term referring to several related processes such as a spreading tendency to use a genetic model of disease explanation, a growing influence of genetics in medical practice, and the slow changing of individual and societal attitudes towards reproduction, prevention and control of disease. These processes can be demonstrated in medical literature on preventive genetic screening and counselling programs for beta-thalassaemia in Cyprus, the United Kingdom and Canada. The preventive possibilities of the new genetic and diagnostic technologies have been quickly understood and advocated by health professionals, and their educational strategies have created a web of social control, in marked contrast to the alleged voluntary decision-making process and free choice. Genetic diagnostic technologies have led to considerable changes in control and management of beta-thalassaemia, and have generated a number of unresolved incongruities.

Hoedemaekers, Rogeer. Predictive genetic screening and the concept of risk. *In:* Clarke, Angus, ed. The Genetic Testing of Children. Washington, DC: BIOS Scientific Publishers; 1998: 245-264. 31 refs. ISBN 1-85996-146-0. BE62766.
 communication; comprehension; decision making; employment; family members; *genetic counseling; genetic disorders; *genetic information; genetic predisposition; *genetic screening; industry; informal social control; insurance; psychological stress; *risk; *risks and benefits;

BE = bioethics accession number   fn. = footnotes   refs. = references

social discrimination; stigmatization; *terminology; *uncertainty; values; *harms

Huggins, M.; Hahn, C.; Costa, T. Staying informed and recontacting patients about research advances: a study of patient attitudes. [Abstract]. *American Journal of Human Genetics.* 1996 Oct; 59(4): A335. BE60094.
*attitudes; *genetic counseling; genetic disorders; *genetic research; patient care team; *patient education; *patients; physicians; survey; *recontact; Toronto

Karlinsky, Harry. Genetic testing and counseling for early-onset autosomal-dominant Alzheimer disease. *In:* Post, Stephen G.; Whitehouse, Peter J., eds. Genetic Testing for Alzheimer Disease: Ethical and Clinical Issues. Baltimore, MD: Johns Hopkins University Press; 1998: 103–117. 19 refs. ISBN 0-8018-5840-2. BE60719.
adults; communication; competence; *dementia; diagnosis; disclosure; family members; *genetic counseling; *genetic screening; informed consent; psychological stress; risks and benefits; third party consent

Kash, Kathryn M. Psychosocial and ethical implications of defining genetic risk for cancers. *Annals of the New York Academy of Sciences.* 1995 Sep 30; 768: 41–52. 26 refs. BE59172.
attitudes; *breast cancer; *cancer; comprehension; confidentiality; disclosure; employment; family members; females; *genetic counseling; *genetic predisposition; *genetic screening; health insurance; informed consent; mass screening; motivation; *psychological stress; risk; social discrimination; United States

Kessler, Seymour. Genetic counseling is directive? Look again. [Letter]. *American Journal of Human Genetics.* 1997 Aug; 61(2): 466–467. 12 refs. BE60178.
coercion; communication; *directive counseling; *genetic counseling

King, David. The persistence of eugenics. *GenEthics News.* 1998 Feb–Mar; No. 22: 6–8. 4 refs. BE61094.
*attitudes; behavioral genetics; *directive counseling; *eugenics; *genetic counseling; genetic determinism; genetic screening; *genetics; *health personnel; historical aspects; informal social control; international aspects; investigators; parents; prenatal diagnosis; reproduction; selective abortion; social control; Twentieth Century

Lafayette, DeeDee; Abuelo, Dianne; Passero, Mary Ann, et al. Attitudes toward cystic fibrosis carrier and prenatal testing and utilization of carrier testing among relatives of individuals with cystic fibrosis. *Journal of Genetic Counseling.* 1999 Feb; 8(1): 17–36. 57 refs. BE61642.
*attitudes; *carriers; *cystic fibrosis; *family members; family planning; *genetic counseling; *genetic screening; *knowledge, attitudes, practice; *prenatal diagnosis; quality of life; *selective abortion; survey; Rhode Island

Lucassen, Anneke. Ethical issues in genetics of mental disorders. *Lancet.* 1998 Sep 26; 352(9133): 1004–1005. 8 refs. BE60793.
dementia; disclosure; family members; *genetic counseling; genetic disorders; *genetic predisposition; genetic research; *genetic screening; *mentally ill; preventive medicine; risk; risks and benefits; selective abortion; stigmatization

McGowan, Ruth. Beyond the disorder: one parent's reflection on genetic counselling. *Journal of Medical Ethics.* 1999 Apr; 25(2): 195–199. 3 refs. BE61925.
*attitudes; carriers; children; compassion; confidentiality; diagnosis; disclosure; *emotions; family members; family relationship; *genetic counseling; *genetic disorders; genetic

screening; *mothers; parents; *patient satisfaction; prenatal diagnosis; psychological stress; selective abortion; terminology; truth disclosure
As a mother of two sons with adrenoleukodystrophy the author of this paper writes about her experiences of genetic counselling following the diagnosis. She discusses the dilemmas, emotions and aftermath this knowledge has brought to her family and the roles she played. Personal concerns are raised about the values guiding genetic counselling which, she found, focused on the technical details without considering the ethical implications arising from the new knowledge or the emotional dilemmas of prenatal testing. Some consequences of choice and the value of hope are discussed. She concludes by challenging genetic counsellors to deliver a service which not only provides technical information but is cognisant of the ethical considerations this information may foist upon a family.

Malkin, D.; Australie, K.; Shuman, C., et al. Parental attitudes to genetic counseling and predictive testing for childhood cancer. [Abstract]. *American Journal of Human Genetics.* 1996 Oct; 59(4): A7. BE60092.
*attitudes; cancer; children; *genetic counseling; *genetic predisposition; *genetic screening; *parents; risk; survey; Toronto

Mao, Xin. Chinese geneticists approach ethics. [Letter]. *Journal of Medical Ethics.* 1998 Jan; 35(1): 83. 14 refs. BE61126.
*attitudes; confidentiality; developing countries; *directive counseling; disclosure; eugenics; *genetic counseling; genetic disorders; genetic predisposition; genetic research; *genetic screening; genetic services; genetics; guidelines; *health personnel; international aspects; investigators; *non–Western World; *prenatal diagnosis; *selective abortion; sex determination; survey; Western World; *China

Mao, Xin. Ethics and genetics in China: an inside story. [Letter]. *Nature Genetics.* 1997 Sep; 17(1): 20. 5 refs. BE60439.
*attitudes; cultural pluralism; ethical relativism; *eugenics; *genetic counseling; *genetic research; *genetics; health personnel; historical aspects; international aspects; investigators; paternalism; politics; values; *China

Müller, H.J.; Deonna, Th.; Abbt, I., et al. Medical-ethical guidelines for genetic investigations in humans. *Schweizerische Medizinische Wochenschrift.* 1994 Jun 4; 124(22): 974–979. 5 refs. BE59774.
confidentiality; disclosure; employment; *genetic counseling; genetic disorders; genetic predisposition; genetic research; *genetic screening; informed consent; insurance; physicians; *practice guidelines; *prenatal diagnosis; professional organizations; selective abortion; right not to know; *Swiss Academy of Medical Sciences

Neilson, Jane. A patient's perspective on genetic counseling and predictive testing for Alzheimer's disease. *Journal of Genetic Counseling.* 1999 Feb; 8(1): 37–46. BE61643.
attitudes; confidentiality; *dementia; *emotions; *genetic counseling; *genetic screening; patients

Nippert, I.; Horst, J.; Wolff, G., et al. Ethical issues in genetic service provision: attitudes of human geneticists in Germany. [Abstract]. *American Journal of Human Genetics.* 1996 Oct; 59(4): A338. BE60095.
adults; alcohol abuse; allowing to die; *attitudes; autonomy; cancer; children; confidentiality; disclosure; Down syndrome; family members; *genetic counseling; genetic disorders; genetic predisposition; *genetic screening; genetic services; *health personnel; Huntington disease; informed

consent; prenatal diagnosis; referral and consultation; spina bifida; survey; ELSI-funded publication; *Germany

Nuffield Council on Bioethics. Mental Disorders and Genetics: The Ethical Context. London: The Council; 1998 Sep. 117 p. Includes references. ISBN 0-9522701-3-7. BE60716.
adoption; advisory committees; carriers; children; competence; confidentiality; dementia; directive counseling; disclosure; drugs; education; employment; eugenics; family members; gene therapy; *genetic counseling; genetic information; *genetic predisposition; *genetic research; *genetic screening; goals; *guidelines; human experimentation; Huntington disease; informed consent; insurance; legal aspects; *mentally disabled; mentally ill; public policy; reproduction; social discrimination; stigmatization; twins; diagnostic kits; pedigree studies; right not to know; Great Britain; *Nuffield Council on Bioethics

Pentz, Rebecca D. Genetic counseling: guidance for chilling choices. *In:* Demy, Timothy J.; Stewart, Gary P., eds. Genetic Engineering: A Christian Response: Crucial Considerations in Shaping Life. Grand Rapids, MI: Kregel Publications; 1999: 188–195. 3 fn. ISBN 0-8254-2357-0. BE61367.
breast cancer; *Christian ethics; chromosome abnormalities; costs and benefits; decision making; directive counseling; disabled; employment; family members; *gene therapy; *genetic counseling; *genetic enhancement; genetic information; *genetic screening; germ cells; health personnel; insurance; pastoral care; patients; prenatal diagnosis; prolongation of life; quality of life; *risks and benefits; social discrimination; theology; values

Peshkin, Beth N.; Lerman, Caryn. Genetic counselling for hereditary breast cancer. *Lancet.* 1999 Jun 26; 353(9171): 2176–2177. 10 refs. BE62268.
attitudes; *breast cancer; disclosure; empirical research; females; *genetic counseling; *genetic predisposition; *genetic screening; informed consent; psychological stress; risk

Pörn, Ingmar. The meaning of 'rights' in the right to know debate. *In:* Chadwick, Ruth; Levitt, Mairi; Shickle, Darren, eds. The Right to Know and the Right Not to Know. Brookfield, VT: Ashgate; 1997: 37–42. 9 refs. 5 fn. ISBN 1-85972-424-8. BE62187.
*autonomy; *genetic counseling; *genetic information; *genetic screening; *moral obligations; philosophy; *rights; truth disclosure; right not to know

Quaid, Kimberly A. Implications of genetic susceptibility testing with apolipoprotein E. *In:* Post, Stephen G.; Whitehouse, Peter J., eds. Genetic Testing for Alzheimer Disease: Ethical and Clinical Issues. Baltimore, MD: Johns Hopkins University Press; 1998: 118–139. 75 refs. ISBN 0-8018-5840-2. BE60720.
autonomy; breast cancer; comprehension; *dementia; directive counseling; *genetic counseling; genetic predisposition; *genetic screening; genetic services; health personnel; Huntington disease; industry; late-onset disorders; mass screening; paternalism; professional competence; psychological stress; refusal to treat; risk; risks and benefits; uncertainty

Shapira, Amos. 'Wrongful life' lawsuits for faulty genetic counselling: should the impaired newborn be entitled to sue? *Journal of Medical Ethics.* 1998 Dec; 24(6): 369–375. 4 fn. BE60785.
compensation; congenital disorders; *disabled; disclosure; *genetic counseling; genetic screening; health personnel; *legal aspects; *legal liability; *negligence; *newborns; parents; prenatal diagnosis; public health; public policy; right to die; selective abortion; value of life; wedge argument;

*wrongful life; *Israel
A "wrongful life" suit is based on the purported tortious liability of a genetic counsellor towards an infant with hereditary defects, with the latter asserting that he or she would not have been born at all if not for the counsellor's negligence. This negligence allegedly lies in the failure on the part of the defendant adequately to advice the parents or to conduct properly the relevant testing and thereby prevent the child's conception or birth (where unimpaired life was not possible). This paper will offer support for the thesis that it would be both feasible and desirable to endorse "wrongful life" compensation actions. The genetic counsellor owed a duty of due professional care to the impaired newborn who now claims that but for the counsellor's negligence, he or she would not have been born at all. The plaintiff's defective life (where healthy life was never an option) constitutes a compensable injury. A sufficient causal link may exist between the plaintiff's injury and the defendant's breach of duty of due professional care and an appropriate measure of damages can be allocated to the disabled newborn. Sanctioning a "wrongful life" cause of action does not necessarily entail abandoning valuable constraints with regard to abortion and euthanasia. Nor does it inevitably lead to an uncontrolled slide down a "slippery slope".

Silvers, Anita. On not iterating women's disability: a crossover perspective on genetic dilemmas. *In:* Donchin, Anne; Purdy, Laura M., eds. Embodying Bioethics: Recent Feminist Advances. Lanham, MD: Rowman and Littlefield; 1999: 177–202. 65 fn. ISBN 0-8476-8924-7. BE61021.
*autonomy; *bioethics; children; directive counseling; *disabled; disadvantaged; *females; *feminist ethics; *genetic counseling; *hearing disorders; models, theoretical; parent child relationship; parents; *physically disabled; quality of life; social discrimination; social interaction; suffering; *values; Americans with Disabilities Act 1990; United States

Smith, David H.; Quaid, Kimberly A.; Dworkin, Roger B., et al. Early Warning: Cases and Ethical Guidance for Presymptomatic Testing in Genetic Disease. Bloomington, IN: Indiana University Press; 1998. 188 p. (Medical ethics series). Bibliography: p. 171–182. ISBN 0-253-33401-2. BE59667.
adolescents; adoption; adults; anonymous testing; autonomy; beneficence; *case studies; casuistry; children; competence; confidentiality; dangerousness; deception; directive counseling; disclosure; dissent; duty to warn; employment; family members; family relationship; *genetic counseling; *genetic disorders; genetic information; genetic predisposition; genetic research; *genetic screening; *guidelines; health personnel; *Huntington disease; informed consent; insurance; laboratories; *late-onset disorders; *moral obligations; paternalism; patients; prenatal diagnosis; professional ethics; psychological stress; refusal to treat; risks and benefits; selective abortion; truth disclosure; ELSI-funded publication; incidental findings; right not to know

Swiglo, B.A.; Lebel, R.R. Re-contact to advise of testing available to detect high risk for carcinoma: response to letters sent to persons initially ascertained for other genetic reasons. [Abstract]. *American Journal of Human Genetics.* 1997 Oct; 61(4): A390. BE59400.
*cancer; *family members; *genetic counseling; *genetic predisposition; genetic screening; prenatal diagnosis; program descriptions; *incidental findings; *recontact

Wachbroit, Robert. Rethinking medical confidentiality: the impact of genetics. *Suffolk University Law Review.* 1993 Winter; 27(4): 1391–1410. 23 fn. BE61596.

BE = bioethics accession number   fn. = footnotes   refs. = references

autonomy; *confidentiality; *disclosure; *duty to warn; *family members; *genetic counseling; genetic disorders; *genetic information; genetic predisposition; genetic screening; health personnel; injuries; moral obligations; *patients; *privacy; professional patient relationship; public health; *standards; trust; NCHGR-funded publication; right not to know

Wertz, D.C. Is there a "women's ethic" in genetics? A survey of ASHG and NSGC. [Abstract]. *American Journal of Human Genetics.* 1996 Oct; 59(4): A340. BE60097.
adults; *attitudes; children; comparative studies; *directive counseling; *females; *genetic counseling; genetic disorders; *genetic screening; *health personnel; late-onset disorders; *males; *physicians; *prenatal diagnosis; selective abortion; sex determination; survey; United States

Wertz, Dorothy C. Chinese genetics and ethics. [Letter]. *Nature Medicine.* 1999 Mar; 5(3): 247. BE62538.
*attitudes; coercion; *genetic counseling; genetic disorders; government regulation; *health personnel; prenatal diagnosis; selective abortion; *China

Wertz, Dorothy C.; Fletcher, John C.; Berg, Kåre, et al.; World Health Organization. Hereditary Diseases Programme. Guidelines on Ethical Issues in Medical Genetics and the Provision of Genetics Services. Geneva: World Health Organization; 1995. 119 p. Bibliography: p. 83-91; international bibliography: annex p. 1-13. BE62200.
adults; anonymous testing; behavioral genetics; competence; confidentiality; conflict of interest; cultural pluralism; directive counseling; disclosure; DNA data banks; education; embryo research; epidemiology; family members; financial support; gene therapy; *genetic counseling; genetic disorders; genetic enhancement; genetic predisposition; genetic research; genetic screening; *genetic services; *guidelines; health personnel; informed consent; investigators; mass media; mass screening; minors; newborns; prenatal diagnosis; professional ethics; professional patient relationship; reproduction; resource allocation; selective abortion; recontact

Wertz, Dorothy C. International perspectives on ethics and human genetics. *Suffolk University Law Review.* 1993 Winter; 27(4): 1411-1456. 102 fn. BE60738.
abortion, induced; *attitudes; autonomy; children; confidentiality; consensus; developing countries; directive counseling; disclosure; employment; family members; *genetic counseling; genetic disorders; genetic information; *genetic screening; genetic services; health personnel; informed consent; *international aspects; intersexuality; legal aspects; non-Western World; parent child relationship; *prenatal diagnosis; privacy; psychological stress; reproductive technologies; sex determination; survey; values; Western World; women's rights; United States

Wertz, Dorothy C. The difficulties of recruiting minorities to studies of ethics and values in genetics. *Community Genetics.* 1998; 1(3): 175-179. 12 refs. BE62367.
adoption; *attitudes; autonomy; *blacks; comparative studies; confidentiality; directive counseling; disclosure; *genetic counseling; genetic disorders; genetic information; genetic research; *genetic screening; genetic services; *health personnel; medical specialties; *minority groups; paternalism; *patients; physicians; prenatal diagnosis; *public opinion; reproductive technologies; selective abortion; sex determination; survey; values; *United States

White, Mary Terrell. Making responsible decisions: an interpretive ethic for genetic decisionmaking. *Hastings Center Report.* 1999 Jan-Feb; 29(1): 14-21. 7 refs. BE61631.
accountability; autonomy; communication; cultural

pluralism; decision making; *directive counseling; disabled; eugenics; future generations; *genetic counseling; genetic disorders; genetic information; genetic screening; goals; *health personnel; moral obligations; normality; parents; prenatal diagnosis; professional patient relationship; *professional role; reproduction; selective abortion; social interaction; technical expertise; values; Niebuhr, Richard
It is widely thought that genetic counselors should work with parents "nondirectively": they should keep parents informed and support their decisions. But this view misconceives human decisionmaking by failing to recognize that value choices are constructed within and constrained by a community. Acknowledging that decisions involve interaction with and responsibility toward others leads to a "dialogical" model of counseling, in which genetic counselors may question and guide parents' decisions.

Wilfond, Benjamin S.; Rothenberg, Karen H.; Thomson, Elizabeth J., et al.; U.S. National Institutes of Health. Cancer Genetics Studies Consortium. Cancer genetic susceptibility testing: ethical and policy implications for future research and clinical practice. *Journal of Law, Medicine and Ethics.* 1997 Winter; 25(4): 243-251. 38 fn. Commented on by E. Kodish, p. 252-255. BE62669.
advisory committees; breast cancer; *cancer; children; confidentiality; costs and benefits; decision making; disclosure; empirical research; *evaluation; family relationship; females; *genetic counseling; genetic information; *genetic predisposition; *genetic screening; genetic services; health insurance reimbursement; informed consent; late-onset disorders; managed care programs; parents; preimplantation diagnosis; prenatal diagnosis; privacy; *public policy; risk; *risks and benefits; social impact; colon cancer; *Cancer Genetics Studies Consortium; National Institutes of Health; United States

GENETIC ENGINEERING *See* GENE THERAPY, GENETIC INTERVENTION, RECOMBINANT DNA RESEARCH

GENETIC INTERVENTION

See also EUGENICS, CLONING, GENE THERAPY, GENETIC COUNSELING, GENETIC SCREENING, GENOME MAPPING, GENETIC RESEARCH, RECOMBINANT DNA RESEARCH

Agar, Nicholas. Liberal eugenics. *Public Affairs Quarterly.* 1998 Apr; 12(2): 137-155. 31 fn. BE62387.
children; *eugenics; *freedom; *future generations; *genetic enhancement; *genetic intervention; goals; human rights; intelligence; justice; *parents; *quality of life; regulation; reproduction; risks and benefits; values; liberalism

Anderson, J. Kerby. Genetic engineering. In: his Moral Dilemmas: Biblical Perspectives on Contemporary Ethical Issues. Nashville, TN: Word Publishing; 1998: 33-43, 229-230. 18 fn. ISBN 0-8499-1446-9. BE62393.
*Christian ethics; cloning; genetic counseling; genetic disorders; *genetic intervention; genetic research; prenatal diagnosis; recombinant DNA research; reproduction

Andrews, Lori B. The Clone Age: Adventures in the New World of Reproductive Technology. New York, NY: Henry Holt; 1999. 264 p. Notes on sources: p. 263-264. ISBN 0-8050-6080-4. BE61832.
artificial insemination; cloning; cryopreservation; disclosure; economics; embryo transfer; eugenics; genetic disorders; genetic enhancement; genetic information; *genetic

intervention; genetic research; genetic screening; genome mapping; health facilities; historical aspects; in vitro fertilization; *industry; infertility; international aspects; legal aspects; misconduct; motivation; multiple pregnancy; ovum donors; parent child relationship; patents; physicians; posthumous reproduction; preimplantation diagnosis; prenatal diagnosis; regulation; remuneration; *reproductive technologies; risks and benefits; selective abortion; semen donors; social impact; surrogate mothers

Appleyard, Bryan. Brave New Worlds: Staying Human in the Genetic Future. New York, NY: Viking; 1998. 198 p. Bibliography: p. 183–186. ISBN 0–670–86989–9. BE60356.
> *attitudes; behavioral genetics; biology; cloning; dehumanization; ecology; *eugenics; evolution; freedom; gene therapy; genetic counseling; genetic determinism; genetic disorders; *genetic intervention; genetic predisposition; genetic research; genetic screening; *genetics; genome mapping; historical aspects; humanism; investigators; life extension; minority groups; morality; National Socialism; normality; politics; preimplantation diagnosis; prenatal diagnosis; preventive medicine; public opinion; public policy; *recombinant DNA research; reproduction; *risks and benefits; *science; selective abortion; self regulation; social control; social discrimination; *social impact; transgenic organisms; value of life; *values; nature; Asilomar Conference

Bagness, Carmel. Genetics, the Fetus and Our Future. Hale, Cheshire, England: Hochland and Hochland; 1998. 105 p. Includes references. ISBN 1–898507–65–1. BE59721.
> aborted fetuses; cadavers; confidentiality; criminal law; disabled; embryo disposition; *embryo research; *embryos; eugenics; fetuses; gene therapy; genetic disorders; genetic enhancement; *genetic intervention; genetic materials; genome mapping; germ cells; legal aspects; moral obligations; multiple pregnancy; ovum donors; patents; personhood; preimplantation diagnosis; property rights; recombinant DNA research; regulation; remuneration; *reproductive technologies; research embryo creation; *risks and benefits; selective abortion; semen donors; social discrimination; social impact; torts; Great Britain; Human Genome Project

Balls, Michael. The precautionary principle should be used with caution -- and should be applied to animal experimentation and genetic manipulation, not merely to protection of the environment. [Editorial]. *ATLA: Alternatives to Laboratory Animals.* 1999 Jan–Feb; 27(1): 1–5. 12 refs. BE62543.
> *animal experimentation; animal organs; cloning; *ecology; evaluation; federal government; *genetic intervention; genome mapping; government regulation; health hazards; organ transplantation; politics; *public policy; research design; risks and benefits; standards; toxicity; transgenic animals; prudence; Great Britain; United States

Balls, Michael. The production of genetically modified animals and humans: an inescapable moral challenge to scientists and laypeople alike. [Editorial]. *ATLA: Alternatives to Laboratory Animals.* 1998 Jan–Feb; 26(1): 1–2. 5 refs. BE59788.
> *cloning; government regulation; hybrids; primates; risks and benefits; *transgenic animals

Barnaby, Wendy. Biological weapons and genetic engineering. *GenEthics News.* 1997 Jun–Jul; No. 18: 4–5. BE60819.
> *biological warfare; *genetic intervention; genetic research; international aspects; microbiology; minority groups; United States

Barton, John; Crandon, John; Kennedy, Donald, et al.

A model protocol to assess the risks of agricultural introductions: a risk–based approach to rationalizing field trial regulations. *Nature Biotechnology.* 1997 Sep; 15(9): 845–848. 9 refs. BE62021.
> *ecology; *evaluation; genetic intervention; genetic research; government regulation; international aspects; *risk; *transgenic organisms; *agriculture; *transgenic plants

Birmingham, Karen. UK leads on science and technology bioethics. [News]. *Nature Medicine.* 1998 Jun; 4(6): 651–652. BE59729.
> accountability; *bioethical issues; DNA data banks; *DNA fingerprinting; embryo research; forensic medicine; gene therapy; *genetic intervention; government regulation; *international aspects; law enforcement; prisoners; *public policy; *regulation; reproductive technologies; science; *Great Britain; United States

Buchanan, Allen. Choosing who will be disabled: genetic intervention and the morality of inclusion. *In:* Paul, Ellen Frankel; Miller, Fred D.; Paul, Jeffrey, eds. Scientific Innovation, Philosophy, and Public Policy. New York, NY: Cambridge University Press; 1996: 18–46. 21 fn. ISBN 0–521–58994–0. BE62742.
> beneficence; *disabled; eugenics; fetuses; gene therapy; genetic disorders; genetic enhancement; *genetic intervention; genetic research; *justice; moral policy; political activity; public policy; quality of life; resource allocation; rights; selective abortion; stigmatization; value of life; values

Butler, Declan. Human genome declaration looks set for United Nations approval. [News]. *Nature.* 1998 Nov 26; 396(6709): 297. BE59535.
> cloning; gene therapy; *genetic intervention; *genome mapping; germ cells; *human rights; *international aspects; Unesco; *United Nations; *Universal Declaration on the Human Genome and Human Rights

Butler, Declan; Reichhardt, Tony. Long–term effect of GM crops serves up food for thought. *Nature.* 1999 Apr 22; 398(6729): 651–656. BE61397.
> ecology; *food; genetic intervention; genetic research; government regulation; health hazards; industry; international aspects; legal aspects; risk; toxicity; transgenic organisms; *agriculture; *transgenic plants; Europe; Japan

Byk, Christian. A map to a new treasure island: the human genome and the concept of common heritage. *Journal of Medicine and Philosophy.* 1998 Jun; 23(3): 234–246. 14 refs. BE59288.
> advisory committees; autonomy; confidentiality; democracy; ecology; future generations; gene therapy; *genetic information; *genetic intervention; *genetic research; genome mapping; *guidelines; historical aspects; *human rights; *international aspects; investigators; legal aspects; moral obligations; obligations of society; privacy; public policy; regulation; rights; risks and benefits; social discrimination; values; vulnerable populations; International Bioethics Committee (Unesco); Twentieth Century; Unesco; *Universal Declaration on the Protection of the Human Genome (Unesco)

While the 1970's have been called the environmental years, the 1990's could be seen as the genome years. As the challenge to map and to sequence the human genome mobilized the scientific community, risks and benefits of information and uses that would derive from this project have also raised ethical issues at the international level. The particular interest of the 1997 UNESCO Declaration relies on the fact that it emphasizes both the scientific importance of genetics and the appropriate reinforcement of human rights in this area. It considers the human genome, at least symbolically, as the common heritage of humanity.

BE = bioethics accession number   fn. = footnotes   refs. = references

Claes, Tom. Cultural background of the ethical and social debate about biotechnology. *In:* Sterckx, Sigrid, ed. Biotechnology, Patents and Morality. Proceedings of an International Workshop, "Biotechnology, Patents and Morality: Towards a Consensus," held in Ghent, Belgium, 17–19 Jan 1996. Brookfield, VT: Ashgate; 1997: 121–127. ISBN 1-84014-158-1. BE62240.
 *genetic intervention; natural law; patents; religion; risks and benefits; secularism; speciesism; *transgenic animals; values; *biotechnology

Coghlan, Andy. Named and shamed: genetic engineers who flouted the rules are brought to book. [News]. *New Scientist.* 1998 Apr 4; 158(2128): 4. BE59716.
 disclosure; *ecology; *genetic intervention; *government regulation; *industry; investigators; research institutes; *scientific misconduct; transgenic organisms; *agriculture; *transgenic plants; Advisory Committee on Releases to the Environment (Great Britain); *Great Britain

Cook, Robin. Chromosome 6. [Fiction]. New York, NY: Berkley Books; 1997. 460 p. ISBN 0-425-16124-2. BE60706.
 animal experimentation; animal organs; cloning; *genetic intervention; industry; organ transplantation; *Africa

Demy, Timothy J.; Stewart, Gary P., eds. Genetic Engineering: A Christian Response: Crucial Considerations in Shaping Life. Grand Rapids, MI: Kregel Publications; 1999. 320 p. (Christian response series). Includes references. ISBN 0-8254-2357-0. BE61359.
 accountability; autonomy; behavioral genetics; *Christian ethics; cloning; compassion; embryo research; embryos; ethical relativism; eugenics; gene therapy; genetic counseling; *genetic determinism; genetic disorders; genetic enhancement; *genetic intervention; genetic predisposition; genetic research; genetic screening; genome mapping; hospices; human rights; involuntary sterilization; justice; mentally disabled; *moral policy; newborns; patents; personhood; policy analysis; postmodernism; prenatal diagnosis; *Protestant ethics; reproductive technologies; *Roman Catholic ethics; selective abortion; suffering; *theology; transgenic organisms; twinning; *value of life; Alabama; Christian Fundamentalists; Evangelical Christians; Lousiana; Social Darwinism; Twentieth Century; United States

de Pomerai, David I. Are there limits to animal transgenesis? *European Journal of Genetics in Society.* 1997; 3(1): 4–12. 50 refs. BE61451.
 animal experimentation; animal rights; animal testing alternatives; Christian ethics; methods; patents; public opinion; suffering; *transgenic animals; trends

De Tavernier, Johan. Biotechnology policy and ethics. *In:* Sterckx, Sigrid, ed. Biotechnology, Patents and Morality. Proceedings of an International Workshop, "Biotechnology, Patents and Morality: Towards a Consensus," held in Ghent, Belgium, 17–19 Jan 1996. Brookfield, VT: Ashgate; 1997: 114–120. ISBN 1-84014-158-1. BE62239.
 animal rights; common good; ecology; food; *genetic intervention; moral obligations; *moral policy; risk; *risks and benefits; social impact; speciesism; suffering; *transgenic animals; values; agriculture; *biotechnology; environmental ethics; transgenic plants

Dickson, David. Proceed with caution, says UK report on ethics of GM foods. [News]. *Nature.* 1999 Jun 3; 399(6735): 396. BE62270.
 advisory committees; developing countries; dissent; ecology; *food; genetic intervention; *government regulation; industry; patents; public policy; agriculture; biotechnology;

*transgenic plants; *Genetically Modified Crops: The Ethical and Social Issues; *Great Britain; *Nuffield Council on Bioethics

Dronamraju, Krishna R. Biological and Social Issues in Biotechnology Sharing. Brookfield, VT: Ashgate; 1998. 165 p. Bibliography: p. 157–162. ISBN 1-84014-897-7. BE60744.
 developing countries; DNA sequences; drug industry; drugs; ecology; economics; federal government; gene therapy; genetic diversity; *genetic intervention; *genetic research; *international aspects; microbiology; *patents; *property rights; public policy; recombinant DNA research; regulation; transgenic animals; agriculture; *technology transfer; *transgenic plants; National Institutes of Health; United States

Eisenberg, Vered H.; Schenker, Joseph G. Genetic engineering: moral aspects and control of practice. *Journal of Assisted Reproduction and Genetics.* 1997 Jul; 14(6): 297–316. 98 refs. BE62404.
 AIDS; cancer; Christian ethics; cloning; eugenics; *gene therapy; genetic enhancement; *genetic intervention; germ cells; government regulation; human experimentation; informed consent; international aspects; Islamic ethics; Jewish ethics; resource allocation; risks and benefits

Engelhardt, H. Tristram. Germ–line genetic engineering and moral diversity: moral controversies in a post–Christian world. *In:* Paul, Ellen Frankel; Miller, Fred D.; Paul, Jeffrey, eds. Scientific Innovation, Philosophy, and Public Policy. New York, NY: Cambridge University Press; 1996: 47–62. 23 fn. ISBN 0–521–58994–0. BE62743.
 beneficence; *cultural pluralism; *gene therapy; genetic enhancement; *genetic intervention; *germ cells; goals; health; *human characteristics; medicine; *moral policy; morality; philosophy; public policy; *secularism; theology; values

European Commission. Group of Advisers to the European Commission on the Ethical Implications of Biotechnology. Luxembourg: Office for Official Publications of the European Communities; 1996. 24 p. Includes summaries of GAEIB opinions on (1) bovine somatotrophin or BST; (2) manufacture of human blood and human plasma products; (3) legal protection of biological inventions; (4) gene therapy; (5) labelling of food derived from modern biotechnology; (6) prenatal diagnosis; and (7) the genetic modification of animals. ISBN 98–827–7350–7. BE59459.
 *advisory committees; bioethical issues; biomedical technologies; committee membership; food; gene therapy; *genetic intervention; germ cells; human rights; *international aspects; *organization and administration; patents; prenatal diagnosis; regulation; science; transgenic animals; *Europe; *European Commission; *Group of Advisers on the Ethical Implications of Biotechnology (European Commission)

European Parliament. Scientific and Technological Options Assessment (STOA) Programme Contractor. Bioethics in Europe. Final Report, July 1992. Luxembourg: European Parliament, Directorate General for Research; 1992 Sep 8. 257 p. Includes references. Pub. No. PE 158.453. BE62499.
 advisory committees; attitudes; *bioethical issues; bioethics; biological warfare; *biomedical technologies; *comparative studies; *ecology; embryo research; fetal research; fetal tissue donation; food; gene therapy; *genetic intervention; genetic screening; genome mapping; germ cells; government regulation; hormones; in vitro fertilization; *international aspects; patents; preimplantation diagnosis; prenatal diagnosis; professional organizations; public opinion; *public

policy; recombinant DNA research; reproductive technologies; risks and benefits; *social impact; technology assessment; transgenic animals; transgenic organisms; agriculture; *biotechnology; *Denmark; *Europe; European Community; *European Parliament; *France; *Germany; *Great Britain; *Greece; *Italy; *Spain

Fagan, John. Genetic Engineering: The Hazards -- Vedic Engineering: The Solutions. Fairfield, IA: Maharish: International University Press; 1995. 172 p. 50 refs. ISBN 0-923569-18-9. BE60504.
　　*alternative therapies; *ecology; evolution; gene pool; gene therapy; *genetic intervention; genetic screening; germ cells; health; health hazards; preventive medicine; *recombinant DNA research; *risks and benefits; transgenic organisms; agriculture; *Ayurveda

Fretz, Leo. Biotechnology and the public debate: some philosophical reflections. *In:* Sterckx, Sigrid, ed. Biotechnology, Patents and Morality. Proceedings of an International Workshop, "Biotechnology, Patents and Morality: Towards a Consensus," held in Ghent, Belgium, 17-19 Jan 1996. Brookfield, VT: Ashgate; 1997: 257-265. 13 fn. ISBN 1-84014-158-1. BE62243.
　　consensus; deontological ethics; ecology; *evaluation; *genetic intervention; genetic predisposition; genetic research; health hazards; insurance; investigators; public opinion; *public participation; risk; *risks and benefits; social discrimination; technical expertise; teleological ethics; *transgenic animals; *biotechnology; Europe

Garcia, Sandra Anderson. Sociocultural and legal implications of creating and sustaining life through biomedical technology. *Journal of Legal Medicine.* 1996 Dec; 17(4): 469-525. 220 fn. BE61244.
　　abortion, induced; allowing to die; bioethics; biomedical research; *biomedical technologies; cultural pluralism; decision making; determination of death; disadvantaged; fetal research; futility; genetic counseling; *genetic intervention; genetic screening; genome mapping; intensive care units; international aspects; investigators; justice; law; legal aspects; minority groups; misconduct; newborns; physicians; political activity; prolongation of life; public policy; religion; reproduction; *reproductive technologies; resource allocation; rights; science; selection for treatment; socioeconomic factors; withholding treatment; United States

Genetics Forum (London). The Case Against Patents in Genetic Engineering: A Special Report from the Genetics Forum. London: Genetics Forum; 1996 Apr. 28 p. 21 fn. ISBN 0-9528201-0-2. BE60709.
　　alternatives; developing countries; genes; genetic diversity; *genetic intervention; genetic research; human rights; industry; *international aspects; *legal aspects; *patents; regulation; *transgenic organisms; agriculture; nature; *Europe; European Commission; European Parliament; European Patent Convention; European Patent Office; European Union; Great Britain; Patent and Trademark Office; United States

Gillon, Raanan. Ethical issues. *In:* Weber, Walter; Mulvihill, John J.; Narod, Steven A., eds. Familial Cancer Management. Boca Raton, FL: CRC Press; 1996: 142-158. 26 refs. BE61799.
　　*cancer; confidentiality; deception; directive counseling; disclosure; dissent; employment; *family members; gene therapy; genetic counseling; genetic disorders; genetic information; *genetic intervention; *genetic predisposition; *genetic screening; informed consent; insurance; justice; mandatory testing; *patient care; physician patient relationship; preventive medicine; rights; risks and benefits; selective abortion; social discrimination; stigmatization; surgery; transgenic organisms; wedge argument; incidental findings; Great Britain

Glover, Eric. French panel calls for closer monitoring of genetic modification. [News]. *Nature.* 1998 Jul 2; 394(6688): 4. BE59888.
　　*advisory committees; biomedical research; consensus; ecology; *genetic intervention; *public participation; public policy; public sector; *recombinant DNA research; *regulation; risks and benefits; *transgenic organisms; agriculture; *France

Golub, Edward S. Finding a vocabulary for the extrascientific significance of technology. *Nature Biotechnology.* 1997 May; 15(5): 394. BE62015.
　　*cloning; confidentiality; genetic determinism; genetic information; *genetic intervention; investigators; public opinion; risks and benefits; *social impact; technology assessment

Gordon, Jon W. Genetic enhancement in humans. *Science.* 1999 Mar 26; 283(5410): 2023-2024. 12 fn. BE61032.
　　animal experimentation; embryo research; eugenics; evaluation; evolution; future generations; gene pool; gene therapy; *genetic enhancement; *genetic intervention; genetic research; germ cells; human experimentation; informed consent; methods; *public policy; reproductive technologies; risks and benefits; social impact; stem cells; *gene transfer

Gosden, Roger. Designing Babies: The Brave New World of Reproductive Technology. New York, NY: W.H. Freeman; 1999. 260 p. Bibliography: p. 247-254. ISBN 0-7167-3299-8. BE62625.
　　age factors; attitudes; autonomy; cloning; congenital disorders; embryos; eugenics; evolution; family planning; females; gene therapy; genetic disorders; *genetic enhancement; *genetic intervention; genetic screening; genetics; germ cells; government regulation; historical aspects; males; methods; parent child relationship; preimplantation diagnosis; prenatal diagnosis; privacy; public policy; reproduction; *reproductive technologies; *risks and benefits; science; selective abortion; sex determination; sex preselection; social control; social impact; surrogate mothers

Hill, Ruaraidh; Stanisstreet, Martin; Boyes, Edward, et al. Animal experimentation needs dissection. [Letter]. *Nature.* 1998 Jan 8; 391(6663): 117. BE59186.
　　*animal experimentation; attitudes; pain; public opinion; students; *transgenic animals; universities

Hobsons Publishing PLC. Genes, Diseases and Dilemmas: A Resource Book for A-Level General Studies and 16-19 Entitlement Curriculum. [Teachers' notes and student booklet; sponsored by the Association of the British Pharmaceutical Industry (ABPI)]. Cambridge, England: Hobsons Scientific Publishing; 1993. 27 p. (Issues series). ISBN 1-85324-893-3. BE59249.
　　confidentiality; gene therapy; genetic counseling; *genetic disorders; genetic enhancement; genetic information; *genetic intervention; genetic predisposition; genetic screening; *genetics; genome mapping; public opinion; schools; selective abortion; transgenic animals; truth disclosure; secondary schools; Great Britain

Hollinger, Dennis P. A theology of healing and genetic engineering. *In:* Demy, Timothy J.; Stewart, Gary P., eds. Genetic Engineering: A Christian Response: Crucial Considerations in Shaping Life. Grand Rapids, MI: Kregel Publications; 1999: 294-303. 11 fn. ISBN 0-8254-2357-0. BE61372.
　　*Christian ethics; dehumanization; economics; eugenics; *gene therapy; *genetic disorders; genetic enhancement; *genetic intervention; *intention; *moral policy; *motivation; religion; social discrimination; theology; value of life; dignity; empowerment; *faith healing

---

Holtug, Nils. Creating and patenting new life forms. *In:* Kuhse, Helga; Singer, Peter, eds. A Companion to Bioethics. Malden, MA: Blackwell; 1998: 206–214. 21 refs. ISBN 0–631–19737–0. BE59496.
  animal rights; ethical analysis; gene therapy; genetic enhancement; *genetic intervention; microbiology; *moral policy; *patents; recombinant DNA research; risks and benefits; suffering; *transgenic animals; *transgenic organisms; values; transgenic plants

Holtug, Nils. Does justice require genetic enhancements? *Journal of Medical Ethics.* 1999 Apr; 25(2): 137–143. 15 fn. BE61917.
  *compensation; cosmetic surgery; disabled; disease; enhancement technologies; *gene therapy; *genetic disorders; *genetic enhancement; *goals; government financing; growth disorders; health; health care; hormones; *justice; *medicine; *moral policy; normality; patient care; preventive medicine; psychological stress; public policy; resource allocation; social discrimination
  It is argued that justice in some cases provides a pro tanto reason genetically to enhance victims of the genetic lottery. Various arguments -- both to the effect that justice provides no such reason and to the effect that while there may be such reasons, they are overridden by certain moral constraints -- are considered and rejected. Finally, it is argued that justice provides stronger reasons to perform more traditional medical tasks (treatments), and that therefore genetic enhancements should not play an important role in a public health care system.

Käppeli, Othmar; Auberson, Lillian. Biotech battlelines. [Letter]. *Nature.* 1998 Jul 2; 394(6688): 10. BE59934.
  attitudes; emotions; *genetic intervention; government regulation; *investigators; mass media; morality; *political activity; public opinion; *public participation; public policy; *recombinant DNA research; risks and benefits; transgenic organisms; *Switzerland

Kaye, Howard L. Anxiety and genetic manipulation: a sociological view. *Perspectives in Biology and Medicine.* 1998 Summer; 41(4): 483–490. 27 refs. BE61110.
  attitudes; autonomy; bioethics; *cloning; *dehumanization; emotions; eugenics; family relationship; future generations; *genetic determinism; genetic identity; *genetic intervention; interdisciplinary communication; *morality; *psychological stress; *public opinion; reproductive technologies; science; self concept; *social impact; social sciences; value of life; *values; dignity; sociology

Kin, Curtis A. Coming soon to the "genetic supermarket" near you. [Note]. *Stanford Law Review.* 1996 Jul; 48(6): 1573–1604. 159 fn. BE62176.
  biomedical technologies; children; drugs; *enhancement technologies; federal government; gene therapy; *genetic enhancement; *government regulation; *growth disorders; *hormones; industry; legal aspects; *normality; recombinant DNA research; risks and benefits; *biotechnology; Food and Drug Administration; *United States

Klaffke, Oliver. The sacred and the profane: Swiss attitudes to genetic engineering have deep cultural roots. [News]. *New Scientist.* 1998 Jun 6; 158(2137): 61. BE59160.
  *attitudes; *ecology; *genetic intervention; government regulation; *historical aspects; public opinion; public participation; public policy; transgenic organisms; *values; nature; *Europe; France; Germany; Italy; Switzerland

Lagay, Faith L. Science, rhetoric, and public discourse in genetic research. *Cambridge Quarterly of Healthcare Ethics.* 1999 Spring; 8(2): 226–237. 33 fn. BE61238.
  alcohol abuse; bioethical issues; *consensus; *cultural pluralism; *decision making; *democracy; emotions; *gene therapy; genetic disorders; *genetic enhancement; *genetic intervention; genetic predisposition; *genetic research; justice; models, theoretical; moral policy; normality; obligations of society; philosophy; postmodernism; public participation; *public policy; values; virtues; needs; rationality; *rhetoric

Leffel, Jim. Genetics and human rights in a postmodern age. *In:* Demy, Timothy J.; Stewart, Gary P., eds. Genetic Engineering: A Christian Response: Crucial Considerations in Shaping Life. Grand Rapids, MI: Kregel Publications; 1999: 126–138. 39 fn. ISBN 0–8254–2357–0. BE61364.
  autonomy; behavioral genetics; *Christian ethics; cloning; commodification; *cultural pluralism; dehumanization; embryo research; employment; *ethical relativism; eugenics; gene therapy; *genetic determinism; *genetic intervention; genetic materials; genetic research; genetic screening; health insurance; historical aspects; *human rights; humanism; patents; *personhood; *postmodernism; preimplantation diagnosis; prenatal diagnosis; property rights; secularism; selective abortion; sex determination; social discrimination; social problems; theology; transgenic organisms; *value of life; dignity; Social Darwinism; United States

Lemkow, Louis. Public Attitudes to Genetic Engineering: Some European Perspectives. Shankill, Ireland: European Foundation for the Improvement of Living and Working Conditions; 1993. 44 p. Bibliography: p. 41–44. ISBN 9282640027. BE62141.
  decision making; drugs; ecology; empirical research; females; food; *genetic intervention; genetic research; *international aspects; knowledge, attitudes, practice; males; occupational exposure; *public opinion; public participation; public policy; regulation; *risks and benefits; social impact; socioeconomic factors; survey; transgenic organisms; agriculture; *Europe; European Economic Community; France; Germany; Great Britain; Spain

Lemonick, Michael D. Designer babies. *Time.* 1999 Jan 11; 153(1): 64–67. BE60312.
  eugenics; genetic disorders; *genetic enhancement; in vitro fertilization; methods; *preimplantation diagnosis; prenatal diagnosis; public opinion; selective abortion; *sex preselection; social impact; United States

Lucassen, Emy. The ethics of genetic engineering. *Journal of Applied Philosophy.* 1996; 13(1): 51–61. 15 fn. BE59554.
  deontological ethics; ecology; ethical analysis; genetic diversity; *genetic intervention; *microbiology; *moral policy; *recombinant DNA research; risks and benefits; *transgenic organisms; agriculture; nature

McGee, Glenn. Ethics and the future of genetic testing. *In:* Smith, Edward; Sapp, Walter, eds. Plain Talk about the Human Genome Project: A Tuskegee University Conference on Its Promise and Perils ... and Matters of Race. Tuskegee, AL: Tuskegee University Press; 1997: 151–158. 7 refs. ISBN 1–891196–01–4. BE61742.
  children; decision making; enhancement technologies; gene therapy; *genetic enhancement; *genetic intervention; genetic research; genetic screening; intelligence; motivation; normality; parents; risks and benefits; transgenic organisms

McGee, Glenn. Genetic enhancement of families. *In:* McGee, Glenn, ed. Pragmatic Bioethics. Nashville, TN: Vanderbilt University Press; 1999: 168–180, 279–280. 20 fn. ISBN 0–8265–1321–2. BE60670.
  behavior control; behavioral genetics; eugenics; gene therapy; genetic diversity; *genetic enhancement; *genetic intervention; genetic research; parent child relationship; *parents; risks and benefits

---

McLean, Margaret R. When what we know outstrips what we can do. *Issues in Ethics (Markkula Center for Applied Ethics).* 1998 Spring–Summer; 9(2): 6–10. BE62037.
confidentiality; family members; genetic counseling; genetic enhancement; genetic information; *genetic intervention; *genetic screening; genome mapping; *Huntington disease; justice; resource allocation; right not to know

Maclean, Norman. Transgenic animals in perspective. *In:* Maclean, Norman, ed. Animals with Novel Genes. New York, NY: Cambridge University Press; 1994: 1–20. 35 refs. ISBN 0-521-43256-1. BE61374.
drugs; ecology; food; gene therapy; government regulation; health hazards; *methods; recombinant DNA research; *risks and benefits; stem cells; terminology; *transgenic animals

Marlier, Eric. Opinions of Europeans on Biotechnology in 1991: Report Undertaken on Behalf of the Directorate-General for Science, Research and Development of the Commission of the European Communities. Brussels, Belgium: INRA (Europe). European Coordination Office; 1991. 98 p. Eurobarometer 35.1. BE59260.
drugs; ecology; food; *genetic intervention; genetic research; government regulation; health hazards; international aspects; knowledge, attitudes, practice; microbiology; *public opinion; *risks and benefits; *social control; social impact; survey; transgenic plants; Belgium; Denmark; *Europe; European Community; France; Germany; Great Britain; Greece; Ireland; Italy; Luxembourg; Netherlands; Portugal; Spain

Masood, Ehsan. Britain opens biotech regulation to greater public involvement. [News]. *Nature.* 1999 May 27; 399(6734): 287–288. BE62269.
advisory committees; attitudes; decision making; ecology; *food; genetic intervention; *government regulation; industry; information dissemination; investigators; political activity; professional organizations; public health; *public opinion; *public participation; *public policy; risks and benefits; social impact; agriculture; *biotechnology; *transgenic plants; Agricultural and Environment Biotechnology Commission (Great Britain); Food Standards Agency (Great Britain); *Great Britain; Human Genetics Commission (Great Britain); Nuffield Council on Bioethics

Meade, Harry M. Dairy gene. *Sciences.* 1997 Sep–Oct; 37(5): 20–25. BE61519.
*cloning; drug industry; drugs; *economics; *methods; *risks and benefits; *transgenic animals

Melnick, Vijaya L. The brave new world of DNA: transcendence or transgression? *In:* Smith, Edward; Sapp, Walter, eds. Plain Talk about the Human Genome Project: A Tuskegee University Conference on Its Promise and Perils ... and Matters of Race. Tuskegee, AL: Tuskegee University Press; 1997: 197–200. 3 refs. ISBN 1-8911196-01-4. BE61747.
disabled; *disease; *genetic disorders; *genetic intervention; *health; mental health; *normality; socioeconomic factors

Mepham, T. Ben; Combes, Robert D.; Balls, Michael, et al. The Use of Transgenic Animals in the European Union: The Report and Recommendations of ECVAM [European Centre for the Validation of Alternative Methods] Workshop 28. *ATLA: Alternatives to Laboratory Animals.* 1998 Jan–Feb; 26(1): 21–43. 81 refs. Report on ECVAM workshop 28 held in Southwell, Nottinghamshire, England, 7–11 Apr 1997. BE59892.
*animal experimentation; animal organs; animal testing alternatives; biomedical research; *guidelines; *international

aspects; methods; public opinion; regulation; risks and benefits; toxicity; *transgenic animals; agriculture; *Europe; *European Union

Miller, Henry I. Policy Controversy in Biotechnology: An Insider's View. Austin, TX: R.G. Landes; 1997. 221 p. (Biotechnology intelligence unit). Includes references. ISBN 1-57059-408-2. BE62779.
drugs; *federal government; food; gene therapy; genetic intervention; *government regulation; human experimentation; international aspects; microbiology; *politics; *public policy; *recombinant DNA research; risk; science; agriculture; *biotechnology; Department of Agriculture; Environmental Protection Agency; Food and Drug Administration; National Institutes of Health; *United States

Milunsky, Aubrey. The "new" genetics: from research to reality. *Suffolk University Law Review.* 1993 Winter; 27(4): 1307–1325. 61 fn. BE60736.
carriers; confidentiality; DNA data banks; economics; employment; gene therapy; genetic disorders; *genetic intervention; genetic predisposition; *genetic screening; genome mapping; industry; informed consent; insurance; laboratories; legal aspects; preimplantation diagnosis; prenatal diagnosis; public policy; sex preselection; social discrimination; United States

Newson, Ainsley; Williamson, Robert. Should we undertake genetic research on intelligence? *Bioethics.* 1999 Jul; 13(3–4): 327–342. 36 fn. BE61883.
*behavioral genetics; eugenics; family relationship; genes; *genetic enhancement; genetic information; *genetic research; genetic screening; *intelligence; resource allocation; risks and benefits; social discrimination; social impact; values
Although the concept of intelligence is difficult to define, research has provided evidence for a significant genetic component. Attempts are now being made to use molecular genetic approaches to identify genes contributing to intelligence, and to determine the ways in which they interact with environmental variables. This research is then likely to determine the developmental pathways of intelligence, in an effort to understand mental handicap and learning disorders and develop new treatment strategies. This paper reviews research on the genetic basis of intelligence, and discusses the ethical concerns, including the role of genetic information, the value we place on intelligence and the allocation of resources. It will be argued that the objections raised are problematic, and that because of the value of this knowledge and the prospect of improving lives, this research is morally required. We will then provide a brief analysis of the issues raised by enhancement of intelligence using genetic technology, and will argue that there is no intrinsic difference between this and other means of optimising intelligence.

O'Mathúna, Dónal P. Applying justice to genetics. *In:* Demy, Timothy J.; Stewart, Gary P., eds. Genetic Engineering: A Christian Response: Crucial Considerations in Shaping Life. Grand Rapids, MI: Kregel Publications; 1999: 50–69. 53 fn. ISBN 0-8254-2357-0. BE61360.
autonomy; behavioral genetics; *Christian ethics; cultural pluralism; *disabled; disadvantaged; ethical relativism; eugenics; family relationship; gene therapy; *genetic determinism; *genetic disorders; genetic enhancement; genetic information; *genetic intervention; genetic screening; *justice; *moral obligations; *obligations of society; parent child relationship; prenatal diagnosis; reproduction; selective abortion; *social discrimination; social problems; theology; utilitarianism; *value of life; *values; virtues; wrongful life; United States

---

BE = bioethics accession number   fn. = footnotes   refs. = references

Pearson, Graham S. How to make microbes safer. *Nature.* 1998 Jul 16; 394(6690): 217-218. BE59154.
*biological warfare; ecology; genetic intervention; guidelines; health hazards; *international aspects; *microbiology; recombinant DNA research; *regulation; risks and benefits; *transgenic organisms

Rappaport, Shabtai A. Genetic engineering: technology, creation, and interference. *Jewish Medical Ethics.* 1997 Jan; 3(1): 3-4. 8 fn. BE59245.
gene therapy; *genetic intervention; hybrids; *Jewish ethics

Resnik, David B.; Steinkraus, Holly B.; Langer, Pamela J. Human Germline Gene Therapy: Scientific, Moral and Political Issues. Austin, TX: R.G. Landes; 1999. 189 p. (Medical intelligence unit; 9). Includes references. ISBN 1-57059-586-0. BE61052.
alternatives; artificial insemination; autonomy; beneficence; children; confidentiality; embryo transfer; eugenics; future generations; gene pool; *gene therapy; genetic determinism; genetic disorders; genetic diversity; genetic enhancement; *genetic intervention; genetic screening; *germ cells; government regulation; human characteristics; human rights; in vitro fertilization; injuries; justice; legal rights; methods; moral obligations; *moral policy; natural law; parents; patents; preimplantation diagnosis; prenatal diagnosis; preventive medicine; privacy; *public policy; risk; *risks and benefits; selection for treatment; selective abortion; social discrimination; *social impact; socioeconomic factors; utilitarianism

Richter, Gerd; Bacchetta, Matthew D. Interventions in the human genome: some moral and ethical considerations. *Journal of Medicine and Philosophy.* 1998 Jun; 23(3): 303-317. 35 refs. BE59294.
autonomy; children; costs and benefits; disclosure; embryo research; *ethical analysis; eugenics; future generations; *gene therapy; *genetic enhancement; *genetic intervention; *germ cells; human experimentation; informed consent; intention; international aspects; justice; *methods; *moral policy; parental consent; preimplantation diagnosis; preventive medicine; public policy; regulation; risk; *risks and benefits; stem cells; Germany
In the debate regarding the different possibilities for gene therapy, it is presupposed that the manipulations are limited to the nuclear genome (nDNA). Given recent advances in genetics, mitochondrial genome (mtDNA) and diseases must be considered as well. In this paper, we propose a three dimensional framework for the ethical debate of gene therapy where we add the genomic type (nDNA vs. mtDNA) as a third dimension to be considered beside the paradigmatic dimensions of target cell (somatic vs. germ-line) and purpose (therapeutic vs. enhancement). Somatic gene therapy can be viewed today as generally accepted, and we review the contemporary arguments surrounding it on the basis of bioethical-pragmatic, socio-political and deontological classifications. Many of the supposed ethical questions of somatic gene therapy today are not new; they are well-known issues of research ethics. We also critically summarize the different international perspectives and the German ethical discussion regarding manipulations of germ-line cells.

Rifkin, Jeremy. Who will decide between defect and perfect? *Washington Post.* 1998 Apr 19: C4. BE59370.
*eugenics; future generations; genetic disorders; *genetic enhancement; *genetic intervention; *germ cells; normality

Robinson, John H.; Berry, Roberta M.; McDonnell, Kevin, eds. Reproduction. *In: their* A Health Law Reader: An Interdisciplinary Approach. Durham, NC: Carolina Academic Press; 1999: 73-180. 38 fn. ISBN

0-89089-907-X. BE62292.
*abortion, induced; attitudes; autonomy; children; cloning; *commodification; dehumanization; disabled; eugenics; family relationship; feminist ethics; fetuses; *freedom; gene therapy; *genetic intervention; genetic screening; government regulation; legal aspects; minority groups; *moral policy; morality; parent child relationship; personhood; prenatal diagnosis; *public policy; *reproduction; *reproductive technologies; rights; selective abortion; sex determination; sexuality; Supreme Court decisions; surrogate mothers; value of life; Roe v. Wade; United States

Saatkamp, Herman J. Genetics and pragmatism. *In:* McGee, Glenn, ed. Pragmatic Bioethics. Nashville, TN: Vanderbilt University Press; 1999: 152-167, 278-279. 8 fn. ISBN 0-8265-1321-2. BE60669.
autonomy; behavioral genetics; decision making; education; *eugenics; freedom; future generations; genetic counseling; genetic determinism; genetic disorders; genetic enhancement; genetic information; *genetic intervention; genetic research; genetic screening; *genetics; genome mapping; moral obligations; parents; philosophy; preimplantation diagnosis; prenatal diagnosis; social control; teleological ethics; *pragmatism

Saegusa, Asako; Nathan, Richard. Japan renews gene therapy efforts ... and plans transgenic medicine guidelines. [News]. *Nature Medicine.* 1998 Nov; 4(11): 1213. BE62158.
cancer; *drugs; *gene therapy; government regulation; guidelines; *human experimentation; industry; recombinant DNA research; *transgenic animals; universities; *Japan; Ministry of Health and Welfare (Japan); National Institute of Health Sciences (Japan); Tokyo University

Sahai, Suman. Bogus debate on bioethics. *Economic and Political Weekly (Bombay).* 1996 Dec 14; 31(50): 3231-3232. BE60696.
attitudes; bioethics; cultural pluralism; *developing countries; ecology; food; *genetic intervention; *genetic research; Hindu ethics; international aspects; non-Western World; *risks and benefits; socioeconomic factors; *transgenic organisms; Western World; agriculture; transgenic plants; *India

Sass, Hans-Martin. Introduction: why protect the human genome? *Journal of Medicine and Philosophy.* 1998 Jun; 23(3): 227-233. 17 refs. BE59287.
autonomy; beneficence; cloning; eugenics; gene therapy; *genetic information; *genetic intervention; genetic materials; *genetic research; genetic screening; genome mapping; germ cells; guidelines; health education; *human rights; international aspects; patents; regulation; risks and benefits; Europe; Germany; Unesco; Universal Declaration on the Protection of the Human Genome (Unesco)

Schatz, Gottfried. The Swiss vote on gene technology. *Science.* 1998 Sep 18; 281(5384): 1810-1811. 6 fn. BE59943.
animal experimentation; *attitudes; cultural pluralism; ecology; *genetic intervention; humanities; interdisciplinary communication; investigators; males; mass media; patents; *political activity; public opinion; *public participation; public policy; *recombinant DNA research; *science; social dominance; transgenic animals; *transgenic organisms; *Gene Protection Initiative (Switzerland); *Switzerland

Schatz, Ulrich. Patents and morality. *In:* Sterckx, Sigrid, ed. Biotechnology, Patents and Morality. Proceedings of an International Workshop, "Biotechnology, Patents and Morality: Towards a Consensus," held in Ghent, Belgium, 17-19 Jan 1996. Brookfield, VT: Ashgate; 1997: 159-170. 2 fn. ISBN 1-84014-158-1. BE62242.
body parts and fluids; DNA sequences; gene therapy; genes;

BE = bioethics accession number   fn. = footnotes   refs. = references

*genetic intervention; germ cells; health hazards; industry; *international aspects; *legal aspects; moral policy; morality; *patents; *regulation; suffering; transgenic animals; *biotechnology; European Patent Convention; European Patent Office

Schiermeier, Quirin. Germans mix support and scepticism for genetic engineering. [News]. *Nature.* 1998 May 28; 393(6683): 299. BE59886.
 *attitudes; eugenics; *genetic intervention; government regulation; industry; investigators; *public opinion; *recombinant DNA research; trust; *Germany

Schiermeier, Quirin. Swiss reject curbs on genetic engineering. [News]. *Nature.* 1998 Jun 11; 393(6685): 507. BE59887.
 advisory committees; animal experimentation; ecology; *genetic intervention; *government regulation; industry; investigators; legal liability; mass media; *political activity; *public participation; public policy; *recombinant DNA research; research institutes; transgenic organisms; national ethics committees; *Switzerland

Schwartz, William B. Life Without Disease: The Pursuit of Medical Utopia. Berkeley, CA: University of California Press; 1998. 178 p. Includes references. ISBN 0-520-21467-6. BE59738.
 anesthesia; biomedical research; *biomedical technologies; cloning; costs and benefits; drugs; *economics; fraud; gene therapy; genetic disorders; *genetic intervention; health care; *health care delivery; health insurance; health maintenance organizations; hospitals; international aspects; legal aspects; life extension; malpractice; *managed care programs; physicians; preventive medicine; *public policy; quality of health care; *resource allocation; *trends; Canada; Europe; Great Britain; *United States

Shattuck, Roger. Knowledge exploding: science and technology. *In: his* Forbidden Knowledge: From Prometheus to Pornography. San Diego, CA: Harcourt Brace; 1996: 173-225. 12 fn. ISBN 0-15-600551-4. BE61060.
 behavioral genetics; case studies; *eugenics; evolution; expert testimony; freedom; gene therapy; *genetic intervention; *genetic research; genetic screening; *genome mapping; germ cells; government regulation; historical aspects; international aspects; investigators; involuntary sterilization; legal aspects; mentally retarded; National Socialism; nuclear warfare; prenatal diagnosis; recombinant DNA research; *risks and benefits; *science; self regulation; social impact; Supreme Court decisions; wrongful life; *knowledge; Asilomar Conference; Buck v. Bell; Manhattan Project; Twentieth Century

Smith, George P. Developing a Standard for Advancing Genetic Health and Scientific Investigation. Available from the author, 3600 John McCormack Rd., NE, Washington, DC 20064; 1997. 17 p. 67 fn. BE59457.
 biomedical technologies; eugenics; freedom; gene therapy; genetic enhancement; genetic information; *genetic intervention; genetic screening; human rights; industry; international aspects; investigators; law; legislation; patents; privacy; public policy; recombinant DNA research; regulation; reproductive technologies; *risks and benefits; science; social control; social discrimination; state interest; transgenic organisms; Genetic Privacy Act; United States

Smith, George P. Pathways to immortality in the new millenium: human responsibility, theological direction, or legal mandate. *Saint Louis University Public Law Review.* 1996; 15(2): 447-469. 133 fn. BE59920.
 assisted suicide; *biomedical technologies; cloning; *cryopreservation; decision making; determination of death; eugenics; freedom; *genetic intervention; genetic research; historical aspects; killing; *legal aspects; *life extension;

religion; reproduction; reproductive technologies; right to die; risks and benefits; science; terminally ill; California; Donaldson v. Van de Kamp

Sterckx, Sigrid, ed. Biotechnology, Patents and Morality. Brookfield, VT: Ashgate; 1997. 324 p. Includes references. Proceedings of an International Workshop, "Biotechnology, Patents and Morality: Towards a Consensus," held in Ghent, Belgium, 17-19 Jan 1996. ISBN 1-84014-158-1. BE62236.
 attitudes; evaluation; genetic disorders; *genetic intervention; genetic screening; international aspects; knowledge, attitudes, practice; legal aspects; *moral policy; morality; *patents; prenatal diagnosis; public opinion; public participation; *public policy; regulation; risk; *risks and benefits; transgenic animals; *transgenic organisms; agriculture; *biotechnology; transgenic plants; *Europe; United States

Svatos, Michele. Patents and morality: a philosophical commentary on the conference 'Biotechnology, patents and morality.' *In:* Sterckx, Sigrid, ed. Biotechnology, Patents and Morality. Proceedings of an International Workshop, "Biotechnology, Patents and Morality: Towards a Consensus," held in Ghent, Belgium, 17-19 Jan 1996. Brookfield, VT: Ashgate; 1997: 291-306. 14 fn. ISBN 1-84014-158-1. BE62244.
 costs and benefits; developing countries; economics; genes; *genetic intervention; genome mapping; germ cells; incentives; industry; information dissemination; international aspects; legal aspects; microbiology; *patents; property rights; regulation; social impact; transgenic animals; utilitarianism; agriculture; *biotechnology; transgenic plants; Europe; National Institutes of Health; United States

Tagliaferro, Linda. Genetic Engineering: Progress or Peril? [Juvenile literature]. Minneapolis, MN: Lerner Publications; 1997. 128 p. (Pro/Con). Bibliography: p. 122-124. ISBN 0-8225-2620-7. BE62343.
 DNA fingerprinting; eugenics; gene therapy; *genetic intervention; genetic screening; genome mapping; germ cells; government regulation; health hazards; patents; prenatal diagnosis; recombinant DNA research; *risks and benefits; selective abortion; transgenic animals; agriculture; transgenic plants; United States

Taylor, Robert. Superhumans. *New Scientist.* 1998 Oct 3; 160(2154): 24-29. 4 refs. BE61940.
 cloning; DNA sequences; *gene therapy; genetic disorders; genetic enhancement; *genetic intervention; *germ cells; government regulation; hybrids; intelligence; methods; *risks and benefits; stem cells; transgenic animals; United States

Turney, Jon. Frankenstein's Footsteps: Science, Genetics and Popular Culture. New Haven, CT: Yale University Press; 1998. 276 p. Bibliography: p. 249-270. ISBN 0-300-07417-4. BE61055.
 animal experimentation; *attitudes; bioethics; *biology; biomedical research; biomedical technologies; cloning; embryo research; eugenics; genes; *genetic intervention; *genetic research; genetics; genome mapping; *historical aspects; human body; in vitro fertilization; international aspects; investigators; *literature; mass media; nuclear warfare; *public opinion; *recombinant DNA research; regulation; reproductive technologies; risks and benefits; *science; social impact; knowledge; Brave New World (Huxley, A.); Dr. Jekyll and Mr. Hyde (Stevenson, R.L.); *Frankenstein (Shelley, M.); Great Britain; In His Image (Rorvik, D.); *Nineteenth Century; R.U.R. (Capek, K.); The Island of Dr. Moreau (Wells, H.G.); *Twentieth Century; United States

Unesco. Universal Declaration on the Human Genome and Human Rights [UNESCO Document 27 V / 45, adopted by the Thirty-first General Assembly of UNESCO,

Paris, 11 November 1997]. *Journal of Medicine and Philosophy.* 1998 Jun; 23(3): 334–341. BE59297.
  confidentiality; developing countries; ethical review; freedom; *genetic intervention; *genetic research; *genome mapping; *guidelines; *human rights; information dissemination; informed consent; *international aspects; public policy; risks and benefits; Unesco; United Nations; *Universal Declaration on the Human Genome and Human Rights

Unesco. International Bioethics Committee.
Proceedings of the Fourth Session, October 1996. Volume I. Paris: The Committee; 1998. 164 p. Includes references. BE61056.
  advisory committees; AIDS; autonomy; beneficence; *bioethical issues; committee membership; drugs; ecology; economics; food; *genetic intervention; *genetic research; *genome mapping; government regulation; *guidelines; *human experimentation; *human rights; *international aspects; investigators; justice; moral obligations; random selection; recombinant DNA research; regulation; remuneration; research subjects; risks and benefits; selection of subjects; standards; transgenic organisms; vulnerable populations; women's health; agriculture; *transgenic plants; Declaration of Helsinki; *International Bioethics Committee (Unesco); Unesco; United Nations; *Universal Declaration on the Human Genome and Human Rights (Unesco)

Unesco. International Bioethics Committee.
Proceedings of the Fourth Session, October 1996. Volume II. Paris: The Committee; 1998. 94 p. Includes references. Papers in English and in French. BE61057.
  adults; advisory committees; autonomy; *bioethical issues; children; females; food; guidelines; *human experimentation; *human rights; immunization; informed consent; *international aspects; nontherapeutic research; privacy; random selection; regulation; research ethics committees; research subjects; therapeutic research; transgenic organisms; women's health; women's rights; agriculture; *transgenic plants; Argentina; Belmont Report; China; Colombia; Great Britain; International Bioethics Committee (Unesco); National Commission for the Protection of Human Subjects; Sweden; Tunisia; Unesco; United States

Van Overwalle, Geertrui. Biotechnology patents in Europe: from law to ethics. *In:* Sterckx, Sigrid, ed. Biotechnology, Patents and Morality. Proceedings of an International Workshop, "Biotechnology, Patents and Morality: Towards a Consensus," held in Ghent, Belgium, 17–19 Jan 1996. Brookfield, VT: Ashgate; 1997: 139–148. 2 fn. ISBN 1-84014-158-1. BE62241.
  evaluation; *genetic intervention; industry; *international aspects; legal aspects; microbiology; morality; *patents; recombinant DNA research; *regulation; transgenic animals; *transgenic organisms; *biotechnology; transgenic plants; *Europe; European Patent Convention; European Patent Office

Vermeersch, Etienne. Ethical aspects of genetic engineering. *In:* Sterckx, Sigrid, ed. Biotechnology, Patents and Morality. Proceedings of an International Workshop, "Biotechnology, Patents and Morality: Towards a Consensus," held in Ghent, Belgium, 17–19 Jan 1996. Brookfield, VT: Ashgate; 1997: 107–113. 1 fn. ISBN 1-84014-158-1. BE62238.
  *genetic intervention; historical aspects; moral obligations; patents; property rights; recombinant DNA research; risks and benefits; science; technology assessment; transgenic organisms; *biotechnology

Wade, Nicholas. Clinton asks study of bid to form part–human, part–cow cells. [News]. *New York Times.* 1998 Nov 15: 31. BE59321.
  advisory committees; *embryo research; *federal government; government financing; government regulation;

*hybrids; politics; *public policy; research embryo creation; *stem cells; National Bioethics Advisory Commission; United States

Wade, Nicholas. Ethics panel is guarded about hybrid of cow cells. [News]. *New York Times.* 1998 Nov 21: A9. BE60643.
  advisory committees; embryo research; *hybrids; industry; *stem cells; tissue donation; *National Bioethics Advisory Commission; United States

Wade, Nicholas. Human–cow hybrid cells are topic of ethics panel. [News]. *New York Times.* 1998 Nov 18: A27. BE60642.
  adults; advisory committees; cloning; *hybrids; industry; *stem cells; tissue donation; National Bioethics Advisory Commission; United States

Wade, Nicholas. Researchers claim embryonic cell mix of human and cow. [News]. *New York Times.* 1998 Nov 12: A1, A26. BE62599.
  autoexperimentation; cloning; *embryo research; embryos; *hybrids; industry; investigators; research embryo creation; *stem cells; Advanced Cell Technology; Cibelli, Jose

Watson, James D. All for the good: why genetic engineering must soldier on. *Time.* 1999 Jan 11; 153(1): 91. BE60318.
  future generations; *genetic intervention; germ cells; health; recombinant DNA research; *risks and benefits

Wolpert, Lewis. Is science dangerous? *Nature.* 1999 Mar 25; 398(6725): 281–282. 4 refs. BE61395.
  behavioral genetics; cloning; conflict of interest; decision making; disclosure; employment; eugenics; food; *genetic intervention; *genetic research; *investigators; moral obligations; obligations to society; prenatal diagnosis; public participation; *risks and benefits; *science; transgenic organisms; whistleblowing; research ethics; transgenic plants

Wright, Robert. Who gets the good genes? *Time.* 1999 Jan 11; 153(1): 67. BE60313.
  decision making; *eugenics; *genetic enhancement; genetic intervention; government regulation; parents; preimplantation diagnosis; prenatal diagnosis; selective abortion; socioeconomic factors; Brave New World (Huxley, A.)

EC ethics group established. [News]. *Nature Biotechnology.* 1998 Feb; 16(2): 121. BE62042.
  *advisory committees; *genetic intervention; *international aspects; organization and administration; *Europe; *European Commission; *European Group on Ethics, Science and Biotechnology; Group of Advisers on the Ethical Implications of Biotechnology (European Commission)

French public say 'non' to modified organisms. [News]. *Nature.* 1998 Oct 22; 395(6704): 736. BE60306.
  *public opinion; *transgenic organisms; *France

GM foods debate needs a recipe for restoring trust. [Editorial]. *Nature.* 1999 Apr 22; 398(6729): 639. BE61396.
  ecology; *food; health hazards; industry; international aspects; *regulation; risk; risks and benefits; transgenic organisms; uncertainty; agriculture; *transgenic plants; Europe; United States

GENETIC RESEARCH

See also BIOMEDICAL RESEARCH, GENOME MAPPING, HUMAN EXPERIMENTATION,

---

BE = bioethics accession number   fn. = footnotes   refs. = references

PATENTING LIFE FORMS, RECOMBINANT DNA RESEARCH

Alper, Joseph. A man in a hurry: stem cells. [Profile of Michael West]. *Science.* 1999 Mar 5; 283(5407): 1434–1435. BE61401.
*biomedical research; cloning; embryo research; genetic intervention; *genetic research; hybrids; industry; investigators; life extension; *stem cells; Advanced Cell Technology Inc.; *West, Michael

Andersen, Bogi. Icelandic health records. [Letter]. *Science.* 1998 Dec 11; 282(5396): 1993. BE61308.
confidentiality; *DNA data banks; *genetic information; *genetic research; *industry; information dissemination; informed consent; *medical records; patients' rights; population genetics; public policy; research ethics committees; *deCODE Genetics; *Iceland

Andersen, Bogi; Arnason, Einar. Iceland's database is ethically questionable. *BMJ (British Medical Journal).* 1999 Jun 5; 318(7197): 1565. BE62325.
confidentiality; *data banks; DNA data banks; ethical review; *genetic information; *genetic research; *industry; informed consent; *medical records; *public policy; *deCODE Genetics; *Iceland

Ault, Alicia. Drug industry hopes to moderate genetic privacy laws. [News]. *Nature Medicine.* 1998 Jan; 4(1): 6. BE59979.
*confidentiality; *drug industry; *genetic information; *genetic research; *government regulation; informed consent; privacy; professional organizations; property rights; state government; Pharmaceutical Research and Manufacturers of America (PhRMA)

Avise, John C. The Genetic Gods: Evolution and Belief in Human Affairs. Cambridge, MA: Harvard University Press; 1998. 279 p. 334 fn. ISBN 0–674–34625–4. BE60009.
behavioral genetics; biology; chromosome abnormalities; *evolution; genetic determinism; genetic disorders; genetic information; genetic intervention; genetic materials; *genetic research; *genetics; intelligence; morality; patents; property rights; recombinant DNA research; religion; science; sociobiology; terminology; theology

Berger, Abi. Private company wins rights to Icelandic gene database. [News]. *BMJ (British Medical Journal).* 1999 Jan 2; 318(7175): 11. BE62606.
confidentiality; *data banks; *DNA data banks; drug industry; *genetic information; *genetic research; *industry; legislation; *medical records; organizational policies; physicians; politics; *population genetics; privacy; professional organizations; public policy; Association of Icelanders for Ethical Science; *deCODE Genetics; *Iceland; Icelandic Medical Association

British Diabetic Association. Ethical issues in research into prevention of insulin–dependent diabetes mellitus (IDDM). [Editorial]. *Diabetic Medicine.* 1996 May; 13(5): 399–400. 2 refs. BE60428.
biomedical research; *diabetes; disclosure; *genetic predisposition; *genetic research; genetic screening; human experimentation; *newborns; parental consent; preventive medicine; professional organizations; British Diabetic Association; Great Britain

Butler, Declan. WHO's bioethics code likely to stir debate. [News]. *Nature.* 1999 Mar 18; 398(6724): 179. BE61961.
bioethical issues; developing countries; employment; ethical review; gene therapy; genes; genetic enhancement; genetic information; *genetic research; genome mapping; germ cells; *guidelines; insurance; *international aspects; patents; *population genetics; regulation; risks and benefits; social impact; community consent; *World Health Organization

Byk, Christian. A map to a new treasure island: the human genome and the concept of common heritage. *Journal of Medicine and Philosophy.* 1998 Jun; 23(3): 234–246. 14 refs. BE59288.
advisory committees; autonomy; confidentiality; democracy; ecology; future generations; gene therapy; *genetic information; *genetic intervention; *genetic research; genome mapping; *guidelines; historical aspects; *human rights; *international aspects; investigators; legal aspects; moral obligations; obligations of society; privacy; public policy; regulation; rights; risks and benefits; social discrimination; values; vulnerable populations; International Bioethics Committee (Unesco); Twentieth Century; Unesco; *Universal Declaration on the Protection of the Human Genome (Unesco)

While the 1970's have been called the environmental years, the 1990's could be seen as the genome years. As the challenge to map and to sequence the human genome mobilized the scientific community, risks and benefits of information and uses that would derive from this project have also raised ethical issues at the international level. The particular interest of the 1997 UNESCO Declaration relies on the fact that it emphasizes both the scientific importance of genetics and the appropriate reinforcement of human rights in this area. It considers the human genome, at least symbolically, as the common heritage of humanity.

Cahill, Lisa Sowle. The new biotech world order. [Symposium: human primordial stem cells]. *Hastings Center Report.* 1999 Mar–Apr; 29(2): 45–48. 9 fn. BE61666.
advisory committees; autonomy; *biomedical research; biomedical technologies; commodification; *common good; economics; *embryo research; ethics committees; federal government; financial support; freedom; *genetic research; genetic services; government financing; human rights; *industry; informed consent; *international aspects; *justice; organizational policies; *regulation; resource allocation; *stem cells; values; Geron Corp.; Geron Ethics Advisory Board; United States

Campbell, Courtney S. Religion and the body in medical research. *Kennedy Institute of Ethics Journal.* 1998 Sep; 8(3): 275–305. 36 refs. 2 fn. BE60168.
advisory committees; altruism; American Indians; attitudes; *autopsies; *biomedical research; *body parts and fluids; *cadavers; commodification; *common good; confidentiality; cultural pluralism; fetal tissue donation; genetic information; *genetic research; genome mapping; *gifts; *human body; informed consent; investigators; Islamic ethics; Jewish ethics; medical education; metaphor; moral obligations; *nontherapeutic research; *organ donation; organ transplantation; property rights; Protestant ethics; *religious ethics; remuneration; Roman Catholic ethics; science; self concept; *theology; *tissue banks; *tissue donation; transplant recipients; values; National Bioethics Advisory Commission

Religious discussion of human organs and tissues has concentrated largely on donation for therapeutic purposes. The retrieval and use of human tissue samples in diagnostic, research, and education contexts have, by contrast, received very little direct theological attention. Initially undertaken at the behest of the National Bioethics Advisory Commission, this essay seeks to explore the theological and religious questions embedded in nontherapeutic use of human tissue. It finds that the "donation paradigm" typically invoked in religious discourse to justify uses of the body for therapeutic reasons is inadequate in the context of nontherapeutic research, while the "resource paradigm" implicit in scientific discourse presumes a reductionist account of the body that runs contrary to important religious values about embodiment. The essay proposes a "contribution paradigm" that provides a religious perspective within which research on human tissue can be both justified and limited.

Caulfield, Timothy. The commercialization of human genetics: profits and problems. *Molecular Medicine Today.* 1998 Apr; 4(4): 148–150. 36 refs. BE62663.
  eugenics; financial support; *genetic research; genetic screening; genetic services; *industry; information dissemination; patents; risks and benefits; universities; biotechnology; United States

Chatterji, Somnath; Jain, Sanjeev; Brahmachari, Samir K., et al. International collaboration in genetics research. [Letter]. *Nature Genetics.* 1997 Feb; 15(2): 124. 7 refs. BE60399.
  *developing countries; *genetic diversity; *genetic materials; *genetic research; government regulation; *international aspects; *minority groups; patents; *population genetics; *India

Coghlan, Andy. Selling the family secrets. [News]. *New Scientist.* 1998 Dec 5; 160(2163): 20–21. BE61543.
  attitudes; data banks; disclosure; *DNA data banks; *genetic information; *genetic research; *industry; informed consent; international aspects; investigators; legislation; medical records; physicians; population genetics; privacy; public policy; Data Protection Commissioners (European Union); *deCODE Genetics; *Iceland

Coghlan, Andy. The price of profit. [News]. *New Scientist.* 1998 May 16; 158(2134): 20–21. BE59605.
  *DNA sequences; federal government; *genetic research; *genome mapping; government financing; *industry; information dissemination; investigational drugs; organizational policies; *patents; *property rights; research institutes; risks and benefits; social impact; National Institutes of Health; United States

Cohen, Philip. Totems and taboos: an Apache tribe has signed a historic deal with geneticists. [News]. *New Scientist.* 1998 Aug 29; 159(2149): 5. BE61793.
  *American Indians; anonymous testing; confidentiality; *genetic research; informed consent; *population genetics; United States

Creskoff, Katharine. Scientific imperialism or service to humanity? The complexities of the Human Genome Diversity Project. *Princeton Journal of Bioethics.* 1998 Spring; 1(1): 6–22. 25 refs. BE62487.
  anthropology; blood specimen collection; cultural pluralism; developing countries; disadvantaged; DNA data banks; *genetic diversity; genetic information; genetic predisposition; *genetic research; *genome mapping; goals; informed consent; international aspects; *minority groups; patents; *population genetics; property rights; *risks and benefits; social discrimination; tissue banks; community consent; *Human Genome Diversity Project

Currie, Rebecca. MRC funds large-scale human genetic database. [News]. *Nature Medicine.* 1998 Dec; 4(12): 1346. BE61529.
  confidentiality; disclosure; *DNA data banks; genetic predisposition; *genetic research; genome mapping; government financing; industry; informed consent; property rights; *public policy; tissue banks; *Great Britain; *Medical Research Council (Great Britain); National Health Service

Cutrer, William; Glahn, Sandra. Dealing with genetic reality: theological and clinical perspectives. *In:* Demy, Timothy J.; Stewart, Gary P., eds. Genetic Engineering:

A Christian Response: Crucial Considerations in Shaping Life. Grand Rapids, MI: Kregel Publications; 1999: 154–169. 11 fn. ISBN 0-8254-2357-0. BE61366.
  autonomy; beginning of life; beneficence; *Christian ethics; cloning; decision making; deontological ethics; *embryo research; embryos; ethical analysis; gene therapy; genetic disorders; genetic enhancement; genetic information; *genetic research; intention; justice; killing; moral complicity; moral policy; personhood; preimplantation diagnosis; *reproductive technologies; *risks and benefits; value of life; virtues; Human Embryo Research Panel; United States

Dan, Zhang; Lei, Xiong. Chinese center sues over study coverage. [News]. *Science.* 1999 Mar 26; 283(5410): 1990–1992. BE61132.
  aged; *blood specimen collection; deception; disclosure; DNA data banks; *genetic materials; *genetic research; human experimentation; informed consent; international aspects; investigators; legal aspects; *mass media; patents; scientific misconduct; *survey; *longevity; Beijing University; *China; China Research Center on Aging; Tong, Zeng; Zeng, Yi

DeRenzo, Evan G.; Biesecker, Leslie G.; Meltzer, Noah. Genetics and the dead: implications for genetics research with samples from deceased persons. *American Journal of Medical Genetics.* 1997 Mar 31; 69(3): 332–334. 12 refs. BE59523.
  body parts and fluids; breast cancer; *cadavers; case studies; confidentiality; disclosure; DNA data banks; ethical review; family members; federal government; genetic information; *genetic materials; *genetic research; genetic screening; government regulation; human experimentation; informed consent; *research ethics committees; risks and benefits; tissue donation; pedigree studies; United States

Dickson, David. Back on track: the rebirth of human genetics in China. [News]. *Nature.* 1998 Nov 26; 396(6709): 303–306. Includes inset articles, "Mining a rich seam of genetic diversity," p. 304 and "A crash course in ethical behaviour," p. 306. BE59437.
  communism; eugenics; *genetic diversity; genetic information; genetic intervention; *genetic research; genetics; *genome mapping; government regulation; historical aspects; industry; international aspects; investigators; minority groups; patents; political systems; *population genetics; private sector; public policy; *China

Dickson, David. China brings in regulations to put a stop to 'genetic piracy'. [News]. *Nature.* 1998 Sep 3; 395(6697): 5. BE59889.
  economics; *genetic information; *genetic materials; *genetic research; genome mapping; *government regulation; informed consent; international aspects; investigators; patents; population genetics; property rights; research institutes; research subjects; tissue donation; *China

Dodson, Michael; Williamson, Robert. Indigenous peoples and the morality of the Human Genome Diversity Project. *Journal of Medical Ethics.* 1999 Apr; 25(2): 204–208. 8 refs. BE61927.
  blood specimen collection; cultural pluralism; deception; decision making; disadvantaged; DNA data banks; drug industry; financial support; *genetic diversity; *genetic materials; genetic predisposition; *genetic research; *genome mapping; government financing; informed consent; international aspects; investigator subject relationship; investigators; *justice; *minority groups; moral obligations; *moral policy; *population genetics; property rights; risks and benefits; social discrimination; tissue banks; tissue donation; values; *aborigines; *community consent; research ethics; Australia; *Human Genome Diversity Project

In addition to the aim of mapping and sequencing one human's genome, the Human Genome Project also

---

intends to characterise the genetic diversity of the world's peoples. The Human Genome Diversity Project raises political, economic and ethical issues. These intersect clearly when the genomes under study are those of indigenous peoples who are already subject to serious economic, legal and/or social disadvantage and discrimination. The fact that some individuals associated with the project have made dismissive comments about indigenous peoples has confused rather than illuminated the deeper issues involved, as well as causing much antagonism among indigenous peoples. There are more serious ethical issues raised by the project for all geneticists, including those who are sympathetic to the problems of indigenous peoples. With particular attention to the history and attitudes of Australian indigenous peoples, we argue that the Human Genome Diversity Project can only proceed if those who further its objectives simultaneously: respect the cultural beliefs of indigenous peoples; publicly support the efforts of indigenous peoples to achieve respect and equality; express respect by a rigorous understanding of the meaning of equitable negotiation of consent, and ensure that both immediate and long term economic benefits from the research flow back to the groups taking part.

Dove, Alan. Genetics research on the town hall agenda, courtesy of ELSI. [News]. *Nature Medicine.* 1998 May; 4(5): 541. BE59727.
  decision making; federal government; *genetic research; government financing; *public participation; *public policy; state government; National Human Genome Research Institute; NHGRI Program on Ethical, Legal, and Social Implications (ELSI); United States; Vermont

Dronamraju, Krishna R. Biological and Social Issues in Biotechnology Sharing. Brookfield, VT: Ashgate; 1998. 165 p. Bibliography: p. 157–162. ISBN 1-84014-897-7. BE60744.
  developing countries; DNA sequences; drug industry; drugs; ecology; economics; federal government; gene therapy; genetic diversity; *genetic intervention; *genetic research; *international aspects; microbiology; *patents; *property rights; public policy; recombinant DNA research; regulation; transgenic animals; agriculture; *technology transfer; *transgenic plants; National Institutes of Health; United States

Duncan, Nigel. World Medical Association opposes Icelandic gene database. [News]. *BMJ (British Medical Journal).* 1999 Apr 24; 318(7191): 1096. BE62421.
  confidentiality; *data banks; DNA data banks; *genetic information; genetic research; government regulation; industry; informed consent; international aspects; *medical records; *organizational policies; *physicians; professional organizations; *public policy; *Iceland; *Icelandic Medical Association; *World Medical Association

Durán, Deborah Guadalupe. Lack of Hispanics' involvement in research -- is it Hispanics or scientists? *Community Genetics.* 1998; 1(3): 183–189. 22 refs. BE62368.
  *attitudes; behavioral research; *biomedical research; cultural pluralism; *genetic research; health; *Hispanic Americans; *investigators; population genetics; *science; selection of subjects; socioeconomic factors; trust; United States

Enserink, Martin. Iceland OKs private health databank. [News]. *Science.* 1999 Jan 1; 283(5398): 13. BE60816.
  attitudes; confidentiality; *data banks; DNA data banks; *genetic information; *genetic research; *industry; information dissemination; informed consent; investigators; legislation; *medical records; *public policy; deCODE

Genetics; *Iceland

Enserink, Martin. Opponents criticize Iceland's database. [News]. *Science.* 1998 Oct 30; 282(5390): 859. BE61714.
  attitudes; computers; confidentiality; *data banks; DNA data banks; *genetic information; *genetic research; government regulation; *industry; informed consent; international aspects; investigators; legislation; *medical records; organizational policies; physicians; population genetics; privacy; professional organizations; *public policy; computer security; deCODE Genetics; *Iceland; Icelandic Medical Association

Faraone, Stephen V.; Gottesman, Irving I.; Tsuang, Ming T. Fifty years of the Nuremberg Code: a time for retrospection and introspection. [Editorial]. *American Journal of Medical Genetics.* 1997 Jul 25; 74(4): 345–347. 16 refs. Includes text of the Nuremberg Code. BE59128.
  codes of ethics; eugenics; *genetic research; *genetics; genome mapping; historical aspects; *human experimentation; *investigators; involuntary euthanasia; involuntary sterilization; medical ethics; *misconduct; National Socialism; *physicians; *psychiatry; Germany; Nuremberg Code; Twentieth Century

Fears, Robin; Poste, George. Building population genetics resources using the U.K. NHS. *Science.* 1999 Apr 9; 284(5412): 267–268. 15 fn. BE61402.
  confidentiality; *data banks; *DNA data banks; epidemiology; *genetic information; *genetic research; government financing; *health care delivery; *industry; informed consent; medical records; *population genetics; *private sector; *public policy; *public sector; regulation; research subjects; *resource allocation; tissue banks; pedigree studies; *Great Britain; *National Health Service

Foster, Morris W.; Eisenbraun, Ann J.; Carter, Thomas H. Communal discourse as a supplement to informed consent for genetic research. *Nature Genetics.* 1997 Nov; 17(3): 277–279. 36 refs. BE59978.
  American Indians; *communication; decision making; family relationship; *genetic research; health care; *informed consent; investigator subject relationship; *population genetics; research subjects; risks and benefits; stigmatization; community consent

Fox, Jeffrey L. Forget Washington: state laws threaten to restrict genetic research, too. [News]. *Journal of NIH Research.* 1997 Nov; 9(11): 19–20. BE59757.
  cloning; confidentiality; federal government; *genetic information; genetic predisposition; *genetic research; *genetic screening; *government regulation; health insurance; industry; *privacy; *property rights; social discrimination; *state government; Health Insurance Portability and Accountability Act 1996; National Institutes of Health; *United States

Genetics Forum (London). Public oppose insurers' genetic test policy. *Splice of Life.* 1997 Apr; 3(5): 10–11. BE59661.
  disclosure; donors; drug industry; *genetic information; *genetic research; *genetic screening; *industry; informed consent; insurance selection bias; *life insurance; *public opinion; survey; tissue donation; Great Britain

Glass, Kathleen Cranley; Weijer, Charles; Lemmens, Trudo, et al. Structuring the review of human genetics protocols, Part II: diagnostic and screening studies. *IRB: A Review of Human Subjects Research.* 1997 May–Aug; 19(3–4): 1–13. 72 refs. BE60213.
  confidentiality; conflict of interest; diagnosis; disclosure; DNA data banks; *ethical review; genetic counseling; genetic diversity; genetic information; genetic predisposition; *genetic research; *genetic screening; *guidelines; *human

---

BE = bioethics accession number   fn. = footnotes   refs. = references

experimentation; informed consent; insurance; international aspects; investigators; laboratories; mass screening; medical records; minority groups; patents; prenatal diagnosis; research design; *research ethics committees; research subjects; risks and benefits; selection of subjects; standards; uncertainty; vulnerable populations

Great Britain. Advisory Committee on Genetic Testing. Genetic research and ethics. *Bulletin of Medical Ethics.* 1999 Feb; No. 145: 21–24. BE61893.

adolescents; advisory committees; carriers; children; confidentiality; disclosure; ethical review; genetic disorders; genetic predisposition; *genetic research; *genetic screening; *guidelines; informed consent; late-onset disorders; public policy; research design; research ethics committees; research subjects; risk; tissue banks; *Advisory Committee on Genetic Testing (Great Britain); Great Britain

Greely, Henry T. Genomics research and human subjects. [Editorial]. *Science.* 1998 Oct 23; 282(5389): 625. BE59646.

DNA data banks; *genetic research; *human experimentation; informed consent; research subjects; tissue banks; trust

Hodgson, John. A genetic heritage betrayed or empowered? *Nature Biotechnology.* 1998 Nov; 16(11): 1017–1021. 2 refs. BE62412.

confidentiality; data banks; dissent; *DNA data banks; financial support; genetic information; *genetic research; *industry; information dissemination; informed consent; investigators; *medical records; physicians; population genetics; presumed consent; property rights; public opinion; public policy; risks and benefits; *deCODE Genetics; *Iceland

Hodgson, John. New "deCODE bill" restarts controversy. [News]. *Nature Biotechnology.* 1998 Sep; 16(9): 816. BE62026.

attitudes; *data banks; *DNA data banks; *genetic research; industry; informed consent; investigators; legislation; medical records; presumed consent; deCODE Genetics; *Iceland

Huggins, M.; Hahn, C.; Costa, T. Staying informed and recontacting patients about research advances: a study of patient attitudes. [Abstract]. *American Journal of Human Genetics.* 1996 Oct; 59(4): A335. BE60094.

*attitudes; *genetic counseling; genetic disorders; *genetic research; patient care team; *patient education; *patients; physicians; survey; *recontact; Toronto

Jackson, Fatimah. Assessing the Human Genome Project: an African–American and bioanthropological critique. *In:* Smith, Edward; Sapp, Walter, eds. Plain Talk about the Human Genome Project: A Tuskegee University Conference on Its Promise and Perils ... and Matters of Race. Tuskegee, AL: Tuskegee University Press; 1997: 95–103. 10 refs. ISBN 1-891196-01-4. BE61738.

*blacks; *genetic diversity; *genetic research; *genome mapping; health care; international aspects; minority groups; non-Western World; population genetics; research design; risks and benefits; *selection of subjects; social discrimination; Western World; whites; Africa; African American Manifesto on Genomic Studies (1994); *Human Genome Project; United States

Jayaraman, K.S. Will new guidelines protect or expose the Indian gene pool? [News]. *Nature Medicine.* 1998 Jun; 4(6): 653. BE59730.

*gene pool; genetic diversity; *genetic materials; *genetic research; government regulation; *guidelines; international aspects; population genetics; *regulation; *India; Indian Council of Medical Research; National Facility for

Functional Genomics (India)

Kerr, Anne; Cunningham–Burley, Sarah; Amos, Amanda. Drawing the line: an analysis of lay people's discussions about the new genetics. *Public Understanding of Science.* 1998 Apr; 7(2): 113–133. 14 fn. BE60906.

autonomy; behavioral genetics; children; cystic fibrosis; decision making; Down syndrome; eugenics; genetic counseling; genetic disorders; *genetic research; *genetic screening; *genetics; homosexuals; *knowledge, attitudes, practice; physicians; *prenatal diagnosis; *public opinion; *public participation; quality of life; selective abortion; socioeconomic factors; stigmatization; suffering; survey; focus groups; qualitative research; Scotland

Kerr, Anne; Cunningham–Burley, Sarah; Amos, Amanda. The new genetics and health: mobilizing lay expertise. *Public Understanding of Science.* 1998 Jan; 7(1): 41–60. 24 fn. BE60905.

behavioral genetics; comprehension; disabled; eugenics; genetic disorders; *genetic research; *genetic screening; *genetics; *knowledge, attitudes, practice; prenatal diagnosis; *public opinion; *public participation; public policy; selective abortion; socioeconomic factors; survey; *technical expertise; focus groups; qualitative research; Scotland

Kolehmainen, Sophia. Iceland's genetic $ell–out. *GeneWATCH.* 1999 Feb; 12(1): 12–13. BE62371.

*data banks; disclosure; dissent; *DNA data banks; economics; *genetic information; *genetic research; *industry; *legal aspects; *medical records; population genetics; privacy; private sector; *property rights; public opinion; *risks and benefits; social discrimination; refusal to participate; Council for Responsible Genetics; *deCODE Genetics; *Iceland

Lagay, Faith L. Science, rhetoric, and public discourse in genetic research. *Cambridge Quarterly of Healthcare Ethics.* 1999 Spring; 8(2): 226–237. 33 fn. BE61238.

alcohol abuse; bioethical issues; *consensus; *cultural pluralism; *decision making; *democracy; emotions; *gene therapy; genetic disorders; *genetic enhancement; *genetic intervention; genetic predisposition; *genetic research; justice; models, theoretical; moral policy; normality; obligations of society; philosophy; postmodernism; public participation; *public policy; values; virtues; needs; rationality; *rhetoric

Lapham, E.V.; Kozma, C.; Weiss, J.O. Consumer experience in genetic research. [Abstract]. *American Journal of Human Genetics.* 1997 Oct; 61(4): A189. *genetic research BE59394.

attitudes; family members; genetic counseling; genetic disorders; *genetic research; informed consent; *patient participation; patients; research subjects; survey; District of Columbia; Maryland

Lewontin, R.C. People are not commodities. *New York Times.* 1999 Jan 23: A19. BE60373.

*commodification; *data banks; *DNA data banks; *genetic research; *industry; information dissemination; informed consent; international aspects; *medical records; population genetics; presumed consent; property rights; public policy; deCODE Genetics; *Iceland

Lin–Fu, Jane S. Advances in genetics: issues for US racial and ethnic minorities: an Asian American and Pacific Islander perspective. *Community Genetics.* 1998; 1(3): 124–129. 27 refs. BE62283.

aliens; *Asian Americans; cultural pluralism; genetic disorders; *genetic research; *genetic services; *minority groups; population genetics; public policy; resource allocation; *social discrimination; socioeconomic factors; stigmatization; emigration and immigration; *United States

---

BE = bioethics accession number   fn. = footnotes   refs. = references

Lyall, Sarah. A country unveils its gene pool and debate flares. [News]. *New York Times.* 1999 Feb 16: F1, F4. BE62600.
> attitudes; confidentiality; *data banks; *DNA data banks; drug industry; economics; *genetic information; *genetic research; *industry; informed consent; *medical records; *population genetics; presumed consent; privacy; risks and benefits; deCODE Genetics; *Iceland

Mao, Xin. Ethics and genetics in China: an inside story. [Letter]. *Nature Genetics.* 1997 Sep; 17(1): 20. 5 refs. BE60439.
> *attitudes; cultural pluralism; ethical relativism; *eugenics; *genetic counseling; *genetic research; *genetics; health personnel; historical aspects; international aspects; investigators; paternalism; politics; values; *China

Marshall, Eliot. Claim of human–cow embryo greeted with skepticism. [News]. *Science.* 1998 Nov 20; 282(5393): 1390–1391. BE59647.
> cloning; embryo research; *genetic research; *hybrids; *industry; stem cells; nuclear transplantation; *Advanced Cell Technology Inc.

Marshall, Eliot. DNA studies challenge the meaning of race. [News]. *Science.* 1998 Oct 23; 282(5389): 654–655. BE59700.
> behavioral genetics; DNA data banks; evolution; federal government; *genetic diversity; *genetic research; *genome mapping; *international aspects; minority groups; *population genetics; public policy; *research design; stigmatization; Human Genome Diversity Project; National Human Genome Research Institute; United States

Marshall, Eliot. Panel proposes tighter rules for tissue studies. [News]. *Science.* 1998 Dec 18; 282(5397): 2165–6. BE59648.
> advisory committees; DNA data banks; donors; federal government; *genetic materials; *genetic research; government regulation; *informed consent; privacy; research ethics committees; stigmatization; *tissue banks; *tissue donation; *National Bioethics Advisory Commission; United States

Masood, Ehsan. Iceland poised to sell exclusive rights to national health data. [News]. *Nature.* 1998 Dec 3; 396(6710): 395. BE59644.
> attitudes; *data banks; DNA data banks; economics; financial support; genetic information; *genetic research; *industry; information dissemination; informed consent; international aspects; investigators; legislation; *medical records; nurses; physicians; population genetics; *property rights; research subjects; deCODE Genetics; *Iceland

Mawer, Simon. Iceland, the nation of clones. *New York Times.* 1999 Jan 23: A19. BE60645.
> drug industry; economics; *genetic research; *genome mapping; *population genetics; *Iceland

Merz, Jon F.; Leonard, Debra G.B.; Miller, Elizabeth R. IRB review and consent in human tissue research. *Science.* 1999 Mar 12; 283(5408): 1647–1648. 18 fn. BE61033.
> authorship; biomedical research; comparative studies; editorial policies; *ethical review; federal government; financial support; *genetic research; government regulation; *guideline adherence; guidelines; *human experimentation; *informed consent; investigators; literature; patient care; records; *research ethics committees; research subjects; science; survey; tissue banks; *tissue donation; pathology; pedigree studies; American Journal of Clinical Pathology; American Journal of Human Genetics; American Journal of Pathology; Human Molecular Genetics; Journal of Medical Genetics; Molecular Diagnosis; Nature; Nature

Genetics; Office for Protection from Research Risks; Science; *United States

Merz, Jon F.; Sankar, Pamela; Taube, Sheila E., et al. Use of human tissues in research: clarifying clinician and researcher roles and information flows. *Journal of Investigative Medicine.* 1997 Jun; 45(5): 252–257. 36 refs. BE62405.
> confidentiality; epidemiology; genetic information; *genetic materials; *genetic research; *informed consent; medical records; research subjects; *tissue banks; tissue donation; pedigree studies; recontact

Mittman, Ilana Suez; Secundy, Marion Gray. A national dialogue on genetics and minority issues. *Community Genetics.* 1998; 1(3): 190–200. 6 refs. BE62369.
> attitudes; biomedical research; education; financial support; genetic counseling; *genetic research; genetic screening; *genetic services; genome mapping; guidelines; health; health personnel; human experimentation; informed consent; investigators; *minority groups; public participation; public policy; risk; science; selection of subjects; social discrimination; socioeconomic factors; stigmatization; trust; needs; United States

National Bioethics Advisory Commission. Genetics Subcommittee. Transcript of the National Bioethics Advisory Commission Genetics Subcommittee Meeting held on 23 Nov 1997, in Bethesda, Maryland. Rockville, MD: The Commission; 1997 Nov 23. 201 p. BE62751.
> advisory committees; confidentiality; *DNA data banks; genetic information; *genetic materials; *genetic research; informed consent; privacy; *public policy; research ethics committees; tissue banks; *tissue donation; *National Bioethics Advisory Commission; United States

Nayfield, Susan G. Ethical and scientific considerations for chemoprevention research in cohorts at genetic risk for breast cancer. *Journal of Cellular Biochemistry. Supplement.* 1996; 25: 123–130. 42 refs. BE60247.
> *breast cancer; cancer; confidentiality; counseling; *drugs; employment; family members; females; genetic counseling; *genetic predisposition; *genetic research; *genetic screening; health insurance; *human experimentation; informed consent; organizational policies; placebos; *preventive medicine; privacy; records; *research design; research subjects; *risk; *risks and benefits; selection of subjects; social discrimination; stigmatization; ovaries; American Society of Clinical Oncology; American Society of Human Genetics; United States

Nelkin, Dorothy; Andrews, Lori. Homo economicus: commercialization of body tissue in the age of biotechnology. *Hastings Center Report.* 1998 Sep–Oct; 28(5): 30–39. 64 fn. BE59552.
> advertising; *biomedical research; blood donation; *body parts and fluids; cadavers; *commodification; conflict of interest; *cord blood; dehumanization; DNA data banks; DNA sequences; *economics; embryos; entrepreneurship; eugenics; financial support; gene therapy; genes; genetic diversity; *genetic materials; *genetic research; historical aspects; *human body; incentives; *industry; informed consent; international aspects; investigators; minority groups; misconduct; organ donation; *patents; physicians; population genetics; *property rights; public policy; social discrimination; stem cells; *tissue banks; tissue donation; trends; trust; universities; vulnerable populations; cell lines; Human Genome Diversity Project; Moore v. Regents of the University of California; United States

The human body is becoming hot property, a resource to be "mined," "harvested," patented, and traded commercially for profit as well as scientific and therapeutic advances. Under the new entrepreneurial approach to the body old tensions take on new

---

BE = bioethics accession number   fn. = footnotes   refs. = references

dimensions -- about consent, the fair distribution of tissues and products developed from them, the individual and cultural values represented by the body, and public policy governing the use of organs and tissues.

Newson, Ainsley; Williamson, Robert. Should we undertake genetic research on intelligence? *Bioethics.* 1999 Jul; 13(3-4): 327-342. 36 fn. BE61883.
 *behavioral genetics; eugenics; family relationship; genes; *genetic enhancement; genetic information; *genetic research; genetic screening; *intelligence; resource allocation; risks and benefits; social discrimination; social impact; values

Although the concept of intelligence is difficult to define, research has provided evidence for a significant genetic component. Attempts are now being made to use molecular genetic approaches to identify genes contributing to intelligence, and to determine the ways in which they interact with environmental variables. This research is then likely to determine the developmental pathways of intelligence, in an effort to understand mental handicap and learning disorders and develop new treatment strategies. This paper reviews research on the genetic basis of intelligence, and discusses the ethical concerns, including the role of genetic information, the value we place on intelligence and the allocation of resources. It will be argued that the objections raised are problematic, and that because of the value of this knowledge and the prospect of improving lives, this research is morally required. We will then provide a brief analysis of the issues raised by enhancement of intelligence using genetic technology, and will argue that there is no intrinsic difference between this and other means of optimising intelligence.

Nuffield Council on Bioethics. Mental Disorders and Genetics: The Ethical Context. London: The Council; 1998 Sep. 117 p. Includes references. ISBN 0-9522701-3-7. BE60716.
 adoption; advisory committees; carriers; children; competence; confidentiality; dementia; directive counseling; disclosure; drugs; education; employment; eugenics; family members; gene therapy; *genetic counseling; genetic information; *genetic predisposition; *genetic research; *genetic screening; goals; *guidelines; human experimentation; Huntington disease; informed consent; insurance; legal aspects; *mentally disabled; mentally ill; public policy; reproduction; social discrimination; stigmatization; twins; diagnostic kits; pedigree studies; right not to know; Great Britain; *Nuffield Council on Bioethics

Ostrer, Harry; Scheuermann, Richard H.; Picker, Louis J. Benefits and dangers of genetic tests. [Letters]. *Nature.* 1998 Mar 5; 392(6671): 14. 6 refs. BE59237.
 advisory committees; breast cancer; DNA data banks; epidemiology; genetic predisposition; *genetic research; *genetic screening; human experimentation; informed consent; Jews; minority groups; *population genetics; *public policy; risks and benefits; *tissue banks; tissue donation; National Bioethics Advisory Commission; United States

Peters, Ted. Should we patent God's creation? *Dialog: A Journal of Theology.* 1996 Spring; 35(2): 117-132. 37 fn. BE61449.
 biomedical technologies; clergy; commodification; *DNA sequences; federal government; financial support; genes; genetic intervention; *genetic research; genome mapping; government financing; industry; information dissemination; *patents; political activity; private sector; *public policy; public sector; recombinant DNA research; religious ethics; risks and benefits; stem cells; theology; *transgenic animals; cell lines; National Institutes of Health; United States; Venter, Craig

Reilly, Philip R.; Page, David C. We're off to see the genome. *Nature Genetics.* 1998 Sep; 20(1): 15-17. 1 ref. BE61711.
 behavioral genetics; confidentiality; *DNA data banks; DNA fingerprinting; drug industry; federal government; genetic diversity; *genetic information; *genetic research; genetic screening; genome mapping; government regulation; informed consent; investigators; law enforcement; mass screening; newborns; population genetics; public opinion; research subjects; *risks and benefits; social discrimination; *social impact; state government; community consent; United States

Roscam Abbing, Henriette D.C. New developments in international health law. *European Journal of Health Law.* 1998 Jun; 5(2): 155-169. Includes text of the Universal Declaration on the Human Genome and Human Rights, p. 163-167. BE60901.
 animal organs; *cloning; communicable diseases; genetic intervention; *genetic research; *genome mapping; *guidelines; *human rights; *international aspects; *regulation; risks and benefits; *tissue transplantation; Council of Europe; *Europe; European Union; Unesco; *Universal Declaration on the Human Genome and Human Rights; World Health Organization

Rothenberg, Karen H.; Rutkin, Amy B. Toward a framework of mutualism: the Jewish community in genetics research. *Community Genetics.* 1998; 1(3): 148-153. 40 refs. BE62286.
 breast cancer; cancer; employment; females; *genetic predisposition; *genetic research; genetic screening; informed consent; insurance; *Jews; research subjects; risks and benefits; *social discrimination; stigmatization; Tay Sachs disease; trust; United States

Sahai, Suman. Bogus debate on bioethics. *Economic and Political Weekly (Bombay).* 1996 Dec 14; 31(50): 3231-3232. BE60696.
 attitudes; bioethics; cultural pluralism; *developing countries; ecology; food; *genetic intervention; *genetic research; Hindu ethics; international aspects; non-Western World; *risks and benefits; socioeconomic factors; *transgenic organisms; Western World; agriculture; transgenic plants; *India

Sass, Hans-Martin. Genotyping in clinical trials: towards a principle of informed request. *Journal of Medicine and Philosophy.* 1998 Jun; 23(3): 288-296. 21 refs. BE59292.
 *autonomy; confidentiality; consent forms; contracts; *DNA data banks; DNA fingerprinting; epidemiology; family members; *genetic information; genetic materials; genetic predisposition; *genetic research; genetic screening; human experimentation; *informed consent; investigator subject relationship; paternalism; privacy; property rights; research subjects; *risks and benefits; social discrimination; standards; tissue banks; pedigree studies

This paper reviews the usefulness of bioethical instruments such as the informed consent principle to handle ethical and political challenges of clinical trials in genotyping and DNA-banking and discusses an informed request model as well as other contractual relations between research institutions, patients, and their families.

Sass, Hans-Martin. Introduction: why protect the human genome? *Journal of Medicine and Philosophy.* 1998 Jun; 23(3): 227-233. 17 refs. BE59287.
 autonomy; beneficence; cloning; eugenics; gene therapy; *genetic information; *genetic intervention; genetic materials; *genetic research; genetic screening; genome mapping; germ cells; guidelines; health education; *human rights; international aspects; patents; regulation; risks and benefits; Europe; Germany; Unesco; Universal Declaration on the Protection of the Human Genome (Unesco)

BE = bioethics accession number   fn. = footnotes   refs. = references

Schrock, Charles R.; Botkin, Jeffrey R.; McMahon, William M., et al. Permission and confidentiality in publishing pedigrees. [Letter and response]. *JAMA.* 1998 Dec 2; 280(21): 1826–1827. 3 refs. BE61242.
*confidentiality; *editorial policies; *family members; *genetic information; *genetic research; guidelines; *informed consent; investigator subject relationship; *patients; research subjects; medical illustration; *pedigree studies; publishing; International Committee of Medical Journal Editors

Schüklenk, Udo. India fears patent and ethics abuses. [News]. *Nature Biotechnology.* 1997 Jul; 15(7): 613. Report on the Indian National Academy of Sciences bioethics symposium held in Goa, India, 22–25 May, 1997. BE62039.
developing countries; drug industry; genetic diversity; genetic materials; *genetic research; *genome mapping; informed consent; international aspects; *patents; property rights; research subjects; *India

Schwartz, John. For sale in Iceland: a nation's genetic code. [News]. *Washington Post.* 1999 Jan 12: A1, A4. BE59875.
attitudes; *DNA data banks; *genetic information; *genetic research; industry; investigators; medical records; physicians; *population genetics; privacy; property rights; public policy; risks and benefits; deCODE Genetics; European Union; *Iceland; Roche Holding AG

Sharp, Richard R.; Barrett, J. Carl. The Environmental Genome Project and bioethics. *Kennedy Institute of Ethics Journal.* 1999 Jun; 9(2): 175–188. 58 refs. 1 fn. BE62385.
confidentiality; disclosure; DNA data banks; ecology; genetic determinism; genetic information; genetic intervention; *genetic predisposition; *genetic research; genetic screening; *genome mapping; *health hazards; informed consent; population genetics; privacy; research subjects; risks and benefits; tissue donation; *Environmental Genome Project; National Institute of Environmental Health Sciences; United States

Shattuck, Roger. Knowledge exploding: science and technology. *In: his* Forbidden Knowledge: From Prometheus to Pornography. San Diego, CA: Harcourt Brace; 1996: 173–225. 12 fn. ISBN 0–15–600551–4. BE61060.
behavioral genetics; case studies; *eugenics; evolution; expert testimony; freedom; gene therapy; *genetic intervention; *genetic research; genetic screening; *genome mapping; germ cells; government regulation; historical aspects; international aspects; investigators; involuntary sterilization; legal aspects; mentally retarded; National Socialism; nuclear warfare; prenatal diagnosis; recombinant DNA research; *risks and benefits; *science; self regulation; social impact; Supreme Court decisions; wrongful life; *knowledge; Asilomar Conference; Buck v. Bell; Manhattan Project; Twentieth Century

Shickle, Darren. Do 'all men desire to know'? A right of society to choose not to know about the genetics of personality traits. *In:* Chadwick, Ruth; Levitt, Mairi; Shickle, Darren, eds. The Right to Know and the Right Not to Know. Brookfield, VT: Ashgate; 1997: 69–77. 22 refs. ISBN 1–85972–424–8. BE62190.
autonomy; *behavioral genetics; common good; decision making; genetic enhancement; genetic predisposition; *genetic research; government financing; government regulation; investigators; normality; *public participation; recombinant DNA research; *science; self regulation; *social control; right not to know

Sponholz, Gerlinde; Baitsch, Helmut; Ahr, Willfried,

et al. Genetic medicine: a new Copernican turning point? *In:* Hanson, Mark J.; Callahan, Daniel, eds. The Goals of Medicine: The Forgotten Issue in Health Care Reform. Washington, DC: Georgetown University Press; 1999: 162–173. 7 fn. ISBN 0–87840–707–3. BE60524.
eugenics; genetic counseling; genetic predisposition; *genetic research; genetic screening; genetics; goals; international aspects; *medicine; physician patient relationship; prenatal diagnosis; public policy; resource allocation; risks and benefits; social impact; values

Sullivan, Patrick. Move to market gene pool angers Iceland's MDs. *Canadian Medical Association Journal.* 1999 Aug 10; 161(3): 305. 1 ref. BE62309.
*attitudes; confidentiality; *data banks; *DNA data banks; genetic information; *genetic research; *industry; *medical records; organizational policies; *physicians; population genetics; privacy; professional organizations; *public policy; deCODE Genetics; *Iceland; *Icelandic Medical Association; World Medical Association

Thomas, Sandy; Caldicott, Fiona; Barchard, Chris, et al. Restrict genetic susceptibility tests. [Letter]. *Nature.* 1998 Sep 24; 395(6700): 317. 1 ref. BE60147.
advisory committees; competence; disclosure; genetic information; *genetic predisposition; *genetic research; *genetic screening; informed consent; mental health; *mentally ill; *nontherapeutic research; public policy; regulation; risks and benefits; selection of subjects; stigmatization; *Nuffield Council on Bioethics

Thomson, Elizabeth. The Ethical, Legal, and Social Implications Program at the National Human Genome Research Institute, NIH. *In:* Smith, Edward; Sapp, Walter, eds. Plain Talk about the Human Genome Project: A Tuskegee University Conference on Its Promise and Perils ... and Matters of Race. Tuskegee, AL: Tuskegee University Press; 1997: 123–130. 8 refs. 5 fn. ISBN 1–891196–01–4. BE61740.
advisory committees; ethical review; federal government; *genetic research; *genome mapping; government financing; government regulation; *program descriptions; research institutes; *Human Genome Project; *NHGRI Program on Ethical, Legal, and Social Implications (ELSI); *NIH–DOE Working Group on Ethical, Legal, and Social Implications (ELSI); *United States

Turney, Jon. Frankenstein's Footsteps: Science, Genetics and Popular Culture. New Haven, CT: Yale University Press; 1998. 276 p. Bibliography: p. 249–270. ISBN 0–300–07417–4. BE61055.
animal experimentation; *attitudes; bioethics; *biology; biomedical research; biomedical technologies; cloning; embryo research; eugenics; genes; *genetic intervention; *genetic research; genetics; genome mapping; *historical aspects; human body; in vitro fertilization; international aspects; investigators; *literature; mass media; nuclear warfare; *public opinion; *recombinant DNA research; regulation; reproductive technologies; risks and benefits; *science; social impact; knowledge; Brave New World (Huxley, A.); Dr. Jekyll and Mr. Hyde (Stevenson, R.L.); *Frankenstein (Shelley, M.); Great Britain; In His Image (Rorvik, D.); *Nineteenth Century; R.U.R. (Capek, K.); The Island of Dr. Moreau (Wells, H.G.); *Twentieth Century; United States

Unesco. Universal declaration on the human genome and human rights (revised draft). *Bulletin of Medical Ethics.* 1997 Mar; No. 126: 9–11. BE60445.
developing countries; genetic disorders; *genetic research; *genome mapping; *guidelines; *human rights; information dissemination; informed consent; *international aspects; *organizational policies; public policy; research subjects; risks and benefits; Unesco; United Nations; *Universal

---

BE = bioethics accession number   fn. = footnotes   refs. = references

Declaration on the Human Genome and Human Rights

Unesco. Universal Declaration on the Human Genome and Human Rights [UNESCO Document 27 V / 45, adopted by the Thirty-first General Assembly of UNESCO, Paris, 11 November 1997]. *Journal of Medicine and Philosophy.* 1998 Jun; 23(3): 334–341. BE59297.
    confidentiality; developing countries; ethical review; freedom; *genetic intervention; *genetic research; *genome mapping; *guidelines; *human rights; information dissemination; informed consent; *international aspects; public policy; risks and benefits; Unesco; United Nations; *Universal Declaration on the Human Genome and Human Rights

Unesco. International Bioethics Committee.
Proceedings of the Fourth Session, October 1996. Volume I. Paris: The Committee; 1998. 164 p. Includes references. BE61056.
    advisory committees; AIDS; autonomy; beneficence; *bioethical issues; committee membership; drugs; ecology; economics; food; *genetic intervention; *genetic research; *genome mapping; government regulation; *guidelines; *human experimentation; *human rights; *international aspects; investigators; justice; moral obligations; random selection; recombinant DNA research; regulation; remuneration; research subjects; risks and benefits; selection of subjects; standards; transgenic organisms; vulnerable populations; women's health; agriculture; *transgenic plants; Declaration of Helsinki; *International Bioethics Committee (Unesco); Unesco; United Nations; *Universal Declaration on the Human Genome and Human Rights (Unesco)

Wadman, Meredith. DuPont opens up access to genetics tool. [News]. *Nature.* 1998 Aug 27; 394(6696): 819. BE60395.
    contracts; federal government; genetic intervention; *genetic research; *industry; patents; *property rights; research institutes; universities; technology transfer; *DuPont Pharmaceuticals; *National Institutes of Health; United States

Wallace, Robert W. The Human Genome Diversity Project: medical benefits versus ethical concerns. *Molecular Medicine Today.* 1998 Feb; 4(2): 59–62. 13 refs. BE61813.
    anthropology; developing countries; DNA data banks; ethical review; federal government; *genetic diversity; genetic information; genetic materials; *genetic research; *genome mapping; government financing; guidelines; industry; informed consent; *international aspects; minority groups; patents; *population genetics; privacy; public policy; *risks and benefits; tissue banks; deCODE Genetics; *Human Genome Diversity Project; Iceland; *National Institutes of Health; National Research Council; National Science Foundation; United States

Walsh, Marie E.; Graber, Glenn C.; Wolfe, Amy K. University-industry relationships in genetic research: potential opportunities and pitfalls. *Accountability in Research.* 1997; 5(4): 265–282. 43 refs. BE60424.
    *conflict of interest; contracts; education; employment; *faculty; federal government; *financial support; *genetic research; gifts; government financing; guidelines; *industry; institutional policies; *investigators; patents; peer review; risks and benefits; scientific misconduct; *universities; *technology transfer; United States; University of Tennessee

Wexler, Alice. Mapping Fate: A Memoir of Family, Risk, and Genetic Research. Berkeley, CA: University of California Press; 1995. 321 p. 163 fn. ISBN 0-520-20741-6. BE60571.
    deception; decision making; *emotions; family members; *family relationship; financial support; *genetic research; genetic screening; genome mapping; *Huntington disease; patient advocacy; *patients; *political activity; psychological stress; stigmatization; truth disclosure; Hereditary Disease Foundation; Huntington's Disease Collaborative Research Group; *Wexler, Alice; *Wexler, Lenore; *Wexler, Milton; *Wexler, Nancy

Wilcox, Allen J.; Taylor, Jack A.; Sharp, Richard R., et al. Genetic determinism and the overprotection of human subjects. [Letter]. *Nature Genetics.* 1999 Apr; 21(4): 362. 8 refs. BE62413.
    disclosure; epidemiology; federal government; *genetic determinism; genetic predisposition; *genetic research; guidelines; *human experimentation; *informed consent; minors; research subjects; risk; National Institutes of Health; United States

Williamson, Robert. What's 'new' about 'genetics'? [Editorial]. *Journal of Medical Ethics.* 1999 Apr; 25(2): 75–76. BE61906.
    attitudes; cloning; eugenics; genetic determinism; genetic information; genetic intervention; *genetic research; genetics; genome mapping

Wingerson, Lois. Unnatural Selection: The Promise and Power of Human Gene Research. New York, NY: Bantam Books; 1998. 399 p. Includes references. ISBN 0-553-09709-1. BE59741.
    advisory committees; behavioral genetics; carriers; confidentiality; embryo research; eugenics; evolution; federal government; genes; genetic counseling; genetic disorders; genetic diversity; genetic predisposition; *genetic research; *genetic screening; *genetics; genome mapping; health insurance; informed consent; Jews; managed care programs; minority groups; preimplantation diagnosis; *prenatal diagnosis; property rights; public policy; risks and benefits; selective abortion; social discrimination; stigmatization; Human Embryo Research Panel; Human Genome Project; NCHGR Program on Ethical, Legal, and Social Implications (ELSI); United States

Wolpert, Lewis. Is science dangerous? *Nature.* 1999 Mar 25; 398(6725): 281–282. 4 refs. BE61395.
    behavioral genetics; cloning; conflict of interest; decision making; disclosure; employment; eugenics; food; *genetic intervention; *genetic research; *investigators; moral obligations; obligations to society; prenatal diagnosis; public participation; *risks and benefits; *science; transgenic organisms; whistleblowing; research ethics; transgenic plants

Can ELSI's principles inform consensus? [Editorial]. *Nature Biotechnology.* 1996 Jun; 14(6): 677. BE61398.
    advisory committees; federal government; genetic information; *genetic research; *genetic screening; genome mapping; informed consent; privacy; *public policy; tissue banks; tissue donation; bundled consent; *NIH-DOE Working Group on Ethical, Legal, and Social Implications (ELSI); *Task Force on Genetic Testing; *United States

Genome Vikings. [Editorial]. *Nature Genetics.* 1998 Oct; 20(2): 99–101. BE61621.
    confidentiality; *data banks; DNA data banks; economics; *genetic information; *genetic research; government regulation; *industry; informed consent; investigators; legislation; medical records; *population genetics; presumed consent; property rights; public policy; research subjects; risks and benefits; tissue banks; *deCODE Genetics

Privacy matters. [Editorial]. *Nature Genetics.* 1998 Jul; 19(3): 207–208. 3 refs. BE61710.
    *confidentiality; disclosure; *editorial policies; family members; *genetic information; *genetic research; genetic screening; guideline adherence; guidelines; *informed consent; investigators; privacy; *research subjects; *pedigree studies; publishing; International Committee of Medical Journal Editors; National Institutes of Health; Office for Protection from Research Risks

---

BE = bioethics accession number   fn. = footnotes   refs. = references

Swimming or drowning? Can Iceland show the world how to commercialise a gene pool? [Editorial]. *New Scientist*. 1998 Dec 5; 160(2163): 3. BE61542.

data banks; *DNA data banks; gene pool; *genetic research; government regulation; *industry; informed consent; medical records; population genetics; privacy; public policy; *Iceland

GENETIC SCREENING

See also DNA FINGERPRINTING, GENETIC COUNSELING, GENETIC INTERVENTION, GENETIC SERVICES, GENOME MAPPING, MASS SCREENING, PRENATAL DIAGNOSIS

Allen, Katrina; Williamson, Robert. Should we genetically test everyone for haemochromatosis? *Journal of Medical Ethics*. 1999 Apr; 25(2): 209–214. 28 refs. BE61928.

adolescents; adults; age factors; carriers; costs and benefits; genetic counseling; genetic information; *genetic screening; health education; *late-onset disorders; *mass screening; newborns; patient care; preventive medicine; psychological stress; *public policy; *risks and benefits; social discrimination; stigmatization; truth disclosure; *hemochromatosis; Australia

The increasing availability of DNA–based diagnostic tests has raised issues about whether these should be applied to the population at large in order to identify, treat or prevent a range of diseases. DNA tests raise concerns in the community for several reasons. There is the possibility of stigmatisation and discrimination between those who test positive and those who don't. High-risk individuals may be identified for whom no proven effective intervention is possible, or conversely may test "positive" for a disease that does not eventuate. Controversy concerning prenatal diagnosis and termination of affected pregnancies may arise. Haemochromatosis, however, is a disease that is not only treatable but also preventable if those at high risk are identified presymptomatically. This paper will identify and discuss key issues regarding DNA–based population screening for haemochromatosis, and argue that population–based genetic screening for haemochromatosis should be supported when a number of contentious issues are addressed. In the context of a health system with limited resources haemochromatosis is the paradigm of a disorder where there is an ethical and clinical imperative to encourage presymptomatic DNA testing for all in ethnically relevant communities.

American College of Obstetricians and Gynecologists. Committee on Obstetrics: Maternal and Fetal Medicine. Current status of cystic fibrosis carrier screening. ACOG Committee Opinion No. 101. *ACOG Committee Opinions*. 1991 Nov; No. 101: 2 p. 10 refs. BE60342.

*carriers; *cystic fibrosis; *genetic screening; guidelines; obstetrics and gynecology; *organizational policies; physicians; professional organizations; *American College of Obstetricians and Gynecologists; National Institutes of Health; United States

Anderson, Gwen. Nondirectiveness in prenatal genetics: patients read between the lines. *Nursing Ethics*. 1999 Mar; 6(2): 126–136. 33 refs. BE61932.

age factors; *attitudes; communication; congenital disorders; costs and benefits; decision making; *directive counseling; disclosure; fathers; females; *genetic counseling; genetic information; *genetic screening; genetic services; health personnel; males; marital relationship; married persons; moral obligations; narrative ethics; nurses; nursing research;

*patients; *pregnant women; *prenatal diagnosis; professional patient relationship; quality of life; selective abortion; suffering; uncertainty; *values; qualitative research; right not to know

Andrews, Lori B. Genetic privacy: from the laboratory to the legislature. *Genome Research*. 1995 Oct; 5(3): 209–213. 17 refs. BE60876.

*confidentiality; disclosure; employment; *genetic information; genetic research; *genetic screening; health insurance; informed consent; *legal aspects; privacy; public policy; self concept; social discrimination; stigmatization; ELSI–funded publication; right not to know; United States

Andrews, Lori B. Prenatal screening and the culture of motherhood. *Hastings Law Journal*. 1996 Apr; 47(4): 967–1006. 185 fn. BE59844.

autonomy; carriers; coercion; decision making; directive counseling; disabled; employment; family relationship; females; genetic disorders; genetic information; *genetic screening; genetic services; insurance selection bias; legal rights; mandatory testing; marital relationship; mass screening; *methods; mother fetus relationship; mothers; parent child relationship; policy analysis; *pregnant women; *prenatal diagnosis; privacy; psychological stress; *public policy; risks and benefits; selective abortion; self concept; social discrimination; *social impact; state interest; treatment refusal; ELSI–funded publication; Fourth Amendment; United States

Andrykowski, Michael A.; Lightner, Robin; Studts, Jamie L., et al. Hereditary cancer risk notification and testing: how interested is the general population? *Journal of Clinical Oncology*. 1997 May; 15(5): 2139–2148. 32 refs. BE59532.

adults; age factors; *attitudes; *cancer; *disclosure; family members; females; *genetic predisposition; *genetic screening; health; males; *public opinion; risk; socioeconomic factors; survey; Kentucky

Annas, George J. Genetic prophecy and genetic privacy. *Trial*. 1996 Jan; 32(1): 18–20, 22–25. 13 refs. BE61733.

adults; disclosure; *DNA data banks; employment; family members; federal government; *genetic information; genetic predisposition; genetic research; *genetic screening; government regulation; insurance; late-onset disorders; legal aspects; *legislation; minors; *privacy; public policy; social discrimination; tissue banks; *Genetic Privacy Act (1995 bill); United States

Austad, Torleiv. The right not to know -- worthy of preservation any longer? An ethical perspective. *Clinical Genetics*. 1996 Aug; 50(2): 85–88. BE59381.

autonomy; *disclosure; *family members; *genetic information; *genetic predisposition; genetic research; *genetic screening; human rights; informed consent; misconduct; *moral obligations; obligations to society; patients; *physicians; *rights; *right not to know

Barber, John C.K. "Code of practice and guidance on human genetic testing services supplied direct to the public": Advisory Committee on Genetic Testing. *Journal of Medical Genetics*. 1998 Jun; 35(6): 443–445. 8 refs. BE61252.

advisory committees; confidentiality; disclosure; genetic counseling; *genetic screening; *genetic services; guidelines; informed consent; *laboratories; physicians; records; *standards; *Advisory Committee on Genetic Testing (Great Britain); *Great Britain

Bayertz, Kurt. What's special about molecular genetic diagnostics? *Journal of Medicine and Philosophy*. 1998 Jun; 23(3): 247–254. 10 refs. BE59289.

coercion; *diagnosis; gene therapy; genetic disorders; genetic information; genetic predisposition; *genetic screening;

BE = bioethics accession number   fn. = footnotes   refs. = references

health; insurance; late-onset disorders; *mass screening; preventive medicine; risks and benefits; social control; social discrimination; *social impact

In its first part, this paper seeks to make plausible (a) that molecular genetic diagnostics differs in ethically relevant ways from traditional types of medical diagnostics and (b) that the consequences of introducing this technology in broad screening-programs to detect widespread genetic diseases in a population which is not at high risk may change our understanding of health and disease in a problematic way. In its second part, the paper discusses some aspects of public control of scientific and technological innovations in the field of molecular genetic diagnostics.

Bernard, Lynn E.; McGillivray, Barbara; Van Allen, Margot I., et al. Duty to re-contact: a study of families at risk for Fragile X. *Journal of Genetic Counseling.* 1999 Feb; 8(1): 3-15. 11 refs. BE61641.

> *attitudes; carriers; *chromosome abnormalities; disclosure; *family members; *genetic counseling; genetic predisposition; *genetic screening; mentally retarded; motivation; *patients; prevalence; risks and benefits; survey; *recontact; British Columbia; Fragile X syndrome

Berry, Roberta M. The Human Genome Project and the end of insurance. *University of Florida Journal of Law and Public Policy.* 1996 Spring; 7(2): 205-256. 177 fn. BE59315.

> confidentiality; economics; *genetic information; *genetic screening; *genome mapping; government regulation; historical aspects; industry; *insurance; insurance selection bias; justice; national health insurance; policy analysis; privacy; *public policy; risk; social discrimination; *social impact; *Human Genome Project; United States

Binedell, Julia. Adolescent requests for predictive genetic testing. *In:* Clarke, Angus, ed. The Genetic Testing of Children. Washington, DC: BIOS Scientific Publishers; 1998: 123-132. 42 refs. ISBN 1-85996-146-0. BE62759.

> *adolescents; children; *competence; comprehension; decision making; empirical research; family members; family relationship; *genetic screening; guidelines; informed consent; *late-onset disorders; risks and benefits; uncertainty; harms; Children Act 1989 (Great Britain); Great Britain

Binstock, Robert H.; Murray, Thomas H. Genetics and long-term-care insurance: ethical and policy issues. *In:* Post, Stephen G.; Whitehouse, Peter J., eds. Genetic Testing for Alzheimer Disease: Ethical and Clinical Issues. Baltimore, MD: Johns Hopkins University Press; 1998: 155-176. 44 refs. ISBN 0-8018-5840-2. BE60722.

> aged; *dementia; *economics; family members; federal government; *genetic information; genetic predisposition; *genetic screening; government financing; government regulation; *health insurance; health insurance reimbursement; home care; industry; insurance selection bias; *justice; *long-term care; *moral policy; nursing homes; obligations of society; *public policy; risk; socioeconomic factors; state government; trends; Medicaid; United States

Boetzkes, Elisabeth. Genetic knowledge and third-party interests. *Cambridge Quarterly of Healthcare Ethics.* 1999 Summer; 8(3): 386-392. 12 fn. BE62481.

> carriers; children; communitarianism; *confidentiality; decision making; *disclosure; *family members; females; genetic disorders; *genetic information; genetic predisposition; *genetic screening; health personnel; informed consent; moral obligations; professional patient relationship; reproduction; standards; values; *harms; *negotiation

Bowman, James E. Minority health issues and genetics.

Community Genetics. 1998; 1(3): 142-144. 10 refs. BE62284.

> blacks; deception; developing countries; employment; federal government; *genetic screening; Hispanic Americans; human experimentation; international aspects; legal aspects; *minority groups; prenatal diagnosis; *public policy; selective abortion; sickle cell anemia; *social discrimination; syphilis; *United States

Bowman, James E. To screen or not to screen: when should screening be offered? *Community Genetics.* 1998; 1(3): 145-147. 8 refs. BE62285.

> blacks; confidentiality; disadvantaged; disclosure; employment; genetic counseling; genetic information; *genetic screening; insurance; Jews; mass screening; phenylketonuria; *prenatal diagnosis; sickle cell anemia; single persons; social discrimination; Tay Sachs disease; United States

Brindle, Lucy. Exploring the approach of psychology as a discipline to the childhood testing debate: issues of theory, empiricism and power. *In:* Clarke, Angus, ed. The Genetic Testing of Children. Washington, DC: BIOS Scientific Publishers; 1998: 183-193. 29 refs. ISBN 1-85996-146-0. BE62763.

> attitudes; autonomy; behavioral research; *children; decision making; *empirical research; *evidence-based medicine; genetic counseling; *genetic screening; health personnel; parents; *psychology; values; rationality

British Medical Association. Human Genetics: Choice and Responsibility. New York, NY: Oxford University Press; 1998. 236 p. 227 fn. Appendixes provide names and addresses of regional genetics centers in the United Kingdom and of concerned organizations in the UK and elsewhere. ISBN 0-19-288055-1. BE61351.

> adolescents; adults; advisory committees; carriers; children; cloning; competence; confidentiality; decision making; disabled; disclosure; employment; eugenics; family members; gene therapy; *genetic counseling; genetic disorders; genetic information; genetic predisposition; genetic research; *genetic screening; *genetic services; *genetics; government financing; guidelines; health personnel; informed consent; insurance; late-onset disorders; mass screening; moral obligations; *organizational policies; parents; patients; physicians; prenatal diagnosis; primary health care; professional ethics; professional organizations; registries; regulation; risks and benefits; terminology; incidental findings; paternity; *British Medical Association; Great Britain; National Health Service

Brooks, Alex. Mentally ill patients need protection from inappropriate genetic testing. [News]. *BMJ (British Medical Journal).* 1998 Oct 3; 317(7163): 903. BE60850.

> advisory committees; children; dementia; disclosure; family members; genetic information; genetic predisposition; *genetic screening; *mentally ill; *public policy; *Great Britain; *Nuffield Council on Bioethics

Brower, Vicki. Insurers keep genetic test options open. [News]. *Nature Biotechnology.* 1997 Aug; 15(8): 708-709. BE62020.

> breast cancer; *cancer; family members; federal government; females; *genetic predisposition; *genetic screening; *industry; *insurance; males; *risk; social discrimination; United States

Brower, Vicki. Lawyers, physicians seek genomics rules. [News]. *Nature Biotechnology.* 1997 Jan; 15(1): 10. BE62038.

> breast cancer; *genetic information; *genetic screening; government regulation; guidelines; human rights; industry; *international aspects; lawyers; physicians; *regulation; risks and benefits; diagnostic kits; Advisory Committee on Genetic Testing (Great Britain); Global Lawyers and

---

BE = bioethics accession number   fn. = footnotes   refs. = references

Physicians; International Bar Association; Program in Genomics, Ethics and Society (Stanford University)

Brown, Barry. Genetic testing, access to genetic data and discrimination: conceptual legislative models. *Suffolk University Law Review.* 1993 Winter; 27(4): 1573–1592. 79 fn. BE60739.
   *confidentiality; disclosure; employment; genetic counseling; genetic disorders; genetic research; *genetic screening; informed consent; insurance; *legal aspects; mandatory programs; *model legislation; newborns; parental consent; parents; *social discrimination; voluntary programs; United States

Brunner, Eric. Gene tests survey: results. *Splice of Life.* 1996 Dec; 3(3): 7–8. BE60108.
   *attitudes; biomedical research; blood specimen collection; confidentiality; disclosure; employment; genetic counseling; genetic information; genetic materials; genetic predisposition; *genetic screening; health insurance; industry; medical records; patents; regulation; social discrimination; standards; survey; tissue donation

Burgess, Michael M.; Laberge, Claude M.; Knoppers, Bartha Maria. Bioethics for clinicians: 14. Ethics and genetics in medicine. *Canadian Medical Association Journal.* 1998 May 19; 158(10): 1309–1313. 42 refs. BE59832.
   confidentiality; duty to warn; family members; *genetic counseling; *genetic information; *genetic predisposition; *genetic screening; guidelines; health personnel; informed consent; insurance; knowledge, attitudes, practice; late–onset disorders; legal aspects; physicians; prenatal diagnosis; psychological stress; risk; social discrimination; Canada

Campbell, Courtney S. Can what you don't know hurt you?: the case of genetic screening for breast cancer. *In:* Smith, Edward; Sapp, Walter, eds. Plain Talk about the Human Genome Project: A Tuskegee University Conference on Its Promise and Perils ... and Matters of Race. Tuskegee, AL: Tuskegee University Press; 1997: 117–122. ISBN 1-891196-01-4. BE61739.
   autonomy; *breast cancer; decision making; females; genetic counseling; genetic information; *genetic predisposition; *genetic screening; health insurance; industry; *risks and benefits; social discrimination; uncertainty; right not to know

Campbell, Harry; Boyd, Kenneth. Screening and the new genetics: a public health perspective on the ethical debate. [Letter]. *Journal of Public Health Medicine.* 1996 Dec; 18(4): 485–486. 9 refs. BE60691.
   autonomy; costs and benefits; cystic fibrosis; eugenics; *genetic screening; mass screening; *prenatal diagnosis; public health; public policy

Canadian Nurses Association. The Role of the Nurse in Reproductive and Genetic Technologies. [Policy statement]. Issued by the Canadian Nurses Association, 50 Driveway, Ottawa, ON, Canada; 1996 Jun. 2 p. 4 refs. 2 fn. Approved by the CNA Board of Directors Jun 1996. BE62000.
   counseling; *genetic screening; *nurse's role; nurses; *organizational policies; professional organizations; *reproductive technologies; Canada; *Canadian Nurses Association

Cappelli, M.; Surh, L.; Verma, S., et al. Canadian women's attitudes towards breast cancer gene testing. [Abstract]. *American Journal of Human Genetics.* 1997 Oct; 61(4): A187. BE59393.
   *attitudes; *breast cancer; comparative studies; drugs; *females; *genetic screening; *patients; preventive medicine; surgery; survey; Canada

Chadwick, Ruth; ten Have, Henk; Husted, Jörgen, et al. Genetic screening and ethics: European perspectives. *Journal of Medicine and Philosophy.* 1998 Jun; 23(3): 255–273. 15 refs. BE59290.
   adults; advisory committees; attitudes; carriers; comparative studies; data banks; decision making; directive counseling; disabled; disclosure; eugenics; family members; females; future generations; gene pool; genetic counseling; genetic disorders; genetic predisposition; *genetic screening; genetic services; goals; health; informed consent; *international aspects; justice; legislation; males; mass screening; moral policy; newborns; normality; pregnant women; prenatal diagnosis; public health; public policy; registries; risks and benefits; selective abortion; social discrimination; stigmatization; suffering; survey; thalassemia; right not to know; Austria; Council of Europe; Cyprus; Danish Council of Ethics; Denmark; *Europe; European Union; Finland; France; Germany; Great Britain; Greece; Health Council (Netherlands); Ireland; Italy; Ministry of Health and Social Affairs (Norway); National Ethics Advisory Committee (France); Netherlands; Norway; Nuffield Council on Bioethics
Analysis and comparison of genetic screening programs shows that the extent of development of programs varies widely across Europe. Regional variations are due not only to genetic disease patterns but also reflect the novelty of genetic services. In most countries, the focus for genetic screening programs has been pregnant women and newborn children. Newborn children are screened only for disorders which are treatable. Prenatal screening when provided is for conditions for which termination may be offered. The only population screening programs for adults are those for thalassaemia carrier status in Cyprus, Greece and Italy. Social responses to genetic screening range from acceptance to hostility. There is a fundamental tension between individual and community in the debates in various European countries about implementation of screening programs. Opposition to genetic screening is frequently expressed in terms of arguments about "eugenics" with insufficient regard to the meaning of the term and its implications. Only a few countries have introduced explicit legislation on genetic screening. Legislation to address discrimination may provide more safeguards than legislation protecting genetic information itself.

Chadwick, Ruth; Levitt, Mairi. Mass media and public discussion in bioethics. *In:* Chadwick, Ruth; Levitt, Mairi; Shickle, Darren, eds. The Right to Know and the Right Not to Know. Brookfield, VT: Ashgate; 1997: 79–86. 10 refs. 1 fn. ISBN 1-85972-424-8. BE62191.
   bioethical issues; genetic research; *genetic screening; *information dissemination; *institutional ethics; *journalism; *mass media; paternalism; prenatal diagnosis; public participation; *risks and benefits; right not to know; Great Britain

Chadwick, Ruth. The philosophy of the right to know and the right not to know. *In:* Chadwick, Ruth; Levitt, Mairi; Shickle, Darren, eds. The Right to Know and the Right Not to Know. Brookfield, VT: Ashgate; 1997: 13–22. 13 refs. ISBN 1-85972-424-8. BE62184.
   autonomy; communitarianism; confidentiality; disclosure; *ethical analysis; family members; genetic counseling; genetic disorders; *genetic information; genetic predisposition; *genetic screening; insurance; mass screening; moral obligations; patients; privacy; reproduction; *rights; teleological ethics; *truth disclosure; utilitarianism; duty to know; *right not to know

Chadwick, Ruth; Levitt, Mairi; Shickle, Darren, eds. The Right to Know and the Right Not to Know. Brookfield, VT: Ashgate; 1997. 101 p. (Avebury series in philosophy). 133 refs. 20 fn. ISBN 1-85972-424-8. BE62183.

autonomy; behavioral genetics; confidentiality; disclosure; ethical analysis; family members; genetic counseling; *genetic information; genetic research; *genetic screening; genetics; historical aspects; information dissemination; legal aspects; mass media; moral obligations; paternalism; privacy; public participation; public policy; rights; risks and benefits; science; social control; socioeconomic factors; terminology; truth disclosure; *right not to know; Euroscreen Project

Christianson, David J. Insurance concerns: are the fears exaggerated? *In:* Smith, Edward; Sapp, Walter, eds. Plain Talk about the Human Genome Project: A Tuskegee University Conference on its Promise and Perils ... and Matters of Race. Tuskegee, AL: Tuskegee University Press; 1997: 169-177. ISBN 1-891196-01-4. BE61744.

*economics; *genetic information; genetic predisposition; *genetic screening; *industry; *insurance selection bias; justice; *life insurance; mandatory testing; mortality; *risk; social discrimination; United States

Clark, William R. The ethics of molecular medicine. *In: his:* The New Healers: The Promise and Problems of Molecular Medicine in the Twenty-First Century. New York, NY: Oxford University Press; 1997: 207-231, 236. 8 refs. ISBN 0-19-511730-1. BE60572.

confidentiality; containment; disclosure; DNA data banks; *DNA fingerprinting; donors; employment; ethical review; forensic medicine; future generations; *gene therapy; genetic counseling; genetic disorders; genetic enhancement; *genetic information; genetic materials; genetic predisposition; *genetic screening; genome mapping; germ cells; government regulation; guidelines; *health insurance; informed consent; insurance selection bias; late-onset disorders; legislation; methods; preimplantation diagnosis; privacy; public policy; recombinant DNA research; *risks and benefits; social discrimination; NIH/DOE Working Group on Ethical, Legal, and Social Issues (ELSI); United States

Clarke, Angus. Genetic screening and counselling. *In:* Kuhse, Helga; Singer, Peter, eds. A Companion to Bioethics. Malden, MA: Blackwell; 1998: 215-228. 42 refs. ISBN 0-631-19737-0. BE59497.

adults; autonomy; carriers; children; confidentiality; disclosure; family members; *genetic counseling; genetic disorders; genetic information; genetic predisposition; *genetic screening; goals; informed consent; late-onset disorders; mass screening; newborns; parental consent; prenatal diagnosis; psychological stress; public health; risks and benefits; social discrimination

Clarke, Angus; Michie, Susan. Parents' responses to predictive genetic testing in their children. [Letter and response]. *Journal of Medical Genetics.* 1997 Feb; 34(2): 174-175. 5 refs. BE60390.

age factors; attitudes; *children; decision making; empirical research; genetic counseling; *genetic screening; late-onset disorders; parental consent; parents; risks and benefits

Clarke, Angus, ed. The Genetic Testing of Children. Washington, DC: BIOS Scientific Publishers; 1998. 334 p. 693 refs. Based on papers presented at a meeting, held in London in June 1996, organised by EUROSCREEN, the British Medical Association, and the Genetics Interest Group. ISBN 1-85996-146-0. BE62755.

adolescents; age factors; *attitudes; autonomy; cancer; carriers; *children; chromosomal disorders; competence; cystic fibrosis; dementia; Duchenne muscular dystrophy; empirical research; family relationship; genetic counseling; genetic disorders; genetic information; genetic predisposition; *genetic screening; genetics; health personnel; Huntington disease; industry; international aspects; *knowledge, attitudes, practice; late-onset

disorders; newborns; organizational policies; parents; paternalism; patients; physicians; prenatal diagnosis; preventive medicine; professional organizations; psychology; public opinion; rights; risk; *risks and benefits; socioeconomic factors; truth disclosure; uncertainty; harms

Clarke, M.P. There are ethical issues in ophthalmology. *BMJ (British Medical Journal).* 1999 Apr 24; 318(7191): 1153. BE62365.

carriers; case studies; children; deception; *eye diseases; family members; genetic counseling; *genetic screening; ophthalmology; right not to know

Clayton, Ellen Wright. Issues in state newborn screening programs. *Pediatrics.* 1992 Oct; 90(4): 641-646. 69 refs. BE60222.

autonomy; confidentiality; congenital disorders; *costs and benefits; decision making; diagnosis; *disclosure; DNA data banks; genetic counseling; *genetic screening; government financing; health insurance reimbursement; *mandatory testing; *mass screening; *newborns; parental consent; *parents; patient care; privacy; prognosis; psychological stress; public policy; records; reproduction; *risks and benefits; *state government; time factors; treatment outcome; right not to know; *United States

Cohen, Cynthia B. Moving away from the Huntington's disease paradigm in the predictive genetic testing of children. *In:* Clarke, Angus, ed. The Genetic Testing of Children. Washington, DC: BIOS Scientific Publishers; 1998: 133-143. 35 refs. ISBN 1-85996-146-0. BE62760.

adolescents; autonomy; beneficence; breast cancer; *children; comprehension; decision making; dementia; disclosure; family relationship; genetic counseling; genetic information; *genetic screening; Huntington disease; *late-onset disorders; parent child relationship; parents; psychological stress; *risks and benefits; social discrimination; social impact; stigmatization; uncertainty; right not to know

Cook, E. David. Genetics and the British insurance industry. *Journal of Medical Ethics.* 1999 Apr; 25(2): 157-162. 10 fn. BE61920.

confidentiality; disclosure; employment; family members; *genetic information; genetic predisposition; *genetic screening; government regulation; *guidelines; *industry; informed consent; *insurance; insurance selection bias; mediation; medical records; *organizational policies; physicians; public policy; referral and consultation; risk; *self regulation; social discrimination; *standards; *Association of British Insurers; *Great Britain

Genetics and genetic testing raise key issues for insurance and employment. Governmental and public concern galvanised the British insurance industry into developing a code of practice. The history of the development of the code, issues of genetic discrimination, access to medical information, consent and the dangers of withholding information and the impact on the equity of pooled risk are explored. Proactive steps by the Association of British Insurers suggest that moral reflection not legislation is the way forward.

Croyle, Robert T.; Achilles, Jennifer S.; Lerman, Caryn. Psychologic aspects of cancer genetic testing: a research update for clinicians. *Cancer.* 1997 Aug 1; 80(3, Suppl.): 569-575. 27 refs. Presented at the American Cancer Society Workshop on Heritable Cancer Syndromes and Genetic Testing, Chicago, IL, 7-8 Oct 1996. BE60889.

attitudes; behavioral research; breast cancer; *cancer; *empirical research; evaluation; family members; genetic counseling; *genetic predisposition; *genetic screening; informed consent; patients; primary health care;

BE = bioethics accession number   fn. = footnotes   refs. = references

*psychological stress; *risks and benefits; self concept; socioeconomic factors

Dalby, Shirley. Commercial testing. *In:* Clarke, Angus, ed. The Genetic Testing of Children. Washington, DC: BIOS Scientific Publishers; 1998: 265–270. ISBN 1-85996-146-0. BE62767.
advertising; *attitudes; children; genetic counseling; genetic information; *genetic screening; *genetic services; health insurance reimbursement; *industry; information dissemination; physicians; *private sector; psychological stress; public opinion; public sector; regulation; survey; private practice; Genetic Interest Group (Great Britain); Great Britain; National Health Service

Decruyenaere, Marleen; Evers–Kiebooms, Gerry; Boogaerts, Andrea, et al. Non-participation in predictive testing for Huntington's disease: individual decision-making, personality and avoidant behaviour in the family. *European Journal of Human Genetics.* 1997 Nov-Dec; 5(6): 351–363. 48 refs. BE62252.
*attitudes; *decision making; *genetic screening; *Huntington disease; *motivation; psychological stress; risk; risks and benefits; siblings; survey; personality; *refusal to participate; severity of illness index; *Belgium

Dickenson, Donna L.; Geller, Gail. Can children and young people consent to be tested for adult onset genetic disorders? [and] Weighing burdens and benefits rather than competence. [Article and commentary]. *BMJ (British Medical Journal).* 1999 Apr 17; 318(7190): 1063–1066. 36 refs. BE62451.
*adolescents; autonomy; cancer; case studies; children; *competence; genetic counseling; genetic predisposition; *genetic screening; genetic services; guidelines; health facilities; Huntington disease; *informed consent; *institutional policies; *late-onset disorders; legal aspects; parental consent; paternalism; professional organizations; *risks and benefits; Great Britain

Dickson, David. Panel urges caution on genetic testing for mental disorders. [News]. *Nature.* 1998 Sep 24; 395(6700): 309. BE60297.
adults; advisory committees; children; *dementia; *genetic predisposition; genetic research; *genetic screening; *mentally ill; regulation; research subjects; schizophrenia; *Great Britain; *Nuffield Council on Bioethics

Draper, Heather; Chadwick, Ruth. Beware! Preimplantation genetic diagnosis may solve some old problems but it also raises new ones. *Journal of Medical Ethics.* 1999 Apr; 25(2): 114–120. 6 fn. BE61913.
abortion, induced; autonomy; beginning of life; case studies; children; *decision making; disabled; Down syndrome; *embryo transfer; embryos; *genetic disorders; *genetic screening; hearing disorders; *in vitro fertilization; legal aspects; *moral obligations; *moral policy; motivation; *parents; *physicians; pregnant women; *preimplantation diagnosis; prenatal diagnosis; property rights; *quality of life; *reproduction; rights; risks and benefits; value of life

Preimplantation genetic diagnosis (PIGD) goes some way to meeting the clinical, psychological and ethical problems of antenatal testing. We should guard, however, against the assumption that PIGD is the answer to all our problems. It also presents some new problems and leaves some old problems untouched. This paper will provide an overview of how PIGD meets some of the old problems but will concentrate on two new challenges for ethics (and, indeed, law). First we look at whether we should always suppose that it is wrong for a clinician to implant a genetically abnormal zygote. The second concern is particularly important in the UK. The Human Fertilisation and Embryology

Act (1990) gives clinicians a statutory obligation to consider the interests of the future children they help to create using in vitro fertilisation (IVF) techniques. Does this mean that because PIGD is based on IVF techniques the balance of power for determining the best interests of the future child shifts from the mother to the clinician?

Dworkin, Mark; Young, Melissa. Gene Blues: Dilemmas of DNA Testing. [Videorecording]. Oley, PA: Bullfrog Films; 1997. 1 videocassette; 30 min.; sd.; color; VHS. BE62128.
breast cancer; cystic fibrosis; disabled; DNA data banks; DNA fingerprinting; employment; eugenics; gene therapy; genetic counseling; genetic disorders; genetic information; genetic predisposition; genetic research; *genetic screening; genetics; health care delivery; health insurance; industry; insurance selection bias; law enforcement; military personnel; normality; prenatal diagnosis; risks and benefits; sickle cell anemia; social discrimination; United States

Episcopal Diocese of Washington, D.C. Committee on Medical Ethics (Chair: Cynthia B. Cohen). Wrestling with the Future: Our Genes and Our Choices. Harrisburg, PA: Morehouse Publishing; 1998. 132 p. Bibliography: p. 125–127. ISBN 0-8192-1762-X. BE61310.
adolescents; adults; carriers; case studies; children; chromosome abnormalities; clergy; confidentiality; congenital disorders; decision making; disclosure; employment; family members; family relationship; genetic counseling; genetic disorders; genetic information; genetic intervention; genetic predisposition; *genetic screening; health insurance; health personnel; informed consent; late-onset disorders; morality; newborns; parents; pastoral care; preimplantation diagnosis; *prenatal diagnosis; privacy; *Protestant ethics; psychological stress; reproduction; *risks and benefits; *selective abortion; sex determination; social discrimination; stigmatization; theology; uncertainty; *Anglican Church; *Episcopal Church; United States

Evers–Kiebooms, Gerry. Adolescents' opinions about genetic risk and genetic testing. *In:* Sterckx, Sigrid, ed. Biotechnology, Patents and Morality. Proceedings of an International Workshop, "Biotechnology, Patents and Morality: Towards a Consensus," held in Ghent, Belgium, 17–19 Jan 1996. Brookfield, VT: Ashgate; 1997: 85–95. 8 refs. ISBN 1-84014-158-1. BE62237.
*adolescents; *attitudes; congenital disorders; genetic counseling; *genetic disorders; *genetic screening; *knowledge, attitudes, practice; mentally disabled; physically disabled; *prenatal diagnosis; *risk; risks and benefits; selective abortion; survey; Belgium

Fanos, Joanna H. Developmental tasks of childhood and adolescence: implications for genetic testing. *American Journal of Medical Genetics.* 1997 Jul 11; 71(1): 22–28. 45 refs. BE59522.
*adolescents; carriers; *children; comprehension; emotions; family relationship; genetic counseling; genetic disorders; genetic predisposition; *genetic screening; late-onset disorders; parent child relationship; *psychological stress; *psychology; *risks and benefits; self concept; sexuality; siblings

Fleck, Leonard. Justice, rights, and Alzheimer disease genetics. *In:* Post, Stephen G.; Whitehouse, Peter J., eds. Genetic Testing for Alzheimer Disease: Ethical and Clinical Issues. Baltimore, MD: Johns Hopkins University Press; 1998: 190–208. 15 refs. ISBN 0-8018-5840-2. BE60724.
age factors; artificial organs; beneficence; *biomedical technologies; breast cancer; costs and benefits; cystic fibrosis; decision making; *dementia; fetal therapy; gene therapy;

BE = bioethics accession number   fn. = footnotes   refs. = references

genetic counseling; genetic disorders; genetic predisposition; *genetic screening; *genetic services; germ cells; *government financing; health care; hearts; *justice; late-onset disorders; *moral obligations; *moral policy; *obligations of society; organ transplantation; preimplantation diagnosis; prenatal diagnosis; public participation; *resource allocation; rights; risks and benefits; selection for treatment; standards; therapeutic research

Fletcher, J.C.; Wertz, D.C. Refusal of employment or insurance. [Abstract]. *American Journal of Human Genetics.* 1997 Oct; 61(4): A56. BE59391.
*employment; genetic counseling; *genetic predisposition; *genetic screening; genetic services; *health insurance; health personnel; *insurance selection bias; *life insurance; physicians; *social discrimination; survey; United States

Fox, Jeffrey L. Forget Washington: state laws threaten to restrict genetic research, too. [News]. *Journal of NIH Research.* 1997 Nov; 9(11): 19–20. BE59757.
cloning; confidentiality; federal government; *genetic information; genetic predisposition; *genetic research; *genetic screening; *government regulation; health insurance; industry; *privacy; *property rights; social discrimination; *state government; Health Insurance Portability and Accountability Act 1996; National Institutes of Health; *United States

Garber, Judy E.; Offit, Kenneth; Olopade, O.I. (Funmi), et al. The American Society of Clinical Oncology position on genetic testing: implications for health care providers: workshop no. 4. *Cancer.* 1997 Aug 1; 80(3, Suppl.): 632–634. 1 ref. Presented at the American Cancer Society Workshop on Heritable Cancer Syndromes and Genetic Testing, Chicago, IL, 7–8 Oct 1996. BE60893.
*cancer; genetic counseling; *genetic predisposition; genetic research; *genetic screening; genetic services; informed consent; laboratories; *organizational policies; physicians; professional competence; professional organizations; standards; *American Cancer Society; *American Society of Clinical Oncology; National Cancer Genetics Network

Genetics Forum (London). Public oppose insurers' genetic test policy. *Splice of Life.* 1997 Apr; 3(5): 10–11. BE59661.
disclosure; donors; drug industry; *genetic information; *genetic research; *genetic screening; *industry; informed consent; insurance selection bias; *life insurance; *public opinion; survey; tissue donation; Great Britain

Gevers, Sjef. Population screening: the role of the law. *European Journal of Health Law.* 1998 Mar; 5(1): 7–18. 16 fn. BE61255.
carriers; competence; confidentiality; congenital disorders; disclosure; epidemiology; family members; *genetic screening; *government regulation; guidelines; informed consent; international aspects; *legal aspects; *legislation; *mass screening; prenatal diagnosis; preventive medicine; public health; risks and benefits; selective abortion; standards; third party consent; right not to know; *Act on Population Screening (Netherlands); *Netherlands

Gillon, Raanan. Ethical issues. *In:* Weber, Walter; Mulvihill, John J.; Narod, Steven A., eds. Familial Cancer Management. Boca Raton, FL: CRC Press; 1996: 142–158. 26 refs. BE61799.
*cancer; confidentiality; deception; directive counseling; disclosure; dissent; employment; *family members; gene therapy; genetic counseling; genetic disorders; genetic information; *genetic intervention; *genetic predisposition; *genetic screening; informed consent; insurance; justice; mandatory testing; *patient care; physician patient relationship; preventive medicine; rights; risks and benefits; selective abortion; social discrimination; stigmatization;

surgery; transgenic organisms; wedge argument; incidental findings; Great Britain

Gillott, John. Childhood testing for carrier status: the perspectives of the Genetic Interest Group. *In:* Clarke, Angus, ed. The Genetic Testing of Children. Washington, DC: BIOS Scientific Publishers; 1998: 97–102. 6 refs. ISBN 1-85996-146-0. BE62758.
*adolescents; autonomy; *carriers; *children; consensus; decision making; dissent; family relationship; genetic disorders; genetic information; *genetic screening; *guidelines; informed consent; late-onset disorders; organizational policies; parents; professional organizations; *risks and benefits; truth disclosure; uncertainty; harms; right not to know; support groups; Clinical Genetics Society (Great Britain); *Genetic Interest Group (Great Britain); Great Britain

Gin, Brian R. Genetic discrimination: Huntington's disease and the Americans with Disabilities Act. [Note]. *Columbia Law Review.* 1997 Jun; 97(5): 1406–1434. 146 fn. BE61214.
*disabled; employment; genetic disorders; genetic screening; HIV seropositivity; *Huntington disease; *late-onset disorders; *legal aspects; legislation; reproduction; *social discrimination; *Americans with Disabilities Act 1990; Equal Employment Opportunity Commission; *United States

Glass, Kathleen Cranley; Weijer, Charles; Lemmens, Trudo, et al. Structuring the review of human genetics protocols, Part II: diagnostic and screening studies. *IRB: A Review of Human Subjects Research.* 1997 May–Aug; 19(3–4): 1–13. 72 refs. BE60213.
confidentiality; conflict of interest; diagnosis; disclosure; DNA data banks; *ethical review; genetic counseling; genetic diversity; genetic information; genetic predisposition; *genetic research; *genetic screening; *guidelines; *human experimentation; informed consent; insurance; international aspects; investigators; laboratories; mass screening; medical records; minority groups; patents; prenatal diagnosis; research design; *research ethics committees; research subjects; risks and benefits; selection of subjects; standards; uncertainty; vulnerable populations

Golden, Frederic. Good eggs, bad eggs: the growing power of prenatal genetic tests is raising thorny new questions about ethics, fairness and privacy. *Time.* 1999 Jan 11; 153(1): 56–59. BE60309.
congenital disorders; decision making; disclosure; employment; family members; fetuses; genetic counseling; genetic disorders; *genetic information; genetic predisposition; *genetic screening; health insurance; late-onset disorders; parents; preimplantation diagnosis; *prenatal diagnosis; public opinion; selective abortion; *social discrimination; truth disclosure; United States

Goldworth, Amnon. Informed consent in the genetic age. *Cambridge Quarterly of Healthcare Ethics.* 1999 Summer; 8(3): 393–400. 15 fn. BE62482.
*autonomy; breast cancer; *cancer; *confidentiality; cultural pluralism; *disclosure; family members; genetic counseling; *genetic information; genetic predisposition; *genetic screening; *informed consent; physician patient relationship; risk; risks and benefits; standards; trust

Great Britain. Advisory Committee on Genetic Testing. Genetic research and ethics. *Bulletin of Medical Ethics.* 1999 Feb; No. 145: 21–24. BE61893.
adolescents; advisory committees; carriers; children; confidentiality; disclosure; ethical review; genetic disorders; genetic predisposition; *genetic research; *genetic screening; *guidelines; informed consent; late-onset disorders; public policy; research design; research ethics committees; research subjects; risk; tissue banks; *Advisory Committee on Genetic Testing (Great Britain); Great Britain

---

Great Britain. Health Departments of the United Kingdom. Advisory Committee on Genetic Testing. Code of practice on human genetic testing services supplied direct to the public. *Community Genetics.* 1998; 1(1): 48. 2 fn. BE61491.
> carriers; confidentiality; disclosure; genetic counseling; *genetic screening; *genetic services; *government regulation; *guidelines; home care; *laboratories; physicians; public policy; *standards; *diagnostic kits; Advisory Committee on Genetic Testing (Great Britain); *Great Britain

Great Britain. Parliament. House of Commons. Science and Technology Committee. Association of British Insurers' Policy Statement on Life Insurance and Genetics. Second Report. London: The Stationery Office; 1997 Feb 19. 7 p. 7 fn. HC 328. Report together with the proceedings of the Committee. BE59418.
> advisory committees; confidentiality; *disclosure; *genetic information; *genetic screening; *industry; insurance selection bias; *life insurance; *organizational policies; public policy; *Association of British Insurers; *Great Britain; House of Commons Select Committee on Science and Technology

Grody, Wayne W.; Pyeritz, Reed E. Report card on molecular genetic testing: room for improvement? [Editorial]. *JAMA.* 1999 Mar 3; 281(9): 845–847. 19 refs. BE60241.
> administrators; confidentiality; duty to warn; *evaluation; family members; genetic counseling; *genetic screening; *genetic services; guideline adherence; health personnel; informed consent; institutional policies; *laboratories; professional competence; professional organizations; regulation; self regulation; *standards; *quality assurance; American College of Medical Genetics Laboratory Practice Committee Standards and Guidelines; College of American Pathologists; *United States

Hallowell, Christopher. Playing the odds: health insurers want to know what's in your DNA. *Time.* 1999 Jan 11; 153(1): 60. BE60310.
> *disclosure; employment; federal government; *genetic information; genetic predisposition; *genetic screening; *health insurance; insurance selection bias; legislation; medical records; *social discrimination; state government; United States

Handelin, Barbara; Wachbroit, Robert; Billings, Paul, et al. Genetic testing and individual rights. [Proceedings of the International Symposium on Law and Science at the Crossroads: Biomedical Technology, Ethics, Public Policy, and the Law; panel discussion]. *Suffolk University Law Review.* 1993 Winter; 27(4): 1477–1497. Moderator: Barry Brown. BE60702.
> behavioral genetics; confidentiality; disclosure; DNA data banks; DNA fingerprinting; family members; genetic disorders; *genetic information; genetic predisposition; genetic research; *genetic screening; genetic services; *industry; informed consent; laboratories; preimplantation diagnosis; privacy; standards; stigmatization; tissue banks

Harper, Peter S. What do we mean by genetic testing? *Journal of Medical Genetics.* 1997 Sep; 34(9): 749–752. 11 refs. BE59931.
> economics; genetic disorders; genetic predisposition; *genetic screening; genetic services; Huntington disease; industry; late-onset disorders; regulation; risks and benefits; terminology; trends

Hasadsri, Linda. The multi-faceted implications of preimplantation genetic testing. *Princeton Journal of Bioethics.* 1998 Spring; 1(1): 76–82. 8 refs. BE62494.
> disabled; embryos; eugenics; genetic disorders; *genetic

screening; late-onset disorders; moral obligations; normality; *preimplantation diagnosis; *risks and benefits; selective abortion; social discrimination

Henn, Wolfram. Genetic screening with the DNA chip: a new Pandora's box? *Journal of Medical Ethics.* 1999 Apr; 25(2): 200–203. 25 refs. BE61926.
> eugenics; genetic disorders; genetic predisposition; *genetic screening; industry; international aspects; late-onset disorders; mass screening; *methods; moral policy; preimplantation diagnosis; prenatal diagnosis; regulation; *risks and benefits; *social impact; *DNA chips

The ethically controversial option of genetic population screening used to be restricted to a small number of rather rare diseases by methodological limitations which are now about to be overcome. With the new technology of DNA microarrays ("DNA chip"), emerging from the synthesis of microelectronics and molecular biology, methods are now at hand for the development of mass screening programmes for a wide spectrum of genetic traits. Thus, the DNA chip may be the key technology for a refined preventive medicine as well as a new dimension of eugenics. The forthcoming introduction of the DNA chip technology into medical practice urgently requires an internationally consistent framework of ethical standards and legal limitations if we do not want it to become a new Pandora's box.

Herman, Joan. Genetic testing and insurance: a question of balance. *In:* Smith, Edward; Sapp; Walter, eds. Plain Talk about the Human Genome Project: A Tuskegee University Conference on Its Promise and Perils ... and Matters of Race. Tuskegee, AL: Tuskegee University Press; 1997: 179–185. ISBN 1-891196-01-4. BE61745.
> confidentiality; *economics; genetic information; *genetic screening; government regulation; *health insurance; *industry; *insurance selection bias; *risk; state government

Hodge, James G. Privacy and antidiscrimination issues: genetics legislation in the United States. *Community Genetics.* 1998; 1(3): 169–174. 70 refs. BE62287.
> carriers; *confidentiality; disclosure; employment; *genetic information; genetic predisposition; *genetic screening; *government regulation; insurance; *legislation; medical records; *privacy; *social discrimination; *state government; *United States

Hodge, Susan E. Paternalistic and protective? [Letter]. *Journal of Genetic Counseling.* 1995 Dec; 4(4): 351–352. 1 ref. BE60452.
> autonomy; confidentiality; *directive counseling; disclosure; family members; *genetic counseling; *genetic screening; *Huntington disease; informed consent; paternalism; *twins

Hoedemaekers, Rogeer; ten Have, Henk. Geneticization: the Cyprus paradigm. *Journal of Medicine and Philosophy.* 1998 Jun; 23(3): 274–287. 17 refs. BE59291.
> *attitudes; carriers; *coercion; decision making; *directive counseling; economics; eugenics; *genetic counseling; *genetic screening; genetic services; genetics; *goals; health education; *health personnel; international aspects; *mass screening; parents; paternalism; *prenatal diagnosis; prevalence; preventive medicine; public health; public opinion; quality of life; *selective abortion; social control; stigmatization; *thalassemia; *Cyprus; Great Britain; Quebec

Geneticization is a broad term referring to several related processes such as a spreading tendency to use a genetic model of disease explanation, a growing influence of genetics in medical practice, and the slow changing of individual and societal attitudes towards reproduction, prevention and control of disease. These processes can be demonstrated in medical literature on preventive genetic screening and counselling programs for beta-thalassaemia in Cyprus, the United Kingdom and Canada. The preventive possibilities of the new genetic and diagnostic technologies have been quickly understood and advocated by health professionals, and their educational strategies have created a web of social control, in marked contrast to the alleged voluntary decision-making process and free choice. Genetic diagnostic technologies have led to considerable changes in control and management of beta-thalassaemia, and have generated a number of unresolved incongruities.

Hoedemaekers, Rogeer. Predictive genetic screening and the concept of risk. *In:* Clarke, Angus, ed. The Genetic Testing of Children. Washington, DC: BIOS Scientific Publishers; 1998: 245-264. 31 refs. ISBN 1-85996-146-0. BE62766.
   communication; comprehension; decision making; employment; family members; *genetic counseling; genetic disorders; *genetic information; genetic predisposition; *genetic screening; industry; informal social control; insurance; psychological stress; *risk; *risks and benefits; social discrimination; stigmatization; *terminology; *uncertainty; values; *harms

Holland, Julie. Should parents be permitted to authorize genetic testing for their children? *Family Law Quarterly.* 1997 Summer; 31(2): 321-353. 188 fn. BE62162.
   *autonomy; *carriers; confidentiality; employment; genetic counseling; genetic disorders; genetic information; *genetic screening; human experimentation; informed consent; insurance selection bias; *late-onset disorders; legal aspects; legal rights; *minors; *parental consent; patient care; privacy; psychological stress; *risks and benefits; social discrimination; standards; *right not to know

Holtzman, Neil A. The UK's policy on genetic testing services supplied direct to the public -- two spheres and two tiers. *Community Genetics.* 1998; 1(1): 49-52. 20 refs. BE61492.
   advisory committees; *carriers; genetic counseling; genetic disorders; *genetic screening; *genetic services; government financing; *government regulation; *guidelines; home care; indigents; industry; justice; *laboratories; mass screening; private sector; *public policy; public sector; social discrimination; *socioeconomic factors; standards; *diagnostic kits; personal financing; Advisory Committee on Genetic Testing (Great Britain); *Great Britain; National Health Service

Hubbard, Ruth. Predictive genetics and the construction of the healthy ill. *Suffolk University Law Review.* 1993 Winter; 27(4): 1209-1224. 31 fn. BE60699.
   decision making; diagnosis; disabled; disease; family members; genetic disorders; genetic predisposition; *genetic screening; genetics; health; health care; industry; mass screening; parents; prenatal diagnosis; selective abortion; social discrimination; socioeconomic factors

Human Genetics Advisory Commission (Great Britain). The Implications of Genetic Testing for Insurance. [Report]. London: The Commission [online]. Internet Web site: http://www.dti.gov.uk/hgac/papers/papers—b.htm [1998 December 7]; 1997 Dec. 32 p. 18 refs. HGAC papers. BE59318.
   advisory committees; confidentiality; disclosure; genetic information; genetic predisposition; *genetic screening; government regulation; industry; insurance selection bias; *life insurance; risk; social discrimination; survey; uncertainty; *Great Britain; Human Genetics Advisory Commission (Great Britain)

Human Genetics Advisory Commission (Great Britain).

The Implications of Genetic Testing for Life Insurance. [Paper; request for responses]. London: The Commission [online]. Internet Web site: http://www.dti.gov.uk/hgac/papers/papers—a.htm [1998 December 7]; 1997 Jul 9. 9 p. HGAC papers. BE59319.
   advisory committees; confidentiality; genetic information; *genetic screening; guidelines; industry; insurance selection bias; *life insurance; risk; Association of British Insurers; *Great Britain; *Human Genetics Advisory Commission (Great Britain)

Human Genome Education [HuGEM] Project. The HuGEM Project: I. An Overview of the Human Genome Project and Its Ethical, Legal and Social Issues (19 min.); II. Opportunities and Challenges of the Human Genome Project (24 min.); III. Issues of Genetic Privacy and Discrimination (45 min.); IV. Genetic Testing Across the Lifespan (30 min.); V. Working Together to Improve Genetic Services (28 min.). Available from the Georgetown University Child Development Center, 3307 M St., NW, Suite 401, Washington, DC 20007; (202) 687-8803; 1996. 5 videocassettes; 146 min. total (19-45 min. each); sd., color; VHS. Videocassettes accompanied by a 68-page manual authored by E.V. Lapham et al. The HuGEM Project is a collaboration between the Georgetown University Child Development Center, a division of the Dept. of Pediatrics, Georgetown University Medical Center, and the Alliance of Genetic Support Groups. BE62800.
   children; confidentiality; disclosure; employment; family members; gene therapy; genetic counseling; *genetic disorders; genetic information; genetic predisposition; *genetic screening; *genetic services; *genome mapping; guidelines; health insurance; health personnel; newborns; patients; prenatal diagnosis; privacy; risks and benefits; social discrimination; technical expertise; ELSI-funded publication; Human Genome Project; United States

Husted, Jørgen. Autonomy and a right not to know. *In:* Chadwick, Ruth; Levitt, Mairi; Shickle, Darren, eds. The Right to Know and the Right Not to Know. Brookfield, VT: Ashgate; 1997: 55-68. 10 refs. 2 fn. ISBN 1-85972-424-8. BE62189.
   *autonomy; beneficence; *confidentiality; decision making; directive counseling; *disclosure; duty to warn; *family members; genetic counseling; *genetic information; *genetic screening; informed consent; *paternalism; physicians; privacy; truth disclosure; values; *right not to know; Great Britain; Nuffield Council on Bioethics

Jaeger, A.S.; Goode, E.L.; Boyle, J.M. Attitudes and opinions towards genetic testing among US Hispanics. [Abstract]. *American Journal of Human Genetics.* 1997 Oct; 61(4): A221. BE59396.
   *attitudes; cancer; genetic counseling; *genetic screening; *Hispanic Americans; survey; United States

James, C.A.; Bernhardt, B.A.; Doksum, T., et al. Attitudes toward BRCA1 testing among physicians and medical students. [Abstract]. *American Journal of Human Genetics.* 1996 Oct; 59(4): A7. BE60091.
   age factors; *attitudes; *breast cancer; family practice; females; genetic counseling; *genetic screening; informed consent; internal medicine; mass screening; *medical education; medical schools; medical specialties; obstetrics and gynecology; *physicians; pregnant women; prenatal diagnosis; *students; surgery; survey; Maryland

Jones, Ian; Craddock, Nick. Ethical issues in genetics of mental disorders. [Letter]. *Lancet.* 1998 Nov 28; 352(9142): 1788. 4 refs. BE60802.
   *genetic predisposition; *genetic screening; *mentally ill;

risks and benefits; *stigmatization

Jones, Valerie A. In the same boat. *JAMA*. 1998 Nov 4; 280(17): 1537–1538. 5 refs. One of three winning essays in the fourth annual (1998) John Conley Ethics Essay Contest for Medical Students. BE59634.
confidentiality; decision making; dementia; economics; genetic counseling; *genetic predisposition; *genetic screening; informed consent; legal aspects; physicians; psychological stress; risks and benefits

Juengst, Eric T. The ethical implications of Alzheimer disease risk testing for other clinical uses of APOE genotyping. *In:* Post, Stephen G.; Whitehouse, Peter J., eds. Genetic Testing for Alzheimer Disease: Ethical and Clinical Issues. Baltimore, MD: Johns Hopkins University Press; 1998: 177–189. 22 refs. ISBN 0-8018-5840-2. BE60723.
beneficence; *dementia; *disclosure; genetic counseling; genetic predisposition; *genetic screening; heart diseases; informed consent; moral obligations; patient education; physicians; risk; risks and benefits; social discrimination; truth disclosure; uncertainty; *incidental findings; recontact

Julian-Reyneir, C.; Eisinger, F.; Aurran, Y., et al. Attitudes about breast cancer genetics and preventive strategies: a national survey of French medical and surgical gynecologists. [Abstract]. *American Journal of Human Genetics*. 1997 Oct; 61(4): A222. BE59397.
*attitudes; *breast cancer; females; genetic counseling; *genetic screening; males; obstetrics and gynecology; *physicians; preventive medicine; surgery; survey; *France

Kahn, Jeffrey. Ethical issues in genetic testing for Alzheimer's disease. *Geriatrics*. 1997 Sep; 52(Suppl. 2): S30–S32. 7 refs. BE60536.
*dementia; employment; genetic counseling; genetic information; genetic predisposition; genetic research; *genetic screening; informed consent; insurance; privacy; risk

Karanjawala, Zarir E.; Collins, Francis S. Genetics in the context of medical practice. *JAMA*. 1998 Nov 4; 280(17): 1533–1534. 14 refs. BE59632.
confidentiality; genetic counseling; genetic information; *genetic screening; genome mapping; government regulation; health insurance; physicians; *primary health care; professional competence; United States

Karlinsky, Harry. Genetic testing and counseling for early-onset autosomal-dominant Alzheimer disease. *In:* Post, Stephen G.; Whitehouse, Peter J., eds. Genetic Testing for Alzheimer Disease: Ethical and Clinical Issues. Baltimore, MD: Johns Hopkins University Press; 1998: 103–117. 19 refs. ISBN 0-8018-5840-2. BE60719.
adults; communication; competence; *dementia; diagnosis; disclosure; family members; *genetic counseling; *genetic screening; informed consent; psychological stress; risks and benefits; third party consent

Kash, Kathryn M. Psychosocial and ethical implications of defining genetic risk for cancers. *Annals of the New York Academy of Sciences*. 1995 Sep 30; 768: 41–52. 26 refs. BE59172.
attitudes; *breast cancer; *cancer; comprehension; confidentiality; disclosure; employment; family members; females; *genetic counseling; *genetic predisposition; *genetic screening; health insurance; informed consent; mass screening; motivation; *psychological stress; risk; social discrimination; United States

Kennedy, Ian. Illness and treatment: meaning for purposes of insurance contract: Katskee v. Blue Cross/Blue

Shield. [Comment]. *Medical Law Review*. 1995 Summer; 3(2): 224–227. BE59258.
breast cancer; *cancer; contracts; *disease; genetic counseling; *genetic predisposition; health; *health insurance reimbursement; *legal aspects; preventive medicine; *surgery; terminology; Great Britain; *Katskee v. Blue Cross/Blue Shield; Nebraska

Kerr, Anne; Cunningham-Burley, Sarah; Amos, Amanda. Drawing the line: an analysis of lay people's discussions about the new genetics. *Public Understanding of Science*. 1998 Apr; 7(2): 113–133. 14 fn. BE60906.
autonomy; behavioral genetics; children; cystic fibrosis; decision making; Down syndrome; eugenics; genetic counseling; genetic disorders; *genetic research; *genetic screening; *genetics; homosexuals; *knowledge, attitudes, practice; physicians; *prenatal diagnosis; *public opinion; *public participation; quality of life; selective abortion; socioeconomic factors; stigmatization; suffering; survey; focus groups; qualitative research; Scotland

Kerr, Anne; Cunningham-Burley, Sarah; Amos, Amanda. The new genetics and health: mobilizing lay expertise. *Public Understanding of Science*. 1998 Jan; 7(1): 41–60. 24 fn. BE60905.
behavioral genetics; comprehension; disabled; eugenics; genetic disorders; *genetic research; *genetic screening; *genetics; *knowledge, attitudes, practice; prenatal diagnosis; *public opinion; *public participation; public policy; selective abortion; socioeconomic factors; survey; *technical expertise; focus groups; qualitative research; Scotland

Kim, Hyang Nina. Prescription for prophecy: confronting the ambiguity of susceptibility testing. *JAMA*. 1998 Nov 4; 280(17): 1535–1536. 7 refs. One of three winning essays in the fourth annual (1998) John Conley Ethics Essay Contest for Medical Students. BE59633.
*communication; decision making; emotions; genetic counseling; genetic information; *genetic predisposition; *genetic screening; informed consent; physicians; risks and benefits; self concept; uncertainty

King, David S. Preimplantation genetic diagnosis and the 'new' eugenics. *Journal of Medical Ethics*. 1999 Apr; 25(2): 176–182. 33 refs. BE61923.
carriers; coercion; congenital disorders; decision making; directive counseling; disabled; embryo disposition; embryo transfer; embryos; *eugenics; gene pool; genetic counseling; genetic disorders; genetic predisposition; *genetic screening; goals; government regulation; health personnel; in vitro fertilization; informal social control; international aspects; knowledge, attitudes, practice; *moral policy; normality; parent child relationship; parents; physicians; *preimplantation diagnosis; prenatal diagnosis; public policy; selective abortion; social discrimination; *social impact; socioeconomic factors; trends
Preimplantation genetic diagnosis (PID) is often seen as an improvement upon prenatal testing. I argue that PID may exacerbate the eugenic features of prenatal testing and make possible an expanded form of free-market eugenics. The current practice of prenatal testing is eugenic in that its aim is to reduce the numbers of people with genetic disorders. Due to social pressures and eugenic attitudes held by clinical geneticists in most countries, it results in eugenic outcomes even though no state coercion is involved. I argue that technological advances may soon make PID widely accessible. Because abortion is not involved, and multiple embryos are available, PID is radically more effective as a tool of genetic selection. It will also make possible selection on the basis of non-pathological characteristics, leading, potentially, to a full-blown free-market eugenics. For these reasons, I argue that PID should be strictly

---

regulated.

Kinghorn, Warren. Indecision. [Excerpt]. *JAMA.* 1998 Nov 4; 280(17): 1538. Excerpt from one of three winning essays in the fourth annual (1998) John Conley Ethics Essay Contest for Medical Students. Full text available on the MS/JAMA Website, at http://www.ama–assn.org/mss. BE59652.
> decision making; *genetic predisposition; *genetic screening; Huntington disease; moral obligations; patients; reproduction

Kleinert, Sabine. Validation of genetic tests for insurance in UK. [News]. *Lancet.* 1998 Nov 14; 352(9140): 1608. BE59658.
> advisory committees; confidentiality; disclosure; genetic disorders; *genetic screening; industry; *insurance; public policy; *regulation; self regulation; standards; voluntary programs; Association of British Insurers; *Great Britain

Kodish, Eric. Commentary: risks and benefits, testing and screening, cancer, genes and dollars. *Journal of Law, Medicine and Ethics.* 1997 Winter; 25(4): 252–255. 22 fn. Commentary on B.S. Wilfond, et al., p. 243–251. BE62670.
> advisory committees; breast cancer; *cancer; confidentiality; economics; genetic information; *genetic predisposition; *genetic screening; genetic services; industry; public policy; risk; *risks and benefits; Cancer Genetics Studies Consortium; National Institutes of Health; United States

Koenig, Barbara A.; Greely, Henry T.; McConnell, Laura M., et al. Genetic testing for BRCA1 and BRCA2: recommendations of the Stanford Program in Genomics, Ethics, and Society. *Journal of Women's Health.* 1998 Jun; 7(5): 531–545. 45 refs. Authors include also members of the Breast Cancer Working Group of the Stanford Program in Genomics, Ethics, and Society. BE62211.
> adults; *breast cancer; carriers; confidentiality; DNA sequences; education; federal government; females; genetic counseling; genetic information; *genetic predisposition; genetic research; *genetic screening; genetic services; government regulation; *guidelines; health insurance reimbursement; health personnel; informed consent; laboratories; legal liability; males; mass screening; minors; patents; prenatal diagnosis; privacy; professional organizations; risk; risks and benefits; *standards; state government; *Stanford Program in Genomics, Ethics, and Society; United States

Kurtz, Zarrina. Appropriate paternalism and the best interests of the child. *In:* Clarke, Angus, ed. The Genetic Testing of Children. Washington, DC: BIOS Scientific Publishers; 1998: 237–243. 8 refs. ISBN 1–85996–146–0. BE62765.
> *children; costs and benefits; decision making; disclosure; genetic information; *genetic screening; genetic services; *parents; *paternalism; public policy; resource allocation; rights; risks and benefits; *state interest; utilitarianism; Children Act 1989 (Great Britain); *Great Britain

Lafayette, DeeDee; Abuelo, Dianne; Passero, Mary Ann, et al. Attitudes toward cystic fibrosis carrier and prenatal testing and utilization of carrier testing among relatives of individuals with cystic fibrosis. *Journal of Genetic Counseling.* 1999 Feb; 8(1): 17–36. 57 refs. BE61642.
> *attitudes; *carriers; *cystic fibrosis; *family members; family planning; *genetic counseling; *genetic screening; *knowledge, attitudes, practice; *prenatal diagnosis; quality of life; *selective abortion; survey; Rhode Island

Lerman, Caryn; Hughes, Chanita; Trock, Bruce J., et

al. Genetic testing in families with hereditary nonpolyposis colon cancer. *JAMA.* 1999 May 5; 281(17): 1618–1622. 34 refs. BE61904.
> *cancer; depressive disorder; diagnosis; evaluation studies; *family members; females; genetic counseling; *genetic predisposition; *genetic screening; health education; insurance; males; preventive medicine; psychological stress; registries; *risk; risks and benefits; social discrimination; socioeconomic factors; statistics; survey; *colon cancer; *refusal to participate; right to know; United States

CONTEXT: Genetic testing for hereditary nonpolyposis colon cancer (HNPCC) is available, but the rates of acceptance of testing or barriers to participation are not known. OBJECTIVE: To investigate rates and predictors of utilization of genetic testing for HNPCC. DESIGN: Cohort study conducted between July 1996 and July 1998. SETTING: Hereditary nonpolyposis colon cancer family registry. PARTICIPANTS: Adult male and female members (n = 208) of 4 extended HNPCC families contacted for a baseline telephone interview. INTERVENTIONS: Family education and individual genetic counseling. MAIN OUTCOME MEASURE: Participant acceptance of HNPCC test results. RESULTS: Of the 208 family members, 90 (43%) received test results and 118 (57%) declined. Of 139 subjects (67%) who completed a baseline telephone interview, 84 (60%) received test results and 55 (40%) declined. Of the 84 subjects who received test results, 35 (42%) received information indicating that they had HNPCC–associated mutations and 49 (58%) that they did not. Test acceptors had higher education levels (odds ratio [OR], 3.74; 95% confidence interval [CI], 2.49-5.61) and were more likely to have participated in a previous genetic linkage study (OR, 4.30; 95% CI, 1.84-10.10). The presence of depression symptoms significantly reduced rates of HNPCC test use (OR, 0.34; 95% CI, 0.17-0.66). Although rates of test use were identical among men and women, the presence of depression symptoms resulted in a 4–fold decrease in test use among women (OR, 0.25; 95% CI, 0.08-0.80) and a smaller, nonsignificant reduction among men (OR, 0.49; 95% CI, 0.19-1.27). CONCLUSIONS: Despite having significantly elevated risks of developing colon cancer, a relatively small proportion of HNPCC family members are likely to use genetic testing. Barriers to test acceptance may include less formal education and the presence of depression symptoms, especially among women. Additional research is needed to generalize these findings to different clinical settings and racially diverse populations.

Levitt, Mairi. A sociological perspective on genetic screening. *European Journal of Genetics in Society.* 1997; 3(2): 19–21. 17 fn. BE61453.
> attitudes; autonomy; behavioral genetics; carriers; decision making; directive counseling; females; genetic counseling; *genetic screening; males; risks and benefits; social discrimination; *social impact; sociology

Levitt, Mairi. Sociological perspectives on the right to know and the right not to know. *In:* Chadwick, Ruth; Levitt, Mairi; Shickle, Darren, eds. The Right to Know and the Right Not to Know. Brookfield, VT: Ashgate; 1997: 29–36. 16 refs. 3 fn. ISBN 1–85972–424–8. BE62186.
> autonomy; disadvantaged; genetic counseling; *genetic information; *genetic screening; health promotion; mass screening; paternalism; rights; *risks and benefits; self induced illness; social sciences; *socioeconomic factors; *truth disclosure; right not to know; Great Britain

Lin, Jonathan H. Divining and altering the future:

BE = bioethics accession number　　　fn. = footnotes　　　refs. = references

implications from the Human Genome Project. [Editorial]. *JAMA.* 1998 Nov 4; 280(17): 1532. 2 refs. BE59631.
> gene therapy; *genetic predisposition; *genetic screening; genome mapping; patient care; patients; physicians; risks and benefits

Lisko, Elaine A. Genetic information and long-term care insurance. *Health Law News.* 1998 Sep; 12(1): 3, 12–13. BE59898.
> aged; dementia; *genetic information; *genetic predisposition; *genetic screening; *government regulation; *health insurance; *insurance selection bias; legislation; *long-term care; nursing homes; social discrimination; state government; *United States

Low, Lawrence; King, Suzanne; Wilkie, Tom. Genetic discrimination in life insurance: empirical evidence from a cross sectional survey of genetic support groups in the United Kingdom. *BMJ (British Medical Journal).* 1998 Dec 12; 317(7173): 1632–1635. 17 refs. BE60234.
> carriers; comparative studies; control groups; cystic fibrosis; Duchenne muscular dystrophy; *family members; *genetic disorders; *genetic information; genetic predisposition; *genetic screening; Huntington disease; industry; *insurance selection bias; *knowledge, attitudes, practice; late–onset disorders; *life insurance; risk; *social discrimination; survey; muscular dystrophy; Disability Discrimination Act 1995 (Great Britain); *Great Britain; Wellcome Trust

OBJECTIVES: To gather empirical evidence on any discrimination based on genetic information shown by the insurance industry in the United Kingdom and to assess how society is likely to handle future genetic information from tests for polygenic multifactorial conditions. DESIGN: Postal questionnaire survey. SUBJECTS: Sample (n=7000) of members from seven British support groups for families with genetic disorders and a representative sample (n=1033) of the general public who answered questions on applying for life insurance as part of an omnibus survey. MAIN OUTCOME MEASURES: Subjects were asked about their experiences with insurers, the medical profession, employers, and social services. Experiences with insurers are reported here. RESULTS: Altogether 33.4% of the study group had problems when applying for life insurance compared with 5% of applicants in the omnibus survey. Thirteen per cent of study respondents from subgroups who represented no adverse actuarial risk on genetic grounds reported that their treatment by insurers seemed to represent unjustified genetic discrimination. CONCLUSIONS: Life insurers may not be operating a consistent policy for assessing genetic information or acting in accord with the actuarial risks brought to them. The inconsistency suggests error rather than a corporate policy of discrimination based on genetic characteristics. Any future proposals for genetic testing for common or multifactorial disorders should be examined carefully.

Lucassen, Anneke. Ethical issues in genetics of mental disorders. *Lancet.* 1998 Sep 26; 352(9133): 1004–1005. 8 refs. BE60793.
> dementia; disclosure; family members; *genetic counseling; genetic disorders; *genetic predisposition; genetic research; *genetic screening; *mentally ill; preventive medicine; risk; risks and benefits; selective abortion; stigmatization

McConnell, L.M.; Koenig, B.A.; Greely, H.T., et al.; Stanford Program in Genomics, Ethics and Society. Alzheimer Disease Working Group. Genetic testing and Alzheimer disease: has the time come? *Nature Medicine.* 1998 Jul; 4(7): 757–759. 13 refs. BE59771.
> *dementia; diagnosis; family members; genetic counseling; *genetic predisposition; *genetic screening; *guidelines; late–onset disorders; preventive medicine; *risks and benefits; *Alzheimer Working Group of the Stanford Program in Genomics, Ethics and Society

McGleenan, Tony. Rights to know and not to know: is there a need for a genetic privacy law? *In:* Chadwick, Ruth; Levitt, Mairi; Shickle, Darren, eds. The Right to Know and the Right Not to Know. Brookfield, VT: Ashgate; 1997: 43–54. 19 refs. 9 fn. ISBN 1–85972–424–8. BE62188.
> common good; *confidentiality; constitutional law; *disclosure; DNA data banks; *genetic information; genetic research; *genetic screening; informed consent; law enforcement; *legal aspects; *legal rights; legislation; *model legislation; moral policy; *privacy; *public policy; social discrimination; Supreme Court decisions; tissue donation; torts; truth disclosure; right not to know; *Genetic Privacy Act (1995 bill); United States

McGovern, Margaret M.; Benach, Marta O.; Wallenstein, Sylvan, et al. Quality assurance in molecular genetic testing laboratories. *JAMA.* 1999 Mar 3; 281(9): 835–840. 18 refs. BE60240.
> administrators; confidentiality; *evaluation; evaluation studies; genetic counseling; *genetic screening; *genetic services; guideline adherence; health personnel; informed consent; institutional policies; *laboratories; professional competence; regulation; *standards; statistics; survey; *quality assurance; American College of Medical Genetics Laboratory Practice Committee Standards and Guidelines; *United States

CONTEXT: Specific regulation of laboratories performing molecular genetic tests may be needed to ensure standards and quality assurance (QA) and safeguard patient rights to informed consent and confidentiality. However, comprehensive analysis of current practices of such laboratories, important for assessing the need for regulation and its impact on access to testing, has not been conducted. OBJECTIVE: To collect and analyze data regarding availability of clinical molecular genetic testing, including personnel standards and laboratory practices. DESIGN: A mail survey in June 1997 of molecular genetic testing laboratory directors and assignment of a QA score based on responses to genetic testing process items. SETTING: Hospital–based, independent, and research–based molecular genetic testing laboratories in the United States. PARTICIPANTS: Directors of molecular genetic testing laboratories (n = 245; response rate, 74.9%). MAIN OUTCOME MEASURE: Laboratory process QA score, using the American College of Medical Genetics Laboratory Practice Committee standards. RESULTS: The 245 responding laboratories reported availability of testing for 94 disorders. Personnel qualifications varied, although all directors had doctoral degrees. The mean QAscore was 90% (range, 44%–100%) with 36 laboratories (15%) scoring lower than 70%. Higher scores were associated with test menu size of more than 4 tests (P = .01), performance of more than 30 analyses annually (P = .01), director having a PhD vs MD degree (P = .002), director board certification (P = .03), independent (P less than .001) and hospital (P = .01) laboratories vs research laboratory, participation in proficiency testing (P less than .001), and Clinical Laboratory Improvement Amendment certification (P = .006). Seventy percent of laboratories provided access to genetic counseling, 69% had a confidentiality policy, and 45% required informed consent prior to testing. CONCLUSION: The finding that a number of laboratories had QA scores that may reflect suboptimal laboratory practices suggests that

---

BE = bioethics accession number   fn. = footnotes   refs. = references

both personnel qualification and laboratory practice standards are most in need of improvement to ensure quality in clinical molecular genetic testing laboratories.

MacKay, Charles; Murphy, Patricia D.; Smith, Robert A., et al. Industry, ethics, and general medicine: workshop no. 5. *Cancer.* 1997 Aug 1; 80(3, Suppl.): 635. Presented at the American Cancer Society Workshop on Heritable Cancer Syndromes and Genetic Testing, Chicago, IL, 7–8 Oct 1996. BE60894.
  advertising; confidentiality; genetic counseling; genetic information; *genetic screening; laboratories; *organizational policies; standards; *American Cancer Society

McLean, Margaret R. When what we know outstrips what we can do. *Issues in Ethics (Markkula Center for Applied Ethics).* 1998 Spring–Summer; 9(2): 6–10. BE62037.
  confidentiality; family members; genetic counseling; genetic enhancement; genetic information; *genetic intervention; *genetic screening; genome mapping; *Huntington disease; justice; resource allocation; right not to know

McLean, Sheila A.M. The genetic testing of children: some legal and ethical concerns. *In:* Clarke, Angus, ed. The Genetic Testing of Children. Washington, DC: BIOS Scientific Publishers; 1998: 17–26. 22 refs. ISBN 1-85996-146-0. BE62756.
  autonomy; *children; competence; confidentiality; diagnosis; family members; genetic counseling; genetic disorders; genetic information; *genetic screening; informed consent; late–onset disorders; legal aspects; moral obligations; parental consent; parents; privacy; *risks and benefits; social discrimination

Magnus, David. Disease gene patenting: the clinician's dilemma. *Cambridge Quarterly of Healthcare Ethics.* 1998 Fall; 7(4): 433–435. 5 fn. BE59146.
  diagnosis; disclosure; economics; *genes; genetic disorders; genetic information; *genetic screening; genetic services; *genome mapping; legal aspects; methods; *patents; physicians; property rights; public policy; risks and benefits; United States

Maldonato, A. Ethical aspects in the prediction of Type I diabetes. *Diabetes, Nutrition and Metabolism.* 1996 Dec; 9(6): 325–329. 29 refs. BE59242.
  bioethics; *diabetes; disclosure; family members; genetic counseling; genetic information; *genetic predisposition; *genetic screening; insurance selection bias; patient care; patient education; preventive medicine; psychological stress; *risks and benefits; therapeutic research

Malkin, D.; Australie, K.; Shuman, C., et al. Parental attitudes to genetic counseling and predictive testing for childhood cancer. [Abstract]. *American Journal of Human Genetics.* 1996 Oct; 59(4): A7. BE60092.
  *attitudes; cancer; children; *genetic counseling; *genetic predisposition; *genetic screening; *parents; risk; survey; Toronto

Mao, Xin. Chinese geneticists approach ethics. [Letter]. *Journal of Medical Ethics.* 1998 Jan; 35(1): 83. 14 refs. BE61126.
  *attitudes; confidentiality; developing countries; *directive counseling; disclosure; eugenics; *genetic counseling; genetic disorders; genetic predisposition; genetic research; *genetic screening; genetic services; genetics; guidelines; *health personnel; international aspects; investigators; *non–Western World; *prenatal diagnosis; *selective abortion; sex determination; survey; Western World; *China

Marshall, Andrew. Genetic tests forge ahead, despite scientific concerns. [News]. *Nature Biotechnology.* 1996 Dec; 14(13): 1642–1643. BE61400.
  *breast cancer; carriers; continuing education; diagnosis; *economics; federal government; genetic counseling; *genetic predisposition; *genetic screening; genetic services; *government regulation; *industry; patient education; physicians; preventive medicine; risk; surgery; *diagnostic kits; Food and Drug Administration; Health Care Financing Administration; *United States

Marshall, Eliot. Beryllium screening raises ethical issues. [News]. *Science.* 1999 Jul 9; 285(5425): 178–179. BE62524.
  data banks; *employment; *genetic predisposition; *genetic screening; *health hazards; *occupational exposure; lung diseases; United States

Martinez, William. Genetic testing of children and adolescents: ethical, legal and psychosocial implications. *Princeton Journal of Bioethics.* 1998 Spring; 1(1): 65–75. 7 refs. BE62493.
  *adolescents; adoption; carriers; *children; competence; decision making; disclosure; genetic counseling; *genetic screening; Huntington disease; informed consent; legal aspects; parent child relationship; parental consent; parents; psychological stress; reproduction; *risks and benefits; self concept; social discrimination

Mecsas–Faxon, S.; Tishler, S.; Pauker, S.P. Cancer genetics program within an HMO: a model of confidential service. [Abstract]. *American Journal of Human Genetics.* 1997 Oct; 61(4): A224. BE59398.
  *cancer; confidentiality; genetic counseling; genetic predisposition; genetic research; *genetic screening; *genetic services; health insurance reimbursement; *health maintenance organizations; medical records; program descriptions; *Harvard Pilgrim Health Care; Massachusetts

Merrill, Sonya. Genetic screening: suffering and sovereignty. *In:* Demy, Timothy J.; Stewart, Gary P., eds. Genetic Engineering: A Christian Response: Crucial Considerations in Shaping Life. Grand Rapids, MI: Kregel Publications; 1999: 304–313. 7 fn. ISBN 0-8254-2357-0. BE61373.
  *biomedical technologies; *Christian ethics; compassion; gene therapy; genetic disorders; genetic predisposition; *genetic screening; genome mapping; *goals; intention; mandatory testing; moral obligations; moral policy; motivation; newborns; pain; prenatal diagnosis; preventive medicine; selective abortion; *suffering; *theology

Meyer, Roberta B. Justification for permitting life insurers to continue to underwrite on the basis of genetic information and genetic test results. *Suffolk University Law Review.* 1993 Winter; 27(4): 1271–1305. 180 fn. BE60735.
  federal government; *genetic information; *genetic screening; government regulation; industry; *insurance selection bias; *legal aspects; legislation; *life insurance; *risk; *social discrimination; state government; United States

Middleton, A.; Hewison, J.; Mueller, R.F. A pilot study of attitudes of deaf and hearing parents towards issues surrounding genetic testing for deafness. [Abstract]. *American Journal of Human Genetics.* 1997 Oct; 61(4): A190. BE59395.
  *attitudes; comparative studies; *genetic disorders; *genetic screening; *hearing disorders; *parents; *physically disabled; *prenatal diagnosis; *selective abortion; survey; Great Britain

Mieth, Dietmar. Reflections on genetic testing in childhood. *In:* Clarke, Angus, ed. The Genetic Testing

BE = bioethics accession number   fn. = footnotes   refs. = references

of Children. Washington, DC: BIOS Scientific Publishers; 1998: 37–45. 13 refs. ISBN 1–85996–146–0. BE62757.

*children; cystic fibrosis; diagnosis; disclosure; family members; genetic counseling; genetic information; *genetic screening; goals; infants; mass screening; parents; patient care; rights; *risks and benefits; uncertainty

Miles, Steven. Managed care issues in genetic testing for Alzheimer disease. *In:* Post, Stephen G.; Whitehouse, Peter J., eds. Genetic Testing for Alzheimer Disease: Ethical and Clinical Issues. Baltimore, MD: Johns Hopkins University Press; 1998: 209–221. 38 refs. ISBN 0–8018–5840–2. BE60725.

anonymous testing; chronically ill; costs and benefits; data banks; *dementia; diagnosis; epidemiology; federal government; genetic counseling; genetic information; genetic predisposition; *genetic screening; government financing; government regulation; health insurance; informed consent; insurance selection bias; justice; long-term care; *managed care programs; medical records; population genetics; private sector; public policy; resource allocation; risk; social discrimination; United States

Milunsky, Aubrey. The "new" genetics: from research to reality. *Suffolk University Law Review.* 1993 Winter; 27(4): 1307–1325. 61 fn. BE60736.

carriers; confidentiality; DNA data banks; economics; employment; gene therapy; genetic disorders; *genetic intervention; genetic predisposition; *genetic screening; genome mapping; industry; informed consent; insurance; laboratories; legal aspects; preimplantation diagnosis; prenatal diagnosis; public policy; sex preselection; social discrimination; United States

Mlot, C. Panel backs widening net of genetic test. [News]. *Science News.* 1997 Apr 26; 151(17): 253. BE61645.

advisory committees; carriers; *cystic fibrosis; genetic counseling; *genetic screening; health insurance reimbursement; mass screening; public policy; voluntary programs; National Institutes of Health; United States

Morrison, P.J. Implications of genetic testing for insurance in the UK. *Lancet.* 1998 Nov 21; 352(9141): 1647–1648. 8 refs. BE60799.

advisory committees; breast cancer; confidentiality; genetic disorders; genetic information; *genetic screening; *government regulation; guidelines; industry; *insurance; insurance selection bias; social discrimination; right not to know; Advisory Committee on Genetic Testing (Great Britain); Association of British Insurers; *Great Britain; Human Genetics Advisory Commission (Great Britain)

Motluk, Alison. Insurers fight shy of gene tests. [News]. *New Scientist.* 1997 Feb 22; 153(2070): 7. BE59712.

disclosure; *genetic information; *genetic screening; industry; *life insurance; self regulation; Association of British Insurers; *Great Britain

Müller, H.J.; Deonna, Th.; Abbt, I., et al. Medical–ethical guidelines for genetic investigations in humans. *Schweizerische Medizinische Wochenschrift.* 1994 Jun 4; 124(22): 974–979. 5 refs. BE59774.

confidentiality; disclosure; employment; *genetic counseling; genetic disorders; genetic predisposition; genetic research; *genetic screening; informed consent; insurance; physicians; *practice guidelines; *prenatal diagnosis; professional organizations; selective abortion; right not to know; *Swiss Academy of Medical Sciences

Murray, Robert. The ethics of predictive genetic screening: are the benefits worth the risks? *In:* Smith, Edward; Sapp, Walter, eds. Plain Talk about the Human Genome Project: A Tuskegee University Conference on

Its Promise and Perils ... and Matters of Race. Tuskegee, AL: Tuskegee University Press; 1997: 139–150. 8 refs. ISBN 1–891196–01–4. BE61741.

autonomy; blacks; confidentiality; family members; federal government; genetic information; *genetic screening; guidelines; historical aspects; justice; mass screening; public policy; *risks and benefits; sickle cell anemia; social discrimination; stigmatization; Twentieth Century; United States

Murray, Thomas. Genetic discrimination in health insurance and why it is wrong. *In:* Smith, Edward; Sapp, Walter, eds. Plain Talk about the Human Genome Project: A Tuskegee University Conference on Its Promise and Perils ... and Matters of Race. Tuskegee, AL: Tuskegee University Press; 1997: 159–168. 5 refs. ISBN 1–891196–01–4. BE61743.

advisory committees; confidentiality; federal government; *genetic information; *genetic screening; government regulation; health care; *health insurance; industry; insurance selection bias; *justice; risk; state government; NCHGR Program on Ethical, Legal, and Social Implications (ELSI); *Task Force on Genetic Information and Insurance; *United States

Nagy, Anne–Marie; De Man, Xavier; Ruibal, Nike, et al. Scientific and ethical issues of preimplantation diagnosis. [Editorial]. *Annals of Medicine.* 1998 Feb; 30(1): 1–6. 35 refs. BE62401.

chromosome abnormalities; genetic disorders; genetic predisposition; *genetic screening; methods; *preimplantation diagnosis; sex preselection

Nayfield, Susan G. Ethical and scientific considerations for chemoprevention research in cohorts at genetic risk for breast cancer. *Journal of Cellular Biochemistry. Supplement.* 1996; 25: 123–130. 42 refs. BE60247.

*breast cancer; cancer; confidentiality; counseling; *drugs; employment; family members; females; genetic counseling; *genetic predisposition; *genetic research; *genetic screening; health insurance; *human experimentation; informed consent; organizational policies; placebos; *preventive medicine; privacy; records; *research design; research subjects; *risk; *risks and benefits; selection of subjects; social discrimination; stigmatization; ovaries; American Society of Clinical Oncology; American Society of Human Genetics; United States

Neilson, Jane. A patient's perspective on genetic counseling and predictive testing for Alzheimer's disease. *Journal of Genetic Counseling.* 1999 Feb; 8(1): 37–46. BE61643.

attitudes; confidentiality; *dementia; *emotions; *genetic counseling; *genetic screening; patients

New England Regional Genetics Group. New England Regional Genetics Group (NERGG) policy statement on screening for cystic fibrosis. *Genetic Resource.* 1991; 6(1): 67–68. BE60449.

carriers; *cystic fibrosis; genetic counseling; *genetic screening; mass screening; standards; United States

Nippert, I.; Horst, J.; Wolff, G., et al. Ethical issues in genetic service provision: attitudes of human geneticists in Germany. [Abstract]. *American Journal of Human Genetics.* 1996 Oct; 59(4): A338. BE60095.

adults; alcohol abuse; allowing to die; *attitudes; autonomy; cancer; children; confidentiality; disclosure; Down syndrome; family members; *genetic counseling; genetic disorders; genetic predisposition; *genetic screening; genetic services; *health personnel; Huntington disease; informed consent; prenatal diagnosis; referral and consultation; spina bifida; survey; ELSI-funded publication; *Germany

---

BE = bioethics accession number   fn. = footnotes   refs. = references

Nuffield Council on Bioethics. Mental Disorders and Genetics: The Ethical Context. London: The Council; 1998 Sep. 117 p. Includes references. ISBN 0-9522701-3-7. BE60716.
> adoption; advisory committees; carriers; children; competence; confidentiality; dementia; directive counseling; disclosure; drugs; education; employment; eugenics; family members; gene therapy; *genetic counseling; genetic information; *genetic predisposition; *genetic research; *genetic screening; goals; *guidelines; human experimentation; Huntington disease; informed consent; insurance; legal aspects; *mentally disabled; mentally ill; public policy; reproduction; social discrimination; stigmatization; twins; diagnostic kits; pedigree studies; right not to know; Great Britain; *Nuffield Council on Bioethics

Ostrer, Harry; Scheuermann, Richard H.; Picker, Louis J. Benefits and dangers of genetic tests. [Letters]. *Nature.* 1998 Mar 5; 392(6671): 14. 6 refs. BE59237.
> advisory committees; breast cancer; DNA data banks; epidemiology; genetic predisposition; *genetic research; *genetic screening; human experimentation; informed consent; Jews; minority groups; *population genetics; *public policy; risks and benefits; *tissue banks; tissue donation; National Bioethics Advisory Commission; United States

Patenaude, Andrea Farkas. Cancer susceptibility testing: risks, benefits and personal beliefs. *In:* Clarke, Angus, ed. The Genetic Testing of Children. Washington, DC: BIOS Scientific Publishers; 1998: 145-156. 47 refs. ISBN 1-85996-146-0. BE62761.
> *cancer; *children; comprehension; empirical research; genetic counseling; genetic disorders; *genetic predisposition; *genetic screening; knowledge, attitudes, practice; late-onset disorders; parents; preventive medicine; *risk; social discrimination; colon cancer

Penticuff, Joy Hinson. Ethical dimensions in genetic screening: a look into the future. *Journal of Obstetric, Gynecologic and Neonatal Nursing.* 1996 Nov-Dec; 25(9): 785-789. 8 refs. BE61560.
> carriers; confidentiality; embryos; employment; genetic counseling; *genetic disorders; genetic information; *genetic predisposition; *genetic screening; informed consent; insurance selection bias; late-onset disorders; mass screening; newborns; nurses; preimplantation diagnosis; prenatal diagnosis; selective abortion; social discrimination; uncertainty; voluntary programs; wrongful life; United States

Pentz, Rebecca D. Genetic counseling: guidance for chilling choices. *In:* Demy, Timothy J.; Stewart, Gary P., eds. Genetic Engineering: A Christian Response: Crucial Considerations in Shaping Life. Grand Rapids, MI: Kregel Publications; 1999: 188-195. 3 fn. ISBN 0-8254-2357-0. BE61367.
> breast cancer; *Christian ethics; chromosome abnormalities; costs and benefits; decision making; directive counseling; disabled; employment; family members; *gene therapy; *genetic counseling; *genetic enhancement; genetic information; *genetic screening; germ cells; health personnel; insurance; pastoral care; patients; prenatal diagnosis; prolongation of life; quality of life; *risks and benefits; social discrimination; theology; values

Persson, Ingmar. Equality and selection for existence. *Journal of Medical Ethics.* 1999 Apr; 25(2): 130-136. 3 refs. BE61916.
> *beginning of life; congenital disorders; *disabled; embryo disposition; *embryo transfer; *embryos; genetic determinism; *genetic disorders; *genetic screening; germ cells; in vitro fertilization; *justice; *moral policy; personhood; *preimplantation diagnosis; public policy; *quality of life; rights; self concept; social interaction; *social

worth; speciesism; *utilitarianism; *value of life
It is argued that the policy of excluding from further life some human gametes and pre-embryos as "unfit" for existence is not at odds with a defensible idea of human equality. Such an idea must be compatible with the obvious fact that the "functional" value of humans differs, that their "use" to themselves and others differs. A defensible idea of human equality is instead grounded in the fact that as this functional difference is genetically determined, it is nothing which makes humans deserve or be worthy of being better or worse off. Rather, nobody is worth a better life than anyone else. This idea of equality is, however, not applicable to gametes and pre-embryos, since they are not human beings, but something out of which human beings develop.

Peshkin, Beth N.; Lerman, Caryn. Genetic counselling for hereditary breast cancer. *Lancet.* 1999 Jun 26; 353(9171): 2176-2177. 10 refs. BE62268.
> attitudes; *breast cancer; disclosure; empirical research; females; *genetic counseling; *genetic predisposition; *genetic screening; informed consent; psychological stress; risk

Pokorski, Robert J.; Sanderson, Patricia; Bennett, Nancy, et al. Insurance issues and genetic testing: challenges and recommendations: workshop no. 1. *Cancer.* 1997 Aug 1; 80(3, Suppl.): 627. Presented at the American Cancer Society Workshop on Heritable Cancer Syndromes and Genetic Testing, Chicago, IL, 7-8 Oct 1996. BE60892.
> confidentiality; *genetic information; genetic research; *genetic screening; health insurance reimbursement; informed consent; *insurance; insurance selection bias; organizational policies; social discrimination; American Cancer Society; Workshop on Heritable Cancer Syndromes and Genetic Testing

Pokorski, Robert J. Insurance underwriting in the genetic era. *Cancer.* 1997 Aug; 80(3, Suppl.): 587-599. 72 refs. Presented at the American Cancer Society Workshop on Heritable Genetic Syndromes and Genetic Testing, Chicago, IL, 7-8 Oct 1996. BE60890.
> cancer; confidentiality; deception; dementia; disclosure; economics; *genetic information; *genetic predisposition; *genetic screening; industry; *insurance; *insurance selection bias; life insurance; long-term care; patients; physicians; *risk; social discrimination

Pörn, Ingmar. The meaning of 'rights' in the right to know debate. *In:* Chadwick, Ruth; Levitt, Mairi; Shickle, Darren, eds. The Right to Know and the Right Not to Know. Brookfield, VT: Ashgate; 1997: 37-42. 9 refs. 5 fn. ISBN 1-85972-424-8. BE62187.
> *autonomy; *genetic counseling; *genetic information; *genetic screening; *moral obligations; philosophy; *rights; truth disclosure; right not to know

Post, Stephen G.; Whitehouse, Peter J., eds. Genetic Testing for Alzheimer Disease: Ethical and Clinical Issues. Baltimore, MD: Johns Hopkins University Press; 1998. 284 p. 605 refs. ISBN 0-8018-5840-2. BE60718.
> age factors; aged; cultural pluralism; *dementia; diagnosis; economics; education; genetic counseling; genetic predisposition; genetic research; *genetic screening; genetic services; genetics; health insurance; justice; long-term care; managed care programs; mass screening; methods; minority groups; moral policy; obligations of society; patents; patient care; physicians; prenatal diagnosis; primary health care; professional competence; public policy; resource allocation; review; social discrimination; values; United States

Quaid, Kimberly A. Implications of genetic susceptibility

testing with apolipoprotein E. *In:* Post, Stephen G.; Whitehouse, Peter J., eds. Genetic Testing for Alzheimer Disease: Ethical and Clinical Issues. Baltimore, MD: Johns Hopkins University Press; 1998: 118–139. 75 refs. ISBN 0-8018-5840-2. BE60720.
> autonomy; breast cancer; comprehension; *dementia; directive counseling; *genetic counseling; genetic predisposition; *genetic screening; genetic services; health personnel; Huntington disease; industry; late–onset disorders; mass screening; paternalism; professional competence; psychological stress; refusal to treat; risk; risks and benefits; uncertainty

Regan, Priscilla M. Genetic testing and workplace surveillance: implications for privacy. *In:* Lyon, David; Zureik, Elia, eds. Computers, Surveillance, and Privacy. Minneapolis, MN: University of Minnesota Press; 1996: 21–46. 54 refs. 10 fn. ISBN 0-8166-2653-7. BE62133.
> computer communication networks; *confidentiality; *employment; evaluation; genetic information; genetic predisposition; *genetic screening; insurance; legal aspects; *privacy; public opinion; *public policy; records; *values; United States

Reilly, Philip R. Carrier screening for cystic fibrosis: a commentary on current legal and social policy issues. *Genetic Resource.* 1991; 6(1): 65–66. BE60448.
> *carriers; *cystic fibrosis; genetic counseling; *genetic screening; pregnant women; primary health care

Reilly, Philip R. Public policy and legal issues raised by advances in genetic screening and testing. *Suffolk University Law Review.* 1993 Winter; 27(4): 1327–1357. 54 fn. BE60737.
> adoption; carriers; children; *confidentiality; *disclosure; duty to warn; economics; employment; family members; genetic disorders; *genetic information; *genetic screening; government regulation; health care delivery; health insurance reimbursement; industry; insurance selection bias; *legal aspects; life insurance; parent child relationship; pregnant women; prenatal diagnosis; *public policy; social discrimination; state government; twins; United States

Richards, Martin. The genetic testing of children: adult attitudes and children's understanding. *In:* Clarke, Angus, ed. The Genetic Testing of Children. Washington, DC: BIOS Scientific Publishers; 1998: 157–168. 44 refs. ISBN 1-85996-146-0. BE62762.
> adults; *attitudes; cancer; *children; *comprehension; decision making; diagnosis; empirical research; family relationship; genetic information; *genetic screening; *genetics; *late–onset disorders; parents; public opinion; public policy; rights; risks and benefits; social discrimination; students; *colon cancer; Great Britain; Wales

Roche, Patricia; Glantz, Leonard H.; Annas, George J. The Genetic Privacy Act: a proposal for national legislation. *In:* Smith, Edward; Sapp, Walter, eds. Plain Talk about the Human Genome Project: A Tuskegee University Conference on Its Promise and Perils ... and Matters of Race. Tuskegee, AL: Tuskegee University Press; 1997: 187–196. 28 fn. ISBN 1-891196-01-4. BE61746.
> competence; *confidentiality; disclosure; *DNA data banks; federal government; *genetic information; *genetic screening; genome mapping; *government regulation; guidelines; informed consent; *legislation; minors; pregnant women; preimplantation diagnosis; prenatal diagnosis; *privacy; risks and benefits; third party consent; tissue banks; DNA analysis; *Genetic Confidentiality and Nondiscrimination Act (1996 bill); *Genetic Privacy Act (1995 bill); United States

Rodriguez, Eduardo. Genetic discrimination and health

care: ethical reflections. *Linacre Quarterly.* 1996 Nov; 63(4): 30–36. 14 fn. BE59304.
> disabled; *genetic information; *genetic screening; genome mapping; health care reform; *health insurance; human rights; insurance selection bias; personhood; prenatal diagnosis; *Roman Catholic ethics; selective abortion; *social discrimination; stigmatization; theology; value of life; United States

Rothstein, Mark A. Preventing the discovery of plaintiff genetic profiles by defendants seeking to limit damages in personal injury litigation. *Indiana Law Journal.* 1996 Fall; 71(4): 877–910. 218 fn. BE62666.
> compensation; *confidentiality; *disclosure; economics; *genetic information; genetic predisposition; genetic screening; late–onset disorders; *legal aspects; legal liability; mandatory testing; medical records; *torts; *life expectancy; United States

Saegusa, Asako. Japanese university approves genetic tests on in vitro embryos. [News]. *Nature.* 1999 Feb 11; 397(6719): 461. BE60397.
> Duchenne muscular dystrophy; ethical review; *genetic screening; guidelines; in vitro fertilization; physicians; political activity; *preimplantation diagnosis; professional organizations; research ethics committees; universities; *Japan; Japan Society of Obstetrics and Gynecology; Kagoshima University Medical School

Schoonmaker, M.; Bernhardt, B.; Holtzman, N.A. Coverage of new genetic technologies: what matters to insurers? [Abstract]. *American Journal of Human Genetics.* 1996 Oct; 59(4): A3. BE60090.
> breast cancer; carriers; costs and benefits; cystic fibrosis; gene therapy; genetic predisposition; *genetic screening; *health insurance; *health insurance reimbursement; *industry; mass screening; organizational policies; pregnant women; survey; United States

Seppa, Nathan. Cancer tests can heighten anxiety. [News]. *Science News.* 1998 Nov 14; 154(20): 316. BE61546.
> *breast cancer; diagnosis; females; *genetic screening; males; preventive medicine; *psychological stress; risks and benefits; mammography

Severin, Matthew J. Breast carcinoma litigation: medical questions, legal answers. *Cancer.* 1997 Aug 1; 80(3, Suppl.): 600–605. 22 refs. Presented at the American Cancer Society Workshop on Heritable Cancer Syndromes and Genetic Testing, Chicago, IL, 7–8 Oct 1996. BE60891.
> *breast cancer; diagnosis; family members; genetic predisposition; *genetic screening; health insurance; health insurance reimbursement; *legal aspects; legal liability; negligence; patient care; physicians; social discrimination; standards; United States

Skene, Loane. Patients' rights or family responsibilities? Two approaches to genetic testing. *Medical Law Review.* 1998 Spring; 6(1): 1–41. 117 fn. BE62169.
> autonomy; comparative studies; contracts; *disclosure; duty to warn; *family members; genetic counseling; genetic disorders; *genetic information; genetic predisposition; genetic research; *genetic screening; *guidelines; health care delivery; health insurance; informed consent; *international aspects; legislation; life insurance; medical records; models, theoretical; *moral obligations; patients; physicians; *privacy; property rights; *public policy; *regulation; *rights; state government; tissue banks; tissue donation; *Australia; Canada; Council of Europe; Great Britain; *United States

Skene, Loane; Charlesworth, Max. The new genetics: legal and ethical implications for medicine. [Editorial].

BE = bioethics accession number   fn. = footnotes   refs. = references

Medical Journal of Australia. 1996 Sep 16; 165(6): 301–302. 8 refs. BE62072.
confidentiality; disclosure; duty to warn; family members; *genetic information; *genetic screening; guidelines; informed consent; insurance; legal aspects; prenatal diagnosis; public policy; social discrimination; Australia

Smith, David H.; Quaid, Kimberly A.; Dworkin, Roger B., et al. Early Warning: Cases and Ethical Guidance for Presymptomatic Testing in Genetic Disease. Bloomington, IN: Indiana University Press; 1998. 188 p. (Medical ethics series). Bibliography: p. 171–182. ISBN 0-253-33401-2. BE59667.
adolescents; adoption; adults; anonymous testing; autonomy; beneficence; *case studies; casuistry; children; competence; confidentiality; dangerousness; deception; directive counseling; disclosure; dissent; duty to warn; employment; family members; family relationship; *genetic counseling; *genetic disorders; genetic information; genetic predisposition; genetic research; *genetic screening; *guidelines; health personnel; *Huntington disease; informed consent; insurance; laboratories; *late-onset disorders; *moral obligations; paternalism; patients; prenatal diagnosis; professional ethics; psychological stress; refusal to treat; risks and benefits; selective abortion; truth disclosure; ELSI-funded publication; incidental findings; right not to know

Smith, George P. Harnessing the human genome through legislative constraint. *European Journal of Health Law.* 1998 Mar; 5(1): 53–65. 65 fn. BE61256.
confidentiality; employment; federal government; genetic disorders; *genetic information; genetic predisposition; genetic research; *genetic screening; insurance; late-onset disorders; *legal aspects; legislation; privacy; social discrimination; state government; United States

Sommerville, Ann; English, Veronica. Genetic privacy: orthodoxy or oxymoron? *Journal of Medical Ethics.* 1999 Apr; 25(2): 144–150. 14 refs. BE61918.
*autonomy; *beneficence; *communitarianism; *confidentiality; decision making; directive counseling; *disclosure; *duty to warn; *family members; freedom; genetic counseling; genetic disorders; *genetic information; *genetic screening; informed consent; married persons; *moral obligations; *moral policy; paternalism; *patients; physician patient relationship; *physicians; *privacy; prognosis; reproduction; rights; risk; risks and benefits; teleological ethics; treatment refusal; truth disclosure; values; harms; *right not to know

In this paper we question whether the concept of "genetic privacy" is a contradiction in terms. And, if so, whether the implications of such a conclusion, inevitably impact on how society comes to perceive privacy and responsibility generally. Current law and ethical discourse place a high value on self-determination and the rights of individuals. In the medical sphere, the recognition of patient "rights" has resulted in health professionals being given clear duties of candour and frankness. Dilemmas arise, however, when patients decline to know relevant information or, knowing it, refuse to share it with others who may also need to know. This paper considers the notions of interconnectedness and responsibility to others which are brought to the fore in the genetic sphere and which challenge the primacy afforded to personal autonomy. It also explores the extent to which an individual's perceived moral obligations can or should be enforced.

Steinbock, Bonnie. Prenatal genetic testing for Alzheimer disease. *In:* Post, Stephen G.; Whitehouse, Peter J., eds. Genetic Testing for Alzheimer Disease: Ethical and Clinical Issues. Baltimore, MD: Johns Hopkins University Press; 1998: 140–151. 17 refs. ISBN

0-8018-5840-2. BE60721.
autonomy; *dementia; disabled; genetic counseling; genetic disorders; *genetic screening; late-onset disorders; moral policy; parents; physicians; pregnant women; *prenatal diagnosis; selective abortion; sex determination

Stepanuk, Natalie Anne. Genetic information and third party access to information: New Jersey's pioneering legislation as a model for federal privacy protection of genetic information. [Comment]. *Catholic University Law Review.* 1998 Spring; 47(3): 1105–1144. 239 fn. BE62036.
*confidentiality; *disclosure; duty to warn; employment; family members; federal government; genetic disorders; *genetic information; genetic predisposition; genetic research; *genetic screening; *government regulation; health insurance; *legal aspects; legislation; medical records; physician patient relationship; *privacy; *property rights; *social discrimination; state government; *Genetic Privacy Act 1996 (NJ); *New Jersey

Stoller, David. Prenatal genetic screening: the enigma of selective abortion. *Journal of Law and Health.* 1997–98; 12(1): 121–140. 111 fn. BE61137.
abortion, induced; congenital disorders; dehumanization; disabled; eugenics; federal government; fetuses; genetic counseling; genetic disorders; genetic enhancement; *genetic screening; genome mapping; government regulation; *legal aspects; *prenatal diagnosis; *selective abortion; sex determination; state government; state interest; stigmatization; Supreme Court decisions; viability; *United States

Tabarrok, Alexander. Genetic testing: an economic and contractarian analysis. *Journal of Health Economics.* 1994 Mar; 13(1): 75–91. 35 refs. 21 fn. BE59804.
confidentiality; decision making; disclosure; *economics; employment; genetic disorders; genetic predisposition; *genetic screening; government regulation; *health insurance; informed consent; *insurance selection bias; legal aspects; policy analysis; *risk; United States

Takala, Tuija. The right to genetic ignorance confirmed. *Bioethics.* 1999 Jul; 13(3–4): 288–293. 15 fn. BE61879.
*autonomy; children; decision making; family members; genetic disorders; *genetic information; *genetic screening; *moral obligations; moral policy; reproduction; *rights; suffering; *truth disclosure; harms; *right not to know

One of the much debated issues around the evolving human genetics is the question of the right to know versus the right not to know. The core question of this theme is whether an *individual* has the right to know about her own genetic constitution and further, does she also have the right to remain in ignorance. Within liberal traditions it is usually held that people, if they so wish, have the right to all the knowledge available about themselves. This right is based on the value of autonomy or on the right of self-determination, and it is sometimes partly justified as a countermeasure to the authorities' control over people. I do not wish to deny the right to genetic knowledge (about oneself). I think that its existence is self-evident. The argument I want to put forth in this paper is that in liberal societies we should acknowledge people's right to remain in ignorance as well. The only reason for not doing this would be that grave harm to others would follow if people were allowed to make these seemingly self-regarding decisions. Arguments presented against the right to ignorance are two-fold. First there are those arguing against the right to ignorance on the grounds of harm to others, that is, philosophers who do not deny people's right to ignorance in self-related matters but wish to state that genetic ignorance causes harm to others, and this is one of the most commonly accepted reasons for

BE = bioethics accession number   fn. = footnotes   refs. = references

restricting people's freedom. The other line of argument flows from the Kantian view that not even merely self-regarding foolishness (in the eyes of others) should be allowed.

Tapper, Melbourne. In the Blood: Sickle Cell Anemia and the Politics of Race. Philadelphia, PA: University of Pennsylvania Press; 1999. 163 p. (Critical histories). 316 fn. ISBN 0-8122-3471-5. BE60752.
> anthropology; *blacks; eugenics; federal government; *genetic screening; historical aspects; mandatory programs; mass screening; public policy; *sickle cell anemia; social discrimination; stigmatization; whites; Africa; Twentieth Century; *United States

Telling, Douglas Cushman. Science in Politics: Eugenics, Sterilization, and Genetic Screening. Ann Arbor, MI: UMI Dissertation Services; 1988. 264 p. Bibliography: p. 251-264. Dissertation, Ph.D. in Political Science, University of Massachusetts, 1988. Order No. 8906337. BE61053.
> bioethical issues; carriers; coercion; employment; *eugenics; fetuses; *genetic screening; government regulation; health hazards; historical aspects; industry; involuntary sterilization; legal aspects; legal liability; newborns; normality; *politics; prenatal diagnosis; *public policy; reproduction; reproductive technologies; science; selective abortion; *social control; social discrimination; socioeconomic factors; state government; *sterilization (sexual); trends; wrongful life; Galton, Francis; Muller, Hermann; Osborn, Frederick; Sanger, Margaret; Twentieth Century; *United States

ten Have, Henk. Living with the future: genetic information and human existence. *In:* Chadwick, Ruth; Levitt, Mairi; Shickle, Darren, eds. The Right to Know and the Right Not to Know. Brookfield, VT: Ashgate; 1997: 87-95. 13 refs. ISBN 1-85972-424-8. BE62192.
> autonomy; coercion; directive counseling; genetic counseling; *genetic information; genetic research; *genetic screening; goals; health promotion; incentives; *mass media; normality; prenatal diagnosis; selective abortion; self induced illness; right not to know

Thomas, Sandy; Caldicott, Fiona; Barchard, Chris, et al. Restrict genetic susceptibility tests. [Letter]. *Nature.* 1998 Sep 24; 395(6700): 317. 1 ref. BE60147.
> advisory committees; competence; disclosure; genetic information; *genetic predisposition; *genetic research; *genetic screening; informed consent; mental health; *mentally ill; *nontherapeutic research; public policy; regulation; risks and benefits; selection of subjects; stigmatization; *Nuffield Council on Bioethics

Thomson, B. Time for reassessment of use of all medical information by UK insurers. *Lancet.* 1998 Oct 10; 352(9135): 1216-1218. 15 refs. BE60795.
> confidentiality; genetic disorders; *genetic information; *genetic screening; health insurance; industry; *insurance; international aspects; legal rights; life insurance; medical records; public policy; rights; social discrimination; right not to know; Association of British Insurers; Europe; *Great Britain; United States

Trippitelli, Carol Lynn; Jamison, Kay R.; Folstein, Marshal F., et al. Pilot study on patients' and spouses' attitudes toward potential genetic testing for bipolar disorder. *American Journal of Psychiatry.* 1998 Jul; 155(7): 899-904. BE59826.
> adults; *attitudes; comparative studies; confidentiality; decision making; *depressive disorder; disclosure; *family members; genetic information; *genetic predisposition; *genetic screening; insurance; *married persons; *mentally ill; minors; motivation; *patients; *prenatal diagnosis; reproduction; risks and benefits; selective abortion; survey;

Johns Hopkins University; Maryland

Troy, Edwin S. Flores. The Genetic Privacy Act: an analysis of privacy and research concerns. *Journal of Law, Medicine and Ethics.* 1997 Winter; 25(4): 256-272. 150 fn. BE62671.
> *confidentiality; consent forms; *disclosure; DNA data banks; eugenics; federal government; genes; genetic disorders; *genetic information; genetic materials; genetic predisposition; genetic research; *genetic screening; *government regulation; guidelines; informed consent; insurance; law enforcement; *legal aspects; legal liability; *legislation; physicians; preventive medicine; *privacy; risks and benefits; social discrimination; state government; terminology; tissue banks; trends; *Genetic Privacy Act; *United States

U.S. Court of Appeals, Ninth Circuit. Norman-Bloodsaw v. Lawrence Berkeley Laboratory. *Federal Reporter, 3d Series.* 1998 Feb 3 (date of decision). 135: 1260-1276. BE62345.
> blacks; constitutional law; due process; *employment; federal government; females; *genetic screening; *legal rights; *mass screening; pregnant women; *privacy; research institutes; sickle cell anemia; social discrimination; state government; syphilis; California; Civil Rights Act 1964; Fifth Amendment; Fourteenth Amendment; Fourth Amendment; *Norman-Bloodsaw v. Lawrence Berkeley Laboratory; United States

The U.S. Court of Appeals for the Ninth Circuit overturned the lower court's dismissal and allowed clerical or administrative workers to sue their employer for testing for "highly private and sensitive medical genetic information such as syphilis, sickle cell trait, and pregnancy" without either their consent or their knowledge during a general employee health examination. The court noted that "the most basic violation possible" of constitutional privacy interests involves the performance of unauthorized testing for medical information and that such testing may be viewed as illegal search under the Fourth Amendment in addition to violation of due process under the Fifth or Fourteenth Amendments. Because there are "few subject areas more personal and more likely to implicate privacy interests than that of one's health or genetic make-up," the court concluded that the unauthorized testing constituted a significant invasion of the right to privacy under the Fourth Amendment. The court reasoned that neither consent to a general medical examination nor consent to providing blood or urine samples abolishes the privacy right not to be tested for intimate, personal matters involving one's health. Also, because black employees were singled out for sickle cell trait testing and female employees for pregnancy testing, the employer discriminated against them concerning terms or conditions of employment, thus violating Title VII of the Civil Rights Act. (KIE abstract)

U.S. Department of Health and Human Services. Secretary's Advisory Committee on Genetic Testing. A Public Consultation on Oversight of Genetic Tests, December 1, 1999 – January 31, 2000. Issued by the Committee, 6000 Executive Blvd., Suite 302, Bethesda, MD 20892, http://www4.od.nih.gov/oba/sacgt.htm; 1999 Dec. 39 p. BE62498.
> advisory committees; behavioral genetics; carriers; confidentiality; *evaluation; *federal government; genetic disorders; genetic predisposition; genetic research; *genetic screening; genetic services; *government regulation; human experimentation; information dissemination; informed consent; laboratories; mass screening; minority groups; newborns; organization and administration; prenatal diagnosis; private sector; professional organizations; *public

---

BE = bioethics accession number   fn. = footnotes   refs. = references

participation; public policy; *regulation; risk; *risks and benefits; social discrimination; *standards; state government; stigmatization; terminology; quality assurance; Centers for Disease Control and Prevention; *Department of Health and Human Services; Food and Drug Administration; Health Care Financing Administration; National Institutes of Health; NIH-DOE Working Group on Ethical, Legal, and Social Implications (ELSI); *Secretary's Advisory Committee on Genetic Testing (DHHS); Task Force on Genetic Testing; *United States

U.S. Department of Health and Human Services. Secretary's Advisory Committee on Genetic Testing. A Public Consultation on Oversight of Genetic Tests, December 1, 1999 – January 31, 2000: Summary. Issued by the Committee, 6000 Executive Blvd., Suite 302, Bethesda, MD 20892, http://www4.od.nih.gov/oba/sacgt.htm; 1999 Dec. 8 p. BE62497.
　　advisory committees; confidentiality; ethical review; *evaluation; *federal government; genetic counseling; genetic research; *genetic screening; genetic services; *government regulation; human experimentation; information dissemination; laboratories; *public participation; public policy; *regulation; *risks and benefits; standards; tissue banks; quality assurance; Department of Health and Human Services; *Secretary's Advisory Committee on Genetic Testing (DHHS); *United States

Ulrich, C.M.; Kristal, A.R.; Durfy, S.J., et al. Attitudes toward genetic testing for cancer risk among Washington State residents. [Abstract]. *American Journal of Human Genetics.* 1996 Oct; 59(4): A340. BE60096.
　　breast cancer; *cancer; confidentiality; disclosure; employment; females; genetic information; *genetic predisposition; *genetic screening; health insurance; males; physicians; privacy; psychological stress; *public opinion; survey; prostate cancer; *Washington

Uzych, Leo; Rischitelli, Gary. Genetic testing data. [Letter and response]. *Journal of Occupational and Environmental Medicine.* 1996 Jan; 38(1): 13–14. 9 refs. BE61442.
　　confidentiality; disclosure; *employment; *genetic screening; industry; occupational medicine; physicians; social discrimination; United States

Vineis, Paolo. Ethical issues in genetic screening for cancer. *Annals of Oncology.* 1997 Oct; 8(10): 945–949. 17 refs. BE60029.
　　autonomy; beneficence; breast cancer; *cancer; employment; family members; future generations; *genetic predisposition; *genetic screening; health hazards; informed consent; justice; minority groups; moral obligations; moral policy; occupational exposure; patients; preventive medicine; principle-based ethics; risk; *risks and benefits; social discrimination; uncertainty; right not to know

Walsh, Julia. Reproductive rights and the Human Genome Project. *Southern California Review of Law and Women's Studies.* 1994 Fall; 4(1): 145–181. 154 fn. BE62684.
　　autonomy; coercion; decision making; disclosure; eugenics; genetic information; *genetic screening; genome mapping; government financing; government regulation; health personnel; informed consent; legal rights; mandatory testing; mass screening; *pregnant women; *prenatal diagnosis; privacy; risks and benefits; selective abortion; social control; state government; voluntary programs; *women's rights; United States

Weiss, J.O.; Kozma, C.; Lapham, E.V. Whom would you trust with your genetic information? [Abstract]. *American Journal of Human Genetics.* 1997 Oct; 61(4): A24. BE59390.
　　*attitudes; clergy; *confidentiality; *disclosure; employment;

*family members; genetic disorders; *genetic information; genetic predisposition; genetic research; *genetic screening; insurance; *patients; survey; District of Columbia

Welch, H. Gilbert; Burke, Wylie. Uncertainties in genetic testing for chronic disease. *JAMA.* 1998 Nov 4; 280(17): 1525–1527. 27 refs. BE59630.
　　age factors; chronically ill; genetic counseling; *genetic predisposition; genetic research; *genetic screening; late-onset disorders; patient care; preventive medicine; research design; risk; time factors; *uncertainty

Welkenhuysen, Myriam; Evers-Kiebooms, Gerry; Decruyenaere, Marleen, et al. Adolescents' attitude towards carrier testing for cystic fibrosis and its relative stability over time. *European Journal of Human Genetics.* 1996; 4(1): 52–62. 28 refs. BE60534.
　　*adolescents; *attitudes; *carriers; *cystic fibrosis; disclosure; *genetic screening; *knowledge, attitudes, practice; mass screening; risks and benefits; self concept; survey; time factors; Belgium

Wertz, D.C. Is there a "women's ethic" in genetics? A survey of ASHG and NSGC. [Abstract]. *American Journal of Human Genetics.* 1996 Oct; 59(4): A340. BE60097.
　　adults; *attitudes; children; comparative studies; *directive counseling; *females; *genetic counseling; genetic disorders; *genetic screening; *health personnel; late-onset disorders; *males; *physicians; *prenatal diagnosis; selective abortion; sex determination; survey; United States

Wertz, Dorothy. Genetics and eugenics. [Letter]. *New Scientist.* 1999 Feb 13; 161(2173): 55–56. BE61796.
　　*attitudes; comparative studies; employment; eugenics; *genetic screening; *health personnel; international aspects; non-Western World; Western World; *China; Great Britain; United States

Wertz, Dorothy C. International perspectives. *In:* Clarke, Angus, ed. The Genetic Testing of Children. Washington, DC: BIOS Scientific Publishers; 1998: 271–287. 43 refs. ISBN 1-85996-146-0. BE62768.
　　adolescents; age factors; alcohol abuse; *attitudes; *autonomy; cancer; carriers; *children; dementia; genetic disorders; genetic information; genetic predisposition; *genetic screening; *genetics; *health personnel; Huntington disease; *international aspects; *knowledge, attitudes, practice; late-onset disorders; organizational policies; *parents; *patients; *physicians; preventive medicine; primary health care; professional organizations; psychological stress; *public opinion; risks and benefits; statistics; stigmatization; survey; truth disclosure; harms; hypercholesterolemia; refusal to participate; right not to know; Asia; Australia; Canada; Europe; *Great Britain; Latin America; Middle East; South Africa; *United States

Wertz, Dorothy C. International perspectives on ethics and human genetics. *Suffolk University Law Review.* 1993 Winter; 27(4): 1411–1456. 102 fn. BE60738.
　　abortion, induced; *attitudes; autonomy; children; confidentiality; consensus; developing countries; directive counseling; disclosure; employment; family members; *genetic counseling; genetic disorders; genetic information; *genetic screening; genetic services; health personnel; informed consent; *international aspects; intersexuality; legal aspects; non-Western World; parent child relationship; *prenatal diagnosis; privacy; psychological stress; reproductive technologies; sex determination; survey; values; Western World; women's rights; United States

Wertz, Dorothy C. The difficulties of recruiting minorities to studies of ethics and values in genetics. *Community Genetics.* 1998; 1(3): 175–179. 12 refs. BE62367.
　　adoption; *attitudes; autonomy; *blacks; comparative

BE = bioethics accession number   fn. = footnotes   refs. = references

studies; confidentiality; directive counseling; disclosure; *genetic counseling; genetic disorders; genetic information; genetic research; *genetic screening; genetic services; *health personnel; medical specialties; *minority groups; paternalism; *patients; physicians; prenatal diagnosis; *public opinion; reproductive technologies; selective abortion; sex determination; survey; values; *United States

Wiggins, S.; Green, T.; Adam, S., et al. A long term (ca 5 years) prospective assessment of psychological consequences of predictive testing for Huntington disease (HD). [For the Canadian Collaborative Study of Predictive Testing]. *American Journal of Human Genetics.* 1996 Oct; 59(4): A7. BE60093.
  *genetic screening; *Huntington disease; *patients; *psychological stress; *risks and benefits; survey; time factors; follow-up studies; Canada

Wilfond, Benjamin S.; Rothenberg, Karen H.; Thomson, Elizabeth J., et al.; U.S. National Institutes of Health. Cancer Genetics Studies Consortium. Cancer genetic susceptibility testing: ethical and policy implications for future research and clinical practice. *Journal of Law, Medicine and Ethics.* 1997 Winter; 25(4): 243-251. 38 fn. Commented on by E. Kodish, p. 252-255. BE62669.
  advisory committees; breast cancer; *cancer; children; confidentiality; costs and benefits; decision making; disclosure; empirical research; *evaluation; family relationship; females; *genetic counseling; genetic information; *genetic predisposition; *genetic screening; genetic services; health insurance reimbursement; informed consent; late-onset disorders; managed care programs; parents; preimplantation diagnosis; prenatal diagnosis; privacy; *public policy; risk; *risks and benefits; social impact; colon cancer; *Cancer Genetics Studies Consortium; National Institutes of Health; United States

Wilkie, Tom. Genetics and insurance in Britain: why more than just the Atlantic divides the English-speaking nations. *Nature Genetics.* 1998 Oct; 20(2): 119-121. 7 refs. BE61622.
  advisory committees; aged; *confidentiality; *disclosure; genetic disorders; *genetic information; *genetic screening; industry; insurance; international aspects; *life insurance; long-term care; national health insurance; *public policy; *Association of British Insurers; *Great Britain; *Human Genetics Advisory Commission (Great Britain); United States

Wingerson, Lois. Unnatural Selection: The Promise and Power of Human Gene Research. New York, NY: Bantam Books; 1998. 399 p. Includes references. ISBN 0-553-09709-1. BE59741.
  advisory committees; behavioral genetics; carriers; confidentiality; embryo research; eugenics; evolution; federal government; genes; genetic counseling; genetic disorders; genetic diversity; genetic predisposition; *genetic research; *genetic screening; *genetics; genome mapping; health insurance; informed consent; Jews; managed care programs; minority groups; preimplantation diagnosis; *prenatal diagnosis; property rights; public policy; risks and benefits; selective abortion; social discrimination; stigmatization; Human Embryo Research Panel; Human Genome Project; NCHGR Program on Ethical, Legal, and Social Implications (ELSI); United States

Zallen, Doris Teichler. Does It Run in the Family? A Consumer's Guide to DNA Testing for Genetic Disorders. New Brunswick, NJ: Rutgers University Press; 1997. 201 p. Bibliography: p. 185-187. Appendixes include a list of resources for consumers. ISBN 0-8135-2446-6. BE60754.
  cancer; carriers; children; decision making; dementia;

economics; employment; family members; gene therapy; genetic counseling; genetic disorders; genetic information; genetic predisposition; genetic research; *genetic screening; genetic services; genetics; information dissemination; insurance; late-onset disorders; prenatal diagnosis; risk; selective abortion; social discrimination; right not to know

Zimmern, R.L. Genetic testing: a conceptual exploration. *Journal of Medical Ethics.* 1999 Apr; 25(2): 151-156. 10 refs. BE61919.
  advisory committees; confidentiality; diagnosis; DNA data banks; genetic counseling; genetic disorders; *genetic information; genetic predisposition; *genetic screening; government regulation; guidelines; methods; moral policy; public policy; *regulation; risk; social discrimination; *terminology; tissue banks; Advisory Committee on Genetic Testing (Great Britain); Great Britain; Task Force on Genetic Testing; United States
This paper attempts to explore a number of conceptual issues surrounding genetic testing. It looks at the meaning of the terms, genetic information and genetic testing in relation to the definition set out by the Advisory Committee on Genetic Testing in the UK, and by the Task Force on Genetic Testing in the USA. It argues that the special arrangements that may be required for the regulation of genetic tests should not be determined by reference to the nature or technology of the test, but by considering those morally relevant features that justify regulation. Failure to do so will lead to the regulation of genetic tests that need not be regulated, and would fail to cover other tests which should be regulated. The paper also argues that there is little in the nature of the properties of gene tests, using DNA or chromosomes, that in itself justifies a special approach.

Zweig, Franklin M.; Walsh, Joseph T.; Freeman, Daniel M. Adjudicating neurogenetics at the crossroads: privacy, adoption, and the death sentence. *Judges' Journal.* 1997 Summer; 36(3): 52-55, 57-58, 90-93. 14 fn. BE59806.
  *adoption; *behavior disorders; *behavioral genetics; capital punishment; case studies; *confidentiality; *criminal law; federal government; *genetic information; *genetic predisposition; *genetic screening; government regulation; killing; *law enforcement; legislation; mandatory testing; parents; prisoners; *privacy; public policy; records; social discrimination; state government; *violence; Colorado; Connecticut; *United States

Appendix 2: EUROSCREEN survey of attitudes to the genetic testing of children among members of the European Society of Human Genetics.*In:* Clarke, Angus, ed. The Genetic Testing of Children. Washington, DC: BIOS Scientific Publishers; 1998: 321-328. ISBN 1-85996-146-0. BE62769.
  age factors; *attitudes; breast cancer; carriers; *children; comparative studies; consensus; cystic fibrosis; fathers; females; *genetic screening; *genetics; health facilities; *health personnel; Huntington disease; institutional policies; international aspects; males; mass screening; newborns; prenatal diagnosis; survey; fragile X syndrome; questionnaires; right not to know; *Europe; European Society of Human Genetics; European Union; *Euroscreen Project

Banking Our Genes: DNA Data on the Information Highway. [Videorecording].Boston, MA: Fanlight Productions; 1995. 1 videocassette; 33 min.; sd.; color; VHS. Producers: Dan Small and Jean E. McEwen. Produced under a grant from the Human Genome Project, U.S. Department of Energy, Ethical, Legal and Social Implications Program, Copyright by the Eunice Kennedy Shriver Center, Waltham, MA. ISBN 1-57295-155-9. Order No. CS-155. BE62711.

BE = bioethics accession number   fn. = footnotes   refs. = references

computer communication networks; confidentiality; disclosure; *DNA data banks; *DNA fingerprinting; *forensic medicine; genetic disorders; *genetic information; genetic materials; genetic predisposition; *genetic screening; insurance; military personnel; *privacy; social discrimination; state government; *tissue banks; ELSI-funded publication; United States

Blood tests of workers restricted by court. [News]. *New York Times.* 1998 Feb 5: A19. BE59563.
  *employment; federal government; *genetic screening; *legal rights; *mass screening; *privacy; syphilis; California; *Lawrence Berkeley National Laboratory; United States

Can ELSI's principles inform consensus? [Editorial]. *Nature Biotechnology.* 1996 Jun; 14(6): 677. BE61398.
  advisory committees; federal government; genetic information; *genetic research; *genetic screening; genome mapping; informed consent; privacy; *public policy; tissue banks; tissue donation; bundled consent; *NIH–DOE Working Group on Ethical, Legal, and Social Implications (ELSI); *Task Force on Genetic Testing; *United States

Employment entrance exam; genetic/medical tests; applicants' consent; statute of limitations: Norman–Bloodsaw v. Lawrence Berkeley Lab. *Mental and Physical Disability Law Reporter.* 1998 Mar–Apr; 22(2): 233. BE61465.
  *employment; *genetic screening; informed consent; *legal aspects; legislation; mass screening; *Americans with Disabilities Act 1990; California; *Norman–Bloodsaw v. Lawrence Berkeley Laboratory; *United States

Legislative insurance against genetic discrimination is insurance for biotechnology. [Editorial]. *Nature Biotechnology.* 1996 May; 14(5): 547. BE61966.
  employment; federal government; genetic information; *genetic predisposition; *genetic screening; health insurance; *industry; *legislation; managed care programs; rights; *social discrimination; state government; uncertainty; *diagnostic kits; United States

What price perfection? [Editorial]. *New Scientist.* 1997 Feb 22; 153(2070): 3. BE59711.
  *eugenics; genetic predisposition; genetic research; *genetic screening; homosexuals; *prenatal diagnosis; selective abortion

GENETIC SERVICES

See also GENE THERAPY, GENETIC COUNSELING, GENETIC SCREENING

Barber, John C.K. "Code of practice and guidance on human genetic testing services supplied direct to the public": Advisory Committee on Genetic Testing. *Journal of Medical Genetics.* 1998 Jun; 35(6): 443–445. 8 refs. BE61252.
  advisory committees; confidentiality; disclosure; genetic counseling; *genetic screening; *genetic services; guidelines; informed consent; *laboratories; physicians; records; *standards; *Advisory Committee on Genetic Testing (Great Britain); *Great Britain

Baumiller, Robert C.; Comley, Sarah; Cunningham, George, et al.; Council of Regional Networks [for Genetic Services] Committee on Ethics. Code of ethical principles for genetics professionals. *American Journal of Medical Genetics.* 1996 Oct 28; 65(3): 177–178. Accepted by the Council of Regional Networks Steering Committee 14 Apr 1994. BE59526.
  *codes of ethics; genetic counseling; genetic research; genetic screening; *genetic services; *health personnel;

interprofessional relations; obligations to society; *professional ethics; professional organizations; professional patient relationship; *Council of Regional Networks for Genetic Services; United States

Baumiller, Robert C.; Cunningham, George; Fisher, Nancy, et al.; Council of Regional Networks [for Genetic Services] Committee on Ethics. Code of ethical principles for genetics professionals: an explication. *American Journal of Medical Genetics.* 1996 Oct 28; 65(3): 179–183. 4 refs. Approved by the Council of Regional Networks Executive Committee 9 Oct 1995. BE59527.
  autonomy; *codes of ethics; communication; confidentiality; directive counseling; genetic counseling; genetic research; genetic screening; *genetic services; *health personnel; information dissemination; interprofessional relations; laboratories; obligations to society; professional competence; *professional ethics; professional organizations; professional patient relationship; standards; tissue banks; *Council of Regional Networks for Genetic Services; United States

Beech, Beverley A. Lawrence; Anderson, Gwen. 'We went through psychological hell': a case report of prenatal diagnosis. [Case study and commentaries]. *Nursing Ethics.* 1999 May; 6(3): 250–256. 12 refs. BE61769.
  age factors; amniocentesis; case studies; communication; congenital disorders; disclosure; Down syndrome; *genetic services; informed consent; interdisciplinary communication; interprofessional relations; *medical errors; patient advocacy; patient care team; *pregnant women; *prenatal diagnosis; professional patient relationship; *psychological stress; *quality of health care; risks and benefits; selective abortion; continuity of patient care; Australia

British Medical Association. Human Genetics: Choice and Responsibility. New York, NY: Oxford University Press; 1998. 236 p. 227 fn. Appendixes provide names and addresses of regional genetics centers in the United Kingdom and of concerned organizations in the UK and elsewhere. ISBN 0-19-288055-1. BE61351.
  adolescents; adults; advisory committees; carriers; children; cloning; competence; confidentiality; decision making; disabled; disclosure; employment; eugenics; family members; gene therapy; *genetic counseling; genetic disorders; genetic information; genetic predisposition; genetic research; *genetic screening; *genetic services; *genetics; government financing; guidelines; health personnel; informed consent; insurance; late-onset disorders; mass screening; moral obligations; *organizational policies; parents; patients; physicians; prenatal diagnosis; primary health care; professional ethics; professional organizations; registries; regulation; risks and benefits; terminology; incidental findings; paternity; *British Medical Association; Great Britain; National Health Service

Chadwick, Ruth. Dimensions of quality in genetic services -- an ethical comment. *European Journal of Human Genetics.* 1997; 5(Suppl. 2): 22–24. 7 refs. BE62208.
  autonomy; costs and benefits; *evaluation; *genetic counseling; genetic disorders; genetic information; genetic screening; *genetic services; goals; international aspects; justice; patient satisfaction; prenatal diagnosis; public health; quality of health care; resource allocation; social discrimination; stigmatization; right not to know; Europe

Dalby, Shirley. Commercial testing. *In:* Clarke, Angus, ed. The Genetic Testing of Children. Washington, DC: BIOS Scientific Publishers; 1998: 265–270. ISBN 1-85996-146-0. BE62767.
  advertising; *attitudes; children; genetic counseling; genetic information; *genetic screening; *genetic services; health insurance reimbursement; *industry; information dissemination; physicians; *private sector; psychological

stress; public opinion; public sector; regulation; survey; private practice; Genetic Interest Group (Great Britain); Great Britain; National Health Service

Fitzpatrick, J.; Hahn, C.; Costa, T., et al. The duty to recontact: attitudes of genetics service providers. [Abstract]. *American Journal of Human Genetics.* 1997 Oct; 61(4): A57. BE59392.
*attitudes; *genetic counseling; genetic research; *genetic services; *health personnel; legal obligations; moral obligations; physicians; standards; survey; *recontact; Canada; United States

Fleck, Leonard. Justice, rights, and Alzheimer disease genetics. *In:* Post, Stephen G.; Whitehouse, Peter J., eds. Genetic Testing for Alzheimer Disease: Ethical and Clinical Issues. Baltimore, MD: Johns Hopkins University Press; 1998: 190–208. 15 refs. ISBN 0-8018-5840-2. BE60724.
age factors; artificial organs; beneficence; *biomedical technologies; breast cancer; costs and benefits; cystic fibrosis; decision making; *dementia; fetal therapy; gene therapy; genetic counseling; genetic disorders; genetic predisposition; *genetic screening; *genetic services; germ cells; *government financing; health care; hearts; *justice; late-onset disorders; *moral obligations; *moral policy; *obligations of society; organ transplantation; preimplantation diagnosis; prenatal diagnosis; public participation; *resource allocation; rights; risks and benefits; selection for treatment; standards; therapeutic research

Goerl, Hans S. Who's that fish on my line? The dangers of electronic distribution of genetic information. *In:* Smith, Edward; Sapp, Walter, eds. Plain Talk about the Human Genome Project: A Tuskegee University Conference on Its Promise and Perils ... and Matters of Race. Tuskegee, AL: Tuskegee University Press; 1997: 201–203. ISBN 1-891196-01-4. BE61748.
*computer communication networks; confidentiality; genetic counseling; *genetic information; genetic research; genetic screening; *genetic services; *information dissemination; *patient education; peer review; Internet

Great Britain. Health Departments of the United Kingdom. Advisory Committee on Genetic Testing. Code of practice on human genetic testing services supplied direct to the public. *Community Genetics.* 1998; 1(1): 48. 2 fn. BE61491.
carriers; confidentiality; disclosure; genetic counseling; *genetic screening; *genetic services; *government regulation; *guidelines; home care; *laboratories; physicians; public policy; *standards; *diagnostic kits; Advisory Committee on Genetic Testing (Great Britain); *Great Britain

Grody, Wayne W.; Pyeritz, Reed E. Report card on molecular genetic testing: room for improvement? [Editorial]. *JAMA.* 1999 Mar 3; 281(9): 845–847. 19 refs. BE60241.
administrators; confidentiality; duty to warn; *evaluation; family members; genetic counseling; *genetic screening; *genetic services; guideline adherence; health personnel; informed consent; institutional policies; *laboratories; professional competence; professional organizations; regulation; self regulation; *standards; *quality assurance; American College of Medical Genetics Laboratory Practice Committee Standards and Guidelines; College of American Pathologists; *United States

Holtzman, Neil A. The UK's policy on genetic testing services supplied direct to the public -- two spheres and two tiers. *Community Genetics.* 1998; 1(1): 49–52. 20 refs. BE61492.
advisory committees; *carriers; genetic counseling; genetic

disorders; *genetic screening; *genetic services; government financing; *government regulation; *guidelines; home care; indigents; industry; justice; *laboratories; mass screening; private sector; *public policy; public sector; social discrimination; *socioeconomic factors; standards; *diagnostic kits; personal financing; Advisory Committee on Genetic Testing (Great Britain); *Great Britain; National Health Service

Human Genome Education [HuGEM] Project. The HuGEM Project: I. An Overview of the Human Genome Project and Its Ethical, Legal and Social Issues (19 min.); II. Opportunities and Challenges of the Human Genome Project (24 min.); III. Issues of Genetic Privacy and Discrimination (45 min.); IV. Genetic Testing Across the Lifespan (30 min.); V. Working Together to Improve Genetic Services (28 min.). Available from the Georgetown University Child Development Center, 3307 M St., NW, Suite 401, Washington, DC 20007; (202) 687–8803; 1996. 5 videocassettes; 146 min. total (19–45 min. each); sd., color; VHS. Videocassettes accompanied by a 68-page manual authored by E.V. Lapham et al. The HuGEM Project is a collaboration between the Georgetown University Child Development Center, a division of the Dept. of Pediatrics, Georgetown University Medical Center, and the Alliance of Genetic Support Groups. BE62800.
children; confidentiality; disclosure; employment; family members; gene therapy; genetic counseling; *genetic disorders; genetic information; genetic predisposition; *genetic screening; *genetic services; *genome mapping; guidelines; health insurance; health personnel; newborns; patients; prenatal diagnosis; privacy; risks and benefits; social discrimination; technical expertise; ELSI–funded publication; Human Genome Project; United States

Lin-Fu, Jane S. Advances in genetics: issues for US racial and ethnic minorities: an Asian American and Pacific Islander perspective. *Community Genetics.* 1998; 1(3): 124–129. 27 refs. BE62283.
aliens; *Asian Americans; cultural pluralism; genetic disorders; *genetic research; *genetic services; *minority groups; population genetics; public policy; resource allocation; *social discrimination; socioeconomic factors; stigmatization; emigration and immigration; *United States

McGovern, Margaret M.; Benach, Marta O.; Wallenstein, Sylvan, et al. Quality assurance in molecular genetic testing laboratories. *JAMA.* 1999 Mar 3; 281(9): 835–840. 18 refs. BE60240.
administrators; confidentiality; *evaluation; evaluation studies; genetic counseling; *genetic screening; *genetic services; guideline adherence; health personnel; informed consent; institutional policies; *laboratories; professional competence; regulation; *standards; statistics; survey; *quality assurance; American College of Medical Genetics Laboratory Practice Committee Standards and Guidelines; *United States

CONTEXT: Specific regulation of laboratories performing molecular genetic tests may be needed to ensure standards and quality assurance (QA) and safeguard patient rights to informed consent and confidentiality. However, comprehensive analysis of current practices of such laboratories, important for assessing the need for regulation and its impact on access to testing, has not been conducted. OBJECTIVE: To collect and analyze data regarding availability of clinical molecular genetic testing, including personnel standards and laboratory practices. DESIGN: A mail survey in June 1997 of molecular genetic testing laboratory directors and assignment of a QA score based on responses to genetic testing process items. SETTING: Hospital-based, independent, and research-based

---

BE = bioethics accession number   fn. = footnotes   refs. = references

molecular genetic testing laboratories in the United States. PARTICIPANTS: Directors of molecular genetic testing laboratories (n = 245; response rate, 74.9%). MAIN OUTCOME MEASURE: Laboratory process QA score, using the American College of Medical Genetics Laboratory Practice Committee standards. RESULTS: The 245 responding laboratories reported availability of testing for 94 disorders. Personnel qualifications varied, although all directors had doctoral degrees. The mean QAscore was 90% (range, 44%-100%) with 36 laboratories (15%) scoring lower than 70%. Higher scores were associated with test menu size of more than 4 tests (P = .01), performance of more than 30 analyses annually (P = .01), director having a PhD vs MD degree (P = .002), director board certification (P = .03), independent (P less than .001) and hospital (P = .01) laboratories vs research laboratory, participation in proficiency testing (P less than .001), and Clinical Laboratory Improvement Amendment certification (P = .006). Seventy percent of laboratories provided access to genetic counseling, 69% had a confidentiality policy, and 45% required informed consent prior to testing. CONCLUSION: The finding that a number of laboratories had QA scores that may reflect suboptimal laboratory practices suggests that both personnel qualification and laboratory practice standards are most in need of improvement to ensure quality in clinical molecular genetic testing laboratories.

McNally, Ruth. Eugenics here and now. *In:* Glasner, Peter; Rothman, Harry, eds. Genetic Imaginations: Ethical, Legal and Social Issues in Human Genome Research. Brookfield, VT: Ashgate; 1998: 69-82. 23 refs. Based on a paper presented at a workshop hosted by the Centre for Social and Economic Research at the University of the West of England; reprinted from *The Genetic Engineer and Biotechnologist*, 1995; 15(2-3). ISBN 1-84014-356-8. BE60019.
    attitudes; congenital disorders; disabled; *eugenics; genetic counseling; *genetic disorders; genetic enhancement; genetic predisposition; genetic screening; *genetic services; genome mapping; international aspects; prenatal diagnosis; public policy; risk; *selective abortion; social impact; wrongful life; *Great Britain; National Health Service

Mecsas-Faxon, S.; Tishler, S.; Pauker, S.P. Cancer genetics program within an HMO: a model of confidential service. [Abstract]. *American Journal of Human Genetics*. 1997 Oct; 61(4): A224. BE59398.
    *cancer; confidentiality; genetic counseling; genetic predisposition; genetic research; *genetic screening; *genetic services; health insurance reimbursement; *health maintenance organizations; medical records; program descriptions; *Harvard Pilgrim Health Care; Massachusetts

Mittman, Ilana Suez; Secundy, Marion Gray. A national dialogue on genetics and minority issues. *Community Genetics*. 1998; 1(3): 190-200. 6 refs. BE62369.
    attitudes; biomedical research; education; financial support; genetic counseling; *genetic research; genetic screening; *genetic services; genome mapping; guidelines; health; health personnel; human experimentation; informed consent; investigators; *minority groups; public participation; public policy; risk; science; selection of subjects; social discrimination; socioeconomic factors; stigmatization; trust; needs; United States

Wertz, Dorothy C.; Fletcher, John C.; Berg, Kåre, et al.; World Health Organization. Hereditary Diseases Programme. Guidelines on Ethical Issues in Medical Genetics and the Provision of Genetics Services.

Geneva: World Health Organization; 1995. 119 p. Bibliography: p. 83-91; international bibliography: annex p. 1-13. BE62200.
    adults; anonymous testing; behavioral genetics; competence; confidentiality; conflict of interest; cultural pluralism; directive counseling; disclosure; DNA data banks; education; embryo research; epidemiology; family members; financial support; gene therapy; *genetic counseling; genetic disorders; genetic enhancement; genetic predisposition; genetic research; genetic screening; *genetic services; *guidelines; health personnel; informed consent; investigators; mass media; mass screening; minors; newborns; prenatal diagnosis; professional ethics; professional patient relationship; reproduction; resource allocation; selective abortion; recontact

Wertz, Dorothy C. Guidelines point the way on genetics ethics. [Letter]. *Nature*. 1999 May 27; 399(6734): 297. BE62567.
    cloning; *genetic services; *guidelines; *international aspects; *International Guidelines on Ethical Issues in Medical Genetics and Genetic Services; *World Health Organization

World Health Organization. Human Genetics Programme. Proposed International Guidelines on Ethical Issues in Medical Genetics and Genetic Services: Report of a WHO Meeting on Ethical Issues in Medical Genetics, Geneva, 15-16 December 1997. Geneva: World Health Organization; 1998. 15 p. 5 refs. WHO/HGN/GL/ETH/98.1. BE62196.
    autonomy; beneficence; confidentiality; disclosure; *DNA data banks; *genetic counseling; genetic information; genetic predisposition; *genetic screening; *genetic services; *genetics; *guidelines; informed consent; international aspects; justice; late-onset disorders; *prenatal diagnosis; professional ethics; resource allocation; tissue banks; voluntary programs; World Health Organization

GENOME MAPPING

See also GENETIC INTERVENTION, GENETIC RESEARCH, GENETIC SCREENING

Barns, Ian. The Human Genome Project and the self. *Soundings*. 1994 Spring-Summer; 77(1-2): 99-128. 62 fn. BE61591.
    capitalism; commodification; dehumanization; genetic research; genetic screening; *genome mapping; *humanism; investigators; literature; mass media; metaphor; morality; motivation; philosophy; recombinant DNA research; risks and benefits; science; self concept; theology; virtues; motion pictures; Blade Runner; Life Story (BBC motion picture); Mapping Our Genes (Wingerson, L.); New Scientist

Belkin, Lisa. Splice Einstein and Sammy Glick, add a little Magellan: banking on genes. *New York Times Magazine*. 1998 Aug 23: 26-31, 56, 58, 60-61. BE60647.
    economics; *entrepreneurship; *financial support; *genome mapping; industry; investigators; private sector; public sector; United States; *Venter, Craig

Berry, Roberta M. The Human Genome Project and the end of insurance. *University of Florida Journal of Law and Public Policy*. 1996 Spring; 7(2): 205-256. 177 fn. BE59315.
    confidentiality; economics; *genetic information; *genetic screening; *genome mapping; government regulation; historical aspects; industry; *insurance; insurance selection bias; justice; national health insurance; policy analysis; privacy; *public policy; risk; social discrimination; *social impact; *Human Genome Project; United States

BE = bioethics accession number   fn. = footnotes   refs. = references

Bosch, Xavier. Geneticists discuss ethics of human genome project. [News]. *Lancet.* 1998 Oct 31; 352(9138): 1448. Summary of the Fourth International Meeting on the Human Genome Project, held in Valencia, Spain, 19–21 Oct 1998. BE59436.
> cloning; genes; genetic information; *genome mapping; *international aspects; patents; reproductive technologies; social discrimination; *Human Genome Project

Boshammer, Susanne; Kayss, Matthias; Runtenberg, Christa, et al. Discussing HUGO: the German debate on the ethical implications of the Human Genome Project. *Journal of Medicine and Philosophy.* 1998 Jun; 23(3): 324–333. 38 refs. BE59296.
> *attitudes; autonomy; bioethics; costs and benefits; ethicists; eugenics; genetic identity; genetic intervention; genetic research; *genome mapping; informal social control; morality; resource allocation; risks and benefits; social impact; technical expertise; wedge argument; dignity; *Germany; *Human Genome Project

The current German criticism of HUGO centers around the term 'human dignity'; consenquentialist and autonomy-based arguments are used. The debate culminates in questioning the integrity of bioethics as a scholarly discipline and has created a heterogeneous coalition of disparate political and social groups that oppose any research that would facilitate genetic pre-selection of human characteristics.

Botstein, David. Of genes and genomes. *In:* Smith, Edward; Sapp, Walter, eds. Plain Talk about the Human Genome Project: A Tuskegee University Conference on Its Promise and Perils ... and Matters of Race. Tuskegee, AL: Tuskegee University Press; 1997: 207–214. ISBN 1-891196-01-4. BE61749.
> cancer; gene therapy; genetic enhancement; genetic predisposition; *genome mapping; goals; methods; risks and benefits; Human Genome Project

Burris, John; Cook-Deegan, Robert; Alberts, Bruce. The Human Genome Project after a decade: policy issues. *Nature Genetics.* 1998 Dec; 20(4): 333–335. 6 refs. BE61623.
> advisory committees; attitudes; economics; ethical review; evaluation; federal government; financial support; *genome mapping; government financing; industry; information dissemination; international aspects; investigators; patents; public policy; risks and benefits; Department of Energy; *Human Genome Project; National Institutes of Health; *National Research Council; NIH-DOE Working Group on Ethical, Legal, and Social Implications (ELSI); *Office of Technology Assessment; United States

Butler, Declan. Human genome declaration looks set for United Nations approval. [News]. *Nature.* 1998 Nov 26; 396(6709): 297. BE59535.
> cloning; gene therapy; *genetic intervention; *genome mapping; germ cells; *human rights; *international aspects; Unesco; *United Nations; *Universal Declaration on the Human Genome and Human Rights

Cantor, Charles R. How will the Human Genome Project improve our quality of life? *Nature Biotechnology.* 1998 Mar; 16(3): 212–213. BE62024.
> cloning; confidentiality; gene therapy; genetic disorders; genetic diversity; genetic information; genetic predisposition; genetic screening; *genome mapping; germ cells; human experimentation; patient care; *risks and benefits; *social impact

Caplan, Arthur L. What's so special about the human genome? *Cambridge Quarterly of Healthcare Ethics.* 1998 Fall; 7(4): 422–424. 14 fn. Commentary on G. McGee,

p. 417–421. BE59143.
> commodification; common good; DNA sequences; economics; *genes; genetic information; *genome mapping; human body; morality; *patents; property rights; public policy; risks and benefits; *value of life; technology transfer; United States

Coghlan, Andy. The price of profit. [News]. *New Scientist.* 1998 May 16; 158(2134): 20–21. BE59605.
> *DNA sequences; federal government; *genetic research; *genome mapping; government financing; *industry; information dissemination; investigational drugs; organizational policies; *patents; *property rights; research institutes; risks and benefits; social impact; National Institutes of Health; United States

Collins, Francis S.; Patrinos, Ari; Jordan, Elke, et al. New goals for the U.S. Human Genome Project: 1998–2003. *Science.* 1998 Oct 23; 282(5389): 682–689. 7 fn. Written with the members of the DOE and NIH planning groups. BE59525.
> DNA data banks; DNA sequences; education; federal government; financial support; genetic research; *genome mapping; *goals; government financing; information dissemination; international aspects; investigators; methods; peer review; private sector; *public policy; social impact; Department of Energy; *Human Genome Project; National Institutes of Health; NIH-DOE Working Group on Ethical, Legal, and Social Implications (ELSI); United States

The Human Genome Project has successfully completed all the major goals in its current 5-year plan, covering the period 1993–98. A new plan, for 1998–2003, is presented, in which human DNA sequencing will be the major emphasis. An ambitious schedule has been set to complete the full sequence by the end of 2003, 2 years ahead of previous projections. In the course of completing the sequence, a "working draft" of the human sequence will be produced by the end of 2001. The plan also includes goals for sequencing technology development; for studying human genome sequence variation; for developing technology for functional genomics; for completing the sequence of Caenorhabditis elegans and Drosophila melanogaster and starting the mouse genome; for studying the ethical, legal, and social implications of genome research; for bioinformatics and computational studies; and for training of genome scientists.

Collins, Francis S. Shattuck Lecture -- medical and societal consequences of the Human Genome Project. *New England Journal of Medicine.* 1999 Jul 1; 341(1): 28–37. 45 refs. Presented as the 109th Shattuck Lecture to the Annual Meeting of the Massachusetts Medical Society, Boston, May 8, 1999. BE62433.
> confidentiality; DNA data banks; federal government; genetic information; genetic predisposition; genetic research; genetic screening; *genome mapping; goals; government financing; government regulation; historical aspects; information dissemination; medicine; preventive medicine; public policy; review; social discrimination; *social impact; genetic medicine; *Human Genome Project; United States

Creskoff, Katharine. Scientific imperialism or service to humanity? The complexities of the Human Genome Diversity Project. *Princeton Journal of Bioethics.* 1998 Spring; 1(1): 6–22. 25 refs. BE62487.
> anthropology; blood specimen collection; cultural pluralism; developing countries; disadvantaged; DNA data banks; *genetic diversity; genetic information; genetic predisposition; *genetic research; *genome mapping; goals; informed consent; international aspects; *minority groups; patents; *population genetics; property rights; *risks and benefits; social discrimination; tissue banks; community consent; *Human Genome Diversity Project

---

BE = bioethics accession number   fn. = footnotes   refs. = references

Cutter, Mary Ann G.; Drexler, Edward; McCullough, Laurence B., et al. Mapping and Sequencing the Human Genome: Science, Ethics, and Public Policy. Colorado Springs, CO: BSCS, the Colorado College; Chicago, IL: American Medical Association; 1992. 94 p. 39 refs. A free monograph for the high school biology classroom. BE60011.

> alcohol abuse; carriers; case studies; *curriculum; cystic fibrosis; DNA sequences; education; employment; ethical analysis; genetic counseling; genetic disorders; genetic predisposition; genetic screening; *genome mapping; Huntington disease; mass screening; methods; public policy; social discrimination; *social impact; *teaching methods; secondary schools; Human Genome Project; United States

Dickson, David. Back on track: the rebirth of human genetics in China. [News]. *Nature.* 1998 Nov 26; 396(6709): 303–306. Includes inset articles, "Mining a rich seam of genetic diversity," p. 304 and "A crash course in ethical behaviour," p. 306. BE59437.

> communism; eugenics; *genetic diversity; genetic information; genetic intervention; *genetic research; genetics; *genome mapping; government regulation; historical aspects; industry; international aspects; investigators; minority groups; patents; political systems; *population genetics; private sector; public policy; *China

Dodson, Michael; Williamson, Robert. Indigenous peoples and the morality of the Human Genome Diversity Project. *Journal of Medical Ethics.* 1999 Apr; 25(2): 204–208. 8 refs. BE61927.

> blood specimen collection; cultural pluralism; deception; decision making; disadvantaged; DNA data banks; drug industry; financial support; *genetic diversity; *genetic materials; genetic predisposition; *genetic research; *genome mapping; government financing; informed consent; international aspects; investigator subject relationship; investigators; *justice; *minority groups; moral obligations; *moral policy; *population genetics; property rights; risks and benefits; social discrimination; tissue banks; tissue donation; values; *aborigines; *community consent; research ethics; Australia; *Human Genome Diversity Project

In addition to the aim of mapping and sequencing one human's genome, the Human Genome Project also intends to characterise the genetic diversity of the world's peoples. The Human Genome Diversity Project raises political, economic and ethical issues. These intersect clearly when the genomes under study are those of indigenous peoples who are already subject to serious economic, legal and/or social disadvantage and discrimination. The fact that some individuals associated with the project have made dismissive comments about indigenous peoples has confused rather than illuminated the deeper issues involved, as well as causing much antagonism among indigenous peoples. There are more serious ethical issues raised by the project for all geneticists, including those who are sympathetic to the problems of indigenous peoples. With particular attention to the history and attitudes of Australian indigenous peoples, we argue that the Human Genome Diversity Project can only proceed if those who further its objectives simultaneously: respect the cultural beliefs of indigenous peoples; publicly support the efforts of indigenous peoples to achieve respect and equality; express respect by a rigorous understanding of the meaning of equitable negotiation of consent, and ensure that both immediate and long term economic benefits from the research flow back to the groups taking part.

Fitzgerald, Jennifer. Geneticizing disability: the Human Genome Project and the commodification of self. *Issues in Law and Medicine.* 1998 Fall; 14(2): 147–163. 61 fn. BE62010.

> attitudes; *commodification; decision making; directive counseling; *disabled; economics; genetic counseling; genetic determinism; genetic disorders; *genetic identity; genetic information; *genome mapping; normality; obligations of society; parent child relationship; parents; prenatal diagnosis; science; selective abortion; self concept; *social impact; *stigmatization; *values

Fleissner, Erwin. Race and the human genome. [Book review essay]. *Hastings Center Report.* 1999 Jul–Aug; 29(4): 40–42. BE62485.

> *genetic diversity; genetic information; genetic predisposition; *genome mapping; health care; health insurance; minority groups; population genetics; risks and benefits; social discrimination; *Human Genome Project; *Plain Talk about the Human Genome Project (Smith, E.; Sapp, W., eds.); United States

Glasner, Peter; Rothman, Harry, eds. Genetic Imaginations: Ethical, Legal and Social Issues in Human Genome Research. Brookfield, VT: Ashgate; 1998. 140 p. (Avebury series in philosophy). Includes references. Papers based on a workshop hosted by the Centre for Social and Economic Research at the University of the West of England; reprinted from *The Genetic Engineer and Biotechnologist*, 1995; 15(2–3): 83–187. ISBN 1-84014-356-8. BE60018.

> congenital disorders; eugenics; evaluation; financial support; gene therapy; genetic screening; *genome mapping; industry; international aspects; methods; organization and administration; public participation; *public policy; selective abortion; *social impact; wrongful life; France; *Great Britain; *Human Genome Project; Medical Research Council (Great Britain); United States

Grisolía, Santiago. Ethical and social aspects of the Human Genome Project. [Meeting report]. *Impact of Science on Society.* 1991; 41[1(161)]: 37–43. Brief report on the First (1988) and Second (1990) Workshops on International Cooperation for the Human Genome Project held in Valencia, Spain. BE59801.

> eugenics; gene therapy; *genome mapping; *international aspects; risks and benefits; *Declaration of Valencia; *Human Genome Project; Spain; Unesco

Human Genome Education [HuGEM] Project. The HuGEM Project: I. An Overview of the Human Genome Project and Its Ethical, Legal and Social Issues (19 min.); II. Opportunities and Challenges of the Human Genome Project (24 min.); III. Issues of Genetic Privacy and Discrimination (45 min.); IV. Genetic Testing Across the Lifespan (30 min.); V. Working Together to Improve Genetic Services (28 min.). Available from the Georgetown University Child Development Center, 3307 M St., NW, Suite 401, Washington, DC 20007; (202) 687-8803; 1996. 5 videocassettes; 146 min. total (19–45 min. each); sd., color; VHS. Videocassettes accompanied by a 68-page manual authored by E.V. Lapham et al. The HuGEM Project is a collaboration between the Georgetown University Child Development Center, a division of the Dept. of Pediatrics, Georgetown University Medical Center, and the Alliance of Genetic Support Groups. BE62800.

> children; confidentiality; disclosure; employment; family members; gene therapy; genetic counseling; *genetic disorders; genetic information; genetic predisposition; *genetic screening; *genetic services; *genome mapping; guidelines; health insurance; health personnel; newborns; patients; prenatal diagnosis; privacy; risks and benefits; social discrimination; technical expertise; ELSI-funded publication; Human Genome Project; United States

Iles, Alastair T. The Human Genome Project: a challenge

BE = bioethics accession number   fn. = footnotes   refs. = references

to the human rights framework. *Harvard Human Rights Journal.* 1996 Spring; 9: 27–60. 125 fn. BE59301.

> autonomy; coercion; communitarianism; covenant; cultural pluralism; developing countries; disadvantaged; employment; eugenics; freedom; gene therapy; genetic counseling; genetic information; genetic research; genetic screening; genetic services; *genome mapping; government regulation; guidelines; health care; *human rights; industry; insurance; *international aspects; investigators; justice; minority groups; policy analysis; private sector; public policy; public sector; risks and benefits; *social control; social discrimination; social dominance; social impact; socioeconomic factors; *standards; liberalism; Council of Europe; Declaration on the Protection of the Human Genome; *Human Genome Project; International Covenant on Civil and Political Rights; International Covenant on Economic, Social and Cultural Rights; Unesco; United Nations; Universal Declaration of Human Rights

Jackson, Fatimah. Assessing the Human Genome Project: an African–American and bioanthropological critique. *In:* Smith, Edward; Sapp, Walter, eds. Plain Talk about the Human Genome Project: A Tuskegee University Conference on Its Promise and Perils ... and Matters of Race. Tuskegee, AL: Tuskegee University Press; 1997: 95–103. 10 refs. ISBN 1–891196–01–4. BE61738.

> *blacks; *genetic diversity; *genetic research; *genome mapping; health care; international aspects; minority groups; non–Western World; population genetics; research design; risks and benefits; *selection of subjects; social discrimination; Western World; whites; Africa; African American Manifesto on Genomic Studies (1994); *Human Genome Project; United States

Juengst, Eric T. Self–critical federal science? The ethics experiment within the U.S. Human Genome Project. *In:* Paul, Ellen Frankel; Miller, Fred D.; Paul, Jeffrey, eds. Scientific Innovation, Philosophy, and Public Policy. New York, NY: Cambridge University Press; 1996: 63–95. 69 fn. ISBN 0–521–58994–0. BE62744.

> administrators; advisory committees; *evaluation; federal government; genetic information; genetic predisposition; genetic research; genetic screening; genetic services; *genome mapping; goals; government financing; government regulation; policy analysis; privacy; *program descriptions; *public policy; resource allocation; social discrimination; *social impact; *Human Genome Project; National Institutes of Health; *NCHGR Program on Ethical, Legal, and Social Implications (ELSI); *United States

King, Patricia. The dilemma of difference. *In:* Smith, Edward; Sapp, Walter, eds. Plain Talk about the Human Genome Project: A Tuskegee University Conference on Its Promise and Perils ... and Matters of Race. Tuskegee, AL: Tuskegee University Press; 1997: 75–81. 7 refs. ISBN 1–891196–01–4. BE61736.

> bioethics; *blacks; disadvantaged; eugenics; genetic information; *genome mapping; health care delivery; historical aspects; human experimentation; informed consent; justice; reproduction; risks and benefits; social control; *social discrimination; syphilis; *Human Genome Project; Tuskegee Syphilis Study; United States

Kluger, Jeffrey. Who owns our genes? *Time.* 1999 Jan 11; 153(1): 51. BE60308.

> *DNA sequences; genes; *genome mapping; legal aspects; *patents; property rights; Patent and Trademark Office; United States

Lemonick, Michael D.; Thompson, Dick. Racing to map our DNA. [News]. *Time.* 1999 Jan 11; 153(1): 44–51. BE60307.

> disclosure; DNA sequences; employment; federal government; genes; *genetic information; *genome mapping; government financing; industry; insurance; international

aspects; investigators; *methods; patents; private sector; public opinion; Human Genome Project; National Center for Human Genome Research; United States

McGee, Glenn. Gene patents can be ethical. *Cambridge Quarterly of Healthcare Ethics.* 1998 Fall; 7(4): 417–421. 4 fn. Commented on by A.L. Kaplan, p. 422–424, and by J.F. Merz and M.K. Cho, p. 425–428. BE59142.

> diagnosis; DNA sequences; *genes; genetic disorders; genetic information; genetic research; genetic screening; *genome mapping; information dissemination; investigators; methods; *patents; public policy; risks and benefits; United States

Magnus, David. Disease gene patenting: the clinician's dilemma. *Cambridge Quarterly of Healthcare Ethics.* 1998 Fall; 7(4): 433–435. 5 fn. BE59146.

> diagnosis; disclosure; economics; *genes; genetic disorders; genetic information; *genetic screening; genetic services; *genome mapping; legal aspects; methods; *patents; physicians; property rights; public policy; risks and benefits; United States

Marshall, Eliot. A second private genome project. [News]. *Science.* 1998 Aug 21; 281(5380): 1121. BE59941.

> *DNA data banks; *drug industry; drugs; genetic predisposition; genetic research; *genome mapping; *private sector; California; *Incyte Pharmaceuticals Inc.

Marshall, Eliot. DNA studies challenge the meaning of race. [News]. *Science.* 1998 Oct 23; 282(5389): 654–655. BE59700.

> behavioral genetics; DNA data banks; evolution; federal government; *genetic diversity; *genetic research; *genome mapping; *international aspects; minority groups; *population genetics; public policy; *research design; stigmatization; Human Genome Diversity Project; National Human Genome Research Institute; United States

Marshall, Eliot. Drug firms to create public database of genetic mutations. [News]. *Science.* 1999 Apr 16; 284(5413): 406–407. BE61771.

> *data banks; *drug industry; *financial support; *genome mapping; *information dissemination; private sector; public sector; Great Britain

Mawer, Simon. Iceland, the nation of clones. *New York Times.* 1999 Jan 23: A19. BE60645.

> drug industry; economics; *genetic research; *genome mapping; *population genetics; *Iceland

Merz, Jon F.; Cho, Mildred K. Disease genes are not patentable: a rebuttal of McGee. *Cambridge Quarterly of Healthcare Ethics.* 1998 Fall; 7(4): 425–428. 8 fn. Commentary on G. McGee, p. 417–421. BE59144.

> diagnosis; DNA sequences; *genes; genetic disorders; genetic screening; *genome mapping; industry; legal aspects; methods; *patents; property rights; public policy; risks and benefits; United States

Murphy, Timothy F. Mapping the human genome. *In:* Kuhse, Helga; Singer, Peter, eds. A Companion to Bioethics. Malden, MA: Blackwell; 1998: 198–205. 17 refs. ISBN 0–631–19737–0. BE59495.

> DNA data banks; DNA sequences; eugenics; genetic information; genetic research; genetic screening; *genome mapping; international aspects; justice; moral policy; patents; resource allocation; risks and benefits; social discrimination; social impact; tissue banks; *Human Genome Project

Roscam Abbing, Henriette D.C. New developments in international health law. *European Journal of Health Law.* 1998 Jun; 5(2): 155–169. Includes text of the Universal Declaration on the Human Genome and Human Rights,

---

p. 163–167. BE60901.
    animal organs; *cloning; communicable diseases; genetic intervention; *genetic research; *genome mapping; *guidelines; *human rights; *international aspects; *regulation; risks and benefits; *tissue transplantation; Council of Europe; *Europe; European Union; Unesco; *Universal Declaration on the Human Genome and Human Rights; World Health Organization

Rosner, Mary; Johnson, T.R. Telling stories: metaphors of the Human Genome Project. *Hypatia.* 1995 Fall; 10(4): 104–129. 62 refs. BE61677.
    disease; eugenics; *feminist ethics; genetic disorders; genetic diversity; *genome mapping; goals; *investigators; males; *metaphor; normality; *science; *social dominance; *values; Western World; nature; *Human Genome Project

Rural Advancement Foundation International (RAFI). Endangered or endangering indigenous peoples? *Splice of Life.* 1996 Dec; 3(3): 5–6. BE60107.
    blood specimen collection; confidentiality; disclosure; DNA sequences; *genetic diversity; *genetic materials; *genome mapping; informed consent; *international aspects; *minority groups; patents; *population genetics; tissue banks; cell lines; Hagahai; *Human Genome Diversity Project; Papua New Guinea

Schüklenk, Udo. India fears patent and ethics abuses. [News]. *Nature Biotechnology.* 1997 Jul; 15(7): 613. Report on the Indian National Academy of Sciences bioethics symposium held in Goa, India, 22–25 May, 1997. BE62039.
    developing countries; drug industry; genetic diversity; genetic materials; *genetic research; *genome mapping; informed consent; international aspects; *patents; property rights; research subjects; *India

Sharp, Richard R.; Barrett, J. Carl. The Environmental Genome Project and bioethics. *Kennedy Institute of Ethics Journal.* 1999 Jun; 9(2): 175–188. 58 refs. 1 fn. BE62385.
    confidentiality; disclosure; DNA data banks; ecology; genetic determinism; genetic information; genetic intervention; *genetic predisposition; *genetic research; genetic screening; *genome mapping; *health hazards; informed consent; population genetics; privacy; research subjects; risks and benefits; tissue donation; *Environmental Genome Project; National Institute of Environmental Health Sciences; United States

Shattuck, Roger. Knowledge exploding: science and technology. *In: his* Forbidden Knowledge: From Prometheus to Pornography. San Diego, CA: Harcourt Brace; 1996: 173–225. 12 fn. ISBN 0-15-600551-4. BE61060.
    behavioral genetics; case studies; *eugenics; evolution; expert testimony; freedom; gene therapy; *genetic intervention; *genetic research; genetic screening; *genome mapping; germ cells; government regulation; historical aspects; international aspects; investigators; involuntary sterilization; legal aspects; mentally retarded; National Socialism; nuclear warfare; prenatal diagnosis; recombinant DNA research; *risks and benefits; *science; self regulation; social impact; Supreme Court decisions; wrongful life; *knowledge; Asilomar Conference; Buck v. Bell; Manhattan Project; Twentieth Century

Smith, Edward; Sapp, Walter, eds. Plain Talk about the Human Genome Project: A Tuskegee University Conference on Its Promise and Perils...and Matters of Race. Tuskegee, AL: Tuskegee University Press; 1997. 292 p. Includes references. Papers from a conference held at Tuskegee University, 26–28 Sep 1996. ISBN 1-891196-01-4. BE61735.
    behavioral genetics; blacks; breast cancer; confidentiality; economics; education; eugenics; federal government; gene therapy; genetic determinism; genetic diversity; genetic enhancement; genetic information; genetic intervention; genetic predisposition; genetic research; genetic screening; genetic services; *genome mapping; goals; government regulation; historical aspects; human experimentation; hypertension; industry; insurance; international aspects; justice; legislation; privacy; risks and benefits; scientific misconduct; selection of subjects; sickle cell anemia; social control; social discrimination; social impact; values; *Human Genome Project; NCHGR Program on Ethical, Legal, and Social Implications (ELSI); Tuskegee Syphilis Study; United States

Smith, G. Kenneth; Kettelberger, Denise M. Patents and the Human Genome Project. *AIPLA Quarterly Journal (American Intellectual Property Law Association).* 1994; 22(1): 27–64. 254 fn. BE59787.
    DNA data banks; *DNA sequences; federal government; genetic research; *genome mapping; government financing; industry; *international aspects; interprofessional relations; investigators; legal aspects; *patents; property rights; *public policy; Europe; Great Britain; Human Genome Organization (HUGO); *Human Genome Project; Japan; National Institutes of Health; Patent and Trademark Office; *United States

Straus, Joseph. Patenting human genes in Europe -- past developments and prospects for the future. *IIC: International Review of Industrial Property and Copyright Law.* 1995 Dec; 26(6): 920–950. 125 fn. BE62710.
    disclosure; DNA sequences; drug industry; *genes; genome mapping; industry; international aspects; *legal aspects; morality; *patents; regulation; *Europe; European Parliament; European Patent Convention; European Patent Office

Thomson, Elizabeth. The Ethical, Legal, and Social Implications Program at the National Human Genome Research Institute, NIH. *In:* Smith, Edward; Sapp, Walter, eds. Plain Talk about the Human Genome Project: A Tuskegee University Conference on Its Promise and Perils ... and Matters of Race. Tuskegee, AL: Tuskegee University Press; 1997: 123–130. 8 refs. 5 fn. ISBN 1-891196-01-4. BE61740.
    advisory committees; ethical review; federal government; *genetic research; *genome mapping; government financing; government regulation; *program descriptions; research institutes; *Human Genome Project; *NHGRI Program on Ethical, Legal, and Social Implications (ELSI); *NIH-DOE Working Group on Ethical, Legal, and Social Implications (ELSI); *United States

Tribble, Jack L. Gene patents -- a pharmaceutical perspective. *Cambridge Quarterly of Healthcare Ethics.* 1998 Fall; 7(4): 429–432. 14 fn. BE59145.
    biomedical research; diagnosis; DNA sequences; *drug industry; federal government; *genes; genetic screening; *genome mapping; information dissemination; investigators; legal aspects; methods; organizational policies; *patents; property rights; public policy; standards; European Union; *Merck Inc.; United States

Unesco. Universal declaration on the human genome and human rights (revised draft). *Bulletin of Medical Ethics.* 1997 Mar; No. 126: 9–11. BE60445.
    developing countries; genetic disorders; *genetic research; *genome mapping; *guidelines; *human rights; information dissemination; informed consent; *international aspects; *organizational policies; public policy; research subjects; risks and benefits; Unesco; United Nations; *Universal Declaration on the Human Genome and Human Rights

Unesco. Universal Declaration on the Human Genome and

Human Rights [UNESCO Document 27 V / 45, adopted by the Thirty-first General Assembly of UNESCO, Paris, 11 November 1997]. *Journal of Medicine and Philosophy*. 1998 Jun; 23(3): 334–341. BE59297.
confidentiality; developing countries; ethical review; freedom; *genetic intervention; *genetic research; *genome mapping; *guidelines; *human rights; information dissemination; informed consent; *international aspects; public policy; risks and benefits; Unesco; United Nations; *Universal Declaration on the Human Genome and Human Rights

Unesco. International Bioethics Committee. Proceedings of the Fourth Session, October 1996. Volume I. Paris: The Committee; 1998. 164 p. Includes references. BE61056.
advisory committees; AIDS; autonomy; beneficence; *bioethical issues; committee membership; drugs; ecology; economics; food; *genetic intervention; *genetic research; *genome mapping; government regulation; *guidelines; *human experimentation; *human rights; *international aspects; investigators; justice; moral obligations; random selection; recombinant DNA research; regulation; remuneration; research subjects; risks and benefits; selection of subjects; standards; transgenic organisms; vulnerable populations; women's health; agriculture; *transgenic plants; Declaration of Helsinki; *International Bioethics Committee (Unesco); Unesco; United Nations; *Universal Declaration on the Human Genome and Human Rights (Unesco)

Wallace, Robert W. The Human Genome Diversity Project: medical benefits versus ethical concerns. *Molecular Medicine Today*. 1998 Feb; 4(2): 59–62. 13 refs. BE61813.
anthropology; developing countries; DNA data banks; ethical review; federal government; *genetic diversity; genetic information; genetic materials; *genetic research; *genome mapping; government financing; guidelines; industry; informed consent; *international aspects; minority groups; patents; *population genetics; privacy; public policy; *risks and benefits; tissue banks; deCODE Genetics; *Human Genome Diversity Project; Iceland; *National Institutes of Health; National Research Council; National Science Foundation; United States

HEALTH

See also MENTAL HEALTH, OCCUPATIONAL HEALTH, PUBLIC HEALTH

Albert, Steven M.; Frank, Lori; Kleinman, Leah, et al. Defining and measuring quality of life in medicine. [Letters and response]. *JAMA*. 1998 Feb 11; 279(6): 429–431. 19 refs. BE59232.
cultural pluralism; disabled; disease; *evaluation; *health; health services research; *patient participation; physicians; *quality of life; treatment outcome; *values

Andrulis, Dennis P. Access to care is the centerpiece in the elimination of socioeconomic disparities in health. *Annals of Internal Medicine*. 1998 Sep 1; 129(5): 412–416. 30 refs. BE59131.
children; empirical research; federal government; government financing; *health; *health care delivery; health insurance; *indigents; mortality; primary health care; public policy; quality of health care; quality of life; *socioeconomic factors; state government; personal financing; United States
Many health care professionals have sustained an almost single-minded conviction that disparities in access to health care across socioeconomic groups are the key reason for the major discrepancies in health status between wealthy persons and poor persons. Others, however, have argued that a host of factors work to create major impediments and that reducing or

eliminating financial barriers to health care in particular will do little to reduce discrepancies in health status. This paper, while acknowledging the spectrum of contributing factors, argues that the elimination of financially based differences in access is central to any effort to create equity in outcomes across socioeconomic groups. Through selected review of the many studies on health insurance, access, outcomes, and socioeconomic status, it establishes that a core links affected populations, their difficulty in financing health care, and the threat to their well-being. In so doing, it cites findings that strongly associate lack of insurance (especially for persons who live in poverty), inability to obtain services, and adverse health outcomes. It also uses the example of Medicaid and other coverage for HIV-infected persons in particular as an important positive instance in which leveling the discrepancies in health care across socioeconomic groups can move toward creating quality in access and outcomes. The competitive pressures in today's health care environment threaten to drive socioeconomic groups further apart, especially insured and uninsured persons. However, the recent enactment of state actions, especially the State Child Health Insurance Program, represent powerful examples of health insurance expansion that have lessons for policymakers at all levels for the monitoring and reduction of socioeconomic disparities.

Annas, George J. Human rights and health -- the Universal Declaration of Human Rights at 50. *New England Journal of Medicine*. 1998 Dec 10; 339(24): 1778–1781. 26 refs. BE60040.
AIDS; capitalism; democracy; developing countries; economics; education; guidelines; *health; *health care; health promotion; historical aspects; *human rights; *international aspects; law; medical ethics; misconduct; natural law; obligations of society; obligations to society; physicians; political activity; prisoners; professional organizations; *public health; public policy; socialism; socioeconomic factors; torture; war; women's rights; Amnesty International; Consortium for Health and Human Rights; Global Lawyers and Physicians; Physicians for Social Responsibility; Physicians for the Prevention of Nuclear War; Physicians of the World; Twentieth Century Doctors without Borders; United Nations; *Universal Declaration of Human Rights

Barragan, Javier Lozano. The demands of health and morality: the health paradigm in WHO. *Dolentium Hominum: Church and Health in the World*. 1997; 36(12th Yr., No. 3): 36–42. 28 fn. BE60598.
Christian ethics; ecology; *health; health care; health care delivery; health education; human rights; *international aspects; morality; quality of life; reproduction; Roman Catholic ethics; women's rights; Declaration of Alma-Ata; Unesco; United Nations; *World Health Organization

Benatar, Solomon R. Global disparities in health and human rights: a critical commentary. *American Journal of Public Health*. 1998 Feb; 88(2): 295–300. 81 refs. Commented on by M.A. Somerville, p. 301–303. BE60776.
capitalism; *developing countries; disadvantaged; ecology; economics; government financing; *health; health care; *human rights; *international aspects; justice; *moral obligations; *non-Western World; *obligations of society; public policy; resource allocation; *socioeconomic factors; war; *Western World; Africa
Widening disparities in health and human rights at a global level represent the dark side of progress associated with escalation of economic and military exploitation and exponential population growth in the 20th century. Even the most basic universal human rights cannot be

---

BE = bioethics accession number   fn. = footnotes   refs. = references

achieved for all under these circumstances. The goal of improved population health will be similarly elusive while medical care is commodified and exploited for commercial gain in the marketplace. Recognition of the powerful forces that polarize our world and commitment to reversing them are essential for the achievement of human rights for all, for the improvement of public health, and for the peaceful progress required to protect the "rational self-interest" of the most privileged people on earth against the escalation of war, disease, and other destructive forces arising from widespread poverty and ecological degradation.

Bernheim, Jan L. How to get serious answers to the serious question: "How have you been?": subjective quality of life (QOL) as an individual experiential emergent construct. *Bioethics.* 1999 Jul; 13(3-4): 272-287. 31 refs. 5 fn. BE61878.
     drugs; *evaluation; *health; health care; *health services research; *quality of life; recall; research design; self concept; therapeutic research; treatment outcome; values; questionnaires

Medical, scientific and societal progress has been such that, in a universalist humanist perspective such as the WHO's, it has become an ethical imperative for the primary endpoints in evidence based health care research to be expressed in e.g. Quality Adjusted Life Years (QALYs). The classical endpoints of discrete health-related functions and duration of survival are increasingly perceived as unacceptably reductionistic. The major problem in 'felicitometrics' is the measurement of the 'quality' term in QALYs. That the mental, physical and social domains, each containing many dimensions and items, all contribute to QOL is uncontroversial. What is controversial, is the weight of the different dimensions in overall QOL. It has been shown to be very different between different patient populations. In human individuals, assuredly complex systems, the many dimensions and items of QOL observably *interact*, probably sometimes in *chaotic* ways. In these conditions, the weights of isolated items in individuals become for all practical purposes meaningless. Therefore, the much used multi-item questionnaires at best describe, but do not evaluate QOL, neither in individuals, nor in populations. For example, allergic patients treated with cetirizine scored better than those on placebo on all dimensions of the SF-36, a standard QOL questionnaire. Here there is no serious doubt that the treatment improved QOL, because it is highly unlikely that any important dimension on which the patient groups would have scored otherwise is missing in the SF-36. However, whether piracetam treatment of acute stroke, which improved the surrogate endpoints neurological and functional scores, also improved QOL is plausible, but will be proven only when comprehensive QOL measurement will have been done. And suppose in randomised populations of end-stage metastatic solid cancer patients, one would compare palliative last-line chemotherapy with only palliative care, and one would, as can be expected, find no significant differences in average survival, and chemotherapy superior for the mental domain, but inferior for the physical comfort domain: we would not know which treatment, on aggregate, would be the better. The problem is that QOL is an individual and *emergent* construct, the resultant of a great many interactions, and of a different order than its contributing components. Overall QOL can therefore best be captured only as the Gestalt of a global self-assessment. Just as people in everyday life, while acting under uncertainty, make global assessments all the time, so they

can seriously answer the serious question: 'How have you been?' A solemn, practical, non peer-relativistic, non-cultural, experiential, and well tolerated way to obtain such responses is Anamnestic Comparative Self Assessment (ACSA), in which the subjects' memories of the best and the worst times in their life experience define their individual scale of QOL. ACSA is thus both exquisitely idiosyncratic, and yet can in a universalist humanistic perspective be considered generic. Using both a multi-item questionnaire *and* a global assessment allows by one logistic regression, to estimate the weights of the dimensions and items in populations, and thus identify those whose improvement would most contribute to the QOL of the greatest number. A combined approach to measurement of QOL is necessary to maximise the utility of QOL interventions.

Bordo, Susan. *Braveheart, Babe,* and the contemporary body. *In:* Parens, Erik, ed. Enhancing Human Traits: Ethical and Social Implications. Washington, DC: Georgetown University Press; 1998: 189-221. 16 fn. ISBN 0-87840-703-0. BE59753.
     advertising; age factors; autonomy; biomedical technologies; capitalism; coercion; communication; *cosmetic surgery; *enhancement technologies; females; *feminist ethics; freedom; *health; *human body; males; *mass media; *normality; pain; physician's role; *self concept; *values; beauty; empowerment; *self care; United States

Borrmans, Maurice. Health, illness, and healing in the great religions: IV. Islam. *Dolentium Hominum: Church and Health in the World.* 1998; No. 37 [yr. 13(1)]: 118-120. 15 fn. BE61782.
     abortion, induced; euthanasia; *health; *health care; historical aspects; *Islamic ethics; medical education; physicians; reproductive technologies; rights; sterilization (sexual); suffering; theology; Declaration of the Rights of Man in Islam

Callahan, Daniel. Age, sex, and resource allocation. *In:* Walker, Margaret Urban, ed. Mother Time: Women, Aging, and Ethics. Lanham, MD: Rowman and Littlefield; 1999: 189-199. 9 fn. ISBN 0-8476-9260-4. BE61900.
     age factors; *aged; biomedical technologies; chronically ill; disabled; disadvantaged; *economics; federal government; *females; *government financing; *health care; *health care reform; health promotion; home care; justice; long-term care; males; mortality; public policy; quality of life; rehabilitation; *resource allocation; social discrimination; *women's health; *women's health services; Medicare; *United States

Callahan, Joan C. Menopause: taking the cures or curing the takes? *In:* Walker, Margaret Urban, ed. Mother Time: Women, Aging, and Ethics. Lanham, MD: Rowman and Littlefield; 1999: 151-174. 48 fn. ISBN 0-8476-9260-4. BE61898.
     adults; advertising; *age factors; cosmetic surgery; disclosure; drug industry; drugs; *females; *hormones; informed consent; *normality; *patient care; physicians; *risks and benefits; stigmatization; Western World; *women's health; *estrogen replacement therapy; *menopause; American Heart Association

Coward, Harold; Ratanakul, Pinit, eds. A Cross-Cultural Dialogue on Health Care Ethics. Waterloo, ON: Wilfrid Laurier University Press; 1999. 274 p. Includes references. This book is the result of the work of a Canada-Thailand interdisciplinary research team of the Centre for Studies in Religion and Society at the University of Victoria in Canada. ISBN 0-88920-325-3. BE62785.

BE = bioethics accession number   fn. = footnotes   refs. = references

alternative therapies; American Indians; attitudes to death; autonomy; *bioethical issues; Buddhist ethics; *cultural pluralism; *decision making; disease; ecology; family relationship; *health; *health care; *health care delivery; informed consent; international aspects; minority groups; minors; patient participation; physician patient relationship; public participation; *public policy; religion; risks and benefits; standards; terminal care; treatment refusal; *values; Confucian ethics; Taoist ethics; Canada; China; Thailand

D'Agostino, Francesco. The person and the right to health. *Dolentium Hominum: Church and Health in the World.* 1998; No. 37 [yr. 13(1)]: 29–30. 4 fn. BE61775.
*health; *human rights; international aspects

de Beaufort, Inez. Individual responsibility for health. *In:* Bennett, Rebecca; Erin, Charles A., eds. HIV and AIDS: Testing, Screening, and Confidentiality. New York, NY: Oxford University Press; 1999: 107–124. 15 fn. ISBN 0-19-823801-0. BE62717.
AIDS; alcohol abuse; autonomy; economics; *health; health care; health insurance; justice; *moral obligations; obligations of society; organ transplantation; physicians; *resource allocation; selection for treatment; *self induced illness; smoking; withholding treatment; personal financing; Netherlands

Dhavamoni, Mariasusai. Health, illness, and healing in the great religions: II. Hinduism. *Dolentium Hominum: Church and Health in the World.* 1998; No. 37 [yr. 13(1)]: 112–115. 12 fn. BE61780.
alternative therapies; disease; *health; health care; *Hindu ethics; human body; medicine; nutrition; preventive medicine; quality of life; values; India

Epstein, Andrew E. Lifestyle and ethical issues: driving and occupational aspects. *In:* Dunbar, Sandra B.; Ellenbogen, Kenneth A.; Epstein, A.E., eds. Sudden Cardiac Death: Past, Present, and Future. Armonk, NY: Futura; 1997: 321–334. 35 refs. ISBN 0-8799-3666-5. BE60021.
age factors; alcohol abuse; behavior control; confidentiality; dangerousness; duty to warn; employment; government regulation; guidelines; *health; *heart diseases; insurance; morbidity; *mortality; physicians; professional organizations; public health; *risk; *traffic accidents; myocardial infarction; American Heart Association; North American Society of Pacing and Electrophysiology; United States

Freeman, David L.; Abrams, Judith Z., eds. Illness and Health in the Jewish Tradition: Writings from the Bible to Today. Philadelphia, PA: Jewish Publication Society; 1999. 291 p. 153 fn. Sourcebook of writings on health, illness, and recovery. ISBN 0-8276-0673-7. BE62731.
attitudes to death; *caring; compassion; females; *health; *Jewish ethics; literature; medicine; moral obligations; patients; physician patient relationship; physicians; *suffering; trust; *value of life; virtues; sick role

Frenk, Julio. Medical care and health improvement: the critical link. [Editorial]. *Annals of Internal Medicine.* 1998 Sep 1; 129(5): 419–420. 5 refs. BE59132.
*health; *health care delivery; historical aspects; indigents; public health; resource allocation; socioeconomic factors; treatment outcome; self care

Fuss, Michael. Health, illness, and healing in the great religions: I. Buddhism. *Dolentium Hominum: Church and Health in the World.* 1998; No. 37 [yr. 13(1)]: 108–111. 7 refs. 26 fn. BE61779.
alternative therapies; *Buddhist ethics; compassion; disease; *health; health care; international aspects; suffering; theology; China; India

Gadow, Sally. Whose body? Whose story? The question about narrative in women's health care. *Soundings.* 1994 Fall–Winter; 77(3–4): 295–307. 30 fn. BE61592.
autonomy; beneficence; biomedical technologies; childbirth; coercion; cosmetic surgery; dehumanization; females; human body; metaphor; *narrative ethics; paternalism; self concept; social dominance; social interaction; *women's health; women's health services; *relational ethics

Gibeau, Anne M. Female genital mutilation: when a cultural practice generates clinical and ethical dilemmas. *Journal of Obstetric, Gynecologic and Neonatal Nursing.* 1998 Jan–Feb; 27(1): 85–91. 17 refs. BE62059.
autonomy; *circumcision; *cultural pluralism; ethical relativism; *females; health personnel; human rights; informed consent; international aspects; legal aspects; non-Western World; refusal to treat; religion; sexuality; values; Western World; *women's health; Africa; United States

Gillespie, Rosemary. Women, the body and brand extension in medicine: cosmetic surgery and the paradox of choice. *Women and Health.* 1996; 24(4): 69–85. 54 refs. BE59443.
advertising; autonomy; *commodification; *cosmetic surgery; economics; *females; *feminist ethics; human body; industry; *informal social control; males; minority groups; *self concept; social dominance; sociology of medicine; *values; *women's health; beauty; *empowerment; rationality

Goodman, Kenneth W. A DiMaggio rule on medical privacy. *New York Times.* 1998 Dec 30: A17. BE60969.
*confidentiality; *disclosure; famous persons; *health; mass media; physicians; privacy

Gostin, Lawrence O.; Feldblum, Chai; Webber, David W. Disability discrimination in America: HIV/AIDS and other health conditions. *JAMA.* 1999 Feb 24; 281(8): 745–752. 78 refs. Includes a table of state legislation protecting persons with HIV infection against discrimination. BE60945.
AIDS; AIDS serodiagnosis; carriers; dentistry; *disabled; *employment; *federal government; genetic disorders; genetic predisposition; *government regulation; health personnel; *HIV seropositivity; *judicial action; *legal aspects; *legislation; mentally disabled; morbidity; occupational exposure; physically disabled; *refusal to treat; reproduction; risk; *social discrimination; *standards; *state government; *Supreme Court decisions; *Americans with Disabilities Act 1990; *Bragdon v. Abbott; Rehabilitation Act 1973; *United States

The Americans With Disabilities Act (ADA) was widely hailed at the time of its enactment in 1990 as providing broad protection against disability discrimination, including discrimination against individuals infected with the human immunodeficiency virus (HIV). In the years since its enactment, however, courts frequently interpreted the ADA as providing far less protection than was initially anticipated. The Supreme Court's first case involving HIV and the acquired immunodeficiency syndrome, Bragdon v Abbott, addressed this trend by ruling that a woman with asymptomatic HIV infection is protected from discrimination in accessing dental services. In doing so, the Court endorsed an interpretation of the ADA that is broadly protective for individuals with disabilities. The Court also ruled that health care professionals may legally refuse to treat a patient because of concern that the patient poses a direct threat to safety only if there is an objective, scientific basis for concluding that the threat to safety is significant. In addition to the ADA, state laws frequently prohibit disability discrimination and apply to some employers

---

BE = bioethics accession number   fn. = footnotes   refs. = references

and others not regulated by federal law. A state–by–state survey of those laws demonstrates that, consistent with Bragdon v Abbott, individuals with asymptomatic HIV have widespread protection on the state level.

Gracia, Diego. What kind of values? A historical perspective on the ends of medicine. *In:* Hanson, Mark J.; Callahan, Daniel, eds. The Goals of Medicine: The Forgotten Issue in Health Care Reform. Washington, DC: Georgetown University Press; 1999: 88–100. 19 fn. ISBN 0–87840–707–3. BE60519.
> ancient history; autonomy; beneficence; bioethics; disease; *goals; *health; *historical aspects; justice; *medicine; morality; pain; principle–based ethics; religious ethics; suffering; trends; *values

Graham, Wendy J.; Newell, Marie–Louise. Seizing the opportunity: collaborative initiatives to reduce HIV and maternal mortality. *Lancet.* 1999 Mar 6; 353(9155): 836–839. 36 refs. BE61222.
> AIDS; cesarean section; childbirth; children; contraception; costs and benefits; *developing countries; drugs; economics; females; health care delivery; health education; *HIV seropositivity; infants; *maternal health; *morbidity; *mortality; *mothers; newborns; patient care; patient education; *pregnant women; prevalence; preventive medicine; quality of health care; resource allocation; sexually transmitted diseases; social impact; *women's health; *women's health services; breast feeding; Africa; AZT; Inter–Agency Group for Safe Motherhood; UNAIDS

Grisso, Jeane Ann; Battistini, Michelle; Ryan, Lesley. Women's health textbooks: codifying science and calling for change. *Annals of Internal Medicine.* 1998 Dec 1; 129(11): 916–918. 10 refs. BE59328.
> evaluation; females; health care delivery; *literature; medical education; medicine; physician patient relationship; primary health care; socioeconomic factors; terminology; *women's health; *women's health services

Gudorf, Christine E. Gender and culture in the globalization of bioethics. *Saint Louis University Public Law Review.* 1996; 15(2): 331–351. 122 fn. BE59913.
> autonomy; beneficence; *bioethics; children; *circumcision; *coercion; *common good; contraception; *cultural pluralism; developing countries; ecology; *females; *feminist ethics; human rights; injuries; *international aspects; involuntary sterilization; justice; males; non–Western World; obligations to society; physicians; *population control; public policy; religion; reproduction; risks and benefits; sexuality; social control; Western World; *women's health

Häggman–Laitila, Arja. The authenticity and ethics of phenomenological research: how to overcome the researcher's own views. *Nursing Ethics.* 1999 Jan; 6(1): 12–22. 37 refs. BE60151.
> attitudes; *behavioral research; *communication; comprehension; *health; *investigator subject relationship; *investigators; nursing ethics; *nursing research; professional ethics; psychology; *research design; research subjects; *qualitative research

Hester, D. Micah. The place of community in medical encounters. *Journal of Medicine and Philosophy.* 1998 Aug; 23(4): 369–383. 19 refs. 7 fn. BE60629.
> autonomy; chronically ill; *communication; communitarianism; disabled; *disease; *health; humanism; narrative ethics; paternalism; patient care; *patient participation; *physician patient relationship; physician's role; *self concept; social dominance; *social interaction

Disease and injury creates a break between the individual and the community which compromises the individual's status within the community as well as the integrity of the self as a "product" of social interaction. Our "everyday" activities are called into question since our ability to fulfill obligations and to achieve many of our ends is diminished through the weakening of our bodies. In light of this account of disease, healing is about restoring the individual to a state of vital functioning, and vital functioning entails communal participation. As John Dewey points out, health as "living healthily" can be understood only in context of each patient's pursuits which are always social and communal. But, if living in community with others is the end–in–view for medical encounters, it too must be implicated in the means to that end. A patient who is given the opportunity to participate as a member of the health care community has already begun within the medical encounter itself to live healthily. It follows, then, that we must work to promote new attitudes within health care towards aiding in the effective agency and participation of patients in their healing process -- i.e., we must see community as healing.

Holm, Søren. Is society responsible for my health? *In:* Bennett, Rebecca; Erin, Charles A., eds. HIV and AIDS: Testing, Screening, and Confidentiality. New York, NY: Oxford University Press; 1999: 125–139. 23 fn. ISBN 0–19–823801–0. BE62718.
> AIDS; *health; *health care delivery; justice; moral obligations; *obligations of society; *resource allocation; self induced illness; state medicine; needs

Joblin, Joseph. Health and the distribution of resources. *Dolentium Hominum: Church and Health in the World.* 1998; No. 37 [yr. 13(1)]: 63–68. 30 fn. BE61777.
> biomedical technologies; common good; developing countries; economics; *health; *health care; *human rights; indigents; international aspects; justice; morality; obligations of society; public policy; *resource allocation; *Roman Catholic ethics; socioeconomic factors; Western World

Jones, Nikki. Culture and reproductive health: challenges for feminist philanthrophy. *In:* Donchin, Anne; Purdy, Laura M., eds. Embodying Bioethics: Recent Feminist Advances. Lanham, MD: Rowman and Littlefield; 1999: 223–237. 46 fn. ISBN 0–8476–8924–7. BE61023.
> childbirth; circumcision; cultural pluralism; *developing countries; females; feminist ethics; human rights; injuries; international aspects; justice; morbidity; mortality; *reproduction; sexuality; social discrimination; values; *women's health; Nigeria; Philippines

Juengst, Eric T. What does *enhancement* mean? *In:* Parens, Erik, ed. Enhancing Human Traits: Ethical and Social Implications. Washington, DC: Georgetown University Press; 1998: 29–47. 27 fn. ISBN 0–87840–703–0. BE59744.
> *biomedical technologies; disease; *enhancement technologies; genetic enhancement; *goals; *health; *health care; justice; *medicine; *moral policy; *normality; patient care; preventive medicine; psychoactive drugs; public policy; risks and benefits; self concept; terminology; *values; NHGRI–funded publication

Krieger, Nancy; Sidney, Stephen; Coakley, Eugenie. Racial discrimination and skin color in the CARDIA study: implications for public health research. *American Journal of Public Health.* 1998 Sep; 88(9): 1308–1313. 61 refs. BE62554.
> *attitudes; *blacks; *emotions; employment; females; *health; health care; Hispanic Americans; law enforcement; males; *minority groups; *public health; *research design; schools; self concept; *social discrimination; *socioeconomic factors; survey; whites; Coronary Artery Risk Development in Young Adults (CARDIA) Study; United States

OBJECTIVES: This study assessed whether skin color

BE = bioethics accession number   fn. = footnotes   refs. = references

and ways of handling anger can serve as markers for experiences of racial discrimination and responses to unfair treatment in public health research. METHODS: Survey data on 1844 Black women and Black men (24 to 42 years old), collected in the year 5 (1990–1991) and year 7 (1992–1993) examinations of the Coronary Artery Risk Development in Young Adults (CARDIA) study, were examined. RESULTS: Skin color was not associated with self-reported experiences of racial discrimination in 5 of 7 specified situations (getting a job, at work, getting housing, getting medical care, in a public setting). Only moderate associations existed between darker skin color and being working class, having low income or low education, and being male (risk ratios under 2). Comparably moderate associations existed between internalizing anger and typically responding to unfair treatment as a fact of life or keeping such treatment to oneself. CONCLUSIONS: Self-reported experiences of racial discrimination and responses to unfair treatment should be measured directly in public health research; data on skin color and ways of handling anger are not sufficient.

Lasby, Clarence G. Eisenhower's Heart Attack: How Ike Beat Heart Disease and Held on to the Presidency. Lawrence, KS: University Press of Kansas; 1997. 384 p. Bibliography: p. 369–376. ISBN 0–7006–0822–2. BE60508.
> *confidentiality; *deception; disclosure; *famous persons; *health; *heart diseases; historical aspects; mass media; patient care; physicians; *politics; professional competence; *Eisenhower, Dwight; *Twentieth Century; United States

McCally, Michael; Haines, Andrew; Fein, Oliver, et al. Poverty and ill health: physicians can, and should, make a difference. *Annals of Internal Medicine.* 1998 Nov 1; 129(9): 726–733. 57 refs. BE59322.
> developing countries; ecology; economics; *health; health care; health promotion; *indigents; *international aspects; moral obligations; *mortality; obligations to society; physician patient relationship; *physician's role; public health; public policy; social problems; *socioeconomic factors; United States

A growing body of research confirms the existence of a powerful connection between socioeconomic status and health. This research has implications for both clinical practice and public policy and deserves to be more widely understood by physicians. Absolute poverty, which implies a lack of resources deemed necessary for survival, is self-evidently associated with poor health, particularly in less developed countries. Over the past two decades, economic decline or stagnation has reduced the incomes of 1.6 billion people. Strong evidence now indicates that relative poverty, which is defined in relation to the average resources available in a society, is also a major determinant of health in industrialized countries. For example, persons in U.S. states with income distributions that are more equitable have longer life expectancies than persons in less egalitarian states. There are numerous possible approaches to improving the health of poor populations. The most essential task is to ensure the satisfaction of basic human needs: shelter, clean air, safe drinking water, and adequate nutrition. Other approaches include reducing barriers to the adoption of healthier modes of living and improving access to appropriate and effective health and social services. Physicians as clinicians, educators, research scientists, and advocates for policy change can contribute to all of these approaches. Physicians and other health professionals should understand poverty and its effects on health and should endeavor to influence policymakers nationally and internationally to reduce the burden of ill health that is a consequence of poverty.

McDonald, Michael. Health, health care, and culture: diverse meanings, shared agendas. *In:* Coward, Harold; Ratanakul, Pinit, eds. A Cross-Cultural Dialogue on Health Care Ethics. Waterloo, ON: Wilfrid Laurier University Press; 1999: 92–112. 32 refs. 24 fn. ISBN 0–88920–325–3. BE62787.
> *cultural pluralism; disease; goals; *health; *health care; justice; obligations of society; philosophy; terminology; needs

McKenny, Gerald P. Enhancements and the ethical significance of vulnerability. *In:* Parens, Erik, ed. Enhancing Human Traits: Ethical and Social Implications. Washington, DC: Georgetown University Press; 1998: 222–237. 15 fn. ISBN 0–87840–703–0. BE59754.
> *biomedical technologies; *enhancement technologies; goals; *health; *human body; medicine; moral obligations; moral policy; normality; *philosophy; postmodernism; self concept; values; virtues; Aristotle; Levinas, Emmanuel; Stoicism

Mann, Jonathan. Health and human rights: broadening the agenda for health professionals. [Editorial]. *Health and Human Rights.* 1996; 2(1): 1–5. 4 refs. BE62084.
> *health; health personnel; health promotion; *human rights; international aspects; misconduct; *public health; public policy

Mann, Jonathan, M.; Gruskin, Sofia; Grodin, Michael A., et al, eds. Health and Human Rights: A Reader. New York, NY: Routledge; 1999. 505 p. Includes references. ISBN 0–415–92102–3. BE62050.
> AIDS; circumcision; developing countries; family planning; females; genetic diversity; genetic research; *health; health care; HIV seropositivity; homosexuals; *human experimentation; *human rights; informed consent; *international aspects; killing; mass screening; medicine; minority groups; misconduct; National Socialism; newborns; patient advocacy; *physicians; *political activity; pregnant women; *public health; public policy; scientific misconduct; sexuality; social discrimination; *social impact; socioeconomic factors; tuberculosis; war; women's health; genocide; Doctors of the World; Doctors without Borders; International Covenant on Civil and Political Rights; International Covenant on Economic, Social and Cultural Rights; International Red Cross and Red Crescent Movement; Physicians for Human Rights; Universal Declaration of Human Rights

Marchand, Sarah; Wikler, Daniel; Landesman, Bruce. Class, health and justice. *Milbank Quarterly.* 1998; 76(3): 449–467. 24 refs. BE59641.
> goals; *health; health care; health care delivery; indigents; international aspects; *justice; *moral policy; *obligations of society; *resource allocation; self induced illness; *socioeconomic factors; standards; egalitarianism

Class inequalities in health are intuitively unjust. Although the link between social class and health status has been fully documented, the precise nature of the injustice has not been made clear. Four alternative views are presented, corresponding to four goals: (1) maximizing the sum total of health; (2) equalizing the health status of higher and lower social classes; (3) maximizing the health status of the lowest social class; and (4) maximizing the health status of the sickest individuals in society. The nature of the injustice is further obscured by several theoretical and empirical questions, like the degree and significance of personal responsibility for illness and the relation of the degree

---

BE = bioethics accession number   fn. = footnotes   refs. = references

of economic inequality to sum total of health.

Melnick, Vijaya L. The brave new world of DNA: transcendence or transgression? *In:* Smith, Edward; Sapp, Walter, eds. Plain Talk about the Human Genome Project: A Tuskegee University Conference on Its Promise and Perils ... and Matters of Race. Tuskegee, AL: Tuskegee University Press; 1997: 197–200. 3 refs. ISBN 1–8911196–01–4. BE61747.
> disabled; *disease; *genetic disorders; *genetic intervention; *health; mental health; *normality; socioeconomic factors

Mirsky, Judith; Radlett, Marty, eds.; Panos Institute. Private Decisions, Public Debate: Women, Reproduction and Population. London: Panos Publications; 1994. 185 p. Includes references. Jounalists' case studies from India, Tanzania, South Korea, Burkina Faso, Philippines, Brazil, Ghana, Ethiopia, Thailand, Pakistan, Chile, and Egypt. ISBN 1–870670–34–5. BE59736.
> abortion, induced; cesarean section; childbirth; circumcision; *contraception; *developing countries; education; employment; *family planning; *females; HIV seropositivity; illegal abortion; infertility; *international aspects; males; nurse midwives; politics; population control; reproduction; Roman Catholics; sex determination; sexually transmitted diseases; social discrimination; socioeconomic factors; sterilization (sexual); *women's health; women's health services; *women's rights; *Brazil; *Burkina Faso; *Chile; *Egypt; *Ethiopia; *Ghana; *India; *Korea; *Pakistan; *Philippines; *Tanzania; *Thailand

Moore, Kirsten; Randolph, Kate; Toubia, Nahid, et al. The synergistic relationship between health and human rights: a case study using female genital mutilation. *Health and Human Rights.* 1997; 2(2): 137–146. 3 fn. Article based on a report by E. Kirberger of a workshop organized in 1995 by the Research, Action & Information Network for Bodily Integrity of Women (RAINBO). BE62090.
> abortion, induced; *circumcision; cultural pluralism; *females; *human rights; Islamic ethics; patient advocacy; *physician's role; physicians; political activity; public policy; *women's health; women's rights; Africa; *Egypt; United States

Morris, David B. Illness and Culture in the Postmodern Age. Berkeley, CA: University of California Press; 1998. 345 p. 506 fn. ISBN 0–520–20869–2. BE59867.
> AIDS; chronically ill; cultural pluralism; death; depressive disorder; disabled; *disease; drugs; ecology; emotions; *health; health care; historical aspects; human body; medicine; metaphor; morbidity; *narrative ethics; *pain; patient care; philosophy; *postmodernism; psychological stress; *suffering; terminal care; trends; women's health; Twentieth Century

Nordenfelt, Lennart. On medicine and other means of health enhancement: towards a conceptual framework. *In:* Hanson, Mark J.; Callahan, Daniel, eds. The Goals of Medicine: The Forgotten Issue in Health Care Reform. Washington, DC: Georgetown University Press; 1999: 69–87. 9 refs. ISBN 0–87840–707–3. BE60518.
> ecology; goals; health; *health care; health education; health personnel; *health promotion; hospitals; medical specialties; *medicine; patient care; philosophy; physician patient relationship; physician's role; preventive medicine; primary health care; public health; rehabilitation

Nordin, Ingemar. The limits of medical practice. *Theoretical Medicine and Bioethics.* 1999 Apr; 20(2): 105–123. 16 fn. BE62213.
> cosmetic surgery; decision making; *goals; *health; *health

care; *health personnel; health promotion; *medicine; models, theoretical; nurse's role; patient care; patient care team; patients; philosophy; physical restraint; *physician's role; physicians; politics; professional organizations; *professional role; *public health; resource allocation; social control; *social problems; technical expertise

Parens, Erik, ed. Enhancing Human Traits: Ethical and Social Implications. Washington, DC: Georgetown University Press; 1998. 258 p. (Hastings Center studies in ethics). 316 fn. ISBN 0–87840–703–0. BE59743.
> advertising; age factors; autonomy; behavior control; *biomedical technologies; blacks; cosmetic surgery; disabled; disease; *enhancement technologies; females; feminist ethics; genetic enhancement; goals; growth disorders; *health; *health care; health insurance reimbursement; hormones; human body; immunization; justice; literature; mass media; medicine; mental health; moral complicity; *moral policy; *normality; patient care; physicians; preventive medicine; psychoactive drugs; psychological stress; public policy; quality of life; resource allocation; review; self concept; social control; suffering; uncertainty; values; beauty; Hastings Center; Project on the Prospect of Technologies Aimed at the Enhancement of Human Capabilities and Traits; United States

Piattelli, Abramo Alberto. Health, illness, and healing in the great religions: III. Judaism. *Dolentium Hominum: Church and Health in the World.* 1998; No. 37 [yr. 13(1)]: 116–117. BE61781.
> disease; food; *health; health care; *Jewish ethics; preventive medicine; theology; value of life

Pincus, Theodore; Esther, Robert; DeWalt, Darren A., et al. Social conditions and self-management are more powerful determinants of health than access to care. *Annals of Internal Medicine.* 1998 Sep 1; 129(5): 406–411. 80 refs. BE59130.
> education; empirical research; employment; *health; *health care delivery; *morbidity; *mortality; patient education; physician's role; prevalence; resource allocation; *socioeconomic factors; statistics; treatment outcome; ambulatory care; *self care; Great Britain; United States

Professional organizations advocate universal access to medical care as a primary approach to improving health in the population. Access to medical services is critical to outcomes of acute processes managed in an inpatient hospital, the setting of most medical education, research, and training, but seems to be limited in its capacity to affect outcomes of outpatient care, the setting of most medical activities. Persistent and widening disparities in health according to socioeconomic status provide evidence of limitations of access to care. First, job classification, a measure of socioeconomic status, was a better predictor of cardiovascular death than cholesterol level, blood pressure, and smoking combined in employed London civil servants with universal access to the National Health Service. Second, disparities in health according to socioeconomic status widened between 1970 and 1980 in the United Kingdom despite universal access (similar trends were seen in the United States). Third, in the United States, noncompletion of high school is a greater risk factor than biological factors for development of many diseases, an association that is explained only in part by age, ethnicity, sex, or smoking status. Fourth, level of formal education predicted cardiovascular mortality better than random assignment to active drug or placebo over 3 years in a clinical trial that provides optimal access to care. Increased recognition of limitations of universal access by physicians and their professional societies may enhance efforts to improve the health of the population.

BE = bioethics accession number   fn. = footnotes   refs. = references

Rogers, Wendy A. Menopause: is this a disease and should we treat it? *In:* Donchin, Anne; Purdy, Laura M., eds. Embodying Bioethics: Recent Feminist Advances. Lanham, MD: Rowman and Littlefield; 1999: 203–219. 49 refs. 15 fn. ISBN 0-8476-8924-7. BE61022.
> age factors; aged; costs and benefits; *disease; drugs; *females; feminist ethics; *hormones; *normality; obstetrics and gynecology; patient care; risks and benefits; *women's health; *estrogen replacement therapy; *menopause; Australia

Saigal, Saroj; Stoskopf, Barbara L.; Feeny, David, et al. Differences in preferences for neonatal outcomes among health care professionals, parents, and adolescents. *JAMA.* 1999 Jun 2; 281(21): 1991–1997. 34 refs. BE62313.
> *adolescents; allowing to die; *attitudes; comparative studies; control groups; *decision making; disabled; *health; intensive care units; *low birth weight; *newborns; normality; *nurses; *parents; patient satisfaction; *physicians; *prolongation of life; *quality of life; survey; *treatment outcome; *value of life; neonatology; Canada

CONTEXT: In neonatal intensive care, parents make important clinical management decisions in conjunction with health care professionals. Yet little information is available on whether preferences of health care professionals and parents for the resulting health outcomes differ. OBJECTIVE: To measure and compare preferences for selected health states from the perspectives of health care professionals (ie, neonatologists and neonatal nurses), parents of extremely low-birth-weight (ELBW) or normal birth-weight infants, and adolescents who were either ELBW or normal birth-weight infants. DESIGN: Cross-sectional cohort study. SETTING AND PARTICIPANTS: A total of 742 participants were recruited and interviewed between 1993 and 1995, including 100 neonatologists from hospitals throughout Canada; 103 neonatal nurses from 3 regional neonatal intensive care units; 264 adolescents (aged 12–16 years), including 140 who were ELBW infants and 124 sociodemographically matched term controls; and 275 parents of the recruited adolescents. MAIN OUTCOME MEASURE: Preferences (utilities) for 4 to 5 hypothetical health states of children were obtained by direct interviews using the standard gamble method. RESULTS: Overall, neonatologists and nurses had similar preferences for the 5 health states, and a similar proportion rated some health states as worse than death (59% of neonatologists and 68% of nurses; P=.20). Health care professionals rated the health states lower than did parents of ELBW and term infants (P less than .001). Overall, 64% of health care professionals and 45% of parents rated 1 or more health states to be worse than death (P less than .001). Differences in mean utility scores between health care professionals and parents and adolescent respondents were most pronounced for the 2 most severely disabled health states (P less than .001). CONCLUSIONS: When asked to rate the health-related quality of life for the hypothetical conditions of children, health care professionals tend to provide lower utility scores than do adolescents and their parents. These findings have implications for decision making in the neonatal intensive care unit.

Schaffner, Kenneth F. Coming home to Hume: a sociobiological foundation for a concept of 'health' and morality. *Journal of Medicine and Philosophy.* 1999 Aug; 24(4): 365–375. 20 refs. 8 fn. BE62614.
> communitarianism; *disease; goals; *health; human characteristics; medicine; *philosophy; *sociobiology; values; Boorse, Christopher; Hume, David

Assessing the normative status of concepts of health and disease involves one in questions regarding the relationship between fact and value. Some have argued that Christopher Boorse's conception of health and disease lacks such a valuational element because it cannot account for types of harms which, while disvalued, do not have evolutionarily dysfunctional consequences. I take Boorse's account and incorporate some Humean-like sociobiological assumptions in order to respond to this challenge. The possession of moral sentiments, I argue, offers an evolutionary advantage (thus falling within Boorse's definition of normal functional abilities). However, this does not amount to emotivism: on the contrary, these sentiments can be the basis of a value system. This value structure introduces the concept of sympathizing with a fellow being's suffering as the basis of a normative dimension to disease. For example, it holds the disvalue of disease to lie in the fact that disease involves suffering and functional limitations. The naturalistic Humean type of account presented here thus jumps the normative-descriptive divide. When Boorse's account is extended to include social sentiments and behaviors, a conception of health emerges which is broader than Boorse's or Kass's, but narrower than the WHO's.

Sheldon, Sally; Wilkinson, Stephen. Female genital mutilation and cosmetic surgery: regulating non-therapeutic body modification. *Bioethics.* 1998 Oct; 12(4): 263–285. 59 fn. BE62276.
> *adults; *circumcision; coercion; comparative studies; *cosmetic surgery; *cultural pluralism; double effect; *females; freedom; *government regulation; human rights; informal social control; informed consent; *injuries; international aspects; legal aspects; males; minority groups; *moral policy; non-Western World; *public policy; *risks and benefits; sexuality; social dominance; *values; Western World; *women's health; Great Britain

In the UK, female genital mutilation is unlawful, not only when performed on minors, but also when performed on adult women. The aim of our paper is to examine several arguments which have been advanced in support of this ban and to assess whether they are sufficient to justify banning female genital mutilation for competent, consenting women. We proceed by comparing female genital mutilation, which is banned, with cosmetic surgery, towards which the law has taken a very permissive stance. We then examine the main arguments for the prohibition of the former, assessing in each case both (a) whether the argument succeeds in justifying the ban and, if so, (b) whether a parallel argument would not also support a ban on the latter. We focus on the following arguments. Female genital mutilation should be unlawful because: (1) no woman could validly consent to it; (2) it is an oppressive and sexist practice; (3) it involves the intentional infliction of injury; (4) it causes offence. Our view is that arguments (3) and (4) are unsound and that, although arguments (1) and (2) may be sound, they support not only a ban on female genital mutilation, but also one on (some types of) cosmetic surgery. Hence, we conclude that the present legal situation in the UK is ethically unsustainable in one of the following ways. Either the ban on female genital mutilation is unjustified because arguments (1) and (2) are not in fact successful; or the law's permissive attitude towards cosmetic surgery is unjustified because arguments (1) and (2) are in fact successful and apply equally to female genital mutilation and (certain forms of) cosmetic surgery. The people of the countries where female genital mutilation is practised resent references to 'barbaric practices imposed on

---

BE = bioethics accession number   fn. = footnotes   refs. = references

women by male-dominated primitive societies', especially when they look at the Western world and see women undergoing their own feminization rites intended to increase sexual desirability: medically dangerous forms of cosmetic plastic surgery, for instance....

Silvers, Anita. A fatal attraction to normalizing: treating disabilities as deviations from "species-typical" functioning. *In:* Parens, Erik, ed. Enhancing Human Traits: Ethical and Social Implications. Washington, DC: Georgetown University Press; 1998: 95–123. 43 fn. ISBN 0–87840–703–0. BE59747.
   *biomedical technologies; community services; cosmetic surgery; costs and benefits; *disabled; disease; *enhancement technologies; genetic intervention; genetic predisposition; *health; *health care; hearing disorders; *justice; medicine; *normality; obligations of society; *physically disabled; public policy; *quality of life; *resource allocation; Daniels, Norman

Sloan, R.P.; Bagiella, E.; Powell, T. Religion, spirituality, and medicine. *Lancet.* 1999 Feb 20; 353(9153): 664–667. 39 refs. BE61086.
   alternative therapies; attitudes; *counseling; *empirical research; *health; health promotion; medical education; medicine; morbidity; mortality; pastoral care; *patient care; physician patient relationship; *physician's role; physicians; public opinion; quality of life; *religion; *research design; risks and benefits; treatment outcome

Somerville, Margaret A. Making health, not war –– musings on global disparities in health and human rights: a critical commentary by Solomon R. Benatar. *American Journal of Public Health.* 1998 Feb; 88(2): 301–303. 11 refs. Commentary on S.R. Benatar, p. 295–300. BE60777.
   conscience; developing countries; government financing; *health; health care; *human rights; *international aspects; *moral obligations; non-Western World; *obligations of society; politics; public policy; suffering; Western World; guilt

Stephenson, Peter. Expanding notions of culture for cross-cultural ethics in health and medicine. *In:* Coward, Harold; Ratanakul, Pinit, eds. A Cross-Cultural Dialogue on Health Care Ethics. Waterloo, ON: Wilfrid Laurier University Press; 1999: 68–91. 47 refs. 2 fn. ISBN 0–88920–325–3. BE62786.
   age factors; aged; American Indians; anthropology; attitudes to death; bioethical issues; bioethics; *cultural pluralism; disadvantaged; drugs; epidemiology; evolution; females; *health; *health care; iatrogenic disease; medicine; minority groups; morbidity; mortality; non-Western World; public health; social dominance; *socioeconomic factors; Western World; women's health; Canada; United States

Tapper, Melbourne. In the Blood: Sickle Cell Anemia and the Politics of Race. Philadelphia, PA: University of Pennsylvania Press; 1999. 163 p. (Critical histories). 316 fn. ISBN 0–8122–3471–5. BE60752.
   anthropology; *blacks; eugenics; federal government; *genetic screening; historical aspects; mandatory programs; mass screening; public policy; *sickle cell anemia; social discrimination; stigmatization; whites; Africa; Twentieth Century; *United States

Verweij, Marcel. Medicalization as a moral problem for preventative medicine. *Bioethics.* 1999 Apr; 13(2): 89–113. 35 fn. BE61671.
   autonomy; behavior control; beneficence; goals; *health; *health promotion; iatrogenic disease; mass screening; medicine; moral obligations; *moral policy; parents; patients; pregnant women; *preventive medicine; public health; *risks and benefits; self induced illness; social control; social impact; social problems; values

Preventive medicine is sometimes criticised as it contributes to medicalization of normal life. The concept 'medicalization' has been introduced by Zola to refer to processes in which the labels 'health' and 'ill' are made relevant for more and more aspects of human life. If preventive medicine contributes to medicalization, would that be morally problematic? My thesis is that such a contribution is indeed morally problematic. The concept is sometimes used to express moral intuitions regarding the practice of prevention and health promotion. Through analysis of these intuitions as well as some other moral concerns, I give an explication of the moral problems of medicalization within the context of preventive medicine.

Wendell, Susan. Old women out of control: some thoughts on aging, ethics, and psychosomatic medicine. *In:* Walter, Margaret Urban, ed. Mother Time: Women, Aging, and Ethics. Lanham, MD: Rowman and Littlefield; 1999: 133–149. 24 refs. 4 fn. ISBN 0–8476–9260–4. BE61897.
   adults; *age factors; aged; attitudes; chronically ill; *diagnosis; disabled; *females; health; *medical errors; *mental health; morbidity; normality; patient care; physicians; *psychiatric diagnosis; *self concept; social discrimination; socioeconomic factors; sociology of medicine; stigmatization; *women's health; menopause; *psychosomatic medicine; North America

HEALTH CARE

See also BIOMEDICAL TECHNOLOGIES, PATIENT CARE

Andrulis, Dennis P. Access to care is the centerpiece in the elimination of socioeconomic disparities in health. *Annals of Internal Medicine.* 1998 Sep 1; 129(5): 412–416. 30 refs. BE59131.
   children; empirical research; federal government; government financing; *health; *health care delivery; health insurance; *indigents; mortality; primary health care; public policy; quality of health care; quality of life; *socioeconomic factors; state government; personal financing; United States
Many health care professionals have sustained an almost single-minded conviction that disparities in access to health care across socioeconomic groups are the key reason for the major discrepancies in health status between wealthy persons and poor persons. Others, however, have argued that a host of factors work to create major impediments and that reducing or eliminating financial barriers to health care in particular will do little to reduce discrepancies in health status. This paper, while acknowledging the spectrum of contributing factors, argues that the elimination of financially based differences in access is central to any effort to create equity in outcomes across socioeconomic groups. Through selected review of the many studies on health insurance, access, outcomes, and socioeconomic status, it establishes that a core links affected populations, their difficulty in financing health care, and the threat to their well-being. In so doing, it cites findings that strongly associate lack of insurance (especially for persons who live in poverty), inability to obtain services, and adverse health outcomes. It also uses the example of Medicaid and other coverage for HIV-infected persons in particular as an important positive instance in which leveling the discrepancies in health care across socioeconomic groups can move toward creating quality in access and outcomes. The competitive pressures in today's health care environment threaten to drive socioeconomic groups further apart,

---

BE = bioethics accession number   fn. = footnotes   refs. = references

especially insured and uninsured persons. However, the recent enactment of state actions, especially the State Child Health Insurance Program, represent powerful examples of health insurance expansion that have lessons for policymakers at all levels for the monitoring and reduction of socioeconomic disparities.

Barrow, Chelmer L.; Easley, Kirk A. The role of gender and race on the time delay for emergency department patients complaining of chest pain to be evaluated by a physician. *Saint Louis University Public Law Review.* 1996; 15(2): 267–277. 38 fn. Commented on by J. Barrow, p. 278–302. BE59910.
    *age factors; *blacks; comparative studies; *emergency care; *females; health care delivery; *heart diseases; *hospitals; institutional policies; *males; *quality of health care; *selection for treatment; social discrimination; *time factors; *whites; myocardial infarction; retrospective studies

Barrow, Jackie. Implications of the Emergency Medical Treatment and Active Labor Act (EMTALA) on differences based on race and gender in the treatment of patients presenting to a hospital emergency department with chest pain. *Saint Louis University Public Law Review.* 1996; 15(2): 278–302. 165 fn. Commentary on C.L. Barrow and K.A. Easley, p. 267–277. BE59911.
    age factors; blacks; *emergency care; federal government; females; *government regulation; heart diseases; *hospitals; indigents; institutional ethics; institutional policies; *legal aspects; legislation; males; minority groups; patient transfer; *quality of health care; *selection for treatment; social discrimination; *socioeconomic factors; standards; *Emergency Medical Treatment and Active Labor Act 1986; Medicare; *United States

Benatar, Solomon R.; Tavistock Group. Shared ethical principles for everybody in health care: a working draft from the Tavistock group. A shared statement of ethical principles for those who shape and give health care. *BMJ (British Medical Journal).* 1999 Jan 23; 318(7178): 249–251. Other members of the Tavistock Group are Donald M. Berwick, Maureen Bisognano, James Dalton, Frank Davidoff, Julio Frenk, Howard Hiatt, Brian Hurwitz, Penny Janeway, Margaret H. Marshall, Richard Norling, Mary Roch Rocklage, Hilary Scott, Amartya Sen, Richard Smith, and Ann Sommerville. BE60329.
    *codes of ethics; confidentiality; *consensus; economics; *guidelines; *health care; *health care delivery; health personnel; human rights; institutional ethics; *interdisciplinary communication; international aspects; obligations of society; patient advocacy; preventive medicine; *professional ethics; public health; quality of health care; resource allocation; Great Britain; Tavistock Group

Blue, Arthur; Keyserlingk, Edward; Rodney, Patricia, et al. A critical view of North American health policy. *In:* Coward, Harold; Ratanakul, Pinit, eds. A Cross-Cultural Dialogue on Health Care Ethics. Waterloo, ON: Wilfrid Laurier University Press; 1999: 215–225. 57 refs. ISBN 0–88920–325–3. BE62795.
    American Indians; geographic factors; guidelines; *health care delivery; health personnel; international aspects; justice; legal aspects; public participation; *public policy; resource allocation; risks and benefits; socioeconomic factors; *Canada; Oregon; *United States

Borrmans, Maurice. Health, illness, and healing in the great religions: IV. Islam. *Dolentium Hominum: Church and Health in the World.* 1998; No. 37 [yr. 13(1)]: 118–120. 15 fn. BE61782.
    abortion, induced; euthanasia; *health; *health care;

historical aspects; *Islamic ethics; medical education; physicians; reproductive technologies; rights; sterilization (sexual); suffering; theology; Declaration of the Rights of Man in Islam

Boyd, Kenneth. Old age, something to look forward to. *In:* Hanson, Mark J.; Callahan, Daniel, eds. The Goals of Medicine: The Forgotten Issue in Health Care Reform. Washington, DC: Georgetown University Press; 1999: 152–161. 21 fn. ISBN 0–87840–707–3. BE60523.
    age factors; *aged; attitudes; economics; family members; *goals; health; *health care; health promotion; life extension; long-term care; *medicine; morbidity; patient care; resource allocation; selection for treatment; adult offspring; dependency; Great Britain

Bulger, Roger J. The Quest for Mercy: The Forgotten Ingredient in Health Care Reform. Charlottesville, VA: Carden Jennings; 1998. 117 p. Bibliography: p. 113–117. ISBN 1–891524–01–1. BE61309.
    attitudes to death; autonomy; caring; codes of ethics; common good; communication; compassion; disease; emotions; empathy; *health care reform; interprofessional relations; managed care programs; mass media; medical education; medical ethics; medicine; motivation; palliative care; patient care; patients; *physician patient relationship; physicians; placebos; prolongation of life; psychology; public health; self concept; social impact; sociology of medicine; suffering; values; Hippocratic Oath; *United States

Cassell, Eric J. Pain, suffering, and the goals of medicine. *In:* Hanson, Mark J.; Callahan, Daniel, eds. The Goals of Medicine: The Forgotten Issue in Health Care Reform. Washington, DC: Georgetown University Press; 1999: 101–117. 8 fn. ISBN 0–87840–707–3. BE60520.
    chronically ill; disease; *goals; health; *health care; historical aspects; *medicine; *pain; patient care; personhood; psychological stress; public health; self concept; *suffering; sick role

Cassidy, Judy. Calvary Hospital focuses on ethics: integrating clinical and organizational ethics meets needs of a changing healthcare system. *Health Progress.* 1998 Nov–Dec; 79(6): 48–50, 52. BE61480.
    clinical ethics; ethics committees; guidelines; health care delivery; *institutional ethics; institutional policies; managed care programs; palliative care; program descriptions; referral and consultation; *religious hospitals; *Roman Catholic ethics; values; *Calvary Hospital (Bronx, NY); Ethical and Religious Directives for Catholic Health Care Services

Churchill, Larry R. Looking to Hume for justice: on the utility of Hume's view of justice for American health care reform. *Journal of Medicine and Philosophy.* 1999 Aug; 24(4): 352–364. 18 refs. 1 fn. BE62613.
    beneficence; common good; ethical theory; *health care delivery; *health care reform; historical aspects; human characteristics; *justice; philosophy; religion; theology; Eighteenth Century; *Hume, David; Rawls, John; Twentieth Century; United States
This essay argues that Hume's theory of justice can be useful in framing a more persuasive case for universal access in health care. Theories of justice derived from a Rawlsian social contract tradition tend to make the conditions for deliberation on justice remote from the lives of most persons, while religiously-inspired views require superhuman levels of benevolence. By contrast, Hume's theory derives justice from the prudent reflections of socially-encumbered selves. This provides a more accessible moral theory and a more realistic path to the establishment of universal access.

BE = bioethics accession number   fn. = footnotes   refs. = references

Collins, Michael F. The role of Catholic hospitals in the new millennium. *Dolentium Hominum: Church and Health in the World.* 1998; No. 37 [yr. 13(1)]: 85–89. 13 refs. BE61778.
> biomedical research; caring; disadvantaged; economics; *health care delivery; indigents; *institutional ethics; medical education; pastoral care; *religious hospitals; *Roman Catholic ethics; values; business ethics; dignity; health facility mergers; United States

Coward, Harold; Ratanakul, Pinit, eds. A Cross-Cultural Dialogue on Health Care Ethics. Waterloo, ON: Wilfrid Laurier University Press; 1999. 274 p. Includes references. This book is the result of the work of a Canada–Thailand interdisciplinary research team of the Centre for Studies in Religion and Society at the University of Victoria in Canada. ISBN 0-88920-325-3. BE62785.
> alternative therapies; American Indians; attitudes to death; autonomy; *bioethical issues; Buddhist ethics; *cultural pluralism; *decision making; disease; ecology; family relationship; *health; *health care; *health care delivery; informed consent; international aspects; minority groups; minors; patient participation; physician patient relationship; public participation; *public policy; religion; risks and benefits; standards; terminal care; treatment refusal; *values; Confucian ethics; Taoist ethics; Canada; China; Thailand

Culpepper, Larry; Gilbert, Thomas T. Evidence and ethics. *Lancet.* 1999 Mar 6; 353(9155): 829–831. 10 refs. BE61220.
> biomedical technologies; chronically ill; costs and benefits; *decision making; diagnosis; *evidence-based medicine; *family practice; health care; health services research; human experimentation; iatrogenic disease; *medical specialties; medicine; patient advocacy; *patient care; patient participation; physician patient relationship; *physicians; practice guidelines; *primary health care; quality of life; random selection; research design; *resource allocation; *risks and benefits; treatment outcome; uncertainty; *values

Donovan, Patricia. Hospital mergers and reproductive health care. *Family Planning Perspectives.* 1996 Nov–Dec; 28(6): 281–284. 21 fn. BE61811.
> *abortion, induced; community services; *contraception; economics; *family planning; geographic factors; government regulation; *hospitals; indigents; *institutional policies; legal aspects; political activity; prenatal diagnosis; referral and consultation; *religious hospitals; *Roman Catholic ethics; state government; trends; voluntary sterilization; *women's health services; *community hospitals; *health facility mergers; American Civil Liberties Union; Montana; New York; *United States

Eijk, W.J. Ethical models for health management. *Dolentium Hominum: Church and Health in the World.* 1998; No. 37 [yr. 13(1)]: 58–62. 31 fn. BE61776.
> aged; alternative therapies; assisted suicide; biomedical technologies; costs and benefits; disabled; enhancement technologies; euthanasia; *health care delivery; human body; managed care programs; organization and administration; patients; personhood; quality adjusted life years; quality of life; religion; Roman Catholic ethics; selection for treatment; social discrimination; treatment refusal; value of life; virtues

Fisher, Elliott S.; Welch, H. Gilbert. Avoiding the unintended consequences of growth in medical care: how might more be worse? *JAMA.* 1999 Feb 3; 281(5): 446–453. 75 refs. BE60239.
> *biomedical technologies; chronically ill; decision making; *diagnosis; disease; drugs; economics; *health care; health care delivery; health services research; iatrogenic disease; mass screening; *medicine; morbidity; mortality; *patient care; prevalence; resource allocation; *risks and benefits; stigmatization; surgery; *technology assessment; treatment

outcome; trends; uncertainty; *health services misuse
The United States has experienced dramatic growth in both the technical capabilities and share of resources devoted to medical care. While the benefits of more medical care are widely recognized, the possibility that harm may result from growth has received little attention. Because harm from more medical care is unexpected, findings of harm are discounted or ignored. We suggest that such findings may indicate a more general problem and deserve serious consideration. First, we delineate 2 levels of decision making where more medical care may be introduced: (1) decisions about whether or not to use a discrete diagnostic or therapeutic intervention and (2) decisions about whether to add system capacity, e.g., the decision to purchase another scanner or employ another physician. Second, we explore how more medical care at either level may lead to harm. More diagnosis creates the potential for labeling and detection of pseudodisease -- disease that would never become apparent to patients during their lifetime without testing. More treatment may lead to tampering, interventions to correct random rather than systematic variation, and lower treatment thresholds, where the risks outweigh the potential benefits. Because there are more diagnoses to treat and more treatments to provide, physicians may be more likely to make mistakes and to be distracted from the issues of greatest concern to their patients. Finally, we turn to the fundamental challenge -- reducing the risk of harm from more medical care. We identify 4 ways in which inadequate information and improper reasoning may allow harmful practices to be adopted -- a constrained model of disease, excessive extrapolation, a missing level of analysis, and the assumption that more is better.

Frenk, Julio. Medical care and health improvement: the critical link. [Editorial]. *Annals of Internal Medicine.* 1998 Sep 1; 129(5): 419–420. 5 refs. BE59132.
> *health; *health care delivery; historical aspects; indigents; public health; resource allocation; socioeconomic factors; treatment outcome; self care

Gostin, Lawrence O.; Hadley, Jack. Health services research: public benefits, personal privacy, and proprietary interests. [Editorial]. *Annals of Internal Medicine.* 1998 Nov 15; 129(10): 833–835. 15 refs. BE59325.
> computer communication networks; *confidentiality; data banks; disclosure; economics; federal government; government regulation; *health services research; industry; informed consent; managed care programs; medical records; *privacy; private sector; standards; Health Insurance Portability and Accountability Act 1996; United States

Grisso, Jeane Ann; Battistini, Michelle; Ryan, Lesley. Women's health textbooks: codifying science and calling for change. *Annals of Internal Medicine.* 1998 Dec 1; 129(11): 916–918. 10 refs. BE59328.
> evaluation; females; health care delivery; *literature; medical education; medicine; physician patient relationship; primary health care; socioeconomic factors; terminology; *women's health; *women's health services

Hamajima, Nobuyuki; Tajima, Kazuo. Patients' views on reference to clinical data. *Journal of Epidemiology.* 1997 Mar; 7(1): 17–19. 10 refs. BE60190.
> age factors; *attitudes; cancer; epidemiology; females; *health services research; *hospitals; males; *medical records; *patients; *privacy; quality of health care; survey; Aichi Cancer Center Hospital; *Japan

Hamel, Ron. A question of value. *Health Progress.* 1997

May–Jun; 78(3): 24–26, 32. BE59685.
administrators; employment; health facilities; *institutional ethics; organization and administration; *religious hospitals; *Roman Catholic ethics; values

Hanson, Mark J.; Callahan, Daniel, eds. The Goals of Medicine: The Forgotten Issue in Health Care Reform. Washington, DC: Georgetown University Press; 1999. 239 p. (Hastings Center studies in ethics). 152 fn. ISBN 0-87840-707-3. BE60516.
aged; biomedical technologies; economics; genetic research; *goals; health; *health care; health promotion; historical aspects; international aspects; medical education; medical ethics; *medicine; pain; physician patient relationship; physician's role; preventive medicine; public health; suffering; trends; values; folk medicine; Goals of Medicine Project (Hastings Center)

Holm, Søren. Is society responsible for my health? *In:* Bennett, Rebecca; Erin, Charles A., eds. HIV and AIDS: Testing, Screening, and Confidentiality. New York, NY: Oxford University Press; 1999: 125–139. 23 fn. ISBN 0-19-823801-0. BE62718.
AIDS; *health; *health care delivery; justice; moral obligations; *obligations of society; *resource allocation; self induced illness; state medicine; needs

Juengst, Eric T. What does *enhancement* mean? *In:* Parens, Erik, ed. Enhancing Human Traits: Ethical and Social Implications. Washington, DC: Georgetown University Press; 1998: 29–47. 27 fn. ISBN 0-87840-703-0. BE59744.
*biomedical technologies; disease; *enhancement technologies; genetic enhancement; *goals; *health; *health care; justice; *medicine; *moral policy; *normality; patient care; preventive medicine; psychoactive drugs; public policy; risks and benefits; self concept; terminology; *values; NHGRI-funded publication

Kane, Rosalie A.; Kane, Robert L.; Ladd, Richard C. The Heart of Long-Term Care. New York, NY: Oxford University Press; 1998. 328 p. Includes references. ISBN 0-19-512238-0. BE62732.
accountability; *aged; allied health personnel; alternatives; chronically ill; community services; disabled; family members; federal government; goals; government financing; health care delivery; health insurance; home care; international aspects; *long-term care; managed care programs; nursing homes; public policy; residential facilities; state government; case managers; personal financing; quality assurance; *United States

Kavanaugh, John F. Ethical commitments in health care systems. *America.* 1998 Nov 7; 179(14): 20. BE62274.
*abortion, induced; *contraception; embryo research; euthanasia; fetal research; health care delivery; hospitals; *institutional ethics; *religious hospitals; reproduction; *Roman Catholic ethics; sterilization (sexual); *health facility mergers; Ethical and Religious Directives for Catholic Health Care Services; United States

Keenan, James F. Institutional cooperation and the ethical and religious directives. *Linacre Quarterly.* 1997 Aug; 64(3): 53–76. 38 fn. BE59311.
abortion, induced; coercion; common good; contraception; *cultural pluralism; health care delivery; health personnel; hospitals; *institutional ethics; *institutional policies; intention; *interprofessional relations; *moral complicity; morality; organization and administration; *religious hospitals; reproductive technologies; *Roman Catholic ethics; sterilization (sexual); *health facility mergers; *Ethical and Religious Directives for Catholic Health Care Services; National Conference of Catholic Bishops; United States

Kopelman, Loretta M.; Palumbo, Michael G. The U.S. health delivery system: inefficient and unfair to children. *American Journal of Law and Medicine.* 1997; 23(2–3): 319–337. 103 fn. BE62503.
age factors; biomedical technologies; *children; decision making; *economics; *ethical theory; *health care; *health care delivery; health insurance; immunization; indigents; infants; *justice; libertarianism; morbidity; mortality; obligations of society; parents; patient advocacy; physicians; preventive medicine; primary health care; public policy; *resource allocation; selection for treatment; standards; uncertainty; utilitarianism; egalitarianism; needs; *United States

Lagnado, Lucette. Their role growing, Catholic hospitals juggle doctrine and medicine. *Wall Street Journal.* 1999 Feb 4: A1, A8. BE61011.
abortion, induced; contraception; *ethicist's role; *ethics consultation; *health care delivery; *hospitals; *institutional policies; political activity; program descriptions; referral and consultation; *religious hospitals; *Roman Catholic ethics; sterilization (sexual); therapeutic abortion; ambulatory care; *health facility mergers; Daughters of Charity National Health System; Florida; New York; Niagara Falls Memorial Hospital; Tennessee

McDonald, Michael. Health, health care, and culture: diverse meanings, shared agendas. *In:* Coward, Harold; Ratanakul, Pinit, eds. A Cross–Cultural Dialogue on Health Care Ethics. Waterloo, ON: Wilfrid Laurier University Press; 1999: 92–112. 32 refs. 24 fn. ISBN 0-88920-325-3. BE62787.
*cultural pluralism; disease; goals; *health; *health care; justice; obligations of society; philosophy; terminology; needs

Mooney, Gavin; Jan, Stephen. Vertical equity: weighing outcomes? or establishing procedures? *Health Policy.* 1997 Jan; 39(1): 79–87. 18 refs. BE59797.
*communitarianism; decision making; economics; goals; health; *health care; *justice; *obligations of society; public participation; *resource allocation; rights; socioeconomic factors; treatment outcome; utilitarianism; values; Broome, John

Nordenfelt, Lennart. On medicine and other means of health enhancement: towards a conceptual framework. *In:* Hanson, Mark J.; Callahan, Daniel, eds. The Goals of Medicine: The Forgotten Issue in Health Care Reform. Washington, DC: Georgetown University Press; 1999: 69–87. 9 refs. ISBN 0-87840-707-3. BE60518.
ecology; goals; health; *health care; health education; health personnel; *health promotion; hospitals; medical specialties; *medicine; patient care; philosophy; physician patient relationship; physician's role; preventive medicine; primary health care; public health; rehabilitation

Nordin, Ingemar. The limits of medical practice. *Theoretical Medicine and Bioethics.* 1999 Apr; 20(2): 105–123. 16 fn. BE62213.
cosmetic surgery; decision making; *goals; *health; *health care; *health personnel; health promotion; *medicine; models, theoretical; nurse's role; patient care; patient care team; patients; philosophy; physical restraint; *physician's role; physicians; politics; professional organizations; *professional role; *public health; resource allocation; social control; *social problems; technical expertise

Olsen, Douglas P. Ethical responsibility in health care reform dialogue. [Editorial]. *NursingConnections.* 1996 Summer; 9(2): 17–22. 9 refs. BE59188.
economics; guidelines; *health care reform; health personnel; *nurses; obligations to society; political activity; quality of

health care; social impact; United States

Parens, Erik, ed. Enhancing Human Traits: Ethical and Social Implications. Washington, DC: Georgetown University Press; 1998. 258 p. (Hastings Center studies in ethics). 316 fn. ISBN 0–87840–703–0. BE59743.
  advertising; age factors; autonomy; behavior control; *biomedical technologies; blacks; cosmetic surgery; disabled; disease; *enhancement technologies; females; feminist ethics; genetic enhancement; goals; growth disorders; *health; *health care; health insurance reimbursement; hormones; human body; immunization; justice; literature; mass media; medicine; mental health; moral complicity; *moral policy; *normality; patient care; physicians; preventive medicine; psychoactive drugs; psychological stress; public policy; quality of life; resource allocation; review; self concept; social control; suffering; uncertainty; values; beauty; Hastings Center; Project on the Prospect of Technologies Aimed at the Enhancement of Human Capabilities and Traits; United States

Pellegrino, Edmund D. The goals and ends of medicine: how are they to be defined? *In:* Hanson, Mark J.; Callahan, Daniel, eds. The Goals of Medicine: The Forgotten Issue in Health Care Reform. Washington, DC: Georgetown University Press; 1999: 55–68. 18 fn. ISBN 0–87840–707–3. BE60517.
  *goals; *health care; *medical ethics; *medicine; moral obligations; obligations to society; patient advocacy; philosophy; physician patient relationship; *physician's role; preventive medicine; public policy; technical expertise; trust; *values; Goals of Medicine Project (Hastings Center)

Pincus, Theodore; Esther, Robert; DeWalt, Darren A., et al. Social conditions and self–management are more powerful determinants of health than access to care. *Annals of Internal Medicine.* 1998 Sep 1; 129(5): 406–411. 80 refs. BE59130.
  education; empirical research; employment; *health; *health care delivery; *morbidity; *mortality; patient education; physician's role; prevalence; resource allocation; *socioeconomic factors; statistics; treatment outcome; ambulatory care; *self care; Great Britain; United States
Professional organizations advocate universal access to medical care as a primary approach to improving health in the population. Access to medical services is critical to outcomes of acute processes managed in an inpatient hospital, the setting of most medical education, research, and training, but seems to be limited in its capacity to affect outcomes of outpatient care, the setting of most medical activities. Persistent and widening disparities in health according to socioeconomic status provide evidence of limitations of access to care. First, job classification, a measure of socioeconomic status, was a better predictor of cardiovascular death than cholesterol level, blood pressure, and smoking combined in employed London civil servants with universal access to the National Health Service. Second, disparities in health according to socioeconomic status widened between 1970 and 1980 in the United Kingdom despite universal access (similar trends were seen in the United States). Third, in the United States, noncompletion of high school is a greater risk factor than biological factors for development of many diseases, an association that is explained only in part by age, ethnicity, sex, or smoking status. Fourth, level of formal education predicted cardiovascular mortality better than random assignment to active drug or placebo over 3 years in a clinical trial that provides optimal access to care. Increased recognition of limitations of universal access by physicians and their professional societies may enhance efforts to improve the health of the population.

Randall, Vernellia R. Slavery, segregation and racism: trusting the health care system ain't always easy! An African American perspective on bioethics. *Saint Louis University Public Law Review.* 1996; 15(2): 191–235. 264 fn. BE59908.
  abortion, induced; *bioethical issues; *bioethics; *blacks; contraception; *cultural pluralism; eugenics; family planning; females; genetic screening; *health care; *health care delivery; health hazards; historical aspects; human experimentation; indigents; involuntary sterilization; males; managed care programs; mass screening; morbidity; mortality; occupational exposure; organ donation; organ transplantation; prisoners; quality of health care; reproductive technologies; resource allocation; scientific misconduct; selection for treatment; sickle cell anemia; *social discrimination; stigmatization; *trust; values; violence; genocide; slavery; Nineteenth Century; Twentieth Century; *United States

Reinders, Hans S. Euthanasia and justice: response to "Euthanasia and health reform in Canada" by Michael Stingl (*CQ* Vol. 7, No. 4). *Cambridge Quarterly of Healthcare Ethics.* 1999 Spring; 8(2): 238–240. BE61239.
  aged; autonomy; coercion; health care delivery; *health care reform; justice; motivation; primary health care; public policy; *quality of health care; quality of life; right to die; suffering; terminal care; values; *voluntary euthanasia; Canada; Netherlands

Rigali, Justin; Law, Bernard; Mahony, Roger, et al. Proposed sale of two Catholic hospitals to for–profit chain. *Origins.* 1997 Nov 6; 27(21): 362–364. BE59970.
  attitudes; clergy; economics; health care delivery; *institutional ethics; *proprietary hospitals; *religious hospitals; *Roman Catholic ethics; teaching hospitals; Missouri; *Queen of Angels–Hollywood Presbyterian Medical Center; *St. Louis University Hospital; Tenet Healthcare Corp.

Rix, Gary; Cutting, Keith. Clinical audit, the case for ethical scrutiny? *International Journal of Health Care Quality Assurance.* 1996; 9(6): 18–20. 8 refs. BE62254.
  confidentiality; ethical review; guidelines; health services research; human experimentation; nurses; *quality of health care; research design; *standards; *medical audit; *Great Britain

Roberts, Laura Weiss; Battaglia, John; Smithpeter, Margaret, et al. An office on Main Street: health care dilemmas in small communities. *Hastings Center Report.* 1999 Jul–Aug; 29(4): 28–37. 35 fn. Includes inset article, "The problems of rural care: four new studies," p. 30–31. BE62467.
  *clinical ethics; community services; confidentiality; conflict of interest; cultural pluralism; *geographic factors; health; *health care delivery; mental health; *patient care; physician patient relationship; physicians; psychological stress; resource allocation; scarcity; social interaction; *socioeconomic factors; values; *rural population; United States

Sabin, James E. Fairness as a problem of love and the heart: a clinician's perspective on priority setting. *BMJ (British Medical Journal).* 1998 Oct 10; 317(7164): 1002–1004. 11 refs. Presented at the Second International Conference on Priorities in Health Care held in London, 8–10 October 1998. BE60832.
  communication; disclosure; *health care delivery; justice; managed care programs; mentally ill; obligations to society; patient advocacy; physician patient relationship; *physician's role; *physicians; public policy; *resource allocation; trust; *United States

Saha, Somnath; Komaromy, Miriam; Koepsell, Thomas

BE = bioethics accession number   fn. = footnotes   refs. = references

D., et al. Patient–physician racial concordance and the perceived quality and use of health care. *Archives of Internal Medicine.* 1999 May 10; 159(9): 997–1004. 42 refs. BE61389.

*attitudes; *blacks; comparative studies; cultural pluralism; evaluation; health care delivery; *Hispanic Americans; *minority groups; patient care; *patient satisfaction; *patients; *physician patient relationship; *physicians; preventive medicine; *quality of health care; socioeconomic factors; survey; *whites; *United States

BACKGROUND: Patients from racial and ethnic minority groups use fewer health care services and are less satisfied with their care than patients from the majority white population. These disparities may be attributable in part to racial or cultural differences between patients and their physicians. OBJECTIVE: To determine whether racial concordance between patients and physicians affects patients' satisfaction with and use of health care. METHODS: We analyzed data from the 1994 Commonwealth Fund's Minority Health Survey, a nationwide, telephone survey of noninstitutionalized adults. For the 2201 white, black, and Hispanic respondents who reported having a regular physician, we examined the association between patient–physician racial concordance and patients' ratings of their physicians, satisfaction with health care, reported receipt of preventive care, and reported receipt of needed medical care. RESULTS: Black respondents with black physicians were more likely than those with nonblack physicians to rate their physicians as excellent (adjusted odds ratio [OR], 2.40; 95% confidence interval [CI], 1.55–3.72) and to report receiving preventive care (adjusted OR, 1.74; 95% CI, 1.01–2.98) and all needed medical care (adjusted OR, 2.94; 95% CI, 1.10–7.87) during the previous year. Hispanics with Hispanic physicians were more likely than those with non-Hispanic physicians to be very satisfied with their health care overall (adjusted OR, 1.74; 95% CI, 1.01–2.99). CONCLUSIONS: Our findings confirm the importance of racial and cultural factors in the patient–physician relationship and reaffirm the role of black and Hispanic physicians in caring for black and Hispanic patients. Improving cultural competence among physicians may enhance the quality of health care for minority populations. In the meantime, by reducing the number of underrepresented minorities entering the US physician workforce, the reversal of affirmative action policies may adversely affect the delivery of health care to black and Hispanic Americans.

Seedhouse, David. Ethics: The Heart of Health Care. Second Edition. New York, NY: Wiley; 1998. 232 p. Bibliography: p. 221–223. ISBN 0-471-97592-3. BE62100.

autonomy; case studies; codes of ethics; costs and benefits; deontological ethics; *ethical analysis; ethical relativism; ethical theory; *ethics; health; *health care; *health personnel; interprofessional relations; justice; law; methods; *moral policy; *morality; patient participation; personhood; principle-based ethics; *professional ethics; professional patient relationship; quality adjusted life years; resource allocation; teleological ethics; utilitarianism; values

Seward, P. John. Restoring the ethical balance in health care. *Health Affairs.* 1997 May–Jun; 16(3): 195–197. BE61329.

*accountability; economics; *health care delivery; managed care programs; medical ethics; *organizational policies; patient advocacy; physician patient relationship; *physicians; professional organizations; quality of health care; *standards; *American Medical Association; United States

Shaw, Allen B. Age as a basis for healthcare rationing: support for agist policies. *Drugs and Aging.* 1996 Dec; 9(6): 403–405. 21 refs. BE60379.

*age factors; *aged; *health care; justice; moral policy; public policy; *resource allocation; *selection for treatment; social discrimination; Great Britain

Silvers, Anita. A fatal attraction to normalizing: treating disabilities as deviations from "species-typical" functioning. *In:* Parens, Erik, ed. Enhancing Human Traits: Ethical and Social Implications. Washington, DC: Georgetown University Press; 1998: 95–123. 43 fn. ISBN 0-87840-703-0. BE59747.

*biomedical technologies; community services; cosmetic surgery; costs and benefits; *disabled; disease; *enhancement technologies; genetic intervention; genetic predisposition; *health; *health care; hearing disorders; *justice; medicine; *normality; obligations of society; *physically disabled; public policy; *quality of life; *resource allocation; Daniels, Norman

Smith, David Barton. Addressing racial inequities in health care: civil rights monitoring and report cards. *Journal of Health Politics, Policy and Law.* 1998 Feb; 23(1): 75–105. 74 refs. BE59778.

*blacks; cadavers; economics; *federal government; government financing; *government regulation; health; health care; *health care delivery; historical aspects; hospitals; legal rights; medical education; medical schools; minority groups; nursing homes; patient admission; patient care; physicians; public policy; quality of health care; self regulation; *social discrimination; standards; Civil Rights Act 1964; Department of Health and Human Services; Department of Health, Education, and Welfare; Medicare; Twentieth Century; *United States

Large racial inequities in health care use continue to be reported, raising concerns about discrimination. Historically, the health system, with its professionally dominated, autonomous, voluntary organizational structure, has presented special challenges to civil rights efforts. De jure racial segregation in the United States gave way to a period of aggressive litigation and enforcement from 1954 until 1968 and then to the current period of relative inactivity. A combination of factors -- declining federal resources and organizational capacity to address more subtle forms of discriminatory practices in health care settings, increasingly restrictive interpretations by the courts, and the lack of any systematic mechanisms for the statistical monitoring of providers -- offers little assurance that discrimination does not continue to play a role in accounting for discrepancies in use. The current rapid transformation of health care into integrated delivery systems driven by risk-based financing presents both new opportunities and new threats. Adequate regulation, markets, and management for such systems impose new requirements for comparative systematic statistical assessment of performance. My conclusion illustrates ways that current "report card" approaches to monitoring performance of such systems could be used to monitor, correct, and build trust in equitable treatment.

Smith, David H. Communication as a reflection of, and a source for, values in health. *Journal of Applied Communication Research.* 1988 Spring; 16(1): 29–38. 20 refs. 2 fn. BE59803.

bioethics; *communication; emotions; health; health care; *health promotion; interdisciplinary communication; moral obligations; obligations to society; physician patient relationship; self induced illness; social interaction; social sciences; trust; *values

Smith, Richard; Hiatt, Howard; Berwick, Donald. A

---

shared statement of ethical principles for those who shape and give health care: a working draft from the Tavistock Group. *Annals of Internal Medicine.* 1999 Jan 19; 130(2): 143–147. 1 ref. BE62602.

> administrators; *codes of ethics; *consensus; economics; goals; *guidelines; *health care; *health care delivery; health facilities; *health personnel; human rights; institutional ethics; *interdisciplinary communication; *international aspects; interprofessional relations; managed care programs; moral obligations; obligations to society; patient advocacy; *professional ethics; public health; resource allocation; *Tavistock Group

Health care delivery in many countries has expanded over the past 150 years from a largely social service delivered by individual practitioners to an intricate network of services provided by teams of professionals. The problems of increasing resource consumption, financial constraints, complexity, and poor system design that have emerged as consequences of these changes have exacerbated many of the ethical tensions inherent in health care and have created new ones. Many groups of professionals that give and affect health care have established separate codes of ethics for their own disciplines, but no shared code exists that might bring all stakeholders in health care into a more consistent moral framework. A multidisciplinary group therefore recently met at Tavistock Square in London in an effort to prepare such a shared code. The result was not a code but a more basic and generic statement of ethical principles. The intent and hope is that it will offer clear guidance for tough calls in real world settings. It is presented here not as a finished work, but as a draft to elicit comment, critique, suggestions for revision, and, especially, ideas for implementation.

Smith, Richard; Hiatt, Howard; Berwick, Donald. Shared ethical principles for everybody in health care: a working draft from the Tavistock group. Introduction. *BMJ (British Medical Journal).* 1999 Jan 23; 318(7178): 248–249. 1 ref. BE60328.

> *codes of ethics; *consensus; *guidelines; *health care; health care delivery; health personnel; institutional ethics; *interdisciplinary communication; *international aspects; *professional ethics; Great Britain; Tavistock Group

Stephenson, Peter. Expanding notions of culture for cross–cultural ethics in health and medicine. *In:* Coward, Harold; Ratanakul, Pinit, eds. A Cross–Cultural Dialogue on Health Care Ethics. Waterloo, ON: Wilfrid Laurier University Press; 1999: 68–91. 47 refs. 2 fn. ISBN 0–88920–325–3. BE62786.

> age factors; aged; American Indians; anthropology; attitudes to death; bioethical issues; bioethics; *cultural pluralism; disadvantaged; drugs; epidemiology; evolution; females; *health; *health care; iatrogenic disease; medicine; minority groups; morbidity; mortality; non–Western World; public health; social dominance; *socioeconomic factors; Western World; women's health; Canada; United States

Townes, Emilie M. Breaking the Fine Rain of Death: African American Health Issues and a Womanist Ethic of Care. New York, NY: Continuum; 1998. 214 p. 433 fn. ISBN 0–8264–1121–5. BE59668.

> AIDS; biomedical research; *blacks; *caring; disadvantaged; drug abuse; females; feminist ethics; government financing; health; *health care; *health care delivery; health insurance; historical aspects; HIV seropositivity; human experimentation; males; managed care programs; morbidity; mortality; paternalism; public health; religion; scientific misconduct; selection of subjects; sexuality; *social discrimination; *socioeconomic factors; sociology of medicine; trust; women's health; slavery; Medicaid; Medicare; Nineteenth Century; Tuskegee Syphilis Study; Twentieth Century; *United States

Tuohey, John F. Covenant model of corporate compliance. *Health Progress.* 1998 Jul–Aug; 79(4): 70–75. 15 fn. BE61617.

> accountability; covenant; ethics committees; federal government; goals; government financing; *institutional ethics; *institutional policies; moral obligations; moral policy; obligations to society; *religious hospitals; *Roman Catholic ethics; business ethics; Medicare; Mercy Health System (OK); United States

Verweij, Marcel. Medicalization as a moral problem for preventative medicine. *Bioethics.* 1999 Apr; 13(2): 89–113. 35 fn. BE61671.

> autonomy; behavior control; beneficence; goals; *health; *health promotion; iatrogenic disease; mass screening; medicine; moral obligations; *moral policy; patients; pregnant women; *preventive medicine; public health; *risks and benefits; self induced illness; social control; social impact; social problems; values

Preventive medicine is sometimes criticised as it contributes to medicalization of normal life. The concept 'medicalization' has been introduced by Zola to refer to processes in which the labels 'health' and 'ill' are made relevant for more and more aspects of human life. If preventive medicine contributes to medicalization, would that be morally problematic? My thesis is that such a contribution is indeed morally problematic. The concept is sometimes used to express moral intuitions regarding the practice of prevention and health promotion. Through analysis of these intuitions as well as some other moral concerns, I give an explication of the moral problems of medicalization within the context of preventive medicine.

Veterans Affairs National Headquarters. Bioethics Committee. Ethical Considerations in Equitable Allocation and Distribution of Limited Health Care Resources: Report. Issued by the VA National Center for Clinical Ethics, White River Junction, VT 05009; 1996 Jan. 15 p. 43 refs. BE59264.

> biomedical technologies; case studies; decision making; federal government; *guidelines; *health care; *institutional policies; justice; *public hospitals; rehabilitation; *resource allocation; selection for treatment; *standards; United States; *Veterans Health Administration

Weisman, Carol S.; Khoury, Amal J.; Cassirer, Christopher, et al. The implications of affiliations between Catholic and non–Catholic health care organizations for availability of reproductive health services. *Women's Health Issues.* 1999 May–Jun; 9(3): 121–134. 19 refs. BE62419.

> abortion, induced; contraception; *health facilities; obstetrics and gynecology; organization and administration; referral and consultation; *religious hospitals; *reproduction; reproductive technologies; Roman Catholic ethics; *Roman Catholics; sterilization (sexual); *women's health services; *health facility mergers; nonprofit organizations; United States

Wells, Barron; Spinks, Nelda. The context of ethics in the health care industry. *Health Manpower Management.* 1996; 22(1): 21–29. 8 refs. BE59338.

> *administrators; *advertising; aged; disabled; drug industry; drugs; economics; *employment; females; *health care delivery; *health facilities; *institutional ethics; medical fees; minority groups; *misconduct; social discrimination; standards; *business ethics; quality assurance; United States

Wikler, Daniel; Marchand, Sarah. Macro–allocation: dividing up the health care budget. *In:* Kuhse, Helga; Singer, Peter, eds. A Companion to Bioethics. Malden, MA: Blackwell; 1998: 306–315. 19 refs. ISBN

BE = bioethics accession number   fn. = footnotes   refs. = references

0–631–19737–0. BE59505.
   costs and benefits; decision making; economics; health;
   *health care; justice; moral policy; public participation;
   public policy; quality adjusted life years; quality of life;
   *resource allocation; self induced illness

Williams, Alan. Intergenerational equity: an exploration
of the 'fair innings' argument. *Health Economics.* 1997
Mar–Apr; 6(2): 117–132. 28 fn. BE59337.
   *age factors; aged; health; *health care; international aspects;
   *justice; prolongation of life; *quality adjusted life years;
   quality of life; *resource allocation; selection for treatment;
   *socioeconomic factors; Great Britain

Witte, Kim. The manipulative nature of health
communication research: ethical issues and guidelines.
American Behavioral Scientist. 1994 Nov; 38(2): 285–293.
26 refs. BE61210.
   *behavior control; common good; *communication; decision
   making; goals; guidelines; *health education; health hazards;
   *health promotion; informal social control; information
   dissemination; preventive medicine; public participation;
   risk; standards

Institutionalised racism in health care. [Editorial]. *Lancet.*
1999 Mar 6; 353(9155): 765. BE61005.
   biomedical research; blacks; *health care delivery; *minority
   groups; morbidity; mortality; physicians; resource allocation;
   selection for treatment; *social discrimination;
   socioeconomic factors; stigmatization; whites; Great Britain;
   United States

HEALTH CARE/ECONOMICS

**Ad Hoc Committee on Health Care Issues and the
Church.** The non–profit nature of Catholic health care
ministry. *Dolentium Hominum: Church and Health in the
World.* 1997; 36(12th Yr., No. 3): 44. BE60599.
   *health care; *organization and administration; property
   rights; *proprietary hospitals; *religious hospitals; *Roman
   Catholic ethics; health facility mergers; *nonprofit
   organizations; United States

Alexander, Elizabeth; Brody, Howard. Ethics by the
numbers: monitoring physicians' integrity in managed
care. *Journal of Clinical Ethics.* 1998 Fall; 9(3): 297–305.
17 fn. BE61338.
   comparative studies; *conflict of interest; economics;
   gatekeeping; *government financing; *health insurance
   reimbursement; *incentives; *managed care programs;
   patient advocacy; *physicians; *primary health care; quality
   of health care; *referral and consultation; remuneration;
   resource allocation; *capitation fee; *physician's practice
   patterns; Michigan

Asch, Steven; Frayne, Susan; Waitzkin, Howard. To
discharge or not to discharge: ethics of care for an
undocumented immigrant. *Journal of Health Care for the
Poor and Underserved.* 1995; 6(1): 3–9. 27 refs. BE60569.
   *aliens; autonomy; beneficence; case studies; decision
   making; gatekeeping; government financing; health care
   delivery; hospitals; indigents; justice; *kidney diseases; legal
   aspects; *patient discharge; *physicians; public policy;
   *refusal to treat; *renal dialysis; *resource allocation;
   *selection for treatment; United States

Baker, Robert. American independence and the right to
emergency care. *JAMA.* 1999 Mar 3; 281(9): 859–860.
12 refs. BE60244.
   administrators; codes of ethics; economics; *emergency care;
   historical aspects; *legal aspects; *legal rights; legislation;
   *managed care programs; *medical ethics; *moral
   obligations; patient advocacy; *patients' rights; physician
   patient relationship; *physicians; professional organizations;

refusal to treat; *utilitarianism; *business ethics; *Patients'
   Bill of Rights; *United States

**Beecham, Linda; Dorozynski, Alexander; Sheldon,
Tony, et al.** Viagra falls: the debate over rationing
continues -- Britain, France, Netherlands, Italy,
Switzerland, Spain, United States, Germany, Israel. *BMJ
(British Medical Journal).* 1998 Sep 26; 317(7162):
836–838. BE59650.
   *drugs; gatekeeping; *government financing; health care;
   *health insurance reimbursement; *international aspects;
   *males; national health insurance; *patient care; physicians;
   private sector; public policy; resource allocation; selection
   for treatment; sexuality; *impotence; personal financing;
   France; Germany; Great Britain; Israel; Italy; Netherlands;
   Spain; Switzerland; United States; *Viagra

Bernard, David B.; Shulkin, David J. The media vs
managed health care: are we seeing a full court press?
Archives of Internal Medicine. 1998 Oct 26; 158(19):
2109–2111. 9 refs. BE59578.
   *editorial policies; *evaluation; *information dissemination;
   *managed care programs; *mass media; motivation; patient
   satisfaction; physicians; public opinion; social impact; survey;
   *United States

BACKGROUND: Despite the fact that medical
coverage for many Americans is shifting rapidly from
traditional insurance to managed care, studies suggest
that most citizens have limited knowledge or
understanding of the implication of this change.
OBJECTIVE: To evaluate the predominant message
being portrayed by the lay press on managed care.
METHODS: We conducted a review of newspaper
articles dealing with managed care from several leading
national newspapers. Surveys, editorials, letters to the
editor, or nonclinical articles were excluded. The articles
were examined to evaluate their likely effect on the
reader's willingness to join a managed care organization,
and were scored using a standardized survey instrument.
The final analysis included data from 85 articles from
an original pool of 277. RESULTS: In only 8% of cases,
the articles were considered likely to have had a positive
influence on the reader and, thus, encourage them to
join or remain with a managed care organization. More
important, in fully two thirds of cases, we believed the
articles portrayed so unfavorable a message that the
reader was less likely to join, or might even decide to
leave, a managed care organization. The articles dealt
most frequently (67%) with patient concerns with
managed care, focused mainly on cost and quality issues,
and managed care representatives were the people whose
opinions were most commonly (53%) solicited.
CONCLUSIONS: It seems highly likely that public
perception of managed health care will be influenced
by the strongly negative representation being portrayed
by the newspapers. While debate over the good vs bad
features of managed care continues, available evidence
suggests this form of health care coverage continues to
grow. The press is likely to remain an important source
by which information about managed care is transmitted
to the public and will certainly influence public decision
making on the issue. If the current negative
representation continues, we may soon begin to see a
widespread backlash of public opinion opposing this
form of health care.

Binstock, Robert H.; Murray, Thomas H. Genetics and
long–term–care insurance: ethical and policy issues. *In:*
Post, Stephen G.; Whitehouse, Peter J., eds. Genetic
Testing for Alzheimer Disease: Ethical and Clinical
Issues. Baltimore, MD: Johns Hopkins University Press;
1998: 155–176. 44 refs. ISBN 0–8018–5840–2. BE60722.

BE = bioethics accession number   fn. = footnotes   refs. = references

aged; *dementia; *economics; family members; federal government; *genetic information; genetic predisposition; *genetic screening; government financing; government regulation; *health insurance; health insurance reimbursement; home care; industry; insurance selection bias; *justice; *long-term care; *moral policy; nursing homes; obligations of society; *public policy; risk; socioeconomic factors; state government; trends; Medicaid; United States

Binstock, Robert H. Old-age-based rationing: from rhetoric to risk? *Generations (American Society on Aging).* 1994 Winter; 18(4): 37–41. 41 refs. BE60550.
    *age factors; *aged; *economics; federal government; government financing; *health care delivery; justice; *public policy; quality of life; *resource allocation; *selection for treatment; terminal care; wedge argument; withholding treatment; Medicare; *United States

Black, Douglas. Medicalised erections on demand? [Editorial]. *Journal of Medical Ethics.* 1999 Feb; 25(1): 5–7. 2 refs. BE61133.
    decision making; drug industry; *drugs; *government financing; government regulation; health; health care; *health insurance reimbursement; international aspects; *males; *patient care; physicians; politics; public policy; quality of life; resource allocation; sexuality; *impotence; needs; personal financing; Great Britain; National Health Service; *Viagra

Black, Peter. Managed care and the patient: surgical, ethical and legal considerations. *Journal of Clinical Neuroscience.* 1997 Apr; 4(2): 149–151. 10 refs. BE59555.
    economics; gatekeeping; legal aspects; *managed care programs; medical ethics; patient advocacy; patient discharge; physician patient relationship; referral and consultation; *surgery; United States

Blake, Robert L.; Early, Elizabeth K. Patients' attitudes about gifts to physicians from pharmaceutical companies. *Journal of the American Board of Family Practice.* 1995 Nov–Dec; 8(6): 457–464. 21 refs. BE61561.
    advertising; *attitudes; *conflict of interest; continuing education; decision making; *drug industry; *drugs; economics; *financial support; *gifts; guidelines; incentives; *knowledge, attitudes, practice; *patient care; *patients; *physicians; professional organizations; survey; Missouri

Bodenheimer, Thomas. Disease management –– promises and pitfalls. *New England Journal of Medicine.* 1999 Apr 15; 340(15): 1202–1205. 28 refs. BE61031.
    *chronically ill; conflict of interest; contracts; *costs and benefits; diabetes; *drug industry; drugs; *economics; entrepreneurship; health care delivery; health maintenance organizations; *managed care programs; *patient care; patient care team; patient education; physician patient relationship; *primary health care; quality of health care; risks and benefits; United States

Bodenheimer, Thomas. The American health care system: physicians and the changing medical marketplace. *New England Journal of Medicine.* 1999 Feb 18; 340(7): 584–588. 38 refs. BE60995.
    contracts; *economics; gatekeeping; *health care delivery; health maintenance organizations; incentives; interprofessional relations; *managed care programs; medical specialties; organization and administration; patient satisfaction; physician patient relationship; *physicians; primary health care; quality of health care; referral and consultation; remuneration; sociology of medicine; time factors; withholding treatment; capitation fee; *United States

Brody, Howard. Ethics in managed care: a matter of focus, a matter of integrity. *Michigan Medicine.* 1998 Dec; 97(12): 28–32. BE61487.
    *conflict of interest; incentives; *managed care programs;

medical ethics; patient advocacy; *physicians; quality of health care; *remuneration; resource allocation; integrity; United States

Brody, Howard; Miller, Franklin G. The internal morality of medicine: explication and application to managed care. *Journal of Medicine and Philosophy.* 1998 Aug; 23(4): 384–410. 58 refs. 16 fn. BE60630.
    assisted suicide; bioethics; capital punishment; conflict of interest; conscience; contraception; contracts; cosmetic surgery; disclosure; drugs; economics; entrepreneurship; family members; family relationship; gatekeeping; *goals; incentives; *managed care programs; *medical ethics; *medicine; misconduct; models, theoretical; *moral obligations; morality; obligations to society; patient advocacy; patient care; physician patient relationship; *physician's role; *physicians; postmodernism; primary health care; professional competence; professional ethics; quality of health care; resource allocation; sexuality; sports medicine; trust; values; voluntary sterilization; withholding treatment; gag clauses; health services misuse; undertreatment

Some ethical issues facing contemporary medicine cannot be fully understood without addressing medicine's internal morality. Medicine as a profession is characterized by certain moral goals and morally acceptable means for achieving those goals. The list of appropriate goals and means allows some medical actions to be classified as clear violations of the internal morality, and others as borderline or controversial cases. Replies are available for common objections, including the superfluity of internal morality for ethical analysis, the argument that internal morality is merely an apology for medicine's traditional power and authority, and the claim that there is no single, "core" internal morality. The value of addressing the internal morality of medicine may be illustrated by a detailed investigation of ethical issues posed by managed care. Managed care poses some fundamental challenges for medicine's internal morality, but also calls for thoughtful reflection and reconsideration of some traditionally held moral views on patient fidelity in particular.

Brown, Murray G. Rationing health care in Canada. *Annals of Health Law.* 1993; 2: 101–119. 22 fn. BE59829.
    compassion; costs and benefits; decision making; *economics; *government financing; *health care delivery; hospitals; justice; *national health insurance; organization and administration; physicians; private sector; *public policy; public sector; *resource allocation; treatment outcome; *values; needs; *Canada

Buchanan, Allen. Managed care: rationing without justice, but not unjustly. *Journal of Health Politics, Policy and Law.* 1998 Aug; 23(4): 617–634. 16 refs. Commented on by S.D. Goold, p. 687–695. BE59780.
    contracts; costs and benefits; decision making; disadvantaged; disclosure; economics; ethical theory; gatekeeping; *health care; *health care delivery; health insurance; *institutional ethics; *justice; *managed care programs; *moral obligations; *moral policy; *physician's role; *private sector; proprietary health facilities; public participation; *public sector; *quality of health care; *resource allocation; *rights; *standards; terminology; *withholding treatment; *United States

Three ethical criticisms of managed care are often voiced: (1) by "skimming the cream" of the patient population, managed care organizations fail to discharge their obligations to improve access, or at least, to not worsen it; (2) managed care organizations engage in rationing, thereby depriving patients of care to which they are entitled; and (3) by pressuring physicians to ration care, managed care organizations interfere with physicians' fulfillment of their fiduciary obligations to

---

provide the best care for each patient. This article argues that each of these criticisms is misconceived. The first rests on the false assumption that the health care system includes a workable division of responsibility regarding access that assigns obligations concerning access to managed care organizations. The second and third criticisms wrongly assume that we in the United States have taken the first step toward assuring equitable access to care for all, articulating a standard for what counts as an "adequate level of care" to which all are entitled. These three misguided criticisms obscure the most fundamental ethical flaw of managed care: the fact that it operates in an institutional setting within which no connection can be made between the activity of rationing and the basic requirements of justice.

Buchanan, Robert J. Tuberculosis and HIV infection: utilization of public programs to fund treatment. *AIDS and Public Policy Journal.* 1997 Winter; 12(4): 122–136. 54 fn. Includes tables of states in which state or local health departments provide care or services to people with tuberculosis. BE59299.
> AIDS; communicable diseases; community services; drugs; *government financing; *health care delivery; HIV seropositivity; home care; indigents; municipal government; *patient care; prevalence; *public health; *public policy; *state government; survey; *tuberculosis; case managers; Medicaid; Medicare; Ryan White Comprehensive AIDS Resources Emergency Act; *United States

Burton, Thomas M. A prostate researcher tested firm's product -- and sat on its board. [News]. *Wall Street Journal.* 1998 Mar 19: A1, A8. BE59671.
> *biomedical research; *conflict of interest; disclosure; *drug industry; drugs; editorial policies; *financial support; fraud; investigators; medical devices; *misconduct; *physicians; *remuneration; surgery; *therapeutic research; *Oesterling, Joseph; University of Michigan

Callahan, Daniel. Age, sex, and resource allocation. *In:* Walker, Margaret Urban, ed. Mother Time: Women, Aging, and Ethics. Lanham, MD: Rowman and Littlefield; 1999: 189–199. 9 fn. ISBN 0–8476–9260–4. BE61900.
> age factors; *aged; biomedical technologies; chronically ill; disabled; disadvantaged; *economics; federal government; *females; *government financing; *health care; *health care reform; health promotion; home care; justice; long–term care; males; mortality; public policy; quality of life; rehabilitation; *resource allocation; social discrimination; *women's health; *women's health services; Medicare; *United States

Callahan, Daniel. Must the young and old struggle over health care resources? *Journal Of Long Term Home Health Care.* 1996 Fall; 15(4): 4–14. Edited version of the annual Iago Galdston Lecture, presented at the New York Academy of Medicine on 3 Jun 1996. BE60947.
> *age factors; *aged; biomedical technologies; children; *economics; *health care; long–term care; moral obligations; obligations of society; public policy; *resource allocation; social impact; trends; withholding treatment; Medicare; United States

Chin, Marshall H. Health outcomes and managed care: discussing the hidden issues. *American Journal Of Managed Care.* 1997 May; 3(5): 756–762. 42 refs. BE60027.
> autonomy; costs and benefits; evidence-based medicine; gatekeeping; guidelines; *health care reform; health insurance; *health services research; incentives; indigents; institutional ethics; *managed care programs; obligations to society; patient satisfaction; patients; physicians; policy

analysis; practice guidelines; preventive medicine; professional autonomy; *public policy; *quality of health care; referral and consultation; remuneration; resource allocation; treatment outcome; uncertainty; values; vulnerable populations; withholding treatment; utilization review; United States

Chisholm, John. Viagra: a botched test case for rationing. [Editorial]. *BMJ (British Medical Journal).* 1999 Jan 30; 318(7179): 273–274. 12 refs. BE60578.
> *drugs; *government financing; *males; patient care; *public policy; *resource allocation; selection for treatment; sexuality; *impotence; *Great Britain; National Health Service; *Viagra

Churchill, Larry R. Mapping the ethical terrain of managed care. *NCCE News (Veterans Health Administration National Center for Clinical Ethics).* 1998 Winter; 6(1): 1–2, 10–11. 7 refs. BE59850.
> conflict of interest; economics; health care delivery; *managed care programs; medical ethics; patient advocacy; patients' rights; physician patient relationship; physicians; trust; business ethics; United States

Cong, Yali. Ethical challenges in critical care medicine: a Chinese perspective. *Journal of Medicine and Philosophy.* 1998 Dec; 23(6): 581–600. 21 refs. 1 fn. BE62067.
> allowing to die; bioethics; *critically ill; decision making; *economics; family members; geographic factors; government financing; *health care delivery; hospitals; *intensive care units; justice; legal aspects; medical devices; non–Western World; patient admission; physician patient relationship; physicians; public policy; *resource allocation; values; personal financing; *China

The major ethical challenges for critical care medicine in China include the high cost of patient care in the ICU, the effect of payment mechanisms on access to critical care, the fact that much more money is spent on patients who die than on ones who live, the extent to which an attempt to rescue and save a patient is made, and the great geographical disparity in distribution of critical care. The ethical problems surrounding critical care medicine bear much relation to the culture, public policy and health care system in China. The essay concludes that China should allocate more resources to ordinary medical services rather than to critical care medicine.

Cunningham, Peter J.; Grossman, Joy M.; St. Peter, Robert F., et al. Managed care and physicians' provision of charity care. *JAMA.* 1999 Mar 24–31; 281(12): 1087–1092. 26 refs. BE60946.
> evaluation studies; *indigents; *managed care programs; *patient care; *physicians; *remuneration; statistics; survey; *uncompensated care; United States

CONTEXT: Health system changes may be affecting the ability of physicians to provide care with little or no compensation from patients who are uninsured and under–insured and may result in decreased access to physicians for uninsured persons. OBJECTIVE: To examine the association between managed care and physicians' provision of charity care. DESIGN: The 1996–1997 Community Tracking Study physician survey. SETTING AND PARTICIPANTS: A nationally representative sample of 10881 physicians from 60 randomly selected communities. MAIN OUTCOME MEASURE: The number of hours in the month prior to the interview that the physician provided care for free or at reduced fees because of the financial need of the patient. RESULTS: Overall, 77.3% of respondents provided an average of 10.3 hours of charity care per week. Physicians who derive at least 85% of their practice revenue from managed care plans were considerably less likely to provide charity care and spend fewer hours providing charity care than physicians with little involvement in managed care plans (P = .01). In addition, physicians who practice in areas with high managed care penetration provided fewer hours of charity care than physicians in other areas, regardless of their own level of involvement with managed care (P less than .01). Differences in charity care provision were also shown for other important factors, including ownership of the practice and practice arrangements (more charity care occurred in solo and 2-physician practices; P less than .01). CONCLUSION: Physicians involved with managed care plans and those who practice in areas with high managed care penetration tend to provide less charity care.

Daniel, C. Ralph; Elewski, Boni E.; Scher, Richard K. Proposed guidelines for speakers discussing medications and other products. *Cutis.* 1997 May; 59(5): 271-272. 4 refs. BE59530.

> advertising; conflict of interest; *continuing education; disclosure; *drug industry; drugs; faculty; *financial support; *gifts; *guidelines; *medical education; *physicians; dermatology; United States

Deutsch, Lisa B. Medicaid payment for organ transplants: the extent of mandated coverage. *Columbia Journal of Law and Social Problems.* 1997 Winter; 30(2): 185-213. 127 fn. BE61254.

> economics; federal government; *government financing; indigents; judicial action; justice; *legal aspects; *organ transplantation; *public policy; resource allocation; *state government; *Medicaid; Social Security Act; *United States; *Wisconsin

Diekema, Douglas S. Children first: the need to reform financing of health care services for children. [Editorial]. *Journal of Health Care for the Poor and Underserved.* 1996; 7(1): 3-14. 48 refs. BE60388.

> adolescents; age factors; beneficence; *children; employment; *financial support; government financing; health care; *health care reform; health insurance; *indigents; justice; libertarianism; moral obligations; *obligations of society; resource allocation; socioeconomic factors; Medicaid; *United States

Dyer, Clare. Transsexuals win case for NHS funded surgery. [News]. *BMJ (British Medical Journal).* 1999 Jan 9; 318(7176): 75. BE62607.

> *government financing; *health care; *legal aspects; *legal rights; resource allocation; *surgery; *transsexualism; *Great Britain; *National Health Service

Emanuel, Ezekiel J.; Goldman, Lee. Protecting patient welfare in managed care: six safeguards. *Journal of Health Politics, Policy and Law.* 1998 Aug; 23(4): 635-659. 71 refs. Commented on by S.D. Goold, p. 687-695. BE59781.

> *accountability; *conflict of interest; decision making; *disclosure; due process; *economics; entrepreneurship; *guidelines; health care delivery; *incentives; *institutional policies; *managed care programs; mandatory programs; medical ethics; organization and administration; patient participation; physician self-referral; physician's role; *physicians; *practice guidelines; quality of health care; *regulation; remuneration; resource allocation; *review committees; self regulation; *standards; trust; withholding treatment; health services misuse; managed competition; quality assurance; *United States

The public is very suspicious and fearful that managed care threatens their health because of its interest in reducing costs. Because physicians' decisions control 75 percent of all health care spending, managed care organizations are focusing their cost-cutting strategies on influencing physician decision making through financial incentives and guidelines. These two techniques have had some important contributions, especially in enhancing efficiency and standardizing care to a high level. Nevertheless, they pose a threat -- and are perceived by the public to pose a threat -- to patients' health and well-being. How can we mitigate the threats to patient welfare posed by financial incentives and guidelines? We propose and analyze six safeguards. These safeguards are not an attempt to revive the fee-for-service system, but an effort to make managed care ethical and to focus it on improving patient welfare. They are designed to work together to ensure that patient welfare remains the primary focus of managed care organizations; they try to create institutional structures that emphasize quality over mere cost reductions.

Epstein, Richard A.; Lindsay, Donald G.; Lally, James F., et al. Articulating a social ethic for health care. [Letters and response]. *JAMA.* 1998 Mar 11; 279(10): 745-746. 3 refs. BE59226.

> children; freedom; health care; *health care delivery; health care reform; *indigents; quality of health care; resource allocation; socioeconomic factors; United States

Evans, Roger W. Liver transplantation in a managed care environment. *Liver Transplantation and Surgery.* 1995 Jan; 1(1): 61-75. 75 refs. BE60903.

> biomedical research; biomedical technologies; *costs and benefits; *economics; geographic factors; goals; health care; health care reform; health facilities; justice; *livers; *managed care programs; *organ transplantation; physicians; practice guidelines; prognosis; *resource allocation; risk; *selection for treatment; transplant recipients; treatment outcome; trends; *United States

Fein, Esther B. Calling infertility a disease, couples battle with insurers. [News]. *New York Times.* 1998 Feb 22: 1, 34. BE59611.

> drugs; embryo transfer; *health insurance reimbursement; in vitro fertilization; *infertility; *reproductive technologies; personal financing; United States

Feldman, Debra S.; Novack, Dennis H.; Gracely, Edward. Effects of managed care on physician-patient relationships, quality of care, and the ethical practice of medicine. *Archives of Internal Medicine.* 1998 Aug 10-24; 158(15): 1626-1632. 54 refs. BE59173.

> *attitudes; communication; confidentiality; *conflict of interest; decision making; disclosure; economics; females; gatekeeping; incentives; informed consent; males; *managed care programs; medical ethics; medical specialties; patient advocacy; patient care; patient participation; *physician patient relationship; *physicians; preventive medicine; *primary health care; professional autonomy; *quality of health care; referral and consultation; *social impact; survey; time factors; trust; continuity of patient care; Pennsylvania; United States

BACKGROUND: Survey studies have shown that physicians believe managed care is having significant impact on many of their professional obligations. METHODS: Primary care physicians were asked about the impact of managed care on: (1) physician-patient relationships, (2) the ability of physicians to carry out their professional ethical obligations, and (3) quality of patient care. In 1996 we surveyed 1011 primary care physicians in Pennsylvania. The survey group's responses were graded on a Likert scale. Space was provided for respondents to include written comments. The SPSS statistical software (SPSS Inc, Chicago, Ill)

BE = bioethics accession number   fn. = footnotes   refs. = references

was used to analyze the data. RESULTS: The response rate was 55%. Most respondents indicated that under managed care physicians are less able to avoid conflicts of interest and less able to place the best interests of patients first. The majority responded that quality of health care is compromised by limitations in location of diagnostic tests, length of hospital stay, and choice of specialists. A significant minority (27%-49%) noted a decrease in the physician's ability to carry out ethical obligations, to respect patient autonomy, and to respect confidentiality in physician–patient communication. Most physicians expressed that managed care made no impact on ability to obtain informed consent or to provide information. There were small but statistically significant sex differences, with female physicians more negative toward managed care. CONCLUSIONS: Many physicians surveyed believe managed care has significant negative effects on the physician–patient relationship, the ability to carry out ethical obligations, and on quality of patient care. These results have implications for health care system reform efforts.

Feldman, Miriam K. The doctor–patient bond: covenant or business contract? *Minnesota Medicine.* 1997 Sep; 80(9): 12–16. BE59932.
  *conflict of interest; decision making; disclosure; economics; gatekeeping; *managed care programs; *physician patient relationship; physicians; public opinion; *trust; withholding treatment; *Minnesota; United States

Finestone, Albert J.; Feldman, Debra; Beasley, John W., et al. Gatekeeping: good or bad, but never indifferent. [Letters and response]. *JAMA.* 1998 Mar 25; 279(12): 908–910. 6 refs. BE59233.
  accountability; *attitudes; decision making; *economics; *gatekeeping; incentives; *managed care programs; organization and administration; patient advocacy; patient care; physician patient relationship; *physician's role; *physicians; preventive medicine; primary health care; professional autonomy; quality of health care; referral and consultation; remuneration; *resource allocation; *risks and benefits; trust; United States

Forret, Patricia; McGuire, Beverly. Ethical guidelines for managed care contract negotiations. *Journal of Health Care Finance.* 1996 Winter; 23(2): 38–45. BE59777.
  abortion, induced; common good; confidentiality; *contracts; economics; employment; ethics committees; evaluation; *guidelines; indigents; *institutional ethics; justice; *managed care programs; moral obligations; organization and administration; quality of health care; *religious hospitals; *Roman Catholic ethics; value of life; values; Eastern Mercy Health System (PA); Mercy Health System (OH)

Fuchs, Victor; Iglehart, John K. Physicians as agents of social control: the thoughts of Victor Fuchs. [Interview]. *Health Affairs.* 1998 Jan–Feb; 17(1): 90–96. 5 refs. BE59179.
  administrators; biomedical research; costs and benefits; cultural pluralism; decision making; *economics; employment; evidence-based medicine; financial support; goals; government financing; health care; *health care delivery; health care reform; health insurance; health promotion; international aspects; managed care programs; medical education; medical ethics; national health insurance; obligations of society; physician patient relationship; *physician's role; public policy; resource allocation; social control; *sociology of medicine; technology assessment; *trends; *values; business ethics; nonprofit organizations; Europe; Medicare; *United States

Fuchs, Victor R. Who Shall Live? Health, Economics,

and Social Choice. Expanded Edition. River Edge, NJ: World Scientific; 1998. 278 p. (Economic ideas leading to the 21st century; v.3). Includes references. Six complementary papers dealing with national health insurance, poverty and health, and other policy issues, including Fuchs's 1996 presidential address to the American Economic Association, accompanying the original 1974 text. ISBN 981–02–3201–2. BE62770.
  age factors; biomedical technologies; costs and benefits; *decision making; drug industry; drugs; *economics; employment; females; health; *health care delivery; *health care reform; health insurance; health maintenance organizations; historical aspects; hospitals; indigents; international aspects; males; morbidity; mortality; *national health insurance; organization and administration; physician's role; physicians; *public policy; *resource allocation; socioeconomic factors; values; *United States

Gervais, Karen G.; Priester, Reinhard; Vawter, Dorothy E., et al, eds. Ethical Challenges in Managed Care: A Casebook. Washington, DC: Georgetown University Press; 1999. 372 p. Includes references. ISBN 0–87840–719–7. BE60175.
  administrators; aged; alternative therapies; biomedical research; case studies; children; chronically ill; clinical ethics; conflict of interest; costs and benefits; critically ill; cultural pluralism; economics; emergency care; health care; health insurance reimbursement; hospitals; incentives; *institutional ethics; justice; *managed care programs; medical education; mentally ill; moral obligations; nurses; nursing homes; obligations to society; patient advocacy; patient care; patient transfer; physicians; primary health care; public health; quality of health care; referral and consultation; rehabilitation; religion; remuneration; resource allocation; standards; business ethics; capitation fee; investigational therapies; United States

Ginzberg, Eli. The uncertain future of managed care. *New England Journal of Medicine.* 1999 Jan 14; 340(2): 144–146. 2 refs. BE60985.
  aged; alternatives; *economics; employment; federal government; government financing; health care delivery; health insurance; indigents; *managed care programs; organizational policies; patients' rights; physicians; political activity; remuneration; resource allocation; *trends; withholding treatment; universal coverage; Medicaid; Medicare; *United States

Ginzberg, Eli. US health system reform in the early 21st century. *JAMA.* 1998 Nov 4; 280(17): 1539. 4 refs. BE59635.
  *economics; federal government; government financing; *health care reform; managed care programs; national health insurance; public policy; state government; trends; personal financing; *Twenty-First Century; *United States

Glantz, Leonard H.; Annas, George J.; Grodin, Michael A., et al. Research in developing countries: taking "benefit" seriously. *Hastings Center Report.* 1998 Nov–Dec; 28(6): 38–42. 18 fn. BE61285.
  *developing countries; drugs; *economics; *financial support; guidelines; *health care; HIV seropositivity; *human experimentation; *international aspects; pregnant women; preventive medicine; *risks and benefits; standards; Africa; AZT

Glasser, Ronald J. The doctor is not in: on the managed failure of managed health care. *Harper's Magazine.* 1998 Mar; 296(1774): 35–41. 3 fn. BE59989.
  administrators; aged; biomedical technologies; *economics; gatekeeping; goals; *health maintenance organizations; industry; insurance selection bias; *managed care programs; physicians; remuneration; self induced illness; *values; withholding treatment; health services misuse; United States

---

BE = bioethics accession number   fn. = footnotes   refs. = references

Gold, Rachel Benson; Richards, Cory L. Managed care and unintended pregnancy. *Women's Health Issues.* 1998 May–Jun; 8(3): 134–147. 18 refs. BE60444.
> confidentiality; *contraception; *family planning; federal government; *females; government financing; government regulation; *health insurance reimbursement; health maintenance organizations; *managed care programs; obstetrics and gynecology; primary health care; *public policy; state government; *women's health services; Medicaid; United States

Gonen, Julianna S. Managed care and unintended pregnancy: testing the limits of prevention. *Women's Health Issues.* 1999 Mar–Apr; 9(2, Suppl.): 26S–35S. 24 refs. BE61969.
> *adolescents; adults; confidentiality; *contraception; costs and benefits; *family planning; federal government; government financing; health insurance; *health insurance reimbursement; health maintenance organizations; *managed care programs; methods; organizational policies; parental consent; parental notification; *public policy; *quality of health care; religious hospitals; Roman Catholics; state government; statistics; *women's health services; Medicaid; United States

Goold, Susan Dorr. Money and trust: relationships between patients, physicians, and health plans. *Journal of Health Politics, Policy and Law.* 1998 Aug; 23(4): 687–695. 8 refs. Commentary on D. Mechanic, "The functions and limitations of trust in the provision of medical care," p. 661–686; on A. Buchanan, "Managed care: rationing without justice, but not unjustly," p. 617–634; and on E.J. Ezekiel and L. Goldman, "Protecting patient welfare in managed care: six safeguards," p. 635–659. BE59783.
> accountability; conflict of interest; contracts; decision making; disclosure; *economics; evaluation; guidelines; health care delivery; health insurance; *incentives; institutional ethics; justice; *managed care programs; moral obligations; organization and administration; patient participation; physician patient relationship; *physicians; professional competence; professional organizations; quality of health care; regulation; remuneration; resource allocation; review committees; *trust

In response to three articles on managed care by Allen Buchanan, David Mechanic, and Ezekiel Emanual and Lee Goldman (this issue), I discuss doctor–patient and organization–member trust and the moral obligations of those relationships. Trust in managed care organizations (providers of and payers for health care) stands in stark contrast to the current contractual model of health insurance purchase, but is more coherent with consumer expectations and with the provider role of such organizations. Such trust is likely to differ from that between doctors and patients. Financial reimbursement systems for physicians, one example of organizational change in our health system, can be evaluated for their impact on both kinds of trust according to their intrusiveness, openness, and goals. Although involving managed care enrollees in value–laden decisions that affect them is commendable, restrictions on or regulation of physician incentive systems may be better accomplished on a national level.

Gray, Gwen. Access to medical care under strain: new pressures in Canada and Australia. *Journal of Health Politics, Policy and Law.* 1998 Dec; 23(6): 905–947. 113 refs. BE59785.
> comparative studies; *economics; government financing; health; *health care delivery; health insurance; indigents; *international aspects; justice; national health insurance; politics; *private sector; public policy; *public sector; social impact; socioeconomic factors; trends; personal financing; *Australia; *Canada; Europe; Organization for Economic Cooperation and Development; United States

Health policy changes intended to achieve cost control in OECD countries run the risk of reintroducing financial barriers to health care. However, although the problems faced are similar, different countries are dealing with the situation in different ways. For example, Canada and Australia, which share many similarities, have taken quite different policy paths in the last decade: Canada has preserved universal access, whereas Australian policy is promoting a two–tier system through the provision of public subsidies for private insurance. The evidence is that country–specific factors such as institutional arrangements, attitudes, and values intersect with economic and financial factors to shape policy outcomes. Moreover, the Canadian and Australian experiences suggest that in relation to access issues, attitudes and values are the key policy determinants.

Griffith, David. Reasons for not seeing drug representatives: lightening workload, cutting costs, and improving quality. [Editorial]. *BMJ (British Medical Journal).* 1999 Jul 10; 319(7202): 69–70. 9 refs. BE62151.
> advertising; alternatives; communication; *conflict of interest; *drug industry; *drugs; *economics; information dissemination; motivation; *patient care; *physicians; quality of health care; time factors; *physician's practice patterns; Great Britain

Gross, Jane. The fight to cover infertility: suit says employer's refusal to pay is form of bias. [News]. *New York Times.* 1998 Dec 7: B1, B6. BE60367.
> *employment; *health insurance reimbursement; infertility; *legal aspects; *reproductive technologies; social discrimination; Equal Employment Opportunity Commission; New York; Saks, Rochelle; United States

Grumbach, Kevin; Osmond, Dennis; Vranizan, Karen, et al. Primary care physicians' experience of financial incentives in managed–care systems. *New England Journal of Medicine.* 1998 Nov 19; 339(21): 1516–1521. 12 refs. BE60039.
> *attitudes; coercion; *economics; *incentives; *knowledge, attitudes, practice; *managed care programs; patient satisfaction; *physicians; *primary health care; quality of health care; referral and consultation; statistics; survey; withholding treatment; *California

BACKGROUND: Managed–care organizations' use of financial incentives to influence the practice of primary care physicians is controversial. We studied the prevalence and effects of these incentives. METHODS: We surveyed a probability sample of primary care physicians practicing in the largest urban counties in California in 1996. The physicians were asked about the types of incentives they encountered, the amount of income that was keyed to incentives, their experience of pressure in their practices, and the ways in which such pressure affected patient care. RESULTS: Data were analyzed for 766 physicians involved in managed–care systems. Thirty–eight percent of these physicians reported that their arrangements with the managed–care system included some type of incentive in the form of a bonus. Fifty–seven percent of the physicians reported that they felt pressure from the managed–care organization to limit referrals (17 percent said they believed such pressure compromised patient care), and 75 percent felt pressure to see more patients per day (24 percent believed such pressure compromised patient care). The physicians who reported that their financial arrangements included an incentive based on referrals were more likely than others to have felt pressured to limit referrals in a manner that compromised care (adjusted odds ratio 2.5; 95 percent confidence

---

BE = bioethics accession number   fn. = footnotes   refs. = references

interval, 1.2 to 5.0), and physicians with an incentive based on productivity were more likely to have felt pressure to see more patients that they believed compromised care (adjusted odds ratio, 2.1; 95 percent confidence interval, 1.2 to 3.8). The physicians whose health care systems used incentives keyed to productivity were less likely than others to be very satisfied with their practices (adjusted odds ratio, 0.4; 95 percent confidence interval, 0.2 to 0.6), whereas those whose systems included incentives related to the quality of care or patients' satisfaction were more likely to be very satisfied (adjusted odds ratio, 1.8; 95 percent confidence interval, 1.1 to 3.0). CONCLUSIONS: Many managed-care organizations include financial incentives for primary care physicians that are indexed to various measures of performance. Incentives that depend on limiting referrals or on greater productivity apply selective pressure to physicians in ways that are believed to compromise care. Incentives that depend on the quality of care and patients' satisfaction are associated with greater job satisfaction among physicians.

Grumbach, Kevin; Selby, Joe V.; Damberg, Cheryl, et al. Resolving the gatekeeper conundrum: what patients value in primary care and referrals to specialists. *JAMA.* 1999 Jul 21; 282(3): 261-266. 32 refs. BE61752.
  *attitudes; *gatekeeping; *managed care programs; medical specialties; *patient satisfaction; *patients; *physician's role; physicians; *primary health care; quality of health care; *referral and consultation; survey; trust; California
CONTEXT: Few data are available regarding how patients view the role of primary care physicians as "gatekeepers" in managed care systems. OBJECTIVE: To determine the extent to which patients value the role of their primary care physicians as first-contact care providers and coordinators of referrals, whether patients perceive that their primary care physicians impede access to specialists, and whether problems in gaining access to specialists are associated with a reduction in patients' trust and confidence in their primary care physicians. DESIGN, SETTING, AND PATIENTS: Cross-sectional survey mailed in the fall of 1997 to 12707 adult patients who were members of managed care plans and received care from 10 large physician groups in California. The response rate among eligible patients was 71%. A total of 7718 patients (mean age, 66.7 years; 32 % female) were eligible for analysis. MAIN OUTCOME MEASURES: Questionnaire items addressed 3 main topics: (1) patient attitudes toward the first-contact and coordinating role of their primary care physicians, (2) patients' ratings of their primary care physicians (trust and confidence in and satisfaction with), and (3) patient perceptions of barriers to specialty referrals. Referral barriers were analyzed as predictors of patients' ratings of their physicians. RESULTS: Almost all patients valued the role of a primary care physician as a source of first-contact care (94%) and coordinator of referrals (89%). Depending on the specific medical problem, 75% to 91% of patients preferred to seek care initially from their primary care physicians rather than specialists. Twenty-three percent reported that their primary care physicians or medical groups interfered with their ability to see specialists. Patients who had difficulty obtaining referrals were more likely to report low trust (adjusted odds ratio [OR], 2.7; 95% confidence interval [CI], 2.1-3.5), low confidence (OR, 2.2; 95% CI, 1.6-2.9), and low satisfaction (OR, 3.3; 95% CI, 2.6-4.2) with their primary care physicians. CONCLUSIONS: Patients value the first-contact and coordinating role of primary care physicians. However, managed care policies that emphasize primary care

physicians as gatekeepers impeding access to specialists undermine patients' trust and confidence in their primary care physicians.

Guyatt, Gordon. Determining an ethical stance: pharmaceutical industry involvement and family medicine residency training. [Editorial]. *Canadian Family Physician.* 1997 Nov; 43: 1898-1900, 1905-1907. 15 refs. Text in English and in French. BE62207.
  alternatives; attitudes; *conflict of interest; *drug industry; drugs; *family practice; financial support; *gifts; information dissemination; institutional policies; *internship and residency; patient care; *physicians; Canada

Halkitis, Perry N.; Dooha, Susan M. The perceptions and experiences of managed care by HIV-positive individuals in New York City. *AIDS and Public Policy Journal.* 1998 Summer; 13(2): 75-84. 23 fn. BE61345.
  *AIDS; *attitudes; communication; comparative studies; disclosure; economics; health insurance; *HIV seropositivity; homosexuals; males; *managed care programs; patient care; patient education; *patient satisfaction; *patients; physicians; primary health care; quality of health care; referral and consultation; stigmatization; survey; case managers; fee-for-service plans; personal financing; qualitative research; Gay Men's Health Crisis; Medicaid; *New York City

Hall, Mark A.; Smith, Teresa Rust; Naughton, Michelle, et al. Judicial protection of managed care consumers: an empirical study of insurance coverage disputes. *Seton Hall Law Review.* 1996; 26: 1055-1068. 13 fn. BE59855.
  contracts; decision making; federal government; *health insurance reimbursement; *judicial action; legislation; *managed care programs; private sector; public sector; statistics; survey; Employee Retirement Income Security Act (ERISA); *United States

Hanford, Jack T. Mental health and managed care. *Journal of Religion and Health.* 1998 Summer; 37(2): 159-165. 13 refs. BE61977.
  health care delivery; *managed care programs; mental health; patient advocacy; professional patient relationship; quality of health care; regulation; withholding treatment; *mental health services; Medicare; United States

Hansen, Jennie Chin; Lynch, Marty; Estes, Carroll L. Is managed care good for older persons: Yes [and] No. *In:* Scharlach, Andrew E.; Kaye, Lenard W., eds. Controversial Issues in Aging. Boston, MA: Allyn and Bacon; 1997: 114-124. 3 refs. ISBN 0-205-19381-1. BE60964.
  *aged; community services; *costs and benefits; *economics; *evaluation; gatekeeping; health care delivery; health facilities; health maintenance organizations; home care; incentives; indigents; long-term care; *managed care programs; *patient care; patient care team; physicians; preventive medicine; primary health care; program descriptions; proprietary health facilities; *quality of health care; referral and consultation; resource allocation; withholding treatment; continuity of patient care; utilization review; Medicaid; Medicare; Program of All-inclusive Care for the Elderly (PACE); United States

Hanson, Kristina W. Public opinion and the mental health parity debate: lessons from the survey literature. *Psychiatric Services.* 1998 Aug; 49(8): 1059-1066. 13 refs. BE59842.
  costs and benefits; *drug abuse; *empirical research; health care reform; *health insurance reimbursement; health services research; information dissemination; *knowledge, attitudes, practice; *mental health; *mentally ill; patient care; *public opinion; public policy; research design; United States

---

BE = bioethics accession number   fn. = footnotes   refs. = references

Harvey, John Collins. Doctors, ethics, and managed care. *Linacre Quarterly.* 1996 Nov; 63(4): 84–93. BE59307.
administrators; common good; conflict of interest; decision making; *economics; gatekeeping; health care; health care delivery; health insurance; historical aspects; incentives; justice; *managed care programs; medical ethics; *moral obligations; obligations of society; patient advocacy; physician patient relationship; *physician's role; proprietary health facilities; quality of health care; resource allocation; rights; *Roman Catholic ethics; withholding treatment; capitation fee; case managers; utilization review; Eighteenth Century; Gregory, John; Medicaid; Medicare; Nineteenth Century; Twentieth Century; *United States

Hillman, Alan L. Mediators of patient trust. [Editorial]. *JAMA.* 1998 Nov 18; 280(19): 1703–1704. 4 refs. BE59654.
attitudes; conflict of interest; incentives; knowledge, attitudes, practice; *managed care programs; patient advocacy; patients; *physician patient relationship; physicians; *remuneration; survey; *trust; capitation fee; United States

Hilzenrath, David S. Healing vs. honesty? For doctors, managed care's cost controls pose moral dilemma. [News]. *Washington Post.* 1998 Mar 15: H1, H6–H7. BE59622.
*conflict of interest; conscience; *deception; economics; employment; *health maintenance organizations; hospitals; *managed care programs; medical education; patient admission; *patient advocacy; patient care; physician patient relationship; *physicians; professional autonomy; surgery; trust; withholding treatment; United States

Himmelstein, David U.; Woolhandler, Steffie. The silence of the doctors: fifty years after Nuremberg. [Editorial]. *Journal of General Internal Medicine.* 1998 Jun; 13(6): 422–423. 5 refs. BE61459.
chronically ill; conflict of interest; *economics; historical aspects; incentives; involuntary euthanasia; killing; *managed care programs; medical ethics; misconduct; *moral complicity; National Socialism; patient advocacy; *physicians; proprietary health facilities; Netherlands; Twentieth Century; *United States

Hoffmann, Diane E. Pain management and palliative care in the era of managed care: issues for health insurers. *Journal of Law, Medicine and Ethics.* 1998 Winter; 26(4): 267–289. 126 fn. BE61163.
*administrators; aged; alternatives; anesthesia; attitudes; biomedical technologies; *chronically ill; *costs and benefits; diagnosis; drug abuse; *drugs; *economics; fraud; health facilities; *health insurance; *health insurance reimbursement; hospices; *managed care programs; medical devices; medical specialties; mental health; opioid analgesics; *organizational policies; *pain; *palliative care; *patient care; physicians; practice guidelines; public policy; *quality of health care; referral and consultation; resource allocation; surgery; survey; *terminal care; *terminally ill; therapeutic research; treatment outcome; acupuncture; biofeedback (psychology); *undertreatment; American Association of Health Plans; *Blue Cross–Blue Shield; Medicare; *United States

Holmes, Helen Bequaert. Closing the gaps: an imperative for feminist bioethics. *In:* Donchin, Anne; Purdy, Laura M., eds. Embodying Bioethics: Recent Feminist Advances. Lanham, MD: Rowman and Littlefield; 1999: 45–63. 50 refs. 16 fn. ISBN 0-8476-8924-7. BE61014.
autonomy; bioethical issues; *bioethics; clinical ethics committees; conflict of interest; *disadvantaged; employment; ethicist's role; ethicists; ethics consultation; *evaluation; females; *feminist ethics; *health care; health personnel; interprofessional relations; *justice; managed care

programs; medicine; minority groups; physicians; social dominance; social impact; *socioeconomic factors; *values; United States

Holt, Natalie. The business of medicine: the professionalization/commercialization boundary in nineteenth-century medical practice. *Pharos.* 1998 Winter; 61(1): 32–37. 17 refs. BE59987.
advertising; deception; drugs; *economics; entrepreneurship; *health care delivery; *historical aspects; interprofessional relations; literature; medical education; medical ethics; *medical fees; *medicine; misconduct; pharmacists; physician patient relationship; *physicians; life style; *practice management; *Nineteenth Century; *United States

Iglehart, John K. The American health care system: Medicaid. *New England Journal of Medicine.* 1999 Feb 4; 340(5): 403–408. 41 refs. BE60992.
adults; aged; children; disabled; *economics; *federal government; financial support; *government financing; *health care delivery; health care reform; health insurance; *indigents; managed care programs; organization and administration; physicians; public hospitals; public policy; quality of health care; remuneration; *state government; statistics; *trends; Health Care Financing Administration; *Medicaid; *United States

Iglehart, John K. The American health care system: Medicare. *New England Journal of Medicine.* 1999 Jan 28; 30(4): 327–332. 38 refs. BE60989.
*aged; disabled; *economics; family practice; *federal government; *government financing; *health care delivery; health care reform; health insurance; managed care programs; medical education; medical fees; medical specialties; organization and administration; physicians; political activity; politics; public opinion; statistics; *trends; End Stage Renal Disease Program; Health Care Financing Administration; *Medicare; *United States

Ikemoto, Lisa C. When a hospital becomes Catholic. *Mercer Law Review.* 1996 Summer; 47(4): 1087–1134. 234 fn. BE62750.
*community services; conscience; *economics; federal government; government financing; government regulation; *health care delivery; indigents; institutional policies; *legal aspects; political activity; private sector; professional organizations; *public participation; *refusal to treat; *religious hospitals; reproduction; *Roman Catholic ethics; *social impact; socioeconomic factors; state government; *women's health services; *health facility mergers; *rural population; Catholic Health Association; Ethical and Religious Directives for Catholic Health Care Services; *United States

Jacobs, Lawrence; Marmor, Theodore; Oberlander, Jonathan. The Oregon Health Plan and the political paradox of rationing: what advocates and critics have claimed and what Oregon did. *Journal of Health Politics, Policy and Law.* 1999 Feb; 24(1): 161–180. 20 refs. 5 fn. BE61756.
decision making; *economics; *evaluation; goals; *government financing; *health care delivery; *health care reform; health insurance; *indigents; managed care programs; organ transplantation; policy analysis; political activity; *politics; public participation; *public policy; *resource allocation; standards; state government; withholding treatment; negotiation; universal coverage; *Oregon; *Oregon Health Plan; United States
The article proceeds in three sections. First, we very briefly review the original proposals and ensuing (and misleading) debate over rationing in Oregon. Next, we explore how the politics of rationing unfolded in Oregon from the enactment of OHP to its implementation. Finally, we consider the character of Oregon's innovation and the broader lessons that it holds for

---

BE = bioethics accession number   fn. = footnotes   refs. = references

reform efforts elsewhere.

Jost, Timothy S. Public financing of pain management: leaky umbrellas and ragged safety nets. *Journal of Law, Medicine and Ethics.* 1998 Winter; 26(4): 290–307. 194 fn. BE61164.
   aged; alternatives; biomedical technologies; *chronically ill; costs and benefits; *drugs; economics; federal government; fraud; *government financing; hospices; hospitals; indigents; managed care programs; medical devices; nursing homes; opioid analgesics; *pain; *palliative care; *patient care; patients; quality of health care; state government; suffering; *terminal care; *terminally ill; time factors; utilization review; *Medicaid; *Medicare; *United States

Jurevic, Amy. Disparate impact under Title VI: discrimination, by any other name, will still have the same impact. *Saint Louis University Public Law Review.* 1996; 15(2): 237–265. 260 fn. BE59909.
   *blacks; economics; federal government; females; *government financing; *government regulation; *health care delivery; hospitals; *indigents; institutional policies; *legal aspects; minority groups; morbidity; public policy; *resource allocation; selection for treatment; *social discrimination; *social impact; standards; state government; obesity; Civil Rights Act 1964; Department of Health and Human Services; *Medicaid; *Oregon; *Oregon Health Plan; *United States

Kahn, Charles N. Patients' rights proposals: the insurers' perspective. *JAMA.* 1999 Mar 3; 281(9): 858. 8 refs. BE60243.
   costs and benefits; economics; employment; federal government; *government regulation; *health insurance; *legal aspects; legislation; *managed care programs; *patients' rights; quality of health care; self regulation; state government; Patients' Bill of Rights; United States

Kalb, Paul E. Health care fraud and abuse. *JAMA.* 1999 Sep 22–29; 282(12): 1163–1168. 63 refs. BE62659.
   conflict of interest; *economics; federal government; *fraud; government financing; *government regulation; *health insurance reimbursement; health personnel; *law enforcement; legal liability; legislation; *physician self-referral; *remuneration; state government; whistleblowing; Ethics in Patient Referral Act 1998; False Claims Act; *United States
   In recent years, health care fraud and abuse have become major issues, in part because of the rising cost of health care, industry consolidation, the emergence of private "whistle-blowers," and a change in the concept of fraud to include an emerging concern about quality of care. The 3 types of conduct that are generally prohibited by health care fraud laws are false claims, kickbacks, and self-referrals. False claims are subject to several criminal, civil, and administrative prohibitions, notably the federal civil False Claims Act. Kickbacks, or inducements with the intent to influence the purchase or sale of health care-related goods or services, are prohibited under the federal Anti-Kickback statute as well as by state laws. Finally, self-referrals -- the referral of patients to an entity with which the referring physician has a financial relationship -- are outlawed by the Ethics in Patient Referral Act as well as numerous state statutes. Consequences of violations of these laws can include, in addition to imprisonment and fines, civil monetary penalties, loss of licensure, loss of staff privileges, and exclusion from participation in federal health care programs. Federal criminal and civil statutes are enforced by the US Department of Justice; administrative actions are pursued by the Department of Health and Human Services' Office of Inspector General; and all state actions are pursued by the

individual states. In addition, private whistle-blowers may, acting in the name of the United States, file suit against an entity under the False Claims Act. Enforcement of health care fraud and abuse laws has become increasingly commonplace and now affects many mainstream providers. This trend is likely to continue.

Kao, Audiey C.; Green, Diane C.; Zaslavsky, Alan M., et al. The relationship between method of physician payment and patient trust. *JAMA.* 1998 Nov 18; 280(19): 1708–1714. 64 refs. BE59655.
   *attitudes; health insurance; health maintenance organizations; incentives; knowledge, attitudes, practice; *managed care programs; medical fees; *patients; *physician patient relationship; primary health care; *remuneration; social impact; survey; *trust; capitation fee; United States
   CONTEXT: Trust is the cornerstone of the patient–physician relationship. Payment methods that place physicians at financial risk have raised concerns about patients' trust in physicians to act in patients' best interests. OBJECTIVE: To evaluate the extent to which methods of physician payment are related to patient trust. DESIGN: Cross-sectional telephone interview survey done between January and June 1997. SETTING: Health plans of a large national insurer in Atlanta, Ga, the Baltimore, Md–Washington, DC, area, and Orlando, Fla. PARTICIPANTS: A total of 2086 adult managed care and indemnity patients. MAIN OUTCOME MEASURE: A 10-item scale (alpha = .94) assessing patients' trust in physicians. RESULTS: More fee-for-service (FFS) indemnity patients (94%) completely or mostly trust their physicians to "put their health and well-being above keeping down the health plan's costs" than salary (77%), capitated (83%), or FFS managed care patients (85%) (P less than .001 for pairwise comparisons). In multivariate analyses that adjusted for potentially confounding factors, FFS indemnity patients also had higher scores on the 10-item trust scale than salary (P less than .001), capitated (P less than .001), or FFS managed care patients (P less than .01). The effects of payment method on patient trust were reduced when a measure based on patients' reports about physician behavior (eg, Does your physician take enough time to answer your questions?) was included in the regression analyses, but the differences remained statistically significant, except for the comparison between FFS managed care and FFS indemnity patients (P = .08). Patients' perceptions of how their physicians were paid were not independently associated with trust, but the 37.7% who said they did not know how their physicians were paid had higher levels of trust than other patients (P less than .01). A total of 30.2% of patients were incorrect about their physicians' method of payment. CONCLUSIONS: Most patients trusted their physicians, but FFS indemnity patients have higher levels of trust than salary, capitated, or FFS managed care patients. Patients' reports of physician behavior accounted for part of the variation in patients' trust in physicians who are paid differently. The impact of payment methods on patient trust may be mediated partly by physician behavior.

Kapp, Marshall B. Can managed care be managed? *Pharos.* 1998 Spring; 61(2): 15–17. 21 refs. BE59985.
   alternatives; autonomy; beneficence; conflict of interest; contracts; disclosure; *economics; *health care delivery; health personnel; incentives; informed consent; justice; *legal liability; malpractice; *managed care programs; *physicians; *quality of health care; resource allocation; utilitarianism; United States

---

BE = bioethics accession number   fn. = footnotes   refs. = references

Keffer, M. Jan. Ethical decisions with limited resources: how is that possible? *Nursing Case Management.* 1997 Sep–Oct; 2(5): 196–202. 3 refs. Article followed by continuing education test questions, p. 201–202. BE59439.
> autonomy; beneficence; chronically ill; critically ill; *decision making; ethical analysis; gatekeeping; health care delivery; *health maintenance organizations; health personnel; managed care programs; moral obligations; patient care; resource allocation; terminal care; terminally ill; *case managers

Kegley, Jacquelyn Ann K. Community, autonomy, and managed care. *In:* McGee, Glenn, ed. Pragmatic Bioethics. Nashville, TN: Vanderbilt University Press; 1999: 204–227, 281–283. 31 fn. ISBN 0-8265-1321-2. BE60673.
> *autonomy; beneficence; biomedical technologies; caring; commodification; *common good; communication; cultural pluralism; decision making; disadvantaged; disease; *economics; freedom; health; *health care delivery; health education; informed consent; justice; *managed care programs; minority groups; paternalism; patient advocacy; patient care team; quality of health care; *resource allocation; social problems; trends; virtues; community consent; loyalty; quality assurance; *United States

Kennedy, Randy. U.S. agency says employer should pay for a woman's infertility treatments. [News]. *New York Times.* 1999 Apr 29: B3. BE61697.
> *employment; federal government; *health insurance reimbursement; infertility; *legal aspects; *reproductive technologies; social discrimination; *Equal Employment Opportunity Commission; New York; Saks, Rochelle; *United States

Khanna, Vikram; Silverman, Henry; Schwartz, Jack. Disclosure of operating practices by managed-care organizations to consumers of healthcare: obligations of informed consent. *Journal of Clinical Ethics.* 1998 Fall; 9(3): 291–296. 27 fn. BE61337.
> autonomy; beneficence; conflict of interest; *disclosure; economics; federal government; government regulation; incentives; *informed consent; institutional ethics; legislation; *managed care programs; *organizational policies; patients; physician patient relationship; physicians; state government; withholding treatment; capitation fee; Employee Retirement Income Security Act 1974 (ERISA); Maryland; United States

Kilborn, Peter T. Pressure growing to cover the cost of birth control. [News]. *New York Times.* 1998 Aug 2: 1, 30. BE60967.
> *contraception; drugs; employment; federal government; government regulation; *health insurance reimbursement; males; patient advocacy; *political activity; private sector; Roman Catholic ethics; sexuality; state government; Right to Life Movement; *United States

Kilner, John F.; Orr, Robert D.; Shelly, Judith Allen, eds. The Changing Face of Health Care: A Christian Appraisal of Managed Care, Resource Allocation, and Patient–Caregiver Relationships. Grand Rapids, MI: Eerdmans, Paternoster Press; 1998. 314 p. (Horizons in bioethics series). Includes references. ISBN 0-8028-4533-9. BE60357.
> administrators; alternative therapies; *Christian ethics; codes of ethics; compassion; covenant; *economics; financial support; gatekeeping; health; health care; *health care delivery; *health care reform; incentives; indigents; institutional ethics; justice; long-term care; malpractice; *managed care programs; medical ethics; mental health; minority groups; moral obligations; nurses; physicians; professional ethics; professional patient relationship;

resource allocation; social impact; theology; trends; business ethics; Good Samaritanism; Great Britain; Hippocratic Oath; *United States

Kolata, Gina. Where marketing and medicine meet. [News]. *New York Times.* 1998 Feb 10: A14. BE59363.
> advertising; *conflict of interest; financial support; *gifts; heart diseases; *industry; *medical devices; medical specialties; *physicians; surgery; *cardiology

Kopelman, Loretta M. Help from Hume reconciling professionalism and managed care. *Journal of Medicine and Philosophy.* 1999 Aug; 24(4): 396–410. 28 refs. 8 fn. BE62616.
> age factors; beneficence; friends; *health care delivery; humanism; *justice; *managed care programs; medical ethics; minority groups; *moral obligations; moral policy; *obligations to society; *patient advocacy; philosophy; physician patient relationship; *physicians; *resource allocation; selection for treatment; social discrimination; socioeconomic factors; trust; *Hume, David; Rachels, James

Health care systems are widely criticized for limiting doctors' roles as patient–advocates. Yet unrestricted advocacy can be unfairly partial, costly, and prejudicial. This essay considers three solutions to the problem of how to reconcile the demands of a just health care system for all patients, with the value of advocacy for some. Two views are considered and rejected, one supporting unlimited advocacy and another defending strict impartiality. A third view suggested by Hume's moral theory seeks to square the moral demands of professional advocacy and just health care systems. A moral basis for limited advocacy exists when it can be justified from a general or moral vantage. Consequently, ethical aspects of professionalism are not necessarily on a collision course with health care systems incorporating managed care. This solution is compatible with goals regarding the importance of humanistic education and professionalism to build patients' trust.

Kopelman, Loretta M.; Palumbo, Michael G. The U.S. health delivery system: inefficient and unfair to children. *American Journal of Law and Medicine.* 1997; 23(2–3): 319–337. 103 fn. BE62503.
> age factors; biomedical technologies; *children; decision making; *economics; *ethical theory; *health care; *health care delivery; health insurance; immunization; indigents; infants; *justice; libertarianism; morbidity; mortality; obligations of society; parents; patient advocacy; physicians; preventive medicine; primary health care; public policy; *resource allocation; selection for treatment; standards; uncertainty; utilitarianism; egalitarianism; needs; *United States

Kosseff, Andrew L.; Gurewich, Victor; Moore, Michael R., et al. Managed care ethics. [Letters and response]. *Annals of Internal Medicine.* 1998 Oct 15; 129(8): 672–674. 3 refs. BE60076.
> common good; conflict of interest; *decision making; *economics; *incentives; *managed care programs; medical ethics; *patient advocacy; physician patient relationship; *physicians; quality of health care; remuneration; *resource allocation; trust; withholding treatment; United States

Krainacker, David A.; Mondragon, Delfi. Ethical responsibilities in a managed care system. *Nebraska Medical Journal.* 1995 Oct; 80(10): 306–308. 17 refs. BE62414.
> health; health care; health insurance; institutional ethics; *managed care programs; medical specialties; patients; physicians; primary health care; rights; United States

Kuczewski, Mark G.; DeVita, Michael. Managed care

BE = bioethics accession number   fn. = footnotes   refs. = references

and end-of-life decisions: learning to live ungagged. *Archives of Internal Medicine.* 1998 Dec 7–21; 158(22): 2424–2428. 13 refs. BE61277.

allowing to die; case studies; *communication; decision making; *disclosure; economics; ethicists; *family members; *health insurance reimbursement; hospices; informed consent; *managed care programs; medical records; *patient care team; patient transfer; *physician's role; professional family relationship; *professional role; social workers; technical expertise; *terminal care; time factors; *case managers

Kuttner, Robert. The American health care system: employer-sponsored health coverage. *New England Journal of Medicine.* 1999 Jan 21; 340(3): 248–252. 12 refs. BE60988.

aged; *economics; *employment; family members; *health care delivery; *health insurance; health insurance reimbursement; hospitals; incentives; managed care programs; organizational policies; physicians; resource allocation; statistics; *trends; withholding treatment; personal financing; *United States

Kuttner, Robert. The American health care system: health insurance coverage. *New England Journal of Medicine.* 1999 Jan 14; 340(2): 163–168. 37 refs. BE60986.

aged; aliens; children; drugs; *economics; employment; federal government; *health care delivery; *health insurance; health insurance reimbursement; indigents; managed care programs; minority groups; public policy; state government; statistics; *trends; continuity of patient care; personal financing; Health Insurance Portability and Accountability Act 1996; *Medicaid; *Medicare; *United States

Kuttner, Robert. The American health care system: Wall Street and health care. *New England Journal of Medicine.* 1999 Feb 25; 340(8): 664–668. 16 refs. BE60949.

biomedical technologies; drug industry; *economics; *health care delivery; health insurance; health maintenance organizations; home care; hospitals; *industry; managed care programs; medical devices; physicians; *private sector; professional autonomy; proprietary health facilities; social impact; *statistics; *trends; withholding treatment; nonprofit organizations; practice management; Medicaid; Medicare; *United States

La Puma, John. Satisfying managed care patients through ethics consultation. *SBC Newsletter (Society for Bioethics Consultation).* 1996 Spring: 12–13. Reprinted from *Managed Care,* 1995 Oct; 4(10): 53–54. BE60418.

attitudes; *ethics consultation; goals; *managed care programs; patient advocacy; patient care; *patient satisfaction; patients; physicians; resource allocation

Lagnado, Lucette. Transplant patients ply an illicit market for vital medicines. [News]. *Wall Street Journal.* 1999 Jun 21: 1, A8. BE62450.

*drugs; *economics; health insurance reimbursement; health personnel; hospitals; institutional policies; legal aspects; *misconduct; motivation; *organ transplantation; *patient care; patients; *transplant recipients; Medicaid; Medicare; United States

Lamm, Richard D. Marginal medicine. *JAMA.* 1998 Sep 9; 280(10): 931–933. 14 refs. BE60284.

beneficence; *common good; disadvantaged; goals; *government financing; health; *health care delivery; health insurance; *managed care programs; medical ethics; moral obligations; obligations to society; patient advocacy; patient care; *physician's role; *public policy; *resource allocation; needs; United States

Lamm, Richard D. Redrawing the ethics map. *Hastings Center Report.* 1999 Mar–Apr; 29(2): 28–29. 5 refs.

BE61659.

caring; *common good; *costs and benefits; economics; health; health care; *health care delivery; indigents; justice; medical ethics; patient advocacy; physicians; *public policy; *resource allocation; social problems; United States

Larkin, Gregory Luke; Weber, James E.; Derse, Arthur R. Universal emergency access under managed care: universal doubt or mission impossible? *Cambridge Quarterly of Healthcare Ethics.* 1999 Spring; 8(2): 213–225. 70 fn. BE61237.

accountability; allied health personnel; communitarianism; conflict of interest; *economics; *emergency care; federal government; gatekeeping; government financing; government regulation; health insurance reimbursement; *health maintenance organizations; home care; hospitals; incentives; indigents; institutional ethics; legal obligations; *managed care programs; moral obligations; patient admission; physicians; proprietary health facilities; public policy; quality of health care; resource allocation; standards; state government; uncompensated care; Emergency Medical Treatment and Active Labor Act 1986; *United States

Leichter, Howard M. Oregon's bold experiment: whatever happened to rationing? *Journal of Health Politics, Policy and Law.* 1999 Feb; 24(1): 147–160. 17 refs. 18 fn. BE61755.

*evaluation; *government financing; *health care delivery; health care reform; *indigents; *managed care programs; *public policy; *resource allocation; standards; state government; withholding treatment; *Medicaid; *Oregon; *Oregon Health Plan

In 1994 Oregon began rationing health care for its Medicaid population, offering health policy makers and analysts around the country a view of one alternative future for health care delivery. The question now, four years after the experiment began, is what does that future look like? The short answer is that it does not look all that different from the present, but it looks different enough to offer important lessons to other states and the federal government. The Oregon experiment, including the prioritization of services and the aggressive use of managed care, has facilitated the expansion of health care coverage to over 100,000 additional Oregonians, helped decrease the percentage of the uninsured as well as reduce uncompensated care in hospitals, reduced the use of hospital emergency rooms, and reduced cost shifting. By most measures, the Oregon experiment appears to be a success.

Levi, Jeffrey. Can access to care for people living with HIV be expanded? *AIDS and Public Policy Journal.* 1998 Summer; 13(2): 56–74. 44 fn. BE61344.

*AIDS; community services; drugs; federal government; *government financing; guidelines; *health care delivery; *HIV seropositivity; indigents; mortality; patient care; *public policy; quality of health care; resource allocation; standards; state government; statistics; Department of Health and Human Services; Department of Housing and Urban Development; Department of Veterans Affairs; Medicaid; Medicare; Ryan White Comprehensive AIDS Resources Emergency Act 1990; *United States

Levine, Carol. The loneliness of the long-term care giver. [Personal narrative]. *New England Journal of Medicine.* 1999 May 20; 340(20): 1587–1590. 10 refs. BE62031.

advance care planning; *chronically ill; *communication; *community services; decision making; *disabled; *economics; education; *family members; goals; *health care delivery; health insurance reimbursement; *home care; injuries; *long-term care; managed care programs; mentally disabled; moral obligations; *obligations of society; *patient care; physically disabled; *professional family relationship; psychological stress; public policy; rehabilitation; *social

---

BE = bioethics accession number   fn. = footnotes   refs. = references

support; Medicare; United States

Levine, Robert A.; Lieberson, Alan. Physicians' perceptions of managed care. *American Journal Of Managed Care.* 1998 Feb; 4(2): 171–180. 37 fn. BE61554.
>   advance directives; allowing to die; alternatives; *attitudes; *contracts; decision making; disclosure; economics; futility; gatekeeping; government regulation; incentives; *knowledge, attitudes, practice; *legal aspects; legal liability; *managed care programs; medical ethics; *moral obligations; patient advocacy; *physicians; quality of health care; remuneration; resuscitation orders; survey; withholding treatment; gag clauses; questionnaires; Connecticut

Levinsky, Norman G. Can we afford medical care for Alice C? *Lancet.* 1998 Dec 5; 352(9143): 1849–1851. 13 refs. BE60805.
>   *age factors; *aged; allowing to die; biomedical technologies; case studies; *economics; futility; government financing; *health care; hospitals; intensive care units; justice; mortality; patient admission; prolongation of life; *public policy; quality of life; *resource allocation; social discrimination; socioeconomic factors; Medicare; *United States

Light, Donald. Saving John Worthy. [Letter]. *Hastings Center Report.* 1999 May–Jun; 29(3): 5. BE61405.
>   *decision making; *emergency care; gatekeeping; *health care delivery; health maintenance organizations; international aspects; *managed care programs; *organization and administration; physician patient relationship; primary health care; *quality of health care; referral and consultation; personal financing; United States

Light, Donald W. Good managed care needs universal health insurance. *Annals of Internal Medicine.* 1999 Apr 20; 130(8): 686–689. 27 refs. BE61603.
>   economics; employment; government regulation; *health care delivery; *health insurance; justice; *managed care programs; patients' rights; public policy; *quality of health care; trends; *universal coverage; United States

Although the increase of corporate managed care has helped to reduce excesses and costs, continued gains in cost-effectiveness depend on good clinically managed care. Benefits of clinically managed care depend on stable contracts and universal coverage. Instead, employers are decreasing coverage and creating a market of "lemons" in which low-cost plans are rewarded for cost-cutting tactics. These tactics have spawned movements that demand rights for patients and providers. Choosing to shore up those rights, however, will increase the number of uninsured persons. This tragic choice, which no other industrialized nation has permitted, will not be resolved until some form of universal health insurance is implemented.

Loewy, Erich H.; Loewy, Roberta Springer. Ethics and managed care: reconstructing a system and refashioning a society. [Editorial]. *Archives of Internal Medicine.* 1998 Dec 7–21; 158(22): 2419–2422. 11 refs. BE61276.
>   accountability; administrators; case studies; coercion; common good; democracy; *disclosure; economics; gatekeeping; *health care reform; health facilities; health insurance reimbursement; justice; *managed care programs; moral obligations; obligations of society; *patient advocacy; patient care; patient discharge; patient transfer; physician patient relationship; *physician's role; *physicians; quality of health care; United States

Lund, Nelson. Two precipices, one chasm: the economics of physician-assisted suicide and euthanasia. *Hastings Constitutional Law Quarterly.* 1997 Summer; 24(4): 903–946. 119 fn. BE62165.
>   abortion, induced; active euthanasia; allowing to die;

artificial feeding; *assisted suicide; biomedical research; codes of ethics; coercion; decision making; dehumanization; *economics; family members; government financing; government regulation; guideline adherence; guidelines; *health care delivery; health insurance; incentives; involuntary euthanasia; *legal aspects; managed care programs; medical ethics; persistent vegetative state; physician patient relationship; *physicians; *public policy; quality of life; resource allocation; right to die; social impact; state government; *Supreme Court decisions; trust; voluntary euthanasia; vulnerable populations; *wedge argument; withholding treatment; *duty to die; *Hippocratic Oath; Netherlands; Roe v. Wade; *United States; Vacco v. Quill; Washington v. Glucksberg

Lysaker, John T.; Sullivan, Michael. Untying the gag: reason in the world of health care reform. *In:* McGee, Glenn, ed. Pragmatic Bioethics. Nashville, TN: Vanderbilt University Press; 1999: 228–245, 283–287. 39 fn. ISBN 0-8265-1321-2. BE60674.
>   capitalism; commodification; democracy; disclosure; *economics; health care; *health care reform; health maintenance organizations; *incentives; indigents; *managed care programs; models, theoretical; physician patient relationship; *physicians; professional autonomy; regulation; remuneration; standards; trends; *gag clauses; *United States

McCullough, Laurence B. Ethics in the management of health care organizations. *Physician Executive.* 1993 Nov–Dec; 19(6): 72–76. 4 refs. BE60638.
>   administrators; autonomy; beneficence; clinical ethics; *economics; ethics; *health care delivery; historical aspects; *hospitals; *institutional ethics; medical ethics; morality; organization and administration; patient advocacy; physicians; practice guidelines; *professional ethics; public policy; quality of health care; remuneration; resource allocation; trends; virtues; business ethics; preventive ethics; Eighteenth Century; Great Britain; Percival, Thomas; Twentieth Century; United States

McQuillen, Michael P.; Menken, Matthew; Hachinski, Vladimir. Managed care and managed death: peas from the same pod? [Article and commentaries]. *Archives of Neurology.* 1997 Mar; 54(3): 326–330. 45 refs. BE60326.
>   active euthanasia; allowing to die; *assisted suicide; autonomy; economics; empirical research; intention; killing; legal aspects; *managed care programs; palliative care; physician's role; physicians; public opinion; resource allocation; right to die; terminology; treatment outcome; utilitarianism; neurology; United States

McSherry, James; Dickie, Gordon L. Swords to ploughshares: gatekeepers turned advocates. [Editorial]. *Canadian Family Physician.* 1998 May; 44: 955–956. 5 refs. BE61851.
>   costs and benefits; *economics; *gatekeeping; health care delivery; incentives; *patient advocacy; *physician's role; *physicians; *primary health care; *resource allocation; Canada

Makover, Michael E. Mismanaged Care: How Corporate Medicine Jeopardizes Your Health. Amherst, NY: Prometheus Books; 1998. 300 p. Bibliography: p. 289–294. ISBN 1-57392-248-X. BE60749.
>   administrators; aged; allied health personnel; alternative therapies; conflict of interest; disclosure; economics; federal government; gatekeeping; goals; government regulation; health care reform; health insurance; health maintenance organizations; malpractice; *managed care programs; physician patient relationship; physicians; practice guidelines; privacy; professional competence; proprietary health facilities; quality of health care; referral and consultation; remuneration; resource allocation; withholding treatment; Clinton Health Security Plan; Medicaid; Medicare; *United States

---

BE = bioethics accession number   fn. = footnotes   refs. = references

Malone, Ruth E. Policy as product: morality and metaphor in health policy discourse. *Hastings Center Report.* 1999 May–Jun; 29(3): 16–22. 29 fn. BE61408.
    bioethics; *commodification; *economics; goals; *health care; medicine; *metaphor; *moral policy; *public policy; socioeconomic factors; *terminology; values; United States
Where we once spoke in military terms, we now often wield the language of the market: health care is a "product" and we are its "providers" and "consumers." The market metaphor constrains in various ways our vision of the goals we pursue in making health policy, of the options available to us in pursuing them, indeed -- because policy implies a certain view of moral agency -- of the way we relate to each other.

Margolis, Lewis H.; Rosner, Fred; Reynolds, Susan, et al. Personal use of drug samples by physicians and office staff. [Letters and responses]. *JAMA.* 1997 Nov 19; 278(19): 1567–1569. 13 refs. BE59340.
    *advertising; conflict of interest; *drug industry; *drugs; economics; family members; financial support; *gifts; medical ethics; *organizational policies; *patient care; *physicians; professional organizations; risks and benefits; *self care; American Medical Association

Mariner, Wendy K. Going Hollywood with patient rights in managed care. *JAMA.* 1999 Mar 3; 281(9): 861. 5 refs. BE60245.
    accountability; *contracts; federal government; *government regulation; *legal aspects; legislation; *managed care programs; mass media; *patients' rights; quality of health care; state government; Patients' Bill of Rights; *United States

Mechanic, David. Muddling through elegantly: finding the proper balance in rationing. *Health Affairs.* 1997 Sep–Oct; 16(5): 83–92. 17 fn. BE59178.
    administrators; biomedical technologies; costs and benefits; cultural pluralism; decision making; *economics; evidence-based medicine; gatekeeping; government regulation; *health care delivery; international aspects; justice; managed care programs; *methods; national health insurance; physicians; political activity; politics; public opinion; *public policy; *resource allocation; socioeconomic factors; values; capitation fee; case managers; *Great Britain; Medicaid; National Health Service; Oregon Health Plan; *United States

Mechanic, David. The functions and limitations of trust in the provision of medical care. *Journal of Health Politics, Policy and Law.* 1998 Aug; 23(4): 661–686. 53 refs. Commented on by S.D. Goold, p. 687–695. BE59782.
    communication; confidentiality; conflict of interest; decision making; *disclosure; *economics; evaluation; gatekeeping; health care delivery; incentives; informed consent; international aspects; *managed care programs; medical errors; negligence; organization and administration; patient advocacy; patient participation; patient satisfaction; *physician patient relationship; physician self-referral; *physicians; professional autonomy; professional competence; public opinion; quality of health care; referral and consultation; *regulation; resource allocation; standards; *trust; withholding treatment; gag clauses; quality assurance; Great Britain; United States
Trust, the expectation that institutions and professionals will act in one's interests, contributes to the effectiveness of medical care. With the rapid privatization of medical care and the growth of managed care, trust may be diminished. Five important aspects of trust are examined: technical and interpersonal competence, physician agency, physician control, confidentiality, and open communication and disclosure. In each case, changing health care arrangements increase the risks of trusting

and encourage regulatory interventions that substitute for some aspects of trust. With the increased size and centralization of health care plans, inevitable errors are attributed to health plans rather than to failures of individual judgment. Such generalized criticisms exacerbate distrust and encourage micromanagement of medical care processes.

Menendez, Roger; Zwelling–Aamot, Marcy L.; White, T. Michael, et al. A new ethic for medicine? [Letters and response]. *New England Journal of Medicine.* 1998 Oct 29; 339(18): 1326–1328. 5 refs. BE60148.
    common good; *conflict of interest; *economics; incentives; *managed care programs; medical ethics; moral obligations; *patient advocacy; physician patient relationship; *physicians; professional autonomy; quality of health care; remuneration; resource allocation; withholding treatment; capitation fee; United States

Menzel, Paul; Gold, Marthe R.; Nord, Erik, et al. Toward a broader view of values in cost–effectiveness analysis of health. *Hastings Center Report.* 1999 May–Jun; 29(3): 7–15. 31 fn. BE61407.
    age factors; bioethics; chronically ill; *costs and benefits; critically ill; disabled; *economics; health; *health care; justice; public participation; quality adjusted life years; quality of life; *resource allocation; selection for treatment; social discrimination; time factors; treatment outcome; utilitarianism; value of life; *values; hope; severity of illness index
By registering different health benefits on a common scale, CEA allows us to assess the relative social importance of different health care interventions and opens the way for the allocation decisions of health care policy. If it is really to be effective, however, CEA must be recalibrated so that it better reflects some of our widely held beliefs about the merits of different kinds of treatment.

Miles, Steven. Managed care issues in genetic testing for Alzheimer disease. *In:* Post, Stephen G.; Whitehouse, Peter J., eds. Genetic Testing for Alzheimer Disease: Ethical and Clinical Issues. Baltimore, MD: Johns Hopkins University Press; 1998: 209–221. 38 refs. ISBN 0-8018-5840-2. BE60725.
    anonymous testing; chronically ill; costs and benefits; data banks; *dementia; diagnosis; epidemiology; federal government; genetic counseling; genetic information; genetic predisposition; *genetic screening; government financing; government regulation; health insurance; informed consent; insurance selection bias; justice; long-term care; *managed care programs; medical records; population genetics; private sector; public policy; resource allocation; risk; social discrimination; United States

Miller, Tracy E. Center stage on the patient protection agenda: grievance and appeal rights. *Journal of Law, Medicine and Ethics.* 1998 Summer; 26(2): 89–99. 77 fn. BE62676.
    disclosure; *due process; federal government; *government regulation; institutional policies; *legal rights; legislation; *managed care programs; patient advocacy; *patients' rights; *physician's role; public policy; *quality of health care; self regulation; standards; state government; *withholding treatment; utilization review; Medicare; *United States

Miller, Tracy E.; Sage, William M. Disclosing physician financial incentives. *JAMA.* 1999 Apr 21; 281(15): 1424–1430. 67 refs. BE61902.
    accountability; autonomy; conflict of interest; *disclosure; *economics; federal government; gatekeeping; *government regulation; *incentives; informed consent; legal aspects; legal obligations; *managed care programs; mandatory programs;

---

moral obligations; organizational policies; patients; patients' rights; physician patient relationship; *physicians; professional organizations; *public policy; remuneration; state government; trust; withholding treatment; empowerment; undertreatment; American Medical Association; Medicaid; Medicare; *United States

Federal and state regulatory initiatives as well as court decisions increasingly require managed care organizations to disclose physician financial incentives and have raised the issue of disclosure by physicians themselves. These mandates are based on ethical and legal principles arising from the patient–physician relationship and the relationship between health plan sponsors and enrollees. Disclosing incentives also serves important policy objectives: it can inform enrollees' choice of plan, reinforce enrollees' capacity to understand and exercise other rights under managed care, and discourage use of compensation methods that might compromise patients' access to treatment. However, significant conceptual and practical questions remain about implementing a disclosure mandate. Unresolved issues include the timing, content, and scope of disclosure, the relationship of disclosure to patients' substantive rights, and the impact of disclosure on trust between patients and physicians. These uncertainties exemplify the challenges facing policymakers, plans, and physicians as they determine how best to inform patients about managed care.

Mitka, Mike. Do-it-yourself report on patient privacy. [News]. *JAMA.* 1998 Dec 9; 280(22): 1897. BE59691.
　　accountability; *confidentiality; disclosure; government regulation; health facilities; health services research; informed consent; institutional policies; law enforcement; *managed care programs; medical records; organizational policies; physicians; privacy; professional organizations; self regulation; standards; American Medical Association; Joint Commission on Accreditation of Healthcare Organizations; National Committee for Quality Assurance; United States

Morreim, E. Haavi. Managed care, ethics, and academic health centers: maximizing potential, minimizing drawbacks. *Academic Medicine.* 1997 May; 72(5): 332–340. 141 refs. BE59879.
　　*conflict of interest; *economics; faculty; gatekeeping; *goals; guidelines; health promotion; *hospitals; incentives; interprofessional relations; *managed care programs; medical education; medical specialties; physicians; practice guidelines; primary health care; professional autonomy; remuneration; standards; capitation fee; investigational therapies; physician's practice patterns; *teaching hospitals; utilization review; United States

Morreim, E. Haavi. To tell the truth: disclosing the incentives and limits of managed care. *American Journal Of Managed Care.* 1997 Jan; 3(1): 35–43. 52 refs. BE60026.
　　autonomy; conflict of interest; contracts; *disclosure; *economics; *forms; gatekeeping; guidelines; *incentives; informed consent; institutional ethics; *institutional policies; legal obligations; *managed care programs; moral obligations; patient advocacy; patients; physicians; practice guidelines; *quality of health care; referral and consultation; remuneration; standards; withholding treatment; gag clauses; utilization review; United States

Moses, Hamilton. Managing managed care. *Clinical Performance and Quality Health Care.* 1996 Oct–Dec; 4(4): 200–202. BE62108.
　　*administrators; conflict of interest; *economics; *incentives; *managed care programs; *organization and administration; *physicians; values

Murphy, Michael J.; DeBernardo, Caren R.;

Shoemaker, Wendy E. Impact of managed care on independent practice and professional ethics: a survey of independent practitioners. *Professional Psychology: Research and Practice.* 1998 Feb; 29(1): 43–51. 18 refs. BE59209.
　　codes of ethics; confidentiality; deception; *decision making; disclosure; economics; health insurance reimbursement; *health personnel; incentives; *knowledge, attitudes, practice; *managed care programs; patient advocacy; patient care; professional autonomy; professional ethics; professional organizations; psychiatric diagnosis; psychoactive drugs; *psychology; *psychotherapy; *quality of health care; social impact; survey; utilization review; American Psychological Association; *United States

Nadelson, Carol C. Ethics and empathy in a changing health care system. *Pharos.* 1996 Fall; 59(4): 29–32. 16 refs. BE59698.
　　accountability; compassion; confidentiality; *economics; *empathy; gatekeeping; *health care delivery; managed care programs; medical ethics; medical records; obligations of society; patient advocacy; patient compliance; *physician patient relationship; *physicians; resource allocation; sociology of medicine; *trends; trust; United States

O'Brien, Daniel. Working for the common good: Catholic healthcare's opportunity to shape values–based managed care. *Health Progress.* 1997 Jan–Feb; 78(1): 40–42, 47. 8 fn. BE60212.
　　*common good; economics; health care; health care delivery; *managed care programs; proprietary health facilities; *Roman Catholic ethics; values; *health facility mergers

Orentlicher, David. Paying physicians more to do less: financial incentives to limit care. *University of Richmond Law Review.* 1996 Jan; 30(1): 155–197. 146 fn. BE59860.
　　alternatives; biomedical technologies; costs and benefits; decision making; *economics; federal government; government regulation; health maintenance organizations; *incentives; *managed care programs; medical education; patient advocacy; patient care; patients; physician patient relationship; *physicians; practice guidelines; professional autonomy; quality of health care; referral and consultation; *remuneration; *resource allocation; risks and benefits; withholding treatment; capitation fee; utilization review; United States

Packer, Samuel. Capitated care is unethical. *Archives of Ophthalmology.* 1997 Sep; 115(9): 1195–1196. 14 refs. BE60030.
　　autonomy; beneficence; commodification; *conflict of interest; employment; incentives; *managed care programs; medicine; patient advocacy; physician patient relationship; *physician's role; *physicians; professional autonomy; *remuneration; resource allocation; sociology of medicine; trust; withholding treatment; *capitation fee; United States

Perone, Nicola; Chervenak, Frank A.; McCullough, Laurence B., et al. Physicians should not be allowed to enter into contractual agreements with managed care companies that do not meet basic ethical standards. [Letter and response]. *American Journal of Obstetrics and Gynecology.* 1997 Aug; 177(2): 481–482. 2 refs. BE59374.
　　accountability; contracts; *managed care programs; physicians; regulation; standards

Peterson, Mark A. Managed care: ethics, trust, and accountability. [Editorial]. *Journal of Health Politics, Policy and Law.* 1998 Aug; 23(4): 611–615. 8 refs. BE59779.
　　accountability; government regulation; *managed care programs; state government; trust; *United States

---

BE = bioethics accession number　　　fn. = footnotes　　　refs. = references

Petrila, John. Ethics, money, and the problem of coercion in managed behavioral health care. *Saint Louis University Law Journal.* 1996 Spring; 40(2): 359–405. 145 fn. BE60063.
   chronically ill; coercion; community services; *conflict of interest; dangerousness; *health care delivery; *health insurance reimbursement; incentives; involuntary commitment; *legal aspects; *legal liability; legal obligations; malpractice; *managed care programs; mental institutions; *mentally ill; moral obligations; *patient advocacy; *patient care; *patient discharge; physician patient relationship; *physicians; practice guidelines; private sector; public sector; quality of health care; remuneration; risk; standards; voluntary admission; withholding treatment; capitation fee; *continuity of patient care; Medicaid; United States

Phillips, Donald F. Erecting an ethical framework for managed care. [Meeting report]. *JAMA.* 1998 Dec 23–30; 280(24): 2060–2062. Report on an American Society of Law, Medicine and Ethics conference held in Cambridge, MA, in Oct 1998. BE59583.
   accountability; decision making; government regulation; health care delivery; health maintenance organizations; incentives; *institutional ethics; legal aspects; *managed care programs; moral obligations; *organization and administration; patient advocacy; patient participation; physicians; *quality of health care; *American Society of Law, Medicine and Ethics; United States

Plutko, Lawrence A. Pursuing justice in an era of managed care: Seattle-based system makes room for the underserved and uninsured. *Health Progress.* 1997 Jan–Feb; 78(1): 37–39, 48. 9 fn. BE60211.
   disadvantaged; health care delivery; justice; *managed care programs; program descriptions; *Roman Catholic ethics; Oregon; *Sisters of Providence Health System (Seattle, WA); Washington

Rai, Arti K. Reflective choice in health care: using information technology to present allocation options. *American Journal of Law and Medicine.* 1999; 25(2–3): 387–402. 122 fn. BE62510.
   autonomy; biomedical technologies; computer communication networks; *contracts; costs and benefits; counseling; decision making; *disclosure; evaluation; government regulation; *health insurance reimbursement; incentives; *information dissemination; *managed care programs; *patient participation; practice guidelines; quality adjusted life years; *resource allocation; personal financing; Internet; United States

Ramsey, Scott D.; Hillman, Alan L.; Pauly, Mark V. The effects of health insurance on access to new medical technologies. *International Journal of Technology Assessment in Health Care.* 1997 Spring; 13(2): 357–367. 26 refs. BE61147.
   *biomedical technologies; bone marrow; comparative studies; *economics; *health insurance; health maintenance organizations; health services research; heart diseases; kidney diseases; leukemia; *managed care programs; patient care; selection for treatment; statistics; tissue transplantation; angioplasty; *fee-for-service plans; proprietary organizations; *utilization review; Blue Cross-Blue Shield; California; Medicaid; Medicare

Reay, Trish. Allocating scarce resources in a publicly funded health system: ethical considerations of a Canadian managed care proposal. *Nursing Ethics.* 1999 May; 6(3): 240–249. 25 refs. BE61768.
   conflict of interest; *decision making; federal government; *gatekeeping; government financing; health care delivery; *health care reform; incentives; justice; *managed care programs; moral obligations; patient advocacy; *physicians; public participation; *public policy; remuneration; *resource allocation; rights; capitation fee; *Alberta; *Canada

Robbins, Dennis. Integrating Managed Care and Ethics: Transforming Challenges into Positive Outcomes. New York, NY: McGraw-Hill; 1998. 327 p. Bibliography: p. 295–319. ISBN 0–07–053083–1. BE62398.
   accountability; advance directives; case studies; clinical ethics committees; confidentiality; decision making; disclosure; economics; employment; evidence-based medicine; gatekeeping; government regulation; health care delivery; home care; incentives; informed consent; institutional ethics; legal aspects; legal liability; long-term care; *managed care programs; medical records; organization and administration; patient advocacy; physician patient relationship; physicians; quality of health care; referral and consultation; review; terminal care; trends; withholding treatment; United States

Root, Jane; Stableford, Sue. Easy-to-read consumer communications: a missing link in Medicaid managed care. *Journal of Health Politics, Policy and Law.* 1999 Feb; 24(1): 1–26. 52 refs. BE61753.
   adults; *communication; *comprehension; *disadvantaged; education; *health education; *information dissemination; legal aspects; *managed care programs; program descriptions; public policy; terminology; Center for Health Care Strategies; *Medicaid; United States
Effective consumer communication is key to successfully moving Medicaid recipients into managed care systems and realizing the promised cost savings from the upheaval. Yet, little attention has been paid to educating these consumers with easy-to-read materials. The Maine Area Health Education Center (AHEC) Health Literacy Center, with the support of the Center for Health Care Strategies, Inc., addressed the problem by offering three national skills training workshops called Writing for the Medicaid Market. The training was marketed to public and private organizations providing Medicaid managed care services, including state Medicaid officials, health benefit counselor staff (enrollment brokers), managed care plan (HMO) staff, and consumer advocates. The training addressed the core issue in health literacy: the mismatch between the low literacy skills of the target population and the high reading level of most health and managed care materials. Posttraining survey data revealed that training was successful in skill building, but also that it addressed only the tip of the iceberg. Faulty and/or nonexistent communication planning limits the success not only of Medicaid, but of other large health and social programs as well. The authors outline the broad scope of the national health literacy problem, share their posttraining survey data, discuss lessons extrapolated from both their data and their experience, and propose a national agenda to address a vast and generally ignored public problem.

Rosenbaum, Sara; Frankford, David M.; Moore, Brad, et al. Who should determine when health care is medically necessary? *New England Journal of Medicine.* 1999 Jan 21; 340(3): 229–232. 19 refs. BE60987.
   conflict of interest; consensus; contracts; costs and benefits; *decision making; economics; evidence-based medicine; goals; *health insurance; *health insurance reimbursement; *industry; legal aspects; *patient care; patients; *physicians; practice guidelines; *standards; therapeutic research; treatment outcome; values; needs; Employee Retirement Income Security Act 1974 (ERISA); United States

Rosenheck, Robert; Armstrong, Moe; Callahan, Daniel, et al. Obligation to the least well off in setting mental health service priorities: a consensus statement. *Psychiatric Services.* 1998 Oct; 49(10): 1273–1274, 1290. 13 refs. BE61446.
   community services; consensus; *costs and benefits; decision making; *economics; federal government; *health care

---

BE = bioethics accession number   fn. = footnotes   refs. = references

delivery; justice; mental health; *mentally ill; *obligations of society; psychiatry; *public policy; *resource allocation; schizophrenia; *selection for treatment; values; *mental health services; *seriously ill; United States; *Veterans Health Administration

Rosenthal, Elisabeth. West's medicine is raising bills for China's sick. [News]. *New York Times.* 1998 Nov 19: A1, A12. BE61119.
conflict of interest; *drug industry; *drugs; *economics; *health care; hospitals; *incentives; institutional policies; international aspects; misconduct; physicians; remuneration; Western World; *China

Royal College of Physicians. Setting Priorities in the NHS: A Framework for Decision-Making. A Report of the Royal College of Physicians. London: Royal College of Physicians of London; 1995 Sep. 38 p. 50 refs. This report was approved by the Royal College of Physicians on 15 Jun 1995. ISBN 1-86016-020-4. BE59460.
administrators; advisory committees; biomedical research; common good; continuing education; costs and benefits; *decision making; *economics; education; evidence-based medicine; goals; *health care delivery; health promotion; health services research; justice; medical education; organization and administration; *organizational policies; patient care; patient care team; patient participation; *physician's role; physicians; preventive medicine; primary health care; private sector; professional organizations; *public participation; *public policy; *quality of health care; referral and consultation; *resource allocation; state medicine; time factors; treatment outcome; vulnerable populations; capitation fee; needs; *Great Britain; National Council for Health Care Priorities (Great Britain); *National Health Service; *Royal College of Physicians

Royal Dutch Medical Association. Medical Ethics Committee. Making Choices Professionally. Issued by the Association: Koninklijke Nederlandsche Maatschappij tot bevordering der Geneeskunst, P.O. Box 20051, 3502 LB, Utrecht, The Netherlands; 1992 Aug. 30 p. 21 fn. Translated from the Dutch by M.J. Tattersall-Evers. BE59261.
decision making; *economics; health care; *health care delivery; health care reform; national health insurance; *physician's role; *physicians; *professional autonomy; quality of health care; resource allocation; selection for treatment; self induced illness; *Netherlands

Russell, Paul S. Understanding resource use in liver transplantation. [Editorial]. *JAMA.* 1999 Apr 21; 281(15): 1431–1432. 9 refs. BE61903.
*economics; evaluation; hospitals; *livers; mortality; *organ transplantation; *public policy; *resource allocation; *scarcity; *selection for treatment; transplant recipients; treatment outcome; length of stay; severity of illness index; United States

Sackett, David. The Doctor's (Ethical and Economic) Dilemma: A Description of the Dilemmas Faced by a Physician Who Tries to Serve Both Individual Patients and Society. Office of Health Economics [OHE] Annual Lecture 1996. London: Office of Health Economics; 1996 Aug. 20 p. 9 refs. ISBN 0901-387-983. BE59419.
allowing to die; autonomy; beneficence; biomedical research; biomedical technologies; case studies; costs and benefits; *decision making; *economics; *evidence-based medicine; guideline adherence; guidelines; human experimentation; justice; *moral obligations; *obligations to society; *patient advocacy; patient care; *physicians; prolongation of life; quality of life; refusal to treat; *resource allocation; risks and benefits; selection for treatment; technical expertise; withholding treatment; *Great Britain; *National Health Service

Sage, William M. Fraud and abuse law. [Editorial]. *JAMA.* 1999 Sep 22–29; 282(12): 1179–1181. 9 refs. BE62661.
*economics; federal government; *fraud; government financing; *government regulation; health insurance reimbursement; health personnel; law enforcement; managed care programs; physician self-referral; remuneration; whistleblowing; Medicare; *United States

Sandquist, Michael A. Do not go gently. *Pharos.* 1996 Fall; 59(4): 14–17. 11 refs. BE59696.
altruism; capitalism; decision making; diagnosis; disclosure; *economics; ethics; *freedom; *government financing; government regulation; health care; *health care delivery; health insurance; health maintenance organizations; hospitals; indigents; managed care programs; medicine; morality; patient care; physician patient relationship; *physicians; *professional autonomy; remuneration; rights; social impact; *trends; withholding treatment; Medicaid; Medicare; *United States

Schmacke, Norbert. Overdramatization of the burdens on health and social services: a continuing debate in the history of German medicine. *International Journal of Health Services.* 1997; 27(3): 559–574. 40 refs. This article is a revised and extended version of a lecture given on 24 Mar 1988, in the context of an exhibition on the government-planned and executed elimination of "lives unworthy of living" in National Socialism. Translated by Sean Mullan and Jutta Rateike-Fear. BE60082.
advisory committees; *aged; AIDS; attitudes; *chronically ill; dementia; *disabled; *economics; *eugenics; euthanasia; *health care delivery; health care reform; health insurance; *historical aspects; homosexuals; killing; *National Socialism; patient care; physicians; political systems; psychiatry; social worth; socioeconomic factors; sociology of medicine; *stigmatization; terminal care; *trends; *Germany; *Twentieth Century; United States

Schwartz, William B. Life Without Disease: The Pursuit of Medical Utopia. Berkeley, CA: University of California Press; 1998. 178 p. Includes references. ISBN 0-520-21467-6. BE59738.
anesthesia; biomedical research; *biomedical technologies; cloning; costs and benefits; drugs; *economics; fraud; gene therapy; genetic disorders; *genetic intervention; health care; *health care delivery; health insurance; health maintenance organizations; hospitals; international aspects; legal aspects; life extension; malpractice; *managed care programs; physicians; preventive medicine; *public policy; quality of health care; *resource allocation; *trends; Canada; Europe; Great Britain; *United States

Seedhouse, David. Death's moral sting. [Editorial]. *Health Care Analysis.* 1998 Dec; 6(4): 273–276. 12 fn. BE61585.
attitudes; attitudes to death; bioethics; *dehumanization; *economics; *health care delivery; incentives; informed consent; medical education; patient care; *physician patient relationship; physicians; privacy; prognosis; quality of life; social discrimination; *sociology of medicine; suffering; terminal care; truth disclosure; *values

Sellers, Phil; North Carolina Medical Society. Bioethics Committee. The role of the medical profession in a managed care environment. Statement of the Bioethics Committee of the North Carolina Medical Society. [Policy statement and commentaries]. *North Carolina Medical Journal.* 1998 Mar–Apr; 59(2): 96–100. 3 refs. Commentaries by P. Sellers, D. Menscer, J. Glasson, S.M. Atkinson, and C. Kirschenbaum. BE60493.
*economics; health care reform; *health insurance; indigents; *managed care programs; *organizational policies; patient advocacy; physician patient relationship; *physician's role; *physicians; professional organizations; quality of health

care; *North Carolina Medical Society; United States

Shalala, Donna E. A Patients' Bill of Rights: the medical student's role. *JAMA.* 1999 Mar 3; 281(9): 857. 4 refs. BE60246.
    advisory committees; alternatives; disclosure; emergency care; federal government; government regulation; *health care delivery; incentives; insurance selection bias; *legal aspects; legislation; *managed care programs; medical education; *patients' rights; physicians; public policy; quality of health care; referral and consultation; students; withholding treatment; gag clauses; *Patients' Bill of Rights; *President's Advisory Commission on Consumer Protection and Quality in the Health Care Industry; *United States

Shapiro, Daniel. Why even egalitarians should favor market health insurance. *Social Philosophy and Policy.* 1998 Summer; 15(2): 84–132. 103 fn. BE61258.
    accountability; autonomy; democracy; economics; employment; federal government; *freedom; government financing; government regulation; health; health care; *health insurance; hospitals; indigents; insurance; *justice; managed care programs; *mandatory programs; *national health insurance; obligations of society; philosophy; policy analysis; political systems; *private sector; public policy; public sector; remuneration; resource allocation; rights; risk; self induced illness; socioeconomic factors; state government; values; *voluntary programs; *egalitarianism; Blue Cross–Blue Shield; Daniels, Norman; Dworkin, Ronald; Medicaid; Medicare; United States

Shaul, Randi Zlotnik; Mendelssohn, David C. Scarce resource allocation decisions: issues of physician conflict and liability. *Humane Health Care International.* 1997 Spring; 13(1): 25–28. 35 refs. BE59960.
    accountability; administrators; *conflict of interest; disclosure; *economics; *gatekeeping; informed consent; kidney diseases; *legal liability; negligence; patient advocacy; physician patient relationship; *physician's role; *physicians; public policy; *renal dialysis; *resource allocation; selection for treatment; social discrimination; standards; time factors; Canada; *Ontario

Sheldon, Tony. Dutch regulate sponorship of hospitals. [News]. *BMJ (British Medical Journal).* 1999 Jun 19; 318(7199): 1644. BE62532.
    codes of ethics; conflict of interest; *drug industry; *financial support; *hospitals; *industry; *regulation; voluntary programs; *Netherlands

Showstack, Jonathan; Katz, Patricia P.; Lake, John R., et al.; National Institute of Diabetes and Digestive and Kidney Diseases. Liver Transplantation Database Group. Resource utilization in liver transplantation: effects of patient characteristics and clinical practice. *JAMA.* 1999 Apr 21; 281(15): 1381–1386. 29 refs. BE61901.
    adults; age factors; alcohol abuse; comparative studies; critically ill; *economics; *evaluation; *hospitals; intensive care units; *livers; *organ transplantation; *resource allocation; selection for treatment; *transplant recipients; length of stay; severity of illness index; *utilization review; California; *Mayo Clinic; Minnesota; Nebraska; *University of California, San Francisco; *University of Nebraska, Omaha
    CONTEXT: Liver transplantation is among the most costly of medical services, yet few studies have addressed the relationship between the resources utilized for this procedure and specific patient characteristics and clinical practices. OBJECTIVE: To assess the association of pretransplant patient characteristics and clinical practices with hospital resource utilization. DESIGN: Prospective cohort of patients who received liver transplants between January 1991 and July 1994. SETTING: University of

California, San Francisco; Mayo Clinic, Rochester, Minn; and the University of Nebraska, Omaha. PATIENTS: Seven hundred eleven patients who received single-organ liver transplants, were at least 16 years old, and had nonfulminant liver disease. MAIN OUTCOME MEASURE: Standardized resource utilization derived from a database created by matching all services to a single price list. RESULTS: Higher adjusted resource utilization was associated with donor age of 60 years or older (28% [$53813] greater mean resource utilization; P=.005); recipient age of 60 years or older (17% [$32795]; P=.01); alcoholic liver disease (26% [$49596]; P=.002); Child–Pugh class C (41% [$67 658]; P less than .001); care from the intensive care unit at time of transplant (42% [$77833]; P less than .001); death in the hospital (35% [$67 076]; P less than .001); and having multiple liver transplants during the index hospitalization (154% increase [$474 740 vs $186 726 for 1 transplant]; P less than .001). Adjusted length of stay and resource utilization also differed significantly among transplant centers. CONCLUSIONS: Clinical, economic, and ethical dilemmas in liver transplantation are highlighted by these findings. Recipients who were older, had alcoholic liver disease, or were severely ill were the most expensive to treat; this suggests that organ allocation criteria may affect transplant costs. Clinical practices and resource utilization varied considerably among transplant centers; methods to reduce variation in practice patterns, such as clinical guidelines, might lower costs while maintaining quality of care.

Silva, Mary Cipriano. Ethics of consumer rights in managed care. *NursingConnections.* 1997 Summer; 10(2): 24–26. 3 refs. BE59189.
    disclosure; drugs; economics; gatekeeping; legal rights; legislation; *managed care programs; patient care; *patients' rights; quality of health care; referral and consultation; state government; withholding treatment; drug formularies; Managed Care Consumer Protection Act; United States

Simon, Steven R.; Pan, Richard J.D.; Sullivan, Amy M., et al. Views of managed care: a survey of students, residents, faculty, and deans at medical schools in the United States. *New England Journal of Medicine.* 1999 Mar 25; 340(12): 928–936. 23 refs. BE61030.
    *administrators; *attitudes; biomedical research; chronically ill; comparative studies; conflict of interest; curriculum; evaluation; *faculty; health care delivery; internal medicine; *internship and residency; interprofessional relations; knowledge, attitudes, practice; *managed care programs; *medical education; *medical schools; *medical specialties; national health insurance; patient care; pediatrics; physician patient relationship; *physicians; *primary health care; quality of health care; remuneration; *students; survey; terminal care; continuity of patient care; fee-for-service plans; *United States
    BACKGROUND AND METHODS: Views of managed care among academic physicians and medical students in the United States are not well known. In 1997, we conducted a telephone survey of a national sample of medical students (506 respondents), residents (494), faculty members (728), department chairs (186), directors of residency training in internal medicine and pediatrics (143), and deans (105) at U.S. medical schools to determine their experiences in and perspectives on managed care. The overall rate of response was 80.1 percent. RESULTS: Respondents rated their attitudes toward managed care on a 0-to-10 scale, with 0 defined as "as negative as possible" and 10 as "as positive as possible." The expressed attitudes toward managed care were negative, ranging from a low mean (+/-SD) score of 3.9+/-1.7 for residents to a high of 5.0+/-1.3 for

---

deans. When asked about specific aspects of care, fee-for-service medicine was rated better than managed care in terms of access (by 80.2 percent of respondents), minimizing ethical conflicts (74.8 percent), and the quality of the doctor-patient relationship (70.6 percent). With respect to the continuity of care, 52.0 percent of respondents preferred fee-for-service medicine, and 29.3 percent preferred managed care. For care at the end of life, 49.1 percent preferred fee-for-service medicine, and 20.5 percent preferred managed care. With respect to care for patients with chronic illness, 41.8 percent preferred fee-for-service care, and 30.8 percent preferred managed care. Faculty members, residency-training directors, and department chairs responded that managed care had reduced the time they had available for research (63.1 percent agreed) and teaching (58.9 percent) and had reduced their income (55.8 percent). Overall, 46.6 percent of faculty members, 26.7 percent of residency-training directors, and 42.7 percent of department chairs reported that the message they delivered to students about managed care was negative. CONCLUSIONS: Negative views of managed care are widespread among medical students, residents, faculty members, and medical school deans.

Sorell, Tom, ed. Health Care, Ethics and Insurance. New York, NY: Routledge; 1998. 240 p. (Professional ethics). Includes references. ISBN 0-415-16284-X. BE61424.
AIDS serodiagnosis; confidentiality; disabled; disclosure; freedom; genetic screening; government financing; health care; health care delivery; *health insurance; justice; life insurance; long-term care; obligations of society; *private sector; public sector; quality of health care; resource allocation; social discrimination; needs; *Great Britain

Steinbrook, Robert. Caring for people with human immunodeficiency virus infection. [Editorial]. *New England Journal of Medicine.* 1998 Dec 24; 339(26): 1926-1928. 15 refs. BE60262.
adults; *AIDS; children; *disadvantaged; *drugs; *economics; federal government; *government financing; *health care delivery; *HIV seropositivity; mortality; *patient care; prevalence; *public policy; state government; statistics; Department of Veterans Affairs; Medicaid; Medicare; *United States

Stoddard, Joan C.; Billings, Paul R.; Astrue, Michael J., et al. Health care providers, insurers, and individual patients; the right to treatment; economic and policy issues. [Proceedings of the International Symposium on Law and Science at the Crossroads: Biomedical Technology, Ethics, Public Policy, and the Law; panel discussion]. *Suffolk University Law Review.* 1993 Winter; 27(4): 1499-1523. Moderators: Linda C. Fentiman and Raja B. Khauli. BE60703.
AIDS; biomedical technologies; bone marrow; conflict of interest; decision making; DNA data banks; gene therapy; genetic disorders; genetic predisposition; genetic research; genetic screening; *health insurance reimbursement; informed consent; insurance; investigators; legal aspects; organ donation; *organ transplantation; parental consent; patient compliance; prognosis; resource allocation; selection for treatment; social discrimination; social worth; technology assessment; therapeutic research; *tissue transplantation; transplant recipients; treatment outcome; *investigational therapies; United States

Stolberg, Sheryl Gay. New rules will force doctors to disclose ties to drug industry. [News]. *New York Times.* 1998 Feb 3: A12. BE59669.
*biomedical research; *conflict of interest; *disclosure; *drug industry; *drugs; federal government; financial support; *government regulation; *incentives; *investigators;

*mandatory reporting; medical devices; *physicians; *therapeutic research; *Food and Drug Administration; United States

Studdert, David M. Direct contracts, data sharing and employee risk selection: new stakes for patient privacy in tomorrow's health insurance markets. *American Journal of Law and Medicine.* 1999; 25(2-3): 233-265. 242 fn. BE62508.
compensation; computers; *confidentiality; conflict of interest; *contracts; disabled; *disclosure; economics; *employment; federal government; government regulation; health care delivery; *health insurance; *incentives; insurance selection bias; *legal aspects; legislation; *managed care programs; occupational medicine; *organization and administration; patient care; *physicians; *privacy; risk; social discrimination; state government; Americans with Disabilities Act 1990; *United States

Sullivan, William M. What is left of professionalism after managed care? *Hastings Center Report.* 1999 Mar-Apr; 29(2): 7-13. 12 fn. BE61655.
capitalism; contracts; *economics; federal government; government financing; government regulation; health care; *health care reform; historical aspects; industry; institutional ethics; lawyers; *managed care programs; moral obligations; national health insurance; *obligations to society; *physician's role; physicians; *professional autonomy; professional organizations; public policy; *self regulation; social control; *sociology of medicine; technical expertise; *trends; trust; business ethics; Nineteenth Century; *Twentieth Century; *United States
Modern American medicine has wedded scientific advance to a small business model of the individual practitioner, defining professionalism as technical understanding. If the profession is to survive, it must draw on older ideals of the learned professions as acting on behalf of the community, and reinvigorate a civic understanding of professional life.

Sulmasy, Daniel P. Cancer, managed care, and therapeutic research: an ethicist's view. *HMO Practice.* 1997 Jun; 11(2): 59-62. 7 refs. BE61558.
*cancer; common good; government financing; *health insurance reimbursement; *health maintenance organizations; hospitals; human experimentation; institutional ethics; investigators; *justice; moral obligations; *moral policy; patient advocacy; peer review; physicians; research institutes; selection of subjects; *therapeutic research; United States

Tabarrok, Alexander. Genetic testing: an economic and contractarian analysis. *Journal of Health Economics.* 1994 Mar; 13(1): 75-91. 35 refs. 21 fn. BE59804.
confidentiality; decision making; disclosure; *economics; employment; genetic disorders; genetic predisposition; *genetic screening; government regulation; *health insurance; informed consent; *insurance selection bias; legal aspects; policy analysis; *risk; United States

U.S. Congress. Senate. A bill to improve the access and choice of patients to quality, affordable health care [Patients' Bill of Rights Act of 1998]. S. 2330, 105th Cong., 2d Sess. Introduced by Trent Lott for Don Nickles, for himself, and others.; 1998 Jul 17 (first reading). 185 p. Read the second time and placed on the calendar 20 Jul 1998. BE59925.
accountability; alternatives; biomedical research; confidentiality; *disclosure; emergency care; *health care delivery; *health insurance; health maintenance organizations; health services research; information dissemination; *legal aspects; legislation; medical records; patient access to records; patient care; *patients' rights; physicians; *quality of health care; referral and consultation; women's health; *women's health services; continuity of

---

BE = bioethics accession number   fn. = footnotes   refs. = references

patient care; Centers for Disease Control and Prevention; Employee Retirement Income Security Act 1974 (ERISA); National Institutes of Health; Office of Research on Women's Health; *Patients' Bill of Rights Act (1998 bill); *United States

Visser, A.A. Oranjemed -- Bloemfontein Protocols preamble. *Journal of the Dental Association of South Africa.* 1996 Nov; 51(11): 673–677. BE61865.

accountability; codes of ethics; confidentiality; conflict of interest; contracts; dentistry; disclosure; gatekeeping; guidelines; health personnel; informed consent; *managed care programs; patient participation; physicians; professional organizations; regulation; standards; Oranjemed Independent Practitioners' Association; *South Africa

Vrbová, H.; Holmerová, I.; Hrubantová, L. Business ethics as a novel issue in health care economics. *Sborník Lékarský.* 1997; 98(3): 225–232. 6 refs. BE62418.

accountability; common good; community services; *economics; *health care delivery; health care reform; health insurance; patient participation; physician patient relationship; quality of health care; *resource allocation; trust; vulnerable populations; *Czech Republic

Wasson, John H.; Bubolz, Thomas A.; Lynn, Joanne, et al. Can we afford comprehensive, supportive care for the very old? *Journal of the American Geriatrics Society.* 1998 Jul; 46(7): 829–832. 20 refs. BE62258.

*aged; *community services; *economics; government financing; health care; *health care delivery; health services research; *home care; *hospitals; managed care programs; mortality; patient admission; patient care; *resource allocation; *health services misuse; *Medicare; *United States

Watson, Sidney Dean. In search of the story: physicians and charity care. *Saint Louis University Public Law Review.* 1996; 15(2): 353–369. 92 fn. BE59914.

*altruism; *bioethical issues; *bioethics; caring; case studies; economics; emergency care; ethicists; *health care delivery; hospitals; *indigents; literature; medical education; medical ethics; methods; minority groups; *moral obligations; *narrative ethics; obligations of society; *patient care; patient compliance; patient transfer; physician patient relationship; *physicians; *refusal to treat; remuneration; social problems; *socioeconomic factors; Medicaid; United States

Weiss, Stefan C. Defining a "patients' bill of rights" for the next century. [Editorial]. *JAMA.* 1999 Mar 3; 281(9): 856. 4 refs. BE60242.

*economics; *health care delivery; *legal aspects; *managed care programs; *patients' rights; physicians; public policy; quality of health care; refusal to treat; *Patients' Bill of Rights; *United States

Wildman, Martin. Quality and the invisible man. [Personal view]. *BMJ (British Medical Journal).* 1998 Dec 12; 317(7173): 1667. BE60266.

*disadvantaged; *economics; *emergency care; *quality of health care; resource allocation; Great Britain; National Health Service

Winerip, Michael. Bedlam on the streets. *New York Times Magazine.* 1999 May 23: 42–49, 56, 65–66, 70. BE61010.

accountability; *community services; *dangerousness; *deinstitutionalized persons; *economics; government financing; *health care delivery; mental institutions; *mentally ill; mentally retarded; municipal government; outpatient commitment; patient compliance; patient discharge; patient transfer; psychoactive drugs; *public policy; residential facilities; schizophrenia; state government; *violence; voluntary admission; *homeless persons; New York City; *United States

Wong, Kenman L. Medicine and the Marketplace: The Moral Dimensions of Managed Care. Notre Dame, IN: University of Notre Dame Press; 1998. 219 p. Includes references. ISBN 0–268–01440–X. BE61847.

accountability; alternatives; conflict of interest; disclosure; *economics; gatekeeping; *health care delivery; health care reform; health insurance reimbursement; health maintenance organizations; incentives; *institutional ethics; justice; legal aspects; *managed care programs; physician patient relationship; physicians; referral and consultation; remuneration; resource allocation; risks and benefits; *business ethics; gag clauses; investigational therapies; nonprofit organizations; proprietary organizations; United States

Zuger, Abigail. Doctors' offices turn into salesrooms. [News]. *New York Times.* 1999 Mar 30: F1, F11. BE60875.

*alternative therapies; coercion; *conflict of interest; dissent; *drugs; *economics; *entrepreneurship; managed care programs; organizational policies; *patient care; *physicians; professional organizations; remuneration; American Medical Association; United States

Health care in America: your money or your life. *Economist.* 1998 Mar 7–13; 346(8058): 23–24, 26. BE60896.

*economics; federal government; government regulation; health care delivery; *managed care programs; preventive medicine; public opinion; quality of health care; risks and benefits; withholding treatment; *United States

Patients or profits? *Economist.* 1998 Mar 7–13; (346)8058: 15. BE60895.

*economics; government regulation; *health care delivery; health care reform; health insurance; managed care programs; *public policy; *United States

HEALTH CARE/FOREIGN COUNTRIES

Aarons, Derrick E. Medicine and its alternatives: health care priorities in the Caribbean. *Hastings Center Report.* 1999 Jul–Aug; 29(4): 23–27. 23 fn. BE62466.

*alternative therapies; biomedical technologies; *developing countries; drugs; goals; *health care; health personnel; interprofessional relations; legal aspects; medical ethics; primary health care; regulation; *socioeconomic factors; standards; *folk medicine; *Caribbean Region

In the Caribbean as in many other areas costly biomedical resources and personnel are limited, and more and more people are turning to alternative medicine and folk practitioners for health care. To meet the goal of providing health care for all, research on nonbiomedical therapies is needed, along with legal recognition of folk practitioners to establish standards of practice.

Abraham, John; Sheppard, Julie. Democracy, technocracy, and the secret state of medicines control: expert and nonexpert perspectives. *Science, Technology, and Human Values.* 1997 Spring; 22(2): 139–167. 38 refs. 2 fn. BE59854.

accountability; attitudes; committee membership; confidentiality; consensus; *decision making; drug abuse; *drug industry; *drugs; *government regulation; health personnel; investigators; mass media; patient care; physician's role; professional role; psychoactive drugs; public opinion; *public participation; public policy; risk; risks and benefits; science; survey; *technical expertise; trust; uncertainty; *values; questionnaires; Committee on the Safety of Medicines (Great Britain); *Great Britain; Medicines Commission (Great Britain)

Begum, Hasna. Health care, ethics and nursing in Bangladesh: a personal perspective. *Nursing Ethics.* 1998

Nov; 5(6): 535–541. 2 refs. BE60814.
abortion, induced; cloning; *developing countries; ecology; family planning; females; genetic information; *health care delivery; health insurance; intensive care units; *nurses; nursing education; quality of health care; reproductive technologies; *socioeconomic factors; terminal care; women's rights; *Bangladesh

Breen, Kerry J.; Plueckhahn, Vernon D.; Cordner, Stephen M. Ethics, Law and Medical Practice. St. Leonards, NSW, Australia: Allen and Unwin; 1997. 367 p. Includes references. Appendices include the Australian Medical Association code of ethics, NHMRC (National Health and Medical Research Council) statement on human experimentation, NHMRC general guidelines for medical practitioners on providing information to patients, and NHMRC recommendations for the donation of cadaveric organs and tissues for transplantation. ISBN 1-86448-407-1. BE59722.
abortion, induced; active euthanasia; allowing to die; autonomy; beneficence; communication; computers; confidentiality; determination of death; drugs; employment; government regulation; *health care delivery; human experimentation; informed consent; interprofessional relations; involuntary commitment; *legal aspects; legal liability; mandatory reporting; medical education; *medical ethics; medical records; mentally ill; misconduct; negligence; organization and administration; parent child relationship; *patient care; physician patient relationship; physicians; professional competence; reproductive technologies; resource allocation; self regulation; sexuality; standards; third party consent; treatment refusal; virtues; withholding treatment; physician impairment; self care; *Australia

Brooks, Alex. Viagra is licensed in Europe, but rationed in Britain. [News]. *BMJ (British Medical Journal).* 1998 Sep 19; 317(7161): 765. BE60827.
*drugs; *government financing; males; patient care; *public policy; *resource allocation; selection for treatment; sexuality; *impotence; *Great Britain; *National Health Service; *Viagra

Brown, Murray G. Rationing health care in Canada. *Annals of Health Law.* 1993; 2: 101–119. 22 fn. BE59829.
compassion; costs and benefits; decision making; *economics; *government financing; *health care delivery; hospitals; justice; *national health insurance; organization and administration; physicians; private sector; *public policy; public sector; *resource allocation; treatment outcome; *values; needs; *Canada

Brown, Phyllida. WHO urges "coverage for all, not coverage of everything." [News]. *BMJ (British Medical Journal).* 1999 May 15; 318(7194): 1305. BE62515.
health; *health care; *international aspects; *obligations of society; preventive medicine; public health; public policy; resource allocation; standards; *World Health Organization

Buetow, Stephen. The scope for the involvement of patients in their consultations with health professionals: rights, responsibilities and preferences of patients. *Journal of Medical Ethics.* 1998 Aug; 24(4): 243–247. 53 refs. BE61289.
*accountability; common good; decision making; *health care delivery; *moral obligations; patient care; *patient participation; *patients; *patients' rights; *professional patient relationship; *Great Britain; National Health Service; Patient's Charter (Great Britain)
The degree and nature of patient involvement in consultations with health professionals influences problem and needs recognition and management, and public accountability. This paper suggests a framework for understanding the scope for patient involvement in such consultations. Patients are defined as co-producers

of formal health services, whose potential for involvement in consultations depends on their personal rights, responsibilities and preferences. Patients' rights in consultations are poorly defined and, in the National Health Service (NHS), not legally enforceable. The responsibilities of patients are also undefined. I suggest that these are not to deny, of their own volition, the rights of others, which in consultations necessitate mutuality of involvement through information-exchange and shared decision-making. Preferences should be met insofar as they do not militate against responsibilities and rights.

Cheng, F.; Ip, Mary; Wong, K.K., et al. Critical care ethics in Hong Kong: cross-cultural conflicts as East meets West. *Journal of Medicine and Philosophy.* 1998 Dec; 23(6): 616–627. 16 refs. BE62069.
aged; *allowing to die; autonomy; critically ill; decision making; family members; futility; *health care delivery; hospitals; *intensive care units; morbidity; non-Western World; patient admission; patient discharge; physicians; prolongation of life; resource allocation; resuscitation orders; selection for treatment; values; withholding treatment; *Hong Kong
The practice of critical care medicine has long been a difficult task for most critical care physicians in the densely populated city of Hong Kong, where we face limited resources and a limited number of intensive care beds. Our triage decisions are largely based on the potential of functional reversibility of the patients. Provision of graded care beds may help to relieve some of the demands on the intensive care beds. Decisions to forego futile medical treatment are frequently physician-guided family-based decisions, which is quite contrary to the Western focus on patient autonomy. However, as people acquire knowledge about health care and they become more aware of individual rights, our critical care doctors will be able to narrow the gaps between the different concepts of medical ethics among our professionals as well as in our society. An open and caring attitude from our intensivists will be important in minimizing the cross-cultural conflict on the complex issue of medical futility.

Cong, Yali. Ethical challenges in critical care medicine: a Chinese perspective. *Journal of Medicine and Philosophy.* 1998 Dec; 23(6): 581–600. 21 refs. 1 fn. BE62067.
allowing to die; bioethics; *critically ill; decision making; *economics; family members; geographic factors; government financing; *health care delivery; hospitals; *intensive care units; justice; legal aspects; medical devices; non-Western World; patient admission; physician patient relationship; physicians; public policy; *resource allocation; values; personal financing; *China
The major ethical challenges for critical care medicine in China include the high cost of patient care in the ICU, the effect of payment mechanisms on access to critical care, the fact that much more money is spent on patients who die than on ones who live, the extent to which an attempt to rescue and save a patient is made, and the great geographical disparity in distribution of critical care. The ethical problems surrounding critical care medicine bear much relation to the culture, public policy and health care system in China. The essay concludes that China should allocate more resources to ordinary medical services rather than to critical care medicine.

Davis, Kathy. The rhetoric of cosmetic surgery: luxury or welfare? *In:* Parens, Erik, ed. Enhancing Human Traits: Ethical and Social Implications. Washington, DC: Georgetown University Press; 1998: 124–134. 13

BE = bioethics accession number   fn. = footnotes   refs. = references

fn. ISBN 0–87840–703–0. BE59748.
*cosmetic surgery; decision making; enhancement technologies; females; feminist ethics; *government financing; guidelines; *health care; health care delivery; *health insurance reimbursement; national health insurance; normality; psychological stress; public participation; *public policy; *resource allocation; selection for treatment; state medicine; suffering; beauty; *Netherlands

de Castro, Leonardo D.; Sy, Peter A. Critical care in the Philippines: the "Robin Hood principle" vs. *kagandahang loob. Journal of Medicine and Philosophy.* 1998 Dec; 23(6): 563–580. 14 refs. 2 fn. BE62066.
allowing to die; attitudes; bioethical issues; biomedical technologies; *critically ill; decision making; developing countries; economics; emergency care; extraordinary treatment; *health care delivery; health maintenance organizations; hospitals; indigents; informed consent; international aspects; justice; legal aspects; newborns; non-Western World; nurses; obligations of society; organ donation; physicians; prolongation of life; public policy; religion; *resource allocation; *values; withholding treatment; *charity; technology transfer; *Philippines
Practical medical decisions are closely integrated with ethical and religious beliefs in the Philippines. This is shown in a survey of Filipino physicians' attitudes towards severely compromised neonates. This is also the reason why the ethical analysis of critical care practices must be situated within the context of local culture. Kagandahang loob and kusang loob are indigenous Filipino ethical concepts that provide a framework for the analysis of several critical care practices. The practice of taking-from-the-rich-to-give-to-the-poor in public hospitals is not compatible with these concepts. The legislated definition of death and other aspects of the Philippine Law on Organ Transplants also fail to be compatible with these concepts. Many ethical issues that arise in a critical care setting have their roots outside the seemingly isolated clinical setting. Critical care need not apply only to individuals in a serious clinical condition. Vulnerable populations require critical attention because potent threats to their lives exist in the water that they drink and the air that they breathe. We cannot ignore these threats even as we move inevitably towards a technologically dependent, highly commercialized approach to health management.

Dósa, Agnes. Bioethics and health law in Hungary. *Saint Louis University Public Law Review.* 1996; 15(2): 403–409. 40 fn. BE59916.
*bioethical issues; coercion; decision making; economics; *health care; informed consent; involuntary commitment; *legal aspects; minors; organ donation; paternalism; patient access to records; patients' rights; physician patient relationship; presumed consent; public health; truth disclosure; *Hungary

Doyal, Len. Public participation and the moral quality of healthcare rationing. *Quality in Health Care.* 1998 Jun; 7(2): 98–102. 37 refs. BE62322.
*decision making; *democracy; futility; government financing; *health care delivery; health personnel; *justice; moral policy; patient participation; *public participation; *public policy; *resource allocation; rights; scarcity; needs; *Great Britain; *National Health Service

Dyer, Clare. Transsexuals win case for NHS funded surgery. [News]. *BMJ (British Medical Journal).* 1999 Jan 9; 318(7176): 75. BE62607.
*government financing; *health care; *legal aspects; *legal rights; resource allocation; *surgery; *transsexualism; *Great Britain; *National Health Service

Dyer, Clare. UK Human Rights Act will allow challenges to treatment refusals. [News]. *BMJ (British Medical Journal).* 1998 Nov 14; 317(7169): 1339. BE62646.
*government financing; *health care; human rights; *legal rights; resource allocation; surgery; transsexualism; European Convention on Human Rights; *Great Britain; *National Health Service

Engelhardt, H. Tristram. Critical care: why there is no global bioethics. *Journal of Medicine and Philosophy.* 1998 Dec; 23(6): 643–651. 4 refs. 1 fn. BE62071.
autonomy; *bioethics; critically ill; *cultural pluralism; decision making; developing countries; economics; *ethical relativism; *health care delivery; informed consent; *international aspects; justice; morality; non-Western World; public policy; quality of health care; resource allocation; secularism; standards; third party consent; *values; Western World; egalitarianism; United States
The high technology and the costs involved in critical care disclose the implausibility of applying the American standard version of bioethics in the developing world. The American standard version of bioethics was framed during the rapid secularization of the American culture, the emergence of a new image for the medical profession, the development of high technology medicine, an ever greater demand in resources, and a shift of focus from families and communities to individuals. This all brought with it a particular ideology of health care which promised Americans (1) the best of care, (2) equal care, and (3) physician/patient choice, without (4) runaway costs. This essay argues that this moral project is impossible in practice. This impossibility is especially salient in developing countries. In addition to the fact that it is financially impossible to provide all in the developing world with the standard of care accepted by law, policy, and convention in developed countries, different moral perspectives with different orderings of values will seem more or less plausible in different cultures. Indeed, such an approach would be harmful. A concrete bioethics applicable across the world does not appear possible.

Fan, Ruiping. Critical care ethics in Asia: global or local? *Journal of Medicine and Philosophy.* 1998 Dec; 23(6): 549–562. 12 refs. 3 fn. BE62065.
autonomy; bioethical issues; bioethics; communitarianism; *critically ill; *cultural pluralism; decision making; developing countries; economics; ethical relativism; ethical theory; family members; *health care delivery; informed consent; intensive care units; *international aspects; *justice; libertarianism; morbidity; mortality; non-Western World; *quality of health care; *resource allocation; third party consent; utilitarianism; values; *Asia; China; Hong Kong; Japan; Philippines; Rawls, John; United States

Fears, Robin; Poste, George. Building population genetics resources using the U.K. NHS. *Science.* 1999 Apr 9; 284(5412): 267–268. 15 fn. BE61402.
confidentiality; *data banks; *DNA data banks; epidemiology; *genetic information; *genetic research; government financing; *health care delivery; *industry; informed consent; medical records; *population genetics; *private sector; *public policy; *public sector; regulation; research subjects; *resource allocation; tissue banks; pedigree studies; *Great Britain; *National Health Service

Glantz, Leonard H.; Annas, George J.; Grodin, Michael A., et al. Research in developing countries: taking "benefit" seriously. *Hastings Center Report.* 1998 Nov–Dec; 28(6): 38–42. 18 fn. BE61285.
*developing countries; drugs; *economics; *financial support; guidelines; *health care; HIV seropositivity; *human experimentation; *international aspects; pregnant

---

BE = bioethics accession number   fn. = footnotes   refs. = references

women; preventive medicine; *risks and benefits; standards; Africa; AZT

Graham, Wendy J.; Newell, Marie-Louise. Seizing the opportunity: collaborative initiatives to reduce HIV and maternal mortality. *Lancet.* 1999 Mar 6; 353(9155): 836–839. 36 refs. BE61222.
AIDS; cesarean section; childbirth; children; contraception; costs and benefits; *developing countries; drugs; economics; females; health care delivery; health education; *HIV seropositivity; infants; *maternal health; *morbidity; *mortality; *mothers; newborns; patient care; patient education; *pregnant women; prevalence; preventive medicine; quality of health care; resource allocation; sexually transmitted diseases; social impact; *women's health; *women's health services; breast feeding; Africa; AZT; Inter-Agency Group for Safe Motherhood; UNAIDS

Gray, Gwen. Access to medical care under strain: new pressures in Canada and Australia. *Journal of Health Politics, Policy and Law.* 1998 Dec; 23(6): 905–947. 113 refs. BE59785.
comparative studies; *economics; government financing; health; *health care delivery; health insurance; indigents; *international aspects; justice; national health insurance; politics; *private sector; public policy; *public sector; social impact; socioeconomic factors; trends; personal financing; *Australia; *Canada; Europe; Organization for Economic Cooperation and Development; United States
Health policy changes intended to achieve cost control in OECD countries run the risk of reintroducing financial barriers to health care. However, although the problems faced are similar, different countries are dealing with the situation in different ways. For example, Canada and Australia, which share many similarities, have taken quite different policy paths in the last decade: Canada has preserved universal access, whereas Australian policy is promoting a two-tier system through the provision of public subsidies for private insurance. The evidence is that country-specific factors such as institutional arrangements, attitudes, and values intersect with economic and financial factors to shape policy outcomes. Moreover, the Canadian and Australian experiences suggest that in relation to access issues, attitudes and values are the key policy determinants.

Hill, Wan Ying; Fraser, Ian; Cotton, Philip. Patients' voices, rights and responsibilities: on implementing social audit in primary health care. *Journal of Business Ethics.* 1998 Oct; 17(13): 1481–1497. 59 refs. 23 fn. BE61217.
*accountability; attitudes; decision making; economics; health care delivery; institutional ethics; legal rights; *organization and administration; *patient participation; *patient satisfaction; patients; *patients' rights; pharmacists; physician patient relationship; physicians; *primary health care; resource allocation; review committees; survey; trust; empowerment; Great Britain; *National Health Service; *Patients' Charter (Great Britain); *Scotland

Holm, Søren. Goodbye to the simple solutions: the second phase of priority setting in health care. *BMJ (British Medical Journal).* 1998 Oct 10; 317(7164): 1000–1002. 6 refs. Presented at the Second International Conference on Priorities in Health Care held in London, 8–10 October 1998. BE60831.
decision making; goals; government financing; *health care delivery; international aspects; *public policy; *resource allocation; severity of illness index; Denmark; Norway; *Scandinavia

Klein, Rudolf. Puzzling out priorities: why we must acknowledge that rationing is a political process. [Editorial]. *BMJ (British Medical Journal).* 1998 Oct 10;

317(7164): 959–960. 10 refs. BE60830.
decision making; *health care delivery; international aspects; politics; *public policy; *resource allocation; *Great Britain; National Health Service

Landman, Willem A.; Henley, Lesley D. Equitable rationing of highly specialised health care services for children: a perspective from South Africa. *Journal of Medical Ethics.* 1999 Jun; 25(3): 224–229. 34 fn. BE61854.
*biomedical technologies; *children; chronically ill; costs and benefits; cystic fibrosis; disabled; disease; futility; *government financing; *health care; *health care delivery; intensive care units; *justice; legal rights; leukemia; methods; moral policy; newborns; organ transplantation; palliative care; prevalence; primary health care; *prognosis; *public policy; quality of health care; *random selection; *resource allocation; scarcity; *selection for treatment; utilitarianism; needs; patient abandonment; *waiting lists; *South Africa
The principles of equality and equity, respectively in the Bill of Rights and the white paper on health, provide the moral and legal foundations for future health care for children in South Africa. However, given extreme health care need and scarce resources, the government faces formidable obstacles if it hopes to achieve a just allocation of public health care resources, especially among children in need of highly specialised health care. In this regard, there is a dearth of moral analysis which is practically useful in the South African situation. We offer a set of moral considerations to guide the macro-allocation of highly specialised public health care services among South Africa's children. We also mention moral considerations which should inform micro-allocation.

Landman, Willem A.; Henley, Lesley D. Tensions in setting health care priorities for South Africa's children. *Journal of Medical Ethics.* 1998 Aug; 24(4): 268–273. 30 fn. BE61294.
beneficence; *children; chronically ill; costs and benefits; decision making; health; *health care; justice; legal aspects; long-term care; moral policy; preventive medicine; primary health care; public health; public participation; *public policy; quality of life; *resource allocation; standards; *health planning; needs; *South Africa
The new South African constitution commits the government to guarantee "basic health services" for every child under 18. Primary health care for pregnant women and children under six and elements of essential primary health care have received priority. At present, there is little analysis of the moral considerations involved in making choices about more advanced or costly health care which may, arguably, also be "basic". This paper illustrates some of the tensions in setting priorities for a just macro-allocation of children's health care, given the realities of need and scarce resources, and the commitment to equality of basic opportunities.

Lerner, Paul. Rationalizing the therapeutic arsenal: German neuropsychiatry in World War I. *In:* Berg, Manfred; Cocks, Geoffrey, eds. Medicine and Modernity: Public Health and Medical Care in Nineteenth- and Twentieth-Century Germany. New York, NY: Cambridge University Press; 1997: 121–148. 106 fn. ISBN 0-521-56411-5. BE59268.
*attitudes; coercion; common good; deception; electroconvulsive therapy; *historical aspects; hypnosis; *mental health; *mentally ill; methods; *military personnel; misconduct; obligations to society; *patient care; physician patient relationship; physician's role; *physicians; psychiatric diagnosis; *psychiatry; psychotherapy; *public policy; rehabilitation; social control; social dominance; *war; post-traumatic stress disorders; *Germany; *Twentieth Century; *World War I

Lessard, Hester. The construction of health care and the ideology of the private in Canadian constitutional law. *Annals of Health Law.* 1993; 2: 121-159. 153 fn. BE59830.
*abortion, induced; constitutional law; criminal law; economics; federal government; government regulation; *health care delivery; *historical aspects; hospitals; *legal aspects; legal rights; national health insurance; physicians; pregnant women; *private sector; *public policy; *public sector; *rights; social discrimination; therapeutic abortion; *women's rights; *Canada; Canadian Charter of Rights and Freedoms; Criminal Code of Canada; Nineteenth Century; R. v. Morgentaler; Twentieth Century

Loff, Bebe; Cordner, Stephen. Aboriginal people trade land claim for dialysis. [News]. *Lancet.* 1998 Oct 31; 352(9138): 1451. BE59640.
*health care delivery; *minority groups; public policy; *renal dialysis; Australia; *Northern Territory

Loff, Bebe; Cordner, Stephen. Learning a culture of respect for human rights. [Commentary]. *Lancet.* 1998 Dec 5; 352(9143): 1800. 3 refs. BE60803.
disadvantaged; forensic medicine; *health care delivery; *human rights; *minority groups; *misconduct; *physicians; *prisoners; *social discrimination; torture; *aborigines; *Australia; *South Africa

McCullough, Laurence B. A transcultural, preventive ethics approach to critical-care medicine: restoring the critical care physician's power and authority. *Journal of Medicine and Philosophy.* 1998 Dec; 23(6): 628-642. 9 refs. BE62070.
*allowing to die; autonomy; beneficence; costs and benefits; *critically ill; *cultural pluralism; *decision making; family members; family relationship; futility; iatrogenic disease; institutional policies; *intensive care units; *international aspects; medical specialties; non-Western World; palliative care; *physicians; primary health care; *professional autonomy; prolongation of life; public policy; resource allocation; resuscitation; *values; withholding treatment; Confucian ethics; *preventive ethics; *China; *Hong Kong; *Japan; *Philippines; United States
This article comments on the treatment of critical-care ethics in four preceding articles about critical-care medicine and its ethical challenges in mainland China, Hong Kong, Japan, and the Philippines. These articles show how cultural values can be in both synchrony and conflict in generating these ethical challenges and in the constraints that they place on the response of critical-care ethics to them. To prevent ethical conflict in critical care the author proposes a two-step approach to the ethical justification of critical-care management: (1) the decision to resuscitate and initiate critical-care management, which is based on the obligation to prevent imminent mortality without permanent loss of consciousness; and (2) the decision to continue critical-care management, which is based on the obligation both to prevent imminent death without permanent loss of consciousness and to avoid unnecessary, significant iatrogenic costs to the patient and psychosocial costs to the family when the reduction of mortality risk is marginal. Physicians and hospitals should restore the critical-care physician's authority and power -- against prevailing cultural values, if necessary -- to control when critical-care intervention is offered, when it is recommended to continue, and when it is recommended to be discontinued and the patient allowed to die.

MacLeod, Stuart M.; Bienenstock, John. Evidence-based rationing: Dutch pragmatism or government insensitivity? [Editorial]. *Canadian Medical Association Journal.* 1998 Jan 27; 158(2): 213-214. 5 refs.

BE60582.
economics; *evidence-based medicine; *health care delivery; health services research; *public policy; quality of health care; *resource allocation; values; Canada; *Netherlands

Mechanic, David. Muddling through elegantly: finding the proper balance in rationing. *Health Affairs.* 1997 Sep-Oct; 16(5): 83-92. 17 fn. BE59178.
administrators; biomedical technologies; costs and benefits; cultural pluralism; decision making; *economics; evidence-based medicine; gatekeeping; government regulation; *health care delivery; international aspects; justice; managed care programs; *methods; national health insurance; physicians; political activity; politics; public opinion; *public policy; *resource allocation; socioeconomic factors; values; capitation fee; case managers; *Great Britain; Medicaid; National Health Service; Oregon Health Plan; *United States

Nakata, Yoshinori; Goto, Takahisa; Morita, Shigeho. Serving the emperor without asking: critical care ethics in Japan. *Journal of Medicine and Philosophy.* 1998 Dec; 23(6): 601-615. 12 refs. BE62068.
*allowing to die; case studies; costs and benefits; *critically ill; decision making; family members; futility; *health care delivery; health insurance; hospitals; intensive care units; medical fees; moral obligations; non-Western World; patient admission; physicians; prolongation of life; resource allocation; terminally ill; *values; pragmatism; *Japan
This article is an attempt by Japanese physicians to introduce the practice patterns and moral justification of Japanese critical care to the world. Japanese health care is characterized by the fact that the fee schedule does not reward high technology medicine, such as surgery and critical care. In spite of the low reimbursement, our critical care practice pattern is characterized by continuing futile treatment for terminal patients in the intensive care unit (ICU). This apparently wasteful practice can be explained by fundamental Japanese cultural values, social factors in Japan, the availability of extensive insurance coverage, physicians' psychological factors, lack of cost-benefit considerations and the pragmatic approach the Japanese take to situations. We attempt to make some brief suggestions regarding the improvement of our critical care practices. Although we can not fully present quantitative data to support our argument, this article represents our real-world approaches to the ethical issues in the ICU in Japan.

Newdick, Christopher. Resource allocation in the National Health Service. *American Journal of Law and Medicine.* 1997; 23(2-3): 291-318. 196 fn. BE62502.
aged; costs and benefits; *decision making; evidence-based medicine; futility; *health care delivery; health insurance reimbursement; judicial action; legal aspects; legal liability; long-term care; negligence; *organization and administration; physicians; refusal to treat; *resource allocation; risks and benefits; selection for treatment; self induced illness; social discrimination; state medicine; *Great Britain; *National Health Service

Reay, Trish. Allocating scarce resources in a publicly funded health system: ethical considerations of a Canadian managed care proposal. *Nursing Ethics.* 1999 May; 6(3): 240-249. 25 refs. BE61768.
conflict of interest; *decision making; federal government; *gatekeeping; government financing; health care delivery; *health care reform; incentives; justice; *managed care programs; moral obligations; patient advocacy; *physicians; public participation; *public policy; remuneration; *resource allocation; rights; capitation fee; *Alberta; *Canada

---

BE = bioethics accession number   fn. = footnotes   refs. = references

Rosenthal, Elisabeth. West's medicine is raising bills for China's sick. [News]. *New York Times.* 1998 Nov 19: A1, A12. BE61119.
> conflict of interest; *drug industry; *drugs; *economics; *health care; hospitals; *incentives; institutional policies; international aspects; misconduct; physicians; remuneration; Western World; *China

Royal College of Physicians. Setting Priorities in the NHS: A Framework for Decision-Making. A Report of the Royal College of Physicians. London: Royal College of Physicians of London; 1995 Sep. 38 p. 50 refs. This report was approved by the Royal College of Physicians on 15 Jun 1995. ISBN 1-86016-020-4. BE59460.
> administrators; advisory committees; biomedical research; common good; continuing education; costs and benefits; *decision making; *economics; education; evidence-based medicine; goals; *health care delivery; health promotion; health services research; justice; medical education; organization and administration; *organizational policies; patient care; patient care team; patient participation; *physician's role; physicians; preventive medicine; primary health care; private sector; professional organizations; *public participation; *public policy; *quality of health care; referral and consultation; *resource allocation; state medicine; time factors; treatment outcome; vulnerable populations; capitation fee; needs; *Great Britain; National Council for Health Care Priorities (Great Britain); *National Health Service; *Royal College of Physicians

Royal Dutch Medical Association. Medical Ethics Committee. Making Choices Professionally. Issued by the Association: Koninklijke Nederlandsche Maatschappij tot bevordering der Geneeskunst, P.O. Box 20051, 3502 LB, Utrecht, The Netherlands; 1992 Aug. 30 p. 21 fn. Translated from the Dutch by M.J. Tattersall-Evers. BE59261.
> decision making; *economics; health care; *health care delivery; health care reform; national health insurance; *physician's role; *physicians; *professional autonomy; quality of health care; resource allocation; selection for treatment; self induced illness; *Netherlands

Russian Federation. Principles of the legislation of the Russion Federation on the protection of the health of citizens. Dated 22 Jul 1993. (*Rossijskaja Gazeta*, 18 Aug 1993, p. 4–7). [Summary]. *International Digest of Health Legislation.* 1994. 45(1). 3–6. BE62694.
> abortion, induced; health; *health care; health care delivery; health personnel; *legal rights; obligations of society; patients' rights; public health; reproductive technologies; vulnerable populations; Russia; *Russian Federation

Sackett, David. The Doctor's (Ethical and Economic) Dilemma: A Description of the Dilemmas Faced by a Physician Who Tries to Serve Both Individual Patients and Society. Office of Health Economics [OHE] Annual Lecture 1996. London: Office of Health Economics; 1996 Aug. 20 p. 9 refs. ISBN 0901-387-983. BE59419.
> allowing to die; autonomy; beneficence; biomedical research; biomedical technologies; case studies; costs and benefits; *decision making; *economics; *evidence-based medicine; guideline adherence; guidelines; human experimentation; justice; *moral obligations; *obligations to society; *patient advocacy; patient care; *physicians; prolongation of life; quality of life; refusal to treat; *resource allocation; risks and benefits; selection for treatment; technical expertise; withholding treatment; *Great Britain; *National Health Service

Saltman, Richard B. Equity and distributive justice in European health care reform. *International Journal of Health Services.* 1997; 27(3): 443–453. 21 refs. This article

is modified from a paper presented at the Seminar on Equity by Health Policy, Dec 1996, in Madrid, Spain. BE60081.
> economics; financial support; health; health care; health care delivery; *health care reform; international aspects; *justice; moral obligations; obligations of society; private sector; *public policy; public sector; resource allocation; *socioeconomic factors; *Europe; World Health Organization

Schmacke, Norbert. Overdramatization of the burdens on health and social services: a continuing debate in the history of German medicine. *International Journal of Health Services.* 1997; 27(3): 559–574. 40 refs. This article is a revised and extended version of a lecture given on 24 Mar 1988, in the context of an exhibition on the government-planned and executed elimination of "lives unworthy of living" in National Socialism. Translated by Sean Mullan and Jutta Rateike-Fear. BE60082.
> advisory committees; *aged; AIDS; attitudes; *chronically ill; dementia; *disabled; *economics; *eugenics; euthanasia; *health care delivery; health care reform; health insurance; *historical aspects; homosexuals; killing; *National Socialism; patient care; physicians; political systems; psychiatry; social worth; socioeconomic factors; sociology of medicine; *stigmatization; terminal care; *trends; *Germany; *Twentieth Century; United States

Schmiedebach, Heinz-Peter. The mentally ill patient caught between the state's demands and the professional interests of psychiatrists. *In:* Berg, Manfred; Cocks, Geoffrey, eds. Medicine and Modernity: Public Health and Medical Care in Nineteenth- and Twentieth-Century Germany. New York, NY: Cambridge University Press; 1997: 99–119. 61 fn. ISBN 0-521-56411-5. BE59267.
> *attitudes; chronically ill; *dehumanization; eugenics; food; forensic psychiatry; health care delivery; *historical aspects; involuntary sterilization; medical specialties; *mental health; *mental institutions; *mentally ill; military personnel; mortality; patient care; *physicians; *psychiatry; public health; public policy; resource allocation; *social control; social problems; social worth; socioeconomic factors; *sociology of medicine; *stigmatization; war; prostitution; Darwinism; *Germany; *Nineteenth Century; *Twentieth Century; World War I

Shaul, Randi Zlotnik; Mendelssohn, David C. Scarce resource allocation decisions: issues of physician conflict and liability. *Humane Health Care International.* 1997 Spring; 13(1): 25–28. 35 refs. BE59960.
> accountability; administrators; *conflict of interest; disclosure; *economics; *gatekeeping; informed consent; kidney diseases; *legal liability; negligence; patient advocacy; physician patient relationship; *physician's role; *physicians; public policy; *renal dialysis; *resource allocation; selection for treatment; social discrimination; standards; time factors; Canada; *Ontario

Sheldon, Tony. Dutch regulate sponorship of hospitals. [News]. *BMJ (British Medical Journal).* 1999 Jun 19; 318(7199): 1644. BE62532.
> codes of ethics; conflict of interest; *drug industry; *financial support; *hospitals; *industry; *regulation; voluntary programs; *Netherlands

Sidley, Pat. Doctors contributed to poor health of black South Africans. [News]. *BMJ (British Medical Journal).* 1998 Nov 7; 317(7168): 1269. BE62645.
> biological warfare; *blacks; *health care delivery; *misconduct; moral complicity; nurses; *physicians; prisoners; professional organizations; public policy; *social discrimination; torture; *South Africa

---

BE = bioethics accession number   fn. = footnotes   refs. = references

Singer, Peter A.; Shaul, Randi Zlotnik. Resource allocation in coronary revascularization. *Canadian Journal of Cardiology*. 1997 Dec; 13(Suppl. D): 64D–66D. BE62105.
   constitutional law; costs and benefits; geographic factors; government regulation; guidelines; health care delivery; health facilities; *heart diseases; justice; organizational policies; physicians; professional organizations; *resource allocation; selection for treatment; social discrimination; standards; *surgery; needs; *Canada; Canada Health Act 1984; Canadian Cardiovascular Society; Canadian Charter of Rights and Freedoms; United Network for Organ Sharing

Smith, Richard. Viagra and rationing: let the sunlight in, let the people speak. [Editorial]. *BMJ (British Medical Journal)*. 1998 Sep 19; 317(7161): 760–761. 6 refs. BE60826.
   decision making; *drugs; government financing; males; public participation; *public policy; *resource allocation; sexuality; values; *impotence; *Great Britain; *National Health Service; Rationing Agenda Group (Great Britain); United States; *Viagra

Stingl, Michael; Burgess, Michael M.; Hubert, John, et al. Euthanasia and health reform in Canada. [Article and commentaries]. *Cambridge Quarterly of Healthcare Ethics*. 1998 Fall; 7(4): 348–370. 46 fn. BE59136.
   *active euthanasia; aged; caring; chronically ill; community services; competence; economics; goals; *health care delivery; *health care reform; home care; involuntary euthanasia; *justice; obligations of society; organization and administration; palliative care; primary health care; *public policy; *quality of health care; quality of life; socioeconomic factors; suffering; *terminal care; terminally ill; *voluntary euthanasia; *Canada; Netherlands

ten Have, Henk A.M.J. Consensus formation and healthcare policy. *In:* ten Have, Henk A.M.J.; Sass, Hans–Martin, eds. Consensus Formation in Healthcare Ethics. Boston, MA: Kluwer Academic; 1998: 45–59. 13 refs. ISBN 0–7923–4944–X. BE62587.
   advisory committees; attitudes; autonomy; biomedical technologies; *consensus; costs and benefits; *decision making; economics; health; *health care; *health care delivery; obligations of society; physicians; public opinion; public participation; *public policy; *resource allocation; rights; scarcity; standards; values; Dunning Committee; *Netherlands

Visser, A.A. Oranjemed -- Bloemfontein Protocols preamble. *Journal of the Dental Association of South Africa*. 1996 Nov; 51(11): 673–677. BE61865.
   accountability; codes of ethics; confidentiality; conflict of interest; contracts; dentistry; disclosure; gatekeeping; guidelines; health personnel; informed consent; *managed care programs; patient participation; physicians; professional organizations; regulation; standards; Oranjemed Independent Practitioners' Association; *South Africa

Vrbová, H.; Holmerová, I.; Hrubantová, L. Business ethics as a novel issue in health care economics. *Sbornik Lekarsky*. 1997; 98(3): 225–232. 6 refs. BE62418.
   accountability; common good; community services; *economics; *health care delivery; health care reform; health insurance; patient participation; physician patient relationship; quality of health care; *resource allocation; trust; vulnerable populations; *Czech Republic

Williams, Alan; Evans, J. Grimley. Rationing health care by age: the case for [and] The case against. *BMJ (British Medical Journal)*. 1997 Mar 15; 314(7083): 820–825. BE60232.
   *age factors; *aged; attitudes; common good; costs and benefits; goals; *health care; *justice; moral policy; patient care; quality adjusted life years; quality of life; *resource allocation; risks and benefits; *selection for treatment; social discrimination; social worth; treatment outcome; values; withholding treatment; needs; *Great Britain; *National Health Service

Working Group on Prioritisation in Health Care (Finland). From Values to Choices: Report. Helsinki, Finland: National Research and Development Centre for Welfare and Health (STAKES); 1995. 78 p. Bibliography: p. 72–77. ISBN 951–33–0035–8. BE62777.
   advisory committees; age factors; aged; allowing to die; alternative therapies; biomedical technologies; decision making; developing countries; economics; genetic screening; government financing; health; health care; *health care delivery; health promotion; human rights; international aspects; justice; legislation; obligations of society; patient care; prenatal diagnosis; professional patient relationship; public participation; public policy; quality of life; *resource allocation; selection for treatment; self induced illness; terminal care; values; *Finland; *Working Group on Prioritisation in Health Care

Wright, Stephen G. The distribution of resources in health care. *Professional Nurse (London)*. 1996 Jun; 11(9): 583–586. BE59988.
   adolescents; deinstitutionalized persons; economics; *health care; infertility; low birth weight; mentally ill; newborns; pregnant women; public policy; refusal to treat; reproductive technologies; *resource allocation; selection for treatment; smoking; withholding treatment; *Great Britain; National Health Service

HEALTH CARE RATIONING See RESOURCE ALLOCATION, SELECTION FOR TREATMENT

HEALTH CARE/RIGHTS

Annas, George J. Human rights and health -- the Universal Declaration of Human Rights at 50. *New England Journal of Medicine*. 1998 Dec 10; 339(24): 1778–1781. 26 refs. BE60040.
   AIDS; capitalism; democracy; developing countries; economics; education; guidelines; *health; *health care; health promotion; historical aspects; *human rights; *international aspects; law; medical ethics; misconduct; natural law; obligations of society; obligations to society; physicians; political activity; prisoners; professional organizations; *public health; public policy; socialism; socioeconomic factors; torture; war; women's rights; Amnesty International; Consortium for Health and Human Rights; Global Lawyers and Physicians; Physicians for Social Responsibility; Physicians for the Prevention of Nuclear War; Physicians of the World; Twentieth Century Doctors without Borders; United Nations; *Universal Declaration of Human Rights

Appleyard, James. The rights of children to health care. [Editorial]. *Journal of Medical Ethics*. 1998 Oct; 24(5): 293–294. 5 refs. BE60250.
   *children; developing countries; *health care; health promotion; *human rights; *international aspects; nutrition; patients' rights; physicians; preventive medicine; professional organizations; quality of health care; rehabilitation; Convention on the Rights of the Child; *Declaration on the Rights of the Child to Health Care; United Nations; *World Medical Association

Baker, Robert. American independence and the right to emergency care. *JAMA*. 1999 Mar 3; 281(9): 859–860. 12 refs. BE60244.
   administrators; codes of ethics; economics; *emergency care; historical aspects; *legal aspects; *legal rights; legislation;

*managed care programs; *medical ethics; *moral obligations; patient advocacy; *patients' rights; physician patient relationship; *physicians; professional organizations; refusal to treat; *utilitarianism; *business ethics; *Patients' Bill of Rights; *United States

Buchanan, Allen. Managed care: rationing without justice, but not unjustly. *Journal of Health Politics, Policy and Law.* 1998 Aug; 23(4): 617–634. 16 refs. Commented on by S.D. Goold, p. 687–695. BE59780.
  contracts; costs and benefits; decision making; disadvantaged; disclosure; economics; ethical theory; gatekeeping; *health care; *health care delivery; health insurance; *institutional ethics; *justice; *managed care programs; *moral obligations; *moral policy; *physician's role; *private sector; proprietary health facilities; public participation; *public sector; *quality of health care; *resource allocation; *rights; *standards; terminology; *withholding treatment; *United States
Three ethical criticisms of managed care are often voiced: (1) by "skimming the cream" of the patient population, managed care organizations fail to discharge their obligations to improve access, or at least, to not worsen it; (2) managed care organizations engage in rationing, thereby depriving patients of care to which they are entitled; and (3) by pressuring physicians to ration care, managed care organizations interfere with physicians' fulfillment of their fiduciary obligations to provide the best care for each patient. This article argues that each of these criticisms is misconceived. The first rests on the false assumption that the health care system includes a workable division of responsibility regarding access that assigns obligations concerning access to managed care organizations. The second and third criticisms wrongly assume that we in the United States have taken the first step toward assuring equitable access to care for all, articulating a standard for what counts as an "adequate level of care" to which all are entitled. These three misguided criticisms obscure the most fundamental ethical flaw of managed care: the fact that it operates in an institutional setting within which no connection can be made between the activity of rationing and the basic requirements of justice.

Cust, Kenneth F.T. Justice and rights to health care. *Reason Papers.* 1993 Fall; 18: 153–168. 28 fn. BE59852.
  capitalism; consensus; contracts; economics; freedom; health; *health care; health care delivery; historical aspects; *justice; morbidity; mortality; physicians; resource allocation; *rights; standards; voluntary programs; needs; *Daniels, Norman; *Gauthier, David; Rawls, John

Daniels, Norman. Is there a right to health care and, if so, what does it encompass? *In:* Kuhse, Helga; Singer, Peter, eds. A Companion to Bioethics. Malden, MA: Blackwell; 1998: 316–325. 25 refs. ISBN 0-631-19737-0. BE59506.
  biomedical technologies; decision making; *health care; health care delivery; *justice; libertarianism; moral obligations; *moral policy; *obligations of society; resource allocation; *rights; *standards; utilitarianism

Davidoff, Frank; Reinecke, Robert D. The 28th Amendment. [Editorial]. *Annals of Internal Medicine.* 1999 Apr 20; 130(8): 692–694. 19 refs. BE61604.
  *constitutional amendments; *health care; *health care delivery; human rights; justice; *legal rights; public policy; *United States

Dyer, Clare. Transsexuals win case for NHS funded surgery. [News]. *BMJ (British Medical Journal).* 1999 Jan 9; 318(7176): 75. BE62607.
  *government financing; *health care; *legal aspects; *legal rights; resource allocation; *surgery; *transsexualism; *Great Britain; *National Health Service

Dyer, Clare. UK Human Rights Act will allow challenges to treatment refusals. [News]. *BMJ (British Medical Journal).* 1998 Nov 14; 317(7169): 1339. BE62646.
  *government financing; *health care; human rights; *legal rights; resource allocation; surgery; transsexualism; European Convention on Human Rights; *Great Britain; *National Health Service

Joblin, Joseph. Health and the distribution of resources. *Dolentium Hominum: Church and Health in the World.* 1998; No. 37 [yr. 13(1)]: 63–68. 30 fn. BE61777.
  biomedical technologies; common good; developing countries; economics; *health; *health care; *human rights; indigents; international aspects; justice; morality; obligations of society; public policy; *resource allocation; *Roman Catholic ethics; socioeconomic factors; Western World

Lessard, Hester. The construction of health care and the ideology of the private in Canadian constitutional law. *Annals of Health Law.* 1993; 2: 121–159. 153 fn. BE59830.
  *abortion, induced; constitutional law; criminal law; economics; federal government; government regulation; *health care delivery; *historical aspects; hospitals; *legal aspects; legal rights; national health insurance; physicians; pregnant women; *private sector; *public policy; *public sector; *rights; social discrimination; therapeutic abortion; *women's rights; *Canada; Canadian Charter of Rights and Freedoms; Criminal Code of Canada; Nineteenth Century; R. v. Morgentaler; Twentieth Century

Mariner, Wendy K. Equitable access to biomedical advances: getting beyond the rights impasse. *Connecticut Law Review.* 1989 Spring; 21(3): 571–603. 103 fn. BE62127.
  abortion, induced; AIDS; *biomedical technologies; constitutional law; costs and benefits; drug industry; *drugs; federal government; government financing; *government regulation; *health care; *investigational drugs; justice; *legal aspects; *legal rights; *obligations of society; *organ transplantation; patient advocacy; patient care; patients; political activity; private sector; *public policy; public sector; *resource allocation; *unproven therapies; Food and Drug Administration; *France; Roussel Uclaf; *RU–486; *United States

Russian Federation. Principles of the legislation of the Russion Federation on the protection of the health of citizens. Dated 22 Jul 1993. (*Rossijskaja Gazeta*, 18 Aug 1993, p. 4–7). [Summary]. *International Digest of Health Legislation.* 1994. 45(1). 3–6. BE62694.
  abortion, induced; health; *health care; health care delivery; health personnel; *legal rights; obligations of society; patients' rights; public health; reproductive technologies; vulnerable populations; Russia; *Russian Federation

Zuccaro, Stefano Maria; Palleschi, Massimo; Italian Society of Hospital Geriatricians. Document on the rights of the sick elderly. *Dolentium Hominum: Church and Health in the World.* 1997; 36(12th Yr., No. 3): 32–35. 15 refs. BE60408.
  *aged; autonomy; disclosure; freedom; *health care; health personnel; *organizational policies; patient care; *patients' rights; professional organizations; quality of health care; *rights; social worth; Europe; *Italian Society of Hospital Geriatricians

Treatment; transsexualism; equal protection; deliberate indifference: Farmer v. Hawk. *Mental and Physical Disability Law Reporter.* 1998 Mar–Apr; 22(2): 174. BE61464.
  *equal protection; federal government; hormones; *legal

BE = bioethics accession number   fn. = footnotes   refs. = references

aspects; *legal rights; *patient care; *prisoners; public policy; *transsexualism; Bureau of Prisons; District of Columbia; *Farmer v. Hawk; United States

HEALTH ECONOMICS See HEALTH CARE/ECONOMICS, RESOURCE ALLOCATION

HEALTH PERSONNEL
See under
AIDS/HEALTH PERSONNEL

HOSPICES
See under
TERMINAL CARE/HOSPICES

HOSPITAL ETHICS COMMITTEES See ETHICISTS AND ETHICS COMMITTEES

HOST MOTHERS See SURROGATE MOTHERS

HUMAN EXPERIMENTATION

See also BEHAVIORAL RESEARCH, BIOMEDICAL RESEARCH, EMBRYO AND FETAL RESEARCH, GENETIC RESEARCH
See also under
AIDS/HUMAN EXPERIMENTATION

Altman, Lawrence K. New direction for transplants raises hopes and questions. [Rebuilding the body: a special report]. *New York Times.* 1999 May 2: 1, 46–47. BE61173.
AIDS; *body parts and fluids; cancer; *cosmetic surgery; drugs; economics; *human experimentation; injuries; methods; *organ transplantation; *quality of life; risk; *risks and benefits; *tissue transplantation; transplant recipients; hands; knees

American Medical Association. Council on Ethical and Judicial Affairs. Subject selection for clinical trials. *IRB: A Review of Human Subjects Research.* 1998 Mar–Jun; 20(2–3): 12–15. 13 fn. BE59995.
*altruism; cancer; coercion; *human experimentation; investigational drugs; *motivation; *nontherapeutic research; organizational policies; patient care; professional organizations; *research subjects; *risks and benefits; *selection of subjects; socioeconomic factors; *therapeutic research; volunteers; American Medical Association; United States

Annas, George J.; Grodin, Michael A. Reflections on the fiftieth anniversary of the Doctors' Trial. *Health and Human Rights.* 1996; 2(1): 7–21. 29 fn. BE62085.
force feeding; guidelines; *historical aspects; *human experimentation; *human rights; informed consent; *international aspects; *misconduct; *National Socialism; organizational policies; *physician's role; *physicians; prisoners; professional organizations; registries; self regulation; torture; British Medical Association; Germany; *Nuremberg Code; *Nuremberg Trials; Twentieth Century; World Medical Association

Baker, Robert. A theory of international bioethics: the negotiable and the non-negotiable. *Kennedy Institute of Ethics Journal.* 1998 Sep; 8(3): 233–273. 50 refs. 12 fn. BE60167.
*bioethics; circumcision; clinical ethics; codes of ethics; competence; *contracts; covenant; *cultural pluralism; developing countries; drugs; *ethical relativism; *ethical

theory; federal government; females; *guidelines; HIV seropositivity; *human experimentation; *human rights; informed consent; *international aspects; investigator subject relationship; investigators; legal rights; medical schools; models, theoretical; *morality; National Socialism; philosophy; physicians; placebos; *postmodernism; pregnant women; privacy; professional ethics; professional organizations; regulation; research subjects; retrospective moral judgment; scientific misconduct; *standards; therapeutic research; third party consent; values; culpability; slavery; Council for International Organizations of Medical Sciences; Declaration of Helsinki; European Convention on Human Rights and Biomedicine; Germany; Harvard Medical School; Nuremberg Code; Nuremberg Trials; United States; World Medical Association

The preceding article in this issue of the *Kennedy Institute of Ethics Journal* presents the argument that "moral fundamentalism," the position that international bioethics rests on "basic" or "fundamental" moral priniciples that are universally accepted in all eras and cultures, collapses under a variety of multicultural and postmodern critiques. The present article looks to the contractarian tradition of Hobbes and Locke -- as reinterpreted by David Gauthier, Robert Nozick, and John Rawls -- for an alternative justification for international bioethics. Drawing on the central themes of this tradition, it is argued that international bioethics can be rationally reconstructed as a negotiated moral order that respects culturally and individually defined areas of nonnegotiability. Further, the theory of a negotiated moral order is consistent with traditional ideals about human rights, is flexible enough to absorb the genuine insights of multiculturalism and postmodernism, and yet is strong enough to justify transcultural and transtemporal moral judgments, including the condemnation of the Nazi doctors at Nuremberg. This theory also is consistent with the history of the ethics of human subjects experimentation and offers insights into current controversies such as the controversy over changing the consent rule for experiments in emergency medicine and the controversy over exempting certain clinical trials of inexpensive treatments for preventing the perinatal transmission of AIDS from the ethical standards of the sponsoring country.

Baker, Robert. Negotiating international bioethics: a response to Tom Beauchamp and Ruth Macklin. *Kennedy Institute of Ethics Journal.* 1998 Dec; 8(4): 423–453. 33 refs. 10 fn. BE62377.
accountability; advisory committees; beneficence; *bioethics; circumcision; contracts; *cultural pluralism; *ethical analysis; *ethical relativism; *ethical theory; females; historical aspects; *human experimentation; *human rights; *international aspects; investigators; *morality; National Socialism; nontherapeutic research; philosophy; physicians; *postmodernism; *principle-based ethics; *radiation; research subjects; *retrospective moral judgment; scientific misconduct; sexuality; social discrimination; stigmatization; values; women's rights; *culpability; *Advisory Committee on Human Radiation Experiments; Asia; Europe; Germany; Twentieth Century; United States

Can the bioethical theories that have served American bioethics so well, serve international bioethics as well? In two papers in the previous issue of the *Kennedy Institute of Ethics Journal,* I contend that the form of principlist fundamentalism endorsed by American bioethicists like Tom Beauchamp and Ruth Macklin will not play on an international stage. Deploying techniques of postmodern scholarship, I argue that principlist fundamentalism justifies neither the condemnation of the Nazi doctors at Nuremberg, nor, as the *Report of the Advisory Committee on the Human Radiation*

Experiments (ACHRE) demonstrates, condemnation of Cold War radiation researchers. Principlist fundamentalism thus appears to be philosophy bankrupt. In this issue of the *Journal*, Beauchamp and Macklin reject this claim, arguing that I have misread the ACHRE report and misunderstood Nazism. They also argue that the form of post–postmodern negotiated human rights theory that I proffer is adequate only insofar as it is itself really fundamentalist; insofar as I take postmodernism seriously, however, I mire international bioethics in relativism. In this response, I reaffirm my anti-fundamentalism, provide further evidence in support of my reading of the ACHRE report, and defend my post–postmodern version of rights theory. I also develop criteria for a minimally adequate theoretical framework for international bioethics.

Beauchamp, Tom L. The mettle of moral fundamentalism: a reply to Robert Baker. *Kennedy Institute of Ethics Journal.* 1998 Dec.; 8(4): 389–401. 7 refs. 2 fn. BE62375.
   accountability; advisory committees; *bioethics; contracts; *cultural pluralism; *ethical analysis; *ethical relativism; *ethical theory; historical aspects; *human experimentation; *human rights; informed consent; *international aspects; investigators; *morality; National Socialism; nontherapeutic research; philosophy; physicians; *principle–based ethics; public policy; *radiation; research subjects; *retrospective moral judgment; scientific misconduct; standards; values; culpability; *Advisory Committee on Human Radiation Experiments; Germany; Twentieth Century; United States
This article is a reply to Robert Baker's attempt to rebut moral fundamentalism, while grounding international bioethics in a form of contractarianism. Baker is mistaken in several of his interpretations of the alleged moral fundamentalism and findings of the Advisory Committee on Human Radiation Experiments. He also misunderstands moral fundamentalism generally and wrongly categorizes it as morally bankrupt. His negotiated contract model is, in the final analysis, itself a form of the moral fundamentalism he declares bankrupt.

Bell, Elmerine Allen Whitfield. Testimony of Elmerine Allen Whitfield Bell [concerning human experimentation with plutonium]. *Accountability in Research.* 1998 Jan; 6(1–2): 167–181. Testimony delivered 18 Jan 1994 to the Subcommittee on Energy and Power of the Committee on Energy and Commerce, U.S. House of Representatives. BE61549.
   blacks; compensation; death; deception; disabled; disclosure; family members; federal government; *historical aspects; *human experimentation; indigents; information dissemination; informed consent; injuries; investigators; medical records; *nontherapeutic research; patients; physicians; public policy; *radiation; research subjects; *scientific misconduct; *Allen, Elmer; Department of Energy; *Twentieth Century; United States; *University of California, San Francisco

Burton, Thomas M. A prostate researcher tested firm's product -- and sat on its board. [News]. *Wall Street Journal.* 1998 Mar 19: A1, A8. BE59671.
   *biomedical research; *conflict of interest; disclosure; *drug industry; drugs; editorial policies; *financial support; *fraud; investigators; medical devices; *misconduct; *physicians; *remuneration; surgery; *therapeutic research; *Oesterling, Joseph; University of Michigan

Campbell, Courtney S. Religion and the body in medical research. *Kennedy Institute of Ethics Journal.* 1998 Sep; 8(3): 275–305. 36 refs. 2 fn. BE60168.
   advisory committees; altruism; American Indians; attitudes; *autopsies; *biomedical research; *body parts and fluids; *cadavers; commodification; *common good; confidentiality; cultural pluralism; fetal tissue donation; genetic information; *genetic research; genome mapping; *gifts; *human body; informed consent; investigators; Islamic ethics; Jewish ethics; medical education; metaphor; moral obligations; *nontherapeutic research; *organ donation; organ transplantation; property rights; Protestant ethics; *religious ethics; remuneration; Roman Catholic ethics; science; self concept; *theology; *tissue banks; *tissue donation; transplant recipients; values; National Bioethics Advisory Commission
Religious discussion of human organs and tissues has concentrated largely on donation for therapeutic purposes. The retrieval and use of human tissue samples in diagnostic, research, and education contexts have, by contrast, received very little direct theological attention. Initially undertaken at the behest of the National Bioethics Advisory Commission, this essay seeks to explore the theological and religious questions embedded in nontherapeutic use of human tissue. It finds that the "donation paradigm" typically invoked in religious discourse to justify uses of the body for therapeutic reasons is inadequate in the context of nontherapeutic research, while the "resource paradigm" implicit in scientific discourse presumes a reductionist account of the body that runs contrary to important religious values about embodiment. The essay proposes a "contribution paradigm" that provides a religious perspective within which research on human tissue can be both justified and limited.

de Castro, Leonardo D. Ethical issues in human experimentation. *In:* Kuhse, Helga; Singer, Peter, eds. A Companion to Bioethics. Malden, MA: Blackwell; 1998: 379–389. 18 refs. ISBN 0–631–19737–0. BE59511.
   autonomy; beneficence; biomedical research; coercion; compensation; competence; disadvantaged; disclosure; *human experimentation; incentives; informed consent; injuries; justice; moral complicity; nontherapeutic research; obligations to society; random selection; research subjects; risks and benefits; scientific misconduct; selection of subjects; therapeutic research; third party consent

Dickert, Neal; Grady, Christine. What's the price of a research subject? Approaches to payment for research participation. *New England Journal of Medicine.* 1999 Jul 15; 341(3): 198–203. 27 refs. BE62035.
   comprehension; disadvantaged; federal government; *human experimentation; *incentives; industry; investigator subject relationship; justice; libertarianism; *models, theoretical; motivation; nontherapeutic research; patients; *public policy; regulation; *remuneration; *research subjects; risk; risks and benefits; therapeutic research; *volunteers; vulnerable populations; egalitarianism; United States

Egilman, David; Wallace, Wes; Stubbs, Cassandra, et al. A little too much of the Buchenwald touch? Military radiation research at the University of Cincinnati, 1960–1972. *Accountability in Research.* 1998 Jan; 6(1–2): 63–102. 83 refs. BE61535.
   adults; advisory committees; bone marrow; cancer; children; compensation; competence; conflict of interest; consent forms; death; deception; disadvantaged; disclosure; editorial policies; federal government; government financing; guideline adherence; guidelines; *historical aspects; hospitals; *human experimentation; informed consent; injuries; investigators; military personnel; mortality; *nontherapeutic research; nuclear warfare; *patients; physicians; professional organizations; public policy; *radiation; research design; research ethics committees; research subjects; review committees; risk; *scientific misconduct; selection of subjects; self regulation; therapeutic research; tissue transplantation; universities; withholding treatment; Advisory Committee on Human Radiation Experiments; American College of Radiology; Atomic

---

Energy Commission; *Department of Defense; Ohio; *Saenger, Eugene; *Twentieth Century; *United States; *University of Cincinnati

Eichenwald, Kurt; Kolata, Gina. A doctor's drug studies turn into fraud. [Research for hire: second of two articles]. *New York Times.* 1999 May 17: A1, A16. BE61175.
biomedical research; coercion; *conflict of interest; *drug industry; *drugs; economics; *entrepreneurship; federal government; financial support; *fraud; government regulation; *human experimentation; *incentives; investigators; managed care programs; misconduct; patient care; *physicians; *remuneration; research subjects; *scientific misconduct; *selection of subjects; trends; *private practice; California; *Fiddes, Robert; Food and Drug Administration; Southern California Research Institute; United States

Eichenwald, Kurt; Kolata, Gina. Drug trials hide conflicts for doctors. [Research for hire: first of two articles]. *New York Times.* 1999 May 16: 1, 34. BE61174.
authorship; biomedical research; coercion; *conflict of interest; contracts; disclosure; *drug industry; *drugs; economics; *entrepreneurship; *human experimentation; *incentives; investigators; misconduct; nurses; *physicians; professional competence; *remuneration; research ethics committees; *selection of subjects; trends; universities; *private practice; United States

Faden, Ruth; Guttman, Dan. In response: speaking truth to historiography. *Medical Humanities Review.* 1997 Fall; 11(2): 37–43. 6 fn. Commentary on R. Martensen, p. 21–36. BE59809.
*advisory committees; biomedical research; entrepreneurship; ethical analysis; *evaluation; *federal government; financial support; government financing; government regulation; guidelines; *historical aspects; *human experimentation; informed consent; investigators; motivation; nontherapeutic research; physicians; politics; public participation; *public policy; *radiation; research subjects; *scientific misconduct; universities; *Advisory Committee on Human Radiation Experiments; Twentieth Century; *United States; University of California, Berkeley

Faraone, Stephen V.; Gottesman, Irving I.; Tsuang, Ming T. Fifty years of the Nuremberg Code: a time for retrospection and introspection. [Editorial]. *American Journal of Medical Genetics.* 1997 Jul 25; 74(4): 345–347. 16 refs. Includes text of the Nuremberg Code. BE59128.
codes of ethics; eugenics; *genetic research; *genetics; genome mapping; historical aspects; *human experimentation; *investigators; involuntary euthanasia; involuntary sterilization; medical ethics; *misconduct; National Socialism; *physicians; *psychiatry; Germany; Nuremberg Code; Twentieth Century

Flegel, Kenneth M. Physicians, finder's fees and free, informed consent. [Editorial]. *Canadian Medical Association Journal.* 1997 Nov 15; 157(10): 1373–1374. 9 refs. BE59681.
coercion; *conflict of interest; *disclosure; drug industry; financial support; guidelines; *human experimentation; *incentives; informed consent; investigator subject relationship; physician patient relationship; *physicians; *referral and consultation; *remuneration; *selection of subjects; Canada

Fox, Jeffrey L. Germline gene therapy contemplated. [News]. *Nature Biotechnology.* 1998 May; 16(5): 407. BE62319.
federal government; *gene therapy; *germ cells; government regulation; *human experimentation; United States

Giesen, Dieter. Civil liability of physicians for new methods of treatment and experimentation: a comparative examination. *Medical Law Review.* 1995 Spring; 3(1): 22–52. 135 fn. BE59999.
coercion; comparative studies; control groups; *disclosure; *human experimentation; informed consent; institutionalized persons; *international aspects; *investigators; *legal liability; malpractice; minors; nontherapeutic research; physicians; placebos; random selection; risks and benefits; standards; therapeutic research; third party consent; Canada; Germany; Great Britain; United States

Greely, Henry T. Genomics research and human subjects. [Editorial]. *Science.* 1998 Oct 23; 282(5389): 625. BE59646.
DNA data banks; *genetic research; *human experimentation; informed consent; research subjects; tissue banks; trust

Kaiser, Jocelyn. EPA ponders pesticide tests in humans. [News]. *Science.* 1999 Jan 1; 283(5398): 18–19. BE60817.
advisory committees; ecology; federal government; health hazards; *human experimentation; *nontherapeutic research; *public policy; *toxicity; volunteers; agriculture; *Environmental Protection Agency; Great Britain; *United States

Kornetsky, Susan. Questions and answers regarding clinical research: an educational brochure. *IRB: A Review of Human Subjects Research.* 1998 Jul–Aug; 20(4): 12–13. BE61098.
*children; disclosure; *hospitals; *human experimentation; informed consent; *institutional policies; parental consent; *parents; *patient education; patients' rights; research subjects; *Children's Hospital (Boston)

La Puma, John. Physician rewards for postmarketing surveillance (seeding studies) in the US. [Editorial]. *PharmacoEconomics.* 1995 Mar; 7(3): 187–190. 14 refs. BE59156.
advertising; conflict of interest; *disclosure; *drug industry; *drugs; goals; *human experimentation; incentives; informed consent; *investigators; *physicians; *remuneration; *postmarketing research; United States

Lehrman, Sally. Virus treatment questioned after gene therapy death. [News]. *Nature.* 1999 Oct 7; 401(6753): 517–518. BE62683.
advisory committees; *death; federal government; *gene therapy; government regulation; *human experimentation; livers; *research subjects; risks and benefits; toxicity; Food and Drug Administration; *Gelsinger, Jesse; National Institutes of Health; Recombinant DNA Advisory Committee; United States; *University of Pennsylvania

Luna, Florencia. Corruption and research. *Bioethics.* 1999 Jul; 13(3–4): 262–271. 19 fn. BE61877.
*biomedical research; developing countries; ethical relativism; *human experimentation; incentives; *international aspects; investigators; legal aspects; *misconduct; politics; regulation; remuneration; research design; research ethics committees; *scientific misconduct; selection of subjects; socioeconomic factors; bribes; *multicenter studies

Last year there was a heated debate regarding clinical trials with AZT carried out in developing countries. AIDS vaccine trials also posed various dilemmas and ethical problems. In this paper I will consider the possibility of corruption in bioethics, and international multi-centre research will be taken as an example. International clinical trials will be seen from another perspective. I will try to show that the possibility of systemic corruption should be considered when designing an international multi-centre research trial which may involve countries in very different situations

---

BE = bioethics accession number   fn. = footnotes   refs. = references

regarding corruption. I will analyze three different approaches to this problem and suggest some strategies regarding their capacity to exclude the possibility of corruption.

Macklin, Ruth. A defense of fundamental principles and human rights: a reply to Robert Baker. *Kennedy Institute of Ethics Journal.* 1998 Dec; 8(4): 403-422. 15 refs. 6 fn. BE62376.
    accountability; advisory committees; autonomy; beneficence; *bioethics; circumcision; coercion; communitarianism; *cultural pluralism; dissent; *ethical analysis; *ethical relativism; *ethical theory; females; historical aspects; *human experimentation; *human rights; informed consent; *international aspects; investigators; *misconduct; *morality; *National Socialism; *non-Western World; nontherapeutic research; physicians; *postmodernism; principle-based ethics; *radiation; research subjects; *retrospective moral judgment; *scientific misconduct; values; *Western World; women's rights; *culpability; *Advisory Committee on Human Radiation Experiments; Asia; Germany; Twentieth Century; United States
This article seeks to rebut Robert Baker's contention that attempts to ground international bioethics in fundamental principles cannot withstand the challenges posed by multiculturalism and postmodernism. First, several corrections are provided of Baker's account of the conclusions reached by the Advisory Committee on Human Radiation Experiments. Second, a rebuttal is offered to Baker's claim that an unbridgeable moral gap exists between Western individualism and non-Western communalism. In conclusion, this article argues that Baker's "nonnegotiable primary goods" cannot do the work of "classical human rights" and that the latter framework is preferable from both a practical and a theoretical standpoint.

Mann, Jonathan, M.; Gruskin, Sofia; Grodin, Michael A., et al, eds. Health and Human Rights: A Reader. New York, NY: Routledge; 1999. 505 p. Includes references. ISBN 0-415-92102-3. BE62050.
    AIDS; circumcision; developing countries; family planning; females; genetic diversity; genetic research; *health; health care; HIV seropositivity; homosexuals; *human experimentation; *human rights; informed consent; *international aspects; killing; mass screening; medicine; minority groups; misconduct; National Socialism; newborns; patient advocacy; *physicians; *political activity; pregnant women; *public health; public policy; scientific misconduct; sexuality; social discrimination; *social impact; socioeconomic factors; tuberculosis; war; women's health; genocide; Doctors of the World; Doctors without Borders; International Covenant on Civil and Political Rights; International Covenant on Economic, Social and Cultural Rights; International Red Cross and Red Crescent Movement; Physicians for Human Rights; Universal Declaration of Human Rights

Martensen, Robert. If only it were so: medical physics, U.S. human radiation experiments, and the *Final Report* of the President's Advisory Committee (ACHRE). *Medical Humanities Review.* 1997 Fall; 11(2): 21-36. 26 fn. Commented on by R. Faden and Dan Guttman, p. 37-43. BE59808.
    *advisory committees; *biomedical research; cancer; conflict of interest; disclosure; drug industry; entrepreneurship; ethical analysis; ethical review; ethicist's role; *evaluation; *federal government; *financial support; government financing; government regulation; guidelines; *historical aspects; *human experimentation; informed consent; investigators; justice; motivation; physicians; policy analysis; politics; *public policy; *radiation; research subjects; resource allocation; science; *scientific misconduct; standards; trust; universities; *Advisory Committee on Human Radiation Experiments; Department of Energy;

*Twentieth Century; *United States; University of California, Berkeley

Matz, Robert; Levine, Myron M.; Tacket, Carol O., et al. Recruiting volunteers for a typhoid vaccine. [Letter and response]. *JAMA.* 1998 Nov 4; 280(17): 1480-1481. 8 refs. BE61078.
    altruism; autoexperimentation; communicable diseases; federal government; *human experimentation; *immunization; informed consent; *nontherapeutic research; research subjects; selection of subjects; *volunteers; *typhoid; Food and Drug Administration; United States; *University of Maryland School of Medicine

Miller, Franklin G.; Rosenstein, Donald L.; DeRenzo, Evan G. Professional integrity in clinical research. *JAMA.* 1998 Oct 28; 280(16): 1449-1454. 30 refs. BE59636.
    beneficence; biomedical research; conflict of interest; drugs; financial support; *human experimentation; incentives; informed consent; *investigator subject relationship; *investigators; medical education; medical ethics; models, theoretical; *moral policy; nontherapeutic research; patients; physician patient relationship; *physicians; professional ethics; *professional role; regulation; research subjects; risks and benefits; teaching methods; therapeutic research; volunteers; withholding treatment; *integrity
In response to public concern over abuses in human medical experimentation, the dominant approach to the ethics of clinical research during the past 30 years has been regulation, particularly via institutional review board review and approval of scientific protocols and written consent forms. However, the effectiveness of regulatory mechanisms in ensuring the ethical conduct of clinical research is limited. Little attention has been devoted to the nature and role of professional integrity of physician investigators, a conscientious framework for guiding investigators in the socially important but morally complex activity of clinical research. Professional integrity is vital in forging an ethically sound relationship between investigators and patient volunteers, a relationship that differs in important ways from the patient-physician relationship in standard clinical practice. We examine critically 2 models of the moral identity of physician investigators, the investigator as clinician and the investigator as scientist; in neither of these 2 models can the physician investigator eliminate completely the moral conflicts posed by clinical research. The professional integrity of physician investigators depends on a coherent moral identity that is proper to the enterprise of clinical research. The roles of clinician and scientist must be integrated to manage conscientiously the ethical complexity, ambiguity, and tensions between the potentially competing loyalties of science and care of volunteer patients.

Morgan, G.L. Is there a right to fetal tissue transplantation? *University of Tasmania Law Review.* 1991; 10(2): 129-156. 152 fn. BE62177.
    aborted fetuses; autonomy; disclosure; *fetal tissue donation; government financing; government regulation; health care; *human experimentation; informed consent; investigator subject relationship; investigators; legal aspects; *legal obligations; legal rights; moral obligations; morbidity; mortality; *obligations of society; paternalism; patients; pregnant women; research subjects; *rights; risks and benefits; therapeutic research; *tissue transplantation; Parkinson disease; *Australia

Nilstun, Tore; Ranstam, Jonas. Ethics in orthopedic research. [Editorial]. *Acta Orthopaedica Scandinavica.* 1997 Jun; 68(3): 205-206. 3 refs. BE60476.
    competence; *editorial policies; ethical review; guideline

---

BE = bioethics accession number   fn. = footnotes   refs. = references

adherence; guidelines; *human experimentation; informed consent; research design; research subjects; vulnerable populations; orthopedics; Council for International Organizations of Medical Sciences; Declaration of Helsinki

Richards, Bill. How a corporate feud doomed human trials of promising therapy. [News]. *Wall Street Journal.* 1999 Aug 6: A1, A6. BE62400.
    *biomedical technologies; *bone marrow; *cancer; *economics; federal government; government financing; human experimentation; *industry; legal aspects; leukemia; methods; *patents; terminally ill; *therapeutic research; *tissue transplantation; *Baxter International Inc.; *Cell Pro Inc.; National Institutes of Health; United States

Richter, Gerd. Treatment of metastatic breast cancer -- economic and ethical considerations. *Cancer Investigation.* 1997; 15(4): 335–341. 33 refs. BE59176.
    age factors; autonomy; bone marrow; *breast cancer; conflict of interest; *costs and benefits; *decision making; disclosure; drugs; *economics; evaluation; females; human experimentation; informed consent; investigators; justice; *patient care; patients; physicians; practice guidelines; prognosis; *prolongation of life; quality adjusted life years; *quality of life; random selection; research design; *resource allocation; risks and benefits; *terminally ill; *therapeutic research; tissue transplantation; toxicity; *treatment outcome; values; vulnerable populations; chemotherapy; United States

Savulescu, Julian. On the commercial exploitation of participants of research. [Letter]. *Journal of Medical Ethics.* 1997 Dec; 23(6): 392. 1 ref. BE59383.
    *compensation; *drug industry; financial support; human experimentation; injuries; *remuneration; *research subjects

Silva, Mary Cipriano. New ANA [American Nurses Association] guidelines for ethics in nursing research. *NursingConnections.* 1996 Summer; 9(2): 28–33. 5 refs. BE59190.
    animal experimentation; autonomy; beneficence; competence; confidentiality; *guidelines; *human experimentation; human rights; informed consent; investigators; justice; moral obligations; nurses; *nursing ethics; *nursing research; privacy; professional competence; professional organizations; research subjects; risks and benefits; scientific misconduct; selection of subjects; whistleblowing; American Nurses Association

Sugarman, Jeremy; Kass, Nancy E.; Goodman, Steven N., et al. What patients say about medical research. *IRB: A Review of Human Subjects Research.* 1998 Jul–Aug; 20(4): 1–7. 21 refs. BE61095.
    advisory committees; altruism; *attitudes; biomedical research; blacks; cancer; coercion; communication; *comprehension; consent forms; decision making; diagnosis; epidemiology; evaluation studies; heart diseases; *human experimentation; informed consent; *motivation; nontherapeutic research; *patient participation; *patients; physicians; remuneration; *research subjects; risk; risks and benefits; socioeconomic factors; survey; terminology; therapeutic research; trust; hope; refusal to participate; Advisory Committee on Human Radiation Experiments; *United States

Sulmasy, Daniel P. Cancer, managed care, and therapeutic research: an ethicist's view. *HMO Practice.* 1997 Jun; 11(2): 59–62. 7 refs. BE61558.
    *cancer; common good; government financing; *health insurance reimbursement; *health maintenance organizations; hospitals; human experimentation; institutional ethics; investigators; *justice; moral obligations; *moral policy; patient advocacy; peer review; physicians; research institutes; selection of subjects; *therapeutic research; United States

Szulc, R. Ethics and research. [Editorial]. *European Journal of Anaesthesiology.* 1996 Mar; 13(2): 93–94. 7 refs. BE60380.
    goals; guidelines; *human experimentation; research design; research ethics committees; risks and benefits; science

Taimi, Kitty. A new challenge for IRBs: medical surveillance for former DOE workers. *Protecting Human Subjects.* 1997 Fall: 6–8. BE60061.
    *employment; *epidemiology; *ethical review; federal government; health; human experimentation; nuclear warfare; *occupational exposure; program descriptions; public policy; *radiation; research design; research ethics committees; expedited review; *Department of Energy; United States

U.S. General Accounting Office. Department of Energy: Information on DOE's Human Tissue Analysis Work. Fact Sheet for Congressional Requesters. Washington, DC: U.S. General Accounting Office; 1995 May. 45 p. GAO/RCED-95-109FS. BE59262.
    federal government; historical aspects; human experimentation; informed consent; *nontherapeutic research; public policy; *radiation; research subjects; statistics; tissue banks; *Department of Energy; Twentieth Century; United States

Unesco. International Bioethics Committee.
    Proceedings of the Fourth Session, October 1996. Volume I. Paris: The Committee; 1998. 164 p. Includes references. BE61056.
    advisory committees; AIDS; autonomy; beneficence; *bioethical issues; committee membership; drugs; ecology; economics; food; *genetic intervention; *genetic research; *genome mapping; government regulation; *guidelines; *human experimentation; *human rights; *international aspects; investigators; justice; moral obligations; random selection; recombinant DNA research; regulation; remuneration; research subjects; risks and benefits; selection of subjects; standards; transgenic organisms; vulnerable populations; women's health; agriculture; *transgenic plants; Declaration of Helsinki; *International Bioethics Committee (Unesco); Unesco; United Nations; *Universal Declaration on the Human Genome and Human Rights (Unesco)

Unesco. International Bioethics Committee.
    Proceedings of the Fourth Session, October 1996. Volume II. Paris: The Committee; 1998. 94 p. Includes references. Papers in English and in French. BE61057.
    adults; advisory committees; autonomy; *bioethical issues; children; females; food; guidelines; *human experimentation; *human rights; immunization; informed consent; *international aspects; nontherapeutic research; privacy; random selection; regulation; research ethics committees; research subjects; therapeutic research; transgenic organisms; women's health; women's rights; agriculture; *transgenic plants; Argentina; Belmont Report; China; Colombia; Great Britain; International Bioethics Committee (Unesco); National Commission for the Protection of Human Subjects; Sweden; Tunisia; Unesco; United States

Wadman, Meredith. Pesticide tests on humans cause concern. [News]. *Nature.* 1998 Aug 6; 394(6693): 515. Includes inset article by M. Wadman, "California laboratory backs its use of volunteers." BE59939.
    federal government; government regulation; health hazards; *human experimentation; *industry; *nontherapeutic research; risk; state government; *toxicity; volunteers; agriculture; Amvac Chemical Corporation; Environmental Protection Agency; Great Britain; United States; Zeneca Ag Products

Walters, LeRoy B. Testimony of LeRoy Walters [concerning written standards for human experimentation in the years 1945 to 1949]. *Accountability*

BE = bioethics accession number   fn. = footnotes   refs. = references

in Research. 1998 Jan; 6(1–2): 149–166. Testimony delivered 18 Jan 1994 to the Subcommittee on Energy and Power of the Committee on Energy and Commerce, U.S. House of Representatives. BE61548.
> children; codes of ethics; compensation; disclosure; *guidelines; *historical aspects; *human experimentation; human rights; information dissemination; informed consent; injuries; international aspects; investigators; medical ethics; mentally disabled; National Socialism; physicians; prisoners; professional organizations; public policy; radiation; research design; research subjects; scientific misconduct; selection of subjects; *standards; American Medical Association; Geneva Conventions; Germany; Nuremberg Code; *Twentieth Century; United Nations; United States; World Medical Association

Wilkinson, Martin; Moore, Andrew. Inducements revisited. *Bioethics.* 1999 Apr; 13(2): 114–130. 21 fn. BE61672.
> altruism; behavioral research; biomedical research; commodification; contracts; financial support; *freedom; gifts; *human experimentation; *incentives; indigents; investigator subject relationship; investigators; justice; *moral policy; nontherapeutic research; *remuneration; research ethics committees; *research subjects; *risks and benefits; selection of subjects; social impact; volunteers

The paper defends the permissibility of paying inducements to research subjects against objections not covered in an earlier paper in Bioethics. The objections are that inducements would cause inequity, crowd out research, and undesirably commercialize the researcher–subject relationship. The paper shows how these objections presuppose implausible factual and/or normative claims. The final position reached is a qualified defence of freedom of contract which not only supports the permissibility of inducements but also offers guidance to ethics committees in dealing with practical problems that might arise if inducements are offered.

World Medical Association. Proposed revision of the Declaration of Helsinki. *Bulletin of Medical Ethics.* 1999 Apr; No. 147: 18–22. BE61824.
> *codes of ethics; control groups; females; *guidelines; *human experimentation; informed consent; *international aspects; investigators; moral obligations; patient care; physicians; professional organizations; records; research design; research ethics committees; research subjects; rights; third party consent; vulnerable populations; *Declaration of Helsinki; World Medical Association

Declaration of Helsinki -- nothing to declare? [Editorial]. *Lancet.* 1999 Apr 17; 353(9161): 1285. BE62267.
> codes of ethics; control groups; developing countries; *guidelines; *human experimentation; *international aspects; placebos; research design; research subjects; socioeconomic factors; standards; therapeutic research; vulnerable populations; *Declaration of Helsinki; Nuremberg Code; World Medical Association

Helsinki Declaration revising continues. [News]. *Bulletin of Medical Ethics.* 1999 Mar; No. 146: 3–5. BE61818.
> accountability; *codes of ethics; control groups; editorial policies; *guidelines; *human experimentation; information dissemination; *international aspects; investigators; nontherapeutic research; physicians; professional organizations; self regulation; therapeutic research; compassionate use; American Medical Association; *Declaration of Helsinki; World Medical Association

Patients for hire, doctors for sale. [Editorial]. *New York Times.* 1999 May 22: A12. BE62247.
> *conflict of interest; disclosure; *drug industry; fraud; *human experimentation; *incentives; indigents; *investigational drugs; medical ethics; misconduct; patient care; *physicians; *remuneration; research subjects; selection

of subjects; *private practice; United States

Testing new drugs: joining a study can be rewarding -- but risky [and] How to find -- and survive -- a clinical trial. *Consumer Reports.* 1998 Dec; 63(12): 64–65. BE62647.
> advertising; conflict of interest; disclosure; drug industry; *drugs; financial support; *human experimentation; informed consent; mass media; placebos; regulation; remuneration; research ethics committees; research subjects; risk; volunteers; United States

World Medical Association adopts statements, etc., on miscellaneous matters. [Texts of statements and declarations]. *International Digest of Health Legislation.* 1997; 48(1): 92–97. Statements and declarations adopted by the 48th General Assembly of the World Medical Association, held in Somerset West, Republic of South Africa, Oct 1996; including the Declaration of Helsinki as amended Oct 1996. BE59591.
> *bioethical issues; biomedical research; *contraception; *domestic violence; *drugs; *family planning; *guidelines; *human experimentation; informed consent; *international aspects; medical education; nontherapeutic research; *organizational policies; *patient care; *physicians; *professional competence; professional organizations; public policy; quality of health care; research ethics committees; self regulation; therapeutic research; third party consent; women's rights; *antibiotics; *Declaration of Helsinki; *World Medical Association

HUMAN EXPERIMENTATION/ETHICS COMMITTEES

Barnard, Kate. Basingstoke LREC revisited. [Letter and editorial comment]. *Bulletin of Medical Ethics.* 1997 Aug; No. 130: 13–17. BE61717.
> administrators; committee membership; dissent; financial support; *government regulation; health facilities; interprofessional relations; *organization and administration; professional competence; *research ethics committees; standards; *Basingstoke Local Research Ethics Committee; Department of Health (Great Britain); *Great Britain; National Health Service; *North and Mid Hampshire Health Authority

Beasley, John W. Primary care research and protection for human subjects. [Letter]. *JAMA.* 1999 May 12; 281(18): 1697–1698. 6 refs. BE62255.
> *epidemiology; *ethical review; geographic factors; *human experimentation; *primary health care; *regional ethics committees; *research ethics committees; multicenter studies; United States

Bergsma, Jan H. Dutch Union of Medical Ethics Committees. *Bulletin of Medical Ethics.* 1999 Feb; No. 145: 19–20. BE61892.
> education; ethical review; evaluation; human experimentation; organization and administration; professional organizations; *research ethics committees; *Dutch Union of Medical Ethics Committees; *Netherlands

Birmingham, Karen; Cimons, Marlene. Government report highlights the lack of clinical trial protection in the US. [News]. *Nature Medicine.* 1998 Jul; 4(7): 749. BE59769.
> accountability; evaluation; federal government; *government regulation; *human experimentation; *research ethics committees; vulnerable populations; multicenter studies; Department of Health and Human Services; *United States

Biros, Michelle H. Institutional review board approval:

when and why? *Academic Emergency Medicine*. 1998 Feb; 5(2): 91-92. 3 refs. BE62523.
   disclosure; editorial policies; *emergency care; ethical review; federal government; government regulation; *human experimentation; investigators; *research ethics committees; scientific misconduct; expedited review; Academic Emergency Medicine; United States

Brower, Vicki. Boston meeting blasts IRBs. [News]. *Nature Medicine*. 1998 Jan; 4(1): 9. Report of the "Ethical Research in an Ethical Society" meeting held in Boston, MA, in Dec 1997. BE59980.
   economics; ethical review; *evaluation; federal government; government regulation; human experimentation; informed consent; investigators; *research ethics committees; research subjects; universities; United States

Choo, Vivien. Thin line between research and audit. *Lancet*. 1998 Aug 1; 352(9125): 337-338. 11 refs. Comment on R.J.M. Snijders et al., p. 343-346. BE60436.
   *Down syndrome; *editorial policies; *ethical review; *evaluation studies; human experimentation; informed consent; *methods; patient care; pregnant women; *prenatal diagnosis; *research ethics committees; *medical audit; Great Britain; Lancet

Dal-Ré, Rafael; Espada, Julián; Ortega, Rafael. Performance of research ethics committees in Spain: a prospective study of 100 applications for clinical trial protocols on medicines. *Journal of Medical Ethics*. 1999 Jun; 25(3): 268-273. 28 refs. BE61863.
   committee membership; drug industry; *drugs; *ethical review; evaluation studies; *human experimentation; international aspects; organization and administration; *research ethics committees; statistics; *time factors; *multicenter studies; SmithKline Beecham; *Spain
OBJECTIVES: To review the characteristics and performance of research ethics committees in Spain in the evaluation of multicentre clinical trial drug protocols. DESIGN: A prospective study of 100 applications. SETTING: Forty-one committees reviewing clinical trial protocols, involving 50 hospitals in 25 cities. MAIN MEASURES: Protocol-related features, characteristics of research ethics committees and evaluation dynamics. RESULTS: The 100 applications involved 15 protocols (of which 12 were multinational) with 12 drugs. Committees met monthly (except one). They had a mean number of 12 members, requested a mean of six complete dossiers and nine additional copies of the protocol with a mean deadline of 14 days before the meeting. All applications were approved except three (two of the three were open-label long-term safety trials rejected by the same committee), which were approved by the other committees involved. The mean time from submission to approval was 64 days. The mean time from submission to arrival of the approval document at our offices was 85 days. Twenty-five committees raised queries for 38 of the 97 finally approved applications. Impact of evaluation fee, number of members, queries raised and experience of committees on timings were not statistically significant. CONCLUSION: Obtaining ethical approval is time-consuming. There is much diversity in the research ethics committees' performance. A remarkable delay (greater than 20 days) exists between the decision and the arrival of the written approval, suggesting administrative or organisational problems.

Dalyell, Tam. More comment from Westminster [research ethics committees]. [News]. *New Scientist*. 1998 Oct 3; 160(2154): 55. BE62096.
   ethical review; human experimentation; international aspects; *research ethics committees; standards; multicenter studies; European Commission; *Great Britain; National

Health Service

DeRenzo, Evan G.; Biesecker, Leslie G.; Meltzer, Noah. Genetics and the dead: implications for genetics research with samples from deceased persons. *American Journal of Medical Genetics*. 1997 Mar 31; 69(3): 332-334. 12 refs. BE59523.
   body parts and fluids; breast cancer; *cadavers; case studies; confidentiality; disclosure; DNA data banks; ethical review; family members; federal government; genetic information; *genetic materials; *genetic research; genetic screening; government regulation; human experimentation; informed consent; *research ethics committees; risks and benefits; tissue donation; pedigree studies; United States

Dresser, Rebecca. Time for new rules on human subjects research? *Hastings Center Report*. 1998 Nov-Dec; 28(6): 23-24. 4 fn. BE61281.
   accountability; *evaluation; federal government; government financing; *government regulation; *human experimentation; organization and administration; *research ethics committees; standards; *Department of Health and Human Services; Food and Drug Administration; Office for Protection from Research Risks; *United States

Egilman, David; Wallace, Wes; Stubbs, Cassandra, et al. Ethical aerobics: ACHRE's flight from responsibility. *Accountability in Research*. 1998 Jan; 6(1-2): 15-61. 94 refs. BE61534.
   advisory committees; cancer; children; codes of ethics; committee membership; *compensation; *conflict of interest; consensus; disclosure; ethical relativism; *evaluation; *federal government; *historical aspects; *human experimentation; *informed consent; *injuries; international aspects; investigators; legal aspects; medical ethics; military personnel; morbidity; mortality; National Socialism; *nontherapeutic research; patient care; patients; physicians; politics; prisoners; professional organizations; *public policy; *radiation; research subjects; retrospective moral judgment; *risk; *scientific misconduct; *standards; volunteers; culpability; recontact; *Advisory Committee on Human Radiation Experiments; American Medical Association; Cold War; Declaration of Helsinki; Faden, Ruth; Feinberg, Kenneth; Katz, Jay; Nuremberg Code; *Twentieth Century; *United States; World Medical Association

Eichenwald, Kurt. Monitoring of drug tests is faulted. [News]. *New York Times*. 1998 Jun 12: A14. BE59610.
   accountability; drugs; ethical review; evaluation; federal government; *government regulation; *human experimentation; medical devices; *research ethics committees; *Department of Health and Human Services; U.S. Congress; *United States

Evans, Donald; Crossland, Nigel; Graham, I.M.F., et al. Issues for research ethics committees: third installment. [Letters]. *Bulletin of Medical Ethics*. 1998 Feb; No. 135: 13-16. 3 refs. BE61887.
   consent forms; *ethical review; *guidelines; *human experimentation; international aspects; minors; radiation; *research ethics committees; third party consent; *multicenter studies; Department of Health (Great Britain); *Great Britain

Foster, Claire; Holley, Sandra. Ethical review of multi-centre research: a survey of multi-centre researchers in the South Thames region. *Journal of the Royal College of Physicians of London*. 1998 May-Jun; 32(3): 242-245. 6 refs. BE62315.
   *attitudes; comparative studies; *ethical review; evaluation; human experimentation; *investigators; organization and administration; regional ethics committees; research design; *research ethics committees; standards; survey; *multicenter studies; *Great Britain

---

BE = bioethics accession number   fn. = footnotes   refs. = references

Glass, Kathleen Cranley; Weijer, Charles; Lemmens, Trudo, et al. Structuring the review of human genetics protocols, Part II: diagnostic and screening studies. *IRB: A Review of Human Subjects Research.* 1997 May–Aug; 19(3–4): 1–13. 72 refs. BE60213.
    confidentiality; conflict of interest; diagnosis; disclosure; DNA data banks; *ethical review; genetic counseling; genetic diversity; genetic information; genetic predisposition; *genetic research; *genetic screening; *guidelines; *human experimentation; informed consent; insurance; international aspects; investigators; laboratories; mass screening; medical records; minority groups; patents; prenatal diagnosis; research design; *research ethics committees; research subjects; risks and benefits; selection of subjects; standards; uncertainty; vulnerable populations

Greenberg, Daniel S. When institutional review boards fail the system. [News]. *Lancet.* 1999 May 22; 353(9166): 1773. BE62430.
    committee membership; conflict of interest; federal government; *government regulation; human experimentation; misconduct; *research ethics committees; self regulation; universities; Duke University Medical Center; National Institutes of Health; Office for Protection from Research Risks; *United States

Hammerschmidt, Dale E. "There is no substantive due process right to conduct human–subject research": the saga of the Minnesota Gamma Hydroxybutyrate Study. *IRB: A Review of Human Subjects Research.* 1997 May–Aug; 19(3–4): 13–15. 2 fn. BE60214.
    drug abuse; *due process; *ethical review; *human experimentation; informed consent; investigational drugs; *investigators; judicial action; *legal aspects; legal liability; legal rights; punishment; *research ethics committees; research subjects; *scientific misconduct; universities; University of Minnesota

Holley, Sandra; Foster, Claire. Ethical review of multi–centre research: a survey of local research ethics committees in the South Thames region. *Journal of the Royal College of Physicians of London.* 1998 May–Jun; 32(3): 238–241. 17 refs. BE62314.
    attitudes; committee membership; *ethical review; *evaluation; guideline adherence; guidelines; human experimentation; organization and administration; regional ethics committees; *research ethics committees; *standards; survey; *multicenter studies; *Great Britain

Kent, Gerry. Responses by four local research ethics committees to submitted proposals. *Journal of Medical Ethics.* 1999 Jun; 25(3): 274–277. 11 refs. BE61864.
    audiovisual aids; autonomy; beneficence; communication; consent forms; decision making; disclosure; *ethical review; evaluation studies; *human experimentation; information dissemination; informed consent; investigators; research design; *research ethics committees; research subjects; risk; statistics; pamphlets; *Great Britain
    BACKGROUND: There is relatively little research concerning the processes whereby Local Research Ethics Committees discharge their responsibilities towards society, potential participants and investigators. OBJECTIVES: To examine the criteria used by LRECs in arriving at their decisions concerning approval of research protocols through an analysis of letters sent to investigators. DESIGN: Four LRECs each provided copies of 50 letters sent to investigators after their submitted proposals had been considered by the committees. These letters were subjected to a content analysis, in which specific comments and requests for additional information and changes in the protocols were recorded and compared. FINDINGS: Overall 24% of proposals were approved without request for changes or clarifications, but this varied by committee: one

committee approved only 6% of proposals without change or clarification while the others ranged from 26% to 32%. The content analyses of responses indicated that they could be placed into four categories: (i) further information for the committee to aid in their deliberations; (ii) requests for changes to the design or justification for the design used; (iii) changes to the information sheets provided to potential participants; and (iv) changes to consent procedures. Of these, alterations to information sheets were the most common type of request. These four types of response could be seen as safeguarding the wellbeing of potential participants (the principle of non–maleficence), of promoting the scientific validity of the research (the principle of beneficence), and of enhancing the rights of potential participants (the principle of autonomy). CONCLUSIONS: The committees were consistent in the types of requests they made of investigators, which can be seen as attempts to protect participants' rights and ensure the scientific validity of studies. Without an analysis of the proposals sent to the committees, however, it is difficult to account for the variation in the requirements set by the committees before approval was given.

Lapierre, Yvon D.; Weijer, Charles. Placebo: pro and con. *NCEHR Communique (National Council on Ethics in Human Research).* 1997–1998 Winter–Spring; 8(2): 11–15. 24 refs. BE62095.
    competence; drugs; ethical review; *guidelines; *human experimentation; informed consent; *mentally ill; *placebos; psychoactive drugs; *research design; *research ethics committees; risks and benefits; Canada; Code of Conduct for Research Involving Humans; Medical Research Council of Canada

Little, Miles. Research, ethics and conflicts of interest. *Journal of Medical Ethics.* 1999 Jun; 25(3): 259–262. 10 refs. BE61861.
    *advisory committees; biomedical research; *committee membership; *communication; *conflict of interest; cultural pluralism; decision making; disclosure; *ethical review; financial support; *human experimentation; *investigators; organization and administration; peer review; public participation; *research ethics committees; research subjects; resource allocation; social dominance; technical expertise; terminology; trust; values; negotiation
    In this paper, I have tried to develop a critique of committee procedures and conflict of interest within research advisory committees and ethical review committees (ERCs). There are specific features of conflict of interest in medical research. Scientists, communities and the subjects of research all have legitimate stakeholdings. The interests of medical scientists are particularly complex, since they are justified by the moral and physical welfare of their research subjects, while the reputations and incomes of scientists depend on the success of their science. Tensions of this kind must at times produce conflict of interest. It is important to recognise that conflicts of interest may unwittingly lead to manipulation of research subjects and their lay representatives on research committees. It is equally important to recognise distinctions between the legal and moral aspects of conflict of interest. Some practical suggestions are made which may go some way towards resolving these difficulties. They indicate what might be needed to ensure the validity of ethical discourse, and to reduce the risks associated with conflict of interest.

Love, Richard R.; Fost, Norman C. Ethical and regulatory challenges in a randomized control trial of adjuvant treatment for breast cancer in Vietnam. *Journal*

BE = bioethics accession number   fn. = footnotes   refs. = references

of Investigative Medicine. 1997 Oct; 45(8): 423–431. 9 refs. BE62062.
> *breast cancer; cultural pluralism; *developing countries; *disclosure; *ethical relativism; ethical review; females; guidelines; *hormones; *human experimentation; *informed consent; *international aspects; non-Western World; paternalism; patient participation; peer review; *random selection; research design; *research ethics committees; standards; surgery; third party consent; Western World; ovaries; United States; *Vietnam

McHale, J.V. Guidelines for medical research -- some ethical and legal problems. *Medical Law Review.* 1993 Summer; 1(2): 160–185. 123 fn. BE59251.
> accountability; adolescents; adults; children; committee membership; compensation; confidentiality; disclosure; *ethical review; government regulation; *guidelines; *human experimentation; incentives; informed consent; injuries; investigators; legal aspects; mentally disabled; *nontherapeutic research; patients; prisoners; public participation; random selection; remuneration; *research ethics committees; research subjects; risks and benefits; *therapeutic research; volunteers; vulnerable populations; *Department of Health (Great Britain); *Great Britain; National Health Service

Macpherson, Cheryl Cox. Research ethics committees: a regional approach. *Theoretical Medicine and Bioethics.* 1999 Apr; 20(2): 161–179. 40 refs. BE62216.
> accountability; committee membership; *cultural pluralism; *developing countries; *ethical relativism; *ethical review; ethicists; *guidelines; *human experimentation; *international aspects; non-Western World; *organization and administration; public participation; *regional ethics committees; *research ethics committees; socioeconomic factors; values; Western World; multicenter studies; *Caribbean Region; Council for International Organizations of Medical Sciences; *Grenada; *Latin America

Maloney, Dennis M. Federal investigation concludes that institutional review boards are in trouble. *Human Research Report.* 1998 Aug; 13(8): 1–2. BE61726.
> conflict of interest; education; ethical review; *evaluation; federal government; *government regulation; human experimentation; informed consent; legislation; *research ethics committees; technical expertise; Department of Health and Human Services; National Institutes of Health; *U.S. Congress; *United States

Maloney, Dennis M. Report says institutional review boards are conducting inadequate reviews. *Human Research Report.* 1998 Sep; 13(9): 1–2. BE61727.
> disclosure; economics; *ethical review; *evaluation; federal government; *government regulation; human experimentation; informed consent; *research ethics committees; time factors; Department of Health and Human Services; *United States

Meinert, Curtis L. IRBs and randomized clinical trials. *IRB: A Review of Human Subjects Research.* 1998 Mar–Jun; 20(2–3): 9–12. 11 refs. BE59994.
> *ethical review; federal government; government regulation; *human experimentation; injuries; investigational drugs; *random selection; *research ethics committees; research subjects; *risks and benefits; standards; multicenter studies; United States

Merz, Jon F.; Leonard, Debra G.B.; Miller, Elizabeth R. IRB review and consent in human tissue research. *Science.* 1999 Mar 12; 283(5408): 1647–1648. 18 fn. BE61033.
> authorship; biomedical research; comparative studies; editorial policies; *ethical review; federal government; financial support; *genetic research; government regulation; *guideline adherence; guidelines; *human experimentation;

*informed consent; investigators; literature; patient care; records; *research ethics committees; research subjects; science; survey; tissue banks; *tissue donation; pathology; pedigree studies; American Journal of Clinical Pathology; American Journal of Human Genetics; American Journal of Pathology; Human Molecular Genetics; Journal of Medical Genetics; Molecular Diagnosis; Nature; Nature Genetics; Office for Protection from Research Risks; Science; *United States

Miller, Franklin G.; Rosenstein, Donald L. Protocol review within the context of a research program. *IRB: A Review of Human Subjects Research.* 1998 Jul–Aug; 20(4): 7–10. 8 refs. BE61096.
> coercion; *comprehension; consent forms; *disclosure; *ethical review; *human experimentation; information dissemination; informed consent; investigators; motivation; *nontherapeutic research; patient education; *patients; physicians; placebos; *research design; *research ethics committees; research subjects; risks and benefits; *therapeutic research; volunteers

Moreno, Jonathan D. IRBs under the microscope. *Kennedy Institute of Ethics Journal.* 1998 Sep; 8(3): 329–337. 7 refs. BE60170.
> accountability; advisory committees; conflict of interest; education; *ethical review; *evaluation; federal government; *government regulation; guidelines; *human experimentation; investigators; mentally disabled; organization and administration; *research ethics committees; scientific misconduct; selection of subjects; state government; statistics; volunteers; vulnerable populations; Department of Health and Human Services; Maryland; National Bioethics Advisory Commission; National Institutes of Health; New York; U.S. Congress; *United States

Nicholson, Richard H. Unity in diversity. *Hastings Center Report.* 1999 Jan–Feb; 29(1): 6. 1 ref. BE61629.
> *ethical review; evaluation; government financing; *government regulation; *human experimentation; *international aspects; investigators; private sector; *research ethics committees; scientific misconduct; standards; *Europe; *Great Britain; *United States

Nightingale, Stuart L. Categories of research eligible for expedited review by IRBs. [News]. *JAMA.* 1999 Jan 6; 281(1): 27. BE61100.
> *ethical review; federal government; *government regulation; *human experimentation; informed consent; *research ethics committees; *expedited review; *Food and Drug Administration; *United States

Prentice, Ernest D.; Gordon, Bruce. IRB review of adverse events in investigational drug studies. *IRB: A Review of Human Subjects Research.* 1997 Nov–Dec; 19(6): 1–4. 4 refs. BE59990.
> consent forms; costs and benefits; *ethical review; federal government; government regulation; *human experimentation; *investigational drugs; investigators; mandatory reporting; *research ethics committees; research subjects; risk; risks and benefits; *toxicity; Food and Drug Administration; Office for Protection from Research Risks; United States; University of Nebraska Medical Center

Ramsay, Sarah. National body unites UK ethics committees. [News]. *Lancet.* 1999 Mar 20; 353(9157): 993. BE61983.
> advisory committees; *organization and administration; *research ethics committees; *national ethics committees; *Association of Research Ethics Committees (Great Britain); *Great Britain

Smith, Trevor. Ethics in Medical Research: A Handbook of Good Practice. New York, NY: Cambridge

---

University Press; 1999. 403 p. Bibliography: p. 378–390. ISBN 0–521–62619–6. BE62737.
  animal organs; children; compensation; confidentiality; critically ill; drug industry; drugs; epidemiology; ethical review; fetal research; forms; gene therapy; genetic materials; genetic research; *guidelines; *human experimentation; incentives; informed consent; injuries; international aspects; *investigators; medical records; mentally disabled; organ transplantation; *organization and administration; placebos; *professional ethics; *research design; *research ethics committees; research subjects; risks and benefits; selection of subjects; self regulation; volunteers; multicenter studies; questionnaires; Declaration of Helsinki; Great Britain; Internet

Til Occam Ltd. Medical Research Ethics Committee Directory: United Kingdom and Republic of Ireland. 1996 Version. [Looseleaf format]. Surrey Research Park, Guildford, England: Til Occam; 1996. 247 p. Intended to be updated annually. ISBN 0–9523780–1–9. BE61648.
  *organization and administration; *research ethics committees; multicenter studies; *England; *Ireland; *Northern Ireland; *Scotland; *Wales

U.S. Congress. House. Committee on Government Reform and Oversight. Subcommittee on Human Resources. Institutional Review Boards: A System in Jeopardy. Hearing, 11 Jun 1998. Washington, DC: U.S. Government Printing Office; 1999. 179 p. Serial No. 105–166. ISBN 0–16–058021–8. BE62631.
  accountability; advisory committees; children; committee membership; competence; conflict of interest; continuing education; drug industry; *ethical review; *evaluation; federal government; financial support; government financing; government regulation; *human experimentation; industry; informed consent; investigational drugs; investigators; medical devices; mentally disabled; patient advocacy; placebos; public participation; *public policy; research design; *research ethics committees; research subjects; risks and benefits; selection of subjects; technical expertise; universities; vulnerable populations; multicenter studies; Department of Health and Human Services; Food and Drug Administration; National Bioethics Advisory Commission; National Institutes of Health; Office for Protection from Research Risks; *United States

Verdun–Jones, Simon; Weisstub, David N. The regulation of biomedical research experimentation in Canada: developing an effective apparatus for the implementation of ethical principles in a scientific milieu. *Ottawa Law Review.* 1996–1997; 28(2): 297–341. 195 fn. BE62175.
  committee membership; ethical review; *government regulation; guidelines; *human experimentation; international aspects; investigators; *regulation; *research ethics committees; self regulation; *social control; universities; *Canada; Great Britain; Medical Research Council of Canada; National Council on Bioethics in Human Research (Canada); United States

Wadman, Meredith. US research safety system 'in jeopardy.' [News]. *Nature.* 1998 Jun 18; 393(6686): 610. BE59386.
  committee membership; conflict of interest; ethical review; evaluation; financial support; government regulation; human experimentation; industry; *research ethics committees; scientific misconduct; Department of Health and Human Services; Office for Protection from Research Risks; U.S. Congress; *United States

Weijer, Charles. The IRB's role in assessing the generalizability of non–NIH–funded clinical trials. *IRB: A Review of Human Subjects Research.* 1998 Mar–Jun; 20(2–3): 1–5. 19 refs. BE59992.
  age factors; drug industry; *ethical review; federal government; *females; financial support; government financing; government regulation; *guidelines; *human experimentation; investigational drugs; *minority groups; nontherapeutic research; *research design; *research ethics committees; risks and benefits; *selection of subjects; therapeutic research; vulnerable populations; Food and Drug Administration; National Institutes of Health; *NIH Guidelines; United States

White, Mary Terrell. Guidelines for IRB review of international collaborative medical research: a proposal. *Journal of Law, Medicine and Ethics.* 1999 Spring; 27(1): 87–94. 29 fn. BE61509.
  accountability; AIDS; behavioral research; case studies; committee membership; confidentiality; consensus; consent forms; *cultural pluralism; *decision making; developing countries; disclosure; dissent; *ethical relativism; *ethical review; financial support; guideline adherence; *guidelines; *human experimentation; human rights; informed consent; *international aspects; investigators; moral complicity; *non–Western World; professional organizations; research design; *research ethics committees; research subjects; risks and benefits; selection of subjects; socioeconomic factors; standards; trust; values; vulnerable populations; *Western World; integrity; *negotiation; China; Council for International Organizations of Medical Sciences; United States

Hospital failed on human research policy. [News]. *Science.* 1998 Nov 6; 282(5391): 1035. BE59660.
  consent forms; ethical review; federal government; government financing; *government regulation; *hospitals; *human experimentation; institutional policies; investigators; organization and administration; punishment; *research ethics committees; scientific misconduct; Chicago; Department of Health and Human Services; Office for Protection from Research Risks; *Rush–Presbyterian–St. Luke's Medical Center (Chicago)

Research involving human subjects: efforts to resolve current ethical controversies. [Introduction to a set of documents, p. S:279–S:348].*In:* BioLaw: A Legal and Ethical Reporter of Medicine, Health Care, and Bioengineering. Special Sections 2(7–8). Frederick, MD: University Publications of America; 1998 Jul–Aug: S:241–S:277. 76 fn. Followed by recent documents on research involving subjects with mental disorders: "Research Involving Individuals with Questionable Capacity to Consent: Ethical Issues and Practical Considerations for Institutional Review Boards"; Testimony from a House of Representatives Committee Hearing on IRBs; and a draft NBAC report, "Research Involving Subjects with Mental Disorders that May Affect Decision–Making Capacity." BE60173.
  advisory committees; autonomy; beneficence; communitarianism; compensation; competence; cultural pluralism; decision making; developing countries; drugs; ethical relativism; evaluation; federal government; government regulation; guidelines; HIV seropositivity; *human experimentation; informed consent; injuries; international aspects; justice; *mentally disabled; newborns; placebos; pregnant women; preventive medicine; public policy; research design; *research ethics committees; research subjects; resource allocation; risks and benefits; schizophrenia; state government; therapeutic research; trends; *vulnerable populations; withholding treatment; AZT; Federal Policy (Common Rule) for the Protection of Human Subjects 1991; National Bioethics Advisory Commission; United States

HUMAN EXPERIMENTATION/FOREIGN COUNTRIES

Achrekar, Abinash; Gupta, Rajesh; Pichayangkura,

Chart, et al. Informed consent for a clinical trial in Thailand. [Letter and responses]. *New England Journal of Medicine.* 1998 Oct 29; 339(18): 1331–1332. 3 refs. BE60149.
> AIDS; audiovisual aids; *communication; *comprehension; *consent forms; control groups; *developing countries; disclosure; drugs; ethical review; *HIV seropositivity; *human experimentation; *informed consent; *newborns; *placebos; *pregnant women; preventive medicine; random selection; *research design; research subjects; terminology; therapeutic research; AZT; Ministry of Public Health (Thailand); *Thailand

Altman, Lawrence K. Ethics panel urges easing of curbs on AIDS vaccine tests. [News]. *New York Times.* 1998 Jun 28: 6. BE59361.
> advisory committees; AIDS; *developing countries; drugs; ethical relativism; guidelines; *HIV seropositivity; *human experimentation; *immunization; informed consent; *international aspects; placebos; research subjects; United States

Annas, George J.; Grodin, Michael A. Human rights and maternal–fetal HIV transmission prevention trials in Africa. *American Journal of Public Health.* 1998 Apr; 88(4): 560–563. 17 refs. BE60130.
> AIDS; comprehension; *control groups; *developing countries; disadvantaged; drugs; economics; ethical relativism; health care delivery; *HIV seropositivity; *human experimentation; *human rights; informed consent; *international aspects; justice; *moral policy; *newborns; patient care; *placebos; *pregnant women; preventive medicine; public health; *public policy; *research design; research subjects; resource allocation; socioeconomic factors; therapeutic research; Africa; AZT; Centers for Disease Control and Prevention; National Institutes of Health; Thailand; United Nations; United States; Universal Declaration of Human Rights

The human rights issues raised by the conduct of maternal–fetal human immunodeficiency virus transmission trials in Africa are not unique to either acquired immunodeficiency syndrome or Africa, but public discussion of these trials presents an opportunity for the United States and other wealthy nations to take the rights and welfare of impoverished populations seriously. The central issue at stake when developed countries perform research on subjects in developing countries is exploitation. The only way to prevent exploitation of a research population is to insist not only that informed consent be obtained but also that, should an intervention be proven beneficial, the intervention will be delivered to the impoverished population. Human rights are universal and cannot be compromised solely on the basis of beliefs or practices of any one country or group. The challenge to the developed countries is to implement programs to improve the health of the people in developing countries both by improving public health infrastructure and by delivering effective drugs and vaccines to the people.

Aoki, Eiko; Watanabe, Toru. Patients' concerns about clinical trials in Japan. [Letter and response]. *Lancet.* 1999 Mar 20; 353(9157): 1019–1020. 7 refs. BE62154.
> *breast cancer; comparative studies; control groups; disclosure; drugs; ethical review; *human experimentation; *informed consent; peer review; *research design; therapeutic research; *Japan; *National Surgical Adjuvant Study of Breast Cancer (Japan)

Arboleda–Flórez, Julio; Weisstub, David N. Ethical research with the mentally disordered. *Canadian Journal of Psychiatry.* 1997 Jun; 42(5): 485–491. 44 refs. BE59174.
> advance directives; advisory committees; autonomy; coercion; *competence; decision making; guidelines; *human experimentation; incentives; *informed consent; institutionalized persons; involuntary commitment; legal aspects; legislation; mental institutions; *mentally disabled; *nontherapeutic research; public policy; research ethics committees; research subjects; *third party consent; time factors; vulnerable populations; *Canada; Law Reform Commission of Canada; Uniform Mental Health Act 1987 (Canada); United States

Association of the British Pharmaceutical Industry. Clinical Trial Compensation Guidelines. Issued by the Association of the British Pharmaceutical Industry, 12 Whitehall, London SW1A 2DY, England; 1991 Jan. 2 p. 2 refs. Reprinted 1994 Mar. BE60352.
> *compensation; *drug industry; *guidelines; *human experimentation; *injuries; *organizational policies; professional organizations; *research subjects; therapeutic research; *Association of the British Pharmaceutical Industry; *Great Britain

Barnard, Kate. Basingstoke LREC revisited. [Letter and editorial comment]. *Bulletin of Medical Ethics.* 1997 Aug; No. 130: 13–17. BE61717.
> administrators; committee membership; dissent; financial support; *government regulation; health facilities; interprofessional relations; *organization and administration; professional competence; *research ethics committees; standards; *Basingstoke Local Research Ethics Committee; Department of Health (Great Britain); *Great Britain; National Health Service; *North and Mid Hampshire Health Authority

Bayer, Ronald. The debate over maternal–fetal HIV transmission prevention trials in Africa, Asia, and the Caribbean: racist exploitation or exploitation of racism? *American Journal of Public Health.* 1998 Apr; 88(4): 567–570. 9 refs. BE60132.
> AIDS; *control groups; *developing countries; disadvantaged; drugs; ethical relativism; ethical review; financial support; guidelines; *HIV seropositivity; *human experimentation; international aspects; justice; *moral policy; *newborns; patient care; *placebos; *pregnant women; prevalence; preventive medicine; random selection; *research design; research subjects; resource allocation; risks and benefits; *social discrimination; socioeconomic factors; standards; therapeutic research; vulnerable populations; Africa; Asia; AZT; Caribbean Region; Centers for Disease Control and Prevention; Council for International Organizations of Medical Sciences; Declaration of Helsinki; Denmark; France; National Institutes of Health; South Africa; United Nations; United States

Baylis, Françoise; Downie, Jocelyn; Sherwin, Susan. Women and health research: from theory, to practice, to policy. *In:* Donchin, Anne; Purdy, Laura M., eds. Embodying Bioethics: Recent Feminist Advances. Lanham, MD: Rowman and Littlefield; 1999: 253–268. 4 fn. ISBN 0-8476-8924-7. BE61025.
> contraception; *females; *feminist ethics; government regulation; *guidelines; *human experimentation; *political activity; *public policy; *selection of subjects; social discrimination; women's health; women's rights; *Canada; *Feminist Health Care Ethics Research Network; *Tri–Council Policy Statement on Ethical Conduct for Research Involving Humans

Benatar, Solomon R. Imperialism, research ethics, and global health. [Editorial]. *Journal of Medical Ethics.* 1998 Aug; 24(4): 221–222. 14 refs. BE60783.
> control groups; *developing countries; drugs; ethical relativism; government financing; health; HIV seropositivity; *human experimentation; informed consent; *international aspects; investigators; newborns; pregnant women; *research design; research subjects; resource allocation; risks and benefits; scientific misconduct; syphilis;

BE = bioethics accession number   fn. = footnotes   refs. = references

Angell, Marcia; AZT; Declaration of Helsinki; Tuskegee Syphilis Study; United States

Bergsma, Jan H. Dutch Union of Medical Ethics Committees. *Bulletin of Medical Ethics.* 1999 Feb; No. 145: 19–20. BE61892.
education; ethical review; evaluation; human experimentation; organization and administration; professional organizations; *research ethics committees; *Dutch Union of Medical Ethics Committees; *Netherlands

Bernstein, Nina. For subjects in Haiti study, free AIDS care has a price: a special report. *New York Times.* 1999 Jun 6: A1, A10. BE62347.
*AIDS; AIDS serodiagnosis; attitudes; conflict of interest; consent forms; counseling; deception; *developing countries; drugs; financial support; government financing; *human experimentation; immunization; incentives; indigents; informed consent; *international aspects; investigators; patient care; physicians; research design; research subjects; *standards; universities; withholding treatment; sexual partners; Cornell University; *Haiti; United States

Blumenthal, Ralph; Miller, Judith. Japanese germ–war atrocities: a half–century of stonewalling the world. *New York Times.* 1999 Mar 4: A12. BE60974.
*biological warfare; dehumanization; disclosure; federal government; historical aspects; *human experimentation; investigators; military personnel; *misconduct; moral complicity; *prisoners; *public policy; records; *scientific misconduct; torture; China; *Japan; Twentieth Century; United States; *World War II

Bonetta, Laura. Inquiry into clinical trial scandal at Canadian research hospital. [News]. *Nature Medicine.* 1998 Oct; 4(10): 1095. BE61528.
administrators; *biomedical research; conflict of interest; disclosure; *drug industry; drugs; *financial support; *hospitals; *human experimentation; *institutional policies; *investigators; misconduct; regulation; thalassemia; toxicity; *Apotex; *Canada; *deferiprone; *Hospital for Sick Children (Toronto); *Olivieri, Nancy

Cannold, Leslie. "There is no evidence to suggest...": changing the way we judge information for disclosure in the informed consent process. *Hypatia.* 1997 Spring; 12(2): 165–184. 35 refs. 4 fn. This paper is a substantial expansion and reworking of Cannold's "A question of control: the tussle over informed consent in the Melbourne trial of RU 486/PG," in *Healthsharing Women: The Newsletter of the Healthsharing Women's Health Resource Service,* 1994; 5(2): 1–2. BE61678.
abortion, induced; autonomy; *communication; comprehension; *disclosure; drugs; *females; *feminist ethics; HIV seropositivity; *human experimentation; in vitro fertilization; *informed consent; investigators; legal aspects; minority groups; pregnant women; research subjects; risk; *standards; uncertainty; *Australia; RU–486

Cocks, Geoffrey. The old as new: the Nuremberg Doctors' Trial and medicine in modern Germany. *In: his* Treating Mind and Body: Essays in the History of Science, Professions, and Society Under Extreme Conditions. New Brunswick, NJ: Transaction Publishers; 1998: 193–213. 71 fn. ISBN 1–56000–310–3. BE62049.
aliens; disabled; eugenics; guidelines; *historical aspects; *human experimentation; investigators; Jews; killing; *misconduct; moral complicity; *National Socialism; nontherapeutic research; *physicians; politics; prisoners; public health; public policy; *scientific misconduct; social control; social discrimination; social dominance; *sociology of medicine; war; *Germany; Guidelines for Novel Treatment and for the Undertaking of Experiments on Humans 1931 (Germany); Nuremberg Trials; *Twentieth Century; World War II

Cocks, Geoffrey. The old as new: the Nuremberg Doctors' Trial and medicine in modern Germany. *In:* Berg, Manfred; Cocks, Geoffrey, eds. Medicine and Modernity: Public Health and Medical Care in Nineteenth– and Twentieth–Century Germany. New York, NY: Cambridge University Press; 1997: 173–191. 71 fn. ISBN 0–521–56411–5. BE59270.
aliens; disabled; eugenics; guidelines; *historical aspects; *human experimentation; investigators; Jews; killing; *misconduct; moral complicity; *National Socialism; nontherapeutic research; *physicians; politics; prisoners; public health; public policy; *scientific misconduct; social control; social discrimination; social dominance; *sociology of medicine; war; Declaration of Helsinki; *Germany; Nuremberg Code; *Nuremberg Trials; *Twentieth Century; World Medical Association; World War II

Cohen, Jon; Ivinson, Adrian J. Clarifying AIDS vaccine trial guidelines. [Letter and response]. *Nature Medicine.* 1998 Oct; 4(10): 1091. BE61527.
AIDS; consensus; developing countries; dissent; *guidelines; *HIV seropositivity; *human experimentation; *immunization; *international aspects; *patient care; research subjects; standards

Crigger, Bette–Jane. The battle over babies: international research in perinatal HIV transmission. *IRB: A Review of Human Subjects Research.* 1998 Jul–Aug; 20(4): 13–15. 8 refs. BE61099.
AIDS; *control groups; *developing countries; *drugs; ethical review; guidelines; health care delivery; *HIV seropositivity; *human experimentation; international aspects; moral policy; *newborns; *placebos; *pregnant women; preventive medicine; public policy; *research design; research subjects; risks and benefits; socioeconomic factors; therapeutic research; vulnerable populations; Africa; Asia; AZT; Centers for Disease Control and Prevention; Council for International Organizations of Medical Sciences; Declaration of Helsinki; National Institutes of Health; United Nations; United States; World Health Organization

Crouch, Robert A.; Arras, John D. AZT trials and tribulations. *Hastings Center Report.* 1998 Nov–Dec; 28(6): 26–34. 32 fn. BE61283.
control groups; *developing countries; *drugs; *economics; financial support; guidelines; health care; *HIV seropositivity; *human experimentation; indigents; *international aspects; investigators; justice; moral obligations; motivation; newborns; *placebos; *pregnant women; *preventive medicine; public policy; *research design; research subjects; resource allocation; rights; *therapeutic research; Africa; *AZT; Centers for Disease Control and Prevention; Thailand; United States

Dal–Ré, Rafael; Espada, Julián; Ortega, Rafael. Performance of research ethics committees in Spain: a prospective study of 100 applications for clinical trial protocols on medicines. *Journal of Medical Ethics.* 1999 Jun; 25(3): 268–273. 28 refs. BE61863.
committee membership; drug industry; *drugs; *ethical review; evaluation studies; *human experimentation; international aspects; organization and administration; *research ethics committees; statistics; *time factors; *multicenter studies; SmithKline Beecham; *Spain
OBJECTIVES: To review the characteristics and performance of research ethics committees in Spain in the evaluation of multicentre clinical trial drug protocols. DESIGN: A prospective study of 100 applications. SETTING: Forty–one committees reviewing clinical trial protocols, involving 50 hospitals in 25 cities. MAIN MEASURES: Protocol–related features, characteristics of research ethics committees and evaluation dynamics. RESULTS: The 100 applications involved 15 protocols (of which 12 were multinational) with 12 drugs.

BE = bioethics accession number   fn. = footnotes   refs. = references

Committees met monthly (except one). They had a mean number of 12 members, requested a mean of six complete dossiers and nine additional copies of the protocol with a mean deadline of 14 days before the meeting. All applications were approved except three (two of the three were open-label long-term safety trials rejected by the same committee), which were approved by the other committees involved. The mean time from submission to approval was 64 days. The mean time from submission to arrival of the approval document at our offices was 85 days. Twenty-five committees raised queries for 38 of the 97 finally approved applications. Impact of evaluation fee, number of members, queries raised and experience of committees on timings were not statistically significant. CONCLUSION: Obtaining ethical approval is time-consuming. There is much diversity in the research ethics committees' performance. A remarkable delay (greater than 20 days) exists between the decision and the arrival of the written approval, suggesting administrative or organisational problems.

Dalyell, Tam. More comment from Westminster [research ethics committees]. [News]. *New Scientist.* 1998 Oct 3; 160(2154): 55. BE62096.
    ethical review; human experimentation; international aspects; *research ethics committees; standards; multicenter studies; European Commission; *Great Britain; National Health Service

Davidson, Sylvia. New European clinical trial regulations are "unacceptable" to industry. [News]. *Nature Biotechnology.* 1998 Feb; 16(2): 127. BE62023.
    confidentiality; data banks; *drug industry; ethical review; *government regulation; guidelines; *human experimentation; *international aspects; investigational drugs; professional organizations; research ethics committees; *Europe; *European Commission; *European Federation of Pharmaceutical Industries and Associations; International Conference on Harmonization; Japan; United States

Day, Michael. How the West gets well. *New Scientist.* 1997 May 17; 154(2082): 14-15. BE59713.
    cancer; *developing countries; drug industry; drugs; economics; females; guidelines; *HIV seropositivity; *human experimentation; informed consent; *international aspects; nontherapeutic research; patient care; placebos; pregnant women; withholding treatment; Africa; India; United States

del Rio, Carlos. Is ethical research feasible in developed and developing countries? *Bioethics.* 1998 Oct; 12(4): 328-330. 5 refs. Commentary on D.B. Resnik, "The ethics of HIV research in developing nations," p. 286-306. BE62281.
    advisory committees; AIDS; control groups; *developing countries; drugs; economics; guidelines; health care delivery; *HIV seropositivity; *human experimentation; informed consent; *international aspects; moral policy; newborns; non-Western World; placebos; pregnant women; preventive medicine; public participation; public policy; *research design; research subjects; therapeutic research; Western World; AZT; Council for International Organizations of Medical Sciences; World Health Organization

Des Jarlais, Don C.; Vanischseni, Suphak; Marmor, Michael, et al. HIV vaccine trials. [Letters and response]. *Science.* 1998 Mar 6; 279(5356): 1433-1436. 5 refs. BE59440.
    contraception; control groups; *developing countries; economics; *ethical relativism; guidelines; *HIV seropositivity; *human experimentation; immunization; international aspects; medical devices; methods; placebos; pregnant women; preventive medicine; research design;

standards; therapeutic research; Africa; United States

Desvarieux, Moïse; Turner, Marie T.; Whalen, Christopher C., et al. Questions about a placebo-controlled trial of preventive therapy for tuberculosis in HIV-infected Ugandans. [Letters and responses]. *New England Journal of Medicine.* 1998 Mar 19; 338(12): 841-843. 11 refs. BE59438.
    communicable diseases; control groups; *developing countries; drugs; historical aspects; *HIV seropositivity; *human experimentation; informed consent; international aspects; *placebos; preventive medicine; *random selection; research design; research ethics committees; scientific misconduct; therapeutic research; *tuberculosis; withholding treatment; Case Western Reserve University; Haiti; Tuskegee Syphilis Study; *Uganda; United States

Dickson, David. British MRC reprimanded over clinical test record. [News]. *Nature Medicine.* 1998 Jul; 4(7): 752. BE59770.
    compensation; *disclosure; evaluation; government regulation; guidelines; historical aspects; hormones; *human experimentation; *informed consent; investigators; radiation; research subjects; risk; scientific misconduct; Creutzfeldt-Jakob syndrome; *Great Britain; *Medical Research Council (Great Britain); Twentieth Century

Dyer, Owen. GP found guilty of forging trial consent forms. [News]. *BMJ (British Medical Journal).* 1998 Nov 28; 317(7171): 1475. BE60954.
    *consent forms; *fraud; *human experimentation; *informed consent; *physicians; punishment; *scientific misconduct; *Bochsler, James; *General Medical Council (Great Britain); *Great Britain

Emanuel, Ezekiel J. A world of research subjects. [Introduction to a set of articles by R.A. Crouch and J.D. Arras; by C. Grady; by L.H. Glantz, G.J. Annas, M.A. Grodin, and W.K. Mariner; and by C. Levine]. *Hastings Center Report.* 1998 Nov-Dec; 28(6): 25. BE61282.
    *developing countries; drugs; financial support; HIV seropositivity; *human experimentation; *international aspects; justice; patient care; pregnant women; research design; research subjects; therapeutic research; vulnerable populations; United States

European Commission. Proposal for a good clinical practice directive. [Official statement]. *Bulletin of Medical Ethics.* 1998 Feb; No. 135: 6-11. BE61886.
    committee membership; *drugs; ethical review; government regulation; *guidelines; *human experimentation; information dissemination; informed consent; *international aspects; research ethics committees; research subjects; *standards; multicenter studies; *Europe; *European Commission; European Union

Evans, Donald; Crossland, Nigel; Graham, I.M.F., et al. Issues for research ethics committees: third installment. [Letters]. *Bulletin of Medical Ethics.* 1998 Feb; No. 135: 13-16. 3 refs. BE61887.
    consent forms; *ethical review; *guidelines; *human experimentation; international aspects; minors; radiation; *research ethics committees; third party consent; *multicenter studies; Department of Health (Great Britain); *Great Britain

Faden, Ruth; Kass, Nancy. HIV research, ethics, and the developing world. [Editorial]. *American Journal of Public Health.* 1998 Apr; 88(4): 548-550. 9 refs. BE60127.
    AIDS; coercion; common good; *control groups; *developing countries; disadvantaged; disclosure; drugs; ethical relativism; ethical review; health care delivery; *HIV seropositivity; *human experimentation; *informed consent;

---

international aspects; *moral policy; *newborns; patient care; *placebos; *pregnant women; preventive medicine; public health; *public policy; random selection; *research design; research subjects; risks and benefits; therapeutic research; retrospective studies; Africa; AZT; United States

Foster, Claire; Holley, Sandra. Ethical review of multi–centre research: a survey of multi–centre researchers in the South Thames region. *Journal of the Royal College of Physicians of London.* 1998 May–Jun; 32(3): 242–245. 6 refs. BE62315.
   *attitudes; comparative studies; *ethical review; evaluation; human experimentation; *investigators; organization and administration; regional ethics committees; research design; *research ethics committees; standards; survey; *multicenter studies; *Great Britain

Fukushima, Masanori. Clinical trials in Japan. *Nature Medicine.* 1995 Jan; 1(1): 12–13. BE59768.
   advisory committees; cancer; comparative studies; conflict of interest; drug industry; financial support; *government regulation; guidelines; *human experimentation; informed consent; international aspects; *investigational drugs; research ethics committees; risks and benefits; Food and Drug Administration; *Japan; *Ministry of Health and Welfare (Japan); United States

Gilhooly, Mary L.M.; Smith, Alexander McCall; Nichols, David, eds.; Scottish Action on Dementia. Rights and Legal Protection Sub–Committee. Dementia: Consent to Treatment, Volume 1 [and] Dementia: Consent to Research, Volume 2. Two Discussion Papers. Edinburgh, Scotland: Scottish Action on Dementia; 1992 Mar. 52 p. (Dementia: human rights series). ISBN 0–948897–14–7. BE59473.
   advance directives; autonomy; behavioral research; clinical ethics committees; *competence; decision making; *dementia; drugs; emergency care; family members; genetic research; *human experimentation; *informed consent; *legal aspects; legal guardians; moral policy; nontherapeutic research; paternalism; *patient care; physicians; research ethics committees; risk; risks and benefits; therapeutic research; *third party consent; treatment refusal; value of life; needs; Mental Health (Scotland) Act 1984; *Scotland

Glantz, Leonard H.; Annas, George J.; Grodin, Michael A., et al. Research in developing countries: taking "benefit" seriously. *Hastings Center Report.* 1998 Nov–Dec; 28(6): 38–42. 18 fn. BE61285.
   *developing countries; drugs; *economics; *financial support; guidelines; *health care; HIV seropositivity; *human experimentation; *international aspects; pregnant women; preventive medicine; *risks and benefits; standards; Africa; AZT

Grady, Christine. Science in the service of healing. *Hastings Center Report.* 1998 Nov–Dec; 28(6): 34–38. 19 fn. BE61284.
   control groups; *developing countries; *drugs; economics; financial support; goals; guidelines; *HIV seropositivity; *human experimentation; *international aspects; newborns; *placebos; *pregnant women; *preventive medicine; *research design; research subjects; Africa; *AZT; Thailand; United States

Graham, Amanda; McDonald, Jim; Association of Canadian Universities for Northern Studies. Board Committee on Revising the Ethical Principles. Ethical Principles for the Conduct of Research in the North. Ottawa, ON: Association of Canadian Universities for Northern Studies; 1998. 28 p. Text in English, in Inuktitut, and in French. ISBN 0–921421–10–9. BE60860.
   American Indians; confidentiality; disclosure; *guidelines;

*human experimentation; informed consent; investigator subject relationship; investigators; *minority groups; privacy; professional organizations; research subjects; risks and benefits; Eskimos; *Arctic Regions; Association of Canadian Universities for Northern Studies; *Canada; Labrador; Northwest Territories; Nunavut; Yukon Territory

Hamilton, Peter. Fatal accident inquiry: death during research. *Bulletin of Medical Ethics.* 1997 Aug; No. 130: 22–24. BE61719.
   aged; anesthesia; consent forms; *death; deception; *disclosure; females; *human experimentation; *informed consent; investigators; legal aspects; pain; research design; research ethics committees; *research subjects; *risks and benefits; sedatives; Moffit, Phyllis; *Scotland

Hannay, Timo. Japan on verge of first gene therapy trial. [News]. *Nature Medicine.* 1995 Jan; 1(1): 9. BE59767.
   advisory committees; *gene therapy; genetic disorders; *government regulation; *human experimentation; international aspects; universities; adenosine deaminase deficiency; *Japan; Ministry of Education, Science and Culture (Japan); Ministry of Health and Welfare (Japan); United States

Hellman, Deborah. Trial and error: can good science be bad medicine? *New Republic.* 1998 Apr 27; 218(17): 14, 16–17. BE61471.
   *developing countries; drugs; federal government; government financing; *HIV seropositivity; *human experimentation; international aspects; newborns; *placebos; *pregnant women; *random selection; *research design; therapeutic research; Africa; Asia; AZT; Centers for Disease Control and Prevention; National Institutes of Health; United States

Hellman, Deborah. Trials on trial. *Philosophy and Public Policy.* 1998 Winter–Spring; 18(1–2): 13–18. 5 refs. BE59814.
   conflict of interest; *control groups; *developing countries; *drugs; *HIV seropositivity; *human experimentation; international aspects; investigators; physicians; *placebos; *pregnant women; public health; *research design; resource allocation; standards; therapeutic research; uncertainty; *AZT; Centers for Disease Control and Prevention; National Institutes of Health; United States

Holley, Sandra; Foster, Claire. Ethical review of multi–centre research: a survey of local research ethics committees in the South Thames region. *Journal of the Royal College of Physicians of London.* 1998 May–Jun; 32(3): 238–241. 17 refs. BE62314.
   attitudes; committee membership; *ethical review; *evaluation; guideline adherence; guidelines; human experimentation; organization and administration; regional ethics committees; *research ethics committees; *standards; survey; *multicenter studies; *Great Britain

Ivinson, Adrian J. Hard–won consensus on AIDS vaccine trial guidelines. [News]. *Nature Medicine.* 1998 Aug; 4(8): 874. BE59731.
   consensus; *developing countries; dissent; drugs; economics; *guidelines; *HIV seropositivity; *human experimentation; *immunization; *international aspects; *patient care; standards; *UNAIDS; World Health Organization

Jones, Judy. Government sets up inquiry into ventilation trial. [News]. *BMJ (British Medical Journal).* 1999 Feb 27; 318(7183): 553. BE60998.
   brain pathology; *deception; human experimentation; mortality; *newborns; *parental consent; *prematurity; public hospitals; random selection; *therapeutic research; *ventilators; *Great Britain; North Staffordshire Hospital

Karim, Quarraisha Abdool; Karim, Salim S. Abdool;

BE = bioethics accession number   fn. = footnotes   refs. = references

Coovadia, Hoosen M., et al. Informed consent for HIV testing in a South African hospital: is it truly informed and truly voluntary? *American Journal of Public Health.* 1998 Apr; 88(4): 637–640. 15 refs. BE60134.
  *AIDS; *AIDS serodiagnosis; coercion; control groups; *counseling; disadvantaged; evaluation studies; *health services research; *HIV seropositivity; human experimentation; *informed consent; *knowledge, attitudes, practice; newborns; *pregnant women; preventive medicine; public hospitals; quality of health care; research design; research ethics committees; research subjects; survey; therapeutic research; voluntary programs; King Edward VIII Hospital (Durban); *South Africa
OBJECTIVE: The purpose of this study was to assess informed consent to human immunodeficiency virus (HIV) testing in a perinatal HIV transmission study in a major referral hospital serving a largely Black population in South Africa. METHODS: First-time antenatal clinic attenders who were randomly selected from those enrolled in the perinatal HIV study (n = 56) answered questionnaires before and after counseling. RESULTS: Knowledge of HIV transmission and prevention, high at the outset, was little improved after counseling. The acceptance rate for HIV testing was high. Despite assurances that participation was voluntary, 88% of the women said they felt compelled to participate in the study. CONCLUSIONS: Informed consent in this setting was truly informed but not truly voluntary.

Karim, Salim S. Abdool. Placebo controls in HIV perinatal transmission trials: a South African's viewpoint. *American Journal of Public Health.* 1998 Apr; 88(4): 564–566. 10 refs. BE60131.
  AIDS; alternatives; autonomy; *control groups; *drugs; economics; ethical review; government financing; health care; *HIV seropositivity; *human experimentation; informed consent; *newborns; nutrition; patient care; *placebos; *pregnant women; *prevalence; preventive medicine; *public policy; *research design; research subjects; resource allocation; sexually transmitted diseases; therapeutic research; breast feeding; AZT; *South Africa

Kempf, Judith. Collecting medical specimens in South America: a dilemma in medical ethics. *Anthropological Quarterly.* 1996 Jul; 69(3): 142–148. 19 refs. BE61212.
  American Indians; *anthropology; attitudes; *autonomy; coercion; communication; comprehension; *cultural pluralism; *developing countries; *epidemiology; *human experimentation; immunization; informed consent; international aspects; *non-Western World; *paternalism; public health; *research design; *research subjects; risk; sociology of medicine; values; *Western World; refusal to participate; Ecuador; *South America

Kennedy, Ian; Sewell, Herb. Xenotransplantation moratorium. [Letter]. *Nature Biotechnology.* 1998 Feb; 16(2): 120. 6 refs. BE62022.
  advisory committees; *animal organs; communicable diseases; *government regulation; *human experimentation; *organ transplantation; *public policy; *risks and benefits; Advisory Group on the Ethics of Xenotransplantation (Great Britain); *Great Britain

Kent, Gerry. Responses by four local research ethics committees to submitted proposals. *Journal of Medical Ethics.* 1999 Jun; 25(3): 274–277. 11 refs. BE61864.
  audiovisual aids; autonomy; beneficence; communication; consent forms; decision making; disclosure; *ethical review; evaluation studies; *human experimentation; information dissemination; informed consent; investigators; research design; *research ethics committees; research subjects; risk; statistics; pamphlets; *Great Britain
BACKGROUND: There is relatively little research concerning the processes whereby Local Research Ethics Committees discharge their responsibilities towards society, potential participants and investigators. OBJECTIVES: To examine the criteria used by LRECs in arriving at their decisions concerning approval of research protocols through an analysis of letters sent to investigators. DESIGN: Four LRECs each provided copies of 50 letters sent to investigators after their submitted proposals had been considered by the committees. These letters were subjected to a content analysis, in which specific comments and requests for additional information and changes in the protocols were recorded and compared. FINDINGS: Overall 24% of proposals were approved without request for changes or clarifications, but this varied by committee: one committee approved only 6% of proposals without change or clarification while the others ranged from 26% to 32%. The content analyses of responses indicated that they could be placed into four categories: (i) further information for the committee to aid in their deliberations; (ii) requests for changes to the design or justification for the design used; (iii) changes to the information sheets provided to potential participants; and (iv) changes to consent procedures. Of these, alterations to information sheets were the most common type of request. These four types of response could be seen as safeguarding the wellbeing of potential participants (the principle of non-maleficence), of promoting the scientific validity of the research (the principle of beneficence), and of enhancing the rights of potential participants (the principle of autonomy). CONCLUSIONS: The committees were consistent in the types of requests they made of investigators, which can be seen as attempts to protect participants' rights and ensure the scientific validity of studies. Without an analysis of the proposals sent to the committees, however, it is difficult to account for the variation in the requirements set by the committees before approval was given.

Kenyon, Georgina. Australian army infected troops and internees in Second World War. [News]. *BMJ (British Medical Journal).* 1999 May 8; 318(7193): 1233. BE62517.
  communicable diseases; drugs; *historical aspects; *human experimentation; Jews; military personnel; *nontherapeutic research; prisoners; *public policy; *scientific misconduct; malaria; *Australia; Twentieth Century; World War II

Kondro, Wayne. Canadian panel calls for review of drug-trial confidentiality agreements. [News]. *Lancet.* 1998 Dec 19–26; 352(9145): 1996. BE60958.
  *biomedical research; confidentiality; *conflict of interest; *contracts; *disclosure; *drug industry; *drugs; *financial support; *hospitals; *human experimentation; *investigators; thalassemia; toxicity; *Apotex; *Canada; *deferiprone; *Hospital for Sick Children (Toronto); *Olivieri, Nancy

Korszniak, N. A review of the use of radio-isotopes in medicine and medical research in Australia (1947–73). *Australasian Radiology.* 1997 May; 41(2): 211–219. 49 refs. BE60230.
  advisory committees; diagnosis; disclosure; federal government; *government regulation; historical aspects; *human experimentation; informed consent; investigators; mass media; minority groups; nontherapeutic research; patient care; patients; *radiation; scientific misconduct; self regulation; state government; therapeutic research; volunteers; *Australia; Declaration of Helsinki; National Health and Medical Research Council (Australia); NHMRC Guidelines; *Papua New Guinea; Radio-isotope Standing Committee (Australia); *Twentieth Century

Larkins, Richard G. Victorian orphans and clinical

---

research. [Editorial]. *Medical Journal of Australia.* 1997 Jul 21; 167(2): 60-61. 12 refs. BE60692.
　　children; guidelines; historical aspects; *human experimentation; immunization; institutionalized persons; regulation; residential facilities; trust; vulnerable populations; *Australia; National Health and Medical Research Council (Australia); Twentieth Century; Victoria

Lemonick, Michael D. Good news at a price : a study finds that AIDS drugs can help poor kids -- but was it ethical? *Time.* 1999 Feb 15; 153(6): 64. BE60961.
　　*developing countries; drugs; *HIV seropositivity; *human experimentation; placebos; *pregnant women; research design; *therapeutic research; treatment outcome; *Africa; South Africa; Tanzania; Uganda

Levine, Carol. Placebos and HIV: lessons learned. *Hastings Center Report.* 1998 Nov-Dec; 28(6): 43-48. 10 fn. BE61286.
　　*developing countries; drug industry; *drugs; economics; ethical review; goals; guidelines; *HIV seropositivity; *human experimentation; informed consent; *international aspects; newborns; *placebos; *pregnant women; *research design; risks and benefits; standards; withholding treatment; Africa; *AZT; Thailand; United States

Lie, Reidar K. Ethics of placebo-controlled trials in developing countries. *Bioethics.* 1998 Oct; 12(4): 307-311. 4 fn. Commentary on D.B. Resnik, "The ethics of HIV research in developing nations," p. 286-306. BE62278.
　　AIDS; *alternatives; control groups; *developing countries; drugs; economics; *HIV seropositivity; *human experimentation; international aspects; *newborns; *placebos; *pregnant women; preventive medicine; random selection; *research design; AZT; Thailand

Loff, Bebe; Cordner, Stephen. World War II malaria trials revisited. [News]. *Lancet.* 1999 May 8; 353(9164): 1597. BE62529.
　　communicable diseases; drugs; *historical aspects; *human experimentation; Jews; military personnel; *nontherapeutic research; prisoners; *public policy; *scientific misconduct; malaria; *Australia; Twentieth Century; World War II

Love, Richard R.; Fost, Norman C. Ethical and regulatory challenges in a randomized control trial of adjuvant treatment for breast cancer in Vietnam. *Journal of Investigative Medicine.* 1997 Oct; 45(8): 423-431. 9 refs. BE62062.
　　*breast cancer; cultural pluralism; *developing countries; *disclosure; *ethical relativism; ethical review; females; guidelines; *hormones; *human experimentation; *informed consent; *international aspects; non-Western World; paternalism; patient participation; peer review; *random selection; research design; *research ethics committees; standards; surgery; third party consent; Western World; ovaries; United States; *Vietnam

Lurie, Peter; Wolfe, Sidney M. Ethics of HIV trials. [Letter]. *Lancet.* 1998 Jan 17; 351(9097): 220. 5 refs. BE59384.
　　*developing countries; drugs; economics; ethical relativism; *HIV seropositivity; *human experimentation; international aspects; newborns; *placebos; *pregnant women; preventive medicine; random selection; research design; time factors; AZT; Centers for Disease Control and Prevention

McHale, J.V. Guidelines for medical research -- some ethical and legal problems. *Medical Law Review.* 1993 Summer; 1(2): 160-185. 123 fn. BE59251.
　　accountability; adolescents; adults; children; committee membership; compensation; confidentiality; disclosure; *ethical review; government regulation; *guidelines; *human experimentation; incentives; informed consent; injuries;

investigators; legal aspects; mentally disabled; *nontherapeutic research; patients; prisoners; public participation; random selection; remuneration; *research ethics committees; research subjects; risks and benefits; *therapeutic research; volunteers; vulnerable populations; *Department of Health (Great Britain); *Great Britain; National Health Service

Macklin, Ruth. International research and ethical imperialism. *In:* her Against Relativism: Cultural Diversity and the Search for Ethical Universals in Medicine. New York, NY: Oxford University Press; 1999: 187-217. 38 fn. ISBN 0-19-511632-1. BE62784.
　　autonomy; behavioral research; confidentiality; consent forms; *cultural pluralism; *developing countries; drugs; *ethical relativism; *ethical review; family members; federal government; government regulation; guidelines; HIV seropositivity; *human experimentation; *human rights; *informed consent; *international aspects; newborns; *non-Western World; placebos; pregnant women; preventive medicine; privacy; research design; research subjects; spousal consent; *standards; sterilization (sexual); third party consent; toxicity; *Western World; community consent; AZT; Bangladesh; China; Declaration of Helsinki; Egypt; Ivory Coast; Latin America; Nigeria; Philippines; quinacrine; Thailand; Uganda; *United States; World Medical Association

Macpherson, Cheryl Cox. Research ethics committees: a regional approach. *Theoretical Medicine and Bioethics.* 1999 Apr; 20(2): 161-179. 40 refs. BE62216.
　　accountability; committee membership; *cultural pluralism; *developing countries; *ethical relativism; *ethical review; ethicists; *guidelines; *human experimentation; *international aspects; non-Western World; *organization and administration; public participation; *regional ethics committees; *research ethics committees; socioeconomic factors; values; Western World; multicenter studies; *Caribbean Region; Council for International Organizations of Medical Sciences; *Grenada; *Latin America

Mann, Jonathan M.; Zion, Deborah; Macpherson, Cheryl Cox, et al. The ethics of AIDS vaccine trials. [Letters and response]. *Science.* 1998 May 29; 280(5368): 1327, 1329-1331. 11 refs. BE59441.
　　*AIDS; codes of ethics; comprehension; *developing countries; drugs; economics; guidelines; HIV seropositivity; *human experimentation; *immunization; informed consent; international aspects; placebos; pregnant women; research design; standards; therapeutic research; vulnerable populations; Africa; Declaration of Helsinki; International Ethical Guidelines for Biomedical Research Involving Human Subjects; United States

Medical Research Council (Great Britain). Responsibility in Investigations on Human Participants and Material and on Personal Information. [Guidance]. London: The Council; 1992 Nov. 15 p. (MRC ethics series). 17 refs. BE59557.
　　behavioral research; body parts and fluids; confidentiality; *guidelines; *human experimentation; informed consent; international aspects; medical records; nontherapeutic research; random selection; research design; research ethics committees; research subjects; therapeutic research; *Great Britain; *Medical Research Council (Great Britain)

Merson, Michael H.; Simonds, R.J.; Rogers, Martha F., et al. Ethics of placebo-controlled trials of zidovudine to prevent the perinatal transmission of HIV in the Third World. [Letters and response; editor's note]. *New England Journal of Medicine.* 1998 Mar 19; 338(12): 836-841. 25 refs. BE59387.
　　conflict of interest; control groups; *developing countries; *drugs; economics; *ethical relativism; federal government; *HIV seropositivity; *human experimentation; informed

consent; international aspects; investigators; justice; newborns; *placebos; *pregnant women; preventive medicine; random selection; *research design; research ethics committees; risks and benefits; scientific misconduct; standards; therapeutic research; Africa; AZT; Centers for Disease Control and Prevention; Ivory Coast; Thailand; United States; World Health Organization

Mitchell, Peter. Alleged unlicensed gene-therapy trial comes to light. [News]. *Lancet.* 1999 Jul 17; 354(9174): 225. BE62662.
  advisory committees; cancer; death; *gene therapy; *government regulation; guideline adherence; *human experimentation; *international aspects; investigators; research subjects; scientific misconduct; *Denmark; Department of Health (Great Britain); *Gene Therapy Advisory Committee (Great Britain); *Great Britain; *Habib, Nagy; *Hammersmith Hospital (London); *Lindkear, Sheen

Mitchell, Peter. Human xenotransplantation trials may be licensed in the UK. [News]. *Lancet.* 1998 Aug 8; 352(9126): 464. BE60268.
  *animal organs; *government regulation; *human experimentation; *organ transplantation; transplant recipients; *Department of Health (Great Britain); *Great Britain; *Xenotransplantation Interim Regulatory Authority (Great Britain)

Morris, Lynn; Martin, Desmond J.; Quinn, Thomas C., et al. The importance of doing HIV research in developing countries. *Nature Medicine.* 1998 Nov; 4(11): 1228–1229. 20 refs. BE62159.
  *AIDS; *biomedical research; *costs and benefits; *developing countries; drugs; economics; *HIV seropositivity; *human experimentation; newborns; patient care; pregnant women; preventive medicine; *resource allocation; *risks and benefits; sexually transmitted diseases; *Africa; AZT

Moss, Sue; Cuckle, Howard. Trial of mammography in women under 50 is ethical. [Letter]. *BMJ (British Medical Journal).* 1998 Dec 5; 317(7172): 1589–1590. 1 ref. BE60976.
  *age factors; *breast cancer; control groups; deception; ethical review; females; *human experimentation; *informed consent; *mass screening; research design; research ethics committees; research subjects; *Great Britain; Medical Research Council (Great Britain); United Kingdom Coordinating Committee on Cancer Research

Mudur, Ganapati. Indian women's groups question contraceptive vaccine research. [News]. *BMJ (British Medical Journal).* 1998 Nov 14; 317(7169): 1340. BE60855.
  *contraception; developing countries; *females; *human experimentation; immunization; *political activity; risks and benefits; *India

Nathan, D.G.; Weatherall, D.J. Academia and industry: lessons from the unfortunate events in Toronto. *Lancet.* 1999 Mar 6; 353(9155): 771–772. 9 refs. BE61219.
  *administrators; *biomedical research; *conflict of interest; developing countries; *disclosure; *drug industry; *drugs; *financial support; *hospitals; *human experimentation; *information dissemination; institutional policies; *investigators; minors; regulation; review committees; *thalassemia; therapeutic research; *toxicity; *universities; whistleblowing; *Apotex; *Canada; *deferiprone; *Hospital for Sick Children (Toronto); *Olivieri, Nancy; University of Toronto

National Council on Bioethics in Human Research (Canada). Facilitating ethical research: promoting informed choice. *NCBHR Communique (National Council on Bioethics in Human Research).* 1996 Dec; 7(2, Suppl.): i–ii, 1–28. 19 refs. Followed by text in French. BE59906.
  age factors; alternatives; coercion; competence; confidentiality; consent forms; disabled; disclosure; *human experimentation; incentives; *informed consent; remuneration; research subjects; risks and benefits; selection of subjects; third party consent; vulnerable populations; *Canada

Nicholson, Richard H. Unity in diversity. *Hastings Center Report.* 1999 Jan–Feb; 29(1): 6. 1 ref. BE61629.
  *ethical review; evaluation; government financing; *government regulation; *human experimentation; *international aspects; investigators; private sector; *research ethics committees; scientific misconduct; standards; *Europe; *Great Britain; *United States

Peart, Nicola; Moore, Andrew. Compensation for injuries suffered by participants in commercially sponsored clinical trials in New Zealand. *Medical Law Review.* 1997 Spring; 5(1): 1–21. 51 fn. BE60003.
  *compensation; control groups; disclosure; *drug industry; drugs; *financial support; *guidelines; *human experimentation; *injuries; *legal aspects; medical errors; patients; research ethics committees; *research subjects; volunteers; Accident, Rehabilitation Compensation Insurance Act 1993 (New Zealand); *New Zealand; *RMI (Research Medicines Industry) Guidelines

Resnik, David B. Replies to commentaries. *Bioethics.* 1998 Oct; 12(4): 331–333. Response to commentaries by R.K. Lie, p. 307–311; by U. Schüklenk, p. 312–319; by J. Thomas, p. 320–327; and by C. Del Rio, p. 328–330 on his article, "The ethics of HIV research in developing nations," p. 286–306. BE62282.
  AIDS; *developing countries; drug industry; drugs; financial support; government financing; health care delivery; *HIV seropositivity; *human experimentation; international aspects; justice; moral policy; *newborns; *placebos; *pregnant women; preventive medicine; public policy; *research design; socioeconomic factors; therapeutic research; AZT

Resnik, David B. The ethics of HIV research in developing nations. *Bioethics.* 1998 Oct; 12(4): 286–306. 62 fn. Commented on by R.K. Lie, p. 307–311; by U. Schüklenk, p. 312–319; by J. Thomas, p. 320–327; and by C. Del Rio, p. 328–330. BE62277.
  AIDS; beneficence; codes of ethics; control groups; *developing countries; drugs; *ethical relativism; *HIV seropositivity; *human experimentation; informed consent; international aspects; justice; metaethics; *moral policy; *newborns; non–Western World; *placebos; *pregnant women; preventive medicine; random selection; *research design; research subjects; socioeconomic factors; *standards; therapeutic research; utilitarianism; Africa; AZT; Centers for Disease Control and Prevention; Declaration of Helsinki; Dominican Republic; National Institutes of Health; Thailand; UNAIDS; World Health Organization
This paper discusses a dispute concerning the ethics of research on preventing the perinatal transmission of HIV in developing nations. Critics of this research argue that it is unethical because it denies a proven treatment to placebo–control groups. Since studies conducted in developed nations would not deny this treatment to subjects, the critics maintain that these experiments manifest a double standard for ethical research and that a single standard of ethics should apply to all research on human subjects. Proponents of the research, however, argue that these charges fail to understand the ethical complexities of research in developing nations, and that study designs can vary according to the social, economic,

---

BE = bioethics accession number   fn. = footnotes   refs. = references

and scientific conditions of research. This essay explores some of the ethical issues raised by this controversial case in order to shed some light on the deeper, meta-ethical questions. The paper argues that standards of ethical research on human subjects are universal but not absolute: there are some general ethical principles that apply to all cases of human subjects research but the application of these principles must take into account factors inherent in particular situations.

Rose, Joanna; Nilsson, Annika. Sweden considers more oversight of research. [News]. *Science.* 1999 Mar 19; 283(5409): 1829. BE62081.
  behavioral research; ethical review; females; financial support; *government regulation; *human experimentation; investigators; peer review; *public policy; research ethics committees; scientific misconduct; *Sweden

Rossel, Peter; Holm, Søren. How does the public perceive the motives of medical researchers for doing research? *Bulletin of Medical Ethics.* 1999 Mar; No. 146: 16–17. 6 refs. BE61820.
  biomedical research; *human experimentation; *investigators; *motivation; patients; physicians; *public opinion; research subjects; survey; trust; *Denmark

Saegusa, Asako. Are Japanese researchers exploiting Thai HIV patients? [News]. *Nature Medicine.* 1998 May; 4(5): 540. BE59726.
  government financing; *HIV seropositivity; *human experimentation; *immunization; *international aspects; investigators; methods; *Japan; Japan Science and Technology Corporation; *Thailand

Saegusa, Asako; Nathan, Richard. Japan renews gene therapy efforts ... and plans transgenic medicine guidelines. [News]. *Nature Medicine.* 1998 Nov; 4(11): 1213. BE62158.
  cancer; *drugs; *gene therapy; government regulation; guidelines; *human experimentation; industry; recombinant DNA research; *transgenic animals; universities; *Japan; Ministry of Health and Welfare (Japan); National Institute of Health Sciences (Japan); Tokyo University

Schüklenk, Udo. Unethical perinatal HIV transmission trials establish bad precedent. *Bioethics.* 1998 Oct; 12(4): 312–319. 21 fn. Commentary on D.B. Resnik, "The ethics of HIV research in developing nations," p. 286–306. BE62279.
  AIDS; alternative therapies; control groups; costs and benefits; *developing countries; drug industry; drugs; economics; ethical analysis; ethical review; guidelines; health care delivery; *HIV seropositivity; *human experimentation; informed consent; international aspects; *moral policy; *newborns; non-Western World; *placebos; *pregnant women; preventive medicine; *research design; research subjects; therapeutic research; Western World; Africa; Asia; AZT; Council for International Organizations of Medical Sciences; Latin America; UNAIDS

Shuchman, Miriam. Independent review adds to controversy at Sick Kids. *Canadian Medical Association Journal.* 1999 Feb 9; 160(3): 386–388. BE62307.
  administrators; *biomedical research; *conflict of interest; contracts; *disclosure; *drug industry; *drugs; *financial support; *hospitals; *human experimentation; institutional policies; *investigators; legal liability; minors; misconduct; review committees; thalassemia; therapeutic research; *toxicity; whistleblowing; *Apotex; *Canada; *deferiprone; *Hospital for Sick Children (Toronto); Naimark, Arnold; *Olivieri, Nancy

Sidley, Pat. South African research into AIDS "cure" severely criticised. [News]. *BMJ (British Medical Journal).* 1997 Mar 15; 314(7083): 771. BE60726.
  administrators; *AIDS; conflict of interest; *drugs; ethical review; government financing; *human experimentation; investigators; research design; *scientific misconduct; *South Africa; University of Pretoria; *Virodene; Visser, Olga; Zuma, Nkosazana

Specter, Michael. Uganda AIDS vaccine test: urgency affects ethics rules. [News]. *New York Times.* 1998 Oct 1: A1, A6. BE60574.
  *AIDS; *developing countries; drugs; economics; HIV seropositivity; *human experimentation; *immunization; informed consent; international aspects; research design; research subjects; risks and benefits; *Uganda

Spurgeon, David. Canadian case questions funding. [News]. *BMJ (British Medical Journal).* 1999 Jan 9; 318(7176): 77. BE60842.
  *biomedical research; confidentiality; conflict of interest; contracts; disclosure; *drug industry; *drugs; *financial support; *hospitals; *human experimentation; institutional policies; *investigators; legal aspects; regulation; therapeutic research; *toxicity; *whistleblowing; *Apotex; *Canada; deferiprone; *Hospital for Sick Children (Toronto); Medical Research Council of Canada; *Olivieri, Nancy

Spurgeon, David. Canadian research councils publish joint code on ethics. [News]. *Nature.* 1998 Oct 1; 395(6701): 420. BE60808.
  advisory committees; *behavioral research; *guidelines; *human experimentation; interdisciplinary communication; *regulation; research ethics committees; *Canada; *Code of Conduct for Research involving Humans; *Medical Research Council of Canada; *Natural Sciences and Engineering Research Council (Canada); *Social Sciences and Humanities Research Council (Canada)

Spurgeon, David. Canadian whistleblower row prompts broader code of conduct. [News]. *Nature.* 1998 Dec 24–31; 396(6713): 715. BE59536.
  *biomedical research; conflict of interest; disclosure; *drug industry; *drugs; *financial support; guidelines; *human experimentation; *investigators; toxicity; whistleblowing; Apotex; *Canada; Hospital for Sick Children (Toronto); *Medical Research Council of Canada; *Olivieri, Nancy

Stolberg, Sheryl Gay. Placebo use is suspended in overseas AIDS trials. [News]. *New York Times.* 1998 Feb 19: A16. BE59368.
  *AIDS; *developing countries; *drugs; economics; federal government; *HIV seropositivity; *human experimentation; *international aspects; *placebos; *pregnant women; *public policy; *research design; *therapeutic research; *AZT; Centers for Disease Control and Prevention; United States

Susser, Mervyn. The prevention of perinatal HIV transmission in the less-developed world. [Editorial]. *American Journal of Public Health.* 1998 Apr; 88(4): 547–548. 11 refs. BE60126.
  AIDS; *control groups; *costs and benefits; *developing countries; disadvantaged; *drugs; *HIV seropositivity; *human experimentation; international aspects; *newborns; *placebos; politics; *pregnant women; preventive medicine; *public policy; *research design; *risks and benefits; therapeutic research; breast feeding; AZT; Centers for Disease Control and Prevention; *France; National Institutes of Health; Thailand; *United Nations; *United States

Tanaka, Yuki. Japanese biological warfare plans and experiments on POWs. *In: his* Hidden Horrors: Japanese War Crimes in World War II. Boulder, CO: Westview Press; 1996: 135–165, 238–242. 72 fn. ISBN 0-8133-2718-0. BE60510.
  *biological warfare; communicable diseases; *dehumanization; *historical aspects; *human

---

experimentation; international aspects; *investigators; killing; military personnel; misconduct; National Socialism; nutrition; *physicians; *prisoners; psychology; public policy; *scientific misconduct; China; *Japan; Manchuria; Rabaul; *Twentieth Century; World War II

Thomas, Joe. Ethical challenges of HIV clinical trials in developing countries. *Bioethics.* 1998 Oct; 12(4): 320–327. 25 fn. Commentary on D.B. Resnik, "The ethics of HIV research in developing nations," p. 286–306. BE62280.
  AIDS; alternative therapies; autonomy; beneficence; conflict of interest; control groups; *developing countries; drug industry; drugs; economics; ethical review; guidelines; *HIV seropositivity; *human experimentation; human rights; international aspects; investigators; justice; moral policy; *newborns; non-Western World; placebos; *pregnant women; preventive medicine; public policy; *research design; research subjects; standards; therapeutic research; AZT; Council for International Organizations of Medical Sciences; Declaration of Helsinki; National Institutes of Health; United States

Til Occam Ltd. Medical Research Ethics Committee Directory: United Kingdom and Republic of Ireland. 1996 Version. [Looseleaf format]. Surrey Research Park, Guildford, England: Til Occam; 1996. 247 p. Intended to be updated annually. ISBN 0-9523780-1-9. BE61648.
  *organization and administration; *research ethics committees; multicenter studies; *England; *Ireland; *Northern Ireland; *Scotland; *Wales

U.S. Department of Health and Human Services. The Conduct of Clinical Trials of Maternal–Infant Transmission of HIV Supported by the United States Department of Health and Human Services in Developing Countries: A Summary of the Needs of Developing Countries, the Scientific Applications, and the Ethical Considerations Assessed by the National Institutes of Health and the Centers for Disease Control and Prevention, 1994–1997. Downloaded from Internet Web site:
http://www.nih.gov/news/mathiv/mathiv.htm and http://www.nih.gov/news/mathiv/whodoc.htm (Appendix) on 6 Dec 1997; 1997 Jul. 10 p. 1 ref. Appendix: Recommendations from the Meeting on Prevention of Mother-to-Infant Transmission of HIV by Use of Antiretrovirals, Geneva, 23–25 June 1994. BE62688.
  *developing countries; drugs; economics; health care; *HIV seropositivity; *human experimentation; *international aspects; *newborns; placebos; *pregnant women; *research design; standards; therapeutic research; withholding treatment; Africa; *AZT; Centers for Disease Control and Prevention; Department of Health and Human Services; National Institutes of Health; Thailand; *United States; World Health Organization

Verdun–Jones, Simon; Weisstub, David N. The regulation of biomedical research experimentation in Canada: developing an effective apparatus for the implementation of ethical principles in a scientific milieu. *Ottawa Law Review.* 1996–1997; 28(2): 297–341. 195 fn. BE62175.
  committee membership; ethical review; *government regulation; guidelines; *human experimentation; international aspects; investigators; *regulation; *research ethics committees; self regulation; *social control; universities; *Canada; Great Britain; Medical Research Council of Canada; National Council on Bioethics in Human Research (Canada); United States

Weindling, Paul. Human experiments in Nazi Germany: reflections on Ernst Klee's book "Auschwitz, die NS-Medizin und ihre Opfer" (1997) and film "Arzte ohne Gewissen" (1996). *Medizinhistorisches Journal.* 1998; 33(2): 161–178. 45 refs. 6 fn. BE61443.
  dentistry; eugenics; health personnel; *historical aspects; *human experimentation; investigators; involuntary euthanasia; literature; mass media; *National Socialism; physicians; public policy; *scientific misconduct; motion pictures; *Germany; *Klee, Ernst; Nuremberg Trials; Twentieth Century

White, Mary Terrell. Guidelines for IRB review of international collaborative medical research: a proposal. *Journal of Law, Medicine and Ethics.* 1999 Spring; 27(1): 87–94. 29 fn. BE61509.
  accountability; AIDS; behavioral research; case studies; committee membership; confidentiality; consensus; consent forms; *cultural pluralism; *decision making; developing countries; disclosure; dissent; *ethical relativism; *ethical review; financial support; guideline adherence; *guidelines; *human experimentation; human rights; informed consent; *international aspects; investigators; moral complicity; *non-Western World; professional organizations; research design; *research ethics committees; research subjects; risks and benefits; selection of subjects; socioeconomic factors; standards; trust; values; vulnerable populations; *Western World; integrity; *negotiation; China; Council for International Organizations of Medical Sciences; United States

Wilfert, Catherine M.; Ammann, Arthur; Bayer, Ronald, et al. Science, ethics, and the future of research into maternal infant transmission of HIV–1: Consensus statement. [For the Perinatal HIV Intervention Research in Developing Countries Workshop Participants]. *Lancet.* 1999 Mar 6; 353(9155): 832–835. 23 refs. BE61221.
  AIDS; alternatives; childbirth; consensus; *control groups; costs and benefits; *developing countries; *drugs; *economics; *guidelines; *HIV seropositivity; *human experimentation; informed consent; international aspects; *moral policy; *mothers; *newborns; nutrition; patient care; *pregnant women; *preventive medicine; public health; quality of health care; *research design; risks and benefits; *socioeconomic factors; standards; therapeutic research; *breast feeding; *Perinatal HIV Intervention Research in Developing Countries Workshop

Zion, Deborah. Ethical considerations of clinical trials to prevent vertical transmission of HIV in developing countries. *Nature Medicine.* 1998 Jan; 4(1): 11–12. 5 refs. BE59981.
  autonomy; coercion; competence; *developing countries; drugs; freedom; *HIV seropositivity; *human experimentation; informed consent; placebos; *pregnant women; *research design; research subjects; AZT

All too human. [News]. *Science.* 1999 Apr 2; 284(5411): 21. BE60857.
  government regulation; *guidelines; *human experimentation; *India; *Indian Council of Medical Research

Government sets up enquiry into adequacy of research controls in North Staffordshire. [News]. *Bulletin of Medical Ethics.* 1999 Feb; No. 145: 3–4. BE61890.
  brain pathology; comparative studies; ethical review; *human experimentation; morbidity; mortality; *newborns; *parental consent; prematurity; research ethics committees; scientific misconduct; *therapeutic research; treatment outcome; *ventilators; *Great Britain; *North Staffordshire Hospital Trust; Southall, David

International Conference on Harmonisation of Technical Requirements for Registration of Pharmaceuticals for Human Use (ICH) adopts Consolidated Guideline on Good Clinical Practice in the Conduct of Clinical Trials

---

BE = bioethics accession number   fn. = footnotes   refs. = references

on Medicinal Products for Human Use. [Introduction and Sections 2 and 3 of the Consolidated Guideline]. *International Digest of Health Legislation.* 1997; 48(2): 231–234. BE59597.
committee membership; *drugs; ethical review; *government regulation; *human experimentation; informed consent; *international aspects; *practice guidelines; records; remuneration; research ethics committees; research subjects; risks and benefits; *standards; European Union; *International Conference on Harmonization; Japan; United States

The perils of paediatric research. [Editorial]. *Lancet.* 1999 Feb 27; 353(9154): 685. BE61029.
alternatives; comparative studies; control groups; ethical review; *human experimentation; intensive care units; investigators; methods; morbidity; mortality; *newborns; *parental consent; physicians; prematurity; research design; research ethics committees; *scientific misconduct; *therapeutic research; treatment outcome; *ventilators; *respiratory distress syndrome; *Great Britain; *North Staffordshire Hospital Trust; *Southall, David

HUMAN EXPERIMENTATION/INFORMED CONSENT

Achrekar, Abinash; Gupta, Rajesh; Pichayangkura, Chart, et al. Informed consent for a clinical trial in Thailand. [Letter and responses]. *New England Journal of Medicine.* 1998 Oct 29; 339(18): 1331–1332. 3 refs. BE60149.
AIDS; audiovisual aids; *communication; *comprehension; *consent forms; control groups; *developing countries; disclosure; drugs; ethical review; *HIV seropositivity; *human experimentation; *informed consent; *newborns; *placebos; *pregnant women; preventive medicine; random selection; *research design; research subjects; terminology; therapeutic research; AZT; Ministry of Public Health (Thailand); *Thailand

Agarwal, Manoj R.; Ferran, Jose; Ost, Katherine, et al. Ethics of 'informed consent' in dementia research -- the debate continues. *International Journal of Geriatric Psychiatry.* 1996 Sep; 11(9): 801–806. 13 refs. BE59447.
*competence; comprehension; *dementia; drugs; evaluation studies; *family members; *informed consent; risks and benefits; survey; *therapeutic research; *third party consent; questionnaires; Great Britain

Alves, Wayne A.; Macciocchi, Stephen N. Ethical considerations in clinical neuroscience: current concepts in neuroclinical trials. *Stroke.* 1996 Oct; 27(10): 1903–1909. 44 refs. BE60623.
*ethical review; federal government; government regulation; *human experimentation; *informed consent; methods; placebos; random selection; *research design; research ethics committees; risks and benefits; therapeutic research; third party consent; deferred consent; *neurosciences; Food and Drug Administration; United States

American Geriatrics Society. Ethics Committee. Informed consent for research on human subjects with dementia. [Position statement]. *Journal of the American Geriatrics Society.* 1998 Oct; 46(10): 1308–1310. Position statement prepared by Greg A. Sachs; reviewed and approved by the American Geriatrics Society Ethics Committee and by the American Geriatrics Society Board of Directors, May 1998. BE62266.
advance directives; competence; decision making; *dementia; ethical review; family members; federal government; government regulation; *human experimentation; *informed consent; nontherapeutic research; *organizational policies; patient participation; professional organizations; public participation; research design; research ethics committees; research subjects; risk; risks and benefits; selection of subjects; state government; therapeutic research; *third party consent; refusal to participate; *American Geriatrics Society; United States

Aoki, Eiko; Watanabe, Toru. Patients' concerns about clinical trials in Japan. [Letter and response]. *Lancet.* 1999 Mar 20; 353(9157): 1019–1020. 7 refs. BE62154.
*breast cancer; comparative studies; control groups; disclosure; drugs; ethical review; *human experimentation; *informed consent; peer review; *research design; therapeutic research; *Japan; *National Surgical Adjuvant Study of Breast Cancer (Japan)

Arboleda–Flórez, Julio; Weisstub, David N. Ethical research with the mentally disordered. *Canadian Journal of Psychiatry.* 1997 Jun; 42(5): 485–491. 44 refs. BE59174.
advance directives; advisory committees; autonomy; coercion; *competence; decision making; guidelines; *human experimentation; incentives; *informed consent; institutionalized persons; involuntary commitment; legal aspects; legislation; mental institutions; *mentally disabled; *nontherapeutic research; public policy; research ethics committees; research subjects; *third party consent; time factors; vulnerable populations; *Canada; Law Reform Commission of Canada; Uniform Mental Health Act 1987 (Canada); United States

Ayd, Frank J. Research on the decisionally impaired: overview and commentary. *Medical–Moral Newsletter.* 1998 Jan–Feb; 35(1–2): 1–8. 12 refs. BE59707.
aged; *competence; critically ill; emergency care; family members; federal government; government regulation; *human experimentation; mentally ill; minors; research subjects; *third party consent; vulnerable populations; United States

Bjørn, Else; Rossel, Peter; Holm, Søren. Can the written information to research subjects be improved? -- an empirical study. *Journal of Medical Ethics.* 1999 Jun; 25(3): 263–267. 19 refs. BE61862.
attitudes; *audiovisual aids; comparative studies; *comprehension; *consent forms; disclosure; drug industry; drugs; *human experimentation; hypertension; information dissemination; *informed consent; patient education; placebos; random selection; *research subjects; sterilization (sexual); volunteers; pamphlets; Denmark
OBJECTIVES: To study whether linguistic analysis and changes in information leaflets can improve readability and understanding. DESIGN: Randomised, controlled study. Two information leaflets concerned with trials of drugs for conditions/diseases which are commonly known were modified, and the original was tested against the revised version. SETTING: Denmark. PARTICIPANTS: 235 persons in the relevant age groups. MAIN MEASURES: Readability and understanding of contents. RESULTS: Both readability and understanding of contents was improved: readability with regard to both information leaflets and understanding with regard to one of the leaflets. CONCLUSION: The results show that both readability and understanding can be improved by increased attention to the linguistic features of the information.

Cannold, Leslie. "There is no evidence to suggest...": changing the way we judge information for disclosure in the informed consent process. *Hypatia.* 1997 Spring; 12(2): 165–184. 35 refs. 4 fn. This paper is a substantial expansion and reworking of Cannold's "A question of control: the tussle over informed consent in the Melbourne trial of RU 486/PG," in *Healthsharing Women: The Newsletter of the Healthsharing Women's*

BE = bioethics accession number   fn. = footnotes   refs. = references

Health Resource Service, 1994; 5(2): 1–2.   BE61678.
abortion, induced; autonomy; *communication; comprehension; *disclosure; drugs; *females; *feminist ethics; HIV seropositivity; *human experimentation; in vitro fertilization; *informed consent; investigators; legal aspects; minority groups; pregnant women; research subjects; risk; *standards; uncertainty; *Australia; RU–486

Dickson, David. British MRC reprimanded over clinical test record. [News]. *Nature Medicine.* 1998 Jul; 4(7): 752. BE59770.
compensation; *disclosure; evaluation; government regulation; guidelines; historical aspects; hormones; *human experimentation; *informed consent; investigators; radiation; research subjects; risk; scientific misconduct; Creutzfeldt-Jakob syndrome; *Great Britain; *Medical Research Council (Great Britain); Twentieth Century

Dove, Alan. No-consent trials raise concern. [News]. *Nature Medicine.* 1999 Mar; 5(3): 250–251. BE62539.
blood transfusions; critically ill; drug industry; economics; *emergency care; federal government; *government regulation; informed consent; mortality; *presumed consent; *therapeutic research; *Food and Drug Administration; *United States

Dyer, Owen. GP found guilty of forging trial consent forms. [News]. *BMJ (British Medical Journal).* 1998 Nov 28; 317(7171): 1475. BE60954.
*consent forms; *fraud; *human experimentation; *informed consent; *physicians; punishment; *scientific misconduct; *Bochsler, James; *General Medical Council (Great Britain); *Great Britain

Edwards, Sarah J.L.; Braunholtz, David A.; Lilford, Richard J., et al. Ethical issues in the design and conduct of cluster randomised controlled trials. *BMJ (British Medical Journal).* 1999 May 22; 318(7195): 1407–1409. 5 refs. BE61394.
control groups; health services research; *human experimentation; *informed consent; *random selection; *research design; *third party consent; Great Britain
In most randomised controlled trials, individual patients are randomised to a treatment or control group, but sometimes this is undesirable or even impossible and groups (clusters) of people may be randomised instead. These are called cluster randomised controlled trials, and although they have been around for a long time, the need for them is likely to increase in line with growing concern to evaluate the delivery of health services, public education, and policy on social care.

Edwards, Sarah J.L.; Lilford, R.J.; Hewison, J. The ethics of randomised controlled trials from the perspectives of patients, the public, and healthcare professionals. *BMJ (British Medical Journal).* 1998 Oct 31; 317(7167): 1209–1212. 47 refs. BE60834.
*attitudes; *comprehension; disclosure; *empirical research; *human experimentation; *informed consent; international aspects; motivation; *patients; physician patient relationship; *physicians; public opinion; *random selection; *research design; *research subjects; therapeutic research

Egilman, David; Wallace, Wes; Stubbs, Cassandra, et al. Ethical aerobics: ACHRE's flight from responsibility. *Accountability in Research.* 1998 Jan; 6(1–2): 15–61. 94 refs. BE61534.
advisory committees; cancer; children; codes of ethics; committee membership; *compensation; *conflict of interest; consensus; disclosure; ethical relativism; *evaluation; *federal government; *historical aspects; *human experimentation; *informed consent; *injuries; international aspects; investigators; legal aspects; medical ethics; military personnel; morbidity; mortality; National Socialism;

*nontherapeutic research; patient care; patients; physicians; politics; prisoners; professional organizations; *public policy; *radiation; research subjects; retrospective moral judgment; *risk; *scientific misconduct; *standards; volunteers; culpability; recontact; *Advisory Committee on Human Radiation Experiments; American Medical Association; Cold War; Declaration of Helsinki; Faden, Ruth; Feinberg, Kenneth; Katz, Jay; Nuremberg Code; *Twentieth Century; *United States; World Medical Association

Faden, Ruth; Kass, Nancy. HIV research, ethics, and the developing world. [Editorial]. *American Journal of Public Health.* 1998 Apr; 88(4): 548–550. 9 refs. BE60127.
AIDS; coercion; common good; *control groups; *developing countries; disadvantaged; disclosure; drugs; ethical relativism; ethical review; health care delivery; *HIV seropositivity; *human experimentation; *informed consent; international aspects; *moral policy; *newborns; patient care; *placebos; *pregnant women; preventive medicine; public health; *public policy; random selection; *research design; research subjects; risks and benefits; therapeutic research; retrospective studies; Africa; AZT; United States

Featherstone, Katie; Donovan, Jenny L. Random allocation or allocation at random? Patients' perspectives of participation in a randomised controlled trial. *BMJ (British Medical Journal).* 1998 Oct 31; 317(7167): 1177–1180. 29 refs. BE60833.
alternatives; *comprehension; evaluation studies; *human experimentation; *informed consent; males; patients; *random selection; recall; *research design; *research subjects; survey; terminology; therapeutic research; *prostatic diseases; qualitative research; Great Britain
OBJECTIVES: To explore trial participants' understandings of randomisation. DESIGN: In this exploratory study, which used qualitative research methods, in-depth, semistructured interviews were carried out with 20 participants from the CLasP randomised controlled trial. Interviews were recorded on audio tape and fully transcribed. Data were analysed by comparing transcripts and describing emergent themes, using a grounded theory approach. SETTING: The CLasP study comprises three linked multicentre, pragmatic randomised controlled trials evaluating the effectiveness and cost effectiveness of laser therapy, standard surgery, and conservative management for men with lower urinary tract symptoms or urinary retention, or both, related to benign prostatic disease. SUBJECTS: 20 participants in the CLasP study were interviewed. Sampling was purposeful: men were included from each of the treatment arms, the two major centres, and at different points in the trial. INTERVENTIONS AND OUTCOME MEASURES: Interviews used a checklist of topics to encourage participants to describe their experiences. Narratives concerning randomisation were compared to identify common themes, retaining the context of the discussion to allow detailed interpretation. RESULTS: Most participants recalled and described aspects of randomisation, such as the involvement of chance, comparison, and concealed allocation. Many found the concept of randomisation difficult, however, and developed alternative lay explanations to make sense of their experiences. Inaccurate patient information and lay interpretations of common trial terms caused confusion. CONCLUSIONS: The provision of clear and accurate patient information is important, but this alone will not ensure consistent interpretation of concepts such as randomisation. Patients may need to discuss the purposes of randomisation in order to understand them fully enough to give truly informed consent.

Foster, Morris W.; Eisenbraun, Ann J.; Carter, Thomas H. Communal discourse as a supplement to informed

---

consent for genetic research. *Nature Genetics*. 1997 Nov; 17(3): 277–279. 36 refs. BE59978.
> American Indians; *communication; decision making; family relationship; *genetic research; health care; *informed consent; investigator subject relationship; *population genetics; research subjects; risks and benefits; stigmatization; community consent

Gilhooly, Mary L.M.; Smith, Alexander McCall; Nichols, David, eds.; Scottish Action on Dementia. Rights and Legal Protection Sub–Committee. Dementia: Consent to Treatment, Volume 1 [and] Dementia: Consent to Research, Volume 2. Two Discussion Papers. Edinburgh, Scotland: Scottish Action on Dementia; 1992 Mar. 52 p. (Dementia: human rights series). ISBN 0–948897–14–7. BE59473.
> advance directives; autonomy; behavioral research; clinical ethics committees; *competence; decision making; *dementia; drugs; emergency care; family members; genetic research; *human experimentation; *informed consent; *legal aspects; legal guardians; moral policy; nontherapeutic research; paternalism; *patient care; physicians; research ethics committees; risk; risks and benefits; therapeutic research; *third party consent; treatment refusal; value of life; needs; Mental Health (Scotland) Act 1984; *Scotland

Grady, Denise. Patient or guinea pig? Dilemma of clinical trials. [News]. *New York Times*. 1999 Jan 5: F1, F4. BE60123.
> attitudes; *disclosure; *drug industry; hepatitis; *human experimentation; *informed consent; investigational drugs; *patients; research design; *research subjects; therapeutic research; Rebetron; Schering–Plough

Guttman, Dan. Disclosure and consent: through the Cold War prism. *Accountability in Research*. 1998 Jan; 6(1–2): 1–14. 22 fn. BE61533.
> advisory committees; consent forms; *disclosure; *federal government; *historical aspects; *human experimentation; information dissemination; *informed consent; *nontherapeutic research; nuclear warfare; *public policy; *radiation; retrospective moral judgment; scientific misconduct; standards; trust; war; Advisory Committee on Human Radiation Experiments; *Atomic Energy Commission; Cold War; Manhattan Project; *Twentieth Century; *United States

Hamilton, Peter. Fatal accident inquiry: death during research. *Bulletin of Medical Ethics*. 1997 Aug; No. 130: 22–24. BE61719.
> aged; anesthesia; consent forms; *death; deception; *disclosure; females; *human experimentation; *informed consent; investigators; legal aspects; pain; research design; research ethics committees; *research subjects; *risks and benefits; sedatives; Moffit, Phyllis; *Scotland

Hilts, Philip J. Psychiatric researchers under fire. [News]. *New York Times*. 1998 May 19: F1, F5. Includes inset article by P.J. Hilts, "Do consent forms tell enough? One case from the front lines," p. F5. BE59613.
> adults; advisory committees; aggression; children; competence; consent forms; deception; federal government; government regulation; *human experimentation; *informed consent; *mentally ill; minority groups; *nontherapeutic research; *psychiatry; psychoactive drugs; risks and benefits; schizophrenia; scientific misconduct; state government; *withholding treatment; National Bioethics Advisory Commission; National Institute of Mental Health; United States

Hilts, Philip J. Study or human experiment? Face–lift project stirs ethical concerns. [News]. *New York Times*. 1998 Jun 21: 25–26. BE59615.
> consent forms; *cosmetic surgery; deception; *disclosure;

ethical review; federal government; government regulation; *human experimentation; *informed consent; *methods; physicians; research design; state government; *Manhattan Eye, Ear and Throat Hospital; New York; United States

Jones, Judy. Government sets up inquiry into ventilation trial. [News]. *BMJ (British Medical Journal)*. 1999 Feb 27; 318(7183): 553. BE60998.
> brain pathology; *deception; human experimentation; mortality; *newborns; *parental consent; *prematurity; public hospitals; random selection; *therapeutic research; *ventilators; *Great Britain; North Staffordshire Hospital

Karim, Quarraisha Abdool; Karim, Salim S. Abdool; Coovadia, Hoosen M., et al. Informed consent for HIV testing in a South African hospital: is it truly informed and truly voluntary? *American Journal of Public Health*. 1998 Apr; 88(4): 637–640. 15 refs. BE60134.
> *AIDS; *AIDS serodiagnosis; coercion; control groups; *counseling; disadvantaged; evaluation studies; *health services research; *HIV seropositivity; human experimentation; *informed consent; *knowledge, attitudes, practice; newborns; *pregnant women; preventive medicine; public hospitals; quality of health care; research design; research ethics committees; research subjects; survey; therapeutic research; voluntary programs; King Edward VIII Hospital (Durban); *South Africa

OBJECTIVE: The purpose of this study was to assess informed consent to human immunodeficiency virus (HIV) testing in a perinatal HIV transmission study in a major referral hospital serving a largely Black population in South Africa. METHODS: First–time antenatal clinic attenders who were randomly selected from those enrolled in the perinatal HIV study (n = 56) answered questionnaires before and after counseling. RESULTS: Knowledge of HIV transmission and prevention, high at the outset, was little improved after counseling. The acceptance rate for HIV testing was high. Despite assurances that participation was voluntary, 88% of the women said they felt compelled to participate in the study. CONCLUSIONS: Informed consent in this setting was truly informed but not truly voluntary.

Kirsch, Michael; Rothschild, Bruce M.; Ridzon, Renée, et al. Patient consent for publication. [Letters and responses]. *JAMA*. 1997 Dec 24–31; 278(24): 2139–2141. 9 refs. BE60135.
> authorship; autonomy; *confidentiality; *disclosure; *editorial policies; *epidemiology; guidelines; health services research; human experimentation; *information dissemination; *informed consent; justice; obligations to society; patient participation; *patients; *privacy; professional organizations; public health; *research subjects; International Committee of Medical Journal Editors

Kodish, Eric D.; Pentz, Rebecca D.; Noll, Robert B., et al. Informed consent in the Childrens Cancer Group: results of preliminary research. [For the Children's Cancer Group]. *Cancer*. 1998 Jun 15; 82(12): 2467–2481. 37 refs. BE61808.
> alternatives; *attitudes; *cancer; *children; coercion; communication; comparative studies; comprehension; consent forms; decision making; *disclosure; emotions; *evaluation; *health personnel; *human experimentation; informed consent; *investigators; nurses; *parental consent; *parents; physicians; professional family relationship; psychological stress; random selection; risks and benefits; survey; *therapeutic research; questionnaires; Children's Cancer Group; United States

Lears, Louise. Research in the emergency department. *Health Care Ethics USA*. 1997 Spring; 5(2): 4–5. 7 refs.

BE = bioethics accession number   fn. = footnotes   refs. = references

BE61723.
   critically ill; *emergency care; federal government; *government regulation; *human experimentation; informed consent; injuries; *presumed consent; risks and benefits; therapeutic research; Food and Drug Administration; United States

Love, Richard R.; Fost, Norman C. Ethical and regulatory challenges in a randomized control trial of adjuvant treatment for breast cancer in Vietnam. *Journal of Investigative Medicine.* 1997 Oct; 45(8): 423–431. 9 refs. BE62062.
   *breast cancer; cultural pluralism; *developing countries; *disclosure; *ethical relativism; ethical review; females; guidelines; *hormones; *human experimentation; *informed consent; *international aspects; non–Western World; paternalism; patient participation; peer review; *random selection; research design; *research ethics committees; standards; surgery; third party consent; Western World; ovaries; United States; *Vietnam

Lynn, Joanne; Muncie, Herbert L.; Magaziner, Jay, et al. Ethical concerns about research on incompetent persons. [Letter and response]. *Journal of the American Geriatrics Society.* 1998 May; 46(5): 660. 1 ref. BE61080.
   *aged; *competence; decision making; *dementia; ethical review; guidelines; *human experimentation; informed consent; nontherapeutic research; research subjects; *risks and benefits; selection of subjects; therapeutic research; *third party consent

Macklin, Ruth. International research and ethical imperialism. *In:* her Against Relativism: Cultural Diversity and the Search for Ethical Universals in Medicine. New York, NY: Oxford University Press; 1999: 187–217. 38 fn. ISBN 0–19–511632–1. BE62784.
   autonomy; behavioral research; confidentiality; consent forms; *cultural pluralism; *developing countries; drugs; *ethical relativism; *ethical review; family members; federal government; government regulation; guidelines; HIV seropositivity; *human experimentation; *human rights; *informed consent; *international aspects; newborns; *non–Western World; placebos; pregnant women; preventive medicine; privacy; research design; research subjects; spousal consent; *standards; sterilization (sexual); third party consent; toxicity; *Western World; community consent; AZT; Bangladesh; China; Declaration of Helsinki; Egypt; Ivory Coast; Latin America; Nigeria; Philippines; quinacrine; Thailand; Uganda; *United States; World Medical Association

Maloney, Dennis M. Proposal on waiver of informed consent poses major issues for research ethics. *Human Research Report.* 1997 Sep; 12(9): 1–3. BE59953.
   disclosure; federal government; *government regulation; *human experimentation; *informed consent; *investigational drugs; *military personnel; patient compliance; research ethics committees; research subjects; risks and benefits; Department of Defense; *Food and Drug Administration; *United States

Marquis, Don. How to resolve an ethical dilemma concerning randomized clinical trials. *New England Journal of Medicine.* 1999 Aug 26; 341(9): 691–693. 17 refs. BE62526.
   alternatives; *decision making; disclosure; evidence–based medicine; *human experimentation; *informed consent; *moral obligations; patient advocacy; *physicians; *random selection; research design; *selection of subjects; therapeutic research; uncertainty

Marshall, Eliot. Panel proposes tighter rules for tissue studies. [News]. *Science.* 1998 Dec 18; 282(5397): 2165–6. BE59648.
   advisory committees; DNA data banks; donors; federal government; *genetic materials; *genetic research; government regulation; *informed consent; privacy; research ethics committees; stigmatization; *tissue banks; *tissue donation; *National Bioethics Advisory Commission; United States

Mazur, Dennis J. Medical Risk and the Right to an Informed Consent in Clinical Care and Clinical Research. Tampa, FL: American College of Physician Executives; 1998. 183 p. Includes references. ISBN 0–924674–64–4. BE59664.
   advertising; communication; competence; conflict of interest; decision making; *disclosure; drug industry; drugs; emergency care; federal government; government regulation; historical aspects; *human experimentation; *informed consent; international aspects; investigator subject relationship; judicial action; *legal aspects; legal liability; legislation; *patient care; patient participation; patients; physician patient relationship; research ethics committees; research subjects; *risk; *risks and benefits; *standards; state government; Canada; Canterbury v. Spence; Eighteenth Century; Great Britain; Nineteenth Century; Twentieth Century; *United States

Merz, Jon F.; Leonard, Debra G.B.; Miller, Elizabeth R. IRB review and consent in human tissue research. *Science.* 1999 Mar 12; 283(5408): 1647–1648. 18 fn. BE61033.
   authorship; biomedical research; comparative studies; editorial policies; *ethical review; federal government; financial support; *genetic research; government regulation; *guideline adherence; guidelines; *human experimentation; *informed consent; investigators; literature; patient care; records; *research ethics committees; research subjects; science; survey; tissue banks; *tissue donation; pathology; pedigree studies; American Journal of Clinical Pathology; American Journal of Human Genetics; American Journal of Pathology; Human Molecular Genetics; Journal of Medical Genetics; Molecular Diagnosis; Nature; Nature Genetics; Office for Protection from Research Risks; Science; *United States

Merz, Jon F.; Sankar, Pamela; Taube, Sheila E., et al. Use of human tissues in research: clarifying clinician and researcher roles and information flows. *Journal of Investigative Medicine.* 1997 Jun; 45(5): 252–257. 36 refs. BE62405.
   confidentiality; epidemiology; genetic information; *genetic materials; *genetic research; *informed consent; medical records; research subjects; *tissue banks; tissue donation; pedigree studies; recontact

Miller, Michelle D. The informed–consent policy of the International Conference on Harmonization of Technical Requirements for Registration of Pharmaceuticals for Human Use: knowledge is the best medicine. [Note]. *Cornell International Law Journal.* 1997; 30(1): 203–244. 318 fn. BE61493.
   autonomy; consensus; *cultural pluralism; disclosure; drug industry; *drugs; federal government; *government regulation; *guidelines; historical aspects; *human experimentation; *informed consent; injuries; *international aspects; nontherapeutic research; paternalism; public participation; research subjects; risks and benefits; scientific misconduct; *standards; therapeutic research; negotiation; Europe; *European Union; *Food and Drug Administration; *International Conference on Harmonization; *Japan; Twentieth Century; *United States

Morin, Karine. The standard of disclosure in human subject experimentation. *Journal of Legal Medicine.* 1998 Jun; 19(2): 157–221. 309 fn. BE61248.
   advisory committees; autonomy; communication; *disclosure; DNA data banks; federal government; genetic research; government regulation; guidelines; *human

experimentation; *informed consent; investigator subject relationship; investigators; *legal aspects; *legal liability; malpractice; nontherapeutic research; patient care; patients; physician patient relationship; physicians; research subjects; risks and benefits; scientific misconduct; *standards; therapeutic research; Food and Drug Administration; National Commission for the Protection of Human Subjects; National Institutes of Health; President's Commission for the Study of Ethical Problems; *United States

Moss, Sue; Cuckle, Howard. Trial of mammography in women under 50 is ethical. [Letter]. *BMJ (British Medical Journal).* 1998 Dec 5; 317(7172): 1589–1590. 1 ref. BE60976.
  *age factors; *breast cancer; control groups; deception; ethical review; females; *human experimentation; *informed consent; *mass screening; research design; research ethics committees; research subjects; *Great Britain; Medical Research Council (Great Britain); United Kingdom Coordinating Committee on Cancer Research

Muncie, Herbert L.; Magaziner, Jay; Hebel, J. Richard, et al. Proxies' decisions about clinical research participation for their charges. *Journal of the American Geriatrics Society.* 1997 Aug; 45(8): 929–933. 19 refs. BE59433.
  *aged; comparative studies; *decision making; evaluation studies; *family members; *human experimentation; informed consent; nontherapeutic research; research subjects; risks and benefits; survey; therapeutic research; *third party consent; Baltimore

National Council on Bioethics in Human Research (Canada). Facilitating ethical research: promoting informed choice. *NCBHR Communique (National Council on Bioethics in Human Research).* 1996 Dec; 7(2, Suppl.): i–ii, 1–28. 19 refs. Followed by text in French. BE59906.
  age factors; alternatives; coercion; competence; confidentiality; consent forms; disabled; disclosure; *human experimentation; incentives; *informed consent; remuneration; research subjects; risks and benefits; selection of subjects; third party consent; vulnerable populations; *Canada

Pfeffer, Naomi; Alderson, Priscilla; Campbell, Harry, et al. Informed consent. [Letters]. *BMJ (British Medical Journal).* 1997 Jul 26; 315(7102): 247–254. 35 refs. BE59224.
  AIDS serodiagnosis; autonomy; beneficence; breast cancer; developing countries; disclosure; editorial policies; ethical review; females; guideline adherence; guidelines; HIV seropositivity; *human experimentation; *informed consent; international aspects; mass screening; parental consent; pregnant women; random selection; research design; scientific misconduct; socioeconomic factors; standards; vulnerable populations

Pinals, Debra A.; Malhotra, Anil K.; Breier, Alan, et al. Informed consent in schizophrenia research. [Letter]. *Psychiatric Services.* 1998 Feb; 49(2): 244. 5 refs. BE60041.
  comparative studies; *competence; *comprehension; *consent forms; control groups; *human experimentation; *informed consent; *mentally ill; *schizophrenia

Sass, Hans-Martin. Genotyping in clinical trials: towards a principle of informed request. *Journal of Medicine and Philosophy.* 1998 Jun; 23(3): 288–296. 21 refs. BE59292.
  *autonomy; confidentiality; consent forms; contracts; *DNA data banks; DNA fingerprinting; epidemiology; family members; *genetic information; genetic materials; genetic predisposition; *genetic research; genetic screening; human experimentation; *informed consent; investigator subject relationship; paternalism; privacy; property rights; research

subjects; *risks and benefits; social discrimination; standards; tissue banks; pedigree studies
This paper reviews the usefulness of bioethical instruments such as the informed consent principle to handle ethical and political challenges of clinical trials in genotyping and DNA-banking and discusses an informed request model as well as other contractual relations between research institutions, patients, and their families.

Schofer, Joel Martin. Violations of informed consent during war. *JAMA.* 1999 May 5; 281(17): 1657. 8 refs. BE62310.
  *biological warfare; decision making; *drugs; federal government; government regulation; human experimentation; *immunization; *informed consent; *investigational drugs; mandatory programs; *military personnel; *preventive medicine; research subjects; risks and benefits; therapeutic research; voluntary programs; *war; chemical warfare; Department of Defense; Food and Drug Administration; *Persian Gulf War; United States

Schrock, Charles R.; Botkin, Jeffrey R.; McMahon, William M., et al. Permission and confidentiality in publishing pedigrees. [Letter and response]. *JAMA.* 1998 Dec 2; 280(21): 1826–1827. 3 refs. BE61242.
  *confidentiality; *editorial policies; *family members; *genetic information; *genetic research; guidelines; *informed consent; investigator subject relationship; *patients; research subjects; medical illustration; *pedigree studies; publishing; International Committee of Medical Journal Editors

Sugarman, Jeremy; McCrory, Douglas C.; Powell, Donald, et al, comps. Empirical research on informed consent: an annotated bibliography. *Hastings Center Report.* 1999 Jan–Feb; 29(1): S1–S42. 9 fn. BE61635.
  adults; aged; competence; comprehension; consent forms; disclosure; *empirical research; human experimentation; *informed consent; patient care; *patients; recall; *research subjects; selection of subjects

Sugarman, Jeremy; McCrory, Douglas C.; Hubal, Robert C. Getting meaningful informed consent from older adults: a structured literature review of empirical research. *Journal of the American Geriatrics Society.* 1998 Apr; 46(4): 517–524. 118 refs. BE60294.
  age factors; *aged; competence; comprehension; consent forms; decision making; disclosure; education; *empirical research; evaluation studies; *human experimentation; *informed consent; literature; methods; *patient care; recall; research design; research subjects; selection of subjects; refusal to participate

Truog, Robert D.; Robinson, Walter; Randolph, Adrienne, et al. Is informed consent always necessary for randomized, controlled trials? *New England Journal of Medicine.* 1999 Mar 11; 340(10): 804–807. 22 refs. BE60950.
  alternatives; autonomy; control groups; ethical review; goals; guidelines; *human experimentation; *informed consent; patient care; patients; *presumed consent; random selection; research ethics committees; research subjects; *risks and benefits; *standards; therapeutic research; uncertainty; United States

Tuthill, Kathryn A. Human experimentation: protecting patient autonomy through informed consent. *Journal of Legal Medicine.* 1997 Jun; 18(2): 221–250. 180 fn. BE61247.
  autonomy; biological warfare; conflict of interest; consent forms; disclosure; drugs; emergency care; federal government; fraud; government regulation; guideline

---

adherence; guidelines; hospitals; *human experimentation; *informed consent; investigational drugs; investigator subject relationship; investigators; *legal aspects; legal liability; malpractice; military personnel; nontherapeutic research; paternalism; patient care; patients; physician patient relationship; physicians; public policy; research ethics committees; research subjects; risks and benefits; scientific misconduct; state government; therapeutic research; *United States

U.S. Food and Drug Administration. Accessibility to new drugs for use in military and civilian exigencies when traditional human efficacy studies are not feasible; determination under the interim rule that informed consent is not feasible for military exigencies; request for comments. *Federal Register.* 1997 Jul 31; 62(147): 40996–41001. BE59405.
    *biological warfare; federal government; *government regulation; *human experimentation; *informed consent; *investigational drugs; *military personnel; public policy; toxicity; volunteers; *war; Department of Defense; *Food and Drug Administration; *Persian Gulf War; United States

Weisstub, David N.; Arboleda–Flórez, Julio. Ethical research with the developmentally disabled. *Canadian Journal of Psychiatry.* 1997 Jun; 42(5): 492–496. 31 refs. BE59175.
    coercion; competence; comprehension; conflict of interest; deinstitutionalized persons; disclosure; guidelines; *human experimentation; *informed consent; institutionalized persons; legislation; *mentally retarded; *nontherapeutic research; patient participation; research subjects; risks and benefits; *third party consent; vulnerable populations; Canada

Wilcox, Allen J.; Taylor, Jack A.; Sharp, Richard R., et al. Genetic determinism and the overprotection of human subjects. [Letter]. *Nature Genetics.* 1999 Apr; 21(4): 362. 8 refs. BE62413.
    disclosure; epidemiology; federal government; *genetic determinism; genetic predisposition; *genetic research; guidelines; *human experimentation; *informed consent; minors; research subjects; risk; National Institutes of Health; United States

Government sets up enquiry into adequacy of research controls in North Staffordshire. [News]. *Bulletin of Medical Ethics.* 1999 Feb; No. 145: 3–4. BE61890.
    brain pathology; comparative studies; ethical review; *human experimentation; morbidity; mortality; *newborns; *parental consent; prematurity; research ethics committees; scientific misconduct; *therapeutic research; treatment outcome; *ventilators; *Great Britain; *North Staffordshire Hospital Trust; Southall, David

Privacy matters. [Editorial]. *Nature Genetics.* 1998 Jul; 19(3): 207–208. 3 refs. BE61710.
    *confidentiality; disclosure; *editorial policies; family members; *genetic information; *genetic research; genetic screening; guideline adherence; guidelines; *informed consent; investigators; privacy; *research subjects; *pedigree studies; publishing; International Committee of Medical Journal Editors; National Institutes of Health; Office for Protection from Research Risks

The perils of paediatric research. [Editorial]. *Lancet.* 1999 Feb 27; 353(9154): 685. BE61029.
    alternatives; comparative studies; control groups; ethical review; *human experimentation; intensive care units; investigators; methods; morbidity; mortality; *newborns; *parental consent; physicians; prematurity; research design; research ethics committees; *scientific misconduct; *therapeutic research; treatment outcome; *ventilators; *respiratory distress syndrome; *Great Britain; *North Staffordshire Hospital Trust; *Southall, David

HUMAN EXPERIMENTATION/MINORS

Arnold, L. Eugene; Stoff, David M.; Cook, Edwin, et al. Biologic procedures: ethical issues in research with children and adolescents. *In:* Hoagwood, Kimberly; Jensen, Peter S.; Fisher, Celia B., eds. Ethical Issues in Mental Health Research with Children and Adolescents. Mahwah, NJ: Lawrence Erlbaum Associates; 1996: 89–111. 62 refs. ISBN 0-8058-1953-3. BE62640.
    *adolescents; age factors; altruism; anesthesia; blood specimen collection; brain; *children; coercion; competence; comprehension; confidentiality; control groups; diagnosis; empirical research; genetic predisposition; *human experimentation; informed consent; *mentally ill; minority groups; nontherapeutic research; parental consent; paternalism; radiation; remuneration; research ethics committees; *risks and benefits; socioeconomic factors; therapeutic research; truth disclosure; incidental findings

Attkisson, C. Clifford; Rosenblatt, Abram; Hoagwood, Kimberly. Research ethics and human subjects protection in child mental health services research and community studies. *In:* Hoagwood, Kimberly; Jensen, Peter S.; Fisher, Celia B., eds. Ethical Issues in Mental Health Research with Children and Adolescents. Mahwah, NJ: Lawrence Erlbaum Associates; 1996: 43–57. 25 refs. ISBN 0-8058-1953-3. BE62637.
    *adolescents; behavioral research; child abuse; *children; community services; confidentiality; dangerousness; duty to warn; epidemiology; ethical review; family members; *health services research; incentives; informed consent; investigator subject relationship; investigators; mandatory reporting; mental health; *mentally ill; parental consent; professional competence; records; research ethics committees; research subjects; United States

Barr, Bernadine Courtright. Spare Children, 1900–1945: Inmates of Orphanages as Subjects of Research in Medicine and in the Social Sciences in America. Ann Arbor, MI: University Microfilms International; 1992. 341 p. Bibliography: p. 325–341. Dissertation, Ph.D. in Education, Stanford University, Jun 1992. Order No. 9302170. BE59732.
    attitudes; *behavioral research; *children; disadvantaged; emotions; epidemiology; historical aspects; *human experimentation; *infants; *institutionalized persons; intelligence; investigators; mentally retarded; normality; parent child relationship; physicians; psychology; *residential facilities; risks and benefits; selection of subjects; socioeconomic factors; diphtheria; Twentieth Century; United States

Clark, Graeme M.; Cowan, Robert S.C.; Dowell, Richard C. Ethical issues. *In:* Clark, Graeme M.; Cowan, Robert S.C.; Dowell, Richard C., eds. Cochlear Implantation for Infants and Children: Advances. San Diego, CA: Singular Publishing Group; 1997: 241–249. 9 refs. ISBN 1-56593-727-9. BE61114.
    age factors; *children; congenital disorders; empirical research; *hearing disorders; infants; informed consent; international aspects; *medical devices; parental consent; *patient care; *physically disabled; *risks and benefits; *surgery; *therapeutic research; treatment outcome; *cochlear implants; Australia; United States

Clark, Reese H. The safe introduction of new technologies into neonatal medicine. *Clinics in Perinatology.* 1996 Sep; 23(3): 519–527. 28 refs. BE60939.
    *biomedical technologies; *evaluation; health personnel; *human experimentation; mortality; *newborns; *patient care; research design; *risks and benefits; technical expertise; *technology assessment; *therapeutic research; treatment outcome; ventilators; extracorporeal membrane oxygenation; multicenter studies

---

BE = bioethics accession number   fn. = footnotes   refs. = references

DeRenzo, Evan G. A bioethicist's perspective. *In:* Hoagwood, Kimberly; Jensen, Peter S.; Fisher, Celia B., eds. Ethical Issues in Mental Health Research with Children and Adolescents. Mahwah, NJ: Lawrence Erlbaum Associates; 1996: 269-286. 57 refs. ISBN 0-8058-1953-3. BE62643.
> *adolescents; *behavior disorders; behavioral research; *children; competence; confidentiality; decision making; empirical research; ethicist's role; federal government; genetic research; genetic screening; government regulation; *human experimentation; informed consent; *mentally ill; nontherapeutic research; review committees; risks and benefits; therapeutic research; third party consent; data monitoring committees; United States

Fisher, Celia B.; Hoagwood, Kimberly; Jensen, Peter S. Casebook on ethical issues in research with children and adolescents with mental disorders. *In:* Hoagwood, Kimberly; Jensen, Peter S.; Fisher, Celia B., eds. Ethical Issues in Mental Health Research with Children and Adolescents. Mahwah, NJ: Lawrence Erlbaum Associates; 1996: 135-266. 188 refs. ISBN 0-8058-1953-3. BE62642.
> *adolescents; aggression; AIDS; alcohol abuse; *behavior disorders; *behavioral research; *case studies; child abuse; *children; competence; confidentiality; control groups; deception; drug abuse; empirical research; forensic psychiatry; genetic screening; HIV seropositivity; homosexuals; *human experimentation; incentives; infants; informed consent; *mentally ill; mentally retarded; minority groups; parent child relationship; parental consent; parents; placebos; privacy; psychoactive drugs; random selection; research design; research subjects; risks and benefits; selection of subjects; suicide; violence; war; withholding treatment; foster care

Fletcher, John C.; Richter, Gerd. Ethical issues of perinatal human gene therapy. *Journal of Maternal-Fetal Medicine.* 1996 Sep-Oct; 5(5): 232-244. 93 refs. BE60136.
> advisory committees; age factors; beneficence; *children; disclosure; embryo research; ethical review; federal government; *fetal research; *fetal therapy; *gene therapy; genetic disorders; genetic enhancement; germ cells; government regulation; growth disorders; historical aspects; hormones; *human experimentation; *infants; informed consent; justice; parents; pregnant women; prenatal diagnosis; privacy; research ethics committees; resource allocation; *risks and benefits; scientific misconduct; selection of subjects; selective abortion; stem cells; thalassemia; adenosine deaminase deficiency; immunologic deficiency syndromes; Germany; National Institutes of Health; Recombinant DNA Advisory Committee; United States

Hoagwood, Kimberly; Jensen, Peter S.; Fisher, Celia B., eds. Ethical Issues in Mental Health Research with Children and Adolescents. Mahwah, NJ: Lawrence Erlbaum Associates; 1996. 313 p. Includes references. ISBN 0-8058-1953-3. BE62634.
> *adolescents; behavior disorders; behavioral research; case studies; child abuse; *children; confidentiality; control groups; family members; family relationship; federal government; government regulation; health services research; *human experimentation; incentives; informed consent; *mentally ill; nontherapeutic research; parental consent; professional family relationship; psychoactive drugs; research design; research ethics committees; risks and benefits; selection of subjects; socioeconomic factors; therapeutic research; Department of Health and Human Services; United States

Jones, Judy. Government sets up inquiry into ventilation trial. [News]. *BMJ (British Medical Journal).* 1999 Feb 27; 318(7183): 553. BE60998.
> brain pathology; *deception; human experimentation;

mortality; *newborns; *parental consent; *prematurity; public hospitals; random selection; *therapeutic research; *ventilators; *Great Britain; North Staffordshire Hospital

Kodish, Eric D.; Pentz, Rebecca D.; Noll, Robert B., et al. Informed consent in the Childrens Cancer Group: results of preliminary research. [For the Children's Cancer Group]. *Cancer.* 1998 Jun 15; 82(12): 2467-2481. 37 refs. BE61808.
> alternatives; *attitudes; *cancer; *children; coercion; communication; comparative studies; comprehension; consent forms; decision making; *disclosure; emotions; *evaluation; *health personnel; *human experimentation; informed consent; *investigators; nurses; *parental consent; *parents; physicians; professional family relationship; psychological stress; random selection; risks and benefits; survey; *therapeutic research; questionnaires; Children's Cancer Group; United States

Kornetsky, Susan. Questions and answers regarding clinical research: an educational brochure. *IRB: A Review of Human Subjects Research.* 1998 Jul-Aug; 20(4): 12-13. BE61098.
> *children; disclosure; *hospitals; *human experimentation; informed consent; *institutional policies; parental consent; *parents; *patient education; patients' rights; research subjects; *Children's Hospital (Boston)

Leonard, Henrietta; Jensen, Peter S.; Vitiello, Benedetto, et al. Ethical issues in psychopharmacological treatment research with children and adolescents. *In:* Hoagwood, Kimberly; Jensen, Peter S.; Fisher, Celia B., eds. Ethical Issues in Mental Health Research with Children and Adolescents. Mahwah, NJ: Lawrence Erlbaum Associates; 1996: 73-88. 32 refs. ISBN 0-8058-1953-3. BE62639.
> *adolescents; behavior disorders; *children; conflict of interest; drug industry; federal government; financial support; government regulation; guidelines; *human experimentation; informed consent; investigators; *mentally ill; *psychoactive drugs; research design; research ethics committees; *risks and benefits; selection of subjects; therapeutic research; treatment outcome; Food and Drug Administration; United States

Maloney, Dennis M. Federal agency proposal will lead to more children serving as research subjects. *Human Research Report.* 1997 Oct; 12(10): 1-2. BE59954.
> *children; *government regulation; *human experimentation; informed consent; investigational drugs; pediatrics; *public policy; research ethics committees; research subjects; vulnerable populations; *Food and Drug Administration; *United States

Maloney, Dennis M. New policy on research with children is part of trend toward including more research subjects. *Human Research Report.* 1998 May; 13(5): 1-2. BE61725.
> federal government; *government regulation; *human experimentation; *minors; *public policy; research ethics committees; selection of subjects; Food and Drug Administration; *National Institutes of Health; Office for Protection from Research Risks; U.S. Congress; *United States

Mason, John Kenyon. Consent to treatment and research in children. *In: his* Medico-Legal Aspects of Reproduction and Parenthood. Second Edition. Brookfield, VT: Ashgate; 1998: 319-339. 83 fn. ISBN 1-84104-065-8. BE61070.
> adolescents; *alternative therapies; animal organs; blood transfusions; *competence; comprehension; decision making; donors; *human experimentation; *informed consent; international aspects; Jehovah's Witnesses; judicial action;

BE = bioethics accession number   fn. = footnotes   refs. = references

*legal aspects; *minors; nontherapeutic research; *organ donation; organ donors; organ transplantation; *parental consent; *parents; *patient care; religion; research subjects; risks and benefits; siblings; state interest; therapeutic research; *tissue donation; *treatment refusal; *Great Britain; United States

Osher, Trina W.; Telesford, Mary. Involving families to improve research. *In:* Hoagwood, Kimberly; Jensen, Peter S.; Fisher, Celia B., eds. Ethical Issues in Mental Health Research with Children and Adolescents. Mahwah, NJ: Lawrence Erlbaum Associates; 1996: 29–39. ISBN 0-8058-1953-3. BE62635.
  *adolescents; behavioral research; *children; confidentiality; control groups; cultural pluralism; deception; decision making; *family members; *family relationship; *human experimentation; investigators; *mentally ill; *professional family relationship; referral and consultation; research design; research ethics committees; risks and benefits; third party consent

Pandit, Jaideep J. Ethical commentaries must be based on sound science. [Letter]. *BMJ (British Medical Journal).* 1998 Dec 5; 317(7172): 1594–1595. 5 refs. BE61130.
  animal experimentation; *human experimentation; *infants; nontherapeutic research; research design; *risks and benefits

Pear, Robert. F.D.A. will require companies to test drugs on children. [News]. *New York Times.* 1998 Nov 28: A1, A10. BE60970.
  adolescents; *children; drug industry; *drugs; federal government; *government regulation; *human experimentation; infants; newborns; parental consent; risks and benefits; therapeutic research; *Food and Drug Administration; United States

Porter, Joan P. Regulatory considerations in research involving children and adolescents with mental disorders. *In:* Hoagwood, Kimberly; Jensen, Peter S.; Fisher, Celia B., eds. Ethical Issues in Mental Health Research with Children and Adolescents. Mahwah, NJ: Lawrence Erlbaum Associates; 1996: 15–28. 10 refs. ISBN 0-8058-1953-3. BE62636.
  *adolescents; *children; confidentiality; federal government; genetic research; *government regulation; *human experimentation; informed consent; *mentally ill; research ethics committees; *Department of Health and Human Services; *United States

Ross, Lainie Friedman. Children, Families, and Health Care Decision Making. New York, NY: Clarendon Press; 1998. 197 p. (Issues in biomedical ethics). Bibliography: p. 177–190. ISBN 0-19-823763-4. BE61944.
  *adolescents; advisory committees; *autonomy; case studies; *children; *competence; *decision making; deontological ethics; directed donation; dissent; family members; *family relationship; federal government; futility; goals; government regulation; guidelines; *human experimentation; legal aspects; *minors; moral development; *moral obligations; nontherapeutic research; *organ donation; *parental consent; *parents; *patient care; pediatrics; personhood; physicians; prolongation of life; quality of life; refusal to treat; rights; risk; risks and benefits; sexuality; siblings; state interest; therapeutic research; *treatment refusal; utilitarianism; *values; liberalism; needs; National Commission for the Protection of Human Subjects; United States

Sereni, Fabio; Selicorni, Angelo. General remarks on the ethical problems of pediatric research. *In:* Burgio, G. Roberto; Lantos, John D., eds. *Primum Non Nocere* Today. Second Edition. New York, NY: Elsevier; 1998: 107–112. 13 refs. 1 fn. ISBN 0-444-82923-7. BE60923.
  fetal research; fetal tissue donation; gene therapy; genetic

screening; *human experimentation; informed consent; late-onset disorders; *minors; nontherapeutic research; parental consent; pediatrics; research ethics committees; risk; technical expertise

Shah, V.S.; Al-Khannan, M.; Quinn, M.W., et al. Is venepuncture in neonatal research ethical? *Archives of Disease in Childhood. Fetal and Neonatal Edition.* 1997 Sep; 77(2): F141–F142. 6 refs. BE59222.
  attitudes; *blood specimen collection; evaluation studies; *mothers; *newborns; *nontherapeutic research; *psychological stress; *risks and benefits; survey; Great Britain

Silverman, William A. Where's the Evidence? Controversies in Modern Medicine. New York, NY: Oxford University Press; 1998. 259 p. Bibliography: p. 225–247. A collection of essays and responses originally published in the journal *Paediatric and Perinatal Epidemiology* between 1987 and 1997. ISBN 0-19-262934-4. BE59723.
  active euthanasia; allowing to die; autonomy; *bioethical issues; biomedical technologies; conflict of interest; congenital disorders; control groups; *decision making; drug industry; *evidence-based medicine; futility; hearts; historical aspects; *human experimentation; informed consent; investigators; low birth weight; *newborns; organ transplantation; pain; parents; *patient care; physicians; *prematurity; prolongation of life; quality of life; *random selection; refusal to treat; *research design; research ethics committees; resource allocation; selection for treatment; social dominance; socioeconomic factors; therapeutic research; treatment outcome; withholding treatment; *neonatology; Great Britain; United States

West, Charles; Pace, Nicholas; Niermeyer, Susan, et al. Hypoxic responses in infants. [Letters and response]. *BMJ (British Medical Journal).* 1998 Sep 5; 317(7159): 675–678. 19 refs. BE59379.
  disclosure; *human experimentation; *infants; *nontherapeutic research; parental consent; research design; *risk; *risks and benefits; intervention studies; Great Britain

West, Doe. Radiation experiments on children at the Fernald and Wrentham schools: lessons for protocols in human subject research. *Accountability in Research.* 1998 Jan; 6(1–2): 103–125. 43 refs. BE61536.
  advisory committees; *children; competence; deception; disclosure; federal government; government financing; guideline adherence; guidelines; *historical aspects; *human experimentation; incentives; informed consent; injuries; *institutionalized persons; investigators; legal guardians; mass media; *mental institutions; *mentally retarded; *nontherapeutic research; nutrition; parental consent; physicians; public hospitals; public policy; *radiation; records; regulation; *residential facilities; retrospective moral judgment; *scientific misconduct; selection of subjects; state government; stigmatization; students; therapeutic research; third party consent; universities; Advisory Committee on Human Radiation Experiments; *Fernald State School (MA); Harvard University; *Massachusetts; Massachusetts Institute of Technology; *Task Force to Review Human Subject Research (MA); *Twentieth Century; United States; *Wrentham State School (MA)

Winerup, Michael. Fighting for Jacob [experimental gene therapy for Canavan disease]. *New York Times Magazine.* 1998 Dec 6: 56–63, 78, 80, 82, 112. BE60648.
  brain; children; congenital disorders; disabled; ethical review; federal government; *gene therapy; *genetic disorders; genetic research; government regulation; *human experimentation; *infants; investigators; marital relationship; *parents; psychological stress; review committees; *surgery; terminally ill; *therapeutic research; treatment outcome;

expedited review; *Canavan disease; Karlin, Lindsay; National Institutes of Health; Seashore, Margretta; *Sontag, Jacob; Sontag, Jordanna; Sontag, Richard; United States; Yale University; Yale-New Haven Hospital

Government sets up enquiry into adequacy of research controls in North Staffordshire. [News]. *Bulletin of Medical Ethics.* 1999 Feb; No. 145: 3-4. BE61890.
    brain pathology; comparative studies; ethical review; *human experimentation; morbidity; mortality; *newborns; *parental consent; prematurity; research ethics committees; scientific misconduct; *therapeutic research; treatment outcome; *ventilators; *Great Britain; *North Staffordshire Hospital Trust; Southall, David

The perils of paediatric research. [Editorial]. *Lancet.* 1999 Feb 27; 353(9154): 685. BE61029.
    alternatives; comparative studies; control groups; ethical review; *human experimentation; intensive care units; investigators; methods; morbidity; mortality; *newborns; *parental consent; physicians; prematurity; research design; research ethics committees; *scientific misconduct; *therapeutic research; treatment outcome; *ventilators; *respiratory distress syndrome; *Great Britain; *North Staffordshire Hospital Trust; *Southall, David

HUMAN EXPERIMENTATION/REGULATION

Baird, Karen L. The new NIH and FDA medical research policies: targeting gender, promoting justice. *Journal of Health Politics, Policy and Law.* 1999 Jun; 24(3): 531-565. 45 refs. 18 fn. BE62425.
    autonomy; congenital disorders; contraception; deception; decision making; drugs; *evaluation; *federal government; *females; fetuses; *government regulation; *guidelines; historical aspects; *human experimentation; informed consent; *justice; minority groups; placebos; *policy analysis; political activity; pregnant women; *public policy; *selection of subjects; social discrimination; toxicity; women's health; women's rights; *Food and Drug Administration; General Accounting Office; *National Institutes of Health; Twentieth Century; U.S. Congress; *United States; Women's Health Initiative
    The National Institutes of Health (NIH) and Food and Drug Administration (FDA) have both recently revised their policies regarding the inclusion of women in clinical trials. Pressured by women's health activists and members of Congress, the NIH has vastly improved its policies; it now requires that women and minorities be included in clinical trials and that an analysis of gender and racial differences be performed. The FDA policy states that women and men should be included in clinical trials if both would receive the drug when marketed and that it expects a gender analysis to be performed. The FDA also lifted its 1977 ban on including women of childbearing potential in the early phases of drug studies. Analyzing these NIH and FDA policies according to a gender justice framework, I find that the NIH has moved significantly toward the institution of gender justice as it applies to medical research policies and that the FDA has taken only small steps toward this goal and lags behind the NIH.

Baker, Robert. A theory of international bioethics: multiculturalism, postmodernism, and the bankruptcy of fundamentalism. *Kennedy Institute of Ethics Journal.* 1998 Sep; 8(3): 201-231. 33 refs. 9 fn. BE60166.
    *accountability; advisory committees; animal experimentation; anthropology; autonomy; *bioethics; codes of ethics; communitarianism; compensation; consensus; *cultural pluralism; dehumanization; *ethical analysis; *ethical relativism; *ethical theory; eugenics; evaluation; *guidelines; historical aspects; *human experimentation; *human rights; informed consent; *international aspects;

investigators; *misconduct; models, theoretical; *morality; *National Socialism; philosophy; physicians; *postmodernism; principle-based ethics; privacy; public policy; *radiation; research subjects; *retrospective moral judgment; *scientific misconduct; standards; terminology; *values; *culpability; slavery; *Advisory Committee on Human Radiation Experiments; Cold War; *Germany; Macklin, Ruth; Nuremberg Code; Nuremberg Trials; Twentieth Century; United States
    The first of two articles analyzing the justifiability of international bioethical codes and of cross-cultural moral judgments reviews "moral fundamentalism," the theory that cross-cultural moral judgments and international bioethical codes are justified by certain "basic" or "fundamental" moral priniciples that are universally accepted in all cultures and eras. Initially propounded by the judges at the 1947 Nuremberg Tribunal, moral fundamentalism has become the received justification of international bioethics, and of cross-temporal and cross-cultural moral judgments. Yet today we are said to live in a multicultural and postmodern world. This article assesses the challenges that multiculturalism and postmodernism pose to fundamentalism and concludes that these challenges render the position philosophically untenable, thereby undermining the received conception of the foundations of international bioethics. The second article, which follows, offers an alternative model -- a model of negotiated moral order -- as a viable justification for international bioethics and for transcultural and transtemporal moral judgments.

Birmingham, Karen; Cimons, Marlene. Government report highlights the lack of clinical trial protection in the US. [News]. *Nature Medicine.* 1998 Jul; 4(7): 749. BE59769.
    accountability; evaluation; federal government; *government regulation; *human experimentation; *research ethics committees; vulnerable populations; multicenter studies; Department of Health and Human Services; *United States

Bonnie, Richard J. Research with cognitively impaired subjects: unfinished business in the regulation of human research. *Archives of General Psychiatry.* 1997 Feb; 54(2): 105-111. 30 refs. BE60377.
    advance directives; advisory committees; autonomy; blacks; competence; federal government; *government regulation; historical aspects; *human experimentation; informed consent; institutionalized persons; *mentally disabled; mentally ill; mentally retarded; psychoactive drugs; research ethics committees; risks and benefits; scientific misconduct; third party consent; vulnerable populations; withholding treatment; Belmont Report; Department of Health and Human Services; Department of Health, Education, and Welfare; National Commission for the Protection of Human Subjects; *United States

Butler, Declan. Europe is urged to hold back on xenotransplant clinical trials. [News]. *Nature.* 1999 Jan 28; 397(6717): 281-282. BE61568.
    *animal organs; attitudes; communicable diseases; *government regulation; *human experimentation; international aspects; investigators; *organ transplantation; public health; risk; *tissue transplantation; *Council of Europe; Europe

Butler, Declan. FDA warns on primate xenotransplants. [News]. *Nature.* 1999 Apr 15; 398(6728): 549. BE62156.
    *animal organs; communicable diseases; federal government; *government regulation; *guidelines; *human experimentation; *organ transplantation; *primates; public health; risk; transplant recipients; swine; Centers for Disease Control and Prevention; *Food and Drug Administration; *United States

---

Capron, Alexander Morgan. Ethical and human–rights issues in research on mental disorders that may affect decision–making capacity. *New England Journal of Medicine.* 1999 May 6; 340(18): 1430–1434. 20 refs. BE62029.
adults; advisory committees; competence; conflict of interest; decision making; federal government; *government regulation; *human experimentation; informed consent; investigators; *mentally ill; minors; *nontherapeutic research; patients; psychoactive drugs; research ethics committees; research institutes; research subjects; risk; scientific misconduct; *therapeutic research; third party consent; withholding treatment; national ethics committees; *National Bioethics Advisory Commission; *United States

Charrow, Robert P. Wheat, guns, and science: human research subjects and the commerce clause. *Journal of NIH Research.* 1997 Nov; 9(11): 55–57. BE59759.
federal government; government financing; *government regulation; *human experimentation; legislation; research ethics committees; research subjects; Federal Policy (Common Rule) for the Protection of Human Subjects 1991; Food and Drug Administration; *Human Research Subject Protections Act (1997 bill); U.S. Congress; *United States

Cohen, Jon. Research shutdown roils Los Angeles VA. [News]. *Science.* 1999 Apr 2; 284(5411): 18–19, 21. BE60847.
administrators; animal experimentation; *federal government; *government regulation; *human experimentation; public hospitals; research ethics committees; *scientific misconduct; Department of Veterans Affairs; Los Angeles; Office for Protection from Research Risks; United States; *West Los Angeles Veterans Affairs Medical Center

Davidson, Sylvia. New European clinical trial regulations are "unacceptable" to industry. [News]. *Nature Biotechnology.* 1998 Feb; 16(2): 127. BE62023.
confidentiality; data banks; *drug industry; ethical review; *government regulation; guidelines; *human experimentation; *international aspects; investigational drugs; professional organizations; research ethics committees; *Europe; *European Commission; *European Federation of Pharmaceutical Industries and Associations; International Conference on Harmonization; Japan; United States

Dresser, Rebecca. Time for new rules on human subjects research? *Hastings Center Report.* 1998 Nov–Dec; 28(6): 23–24. 4 fn. BE61281.
accountability; *evaluation; federal government; government financing; *government regulation; *human experimentation; organization and administration; *research ethics committees; standards; *Department of Health and Human Services; Food and Drug Administration; Office for Protection from Research Risks; *United States

Eichenwald, Kurt. Monitoring of drug tests is faulted. [News]. *New York Times.* 1998 Jun 12: A14. BE59610.
accountability; drugs; ethical review; evaluation; federal government; *government regulation; *human experimentation; medical devices; *research ethics committees; *Department of Health and Human Services; U.S. Congress; *United States

Ferenz, Leonard. Ethical considerations of federal guidelines and models of moral responsibility governing neuropharmacologic research. *In:* Hertzman, Marc; Feltner, Douglas, E., eds. The Handbook of Psychopharmacology Trials: An Overview of Scientific, Political, and Ethical Concerns. New York, NY: New York University Press; 1997: 23–45. 18 refs. ISBN 0–8147–3532–0. BE60505.
*accountability; *autonomy; behavior control; behavior disorders; beneficence; biomedical research; competence; decision making; disclosure; disease; enhancement technologies; ethical review; federal government; freedom; goals; *government regulation; health; *human experimentation; informed consent; investigators; medicine; mental health; mentally ill; moral obligations; moral policy; natural law; normality; *paternalism; *psychoactive drugs; psychotherapy; research design; research ethics committees; research subjects; risks and benefits; self regulation; treatment refusal; trust; Department of Health and Human Services; Food and Drug Administration; Patient Self–Determination Act 1990; *United States

Fox, Marie; McHale, Jean. Xenotransplantation: the ethical and legal ramifications. *Medical Law Review.* 1998 Spring; 6(1): 42–61. 101 fn. BE62170.
advisory committees; animal experimentation; *animal organs; *animal rights; communicable diseases; competence; conscience; disclosure; *government regulation; health personnel; *human experimentation; informed consent; international aspects; legal aspects; organ donation; *organ transplantation; patents; primates; *public health; *public policy; risk; *risks and benefits; scarcity; *speciesism; suffering; transgenic animals; *transplant recipients; swine; Advisory Group on the Ethics of Xenotransplantation (Great Britain); Europe; *Great Britain; Nuffield Council on Bioethics; United States; Xenotransplantation Interim Regulatory Authority (Great Britain)

Fukushima, Masanori. Clinical trials in Japan. *Nature Medicine.* 1995 Jan; 1(1): 12–13. BE59768.
advisory committees; cancer; comparative studies; conflict of interest; drug industry; financial support; *government regulation; guidelines; *human experimentation; informed consent; international aspects; *investigational drugs; research ethics committees; risks and benefits; Food and Drug Administration; *Japan; *Ministry of Health and Welfare (Japan); United States

Grady, Denise. Fraud found in analyzing breast cancer. [News]. *New York Times.* 1999 Feb 6: A13. BE61124.
*breast cancer; federal government; *fraud; *government regulation; *human experimentation; medical records; nurses; *scientific misconduct; National Cancer Institute; *National Surgical Adjuvant Breast and Bowel Project; Office of Research Integrity; Philpot, Thomas; tamoxifen

Hannay, Timo. Japan on verge of first gene therapy trial. [News]. *Nature Medicine.* 1995 Jan; 1(1): 9. BE59767.
advisory committees; *gene therapy; genetic disorders; *government regulation; *human experimentation; international aspects; universities; adenosine deaminase deficiency; *Japan; Ministry of Education, Science and Culture (Japan); Ministry of Health and Welfare (Japan); United States

Hilts, Philip J. Duke's plan ends the ban on research. [News]. *New York Times.* 1999 May 15: A10. BE61699.
federal government; *government regulation; *human experimentation; organization and administration; research ethics committees; *scientific misconduct; self regulation; *universities; *Duke University Medical Center; *Office for Protection from Research Risks; United States

Hilts, Philip J.; Stolberg, Sheryl Gay. Ethics lapses at Duke halt dozens of human experiments. [News]. *New York Times.* 1999 May 13: A26. BE61698.
disclosure; federal government; *government regulation; *human experimentation; informed consent; injuries; nontherapeutic research; organization and administration; research ethics committees; research subjects; *scientific misconduct; universities; volunteers; *Duke University Medical Center; *Office for Protection from Research Risks; United States

---

Hilts, Philip J. V.A. hospital is told to halt all research. [News]. *New York Times.* 1999 Mar 25: A25. BE60872.
    administrators; animal experimentation; *federal government; *government regulation; *human experimentation; informed consent; *mentally ill; psychoactive drugs; *public hospitals; research ethics committees; *scientific misconduct; withholding treatment; Department of Veterans Affairs; Los Angeles; Office for Protection from Research Risks; United States; *West Los Angeles Veterans Affairs Medical Center

Kennedy, Ian; Sewell, Herb. Xenotransplantation moratorium. [Letter]. *Nature Biotechnology.* 1998 Feb; 16(2): 120. 6 refs. BE62022.
    advisory committees; *animal organs; communicable diseases; *government regulation; *human experimentation; *organ transplantation; *public policy; *risks and benefits; Advisory Group on the Ethics of Xenotransplantation (Great Britain); *Great Britain

Korszniak, N. A review of the use of radio-isotopes in medicine and medical research in Australia (1947–73). *Australasian Radiology.* 1997 May; 41(2): 211–219. 49 refs. BE60230.
    advisory committees; diagnosis; disclosure; federal government; *government regulation; historical aspects; *human experimentation; informed consent; investigators; mass media; minority groups; nontherapeutic research; patient care; patients; *radiation; scientific misconduct; self regulation; state government; therapeutic research; volunteers; *Australia; Declaration of Helsinki; National Health and Medical Research Council (Australia); NHMRC Guidelines; *Papua New Guinea; Radio-isotope Standing Committee (Australia); *Twentieth Century

Lears, Louise. Research in the emergency department. *Health Care Ethics USA.* 1997 Spring; 5(2): 4–5. 7 refs. BE61723.
    critically ill; *emergency care; federal government; *government regulation; *human experimentation; informed consent; injuries; *presumed consent; risks and benefits; therapeutic research; Food and Drug Administration; United States

Macilwain, Colin. Proposed restrictions relaxed on research on mentally disabled. [News]. *Nature.* 1998 Oct 22; 395(6704): 731. BE60298.
    advisory committees; federal government; *government regulation; *human experimentation; investigators; *mentally ill; nontherapeutic research; research ethics committees; research subjects; risk; *National Bioethics Advisory Commission; *United States

McNeill, Paul M. Experimentation on human beings. *In:* Kuhse, Helga; Singer, Peter, eds. A Companion to Bioethics. Malden, MA: Blackwell; 1998: 369–378. 9 refs. ISBN 0-631-19737-0. BE59510.
    codes of ethics; *ethical review; guidelines; historical aspects; *human experimentation; *international aspects; *nontherapeutic research; professional organizations; *regulation; research ethics committees; scientific misconduct; Australia; Declaration of Helsinki; Germany; Great Britain; Japan; New Zealand; Nuremberg Code; United States

Maloney, Dennis M. Federal agency proposal will lead to more children serving as research subjects. *Human Research Report.* 1997 Oct; 12(10): 1–2. BE59954.
    *children; *government regulation; *human experimentation; informed consent; investigational drugs; pediatrics; *public policy; research ethics committees; research subjects; vulnerable populations; *Food and Drug Administration; *United States

Maloney, Dennis M. Federal investigation concludes that institutional review boards are in trouble. *Human Research Report.* 1998 Aug; 13(8): 1–2. BE61726.
    conflict of interest; education; ethical review; *evaluation; federal government; *government regulation; human experimentation; informed consent; legislation; *research ethics committees; technical expertise; Department of Health and Human Services; National Institutes of Health; *U.S. Congress; *United States

Maloney, Dennis M. First federal agency to now require treatment for injured research subjects. [News]. *Human Research Report.* 1998 Apr; 13(4): 1–2. BE59956.
    *compensation; contracts; emergency care; employment; federal government; *government regulation; *human experimentation; *injuries; patient care; *research subjects; *Department of Veterans Affairs; *United States

Maloney, Dennis M. New human subject regulations would change certain IRB reviews. [News]. *Human Research Report.* 1998 Jul; 13(7): 1–2. BE59800.
    federal government; *government regulation; *human experimentation; informed consent; *pregnant women; research ethics committees; selection of subjects; *Department of Health and Human Services; *United States

Maloney, Dennis M. New policy on research with children is part of trend toward including more research subjects. *Human Research Report.* 1998 May; 13(5): 1–2. BE61725.
    federal government; *government regulation; *human experimentation; *minors; *public policy; research ethics committees; selection of subjects; Food and Drug Administration; *National Institutes of Health; Office for Protection from Research Risks; U.S. Congress; *United States

Maloney, Dennis M. Proposal on waiver of informed consent poses major issues for research ethics. *Human Research Report.* 1997 Sep; 12(9): 1–3. BE59953.
    disclosure; federal government; *government regulation; *human experimentation; *informed consent; *investigational drugs; *military personnel; patient compliance; research ethics committees; research subjects; risks and benefits; Department of Defense; *Food and Drug Administration; *United States

Maloney, Dennis M. Report says institutional review boards are conducting inadequate reviews. *Human Research Report.* 1998 Sep; 13(9): 1–2. BE61727.
    disclosure; economics; *ethical review; *evaluation; federal government; *government regulation; human experimentation; informed consent; *research ethics committees; time factors; Department of Health and Human Services; *United States

Marshall, Eliot. Panel pulls back report after NIH critique. [News]. *Science.* 1998 Oct 30; 282(5390): 857,859. BE61967.
    advisory committees; competence; dissent; ethical review; federal government; *government regulation; guidelines; *human experimentation; informed consent; investigators; *mentally ill; nontherapeutic research; *public policy; research subjects; risk; selection of subjects; *National Bioethics Advisory Commission; *National Institutes of Health; *United States

Marshall, Eliot. Panel tightens rules on mental disorders. [News]. *Science.* 1998 Nov 27; 282(5394): 1617. BE60302.
    advisory committees; attitudes; competence; federal government; *government regulation; *human experimentation; informed consent; investigators; *mentally ill; nontherapeutic research; patient participation; research ethics committees; research subjects; risk; *National Bioethics Advisory Commission; *United States

---

BE = bioethics accession number   fn. = footnotes   refs. = references

Marshall, Eliot. Shutdown of research at Duke sends a message. [News]. *Science.* 1999 May 21; 284(5418): 1246. BE61773.
  administrators; federal government; government financing; *government regulation; hospitals; *human experimentation; research ethics committees; *scientific misconduct; universities; *Duke University Medical Center; *Office for Protection from Research Risks; United States

Marwick, Charles. Protecting subjects of clinical research. [News]. *JAMA.* 1999 Aug 11; 282(6): 516–517. BE62514.
  advisory committees; federal government; *government regulation; *human experimentation; National Bioethics Advisory Commission; *Office for Protection from Research Risks; *United States

Michels, Robert. Are research ethics bad for our mental health? *New England Journal of Medicine.* 1999 May 6; 340(18): 1427–1430. 20 refs. BE62028.
  advisory committees; committee membership; competence; decision making; *federal government; *government regulation; *human experimentation; informed consent; investigators; *mentally ill; moral obligations; patient advocacy; placebos; psychoactive drugs; *public policy; research ethics committees; research subjects; therapeutic research; third party consent; withholding treatment; *National Bioethics Advisory Commission; *United States

Miller, Michelle D. The informed–consent policy of the International Conference on Harmonization of Technical Requirements for Registration of Pharmaceuticals for Human Use: knowledge is the best medicine. [Note]. *Cornell International Law Journal.* 1997; 30(1): 203–244. 318 fn. BE61493.
  autonomy; consensus; *cultural pluralism; disclosure; drug industry; *drugs; federal government; *government regulation; *guidelines; historical aspects; *human experimentation; *informed consent; injuries; *international aspects; nontherapeutic research; paternalism; public participation; research subjects; risks and benefits; scientific misconduct; *standards; therapeutic research; negotiation; Europe; *European Union; *Food and Drug Administration; *International Conference on Harmonization; *Japan; Twentieth Century; *United States

Mitchell, Peter. Human xenotransplantation trials may be licensed in the UK. [News]. *Lancet.* 1998 Aug 8; 352(9126): 464. BE60268.
  *animal organs; *government regulation; *human experimentation; *organ transplantation; transplant recipients; *Department of Health (Great Britain); *Great Britain; *Xenotransplantation Interim Regulatory Authority (Great Britain)

Moreno, Jonathan; Caplan, Arthur L.; Wolpe, Paul Root; Project on Informed Consent, Human Research Ethics Group (University of Pennsylvania Health System, Center for Bioethics). Updating protections for human subjects involved in research. *JAMA.* 1998 Dec 9; 280(22): 1951–1958. 36 refs. BE59581.
  advance directives; advisory committees; biomedical research; children; committee membership; compensation; competence; conflict of interest; consent forms; dementia; emergency care; *ethical review; *evaluation; federal government; *females; financial support; *government regulation; *guidelines; *human experimentation; information dissemination; informed consent; injuries; investigational drugs; investigators; minority groups; nontherapeutic research; organization and administration; private sector; property rights; *public policy; public sector; research ethics committees; research subjects; risks and benefits; selection of subjects; state government; students; therapeutic research; third party consent; vulnerable populations; multicenter studies; national ethics committees;

Food and Drug Administration; Human Research Ethics Group; National Bioethics Advisory Commission; Office for Protection from Research Risks; *United States

For decades, all federally funded research involving human subjects has been subject to regulations that require the informed consent of the subject and oversight by the local institution. These regulations last underwent major revision in 1981 and have remained unchanged despite significant changes in the nature of clinical science, the financial sources of research support, and the institutional environment in which clinical research is conducted. In the intervening years, doubt has evolved as to whether the regulations currently in place adequately protect the welfare and rights of research subjects in today's clinical research environment and whether the costs, in terms of time, bureaucracy, and delay, are justified by the level of protection afforded. The Human Research Ethics Group, administered by the Center for Bioethics at the University of Pennsylvania Health System, extensively reviewed the status of existing human subjects protections with the aim of making recommendations to improve and reform the regulations. Here, we present recommendations constituting a consensus of the group members for reform in 3 key areas: protecting subject populations with special needs and vulnerabilities, oversight by institutional review boards, and regulatory policy.

Moreno, Jonathan D. IRBs under the microscope. *Kennedy Institute of Ethics Journal.* 1998 Sep; 8(3): 329–337. 7 refs. BE60170.
  accountability; advisory committees; conflict of interest; education; *ethical review; *evaluation; federal government; *government regulation; guidelines; *human experimentation; investigators; mentally disabled; organization and administration; *research ethics committees; scientific misconduct; selection of subjects; state government; statistics; volunteers; vulnerable populations; Department of Health and Human Services; Maryland; National Bioethics Advisory Commission; National Institutes of Health; New York; U.S. Congress; *United States

Morgan, Frank. Babe the magnificent organ donor? The perils and promises surrounding xenotransplantation. [Comment]. *Journal of Contemporary Health Law and Policy.* 1997 Fall; 14(1): 127–160. 260 fn. BE60879.
  *animal organs; animal rights; body parts and fluids; bone marrow; communicable diseases; comparative studies; federal government; *government regulation; *guidelines; *human experimentation; informed consent; legal aspects; *organ transplantation; presumed consent; primates; public health; *public policy; research ethics committees; *risks and benefits; scarcity; tissue transplantation; transgenic animals; transplant recipients; swine; Department of Health and Human Services; *Great Britain; Institute of Medicine; National Organ Transplant Act 1984; Nuffield Council on Bioethics; Public Health Service; *United States

National Bioethics Advisory Commission. Research Involving Persons with Mental Disorders That May Affect Decisionmaking Capacity. Volume I: Report and Recommendations of the National Bioethics Advisory Commission. Rockville, MD: The Commission; 1998 Dec. 88 p. 284 fn. BE60861.
  advance directives; advisory committees; committee membership; *competence; *ethical review; family members; federal government; government regulation; *guidelines; *human experimentation; informed consent; investigators; *mentally ill; nontherapeutic research; *organizational policies; policy analysis; *public policy; research design; research ethics committees; research subjects; review; risks and benefits; third party consent; withholding treatment; *National Bioethics Advisory Commission; United States

---

BE = bioethics accession number   fn. = footnotes   refs. = references

Nease, Donald E.; Doukas, David J. Research privacy or freedom of information? [News]. *Hastings Center Report.* 1999 May–Jun; 29(3): 47. BE61415.
> biomedical research; *confidentiality; disclosure; federal government; freedom; government financing; *government regulation; *human experimentation; *information dissemination; informed consent; legislation; *research subjects; Freedom of Information Act; *United States

Nicholson, Richard H. Unity in diversity. *Hastings Center Report.* 1999 Jan–Feb; 29(1): 6. 1 ref. BE61629.
> *ethical review; evaluation; government financing; *government regulation; *human experimentation; *international aspects; investigators; private sector; *research ethics committees; scientific misconduct; standards; *Europe; *Great Britain; *United States

Nightingale, Stuart L. Categories of research eligible for expedited review by IRBs. [News]. *JAMA.* 1999 Jan 6; 281(1): 27. BE61100.
> *ethical review; federal government; *government regulation; *human experimentation; informed consent; *research ethics committees; *expedited review; *Food and Drug Administration; *United States

Office for Protection from Research Risks Review Panel. Report to the Advisory Committee to the Director, NIH. The Panel [online]. Downloaded from Internet Web site: http://www.nih.gov/grants/oprr/references/060399b.html on 7 Jun 1999; 1999 Jun 3. 16 p. BE60825.
> advisory committees; *animal experimentation; conflict of interest; ethical review; evaluation; *federal government; financial support; government financing; *government regulation; *human experimentation; *organization and administration; private sector; multicenter studies; *Department of Health and Human Services; *National Institutes of Health; *Office for Protection from Research Risks; *United States

Pear, Robert. F.D.A. will require companies to test drugs on children. [News]. *New York Times.* 1998 Nov 28: A1, A10. BE60970.
> adolescents; *children; drug industry; *drugs; federal government; *government regulation; *human experimentation; infants; newborns; parental consent; risks and benefits; therapeutic research; *Food and Drug Administration; United States

Peart, Nicola; Moore, Andrew. Compensation for injuries suffered by participants in commercially sponsored clinical trials in New Zealand. *Medical Law Review.* 1997 Spring; 5(1): 1–21. 51 fn. BE60003.
> *compensation; control groups; disclosure; *drug industry; drugs; *financial support; *guidelines; *human experimentation; *injuries; *legal aspects; medical errors; patients; research ethics committees; *research subjects; volunteers; Accident, Rehabilitation Compensation Insurance Act 1993 (New Zealand); *New Zealand; *RMI (Research Medicines Industry) Guidelines

Porter, Joan P. Regulatory considerations in research involving children and adolescents with mental disorders. *In:* Hoagwood, Kimberly; Jensen, Peter S.; Fisher, Celia B., eds. Ethical Issues in Mental Health Research with Children and Adolescents. Mahwah, NJ: Lawrence Erlbaum Associates; 1996: 15–28. 10 refs. ISBN 0-8058-1953-3. BE62636.
> *adolescents; *children; confidentiality; federal government; genetic research; *government regulation; *human experimentation; informed consent; *mentally ill; research ethics committees; *Department of Health and Human Services; *United States

Rose, Joanna; Nilsson, Annika. Sweden considers more oversight of research. [News]. *Science.* 1999 Mar 19; 283(5409): 1829. BE62081.
> behavioral research; ethical review; females; financial support; *government regulation; *human experimentation; investigators; peer review; *public policy; research ethics committees; scientific misconduct; *Sweden

Rothenberg, Karen H. Gender matters: implications for clinical research and women's health care. *Houston Law Review.* 1996 Symposium; 32(5): 1201–1272. 452 fn. BE59798.
> autonomy; biomedical research; communication; confidentiality; constitutional law; decision making; drugs; equal protection; federal government; *females; fetuses; government financing; *government regulation; *human experimentation; justice; legal liability; legal rights; males; physician patient relationship; pregnant women; prenatal injuries; *public policy; reproduction; *selection of subjects; *social discrimination; spousal consent; spousal notification; state government; Supreme Court decisions; torts; women's health; DHHS Guidelines; Food and Drug Administration; International Union, UAW v. Johnson Controls, Inc.; National Institutes of Health; *United States

Spurgeon, David. Canadian research councils publish joint code on ethics. [News]. *Nature.* 1998 Oct 1; 395(6701): 420. BE60808.
> advisory committees; *behavioral research; *guidelines; *human experimentation; interdisciplinary communication; *regulation; research ethics committees; *Canada; *Code of Conduct for Research involving Humans; *Medical Research Council of Canada; *Natural Sciences and Engineering Research Council (Canada); *Social Sciences and Humanities Research Council (Canada)

Stolberg, Sheryl Gay. New rules will force doctors to disclose ties to drug industry. [News]. *New York Times.* 1998 Feb 3: A12. BE59669.
> *biomedical research; *conflict of interest; *disclosure; *drug industry; *drugs; federal government; financial support; *government regulation; *incentives; *investigators; *mandatory reporting; medical devices; *physicians; *therapeutic research; *Food and Drug Administration; United States

Tunisia. Decree No. 93–1155 of 17 May 1993 promulgating the Code of Medical Ethics. (*Journal Official de la Republique Tunisienne,* 28 May and 1 Jun 1993, No. 40, p. 764–770). [Summary]. *International Digest of Health Legislation.* 1994. 45(1). 53–54. BE62695.
> codes of ethics; *human experimentation; *legal aspects; medical ethics; nontherapeutic research; physicians; therapeutic research; *Tunisia

U.S. General Accounting Office. Scientific Research: Continued Vigilance Critical to Protecting Human Subjects. Report to the Ranking Minority Member, Committee on Governmental Affairs, U.S. Senate. Washington, DC: U.S. General Accounting Office; 1996 Mar. 46 p. GAO/HEHS-96-72. BE59263.
> disclosure; drugs; federal government; *government regulation; *human experimentation; informed consent; research ethics committees; research subjects; vulnerable populations; *Department of Health and Human Services; Food and Drug Administration; National Institutes of Health; Office for Protection from Research Risks; *United States

U.S. General Accounting Office. Scientific Research: Continued Vigilance Critical to Protecting Human Subjects [Testimony: Statement of Sarah F. Jaggar before the Committee on Governmental Affairs, U.S. Senate]. Washington, DC: U.S. General Accounting

---

BE = bioethics accession number   fn. = footnotes   refs. = references

Office; 1996 Mar 12. 9 p. GAO/T-HEHS-96-102. BE59421.

> drugs; ethical review; federal government; *government regulation; *human experimentation; informed consent; research ethics committees; research subjects; scientific misconduct; vulnerable populations; Department of Health and Human Services; *Food and Drug Administration; *Office for Protection from Research Risks; *United States

U.S. National Institutes of Health. Recombinant DNA research: actions under the guidelines; notice. *Federal Register.* 1995 Apr 27; 60(81): 20726–20737. BE59544.

> *advisory committees; confidentiality; containment; *ethical review; federal government; *gene therapy; *government regulation; guidelines; *human experimentation; informed consent; organization and administration; *recombinant DNA research; *Food and Drug Administration; *National Institutes of Health; *NIH Guidelines; Office of Recombinant DNA Activities; Points to Consider: Transfer of Recombinant DNA into Human Subjects; *Recombinant DNA Advisory Committee; *United States

Verdun–Jones, Simon; Weisstub, David N. The regulation of biomedical research experimentation in Canada: developing an effective apparatus for the implementation of ethical principles in a scientific milieu. *Ottawa Law Review.* 1996–1997; 28(2): 297–341. 195 fn. BE62175.

> committee membership; ethical review; *government regulation; guidelines; *human experimentation; international aspects; investigators; *regulation; *research ethics committees; self regulation; *social control; universities; *Canada; Great Britain; Medical Research Council of Canada; National Council on Bioethics in Human Research (Canada); United States

Wadman, Meredith. Higher status for 'research risks' office? [News]. *Nature.* 1999 Feb 18; 397(6720): 550. BE60398.

> conflict of interest; federal government; government financing; *government regulation; *human experimentation; organization and administration; public policy; Department of Health and Human Services; National Institutes of Health; *Office for Protection from Research Risks; *United States

Wadman, Meredith. NIH ethics office clamps down on Duke...as basic scientists feel the pinch in LA. [News]. *Nature.* 1999 May 20; 399(6733): 190. BE61760.

> advisory committees; ethical review; federal government; government financing; *government regulation; hospitals; *human experimentation; investigators; organization and administration; research ethics committees; *scientific misconduct; universities; Department of Veterans Affairs; *Duke University Medical Center; National Bioethics Advisory Commission; National Institutes of Health; *Office for Protection from Research Risks; *United States; *West Los Angeles Veterans Affairs Medical Center

Weiss, Rick. Fertility innovation or exploitation? *Washington Post.* 1998 Feb 9: A1, A12. BE59625.

> biomedical research; cancer; cryopreservation; disclosure; ethical review; females; government regulation; health facilities; *human experimentation; in vitro fertilization; *infertility; informed consent; laboratories; ovum; *private sector; *regulation; *reproductive technologies; research ethics committees; risks and benefits; *self regulation; standards; state government; ovaries; United States

A suitable case for treatment. [Editorial]. *Nature.* 1999 May 20; 399(6733): 183. BE61758.

> government financing; *government regulation; *human experimentation; research ethics committees; *scientific misconduct; universities; *Duke University Medical Center; *Office for Protection from Research Risks; United States

Hospital failed on human research policy. [News]. *Science.* 1998 Nov 6; 282(5391): 1035. BE59660.

> consent forms; ethical review; federal government; government financing; *government regulation; *hospitals; *human experimentation; institutional policies; investigators; organization and administration; punishment; *research ethics committees; scientific misconduct; Chicago; Department of Health and Human Services; Office for Protection from Research Risks; *Rush–Presbyterian–St. Luke's Medical Center (Chicago)

International Conference on Harmonisation of Technical Requirements for Registration of Pharmaceuticals for Human Use (ICH) adopts Consolidated Guideline on Good Clinical Practice in the Conduct of Clinical Trials on Medicinal Products for Human Use. [Introduction and Sections 2 and 3 of the Consolidated Guideline]. *International Digest of Health Legislation.* 1997; 48(2): 231–234. BE59597.

> committee membership; *drugs; ethical review; *government regulation; *human experimentation; informed consent; *international aspects; *practice guidelines; records; remuneration; research ethics committees; research subjects; risks and benefits; *standards; European Union; *International Conference on Harmonization; Japan; United States

Pig in the middle: a moratorium on clinical trials of animal transplantation is justified. [Editorial]. *Nature.* 1999 Jan 28; 397(6717): 279. BE61567.

> *animal organs; communicable diseases; *government regulation; *human experimentation; international aspects; *organ transplantation; public health; risk; transplant recipients; swine; *Council of Europe; Europe

When mental patients are at risk. [Editorial]. *New York Times.* 1999 Mar 31: A24. BE60909.

> *federal government; *government regulation; *human experimentation; *mentally ill; psychoactive drugs; public hospitals; schizophrenia; *scientific misconduct; withholding treatment; Department of Veterans Affairs; Los Angeles; United States; West Los Angeles Veterans Affairs Medical Center

HUMAN EXPERIMENTATION/RESEARCH DESIGN

Achrekar, Abinash; Gupta, Rajesh; Pichayangkura, Chart, et al. Informed consent for a clinical trial in Thailand. [Letter and responses]. *New England Journal of Medicine.* 1998 Oct 29; 339(18): 1331–1332. 3 refs. BE60149.

> AIDS; audiovisual aids; *communication; *comprehension; *consent forms; control groups; *developing countries; disclosure; drugs; ethical review; *HIV seropositivity; *human experimentation; *informed consent; *newborns; *placebos; *pregnant women; preventive medicine; random selection; *research design; research subjects; terminology; therapeutic research; AZT; Ministry of Public Health (Thailand); *Thailand

Alves, Wayne A.; Macciocchi, Stephen N. Ethical considerations in clinical neuroscience: current concepts in neuroclinical trials. *Stroke.* 1996 Oct; 27(10): 1903–1909. 44 refs. BE60623.

> *ethical review; federal government; government regulation; *human experimentation; *informed consent; methods; placebos; random selection; *research design; research ethics committees; risks and benefits; therapeutic research; third party consent; deferred consent; *neurosciences; Food and Drug Administration; United States

Annas, George J.; Grodin, Michael A. Human rights and maternal-fetal HIV transmission prevention trials

---

in Africa. *American Journal of Public Health*. 1998 Apr; 88(4): 560–563. 17 refs. BE60130.

AIDS; comprehension; *control groups; *developing countries; disadvantaged; drugs; economics; ethical relativism; health care delivery; *HIV seropositivity; *human experimentation; *human rights; informed consent; *international aspects; justice; *moral policy; *newborns; patient care; *placebos; *pregnant women; preventive medicine; public health; *public policy; *research design; research subjects; resource allocation; socioeconomic factors; therapeutic research; Africa; AZT; Centers for Disease Control and Prevention; National Institutes of Health; Thailand; United Nations; United States; Universal Declaration of Human Rights

The human rights issues raised by the conduct of maternal–fetal human immunodeficiency virus transmission trials in Africa are not unique to either acquired immunodeficiency syndrome or Africa, but public discussion of these trials presents an opportunity for the United States and other wealthy nations to take the rights and welfare of impoverished populations seriously. The central issue at stake when developed countries perform research on subjects in developing countries is exploitation. The only way to prevent exploitation of a research population is to insist not only that informed consent be obtained but also that, should an intervention be proven beneficial, the intervention will be delivered to the impoverished population. Human rights are universal and cannot be compromised solely on the basis of beliefs or practices of any one country or group. The challenge to the developed countries is to implement programs to improve the health of the people in developing countries both by improving public health infrastructure and by delivering effective drugs and vaccines to the people.

Aoki, Eiko; Watanabe, Toru. Patients' concerns about clinical trials in Japan. [Letter and response]. *Lancet*. 1999 Mar 20; 353(9157): 1019–1020. 7 refs. BE62154.

*breast cancer; comparative studies; control groups; disclosure; drugs; ethical review; *human experimentation; *informed consent; peer review; *research design; therapeutic research; *Japan; *National Surgical Adjuvant Study of Breast Cancer (Japan)

Ashcroft, Richard. Equipoise, knowledge and ethics in clinical research and practice. *Bioethics*. 1999 Jul; 13(3–4): 314–326. 26 fn. BE61882.

decision analysis; *decision making; *human experimentation; patient participation; physicians; random selection; *research design; research subjects; risks and benefits; *uncertainty; values

It is widely maintained that a clinical trial is ethical only if some form of equipoise between the treatments being compared obtains. To be in equipoise between two treatments A and B is to be cognitively indifferent between the statement 'A is strictly more effective than B' and its negation. It is natural to claim that equipoise regarding A and B is necessary for randomised assignment to treatments A and B to be beneficent and non–maleficent and is sufficient for such an assignment to be fair. Cashing this out precisely is difficult, and various forms of equipoise have been discussed which consider whose equipoise is relevant to the decision. This is to make judgement of equipoise something to be managed socially, while its prima facie significance is supposedly cognitive. Recent reconstructions of equipoise–like concepts in epistemology give clues about how to understand equipoise cognitively. In this paper I examine some of this work and discuss how successful it has been. I suggest that while this work is promising, it still has far to go, and that while equipoise remains the best theory we have of the cognitive justification

for clinical trials, it is nonetheless incoherent.

Avins, Andrew L. Can unequal be more fair? Ethics, subject allocation, and randomised clinical trials. *Journal of Medical Ethics*. 1998 Dec; 24(6): 401–408. 50 refs. BE60790.

decision making; *human experimentation; *methods; placebos; *random selection; *research design; selection of subjects; statistics; therapeutic research

Randomised clinical trials provide the most valid means of establishing the efficacy of clinical therapeutics. Ethical standards dictate that patients and clinicians should not consent to randomisation unless there is uncertainty about whether any of the treatment options is superior to the others ("equipoise"). However, true equipoise is rarely present; most randomised trials, therefore, present challenging ethical dilemmas. Minimising the tension between science and ethics is an obligation of investigators and clinicians. This article briefly reviews several techniques for addressing this issue and suggests that unbalanced randomisation, a technique rarely employed in current clinical trial practice, may be useful for enhancing the ethical design of human experimentation.

Bayer, Ronald. The debate over maternal–fetal HIV transmission prevention trials in Africa, Asia, and the Caribbean: racist exploitation or exploitation of racism? *American Journal of Public Health*. 1998 Apr; 88(4): 567–570. 9 refs. BE60132.

AIDS; *control groups; *developing countries; disadvantaged; drugs; ethical relativism; ethical review; financial support; guidelines; *HIV seropositivity; *human experimentation; international aspects; justice; *moral policy; *newborns; patient care; *placebos; *pregnant women; prevalence; preventive medicine; random selection; *research design; research subjects; resource allocation; risks and benefits; *social discrimination; socioeconomic factors; standards; therapeutic research; vulnerable populations; Africa; Asia; AZT; Caribbean Region; Centers for Disease Control and Prevention; Council for International Organizations of Medical Sciences; Declaration of Helsinki; Denmark; France; National Institutes of Health; South Africa; United Nations; United States

Benatar, Solomon R. Imperialism, research ethics, and global health. [Editorial]. *Journal of Medical Ethics*. 1998 Aug; 24(4): 221–222. 14 refs. BE60783.

control groups; *developing countries; drugs; ethical relativism; government financing; health; HIV seropositivity; *human experimentation; informed consent; *international aspects; investigators; newborns; pregnant women; *research design; research subjects; resource allocation; risks and benefits; scientific misconduct; syphilis; Angell, Marcia; AZT; Declaration of Helsinki; Tuskegee Syphilis Study; United States

Cohen, Peter J. The placebo is not dead: three historical vignettes. *IRB: A Review of Human Subjects Research*. 1998 Mar–Jun; 20(2–3): 6–8. 10 refs. BE59993.

drugs; heart diseases; historical aspects; *human experimentation; newborns; *placebos; prematurity; *research design; risks and benefits; surgery; cerebrovascular disorders; eye diseases; sham surgery

Collins, Harry; Pinch, Trevor. ACTing UP: AIDS cures and lay expertise. *In: their* The Golem at Large: What You Should Know About Technology. New York, NY: Cambridge University Press; 1998: 126–150. ISBN 0–521–55141–2. BE61681.

*AIDS; biomedical research; decision making; *drugs; federal government; government regulation; HIV seropositivity; *homosexuals; *human experimentation; investigator subject relationship; patient care; *patient

---

BE = bioethics accession number   fn. = footnotes   refs. = references

participation; physician patient relationship; placebos; *political activity; *public participation; *research design; research subjects; technical expertise; therapeutic research; *ACT UP; Food and Drug Administration; New York City; San Francisco; United States

Crigger, Bette-Jane. The battle over babies: international research in perinatal HIV transmission. *IRB: A Review of Human Subjects Research.* 1998 Jul–Aug; 20(4): 13–15. 8 refs. BE61099.
  AIDS; *control groups; *developing countries; *drugs; ethical review; guidelines; health care delivery; *HIV seropositivity; *human experimentation; international aspects; moral policy; *newborns; *placebos; *pregnant women; preventive medicine; public policy; *research design; research subjects; risks and benefits; socioeconomic factors; therapeutic research; vulnerable populations; Africa; Asia; AZT; Centers for Disease Control and Prevention; Council for International Organizations of Medical Sciences; Declaration of Helsinki; National Institutes of Health; United Nations; United States; World Health Organization

Crouch, Robert A.; Arras, John D. AZT trials and tribulations. *Hastings Center Report.* 1998 Nov–Dec; 28(6): 26–34. 32 fn. BE61283.
  control groups; *developing countries; *drugs; *economics; financial support; guidelines; health care; *HIV seropositivity; *human experimentation; indigents; *international aspects; investigators; justice; moral obligations; motivation; newborns; *placebos; *pregnant women; *preventive medicine; public policy; *research design; research subjects; resource allocation; rights; *therapeutic research; Africa; *AZT; Centers for Disease Control and Prevention; Thailand; United States

del Rio, Carlos. Is ethical research feasible in developed and developing countries? *Bioethics.* 1998 Oct; 12(4): 328–330. 5 refs. Commentary on D.B. Resnik, "The ethics of HIV research in developing nations," p. 286–306. BE62281.
  advisory committees; AIDS; control groups; *developing countries; drugs; economics; guidelines; health care delivery; *HIV seropositivity; *human experimentation; informed consent; *international aspects; moral policy; newborns; non-Western World; placebos; pregnant women; preventive medicine; public participation; public policy; *research design; research subjects; therapeutic research; Western World; AZT; Council for International Organizations of Medical Sciences; World Health Organization

Desvarieux, Moïse; Turner, Marie T.; Whalen, Christopher C., et al. Questions about a placebo-controlled trial of preventive therapy for tuberculosis in HIV-infected Ugandans. [Letters and responses]. *New England Journal of Medicine.* 1998 Mar 19; 338(12): 841–843. 11 refs. BE59438.
  communicable diseases; control groups; *developing countries; drugs; historical aspects; *HIV seropositivity; *human experimentation; informed consent; international aspects; *placebos; preventive medicine; *random selection; research design; research ethics committees; scientific misconduct; therapeutic research; *tuberculosis; withholding treatment; Case Western Reserve University; Haiti; Tuskegee Syphilis Study; *Uganda; United States

de Zoysa, Isabelle; Elias, Christopher J.; Bentley, Margaret E. Ethical challenges in efficacy trials of vaginal microbicides for HIV prevention. *American Journal of Public Health.* 1998 Apr; 88(4): 571–575. 48 refs. BE60133.
  AIDS; AIDS serodiagnosis; community services; control groups; counseling; decision making; *developing countries; *disadvantaged; *drugs; ethical review; *females; guidelines; health education; health promotion; health services research; *HIV seropositivity; *human experimentation; investigators;

justice; *moral policy; *preventive medicine; public participation; *research design; research subjects; resource allocation; *risks and benefits; sexuality; *sexually transmitted diseases; women's health services; *condoms; prostitution

This paper discusses some of the ethical challenges raised by advanced clinical trials designed to assess the safety and efficacy of vaginal microbicides in protecting women from HIV infection. The ethical principles that guide clinical research involving human subjects require that all participants in such trials be provided available measures known to reduce the risk of HIV infection. However, this will reduce the ability of the study to assess the protective effect of the test microbicide. In addition, providing extensive services to trial participants may be construed as an undue inducement if the study is being conducted among vulnerable groups such as sex workers or women from disadvantaged communities. Suggestions are provided to resolve this dilemma in the planning and implementation of HIV prevention services for trial participants.

Edi-Osagie, E.C.O.; Edi-Osagie, N.E.; Lurie, Peter, et al. Ethics and international research. [Letters and response]. *BMJ (British Medical Journal).* 1998 Feb 21; 316(7131): 625–628. 13 refs. BE59378.
  *control groups; *developing countries; drugs; guidelines; *HIV seropositivity; *human experimentation; informed consent; international aspects; newborns; *placebos; *pregnant women; random selection; *research design; risks and benefits; socioeconomic factors; *Africa; AZT; Thailand; United States

Edwards, Sarah J.L.; Braunholtz, David A.; Lilford, Richard J., et al. Ethical issues in the design and conduct of cluster randomised controlled trials. *BMJ (British Medical Journal).* 1999 May 22; 318(7195): 1407–1409. 5 refs. BE61394.
  control groups; health services research; *human experimentation; *informed consent; *random selection; *research design; *third party consent; Great Britain

In most randomised controlled trials, individual patients are randomised to a treatment or control group, but sometimes this is undesirable or even impossible and groups (clusters) of people may be randomised instead. These are called cluster randomised controlled trials, and although they have been around for a long time, the need for them is likely to increase in line with growing concern to evaluate the delivery of health services, public education, and policy on social care.

Edwards, Sarah J.L.; Lilford, R.J.; Hewison, J. The ethics of randomised controlled trials from the perspectives of patients, the public, and healthcare professionals. *BMJ (British Medical Journal).* 1998 Oct 31; 317(7167): 1209–1212. 47 refs. BE60834.
  *attitudes; *comprehension; disclosure; *empirical research; *human experimentation; *informed consent; international aspects; motivation; *patients; physician patient relationship; *physicians; public opinion; *random selection; *research design; *research subjects; therapeutic research

Ernst, E. Towards a risk-benefit evaluation of placebos. *Wiener Medizinische Wochenschrift.* 1998; 148(20): 461–463. 35 refs. BE61625.
  drugs; *evaluation; evidence-based medicine; human experimentation; *patient care; *placebos; research design; *risks and benefits

Faden, Ruth; Kass, Nancy. HIV research, ethics, and the developing world. [Editorial]. *American Journal of Public Health.* 1998 Apr; 88(4): 548–550. 9 refs. BE60127.

BE = bioethics accession number   fn. = footnotes   refs. = references

AIDS; coercion; common good; *control groups; *developing countries; disadvantaged; disclosure; drugs; ethical relativism; ethical review; health care delivery; *HIV seropositivity; *human experimentation; *informed consent; international aspects; *moral policy; *newborns; patient care; *placebos; *pregnant women; preventive medicine; public health; *public policy; random selection; *research design; research subjects; risks and benefits; therapeutic research; retrospective studies; Africa; AZT; United States

Fairchild, Amy L.; Bayer, Ronald. Uses and abuses of Tuskegee. *Science.* 1999 May 7; 284(5416): 919–921. 23 refs. BE61403.
   AIDS serodiagnosis; anonymous testing; *blacks; deception; developing countries; disclosure; *drug abuse; drugs; historical aspects; *HIV seropositivity; *human experimentation; indigents; informed consent; mandatory testing; medical devices; newborns; physicians; placebos; pregnant women; *preventive medicine; public policy; *research design; scientific misconduct; *social discrimination; syphilis; *trust; *vulnerable populations; withholding treatment; *needle-exchange programs; AZT; *Tuskegee Syphilis Study; Twentieth Century; *United States

Featherstone, Katie; Donovan, Jenny L. Random allocation or allocation at random? Patients' perspectives of participation in a randomised controlled trial. *BMJ (British Medical Journal).* 1998 Oct 31; 317(7167): 1177–1180. 29 refs. BE60833.
   alternatives; *comprehension; evaluation studies; *human experimentation; *informed consent; males; patients; *random selection; recall; *research design; *research subjects; survey; terminology; therapeutic research; *prostatic diseases; qualitative research; Great Britain

OBJECTIVES: To explore trial participants' understandings of randomisation. DESIGN: In this exploratory study, which used qualitative research methods, in-depth, semistructured interviews were carried out with 20 participants from the CLasP randomised controlled trial. Interviews were recorded on audio tape and fully transcribed. Data were analysed by comparing transcripts and describing emergent themes, using a grounded theory approach. SETTING: The CLasP study comprises three linked multicentre, pragmatic randomised controlled trials evaluating the effectiveness and cost effectiveness of laser therapy, standard surgery, and conservative management for men with lower urinary tract symptoms or urinary retention, or both, related to benign prostatic disease. SUBJECTS: 20 participants in the CLasP study were interviewed. Sampling was purposeful: men were included from each of the treatment arms, the two major centres, and at different points in the trial. INTERVENTIONS AND OUTCOME MEASURES: Interviews used a checklist of topics to encourage participants to describe their experiences. Narratives concerning randomisation were compared to identify common themes, retaining the context of the discussion to allow detailed interpretation. RESULTS: Most participants recalled and described aspects of randomisation, such as the involvement of chance, comparison, and concealed allocation. Many found the concept of randomisation difficult, however, and developed alternative lay explanations to make sense of their experiences. Inaccurate patient information and lay interpretations of common trial terms caused confusion. CONCLUSIONS: The provision of clear and accurate patient information is important, but this alone will not ensure consistent interpretation of concepts such as randomisation. Patients may need to discuss the purposes of randomisation in order to understand them fully enough to give truly informed consent.

García–Alonso, F.; Guallar, E.; Bakke, O.M., et al. Use and abuse of placebo in phase III trials. *European Journal Of Clinical Pharmacology.* 1998 Apr; 54(2): 101–105. 32 refs. English version of a paper published in Spanish in *Medicina Clinica,* 1997; 109: 797–801. BE61810.
   control groups; depressive disorder; drugs; *guidelines; heart diseases; *human experimentation; informed consent; *placebos; research design; therapeutic research; withholding treatment

Grady, Christine. Science in the service of healing. *Hastings Center Report.* 1998 Nov–Dec; 28(6): 34–38. 19 fn. BE61284.
   control groups; *developing countries; *drugs; economics; financial support; goals; guidelines; *HIV seropositivity; *human experimentation; *international aspects; newborns; *placebos; *pregnant women; *preventive medicine; *research design; research subjects; Africa; *AZT; Thailand; United States

Harper, William. The role of futility judgments in improperly limiting the scope of clinical research. *Journal of Medical Ethics.* 1998 Oct; 24(5): 308–313. 53 fn. BE60251.
   *biomedical research; costs and benefits; critically ill; decision making; disclosure; *futility; hospitals; *investigators; patient discharge; *patient participation; physicians; quality of life; *research design; resuscitation; statistics; *therapeutic research; *time factors; *treatment outcome; value of life; *values; withholding treatment

In medical research, the gathering and presenting of data can be limited in accordance with the futility judgments of the researchers. In that case, research results falling below the threshold of what the researchers deem beneficial would not be reported in detail. As a result, the reported information would tend to be useful only to those who share the valuational assumptions of the researchers. Should this practice become entrenched, it would reduce public confidence in the medical establishment, aggravate factionalism within the research community, and unduly influence treatment decisions. I suggest alternative frameworks for measuring survival outcomes.

Hellman, Deborah. Trial and error: can good science be bad medicine? *New Republic.* 1998 Apr 27; 218(17): 14, 16–17. BE61471.
   *developing countries; drugs; federal government; government financing; *HIV seropositivity; *human experimentation; international aspects; newborns; *placebos; *pregnant women; *random selection; *research design; therapeutic research; Africa; Asia; AZT; Centers for Disease Control and Prevention; National Institutes of Health; United States

Hellman, Deborah. Trials on trial. *Philosophy and Public Policy.* 1998 Winter–Spring; 18(1–2): 13–18. 5 refs. BE59814.
   conflict of interest; *control groups; *developing countries; *drugs; *HIV seropositivity; *human experimentation; international aspects; investigators; physicians; *placebos; *pregnant women; public health; *research design; resource allocation; standards; therapeutic research; uncertainty; *AZT; Centers for Disease Control and Prevention; National Institutes of Health; United States

Hope, Tony. Medical research needs lay involvement. [Editorial]. *Journal of Medical Ethics.* 1998 Oct; 24(5): 291–292. 7 refs. BE60249.
   *biomedical research; costs and benefits; decision making; *futility; hospitals; *investigators; mortality; patient discharge; *patient participation; *public participation;

BE = bioethics accession number   fn. = footnotes   refs. = references

quality of life; *research design; resource allocation; resuscitation; *therapeutic research; time factors; *treatment outcome; *values; Great Britain

Johannes, Laura. Sham surgery is used to test effectiveness of novel operations. [News]. *Wall Street Journal.* 1998 Dec 11: A1. BE59620.
  *brain; cancer; central nervous system diseases; control groups; federal government; financial support; *human experimentation; informed consent; pain; *placebos; *research design; risks and benefits; *surgery; tissue transplantation; treatment outcome; Parkinson disease; *sham surgery; Food and Drug Administration; National Institutes of Health; United States

Karim, Salim S. Abdool. Placebo controls in HIV perinatal transmission trials: a South African's viewpoint. *American Journal of Public Health.* 1998 Apr; 88(4): 564–566. 10 refs. BE60131.
  AIDS; alternatives; autonomy; *control groups; *drugs; economics; ethical review; government financing; health care; *HIV seropositivity; *human experimentation; informed consent; *newborns; nutrition; patient care; *placebos; *pregnant women; *prevalence; preventive medicine; *public policy; *research design; research subjects; resource allocation; sexually transmitted diseases; therapeutic research; breast feeding; AZT; *South Africa

Kempf, Judith. Collecting medical specimens in South America: a dilemma in medical ethics. *Anthropological Quarterly.* 1996 Jul; 69(3): 142–148. 19 refs. BE61212.
  American Indians; *anthropology; attitudes; *autonomy; coercion; communication; comprehension; *cultural pluralism; *developing countries; *epidemiology; *human experimentation; immunization; informed consent; international aspects; *non–Western World; *paternalism; public health; *research design; *research subjects; risk; sociology of medicine; values; *Western World; refusal to participate; Ecuador; *South America

Koepp, Robert; Miles, Stephen H.; Qizilbash, Nawab, et al. Meta–analysis of tacrine for Alzheimer disease: the influence of industry sponsors. [Letter and response]. *JAMA.* 1999 Jun 23–30; 281(24): 2287–2288. 7 refs. BE62210.
  *biomedical research; *conflict of interest; *dementia; *drug industry; *drugs; *financial support; human experimentation; *investigators; patient care; *research design; *therapeutic research; treatment outcome; *metaanalysis; Great Britain; *tacrine; United States

Lapierre, Yvon D.; Weijer, Charles. Placebo: pro and con. *NCEHR Communique (National Council on Ethics in Human Research).* 1997–1998 Winter–Spring; 8(2): 11–15. 24 refs. BE62095.
  competence; drugs; ethical review; *guidelines; *human experimentation; informed consent; *mentally ill; *placebos; psychoactive drugs; *research design; *research ethics committees; risks and benefits; Canada; Code of Conduct for Research Involving Humans; Medical Research Council of Canada

Levine, Carol. Placebos and HIV: lessons learned. *Hastings Center Report.* 1998 Nov–Dec; 28(6): 43–48. 10 fn. BE61286.
  *developing countries; drug industry; *drugs; economics; ethical review; goals; guidelines; *HIV seropositivity; *human experimentation; informed consent; *international aspects; newborns; *placebos; *pregnant women; *research design; risks and benefits; standards; withholding treatment; Africa; *AZT; Thailand; United States

Levine, Robert J.; Dennison, David K. Randomized clinical trials in periodontology: ethical considerations.

Annals of Periodontology. 1997 Mar; 2(1): 83–94. 39 refs. BE62402.
  alternatives; control groups; *dentistry; disclosure; *human experimentation; informed consent; placebos; *random selection; *research design; research subjects; risks and benefits; selection of subjects

Lie, Reidar K. Ethics of placebo–controlled trials in developing countries. *Bioethics.* 1998 Oct; 12(4): 307–311. 4 fn. Commentary on D.B. Resnik, "The ethics of HIV research in developing nations," p. 286–306. BE62278.
  AIDS; *alternatives; control groups; *developing countries; drugs; economics; *HIV seropositivity; *human experimentation; international aspects; *newborns; *placebos; *pregnant women; preventive medicine; random selection; *research design; AZT; Thailand

Love, Richard R.; Fost, Norman C. Ethical and regulatory challenges in a randomized control trial of adjuvant treatment for breast cancer in Vietnam. *Journal of Investigative Medicine.* 1997 Oct; 45(8): 423–431. 9 refs. BE62062.
  *breast cancer; cultural pluralism; *developing countries; *disclosure; *ethical relativism; ethical review; females; guidelines; *hormones; *human experimentation; *informed consent; *international aspects; non–Western World; paternalism; patient participation; peer review; *random selection; research design; *research ethics committees; standards; surgery; third party consent; Western World; ovaries; United States; *Vietnam

Lurie, Peter; Wolfe, Sidney M. Ethics of HIV trials. [Letter]. *Lancet.* 1998 Jan 17; 351(9097): 220. 5 refs. BE59384.
  *developing countries; drugs; economics; ethical relativism; *HIV seropositivity; *human experimentation; international aspects; newborns; *placebos; *pregnant women; preventive medicine; random selection; research design; time factors; AZT; Centers for Disease Control and Prevention

McCarthy, James. Placebo in research on schizophrenia. [Letter]. *Psychiatric Services.* 1998 May; 49(5): 699. 3 refs. BE61445.
  autonomy; beneficence; competence; *human experimentation; informed consent; *mentally ill; *placebos; *psychoactive drugs; *research design; research subjects; risks and benefits; *schizophrenia; withholding treatment

Markman, Maurie. Ethical issues in clinical trials in oncology. *Cleveland Clinic Journal of Medicine.* 1997 May; 64(5): 275–277. 4 refs. BE59228.
  alternatives; *cancer; control groups; disclosure; *drugs; *human experimentation; informed consent; placebos; random selection; *research design; research subjects; risks and benefits; therapeutic research; toxicity

Marquis, Don. How to resolve an ethical dilemma concerning randomized clinical trials. *New England Journal of Medicine.* 1999 Aug 26; 341(9): 691–693. 17 refs. BE62526.
  alternatives; *decision making; disclosure; evidence–based medicine; *human experimentation; *informed consent; *moral obligations; patient advocacy; *physicians; *random selection; research design; *selection of subjects; therapeutic research; uncertainty

Meldrum, Marcia. "A calculated risk": the Salk polio vaccine field trials of 1954. *BMJ (British Medical Journal).* 1998 Oct 31; 317(7167): 1233–1236. 21 refs. BE60836.
  children; *control groups; financial support; health personnel; *historical aspects; *human experimentation; *immunization; investigators; *placebos; *poliomyelitis; public health; public policy; random selection; *research

design; state government; National Foundation for Infantile Paralysis; *Salk, Jonas; *Twentieth Century; *United States

Merson, Michael H.; Simonds, R.J.; Rogers, Martha F., et al. Ethics of placebo-controlled trials of zidovudine to prevent the perinatal transmission of HIV in the Third World. [Letters and response; editor's note]. *New England Journal of Medicine.* 1998 Mar 19; 338(12): 836–841. 25 refs. BE59387.
> conflict of interest; control groups; *developing countries; *drugs; economics; *ethical relativism; federal government; *HIV seropositivity; *human experimentation; informed consent; international aspects; investigators; justice; newborns; *placebos; *pregnant women; preventive medicine; random selection; *research design; research ethics committees; risks and benefits; scientific misconduct; standards; therapeutic research; Africa; AZT; Centers for Disease Control and Prevention; Ivory Coast; Thailand; United States; World Health Organization

Miller, Franklin G.; Rosenstein, Donald L. Protocol review within the context of a research program. *IRB: A Review of Human Subjects Research.* 1998 Jul–Aug; 20(4): 7–10. 8 refs. BE61096.
> coercion; *comprehension; consent forms; *disclosure; *ethical review; *human experimentation; information dissemination; informed consent; investigators; motivation; *nontherapeutic research; patient education; *patients; physicians; placebos; *research design; *research ethics committees; research subjects; risks and benefits; *therapeutic research; volunteers

Nayfield, Susan G. Ethical and scientific considerations for chemoprevention research in cohorts at genetic risk for breast cancer. *Journal of Cellular Biochemistry. Supplement.* 1996; 25: 123–130. 42 refs. BE60247.
> *breast cancer; cancer; confidentiality; counseling; *drugs; employment; family members; females; genetic counseling; *genetic predisposition; *genetic research; *genetic screening; health insurance; *human experimentation; informed consent; organizational policies; placebos; *preventive medicine; privacy; records; *research design; research subjects; *risk; *risks and benefits; selection of subjects; social discrimination; stigmatization; ovaries; American Society of Clinical Oncology; American Society of Human Genetics; United States

Pieters, Toine. Marketing medicines through randomised controlled trials: the case of interferon. *BMJ (British Medical Journal).* 1998 Oct 31; 317(7167): 1231–1233. 22 refs. BE60835.
> biomedical research; *cancer; *drug industry; *drugs; *economics; *financial support; *human experimentation; incentives; investigators; motivation; patient care; physicians; *random selection; *research design; resource allocation; therapeutic research; treatment outcome; *interferon

Pocock, Stuart; White, Ian. Trials stopped early: too good to be true? *Lancet.* 1999 Mar 20; 353(9157): 943–944. 9 refs. BE61461.
> cancer; decision making; *human experimentation; random selection; *research design; review committees; *risks and benefits; *statistics; *therapeutic research; *time factors; uncertainty; data monitoring committees

Resnik, David B. Replies to commentaries. *Bioethics.* 1998 Oct; 12(4): 331–333. Response to commentaries by R.K. Lie, p. 307–311; by U. Schüklenk, p. 312–319; by J. Thomas, p. 320–327; and by C. Del Rio, p. 328–330 on his article, "The ethics of HIV research in developing nations," p. 286–306. BE62282.
> AIDS; *developing countries; drug industry; drugs; financial support; government financing; health care delivery; *HIV seropositivity; *human experimentation; international

aspects; justice; moral policy; *newborns; *placebos; *pregnant women; preventive medicine; public policy; *research design; socioeconomic factors; therapeutic research; AZT

Resnik, David B. The ethics of HIV research in developing nations. *Bioethics.* 1998 Oct; 12(4): 286–306. 62 fn. Commented on by R.K. Lie, p. 307–311; by U. Schüklenk, p. 312–319; by J. Thomas, p. 320–327; and by C. Del Rio, p. 328–330. BE62277.
> AIDS; beneficence; codes of ethics; control groups; *developing countries; drugs; *ethical relativism; *HIV seropositivity; *human experimentation; informed consent; international aspects; justice; metaethics; *moral policy; *newborns; non-Western World; *placebos; *pregnant women; preventive medicine; random selection; *research design; research subjects; socioeconomic factors; *standards; therapeutic research; utilitarianism; Africa; AZT; Centers for Disease Control and Prevention; Declaration of Helsinki; Dominican Republic; National Institutes of Health; Thailand; UNAIDS; World Health Organization

This paper discusses a dispute concerning the ethics of research on preventing the perinatal transmission of HIV in developing nations. Critics of this research argue that it is unethical because it denies a proven treatment to placebo-control groups. Since studies conducted in developed nations would not deny this treatment to subjects, the critics maintain that these experiments manifest a double standard for ethical research and that a single standard of ethics should apply to all research on human subjects. Proponents of the research, however, argue that these charges fail to understand the ethical complexities of research in developing nations, and that study designs can vary according to the social, economic, and scientific conditions of research. This essay explores some of the ethical issues raised by this controversial case in order to shed some light on the deeper, meta-ethical questions. The paper argues that standards of ethical research on human subjects are universal but not absolute: there are some general ethical principles that apply to all cases of human subjects research but the application of these principles must take into account factors inherent in particular situations.

Rosser, Walter W. Application of evidence from randomised controlled trials to general practice. *Lancet.* 1999 Feb 20; 353(9153): 661–664. 31 refs. BE61085.
> chronically ill; control groups; *costs and benefits; *decision making; evaluation; *evidence-based medicine; *family practice; health insurance reimbursement; health promotion; *human experimentation; international aspects; *patient care; *patient participation; physician patient relationship; *physicians; preventive medicine; primary health care; quality of life; *random selection; research design; resource allocation; *risks and benefits; *socioeconomic factors; standards; *values

Schaffner, Kenneth F. Ethical considerations in human investigation involving paradigm shifts: organ transplantation in the 1990s. *IRB: A Review of Human Subjects Research.* 1997 Nov–Dec; 19(6): 5–10. 45 refs. BE59991.
> animal organs; bone marrow; cancer; drugs; ethical review; gene therapy; *human experimentation; kidneys; livers; *organ transplantation; *research design; research ethics committees; transplant recipients; University of Pittsburgh

Schüklenk, Udo. Unethical perinatal HIV transmission trials establish bad precedent. *Bioethics.* 1998 Oct; 12(4): 312–319. 21 fn. Commentary on D.B. Resnik, "The ethics of HIV research in developing nations," p. 286–306. BE62279.
> AIDS; alternative therapies; control groups; costs and

---

benefits; *developing countries; drug industry; drugs; economics; ethical analysis; ethical review; guidelines; health care delivery; *HIV seropositivity; *human experimentation; informed consent; international aspects; *moral policy; *newborns; non-Western World; *placebos; *pregnant women; preventive medicine; *research design; research subjects; therapeutic research; Western World; Africa; Asia; AZT; Council for International Organizations of Medical Sciences; Latin America; UNAIDS

Shapiro, Arthur K.; Shapiro, Elaine. The Powerful Placebo: From Ancient Priest to Modern Physician. Baltimore, MD: Johns Hopkins University Press; 1997. 280 p. Bibliography: p. 239-272. ISBN 0-8018-5569-1. BE62149.
   alternative therapies; ancient history; attitudes; control groups; drugs; empirical research; ethicists; evaluation; fraud; *historical aspects; *human experimentation; international aspects; *patient care; patients; physicians; *placebos; psychoactive drugs; psychotherapy; random selection; *research design; review; risks and benefits; scientific misconduct; surgery; terminology; quackery; Eighteenth Century; Middle Ages; Nineteenth Century; Seventeenth Century; Twentieth Century

Silverman, William A. Where's the Evidence? Controversies in Modern Medicine. New York, NY: Oxford University Press; 1998. 259 p. Bibliography: p. 225-247. A collection of essays and responses originally published in the journal *Paediatric and Perinatal Epidemiology* between 1987 and 1997. ISBN 0-19-262934-4. BE59723.
   active euthanasia; allowing to die; autonomy; *bioethical issues; biomedical technologies; conflict of interest; congenital disorders; control groups; *decision making; drug industry; *evidence-based medicine; futility; hearts; historical aspects; *human experimentation; informed consent; investigators; low birth weight; *newborns; organ transplantation; pain; parents; *patient care; physicians; *prematurity; prolongation of life; quality of life; *random selection; refusal to treat; *research design; research ethics committees; resource allocation; selection for treatment; social dominance; socioeconomic factors; therapeutic research; treatment outcome; withholding treatment; *neonatology; Great Britain; United States

Smith, Trevor. Ethics in Medical Research: A Handbook of Good Practice. New York, NY: Cambridge University Press; 1999. 403 p. Bibliography: p. 378-390. ISBN 0-521-62619-6. BE62737.
   animal organs; children; compensation; confidentiality; critically ill; drug industry; drugs; epidemiology; ethical review; fetal research; forms; gene therapy; genetic materials; genetic research; *guidelines; *human experimentation; incentives; informed consent; injuries; international aspects; *investigators; medical records; mentally disabled; organ transplantation; *organization and administration; placebos; *professional ethics; *research design; *research ethics committees; research subjects; risks and benefits; selection of subjects; self regulation; volunteers; multicenter studies; questionnaires; Declaration of Helsinki; Great Britain; Internet

Stein, C. Michael; Pincus, Theodore. Placebo-controlled studies in rheumatoid arthritis: ethical issues. *Lancet.* 1999 Jan 30; 353(9150): 400-403. 37 refs. BE61084.
   *chronically ill; conflict of interest; *control groups; disclosure; drug industry; *drugs; *guidelines; *human experimentation; hypertension; incentives; informed consent; investigators; morbidity; patient advocacy; patient care; *placebos; *random selection; regulation; remuneration; *research design; research ethics committees; research subjects; risk; time factors; toxicity; treatment outcome; withholding treatment; *rheumatoid arthritis; Food and Drug Administration; United States

Stolberg, Sheryl Gay. Decisive moment on Parkinson's fetal-cell transplants. [News]. *New York Times.* 1999 Apr 20: F2. BE61073.
   aborted fetuses; *brain; central nervous system diseases; control groups; fetal research; fetal tissue donation; government financing; *human experimentation; physicians; *placebos; random selection; *research design; risks and benefits; *surgery; *tissue transplantation; *Parkinson disease; *sham surgery; Freed, Curt; National Institute of Neurological Disorders and Stroke; United States; University of Colorado

Stolberg, Sheryl Gay. Placebo use is suspended in overseas AIDS trials. [News]. *New York Times.* 1998 Feb 19: A16. BE59368.
   *AIDS; *developing countries; *drugs; economics; federal government; *HIV seropositivity; *human experimentation; *international aspects; *placebos; *pregnant women; *public policy; *research design; *therapeutic research; *AZT; Centers for Disease Control and Prevention; United States

Stolberg, Sheryl Gay. Sham surgery returns as a research tool. [News]. *New York Times.* 1999 Apr 25: WK 3. BE61074.
   control groups; deception; drugs; *human experimentation; *placebos; random selection; *research design; risks and benefits; *surgery; treatment outcome; *sham surgery

Susser, Mervyn. The prevention of perinatal HIV transmission in the less-developed world. [Editorial]. *American Journal of Public Health.* 1998 Apr; 88(4): 547-548. 11 refs. BE60126.
   AIDS; *control groups; *costs and benefits; *developing countries; disadvantaged; *drugs; *HIV seropositivity; *human experimentation; international aspects; *newborns; *placebos; politics; *pregnant women; preventive medicine; *public policy; *research design; *risks and benefits; therapeutic research; breast feeding; AZT; Centers for Disease Control and Prevention; *France; National Institutes of Health; Thailand; *United Nations; *United States

Thomas, Joe. Ethical challenges of HIV clinical trials in developing countries. *Bioethics.* 1998 Oct; 12(4): 320-327. 25 fn. Commentary on D.B. Resnik, "The ethics of HIV research in developing nations," p. 286-306. BE62280.
   AIDS; alternative therapies; autonomy; beneficence; conflict of interest; control groups; *developing countries; drug industry; drugs; economics; ethical review; guidelines; *HIV seropositivity; *human experimentation; human rights; international aspects; investigators; justice; moral policy; *newborns; non-Western World; placebos; *pregnant women; preventive medicine; public policy; *research design; research subjects; standards; therapeutic research; AZT; Council for International Organizations of Medical Sciences; Declaration of Helsinki; National Institutes of Health; United States

Tishler, L. Carl; Gordon, Lisa B. Ethical parameters of challenge studies inducing psychosis with ketamine. *Ethics and Behavior.* 1999; 9(3): 211-217. 32 refs. BE62082.
   disclosure; human experimentation; incentives; informed consent; mentally ill; *nontherapeutic research; normality; *psychoactive drugs; remuneration; *research design; *schizophrenia; selection of subjects; *volunteers; *challenge studies
   Researchers routinely induce psychosis in healthy volunteers via ketamine infusion to expand their knowledge of schizophrenia. We question the ethics of the nature and procedures of such studies. We also address safeguards for ethically conducting and reporting such pursuits, including recruitment, screening, available treatment, and follow-up.

BE = bioethics accession number   fn. = footnotes   refs. = references

Tramèr, Martin R.; Reynolds, D. John M.; Moore, R. Andrew, et al. When placebo controlled trials are essential and equivalence trials are inadequate. *BMJ (British Medical Journal).* 1998 Sep 26; 317(7162): 875–880. 59 refs. BE59629.
control groups; drugs; *human experimentation; *placebos; *research design; risks and benefits; ondansetron

U.S. Department of Health and Human Services. The Conduct of Clinical Trials of Maternal–Infant Transmission of HIV Supported by the United States Department of Health and Human Services in Developing Countries: A Summary of the Needs of Developing Countries, the Scientific Applications, and the Ethical Considerations Assessed by the National Institutes of Health and the Centers for Disease Control and Prevention, 1994–1997. Downloaded from Internet Web site: http://www.nih.gov/news/mathiv/mathiv.htm and http://www.nih.gov/news/mathiv/whodoc.htm (Appendix) on 6 Dec 1997; 1997 Jul. 10 p. 1 ref. Appendix: Recommendations from the Meeting on Prevention of Mother-to-Infant Transmission of HIV by Use of Antiretrovirals, Geneva, 23–25 June 1994. BE62688.
*developing countries; drugs; economics; health care; *HIV seropositivity; *human experimentation; *international aspects; *newborns; placebos; *pregnant women; *research design; standards; therapeutic research; withholding treatment; Africa; *AZT; Centers for Disease Control and Prevention; Department of Health and Human Services; National Institutes of Health; Thailand; *United States; World Health Organization

Weijer, Charles. The IRB's role in assessing the generalizability of non–NIH–funded clinical trials. *IRB: A Review of Human Subjects Research.* 1998 Mar–Jun; 20(2-3): 1–5. 19 refs. BE59992.
age factors; drug industry; *ethical review; federal government; *females; financial support; government financing; government regulation; *guidelines; *human experimentation; investigational drugs; *minority groups; nontherapeutic research; *research design; *research ethics committees; risks and benefits; *selection of subjects; therapeutic research; vulnerable populations; Food and Drug Administration; National Institutes of Health; *NIH Guidelines; United States

Welton, A.J.; Vickers, M.R.; Cooper, J.A., et al. Is recruitment more difficult with a placebo arm in randomised controlled trials? A quasirandomised, interview based study. *BMJ (British Medical Journal).* 1999 Apr 24; 318(7191): 1114–1117. 10 refs. BE62301.
altruism; *attitudes; decision making; disclosure; evaluation studies; females; hormones; *human experimentation; informed consent; motivation; *patient participation; *placebos; *random selection; *research design; *research subjects; risks and benefits; selection of subjects; *estrogen replacement therapy; *refusal to participate; Great Britain
OBJECTIVE: To investigate whether including a placebo arm in a clinical trial of hormone replacement therapy influenced women's stated willingness to participate. DESIGN: Quasirandomised, interview based study. Setting: 10 group practices in the Medical Research Council's General Practice Research Framework. PARTICIPANTS: 436 postmenopausal women aged 45-64 who had not had a hysterectomy. MAIN OUTCOME MEASURES: Stated willingness to enter a trial and reasons for the decisions made. RESULTS: Of 218 women told about the trial without a placebo arm, 85 (39%) indicated their willingness to enter compared with 65 (30%) of the 218 women told about the trial with the placebo arm (P=0.06). Part of

this difference was due to explicit reluctance to take a placebo. Altruism and personal benefit were the reasons most frequently given for wanting to take part in a trial. The reasons most frequently cited for not wanting to take part were reluctance to restart periods, not wanting to take unknown or unnecessary tablets, or not wanting to interfere with present good health. CONCLUSION: For preventive trials the inclusion of a placebo arm may reduce patients' willingness to participate.

Wendler, Dave. When should "riskier" subjects be excluded from research participation? *Kennedy Institute of Ethics Journal.* 1998 Sep; 8(3): 307–327. 9 refs. 2 fn. BE60169.
age factors; autonomy; decision making; drugs; *females; fetuses; government regulation; *guidelines; *human experimentation; international aspects; investigators; justice; kidney diseases; males; moral policy; patients; preconception injuries; *pregnant women; prenatal injuries; *research design; research ethics committees; *research subjects; rights; *risk; risks and benefits; *selection of subjects; volunteers; Australia; Great Britain; United States
The exclusion of potential subjects based on increased risks is a common practice in human subjects research. However, there are no guidelines to ensure that this practice is conducted in a systematic and fair way. This gap in the literature and regulation is addressed by a specific account of a "condition on inclusion risks" (CIR), a condition under which potential subjects should be excluded from research on the basis of increased risks. This account provides a general framework for assessing standard exclusions as well as more controversial ones such as the exclusion of pregnant women and women of childbearing potential from certain types of research.

Wilfert, Catherine M.; Ammann, Arthur; Bayer, Ronald, et al. Science, ethics, and the future of research into maternal infant transmission of HIV-1: Consensus statement. [For the Perinatal HIV Intervention Research in Developing Countries Workshop Participants]. *Lancet.* 1999 Mar 6; 353(9155): 832–835. 23 refs. BE61221.
AIDS; alternatives; childbirth; consensus; *control groups; costs and benefits; *developing countries; *drugs; *economics; *guidelines; *HIV seropositivity; *human experimentation; informed consent; international aspects; *moral policy; *mothers; *newborns; nutrition; patient care; *pregnant women; *preventive medicine; public health; quality of health care; *research design; risks and benefits; *socioeconomic factors; standards; therapeutic research; *breast feeding; *Perinatal HIV Intervention Research in Developing Countries Workshop

Zion, Deborah. Ethical considerations of clinical trials to prevent vertical transmission of HIV in developing countries. *Nature Medicine.* 1998 Jan; 4(1): 11–12. 5 refs. BE59981.
autonomy; coercion; competence; *developing countries; drugs; freedom; *HIV seropositivity; *human experimentation; informed consent; placebos; *pregnant women; *research design; research subjects; AZT

HUMAN EXPERIMENTATION/SPECIAL POPULATIONS

Achrekar, Abinash; Gupta, Rajesh; Pichayangkura, Chart, et al. Informed consent for a clinical trial in Thailand. [Letter and responses]. *New England Journal of Medicine.* 1998 Oct 29; 339(18): 1331–1332. 3 refs. BE60149.
AIDS; audiovisual aids; *communication; *comprehension; *consent forms; control groups; *developing countries; disclosure; drugs; ethical review; *HIV seropositivity;

BE = bioethics accession number   fn. = footnotes   refs. = references

*human experimentation; *informed consent; *newborns; *placebos; *pregnant women; preventive medicine; random selection; *research design; research subjects; terminology; therapeutic research; AZT; Ministry of Public Health (Thailand); *Thailand

Adshead, Gwen. Ethics in psychiatric research and practice. *Current Opinion in Psychiatry.* 1996 Sep; 9(5): 348–351. 37 refs. BE60596.
    competence; confidentiality; *human experimentation; informed consent; *mentally ill; misconduct; *patient care; physician patient relationship; *psychiatry; research ethics committees; research subjects; social discrimination

Agarwal, Manoj R.; Ferran, Jose; Ost, Katherine, et al. Ethics of 'informed consent' in dementia research — the debate continues. *International Journal of Geriatric Psychiatry.* 1996 Sep; 11(9): 801–806. 13 refs. BE59447.
    *competence; comprehension; *dementia; drugs; evaluation studies; *family members; *informed consent; risks and benefits; survey; *therapeutic research; *third party consent; questionnaires; Great Britain

Allebeck, Peter. Forensic psychiatric studies and research ethical considerations. *Nordic Journal of Psychiatry.* 1997; 51(Suppl. 39): 53–56. 6 refs. BE60622.
    autonomy; beneficence; competence; *forensic psychiatry; guidelines; *human experimentation; informed consent; international aspects; justice; *mentally disabled; random selection; remuneration; research subjects; Council for International Organizations of Medical Sciences; Declaration of Helsinki; World Health Organization

Altman, Lawrence K. Treating elderly's cancer is frustrating many experts. [News]. *New York Times.* 1998 May 20: A14. BE60469.
    age factors; *aged; *cancer; drugs; *human experimentation; international aspects; *patient care; research subjects; risks and benefits; *selection of subjects; therapeutic research; Italy; United States

Altman, Lawrence K. Who Goes First? The Story of Self-Experimentation in Medicine. With a New Preface. Berkeley, CA: University of California Press; 1998. 430 p. 602 fn. Originally published by Random House, 1987. ISBN 0–520–21281–9. BE61042.
    *autoexperimentation; famous persons; historical aspects; *human experimentation; international aspects; *investigators; motivation; *nontherapeutic research; *physicians; *research subjects; *selection of subjects; volunteers

American College of Obstetricians and Gynecologists. Committee on Ethics. Ethical considerations in research involving pregnant women. ACOG Committee Opinion No. 213, Nov 1998. *Women's Health Issues.* 1999 Jul–Aug; 9(4): 194–198. 14 refs. BE61970.
    conflict of interest; diagnosis; disclosure; ethical review; federal government; females; fetuses; government regulation; *guidelines; *human experimentation; incentives; informed consent; investigators; nontherapeutic research; obstetrics and gynecology; *organizational policies; patient care; physicians; *pregnant women; professional organizations; research design; research subjects; risks and benefits; *selection of subjects; therapeutic research; *American College of Obstetricians and Gynecologists; United States

Annas, George J.; Grodin, Michael A. Human rights and maternal–fetal HIV transmission prevention trials in Africa. *American Journal of Public Health.* 1998 Apr; 88(4): 560–563. 17 refs. BE60130.
    AIDS; comprehension; *control groups; *developing countries; disadvantaged; drugs; economics; ethical relativism; health care delivery; *HIV seropositivity;

*human experimentation; *human rights; informed consent; *international aspects; justice; *moral policy; *newborns; patient care; *placebos; *pregnant women; preventive medicine; public health; *public policy; *research design; research subjects; resource allocation; socioeconomic factors; therapeutic research; Africa; AZT; Centers for Disease Control and Prevention; National Institutes of Health; Thailand; United Nations; United States; Universal Declaration of Human Rights

The human rights issues raised by the conduct of maternal–fetal human immunodeficiency virus transmission trials in Africa are not unique to either acquired immunodeficiency syndrome or Africa, but public discussion of these trials presents an opportunity for the United States and other wealthy nations to take the rights and welfare of impoverished populations seriously. The central issue at stake when developed countries perform research on subjects in developing countries is exploitation. The only way to prevent exploitation of a research population is to insist not only that informed consent be obtained but also that, should an intervention be proven beneficial, the intervention will be delivered to the impoverished population. Human rights are universal and cannot be compromised solely on the basis of beliefs or practices of any one country or group. The challenge to the developed countries is to implement programs to improve the health of the people in developing countries both by improving public health infrastructure and by delivering effective drugs and vaccines to the people.

Arboleda–Flórez, Julio; Weisstub, David N. Ethical research with the mentally disordered. *Canadian Journal of Psychiatry.* 1997 Jun; 42(5): 485–491. 44 refs. BE59174.
    advance directives; advisory committees; autonomy; coercion; *competence; decision making; guidelines; *human experimentation; incentives; *informed consent; institutionalized persons; involuntary commitment; legal aspects; legislation; mental institutions; *mentally disabled; *nontherapeutic research; public policy; research ethics committees; research subjects; *third party consent; time factors; vulnerable populations; *Canada; Law Reform Commission of Canada; Uniform Mental Health Act 1987 (Canada); United States

Arnold, L. Eugene; Stoff, David M.; Cook, Edwin, et al. Biologic procedures: ethical issues in research with children and adolescents. *In:* Hoagwood, Kimberly; Jensen, Peter S.; Fisher, Celia B., eds. Ethical Issues in Mental Health Research with Children and Adolescents. Mahwah, NJ: Lawrence Erlbaum Associates; 1996: 89–111. 62 refs. ISBN 0–8058–1953–3. BE62640.
    *adolescents; age factors; altruism; anesthesia; blood specimen collection; brain; *children; coercion; competence; comprehension; confidentiality; control groups; diagnosis; empirical research; genetic predisposition; *human experimentation; informed consent; *mentally ill; minority groups; nontherapeutic research; parental consent; paternalism; radiation; remuneration; research ethics committees; *risks and benefits; socioeconomic factors; therapeutic research; truth disclosure; incidental findings

Attkisson, C. Clifford; Rosenblatt, Abram; Hoagwood, Kimberly. Research ethics and human subjects protection in child mental health services research and community studies. *In:* Hoagwood, Kimberly; Jensen, Peter S.; Fisher, Celia B., eds. Ethical Issues in Mental Health Research with Children and Adolescents. Mahwah, NJ: Lawrence Erlbaum Associates; 1996: 43–57. 25 refs. ISBN 0–8058–1953–3. BE62637.
    *adolescents; behavioral research; child abuse; *children; community services; confidentiality; dangerousness; duty to warn; epidemiology; ethical review; family members; *health services research; incentives; informed consent; investigator

---

BE = bioethics accession number   fn. = footnotes   refs. = references

subject relationship; investigators; mandatory reporting; mental health; *mentally ill; parental consent; professional competence; records; research ethics committees; research subjects; United States

Ayd, Frank J. Research on the decisionally impaired: overview and commentary. *Medical-Moral Newsletter.* 1998 Jan-Feb; 35(1-2): 1-8. 12 refs. BE59707.
aged; *competence; critically ill; emergency care; family members; federal government; government regulation; *human experimentation; mentally ill; minors; research subjects; *third party consent; vulnerable populations; United States

Baird, Karen L. The new NIH and FDA medical research policies: targeting gender, promoting justice. *Journal of Health Politics, Policy and Law.* 1999 Jun; 24(3): 531-565. 45 refs. 18 fn. BE62425.
autonomy; congenital disorders; contraception; deception; decision making; drugs; *evaluation; *federal government; *females; fetuses; *government regulation; *guidelines; historical aspects; *human experimentation; informed consent; *justice; minority groups; placebos; *policy analysis; political activity; pregnant women; *public policy; *selection of subjects; social discrimination; toxicity; women's health; women's rights; *Food and Drug Administration; General Accounting Office; *National Institutes of Health; Twentieth Century; U.S. Congress; *United States; Women's Health Initiative

The National Institutes of Health (NIH) and Food and Drug Administration (FDA) have both recently revised their policies regarding the inclusion of women in clinical trials. Pressured by women's health activists and members of Congress, the NIH has vastly improved its policies; it now requires that women and minorities be included in clinical trials and that an analysis of gender and racial differences be performed. The FDA policy states that women and men should be included in clinical trials if both would receive the drug when marketed and that it expects a gender analysis to be performed. The FDA also lifted its 1977 ban on including women of childbearing potential in the early phases of drug studies. Analyzing these NIH and FDA policies according to a gender justice framework, I find that the NIH has moved significantly toward the institution of gender justice as it applies to medical research policies and that the FDA has taken only small steps toward this goal and lags behind the NIH.

Bayer, Ronald. The debate over maternal-fetal HIV transmission prevention trials in Africa, Asia, and the Caribbean: racist exploitation or exploitation of racism? *American Journal of Public Health.* 1998 Apr; 88(4): 567-570. 9 refs. BE60132.
AIDS; *control groups; *developing countries; disadvantaged; drugs; ethical relativism; ethical review; financial support; guidelines; *HIV seropositivity; *human experimentation; international aspects; justice; *moral policy; *newborns; patient care; *placebos; *pregnant women; prevalence; preventive medicine; random selection; *research design; research subjects; resource allocation; risks and benefits; *social discrimination; socioeconomic factors; standards; therapeutic research; vulnerable populations; Africa; Asia; AZT; Caribbean Region; Centers for Disease Control and Prevention; Council for International Organizations of Medical Sciences; Declaration of Helsinki; Denmark; France; National Institutes of Health; South Africa; United Nations; United States

Baylis, Françoise; Downie, Jocelyn; Sherwin, Susan. Women and health research: from theory, to practice, to policy. *In:* Donchin, Anne; Purdy, Laura M., eds. Embodying Bioethics: Recent Feminist Advances. Lanham, MD: Rowman and Littlefield; 1999: 253-268.

4 fn. ISBN 0-8476-8924-7. BE61025.
contraception; *females; *feminist ethics; government regulation; *guidelines; *human experimentation; *political activity; *public policy; *selection of subjects; social discrimination; women's health; women's rights; *Canada; *Feminist Health Care Ethics Research Network; *Tri-Council Policy Statement on Ethical Conduct for Research Involving Humans

Blumenthal, Ralph; Miller, Judith. Japanese germ-war atrocities: a half-century of stonewalling the world. *New York Times.* 1999 Mar 4: A12. BE60974.
*biological warfare; dehumanization; disclosure; federal government; historical aspects; *human experimentation; investigators; military personnel; *misconduct; moral complicity; *prisoners; *public policy; records; *scientific misconduct; torture; China; *Japan; Twentieth Century; United States; *World War II

Bonnie, Richard J. Research with cognitively impaired subjects: unfinished business in the regulation of human research. *Archives of General Psychiatry.* 1997 Feb; 54(2): 105-111. 30 refs. BE60377.
advance directives; advisory committees; autonomy; blacks; competence; federal government; *government regulation; historical aspects; *human experimentation; informed consent; institutionalized persons; *mentally disabled; mentally ill; mentally retarded; psychoactive drugs; research ethics committees; risks and benefits; scientific misconduct; third party consent; vulnerable populations; withholding treatment; Belmont Report; Department of Health and Human Services; Department of Health, Education, and Welfare; National Commission for the Protection of Human Subjects; *United States

Boyce, Nell. Psychiatric guinea pigs are left in limbo. [News]. *New Scientist.* 1998 Nov 28; 160(2162): 21. BE61541.
advisory committees; competence; federal government; government regulation; guidelines; *human experimentation; informed consent; *mentally ill; nontherapeutic research; research subjects; National Bioethics Advisory Commission; United States

Cannold, Leslie. "There is no evidence to suggest...": changing the way we judge information for disclosure in the informed consent process. *Hypatia.* 1997 Spring; 12(2): 165-184. 35 refs. 4 fn. This paper is a substantial expansion and reworking of Cannold's "A question of control: the tussle over informed consent in the Melbourne trial of RU 486/PG," in *Healthsharing Women: The Newsletter of the Healthsharing Women's Health Resource Service,* 1994; 5(2): 1-2. BE61678.
abortion, induced; autonomy; *communication; comprehension; *disclosure; drugs; *females; *feminist ethics; HIV seropositivity; *human experimentation; in vitro fertilization; *informed consent; investigators; legal aspects; minority groups; pregnant women; research subjects; risk; *standards; uncertainty; *Australia; RU-486

Capron, Alexander Morgan. Ethical and human-rights issues in research on mental disorders that may affect decision-making capacity. *New England Journal of Medicine.* 1999 May 6; 340(18): 1430-1434. 20 refs. BE62029.
adults; advisory committees; competence; conflict of interest; decision making; federal government; *government regulation; *human experimentation; informed consent; investigators; *mentally ill; minors; *nontherapeutic research; patients; psychoactive drugs; research ethics committees; research institutes; research subjects; risk; scientific misconduct; *therapeutic research; third party consent; withholding treatment; national ethics committees; *National Bioethics Advisory Commission; *United States

---

BE = bioethics accession number   fn. = footnotes   refs. = references

Catalano, Joseph T. The ethics of cadaver experimentation. *Critical Care Nurse.* 1994 Dec; 14(6): 82–85. 8 refs. BE61434.
    administrators; *cadavers; conscience; *continuing education; emergency care; hospitals; human body; institutional policies; interprofessional relations; *nontherapeutic research; *nurses; nursing education; *nursing ethics; presumed consent; property rights; intubation

Chervenak, Frank A.; McCullough, Laurence B. Ethical considerations in research involving pregnant women. *Women's Health Issues.* 1999 Jul–Aug; 9(4): 206–207. 4 refs. BE61973.
    fathers; federal government; females; fetuses; *government regulation; guidelines; *human experimentation; informed consent; obstetrics and gynecology; *organizational policies; physicians; *pregnant women; professional organizations; research subjects; *risks and benefits; *selection of subjects; *American College of Obstetricians and Gynecologists; United States

Clark, Graeme M.; Cowan, Robert S.C.; Dowell, Richard C. Ethical issues. *In:* Clark, Graeme M.; Cowan, Robert S.C.; Dowell, Richard C., eds. Cochlear Implantation for Infants and Children: Advances. San Diego, CA: Singular Publishing Group; 1997: 241–249. 9 refs. ISBN 1-56593-727-9. BE61114.
    age factors; *children; congenital disorders; empirical research; *hearing disorders; infants; informed consent; international aspects; *medical devices; parental consent; *patient care; *physically disabled; *risks and benefits; *surgery; *therapeutic research; treatment outcome; *cochlear implants; Australia; United States

Crigger, Bette–Jane. The battle over babies: international research in perinatal HIV transmission. *IRB: A Review of Human Subjects Research.* 1998 Jul–Aug; 20(4): 13–15. 8 refs. BE61099.
    AIDS; *control groups; *developing countries; *drugs; ethical review; guidelines; health care delivery; *HIV seropositivity; *human experimentation; international aspects; moral policy; *newborns; *placebos; *pregnant women; preventive medicine; public policy; *research design; research subjects; risks and benefits; socioeconomic factors; therapeutic research; vulnerable populations; Africa; Asia; AZT; Centers for Disease Control and Prevention; Council for International Organizations of Medical Sciences; Declaration of Helsinki; National Institutes of Health; United Nations; United States; World Health Organization

Crouch, Robert A.; Arras, John D. AZT trials and tribulations. *Hastings Center Report.* 1998 Nov–Dec; 28(6): 26–34. 32 fn. BE61283.
    control groups; *developing countries; *drugs; *economics; financial support; guidelines; health care; *HIV seropositivity; *human experimentation; indigents; *international aspects; investigators; justice; moral obligations; motivation; newborns; *placebos; *pregnant women; *preventive medicine; public policy; *research design; research subjects; resource allocation; rights; *therapeutic research; Africa; *AZT; Centers for Disease Control and Prevention; Thailand; United States

Davis, Dena S. Medical research with college athletes: some ethical issues. *IRB: A Review of Human Subjects Research.* 1998 Jul–Aug; 20(4): 10–11. 3 fn. BE61097.
    behavioral research; coercion; faculty; *human experimentation; informed consent; minority groups; nontherapeutic research; research subjects; selection of subjects; *sports medicine; *students; therapeutic research; *universities; United States

DeRenzo, Evan G. A bioethicist's perspective. *In:* Hoagwood, Kimberly; Jensen, Peter S.; Fisher, Celia B.,

eds. Ethical Issues in Mental Health Research with Children and Adolescents. Mahwah, NJ: Lawrence Erlbaum Associates; 1996: 269–286. 57 refs. ISBN 0-8058-1953-3. BE62643.
    *adolescents; *behavior disorders; behavioral research; *children; competence; confidentiality; decision making; empirical research; ethicist's role; federal government; genetic research; genetic screening; government regulation; *human experimentation; informed consent; *mentally ill; nontherapeutic research; review committees; risks and benefits; therapeutic research; third party consent; data monitoring committees; United States

de Zoysa, Isabelle; Elias, Christopher J.; Bentley, Margaret E. Ethical challenges in efficacy trials of vaginal microbicides for HIV prevention. *American Journal of Public Health.* 1998 Apr; 88(4): 571–575. 48 refs. BE60133.
    AIDS; AIDS serodiagnosis; community services; control groups; counseling; decision making; *developing countries; *disadvantaged; *drugs; ethical review; *females; guidelines; health education; health promotion; health services research; *HIV seropositivity; *human experimentation; investigators; justice; *moral policy; *preventive medicine; public participation; *research design; research subjects; resource allocation; *risks and benefits; sexuality; *sexually transmitted diseases; women's health services; *condoms; prostitution
This paper discusses some of the ethical challenges raised by advanced clinical trials designed to assess the safety and efficacy of vaginal microbicides in protecting women from HIV infection. The ethical principles that guide clinical research involving human subjects require that all participants in such trials be provided available measures known to reduce the risk of HIV infection. However, this will reduce the ability of the study to assess the protective effect of the test microbicide. In addition, providing extensive services to trial participants may be construed as an undue inducement if the study is being conducted among vulnerable groups such as sex workers or women from disadvantaged communities. Suggestions are provided to resolve this dilemma in the planning and implementation of HIV prevention services for trial participants.

Eckenwiler, Lisa Ann. Women and the Ethics of Clinical Research: Broadening Conceptions of Justice. Ann Arbor, MI: UMI Dissertation Services; 1997. 237 p. Bibliography: p. 212–236. Dissertation, Ph.D. in Philosophy, University of Tennessee, Knoxville, May 1997. UMI No. 9809941. BE61833.
    communication; *communitarianism; cultural pluralism; decision making; democracy; drugs; employment; ethical review; ethical theory; federal government; *females; financial support; government regulation; health care delivery; *human experimentation; *justice; legal aspects; *public policy; research design; research ethics committees; research subjects; risks and benefits; *selection of subjects; *social discrimination; social dominance; socioeconomic factors; vulnerable populations; women's health; Food and Drug Administration; National Institutes of Health; United States

Edi-Osagie, E.C.O.; Edi-Osagie, N.E.; Lurie, Peter, et al. Ethics and international research. [Letters and response]. *BMJ (British Medical Journal).* 1998 Feb 21; 316(7131): 625–628. 13 refs. BE59378.
    *control groups; *developing countries; drugs; guidelines; *HIV seropositivity; *human experimentation; informed consent; international aspects; newborns; *placebos; *pregnant women; random selection; *research design; risks and benefits; socioeconomic factors; *Africa; AZT; Thailand; United States

---

BE = bioethics accession number   fn. = footnotes   refs. = references

Faden, Ruth; Kass, Nancy. HIV research, ethics, and the developing world. [Editorial]. *American Journal of Public Health.* 1998 Apr; 88(4): 548–550. 9 refs. BE60127.
     AIDS; coercion; common good; *control groups; *developing countries; disadvantaged; disclosure; drugs; ethical relativism; ethical review; health care delivery; *HIV seropositivity; *human experimentation; *informed consent; international aspects; *moral policy; *newborns; patient care; *placebos; *pregnant women; preventive medicine; public health; *public policy; random selection; *research design; research subjects; risks and benefits; therapeutic research; retrospective studies; Africa; AZT; United States

Fairchild, Amy L.; Bayer, Ronald. Uses and abuses of Tuskegee. *Science.* 1999 May 7; 284(5416): 919–921. 23 refs. BE61403.
     AIDS serodiagnosis; anonymous testing; *blacks; deception; developing countries; disclosure; *drug abuse; drugs; historical aspects; *HIV seropositivity; *human experimentation; indigents; informed consent; mandatory testing; medical devices; newborns; physicians; placebos; pregnant women; *preventive medicine; public policy; *research design; scientific misconduct; *social discrimination; syphilis; *trust; *vulnerable populations; withholding treatment; *needle–exchange programs; AZT; *Tuskegee Syphilis Study; Twentieth Century; *United States

Fisher, Celia B.; Hoagwood, Kimberly; Jensen, Peter S. Casebook on ethical issues in research with children and adolescents with mental disorders. *In:* Hoagwood, Kimberly; Jensen, Peter S.; Fisher, Celia B., eds. Ethical Issues in Mental Health Research with Children and Adolescents. Mahwah, NJ: Lawrence Erlbaum Associates; 1996: 135–266. 188 refs. ISBN 0–8058–1953–3. BE62642.
     *adolescents; aggression; AIDS; alcohol abuse; *behavior disorders; *behavioral research; *case studies; child abuse; *children; competence; confidentiality; control groups; deception; drug abuse; empirical research; forensic psychiatry; genetic screening; HIV seropositivity; homosexuals; *human experimentation; incentives; infants; informed consent; *mentally ill; mentally retarded; minority groups; parent child relationship; parental consent; parents; placebos; privacy; psychoactive drugs; random selection; research design; research subjects; risks and benefits; selection of subjects; suicide; violence; war; withholding treatment; foster care

Gates, Elena. Two challenges for research ethics: innovative treatment and fetal therapy. *Women's Health Issues.* 1999 Jul–Aug; 9(4): 208–210. 14 refs. BE61974.
     coercion; *fetal research; *fetal therapy; fetuses; *human experimentation; informed consent; nontherapeutic research; obstetrics and gynecology; organizational policies; patient care; physicians; *pregnant women; professional organizations; research subjects; *risks and benefits; *surgery; therapeutic research; treatment refusal; *investigational therapies; American College of Obstetricians and Gynecologists

Gilhooly, Mary L.M.; Smith, Alexander McCall; Nichols, David, eds.; Scottish Action on Dementia. Rights and Legal Protection Sub–Committee. Dementia: Consent to Treatment, Volume 1 [and] Dementia: Consent to Research, Volume 2. Two Discussion Papers. Edinburgh, Scotland: Scottish Action on Dementia; 1992 Mar. 52 p. (Dementia: human rights series). ISBN 0–948897–14–7. BE59473.
     advance directives; autonomy; behavioral research; clinical ethics committees; *competence; decision making; *dementia; drugs; emergency care; family members; genetic research; *human experimentation; *informed consent; *legal aspects; legal guardians; moral policy; nontherapeutic research; paternalism; *patient care; physicians; research

ethics committees; risk; risks and benefits; therapeutic research; *third party consent; treatment refusal; value of life; needs; Mental Health (Scotland) Act 1984; *Scotland

Gorelick, Philip B.; Harris, Yvonne; Burnett, Barbara, et al. The recruitment triangle: reasons why African Americans enroll, refuse to enroll, or voluntarily withdraw from a clinical trial: an interim report from the African–American Antiplatelet Stroke Prevention Study (AAASPS). *Journal of the National Medical Association.* 1998 Mar; 90(3): 141–145. 18 refs. BE62652.
     *attitudes; *blacks; family members; *human experimentation; *motivation; professional patient relationship; *research subjects; scientific misconduct; selection of subjects; survey; therapeutic research; trust; cerebrovascular disorders; refusal to participate; African–American Antiplatelet Stroke Prevention Study; United States

Gottlieb, Scott. NCI defends research involving minority groups. [News]. *Nature Medicine.* 1999 Mar; 5(3): 254. BE62541.
     behavioral research; *biomedical research; *cancer; evaluation; *federal government; *government financing; *human experimentation; indigents; *minority groups; organizational policies; preventive medicine; research institutes; resource allocation; *socioeconomic factors; Institute of Medicine; *National Cancer Institute; *The Unequal Burden of Cancer (Institute of Medicine); *United States

Grady, Christine. Science in the service of healing. *Hastings Center Report.* 1998 Nov–Dec; 28(6): 34–38. 19 fn. BE61284.
     control groups; *developing countries; *drugs; economics; financial support; goals; guidelines; *HIV seropositivity; *human experimentation; *international aspects; newborns; *placebos; *pregnant women; *preventive medicine; *research design; research subjects; Africa; *AZT; Thailand; United States

Graham, Amanda; McDonald, Jim; Association of Canadian Universities for Northern Studies. Board Committee on Revising the Ethical Principles. Ethical Principles for the Conduct of Research in the North. Ottawa, ON: Association of Canadian Universities for Northern Studies; 1998. 28 p. Text in English, in Inuktitut, and in French. ISBN 0–921421–10–9. BE60860.
     American Indians; confidentiality; disclosure; *guidelines; *human experimentation; informed consent; investigator subject relationship; investigators; *minority groups; privacy; professional organizations; research subjects; risks and benefits; Eskimos; *Arctic Regions; Association of Canadian Universities for Northern Studies; *Canada; Labrador; Northwest Territories; Nunavut; Yukon Territory

Hellman, Deborah. Trial and error: can good science be bad medicine? *New Republic.* 1998 Apr 27; 218(17): 14, 16–17. BE61471.
     *developing countries; drugs; federal government; government financing; *HIV seropositivity; *human experimentation; international aspects; newborns; *placebos; *pregnant women; *random selection; *research design; therapeutic research; Africa; Asia; AZT; Centers for Disease Control and Prevention; National Institutes of Health; United States

Hellman, Deborah. Trials on trial. *Philosophy and Public Policy.* 1998 Winter–Spring; 18(1–2): 13–18. 5 refs. BE59814.
     conflict of interest; *control groups; *developing countries; *drugs; *HIV seropositivity; *human experimentation; international aspects; investigators; physicians; *placebos;

BE = bioethics accession number   fn. = footnotes   refs. = references

*pregnant women; public health; *research design; resource allocation; standards; therapeutic research; uncertainty; *AZT; Centers for Disease Control and Prevention; National Institutes of Health; United States

Hilts, Philip J. Psychiatric researchers under fire. [News]. *New York Times.* 1998 May 19: F1, F5. Includes inset article by P.J. Hilts, "Do consent forms tell enough? One case from the front lines," p. F5. BE59613.
adults; advisory committees; aggression; children; competence; consent forms; deception; federal government; government regulation; *human experimentation; *informed consent; *mentally ill; minority groups; *nontherapeutic research; *psychiatry; psychoactive drugs; risks and benefits; schizophrenia; scientific misconduct; state government; *withholding treatment; National Bioethics Advisory Commission; National Institute of Mental Health; United States

Hilts, Philip J. Psychiatric unit's ethics faulted. [News]. *New York Times.* 1998 May 28: A26. BE59614.
federal government; *government regulation; *human experimentation; informed consent; *mentally ill; psychoactive drugs; research institutes; schizophrenia; *scientific misconduct; *withholding treatment; *Office for Protection from Research Risks; *University of Maryland at Baltimore

Hilts, Philip J. V.A. hospital is told to halt all research. [News]. *New York Times.* 1999 Mar 25: A25. BE60872.
administrators; animal experimentation; *federal government; *government regulation; *human experimentation; informed consent; *mentally ill; psychoactive drugs; *public hospitals; research ethics committees; *scientific misconduct; withholding treatment; Department of Veterans Affairs; Los Angeles; Office for Protection from Research Risks; United States; *West Los Angeles Veterans Affairs Medical Center

Hoagwood, Kimberly; Jensen, Peter S.; Fisher, Celia B., eds. Ethical Issues in Mental Health Research with Children and Adolescents. Mahwah, NJ: Lawrence Erlbaum Associates; 1996. 313 p. Includes references. ISBN 0-8058-1953-3. BE62634.
*adolescents; behavior disorders; behavioral research; case studies; child abuse; *children; confidentiality; control groups; family members; family relationship; federal government; government regulation; health services research; *human experimentation; incentives; informed consent; *mentally ill; nontherapeutic research; parental consent; professional family relationship; psychoactive drugs; research design; research ethics committees; risks and benefits; selection of subjects; socioeconomic factors; therapeutic research; Department of Health and Human Services; United States

Kirp, David L. Blood, sweat, and tears: the Tuskegee experiment and the era of AIDS. *Tikkun.* 1995 May–Jun; 10(3): 50–54. BE61473.
*AIDS; *attitudes; *blacks; deception; federal government; historical aspects; homosexuals; *human experimentation; investigators; morbidity; mortality; motivation; nontherapeutic research; physicians; public health; public policy; radiation; research design; research subjects; *scientific misconduct; social discrimination; syphilis; *trust; vulnerable populations; whites; withholding treatment; Centers for Disease Control and Prevention; Foster, Henry; Public Health Service; *Tuskegee Syphilis Study; Twentieth Century; United States

Kolata, Gina; Eichenwald, Kurt. For the uninsured, drug trials are health care. [Stopgap medicine: a special report]. *New York Times.* 1999 Jun 22: A1, C12. BE62248.
chronically ill; coercion; *conflict of interest; deception;

drug industry; *human experimentation; *indigents; *investigational drugs; investigators; managed care programs; patient care; *patients; *physicians; placebos; quality of health care; research subjects; risks and benefits; patient abandonment; *private practice; United States

Kumar, Sanjay. Research into anti–fertility vaccine continues despite protests. [News]. *Lancet.* 1998 Nov 7; 352(9139): 1528. BE60305.
*contraception; developing countries; *females; *human experimentation; immunization; international aspects; political activity; *risks and benefits; scientific misconduct; women's health; India

Lapierre, Yvon D.; Weijer, Charles. Placebo: pro and con. *NCEHR Communique (National Council on Ethics in Human Research).* 1997-1998 Winter–Spring; 8(2): 11–15. 24 refs. BE62095.
competence; drugs; ethical review; *guidelines; *human experimentation; informed consent; *mentally ill; *placebos; psychoactive drugs; *research design; *research ethics committees; risks and benefits; Canada; Code of Conduct for Research Involving Humans; Medical Research Council of Canada

Lehrman, Nathaniel S. The ethics of harmful psychiatric research: a faulty effort to defend them. *Accountability in Research.* 1997; 5(4): 283–288. 36 refs. BE60425.
beneficence; disclosure; *human experimentation; informed consent; *mentally ill; nontherapeutic research; physician patient relationship; *psychoactive drugs; research design; research subjects; *schizophrenia; scientific misconduct; trust; universities; *withholding treatment; Appelbaum, Paul; University of California, Los Angeles

Lemonick, Michael D. Good news at a price : a study finds that AIDS drugs can help poor kids -- but was it ethical? *Time.* 1999 Feb 15; 153(6): 64. BE60961.
*developing countries; drugs; *HIV seropositivity; *human experimentation; placebos; *pregnant women; research design; *therapeutic research; treatment outcome; *Africa; South Africa; Tanzania; Uganda

Leonard, Henrietta; Jensen, Peter S.; Vitiello, Benedetto, et al. Ethical issues in psychopharmacological treatment research with children and adolescents. *In:* Hoagwood, Kimberly; Jensen, Peter S.; Fisher, Celia B., eds. Ethical Issues in Mental Health Research with Children and Adolescents. Mahwah, NJ: Lawrence Erlbaum Associates; 1996: 73–88. 32 refs. ISBN 0-8058-1953-3. BE62639.
*adolescents; behavior disorders; *children; conflict of interest; drug industry; federal government; financial support; government regulation; guidelines; *human experimentation; informed consent; investigators; *mentally ill; *psychoactive drugs; research design; research ethics committees; *risks and benefits; selection of subjects; therapeutic research; treatment outcome; Food and Drug Administration; United States

Levine, Carol. Placebos and HIV: lessons learned. *Hastings Center Report.* 1998 Nov–Dec; 28(6): 43–48. 10 fn. BE61286.
*developing countries; drug industry; *drugs; economics; ethical review; goals; guidelines; *HIV seropositivity; *human experimentation; informed consent; *international aspects; newborns; *placebos; *pregnant women; *research design; risks and benefits; standards; withholding treatment; Africa; *AZT; Thailand; United States

Lie, Reidar K. Ethics of placebo-controlled trials in developing countries. *Bioethics.* 1998 Oct; 12(4): 307–311. 4 fn. Commentary on D.B. Resnik, "The ethics of HIV research in developing nations," p. 286–306. BE62278.

BE = bioethics accession number   fn. = footnotes   refs. = references

AIDS; *alternatives; control groups; *developing countries; drugs; economics; *HIV seropositivity; *human experimentation; international aspects; *newborns; *placebos; *pregnant women; preventive medicine; random selection; *research design; AZT; Thailand

Lurie, Peter; Wolfe, Sidney M. Ethics of HIV trials. [Letter]. *Lancet.* 1998 Jan 17; 351(9097): 220. 5 refs. BE59384.
*developing countries; drugs; economics; ethical relativism; *HIV seropositivity; *human experimentation; international aspects; newborns; *placebos; *pregnant women; preventive medicine; random selection; research design; time factors; AZT; Centers for Disease Control and Prevention

Lynn, Joanne; Muncie, Herbert L.; Magaziner, Jay, et al. Ethical concerns about research on incompetent persons. [Letter and response]. *Journal of the American Geriatrics Society.* 1998 May; 46(5): 660. 1 ref. BE61080.
*aged; *competence; decision making; *dementia; ethical review; guidelines; *human experimentation; informed consent; nontherapeutic research; research subjects; *risks and benefits; selection of subjects; therapeutic research; *third party consent

McCarthy, James. Placebo in research on schizophrenia. [Letter]. *Psychiatric Services.* 1998 May; 49(5): 699. 3 refs. BE61445.
autonomy; beneficence; competence; *human experimentation; informed consent; *mentally ill; *placebos; *psychoactive drugs; *research design; research subjects; risks and benefits; *schizophrenia; withholding treatment

Macilwain, Colin. Proposed restrictions relaxed on research on mentally disabled. [News]. *Nature.* 1998 Oct 22; 395(6704): 731. BE60298.
advisory committees; federal government; *government regulation; *human experimentation; investigators; *mentally ill; nontherapeutic research; research ethics committees; research subjects; risk; *National Bioethics Advisory Commission; *United States

McIntosh, Kenneth. Short (and shorter) courses of zidovudine. [Editorial]. *New England Journal of Medicine.* 1998 Nov 12; 339(20): 1467-1468. 10 refs. BE59344.
childbirth; developing countries; *drugs; *HIV seropositivity; *human experimentation; international aspects; *newborns; placebos; *pregnant women; preventive medicine; *therapeutic research; time factors; treatment outcome; *AZT

Macklin, Ruth. International research and ethical imperialism. *In:* her Against Relativism: Cultural Diversity and the Search for Ethical Universals in Medicine. New York, NY: Oxford University Press; 1999: 187-217. 38 fn. ISBN 0-19-511632-1. BE62784.
autonomy; behavioral research; confidentiality; consent forms; *cultural pluralism; *developing countries; drugs; *ethical relativism; *ethical review; family members; federal government; government regulation; guidelines; HIV seropositivity; *human experimentation; *human rights; *informed consent; *international aspects; newborns; *non-Western World; placebos; pregnant women; preventive medicine; privacy; research design; research subjects; spousal consent; *standards; sterilization (sexual); third party consent; toxicity; *Western World; community consent; AZT; Bangladesh; China; Declaration of Helsinki; Egypt; Ivory Coast; Latin America; Nigeria; Philippines; quinacrine; Thailand; Uganda; *United States; World Medical Association

Maloney, Dennis M. New human subject regulations would change certain IRB reviews. [News]. *Human Research Report.* 1998 Jul; 13(7): 1-2. BE59800.
federal government; *government regulation; *human experimentation; informed consent; *pregnant women; research ethics committees; selection of subjects; *Department of Health and Human Services; *United States

Maloney, Dennis M. Proposal on waiver of informed consent poses major issues for research ethics. *Human Research Report.* 1997 Sep; 12(9): 1-3. BE59953.
disclosure; federal government; *government regulation; *human experimentation; *informed consent; *investigational drugs; *military personnel; patient compliance; research ethics committees; research subjects; risks and benefits; Department of Defense; *Food and Drug Administration; *United States

Marshall, Eliot. NIMH to screen studies for science and human risks. [News]. *Science.* 1999 Jan 22; 283(5401): 464-465. BE60340.
advisory committees; beneficence; *ethical review; federal government; government regulation; *human experimentation; *mentally ill; patient advocacy; psychoactive drugs; *public policy; research design; schizophrenia; scientific misconduct; withholding treatment; *National Institute of Mental Health; *United States

Marshall, Eliot. Panel pulls back report after NIH critique. [News]. *Science.* 1998 Oct 30; 282(5390): 857,859. BE61967.
advisory committees; competence; dissent; ethical review; federal government; *government regulation; guidelines; *human experimentation; informed consent; investigators; *mentally ill; nontherapeutic research; *public policy; research subjects; risk; selection of subjects; *National Bioethics Advisory Commission; *National Institutes of Health; *United States

Marshall, Eliot. Panel tightens rules on mental disorders. [News]. *Science.* 1998 Nov 27; 282(5394): 1617. BE60302.
advisory committees; attitudes; competence; federal government; *government regulation; *human experimentation; informed consent; investigators; *mentally ill; nontherapeutic research; patient participation; research ethics committees; research subjects; risk; *National Bioethics Advisory Commission; *United States

Merkatz, Ruth B. Inclusion of women in clinical trials: a historical overview of scientific, ethical, and legal issues. *Journal of Obstetric, Gynecologic and Neonatal Nursing.* 1998 Jan-Feb; 27(1): 78-84. 27 refs. BE62058.
autonomy; beneficence; drug industry; federal government; *females; guidelines; historical aspects; HIV seropositivity; *human experimentation; *investigational drugs; justice; legal aspects; legal liability; *pregnant women; *public policy; research subjects; risks and benefits; *selection of subjects; women's health; *Food and Drug Administration; *National Institutes of Health; United States

Merson, Michael H.; Simonds, R.J.; Rogers, Martha F., et al. Ethics of placebo-controlled trials of zidovudine to prevent the perinatal transmission of HIV in the Third World. [Letters and response; editor's note]. *New England Journal of Medicine.* 1998 Mar 19; 338(12): 836-841. 25 refs. BE59387.
conflict of interest; control groups; *developing countries; *drugs; economics; *ethical relativism; federal government; *HIV seropositivity; *human experimentation; informed consent; international aspects; investigators; justice; newborns; *placebos; *pregnant women; preventive medicine; random selection; *research design; research ethics committees; risks and benefits; scientific misconduct; standards; therapeutic research; Africa; AZT; Centers for Disease Control and Prevention; Ivory Coast; Thailand; United States; World Health Organization

Michels, Robert. Are research ethics bad for our mental health? *New England Journal of Medicine.* 1999 May 6; 340(18): 1427–1430. 20 refs. BE62028.
   advisory committees; committee membership; competence; decision making; *federal government; *government regulation; *human experimentation; informed consent; investigators; *mentally ill; moral obligations; patient advocacy; placebos; psychoactive drugs; *public policy; research ethics committees; research subjects; therapeutic research; third party consent; withholding treatment; *National Bioethics Advisory Commission; *United States

Mudur, Ganapati. Indian women's groups question contraceptive vaccine research. [News]. *BMJ (British Medical Journal).* 1998 Nov 14; 317(7169): 1340. BE60855.
   *contraception; developing countries; *females; *human experimentation; immunization; *political activity; risks and benefits; *India

Muncie, Herbert L.; Magaziner, Jay; Hebel, J. Richard, et al. Proxies'decisions about clinical research participation for their charges. *Journal of the American Geriatrics Society.* 1997 Aug; 45(8): 929–933. 19 refs. BE59433.
   *aged; comparative studies; *decision making; evaluation studies; *family members; *human experimentation; informed consent; nontherapeutic research; research subjects; risks and benefits; survey; therapeutic research; *third party consent; Baltimore

National Bioethics Advisory Commission. Research Involving Persons with Mental Disorders That May Affect Decisionmaking Capacity. Volume I: Report and Recommendations of the National Bioethics Advisory Commission. Rockville, MD: The Commission; 1998 Dec. 88 p. 284 fn. BE60861.
   advance directives; advisory committees; committee membership; *competence; *ethical review; family members; federal government; government regulation; *guidelines; *human experimentation; informed consent; investigators; *mentally ill; nontherapeutic research; *organizational policies; policy analysis; *public policy; research design; research ethics committees; research subjects; review; risks and benefits; third party consent; withholding treatment; *National Bioethics Advisory Commission; United States

Oberman, Michelle. Real and perceived legal barriers to the inclusion of women in clinical trials. *In:* Dan, Alice J., ed. Reframing Women's Health: Multidisciplinary Research and Practice. Thousand Oaks, CA: Sage Publications; 1994: 266–276. 26 refs. ISBN 0–8039–5860–9. BE60657.
   drug industry; federal government; *females; government regulation; guidelines; *human experimentation; investigational drugs; legal liability; pregnant women; research subjects; risks and benefits; *selection of subjects; *social discrimination; toxicity; Food and Drug Administration; United States

O'Rourke, Dennis. Half Life: A Parable for the Nuclear Age. [Videorecording]. Available from Direct Cinema Ltd., P.O. Box 69799, Los Angeles, CA, 90069, (213)396–4774; 1986. Videocassette; 86 min.; sd., color; VHS. ISBN 1–55974–135–X. Written, directed, and produced by Dennis O'Rourke. BE62227.
   cancer; deception; developing countries; federal government; genetic disorders; health hazards; *human experimentation; injuries; *morbidity; *nontherapeutic research; *nuclear warfare; *public policy; *radiation; *scientific misconduct; Atomic Energy Commission; Department of Energy; *Micronesia; *United States

Osher, Trina W.; Telesford, Mary. Involving families

to improve research. *In:* Hoagwood, Kimberly; Jensen, Peter S.; Fisher, Celia B., eds. Ethical Issues in Mental Health Research with Children and Adolescents. Mahwah, NJ: Lawrence Erlbaum Associates; 1996: 29–39. ISBN 0–8058–1953–3. BE62635.
   *adolescents; behavioral research; *children; confidentiality; control groups; cultural pluralism; deception; decision making; *family members; *family relationship; *human experimentation; investigators; *mentally ill; *professional family relationship; referral and consultation; research design; research ethics committees; risks and benefits; third party consent

Pinals, Debra A.; Malhotra, Anil K.; Breier, Alan, et al. Informed consent in schizophrenia research. [Letter]. *Psychiatric Services.* 1998 Feb; 49(2): 244. 5 refs. BE60041.
   comparative studies; *competence; *comprehension; *consent forms; control groups; *human experimentation; *informed consent; *mentally ill; *schizophrenia

Pincus, Harold Alan; Lieberman, Jeffrey A.; Ferris, Sandy, eds. Ethics in Psychiatric Research: A Resource Manual for Human Subjects Protection. Washington, DC: American Psychiatric Association; 1999. 341 p. Includes references. Appendixes include summaries or text of reports, codes of ethics, federal guidelines, policies, and regulations concerning human subjects research. ISBN 0–89042–281–8. BE62342.
   adolescents; advisory committees; alcohol abuse; autonomy; beneficence; children; competence; comprehension; confidentiality; decision making; disclosure; drug abuse; family members; federal government; government regulation; guidelines; historical aspects; *human experimentation; informed consent; interprofessional relations; investigators; justice; *mentally ill; mentally retarded; moral policy; nontherapeutic research; parental consent; patient advocacy; patient care; physicians; placebos; *psychiatry; psychoactive drugs; public policy; remuneration; research design; research ethics committees; research subjects; risks and benefits; scientific misconduct; selection of subjects; therapeutic research; third party consent; vulnerable populations; withholding treatment; Belmont Report; Declaration of Helsinki; DHHS Guidelines; National Alliance for the Mentally Ill; National Bioethics Advisory Commission; National Commission for the Protection of Human Subjects; Nuremberg Code; President's Commission for the Study of Ethical Problems; Twentieth Century; *United States

Porter, Joan P. Regulatory considerations in research involving children and adolescents with mental disorders. *In:* Hoagwood, Kimberly; Jensen, Peter S.; Fisher, Celia B., eds. Ethical Issues in Mental Health Research with Children and Adolescents. Mahwah, NJ: Lawrence Erlbaum Associates; 1996: 15–28. 10 refs. ISBN 0–8058–1953–3. BE62636.
   *adolescents; *children; confidentiality; federal government; genetic research; *government regulation; *human experimentation; informed consent; *mentally ill; research ethics committees; *Department of Health and Human Services; *United States

Resnik, David B. The ethics of HIV research in developing nations. *Bioethics.* 1998 Oct; 12(4): 286–306. 62 fn. Commented on by R.K. Lie, p. 307–311; by U. Schüklenk, p. 312–319; by J. Thomas, p. 320–327; and by C. Del Rio, p. 328–330. BE62277.
   AIDS; beneficence; codes of ethics; control groups; *developing countries; drugs; *ethical relativism; *HIV seropositivity; *human experimentation; informed consent; international aspects; justice; metaethics; *moral policy; *newborns; non–Western World; *placebos; *pregnant women; preventive medicine; random selection; *research design; research subjects; socioeconomic factors; *standards; therapeutic research; utilitarianism; Africa; AZT; Centers

---

BE = bioethics accession number   fn. = footnotes   refs. = references

for Disease Control and Prevention; Declaration of Helsinki; Dominican Republic; National Institutes of Health; Thailand; UNAIDS; World Health Organization

This paper discusses a dispute concerning the ethics of research on preventing the perinatal transmission of HIV in developing nations. Critics of this research argue that it is unethical because it denies a proven treatment to placebo-control groups. Since studies conducted in developed nations would not deny this treatment to subjects, the critics maintain that these experiments manifest a double standard for ethical research and that a single standard of ethics should apply to all research on human subjects. Proponents of the research, however, argue that these charges fail to understand the ethical complexities of research in developing nations, and that study designs can vary according to the social, economic, and scientific conditions of research. This essay explores some of the ethical issues raised by this controversial case in order to shed some light on the deeper, meta-ethical questions. The paper argues that standards of ethical research on human subjects are universal but not absolute: there are some general ethical principles that apply to all cases of human subjects research but the application of these principles must take into account factors inherent in particular situations.

Roche, Patricia A.; Grodin, Michael A. Why single out pregnant women? Comments on ACOG's recommendations for involving pregnant women in research. *Women's Health Issues.* 1999 Jul–Aug; 9(4): 202–205. BE61972.
autonomy; coercion; conflict of interest; disclosure; federal government; females; fetuses; government regulation; *guidelines; *human experimentation; incentives; informed consent; obstetrics and gynecology; *organizational policies; paternalism; patient care; physicians; *pregnant women; professional organizations; public policy; research subjects; *risks and benefits; *selection of subjects; standards; *American College of Obstetricians and Gynecologists; United States

Rosser, Sue V. Gender bias in clinical research: the difference it makes. *In:* Dan, Alice J., ed. Reframing Women's Health: Multidisciplinary Research and Practice. Thousand Oaks, CA: Sage Publications; 1994: 253–265. 60 refs. ISBN 0–8039–5860–9. BE60656.
biomedical research; disadvantaged; *females; financial support; *human experimentation; informed consent; males; morbidity; research design; research subjects; *selection of subjects; *social discrimination; socioeconomic factors; women's health; women's health services; United States

Rothenberg, Karen H. Gender matters: implications for clinical research and women's health care. *Houston Law Review.* 1996 Symposium; 32(5): 1201–1272. 452 fn. BE59798.
autonomy; biomedical research; communication; confidentiality; constitutional law; decision making; drugs; equal protection; federal government; *females; fetuses; government financing; *government regulation; *human experimentation; justice; legal liability; legal rights; males; physician patient relationship; pregnant women; prenatal injuries; *public policy; reproduction; *selection of subjects; *social discrimination; spousal consent; spousal notification; state government; Supreme Court decisions; torts; women's health; DHHS Guidelines; Food and Drug Administration; International Union, UAW v. Johnson Controls, Inc.; National Institutes of Health; *United States

Schofer, Joel Martin. Violations of informed consent during war. *JAMA.* 1999 May 5; 281(17): 1657. 8 refs. BE62310.
*biological warfare; decision making; *drugs; federal government; government regulation; human

experimentation; *immunization; *informed consent; *investigational drugs; mandatory programs; *military personnel; *preventive medicine; research subjects; risks and benefits; therapeutic research; voluntary programs; *war; chemical warfare; Department of Defense; Food and Drug Administration; *Persian Gulf War; United States

Schüklenk, Udo. Access to Experimental Drugs in Terminal Illness: Ethical Issues. New York, NY: Pharmaceutical Products Press; 1998. 228 p. Bibliography: p. 205–217. ISBN 0–7890–0563–8. BE59923.
*AIDS; alternative therapies; altruism; *autonomy; competence; drug abuse; government regulation; health insurance reimbursement; homosexuals; *human experimentation; informed consent; *investigational drugs; *moral policy; nontherapeutic research; obligations of society; *paternalism; patient compliance; placebos; political activity; research design; risks and benefits; selection of subjects; social discrimination; socioeconomic factors; *terminally ill; *therapeutic research; vulnerable populations; withholding treatment; AZT; Food and Drug Administration; National Institutes of Health; United States

Schüklenk, Udo. Unethical perinatal HIV transmission trials establish bad precedent. *Bioethics.* 1998 Oct; 12(4): 312–319. 21 fn. Commentary on D.B. Resnik, "The ethics of HIV research in developing nations," p. 286–306. BE62279.
AIDS; alternative therapies; control groups; costs and benefits; *developing countries; drug industry; drugs; economics; ethical analysis; ethical review; guidelines; health care delivery; *HIV seropositivity; *human experimentation; informed consent; international aspects; *moral policy; *newborns; non–Western World; *placebos; *pregnant women; preventive medicine; *research design; research subjects; therapeutic research; Western World; Africa; Asia; AZT; Council for International Organizations of Medical Sciences; Latin America; UNAIDS

Sharpe, Virginia A. Ethical considerations? A commentary on ACOG committee opinion 213: "Ethical considerations in research involving pregnant women." *Women's Health Issues.* 1999 Jul–Aug; 9(4): 199–201. BE61971.
conflict of interest; federal government; *females; fetuses; government regulation; *guidelines; *human experimentation; informed consent; investigators; justice; obstetrics and gynecology; *organizational policies; patient care; physicians; *pregnant women; professional organizations; public policy; research subjects; risks and benefits; *selection of subjects; *American College of Obstetricians and Gynecologists; United States

Shavers-Hornaday, Vickie L.; Lynch, Charles F.; Burmeister, Leon F., et al. Why are African Americans under-represented in medical research studies? Impediments to participation. *Ethnicity and Health.* 1997 Mar–Jun; 2(1–2): 31–45. 107 refs. BE59837.
AIDS; *attitudes; *blacks; economics; health care delivery; *human experimentation; investigators; minority groups; physicians; public policy; quality of health care; *research subjects; scientific misconduct; *selection of subjects; social discrimination; syphilis; trust; slavery; Alcohol, Drug and Mental Health Administration; National Institutes of Health; Tuskegee Syphilis Study; United States

Stolberg, Sheryl Gay. Placebo use is suspended in overseas AIDS trials. [News]. *New York Times.* 1998 Feb 19: A16. BE59368.
*AIDS; *developing countries; *drugs; economics; federal government; *HIV seropositivity; *human experimentation; *international aspects; *placebos; *pregnant women; *public policy; *research design; *therapeutic research; *AZT; Centers for Disease Control and Prevention; United States

---

BE = bioethics accession number   fn. = footnotes   refs. = references

Sugarman, Jeremy; McCrory, Douglas C.; Hubal, Robert C. Getting meaningful informed consent from older adults: a structured literature review of empirical research. *Journal of the American Geriatrics Society.* 1998 Apr; 46(4): 517–524. 118 refs. BE60294.
    age factors; *aged; competence; comprehension; consent forms; decision making; disclosure; education; *empirical research; evaluation studies; *human experimentation; *informed consent; literature; methods; *patient care; recall; research design; research subjects; selection of subjects; refusal to participate

Susser, Mervyn. The prevention of perinatal HIV transmission in the less–developed world. [Editorial]. *American Journal of Public Health.* 1998 Apr; 88(4): 547–548. 11 refs. BE60126.
    AIDS; *control groups; *costs and benefits; *developing countries; disadvantaged; *drugs; *HIV seropositivity; *human experimentation; international aspects; *newborns; *placebos; politics; *pregnant women; preventive medicine; *public policy; *research design; *risks and benefits; therapeutic research; breast feeding; AZT; Centers for Disease Control and Prevention; *France; National Institutes of Health; Thailand; *United Nations; *United States

Tanaka, Yuki. Japanese biological warfare plans and experiments on POWs. *In: his* Hidden Horrors: Japanese War Crimes in World War II. Boulder, CO: Westview Press; 1996: 135–165, 238–242. 72 fn. ISBN 0–8133–2718–0. BE60510.
    *biological warfare; communicable diseases; *dehumanization; *historical aspects; *human experimentation; international aspects; *investigators; killing; military personnel; misconduct; National Socialism; nutrition; *physicians; *prisoners; psychology; public policy; *scientific misconduct; China; *Japan; Manchuria; Rabaul; *Twentieth Century; World War II

Thomas, Joe. Ethical challenges of HIV clinical trials in developing countries. *Bioethics.* 1998 Oct; 12(4): 320–327. 25 fn. Commentary on D.B. Resnik, "The ethics of HIV research in developing nations," p. 286–306. BE62280.
    AIDS; alternative therapies; autonomy; beneficence; conflict of interest; *developing countries; drug industry; drugs; economics; ethical review; guidelines; *HIV seropositivity; *human experimentation; human rights; international aspects; investigators; justice; moral policy; *newborns; non–Western World; placebos; *pregnant women; preventive medicine; public policy; *research design; research subjects; standards; therapeutic research; AZT; Council for International Organizations of Medical Sciences; Declaration of Helsinki; National Institutes of Health; United States

Tishler, L. Carl; Gordon, Lisa B. Ethical parameters of challenge studies inducing psychosis with ketamine. *Ethics and Behavior.* 1999; 9(3): 211–217. 32 refs. BE62082.
    disclosure; human experimentation; incentives; informed consent; mentally ill; *nontherapeutic research; normality; *psychoactive drugs; remuneration; *research design; *schizophrenia; selection of subjects; *volunteers; *challenge studies
    Researchers routinely induce psychosis in healthy volunteers via ketamine infusion to expand their knowledge of schizophrenia. We question the ethics of the nature and procedures of such studies. We also address safeguards for ethically conducting and reporting such pursuits, including recruitment, screening, available treatment, and follow–up.

U.S. Department of Health and Human Services. The Conduct of Clinical Trials of Maternal–Infant Transmission of HIV Supported by the United States Department of Health and Human Services in Developing Countries: A Summary of the Needs of Developing Countries, the Scientific Applications, and the Ethical Considerations Assessed by the National Institutes of Health and the Centers for Disease Control and Prevention, 1994–1997. Downloaded from Internet Web site: http://www.nih.gov/news/mathiv/mathiv.htm and http://www.nih.gov/news/mathiv/whodoc.htm (Appendix) on 6 Dec 1997; 1997 Jul. 10 p. 1 ref. Appendix: Recommendations from the Meeting on Prevention of Mother–to–Infant Transmission of HIV by Use of Antiretrovirals, Geneva, 23–25 June 1994. BE62688.
    *developing countries; drugs; economics; health care; *HIV seropositivity; *human experimentation; *international aspects; *newborns; placebos; *pregnant women; *research design; standards; therapeutic research; withholding treatment; Africa; *AZT; Centers for Disease Control and Prevention; Department of Health and Human Services; National Institutes of Health; Thailand; *United States; World Health Organization

U.S. Food and Drug Administration. Accessibility to new drugs for use in military and civilian exigencies when traditional human efficacy studies are not feasible; determination under the interim rule that informed consent is not feasible for military exigencies; request for comments. *Federal Register.* 1997 Jul 31; 62(147): 40996–41001. BE59405.
    *biological warfare; federal government; *government regulation; *human experimentation; *informed consent; *investigational drugs; *military personnel; public policy; toxicity; volunteers; *war; Department of Defense; *Food and Drug Administration; *Persian Gulf War; United States

Wadman, Meredith. Ethical protection for subjects 'could stifle psychiatric research.' [News]. *Nature.* 1998 Aug 20; 394(6695): 713. BE60394.
    advisory committees; biomedical research; government regulation; *human experimentation; medical schools; *mentally ill; nontherapeutic research; professional organizations; *public policy; risks and benefits; third party consent; *Association of American Medical Colleges; National Bioethics Advisory Commission; *United States

Weijer, Charles. Selecting subjects for participation in clinical research: one sphere of justice. *Journal of Medical Ethics.* 1999 Feb; 25(1): 31–36. 34 fn. BE61192.
    aged; biomedical research; drug abuse; *females; government financing; guidelines; health care; HIV seropositivity; *human experimentation; international aspects; *justice; mentally ill; pregnant women; prenatal injuries; research design; research ethics committees; resource allocation; *selection of subjects; social dominance; social worth; therapeutic research; vulnerable populations; women's health; NIH Guidelines; Walzer, Michael
    Recent guidelines from the US National Institutes of Health (NIH) mandate the inclusion of adequate numbers of women in clinical trials. Ought such standards to apply internationally? Walzer's theory of justice is brought to bear on the problem, the first use of the theory in research ethics, and it argues for broad application of the principle of adequate representation. A number of practical conclusions for research ethics committees (RECs) are outlined. Eligibility criteria in clinical trials ought to be justified by trial designers. Research ethics committees ought to question criteria that seem to exclude unnecessarily women from research participation. The issue of adequate representation should be construed broadly, so as to include consideration of the representation of the elderly, persons with HIV, mental illness and substance abuse disorders

---

BE = bioethics accession number   fn. = footnotes   refs. = references

in clinical research.

Weijer, Charles. The IRB's role in assessing the generalizability of non–NIH–funded clinical trials. *IRB: A Review of Human Subjects Research.* 1998 Mar–Jun; 20(2–3): 1–5. 19 refs. BE59992.
    age factors; drug industry; *ethical review; federal government; *females; financial support; government financing; government regulation; *guidelines; *human experimentation; investigational drugs; *minority groups; nontherapeutic research; *research design; *research ethics committees; risks and benefits; *selection of subjects; therapeutic research; vulnerable populations; Food and Drug Administration; National Institutes of Health; *NIH Guidelines; United States

Weisstub, David N.; Arboleda–Flórez, Julio. Ethical research with the developmentally disabled. *Canadian Journal of Psychiatry.* 1997 Jun; 42(5): 492–496. 31 refs. BE59175.
    coercion; competence; comprehension; conflict of interest; deinstitutionalized persons; disclosure; guidelines; *human experimentation; *informed consent; institutionalized persons; legislation; *mentally retarded; *nontherapeutic research; patient participation; research subjects; risks and benefits; *third party consent; vulnerable populations; Canada

Wendler, Dave. When should "riskier" subjects be excluded from research participation? *Kennedy Institute of Ethics Journal.* 1998 Sep; 8(3): 307–327. 9 refs. 2 fn. BE60169.
    age factors; autonomy; decision making; drugs; *females; fetuses; government regulation; *guidelines; *human experimentation; international aspects; investigators; justice; kidney diseases; males; moral policy; patients; preconception injuries; *pregnant women; prenatal injuries; *research design; research ethics committees; *research subjects; rights; *risk; risks and benefits; *selection of subjects; volunteers; Australia; Great Britain; United States
The exclusion of potential subjects based on increased risks is a common practice in human subjects research. However, there are no guidelines to ensure that this practice is conducted in a systematic and fair way. This gap in the literature and regulation is addressed by a specific account of a "condition on inclusion risks" (CIR), a condition under which potential subjects should be excluded from research on the basis of increased risks. This account provides a general framework for assessing standard exclusions as well as more controversial ones such as the exclusion of pregnant women and women of childbearing potential from certain types of research.

West, Doe. Radiation experiments on children at the Fernald and Wrentham schools: lessons for protocols in human subject research. *Accountability in Research.* 1998 Jan; 6(1–2): 103–125. 43 refs. BE61536.
    advisory committees; *children; competence; deception; disclosure; federal government; government financing; guideline adherence; guidelines; *historical aspects; *human experimentation; incentives; informed consent; injuries; *institutionalized persons; investigators; legal guardians; mass media; *mental institutions; *mentally retarded; *nontherapeutic research; nutrition; parental consent; physicians; public hospitals; public policy; *radiation; records; regulation; *residential facilities; retrospective moral judgment; *scientific misconduct; selection of subjects; state government; stigmatization; students; therapeutic research; third party consent; universities; Advisory Committee on Human Radiation Experiments; *Fernald State School (MA); Harvard University; *Massachusetts; Massachusetts Institute of Technology; *Task Force to Review Human Subject Research (MA); *Twentieth Century; United States; *Wrentham State School (MA)

Wilfert, Catherine M.; Ammann, Arthur; Bayer, Ronald, et al. Science, ethics, and the future of research into maternal infant transmission of HIV–1: Consensus statement. [For the Perinatal HIV Intervention Research in Developing Countries Workshop Participants]. *Lancet.* 1999 Mar 6; 353(9155): 832–835. 23 refs. BE61221.
    AIDS; alternatives; childbirth; consensus; *control groups; costs and benefits; *developing countries; *drugs; *economics; *guidelines; *HIV seropositivity; *human experimentation; informed consent; international aspects; *moral policy; *mothers; *newborns; nutrition; patient care; *pregnant women; *preventive medicine; public health; quality of health care; *research design; risks and benefits; *socioeconomic factors; standards; therapeutic research; *breast feeding; *Perinatal HIV Intervention Research in Developing Countries Workshop

Yankauer, Alfred. The neglected lesson of the Tuskegee study. [Letter]. *American Journal of Public Health.* 1998 Sep; 88(9): 1406. 8 refs. BE62555.
    *blacks; editorial policies; *human experimentation; informed consent; *scientific misconduct; *social discrimination; syphilis; withholding treatment; Public Health Service; *Tuskegee Syphilis Study; United States

Zion, Deborah. Ethical considerations of clinical trials to prevent vertical transmission of HIV in developing countries. *Nature Medicine.* 1998 Jan; 4(1): 11–12. 5 refs. BE59981.
    autonomy; coercion; competence; *developing countries; drugs; freedom; *HIV seropositivity; *human experimentation; informed consent; placebos; *pregnant women; *research design; research subjects; AZT

Don't die of recklessness. [Editorial]. *New Scientist.* 1997 Oct 4; 156(2102): 3. BE60458.
    *autoexperimentation; HIV seropositivity; *human experimentation; immunization; *investigators; nontherapeutic research; *physicians; *risk; volunteers

Miss Evers' Boys. [Videorecording; "based on the true story of the infamous Tuskegee Experiment"].New York, NY: HBO Home Video; 1997. 1 videocassette; 118 min.; sd.; color; VHS. HBO in association with Anasazi Productions; a Joseph Sargent film. BE62194.
    *blacks; deception; federal government; government financing; *historical aspects; human experimentation; indigents; informed consent; investigators; *nontherapeutic research; nurses; physicians; public policy; research subjects; *scientific misconduct; *social discrimination; *syphilis; therapeutic research; *withholding treatment; Alabama; Evers, Eunice; *Public Health Service; *Tuskegee Syphilis Study; *Twentieth Century; *United States

Research guidelines issued for persons with mental disorders and impaired capacity to make decisions. [News]. *Psychiatric Services.* 1999 Jan; 50(1): 128–129. BE62076.
    advisory committees; committee membership; *competence; ethical review; government regulation; *guidelines; *human experimentation; informed consent; *mentally ill; organizational policies; professional organizations; psychiatry; *public policy; research design; research ethics committees; research subjects; risks and benefits; third party consent; American Psychiatric Association; *National Bioethics Advisory Commission; United States

Research involving human subjects: efforts to resolve current ethical controversies. [Introduction to a set of documents, p. S:279–S:348].*In:* BioLaw: A Legal and Ethical Reporter of Medicine, Health Care, and Bioengineering. Special Sections 2(7–8). Frederick, MD: University Publications of America; 1998 Jul–Aug: S:241–S:277. 76 fn. Followed by recent documents on

---

BE = bioethics accession number   fn. = footnotes   refs. = references

research involving subjects with mental disorders: "Research Involving Individuals with Questionable Capacity to Consent: Ethical Issues and Practical Considerations for Institutional Review Boards"; Testimony from a House of Representatives Committee Hearing on IRBs; and a draft NBAC report, "Research Involving Subjects with Mental Disorders that May Affect Decision-Making Capacity." BE60173.
   advisory committees; autonomy; beneficence; communitarianism; compensation; competence; cultural pluralism; decision making; developing countries; drugs; ethical relativism; evaluation; federal government; government regulation; guidelines; HIV seropositivity; *human experimentation; informed consent; injuries; international aspects; justice; *mentally disabled; newborns; placebos; pregnant women; preventive medicine; public policy; research design; *research ethics committees; research subjects; resource allocation; risks and benefits; schizophrenia; state government; therapeutic research; trends; *vulnerable populations; withholding treatment; AZT; Federal Policy (Common Rule) for the Protection of Human Subjects 1991; National Bioethics Advisory Commission; United States

When mental patients are at risk. [Editorial]. *New York Times.* 1999 Mar 31: A24. BE60909.
   *federal government; *government regulation; *human experimentation; *mentally ill; psychoactive drugs; public hospitals; schizophrenia; *scientific misconduct; withholding treatment; Department of Veterans Affairs; Los Angeles; United States; West Los Angeles Veterans Affairs Medical Center

IMMUNIZATION

See also PUBLIC HEALTH

Altman, Lawrence K. Ethics panel urges easing of curbs on AIDS vaccine tests. [News]. *New York Times.* 1998 Jun 28: 6. BE59361.
   advisory committees; AIDS; *developing countries; drugs; ethical relativism; guidelines; *HIV seropositivity; *human experimentation; *immunization; informed consent; *international aspects; placebos; research subjects; United States

Altman, Lawrence K. F.D.A. authorizes first full testing for H.I.V. vaccine. [News]. *New York Times.* 1998 Jun 4: A1, A23. BE59362.
   developing countries; drug abuse; drug industry; federal government; *government regulation; *HIV seropositivity; homosexuals; *human experimentation; *immunization; international aspects; placebos; research design; risks and benefits; volunteers; *Food and Drug Administration; Thailand; *United States; Vaxgen Inc.

Beloqui, Jorge; Chokevivat, Vichai; Collins, Chris. HIV vaccine research and human rights: examples from three countries planning efficacy trials. *Health and Human Rights.* 1998; 3(1): 38–58. 21 fn. BE62574.
   compensation; *developing countries; drug industry; economics; ethical review; health care; *HIV seropositivity; *human rights; *immunization; injuries; *international aspects; justice; preventive medicine; public policy; research design; research subjects; risks and benefits; social discrimination; stigmatization; *therapeutic research; volunteers; Brazil; Thailand

Cohen, Jon; Ivinson, Adrian J. Clarifying AIDS vaccine trial guidelines. [Letter and response]. *Nature Medicine.* 1998 Oct; 4(10): 1091. BE61527.
   AIDS; consensus; developing countries; dissent; *guidelines; *HIV seropositivity; *human experimentation; *immunization; *international aspects; *patient care;

research subjects; standards

Cohen, Jon. No consensus on rules for AIDS vaccine trials. [News]. *Science.* 1998 Jul 3; 281(5373): 22–23. BE59940.
   advisory committees; *AIDS; *developing countries; drugs; ethical review; HIV seropositivity; *human experimentation; *immunization; international aspects; investigators; patient care; research design; research subjects; withholding treatment; research ethics; United Nations

Day, Michael. This won't hurt ... have we fully investigated the risks associated with immunisation. [News]. *New Scientist.* 1998 Mar 7; 157(2124): 4. BE59715.
   behavior disorders; children; iatrogenic disease; *immunization; *risks and benefits; Great Britain

Gordon, Todd E.; Zook, Eric G.; Averhoff, Francisco M., et al. Consent for adolescent vaccination: issues and current practices. *Journal of School Health.* 1997 Sep; 67(7): 259–264. 15 refs. BE59637.
   *adolescents; age factors; communicable diseases; *government regulation; hepatitis; *immunization; *informed consent; minors; *parental consent; *state government; survey; *United States

Ivinson, Adrian J. Hard-won consensus on AIDS vaccine trial guidelines. [News]. *Nature Medicine.* 1998 Aug; 4(8): 874. BE59731.
   consensus; *developing countries; dissent; drugs; economics; *guidelines; *HIV seropositivity; *human experimentation; *immunization; *international aspects; *patient care; standards; *UNAIDS; World Health Organization

Lee, J.W.; Melgaard, Bjorn; Hull, Harry F., et al. Ethical dilemmas in polio eradication. *American Journal of Public Health.* 1998 Jan; 88(1): 130–132. 6 refs. BE62551.
   *developing countries; economics; *immunization; *international aspects; *poliomyelitis; primary health care; public health; public policy; *resource allocation; World Health Organization

Mann, Jonathan M.; Zion, Deborah; Macpherson, Cheryl Cox, et al. The ethics of AIDS vaccine trials. [Letters and response]. *Science.* 1998 May 29; 280(5368): 1327, 1329–1331. 11 refs. BE59441.
   *AIDS; codes of ethics; comprehension; *developing countries; drugs; economics; guidelines; HIV seropositivity; *human experimentation; *immunization; informed consent; international aspects; placebos; pregnant women; research design; standards; therapeutic research; vulnerable populations; Africa; Declaration of Helsinki; International Ethical Guidelines for Biomedical Research Involving Human Subjects; United States

Marwick, Charles. IOM committee gazes into new vaccine future. [News]. *JAMA.* 1999 Apr 21; 281(15): 1366–1367. BE61952.
   advisory committees; *communicable diseases; *costs and benefits; *evaluation; *immunization; preventive medicine; *public policy; quality adjusted life years; *Institute of Medicine; United States

Matz, Robert; Levine, Myron M.; Tacket, Carol O., et al. Recruiting volunteers for a typhoid vaccine. [Letter and response]. *JAMA.* 1998 Nov 4; 280(17): 1480–1481. 8 refs. BE61078.
   altruism; autoexperimentation; communicable diseases; federal government; *human experimentation; *immunization; informed consent; *nontherapeutic research; research subjects; selection of subjects; *volunteers;

BE = bioethics accession number   fn. = footnotes   refs. = references

*typhoid; Food and Drug Administration; United States;
*University of Maryland School of Medicine

Meldrum, Marcia. "A calculated risk": the Salk polio
vaccine field trials of 1954. *BMJ (British Medical
Journal)*. 1998 Oct 31; 317(7167): 1233–1236. 21 refs.
BE60836.
children; *control groups; financial support; health
personnel; *historical aspects; *human experimentation;
*immunization; investigators; *placebos; *poliomyelitis;
public health; public policy; random selection; *research
design; state government; National Foundation for Infantile
Paralysis; *Salk, Jonas; *Twentieth Century; *United States

Morris, Kelly. US military face punishment for refusing
anthrax vaccine. [News]. *Lancet.* 1999 Jan 9; 353(9147):
130. BE60981.
*biological warfare; *immunization; mandatory programs;
*military personnel; *punishment; *risks and benefits;
voluntary programs; *refusal to participate; *Canada; Great
Britain; *United States

Myers, Steven Lee. Airman discharged for refusal to take
anthrax vaccine as rebellion grows. [News]. *New York
Times.* 1999 Mar 11: A24. BE60908.
*biological warfare; *immunization; *military personnel;
*punishment; *refusal to participate; Bettendorf, Jeffrey;
United States

Pollak, Michael. Doctors fighting backlash over vaccines.
[News]. *New York Times.* 1999 Apr 27: F7. BE61172.
attitudes; children; communicable diseases; compensation;
federal government; *immunization; injuries; mandatory
programs; parental consent; public opinion; public policy;
registries; *risks and benefits; state government; voluntary
programs; United States

**Redenbaugh, Russell; Phillips, Alan; Fisher, Barbara
Loe, et al.; Children's Defense Fund; U.S. Centers
for Disease Control and Prevention.** Are government
vaccination programs beneficial? *In:* Dudley, William,
ed. Epidemics: Opposing Viewpoints. San Diego, CA:
Greenhaven Press; 1999: 86–134, 174. Bibliography: p.
134; discussion questions: p. 174. ISBN 1-56510-940-6.
BE59825.
*children; compensation; deception; drug industry; federal
government; government financing; *immunization;
informed consent; injuries; legal rights; *mandatory
programs; morbidity; parents; political activity; public
health; *public policy; risk; *risks and benefits; whooping
cough; Nation of Islam; United States

Richey, Warren. A vaccination war erupts in military.
[News]. *Christian Science Monitor.* 1999 Jan 28: 2.
BE61007.
*biological warfare; *immunization; mandatory programs;
*military personnel; punishment; *risks and benefits;
voluntary programs; *refusal to participate; Great Britain;
*United States

Ridway, Derry. No-fault vaccine insurance: lessons from
the National Vaccine Injury Compensation Program.
Journal of Health Politics, Policy and Law. 1999 Feb; 24(1):
59–90. 47 refs. 11 fn. BE61754.
children; communicable diseases; *compensation; *drug
industry; evaluation; expert testimony; *federal government;
iatrogenic disease; *immunization; *injuries; lawyers; *legal
aspects; program descriptions; *public policy; risks and
benefits; social impact; statistics; torts; whooping cough;
*National Vaccine Injury Compensation Program; *United
States
During the first eight years of the National Vaccine
Injury Compensation Program (NVICP), 786 contested
claims were resolved through published judicial

opinions. The likelihood of compensation depended in
part on the closeness of the match between the described
injury and a specified list of acknowledged untoward
vaccine side effects. In addition, the chances of applicant
success were influenced by the applicant's choice of
attorney and expert witnesses, by the assignment of the
Special Master to decide the case, and increasingly over
time, by the applicant's ability to comply with procedural
requirements. The majority of contested claims arose
from pertussis immunizations. For pertussis claims, the
goal of insulating manufacturers from product law
liability suits has been achieved by granting
compensation to applicants whose injuries are not
scientifically recognized effects of the vaccine. In spite
of (or because of) this jarring contradiction between the
legal and medical understanding of causation, vaccine
availability and childhood immunization rates improved
during the early years of the plan. The apparent success
of the program may encourage the substitution of
no-fault compensation plans for tort-based consumer
protection for other products, both medical and
nonmedical.

Saegusa, Asako. Are Japanese researchers exploiting Thai
HIV patients? [News]. *Nature Medicine.* 1998 May; 4(5):
540. BE59726.
government financing; *HIV seropositivity; *human
experimentation; *immunization; *international aspects;
investigators; methods; *Japan; Japan Science and
Technology Corporation; *Thailand

Schofer, Joel Martin. Violations of informed consent
during war. *JAMA.* 1999 May 5; 281(17): 1657. 8 refs.
BE62310.
*biological warfare; decision making; *drugs; federal
government; government regulation; human
experimentation; *immunization; *informed consent;
*investigational drugs; mandatory programs; *military
personnel; *preventive medicine; research subjects; risks and
benefits; therapeutic research; voluntary programs; *war;
chemical warfare; Department of Defense; Food and Drug
Administration; *Persian Gulf War; United States

Sibbald, Barbara. CMA says no to mandatory hepatitis
B vaccination, screening for MDs. *Canadian Medical
Association Journal.* 1998 Jul 14; 159(1): 64–65. BE61129.
autonomy; confidentiality; consensus; dentistry; dissent;
guidelines; *health personnel; *hepatitis; iatrogenic disease;
*immunization; *mandatory programs; mandatory testing;
*mass screening; *organizational policies; *physicians;
privacy; professional organizations; *public policy; surgery;
*voluntary programs; *Canada; Canadian Dental
Association; *Canadian Medical Association; *Health
Canada

Specter, Michael. Uganda AIDS vaccine test: urgency
affects ethics rules. [News]. *New York Times.* 1998 Oct
1: A1, A6. BE60574.
*AIDS; *developing countries; drugs; economics; HIV
seropositivity; *human experimentation; *immunization;
informed consent; international aspects; research design;
research subjects; risks and benefits; *Uganda

Effort to increase child immunization is under attack in
Idaho. [News]. *New York Times.* 1999 Mar 7: 25.
BE60975.
*children; *dissent; government regulation; *immunization;
legislation; parental consent; privacy; *public policy;
*registries; religion; state government; Christian Coalition;
*Idaho

The need of the many ... when individuals suffer for the
sake of society we must compensate them properly.

BE = bioethics accession number   fn. = footnotes   refs. = references

[Editorial]. *New Scientist.* 1998 Mar 7; 157(2124): 3. BE59604.

behavior disorders; *children; *compensation; *immunization; *injuries; obligations of society; public policy; risks and benefits; *Great Britain; United States

IN VITRO FERTILIZATION

See also REPRODUCTIVE TECHNOLOGIES

Bahnsen, Ulrich. Swiss to vote on ban on *in vitro* fertilization. [News]. *Nature.* 1998 Nov 12; 396(6707): 105. BE59659.

embryo research; *government regulation; *in vitro fertilization; ovum donors; political activity; preimplantation diagnosis; *public participation; *reproductive technologies; stem cells; *Switzerland

Byers, Keith Alan. Infertility and in vitro fertilization: a growing need for consumer-oriented regulation of the in vitro fertilization industry. *Journal of Legal Medicine.* 1997 Sep; 18(3): 265-313. 304 fn. BE59838.

advisory committees; AIDS serodiagnosis; communicable diseases; cryopreservation; economics; embryo disposition; embryo research; embryo transfer; federal government; genetic disorders; government financing; *government regulation; *health facilities; *in vitro fertilization; industry; *infertility; legal aspects; legislation; mandatory testing; misconduct; multiple pregnancy; ovum donors; physicians; psychological stress; public opinion; *public policy; quality of health care; remuneration; *reproductive technologies; standards; state government; statistics; treatment outcome; Ethics Advisory Board; Fertility Clinic Success Rate and Certification Act 1992; Human Embryo Research Panel; *United States

Ellenson, David. Artificial fertilization (hafrayyah melakhutit) and procreative autonomy in light of two contemporary Israeli responsa. *In:* Jacob, Walter; Zemer, Moshe, eds. The Fetus and Fertility in Jewish Law: Essays and Responsa. Pittsburgh, PA: Rodef Shalom Press; Freehof Institute of Progressive Halakhah; 1995: 19-38. 23 fn. ISBN 0-929699-07-6. BE61837.

artificial insemination; autonomy; children; drugs; embryo disposition; *embryo transfer; family relationship; genetic identity; genetic intervention; *in vitro fertilization; infertility; *Jewish ethics; married persons; multiple pregnancy; parent child relationship; reproduction; *reproductive technologies; risks and benefits; selective abortion; surrogate mothers; *theology; wedge argument; women's rights; Orthodox Judaism; Reform Judaism

Forster, Heidi P.; Robertson, John. Frozen embryo disposition. [Letter and response]. *Hastings Center Report.* 1999 Mar-Apr; 29(2): 4-5. BE61652.

contracts; *cryopreservation; *decision making; *dissent; *embryo disposition; embryo research; embryo transfer; *embryos; *in vitro fertilization; informed consent; *legal aspects; married persons; ovum donors; property rights; semen donors; divorce; Kass v. Kass; New York

Great Britain. Human Fertilisation and Embryology Authority. Sixth Annual Report [1995-1996]. London: The Authority; 1997. 45 p. Includes references. "This report covers the year beginning 1 Nov 1995 with a foreward look for the year beginning 1 Nov 1996." BE60714.

age factors; artificial insemination; cloning; cryopreservation; *embryo research; embryos; genetic screening; *government regulation; guidelines; *health facilities; HIV seropositivity; *in vitro fertilization; information dissemination; informed consent; posthumous reproduction; preimplantation diagnosis; remuneration; *reproductive technologies; semen donors; sperm;

*standards; statistics; *Great Britain; Human Fertilisation and Embryology Act 1990; *Human Fertilisation and Embryology Authority

Grubb, Andrew. Frozen embryos: rights of inheritance: In Re the Estate of the Late K. [Comment]. *Medical Law Review.* 1997 Spring; 5(1): 121-124. BE59764.

childbirth; *cryopreservation; embryo transfer; *embryos; fathers; fetuses; in vitro fertilization; *legal aspects; *legal rights; newborns; parent child relationship; personhood; *posthumous reproduction; property rights; *Australia; Great Britain; *In re Estate of the Late K; *Tasmania

Hildt, Elisabeth; Mieth, Dietmar, eds. In Vitro Fertilisation in the 1990s: Towards a Medical, Social and Ethical Evaluation. Brookfield, VT: Ashgate; 1998. 370 p. Includes references. This book is a collection of the lectures delivered at the symposium, "IVF in the 90s -- Methods, Contexts, Consequences," which was organized by the European Network for Biomedical Ethics and held in Stuttgart, Germany, 16-19 Jan 1997. ISBN 1-85972-685-2. BE61311.

alternatives; attitudes; autonomy; bioethics; counseling; cultural pluralism; decision making; directive counseling; embryo disposition; embryo research; *embryo transfer; embryos; evaluation; females; gene therapy; government regulation; historical aspects; *in vitro fertilization; infertility; males; moral obligations; multiple pregnancy; patients; preimplantation diagnosis; psychological stress; reproduction; *reproductive technologies; rights; selective abortion; statistics; treatment outcome; dignity; Europe

Mackler, Aaron L. An expanded partnership with God? In vitro fertilization in Jewish ethics. *Journal of Religious Ethics.* 1997 Fall; 25(2): 277-304. 76 refs. 16 fn. BE60304.

cryopreservation; embryo disposition; embryo research; *embryo transfer; embryos; fetal development; fetuses; genetic screening; *in vitro fertilization; *Jewish ethics; *married persons; maternal health; mental health; mothers; multiple pregnancy; *ovum donors; parent child relationship; personhood; *preimplantation diagnosis; prenatal diagnosis; reproduction; *reproductive technologies; risks and benefits; selective abortion; *semen donors; *theology; therapeutic abortion

Massachusetts. Trial Court, Probate and Family Department, Suffolk County. AZ v. BZ. Unpublished redacted copy; 1996. 31 p. Permanent restraining order injunction and findings of fact and conclusions of law on request for restraining order. BE60049.

consent forms; *contracts; *cryopreservation; decision making; *embryo disposition; embryo transfer; *embryos; *in vitro fertilization; informed consent; *legal aspects; *legal rights; *marital relationship; ovum donors; personhood; privacy; property rights; reproduction; semen donors; time factors; unwanted children; *divorce; *AZ v. BZ; Davis v. Davis; Kass v. Kass; *Massachusetts; New York; Tennessee

The Massachusetts Trial Court, Probate and Family Department, for Suffolk County resolved the issue of disposition of cryopreserved embryos prior to entry of a divorce judgment. The court decided in favor of the husband AZ who sought to avoid parenthood, provided that the wife BZ has a reasonable possibility of achieving parenthood through other means. Because BZ had lost both fallopian tubes in ectopic pregnancies, she and her husband AZ conceived twin daughters through in vitro fertilization (IVF) and froze the remaining seven pre-embryos in two vials. Unknown to her husband, BZ underwent an unsuccessful embryo transfer using the embryos from one vial in the month before AZ and BZ separated. Four cryopreserved embryos remained in the last vial. The judge held that a "special status" category best recognizes the dual characteristics of pre-embryos

---

BE = bioethics accession number   fn. = footnotes   refs. = references

as property and as persons. Discussing the issue of procreational autonomy, the judge found that IVF differs from natural reproduction and has none of the concerns about a woman's bodily integrity. Because the disposition agreement signed by both AZ and BZ at the time of ovum harvest is seven years old and subject to an unforeseeable change of circumstances, the court balanced the interests of the gamete providers and those of a subsequent child. (KIE abstract)

Melo–Martín, Immaculada de. Making Babies: Biomedical Technologies, Reproductive Ethics, and Public Policy. Boston, MA: Kluwer Academic; 1998. 199 p. Includes references. ISBN 0–7923–5116–9. BE61842.
 advisory committees; common good; disclosure; ethical theory; *evaluation; *in vitro fertilization; infertility; informed consent; *international aspects; legal aspects; methods; *public policy; *reproductive technologies; *risks and benefits; social impact; *technology assessment; treatment outcome; uncertainty; women's health; Australia; Canada; Europe; Great Britain; Spain; United States

Mor–Yosef, Shlomo. Cost effectiveness of *in vitro* fertilization. *Journal of Assisted Reproduction and Genetics.* 1995 Sep; 12(8): 524–530. 24 refs. BE60565.
 alternatives; *costs and benefits; evaluation; financial support; health insurance reimbursement; hospitals; *in vitro fertilization; international aspects; private sector; public policy; public sector; reproductive technologies; resource allocation; selection for treatment; Canada; Europe; Israel; United States

Murray, Thomas H. Money–back guarantees for IVF: an ethical critique. *Journal of Law, Medicine and Ethics.* 1997 Winter; 25(4): 292–294. 11 fn. Commentary on J.A. Robertson and T.J. Schneyer, p. 283–291. BE62674.
 commodification; contracts; *embryo transfer; health facilities; *in vitro fertilization; *incentives; insurance; justice; medical fees; newborns; *patients; physicians; *remuneration; risk; selection for treatment; *treatment outcome; values; American Medical Association; United States

New York. Supreme Court, Appellate Division, Second Department. Kass v. Kass. *New York Supplement, 2d Series.* 1997 Sep 8 (date of decision). 663: 581–602. BE60051.
 *contracts; *cryopreservation; decision making; dissent; *embryo disposition; embryo research; embryo transfer; *embryos; *in vitro fertilization; informed consent; *legal aspects; legal rights; *marital relationship; ovum donors; personhood; property rights; reproduction; semen donors; *divorce; *Kass v. Kass; New York
 The New York Supreme Court, Appellate Division, enforced an informed consent agreement between husband and wife concerning disposition of cryopreserved embryos, following in vitro fertilization (IVF), for use in scientific research. Maureen and Steven Kass had provided for the use of their frozen pre–zygotes in an IVF consent form, and later affirmed that use in an uncontested divorce agreement. Maureen Kass then changed her mind and sought legal possession and custody of the five pre–embryos for transfer into herself. The trial court had granted her exclusive control based on the determination that a husband's procreative rights in IVF were no greater than those in vivo. The appellate court, however, reversed the trial court and upheld the agreement because the couple's original mutual intent on disposition in the event of a contingency was clear and unequivocal. (KIE abstract)

Robertson, John A.; Schneyer, Theodore J. Professional

self–regulation and shared–risk programs for in vitro fertilization. *Journal of Law, Medicine and Ethics.* 1997 Winter; 25(4): 283–291. 44 fn. Commented on by T.H. Murray, p. 292–294. BE62673.
 age factors; conflict of interest; deception; *embryo transfer; females; guidelines; health facilities; health insurance reimbursement; *in vitro fertilization; *incentives; informed consent; *insurance; legal aspects; malpractice; medical fees; *organizational policies; *patients; physicians; professional organizations; public policy; *remuneration; risk; selection for treatment; *self regulation; *treatment outcome; *American Medical Association; United States

Rohde, David. Black parents prevail in embryo mix–up. [News]. *New York Times.* 1999 Jul 17: B3. BE62446.
 *blacks; children; dissent; *embryo transfer; health facilities; in vitro fertilization; *legal aspects; mothers; *negligence; *parent child relationship; siblings; *whites; *Fasano, Donna; Fasano, Richard; IVF New York (New York City); New York; *Perry-Rogers, Deborah; Rogers, Robert

Simini, Bruno. Italy moves on with in–vitro fertilisation legislation. [News]. *Lancet.* 1999 Jun 5; 353(9168): 1950. BE62681.
 age factors; cloning; cryopreservation; donors; embryo disposition; embryos; females; germ cells; *government regulation; *in vitro fertilization; *legal aspects; legal liability; *legislation; physicians; *reproductive technologies; selection for treatment; *Italy

van Balen, Frank. Development of IVF children. *Developmental Review.* 1998 Mar; 18(1): 30–46. 42 refs. BE60348.
 attitudes; *children; congenital disorders; *empirical research; fathers; *in vitro fertilization; intelligence; international aspects; mothers; multiple pregnancy; *parent child relationship; psychology; *reproductive technologies; semen donors; *treatment outcome

Watts, Jonathan. In–vitro fertilisation guidelines fall behind the times. [News]. *Lancet.* 1999 Jan 23; 353(9149): 303. BE60392.
 *guideline adherence; *guidelines; *in vitro fertilization; married persons; obstetrics and gynecology; *organizational policies; ovum donors; physicians; professional organizations; regulation; *reproductive technologies; semen donors; *Japan; *Japan Society of Obstetrics and Gynecology

Clinic plans to destroy unclaimed embryos. [News]. *New York Times.* 1999 Jul 13: F14. BE62546.
 *cryopreservation; *embryo disposition; *embryos; *health facilities; *in vitro fertilization; institutional policies; *Arizona Institute of Reproductive Medicine; United States

Judge orders divorcing couple's frozen embryos destroyed. [News]. *New York Times.* 1998 Sep 29: B6. BE60968.
 advance directives; contracts; cryopreservation; decision making; *dissent; *embryo disposition; *embryos; *in vitro fertilization; *legal aspects; married persons; *divorce; *New Jersey

No ABA embryo policy. [News]. *Washington Post.* 1998 Feb 3: A5. BE59675.
 *cryopreservation; dissent; *embryo disposition; embryo transfer; *embryos; *in vitro fertilization; lawyers; *legal aspects; *organizational policies; professional organizations; property rights; divorce; *American Bar Association; United States

INFANTICIDE

See also ALLOWING TO DIE/INFANTS, EUTHANASIA

BE = bioethics accession number   fn. = footnotes   refs. = references

INFANTS
See under
   ALLOWING TO DIE/INFANTS

INFORMED CONSENT

See also TREATMENT REFUSAL
See also under
   HUMAN EXPERIMENTATION/INFORMED
   CONSENT

Alberta Law Reform Institute. Advance Directives and Substitute Decision–Making in Personal Healthcare: A Joint Report of the Alberta Law Reform Institute and the Health Law Institute. Edmonton, AB: The Institute; 1993 Mar. 60 p. 94 fn. Report No. 64. ISBN 0–8886–4180–X. BE60502.
   *advance directives; age factors; competence; decision making; emergency care; family members; government regulation; health care; *legal aspects; legislation; model legislation; standards; *third party consent; *Alberta; Alberta Law Reform Institute; British Columbia; Canada; Manitoba; Newfoundland; Ontario; Saskatchewan

Alderson, Priscilla; Goodey, Christopher. Theories of consent. *BMJ (British Medical Journal).* 1998 Nov 7; 317(7168): 1313–1315. 18 refs. BE60837.
   autonomy; coercion; competence; comprehension; decision making; disclosure; emotions; historical aspects; human experimentation; *informed consent; *models, theoretical; patient care; patients; physicians; postmodernism; standards

Alpers, Ann; Lo, Bernard. Avoiding family feuds: responding to surrogate demands for life–sustaining interventions. *Journal of Law, Medicine and Ethics.* 1999 Spring; 27(1): 74–80. 45 fn. BE61507.
   *advance directives; *allowing to die; autonomy; *beneficence; biomedical technologies; case studies; communication; *conscience; consensus; cultural pluralism; *decision making; directive adherence; disclosure; *dissent; *family members; *family relationship; friends; *futility; intention; minority groups; moral obligations; patient care team; *physicians; *professional family relationship; prognosis; *prolongation of life; religion; resuscitation orders; risks and benefits; *suffering; *third party consent; time factors; *values; withholding treatment; integrity; *negotiation; oral directives

American Society for Reproductive Medicine. Ethics Committee. Informed consent and the use of gametes and embryos for research. *Fertility and Sterility.* 1997 Nov; 68(5): 780–781. 1 ref. BE62008.
   disclosure; *donors; embryo disposition; *embryo research; *embryos; *germ cells; *informed consent; investigators; *ovum donors; patients; reproductive technologies; *research embryo creation; research ethics committees; *semen donors; *tissue donation; viability; American Society for Reproductive Medicine

Andrews, Lori B. The sperminator. *New York Times Magazine.* 1999 Mar 28: 62–65. BE60874.
   advance directives; cadavers; coercion; cryopreservation; decision making; directed donation; family members; family relationship; *informed consent; legal aspects; married persons; physicians; *posthumous reproduction; *semen donors; single persons; sperm; tissue donation; *coma; United States

Appelbaum, Paul S.; Grisso, Thomas. Capacities of hospitalized, medically ill patients to consent to treatment. *Psychosomatics.* 1997 Mar–Apr; 38(2): 119–125. 21 refs. BE59193.
   alternatives; comparative studies; *competence; comprehension; control groups; decision making; disclosure; evaluation studies; heart diseases; *hospitals; *informed consent; patient care; *patients; risks and benefits; rationality; United States

Appelbaum, Paul S. Ought we to require emotional capacity as part of decisional competence? *Kennedy Institute of Ethics Journal.* 1998 Dec; 8(4): 377–387. 12 refs. BE62374.
   brain pathology; *competence; comprehension; decision making; *emotions; evaluation; *informed consent; mentally ill; patients; *standards; MacArthur Treatment Competence Study
The preceding commentary by Louis Charland suggests that traditional cognitive views of decision–making competence err in not taking into account patients' emotional capacities. Examined closely, however, Charland's argument fails to escape the cognitive bias that he condemns. However, there may be stronger arguments for broadening the focus of competence assessment to include emotional capacities, centering on the ways in which emotions aid humans in processing information. Before emotional capacities are added to the list of functions essential for decisional competence, though, the feasibility and utility of such a reorientation must be demonstrated.

Artnak, Kathryn E. Informed consent in the elderly: assessing decisional capacity. *Seminars in Perioperative Nursing.* 1997 Jan; 6(1): 59–64. 10 refs. BE59194.
   *aged; attitudes; autonomy; beneficence; case studies; communication; *competence; comprehension; *decision making; disclosure; hospitals; *informed consent; moral obligations; *nurse's role; paternalism; *patient care; quality of life; risks and benefits; social discrimination; time factors; treatment refusal; values

Barton, C. Dennis; Mallik, Harminder S.; Orr, William B., et al. Clinicians' judgment of capacity of nursing home patients to give informed consent. *Psychiatric Services.* 1996 Sep; 47(9): 956–960. 24 refs. BE61530.
   advance directives; *aged; attitudes; *competence; dementia; *evaluation; evaluation studies; *health personnel; *informed consent; institutionalized persons; legal aspects; *nursing homes; third party consent; Maryland

Beecham, Linda. GMC advises doctors on seeking consent. [News]. *BMJ (British Medical Journal).* 1999 Feb 27; 318(7183): 553. BE60997.
   disclosure; *guidelines; *informed consent; patient care; *physicians; *General Medical Council (Great Britain); *Great Britain

Blustein, Jeffrey. Choosing for others as continuing a life story: the problem of personal identity revisited. *Journal of Law, Medicine and Ethics.* 1999 Spring; 27(1): 20–31. 37 fn. Commented on by M.G. Kuczewski, p. 32–36. BE61501.
   *advance directives; autonomy; communitarianism; competence; death; *decision making; dementia; *directive adherence; family members; friends; *moral policy; narrative ethics; patient care; persistent vegetative state; *personhood; philosophy; *self concept; standards; terminal care; *third party consent; time factors; Dresser, Rebecca; Robertson, John

Bogardus, Sidney T.; Holmboe, Eric; Jekel, James F. Perils, pitfalls, and possibilities in talking about medical risk. *JAMA.* 1999 Mar 17; 281(11): 1037–1041. 37 refs. BE61703.
   *communication; comprehension; decision making; *disclosure; *informed consent; patients; *risk; risks and benefits; treatment outcome; uncertainty

---

BE = bioethics accession number   fn. = footnotes   refs. = references

Virtually every course of medical action is associated with some adverse risk to the patient. Discussing these risks with patients is a fundamental duty of physicians both to fulfill a role as trusted adviser and to promote the ethical principle of autonomy (particularly as embodied in the doctrine of informed consent). Discussing medical risk is a difficult task to accomplish appropriately. Challenges stem from gaps in the physician's knowledge about pertinent risks, uncertainty about how much and what kind of information to communicate, and difficulties in communicating risk information in a format that is clearly understood by most patients. For example, a discussion of the risk of undergoing a procedure should be accompanied by a discussion of the risk of not undergoing a procedure. This article describes basic characteristics of risk information, outlines major challenges in communicating risk information, and suggests several ways to communicate risk information to patients in an understandable format. Ultimately, a combination of formats (eg, qualitative, quantitative, and graphic) may best accommodate the widely varying needs, preferences, and abilities of patients. Such communication will help the physician accomplish the fundamental duty of teaching the patient the information necessary to make an informed and appropriate decision.

Brazell, Nancy E. The significance and application of informed consent. *AORN Journal (Association of Operating Room Nurses).* 1997 Feb; 65(2): 377, 379–380, 382, 385–386. 11 refs. 23 fn. BE62102.
> communication; comprehension; decision making; disclosure; ethical theory; historical aspects; *informed consent; legal aspects; medical education; *nurses; patient participation; patients' rights; physicians; standards; *surgery; Eighteenth Century; Great Britain; Twentieth Century; United States

British Medical Association; Royal College of Nursing. The Older Person: Consent and Care: Report of the British Medical Association and the Royal College of Nursing. London: British Medical Association; 1995 Apr. 63 p. 27 refs. ISBN 0-7279-0912-6. BE59169.
> advance directives; *aged; autonomy; communication; competence; confidentiality; *decision making; disclosure; family members; health facilities; human experimentation; *informed consent; institutionalized persons; nurses; patient advocacy; *patient care; patient care team; patients' rights; physical restraint; physicians; *practice guidelines; professional organizations; resuscitation orders; third party consent; treatment refusal; elder abuse; *British Medical Association; *Great Britain; *Royal College of Nursing

Butler, Dennis J.; Edwards, Ann; Tzelepis, Angela, et al. Informed consent for videotaping. [Letter and response]. *Academic Medicine.* 1996 Dec; 71(12): 1276–1277. 1 ref. BE61376.
> *audiovisual aids; *confidentiality; disclosure; *informed consent; internship and residency; *medical education; physician patient relationship; privacy; teaching methods; *video recording

Cale, Gita S. Risk-related standards of competence: continuing the debate over risk-related standards of competence. *Bioethics.* 1999 Apr; 13(2): 131–148. 28 fn. Commentary on I. Wilks, "The debate over risk-related standards of competence," *Bioethics,* 1997 Oct; 11(5): 413–426. BE61673.
> *autonomy; beneficence; *competence; *decision making; evaluation; *informed consent; *moral policy; patient care; patients; *risk; *risks and benefits; *standards; *treatment refusal
> This discussion paper addresses Ian Wilks' defence of

the risk-related standard of competence that appears in *Bioethics 11.* Wilks there argues that the puzzle posed by Mark Wicclair in *Bioethics 5* against Dan Brock's argument in favour of a risk-related standard of competence -- namely that Brock's argument allows for situations of asymmetrical competence -- is not a genuine problem for a risk-related standard of competence. To show this, Wilks presents what he believes to be two examples of real situations in which asymmetrical competence arises. I argue that insofar as Wilks equivocates two senses of competence in his examples -- namely, competence to perform a task and competence in performing a task -- Wilks is unable to illustrate the existence of real situations of asymmetrical competence. By examining the way in which Wilks equivocates two senses of competence in his examples, and by applying the results of this examination to the problem of patient competency within the medical field, I argue that not only does Wilks fail to show that situations of asymmetrical competence exist, but he is also unable to provide a foundation for understanding how the risk-related standard of competence can strike a balance between an individual's autonomy and benevolent intervention. I thus conclude that insofar as Wilks fails to answer the objections raised by Wicclair and others against the risk-related standard of competence, the risk-related standard of competence continues to be undermined by the problem of asymmetrical competence.

Capen, Karen. There's more to Krever's report than the blood issue -- much more. *Canadian Medical Association Journal.* 1998 Jan 13; 158(1): 92–94. 2 refs. BE60593.
> advisory committees; *blood transfusions; communication; disclosure; guidelines; *informed consent; mandatory reporting; patient care; physician patient relationship; physician's role; physicians; public health; standards; Canada; *Krever Report

Chalmers, Don; Schwartz, Robert. Rogers v. Whitaker and informed consent in Australia: a fair dinkum duty of disclosure. *Medical Law Review.* 1993 Summer; 1(2): 139–159. 76 fn. BE59250.
> *disclosure; *informed consent; injuries; *legal aspects; *legal liability; *negligence; patient care; *physicians; *risks and benefits; standards; surgery; *Australia; Canterbury v. Spence; Great Britain; *Rogers v. Whitaker; Sidaway v. Governors of Bethlem Royal Hospital; United States

Chapman, I.H. Informed consent: survey of Auckland, N.Z. anaesthetists' practice and attitudes. *Anaesthesia and Intensive Care.* 1997 Dec; 25(6): 671–674. 8 refs. BE61555.
> *anesthesia; *disclosure; guidelines; *informed consent; *knowledge, attitudes, practice; patient care; patient education; *physicians; risk; survey; *anesthesiology; questionnaires; *Auckland; Medical Council of New Zealand; *New Zealand

Charland, Louis C. Appreciation and emotion: theoretical reflections on the MacArthur Treatment Competence Study. *Kennedy Institute of Ethics Journal.* 1998 Dec; 8(4): 359–376. 45 refs. 5 fn. BE62373.
> alternatives; *competence; comprehension; decision making; *emotions; evaluation; goals; *informed consent; patient care; patients; risks and benefits; *standards; treatment refusal; values; MacArthur Treatment Competence Study
> When emotions are mentioned in the literature on mental competence, it is generally because they are thought to influence competence negatively; that is, they are thought to impede or compromise the cognitive capacities that are taken to underlie competence. The purpose of the present discussion is to explore the

---

BE = bioethics accession number   fn. = footnotes   refs. = references

possibility that emotions might play a more positive role in the determination of competence. Using the MacArthur Treatment Competence Study as an example, it is argued that *appreciation*, a central theoretical concept in many contemporary approaches to competence, has important emotive components that are seldom sufficiently recognized or acknowledged. If true, this means that some leading contemporary accounts of competence need to be revised in order to make more adequate provision for the positive contribution of emotion.

Collopy, Bart J. The moral underpinning of the proxy–provider relationship: issues of trust and distrust. *Journal of Law, Medicine and Ethics.* 1999 Spring; 27(1): 37–45. 25 fn. BE61503.
    *advance directives; advisory committees; autonomy; communication; competence; conflict of interest; *consensus; *decision making; *directive adherence; *family members; *family relationship; friends; motivation; patients; physician patient relationship; physicians; *professional family relationship; *standards; *third party consent; *trust; values; New York State Task Force on Life and the Law; President's Commission for the Study of Ethical Problems

Csillag, Claudio. Brazil abolishes "presumed consent" in organ donation. [News]. *Lancet.* 1998 Oct 24; 352(9137): 1367. BE60270.
    *cadavers; *family members; *legal aspects; *organ donation; *presumed consent; *third party consent; *Brazil

Daar, Judith F. Informed consent: defining limits through therapeutic parameters. *Whittier Law Review.* 1995; 16(1): 187–209. 60 fn. BE59214.
    biomedical research; cancer; *disclosure; economics; HIV seropositivity; iatrogenic disease; incentives; *informed consent; investigators; *legal aspects; legal liability; mortality; patents; patient care; patients; physician patient relationship; physicians; prognosis; property rights; research subjects; *standards; surgery; tissue donation; treatment outcome; truth disclosure; cell lines; *Arato v. Avedon; California; *Faya v. Almaraz; Maryland; Moore v. Regents of the University of California; *United States

Doyal, Len. Moral quality entails a high standard of informed consent. [Editorial]. *Quality in Health Care.* 1998 Jun; 7(2): 63–64. 21 refs. BE62321.
    communication; consent forms; disclosure; government regulation; *informed consent; patient care; quality of health care; standards; treatment refusal; Department of Health (Great Britain); *Great Britain

Dunne, Cara; Warren, Catherine. Lethal autonomy: the malfunction of the informed consent mechanism within the context of prenatal diagnosis of genetic variants. *Issues in Law and Medicine.* 1998 Fall; 14(2): 165–202. 75 fn. BE62011.
    *autonomy; cancer; directive counseling; disclosure; Down syndrome; *eugenics; *genetic counseling; genetic disorders; genetic screening; genome mapping; health personnel; historical aspects; *informed consent; killing; legal liability; mentally retarded; minority groups; National Socialism; physician's role; *prenatal diagnosis; quality of life; selective abortion; social discrimination; sterilization (sexual); wrongful life; Germany; Human Genome Project; Twentieth Century; United States

Elliott, Carl. Patients doubtfully capable or incapable of consent. *In:* Kuhse, Helga; Singer, Peter, eds. A Companion to Bioethics. Malden, MA: Blackwell; 1998: 452–462. 26 refs. ISBN 0–631–19737–0. BE59518.
    adults; altruism; autonomy; brain pathology; children; *competence; decision making; depressive disorder; family

members; human experimentation; *informed consent; mentally disabled; parental consent; patient care; persistent vegetative state; *third party consent

Erin, Charles A. Some comments on the ethics of consent to the use of ovarian tissue from aborted fetuses and dead women. *In:* Harris, John; Holm, Søren, eds. The Future of Human Reproduction: Ethics, Choice, and Regulation. New York, NY: Oxford University Press; 1998: 162–175. 33 fn. ISBN 0–19–823761–8. BE61268.
    *aborted fetuses; advance directives; autonomy; *cadavers; decision making; disclosure; dissent; family members; *fetal tissue donation; germ cells; *informed consent; legal aspects; *ovum donors; parental consent; posthumous reproduction; presumed consent; third party consent; *tissue donation; *ovaries; Great Britain; Human Tissue Act 1961 (Great Britain)

Fins, Joseph J. Commentary: from contract to covenant in advance care planning. *Journal of Law, Medicine and Ethics.* 1999 Spring; 27(1): 46–51. 29 fn. BE61504.
    *advance care planning; *advance directives; allowing to die; artificial feeding; autonomy; case studies; clinical ethics committees; *contracts; *covenant; *decision making; dementia; *directive adherence; family members; *family relationship; friends; living wills; love; marital relationship; moral obligations; patients; physicians; prolongation of life; resuscitation; resuscitation orders; risks and benefits; terminal care; *third party consent; treatment refusal; trust; withholding treatment

Freda, Margaret Comerford; DeVore, Nancy; Valentine–Adams, Nancy, et al. Informed consent for maternal serum alpha–fetoprotein screening in an inner city population: how informed is it? *Journal of Obstetric, Gynecologic and Neonatal Nursing.* 1998 Jan–Feb; 27(1): 99–106. 32 refs. BE62061.
    *comprehension; congenital disorders; disadvantaged; disclosure; *informed consent; knowledge, attitudes, practice; *minority groups; nurse's role; *pregnant women; *prenatal diagnosis; survey; *alpha fetoproteins; prospective studies; qualitative research; *urban population; United States

Freedman, Benjamin. Duty and Healing: Foundations of a Jewish Bioethic. New York, NY: Routledge; 1999. 344 p. (Reflective bioethics). 413 fn. With an introduction by Charles Weijer. ISBN 0–415–92180–5. BE61646.
    aged; allowing to die; artificial feeding; autonomy; *bioethical issues; *bioethics; case studies; coercion; *competence; cosmetic surgery; *decision making; drugs; ethical analysis; *ethicist's role; *ethics consultation; *family members; *family relationship; health; hospitals; human experimentation; *informed consent; *Jewish ethics; mentally ill; methods; *moral obligations; occupational exposure; palliative care; paralysis; parent child relationship; *patient care; physician's role; prolongation of life; quality of life; *rights; risks and benefits; secularism; suffering; terminal care; theology; third party consent; treatment refusal; truth disclosure; uncertainty; value of life; unproven therapies

Frolik, Lawrence A., ed. Health care decision making. *In:* his Aging and the Law: An Interdisciplinary Reader. Philadelphia, PA: Temple University Press; 1999: 295–394. 14 refs. 296 fn. ISBN 1–56639–653–0. BE61059.
    advance care planning; advance directives; *aged; *allowing to die; *assisted suicide; attitudes; *autonomy; chronically ill; clinical ethics; coercion; communication; *competence; critically ill; cultural pluralism; *decision making; disclosure; family members; hospitals; *informed consent; judicial action; *legal aspects; mentally disabled; minority groups; nursing homes; patient advocacy; *patient care; patient care team; patients; persistent vegetative state; physicians; prolongation of life; resource allocation; resuscitation; *right

---

BE = bioethics accession number   fn. = footnotes   refs. = references

to die; standards; suffering; *terminal care; terminally ill; *third party consent; treatment refusal; truth disclosure; voluntary euthanasia; wedge argument; withholding treatment; In re Fiori; In re Milton; Medicaid; Medicare; Pocono Medical Center v. Harley; Study to Understand Prognoses and Preferences for Outcomes and Risks of Treatments (SUPPORT); Uniform Health Care Decisions Act 1993; *United States

Goldworth, Amnon. Informed consent in the genetic age. *Cambridge Quarterly of Healthcare Ethics.* 1999 Summer; 8(3): 393–400. 15 fn. BE62482.
  *autonomy; breast cancer; *cancer; *confidentiality; cultural pluralism; *disclosure; family members; genetic counseling; *genetic information; genetic predisposition; *genetic screening; *informed consent; physician patient relationship; risk; risks and benefits; standards; trust

Griffiths, John R. Consent -- Scots law and the patient's right to know. *Medicine and Law.* 1996; 15(1): 1–6. BE61202.
  compensation; contraception; diagnosis; *disclosure; drugs; eye diseases; infertility; *informed consent; injuries; *legal liability; negligence; patient care; *physicians; psychological stress; risk; risks and benefits; surgery; Cosgrove v. Lothian Health Board; Goorkani v. Tayside Health Board; Ingram v. Ritchie; Moyes v. Lothian Health Board; *Scotland

Hartshorne, J.E. Principles of valid informed consent to treatment in dentistry. *Journal of the Dental Association of South Africa.* 1993 Aug; 48(8): 465–468. BE60694.
  autonomy; competence; comprehension; *dentistry; disclosure; *informed consent; patient care; practice guidelines

Holzer, Jacob C.; Gansler, David A.; Moczynski, Nancy P., et al. Cognitive functions in the informed consent evaluation process: a pilot study. *Journal of the American Academy of Psychiatry and the Law.* 1997; 25(4): 531–540. 22 refs. BE59150.
  comparative studies; *competence; decision making; *evaluation; hospitals; *informed consent; patient care; *patients; psychiatry; survey; cognition disorders; Lemuel Shattuck Hospital (Boston, MA)

Houghton, D.J.; Williams, S.; Bennett, J.D., et al. Informed consent: patients' and junior doctors' perceptions of the consent procedure. *Clinical Otolaryngology.* 1997 Dec; 22(6): 515–518. 11 refs. BE62458.
  *attitudes; competence; consent forms; disclosure; hospitals; *informed consent; *knowledge, attitudes, practice; patient care team; *patient satisfaction; *patients; *physicians; risks and benefits; *surgery; survey; Great Britain; Royal Liverpool Hospital

Illinois. Appellate Court, First District, Fourth Division. In re Estate of Austwick. *North Eastern Reporter, 2d Series.* 1995 Sep 7 (date of decision). 656: 773–779. BE59974.
  aged; competence; *decision making; institutionalized persons; *legal aspects; *legal guardians; nursing homes; patient care; psychoactive drugs; *resuscitation orders; *third party consent; Illinois; *In re Estate of Austwick
The Illinois Appellate Court for the First District held that a public guardian is not authorized to enter a do–not–resuscitate (DNR) order into a ward's medical chart when the ward has the decisional capacity to forgo life–sustaining treatment. Lucille Austwick, an 81–year–old woman in a nursing home, was adjudicated as disabled under the state's probate act and appointed a public guardian. The guardian entered a DNR order into Austwick's chart with her consent. Austwick petitioned the court one year later to have the order

removed. The court here affirmed the trial court's order for removal of the DNR order because the guardian lacked authority to enter the order. Austwick had further argued that her public guardian should be removed for cause because he lacked legal authority when he consented to the DNR order and to psychotropic medication treatment. The court held that the public guardian's erroneous misinterpretation of the probate act was without bad faith and did not prejudice Austwick and, thus, did not warrant removal for cause. (KIE abstract)

Kapp, Marshall B. Commentary: anxieties as a legal impediment to the doctor–proxy relationship. *Journal of Law, Medicine and Ethics.* 1999 Spring; 27(1): 69–73. 31 fn. BE61506.
  administrators; *advance directives; *allowing to die; *decision making; *dissent; emotions; family members; futility; health facilities; information dissemination; institutional policies; knowledge, attitudes, practice; legal aspects; *legal liability; malpractice; motivation; *physicians; *professional family relationship; *prolongation of life; psychological stress; public policy; terminal care; *third party consent; treatment refusal; withholding treatment; risk management; United States

Karlawish, Jason H.T. Shared decision making in critical care: a clinical reality and an ethical necessity. *American Journal of Critical Care.* 1996 Nov; 5(6): 391–396. 29 refs. BE62006.
  allowing to die; communication; comprehension; *critically ill; *decision making; disclosure; family members; futility; *informed consent; *intensive care units; interprofessional relations; *narrative ethics; nurses; *patient care; patient care team; patient participation; physicians; professional family relationship; professional patient relationship; risk; standards; *third party consent; values; *withholding treatment

Khanna, Vikram; Silverman, Henry; Schwartz, Jack. Disclosure of operating practices by managed–care organizations to consumers of healthcare: obligations of informed consent. *Journal of Clinical Ethics.* 1998 Fall; 9(3): 291–296. 27 fn. BE61337.
  autonomy; beneficence; conflict of interest; *disclosure; economics; federal government; government regulation; incentives; *informed consent; institutional ethics; legislation; *managed care programs; *organizational policies; patients; physician patient relationship; physicians; state government; withholding treatment; capitation fee; Employee Retirement Income Security Act 1974 (ERISA); Maryland; United States

Kuczewski, Mark G. Commentary: narrative views of personal identity and substituted judgment in surrogate decision making. *Journal of Law, Medicine and Ethics.* 1999 Spring; 27(1): 32–36. 19 fn. Commentary on J. Blustein, p. 20–31. BE61502.
  *advance directives; allowing to die; autonomy; competence; *decision making; dementia; *directive adherence; family members; friends; legal aspects; living wills; moral policy; narrative ethics; persistent vegetative state; *personhood; philosophy; physicians; prolongation of life; *self concept; standards; terminal care; *third party consent; time factors; withholding treatment; Dresser, Rebecca; Robertson, John

Lloyd, A.J.; Hayes, P.D.; London, N.J.M., et al. Patients' ability to recall risk associated with treatment options. [Research letter]. *Lancet.* 1999 Feb 20; 353(9153): 645. 3 refs. BE61087.
  comprehension; counseling; *disclosure; *informed consent; *patients; preventive medicine; *recall; *risk; *risks and benefits; *surgery; survey; time factors; cerebrovascular disorders; Great Britain

---

BE = bioethics accession number   fn. = footnotes   refs. = references

McFadyen, Anne; Gledhill, Julia; Whitlow, Barry, et al. First trimester ultrasound screening carries ethical and psychological implications. [Editorial]. *BMJ (British Medical Journal).* 1998 Sep 12; 317(7160): 694–695. 11 refs. BE59883.
chromosome abnormalities; congenital disorders; disclosure; fetal development; fetuses; genetic counseling; genetic disorders; *informed consent; mass screening; *pregnant women; *prenatal diagnosis; psychological stress; *risks and benefits; selective abortion; *time factors; treatment refusal; uncertainty; *ultrasonography

Macklin, Ruth. Ethics, informed consent, and assisted reproduction. *Journal of Assisted Reproduction and Genetics.* 1995 Sep; 12(8): 484–490. 17 fn. BE60560.
autonomy; competence; comprehension; contraception; cryopreservation; cultural pluralism; decision making; developing countries; *disclosure; embryo disposition; embryos; ethical relativism; females; in vitro fertilization; infertility; *informed consent; mentally retarded; multiple pregnancy; ovum donors; parent child relationship; physicians; professional competence; *reproductive technologies; risks and benefits; surrogate mothers; treatment outcome; values; Western World

Marta, Jan. Whose consent is it anyway? A poststructuralist framing of the person in medical decision–making. *Theoretical Medicine and Bioethics.* 1998 Aug; 19(4): 353–370. 33 fn. BE60158.
*accountability; *autonomy; beneficence; communication; *competence; decision making; *emotions; *informed consent; mentally ill; *models, theoretical; patient participation; patients; personhood; *physician patient relationship; physician's role; physicians; *psychology; *psychotherapy; self concept; standards; *rationality; *poststructuralism

May, Thomas. Assessing competency without judging merit. *Journal of Clinical Ethics.* 1998 Fall; 9(3): 247–257. 23 fn. BE61333.
alternatives; *autonomy; *competence; comprehension; *decision making; evaluation; *informed consent; patient care; patients; risks and benefits; *standards; treatment outcome; treatment refusal; values

May, William E. Making health care decisions for others. *Ethics and Medics.* 1997 Jun; 22(6): 1–3. BE61720.
active euthanasia; adults; *advance directives; allowing to die; *decision making; *directive adherence; dissent; intention; moral obligations; *Roman Catholic ethics; *third party consent; values; withholding treatment; Ethical and Religious Directives for Catholic Health Care Services

Mazur, Dennis J. Medical Risk and the Right to an Informed Consent in Clinical Care and Clinical Research. Tampa, FL: American College of Physician Executives; 1998. 183 p. Includes references. ISBN 0-924674-64-4. BE59664.
advertising; communication; competence; conflict of interest; decision making; *disclosure; drug industry; drugs; emergency care; federal government; government regulation; historical aspects; *human experimentation; *informed consent; international aspects; investigator subject relationship; judicial action; *legal aspects; legal liability; legislation; *patient care; patient participation; patients; physician patient relationship; research ethics committees; research subjects; *risk; *risks and benefits; *standards; state government; Canada; Canterbury v. Spence; Eighteenth Century; Great Britain; Nineteenth Century; Twentieth Century; *United States

Mezey, Mathy; Mitty, Ethel; Ramsey, Gloria. Assessment of decision–making capacity: nursing's role. *Journal of Gerontological Nursing.* 1997 Mar; 23(3): 28–35.

40 refs. BE60385.
advance directives; aged; *competence; comprehension; *decision making; dementia; depressive disorder; disclosure; *evaluation; *informed consent; legal aspects; *nurse's role; patient care; physicians; standards; treatment refusal

Nieuw, A.D. Informed consent. *Medicine and Law.* 1993; 12(1–2): 125–130. BE60619.
allowing to die; competence; *disclosure; *informed consent; *legal aspects; legal liability; living wills; physicians; risks and benefits; third party consent; treatment refusal; truth disclosure; United States

Olick, Robert S. Deciding for Incompetent Patients: The Nature and Limits of Prospective Autonomy and Advance Directives. Ann Arbor, MI: UMI Dissertation Services; 1996. 374 p. (2 v. in 1). 436 fn. Dissertation, Ph.D. in Philosophy, Georgetown University, Dec 1996. Order No. 9720773. BE62147.
advance care planning; *advance directives; *allowing to die; *autonomy; beneficence; case studies; clinical ethics committees; *competence; consensus; *decision making; dementia; directive adherence; ethical analysis; ethical review; ethical theory; family members; government regulation; guidelines; *intention; legal aspects; legal rights; models, theoretical; *moral policy; paternalism; persistent vegetative state; *personhood; physicians; prolongation of life; risks and benefits; standards; state government; terminally ill; *third party consent; treatment refusal; values; withholding treatment; *integrity; Cruzan v. Director, Missouri Department of Health; In re Quinlan; Patient Self–Determination Act 1990; United States

O'Rourke, Kevin; Sulmasy, Daniel P.; Terry, Peter B., et al. Accuracy of substituted judgments in patients with terminal diagnoses. [Letter and response]. *Annals of Internal Medicine.* 1998 Dec 15; 129(12): 1082–1083. 4 refs. BE60077.
*allowing to die; artificial feeding; *autonomy; *decision making; *family members; *futility; patients; *persistent vegetative state; prognosis; *prolongation of life; *quality of life; risks and benefits; *third party consent; withholding treatment

O'Rourke, Kevin. Surrogate decision making: ethical issues. *Health Care Ethics USA.* 1998 Summer; 6(3): 2–3. 6 refs. BE60820.
allowing to die; *attitudes; consensus; *decision making; dementia; family members; futility; patients; persistent vegetative state; physicians; prognosis; *prolongation of life; terminally ill; *third party consent; values; withholding treatment

Pang, Mei–che Samantha. Protective truthfulness: the Chinese way of safeguarding patients in informed treatment decisions. *Journal of Medical Ethics.* 1999 Jun; 25(3): 247–253. 42 refs. BE61859.
autonomy; *beneficence; competence; confidentiality; cultural pluralism; *decision making; diagnosis; disclosure; empirical research; evaluation studies; *family members; historical aspects; hospitals; *informed consent; *medical ethics; *moral obligations; non–Western World; *nurse patient relationship; *nurses; nursing ethics; nursing research; *paternalism; patient care; patients' rights; *physician patient relationship; physicians; privacy; professional competence; prognosis; psychological stress; survey; terminal care; *third party consent; trust; *truth disclosure; value of life; values; virtues; vulnerable populations; hope; *China
The first part of this paper examines the practice of informed treatment decisions in the protective medical system in China today. The second part examines how health care professionals in China perceive and carry out their responsibilities when relaying information to vulnerable patients, based on the findings of an empirical study that I had undertaken to examine the moral

---

experience of nurses in practice situations. In the Chinese medical ethics tradition, refinement [jing] in skills and sincerity [cheng] in relating to patients are two cardinal virtues that health care professionals are required to possess. This notion of absolute sincerity carries a strong sense of parental protectiveness. The empirical findings reveal that most nurses are ambivalent about telling the truth to patients. Truth-telling would become an insincere act if a patient were to lose hope and confidence in life after learning of his or her disease. In this system of protective medical care, it is arguable as to whose interests are being protected: the patient, the family or the hospital. I would suggest that the interests of the hospital and the family members who legitimately represent the patient's interests are being honoured, but at the expense of the patient's right to know.

Post, Linda Farber; Blustein, Jeffrey; Dubler, Nancy Neveloff. The doctor-proxy relationship: an untapped resource: introduction. *Journal of Law, Medicine and Ethics.* 1999 Spring; 27(1): 5-12. 23 fn. BE61499.

> *advance care planning; *advance directives; allowing to die; alternatives; *communication; consensus; cultural pluralism; *decision making; diagnosis; disclosure; dissent; *family members; family relationship; friends; hospitals; legal aspects; living wills; mediation; medical records; models, theoretical; narrative ethics; patient care; patient education; physician patient relationship; *physicians; *professional family relationship; prognosis; prolongation of life; religion; *third party consent; trust; values; withholding treatment; values histories; United States

Powell, Tia. Extubating Mrs. K: psychological aspects of surrogate decision making. *Journal of Law, Medicine and Ethics.* 1999 Spring; 27(1): 81-86. 21 fn. BE61508.

> *advance directives; *allowing to die; caring; case studies; communication; cultural pluralism; *decision making; *dissent; *emotions; *family members; *family relationship; friends; intensive care units; justice; mediation; minority groups; physicians; *professional family relationship; *prolongation of life; psychological stress; *third party consent; treatment refusal; values; ventilators; withholding treatment; absence of proxy

Raphaely, Den. Informed consent near death: myth and actuality. *Family Systems Medicine.* 1991 Winter; 9(4): 343-370. 18 refs. BE61894.

> *communication; consensus; *decision making; disclosure; family members; *informed consent; *intensive care units; interprofessional relations; nurses; patient care team; physician patient relationship; physicians; terminally ill

Roach, William H.; Aspen Health Law and Compliance Center. Documenting consent to treatment. *In: their* Medical Records and the Law. Third Edition. Gaithersburg, MD: Aspen Publishers; 1998: 62-86. 57 fn. ISBN 0-8342-1104-1. BE62747.

> adults; alternatives; competence; *consent forms; diagnosis; *disclosure; emergency care; health facilities; health personnel; human experimentation; *informed consent; institutional policies; *legal aspects; legal liability; legislation; *medical records; minors; patient care; physicians; presumed consent; prisoners; prognosis; risks and benefits; state government; third party consent; treatment refusal; *United States

Robinson, John H.; Berry, Roberta M.; McDonnell, Kevin, eds. Issues in adult health care. *In: their* A Health Law Reader: An Interdisciplinary Approach. Durham, NC: Carolina Academic Press; 1999: 239-337. 17 fn. ISBN 0-89089-907-X. BE62294.

> adults; altruism; autonomy; cadavers; commodification; competence; computers; *confidentiality; conflict of interest;

data banks; decision making; *disclosure; duty to warn; genetic information; health care delivery; human experimentation; *informed consent; justice; *legal aspects; legal liability; medical records; mentally ill; negligence; *organ donation; organ donors; *organ transplantation; patient care; physician patient relationship; physicians; *privacy; psychotherapy; public health; public policy; quality of health care; remuneration; resource allocation; risks and benefits; social dominance; torts; Tarasoff v. Regents of the University of California; Uniform Anatomical Gift Act; United States

Rosoff, Arnold J. Informed consent in the electronic age. *American Journal of Law and Medicine.* 1999; 25(2-3): 367-386. 73 fn. BE62505.

> audiovisual aids; communication; comprehension; computer communication networks; *computers; disclosure; industry; information dissemination; *informed consent; legal liability; patient care; *patient education; *physician patient relationship; physician's role; risks and benefits; social impact; trends; *telemedicine; Internet

Sabatino, Charles P. The legal and functional status of the medical proxy: suggestions for statutory reform. *Journal of Law, Medicine and Ethics.* 1999 Spring; 27(1): 52-68. 92 fn. BE61505.

> *advance directives; allowing to die; autonomy; comparative studies; conflict of interest; conscience; contracts; *decision making; directive adherence; dissent; evaluation; family members; family relationship; friends; health facilities; historical aspects; institutional policies; judicial action; law; *legal aspects; *legal obligations; legislation; *living wills; model legislation; patient advocacy; patient transfer; physicians; professional family relationship; *public policy; *standards; *state government; terminal care; *third party consent; *United States

Schneider, Carl E. The Practice of Autonomy: Patients, Doctors, and Medical Decisions. New York, NY: Oxford University Press; 1998. 307 p. 1,224 fn. ISBN 0-19-511397-7. BE59665.

> attitudes; *autonomy; bioethics; cancer; caring; chronically ill; *communication; compassion; comprehension; *decision making; disclosure; empirical research; family relationship; health care reform; *informed consent; law; literature; managed care programs; models, theoretical; narrative ethics; organization and administration; paternalism; *patient participation; *patients; *physician patient relationship; practice guidelines; professional autonomy; psychological stress; psychology; self concept; sociology of medicine; survey; terminally ill; time factors; truth disclosure; uncertainty; sick role; Great Britain; United States

Schultz, Elizabeth A. Informed consent: an overview. *CRNA: The Clinical Forum for Nurse Anesthetists.* 1998 Feb; 9(1): 2-9. 25 refs. BE62104.

> alternatives; anesthesia; autonomy; coercion; competence; consent forms; decision making; *disclosure; historical aspects; *informed consent; *legal aspects; paternalism; patients; physicians; psychological stress; risk; risks and benefits; United States

Sharma, Dinesh C. Indian organ donation goes ahead without consent. [News]. *Lancet.* 1999 Mar 27; 353(9158): 1076. BE61985.

> adults; *competence; directed donation; *family members; kidneys; *organ donation; *organ donors; parental consent; physically disabled; renal dialysis; risks and benefits; *siblings; *third party consent; *India

Slovenko, Ralph. Informed consent: information about the physician. *Medicine and Law.* 1994; 13(5-6): 467-472. 28 fn. BE60006.

> *AIDS; alcohol abuse; deception; *disclosure; iatrogenic disease; *informed consent; *internship and residency; *legal

---

liability; malpractice; *physicians; *professional competence; psychotherapy; quality of health care; values; *physician impairment; teaching hospitals; Estate of Behringer v. Medical Center at Princeton; National Practitioner Data Bank; New Jersey; United States

Slovenko, Ralph; Sugarman, Jeremy; McCrory, Douglas C., et al. Why study informed consent? [Letter and response]. *Hastings Center Report.* 1999 Jul–Aug; 29(4): 4. BE62459.
  *empirical research; *informed consent; legal aspects; United States

South Africa. Supreme Court, Cape Provincial Division. Castell v. De Greef. *South Africa Law Reports.* 1994 Feb 17 (date of decision). 1994(4): 408–441. BE59572.
  *disclosure; *informed consent; *legal aspects; negligence; patients; physicians; risk; risks and benefits; *standards; surgery; *Castell v. De Greef; *South Africa
With this decision, the South African Supreme Court established the "reasonable patient" standard for disclosure in providing informed consent. The Court defined a risk as being material if "in the circumstances of the particular case: (a) a reasonable person in the patient's position, if warned of the risk, would be likely to attach significance to it; or (b) the medical practitioner is or should reasonably be aware that the particular patient, if warned of the risk, would be likely to attach significance to it." In determining the standard of care, the Court blended the "reasonable patient" test with the individual patient's "additional needs test." Castell v. De Greef follows Australia's 1993 case, Rogers v. Whitaker and rejects Britain's 1985 case Sidaway v. Bethlem Royal Hospital Governors, which reaffirmed the Bolam principle, that the standard for disclosure is the "reasonable doctor" one. The South African Court viewed the standard as being in accord with the fundamental right of self determination and individual autonomy. The facts in Castell involved a prophylactic subcutaneous double mastectomy and simultaneous breast reconstruction using silicone implants and a transpositional flap procedure. The operation had a 50% rate of complication, which in this case involved necrosis and infection. (KIE abstract)

Spinsanti, Sandro. Obtaining consent from the family: a horizon for clinical ethics. *In:* ten Have, Henk A.M.J.; Sass, Hans–Martin, eds. Consensus Formation in Healthcare Ethics. Boston, MA: Kluwer Academic; 1998: 209–217. 5 refs. 3 fn. ISBN 0-7923-4944-X. BE62596.
  allowing to die; autonomy; beneficence; cancer; caring; case studies; consensus; *decision making; diagnosis; *family members; family relationship; paternalism; patient advocacy; *physician's role; physicians; *professional family relationship; prognosis; prolongation of life; terminal care; terminally ill; *third party consent; *truth disclosure; withholding treatment; *Italy

Stanberry, Ben. The legal and ethical aspects of telemedicine. 3: Telemedicine and malpractice. *Journal of Telemedicine and Telecare.* 1998; 4(2): 72–79. 31 fn. BE62406.
  *computer communication networks; confidentiality; consent forms; emergency care; health personnel; *informed consent; *legal liability; *malpractice; negligence; *patient care; physician patient relationship; professional competence; *referral and consultation; *standards; treatment refusal; *telemedicine; Great Britain

Sugarman, Jeremy; McCrory, Douglas C.; Powell,

Donald, et al, comps. Empirical research on informed consent: an annotated bibliography. *Hastings Center Report.* 1999 Jan–Feb; 29(1): S1–S42. 9 fn. BE61635.
  adults; aged; competence; comprehension; consent forms; disclosure; *empirical research; human experimentation; *informed consent; patient care; *patients; recall; *research subjects; selection of subjects

Sugarman, Jeremy; McCrory, Douglas C.; Hubal, Robert C. Getting meaningful informed consent from older adults: a structured literature review of empirical research. *Journal of the American Geriatrics Society.* 1998 Apr; 46(4): 517–524. 118 refs. BE60294.
  age factors; *aged; competence; comprehension; consent forms; decision making; disclosure; education; *empirical research; evaluation studies; *human experimentation; *informed consent; literature; methods; *patient care; recall; research design; research subjects; selection of subjects; refusal to participate

Tabak, Nili. Informed consent: the nurse's dilemma. *Medicine and Law.* 1996; 15(1): 7–16. 13 refs. BE61203.
  autonomy; decision making; *disclosure; *informed consent; *nurse's role; nursing education; nursing ethics; patient advocacy; *patient care; patients; physician nurse relationship; physician patient relationship; physicians; risks and benefits; *therapeutic research

Veterans Affairs National Headquarters. Bioethics Committee. Surrogate–Written Advance Directives: Report. Issued by the VA National Center for Clinical Ethics, White River Junction, VT 05009; 1996 Jan. 6 p. 9 fn. BE59266.
  *advance directives; *allowing to die; *decision making; family members; federal government; institutional policies; legal guardians; patient care; patient care team; public hospitals; terminally ill; *third party consent; withholding treatment; United States; Veterans Health Administration

Waibel, U.G.; Huber, Ch.; Riccabona, U.M., et al. Medicolegal aspects of patient information before regional anesthesia in Austria. *Acta Anaesthesiologica Scandinavica.* 1997; 111(Suppl.): 229–231. 5 refs. BE62002.
  alternatives; *anesthesia; decision making; *disclosure; *informed consent; *legal aspects; medical records; patient participation; *physicians; risks and benefits; *Austria

White, Becky Cox; Zimbelman, Joel. Abandoning informed consent: an idea whose time has not yet come. *Journal of Medicine and Philosophy.* 1998 Oct; 23(5): 477–499. 57 refs. 26 fn. Commentary on R. Veatch, "Abandoning informed consent," *Hastings Center Report,* 1995 Mar–Apr; 25(2): 5–12. Note: the journal issue cover shows a date of August 1998, which is incorrect. BE62114.
  alternatives; autonomy; beneficence; communication; decision making; disclosure; ethical analysis; goals; historical aspects; *informed consent; medicine; patient care; patient participation; *patients; physician patient relationship; *physicians; privacy; risks and benefits; *values; *Veatch, Robert
In a recent critique of informed consent, Robert Veatch argues that the practice is in principle unable to attain the goals for which it was developed. We argue that Veatch's focus on the theoretical impossibility of determining patients' best interests in misapplied to the practical discipline of medicine, and that he wrongly assumes that the patient-physician communication fails to provide the knowledge needed to insure the patient's best interests. We further argue that Veatch's suggested alternative, value-based patient-professional pairing, is, on his own terms, impossible to implement. Finally, we

---

reexamine the philosophical and practical justifications for informed consent and conclude that the practice should be retained.

Wicclair, Mark R. The continuing debate over risk-related standards of competence. *Bioethics.* 1999 Apr; 13(2): 149-153. 10 fn. Commentary on I. Wilks, "The debate over risk-related standards of competence," *Bioethics*, 1997 Oct; 11(5): 413-426. BE61674.
*competence; *decision making; *informed consent; *moral policy; paternalism; patient care; patients; *risk; *risks and benefits; *standards; *treatment refusal

Wilks, Ian. Asymmetrical competence. *Bioethics.* 1999 Apr; 13(2): 154-159. 4 fn. BE61675.
*competence; *decision making; *informed consent; *moral policy; patient care; patients; *risk; *risks and benefits; *standards; *treatment refusal

Wisconsin. Court of Appeals. Schreiber v. Physicians Insurance Company. *North Western Reporter, 2d Series.* 1998 Feb 17 (date of decision). 579: 730-739. BE61998.
alternatives; *cesarean section; *childbirth; compensation; *decision making; *informed consent; injuries; *legal aspects; *legal liability; malpractice; newborns; *physicians; *pregnant women; refusal to treat; state government; *Schreiber v. Physicians Insurance Company; Wisconsin
Reversing a trial court's determination, the Court of Appeals of Wisconsin held that a physician violated Wisconsin's informed consent law by refusing to honor a patient's request for a cesarean delivery when such a delivery was a viable treatment option. Janice Schreiber initially requested a vaginal delivery but later requested a cesarean delivery three separate times. The court held that the right to select medical treatment also encompasses a right to change one's mind. During the delay that ensued as a result of the physician's failure to deliver by cesarean, Janice's uterus ruptured depriving the child of oxygen that caused her to be born with spastic quadriplegia. The court did not apply its traditional objective test (reasonable person) in determining causation in informed consent breach, instead determining directly whether the damages were a result of the physician's failure to honor the patient's request. The court specially noted that it was not ruling on a case where the physician is ethically opposed to the treatment option or where the treatment option falls outside the physician's practice and experience. (KIE abstract)

Wisconsin. Supreme Court. Schreiber v. Physicians Insurance Company. *North Western Reporter, 2d Series.* 1999 Jan 26 (date of decision). 588: 26-35. BE61999.
alternatives; *cesarean section; *childbirth; compensation; *decision making; *informed consent; injuries; *legal aspects; *legal liability; malpractice; *newborns; *physicians; *pregnant women; refusal to treat; state government; *Schreiber v. Physicians Insurance Company; Wisconsin
The Supreme Court of Wisconsin held that once a patient withdraws consent for a procedure or when medical circumstances change, a physician is obligated to conduct another informed consent discussion. Janice Schreiber consented to a vaginal delivery but later requested a cesarean delivery on three separate occasions. The court held that these separate requests constituted a withdrawal of consent and at the time of the withdrawal there existed medically viable options for treatment which required a new informed consent discussion. The court explicitly rejected the notion that once a procedure has been initiated the time for a decision and discussions relating to that decision have passed. During the delay that ensued as a result of the

physician's failure to deliver by cesarean section, Janice's uterus ruptured depriving the child of oxygen that caused her to be born with spastic quadriplegia. The court applied a subjective test when determining causation instead of the traditional objective (reasonable person) test. The court explicitly held that its ruling did not create a patient right to demand any treatment desired, a requirement that physicians perform procedures they do not consider medically viable, a requirement that physicians perform procedures for which they lack appropriate training, or a requirement that physicians perform procedures to which they are morally opposed. (KIE abstract)

Young, Robert. Informed consent and patient autonomy. *In:* Kuhse, Helga; Singer, Peter, eds. A Companion to Bioethics. Malden, MA: Blackwell; 1998: 441-451. 11 refs. ISBN 0-631-19737-0. BE59517.
alternatives; *autonomy; coercion; competence; decision making; disclosure; *informed consent; legal aspects; patient care; patient participation; risks and benefits; Australia; United States

Zelenik, Jomarie; Post, Linda Farber; Mulvihill, Michael, et al. The doctor-proxy relationship: perception and communication. *Journal of Law, Medicine and Ethics.* 1999 Spring; 27(1): 13-19. 16 fn. BE61500.
*advance care planning; *advance directives; aged; allowing to die; artificial feeding; *attitudes; *communication; comparative studies; *competence; *decision making; *family members; friends; hospitals; *knowledge, attitudes, practice; medical records; *patient care; patient care team; patient participation; *physicians; *professional family relationship; resuscitation orders; statistics; surgery; survey; *third party consent; ventilators; withholding treatment; retrospective studies; Montefiore Medical Center (Bronx, NY); New York City

A birth spurs debate on using sperm after death. [Editorial]. *New York Times.* 1999 Mar 27: All. BE60873.
cadavers; cryopreservation; *informed consent; married persons; *posthumous reproduction; *semen donors; sperm; United States

INFORMED CONSENT/MENTALLY DISABLED

American Geriatrics Society. Ethics Committee. Informed consent for research on human subjects with dementia. [Position statement]. *Journal of the American Geriatrics Society.* 1998 Oct; 46(10): 1308-1310. Position statement prepared by Greg A. Sachs; reviewed and approved by the American Geriatrics Society Ethics Committee and by the American Geriatrics Society Board of Directors, May 1998. BE62266.
advance directives; competence; decision making; *dementia; ethical review; family members; federal government; government regulation; *human experimentation; *informed consent; nontherapeutic research; *organizational policies; patient participation; professional organizations; public participation; research design; research ethics committees; research subjects; risk; risks and benefits; selection of subjects; state government; therapeutic research; *third party consent; refusal to participate; *American Geriatrics Society; United States

Appelbaum, Binyamin C.; Appelbaum, Paul S.; Grisso, Thomas. Competence to consent to voluntary psychiatric hospitalization: a test of a standard proposed by APA. *Psychiatric Services.* 1998 Sep; 49(9): 1193-1196. 15 refs. BE61531.
*competence; *comprehension; consent forms; disclosure; *evaluation; evaluation studies; *informed consent; institutionalized persons; mental institutions; *mentally ill;

BE = bioethics accession number   fn. = footnotes   refs. = references

*recall; *standards; *voluntary admission; American Psychiatric Association; University of Massachusetts Medical Center

Berghmans, Ron L.P. Ethical hazards of the substituted judgement test in decision making concerning the end of life of dementia patients. [Editorial]. *International Journal of Geriatric Psychiatry.* 1997 Mar; 12(3): 283–287. 23 refs. BE59429.
    advance directives; *aged; *allowing to die; autonomy; competence; *decision making; *dementia; family members; *patient care; personhood; physicians; prolongation of life; quality of life; risks and benefits; *third party consent; time factors; treatment refusal; value of life; oral directives; personal identity

Birleson, Peter. Legal rights and responsibilities of adolescents and staff in Victorian Child and Adolescent Mental Health Services. *Australian and New Zealand Journal of Psychiatry.* 1996 Dec; 30(6): 805–812. 14 refs. BE61807.
    *adolescents; behavior disorders; competence; consensus; *decision making; *health personnel; *informed consent; institutionalized persons; involuntary commitment; judicial action; *legal aspects; *legal guardians; legal rights; mental institutions; *mentally ill; *parental consent; *parents; *patient care; physical restraint; professional family relationship; psychoactive drugs; third party consent; treatment refusal; mental health services; Australia; Mental Health Act 1986 (Victoria); *Victoria

Brakman, Sarah-Vaughan; Amari-Vaught, Eileen. Resistance and refusal. [Case study and commentaries]. *Hastings Center Report.* 1999 Jan–Feb; 29(1): 22–23. BE61632.
    anesthesia; autonomy; beneficence; case studies; competence; decision making; dissent; females; health personnel; legal aspects; legal guardians; *mentally retarded; obstetrics and gynecology; preventive medicine; residential facilities; risks and benefits; *third party consent; *treatment refusal

Derse, Arthur R. Making decisions about life-sustaining medical treatment in patients with dementia: the problem of patient decision-making capacity. *Theoretical Medicine and Bioethics.* 1999 Jan; 20(1): 55–67. 42 refs. BE62124.
    *aged; *allowing to die; assisted suicide; autonomy; beneficence; case studies; *compensation; comprehension; *decision making; *dementia; diagnosis; emergency care; heart diseases; human experimentation; *informed consent; patient care; patient participation; *prolongation of life; quality of life; recall; *resuscitation; standards; surgery; third party consent; *treatment refusal; truth disclosure; withholding treatment; rationality

Fellows, Lesley K. Competency and consent in dementia. *Journal of the American Geriatrics Society.* 1998 Jul; 46(7): 922–926. 20 refs. BE62261.
    *advance directives; *aged; autonomy; beneficence; coercion; communication; *competence; *decision making; *dementia; family members; *informed consent; *patient care; patient participation; personhood; physicians; *risks and benefits; self concept; standards; terminal care; *third party consent; time factors; values

Fennell, Phil. Statutory authority to treat, relatives and treatment proxies. *Medical Law Review.* 1994 Spring; 2(1): 30–56. 100 fn. BE59760.
    advisory committees; competence; comprehension; *decision making; disclosure; emergency care; *family members; health personnel; informed consent; *legal aspects; legal liability; legal obligations; *mentally disabled; mentally ill; mentally retarded; patient care; public policy; referral and consultation; risks and benefits; *third party consent; treatment refusal; *Great Britain; *Law Commission (Great Britain)

Freeman, Michael. Deciding for the intellectually impaired. *Medical Law Review.* 1994 Spring; 2(1): 77–91. 75 fn. BE59997.
    abortion, induced; advisory committees; alternatives; artificial feeding; competence; *decision making; *judicial action; *legal aspects; *mentally disabled; nontherapeutic research; patient advocacy; patient care; public policy; risks and benefits; sterilization (sexual); *third party consent; tissue donation; withholding treatment; *Great Britain; *Law Commission (Great Britain)

Gilhooly, Mary L.M.; Smith, Alexander McCall; Nichols, David, eds.; Scottish Action on Dementia. Rights and Legal Protection Sub-Committee. Dementia: Consent to Treatment, Volume 1 [and] Dementia: Consent to Research, Volume 2. Two Discussion Papers. Edinburgh, Scotland: Scottish Action on Dementia; 1992 Mar. 52 p. (Dementia: human rights series). ISBN 0-948897-14-7. BE59473.
    advance directives; autonomy; behavioral research; clinical ethics committees; *competence; decision making; *dementia; drugs; emergency care; family members; genetic research; *human experimentation; *informed consent; *legal aspects; legal guardians; moral policy; nontherapeutic research; paternalism; *patient care; physicians; research ethics committees; risk; risks and benefits; therapeutic research; *third party consent; treatment refusal; value of life; needs; Mental Health (Scotland) Act 1984; *Scotland

Great Britain. England. High Court of Justice. Family Division. Re H (Mental Patients: Diagnosis). *Family Law Reports.* 1992 Jul 1 (date of decision). [1993] 1: 28–33. BE60045.
    anesthesia; brain pathology; competence; decision making; *diagnosis; *judicial action; *legal aspects; *mentally ill; methods; *patient care; physicians; risks and benefits; schizophrenia; *third party consent; *Great Britain; *Re H (Mental Patient: Diagnosis)
England's High Court of Justice, Family Division, dismissed a health authority's application for a judicial declaration that a proposed diagnostic procedure on a mentally ill woman incapable of consent was lawful, because such a declaration "might be an unfortunate signal to others in the future that it was appropriate, as a matter of good medical practice, for the implementation of such procedures to be delayed pending the outcome of a costly application to the court." H, age 25, suffered from schizophrenia. Doctors suspected that she had a brain tumor and wanted to give her a diagnostic CT brain scan. H would require heavy sedation under general anesthesia and an injection of the contrast medium. H hated needles, would likely be non-cooperative, and lacked any capacity for informed consent. Her parents strongly supported the procedure as did the Official Solicitor, who represented H as guardian *ad litem*. The Official Solicitor, however, opposed a judicial application as inappropriate, because the doctors had already decided that the brain scan was in H's best interest. The court found no distinction between therapeutic and diagnostic procedures. In this circumstance the court agreed with the Official Solicitor that a judicial declaration would not be appropriate. The court found that the proposed brain scan was clearly in H's best interests. Accordingly, as the court quoted from *Re F (Sterilisation: Mental Patient)*, "a doctor can lawfully operate on, or give other treatment to, adult patients who are incapable, for one reason or another, of consenting to his doing so, provided that the operation or other treatment is in the best interests of such patients." (KIE abstract).

Great Britain. England. High Court of Justice, Family

Division. Re K, W and H (Minors) (Medical Treatment). *Family Law Reports.* 1992 Sep 10 (date of decision). 1993: 854–859. BE59973.

adolescents; behavior disorders; competence; emergency care; *informed consent; *legal aspects; mental institutions; *mentally ill; *minors; *parental consent; *treatment refusal; Children Act 1989 (Great Britain); *Great Britain; Mental Health Act 1983 (Great Britain); *Re K, W and H (Minors) (Medical Treatment); Re R (A Minor) (Wardship: Medical Treatment)

The Family Division of the High Court of Justice of England's Supreme Court of Judicature refused to rule on a mental hospital's application for clarification of the law regarding consent of minors to receive emergency medication under the Mental Health Act and the Children Act. Three girls, all about 15 years of age, had been admitted for psychiatric care at St. Andrew's Hospital and, prior to their admission, consent for use of medication in emergency situations had been obtained from their parents. After complaints had been received from the girls that they had not consented to receive medication and about other matters, a committee investigation and report followed. The committee recommended that a court ruling be obtained on the issue. The court found the hospital's application "misconceived and unnecessary." Following the Court of Appeal in *Re R (A Minor) (Wardship: Medical Treatment)*, the court held that "a child with *Gillick* competence can consent to treatment, but if he or she declines to do so, consent can be given by someone else who has parental rights or responsibilities." In this case, none of the patients were *Gillick* competent, and even if that was not the case, any refusal of treatment would not put the hospital or doctors at risk for liability because the requisite parental consent had been obtained. (KIE abstract)

Gunn, Michael. The meaning of incapacity. *Medical Law Review.* 1994 Spring; 2(1): 8–29. 93 fn. BE59901.

adults; autonomy; *competence; comprehension; *informed consent; *legal aspects; *mentally disabled; patient care; *standards; third party consent; treatment refusal; *Great Britain; *Law Commission (Great Britain)

Kitamura, Fusako; Tomoda, Atsuko; Tsukada, Kazumi, et al. Method for assessment of competency to consent in the mentally ill: rationale, development, and comparison with the medically ill. *International Journal of Law and Psychiatry.* 1998 Summer; 21(3): 223–244. 35 refs. 18 fn. BE61668.

autonomy; comparative studies; *competence; comprehension; disclosure; due process; *evaluation; *informed consent; involuntary commitment; legal aspects; legal rights; *mentally ill; methods; patient care; patients; treatment refusal; Japan; United States

McCubbin, Michael; Weisstub, David N. Toward a pure best interests model of proxy decision making for incompetent psychiatric patients. *International Journal of Law and Psychiatry.* 1998 Winter; 21(1): 1–30. 202 refs. 12 fn. BE59928.

advance directives; autonomy; beneficence; coercion; common good; *competence; constitutional law; *decision making; family members; federal government; *goals; institutionalized persons; judicial action; *legal aspects; *mentally ill; paternalism; *patient care; physicians; psychiatric wills; psychiatry; psychoactive drugs; review; risks and benefits; *standards; state interest; *third party consent; time factors; treatment refusal; uncertainty; values; U.S. v. Charters; United States; Washington v. Harper

McHale, J.V. Mental incapacity: some proposals for legislative reform. *Journal of Medical Ethics.* 1998 Oct;

24(5): 322–327. 67 fn. BE60254.

adults; advance directives; advisory committees; allowing to die; blood transfusions; *competence; *decision making; evaluation; family members; *informed consent; *judicial action; *legal aspects; *legislation; *mentally disabled; nontherapeutic research; patient care; persistent vegetative state; practice guidelines; *public policy; risks and benefits; *standards; sterilization (sexual); *third party consent; tissue donation; *treatment refusal; withholding treatment; *Who Decides? Making Decisions on Behalf of Mentally Incompetent Patients; Airedale NHS Trust v. Bland; *Great Britain; House of Lords Select Committee on Medical Ethics; *Law Commission (Great Britain); Re C (Adult: Refusal of Treatment); Re F (Mental Patient: Sterilisation); Re T (Adult: Refusal of Medical Treatment)

While the decision of the House of Lords in Re F in [1990] clarified somewhat the law concerning the treatment of the mentally incapacitated adult, many uncertainties remained. This paper explores proposals discussed in a recent government green paper for reform of the law in an area involving many difficult ethical dilemmas.

Marson, Daniel C.; Chatterjee, Anjan; Ingram, Kellie K., et al. Toward a neurologic model of competency: cognitive predictors of capacity to consent in Alzheimer's disease using three different legal standards. *Neurology.* 1996 Mar; 46(3): 666–672. 40 refs. BE60400.

*competence; comprehension; *dementia; *evaluation; *informed consent; legal aspects; patient care; recall; *standards

O'Neill, Patrick. Negotiating Consent in Psychotherapy. New York, NY: New York University Press; 1998. 188 p. (Qualitative studies in psychology). Bibliography: p. 177–183. ISBN 0-8147-6195-X. BE61647.

adolescents; adults; alternatives; attitudes; behavior disorders; child abuse; coercion; *communication; confidentiality; dangerousness; disclosure; duty to warn; food; *health personnel; *informed consent; *knowledge, attitudes, practice; parental consent; patients; prisoners; *professional patient relationship; *psychology; *psychotherapy; sex offenses; survey; anorexia nervosa; bulimia; negotiation; qualitative research

Purtell, Dennis J.; Brakman, Sarah-Vaughan. Autonomy and the mentally disabled. [Letter and response]. *Hastings Center Report.* 1999 Jul–Aug; 29(4): 5. BE62461.

autonomy; beneficence; institutionalized persons; legal guardians; *mentally retarded; obstetrics and gynecology; preventive medicine; risks and benefits; *third party consent; *treatment refusal

Royal College of Psychiatrists. Consent of Non-Volitional Patients and *De Facto* Detention of Informal Patients. Issued by the Royal College of Psychiatrists, 17 Belgrave Sq., London SW1X 8PG, England; 1989 Oct. 23 p. 18 refs. Council Report CR6. Appendixes include "Legal minors" by J. Hendriks, "Assent to operation by medical staff where patient unable to give consent" by Frenchay Health Authority, "Exercising restraint" by B. Pitt, and "Sterilisation of a mentally incapable woman" by D. Brahams. BE60353.

*behavior control; coercion; *competence; consent forms; decision making; dementia; *informed consent; institutionalized persons; legal aspects; *mentally disabled; mentally retarded; minors; organizational policies; *patient care; *physical restraint; professional organizations; sterilization (sexual); third party consent; *Great Britain; *Royal College of Psychiatrists; Scotland

Shapiro, Robyn S. In re Edna MF: case law confusion in surrogate decision making. *Theoretical Medicine and*

Bioethics. 1999 Jan; 20(1): 45–54. 22 refs. 3 fn. BE62123.
advance directives; *allowing to die; artificial feeding; competence; constitutional law; *decision making; *dementia; equal protection; freedom; judicial action; *legal aspects; legal guardians; legal rights; persistent vegetative state; *risks and benefits; terminally ill; *third party consent; withholding treatment; Fourteenth Amendment; *In re Guardianship and Protective Placement of Edna M.; *Wisconsin

Wilson, Petra. The Law Commission's report on mental incapacity: medically vulnerable adults or politically vulnerable law? *Medical Law Review.* 1996 Autumn; 4(3): 227–249. 83 fn. BE61511.
adults; *advance directives; advisory committees; *competence; *decision making; dementia; human experimentation; informed consent; judicial action; *legal aspects; legal guardians; *mentally disabled; mentally retarded; model legislation; patient care; persistent vegetative state; public policy; standards; *third party consent; treatment refusal; *Great Britain; *Law Commission (Great Britain)

INFORMED CONSENT/MINORS

Allen, Keith D.; Hodges, Eric D.; Knudsen, Sharon K. Comparing four methods to inform parents about child behavior management: how to inform for consent. *Pediatric Dentistry.* 1995 May–Jun; 17(3): 180–186. 20 refs. BE62416.
*attitudes; audiovisual aids; *behavior control; *communication; comparative studies; consent forms; *dentistry; *disclosure; informed consent; *methods; *minors; *parental consent; *parents; patient compliance; pediatrics; Nebraska; University of Nebraska Pediatric Dental Clinic

Birleson, Peter. Legal rights and responsibilities of adolescents and staff in Victorian Child and Adolescent Mental Health Services. *Australian and New Zealand Journal of Psychiatry.* 1996 Dec; 30(6): 805–812. 14 refs. BE61807.
*adolescents; behavior disorders; competence; consensus; *decision making; *health personnel; *informed consent; institutionalized persons; involuntary commitment; judicial action; *legal aspects; *legal guardians; legal rights; mental institutions; *mentally ill; *parental consent; *parents; *patient care; physical restraint; professional family relationship; psychoactive drugs; third party consent; treatment refusal; mental health services; Australia; Mental Health Act 1986 (Victoria); *Victoria

Dickenson, Donna L.; Geller, Gail. Can children and young people consent to be tested for adult onset genetic disorders? [and] Weighing burdens and benefits rather than competence. [Article and commentary]. *BMJ (British Medical Journal).* 1999 Apr 17; 318(7190): 1063–1066. 36 refs. BE62451.
*adolescents; autonomy; cancer; case studies; children; *competence; genetic counseling; genetic predisposition; *genetic screening; genetic services; guidelines; health facilities; Huntington disease; *informed consent; *institutional policies; *late–onset disorders; legal aspects; parental consent; paternalism; professional organizations; *risks and benefits; Great Britain

Dickenson, Donna L.; Nicholson, Richard. Children's rights. [Letter and response]. *Hastings Center Report.* 1999 Jan–Feb; 29(1): 5. BE61628.
children; competence; *decision making; *informed consent; international aspects; legal aspects; *minors; parental consent; *treatment refusal; Great Britain; United States

Felsman, Janine P. Eliminating parental consent and

notification for adolescent HIV testing: a legitimate statutory response to the AIDS epidemic. [Note]. *Journal of Law and Policy.* 1996; 5(1): 339–383. 146 fn. BE59302.
*adolescents; *AIDS serodiagnosis; competence; *confidentiality; *counseling; *government regulation; *HIV seropositivity; *informed consent; *legal aspects; legal rights; *parental consent; *parental notification; parents; patient care; privacy; *public policy; social impact; state government; state interest; *voluntary programs; United States

Gordon, Todd E.; Zook, Eric G.; Averhoff, Francisco M., et al. Consent for adolescent vaccination: issues and current practices. *Journal of School Health.* 1997 Sep; 67(7): 259–264. 15 refs. BE59637.
*adolescents; age factors; communicable diseases; *government regulation; hepatitis; *immunization; *informed consent; minors; *parental consent; *state government; survey; *United States

Great Britain. England. High Court of Justice, Family Division. Re K, W and H (Minors) (Medical Treatment). *Family Law Reports.* 1992 Sep 10 (date of decision). 1993: 854–859. BE59973.
adolescents; behavior disorders; competence; emergency care; *informed consent; *legal aspects; mental institutions; *mentally ill; *minors; *parental consent; *treatment refusal; Children Act 1989 (Great Britain); *Great Britain; Mental Health Act 1983 (Great Britain); *Re K, W and H (Minors) (Medical Treatment); Re R (A Minor) (Wardship: Medical Treatment)
The Family Division of the High Court of Justice of England's Supreme Court of Judicature refused to rule on a mental hospital's application for clarification of the law regarding consent of minors to receive emergency medication under the Mental Health Act and the Children Act. Three girls, all about 15 years of age, had been admitted for psychiatric care at St. Andrew's Hospital and, prior to their admission, consent for use of medication in emergency situations had been obtained from their parents. After complaints had been received from the girls that they had not consented to receive medication and about other matters, a committee investigation and report followed. The committee recommended that a court ruling be obtained on the issue. The court found the hospital's application "misconceived and unnecessary." Following the Court of Appeal in *Re R (A Minor) (Wardship: Medical Treatment)*, the court held that "a child with *Gillick* competence can consent to treatment, but if he or she declines to do so, consent can be given by someone else who has parental rights or responsibilities." In this case, none of the patients were *Gillick* competent, and even if that was not the case, any refusal of treatment would not put the hospital or doctors at risk for liability because the requisite parental consent had been obtained. (KIE abstract)

Holland, Julie. Should parents be permitted to authorize genetic testing for their children? *Family Law Quarterly.* 1997 Summer; 31(2): 321–353. 188 fn. BE62162.
*autonomy; *carriers; confidentiality; employment; genetic counseling; genetic disorders; genetic information; *genetic screening; human experimentation; informed consent; insurance selection bias; *late–onset disorders; legal aspects; legal rights; *minors; *parental consent; patient care; privacy; psychological stress; *risks and benefits; social discrimination; standards; *right not to know

Mason, John Kenyon. Consent to treatment and research in children. *In: his* Medico–Legal Aspects of Reproduction and Parenthood. Second Edition. Brookfield, VT: Ashgate; 1998: 319–339. 83 fn. ISBN

1-84104-065-8. BE61070.
adolescents; *alternative therapies; animal organs; blood transfusions; *competence; comprehension; decision making; donors; *human experimentation; *informed consent; international aspects; Jehovah's Witnesses; judicial action; *legal aspects; *minors; nontherapeutic research; *organ donation; organ donors; organ transplantation; *parental consent; *parents; *patient care; religion; research subjects; risks and benefits; siblings; state interest; therapeutic research; *tissue donation; *treatment refusal; *Great Britain; United States

Nicholls, Michael. Keyholders and flak jackets: consent to medical treatment for children. *Family Law.* 1994 Feb; 24: 81–85. BE61826.
adolescents; age factors; competence; decision making; emergency care; *informed consent; judicial action; *legal aspects; *minors; parental consent; parents; patient care; *treatment refusal; *Great Britain

Ross, Lainie Friedman. Children, Families, and Health Care Decision Making. New York, NY: Clarendon Press; 1998. 197 p. (Issues in biomedical ethics). Bibliography: p. 177–190. ISBN 0-19-823763-4. BE61944.
*adolescents; advisory committees; *autonomy; case studies; *children; *competence; *decision making; deontological ethics; directed donation; dissent; family members; *family relationship; federal government; futility; goals; government regulation; guidelines; *human experimentation; legal aspects; *minors; moral development; *moral obligations; nontherapeutic research; *organ donation; *parental consent; *parents; *patient care; pediatrics; personhood; physicians; prolongation of life; quality of life; refusal to treat; rights; risk; risks and benefits; sexuality; siblings; state interest; therapeutic research; *treatment refusal; utilitarianism; *values; liberalism; needs; National Commission for the Protection of Human Subjects; United States

St. Clair, Thomas. Informed consent in pediatric dentistry: a comprehensive overview. *Pediatric Dentistry.* 1995 Mar–Apr; 17(2): 90–97. 92 fn. BE62415.
behavior control; *dentistry; disclosure; informed consent; *legal aspects; *minors; *parental consent; patient compliance; pediatrics; physical restraint; standards; *United States

Scarnecchia, Suellyn; Field, Julie Kunce. Judging girls: decision making in parental consent to abortion cases. *Michigan Journal of Gender and Law.* 1995; 3(41): 75–123. 134 fn. BE59408.
*abortion, induced; *adolescents; *competence; counseling; *decision making; *informed consent; *judicial action; *legal aspects; legislation; *minors; *parental consent; standards; state government; Supreme Court decisions; *Michigan; United States

Williams, L.; Harris, A.; Thompson, M., et al. Consent to treatment by minors attending accident and emergency departments: guidelines. *Journal of Accident and Emergency Medicine.* 1997 Sep; 14(5): 286–289. 2 refs. BE59430.
adolescents; children; competence; critically ill; decision analysis; *emergency care; *guidelines; hospitals; *informed consent; judicial action; *legal aspects; *minors; *parental consent; *parents; physical restraint; *physicians; referral and consultation; third party consent; *treatment refusal; Children Act 1989 (Great Britain); Family Law Reform Act 1969 (Great Britain); *Great Britain

Yamamoto, Loren G. Application of informed consent principles in the emergency department evaluation of febrile children at risk for occult bacteremia. *Hawaii Medical Journal.* 1997 Nov; 56(11): 313–317, 320–322. 50 refs. BE59336.
age factors; alternatives; *attitudes; *children; consent forms; decision making; diagnosis; disclosure; drugs; *emergency care; health insurance; infants; *parental consent; *parents; patient care; physicians; risks and benefits; survey; uncertainty; antibiotics; Hawaii

INSTITUTIONAL REVIEW BOARDS *See* BEHAVIORAL RESEARCH/ETHICS COMMITTEES, HUMAN EXPERIMENTATION/ETHICS COMMITTEES

INVOLUNTARY COMMITMENT

Cascardi, Michele; Poythress, Norman G. Correlates of perceived coercion during psychiatric hospital admission. *International Journal of Law and Psychiatry.* 1997 Fall; 20(4): 445–458. 28 refs. BE59339.
attitudes; *coercion; comparative studies; empirical research; family members; health personnel; incentives; *institutionalized persons; *involuntary commitment; law enforcement; mental institutions; *mentally ill; *patient admission; patient satisfaction; survey; treatment outcome; *voluntary admission; Florida; United States

Chavkin, David F. "For their own good": civil commitment of alcohol and drug–dependent pregnant women. *South Dakota Law Review.* 1992; 37(2): 224–288. 341 fn. BE61350.
*alcohol abuse; alternatives; *coercion; *drug abuse; due process; fetuses; goals; *involuntary commitment; *legal aspects; legal rights; *mandatory programs; outpatient commitment; *pregnant women; *prenatal injuries; social discrimination; standards; treatment refusal; voluntary programs; United States

Kellogg, Sarah C. The due process right to a safe and humane environment for patients in state custody: the voluntary/involuntary distinction. [Note]. *American Journal of Law and Medicine.* 1997; 23(2–3): 339–362. 219 fn. BE62504.
constitutional law; *due process; equal protection; *institutionalized persons; *involuntary commitment; *legal aspects; *legal rights; *mental institutions; *mentally ill; *mentally retarded; *patients' rights; physical restraint; public hospitals; standards; Supreme Court decisions; *voluntary admission; *DeShaney v. Winnebago County Department of Social Services; *United States; *Youngberg v. Romeo

Linburn, Geoffrey E. *Donaldson* revisited: is dangerousness a constitutional requirement for civil commitment? *Journal of the American Academy of Psychiatry and the Law.* 1998; 26(3): 343–351. 36 fn. BE61706.
constitutional amendments; *dangerousness; due process; *involuntary commitment; *legal aspects; *mentally ill; obligations of society; patient care; standards; state interest; *Supreme Court decisions; *O'Connor v. Donaldson; United States

Mordini, Emilio. Mandatory hospitalisation in mental health. *Bulletin of Medical Ethics.* 1997 Nov; No. 133: 18–21. 6 refs. Paper delivered at the 1997 Annual Meeting of the European Association of Centres of Medical Ethics at Coimbra, Portugal, 24–25 Oct 1997. BE59704.
behavior control; coercion; dangerousness; deinstitutionalized persons; historical aspects; hospitals; international aspects; *involuntary commitment; legal aspects; mental institutions; *mentally ill; paternalism; patient care; psychoactive drugs; social discrimination; treatment refusal

---

BE = bioethics accession number   fn. = footnotes   refs. = references

INVOLUNTARY COMMITMENT/FOREIGN COUNTRIES

Bar El, Yair Carlos; Durst, Rimona; Rabinowitz, Jonathan, et al. Implementation of order of compulsory ambulatory treatment in Jerusalem. *International Journal of Law and Psychiatry.* 1998 Winter; 21(1): 65–71. 15 refs. BE59930.
> communication; dangerousness; evaluation studies; health personnel; interprofessional relations; involuntary commitment; law enforcement; *legal aspects; medical records; mental institutions; *mentally ill; *outpatient commitment; patient compliance; standards; Israel; *Jerusalem

Bosch, Xavier. Eating disorders may warrant compulsory hospital admission. [News]. *Lancet.* 1999 Mar 20; 353(9157): 993. BE61958.
> *behavior disorders; coercion; food; *involuntary commitment; judicial action; *legal aspects; parents; patients; treatment refusal; *anorexia nervosa; *bulimia; *Spain

Cohen, Pamela Schwartz. Psychiatric commitment in Japan: international concern and domestic reform. *UCLA Pacific Basin Law Journal.* 1995 Fall; 14(1): 28–74. 234 fn. BE59273.
> advisory committees; committee membership; community services; family members; health care reform; historical aspects; *human rights; *international aspects; *involuntary commitment; lawyers; *legal aspects; legal rights; mental institutions; *mentally ill; *non–Western World; paternalism; patient advocacy; patient care; *patient discharge; *patients' rights; physical restraint; physician patient relationship; *review committees; social discrimination; *standards; stigmatization; third party consent; values; voluntary admission; *International Commission of Jurists; *Japan; *Mental Health Act 1987 (Japan); Principles for the Protection of Persons with Mental Illness; *Psychiatric Review Boards (Japan); Twentieth Century; United Nations

Eastman, Nigel. Public health psychiatry or crime prevention? [Editorial]. *BMJ (British Medical Journal).* 1999 Feb 27; 318(7183): 549–551. 17 refs. BE61975.
> *behavior disorders; *dangerousness; *forensic psychiatry; government regulation; *involuntary commitment; law enforcement; patients; *physician's role; prisoners; public policy; *Great Britain

Glover, Nicola. Community care -- same problems, different epithet? *Journal of Medical Ethics.* 1998 Oct; 24(5): 336–340. 9 refs. BE60256.
> coercion; *community services; dangerousness; *deinstitutionalized persons; evaluation; freedom; *legal aspects; legal guardians; *mentally ill; *outpatient commitment; paternalism; *patient care; patient compliance; psychoactive drugs; time factors; *Great Britain; *Mental Health (Patients in the Community) Act 1995

A negative image of community care prevails. This method of care is perceived to be a relatively novel phenomenon and has received mixed media coverage. The negative image of community care has led to the growing belief that this care method has failed. This failure has largely been ascribed to the lack of powers available to control patients in the community and to the method's relative novelty. However, this paper contends that there are two flaws to the above assertion: first, community care is far from new, and second, the inherent problem is not the lack of powers available to control patients in the community, but, essentially, the absence of a secure and stable environment within the community.

Jaworowski, Solomon; Nachmias, Solomon; Zabow,

Aubrey. Enforced psychiatric treatment of minors in Israel: the interface between the Mental Health Act and the Youth Law. *Israel Journal of Psychiatry and Related Sciences.* 1995; 32(2): 114–119. 14 refs. BE59977.
> adolescents; *behavior disorders; case studies; dangerousness; *involuntary commitment; *legal aspects; *mentally ill; *minors; outpatient commitment; parental consent; *standards; suicide; treatment refusal; *Israel; Law for the Treatment of the Mentally Ill 1991 (Israel); Youth Law (Israel)

Kaltiala–Heino, Riittakerttu; Laippala, Pekka; Salokangas, Raimo K.R. Impact of coercion on treatment outcome. *International Journal of Law and Psychiatry.* 1997 Summer; 20(3): 311–322. 32 refs. BE59689.
> attitudes; *coercion; comparative studies; emotions; freedom; *institutionalized persons; *involuntary commitment; mental institutions; *mentally ill; patient satisfaction; patients; survey; *treatment outcome; *voluntary admission; *Finland

Kjellin, Lars; Andersson, Kristina; Candefjord, Inga–Lill, et al. Ethical benefits and costs of coercion in short–term inpatient psychiatric care. *Psychiatric Services.* 1997 Dec; 48(12): 1567–1570. 12 refs. BE61624.
> *autonomy; beneficence; *coercion; comparative studies; evaluation studies; hospitals; *institutionalized persons; *involuntary commitment; mental health; mental institutions; *mentally ill; *patient care; patient discharge; patient satisfaction; risks and benefits; survey; *treatment outcome; *voluntary admission; *Sweden

Kjellin, Lars; Westrin, Claes–Göran. Involuntary admissions and coercive measures in psychiatric care: registered and reported. *International Journal of Law and Psychiatry.* 1998 Winter; 21(1): 31–42. 20 refs. BE59929.
> *coercion; comparative studies; family members; institutionalized persons; *involuntary commitment; medical records; mental institutions; *mentally ill; nurses; *patient admission; *patient care; patients; physical restraint; psychoactive drugs; standards; survey; time factors; *voluntary admission; *Sweden

Kokkonen, Paula. Coercion and legal protection in psychiatric care in Finland. *Medicine and Law.* 1993; 12(1–2): 113–124. 16 refs. BE60618.
> behavior control; *coercion; dangerousness; institutionalized persons; *involuntary commitment; *legal rights; *mentally ill; patient care; psychiatric diagnosis; psychoactive drugs; referral and consultation; patient isolation; *Finland; Mental Health Act 1990 (Finland)

Kullgren, G.; Jacobsson, L.; Lynöe, N., et al. Practices and attitudes among Swedish psychiatrists regarding the ethics of compulsory treatment. *Acta Psychiatrica Scandinavica.* 1996 May; 93(5): 389–396. 13 refs. BE61553.
> case studies; *coercion; dangerousness; decision making; electroconvulsive therapy; family members; *involuntary commitment; *knowledge, attitudes, practice; medical ethics; *mentally ill; misconduct; paternalism; *patient care; *physical restraint; physician patient relationship; *physicians; presumed consent; psychiatric diagnosis; *psychiatry; psychoactive drugs; sex offenses; sexuality; sterilization (sexual); therapeutic abortion; truth disclosure; *Sweden

Price, David P.T. Civil commitment of the mentally ill: compelling arguments for reform. *Medical Law Review.* 1994 Autumn; 2(3): 321–352. 120 fn. BE60605.
> autonomy; competence; criminal law; dangerousness; *involuntary commitment; *legal aspects; legislation; mental institutions; *mentally ill; paternalism; patient care; social discrimination; *standards; *Great Britain; *Mental Health

---

BE = bioethics accession number   fn. = footnotes   refs. = references

Act 1983 (Great Britain)

Ramsay, Sarah. UK psychiatrists refuse to treat the untreatable. [News]. *Lancet.* 1999 Feb 20; 353(9153): 647. BE61708.
  *dangerousness; *forensic psychiatry; government regulation; *involuntary commitment; law enforcement; *mentally ill; *physician's role; violence; *Great Britain; National Health Service

Detention of potentially dangerous people. [Editorial]. *Lancet.* 1998 Nov 21; 352(9141): 1641. BE61197.
  behavior disorders; *dangerousness; *involuntary commitment; *legal aspects; legal liability; *mentally ill; physicians; psychiatric diagnosis; psychiatry; *Great Britain; Mental Health Act 1983 (Great Britain)

INVOLUNTARY COMMITMENT/MINORS

Jaworowski, Solomon; Nachmias, Solomon; Zabow, Aubrey. Enforced psychiatric treatment of minors in Israel: the interface between the Mental Health Act and the Youth Law. *Israel Journal of Psychiatry and Related Sciences.* 1995; 32(2): 114–119. 14 refs. BE59977.
  adolescents; *behavior disorders; case studies; dangerousness; *involuntary commitment; *legal aspects; *mentally ill; *minors; outpatient commitment; parental consent; *standards; suicide; treatment refusal; *Israel; Law for the Treatment of the Mentally Ill 1991 (Israel); Youth Law (Israel)

Molnar, Beth E. Juveniles and psychiatric institutionalization: toward better due process and treatment review in the United States. *Health and Human Rights.* 1997; 2(2): 99–116. 46 fn. BE62089.
  *behavior control; behavior disorders; child abuse; *due process; health insurance reimbursement; homosexuals; *human rights; international aspects; *involuntary commitment; *legal aspects; mental institutions; *minors; misconduct; operant conditioning; parents; physical restraint; proprietary health facilities; voluntary admission; *Convention on the Rights of the Child; United Nations; *United States

Schmidt, Kelli. "Who are you to say what my best interest is?" Minors' due process rights when admitted by parents for inpatient mental health treatment. [Comment]. *Washington Law Review.* 1996 Oct; 71(4): 1187–1217. 202 fn. BE59417.
  behavior disorders; constitutional law; *due process; freedom; *involuntary commitment; *judicial action; *legal aspects; *legal rights; mental institutions; *mentally ill; *minors; parental consent; privacy; proprietary health facilities; psychiatric diagnosis; Supreme Court decisions; *treatment refusal; voluntary admission; Parham v. J.R.; *State ex rel. T.B. v. CPC Fairfax Hospital; United States; *Washington

INVOLUNTARY STERILIZATION *See* STERILIZATION

JUSTICE *See* HEALTH CARE/RIGHTS, RESOURCE ALLOCATION

LEGAL ASPECTS
  See under
    ABORTION/LEGAL ASPECTS
    ALLOWING TO DIE/LEGAL ASPECTS
    CONFIDENTIALITY/LEGAL ASPECTS
    EUTHANASIA/LEGAL ASPECTS

LIFE EXTENSION

Bova, Ben. The impact of immortality. *In: his* Immortality: How Science Is Extending Your Life Span -- and Changing the World. New York, NY: Avon Books; 1998: 183–251. 24 fn. ISBN 0-380-97518-1. BE62130.
  adults; aged; attitudes; attitudes to death; biomedical research; biomedical technologies; cloning; costs and benefits; economics; gene therapy; genetic determinism; genetic intervention; genetic screening; government financing; insurance; *life extension; mortality; politics; population control; private sector; prolongation of life; religious ethics; reproductive technologies; resource allocation; right to die; risks and benefits; science; *social impact; United States

Klotzko, Arlene Judith. Immortal longings. *New Scientist.* 1998 Dec 5; 160(2163): 49. BE61544.
  *embryo research; government financing; government regulation; industry; *life extension; *stem cells; United States

LIVING WILLS *See* ADVANCE DIRECTIVES

MASS SCREENING

  See also AIDS/TESTING AND SCREENING, GENETIC SCREENING, PUBLIC HEALTH

Allen, Katrina; Williamson, Robert. Should we genetically test everyone for haemochromatosis? *Journal of Medical Ethics.* 1999 Apr; 25(2): 209–214. 28 refs. BE61928.
  adolescents; adults; age factors; carriers; costs and benefits; genetic counseling; genetic information; *genetic screening; health education; *late-onset disorders; *mass screening; newborns; patient care; preventive medicine; psychological stress; *public policy; *risks and benefits; social discrimination; stigmatization; truth disclosure; *hemochromatosis; Australia
The increasing availability of DNA-based diagnostic tests has raised issues about whether these should be applied to the population at large in order to identify, treat or prevent a range of diseases. DNA tests raise concerns in the community for several reasons. There is the possibility of stigmatisation and discrimination between those who test positive and those who don't. High-risk individuals may be identified for whom no proven effective intervention is possible, or conversely may test "positive" for a disease that does not eventuate. Controversy concerning prenatal diagnosis and termination of affected pregnancies may arise. Haemochromatosis, however, is a disease that is not only treatable but also preventable if those at high risk are identified presymptomatically. This paper will identify and discuss key issues regarding DNA-based population screening for haemochromatosis, and argue that population-based genetic screening for haemochromatosis should be supported when a number of contentious issues are addressed. In the context of a health system with limited resources haemochromatosis is the paradigm of a disorder where there is an ethical and clinical imperative to encourage presymptomatic DNA testing for all in ethnically relevant communities.

Bayertz, Kurt. What's special about molecular genetic diagnostics? *Journal of Medicine and Philosophy.* 1998 Jun; 23(3): 247–254. 10 refs. BE59289.
  coercion; *diagnosis; gene therapy; genetic disorders; genetic information; genetic predisposition; *genetic screening; health; insurance; late-onset disorders; *mass screening;

BE = bioethics accession number   fn. = footnotes   refs. = references

preventive medicine; risks and benefits; social control; social discrimination; *social impact

In its first part, this paper seeks to make plausible (a) that molecular genetic diagnostics differs in ethically relevant ways from traditional types of medical diagnostics and (b) that the consequences of introducing this technology in broad screening-programs to detect widespread genetic diseases in a population which is not at high risk may change our understanding of health and disease in a problematic way. In its second part, the paper discusses some aspects of public control of scientific and technological innovations in the field of molecular genetic diagnostics.

Campbell, Harry; Boyd, Kenneth. Screening and the new genetics: a public health perspective on the ethical debate. [Letter]. *Journal of Public Health Medicine.* 1996 Dec; 18(4): 485–486. 9 refs. BE60691.
> autonomy; costs and benefits; cystic fibrosis; eugenics; *genetic screening; mass screening; *prenatal diagnosis; public health; public policy

Cheng, Leo H.H.; Whittington, Richard M. Natural deaths while driving: would screening for risk be ethically justified? *Journal of Medical Ethics.* 1998 Aug; 24(4): 248–251. 13 refs. BE61290.
> aged; autonomy; beneficence; confidentiality; *death; duty to warn; *heart diseases; mandatory programs; *mass screening; *mortality; paternalism; physicians; *preventive medicine; public health; public policy; *risk; survey; *traffic accidents; retrospective studies; Great Britain

OBJECTIVES: To determine the epidemiology and the underlying pathological conditions of natural deaths among motor vehicle drivers. Sudden death while driving may cause damage to properties, other vehicles or road users. Although the Medical Commission on Accident Prevention recommended restrictions to drivers at risk of sudden death due to their medical conditions, these restrictions are useless if they do not result in greater safety to the public. DESIGN: A retrospective study of natural deaths of motor vehicle drivers. SETTING: Natural deaths of motor vehicle drivers reported to the coroner for Birmingham and Solihull. SUBJECTS: 86 consecutive natural deaths of motor vehicle drivers in a five-year period between 1984 and 1988. RESULTS: Of the 86 fatalities reviewed, 80 (93%) sudden deaths were caused by ischaemic heart disease. Fifty vehicles were involved in collision with 32 properties, 20 other vehicles and six pedestrians. Fifty-one out of 80 cardiac deaths had past cardiac history and three had reported chest pain prior to the sudden death. CONCLUSION: An applied normative ethical assessment based on the basic moral principles of autonomy, justice, beneficence and non-maleficence are discussed. We conclude that medical screening of drivers has little benefit for the drivers or other persons.

Clayton, Ellen Wright. Issues in state newborn screening programs. *Pediatrics.* 1992 Oct; 90(4): 641–646. 69 refs. BE60222.
> autonomy; confidentiality; congenital disorders; *costs and benefits; decision making; diagnosis; *disclosure; DNA data banks; genetic counseling; *genetic screening; government financing; health insurance reimbursement; *mandatory testing; *mass screening; *newborns; parental consent; *parents; patient care; privacy; prognosis; psychological stress; public policy; records; reproduction; *risks and benefits; *state government; time factors; treatment outcome; right not to know; *United States

Cuckle, Howard. Rational Down syndrome screening policy. *American Journal of Public Health.* 1998 Apr;

88(4): 558–559. 13 refs. BE60129.
> age factors; chorionic villi sampling; costs and benefits; *decision analysis; *Down syndrome; fetal development; *mass screening; *methods; *pregnant women; *prenatal diagnosis; *public policy; risk; risks and benefits; values; ultrasonography

Frank, Stacy; Esch, Julie Funesti; Margeson, Nancy E. Mandatory HIV testing of newborns: the impact on women. *American Journal of Nursing.* 1998 Oct; 98(10): 49–51. 8 refs. BE61804.
> *AIDS serodiagnosis; counseling; government regulation; *HIV seropositivity; informed consent; *mandatory testing; *mass screening; mothers; *newborns; nurses; patient care; public policy; risks and benefits; state government; *voluntary programs; New York

Gevers, Sjef. Population screening: the role of the law. *European Journal of Health Law.* 1998 Mar; 5(1): 7–18. 16 fn. BE61255.
> carriers; competence; confidentiality; congenital disorders; disclosure; epidemiology; family members; *genetic screening; *government regulation; guidelines; informed consent; international aspects; *legal aspects; *legislation; *mass screening; prenatal diagnosis; preventive medicine; public health; risks and benefits; selective abortion; standards; third party consent; right not to know; *Act on Population Screening (Netherlands); *Netherlands

Heikkilä, Annaleena; Ryynänen, Markku; Kirkinen, Pertti, et al. Results and views of women in population-wide pregnancy screening for trisomy 21 in East Finland. *Fetal Diagnosis and Therapy.* 1997 Mar–Apr; 12(2): 93–96. 22 refs. BE59230.
> age factors; *attitudes; *Down syndrome; *mass screening; *pregnant women; *prenatal diagnosis; survey; *Finland

Hoedemaekers, Rogeer; ten Have, Henk. Geneticization: the Cyprus paradigm. *Journal of Medicine and Philosophy.* 1998 Jun; 23(3): 274–287. 17 refs. BE59291.
> *attitudes; carriers; *coercion; decision making; *directive counseling; economics; eugenics; *genetic counseling; *genetic screening; genetic services; genetics; *goals; health education; *health personnel; international aspects; *mass screening; parents; paternalism; *prenatal diagnosis; prevalence; preventive medicine; public health; public opinion; quality of life; *selective abortion; social control; stigmatization; *thalassemia; *Cyprus; Great Britain; Quebec

Geneticization is a broad term referring to several related processes such as a spreading tendency to use a genetic model of disease explanation, a growing influence of genetics in medical practice, and the slow changing of individual and societal attitudes towards reproduction, prevention and control of disease. These processes can be demonstrated in medical literature on preventive genetic screening and counselling programs for beta-thalassaemia in Cyprus, the United Kingdom and Canada. The preventive possibilities of the new genetic and diagnostic technologies have been quickly understood and advocated by health professionals, and their educational strategies have created a web of social control, in marked contrast to the alleged voluntary decision-making process and free choice. Genetic diagnostic technologies have led to considerable changes in control and management of beta-thalassaemia, and have generated a number of unresolved incongruities.

Malm, H.M. Medical screening and the value of early detection: when unwarranted faith leads to unethical recommendations. *Hastings Center Report.* 1999 Jan–Feb; 29(1): 26–37. 55 fn. BE61634.
> age factors; breast cancer; cancer; costs and benefits;

---

*evaluation studies; *evidence-based medicine; females; guidelines; health promotion; heart diseases; human experimentation; hypertension; informed consent; males; *mass screening; mortality; nutrition; *preventive medicine; professional organizations; random selection; research design; *risks and benefits; statistics; surgery; cholesterol; prostate cancer; United States

Medical screening is justified on the strength of the assumption that the earlier disease is detected, the better it is for the patient. On examination, however, the assumption turns out to be severely flawed, and inadequate anyway, since it is not only the patient with whom we should be concerned, but healthy people as well. Instead of making assumptions about the ill, we should prove a test's overall benefit to the individual taking it before we recommend it.

Millard, Dietra D. Toxicology testing in neonates: is it ethical, and what does it mean? *Clinics in Perinatology.* 1996 Sep; 23(3): 491–507. 84 refs. BE60937.
confidentiality; congenital disorders; disclosure; *drug abuse; fetuses; intensive care units; *mass screening; morbidity; mortality; mothers; *newborns; parent child relationship; patient discharge; physicians; *pregnant women; *prenatal injuries; prevalence; prognosis; risks and benefits; social problems; social workers

Moss, Sue; Cuckle, Howard. Trial of mammography in women under 50 is ethical. [Letter]. *BMJ (British Medical Journal).* 1998 Dec 5; 317(7172): 1589–1590. 1 ref. BE60976.
*age factors; *breast cancer; control groups; deception; ethical review; females; *human experimentation; *informed consent; *mass screening; research design; research ethics committees; research subjects; *Great Britain; Medical Research Council (Great Britain); United Kingdom Coordinating Committee on Cancer Research

Nicholson, Richard H. "Don't die of ignorance." *Hastings Center Report.* 1999 May–Jun; 29(3): 6. 5 refs. BE61406.
breast cancer; cancer; costs and benefits; evaluation; females; genetic screening; health care delivery; *mass screening; physicians; prenatal diagnosis; preventive medicine; public policy; risks and benefits; Europe; Great Britain

Pellissier, James M.; Venta, Enrique R. Introducing patient values into the decision making process for breast cancer screening. *Women and Health.* 1996; 24(4): 47–67. 40 refs. BE59442.
autonomy; *breast cancer; communication; *decision analysis; *decision making; evaluation; *females; *mass screening; models, theoretical; paternalism; *patient participation; *physician patient relationship; practice guidelines; risk; *values; United States

Serra-Prat, Mateu; Gallo, Pedro; Jovell, Albert J., et al. Trade-offs in prenatal detection of Down syndrome. *American Journal of Public Health.* 1998 Apr; 88(4): 551–557. 35 refs. BE60128.
age factors; *alternatives; amniocentesis; comparative studies; costs and benefits; *decision analysis; decision making; *Down syndrome; *mass screening; *methods; *pregnant women; *prenatal diagnosis; *public policy; *risks and benefits; values; ultrasonography; Catalonia; Spain
OBJECTIVES: This paper presents the results of different screening policies for prenatal detection of Down syndrome that would allow decision makers to make informed choices. METHODS: A decision analysis model was built to compare 8 screening policies with regard to a selected set of outcome measures. Probabilities used in the analysis were obtained from official administrative data reports in Spain and Catalonia and from data published in the medical literature. Sensitivity analyses were carried out to test the

robustness of screening policies' results to changes in uptake rates, diagnostic accuracy, and resources consumed. RESULTS: Selected screening policies posed major trades-offs regarding detection rates, false-positive results, fetal loss, and costs of the programs. All outcome measures considered were found quite robust to changes in uptake rates. Sensitivity and specificity rates of screening tests were shown to be the most influential factors in the outcome measures considered. CONCLUSIONS: The disclosed trade-offs emphasize the need to comprehensively inform decision makers about both positive and negative consequences of adopting one screening policy or another.

Sibbald, Barbara. CMA says no to mandatory hepatitis B vaccination, screening for MDs. *Canadian Medical Association Journal.* 1998 Jul 14; 159(1): 64–65. BE61129.
autonomy; confidentiality; consensus; dentistry; dissent; guidelines; *health personnel; *hepatitis; iatrogenic disease; *immunization; *mandatory programs; mandatory testing; *mass screening; *organizational policies; *physicians; privacy; professional organizations; *public policy; surgery; *voluntary programs; *Canada; Canadian Dental Association; *Canadian Medical Association; *Health Canada

U.S. Court of Appeals, Ninth Circuit.
Norman-Bloodsaw v. Lawrence Berkeley Laboratory. *Federal Reporter, 3d Series.* 1998 Feb 3 (date of decision). 135: 1260–1276. BE62345.
blacks; constitutional law; due process; *employment; federal government; females; *genetic screening; *legal rights; *mass screening; pregnant women; *privacy; research institutes; sickle cell anemia; social discrimination; state government; syphilis; California; Civil Rights Act 1964; Fifth Amendment; Fourteenth Amendment; Fourth Amendment; *Norman-Bloodsaw v. Lawrence Berkeley Laboratory; United States
The U.S. Court of Appeals for the Ninth Circuit overturned the lower court's dismissal and allowed clerical or administrative workers to sue their employer for testing for "highly private and sensitive medical genetic information such as syphilis, sickle cell trait, and pregnancy" without either their consent or their knowledge during a general employee health examination. The court noted that "the most basic violation possible" of constitutional privacy interests involves the performance of unauthorized testing for medical information and that such testing may be viewed as illegal search under the Fourth Amendment in addition to violation of due process under the Fifth or Fourteenth Amendments. Because there are "few subject areas more personal and more likely to implicate privacy interests than that of one's health or genetic make-up," the court concluded that the unauthorized testing constituted a significant invasion of the right to privacy under the Fourth Amendment. The court reasoned that neither consent to a general medical examination nor consent to providing blood or urine samples abolishes the privacy right not to be tested for intimate, personal matters involving one's health. Also, because black employees were singled out for sickle cell trait testing and female employees for pregnancy testing, the employer discriminated against them concerning terms or conditions of employment, thus violating Title VII of the Civil Rights Act. (KIE abstract)

Blood tests of workers restricted by court. [News]. *New York Times.* 1998 Feb 5: A19. BE59563.
*employment; federal government; *genetic screening; *legal rights; *mass screening; *privacy; syphilis; California; *Lawrence Berkeley National Laboratory; United States

---

BE = bioethics accession number   fn. = footnotes   refs. = references

MEDICAL CARE *See* HEALTH CARE, PATIENT CARE, TERMINAL CARE

MEDICAL ETHICS

See also BIOETHICS, NURSING ETHICS, PROFESSIONAL ETHICS

Aarons, D. Medical ethics: a sensitization to some important issues. *West Indian Medical Journal.* 1996 Sep; 45(3): 74–77. 15 refs. The 1996 Mike DaSilva Lecture, delivered at the annual symposium of the Medical Association of Jamaica. BE60405.
   bioethical issues; historical aspects; *medical ethics; physician patient relationship; physicians; professional competence; physician impairment

Adams, James; Society for Academic Emergency Medicine. Ethics Committee. Virtue in emergency medicine. *Academic Emergency Medicine.* 1996 Oct; 3(10): 961–966. 25 refs. BE60678.
   altruism; codes of ethics; compassion; *emergency care; historical aspects; justice; *medical ethics; *virtues; courage; integrity; prudence

Applebaum, Arthur Isak. Doctor, schmoctor: practice positivism and its complications. *In: his* Ethics for Adversaries: The Morality of Roles in Public and Professional Life. Princeton, NJ: Princeton University Press; 1999: 45–60. 9 fn. ISBN 0–691–00712–8. BE62129.
   conflict of interest; disclosure; duty to warn; gatekeeping; insurance; lawyers; legal obligations; managed care programs; *medical ethics; *moral obligations; mortality; occupational medicine; patient advocacy; physician patient relationship; *physician's role; professional competence; *professional ethics; *professional role; virtues

Baker, Robert. American independence and the right to emergency care. *JAMA.* 1999 Mar 3; 281(9): 859–860. 12 refs. BE60244.
   administrators; codes of ethics; economics; *emergency care; historical aspects; *legal aspects; *legal rights; legislation; *managed care programs; *medical ethics; *moral obligations; patient advocacy; *patients' rights; physician patient relationship; *physicians; professional organizations; refusal to treat; *utilitarianism; *business ethics; *Patients' Bill of Rights; *United States

Barondess, Jeremiah A. Care of the medical ethos: reflections on Social Darwinism, racial hygiene, and the Holocaust. *Annals of Internal Medicine.* 1998 Dec 1; 129(11): 891–898. 34 refs. BE59326.
   dehumanization; disabled; disadvantaged; *eugenics; evolution; genetics; health care delivery; *historical aspects; human experimentation; international aspects; investigators; involuntary euthanasia; involuntary sterilization; justice; killing; *medical ethics; *medicine; minority groups; *misconduct; *moral complicity; *National Socialism; physician's role; *physicians; prisoners; psychiatry; public health; public policy; science; suffering; values; Darwinism; *Germany; *Twentieth Century; United States

Bettman, Jerome W. Ethics and the American Academy of Ophthalmology in historical perspective. *Ophthalmology.* 1996 Aug; 103(8, Suppl.): S29–S39. 37 refs. BE60403.
   ancient history; codes of ethics; ethics committees; government regulation; *historical aspects; human experimentation; malpractice; managed care programs; *medical ethics; misconduct; *ophthalmology; patient care; physicians; professional autonomy; *professional organizations; *self regulation; *American Academy of Ophthalmology; Eighteenth Century; Middle Ages;

Nineteenth Century; Twentieth Century; United States

Bin Saeed, Khalid Saad. How physician executives and clinicians perceive ethical issues in Saudi Arabian hospitals. *Journal of Medical Ethics.* 1999 Feb; 25(1): 51–56. 12 refs. BE61196.
   *administrators; allowing to die; *attitudes; *bioethical issues; codes of ethics; comparative studies; confidentiality; conflict of interest; continuing education; cultural pluralism; deontological ethics; ethics committees; gifts; *hospitals; *institutional ethics; institutional policies; interprofessional relations; medical education; *medical ethics; misconduct; patient advocacy; patient care; patients' rights; physician patient relationship; *physicians; professional autonomy; prolongation of life; regulation; resource allocation; social discrimination; socioeconomic factors; survey; terminally ill; utilitarianism; values; withholding treatment; *Saudi Arabia

OBJECTIVES: To compare the perceptions of physician executives and clinicians regarding ethical issues in Saudi Arabian hospitals and the attributes that might lead to the existence of these ethical issues. DESIGN: Self-completion questionnaire administered from February to July 1997. SETTING: Different health regions in the Kingdom of Saudi Arabia. PARTICIPANTS: Random sample of 457 physicians (317 clinicians and 140 physician executives) from several hospitals in various regions across the kingdom. RESULTS: There were statistically significant differences in the perceptions of physician executives and clinicians regarding the existence of various ethical issues in their hospitals. The vast majority of physician executives did not perceive that seven of the eight issues addressed by the study were ethical concerns in their hospitals. However, the majority of the clinicians perceived that six of the same eight issues were ethical considerations in their hospitals. Statistically significant differences in the perceptions of physician executives and clinicians were observed in only three out of eight attributes that might possibly lead to the existence of ethical issues. The most significant attribute that was perceived to result in ethical issues was that of hospitals having a multinational staff. CONCLUSION: The study calls for the formulation of a code of ethics that will address specifically the physicians who work in the kingdom of Saudi Arabia. As a more immediate initiative, it is recommended that seminars and workshops be conducted to provide physicians with an opportunity to discuss the ethical dilemmas they face in their medical practice.

Bloche, M. Gregg. Clinical loyalties and the social purposes of medicine. *JAMA.* 1999 Jan 20; 281(3): 268–274. BE60693.
   *beneficence; bioethics; capital punishment; clinical ethics; common good; *conflict of interest; disclosure; economics; forensic psychiatry; gatekeeping; goals; human rights; informed consent; injuries; law; legal aspects; managed care programs; mediation; *medical ethics; medicine; *obligations to society; patient advocacy; patient care; *physician patient relationship; *physician's role; *physicians; professional autonomy; public health; torture; trust; *loyalty; United States

Physicians increasingly face conflicts between the ethic of undivided loyalty to patients and pressure to use clinical methods and judgment for social purposes and on behalf of third parties. The principal legal and ethical paradigms by which these conflicts are managed are inadequate, because they either deny or unsuccessfully finesse the reality of contradiction between fidelity to patients and society's other expectations of medicine. This reality needs to be more squarely acknowledged. The challenge for ethics and law is not to resolve this tension -- an impossible task -- but to mediate it in

---

BE = bioethics accession number   fn. = footnotes   refs. = references

myriad clinical circumstances in a way that preserves the primacy of keeping faith with patients while conceding the legitimacy of society's other expectations of medicine.

Breen, Kerry J.; Plueckhahn, Vernon D.; Cordner, Stephen M. Ethics, Law and Medical Practice. St. Leonards, NSW, Australia: Allen and Unwin; 1997. 367 p. Includes references. Appendices include the Australian Medical Association code of ethics, NHMRC (National Health and Medical Research Council) statement on human experimentation, NHMRC general guidelines for medical practitioners on providing information to patients, and NHMRC recommendations for the donation of cadaveric organs and tissues for transplantation. ISBN 1-86448-407-1. BE59722.
abortion, induced; active euthanasia; allowing to die; autonomy; beneficence; communication; computers; confidentiality; determination of death; drugs; employment; government regulation; *health care delivery; human experimentation; informed consent; interprofessional relations; involuntary commitment; *legal aspects; legal liability; mandatory reporting; medical education; *medical ethics; medical records; mentally ill; misconduct; negligence; organization and administration; parent child relationship; *patient care; physician patient relationship; physicians; professional competence; reproductive technologies; resource allocation; self regulation; sexuality; standards; third party consent; treatment refusal; virtues; withholding treatment; physician impairment; self care; *Australia

Brody, Howard; Miller, Franklin G. The internal morality of medicine: explication and application to managed care. *Journal of Medicine and Philosophy.* 1998 Aug; 23(4): 384–410. 58 refs. 16 fn. BE60630.
assisted suicide; bioethics; capital punishment; conflict of interest; conscience; contraception; contracts; cosmetic surgery; disclosure; drugs; economics; entrepreneurship; family members; family relationship; gatekeeping; *goals; incentives; *managed care programs; *medical ethics; *medicine; misconduct; models, theoretical; *moral obligations; morality; obligations to society; patient advocacy; patient care; physician patient relationship; *physician's role; *physicians; postmodernism; primary health care; professional competence; professional ethics; quality of health care; resource allocation; sexuality; sports medicine; trust; values; voluntary sterilization; withholding treatment; gag clauses; health services misuse; undertreatment
Some ethical issues facing contemporary medicine cannot be fully understood without addressing medicine's internal morality. Medicine as a profession is characterized by certain moral goals and morally acceptable means for achieving those goals. The list of appropriate goals and means allows some medical actions to be classified as clear violations of the internal morality, and others as borderline or controversial cases. Replies are available for common objections, including the superfluity of internal morality for ethical analysis, the argument that internal morality is merely an apology for medicine's traditional power and authority, and the claim that there is no single, "core" internal morality. The value of addressing the internal morality of medicine may be illustrated by a detailed investigation of ethical issues posed by managed care. Managed care poses some fundamental challenges for medicine's internal morality, but also calls for thoughtful reflection and reconsideration of some traditionally held moral views on patient fidelity in particular.

Casarett, David J. Moral perception and the pursuit of medical philosophy. *Theoretical Medicine and Bioethics.* 1999 Apr; 20(2): 125–139. 58 fn. BE62214.

bioethics; clinical ethics; diagnosis; disease; health; *medical ethics; *medicine; moral development; *narrative ethics; patient care; patients; *philosophy; *physician patient relationship; *physicians; self concept; suffering; values; *phenomenology

Dinwiddie, Stephen H.; Yutzy, Sean H. Ethical issues in psychiatric practice. *In:* Guze, Samuel B., ed. Adult Pyschiatry. (Mosby's neurology psychiatry access series). St. Louis, MO: Mosby-Year Book; 1996: 445–453. 2 refs. ISBN 0-8151-3993-4. BE61058.
alcohol abuse; assisted suicide; autonomy; beneficence; competence; confidentiality; conflict of interest; depressive disorder; human experimentation; informed consent; *medical ethics; *mentally ill; organ transplantation; paternalism; *patient care; physician patient relationship; *psychiatry; referral and consultation; risks and benefits; selection for treatment; treatment refusal

Doxiadis, Spyros A. Why medical ethics? *Pediatrician.* 1990; 17(2): 56–58. 2 refs. BE59449.
bioethics; disadvantaged; health promotion; historical aspects; human rights; *medical ethics; medicine; physicians; *preventive medicine; resource allocation

Drane, James F. Decisionmaking and consensus formation in clinical ethics. *In:* ten Have, Henk A.M.J.; Sass, Hans-Martin, eds. Consensus Formation in Healthcare Ethics. Boston, MA: Kluwer Academic; 1998: 143–157. 13 refs. 7 fn. ISBN 0-7923-4944-X. BE62592.
bioethics; casuistry; *clinical ethics; *consensus; cultural pluralism; *decision making; ethical analysis; ethical relativism; *international aspects; medical ethics; methods; patient care; Europe; Latin America; North America

Engelhardt, Dietrich V. The ethics of pediatrics and the ill child in history. *In:* Burgio, G. Roberto; Lantos, John D., eds. Primum Non Nocere Today. Second Edition. New York, NY: Elsevier; 1998: 11–21. 28 refs. ISBN 0-444-82923-7. BE60918.
ancient history; children; Christian ethics; disease; euthanasia; fathers; *historical aspects; infanticide; Islamic ethics; legal rights; *medical ethics; *pediatrics; physicians; secularism; value of life; virtues; Western World

Griffith, Ezra E.H. Ethics in forensic psychiatry: a cultural response to Stone and Appelbaum. *Journal of the American Academy of Psychiatry and the Law.* 1998; 26(2): 171–184. 22 refs. BE59153.
beneficence; *blacks; *conflict of interest; *cultural pluralism; disclosure; *expert testimony; *forensic psychiatry; historical aspects; Jews; justice; law enforcement; *medical ethics; *minority groups; moral obligations; patient advocacy; physician patient relationship; *physician's role; physicians; political activity; social discrimination; *social dominance; whites; United States

Halpern, Abraham L.; Freedman, Alfred M.; Schoenholtz, Jack C., et al. Ethics in forensic psychiatry. [Letter and response]. *American Journal of Psychiatry.* 1998 Apr; 155(4): 575–577. 13 refs. BE60179.
*capital punishment; codes of ethics; *competence; conflict of interest; *expert testimony; *forensic psychiatry; law enforcement; *medical ethics; organizational policies; patient care; physician patient relationship; *physician's role; physicians; professional organizations; psychiatric diagnosis; psychiatry; American Academy of Psychiatry and the Law; American Medical Association; American Psychiatric Association

Harris, John; Holm, Søren. Risk-taking and professional responsibility. *Journal of the Royal Society of Medicine.* 1997 Nov; 90(11): 625–629. 4 refs. BE62428.
AIDS; altruism; communicable diseases; contracts;

BE = bioethics accession number   fn. = footnotes   refs. = references

emergency care; employment; HIV seropositivity; *medical ethics; *moral obligations; *occupational exposure; physicians; *professional ethics; *risk

Jones, Anne Hudson. Narrative based medicine: narrative in medical ethics. *BMJ (British Medical Journal).* 1999 Jan 23; 318(7178): 253–256. 35 refs. BE60331.
    bioethics; casuistry; education; ethicists; humanities; interdisciplinary communication; *literature; medical education; *medical ethics; medicine; methods; *narrative ethics; patient participation; physician patient relationship; physicians; principle-based ethics; professional ethics; teaching methods; virtues

Koehn, Daryl. The Ground of Professional Ethics. New York, NY: Routledge; 1994. 224 p. (Professional ethics). Bibliography: p. 213–219. ISBN 0–415–11667–8. BE61841.
    beneficence; *clergy; common good; confidentiality; conflict of interest; contracts; health; justice; law; *lawyers; *medical ethics; medicine; moral obligations; obligations to society; physician patient relationship; *physicians; *professional ethics; professional role; religion; self regulation; technical expertise; trust

Lascaratos, John; Poulakou–Rebelakou, Effie; Marketos, Spyros. Abandonment of terminally ill patients in the Byzantine era: an ancient tradition? *Journal of Medical Ethics.* 1999 Jun; 25(3): 254–258. 36 fn. BE61860.
    *ancient history; *attitudes to death; Christian ethics; famous persons; futility; goals; *historical aspects; *medical ethics; medicine; physician patient relationship; physician's role; *physicians; *refusal to treat; *terminal care; *terminally ill; *patient abandonment; *rituals; *Byzantium; *Middle Ages
Our research on the texts of the Byzantine historians and chroniclers revealed an apparently curious phenomenon, namely, the abandonment of terminally ill emperors by their physicians when the latter realised that they could not offer any further treatment. This attitude tallies with the mentality of the ancient Greek physicians, who even in Hippocratic times thought the treatment and care of the terminally ill to be a challenge to nature and hubris to the gods. Nevertheless, it is a very curious attitude in the light of the concepts of the Christian Byzantine physicians who, according to the doctrines of the Christian religion, should have been imbued with the spirit of philanthropy and love for their fellowmen. The meticulous analysis of three examples of abandonment of Byzantine emperors, and especially that of Alexius I Comnenus, by their physicians reveals that this custom, following ancient pagan ethics, in those times took on a ritualised form without any significant or real content.

Lowy, Cathy. What is 'ethics'? [Comment]. *Australian and New Zealand Journal of Psychiatry.* 1997 Feb; 31(1): 83–84. Commentary on R. Pargiter and S. Bloch, "The ethics committee of a psychiatric college: its procedures and themes," p. 76–82. BE60278.
    economics; *ethics committees; forensic psychiatry; *medical ethics; organization and administration; *physicians; *professional organizations; *psychiatry; Australia; New Zealand; *Royal Australian and New Zealand College of Psychiatrists

McCullough, Laurence B. Hume's influence on John Gregory and the history of medical ethics. *Journal of Medicine and Philosophy.* 1999 Aug; 24(4): 376–395. 29 refs. 6 fn. BE62615.
    bioethics; caring; clinical ethics; *compassion; confidentiality; empathy; females; feminist ethics; *historical aspects; human experimentation; males; *medical ethics;

misconduct; philosophy; physician patient relationship; sexuality; socioeconomic factors; suffering; *virtues; *Eighteenth Century; *Gregory, John; *Hume, David; Scotland
The concept of medicine as a profession in the English–language literature of medical ethics is of recent vintage, invented by the Scottish physician and medical ethicist, John Gregory (1724–1773). Gregory wrote the first secular, philosophical, clinical, and feminine medical ethics and bioethics in the English language and did so on the basis of Hume's principle of sympathy. This paper provides a brief account of Gregory's invention and the role that Humean sympathy plays in that invention, with reference to key texts in Gregory's work. The paper also considers two interesting and perhaps provocative ways in which Hume can be read through Gregory: first, sympathy as a principle of scientific discovery in Hume's science of man and moral physiology; and sympathy as gendered feminine in Hume's moral philosophy. Hume's principle of sympathy is at the core of Gregory's medical ethics and the histories of Western medical ethics and bioethics pivot on Gregory -- and, therefore, on Hume -- as it does on few other figures.

McCullough, Laurence B. John Gregory and the Invention of Professional Medical Ethics and the Profession of Medicine. Boston, MA: Kluwer Academic; 1998. 347 p. (Philosophy and medicine; 56). Bibliography: p. 313–331. ISBN 0–7923–4917–2. BE62144.
    bioethical issues; bioethics; caring; clinical ethics; empathy; feminist ethics; *historical aspects; literature; *medical ethics; *medicine; moral obligations; paternalism; *philosophy; physician patient relationship; physicians; science; self concept; sociology of medicine; virtues; Bacon, Francis; *Eighteenth Century; *Gregory, John; Hume, David; Scotland

McCullough, Laurence B. John Gregory's Writings on Medical Ethics and Philosophy of Medicine. Boston, MA: Kluwer Academic; 1998. 254 p. (Philosophy and medicine; 57. Classics of medical ethics; 1). Includes references. ISBN 0–7923–5000–6. BE62143.
    bioethics; feminist ethics; *historical aspects; literature; medical education; *medical ethics; *medicine; *philosophy; physician patient relationship; physicians; sociology of medicine; virtues; Bacon, Francis; *Eighteenth Century; Great Britain; *Gregory, John; Hume, David; Scotland

McCullough, Laurence B. Laying medicine open: understanding major turning points in the history of medical ethics. *Kennedy Institute of Ethics Journal.* 1999 Mar; 9(1): 7–23. 15 refs. BE62327.
    *accountability; *bioethics; conflict of interest; economics; entrepreneurship; *evidence-based medicine; *historical aspects; incentives; institutional ethics; managed care programs; *medical ethics; *medicine; moral obligations; physician patient relationship; *physicians; professional competence; quality of health care; resource allocation; virtues; Eighteenth Century; Gregory, John; Scotland; Twentieth Century; United States
At different times during its history medicine has been laid open to accountability for its scientific and moral quality. This phenmenon of laying medicine open has sometimes resulted in major turning points in the history of medical ethics. In this paper, I examine two examples of when the laying open of medicine has generated such turning points: eighteenth–century British medicine and late twentieth–century American medicine. In the eighteenth century, the Scottish physician–philosopher, John Gregory (1724–1773), concerned with the unscientific, entrepreneurial, self-interested nature of then current medical practice, laid medicine open to

---

accountability using the tools of ethics and philosophy of medicine. In the process, Gregory wrote the first professional ethics of medicine in the English-language literature, based on the physician's fiduciary responsibility to the patient. In the late twentieth century, the managed practice of medicine has laid medicine open to accountability for its scientific quality and economic cost. This current laying open of medicine creates the challenge of developing medical ethics and bioethics for population-based medical science and practice.

Murphy, Edmond A.; Butzow, James J.; Suarez-Murias, Edward L. Underpinnings of Medical Ethics. Baltimore, MD: Johns Hopkins University Press; 1997. 480 p. Bibliography: p. 449–462. ISBN 0-8018-5568-3. BE61356.
　　accountability; *decision making; deontological ethics; diagnosis; *disease; ethical analysis; *ethics; eugenics; freedom; intention; law; *medical ethics; *medicine; methods; models, theoretical; morality; *normality; *pain; patient care; *philosophy; physician's role; quality of life; rights; statistics; *suffering; teleological ethics; terminology; uncertainty; value of life; integrity; longevity

Norris, Peggy. Medical Ethics. Southport, Merseyside, England: Christian Theology Trust; 1992. 41 p. (Ethics module; 12). Includes references. ISBN 1-897705-01-8. BE59558.
　　abortion, induced; codes of ethics; embryo disposition; embryo research; eugenics; euthanasia; government regulation; historical aspects; hospices; human experimentation; *medical ethics; misconduct; National Socialism; palliative care; population control; preimplantation diagnosis; reproductive technologies; Germany; Great Britain; Hippocratic Oath

Pang, Mei-che Samantha. Protective truthfulness: the Chinese way of safeguarding patients in informed treatment decisions. *Journal of Medical Ethics.* 1999 Jun; 25(3): 247–253. 42 refs. BE61859.
　　autonomy; *beneficence; competence; confidentiality; cultural pluralism; *decision making; diagnosis; disclosure; empirical research; evaluation studies; *family members; historical aspects; hospitals; *informed consent; *medical ethics; *moral obligations; non-Western World; *nurse patient relationship; *nurses; nursing ethics; nursing research; *paternalism; patient care; patients' rights; *physician patient relationship; physicians; privacy; professional competence; prognosis; psychological stress; survey; terminal care; *third party consent; trust; *truth disclosure; value of life; values; virtues; vulnerable populations; hope; *China

The first part of this paper examines the practice of informed treatment decisions in the protective medical system in China today. The second part examines how health care professionals in China perceive and carry out their responsibilities when relaying information to vulnerable patients, based on the findings of an empirical study that I had undertaken to examine the moral experience of nurses in practice situations. In the Chinese medical ethics tradition, refinement [jing] in skills and sincerity [cheng] in relating to patients are two cardinal virtues that health care professionals are required to possess. This notion of absolute sincerity carries a strong sense of parental protectiveness. The empirical findings reveal that most nurses are ambivalent about telling the truth to patients. Truth-telling would become an insincere act if a patient were to lose hope and confidence in life after learning of his or her disease. In this system of protective medical care, it is arguable as to whose interests are being protected: the patient, the family or the hospital. I would suggest that the interests of the hospital and the family members who legitimately represent the patient's interests are being honoured, but

at the expense of the patient's right to know.

Pargiter, Russell; Bloch, Sidney. The ethics committee of a psychiatric college: its procedures and themes. *Australian and New Zealand Journal of Psychiatry.* 1997 Feb; 31(1): 76–82. 18 refs. Commented on by C. Lowy, p. 83–84. BE60277.
　　codes of ethics; economics; *ethics committees; forensic psychiatry; guidelines; medical education; *medical ethics; organization and administration; *physicians; *professional organizations; *psychiatry; self regulation; Australia; New Zealand; *Royal Australian and New Zealand College of Psychiatrists

Pellegrino, Edmund D. The goals and ends of medicine: how are they to be defined? *In:* Hanson, Mark J.; Callahan, Daniel, eds. The Goals of Medicine: The Forgotten Issue in Health Care Reform. Washington, DC: Georgetown University Press; 1999: 55–68. 18 fn. ISBN 0-87840-707-3. BE60517.
　　*goals; *health care; *medical ethics; *medicine; moral obligations; obligations to society; patient advocacy; philosophy; physician patient relationship; *physician's role; preventive medicine; public policy; technical expertise; trust; *values; Goals of Medicine Project (Hastings Center)

Ross, Saul; Malloy, David Cruise. Biomedical Ethics: Concepts and Cases for Health Care Professionals. Buffalo, NY: Thompson Educational Publishing; 1999. 192 p. Bibliography: p. 186–189 ISBN 1-55077-090-X. BE62148.
　　*bioethical issues; *bioethics; *case studies; decision making; deontological ethics; ethical analysis; *ethical theory; medical education; *medical ethics; moral development; moral policy; physician patient relationship; teleological ethics

Tauber, Alfred I. Confessions of a Medicine Man: An Essay in Popular Philosophy. Cambridge, MA: MIT Press; 1999. 159 p. Includes references. ISBN 0-262-20114-3. BE60753.
　　autonomy; biomedical research; biomedical technologies; decision making; economics; health care; medical education; *medical ethics; *medicine; patient advocacy; *philosophy; *physician patient relationship; physician's role; *physicians; postmodernism; resource allocation; self concept; Nietzsche, Friedrich; United States

Thomasma, David C. Stewardship of the aged: meeting the ethical challenge of ageism. *Cambridge Quarterly of Healthcare Ethics.* 1999 Spring; 8(2): 148–159. 38 fn. BE61232.
　　advance directives; *aged; allowing to die; autonomy; beneficence; biomedical technologies; case studies; casuistry; chronically ill; *clinical ethics; competence; covenant; *decision making; dissent; family members; health personnel; home care; hospitals; justice; legal guardians; long-term care; medicine; nursing homes; paternalism; *patient advocacy; *patient care; *patient participation; physical restraint; *physician patient relationship; prolongation of life; public policy; quality of life; resource allocation; right to die; risks and benefits; selection for treatment; social discrimination; terminal care; terminally ill; treatment refusal; *values; withholding treatment; elder abuse

Trotter, C. Griffin. The medical covenant: a Roycean perspective. *In:* McGee, Glenn, ed. Pragmatic Bioethics. Nashville, TN: Vanderbilt University Press; 1999: 84–96, 266–269. 35 fn. ISBN 0-8265-1321-2. BE60665.
　　autonomy; beneficence; compassion; *covenant; economics; health care; mediation; *medical ethics; *medicine; *models, theoretical; obligations to society; patient care; *philosophy; *physician patient relationship; physician's role; regulation; standards; *virtues; *loyalty; *pragmatism; *Royce, Josiah

---

Weinstock, Robert; Pearlman, Theodore. Letters to the editor [responses to P.S. Appelbaum, "A theory of ethics for forensic psychiatry," *JAAPS* 1997; 25(3): 233-247]. *Journal of the American Academy of Psychiatry and the Law.* 1998; 26(1): 151-157. 10 refs. BE61730.
  capital punishment; confidentiality; conflict of interest; disclosure; expert testimony; *forensic psychiatry; *medical ethics; moral obligations; physician patient relationship; *physician's role; prisoners; professional ethics; professional role; values

Zanobio, Bruno. The ethical dimension of Hippocratic medicine and its specific relationship to Christian morality. *Dolentium Hominum: Church and Health in the World.* 1996; 31(11th Yr., No. 1): 29-32. 37 refs. BE61000.
  *ancient history; *Christian ethics; codes of ethics; deontological ethics; futility; *historical aspects; literature; medical education; *medicine; morality; physician patient relationship; *physicians; refusal to treat; social worth; value of life; Hippocrates; *Hippocratic Oath

MEDICAL ETHICS/CODES OF ETHICS

American Medical Association. Council on Ethical and Judicial Affairs. Code of Medical Ethics: Current Opinions with Annotations, 1998-1999 Edition. Chicago, IL: American Medical Association; 1998. 228 p. ISBN 0-89970-960-5. BE61043.
  abortion, induced; active euthanasia; advance directives; advertising; AIDS serodiagnosis; allowing to die; attitudes; *bioethical issues; biomedical technologies; capital punishment; clinical ethics committees; *codes of ethics; confidentiality; conflict of interest; cord blood; domestic violence; economics; fetal research; futility; gene therapy; genetic counseling; genetic screening; ghost surgery; gifts; health care; HIV seropositivity; human experimentation; interprofessional relations; *medical ethics; medical etiquette; medical records; misconduct; organ donation; *organizational policies; patents; physician patient relationship; *physicians; professional organizations; referral and consultation; remuneration; reproductive technologies; resource allocation; resuscitation orders; social discrimination; sports medicine; physician impairment; *American Medical Association

Crawshaw, Ralph. Cautionary note on reforming medical oaths. *Bulletin of Medical Ethics.* 1997 Nov; No. 133: 13-14. 14 refs. BE59703.
  ancient history; *codes of ethics; historical aspects; *medical ethics; *Hippocratic Oath; Twentieth Century

Guillen, Diego Gracia. The Hippocratic Oath in the development of medicine. *Dolentium Hominum: Church and Health in the World.* 1996; 31(11th Yr., No. 1): 22-28. BE60999.
  ancient history; beneficence; clergy; *codes of ethics; compassion; confidentiality; *historical aspects; justice; legal obligations; love; *medical ethics; *medicine; *moral obligations; morality; obligations to society; physician patient relationship; *physician's role; *professional ethics; *religion; self regulation; technical expertise; *terminology; trust; *virtues; Western World; judges; Aristotle; *Hippocratic Oath; Socrates

Honings, Bonifacio. The Charter for Health Care Workers: a synthesis of Hippocratic ethics and Christian morality. *Dolentium Hominum: Church and Health in the World.* 1996; 31(11th Yr., No. 1): 48-52. 41 fn. BE61002.
  abortion, induced; active euthanasia; allowing to die; beginning of life; beneficence; *Christian ethics; *codes of ethics; empathy; health personnel; marital relationship; *medical ethics; moral obligations; *morality; organ donation; patient education; *physician patient relationship;

*physician's role; professional ethics; reproduction; reproductive technologies; *Roman Catholic ethics; suffering; terminal care; terminally ill; *theology; trust; *value of life; *Charter for Health Care Workers; Hippocrates; *Hippocratic Oath

Kumar, Sanjay. New medical council to create code of ethics for Delhi's doctors. [News]. *Lancet.* 1998 Oct 31; 352(9138): 1453. BE59657.
  *codes of ethics; *medical ethics; misconduct; *physicians; professional competence; *self regulation; *India; *Medical Council of Delhi

Newman, David H. A medical school honor code: what does it mean? *Pharos.* 1997 Spring; 60(2): 2-4. BE60337.
  *codes of ethics; medical education; medical ethics; *medical schools; misconduct; *students; whistleblowing; cheating; Hippocratic Oath

Rodriguez, Gonzalo Herranz. Contemporary ethical codes of professional conduct. *Dolentium Hominum: Church and Health in the World.* 1996; 31(11th Yr., No. 1): 33-36. BE61001.
  altruism; autonomy; beneficence; *Christian ethics; *codes of ethics; *emergency care; indigents; *international aspects; Jewish ethics; *medical ethics; misconduct; *moral obligations; nurses; *patient care; physician patient relationship; *physicians; professional ethics; sexuality; *social discrimination; value of life; values; vulnerable populations; war; dignity; Belgium; Ethical Principles of European Medicine; France; Geneva Declaration; *Good Samaritanism; Great Britain; Hippocratic Oath; International Code of Medical Ethics; Ireland; Italy; Portugal; Spain; United States; World Medical Association

Yakir, Avi; Glick, Shimon M. Medical students' attitudes to the physician's oath. *Medical Education.* 1998 Mar; 32(2): 133-137. 15 refs. BE62317.
  *attitudes; *codes of ethics; *medical education; *medical ethics; moral obligations; *students; survey; time factors; Ben-Gurion University; *Hippocratic Oath; *Israel

World Psychiatric Association approves Declaration of Madrid (25 Aug 1996). [Texts of the Declaration of Madrid and of related Guidelines Concerning Specific Situations]. *International Digest of Health Legislation.* 1997; 48(2): 240-242. BE59600.
  capital punishment; *codes of ethics; confidentiality; euthanasia; *guidelines; human experimentation; informed consent; *international aspects; *medical ethics; mentally ill; organ donation; physician patient relationship; physicians; professional organizations; *psychiatry; psychotherapy; selective abortion; sex determination; torture; *Declaration of Madrid; *World Psychiatric Association

MEDICAL ETHICS/EDUCATION

Beaudoin, Claude; Maheux, Brigitte; Côté, Luc, et al. Clinical teachers as humanistic caregivers and educators: perceptions of senior clerks and second-year residents. *Canadian Medical Association Journal.* 1998 Oct 6; 159(7): 765-769. 19 refs. BE62356.
  *attitudes; comparative studies; evaluation; *faculty; *humanism; *internship and residency; *interprofessional relations; *medical education; medical ethics; medical schools; *physician patient relationship; *physicians; *students; survey; *clinical clerkships; Laval University; Quebec; University of Montreal; University of Sherbrooke

Bickel, Janet. Proceedings of the AAMC Conference on Students' and Residents' Ethical and Professional Development: introduction. *Academic Medicine.* 1996 Jun; 71(6): 622-623. Conference held 27-28 Oct 1995.

BE = bioethics accession number   fn. = footnotes   refs. = references

BE61428.
    internship and residency; *medical education; *medical
    ethics; *moral development; physicians; *students;
    Association of American Medical Colleges

Bickel, Janet. Summaries of break-out sessions [AAMC
Conference on Students' and Residents' Ethical and
Professional Development, 27-28 Oct 1995]. *Academic
Medicine.* 1996 Jun; 71(6): 634-640. 17 refs. BE61430.
    administrators; conflict of interest; curriculum; deception;
    faculty; institutional policies; internship and residency;
    interprofessional relations; *medical education; *medical
    ethics; medical schools; misconduct; *moral development;
    patient care; physicians; sociology of medicine; *students;
    teaching methods; whistleblowing

Block, Susan; Billings, J. Andrew. Nurturing humanism
through teaching palliative care. *Academic Medicine.*
1998 Jul; 73(7): 763-765. 12 refs. BE59880.
    cultural pluralism; curriculum; hospices; *humanism;
    interprofessional relations; *medical education; medical
    ethics; medical schools; *palliative care; patient care team;
    physician patient relationship; professional family
    relationship; students; *terminal care; teaching hospitals

**Branch, William T.; Pels, Richard J.; Hafler, Janet
P.** Medical students' empathic understanding of their
patients. *Academic Medicine.* 1998 Apr; 73(4): 360-362.
BE59876.
    AIDS; compassion; domestic violence; drug abuse;
    *empathy; *medical education; medical ethics; *moral
    development; *physician patient relationship; *students;
    suffering; teaching methods

Buss, Mary K.; Marx, Eric S.; Sulmasy, Daniel P.
The preparedness of students to discuss end-of-life issues
with patients. *Academic Medicine.* 1998 Apr; 73(4):
418-422. 16 refs. BE59878.
    *advance care planning; *advance directives; age factors;
    allowing to die; assisted suicide; communication; ethics
    consultation; *knowledge, attitudes, practice; *medical
    education; medical schools; physician patient relationship;
    *students; survey; *terminal care; *Georgetown University
    School of Medicine; Mayo Medical School

Crausman, Robert S.; Armstrong, John D. Ethically
based medical decision making in the intensive care unit:
residency teaching strategies. *Critical Care Clinics.* 1996
Jan; 12(1): 71-84. 54 refs. BE59278.
    *bioethics; *clinical ethics; communication; curriculum;
    decision making; dissent; ethicists; faculty; family members;
    *intensive care units; interdisciplinary communication;
    *internship and residency; *medical education; *medical
    ethics; patient care; patient care team; physician patient
    relationship; *physicians; teaching methods; uncertainty;
    values

Federman, Daniel D. Protecting the future of medicine
-- from themselves. [Editorial]. *Annals of Internal
Medicine.* 1999 Jan 5; 130(1): 66-67. 6 refs. BE59332.
    AIDS; *communicable diseases; curriculum; faculty;
    *hepatitis; *HIV seropositivity; *medical education; moral
    obligations; *occupational exposure; patient care; preventive
    medicine; risk; *students; *infection control; University of
    California, San Francisco

Higgs, Roger. Do studies of the nature of cases mislead
about the reality of cases? A response to Pattison *et al.*
Journal of Medical Ethics. 1999 Feb; 25(1): 47-50. 13 refs.
BE61195.
    authorship; *bioethics; *case studies; *clinical ethics;
    dehumanization; *education; emotions; evaluation; literature;
    *medical ethics; *teaching methods; values
This article questions whether many are misled by

current case studies. Three broad types of style of case
study are described. A stark style, based on medical case
studies, a fictionalised style in reaction, and a personal
statement made in discussion groups by an original
protagonist. Only the second type fits Pattison's
category. Language remains an important issue, but to
be examined as the case is lived in discussion rather than
as a potentially reductionist study of the case as text.

Hope, R.A.; Fulford, K.W.M.; Yates, Anne. The Oxford
Practice Skills Course: Ethics, Law, and Communication
Skills in Health Care Education. [Instructor's Manual].
New York, NY: Oxford University Press; 1996. 181
p. Includes references. Manual outlines a course in
professional practice skills developed in the University
of Oxford Medical School for clinical medical students.
ISBN 0-19-262754-6. BE59865.
    case studies; clinical ethics; communication; confidentiality;
    *curriculum; informed consent; legal aspects; *medical
    education; *medical ethics; physician patient relationship;
    reproductive technologies; resource allocation; resuscitation
    orders; selection for treatment; *teaching methods; treatment
    refusal; Great Britain; *Oxford Practice Skills Project

**Hundert, Edward M.; Hafferty, Fred; Christakis,
Dimitri.** Characteristics of the informal curriculum and
trainees' ethical choices. *Academic Medicine.* 1996 Jun;
71(6): 624-633. 22 refs. Opening plenary session of the
AAMC Conference on Students' and Residents' Ethical
and Professional Development, 27-28 Oct 1995.
BE61429.
    curriculum; internship and residency; interprofessional
    relations; *medical education; *medical ethics; misconduct;
    *moral development; physicians; sociology of medicine;
    *students; teaching methods; values

Janson, C.G. Thoughts on medical ethics and education.
Pharos. 1997 Fall; 60(4): 31-34. 10 refs. BE60339.
    ancient history; historical aspects; *medical education;
    *medical ethics; philosophy; teaching methods; virtues;
    Marcus Aurelius

London, Leslie; McCarthy, G. Teaching medical students
on the ethical dimensions of human rights: meeting the
challenge in South Africa. *Journal of Medical Ethics.* 1998
Aug; 24(4): 257-262. 22 fn. BE61292.
    blacks; comparative studies; control groups; *curriculum;
    *evaluation; evaluation studies; historical aspects; *human
    rights; *knowledge, attitudes, practice; *medical education;
    *medical ethics; misconduct; physicians; prisoners;
    professional organizations; social discrimination; *students;
    teaching methods; torture; *South Africa; *University of
    Cape Town
SETTING: Previous health policies in South Africa
neglected the teaching of ethics and human rights to
health professionals. In April 1995, a pilot course was
run at the University of Cape Town in which the ethical
dimensions of human rights issues in South Africa were
explored. OBJECTIVES: To compare knowledge and
attitudes of participating students with a group of control
students. DESIGN: Retrospective cohort study.
SUBJECTS: Seventeen fourth-year medical students
who participated in the course and 13 control students
from the same class, matched for gender.
INTERVENTIONS: Students participated in a
one-week module on ethics and human rights. Five
months after the course had been run, students completed
a semi-structured questionnaire exploring their
knowledge and attitudes with regards to ethics and
human rights issues. MAIN OUTCOME MEASURES:
Knowledge scores, attitude scores and various individual
indicators of attitude. RESULTS: Clear benefits for

BE = bioethics accession number   fn. = footnotes   refs. = references

overall knowledge score, for four out of five individual knowledge questions and for one of the attitude questions, were demonstrated. Participating students also appeared to be more convinced of the need for teaching on the ethical dimensions of human rights at postgraduate level and that such teaching should also be integrated in the curriculum. The low response rate amongst controls may have selected students who were more socially conscious, thereby leading to an underestimate of the true impact of the course. CONCLUSION: The evaluation indicates clear benefits of the course for undergraduate students, and supports arguments for the inclusion of such courses in the training of health professionals. This is particularly important given the challenges posed by the Truth and Reconciliation Commission to the health professions to address past complicity in human rights abuses through reorientation of medical training in South Africa.

Ludmerer, Kenneth M. Instilling professionalism in medical education. [Editorial]. *JAMA.* 1999 Sep 1; 282(9): 881–882. 14 refs. BE62658.
　　attitudes; curriculum; economics; faculty; humanism; institutional ethics; interprofessional relations; *medical education; *medical ethics; medical schools; students; teaching methods; *values; virtues; mentors; teaching hospitals

Neufeld, Victor R. Physician as humanist: still an educational challenge. [Editorial]. *Canadian Medical Association Journal.* 1998 Oct 6; 159(7): 787–788. 7 refs. BE62358.
　　attitudes; *communication; empirical research; *faculty; *humanism; internship and residency; interprofessional relations; *medical education; *physician patient relationship; *physicians; public opinion; students; Canada

Newman, David H. A medical school honor code: what does it mean? *Pharos.* 1997 Spring; 60(2): 2–4. BE60337.
　　*codes of ethics; medical education; medical ethics; *medical schools; misconduct; *students; whistleblowing; cheating; Hippocratic Oath

Nordio, S. Beneficence, virtues and ethical committees in pediatrics: epistemology, bioethics and medical pedagogy in pediatrics. *In:* Burgio, G. Roberto; Lantos, John D., eds. *Primum Non Nocere* Today. Second Edition. New York, NY: Elsevier; 1998: 147–158. 53 refs. ISBN 0-444-82923-7. BE60925.
　　adolescents; age factors; autonomy; beneficence; *bioethics; children; clinical ethics committees; cultural pluralism; disclosure; ethical theory; informed consent; *medical education; *medical ethics; newborns; parental consent; paternalism; patient care; *pediatrics; philosophy; physician patient relationship; physicians; principle-based ethics; research ethics committees; teleological ethics; trends; virtues

Schubert–Lehnhardt, Viola. Issues in the study of medical ethics. *Medicine and Law.* 1993; 12(1–2): 33–39. 16 fn. BE60610.
　　curriculum; interdisciplinary communication; *medical education; *medical ethics; students; teaching methods; universities; East Germany; *Germany; Martin Luther University

Swenson, Sara L.; Rothstein, Julie A. Navigating the wards: teaching medical students to use their moral compasses. *Academic Medicine.* 1996 Jun; 71(6): 591–594. 14 refs. BE61426.
　　goals; hospitals; *medical education; *medical ethics; *moral development; *students; *teaching methods; integrity

Swick, Herbert M.; Szenas, Philip; Danoff, Deborah, et al. Teaching professionalism in undergraduate medical education. *JAMA.* 1999 Sep 1; 282(9): 830–832. 10 refs. BE62656.
　　*curriculum; evaluation; faculty; humanism; *medical education; *medical ethics; *medical schools; statistics; survey; teaching methods; *values; *virtues; *United States
　　CONTEXT: There is a growing consensus among medical educators that to promote the professional development of medical students, schools of medicine should provide explicit learning experiences in professionalism. OBJECTIVE: To determine whether and how schools of medicine were teaching professionalism in the 1998–1999 academic year. DESIGN, SETTING, AND PARTICIPANTS: A 2-stage survey was sent to 125 US medical schools in the fall of 1998. A total of 116 (92.3%) responded to the first stage of the survey. The second survey led to a qualitative analysis of curriculum materials submitted by 41 schools. MAIN OUTCOME MEASURES: Presence or absence of learning experiences (didactic or experiential) in undergraduate medical curriculum explicitly intended to promote professionalism in medical students, with curriculum evaluation based on 4 attributes commonly recognized as essential to professionalism: subordination of one's self-interests, adherence to high ethical and moral standards, response to societal needs, and demonstration of evincible core humanistic values. RESULTS: Of the 116 responding medical schools, 104 (89.7%) reported that they offer some formal instruction related to professionalism. Fewer schools have explicit methods for assessing professional behaviors (n = 64 [55.2%]) or conduct targeted faculty development programs (n = 39 [33.6%]). Schools use diverse strategies to promote professionalism, ranging from an isolated white-coat ceremony or other orientation experience (n = 71 [78.9%]) to an integrated sequence of courses over multiple years of the curriculum (n = 25 [27.8%]). Of the 41 schools that provided curriculum materials, 27 (65.9%) addressed subordinating self-interests; 31 (75.6%), adhering to high ethical and moral standards; 17 (41.5%), responding to societal needs; and 22 (53.7%), evincing core humanistic values. CONCLUSIONS: Our results suggest that the teaching of professionalism in undergraduate medical education varies widely. Although most medical schools in the United States now address this important topic in some manner, the strategies used to teach professionalism may not always be adequate.

Wray, Samuel R.; Parshad, Omkar; Young, Lauriann E. Ethics and law in the medical curriculum -- a University of the West Indies perspective. *Medicine and Law.* 1993; 12(1–2): 41–45. 4 refs. BE60611.
　　bioethical issues; *curriculum; *law; *medical education; *medical ethics; teaching methods; *University of the West Indies; West Indies

Yakir, Avi; Glick, Shimon M. Medical students' attitudes to the physician's oath. *Medical Education.* 1998 Mar; 32(2): 133–137. 15 refs. BE62317.
　　*attitudes; *codes of ethics; *medical education; *medical ethics; moral obligations; *students; survey; time factors; Ben-Gurion University; *Hippocratic Oath; *Israel

MENTAL HEALTH
See also under
　　CONFIDENTIALITY/MENTAL HEALTH

BE = bioethics accession number　　　fn. = footnotes　　　refs. = references

de Jong, Judith; Reatig, Natalie. SAMHSA philosophy and statement on ethical principles. *Ethics and Behavior.* 1998; 8(4): 339–343. BE60165.
> accountability; *alcohol abuse; autonomy; beneficence; codes of ethics; cultural pluralism; *drug abuse; federal government; health care delivery; *health promotion; *institutional ethics; justice; *mental health; *mentally ill; minority groups; preventive medicine; rehabilitation; resource allocation; social problems; trust; community consent; *community medicine; intervention studies; *Substance Abuse and Mental Health Services Administration; United States

As the major federal agency responsible for improving the delivery and effectiveness of substance abuse and mental health services to the American public, the Substance Abuse and Mental Health Services Administration (SAMHSA) is aware that its programs deal with especially sensitive issues. As a national leader in advancing effective services to persons with addictive and mental disorders, SAMHSA has stewardship over important interventions affecting personal, community, institutional, and social values. Inherent in SAMHSA's mission and goals is a commitment to protect and promote the human, civil, and legal rights and moral freedoms of those individuals and groups who participate in SAMHSA-funded activities and to demonstrate that Agency policies and procedures are congruent with publicly acceptable ethical principles and standards of conduct. A foundation of mutual trust between SAMHSA officials and participants as well as sensitivity to issues of public accountability will hasten and strengthen progress toward this shared vision.

Elliott, Carl. The tyranny of happiness: ethics and cosmetic psychopharmacology. *In:* Parens, Erik, ed. Enhancing Human Traits: Ethical and Social Implications. Washington, DC: Georgetown University Press; 1998: 177–188. 11 fn. ISBN 0–87840–703–0. BE59752.
> *behavior control; depressive disorder; *emotions; enhancement technologies; literature; *mental health; normality; psychiatry; *psychoactive drugs; psychological stress; *quality of life; *self concept; uncertainty; value of life; *values; Western World; authenticity; Listening to Prozac (Kramer, P.); Percy, Walker; Prozac; Twentieth Century; United States

Fulford, K.W.M. Dissent and dissensus: the limits of consensus formation in psychiatry. *In:* ten Have, Henk A.M.J.; Sass, Hans-Martin, eds. Consensus Formation in Healthcare Ethics. Boston, MA: Kluwer Academic; 1998: 175–192. 36 refs. 1 fn. ISBN 0–7923–4944–X. BE62594.
> *consensus; disease; *dissent; forensic psychiatry; health; historical aspects; medicine; *mental health; philosophy; *psychiatric diagnosis; *psychiatry; *values; Nineteenth Century; Twentieth Century

Hanford, Jack T. Mental health and managed care. *Journal of Religion and Health.* 1998 Summer; 37(2): 159–165. 13 refs. BE61977.
> health care delivery; *managed care programs; mental health; patient advocacy; professional patient relationship; quality of health care; regulation; withholding treatment; *mental health services; Medicare; United States

Hanson, Kristina W. Public opinion and the mental health parity debate: lessons from the survey literature. *Psychiatric Services.* 1998 Aug; 49(8): 1059–1066. 13 refs. BE59842.
> costs and benefits; *drug abuse; *empirical research; health care reform; *health insurance reimbursement; health services research; information dissemination; *knowledge, attitudes, practice; *mental health; *mentally ill; patient care; *public opinion; public policy; research design; United States

Joy, Mark; Hemmings, Gwynneth; Al–Adwani, Andrew, et al. Parity of mental illness, disparity for the mental patient. [Letters and response]. *Lancet.* 1999 Jan 2; 353(9146): 73–74. 8 refs. BE61620.
> advance directives; *behavior control; coercion; competence; dangerousness; involuntary commitment; law enforcement; *mental health; *mentally ill; physicians; prisoners; psychiatric diagnosis; psychiatric wills; psychiatry; schizophrenia; stigmatization; suicide

Lerner, Paul. Rationalizing the therapeutic arsenal: German neuropsychiatry in World War I. *In:* Berg, Manfred; Cocks, Geoffrey, eds. Medicine and Modernity: Public Health and Medical Care in Nineteenth- and Twentieth-Century Germany. New York, NY: Cambridge University Press; 1997: 121–148. 106 fn. ISBN 0–521–56411–5. BE59268.
> *attitudes; coercion; common good; deception; electroconvulsive therapy; *historical aspects; hypnosis; *mental health; *mentally ill; methods; *military personnel; misconduct; obligations to society; *patient care; physician patient relationship; physician's role; *physicians; psychiatric diagnosis; *psychiatry; psychotherapy; *public policy; rehabilitation; social control; social dominance; *war; post-traumatic stress disorders; *Germany; *Twentieth Century; *World War I

Rosenheck, Robert; Armstrong, Moe; Callahan, Daniel, et al. Obligation to the least well off in setting mental health service priorities: a consensus statement. *Psychiatric Services.* 1998 Oct; 49(10): 1273–1274, 1290. 13 refs. BE61446.
> community services; consensus; *costs and benefits; decision making; *economics; federal government; *health care delivery; justice; mental health; *mentally ill; *obligations of society; psychiatry; *public policy; *resource allocation; schizophrenia; *selection for treatment; values; *mental health services; *seriously ill; United States; *Veterans Health Administration

Schmiedebach, Heinz–Peter. The mentally ill patient caught between the state's demands and the professional interests of psychiatrists. *In:* Berg, Manfred; Cocks, Geoffrey, eds. Medicine and Modernity: Public Health and Medical Care in Nineteenth- and Twentieth-Century Germany. New York, NY: Cambridge University Press; 1997: 99–119. 61 fn. ISBN 0–521–56411–5. BE59267.
> *attitudes; chronically ill; *dehumanization; eugenics; food; forensic psychiatry; health care delivery; *historical aspects; involuntary sterilization; medical specialties; *mental health; *mental institutions; *mentally ill; military personnel; mortality; patient care; *physicians; *psychiatry; public health; public policy; resource allocation; *social control; social problems; social worth; socioeconomic factors; *sociology of medicine; *stigmatization; war; prostitution; Darwinism; *Germany; *Nineteenth Century; *Twentieth Century; World War I

Sharkey, Joe. Bedlam: Greed, Profiteering, and Fraud in a Mental Health System Gone Crazy. New York, NY: St. Martin's Press; 1994. 294 p. ISBN 0–312–10421–9. BE62500.
> adolescents; adults; advertising; alcohol abuse; behavior disorders; children; coercion; drug abuse; *fraud; *health insurance reimbursement; involuntary commitment; legal aspects; mental health; *mental institutions; *misconduct; patient admission; *proprietary health facilities; psychiatric diagnosis; *referral and consultation; voluntary admission; *mental health services; National Medical Enterprises; Texas; *United States

---

BE = bioethics accession number   fn. = footnotes   refs. = references

Trickett, Edison J. Toward a framework for defining and resolving ethical issues in the protection of communities involved in primary prevention projects. *Ethics and Behavior.* 1998; 8(4): 321–337. 34 refs. BE60164.

adolescents; *alcohol abuse; aliens; anthropology; behavior disorders; *behavioral research; children; cultural pluralism; disadvantaged; *drug abuse; ecology; education; health education; *health promotion; health services research; informed consent; injuries; investigator subject relationship; *mental health; mentally ill; metaphor; minority groups; patient education; *preventive medicine; professional ethics; psychology; public health; sexually transmitted diseases; social dominance; *social problems; trust; values; *community medicine; *intervention studies

Ethical issues flow from and are embedded in contexts of practice. *Contexts of practice* refer to the diverse social settings where interventions occur. Primary prevention activities require new professional roles in these diverse social settings. These new roles engage the professional in new activities, which in turn allow new ethical issues to arise. This article takes an ecological perspective on ethical issues arising from the enactment of new preventive roles intended to affect groups or communities. Within this perspective, the concepts of context and culture take on special conceptual significance. Four ecological assumptions about preventive interventions intended to affect groups or communities are offered as a means of framing ethical issues in such interventions. Finally, several approaches to developing ecological knowledge about the contexts of practice are presented as ways of furthering our ability to conceptualize and cope with ethical issues in preventive interventions intended to affect groups or communities.

Wendell, Susan. Old women out of control: some thoughts on aging, ethics, and psychosomatic medicine. *In:* Walter, Margaret Urban, ed. Mother Time: Women, Aging, and Ethics. Lanham, MD: Rowman and Littlefield; 1999: 133–149. 24 refs. 4 fn. ISBN 0-8476-9260-4. BE61897.

adults; *age factors; aged; attitudes; chronically ill; *diagnosis; disabled; *females; health; *medical errors; *mental health; morbidity; normality; patient care; physicians; *psychiatric diagnosis; *self concept; social discrimination; socioeconomic factors; sociology of medicine; stigmatization; *women's health; menopause; *psychosomatic medicine; North America

MENTALLY DISABLED

See also BEHAVIOR CONTROL, ELECTROCONVULSIVE THERAPY, INVOLUNTARY COMMITMENT
See under
INFORMED CONSENT/MENTALLY DISABLED
PATIENT CARE/MENTALLY DISABLED
PATIENTS' RIGHTS/MENTALLY DISABLED
STERILIZATION/MENTALLY DISABLED
TREATMENT REFUSAL/MENTALLY DISABLED

MERCY KILLING *See* EUTHANASIA

MINORS

See under
ABORTION/MINORS
BEHAVIORAL RESEARCH/MINORS
CONTRACEPTION/MINORS

HUMAN EXPERIMENTATION/MINORS
INFORMED CONSENT/MINORS
INVOLUNTARY COMMITMENT/MINORS
PATIENT CARE/MINORS
TREATMENT REFUSAL/MINORS

MISCONDUCT *See* FRAUD AND MISCONDUCT

NURSE PATIENT RELATIONSHIP *See* NURSING ETHICS, PROFESSIONAL PATIENT RELATIONSHIP

NURSING CARE *See* PATIENT CARE, TERMINAL CARE

NURSING ETHICS

See also BIOETHICS, MEDICAL ETHICS, PROFESSIONAL ETHICS

Chally, Pamela S.; Loriz, Lillia. Ethics in the trenches: decision making in practice -- a practical model for resolving the types of ethical dilemmas you face daily. *American Journal of Nursing.* 1998 Jun; 98(6): 17–20. 12 refs. BE61801.

aged; autonomy; beneficence; case studies; critically ill; *decision making; intensive care units; justice; models, theoretical; nurses; *nursing ethics; patient admission; patient care; patient discharge; physical restraint; resource allocation; truth disclosure

Davis, Anne J. Global influence of American nursing: some ethical issues. *Nursing Ethics.* 1999 Mar; 6(2): 118–125. 17 refs. BE61931.

autonomy; caring; *cultural pluralism; decision making; *ethical relativism; ethical theory; family members; family relationship; historical aspects; informed consent; *international aspects; non-Western World; nurses; nursing education; *nursing ethics; nursing research; patient participation; patients' rights; principle–based ethics; self concept; *social impact; *social interaction; trends; *values; virtues; Western World; *Japan; *United States

de Raeve, Louise. Maintaining integrity through clinical supervision. *Nursing Ethics.* 1998 Nov; 5(6): 486–496. 17 refs. BE60810.

*administrators; communication; conscience; counseling; *interprofessional relations; nurse patient relationship; *nurses; *nursing ethics; psychological stress; values; *integrity

Dunn, Debra Geller. Bioethics and nursing. *NursingConnections.* 1994 Fall; 7(3): 43–51. 22 refs. BE59811.

bioethics; codes of ethics; *decision making; misconduct; moral development; nurses; *nursing ethics; patient advocacy; whistleblowing

Gastmans, Chris. Care as a moral attitude in nursing. *Nursing Ethics.* 1999 May; 6(3): 214–223. 21 refs. BE61766.

attitudes; *caring; emotions; *moral development; nurse patient relationship; nurse's role; *nurses; *nursing ethics; professional competence

Gastmans, Chris; Dierckx de Casterle, Bernadette; Schotsmans, Paul. Nursing considered as moral practice: a philosophical–ethical interpretation of nursing. *Kennedy Institute of Ethics Journal.* 1998 Mar; 8(1): 43–69. 33 refs. 3 fn. Commented on by C.R. Taylor,

---

BE = bioethics accession number   fn. = footnotes   refs. = references

p. 71–82. BE59354.
altruism; beneficence; *caring; communication; emotions; goals; motivation; *nurse patient relationship; *nurse's role; nurses; *nursing ethics; patient admission; patient care; patient participation; patients; philosophy; professional competence; religion; technical expertise; trust; values; *virtues

Discussions of ethical approaches in nursing have been much enlivened in recent years, for instance by new developments in the theory of care. Nevertheless, many ethical concepts in nursing still need to be clarified. The purpose of this contribution is to develop a fundamental ethical view on nursing care considered as moral practice. Three main components are analyzed more deeply -- i.e., the caring relationship, caring behavior as the integration of virtue and expert activity, and "good care" as the ultimate goal of nursing practice. For the development of this philosophical–ethical interpretation of nursing, we have mainly drawn on the pioneering work of Anne Bishop and John Scudder, Alasdair MacIntyre, Lawrence Blum, and Louis Janssens. We will also show that the European philosophical background offers some original ideas for this endeavor.

Guido, Ginny Wacker. Ethics. *In: her* Legal Issues in Nursing. Second Edition. Stamford, CT: Appleton and Lange; 1997: 355–366. 11 refs. Chapter is followed by a glossary, p. 367–388, and appendixes providing texts of the ANA Code of Ethics, the International Code for Nurses, a Sample Professional Liability Insurance Policy and Model Practice of Nursing Acts, p. 389–397. ISBN 0-8385-5647-7. BE61849.
clinical ethics committees; decision making; ethical analysis; ethical theory; ethics; guidelines; law; legal aspects; nurses; *nursing ethics; principle-based ethics; treatment refusal

Hough, M. Catherine. Ethical dilemmas faced by critical care nurses in clinical practice: walking the line. *Critical Care Clinics.* 1996 Jan; 12(1): 123–133. 20 refs. BE59282.
allowing to die; caring; case studies; *critically ill; deception; *decision making; double effect; drugs; females; futility; intensive care units; males; moral development; narrative ethics; *nurses; *nursing ethics; pain; palliative care; *patient care; physician nurse relationship; physicians; resource allocation; *terminally ill; whistleblowing

McAlpine, Heather; Kristjanson, Linda; Poroch, Davina. Development and testing of the ethical reasoning tool (ERT): an instrument to measure the ethical reasoning of nurses. *Journal of Advanced Nursing.* 1997 Jun; 25(6): 1151–1161. 63 refs. BE60539.
attitudes; communication; decision making; *evaluation; *moral development; nurse patient relationship; nurse's role; *nurses; nursing education; *nursing ethics; nursing research; physician nurse relationship; students; values

Proulx, Amy J. Should you call a code? When a patient's condition is terminal, how do you handle a code? *American Journal of Nursing.* 1998 Jun; 98(6): 41. BE61816.
allowing to die; *decision making; family members; institutional policies; nurses; *nursing ethics; prolongation of life; *resuscitation orders; *terminally ill

Salladay, Susan A. Nursing ethics: growing beyond rules of conduct. *Journal of Christian Nursing.* 1997 Spring; 14(2): 20–23. 26 fn. BE59431.
*Christian ethics; historical aspects; nurse's role; *nursing ethics; values

Scott, P. Anne. Professional ethics: are we on the wrong track? *Nursing Ethics.* 1998 Nov; 5(6): 477–485. 16 refs.

BE60809.
accountability; alternatives; autonomy; behavior control; behavior disorders; case studies; codes of ethics; deception; decision making; interprofessional relations; *misconduct; *nurse's role; *nurses; *nursing ethics; patient care team; physicians; principle-based ethics; psychoactive drugs; *punishment; regulation; standards; treatment refusal; *Great Britain; United Kingdom Central Council for Nursing, Midwifery and Health Visiting

Silva, Mary Cipriano. New ANA [American Nurses Association] guidelines for ethics in nursing research. *NursingConnections.* 1996 Summer; 9(2): 28–33. 5 refs. BE59190.
animal experimentation; autonomy; beneficence; competence; confidentiality; *guidelines; *human experimentation; human rights; informed consent; investigators; justice; moral obligations; nurses; *nursing ethics; *nursing research; privacy; professional competence; professional organizations; research subjects; risks and benefits; scientific misconduct; selection of subjects; whistleblowing; American Nurses Association

Söderberg, Anna; Gilje, Fredricka; Norberg, Astrid. Dignity in situations of ethical difficulty in intensive care. *Intensive and Critical Care Nursing.* 1997 Jun; 13(3): 135–144. 32 refs. BE60479.
allowing to die; caring; conscience; decision making; dehumanization; *intensive care units; *narrative ethics; nurse patient relationship; *nurses; *nursing ethics; *patient care; physician nurse relationship; psychological stress; terminal care; withholding treatment; *dignity; qualitative research; Sweden

Taylor, Carol R. Reflections on "Nursing considered as moral practice." *Kennedy Institute of Ethics Journal.* 1998 Mar; 8(1): 71–82. 12 refs. Commentary on C. Gastmans, B. Dierckx de Casterle, P. Schotsmans, p. 43–69. BE59355.
accountability; altruism; *caring; compassion; empathy; *goals; health; *moral obligations; nurse patient relationship; *nurse's role; nurses; *nursing ethics; nursing research; values; *virtues

This response to the preceding article by Gastmans, Dierckx de Casterle, and Schotsmans challenges the notion of "good care" as the ultimate goal of nursing practice, explores further the possible goals of nursing and how they may be identified, and presents six elements of professional caring along with their related virtues and moral obligations.

Tschudin, Verena; Hunt, Geoffrey; Olsen, Douglas, et al. International Centres for Nursing Ethics [ICNE]. [Editorial]. *Nursing Ethics.* 1999 May; 6(3): 187–188. BE61763.
*international aspects; *nursing ethics; research institutes; Great Britain; *International Centres for Nursing Ethics

Tsuchin, Verena. Special issues facing nurses. *In:* Kuhse, Helga; Singer, Peter, eds. A Companion to Bioethics. Malden, MA: Blackwell; 1998: 463–471. 19 refs. ISBN 0-631-19737-0. BE59519.
caring; codes of ethics; conflict of interest; interprofessional relations; *nurse's role; *nurses; nursing education; *nursing ethics; patient advocacy; patient care; physician nurse relationship; *professional autonomy; whistleblowing

van Hooft, Stan. Acting from the virtue of caring in nursing. *Nursing Ethics.* 1999 May; 6(3): 189–201. 15 refs. BE61764.
*caring; emotions; *moral development; motivation; nurse patient relationship; nurses; *nursing ethics; principle-based ethics; professional competence; *virtues; Kuhse, Helga

---

BE = bioethics accession number   fn. = footnotes   refs. = references

van Hooft, Stan; Gillam, Lynn; Byrnes, Margot. The logic of ethical thinking. *In: their* Facts and Values: An Introduction to Critical Thinking for Nurses. Philadelphia, PA: MacLennan and Petty; 1995: 185–270, 278. 20 refs. 8 fn. ISBN 0-86433-107-X. BE60512.
  accountability; beneficence; caring; conscience; decision making; *ethical analysis; ethics; moral obligations; nurses; *nursing ethics; patient advocacy; patient care; quality of life; rights; risks and benefits; values; dignity

NURSING ETHICS/EDUCATION

Catalano, Joseph T. The ethics of cadaver experimentation. *Critical Care Nurse.* 1994 Dec; 14(6): 82–85. 8 refs. BE61434.
  administrators; *cadavers; conscience; *continuing education; emergency care; hospitals; human body; institutional policies; interprofessional relations; *nontherapeutic research; *nurses; nursing education; *nursing ethics; presumed consent; property rights; intubation

Long, Ann; Slevin, Eamonn. Living with dementia: communicating with an older person and her family. *Nursing Ethics.* 1999 Jan; 6(1): 23–36. 54 refs. BE60152.
  *aged; autonomy; beneficence; *caring; *communication; deception; dehumanization; *dementia; diagnosis; empathy; ethical analysis; family members; family relationship; humanism; *nurse patient relationship; *nurses; *nursing education; nursing research; paternalism; *patient care; *professional family relationship; psychological stress; psychology; social dominance; stigmatization; truth disclosure; adult offspring; University of Ulster (Northern Ireland)

Roberts, E. Francine. Academic misconduct in schools of nursing. *NursingConnections.* 1997 Fall; 10(3): 28–36. 24 refs. BE59191.
  attitudes; faculty; institutional policies; *misconduct; moral development; nurses; *nursing education; *nursing ethics; schools; *students; teaching methods

Webb, John; Warwick, Catherine. Getting it right: the teaching of philosophical health care ethics. *Nursing Ethics.* 1999 Mar; 6(2): 150–156. 4 refs. BE61934.
  bioethical issues; curriculum; ethical analysis; ethical theory; *nursing education; *nursing ethics; *teaching methods

OCCUPATIONAL HEALTH

See also PUBLIC HEALTH

American Association of Occupational Health Nurses; American College of Occupational and Environmental Medicine. AAOHN and ACOEM consensus statement for confidentiality of employee health information. *AAOHN Journal (American Association of Occupational Health Nurses).* 1997 Nov; 45(11): 613. Approved by the Board of Directors of both organizations on 4 May 1997. BE59926.
  *confidentiality; disclosure; employment; informed consent; law enforcement; legal aspects; *medical records; *nurses; *occupational medicine; *organizational policies; *physicians; professional organizations; public health; *American Association of Occupational Health Nurses; *American College of Occupational and Environmental Medicine; United States

Derickson, Alan. Black Lung: Anatomy of a Public Health Disaster. Ithaca, NY: Cornell University Press; 1998. 237 p. 429 fn. ISBN 0-8014-3186-7. BE60743.
  economics; *employment; federal government; *government regulation; health; *health hazards; historical aspects; *industry; legal aspects; morbidity; mortality; *occupational exposure; occupational medicine; physicians; political activity; public policy; state government; *lung diseases; Federal Coal Mine and Safety Act 1969; Nineteenth Century; Twentieth Century; United Mine Workers of America; *United States

Egilman, David; Wallace, Wes; Hom, Candace. Corporate corruption of medical literature: asbestos studies concealed by W.R. Grace & Co. *Accountability in Research.* 1998 Jan; 6(1–2): 127–147. 76 refs. BE61547.
  animal experimentation; biomedical research; cancer; compensation; contracts; *deception; *disclosure; economics; employment; *epidemiology; federal government; financial support; government regulation; *health hazards; *industry; information dissemination; injuries; institutional ethics; insurance; investigators; legal liability; *morbidity; mortality; *occupational exposure; *scientific misconduct; *lung diseases; Montana; National Institutes of Occupational Safety and Health; United States; *W.R. Grace & Co.

Kern, David G.; Kern, Robin K.; Durand, Kate T.H., et al. Secrecy in science: the flock worker's lung investigation. [Letter and response]. *Annals of Internal Medicine.* 1999 Apr 6; 130(7): 616. 6 refs. BE62562.
  biomedical research; confidentiality; contracts; *disclosure; editorial policies; employment; *epidemiology; *health hazards; hospitals; *industry; investigators; *occupational exposure; physicians; toxicity; universities; *lung diseases

Marshall, Eliot. Beryllium screening raises ethical issues. [News]. *Science.* 1999 Jul 9; 285(5425): 178–179. BE62524.
  data banks; *employment; *genetic predisposition; *genetic screening; *health hazards; *occupational exposure; lung diseases; United States

Merrill, William W.; Beckett, William S.; Raymond, Lawrence W., et al. Flock worker's lung. [Letters and response]. *Annals of Internal Medicine.* 1999 Apr 6; 130(7): 615–616. 11 refs. BE62561.
  confidentiality; contracts; diagnosis; *disclosure; *employment; *health hazards; *industry; investigators; legislation; mandatory reporting; *occupational exposure; occupational medicine; physicians; professional ethics; *toxicity; *lung diseases; Toxic Substances Control Act; United States

Studdert, David M. Direct contracts, data sharing and employee risk selection: new stakes for patient privacy in tomorrow's health insurance markets. *American Journal of Law and Medicine.* 1999; 25(2–3): 233–265. 242 fn. BE62508.
  compensation; computers; *confidentiality; conflict of interest; *contracts; disabled; *disclosure; economics; *employment; federal government; government regulation; health care delivery; *health insurance; *incentives; insurance selection bias; *legal aspects; legislation; *managed care programs; occupational medicine; *organization and administration; patient care; *physicians; *privacy; risk; social discrimination; state government; Americans with Disabilities Act 1990; *United States

Taimi, Kitty. A new challenge for IRBs: medical surveillance for former DOE workers. *Protecting Human Subjects.* 1997 Fall: 6–8. BE60061.
  *employment; *epidemiology; *ethical review; federal government; health; human experimentation; nuclear warfare; *occupational exposure; program descriptions; public policy; *radiation; research design; research ethics committees; expedited review; *Department of Energy; United States

---

BE = bioethics accession number   fn. = footnotes   refs. = references

OPERANT CONDITIONING *See* BEHAVIOR CONTROL

ORGAN AND TISSUE DONATION

See also BLOOD DONATION, ORGAN AND TISSUE TRANSPLANTATION

Agich, George J. From Pittsburgh to Cleveland: NHBD [non-heart-beating donor] controversies and bioethics. *Cambridge Quarterly of Healthcare Ethics.* 1999 Summer; 8(3): 269–274. 12 fn. BE62470.
> advance directives; allowing to die; autonomy; bioethical issues; *cadavers; *cardiac death; determination of death; donor cards; *ethicist's role; family members; hospitals; informed consent; *institutional policies; interdisciplinary communication; killing; *mass media; *organ donation; patients; third party consent; trust; withholding treatment; *Cleveland Clinic Foundation; 60 Minutes (CBS News television program)

Akabayashi, Akira. Transplantation from a brain dead donor in Japan. [News]. *Hastings Center Report.* 1999 May–Jun; 29(3): 48. BE61416.
> *brain death; determination of death; donor cards; family members; *legal aspects; legislation; *organ donation; organ transplantation; third party consent; *Japan

American Society for Reproductive Medicine. Ethics Committee. Informed consent and the use of gametes and embryos for research. *Fertility and Sterility.* 1997 Nov; 68(5): 780–781. 1 ref. BE62008.
> disclosure; *donors; embryo disposition; *embryo research; *embryos; *germ cells; *informed consent; investigators; *ovum donors; patients; reproductive technologies; *research embryo creation; research ethics committees; *semen donors; *tissue donation; viability; American Society for Reproductive Medicine

Andrews, Edmund L. German company to leave China over sales of organs. [News]. *New York Times.* 1998 Mar 7: A5. BE60468.
> aliens; cadavers; capital punishment; *health facilities; international aspects; *kidneys; *organ donation; organ transplantation; *prisoners; *remuneration; *renal dialysis; *China; Fresenius Medical Care A.G.; *Germany

Argentina. Law No. 24193 of 24 Mar 1993 on the transplantation of organs and anatomical materials. (*Boletin Oficial de la Repdblica Argentina*, 26 Apr 1993, Section 1, No. 27625, p. 1–5). [Summary]. *International Digest of Health Legislation.* 1994. 45(1). 35–36. BE62689.
> cadavers; compensation; incentives; informed consent; *legal aspects; *organ donation; organ donors; organ transplantation; third party consent; *Argentina

Arnold, Robert M.; Siminoff, Laura A.; Frader, Joel E. Ethical issues in organ procurement: a review for intensivists. *Critical Care Clinics.* 1996 Jan; 12(1): 29–48. 133 refs. BE59276.
> brain death; cadavers; cardiac death; coercion; competence; determination of death; disclosure; family members; health personnel; incentives; informed consent; legal aspects; *organ donation; organ donors; public policy; required request; scarcity; third party consent; ventilators; refusal to donate; United States

Bahnsen, Ulrich. Switzerland adopts transplant guidelines. [News]. *Nature.* 1999 Feb 18; 397(6720): 553. BE61569.
> animal organs; *government regulation; guidelines; legal aspects; *organ donation; *organ transplantation; political activity; remuneration; *Switzerland

Becker, Carl. Money talks, money kills -- the economics of transplantation in Japan and China. *Bioethics.* 1999 Jul; 13(3–4): 236–243. 33 fn. BE61873.
> allowing to die; *brain death; *capital punishment; *determination of death; directed donation; *economics; hospitals; institutional policies; *legal aspects; *motivation; non-Western World; *organ donation; *organ transplantation; *prisoners; *public policy; *China; *Japan
> Japan and China have long resisted the Western trend of organ transplantation from brain-dead patients, based on a 'Confucian' respect for integrity of ancestors' bodies. While their general publics continue to harbor grave doubts about such practices, their medical and political elites are hastening towards the road of organ-harvesting and organ-marketing, largely for economic reasons. This report illustrates the ways that economics is motivating brain-death legislation in Japan and criminal executions in China.

Benedict, James. The use of fetal tissue: a cautious approval. *Christian Century.* 1998 Feb 18; 115(5): 164–165. BE60446.
> *aborted fetuses; *Christian ethics; *fetal tissue donation; risks and benefits

Berger, Jeffrey T. Culture and ethnicity in clinical care. *Archives of Internal Medicine.* 1998 Oct 26; 158(19): 2085–2090. 110 refs. BE59577.
> *advance directives; *alternative therapies; American Indians; Asian Americans; *attitudes; autopsies; blacks; cancer; *cultural pluralism; family relationship; health; Hispanic Americans; knowledge, attitudes, practice; living wills; *minority groups; nutrition; *organ donation; *patient care; physicians; preventive medicine; prolongation of life; socioeconomic factors; *truth disclosure; whites; withholding treatment; United States

Bleich, J. David; Caplan, Arthur L.; Murray, Joseph E., et al. Defining the limits of organ and tissue research and transplantation. [Proceedings of the International Symposium on Law and Science at the Crossroads: Biomedical Technology, Ethics, Public Policy, and the Law; panel discussion]. *Suffolk University Law Review.* 1993 Winter; 27(4): 1457–1476. Moderator: Raja B. Khauli. BE60701.
> aborted fetuses; autonomy; body parts and fluids; *brain death; cadavers; cardiac death; *determination of death; *fetal tissue donation; *organ donation; organ donors; presumed consent; public policy; remuneration; values

Bleich, J. David. Moral debate and semantic sleight of hand. *Suffolk University Law Review.* 1993 Winter; 27(4): 1173–1193. 44 fn. BE60698.
> *aborted fetuses; abortion, induced; beginning of life; *brain death; cultural pluralism; decision making; democracy; *determination of death; fetal research; *fetal tissue donation; fetuses; government financing; legal aspects; legal rights; moral policy; newborns; prolongation of life; public policy; quality of life; religion; religious ethics; standards; state interest; theology; value of life; *values; withholding treatment

Bosch, Xavier. European body to oversee tissue banks. [News]. *Nature Medicine.* 1998 Sep; 4(9): 988. BE62173.
> communicable diseases; *regulation; *tissue banks; *tissue donation; Europe; *European Union

Bosch, Xavier. Spain leads world in organ donation and transplantation. [News]. *JAMA.* 1999 Jul 7; 282(1): 17–18. BE61954.
> body parts and fluids; brain death; cadavers; cardiac death;

BE = bioethics accession number   fn. = footnotes   refs. = references

confidentiality; health personnel; HIV seropositivity; information dissemination; *organ donation; organ donors; *organ transplantation; organizational policies; presumed consent; *public policy; remuneration; selection for treatment; statistics; transplant recipients; National Transplant Organization (Spain); *Spain

Bratton, Letitia B.; Griffin, Linner Ward. A kidney donor's dilemma: the sibling who can donate -- but doesn't. *Social Work in Health Care.* 1994; 20(2): 75-96. 54 fn. BE60224.
altruism; autonomy; coercion; *counseling; *decision making; *directed donation; family relationship; *kidneys; legal aspects; moral obligations; *moral policy; motivation; *organ donation; patient advocacy; psychological stress; *risks and benefits; *siblings; *social workers; transplant recipients; values; *refusal to donate

Broumand, B. Living donors: the Iran experience. *Nephrology, Dialysis, Transplantation.* 1997 Sep; 12(9): 1830-1831. 5 refs. BE60034.
*kidneys; morbidity; mortality; motivation; *organ donation; *organ donors; *remuneration; risks and benefits; statistics; *treatment outcome; *unrelated donors; *Iran

Burgio, G. Roberto; Locatelli, F.; Nespoli, L. Hematopoietic stem cell transplantation in pediatric practice: a bioethical reassessment. *In:* Burgio, G. Roberto; Lantos, John D., eds. *Primum Non Nocere* Today. Second Edition. New York, NY: Elsevier; 1998: 85-99. 64 refs. ISBN 0-444-82923-7. BE60921.
beneficence; *blood donation; *bone marrow; *children; *cord blood; donors; economics; family members; informed consent; intention; justice; moral policy; *newborns; parents; pediatrics; pregnant women; private sector; reproduction; resource allocation; *risks and benefits; siblings; *stem cells; *tissue banks; *tissue donation; tissue transplantation; placentas; unrelated donors

Campbell, Courtney S. Religion and the body in medical research. *Kennedy Institute of Ethics Journal.* 1998 Sep; 8(3): 275-305. 36 refs. 2 fn. BE60168.
advisory committees; altruism; American Indians; attitudes; *autopsies; *biomedical research; *body parts and fluids; *cadavers; commodification; *common good; confidentiality; cultural pluralism; fetal tissue donation; genetic information; *genetic research; genome mapping; *gifts; *human body; informed consent; investigators; Islamic ethics; Jewish ethics; medical education; metaphor; moral obligations; *nontherapeutic research; *organ donation; organ transplantation; property rights; Protestant ethics; *religious ethics; remuneration; Roman Catholic ethics; science; self concept; *theology; *tissue banks; *tissue donation; transplant recipients; values; National Bioethics Advisory Commission
Religious discussion of human organs and tissues has concentrated largely on donation for therapeutic purposes. The retrieval and use of human tissue samples in diagnostic, research, and education contexts have, by contrast, received very little direct theological attention. Initially undertaken at the behest of the National Bioethics Advisory Commission, this essay seeks to explore the theological and religious questions embedded in nontherapeutic use of human tissue. It finds that the "donation paradigm" typically invoked in religious discourse to justify uses of the body for therapeutic reasons is inadequate in the context of nontherapeutic research, while the "resource paradigm" implicit in scientific discourse presumes a reductionist account of the body that runs contrary to important religious values about embodiment. The essay proposes a "contribution paradigm" that provides a religious perspective within which research on human tissue can be both justified and limited.

Caplan, Arthur L. Am I my brother's keeper? *Suffolk University Law Review.* 1993 Winter; 27(4): 1195-1208. 40 fn. BE61593.
altruism; body parts and fluids; cadavers; coercion; competence; conflict of interest; disclosure; *family members; friends; informed consent; international aspects; kidneys; legal aspects; livers; love; mentally disabled; minors; moral obligations; moral policy; motivation; *organ donation; *organ donors; patient advocacy; patient care team; *presumed consent; public policy; remuneration; *required request; *risks and benefits; scarcity; third party consent; tissue donation; transplant recipients; lungs; pancreases; *unrelated donors; United States

Caplan, Arthur L.; Coelho, Daniel H. The Ethics of Organ Transplants: The Current Debate. Amherst, NY: Prometheus Books; 1998. 350 p. Bibliography: p. 347-350. ISBN 1-57392-224-2. BE60916.
aborted fetuses; abortion, induced; alcohol abuse; altruism; anencephaly; animal organs; blacks; brain death; cadavers; cardiac death; coercion; commodification; determination of death; directed donation; disadvantaged; donor cards; economics; family members; fetal tissue donation; health insurance reimbursement; incentives; international aspects; justice; kidneys; legal aspects; livers; *moral policy; *organ donation; organ donors; *organ transplantation; persistent vegetative state; presumed consent; primates; prognosis; *public policy; *remuneration; required request; *resource allocation; retreatment; *selection for treatment; *tissue transplantation; transplant recipients; mandated choice; refusal to donate; *unrelated donors; Medicaid; Medicare; Oregon; Uniform Anatomical Gift Act; United States

Charatan, Fred. Pennsylvania plans to reward organ donation. [News]. *BMJ (British Medical Journal).* 1999 May 22; 318(7195): 1371. BE61951.
cadavers; family members; *government financing; *incentives; *organ donation; *public policy; *remuneration; state government; *Pennsylvania

Childress, James F. The gift of life: ethical issues in organ transplantation. *Bulletin of the American College of Surgeons.* 1996 Mar; 81(3): 8-22. 30 refs. BE60529.
autonomy; body parts and fluids; brain death; *cadavers; communitarianism; decision making; determination of death; donor cards; education; family members; gifts; incentives; justice; legal aspects; libertarianism; mandatory programs; *moral policy; obligations to society; *organ donation; organ transplantation; presumed consent; property rights; *public policy; remuneration; required request; risks and benefits; statistics; third party consent; trust; utilitarianism; voluntary programs; National Organ Transplant Act 1984; Uniform Anatomical Gift Act; United Network for Organ Sharing; *United States

Chugh, Kirpal S.; Jha, Vivekanand. Commerce in transplantation in Third World countries. *Kidney International.* 1996 May; 49(5): 1181-1186. 34 refs. BE61562.
*cadavers; coercion; *commodification; *developing countries; family members; females; health facilities; international aspects; *kidneys; legal aspects; married persons; morbidity; *organ donation; *organ donors; *organ transplantation; organizational policies; prisoners; professional organizations; public policy; *remuneration; scarcity; *socioeconomic factors; statistics; transplant recipients; treatment outcome; *unrelated donors; *Asia; China; *India; Latin America

Clark, Richard E. Bone-marrow donation by mentally incapable adults. *Lancet.* 1998 Dec 5; 352(9143): 1847-1848. 9 refs. BE60804.
adults; *bone marrow; competence; *decision making; directed donation; family relationship; *legal aspects; *mentally retarded; physically disabled; risks and benefits; *siblings; *tissue donation; *Great Britain; *Re Y

BE = bioethics accession number   fn. = footnotes   refs. = references

Coelho, Daniel H.; Caplan, Arthur L. The unclaimed cadaver. *Academic Medicine.* 1997 Sep; 72(9): 741–743. 4 refs. BE59881.
  biomedical research; *cadavers; geographic factors; hospitals; human body; indigents; *institutional policies; *medical education; medical schools; nursing homes; patients; *public policy; socioeconomic factors; state government; *tissue donation; homeless persons; Uniform Anatomical Gift Act; *United States

Crouch, Robert A.; Elliott, Carl. Moral agency and the family: the case of living related organ transplantation. *Cambridge Quarterly of Healthcare Ethics.* 1999 Summer; 8(3): 275–287. 36 fn. BE62471.
  adolescents; autonomy; *children; coercion; common good; competence; *directed donation; emotions; *family members; *family relationship; informed consent; judicial action; kidneys; livers; love; mentally retarded; *minors; moral obligations; *moral policy; motivation; *organ donation; *organ donors; organ transplantation; parent child relationship; parental consent; *parents; psychology; *risks and benefits; *siblings; standards; tissue donation; transplant recipients; United States

Csillag, Claudio. Brazil abolishes "presumed consent" in organ donation. [News]. *Lancet.* 1998 Oct 24; 352(9137): 1367. BE60270.
  *cadavers; *family members; *legal aspects; *organ donation; *presumed consent; *third party consent; *Brazil

Daar, A.S. Paid organ donation -- the Grey Basket concept. [Editorial]. *Journal of Medical Ethics.* 1998 Dec; 24(6): 365–368. 24 refs. BE61251.
  altruism; autonomy; body parts and fluids; cadavers; family members; incentives; international aspects; kidneys; *moral policy; *organ donation; organ donors; physicians; public opinion; public policy; regulation; *remuneration; scarcity

Davison, Alex M. Commercialization in organ donation. [Editorial]. *Nephrology, Dialysis, Transplantation.* 1994; 9(4): 348–349. 3 refs. BE61586.
  cultural pluralism; *developing countries; ethical relativism; indigents; *international aspects; *kidneys; morbidity; *organ donation; *organ donors; *organ transplantation; *remuneration; risk; scarcity; *transplant recipients; treatment outcome; *unrelated donors

Deech, Ruth. Legal and ethical responsibilities of gamete banks. [Article and discussion]. *Human Reproduction.* 1998 May; 13(Suppl. 2): 80–89. BE61483.
  advertising; age factors; confidentiality; counseling; directed donation; disclosure; family members; *government regulation; *guidelines; informed consent; institutional ethics; international aspects; *legislation; *ovum; *ovum donors; registries; remuneration; reproductive technologies; *semen donors; *sperm; *tissue banks; tissue donation; *Great Britain; *Human Fertilisation and Embryology Act 1990; *Human Fertilisation and Embryology Authority

Dekkers, Wim J.M.; ten Have, Henk A.M.J. Biomedical research with human body "parts". *In:* ten Have, Henk A.M.J.; Welie, Jos V.M., eds. Ownership of the Human Body: Philosophical Considerations on the Use of the Human Body and Its Parts in Health Care. Boston, MA: Kluwer Academic; 1998: 49–63. 20 refs. 1 fn. Translated from the Dutch. ISBN 0–7923–5150–9. BE61319.
  *biomedical research; *body parts and fluids; donors; ethical review; fetal tissue donation; genetic materials; human body; human experimentation; informed consent; *organ donation; property rights; remuneration; *tissue donation; cell lines

Drew, Christopher. U.S. says 2 Chinese offered organs from the executed. [News]. *New York Times.* 1998 Feb 24: A1, B5. BE60464.
  body parts and fluids; cadavers; capital punishment; criminal law; hospitals; international aspects; kidneys; *law enforcement; *organ donation; organ transplantation; *prisoners; *remuneration; *China; New York City

Dunstan, G.R. The ethics of organ donation. *British Medical Bulletin.* 1997; 53(4): 921–939. 41 refs. BE62608.
  adults; altruism; animal organs; autonomy; body parts and fluids; bone marrow; cadavers; children; coercion; directed donation; family members; fetal tissue donation; gifts; guidelines; informed consent; intensive care units; international aspects; legal aspects; *organ donation; organ donors; organizational policies; paternalism; physicians; presumed consent; professional organizations; regulation; remuneration; required request; third party consent; *tissue donation; treatment refusal; ventilators; refusal to donate; Great Britain

Dworkin, Gerald; Kennedy, Ian. Human tissue: rights in the body and its parts. *Medical Law Review.* 1993 Autumn; 1(3): 291–319. 78 fn. BE59900.
  *biomedical research; *body parts and fluids; cadavers; embryos; genetic intervention; government regulation; *human body; informed consent; investigators; judicial action; *legal aspects; *legal rights; *organ donation; organ donors; patents; patients; *property rights; public policy; remuneration; third party consent; *tissue donation; Europe; *Great Britain; Moore v. Regents of the University of California; United States

Eckholm, Erik. Arrests put focus on human organs from China. [News]. *New York Times.* 1998 Feb 25: B4. BE60465.
  aliens; body parts and fluids; cadavers; capital punishment; criminal law; hospitals; international aspects; kidneys; *law enforcement; *organ donation; organ transplantation; *prisoners; *remuneration; *China; Hong Kong; New York City; Singapore; Taiwan

Eisenberg, V.H.; Schenker, J.G. Pre-embryo donation: ethical and legal aspects. *International Journal of Gynaecology and Obstetrics.* 1998 Jan; 60(1): 51–57. 39 refs. BE60695.
  age factors; confidentiality; cryopreservation; disclosure; *donors; *embryo transfer; *embryos; international aspects; legal aspects; medical records; *ovum donors; parent child relationship; property rights; registries; religion; remuneration; *reproductive technologies; selection for treatment; *semen donors; single persons; standards; tissue banks

Engelhart, Karlheinz; King, T.T.; Bakran, A., et al. Organ donation and permanent vegetative state. [Letters and response]. *Lancet.* 1998 Jan 17; 351(9097): 211–213. 4 refs. BE59303.
  allowing to die; artificial feeding; *determination of death; drugs; involuntary euthanasia; *killing; National Socialism; *organ donation; *persistent vegetative state; withholding treatment; Great Britain

Englert, Y.; Govaerts, I. Oocyte donation: particular technical and ethical aspects. *Human Reproduction.* 1998 May; 13(Suppl. 2): 90–97. 34 refs. BE61484.
  age factors; artificial insemination; attitudes; comparative studies; confidentiality; counseling; cryopreservation; directed donation; family members; females; in vitro fertilization; informed consent; methods; motivation; *ovum donors; remuneration; semen donors; socioeconomic factors; *tissue donation; Europe; United States

Erin, Charles A. Some comments on the ethics of consent to the use of ovarian tissue from aborted fetuses and dead women. *In:* Harris, John; Holm, Søren, eds. The Future of Human Reproduction: Ethics, Choice, and

---

BE = bioethics accession number   fn. = footnotes   refs. = references

Regulation. New York, NY: Oxford University Press; 1998: 162–175. 33 fn. ISBN 0-19-823761-8. BE61268.
*aborted fetuses; advance directives; autonomy; *cadavers; decision making; disclosure; dissent; family members; *fetal tissue donation; germ cells; *informed consent; legal aspects; *ovum donors; parental consent; posthumous reproduction; presumed consent; third party consent; *tissue donation; *ovaries; Great Britain; Human Tissue Act 1961 (Great Britain)

Fagot-Largeault, Anne. Ownership of the human body: judicial and legislative responses in France. *In:* ten Have, Henk A.M.J.; Welie, Jos V.M., eds. Ownership of the Human Body: Philosophical Considerations on the Use of the Human Body and Its Parts in Healthcare. Boston, MA: Kluwer Academic; 1998: 115–140. 39 refs. 2 fn. ISBN 0-7923-5150-9. BE61321.
abortion, induced; advisory committees; *bioethical issues; blood donation; *body parts and fluids; commodification; contraception; government regulation; historical aspects; *human body; human experimentation; human rights; informed consent; *legal aspects; nontherapeutic research; obligations to society; organ donation; presumed consent; privacy; *property rights; remuneration; sexuality; therapeutic research; women's rights; national ethics committees; *France; National Ethics Advisory Committee (France)

Fasting, Ulla; Christensen, Jan; Glending, Susanne; Amnesty International. Danish Working Group for Children. Children sold for transplants: medical and legal aspects. *Nursing Ethics.* 1998 Nov; 5(6): 518–526. 11 refs. BE60812.
adults; animal organs; *children; *coercion; guidelines; human rights; *international aspects; law enforcement; legal aspects; misconduct; *organ donation; *organ donors; organ transplantation; organizational policies; parents; physicians; *remuneration; scarcity; Convention on the Rights of the Child; *Europe; European Parliament; Eurotransplant; Scandiatransplant; United Nations; World Health Organization

Fentiman, Linda C. Organ donation as national service: a proposed federal organ donation law. *Suffolk University Law Review.* 1993 Winter; 27(4): 1593–1612. 71 fn. BE61597.
federal government; geographic factors; government regulation; health insurance reimbursement; *model legislation; *organ donation; *organ donors; organ transplantation; *presumed consent; *public policy; registries; *remuneration; scarcity; selection for treatment; *tissue donation; tissue transplantation; transplant recipients; refusal to donate; *United States

Fielding, Helen A. Body measures: phenomenological considerations of corporeal ethics. *Journal of Medicine and Philosophy.* 1998 Oct; 23(5): 533–545. 11 refs. 3 fn. Note: the journal issue cover shows a date of August 1998, which is incorrect. BE62117.
audiovisual aids; *bioethics; body parts and fluids; commodification; *human body; mass media; motivation; *organ donation; philosophy; *remuneration; *phenomenology; Dekalog 10: Thou Shall Not Covet Thy Neighbour's Goods; Heidegger, Martin; Kieślowski, Krzysztof; Merleau-Ponty, Maurice
The development of bioethics primarily at the cognitive level further perpetuates the tendency to construe all aspects of our lives, including our bodies, as technical systems. For example, if we consider the moral issue of organ sales without taking our embodiment into account, there appear to be no sound arguments for opposing such sales. However, it is important to consider the aspects of the phenomenal body that challenge rational deliberation by exploring an embodied approach

to the ethical dilemma produced by a proposed kidney exchange as presented in Krzysztof Kieślowski's *Dekalog* films. What is sought is a description of a body-measure that would serve as a critique of strictly cognitive bioethical deliberations.

Fine, Andrea. Fertility business hits Internet, weaving web of controversy. [News]. *Christian Science Monitor.* 1998 Sept 11: 3. BE60640.
*advertising; commodification; *computer communication networks; females; *ovum donors; regulation; *remuneration; risk; *Internet

First, M. Roy. Controversies in organ donation: minority donation and living unrelated renal donors. *Transplantation Proceedings.* 1997 Feb–Mar; 29(1–2): 67–69. 25 refs. BE61574.
*blacks; *cadavers; family members; friends; *kidneys; knowledge, attitudes, practice; married persons; *organ donation; *organ donors; organ transplantation; scarcity; transplant recipients; treatment outcome; lungs; *unrelated donors; United States

Fost, Norman. The unimportance of death. *In:* Youngner, Stuart J.; Arnold, Robert M.; Schapiro, Renie, eds. The Definition of Death: Contemporary Controversies. Baltimore, MD: Johns Hopkins University Press; 1999: 161–178. 39 fn. ISBN 0-8018-5985-9. BE60764.
advisory committees; allowing to die; anencephaly; body parts and fluids; brain; *brain death; cardiac death; *determination of death; *legal aspects; legislation; *organ donation; persistent vegetative state; presumed consent; prolongation of life; *public policy; required request; standards; terminally ill; utilitarianism; withholding treatment; coma; health services misuse; Harvard Committee on Brain Death; United States

France. Decree No. 96-1041 of 2 Dec 1996 on the determination of death prior to the removal of organs, tissues, and cells for therapeutic or scientific purposes, and amending the Public Health Code (Second Part: decrees made after consulting the *Conseil d'Etat*). (*Journal officiel de la Republique fran3aise, Lois et Decrets,* 4 Dec 1996, No. 282, p. 17615). *International Digest of Health Legislation.* 1997; 48(2): 197–198. 1 fn. BE59595.
brain death; *cadavers; *determination of death; *legal aspects; *organ donation; *France

Gillam, Lynn. The 'more-abortions' objection to fetal tissue transplantation. *Journal of Medicine and Philosophy.* 1998 Aug; 23(4): 411–427. 27 refs. 14 fn. BE60631.
*aborted fetuses; *abortion, induced; *deontological ethics; double effect; *ethical analysis; *fetal tissue donation; injuries; *intention; moral complicity; *moral policy; motivation; pregnant women; social impact; utilitarianism; *wedge argument
One common objection to fetal tissue transplantation (FTT) is that, if it were to become a standard form of treatment, it would encourage or entrench the practice of abortion. This claim is at least factually plausible, although it cannot be definitively established. However, even if true, it does not constitute a compelling ethical argument against FTT. The harm allegedly brought about by FTT, when assessed by widely accepted non-consequentialist criteria, has limited moral significance. Even if FTT would cause more abortions to be performed, and abortion is taken to be a serious moral wrong, this is not sufficient in itself to make FTT wrong.

Glick, Shimon. Ethical aspects of organ transplantation.

BE = bioethics accession number   fn. = footnotes   refs. = references

Jewish Medical Ethics. 1997 Jan; 3(1): 11–13. BE59243.
body parts and fluids; determination of death; international aspects; *organ donation; *organ transplantation; resource allocation; selection for treatment; transplant recipients; Israel

Gold, Richard. Owning our bodies: an examination of property law and biotechnology. *San Diego Law Review.* 1995; 32(4): 1167–1247. 320 fn. BE59853.
*biomedical research; *body parts and fluids; commodification; *economics; health; *human body; informed consent; *legal aspects; patents; patients; politics; *property rights; recombinant DNA research; religion; Supreme Court decisions; *tissue donation; transgenic organisms; *values; cell lines; Diamond v. Chakrabarty; Moore v. Regents of the University of California; United States

Grady, Denise. Live donors revolutionize liver care. [News]. *New York Times.* 1999 Aug 2: A1, A12. BE62449.
adults; *directed donation; *family members; *livers; *organ donation; *organ donors; risks and benefits; scarcity; siblings; tissue donation; LaBanca, Felicia; United States; Vilardi, John

Groopman, Jerome. The moral way to pay for human organs. *New York Times.* 1999 May 7: A27. BE61071.
alternatives; body parts and fluids; cadavers; coercion; family members; federal government; geographic factors; health facilities; *incentives; indigents; *organ donation; organ donors; *public policy; *remuneration; resource allocation; state government; volunteers; *Pennsylvania; *United States

Grubb, Andrew. Use of fetal eggs and infertility treatment: Human Fertilisation and Embryology Act 1990, section 3A. [Comment]. *Medical Law Review.* 1995 Summer; 3(2): 203–204. BE59254.
aborted fetuses; criminal law; embryo transfer; embryos; *fetal tissue donation; germ cells; *government regulation; in vitro fertilization; *legislation; *ovum; *reproductive technologies; *Great Britain; *Human Fertilisation and Embryology Act 1990

Gunning, Jennifer. Oocyte donation: the legislative framework in Western Europe. [Article and discussion]. *Human Reproduction.* 1998 May; 13(Suppl. 2): 98–104. 2 refs. BE61485.
aborted fetuses; cadavers; confidentiality; cryopreservation; *government regulation; *international aspects; *legislation; married persons; *ovum donors; *reproductive technologies; single persons; *tissue donation; Austria; Denmark; *Europe; France; Germany; Great Britain; Human Fertilisation and Embryology Act 1990; Norway; Spain; Sweden; Switzerland

Herdman, Roger; Beauchamp, Tom L.; Potts, John T. The Institute of Medicine's report on non–heart–beating organ transplantation. *Kennedy Institute of Ethics Journal.* 1998 Mar; 8(1): 89–90. 1 fn. BE59356.
body parts and fluids; *cadavers; *cardiac death; conflict of interest; decision making; determination of death; disclosure; drugs; family members; federal government; guidelines; health facilities; institutional policies; *organ donation; organ transplantation; physicians; public policy; scarcity; standards; third party consent; treatment outcome; withholding treatment; Department of Health and Human Services; *Institute of Medicine; Organ Procurement and Transplantation Network; *United States
In December 1997, the Institute of Medicine (IOM) released a report on medical and ethical issues in the procurement of non–heart–beating organ donors. This report had been requested in May 1997 by the Department of Health and Human Services (DHHS). We will here describe the genesis of the IOM report,

the medical and moral concerns that led the DHHS to sponsor it, the process of producing it, and its conclusions. The analyses, findings, and recommendations of the report are also reviewed, in particular the central issues that led to suggestions for policy changes.

Herz, Susan E. Two steps to three choices: a new approach to mandated choice. *Cambridge Quarterly of Healthcare Ethics.* 1999 Summer; 8(3): 340–347. 23 fn. BE62477.
autonomy; beneficence; *decision making; education; informed consent; justice; *mandatory programs; moral policy; *organ donation; *public policy; state government; third party consent; *mandated choice; refusal to donate; United States

Hicks, Stephen C. The regulation of fetal tissue transplantation: different legislative models for different purposes. *Suffolk University Law Review.* 1993 Winter; 27(4): 1613–1629. 46 fn. BE61598.
*aborted fetuses; abortion, induced; criminal law; directed donation; embryo disposition; embryo research; embryos; federal government; *fetal research; *fetal tissue donation; government financing; *government regulation; informed consent; *model legislation; nontherapeutic research; organ donation; organ transplantation; remuneration; research ethics committees; state government; therapeutic research; tissue donation; tissue transplantation; abortion, spontaneous; NIH Revitalization Act 1993; Uniform Anatomical Gift Act; *United States

Ikels, Charlotte. Ethical issues in organ procurement in Chinese societies. *China Journal.* 1997 Jul; No. 38: 95–119. 66 fn. BE59198.
aliens; *attitudes; *cadavers; capital punishment; comparative studies; determination of death; family members; females; health insurance; informed consent; international aspects; *kidneys; males; *organ donation; *organ donors; *organ transplantation; physicians; political systems; *presumed consent; *prisoners; *public policy; religion; remuneration; scarcity; siblings; social discrimination; statistics; third party consent; transplant recipients; Confucian ethics; personal financing; refusal to donate; *unrelated donors; *China; *Hong Kong; *Singapore; *Taiwan

Illhardt, Franz J. Ownership of the human body: deontological approaches. *In:* ten Have, Henk A.M.J.; Welie, Jos V.M., eds. Ownership of the Human Body: Philosophical Considerations on the Use of the Human Body and Its Parts in Healthcare. Boston, MA: Kluwer Academic; 1998: 187–206. 37 refs. 5 fn. ISBN 0–7923–5150–9. BE61323.
autonomy; *deontological ethics; determination of death; *human body; informed consent; moral obligations; obligations to society; *organ donation; organ transplantation; philosophy; presumed consent; *property rights; quality of life; regulation; selection for treatment; self concept; teleological ethics; theology; transplant recipients; Europe

Isoniemi, H. Living kidney donation: a surgeon's opinion. *Nephrology, Dialysis, Transplantation.* 1997 Sep; 12(9): 1828–1829. BE60033.
altruism; *attitudes; cadavers; coercion; family members; friends; health; institutional policies; *kidneys; love; married persons; mental health; moral obligations; motivation; *organ donation; *organ donors; *physicians; public policy; *risks and benefits; statistics; surgery; unrelated donors; *Finland

Israeli, Saul. Organ transplants: responsa. *Jewish Medical Ethics.* 1997 Jan; 3(1): 14–17. 41 fn. BE59244.
body parts and fluids; cadavers; donor cards; family

BE = bioethics accession number   fn. = footnotes   refs. = references

members; *Jewish ethics; moral obligations; *organ donation; *organ donors; remuneration; risk; *tissue donation

Jakobsen, A. Living renal transplantation -- the Oslo experience. *Nephrology, Dialysis, Transplantation.* 1997 Sep; 12(9): 1825-1827. 5 refs. BE60032.
altruism; attitudes; coercion; costs and benefits; family members; hospitals; *institutional policies; *kidneys; *organ donation; *organ donors; *organ transplantation; public policy; risks and benefits; statistics; transplant recipients; unrelated donors; *Norway

Jonsson, Lena. The Swedish transplantation law. *International Digest of Health Legislation.* 1997; 48(2): 237-239. BE59598.
aborted fetuses; abortion, induced; autonomy; beneficence; cadavers; decision making; family members; *fetal tissue donation; informed consent; *legal aspects; *organ donation; organ donors; presumed consent; third party consent; tissue donation; *Sweden

Josefson, Deborah. Prisoner wants to donate his second kidney. [News]. *BMJ (British Medical Journal).* 1999 Jan 2; 318(7175): 7. BE60840.
attitudes; beneficence; *directed donation; *family members; *kidneys; *organ donation; physicians; *prisoners; refusal to treat; renal dialysis; transplant recipients; *Patterson, David; Patterson, Renada

Julvez, Jean; Tuppin, Phillippe; Cohen, Sophie. Survey in France of response to xenotransplantation. [Research letter]. *Lancet.* 1999 Feb 27; 353(9154): 726. 4 refs. BE61199.
*allied health personnel; *animal organs; *attitudes; communicable diseases; comparative studies; human experimentation; *nurses; *organ donation; *organ transplantation; *physicians; public opinion; risk; *students; survey; swine; *France; French Transplant Agency

Kefalides, Paul. Solid organ transplantation. 1: Many problems, new solutions. *Annals of Internal Medicine.* 1998 Dec 15; 129(12): 1093-1095. BE59329.
cadavers; kidneys; livers; methods; *organ donation; *organ donors; organ transplantation; scarcity; lungs; pancreases

Kefalides, Paul. Solid organ transplantation. 2: Ethical considerations. *Annals of Internal Medicine.* 1999 Jan 19; 130(2): 169-170. BE62559.
body parts and fluids; cadavers; federal government; government regulation; hospitals; *organ donation; organ donors; *organ transplantation; remuneration; resource allocation; selection for treatment; transplant recipients; Department of Health and Human Services; United States

Kerr, Susan M.; Caplan, Arthur; Polin, Glenn, et al. Postmortem sperm procurement. *Journal of Urology.* 1997 Jun; 157(6): 2154-2158. 9 refs. BE60194.
clinical ethics committees; *cryopreservation; decision making; *health facilities; institutional policies; *knowledge, attitudes, practice; married persons; methods; physicians; *posthumous reproduction; reproductive technologies; *semen donors; *sperm; statistics; survey; time factors; questionnaires; Canada; United States

Khamsi, Firouz; Endman, Maxine W.; Lacanna, Iara C., et al. Some psychological aspects of oocyte donation from known donors on altruistic basis. *Fertility and Sterility.* 1997 Aug; 68(2): 323-327. 12 refs. BE60334.
*altruism; *attitudes; confidentiality; disclosure; emotions; females; gifts; *motivation; *ovum donors; *patients; psychology; social interaction; survey; Ontario

Khauli, Raja B. Issues and controversies surrounding

organ donation and transplantation: the need for laws that ensure equity and optimal utility of a scarce resource. *Suffolk University Law Review.* 1993 Winter; 27(4): 1225-1236. 37 fn. BE60734.
accountability; body parts and fluids; cadavers; economics; family members; incentives; justice; kidneys; legal aspects; legislation; minority groups; *organ donation; *organ transplantation; patient compliance; presumed consent; prognosis; *public policy; remuneration; renal dialysis; required request; *resource allocation; retreatment; scarcity; selection for treatment; treatment outcome; National Organ Transplant Act 1984; Organ Procurement and Transplant Network; United Network for Organ Sharing; United States

Kishore, R.R. Organ donation consanguinity or universality. *Medicine and Law.* 1996; 15(1): 93-104. 15 refs. BE61206.
*altruism; body parts and fluids; cadavers; coercion; directed donation; *family members; gifts; international aspects; legal aspects; motivation; *organ donation; *organ donors; organ transplantation; organizational policies; property rights; *remuneration; resource allocation; scarcity; selection for treatment; transplant recipients; needs; refusal to donate; *unrelated donors; *World Health Assembly

Klen, Rudolf. Aborted embryos -- law and ethics. *Bulletin of Medical Ethics.* 1998 Feb; No. 135: 22-23. BE61889.
*aborted fetuses; abortion, induced; confidentiality; decision making; *embryo disposition; embryo research; fetal research; *fetal tissue donation; government regulation; informed consent; international aspects; pregnant women; tissue banks; tissue transplantation; Czech Republic

Korzick, Karen A.; Terry, Peter B. Cadaveric organ donation: rethinking SPRT [Selection of Potential Recipients of Transplants]. [Editorial]. *Archives of Internal Medicine.* 1999 Mar 8; 159(5): 427-428. 2 refs. Commentary on R.M. Sade, p. 438-442. BE61326.
autonomy; *cadavers; communitarianism; cultural pluralism; *directed donation; disadvantaged; family members; incentives; justice; libertarianism; *moral policy; *motivation; *organ donation; organ donors; organ transplantation; privacy; religion; resource allocation; risks and benefits; selection for treatment; third party consent; *transplant recipients; utilitarianism; egalitarianism

Krauthammer, Charles. Of headless mice...and men: the ultimate cloning horror: human organ farms. *Time.* 1998 Jan 19; 151(2): 76. BE59164.
animal experimentation; body parts and fluids; *cloning; investigators; motivation; *organ donation; personhood; *headless organisms; Seed, Richard

Krauthammer, Charles. Yes, let's pay for organs. *Time.* 1999 May 17; 153(19): 100. BE61041.
body parts and fluids; *cadavers; commodification; *family members; incentives; indigents; kidneys; morality; *organ donation; organ donors; *public policy; *remuneration; state government; dignity; Pennsylvania

Lachs, John. On selling organs. *In: his* The Relevance of Philosophy to Life. Nashville, TN: Vanderbilt University Press; 1995: 195-198. ISBN 0-8265-1262-3. BE60865.
autonomy; body parts and fluids; economics; freedom; government regulation; indigents; moral policy; *organ donation; paternalism; property rights; public policy; *remuneration; state interest

Lafferty, Kevin J.; Furer, Julie J. Legal and medical implications of fetal tissue transplantation. *Suffolk University Law Review.* 1993 Winter; 27(4): 1237-1248. 59 fn. BE61594.
aborted fetuses; diabetes; federal government; *fetal

BE = bioethics accession number   fn. = footnotes   refs. = references

research; *fetal tissue donation; *government financing; *government regulation; *legal aspects; methods; private sector; *public policy; state government; *tissue transplantation; pancreases; United States

Lamb, David. Organ transplants, death, and policies for procurement. *Monist.* 1993 Apr; 76(2): 203–221. 27 refs. BE60221.
altruism; body parts and fluids; *brain death; cadavers; coercion; commodification; cultural pluralism; *determination of death; family members; gifts; human body; intensive care units; international aspects: mentally disabled; minors; moral obligations; *organ donation; *organ donors; organ transplantation; patient transfer; presumed consent; religious ethics; remuneration; required request; resource allocation; risks and benefits; selection for treatment; standards; terminally ill; transplant recipients; ventilators; refusal to donate; Europe; Great Britain; Japan; United States

Lock, Margaret. The problem of brain death: Japanese disputes about bodies and modernity. *In:* Youngner, Stuart J., Arnold, Robert M., Schapiro, Renie, eds. The Definition of Death: Contemporary Controversies. Baltimore, MD: Johns Hopkins University Press; 1999: 239–256. 35 fn. ISBN 0-8018-5985-9. BE60769.
advisory committees; *attitudes to death; *brain death; Buddhist ethics; cardiac death; consensus; *determination of death; diagnosis; *dissent; family members; international aspects; legal aspects; mass media; non-Western World; *organ donation; organ transplantation; organizational policies; persistent vegetative state; physicians; professional organizations; public opinion; *public policy; secularism; values; Western World; Confucian ethics; Brain Death Advisory Council (Japan); *Japan; Japan Society for Transplantation; Patients' Rights Committee (Japan); Special Cabinet Committee on Brain Death and Organ Transplants (Japan)

Lu, Leonard. Commerce in organ transplantation. *Pharos.* 1998 Spring; 61(2): 2–5. 14 refs. BE59984.
age factors; aliens; altruism; autonomy; coercion; commodification; communicable diseases; costs and benefits; health insurance; *incentives; indigents; informed consent; kidney diseases; *kidneys; motivation; *organ donation; *organ donors; property rights; public policy; quality of life; *remuneration; renal dialysis; *risks and benefits; utilitarianism; United States

McDaniels, Andrea. Brazil mandates organ 'donation' for transplants. [News]. *Christian Science Monitor.* 1998 Jan 16: 1, 9. BE60319.
attitudes; cadavers; clergy; dissent; family members; indigents; *legal aspects; *mandatory programs; *organ donation; organizational policies; physicians; *presumed consent; professional organizations; public opinion; *public policy; social discrimination; third party consent; *refusal to donate; *Brazil; Brazilian Association for Organ Transplants

Machado, Nora. Using the Bodies of the Dead: Legal, Ethical and Organisational Dimensions of Organ Transplantation. Brookfield, VT: Ashgate/Dartmouth; 1998. 262 p. Bibliography: p. 241–258. ISBN 1-85521-973-5. BE62581.
altruism; attitudes; autonomy; body parts and fluids; brain death; *cadavers; determination of death; government regulation; hospitals; human body; informed consent; international aspects; legal aspects; *organ donation; organ donors; *organ transplantation; organization and administration; presumed consent; property rights; resource allocation; selection for treatment; *sociology of medicine; statistics; third party consent; transplant recipients; rituals; Europe; *Sweden

Man, Rae. Will Israel be the first to allow organ sales? [News]. *Nature Medicine.* 1998 Apr; 4(4): 376. BE59709.
kidneys; *organ donation; organ donors; public policy; *remuneration; *Israel

Markovitz, Barry; May, Larry. Three patients, two hearts. [Case study and commentaries]. *Hastings Center Report.* 1998 Sep–Oct; 28(5): 20–21. BE59549.
adolescents; adoption; advertising; *cadavers; case studies; critically ill; decision making; *directed donation; geographic factors; hearts; justice; *organ donation; *organ transplantation; parents; *resource allocation; scarcity; *selection for treatment; *transplant recipients

Marshall, Eliot. Panel proposes tighter rules for tissue studies. [News]. *Science.* 1998 Dec 18; 282(5397): 2165–6. BE59648.
advisory committees; DNA data banks; donors; federal government; *genetic materials; *genetic research; government regulation; *informed consent; privacy; research ethics committees; stigmatization; *tissue banks; *tissue donation; *National Bioethics Advisory Commission; United States

Mason, John Kenyon. Consent to treatment and research in children. *In:* his Medico-Legal Aspects of Reproduction and Parenthood. Second Edition. Brookfield, VT: Ashgate; 1998: 319–339. 83 fn. ISBN 1-84104-065-8. BE61070.
adolescents; *alternative therapies; animal organs; blood transfusions; *competence; comprehension; decision making; donors; *human experimentation; *informed consent; international aspects; Jehovah's Witnesses; judicial action; *legal aspects; *minors; nontherapeutic research; *organ donation; organ donors; organ transplantation; *parental consent; *parents; *patient care; religion; research subjects; risks and benefits; siblings; state interest; therapeutic research; *tissue donation; *treatment refusal; *Great Britain; United States

Mason, John Kenyon. Fetal experimentation. *In:* his Medico-Legal Aspects of Reproduction and Parenthood. Second Edition. Brookfield, VT: Ashgate; 1998: 187–206. 62 fn. ISBN 1-84104-065-8. BE61065.
*aborted fetuses; advisory committees; anencephaly; brain; determination of death; *fetal research; *fetal tissue donation; *fetuses; incentives; informed consent; *legal aspects; moral policy; newborns; nontherapeutic research; organ donation; pregnant women; prolongation of life; public policy; research ethics committees; risk; therapeutic research; tissue transplantation; viability; ovaries; Abortion Act 1967 (Great Britain); British Medical Association; *Great Britain; Human Fertilisation and Embryology Act 1990; Human Tissue Act 1961 (Great Britain); Infant Life (Preservation) Act 1929 (Great Britain); Offences Against the Person Act 1861 (Great Britain); Peel Committee Report; Polkinghorne Report

Menikoff, Jerry. Doubts about death: the silence of the Institute of Medicine. *Journal of Law, Medicine and Ethics.* 1998 Summer; 26(2): 157–165. 63 fn. Commented on by J.T. Potts et al., p. 166–168. BE62678.
advisory committees; brain death; *cadavers; *cardiac death; *determination of death; disclosure; *evaluation; *guidelines; informed consent; model legislation; *organ donation; organizational policies; policy analysis; *standards; *time factors; ventilators; *Institute of Medicine; Uniform Determination of Death Act; *United States

Merz, Jon F.; Leonard, Debra G.B.; Miller, Elizabeth R. IRB review and consent in human tissue research. *Science.* 1999 Mar 12; 283(5408): 1647–1648. 18 fn. BE61033.
authorship; biomedical research; comparative studies; editorial policies; *ethical review; federal government;

financial support; *genetic research; government regulation; *guideline adherence; guidelines; *human experimentation; *informed consent; investigators; literature; patient care; records; *research ethics committees; research subjects; science; survey; tissue banks; *tissue donation; pathology; pedigree studies; American Journal of Clinical Pathology; American Journal of Human Genetics; American Journal of Pathology; Human Molecular Genetics; Journal of Medical Genetics; Molecular Diagnosis; Nature; Nature Genetics; Office for Protection from Research Risks; Science; *United States

Merz, Jon F.; Sankar, Pamela; Taube, Sheila E., et al. Use of human tissues in research: clarifying clinician and researcher roles and information flows. *Journal of Investigative Medicine.* 1997 Jun; 45(5): 252–257. 36 refs. BE62405.
confidentiality; epidemiology; genetic information; *genetic materials; *genetic research; *informed consent; medical records; research subjects; *tissue banks; tissue donation; pedigree studies; recontact

Moustarah, Fady. Organ procurement: let's presume consent. *Canadian Medical Association Journal.* 1998 Jan 27; 158(2): 231–234. 14 refs. First prize essay in the 1997 Dr. William Logie Medical Ethics Essay Contest for Canadian undergraduate medical students. BE60583.
autonomy; cadavers; donor cards; family members; informed consent; *organ donation; *presumed consent; *public policy; resource allocation; risks and benefits; scarcity; third party consent; *Canada; United States

National Bioethics Advisory Commission. Genetics Subcommittee. Transcript of the National Bioethics Advisory Commission Genetics Subcommittee Meeting held on 23 Nov 1997, in Bethesda, Maryland. Rockville, MD: The Commission; 1997 Nov 23. 201 p. BE62751.
advisory committees; confidentiality; *DNA data banks; genetic information; *genetic materials; *genetic research; informed consent; privacy; *public policy; research ethics committees; tissue banks; *tissue donation; *National Bioethics Advisory Commission; United States

Nelkin, Dorothy; Andrews, Lori. Homo economicus: commercialization of body tissue in the age of biotechnology. *Hastings Center Report.* 1998 Sep–Oct; 28(5): 30–39. 64 fn. BE59552.
advertising; *biomedical research; blood donation; *body parts and fluids; cadavers; *commodification; conflict of interest; *cord blood; dehumanization; DNA data banks; DNA sequences; *economics; embryos; entrepreneurship; eugenics; financial support; gene therapy; genes; genetic diversity; *genetic materials; *genetic research; historical aspects; *human body; incentives; *industry; informed consent; international aspects; investigators; minority groups; misconduct; organ donation; *patents; physicians; population genetics; *property rights; public policy; social discrimination; stem cells; *tissue banks; *tissue donation; trends; trust; universities; vulnerable populations; cell lines; Human Genome Diversity Project; Moore v. Regents of the University of California; United States
The human body is becoming hot property, a resource to be "mined," "harvested," patented, and traded commercially for profit as well as scientific and therapeutic advances. Under the new entrepreneurial approach to the body old tensions take on new dimensions -- about consent, the fair distribution of tissues and products developed from them, the individual and cultural values represented by the body, and public policy governing the use of organs and tissues.

Nicholson, Michael L.; Bradley, J. Andrew. Renal transplantation from living donors. [Editorial]. *BMJ (British Medical Journal).* 1999 Feb 13; 318(7181): 409–410. 10 refs. BE61027.
family members; *kidneys; married persons; methods; *organ donation; *organ donors; *organ transplantation; *risks and benefits; surgery; transplant recipients; *treatment outcome; unrelated donors; Great Britain

Nieves, Evelyn. Girl awaits father's 2d kidney, and decision by medical ethicists. [News]. *New York Times.* 1998 Dec 5: A1, A11. BE61120.
*altruism; children; clinical ethics committees; decision making; *directed donation; economics; ethicists; *family members; *fathers; *kidneys; *organ donation; *organ donors; prisoners; prognosis; renal dialysis; transplant recipients; Daniel-Patterson, Renada; *Patterson, David

Nys, Herman. Therapeutic use of human organs and tissues under Belgian law. *Medicine and Law.* 1993; 12(1–2): 131–135. 5 refs. BE60620.
age factors; brain death; cadavers; determination of death; donors; family members; *government regulation; *legal aspects; legislation; minors; nontherapeutic research; *organ donation; organ transplantation; presumed consent; third party consent; *tissue donation; tissue transplantation; *Belgium

Ostrer, Harry; Scheuermann, Richard H.; Picker, Louis J. Benefits and dangers of genetic tests. [Letters]. *Nature.* 1998 Mar 5; 392(6671): 14. 6 refs. BE59237.
advisory committees; breast cancer; DNA data banks; epidemiology; genetic predisposition; *genetic research; *genetic screening; human experimentation; informed consent; Jews; minority groups; *population genetics; *public policy; risks and benefits; *tissue banks; tissue donation; National Bioethics Advisory Commission; United States

Palmer, Louis J. Organ Transplants from Executed Prisoners: An Argument for the Creation of Death Sentence Organ Removal Statutes. Jefferson, NC: McFarland; 1999. 156 p. 429 fn. ISBN 0-7864-0673-9. BE61943.
anesthesia; body parts and fluids; brain death; cadavers; *capital punishment; constitutional amendments; *constitutional law; due process; equal protection; federal government; *legal aspects; *mandatory programs; methods; *model legislation; *organ donation; *prisoners; property rights; public policy; punishment; remuneration; scarcity; state government; voluntary programs; China; Great Britain; Uniform Anatomical Gift Act; *United States

Peru. Supreme Decree No. 014–88–SA of 19 May 1988. (*Revista de Legislacifn y Jurisprudencia: Normas Legales,* May–Jun 1988, Vol. 152, p. 167–171). [Summary]. *International Digest of Health Legislation.* 1994. 45(1). 36–37. BE62693.
brain death; cadavers; compensation; informed consent; *legal aspects; *organ donation; organ donors; organ transplantation; registries; tissue banks; *Peru

Portmann, John. Cutting bodies to harvest organs. *Cambridge Quarterly of Healthcare Ethics.* 1999 Summer; 8(3): 288–298. 14 fn. BE62472.
*attitudes; *autonomy; body parts and fluids; *cadavers; *Christian ethics; *emotions; family members; historical aspects; *human body; Jewish ethics; moral obligations; *motivation; *organ donation; Roman Catholic ethics; scarcity; secularism; *surgery; third party consent; values; *refusal to donate; United States

Potts, John T.; Herdman, Roger C.; Beauchamp, Thomas L., et al. Commentary: clear thinking and open discussion guide IOM's report on organ donation. *Journal of Law, Medicine and Ethics.* 1998 Summer; 26(2): 166–168. 10 fn. Commentary on J. Menikoff, p. 157–168.

BE62679.

advisory committees; brain death; *cadavers; *cardiac death; *determination of death; disclosure; *guidelines; informed consent; institutional policies; *organ donation; policy analysis; public policy; standards; *time factors; *Institute of Medicine; *United States

Price, David; Akveld, Hans. Living donor organ transplantation in Europe: re-evaluating its role. *European Journal of Health Law.* 1998 Mar; 5(1): 19–44. 93 fn. BE61215.

adults; body parts and fluids; cadavers; coercion; competence; disclosure; family members; friends; government regulation; informed consent; *international aspects; kidneys; *legal aspects; mentally disabled; minors; *organ donation; *organ donors; physicians; risks and benefits; scarcity; time factors; transplant recipients; treatment outcome; unrelated donors; *Europe

Price, David; Akveld, Hans. Rotterdam Symposium on living organ donation (Rotterdam, 6–7 Nov 1995). [Meeting report]. *International Digest of Health Legislation.* 1997; 48(1): 77–80. BE59590.

coercion; compensation; economics; informed consent; injuries; *international aspects; kidneys; legal aspects; motivation; *organ donation; *organ donors; risks and benefits; unrelated donors; Belgium; *Europe; Great Britain; Netherlands

Rayner, John D. Organ transplantation. *In: his* Jewish Religious Law: A Progressive Perspective. New York, NY: Berghahn Books; 1998: 124–129. ISBN 1-57181-976-2. BE62135.

aborted fetuses; animal organs; body parts and fluids; brain; determination of death; fetal tissue donation; *Jewish ethics; *organ donation; *organ transplantation; prolongation of life; resource allocation; *tissue transplantation; value of life; *Reform Judaism

Resnik, David B. The commodification of human reproductive materials. *Journal of Medical Ethics.* 1998 Dec; 24(6): 388–393. 21 refs. BE60788.

autonomy; *body parts and fluids; *commodification; *embryos; *genes; *genetic materials; *germ cells; human body; moral policy; ovum donors; patents; personhood; property rights; regulation; *remuneration; reproductive technologies; semen donors; tissue donation; transgenic organisms

This essay develops a framework for thinking about the moral basis for the commodification of human reproductive materials. It argues that selling and buying gametes and genes is morally acceptable although there should not be a market for zygotes, embryos, or genomes. Also a market in gametes and genes should be regulated in order to address concerns about the adverse social consequences of commodification.

Rhodes, Rosamond. Organ transplantation. *In:* Kuhse, Helga; Singer, Peter, eds. A Companion to Bioethics. Malden, MA: Blackwell; 1998: 329–340. 18 refs. ISBN 0-631-19737-0. BE59507.

body parts and fluids; brain death; cadavers; determination of death; family members; health facilities; international aspects; justice; moral obligations; moral policy; obligations of society; obligations to society; *organ donation; organ donors; *organ transplantation; presumed consent; public policy; remuneration; resource allocation; risks and benefits; selection for treatment; third party consent; tissue donation; tissue transplantation; transplant recipients

Richard–Hughes, Sharon. Attitudes and beliefs of Afro-Americans related to organ and tissue donation. *International Journal of Trauma Nursing.* 1997 Oct–Dec; 3(4): 119–123. 15 refs. BE60538.

*blacks; *knowledge, attitudes, practice; *organ donation; socioeconomic factors; survey; Southeastern United States

Robertson, John A. Abortion to obtain fetal tissue for transplant. *Suffolk University Law Review.* 1993 Winter; 27(4): 1359–1389. 75 fn. BE61595.

*aborted fetuses; *abortion, induced; advisory committees; anencephaly; attitudes; coercion; constitutional law; criminal law; *decision making; *directed donation; family members; federal government; fetal research; *fetal tissue donation; *government regulation; informed consent; killing; legal aspects; *legal rights; *moral policy; motivation; organ donation; persistent vegetative state; *pregnant women; public policy; remuneration; reproduction; sex determination; state interest; tissue transplantation; transplant recipients; *women's rights; Department of Health and Human Services; National Institutes of Health; United States

Robinson, John H.; Berry, Roberta M.; McDonnell, Kevin, eds. Issues in adult health care. *In: their* A Health Law Reader: An Interdisciplinary Approach. Durham, NC: Carolina Academic Press; 1999: 239–337. 17 fn. ISBN 0-89089-907-X. BE62294.

adults; altruism; autonomy; cadavers; commodification; competence; computers; *confidentiality; conflict of interest; data banks; decision making; *disclosure; duty to warn; genetic information; health care delivery; human experimentation; *informed consent; justice; *legal aspects; legal liability; medical records; mentally ill; negligence; *organ donation; organ donors; *organ transplantation; patient care; physician patient relationship; physicians; *privacy; psychotherapy; public health; public policy; quality of health care; remuneration; resource allocation; risks and benefits; social dominance; torts; Tarasoff v. Regents of the University of California; Uniform Anatomical Gift Act; United States

Robinson, John H.; Berry, Roberta M.; McDonnell, Kevin, eds. Neonates and children. *In: their* A Health Law Reader: An Interdisciplinary Approach. Durham, NC: Carolina Academic Press; 1999: 181–238. 46 fn. ISBN 0-89089-907-X. BE62293.

*allowing to die; *anencephaly; *children; Christian Scientists; *congenital disorders; cultural pluralism; *decision making; determination of death; *disabled; futility; human experimentation; informed consent; *legal aspects; legal liability; legal rights; *newborns; nontherapeutic research; *organ donation; *parents; patient care; personhood; prolongation of life; quality of life; religion; *rights; risks and benefits; social discrimination; standards; therapeutic research; third party consent; *treatment refusal; *value of life; wedge argument; withholding treatment; Americans with Disabilities Act 1990; United States

Roels, L.; Deschoolmeester, G.; Vanrenterghem, Y. A profile of people objecting to organ donation in a country with a presumed consent law: data from the Belgian National Registry. *Transplantation Proceedings.* 1997 Feb–Mar; 29(1–2): 1473–1475. 6 refs. BE61575.

age factors; aliens; *attitudes; cadavers; females; legal aspects; males; minority groups; *organ donation; *presumed consent; public policy; *registries; statistics; *tissue donation; *refusal to donate; *Belgium; Portugal

Ross, Lainie Friedman. Children, Families, and Health Care Decision Making. New York, NY: Clarendon Press; 1998. 197 p. (Issues in biomedical ethics). Bibliography: p. 177–190. ISBN 0-19-823763-4. BE61944.

*adolescents; advisory committees; *autonomy; case studies; *children; *competence; *decision making; deontological ethics; directed donation; dissent; family members; *family relationship; federal government; futility; goals; government regulation; guidelines; *human experimentation; legal aspects; *minors; moral development; *moral obligations; nontherapeutic research; *organ donation; *parental consent;

*parents; *patient care; pediatrics; personhood; physicians; prolongation of life; quality of life; refusal to treat; rights; risk; risks and benefits; sexuality; siblings; state interest; therapeutic research; *treatment refusal; utilitarianism; *values; liberalism; needs; National Commission for the Protection of Human Subjects; United States

Sade, Robert M. Cadaveric organ donation: rethinking donor motivation. *Archives of Internal Medicine.* 1999 Mar 8; 159(5): 438–442. 25 refs. Commented on by K.A. Korzick and P.B. Terry, p. 427–428. BE61327.

advance directives; autonomy; beneficence; blacks; body parts and fluids; *cadavers; cultural pluralism; *directed donation; disadvantaged; *family members; gifts; *incentives; justice; minority groups; *moral policy; *motivation; *organ donation; organ donors; organ transplantation; resource allocation; risks and benefits; scarcity; selection for treatment; third party consent; *transplant recipients; National Organ Transplant Act 1984; Uniform Anatomical Gift Act; United Network for Organ Sharing; United States

Saegusa, Asako. Japan's transplant law 'is too stringent'. [News]. *Nature.* 1999 Mar 11; 398(6723): 95. BE61959.

brain death; family members; government regulation; international aspects; *legal aspects; legislation; minors; *organ donation; organ transplantation; third party consent; *Japan

Sass, Hans-Martin. Ethics of the allocation of highly advanced medical technologies. *Artificial Organs.* 1998 Mar; 22(3): 263–268. 14 refs. BE60080.

advisory committees; animal organs; artificial organs; *biomedical technologies; coercion; cultural pluralism; developing countries; economics; genetic predisposition; genetic screening; health education; health promotion; *incentives; international aspects; *justice; *organ donation; organ donors; *organ transplantation; preventive medicine; regulation; remuneration; *resource allocation; *socioeconomic factors

Schenker, Joseph G. Sperm, oocyte, and pre-embryo donation. *Journal of Assisted Reproduction and Genetics.* 1995 Sep; 12(8): 499–508. 16 refs. BE60562.

aborted fetuses; age factors; artificial insemination; confidentiality; *donors; embryo transfer; *embryos; females; genetic materials; guidelines; in vitro fertilization; infertility; informed consent; males; medical records; ovum; *ovum donors; public policy; religious ethics; remuneration; *reproductive technologies; selection for treatment; *semen donors; single persons; sperm; tissue banks; tissue donation

Schwindt, Richard; Vining, Aidan. Proposal for a mutual insurance pool for transplant organs. *Journal of Health Politics, Policy and Law.* 1998 Oct; 23(5): 725–741. 44 refs. BE59784.

accountability; adults; *body parts and fluids; cadavers; economics; *incentives; *insurance; motivation; *organ donation; organ transplantation; organization and administration; policy analysis; private sector; property rights; public policy; public sector; remuneration; resource allocation; risks and benefits; scarcity; selection for treatment; transplant recipients; trust; voluntary programs; United States

Over the past decade there have been numerous proposals to use market system incentives to attenuate the persistent shortage of transplantable human organs. While shortages have grown, opposition to market-based solutions has remained adamant. Much of the opposition has focused on monetary incentives. This article explores an alternative -- a mutual insurance pool to increase the supply of organs. In the process, criticisms of earlier proposals (specifically the future delivery scheme) are addressed, the operation of an insurance pool is described, and problems associated with insurance

markets are identified and addressed. The article concludes that an insurance pool could overcome public and political resistance to more explicit market-based solutions.

Sever, M.S.; Ecder, T.; Aydin, A.E., et al. Living unrelated (paid) kidney transplantation in Third-World countries: high risk of complications besides the ethical problem. *Nephrology, Dialysis, Transplantation.* 1994; 9(4): 350–354. 35 refs. BE61587.

case studies; *developing countries; *kidneys; legal aspects; *morbidity; *organ donation; *organ donors; *organ transplantation; patient care; *remuneration; risk; risks and benefits; *transplant recipients; treatment outcome; *unrelated donors; *India; Turkey

Sharma, Dinesh C. Indian organ donation goes ahead without consent. [News]. *Lancet.* 1999 Mar 27; 353(9158): 1076. BE61985.

adults; *competence; directed donation; *family members; kidneys; *organ donation; *organ donors; parental consent; physically disabled; renal dialysis; risks and benefits; *siblings; *third party consent; *India

Shenfield, Françoise. Recruitment and counselling of sperm donors: ethical problems. *Human Reproduction.* 1998 May; 13(Suppl. 2): 70–75. 29 refs. BE61482.

advertising; altruism; attitudes; coercion; confidentiality; *counseling; fathers; guidelines; informed consent; international aspects; motivation; remuneration; *semen donors; sperm; *tissue donation; France; Great Britain

Simini, Bruno. US human organ dealer arrested in Italy. [News]. *Lancet.* 1998 Oct 17; 352(9136): 1289. BE61102.

aliens; *body parts and fluids; international aspects; *law enforcement; legal aspects; misconduct; *organ donation; *remuneration; *Italy; United States

Siminoff, Laura A.; Bloch, Alexia. American attitudes and beliefs about brain death: the empirical literature. *In:* Youngner, Stuart J.; Arnold, Robert M.; Schapiro, Renie, eds. The Definition of Death: Contemporary Controversies. Baltimore, MD: Johns Hopkins University Press; 1999: 183–193. 37 refs. ISBN 0-8018-5985-9. BE60765.

*attitudes to death; *brain death; cardiac death; cultural pluralism; *determination of death; donor cards; *empirical research; family members; international aspects; *knowledge, attitudes, practice; minority groups; nurses; *organ donation; physicians; presumed consent; *public opinion; *standards; Japan; *United States

Siminoff, Laura A.; Arnold, Robert. Increasing organ donation in the African-American community: altruism in the face of an untrustworthy system. [Editorial]. *Annals of Internal Medicine.* 1999 Apr 6; 130(7): 607–609. 19 refs. BE62603.

altruism; *attitudes; *blacks; cadavers; donor cards; information dissemination; kidneys; knowledge, attitudes, practice; *organ donation; organ donors; organ transplantation; scarcity; statistics; third party consent; transplant recipients; trust; whites; *United States

Smith, George P. Organ harvesting: salvaging a new beginning. *In: his* Family Values and the New Society: Dilemmas of the 21st Century. Westport, CT: Praeger; 1998: 247–267. 129 fn. ISBN 0-275-96221-0. BE62299.

autopsies; body parts and fluids; brain death; cadavers; cardiac death; coercion; contracts; determination of death; legal aspects; legislation; mandatory programs; *organ donation; organ donors; property rights; public opinion; *public policy; remuneration; required request; resource allocation; third party consent; utilitarianism; voluntary programs; withholding treatment; National Organ

---

BE = bioethics accession number   fn. = footnotes   refs. = references

Transplant Act 1984; Uniform Anatomical Gift Act; United States

Stolberg, Sheryl Gay. Animals as organ donors? Not until they're germ-free. *New York Times.* 1998 Feb 3: F1, F6. BE60463.
animal experimentation; *animal organs; attitudes; communicable diseases; dissent; *government regulation; guidelines; human experimentation; industry; investigators; *organ donation; *organ transplantation; physicians; public health; public opinion; *risk; risks and benefits; therapeutic research; *transgenic animals; *transplant recipients; swine; Food and Drug Administration; Public Health Service; United States

Stolberg, Sheryl Gay. Pennsylvania set to break taboo on reward for organ donation. [News]. *New York Times.* 1999 May 6: A1, A30. BE61075.
body parts and fluids; cadavers; family members; federal government; *incentives; legal aspects; *organ donation; *public policy; state government; National Organ Transplant Act 1984; *Pennsylvania; United States

Swinn, Michael; Emberton, Mark; Ralph, David, et al. Retrieving semen from a dead patient: Utilitarianism in the absence of definitive guidelines; The patient was assaulted; Some ethical concerns were ignored; [and] An ethic of ambivalence. *BMJ (British Medical Journal).* 1998 Dec 5; 317(7172): 1583–1585. 7 refs. BE60233.
advance directives; *brain death; *cadavers; case studies; competence; cryopreservation; family members; informed consent; married persons; physicians; *posthumous reproduction; *semen donors; sperm; third party consent; utilitarianism; Great Britain

Szawarski, Zbigniew. The stick, the eye, and ownership of the body. *In:* ten Have, Henk A.M.J.; Welie, Jos V.M., eds. Ownership of the Human Body: Philosophical Considerations on the Use of the Human Body and Its Parts in Healthcare. Boston, MA: Kluwer Academic; 1998: 81–96. 26 refs. ISBN 0-7923-5150-9. BE61320.
altruism; body parts and fluids; cadavers; commodification; common good; gifts; *human body; *organ donation; philosophy; presumed consent; *property rights; remuneration; self concept; eyes

ten Have, Henk A.M.J.; Welie, Jos V.M., eds. Ownership of the Human Body: Philosophical Considerations on the Use of the Human Body and Its Parts in Healthcare. Boston, MA: Kluwer Academic; 1998. 235 p. (Philosophy and medicine; v. 59). 284 refs. 45 fn. ISBN 0-7923-5150. BE61317.
altruism; autonomy; autopsies; *bioethical issues; biomedical research; blood donation; *body parts and fluids; cadavers; commodification; common good; deontological ethics; ethical theory; historical aspects; *human body; human experimentation; legal aspects; libertarianism; mandatory programs; *moral policy; organ donation; philosophy; postmodernism; *property rights; public policy; religion; remuneration; rights; Roman Catholic ethics; *tissue donation; utilitarianism; voluntary programs; Denmark; Europe; France; Germany; Netherlands

Thorne, Emanuel D. When private parts are made public goods: the economics of market-inalienability. *Yale Journal on Regulation.* 1998 Winter; 15(1): 149–175. 61 fn. BE61525.
altruism; blood donation; *body parts and fluids; directed donation; *economics; incentives; motivation; *organ donation; policy analysis; property rights; public policy; *regulation; *remuneration; resource allocation; risks and benefits; scarcity; Arrow, Kenneth; Titmuss, Richard

Trotter, Griffin. Mandated choice for organ donation.

Health Care Ethics USA. 1997 Spring; 5(2): 2–3. 2 refs. BE61722.
altruism; autonomy; contracts; covenant; *decision making; *mandatory programs; moral obligations; moral policy; obligations to society; *organ donation; public policy; *mandated choice; United States

Uruguay. Decree No. 660/991 of 4 Dec 1991 updating Regulations No. 86/977, made for the implementation of Law No. 14005, for the purpose of determining the technical supervision of the National Organ and Tissue Bank. (*Diario Oficial de la Repdblic Oriental del Uruguay*, 10 Feb 1992, No. 23521, p. 194–A). [Summary]. *International Digest of Health Legislation.* 1994. 45(1). 38. BE62696.
adults; informed consent; *legal aspects; *mandatory programs; *organ donation; registries; *mandated choice; refusal to donate; *Uruguay

Veatch, Robert M. Egalitarian and maximin theories of justice: directed donation of organs for transplant. *Journal of Medicine and Philosophy.* 1998 Oct; 23(5): 456–476. 13 refs. 12 fn. Note: the journal issue cover shows a date of August 1998, which is incorrect. BE62113.
beneficence; *directed donation; ethical analysis; *ethical theory; freedom; health; health care delivery; *justice; *moral policy; *organ donation; *organ transplantation; public policy; *resource allocation; rights; *selection for treatment; self concept; social discrimination; socioeconomic factors; transplant recipients; utilitarianism; whites; *egalitarianism; *Rawls, John; United Network for Organ Sharing; United States
It is common to interpret Rawls's maximin theory of justice as egalitarian. Compared to utilitarian theories, this may be true. However, in special cases practices that distribute resources so as to benefit the worst off actually increase the inequality between the worst off and some who are better off. In these cases the Rawlsian maximin parts company with what is here called true egalitarianism. A policy question requiring a distinction between maximin and "true egalitarian" allocations has arisen in the arena of organ transplantation. This case is examined here as a venue for differentiating maximin and true egalitarian theories. Directed donation is the name given to donations of organs restricted to a particular social group. For example, the family of a member of the Ku Klux Klan donated his organs on the provision that they go only to members of the Caucasian race. While such donations appear to be discriminatory, if certain plausible assumptions are made, they satisfy the maximin criterion. They selectively advantage the recipient of the organs without harming anyone (assuming the organs would otherwise go unused). Moreover, everyone who is lower on the waiting list (who, thereby, could be considered worse off) is advantaged by moving up on the waiting list. This paper examines how maximin and more truly egalitarian theories handle this case arguing that, to the extent that directed donation in unethical, the best account of that conclusion is that an egalitarian principle of justice is to be preferred to the maximin.

Velasco, N.; Drukker, Alfred; Lyon, Sue, et al. Organ donation and kidney sales. [Letters]. *Lancet.* 1998 Aug 8; 352(9126): 483–485. 9 refs. BE60980.
cadavers; developing countries; family members; indigents; international aspects; *kidneys; *organ donation; *organ donors; physicians; quality of life; *remuneration; renal dialysis; risks and benefits; transplant recipients

Vikhanski, Luba. Israel introduces organ swap scheme.

[News]. *Nature Medicine*. 1998 Apr; 4(4): 377. BE59710.
*directed donation; *incentives; *kidneys; *organ donation; organ donors; organ transplantation; *public policy; scarcity; selection for treatment; transplant recipients; *Israel

Watts, Jonathan. Concept of brain death to be accepted in South Korea. [News]. *Lancet*. 1998 Dec 19–26; 352(9145): 1996. BE60272.
*brain death; cadavers; *determination of death; family members; *legal aspects; *organ donation; third party consent; *Korea

Weiss, A.H.; Fortinsky, R.H.; Laughlin, J., et al. Parental consent for pediatric cadaveric organ donation. *Transplantation Proceedings*. 1997 May; 29(3): 1896–1901. 24 refs. BE60200.
altruism; brain death; *cadavers; *children; disclosure; family members; incentives; information dissemination; *knowledge, attitudes, practice; motivation; *organ donation; organ transplantation; *parental consent; *parents; presumed consent; *professional family relationship; remuneration; survey; transplant recipients; *refusal to donate; retrospective studies; California

Wu, John; Sheil, A.G. Ross; Guttmann, Ronald D., et al. Spare parts. [Letters and response]. *Sciences*. 1998 May/Jun; 38(3): 5, 8. BE60105.
*body parts and fluids; cadavers; capital punishment; health personnel; international aspects; misconduct; *organ donation; organ transplantation; organizational policies; physicians; *prisoners; professional organizations; self regulation; *China; Transplantation Society

WuDunn, Sheryl. Death taboo weakening, Japan sees 1st transplant. [News]. *New York Times*. 1999 Mar 1: A8. BE60973.
advance directives; *brain death; cardiac death; *determination of death; hearts; *legal aspects; *organ donation; *organ transplantation; *Japan

An organ donation offer on death row is refused. [News]. *New York Times*. 1998 Sep 9: A23. BE61118.
*capital punishment; *organ donation; *prisoners; public policy; state government; *Nobles, Jonathan; *Texas

Current European laws on gamete donation. *Human Reproduction*. 1998 May; 13(Suppl. 2): 105–134. BE61486.
bone marrow; cadavers; cloning; confidentiality; cryopreservation; embryo research; embryo transfer; gene therapy; genetic counseling; genetic intervention; genetic screening; germ cells; *government regulation; health facilities; hybrids; informed consent; *international aspects; *legislation; organ donation; *ovum donors; posthumous reproduction; preimplantation diagnosis; prenatal diagnosis; *reproductive technologies; *semen donors; sex preselection; *tissue donation; Austria; Denmark; *Europe; France; Germany; Great Britain; Israel; Norway; Portugal; Spain; Sweden; Switzerland

Kevorkian offers organs in assisted–suicide case. [News]. *New York Times*. 1998 Jun 8: A18. BE60474.
*assisted suicide; cadavers; hospitals; *kidneys; *organ donation; patients; physicians; standards; *Kevorkian, Jack; Michigan

Special section: organ transplantation: shaping policy and keeping public trust. [Bibliography]. *Cambridge Quarterly of Healthcare Ethics*. 1999 Summer; 8(3): 348–350. BE62478.
*organ donation; *organ transplantation

ORGAN AND TISSUE TRANSPLANTATION

See also ORGAN AND TISSUE DONATION

Alexander, G. Caleb; Sehgal, Ashwini R. Barriers to cadaveric renal transplantation among blacks, women, and the poor. *JAMA*. 1998 Oct 7; 280(13): 1148–1152. 21 refs. BE60285.
attitudes; blacks; cadavers; comparative studies; females; indigents; *kidneys; males; *organ transplantation; patients; prognosis; referral and consultation; renal dialysis; *resource allocation; *selection for treatment; *socioeconomic factors; *transplant recipients; whites; prospective studies; waiting lists; Indiana; Kentucky; Ohio
CONTEXT: Cadaveric renal transplantation rates differ greatly by race, sex, and income. Previous efforts to lessen these differences have focused on the transplant waiting list. However, the transplantation process involves a series of steps related to medical suitability, interest in transplantation, pretransplant workup, and movement up a waiting list to eventual transplantation. OBJECTIVE: To determine the relative importance of each step in explaining differences in cadaveric renal transplantation rates. DESIGN: Prospective cohort study. SETTING AND PATIENTS: A total of 7125 patients beginning long–term dialysis between January 1993 and December 1996 in Indiana, Kentucky, and Ohio. MAIN OUTCOME MEASURES: Completion of 4 separate steps during each patient–year of follow–up: (A) being medically suitable and possibly interested in transplantation; (B) being definitely interested in transplantation; (C) completing the pretransplant workup; and (D) moving up a waiting list and receiving a transplant. RESULTS: Compared with whites, blacks were less likely to complete steps B (odds ratio [OR], 0.68; 95% confidence interval [CI], 0.61–0.76), C (OR, 0.56; 95% CI, 0.48–0.65), and D (OR, 0.50; 95% CI, 0.40–0.62) after adjustment for age, sex, cause of renal failure, years receiving dialysis, and median income of patient ZIP code. Compared with men, women were less likely to complete each of the 4 steps, with ORs of 0.90, 0.89, 0.80, and 0.82, respectively. Poor individuals were less likely than wealthy individuals to complete steps A, B, and C, with ORs of 0.67, 0.78, and 0.77, respectively. CONCLUSIONS: Barriers at several steps are responsible for sociodemographic differences in access to cadaveric renal transplantation. Efforts to allocate kidneys equitably must address each step of the transplant process.

Altman, Lawrence K. New direction for transplants raises hopes and questions. [Rebuilding the body: a special report]. *New York Times*. 1999 May 2: 1, 46–47. BE61173.
AIDS; *body parts and fluids; cancer; *cosmetic surgery; drugs; economics; *human experimentation; injuries; methods; *organ transplantation; *quality of life; risk; *risks and benefits; *tissue transplantation; transplant recipients; hands; knees

Altman, Lawrence K. 'Role model' with a past clouds medical triumph. [News]. *New York Times*. 1999 Apr 27: F6. BE61171.
body parts and fluids; human experimentation; patient compliance; prisoners; quality of life; selection for treatment; *tissue transplantation; *transplant recipients; *hands; Australia; France; *Hallan, Clint

Ankeny, Rachel A. Recasting the debate on multiple listing for transplantation through consideration of both principles and practice. *Cambridge Quarterly of Healthcare Ethics*. 1999 Summer; 8(3): 330–339. 30 fn. BE62476.
autonomy; body parts and fluids; *geographic factors; hospitals; institutional policies; justice; motivation; *organ transplantation; *patients; public policy; *resource allocation; scarcity; *selection for treatment; socioeconomic

factors; standards; time factors; *transplant recipients; *waiting lists; United Network for Organ Sharing; United States

Bahnsen, Ulrich. Switzerland adopts transplant guidelines. [News]. *Nature.* 1999 Feb 18; 397(6720): 553. BE61569.
   animal organs; *government regulation; guidelines; legal aspects; *organ donation; *organ transplantation; political activity; remuneration; *Switzerland

Bartlett, Rachel. The ethics of xenotransplantation. [Letter]. *Journal of Medical Ethics.* 1998 Dec; 24(6): 414–415. 9 refs. BE60979.
   advisory committees; anencephaly; *animal organs; brain death; communicable diseases; newborns; organ donation; *organ transplantation; persistent vegetative state; presumed consent; public policy; risk; scarcity; Advisory Group on the Ethics of Xenotransplantation (Great Britain); Great Britain; Nuffield Council on Bioethics

Becker, Carl. Money talks, money kills -- the economics of transplantation in Japan and China. *Bioethics.* 1999 Jul; 13(3–4): 236–243. 33 fn. BE61873.
   allowing to die; *brain death; *capital punishment; *determination of death; directed donation; *economics; hospitals; institutional policies; *legal aspects; *motivation; non–Western World; *organ donation; *organ transplantation; *prisoners; *public policy; *China; *Japan
   Japan and China have long resisted the Western trend of organ transplantation from brain–dead patients, based on a 'Confucian' respect for integrity of ancestors' bodies. While their general publics continue to harbor grave doubts about such practices, their medical and political elites are hastening towards the road of organ–harvesting and organ–marketing, largely for economic reasons. This report illustrates the ways that economics is motivating brain–death legislation in Japan and criminal executions in China.

Bollinger, R. Randal. A UNOS [United Network for Organ Sharing] perspective on donor liver allocation. *Liver Transplantation and Surgery.* 1995 Jan; 1(1): 47–55. 6 refs. BE60881.
   dissent; federal government; geographic factors; goals; guidelines; health facilities; *livers; *organ transplantation; *organizational policies; physicians; prognosis; program descriptions; public policy; *resource allocation; scarcity; selection for treatment; standards; statistics; time factors; transplant recipients; voluntary programs; waiting lists; *United Network for Organ Sharing; *United States

Bosch, Xavier. Spain leads world in organ donation and transplantation. [News]. *JAMA.* 1999 Jul 7; 282(1): 17–18. BE61954.
   body parts and fluids; brain death; cadavers; cardiac death; confidentiality; health personnel; HIV seropositivity; information dissemination; *organ donation; organ donors; *organ transplantation; organizational policies; presumed consent; *public policy; remuneration; selection for treatment; statistics; transplant recipients; National Transplant Organization (Spain); *Spain

Bosch, Xavier. Spain releases xenotransplantation guidelines. [News]. *Nature Medicine.* 1998 Aug; 4(8): 876. BE59772.
   *animal organs; *guidelines; human experimentation; *organ transplantation; *public policy; *Spain

Brand, Donald A.; Kliger, Alan S. Planning for a kidney transplant: is my doctor listening? *JAMA.* 1999 Aug 18; 282(7): 691–694. 36 refs. BE62655.
   case studies; *communication; *decision analysis; *decision making; kidney diseases; *kidneys; *organ transplantation; *patients; *physician patient relationship; physicians; quality

of life; renal dialysis; *risks and benefits

Butler, Declan. Europe is urged to hold back on xenotransplant clinical trials. [News]. *Nature.* 1999 Jan 28; 397(6717): 281–282. BE61568.
   *animal organs; attitudes; communicable diseases; *government regulation; *human experimentation; international aspects; investigators; *organ transplantation; public health; risk; *tissue transplantation; *Council of Europe; Europe

Butler, Declan. FDA warns on primate xenotransplants. [News]. *Nature.* 1999 Apr 15; 398(6728): 549. BE62156.
   *animal organs; communicable diseases; federal government; *government regulation; *guidelines; *human experimentation; *organ transplantation; *primates; public health; risk; transplant recipients; swine; Centers for Disease Control and Prevention; *Food and Drug Administration; *United States

Butler, Declan. Transplant panel to play 'honest broker.' [News]. *Nature.* 1999 Apr 22; 398(6729): 643. BE61963.
   *animal organs; ethicists; guidelines; human experimentation; information dissemination; *international aspects; investigators; *organ transplantation; public participation; *risks and benefits; tissue transplantation

Caplan, Arthur L.; Coelho, Daniel H. The Ethics of Organ Transplants: The Current Debate. Amherst, NY: Prometheus Books; 1998. 350 p. Bibliography: p. 347–350. ISBN 1–57392–224–2. BE60916.
   aborted fetuses; abortion, induced; alcohol abuse; altruism; anencephaly; animal organs; blacks; brain death; cadavers; cardiac death; coercion; commodification; determination of death; directed donation; disadvantaged; donor cards; economics; family members; fetal tissue donation; health insurance reimbursement; incentives; international aspects; justice; kidneys; legal aspects; livers; *moral policy; *organ donation; organ donors; *organ transplantation; persistent vegetative state; presumed consent; primates; prognosis; *public policy; remuneration; required request; *resource allocation; retreatment; *selection for treatment; *tissue transplantation; transplant recipients; mandated choice; refusal to donate; *unrelated donors; Medicaid; Medicare; Oregon; Uniform Anatomical Gift Act; United States

Caplan, Arthur L. Wearing your organ transplant on your sleeve. *Hastings Center Report.* 1999 Mar–Apr; 29(2): 52. BE61667.
   body parts and fluids; human experimentation; organ donation; *organ transplantation; *quality of life; risks and benefits; therapeutic research; *hands

Cartwright, Will. The pig, the transplant surgeon and the Nuffield Council. *Medical Law Review.* 1996 Autumn; 4(3): 250–269. 39 fn. BE61512.
   *advisory committees; animal experimentation; *animal organs; *animal rights; consensus; decision making; food; government regulation; human characteristics; human experimentation; *moral policy; morality; organ donation; *organ transplantation; pain; philosophy; primates; risk; risks and benefits; self concept; *speciesism; transgenic animals; values; domestic animals; *swine; Advisory Committee on Xenotransplantation (Great Britain); Great Britain; *Institute of Medical Ethics (Great Britain); *Nuffield Council on Bioethics

Chugh, Kirpal S.; Jha, Vivekanand. Commerce in transplantation in Third World countries. *Kidney International.* 1996 May; 49(5): 1181–1186. 34 refs. BE61562.
   *cadavers; coercion; *commodification; *developing countries; family members; females; health facilities; international aspects; *kidneys; legal aspects; married persons; morbidity; *organ donation; *organ donors; *organ

---

BE = bioethics accession number   fn. = footnotes   refs. = references

transplantation; organizational policies; prisoners; professional organizations; public policy; *remuneration; scarcity; *socioeconomic factors; statistics; transplant recipients; treatment outcome; *unrelated donors; *Asia; China; *India; Latin America

Crigger, Bette-Jane. Xenotransplantation [title supplied]. *Hastings Center Report.* 1999 Jan-Feb; 29(1): 50. Report on the Hastings Center's 1998 Fellows Meeting on ethical and public policy issues in xenotransplantation. BE61638.
    *animal organs; human experimentation; informed consent; *organ transplantation; public policy; risk; *risks and benefits; transgenic animals; swine

Currie, Rebecca. UK moves ahead on the xenotransplantation issue. [News]. *Nature Medicine.* 1998 Sep; 4(9): 988. BE62157.
    *animal organs; communicable diseases; *government regulation; guidelines; human experimentation; *organ transplantation; *tissue transplantation; transplant recipients; swine; *Great Britain; *Xenotransplantation Interim Regulatory Authority (Great Britain)

Davison, Alex M. Commercialization in organ donation. [Editorial]. *Nephrology, Dialysis, Transplantation.* 1994; 9(4): 348-349. 3 refs. BE61586.
    cultural pluralism; *developing countries; ethical relativism; indigents; *international aspects; *kidneys; morbidity; *organ donation; *organ donors; *organ transplantation; *remuneration; risk; scarcity; *transplant recipients; treatment outcome; *unrelated donors

Deutsch, Lisa B. Medicaid payment for organ transplants: the extent of mandated coverage. *Columbia Journal of Law and Social Problems.* 1997 Winter; 30(2): 185-213. 127 fn. BE61254.
    economics; federal government; *government financing; indigents; judicial action; justice; *legal aspects; *organ transplantation; *public policy; resource allocation; *state government; *Medicaid; Social Security Act; *United States; *Wisconsin

Dossetor, John B. Economic, social, racial and age-related considerations in dialysis and transplantation. *Current Opinion in Nephrology and Hypertension.* 1995 Nov; 4(6): 498-501. 39 refs. BE59835.
    *age factors; aged; blacks; cadavers; developing countries; females; *international aspects; kidney diseases; *kidneys; males; *minority groups; organ donation; organ donors; *organ transplantation; remuneration; *renal dialysis; *resource allocation; selection for treatment; *socioeconomic factors; statistics; transplant recipients; treatment outcome; whites

Evans, Roger W. Liver transplantation in a managed care environment. *Liver Transplantation and Surgery.* 1995 Jan; 1(1): 61-75. 75 refs. BE60903.
    biomedical research; biomedical technologies; *costs and benefits; *economics; geographic factors; goals; health care; health care reform; health facilities; justice; *livers; *managed care programs; *organ transplantation; physicians; practice guidelines; prognosis; *resource allocation; risk; *selection for treatment; transplant recipients; treatment outcome; trends; *United States

Finder, Stuart G.; Fox, Mark D.; Frist, William H., et al. The ethicist's role on the transplant team: a study of heart, lung, and liver transplantation programs in the United States. *Clinical Transplantation.* 1993 Dec; 7(6): 559-564. 22 refs. BE60203.
    clinical ethics; *decision making; education; *ethicist's role; *ethics consultation; hearts; hospitals; institutional policies; livers; organ donation; *organ transplantation; *patient care

team; program descriptions; resource allocation; review committees; selection for treatment; self concept; statistics; survey; transplant recipients; lungs; *United States; Vanderbilt University Medical Center

Fox, Marie; McHale, Jean. Xenotransplantation: the ethical and legal ramifications. *Medical Law Review.* 1998 Spring; 6(1): 42-61. 101 fn. BE62170.
    advisory committees; animal experimentation; *animal organs; *animal rights; communicable diseases; competence; conscience; disclosure; *government regulation; health personnel; *human experimentation; informed consent; international aspects; legal aspects; organ donation; *organ transplantation; patents; primates; *public health; *public policy; risk; *risks and benefits; scarcity; *speciesism; suffering; transgenic animals; *transplant recipients; swine; Advisory Group on the Ethics of Xenotransplantation (Great Britain); Europe; *Great Britain; Nuffield Council on Bioethics; United States; Xenotransplantation Interim Regulatory Authority (Great Britain)

France. Order of 6 Nov 1996 approving the Rules for the distribution and allocation of transplants removed from deceased persons for the purpose of organ transplantation. (*Journal officiel de la Republique fran3aise, Lois et Decrets,* 10 Nov 1996, No. 263, pp. 16475-16476). *International Digest of Health Legislation.* 1997; 48(1): 15-18. BE59588.
    adults; *body parts and fluids; cadavers; children; *legal aspects; *organ transplantation; prognosis; *resource allocation; *selection for treatment; time factors; transplant recipients; *France

Glick, Shimon. Ethical aspects of organ transplantation. *Jewish Medical Ethics.* 1997 Jan; 3(1): 11-13. BE59243.
    body parts and fluids; determination of death; international aspects; *organ donation; *organ transplantation; resource allocation; selection for treatment; transplant recipients; Israel

Grubb, Andrew. Medical treatment (child): parental refusal and role of the court -- Re T (A Minor) (Wardship: Medical Treatment). [Comment]. *Medical Law Review.* 1996 Autumn; 4(3): 315-319. BE61515.
    allowing to die; *children; congenital disorders; *decision making; *infants; judicial action; *legal aspects; livers; mothers; *organ transplantation; *parents; surgery; *treatment refusal; *Great Britain; *Re T (A Minor) (Wardship: Medical Treatment)

Himma, Kenneth Einar. A critique of UNOS liver allocation policy. *Cambridge Quarterly of Healthcare Ethics.* 1999 Summer; 8(3): 311-320. 38 fn. Article followed by update on UNOS policy, p. 320. BE62474.
    chronically ill; critically ill; emergency care; ethical analysis; *justice; *livers; mortality; *organ transplantation; *organizational policies; *prognosis; *public policy; *resource allocation; scarcity; *selection for treatment; time factors; transplant recipients; treatment outcome; liver diseases; *needs; survival; waiting lists; *United Network for Organ Sharing; United States

Howard, Louise; Fahy, Tom. Liver transplantation for alcoholic liver disease. [Editorial]. *British Journal of Psychiatry.* 1997 Dec; 171: 497-500. 30 refs. BE59335.
    *alcohol abuse; *livers; *organ transplantation; patient compliance; *prognosis; psychiatric diagnosis; psychiatry; risk; selection for treatment; self induced illness; transplant recipients; *treatment outcome

Ikels, Charlotte. Ethical issues in organ procurement in Chinese societies. *China Journal.* 1997 Jul; No. 38: 95-119. 66 fn. BE59198.
    aliens; *attitudes; *cadavers; capital punishment;

comparative studies; determination of death; family members; females; health insurance; informed consent; international aspects; *kidneys; males; *organ donation; *organ donors; *organ transplantation; physicians; political systems; *presumed consent; *prisoners; *public policy; religion; remuneration; scarcity; siblings; social discrimination; statistics; third party consent; transplant recipients; Confucian ethics; personal financing; refusal to donate; *unrelated donors; *China; *Hong Kong; *Singapore; *Taiwan

Institute of Biology (Great Britain). Institute of Biology Response to the Advisory Group on the Ethics of Xenotransplantation, made to the Department of Health. [Consultation response]. London: Institute of Biology [online]. Downloaded from Internet Web site: http://www.primex.co.uk/iob/d13.html on 16 Jan 1998; 1996 Apr 1. 5 p. 2 refs. BE59573.
    animal experimentation; *animal organs; biomedical research; communicable diseases; genetic intervention; government regulation; hybrids; organ donation; *organ transplantation; organizational policies; professional organizations; public opinion; *risks and benefits; scarcity; transgenic animals; Advisory Group on the Ethics of Xenotransplantation (Great Britain); *Great Britain; *Institute of Biology (Great Britain)

Institute of Biology (Great Britain); British Electrophoresis Society; British Association for Tissue Banks; et al. Xenotransplantation -- Reply to the Government's Response from the Institute of Biology and British Electrophoresis Society (with additional comments from the British Association of Tissue Banks and the Society for Low Temperature Biology). [Consultations]. London: Institute of Biology [online]. Downloaded from Web site: http://www.thomson.com/iob/xenotrans2.html on 16 Jan 1998; 1997 May 6. 2 p. BE59574.
    *animal organs; biomedical research; communicable diseases; government financing; government regulation; human experimentation; organ donation; *organ transplantation; organizational policies; primates; professional organizations; public policy; *risks and benefits; scarcity; standards; infection control; swine; Advisory Group on the Ethics of Xenotransplantation (Great Britain); Department of Health (Great Britain); *Great Britain; Institute of Biology (Great Britain)

Iqbal, Aamir; Holley, Jean L. Ethical issues in end-stage renal disease patients who use illicit intravenous drugs. *Seminars in Dialysis.* 1995 Jan-Feb; 8(1): 35-38. 30 refs. BE59922.
    case studies; *drug abuse; *kidney diseases; kidneys; methods; *organ transplantation; *patient compliance; *renal dialysis; *resource allocation; risks and benefits; *selection for treatment; self induced illness; social worth

Jakobsen, A. Living renal transplantation -- the Oslo experience. *Nephrology, Dialysis, Transplantation.* 1997 Sep; 12(9): 1825-1827. 5 refs. BE60032.
    altruism; attitudes; coercion; costs and benefits; family members; hospitals; *institutional policies; *kidneys; *organ donation; *organ donors; *organ transplantation; public policy; risks and benefits; statistics; transplant recipients; unrelated donors; *Norway

Julvez, Jean; Tuppin, Phillippe; Cohen, Sophie. Survey in France of response to xenotransplantation. [Research letter]. *Lancet.* 1999 Feb 27; 353(9154): 726. 4 refs. BE61199.
    *allied health personnel; *animal organs; *attitudes; communicable diseases; comparative studies; human experimentation; *nurses; *organ donation; *organ transplantation; *physicians; public opinion; risk; *students;

survey; swine; *France; French Transplant Agency

Kefalides, Paul. Solid organ transplantation. 2: Ethical considerations. *Annals of Internal Medicine.* 1999 Jan 19; 130(2): 169-170. BE62559.
    body parts and fluids; cadavers; federal government; government regulation; hospitals; *organ donation; organ donors; *organ transplantation; remuneration; resource allocation; selection for treatment; transplant recipients; Department of Health and Human Services; United States

Kennedy, Ian; Sewell, Herb. Xenotransplantation moratorium. [Letter]. *Nature Biotechnology.* 1998 Feb; 16(2): 120. 6 refs. BE62022.
    advisory committees; *animal organs; communicable diseases; *government regulation; *human experimentation; *organ transplantation; *public policy; *risks and benefits; Advisory Group on the Ethics of Xenotransplantation (Great Britain); *Great Britain

Khauli, Raja B. Issues and controversies surrounding organ donation and transplantation: the need for laws that ensure equity and optimal utility of a scarce resource. *Suffolk University Law Review.* 1993 Winter; 27(4): 1225-1236. 37 fn. BE60734.
    accountability; body parts and fluids; cadavers; economics; family members; incentives; justice; kidneys; legal aspects; legislation; minority groups; *organ donation; *organ transplantation; patient compliance; presumed consent; prognosis; *public policy; remuneration; renal dialysis; required request; *resource allocation; retreatment; scarcity; selection for treatment; treatment outcome; National Organ Transplant Act 1984; Organ Procurement and Transplant Network; United Network for Organ Sharing; United States

Klintmalm, Goran B. Who should receive the liver allograft: the transplant center or the recipient? *Liver Transplantation and Surgery.* 1995 Jan; 1(1): 55-58. 2 refs. BE60882.
    geographic factors; health facilities; kidneys; *livers; *organ transplantation; prognosis; *resource allocation; scarcity; selection for treatment; time factors; transplant recipients; treatment outcome; waiting lists; United Network for Organ Sharing; *United States

Koch, Tom. The Limits of Principle: Deciding Who Lives and What Dies. Westport, CT: Praeger; 1998. 176 p. Bibliography: p. 159-168. ISBN 0-275-96407-8. BE60113.
    allowing to die; amyotrophic lateral sclerosis; *anencephaly; animal rights; *bioethical issues; bioethics; biomedical technologies; consensus; cultural pluralism; *decision making; disabled; Down syndrome; ethical analysis; eugenics; guidelines; historical aspects; intelligence; international aspects; legal aspects; methods; moral policy; newborns; organ donation; *organ transplantation; patient compliance; personhood; prognosis; prolongation of life; *quality of life; renal dialysis; *resource allocation; rights; scarcity; *selection for treatment; selective abortion; social worth; speciesism; transplant recipients; treatment outcome; *value of life; values

Kuczewski, Mark G.; Seiden, Dena J.; Frader, Joel, et al. Retransplantation and the "noncompliant" patient. [Case study and commentaries]. *Cambridge Quarterly of Healthcare Ethics.* 1999 Summer; 8(3): 375-381. BE62479.
    adolescents; alternatives; case studies; communication; competence; counseling; depressive disorder; drugs; ethicists; justice; kidneys; *organ transplantation; *patient compliance; patient participation; professional patient relationship; refusal to treat; renal dialysis; resource allocation; *retreatment; *selection for treatment; socioeconomic factors; transplant recipients

Lafferty, Kevin J.; Furer, Julie J. Legal and medical

BE = bioethics accession number   fn. = footnotes   refs. = references

implications of fetal tissue transplantation. *Suffolk University Law Review.* 1993 Winter; 27(4): 1237-1248. 59 fn. BE61594.
    aborted fetuses; diabetes; federal government; *fetal research; *fetal tissue donation; *government financing; *government regulation; *legal aspects; methods; private sector; *public policy; state government; *tissue transplantation; pancreases; United States

Lagnado, Lucette. Transplant patients ply an illicit market for vital medicines. [News]. *Wall Street Journal.* 1999 Jun 21: 1, A8. BE62450.
    *drugs; *economics; health insurance reimbursement; health personnel; hospitals; institutional policies; legal aspects; *misconduct; motivation; *organ transplantation; *patient care; patients; *transplant recipients; Medicaid; Medicare; United States

Lin, Hung-Mo; Kauffman, H. Myron; McBride, Maureen A., et al. Center-specific graft and patient survival rates: 1997 United Network for Organ Sharing (UNOS) report. *JAMA.* 1998 Oct 7; 280(13): 1153-1160. 28 refs. BE60286.
    age factors; Asian Americans; blacks; cadavers; evaluation studies; females; hearts; *hospitals; kidneys; livers; males; *mortality; organ donation; organ donors; *organ transplantation; retreatment; statistics; survey; *time factors; *transplant recipients; *treatment outcome; whites; lungs; pancreases; United Network for Organ Sharing; United States
    CONTEXT: Multiple comprehensive, risk-adjusted studies evaluating short-term surgical mortality have been reported previously. This report analyzes short-term and long-term outcomes, both nationally and at each individual transplant program, for all solid organ transplantations performed in the United States. OBJECTIVES: To report graft and patient survival rates for all solid organ transplantations, both nationally and at each specific transplant program in the United States, and to compare the expected survival rate with the actual survival rate of each individual program. DESIGN AND SETTING: Multivariate regression analysis of donor and recipient factors affecting graft and patient survival of all kidney, liver, pancreas, heart, lung, and heart-lung transplants reported to the United Network for Organ Sharing from 742 separate transplant programs. PATIENTS: A cohort of 97587 solid organ transplantations performed on 92966 recipients in the United States from January 1988 through April 1994. MAIN OUTCOME MEASURES: Short-term and conditional 3-year national and individual transplant program graft and patient survival rates overall and from 2 separate eras (era 1, January 1988–April 1992; era 2, May 1992–April 1994); comparison of actual center-specific performance with risk-adjusted expected performance and identification of centers with better-than-expected or worse-than-expected survival rates. RESULTS: One-year graft follow-up exceeded 98% and conditional 3-year follow-up exceeded 91% for all organs. Graft and patient survival improved significantly in era 2 compared with era 1 for all cadaver organs except heart, which remained the same. One-year cadaveric graft survival ranged from 81.5% for heart to 61.9% for heart-lung and 3-year conditional graft survival ranged from 91.3% for pancreas to 74.7% for lung. The percentage of programs whose actual 1-year graft survival was not different from or was better than their risk-adjusted expected survival ranged from 98.3% for heart-lung to 75.7% for liver. Most kidney, liver, and heart programs whose actual survival was significantly less than expected performed small numbers (less than the national average) of transplantations per

year. CONCLUSIONS: Graft and patient survival for solid organ transplantations showed improvement over time. Conditional 3-year graft and patient survival rates were approximately 90% for all organs except for lung and heart-lung. The conditional 3-year survival rates were better than 1-year survival rates, indicating the major risk after transplantation occurs in the first year. The majority of transplant programs achieved actual survival rates not significantly different from their expected survival rates. Center effects were most significant within the first year after transplantation and had much less influence on long-term survival outcomes.

McChesney, Lawrence P.; Braithwaite, Susan S. Expectations and outcomes in organ transplantation. *Cambridge Quarterly of Healthcare Ethics.* 1999 Summer; 8(3): 299-310. 18 fn. BE62473.
    allowing to die; committee membership; decision making; economics; hospitals; incentives; information dissemination; informed consent; morbidity; mortality; *organ transplantation; organization and administration; physician patient relationship; *physicians; prognosis; regulation; *resource allocation; risk; *selection for treatment; technical expertise; transplant recipients; *treatment outcome; treatment refusal; United States

Machado, Nora. Using the Bodies of the Dead: Legal, Ethical and Organisational Dimensions of Organ Transplantation. Brookfield, VT: Ashgate/Dartmouth; 1998. 262 p. Bibliography: p. 241-258. ISBN 1-85521-973-5. BE62581.
    altruism; attitudes; autonomy; body parts and fluids; brain death; *cadavers; determination of death; government regulation; hospitals; human body; informed consent; international aspects; legal aspects; *organ donation; organ donors; *organ transplantation; organization and administration; presumed consent; property rights; resource allocation; selection for treatment; *sociology of medicine; statistics; third party consent; transplant recipients; rituals; Europe; *Sweden

Markovitz, Barry; May, Larry. Three patients, two hearts. [Case study and commentaries]. *Hastings Center Report.* 1998 Sep-Oct; 28(5): 20-21. BE59549.
    adolescents; adoption; advertising; *cadavers; case studies; critically ill; decision making; *directed donation; geographic factors; hearts; justice; *organ donation; *organ transplantation; parents; *resource allocation; scarcity; *selection for treatment; *transplant recipients

Meester, Johan De. Eurotransplant allocation procedures: the basics, March 1996. *In:* Lachmann, Rolf; Meuter, Norbert, eds. Zur Gerechtigkeit der Organverteilung: Ein Problem der Transplantationsmedizin aus interdisziplinärer Sicht. Stuttgart, Germany: G. Fischer; 1997: 167-177. 2 refs. ISBN 3-437-21136-6. BE60742.
    age factors; body parts and fluids; international aspects; kidneys; livers; *organ transplantation; program descriptions; *resource allocation; selection for treatment; time factors; transplant recipients; Europe; *Eurotransplant

Mepham, T.B.; Crilly, R.E. Transgenic xenotransplantation: utilitarian and deontological caveats. *In:* van Zutphen, L.F.M.; Balls, M., eds. Animal Alternatives, Welfare and Ethics. New York, NY: Elsevier; 1997: 355-360. 9 refs. ISBN 0-444-82424-3. BE61688.
    alternatives; *animal organs; animal rights; artificial organs; cadavers; *deontological ethics; ethical analysis; justice; organ donation; *organ transplantation; resource allocation; risk; speciesism; transgenic animals; *utilitarianism; wedge argument; swine; Great Britain

---

Milford, Edgar L. Organ transplantation -- barriers, outcomes, and evolving policies. [Editorial]. *JAMA.* 1998 Oct 7; 280(13): 1184-1185. 11 refs. BE60288.
age factors; body parts and fluids; cadavers; critically ill; data banks; federal government; geographic factors; government financing; government regulation; kidneys; mortality; organ donation; *organ transplantation; prognosis; public policy; *resource allocation; *selection for treatment; *socioeconomic factors; time factors; transplant recipients; *treatment outcome; Department of Health and Human Services; End Stage Renal Disease Program; United Network for Organ Sharing; United States

Mitchell, Peter. Human xenotransplantation trials may be licensed in the UK. [News]. *Lancet.* 1998 Aug 8; 352(9126): 464. BE60268.
*animal organs; *government regulation; *human experimentation; *organ transplantation; transplant recipients; *Department of Health (Great Britain); *Great Britain; *Xenotransplantation Interim Regulatory Authority (Great Britain)

Morgan, Frank. Babe the magnificent organ donor? The perils and promises surrounding xenotransplantation. [Comment]. *Journal of Contemporary Health Law and Policy.* 1997 Fall; 14(1): 127-160. 260 fn. BE60879.
*animal organs; animal rights; body parts and fluids; bone marrow; communicable diseases; comparative studies; federal government; *government regulation; *guidelines; *human experimentation; informed consent; legal aspects; *organ transplantation; presumed consent; primates; public health; *public policy; research ethics committees; *risks and benefits; scarcity; tissue transplantation; transgenic animals; transplant recipients; swine; Department of Health and Human Services; *Great Britain; Institute of Medicine; National Organ Transplant Act 1984; Nuffield Council on Bioethics; Public Health Service; *United States

Morgan, G.L. Is there a right to fetal tissue transplantation? *University of Tasmania Law Review.* 1991; 10(2): 129-156. 152 fn. BE62177.
aborted fetuses; autonomy; disclosure; *fetal tissue donation; government financing; government regulation; health care; *human experimentation; informed consent; investigator subject relationship; investigators; legal aspects; *legal obligations; legal rights; moral obligations; morbidity; mortality; *obligations of society; paternalism; patients; pregnant women; research subjects; *rights; risks and benefits; therapeutic research; *tissue transplantation; Parkinson disease; *Australia

Morray, Barbara H. The lottery of life: should organ transplants be used to even the odds? *Dimensions of Critical Care Nursing.* 1995 Sep-Oct; 14(5): 266-272. 19 refs. BE60533.
beneficence; case studies; *child abuse; clinical ethics committees; decision making; *infants; justice; legal guardians; *livers; mothers; nurses; *organ transplantation; parent child relationship; patient compliance; physicians; prognosis; quality of life; resource allocation; risks and benefits; *selection for treatment; *socioeconomic factors; utilitarianism

Mudur, Ganapati. Indian surgeon challenges ban on xenotransplantation. [News]. *BMJ (British Medical Journal).* 1999 Jan 9; 318(7176): 79. BE60843.
*animal organs; criminal law; government regulation; hearts; *legal liability; misconduct; *organ transplantation; *physicians; swine; *Baruah, Dhani Ram; *India

Nakazato, Paul Z. Controversial aspects of the current liver donor allocation system for liver transplantation. *Academic Radiology.* 1995 Mar; 2(3): 244-248. 12 refs. BE62001.
geographic factors; hospitals; *livers; mortality; *organ transplantation; prognosis; *public policy; *resource allocation; retreatment; scarcity; selection for treatment; transplant recipients; treatment outcome; severity of illness index; waiting lists; United Network for Organ Sharing; United States

Nasto, Barbara. Xenotransplantation: proceed with caution. [News]. *Nature Biotechnology.* 1996 Apr; 14(4): 424,426. BE61987.
advisory committees; *animal organs; communicable diseases; federal government; government regulation; guidelines; human experimentation; industry; international aspects; *organ transplantation; primates; public health; *public policy; risk; swine; Centers for Disease Control and Prevention; Food and Drug Administration; *Great Britain; Nuffield Council on Bioethics; *United States

Nicholson, Michael L.; Bradley, J. Andrew. Renal transplantation from living donors. [Editorial]. *BMJ (British Medical Journal).* 1999 Feb 13; 318(7181): 409-410. 10 refs. BE61027.
family members; *kidneys; married persons; methods; *organ donation; *organ donors; *organ transplantation; *risks and benefits; surgery; transplant recipients; *treatment outcome; unrelated donors; Great Britain

Noble, Holcomb B. Of life, death and the rules of liver transplants. [News]. *New York Times.* 1999 Apr 6: F6. BE61072.
economics; guidelines; health insurance reimbursement; *health maintenance organizations; *hepatitis; hospitals; *livers; *organ transplantation; prognosis; *refusal to treat; resource allocation; *selection for treatment; treatment outcome; personal financing; Florida

Payne, William D. The rational development of liver allocation policy. *Liver Transplantation and Surgery.* 1995 Jan; 1(1): 58-61. 2 refs. BE60883.
federal government; geographic factors; health facilities; *livers; *organ transplantation; organizational policies; prognosis; public policy; *resource allocation; selection for treatment; transplant recipients; treatment outcome; waiting lists; United Network for Organ Sharing; *United States

Pinkus, Rosa Lynn. Editorial comment on 'the ethicist's role.' *Clinical Transplantation.* 1993 Dec; 7(6): 565-566. 4 refs. BE60204.
clinical ethics; decision making; *ethicist's role; ethics consultation; *organ transplantation; patient care team; technical expertise; United States

Purtilo, Ruth B. What kind of a good is a donor liver anyway, and why should we care? *Liver Transplantation and Surgery.* 1995 Jan; 1(1): 75-80. 8 refs. BE60884.
body parts and fluids; *common good; democracy; directed donation; *justice; *livers; *organ transplantation; patient advocacy; physicians; *public policy; *resource allocation; scarcity; selection for treatment; transplant recipients; values; United States

Rayner, John D. Organ transplantation. *In: his* Jewish Religious Law: A Progressive Perspective. New York, NY: Berghahn Books; 1998: 124-129. ISBN 1-57181-976-2. BE62135.
aborted fetuses; animal organs; body parts and fluids; brain; determination of death; fetal tissue donation; *Jewish ethics; *organ donation; *organ transplantation; prolongation of life; resource allocation; *tissue transplantation; value of life; *Reform Judaism

Rhodes, Rosamond. Organ transplantation. *In:* Kuhse, Helga; Singer, Peter, eds. A Companion to Bioethics. Malden, MA: Blackwell; 1998: 329-340. 18 refs. ISBN 0-631-19737-0. BE59507.

BE = bioethics accession number   fn. = footnotes   refs. = references

body parts and fluids; brain death; cadavers; determination of death; family members; health facilities; international aspects; justice; moral obligations; moral policy; obligations of society; obligations to society; *organ donation; organ donors; *organ transplantation; presumed consent; public policy; remuneration; resource allocation; risks and benefits; selection for treatment; third party consent; tissue donation; tissue transplantation; transplant recipients

Richards, Bill. How a corporate feud doomed human trials of promising therapy. [News]. *Wall Street Journal.* 1999 Aug 6: A1, A6. BE62400.
   *biomedical technologies; *bone marrow; *cancer; *economics; federal government; government financing; human experimentation; *industry; legal aspects; leukemia; methods; *patents; terminally ill; *therapeutic research; *tissue transplantation; *Baxter International Inc.; *Cell Pro Inc.; National Institutes of Health; United States

Robinson, John H.; Berry, Roberta M.; McDonnell, Kevin, eds. Issues in adult health care. *In: their* A Health Law Reader: An Interdisciplinary Approach. Durham, NC: Carolina Academic Press; 1999: 239–337. 17 fn. ISBN 0-89089-907-X. BE62294.
   adults; altruism; autonomy; cadavers; commodification; competence; computers; *confidentiality; conflict of interest; data banks; decision making; *disclosure; duty to warn; genetic information; health care delivery; human experimentation; *informed consent; justice; *legal aspects; legal liability; medical records; mentally ill; negligence; *organ donation; organ donors; *organ transplantation; patient care; physician patient relationship; physicians; *privacy; psychotherapy; public health; public policy; quality of health care; remuneration; resource allocation; risks and benefits; social dominance; torts; Tarasoff v. Regents of the University of California; Uniform Anatomical Gift Act; United States

Roscam Abbing, Henriette D.C. New developments in international health law. *European Journal of Health Law.* 1998 Jun; 5(2): 155–169. Includes text of the Universal Declaration on the Human Genome and Human Rights, p. 163–167. BE60901.
   animal organs; *cloning; communicable diseases; genetic intervention; *genetic research; *genome mapping; *guidelines; *human rights; *international aspects; *regulation; risks and benefits; *tissue transplantation; Council of Europe; *Europe; European Union; Unesco; *Universal Declaration on the Human Genome and Human Rights; World Health Organization

Russell, Paul S. Understanding resource use in liver transplantation. [Editorial]. *JAMA.* 1999 Apr 21; 281(15): 1431–1432. 9 refs. BE61903.
   *economics; evaluation; hospitals; *livers; mortality; *organ transplantation; *public policy; *resource allocation; *scarcity; *selection for treatment; transplant recipients; treatment outcome; length of stay; severity of illness index; United States

Sachs, David H.; Colvin, Robert B.; Cosimi, A. Benedict, et al. Xenotransplantation -- caution, but no moratorium. [Letter and response]. *Nature Medicine.* 1998 Apr; 4(4): 372–373. 2 refs. BE59694.
   advisory committees; *animal organs; *decision making; government regulation; human experimentation; *organ transplantation; *public participation; public policy; risk; Food and Drug Administration; United States

Sass, Hans–Martin. Ethics of the allocation of highly advanced medical technologies. *Artificial Organs.* 1998 Mar; 22(3): 263–268. 14 refs. BE60080.
   advisory committees; animal organs; artificial organs; *biomedical technologies; coercion; cultural pluralism; developing countries; economics; genetic predisposition; genetic screening; health education; health promotion; *incentives; international aspects; *justice; *organ donation; organ donors; *organ transplantation; preventive medicine; regulation; remuneration; *resource allocation; *socioeconomic factors

Schaffner, Kenneth F. Ethical considerations in human investigation involving paradigm shifts: organ transplantation in the 1990s. *IRB: A Review of Human Subjects Research.* 1997 Nov–Dec; 19(6): 5–10. 45 refs. BE59991.
   animal organs; bone marrow; cancer; drugs; ethical review; gene therapy; *human experimentation; kidneys; livers; *organ transplantation; *research design; research ethics committees; transplant recipients; University of Pittsburgh

Schlaudraff, Udo. Xenotransplantation: benefits and risks to society. *Bulletin of Medical Ethics.* 1999 Mar; No. 146: 13–15. 1 ref. Paper delivered at a symposium sponsored by the Deutsche Forschungsgemeinschaft (German Research Society) at Loccum, Germany, Feb 1999. BE61819.
   accountability; altruism; *animal organs; justice; *organ transplantation; Protestant ethics; resource allocation; *risks and benefits; scarcity

Schmidt, Volker H. The politics of justice and the paradox of justification. *Social Justice Research.* 1998 Mar; 11(1): 3–19. 46 refs. BE59359.
   blacks; cultural pluralism; dissent; ethical analysis; ethical theory; *institutional policies; *justice; kidney diseases; kidneys; minority groups; organ donation; *organ transplantation; *public policy; *resource allocation; *selection for treatment; transplant recipients; treatment outcome; uncertainty; histocompatibility; rationality

Sever, M.S.; Ecder, T.; Aydin, A.E., et al. Living unrelated (paid) kidney transplantation in Third–World countries: high risk of complications besides the ethical problem. *Nephrology, Dialysis, Transplantation.* 1994; 9(4): 350–354. 35 refs. BE61587.
   case studies; *developing countries; *kidneys; legal aspects; *morbidity; *organ donation; *organ donors; *organ transplantation; patient care; *remuneration; risk; risks and benefits; *transplant recipients; treatment outcome; *unrelated donors; *India; Turkey

Sharma, Dinesh C. Indian xenotransplantation surgeon seeks damages from government. [News]. *Lancet.* 1999 Jan 2; 353(9146): 48. BE61563.
   *animal organs; compensation; *criminal law; death; government regulation; hearts; kidneys; legal aspects; *legal liability; misconduct; *organ transplantation; *physicians; transplant recipients; lungs; swine; *Baruah, Dhani Ram; *India; Organ Transplant Act 1994 (India)

Showstack, Jonathan; Katz, Patricia P.; Lake, John R., et al.; National Institute of Diabetes and Digestive and Kidney Diseases. Liver Transplantation Database Group. Resource utilization in liver transplantation: effects of patient characteristics and clinical practice. *JAMA.* 1999 Apr 21; 281(15): 1381–1386. 29 refs. BE61901.
   adults; age factors; alcohol abuse; comparative studies; critically ill; *economics; *evaluation; *hospitals; intensive care units; *livers; *organ transplantation; *resource allocation; selection for treatment; *transplant recipients; length of stay; severity of illness index; *utilization review; California; *Mayo Clinic; Minnesota; Nebraska; *University of California, San Francisco; *University of Nebraska, Omaha
   CONTEXT: Liver transplantation is among the most costly of medical services, yet few studies have addressed the relationship between the resources utilized for this

---

BE = bioethics accession number   fn. = footnotes   refs. = references

procedure and specific patient characteristics and clinical practices. OBJECTIVE: To assess the association of pretransplant patient characteristics and clinical practices with hospital resource utilization. DESIGN: Prospective cohort of patients who received liver transplants between January 1991 and July 1994. SETTING: University of California, San Francisco; Mayo Clinic, Rochester, Minn; and the University of Nebraska, Omaha. PATIENTS: Seven hundred eleven patients who received single-organ liver transplants, were at least 16 years old, and had nonfulminant liver disease. MAIN OUTCOME MEASURE: Standardized resource utilization derived from a database created by matching all services to a single price list. RESULTS: Higher adjusted resource utilization was associated with donor age of 60 years or older (28% [$53813] greater mean resource utilization; P=.005); recipient age of 60 years or older (17% [$32795]; P=.01); alcoholic liver disease (26% [$49596]; P=.002); Child-Pugh class C (41% [$67 658]; P less than .001); care from the intensive care unit at time of transplant (42% [$77833]; P less than .001); death in the hospital (35% [$67 076]; P less than .001); and having multiple liver transplants during the index hospitalization (154% increase [$474 740 vs $186 726 for 1 transplant]; P less than .001). Adjusted length of stay and resource utilization also differed significantly among transplant centers. CONCLUSIONS: Clinical, economic, and ethical dilemmas in liver transplantation are highlighted by these findings. Recipients who were older, had alcoholic liver disease, or were severely ill were the most expensive to treat; this suggests that organ allocation criteria may affect transplant costs. Clinical practices and resource utilization varied considerably among transplant centers; methods to reduce variation in practice patterns, such as clinical guidelines, might lower costs while maintaining quality of care.

Stoddard, Joan C.; Billings, Paul R.; Astrue, Michael J., et al. Health care providers, insurers, and individual patients; the right to treatment; economic and policy issues. [Proceedings of the International Symposium on Law and Science at the Crossroads: Biomedical Technology, Ethics, Public Policy, and the Law; panel discussion]. *Suffolk University Law Review.* 1993 Winter; 27(4): 1499-1523. Moderators: Linda C. Fentiman and Raja B. Khauli. BE60703.
AIDS; biomedical technologies; bone marrow; conflict of interest; decision making; DNA data banks; gene therapy; genetic disorders; genetic predisposition; genetic research; genetic screening; *health insurance reimbursement; informed consent; insurance; investigators; legal aspects; organ donation; *organ transplantation; parental consent; patient compliance; prognosis; resource allocation; selection for treatment; social discrimination; social worth; technology assessment; therapeutic research; *tissue transplantation; transplant recipients; treatment outcome; *investigational therapies; United States

Stolberg, Sheryl Gay. Animals as organ donors? Not until they're germ-free. *New York Times.* 1998 Feb 3: F1, F6. BE60463.
animal experimentation; *animal organs; attitudes; communicable diseases; dissent; *government regulation; guidelines; human experimentation; industry; investigators; *organ donation; *organ transplantation; physicians; public health; public opinion; *risk; risks and benefits; therapeutic research; *transgenic animals; *transplant recipients; swine; Food and Drug Administration; Public Health Service; United States

Stolberg, Sheryl Gay. Decisive moment on Parkinson's fetal-cell transplants. [News]. *New York Times.* 1999 Apr

20: F2. BE61073.
aborted fetuses; *brain; central nervous system diseases; control groups; fetal research; fetal tissue donation; government financing; *human experimentation; physicians; *placebos; random selection; *research design; risks and benefits; *surgery; *tissue transplantation; *Parkinson disease; *sham surgery; Freed, Curt; National Institute of Neurological Disorders and Stroke; United States; University of Colorado

Stolberg, Sheryl Gay. Fight over organs shifts to states from Washington. [News]. *New York Times.* 1999 Mar 11: A1, A26. BE60870.
*body parts and fluids; economics; *federal government; geographic factors; *government regulation; health facilities; organ donation; *organ transplantation; political activity; *resource allocation; scarcity; *state government; time factors; waiting lists; Department of Health and Human Services; *United States

Stolberg, Sheryl Gay. Health secretary urges donor priority for sickest patients. [News]. *New York Times.* 1998 Feb 27: A16. BE60466.
critically ill; federal government; geographic factors; government regulation; livers; *organ transplantation; prognosis; *public policy; *resource allocation; *selection for treatment; *transplant recipients; *Department of Health and Human Services; United Network for Organ Sharing; *United States

Stolberg, Sheryl Gay. Organ transplant panel urges a broad sharing of livers. [News]. *New York Times.* 1999 Jul 21: A14. BE62447.
advisory committees; federal government; *geographic factors; *government regulation; *livers; *organ transplantation; *public policy; *resource allocation; scarcity; selection for treatment; waiting lists; Department of Health and Human Services; *Institute of Medicine; United Network for Organ Sharing; *United States

Tackaberry, Eilleen; Ganz, Peter R.
Xenotransplantation: assessing the unknowns. [Editorial]. *Canadian Medical Association Journal.* 1998 Jul 14; 159(1): 41-43. 13 refs. BE62205.
*animal organs; biomedical research; communicable diseases; government regulation; human experimentation; international aspects; *organ transplantation; public health; risk; risks and benefits; *tissue transplantation; transplant recipients; swine; Canada; United States

Thomasma, David C.; Micetich, Kenneth C.; Brems, John, et al. The ethics of competition in liver transplantation. *Cambridge Quarterly of Healthcare Ethics.* 1999 Summer; 8(3): 321-329. 28 fn. BE62475.
beneficence; economics; federal government; *geographic factors; *government regulation; guidelines; hospitals; institutional policies; *justice; *livers; *misconduct; organ donation; organ donors; *organ transplantation; physicians; prisoners; public policy; *resource allocation; scarcity; *selection for treatment; standards; technical expertise; time factors; *transplant recipients; needs; *waiting lists; Department of Health and Human Services; United Network for Organ Sharing; *United States

Ubel, Peter A.; Caplan, Arthur L. Geographic favoritism in liver transplantation -- unfortunate or unfair? *New England Journal of Medicine.* 1998 Oct 29; 339(18): 1322-1325. 34 refs. BE60300.
cadavers; critically ill; federal government; *geographic factors; *government regulation; hospitals; *justice; *livers; mortality; *organ transplantation; physicians; *prognosis; *public policy; *resource allocation; retreatment; *selection for treatment; self regulation; *standards; state government; time factors; *transplant recipients; treatment outcome; *seriously ill; United Network for Organ Sharing; *United

States

Ubel, Peter A.; Baron, Jonathan; Asch, David A. Social responsibility, personal responsibility, and prognosis in public judgments about transplant allocation. *Bioethics.* 1999 Jan; 13(1): 57–68. 11 fn. BE60888.
*drug abuse; *hearts; *nutrition; *organ transplantation; prognosis; *public opinion; *resource allocation; *selection for treatment; *self induced illness; *smoking; survey; transplant recipients; Pennsylvania

Varekamp, Inge; Meiland, Franka J.M.; Hoos, Aloysia M., et al. The meaning of urgency in the allocation of scarce health care resources; a comparison between renal transplantation and psychogeriatric nursing home care. *Health Policy.* 1998 May; 44(2): 135–148. 20 refs. 1 fn. BE59149.
*aged; critically ill; dementia; evaluation studies; family members; home care; *kidneys; nurses; *nursing homes; *organ transplantation; *patient admission; patient advocacy; patient compliance; physicians; *prognosis; psychological stress; *resource allocation; scarcity; *selection for treatment; *time factors; qualitative research; *Netherlands

Veatch, Robert M. Egalitarian and maximin theories of justice: directed donation of organs for transplant. *Journal of Medicine and Philosophy.* 1998 Oct; 23(5): 456–476. 13 refs. 12 fn. Note: the journal issue cover shows a date of August 1998, which is incorrect. BE62113.
beneficence; *directed donation; ethical analysis; *ethical theory; freedom; health; health care delivery; *justice; *moral policy; *organ donation; *organ transplantation; public policy; *resource allocation; rights; *selection for treatment; self concept; social discrimination; socioeconomic factors; transplant recipients; utilitarianism; whites; *egalitarianism; *Rawls, John; United Network for Organ Sharing; United States

It is common to interpret Rawls's maximin theory of justice as egalitarian. Compared to utilitarian theories, this may be true. However, in special cases practices that distribute resources so as to benefit the worst off actually increase the inequality between the worst off and some who are better off. In these cases the Rawlsian maximin parts company with what is here called true egalitarianism. A policy question requiring a distinction between maximin and "true egalitarian" allocations has arisen in the arena of organ transplantation. This case is examined here as a venue for differentiating maximin and true egalitarian theories. Directed donation is the name given to donations of organs restricted to a particular social group. For example, the family of a member of the Ku Klux Klan donated his organs on the provision that they go only to members of the Caucasian race. While such donations appear to be discriminatory, if certain plausible assumptions are made, they satisfy the maximin criterion. They selectively advantage the recipient of the organs without harming anyone (assuming the organs would otherwise go unused). Moreover, everyone who is lower on the waiting list (who, thereby, could be considered worse off) is advantaged by moving up on the waiting list. This paper examines how maximin and more truly egalitarian theories handle this case arguing that, to the extent that directed donation in unethical, the best account of that conclusion is that an egalitarian principle of justice is to be preferred to the maximin.

Watts, Jonathan. Japan does its first official heart and liver transplantations. [News]. *Lancet.* 1999 Mar 6; 353(9155): 821. BE61039.
*brain death; cadavers; *determination of death; donor

cards; hearts; kidneys; legal aspects; livers; mass media; organ donation; *organ transplantation; public opinion; corneas; *Japan; Organ and Transplant Law 1997 (Japan)

Weiss, Robin A. Xenografts and retroviruses. *Science.* 1999 Aug 20; 285(5431): 1221–1222. 17 refs. BE62525.
*animal organs; *organ transplantation; risk; *risks and benefits

Weiss, Robin A. Xenotransplantation. *BMJ (British Medical Journal).* 1998 Oct 3; 317(7163): 931–934. 22 refs. BE60828.
*animal organs; communicable diseases; hearts; kidneys; *organ transplantation; public health; *risks and benefits; transgenic animals; swine; Great Britain

WuDunn, Sheryl. Death taboo weakening, Japan sees 1st transplant. [News]. *New York Times.* 1999 Mar 1: A8. BE60973.
advance directives; *brain death; cardiac death; *determination of death; hearts; *legal aspects; *organ donation; *organ transplantation; *Japan

An uncalculated risk. [Editorial]. *New Scientist.* 1997 Oct 18; 156(2104): 3. BE60459.
*animal organs; communicable diseases; human experimentation; *organ transplantation; regulation; risks and benefits; swine

Does biomedical research need another moratorium? [Editorial]. *Nature Medicine.* 1998 Feb; 4(2): 131. BE60440.
*animal organs; communicable diseases; federal government; government regulation; human experimentation; *organ transplantation; *risk; risks and benefits; swine; Food and Drug Administration; United States

Improving access to organs. [Editorial]. *New York Times.* 1999 Jul 26: A14. BE62448.
federal government; *geographic factors; *government regulation; health facilities; justice; *organ transplantation; political activity; *resource allocation; time factors; Department of Health and Human Services; U.S. Congress; *United States

In your face: if the idea of a hand transplant seems hard to take, just wait.... [Editorial]. *New Scientist.* 1998 Oct 3; 160(2154): 3. BE61939.
*body parts and fluids; *cosmetic surgery; *organ transplantation; *risks and benefits; hands; *Hallam, Clint

Misguided chauvinisim on organs. [Editorial]. *New York Times.* 1999 Mar 12: A22. BE60871.
*body parts and fluids; *federal government; geographic factors; *government regulation; *organ transplantation; *resource allocation; scarcity; *state government; time factors; waiting lists; *United States

Pig in the middle: a moratorium on clinical trials of animal transplantation is justified. [Editorial]. *Nature.* 1999 Jan 28; 397(6717): 279. BE61567.
*animal organs; communicable diseases; *government regulation; *human experimentation; international aspects; *organ transplantation; public health; risk; transplant recipients; swine; *Council of Europe; Europe

Special section: organ transplantation: shaping policy and keeping public trust. [Bibliography]. *Cambridge Quarterly of Healthcare Ethics.* 1999 Summer; 8(3): 348–350. BE62478.
*organ donation; *organ transplantation

Xenotransplant caution continues. [Editorial]. *Nature.* 1999 Apr 15; 398(6728): 543. BE62155.

BE = bioethics accession number   fn. = footnotes   refs. = references

*animal organs; communicable diseases; federal government; *government regulation; human experimentation; *organ transplantation; *primates; public health; risk; transplant recipients; swine; *Food and Drug Administration; *United States

Xenotransplantation and the "yuk" factor. [Editorial]. *Nature Biotechnology.* 1996 Apr; 14(4): 403–404. BE61964.
    *animal organs; attitudes; *communicable diseases; human experimentation; mass media; *organ transplantation; primates; *risk; uncertainty; swine; Great Britain; *Nuffield Council on Bioethics

Xenotransplantation: International Policy Issues.Paris, France: Organisation for Economic Co–operation and Development; 1999. 114 p. (OECD proceedings). Bibliography: p. 107–114. A summary of the discussions of the joint OECD–New York Academy of Sciences Workshop on "International Issues in Transplantation Biotechnology, Including the Use of Non–human Cells, Tissues and Organs," held in New York, NY, 18–20 March 1998. ISBN 92–64–17030–8. BE62583.
    animal experimentation; *animal organs; body parts and fluids; communicable diseases; developing countries; economics; guidelines; human experimentation; industry; *international aspects; organ donation; *organ transplantation; primates; public health; public policy; regulation; risk; scarcity; statistics; transgenic animals; treatment outcome; swine; Europe; North America

ORGAN PROCUREMENT *See* ORGAN AND TISSUE DONATION

OVUM DONORS *See* REPRODUCTIVE TECHNOLOGIES, SURROGATE MOTHERS

PALLIATIVE CARE *See* TERMINAL CARE

PARENTAL CONSENT *See* ABORTION/MINORS, ALLOWING TO DIE/INFANTS, HUMAN EXPERIMENTATION/MINORS, INFORMED CONSENT/MINORS, TREATMENT REFUSAL/MINORS

PASSIVE EUTHANASIA *See* ALLOWING TO DIE

PATENTING LIFE FORMS

See also GENETIC RESEARCH, RECOMBINANT DNA RESEARCH

Baird, Patricia. Patenting and human genes. *Perspectives in Biology and Medicine.* 1998 Spring; 41(3): 391–408. 35 refs. BE60350.
    developing countries; DNA sequences; economics; *genes; genetic materials; genetic research; industry; information dissemination; *international aspects; legal aspects; minority groups; *patents; Europe; European Patent Office; Human Genome Organization; National Institutes of Health; Patent and Trademark Office; United States

Ciliberti, Rosella. Biotechnological patents and ethical aspects. *Cancer Detection and Prevention.* 1993; 17(2): 313–315. BE62483.
    legal aspects; *patents; public policy; recombinant DNA research; *transgenic organisms; *biotechnology; Italy; National Institute for Cancer Research of Genoa

Elizalde, Jose. The patentability of human genes: an

ethical debate in the European Community. *Journal of Medicine and Philosophy.* 1998 Jun; 23(3): 318–323. 21 refs. BE59295.
    bioethics; ecology; freedom; *genes; genetic intervention; genetic research; government regulation; guidelines; human rights; industry; informed consent; international aspects; justice; legal aspects; *patents; public policy; transgenic organisms; *Europe; *European Community; European Parliament
The European Parliament rejected in 1995 the European Commission proposal to harmonize legal protection of biotechnological inventions. Although it did not seem initially the most contentious of the many issues involved in the current legal and ethical debate around biomedicine and genetics, patenting is now focusing bioethics in Europe.

European Commission. Group of Advisers on the Ethical Implications of Biotechnology. Ethical aspects of patenting inventions involving elements of human origin. *European Journal of Genetics in Society.* 1997; 3(1): 1–3. BE61450.
    advisory committees; *body parts and fluids; DNA sequences; donors; genes; *genetic materials; human body; informed consent; *international aspects; *patents; public policy; *European Commission; *Group of Advisers on the Ethical Implications of Biotechnology (European Commission)

Genetics Forum (London). The Case Against Patents in Genetic Engineering: A Special Report from the Genetics Forum. London: Genetics Forum; 1996 Apr. 28 p. 21 fn. ISBN 0–9528201–0–2. BE60709.
    alternatives; developing countries; genes; genetic diversity; *genetic intervention; genetic research; human rights; industry; *international aspects; *legal aspects; *patents; regulation; *transgenic organisms; agriculture; nature; *Europe; European Commission; European Parliament; European Patent Convention; European Patent Office; European Union; Great Britain; Patent and Trademark Office; United States

Holtug, Nils. Creating and patenting new life forms. *In:* Kuhse, Helga; Singer, Peter, eds. A Companion to Bioethics. Malden, MA: Blackwell; 1998: 206–214. 21 refs. ISBN 0–631–19737–0. BE59496.
    animal rights; ethical analysis; gene therapy; genetic enhancement; *genetic intervention; microbiology; *moral policy; *patents; recombinant DNA research; risks and benefits; suffering; *transgenic animals; *transgenic organisms; values; transgenic plants

Maher, Effat A. Ethical and intellectual property in the biological sciences. *Cellular and Molecular Biology.* 1997 May; 43(3): 263–267. 17 refs. BE60235.
    biomedical technologies; body parts and fluids; developing countries; disclosure; DNA sequences; ecology; genes; genetic materials; information dissemination; *legal aspects; moral policy; *patents; property rights; risks and benefits; *transgenic organisms; *Canada

Marshall, Eliot. Legal fight over patents on life. [News]. *Science.* 1999 Jun 25; 284(5423): 2067, 2069. BE62364.
    *hybrids; *legal aspects; *patents; Newman, Stuart; Patent and Trademark Office; Rifkin, Jeremy; United States

Mitchell, C. Ben. Patenting life: an Evangelical response. *In:* Demy, Timothy J.; Stewart, Gary P., eds. Genetic Engineering: A Christian Response: Crucial Considerations in Shaping Life. Grand Rapids, MI: Kregel Publications; 1999: 88–102. 49 fn. ISBN 0–8254–2357–0. BE61362.
    *body parts and fluids; *commodification; developing countries; DNA sequences; genetic diversity; genetic

---

BE = bioethics accession number   fn. = footnotes   refs. = references

intervention; *genetic materials; *human body; investigators; *justice; *legal aspects; microbiology; minority groups; organizational policies; *patents; *property rights; *Protestant ethics; recombinant DNA research; Supreme Court decisions; *theology; transgenic animals; *transgenic organisms; aborigines; slavery; Council for Responsible Genetics; Diamond v. Chakrabarty; *Evangelical Christians; Hagahai; Human Genome Organization (HUGO); Moore v. Regents of the University of California; Papua New Guinea; Patent and Trademark Office; United States

Nicholson, Richard H. Power corrupts...? *Hastings Center Report.* 1998 Sep–Oct; 28(5): 6. BE59546.
food; *industry; *international aspects; legal aspects; *patents; *transgenic organisms; agriculture; *transgenic plants; *Europe; Great Britain; Monsanto

Peters, Ted. Should we patent God's creation? *Dialog: A Journal of Theology.* 1996 Spring; 35(2): 117–132. 37 fn. BE61449.
biomedical technologies; clergy; commodification; *DNA sequences; federal government; financial support; genes; genetic intervention; *genetic research; genome mapping; government financing; industry; information dissemination; *patents; political activity; private sector; *public policy; public sector; recombinant DNA research; religious ethics; risks and benefits; stem cells; theology; *transgenic animals; cell lines; National Institutes of Health; United States; Venter, Craig

Schatz, Ulrich. Patents and morality. *In:* Sterckx, Sigrid, ed. Biotechnology, Patents and Morality. Proceedings of an International Workshop, "Biotechnology, Patents and Morality: Towards a Consensus," held in Ghent, Belgium, 17–19 Jan 1996. Brookfield, VT: Ashgate; 1997: 159–170. 2 fn. ISBN 1–84014–158–1. BE62242.
body parts and fluids; DNA sequences; gene therapy; genes; *genetic intervention; germ cells; health hazards; industry; *international aspects; *legal aspects; moral policy; morality; *patents; *regulation; suffering; transgenic animals; *biotechnology; European Patent Convention; European Patent Office

Sterckx, Sigrid, ed. Biotechnology, Patents and Morality. Brookfield, VT: Ashgate; 1997. 324 p. Includes references. Proceedings of an International Workshop, "Biotechnology, Patents and Morality: Towards a Consensus," held in Ghent, Belgium, 17–19 Jan 1996. ISBN 1–84014–158–1. BE62236.
attitudes; evaluation; genetic disorders; *genetic intervention; genetic screening; international aspects; knowledge, attitudes, practice; legal aspects; *moral policy; morality; *patents; prenatal diagnosis; public opinion; public participation; *public policy; regulation; risk; *risks and benefits; transgenic animals; *transgenic organisms; agriculture; *biotechnology; transgenic plants; *Europe; United States

Straus, Joseph. Patenting human genes in Europe –– past developments and prospects for the future. *IIC: International Review of Industrial Property and Copyright Law.* 1995 Dec; 26(6): 920–950. 125 fn. BE62710.
disclosure; DNA sequences; drug industry; *genes; genome mapping; industry; international aspects; *legal aspects; morality; *patents; regulation; *Europe; European Parliament; European Patent Convention; European Patent Office

Svatos, Michele. Patents and morality: a philosophical commentary on the conference 'Biotechnology, patents and morality.' *In:* Sterckx, Sigrid, ed. Biotechnology, Patents and Morality. Proceedings of an International Workshop, "Biotechnology, Patents and Morality: Towards a Consensus," held in Ghent, Belgium, 17–19

Jan 1996. Brookfield, VT: Ashgate; 1997: 291–306. 14 fn. ISBN 1–84014–158–1. BE62244.
costs and benefits; developing countries; economics; genes; *genetic intervention; genome mapping; germ cells; incentives; industry; information dissemination; international aspects; legal aspects; microbiology; *patents; property rights; regulation; social impact; transgenic animals; utilitarianism; agriculture; *biotechnology; transgenic plants; Europe; National Institutes of Health; United States

Van Overwalle, Geertrui. Biotechnology patents in Europe: from law to ethics. *In:* Sterckx, Sigrid, ed. Biotechnology, Patents and Morality. Proceedings of an International Workshop, "Biotechnology, Patents and Morality: Towards a Consensus," held in Ghent, Belgium, 17–19 Jan 1996. Brookfield, VT: Ashgate; 1997: 139–148. 2 fn. ISBN 1–84014–158–1. BE62241.
evaluation; *genetic intervention; industry; *international aspects; legal aspects; microbiology; morality; *patents; recombinant DNA research; *regulation; transgenic animals; *transgenic organisms; *biotechnology; transgenic plants; *Europe; European Patent Convention; European Patent Office

Weiss, Rick. What is patently offensive? [News]. *Washington Post.* 1998 May 11: A21. BE59571.
*hybrids; legal aspects; *patents; public policy; stem cells; transgenic organisms; Patent and Trademark Office; Rifkin, Jeremy; United States

PATERNALISM *See* PROFESSIONAL PATIENT RELATIONSHIP

PATIENT ACCESS TO RECORDS

See also CONFIDENTIALITY, TRUTH DISCLOSURE

Birchard, Karen. Irish doctors concerned by information access. [News]. *Lancet.* 1998 Oct 24; 352(9137): 1368. BE60823.
attitudes; children; *confidentiality; disclosure; *government regulation; HIV seropositivity; legal liability; legal rights; legislation; *medical records; parents; *patient access to records; physician patient relationship; physicians; sexual partners; Freedom of Information Act (Ireland); *Ireland

Bosch, Xavier. Spanish patients' access to records boosted. [News]. *Lancet.* 1999 Jul 17; 354(9174): 232. BE62531.
*legal aspects; legal rights; *medical records; *patient access to records; *Catalonia; Spain

de Klerk, Anton. The right of patients to have access to their medical records: the position in South African law. *Medicine and Law.* 1993; 12(1–2): 77–83. 10 refs. BE60614.
disclosure; *legal aspects; legal rights; *medical records; *patient access to records; physicians; property rights; risks and benefits; *South Africa

Grubb, Andrew. Access to medical records –– Breen v. Williams. [Comment]. *Medical Law Review.* 1995 Spring; 3(1): 102–107. BE60606.
disclosure; *legal aspects; *legal rights; *medical records; *patient access to records; physician patient relationship; physicians; property rights; Australia; *Breen v. Williams; *New South Wales

Roach, William H.; Aspen Health Law and Compliance Center. Access to medical record information. *In: their* Medical Records and the Law. Third Edition. Gaithersburg, MD: Aspen Publishers; 1998: 87–139. 291

BE = bioethics accession number   fn. = footnotes   refs. = references

fn. ISBN 0–8342–1104–1. BE62748.
  alcohol abuse; *confidentiality; disclosure; drug abuse; epidemiology; federal government; genetic information; government regulation; health facilities; health personnel; *legal aspects; legislation; *medical records; mentally ill; minors; patient access to records; peer review; *property rights; remuneration; state government; quality assurance; utilization review; *United States

U.S. Congress. House. A bill to establish federal penalties for prohibited uses and disclosures of individually identifiable health information, to establish a right in an individual to inspect and copy their own health information, and for other purposes [Consumer Health and Research technology (CHART) Protection Act]. H.R. 3900, 105th Cong., 2d Sess. Introduced by Christopher Shays.; 1998 May 19. 48 p. Referred to the Committee on Commerce, and in addition to the Committees on Ways and Means and on Government Reform and Oversight. BE62444.
  biomedical research; computers; *confidentiality; criminal law; *disclosure; epidemiology; federal government; government regulation; informed consent; law enforcement; *legal aspects; legislation; *medical records; *patient access to records; state government; *Consumer Health and Research Technology (CHART) Protection Act (1998 bill); *United States

Waller, Adele A.; Alcantara, Oscar L. Ownership of health information in the information age. *Journal of the American Health Information Management Association.* 1998 Mar; 69(3): 28–40. 36 fn. Includes a continuing education quiz, p. 39–40. BE60433.
  *computer communication networks; confidentiality; contracts; *data banks; disclosure; genetic information; health care delivery; health personnel; hospitals; *legal aspects; *medical records; *patient access to records; patients; *property rights; United States

Weiss, Meira. For doctors' eyes only: medical records in two Israeli hospitals. *Culture, Medicine and Psychiatry.* 1997 Sep; 21(3): 283–302. 46 refs. BE60626.
  anthropology; *attitudes; confidentiality; diagnosis; guideline adherence; hospitals; malpractice; *medical records; medicine; motivation; *patient access to records; physician patient relationship; *physicians; property rights; records; social dominance; *sociology of medicine; standards; survey; truth disclosure; *Israel

PATIENT CARE

See also HEALTH CARE, PROFESSIONAL PATIENT RELATIONSHIP, SELECTION FOR TREATMENT, TERMINAL CARE

American College of Obstetricians and Gynecologists. Committee on Ethics. Obstetrician–gynecologists' ethical responsibilities, concerns, and risks pertaining to adoption. ACOG Committee Opinion No. 194. *ACOG Committee Opinions.* 1997 Nov; No. 194: 4 p. 6 refs. BE61298.
  *adoption; alternatives; confidentiality; conflict of interest; counseling; disclosure; infertility; information dissemination; moral obligations; obstetrics and gynecology; *organizational policies; patient education; *physician's role; *physicians; pregnant women; professional organizations; referral and consultation; risks and benefits; unwanted children; *American College of Obstetricians and Gynecologists

Andersen, David; Cavalier, Robert; Covey, Preston K. A Right to Die? The Dax Cowart Case. [CD-ROM computer file]. New York, NY: Routledge; 1996 Jun.

1 computer laser optical disc; sd., col.; 4 – 3/4 in. + user guide and teacher's guide.. Interactive; contains scenes of medical treatment which some may find distressing. Versions available for Windows or Macintosh (single user ISBN 0–415–91753–0, multiple user pack ISBN 0–415–91754–9); contact Routledge (e-mail: info.dax@routledge.com; http://www.routledge.com/routledge.html). BE59871.
  *allowing to die; assisted suicide; *autonomy; beneficence; *burns; case studies; coercion; decision making; dissent; moral obligations; *pain; paternalism; *patient care; patient care team; physically disabled; physician patient relationship; physicians; *prolongation of life; quality of life; rehabilitation; *right to die; *suffering; suicide; teaching methods; treatment outcome; *treatment refusal; *Cowart, Dax

Antle, Beverley J.; Carlin, Kathleen. Enhancing patient participation in team decision making. *Humane Health Care International.* 1997 Spring; 13(1): 32–35. 8 refs. BE59961.
  autonomy; *decision making; evaluation; health personnel; models, theoretical; *patient care; *patient care team; *patient participation; professional patient relationship; patient care planning

Baergen, Ralph; Baergen, Carolyn. Paternalism, risk and patient choice. *Journal of the American Dental Association.* 1997 Apr; 128(4): 481–484. 10 refs. BE60216.
  *autonomy; *beneficence; case studies; competence; comprehension; cosmetic surgery; *decision making; *dentistry; disclosure; *health personnel; injuries; *paternalism; *patient care; patient participation; *patients; professional ethics; professional patient relationship; *refusal to treat; risk; values

Barrow, Chelmer L.; Easley, Kirk A. The role of gender and race on the time delay for emergency department patients complaining of chest pain to be evaluated by a physician. *Saint Louis University Public Law Review.* 1996; 15(2): 267–277. 38 fn. Commented on by J. Barrow, p. 278–302. BE59910.
  *age factors; *blacks; comparative studies; *emergency care; *females; health care delivery; *heart diseases; *hospitals; institutional policies; *males; *quality of health care; *selection for treatment; social discrimination; *time factors; *whites; myocardial infarction; retrospective studies

Barrow, Jackie. Implications of the Emergency Medical Treatment and Active Labor Act (EMTALA) on differences based on race and gender in the treatment of patients presenting to a hospital emergency department with chest pain. *Saint Louis University Public Law Review.* 1996; 15(2): 278–302. 165 fn. Commentary on C.L. Barrow and K.A. Easley, p. 267–277. BE59911.
  age factors; blacks; *emergency care; federal government; females; *government regulation; heart diseases; *hospitals; indigents; institutional ethics; institutional policies; *legal aspects; legislation; males; minority groups; patient transfer; *quality of health care; *selection for treatment; social discrimination; *socioeconomic factors; standards; *Emergency Medical Treatment and Active Labor Act 1986; Medicare; *United States

Berger, Jeffrey T. Culture and ethnicity in clinical care. *Archives of Internal Medicine.* 1998 Oct 26; 158(19): 2085–2090. 110 refs. BE59577.
  *advance directives; *alternative therapies; American Indians; Asian Americans; *attitudes; autopsies; blacks; cancer; *cultural pluralism; family relationship; health; Hispanic Americans; knowledge, attitudes, practice; living wills; *minority groups; nutrition; *organ donation; *patient care; physicians; preventive medicine; prolongation of life; socioeconomic factors; *truth disclosure; whites;

BE = bioethics accession number   fn. = footnotes   refs. = references

withholding treatment; United States

Bignell, C.J. Chaperones for genital examination. [Editorial]. *BMJ (British Medical Journal).* 1999 Jul 17; 319(7203): 137–138. 7 refs. BE62453.
adolescents; adults; *females; institutional policies; knowledge, attitudes, practice; *males; nurses; obstetrics and gynecology; *patient care; patients; *physician patient relationship; physicians; *privacy; sexuality; ambulatory care; *physical examination; Great Britain

Bodenheimer, Thomas. Disease management -- promises and pitfalls. *New England Journal of Medicine.* 1999 Apr 15; 340(15): 1202–1205. 28 refs. BE61031.
*chronically ill; conflict of interest; contracts; *costs and benefits; diabetes; *drug industry; drugs; *economics; entrepreneurship; health care delivery; health maintenance organizations; *managed care programs; *patient care; patient care team; patient education; physician patient relationship; *primary health care; quality of health care; risks and benefits; United States

Boettcher, Brian. Fatal episodes in medical history. [Personal view]. *BMJ (British Medical Journal).* 1998 Dec 5; 317(7172): 1603. BE60265.
alternative therapies; legal liability; medical education; mental institutions; mentally ill; *misconduct; mortality; *patient care; peer review; *physicians; *professional competence; psychiatry; regulation; social impact; standards; *whistleblowing; deep sleep therapy; Australia; Chelmsford Private Hospital (Sydney); Royal Commission into Deep Sleep (Australia)

Breen, Kerry J.; Plueckhahn, Vernon D.; Cordner, Stephen M. Ethics, Law and Medical Practice. St. Leonards, NSW, Australia: Allen and Unwin; 1997. 367 p. Includes references. Appendices include the Australian Medical Association code of ethics, NHMRC (National Health and Medical Research Council) statement on human experimentation, NHMRC general guidelines for medical practitioners on providing information to patients, and NHMRC recommendations for the donation of cadaveric organs and tissues for transplantation. ISBN 1-86448-407-1. BE59722.
abortion, induced; active euthanasia; allowing to die; autonomy; beneficence; communication; computers; confidentiality; determination of death; drugs; employment; government regulation; *health care delivery; human experimentation; informed consent; interprofessional relations; involuntary commitment; *legal aspects; legal liability; mandatory reporting; medical education; *medical ethics; medical records; mentally ill; misconduct; negligence; organization and administration; parent child relationship; *patient care; physician patient relationship; physicians; professional competence; reproductive technologies; resource allocation; self regulation; sexuality; standards; third party consent; treatment refusal; virtues; withholding treatment; physician impairment; self care; *Australia

Brenner, Zara R.; Duffy-Durnin, Karen. Toward restraint-free care. *American Journal of Nursing.* 1998 Dec; 98(12): 16F, 16H–16I. 4 refs. BE61817.
aged; *alternatives; autonomy; costs and benefits; *hospitals; institutional policies; mentally disabled; *nurses; *patient care; *physical restraint; risks and benefits; dignity

Budd, Susan; Sharma, Ursula, eds. The Healing Bond: The Patient–Practitioner Relationship and Therapeutic Responsibility. New York, NY: Routledge; 1994. 239 p. Includes references. ISBN 0-415-09052-0. BE59734.
accountability; *alternative therapies; anthropology; contraception; counseling; family planning; females; health personnel; interprofessional relations; lawyers; legal liability; males; malpractice; moral obligations; negligence; nurse

midwives; *patient care; patient participation; *physician patient relationship; professional autonomy; *professional patient relationship; psychotherapy; referral and consultation; self regulation; sociology of medicine; trust; holistic medicine; quackery; self care; General Medical Council (Great Britain); Great Britain

Cahill, Jo. Patient participation -- a review of the literature. *Journal of Clinical Nursing.* 1998 Mar; 7(2): 119–128. 81 refs. BE60690.
autonomy; decision making; empirical research; hospitals; knowledge, attitudes, practice; literature; nurse patient relationship; nurses; nursing research; paternalism; *patient care; *patient participation; patients; review; trends; Great Britain

Carrillo, J. Emilio; Green, Alexander R.; Betancourt, Joseph R. Cross-cultural primary care: a patient-based approach. *Annals of Internal Medicine.* 1999 May 18; 130(10): 829–834. 44 refs. BE61610.
communication; *cultural pluralism; curriculum; *medical education; *minority groups; patient participation; *physician patient relationship; *primary health care; socioeconomic factors; United States
In today's multicultural society, assuring quality health care for all persons requires that physicians understand how each patient's sociocultural background affects his or her health beliefs and behaviors. Cross-cultural curricula have been developed to address these issues but are not widely used in medical education. Many curricula take a categorical and potentially stereotypic approach to "cultural competence" that weds patients of certain cultures to a set of specific, unifying characteristics. In addition, curricula frequently overlook the importance of social factors on the cross-cultural encounter. This paper discusses a patient-based cross-cultural curriculum for residents and medical students that teaches a framework for analysis of the individual patient's social context and cultural health beliefs and behaviors. The curriculum consists of five thematic units taught in four 2-hour sessions. The goal is to help physicians avoid cultural generalizations while improving their ability to understand, communicate with, and care for patients from diverse backgrounds.

Casper, Monica J. Working on and around human fetuses: the contested domain of fetal surgery. *In:* Berg, Marc; Mol, Annemarie, eds. Differences in Medicine: Unraveling Practices, Techniques, and Bodies. Durham, NC: Duke University Press; 1998: 28–52. 23 fn. ISBN 0-8223-2174-2. BE62132.
conflict of interest; *congenital disorders; decision making; *dissent; fetal research; *fetal therapy; *fetuses; *goals; hospitals; human experimentation; *interdisciplinary communication; *interprofessional relations; investigators; maternal health; *medical specialties; morbidity; mortality; mother fetus relationship; newborns; nurses; *obstetrics and gynecology; patient advocacy; *patient care team; pediatrics; physician patient relationship; *physicians; *pregnant women; prenatal diagnosis; psychological stress; *risks and benefits; selection for treatment; social dominance; *social workers; *sociology of medicine; *surgery; technical expertise; therapeutic research; treatment outcome; negotiation; neonatology; perinatology

Clouser, K. Danner; Hufford, David J.; Morrison, Catherine J. What's in a word? *Alternative Therapies in Health and Medicine.* 1995 Jul; 1(3): 78–79. 7 refs. BE60679.
*alternative therapies; medicine; stigmatization; *terminology

Coulter, Angela; Entwistle, Vikki; Gilbert, David.

Sharing decisions with patients: is the information good enough? *BMJ (British Medical Journal)*. 1999 Jan 30; 318(7179): 318–322. 14 refs. BE60581.
   attitudes; audiovisual aids; *decision making; disclosure; *evaluation; *information dissemination; informed consent; *patient care; *patient education; *patient participation; *patient satisfaction; patients; risks and benefits; *standards; survey; uncertainty; self care; Great Britain; National Health Service

Covinsky, Kenneth E.; Bates, Carol K.; Davis, Roger B., et al. Physicians' attitudes toward using patient reports to assess quality of care. *Academic Medicine*. 1996 Dec; 71(12): 1353–1356. 6 refs. BE61382.
   *attitudes; communication; *evaluation; hospitals; internship and residency; medical specialties; *patient care; *patient participation; *physicians; *quality of health care; survey; teaching hospitals; *Beth Israel Hospital (Boston); Boston

Culpepper, Larry; Gilbert, Thomas T. Evidence and ethics. *Lancet*. 1999 Mar 6; 353(9155): 829–831. 10 refs. BE61220.
   biomedical technologies; chronically ill; costs and benefits; *decision making; diagnosis; *evidence-based medicine; *family practice; health care; health services research; human experimentation; iatrogenic disease; *medical specialties; medicine; patient advocacy; *patient care; patient participation; physician patient relationship; *physicians; practice guidelines; *primary health care; quality of life; random selection; research design; *resource allocation; *risks and benefits; treatment outcome; uncertainty; *values

Davidoff, Frank. Weighing the alternatives: lessons from the paradoxes of alternative medicine. [Editorial]. *Annals of Internal Medicine*. 1998 Dec 15; 129(12): 1068–1070. 20 refs. BE60276.
   *alternative therapies; autonomy; caring; deception; economics; goals; health; health promotion; *patient care; patients; physician patient relationship; prognosis; sociology of medicine; truth disclosure; empowerment; hope; personal financing; self care; United States

DeRenzo, Evan G. Ethical considerations in dysphagia treatment and research: secular and sacred. *In:* Sonies, Barbara C., ed. Dysphagia: A Continuum of Care. Gaithersburg, MD: Aspen Publishing; 1997: 91–106. 28 refs. ISBN 0-8342-0785-0. BE59559.
   adults; advance directives; aged; *artificial feeding; autonomy; beneficence; case studies; children; chronically ill; communication; competence; *cultural pluralism; *decision making; *ethical analysis; ethical theory; *food; health personnel; informed consent; *moral policy; nutrition; *patient care; patients; physicians; public policy; rehabilitation; religion; risks and benefits; social interaction; terminally ill; therapeutic research; third party consent; treatment outcome; treatment refusal; *values; withholding treatment; cerebrovascular disorders; *deglutition disorders

De Ville, Kenneth. Act first and look up the law afterward?: medical malpractice and the ethics of defensive medicine. *Theoretical Medicine and Bioethics*. 1998 Dec; 19(6): 569–589. 96 refs. BE61155.
   beneficence; *decision making; disclosure; economics; informed consent; lawyers; *legal liability; *malpractice; motivation; *patient care; patients; physician patient relationship; *physicians; risk; physician's practice patterns; United States

Dreger, Alice Domurat. Hemaphrodites and the Medical Invention of Sex. Cambridge, MA: Harvard University Press; 1998. 268 p. 682 fn. ISBN 0-674-08927-8. BE62621.
   adults; attitudes; children; cosmetic surgery; counseling; deception; dehumanization; diagnosis; *females; *historical

aspects; homosexuals; hormones; human body; infants; international aspects; *intersexuality; *males; narrative ethics; *normality; parental consent; paternalism; patient care; physician patient relationship; physicians; postmodernism; prevalence; self concept; *sexuality; *sociology of medicine; stigmatization; surgery; terminology; truth disclosure; *France; *Great Britain; *Nineteenth Century; Twentieth Century; United States

Eisinger, F.; Geller, G.; Burke, W., et al. Cultural basis for differences between US and French clinical recommendations for women at increased risk of breast and ovarian cancer. *Lancet*. 1999 Mar 13; 353(9156): 919–920. 14 refs. BE61200.
   advisory committees; *attitudes; *autonomy; *breast cancer; *cancer; communitarianism; comparative studies; consensus; *cultural pluralism; *decision making; *females; *genetic predisposition; genetic screening; government regulation; informed consent; *international aspects; mass screening; *paternalism; *patient care; *patient participation; *physicians; practice guidelines; *preventive medicine; public participation; risk; surgery; time factors; *values; *self care; *France; *United States

Epstein, Ronald M. Mindful practice. *JAMA*. 1999 Sep 1; 282(9): 833–839. 104 refs. BE62657.
   compassion; decision making; diagnosis; emotions; empathy; evidence-based medicine; *knowledge, attitudes, practice; medical education; medical errors; medical ethics; *medicine; *patient care; peer review; physician patient relationship; *physicians; *professional competence; *psychology; self concept; technical expertise; values; mentors; *physician's practice patterns
Mindful practitioners attend in a nonjudgmental way to their own physical and mental processes during ordinary, everyday tasks. This critical self-reflection enables physicians to listen attentively to patients' distress, recognize their own errors, refine their technical skills, make evidence-based decisions, and clarify their values so that they can act with compassion, technical competence, presence, and insight. Mindfulness informs all types of professionally relevant knowledge, including propositional facts, personal experiences, processes, and know-how, each of which may be tacit or explicit. Explicit knowledge is readily taught, accessible to awareness, quantifiable and easily translated into evidence-based guidelines. Tacit knowledge is usually learned during observation and practice, includes prior experiences, theories-in-action, and deeply held values, and is usually applied more inductively. Mindful practitioners use a variety of means to enhance their ability to engage in moment-to-moment self-monitoring, bring to consciousness their tacit personal knowledge and deeply held values, use peripheral vision and subsidiary awareness to become aware of new information and perspectives, and adopt curiosity in both ordinary and novel situations. In contrast, mindlessness may account for some deviations from professionalism and errors in judgment and technique. Although mindfulness cannot be taught explicitly, it can be modeled by mentors and cultivated in learners. As a link between relationship-centered care and evidence-based medicine, mindfulness should be considered a characteristic of good clinical practice.

Ernst, E. Towards a risk-benefit evaluation of placebos. *Wiener Medizinische Wochenschrift*. 1998; 148(20): 461–463. 35 refs. BE61625.
   drugs; *evaluation; evidence-based medicine; human experimentation; *patient care; *placebos; research design; *risks and benefits

Fairman, Julie; Happ, Mary Beth. For their own good?

BE = bioethics accession number   fn. = footnotes   refs. = references

A historical examination of restraint use. *HEC (HealthCare Ethics Committee) Forum.* 1998 Sep–Dec; 10(3–4): 290–299. 36 refs. BE61180.
aged; attitudes; *behavior control; biomedical technologies; government regulation; historical aspects; hospitals; *nurses; nursing education; *patient care; *physical restraint; risks and benefits; United States

Ferrell, Betty R. Pain management: a moral imperative. *American Nurses Association Center for Ethics and Human Rights Communique.* 1996–1997 Winter; 5(2): 4–5. 9 refs. BE60407.
moral obligations; *nurses; *pain; *palliative care; patient advocacy

Fisher, Elliott S.; Welch, H. Gilbert. Avoiding the unintended consequences of growth in medical care: how might more be worse? *JAMA.* 1999 Feb 3; 281(5): 446–453. 75 refs. BE60239.
*biomedical technologies; chronically ill; decision making; *diagnosis; disease; drugs; economics; *health care; health care delivery; health services research; iatrogenic disease; mass screening; *medicine; morbidity; mortality; *patient care; prevalence; resource allocation; *risks and benefits; stigmatization; surgery; *technology assessment; treatment outcome; trends; uncertainty; *health services misuse

The United States has experienced dramatic growth in both the technical capabilities and share of resources devoted to medical care. While the benefits of more medical care are widely recognized, the possibility that harm may result from growth has received little attention. Because harm from more medical care is unexpected, findings of harm are discounted or ignored. We suggest that such findings may indicate a more general problem and deserve serious consideration. First, we delineate 2 levels of decision making where more medical care may be introduced: (1) decisions about whether or not to use a discrete diagnostic or therapeutic intervention and (2) decisions about whether to add system capacity, e.g., the decision to purchase another scanner or employ another physician. Second, we explore how more medical care at either level may lead to harm. More diagnosis creates the potential for labeling and detection of pseudodisease -- disease that would never become apparent to patients during their lifetime without testing. More treatment may lead to tampering, interventions to correct random rather than systematic variation, and lower treatment thresholds, where the risks outweigh the potential benefits. Because there are more diagnoses to treat and more treatments to provide, physicians may be more likely to make mistakes and to be distracted from the issues of greatest concern to their patients. Finally, we turn to the fundamental challenge -- reducing the risk of harm from more medical care. We identify 4 ways in which inadequate information and improper reasoning may allow harmful practices to be adopted -- a constrained model of disease, excessive extrapolation, a missing level of analysis, and the assumption that more is better.

Fisher, Ian. Families providing complex medical care, tubes and all. *New York Times.* 1998 Jun 7: 1, 30. BE60473.
adults; aged; *biomedical technologies; children; *chronically ill; economics; *family members; *home care; managed care programs; psychological stress; risks and benefits; technical expertise; Family and Medical Leave Act; United States

Fleetwood, Janet. Editor's introduction [to a set of nine articles on the use of restraints in healthcare]. *HEC (HealthCare Ethics Committee) Forum.* 1998 Sep–Dec;

10(3–4): 231–234. BE61216.
aged; *behavior control; case studies; children; hospitals; intensive care units; legal aspects; mentally ill; motivation; nursing homes; pain; patient care; patient compliance; *physical restraint; psychological stress; treatment refusal; ventilators

Gates, Elena A. New surgical procedures: can our patients benefit while we learn? [Article and discussion]. *American Journal of Obstetrics and Gynecology.* 1997 Jun; 176(6): 1293–1299. 31 refs. BE59372.
*alternatives; *continuing education; *disclosure; informed consent; medical devices; medical education; medical errors; *methods; obstetrics and gynecology; peer review; physicians; *professional competence; risks and benefits; self regulation; *surgery; *laparoscopy

Gilbert, Bonny. Infertility and the ADA: health insurance coverage for infertility treatment. *Defense Council Journal.* 1996; 63(1): 42–57. 80 fn. BE59349.
*disabled; drugs; economics; federal government; *health insurance reimbursement; *infertility; *legal aspects; legal rights; legislation; *patient care; *reproductive technologies; standards; state government; surgery; *Americans with Disabilities Act 1990; *United States

Gillespie, Rosemary. Women, the body and brand extension in medicine: cosmetic surgery and the paradox of choice. *Women and Health.* 1996; 24(4): 69–85. 54 refs. BE59443.
advertising; autonomy; *commodification; *cosmetic surgery; economics; *females; *feminist ethics; human body; industry; *informal social control; males; minority groups; *self concept; social dominance; sociology of medicine; *values; *women's health; beauty; *empowerment; rationality

Gillon, Raanan. Ethical issues. *In:* Weber, Walter; Mulvihill, John J.; Narod, Steven A., eds. Familial Cancer Management. Boca Raton, FL: CRC Press; 1996: 142–158. 26 refs. BE61799.
*cancer; confidentiality; deception; directive counseling; disclosure; dissent; employment; *family members; gene therapy; genetic counseling; genetic disorders; genetic information; *genetic intervention; *genetic predisposition; *genetic screening; informed consent; insurance; justice; mandatory testing; *patient care; physician patient relationship; preventive medicine; rights; risks and benefits; selective abortion; social discrimination; stigmatization; surgery; transgenic organisms; wedge argument; incidental findings; Great Britain

Gilman, Sander L. Making the Body Beautiful: A Cultural History of Aesthetic Surgery. Princeton, NJ: Princeton University Press; 1999. 396 p. 746 fn. ISBN 0-691-02672-6. BE61680.
body parts and fluids; circumcision; *cosmetic surgery; disease; females; *historical aspects; human body; international aspects; Jews; literature; males; mass media; minority groups; psychology; statistics; stigmatization; syphilis; terminology; transsexualism; Western World; beauty; motion pictures; Enlightenment; Nineteenth Century; Renaissance; Twentieth Century

Goldberg, Susan L. Legal aspects of restraint use in hospitals and nursing homes. *HEC (HealthCare Ethics Committee) Forum.* 1998 Sep–Dec; 10(3–4): 276–289. 30 refs. BE61179.
*behavior control; drugs; federal government; *government regulation; *hospitals; informed consent; legal liability; medical devices; *nursing homes; *patient care; patients' rights; *physical restraint; self regulation; standards; state government; treatment refusal; Joint Commission on Accreditation of Healthcare Organizations; Medicaid; Medicare; Nursing Home Reform Act 1987; United States

---

BE = bioethics accession number   fn. = footnotes   refs. = references

Goldman, Marina. Physical restraints. [Bibliography]. *HEC (HealthCare Ethics Committee) Forum.* 1998 Sep–Dec; 10(3–4): 323–337. BE61184.

aged; alternatives; behavior control; family members; hospitals; mentally ill; nurses; nursing homes; *physical restraint

Goodman, Kenneth W. Critical care computing: outcomes, confidentiality, and appropriate use. *Critical Care Clinics.* 1996 Jan; 12(1): 109–122. 36 refs. BE59281.

allowing to die; *computer communication networks; *computers; *confidentiality; *critically ill; data banks; decision analysis; *decision making; disclosure; epidemiology; evaluation; *futility; health services research; HIV seropositivity; informed consent; intensive care units; medical records; *patient care; physicians; privacy; *prognosis; research subjects; resource allocation; *statistics; *treatment outcome; truth disclosure; *uncertainty; withholding treatment; severity of illness index

Haiken, Elizabeth. Venus Envy: A History of Cosmetic Surgery. Baltimore, MD: Johns Hopkins University Press; 1997. 370 p. 461 fn. ISBN 0-8018-5763-5. BE62626.

aged; attitudes; blacks; *cosmetic surgery; famous persons; females; *historical aspects; males; mass media; medical devices; medical specialties; minority groups; motivation; physicians; professional organizations; public opinion; risks and benefits; self concept; socioeconomic factors; stigmatization; artificial implants; beauty; mammaplasty; *Twentieth Century; United States

Hough, M. Catherine. Ethical dilemmas faced by critical care nurses in clinical practice: walking the line. *Critical Care Clinics.* 1996 Jan; 12(1): 123–133. 20 refs. BE59282.

allowing to die; caring; case studies; *critically ill; deception; *decision making; double effect; drugs; females; futility; intensive care units; males; moral development; narrative ethics; *nurses; *nursing ethics; pain; palliative care; *patient care; physician nurse relationship; physicians; resource allocation; *terminally ill; whistleblowing

Ilani, Zvi; Weinberger, Yaakov, comps. The obligation to heal and medical malpractice. *Jewish Medical Ethics.* 1997 Jan; 3(1): 18–29. 85 fn. Translated from the Hebrew sources by Uriah F. Cheskin and Yitzchak Pechenick. BE59246.

active euthanasia; coercion; communicable diseases; disease; double effect; drugs; indigents; *Jewish ethics; medical fees; medicine; moral obligations; pain; *patient care; *physician's role; professional competence; refusal to treat; risk; strikes; *theology; treatment refusal

Jackson, Jean E. Hippocrates in the bush. *Anthropological Quarterly.* 1996 Jul; 69(3): 120–122. 13 refs. 1 fn. BE61211.

*anthropology; *cultural pluralism; *developing countries; drugs; injuries; *international aspects; *non-Western World; *patient care; *risks and benefits; sociology of medicine; *Western World; withholding treatment; unsolicited intervention; South America

Jacobson, Nora. The socially constructed breast: breast implants and the medical construction of need. *American Journal of Public Health.* 1998 Aug; 88(8): 1254–1261. 81 fn. BE60376.

attitudes; autonomy; breast cancer; *cosmetic surgery; federal government; *females; government regulation; *historical aspects; human experimentation; mass media; *medical devices; physicians; politics; preventive medicine; psychology; public health; rehabilitation; risks and benefits; *sociology of medicine; surgery; *values; women's health; *breast implants; *needs; Food and Drug Administration; Nineteenth Century; *Twentieth Century; United States

When silicone gel breast implants became the subject of a public health controversy in the early 1990s, the most pressing concern was safety. This paper looks at another, less publicized issue: the need for implants. Using a symbolic interactionist approach, the author explores the social construction of the need for implants by tracing the history of the 3 surgical procedures for which implants were used. Stakeholders in this history constructed need as legitimized individual desire, the form of which shifted with changes in the technological and social context.

Jones, Steve; Oswald, Nigel; Date, Jan, et al. Attitudes of patients to medical student participation: general practice consultations on the Cambridge Community-Based Clinical Course. *Medical Education.* 1996 Jan; 30(1): 14–17. 7 refs. BE62316.

*attitudes; community services; *family practice; *medical education; *patient care; *patient satisfaction; *patients; primary health care; *students; survey; *East Bramwell Health Centre (Cambridge, England); Great Britain

Keyserlingk, Edward. Comparing the participation of Native North American and Euro-North American patients in health care decisions. *In:* Coward, Harold; Ratanakul, Pinit, eds. A Cross-Cultural Dialogue on Health Care Ethics. Waterloo, ON: Wilfrid Laurier University Press; 1999: 176–189. 31 refs. 2 fn. ISBN 0-88920-325-3. BE62793.

*alternative therapies; *American Indians; *attitudes; *autonomy; comparative studies; *cultural pluralism; *decision making; empirical research; informed consent; *patient care; *patient participation; physician patient relationship; professional patient relationship; *whites; faith healing; holistic health; Canada; North America

Kim, H. Nina; Gates, Elena; Lo, Bernard. What hysterectomy patients want to know about the roles of residents and medical students in their care. *Academic Medicine.* 1998 Mar; 73(3): 339–341. 4 refs. BE61432.

*attitudes; communication; *disclosure; females; hospitals; informed consent; institutional policies; *internship and residency; medical education; *obstetrics and gynecology; *patient care; *patients; physicians; privacy; quality of health care; recall; *students; surgery; survey; *hysterectomy; teaching hospitals; San Francisco; University of California, San Francisco

Kravitz, Richard L. Ethnic differences in use of cardiovascular procedures: new insights and new challenges. [Editorial]. *Annals of Internal Medicine.* 1999 Feb 2; 130(3): 231–233. 18 refs. BE60927.

*blacks; health insurance; *heart diseases; kidney diseases; *patient care; physician patient relationship; quality of health care; referral and consultation; *selection for treatment; *surgery; *whites; *angioplasty; continuity of patient care; *coronary artery bypass; undertreatment; Los Angeles; New York City; North Carolina

Leape, Lucian L.; Hilborne, Lee H.; Bell, Robert, et al. Underuse of cardiac procedures: do women, ethnic minorities, and the uninsured fail to receive needed revascularization? *Annals of Internal Medicine.* 1999 Feb 2; 130(3): 183–192. 38 refs. BE60926.

blacks; comparative studies; evaluation studies; *females; health insurance; *heart diseases; Hispanic Americans; hospitals; *indigents; *males; medical records; *minority groups; *patient care; proprietary hospitals; public hospitals; referral and consultation; *selection for treatment; *surgery; *angioplasty; *coronary artery bypass; retrospective studies; *undertreatment; Medicaid; Medicare; New York City

BACKGROUND: Women, ethnic minorities, and uninsured persons receive fewer cardiac procedures than affluent white male patients do, but rates of use are crude indicators of quality. The important question is, Do women, minorities, and the uninsured fail to receive cardiac procedures when they need them? OBJECTIVE: To measure receipt of necessary coronary artery bypass graft (CABG) surgery and percutaneous transluminal coronary angioplasty (PTCA) overall; by patient sex, ethnicity, and payer status; and by availability of on–site revascularization. DESIGN: Retrospective, randomized medical record review. SETTING: 13 of the 24 hospitals in New York City that provide coronary angiography. PATIENTS: 631 patients who had coronary angiography in 1992 and met the RAND expert panel criteria for necessary revascularization. MEASUREMENTS: The percentage of patients who had CABG surgery or PTCA was measured, as were variations in use rates by sex, ethnic group, insurance status, and availability of on–site revascularization. Clinical and laboratory data were retrieved from medical records to identify patients who met the panel criteria for necessary revascularization. Receipt of revascularization was determined from state reports, medical records, and information provided by cardiologists. RESULTS: Overall, 74% (95% CI, 71% to 77%) of patients who met the panel criteria for necessary revascularization had CABG surgery or PTCA (underuse rate, 26%). No differences were found in use rates by patient sex, ethnic group, or payer status, but hospitals that provided on–site revascularization had higher use rates (76% [CI, 74% to 79%]) than hospitals that did not provide it (59% [CI, 56% to 65%]) (P less than 0.01). In hospitals that did not provide on–site revascularization, uninsured patients were less likely to have revascularization recommended to them (52% [CI, 32% to 78%]); rates of recommendation for patients with private insurance, Medicare, and Medicaid were 82%, 91%, and 75%, respectively (P = 0.026). CONCLUSIONS: Although revascularization procedures are substantially underused, no variations in rate of use by sex, ethnic group, or payer status were seen among patients treated in hospitals that provide CABG surgery and PTCA. However, underuse was significantly greater in hospitals that do not provide these procedures, particularly among uninsured persons.

Levine, Carol. The loneliness of the long–term care giver. [Personal narrative]. *New England Journal of Medicine.* 1999 May 20; 340(20): 1587–1590. 10 refs. BE62031.
advance care planning; *chronically ill; *communication; *community services; decision making; *disabled; *economics; education; *family members; goals; *health care delivery; health insurance reimbursement; *home care; injuries; *long–term care; managed care programs; mentally disabled; moral obligations; *obligations of society; *patient care; physically disabled; *professional family relationship; psychological stress; public policy; rehabilitation; *social support; Medicare; United States

MacFie, J. Ethical implications of recognizing nutritional support as a medical therapy. *British Journal of Surgery.* 1996 Nov; 83(11): 1567–1568. 15 refs. Based on a lecture given at the World Congress of Gastroenterology in Los Angeles, CA, Oct 1994, and published in *Nutrition* 1995; 11(Suppl. 2): 213–216. BE59529.
allowing to die; *artificial feeding; autonomy; beneficence; critically ill; food; hospitals; *nutrition; *patient care; persistent vegetative state; prognosis; risks and benefits; withholding treatment; Great Britain

Macklin, Ruth. Ethical relativism in a multicultural society. *Kennedy Institute of Ethics Journal.* 1998 Mar; 8(1): 1–22. 15 refs. Adapted from a chapter in a book by the author to be published by Oxford University Press

in 1999. BE59351.
advance directives; aged; aliens; *alternative therapies; American Indians; Asian Americans; attitudes; *autonomy; *beneficence; blacks; cancer; child abuse; circumcision; communication; *cultural pluralism; *decision making; diagnosis; disclosure; ethical analysis; *ethical relativism; *family members; family relationship; females; informed consent; international aspects; Jews; justice; legislation; *minority groups; minors; *moral policy; pain; paternalism; *patient care; patient education; *patients; *physician's role; physicians; prognosis; public health; religion; risks and benefits; terminally ill; truth disclosure; *values; *United States
The multicultural composition of the United States can pose problems for physicians and patients who come from diverse backgrounds. Although respect for cultural diversity mandates tolerance of the beliefs and practices of others, in some situations excessive tolerance can produce harm to patients. Careful analysis is needed to determine which values are culturally relative and which rest on an underlying universal ethical principle. A conception of justice as equality challenges the notion that it is always necessary to respect all of the beliefs and practices of every cultural group.

Markens, Susan; Browner, C.H.; Press, Nancy. Feeding the fetus: on interrogating the notion of maternal–fetal conflict. *Feminist Studies.* 1997 Summer; 23(2): 351–372. 46 fn. BE59795.
attitudes; behavior control; feminist ethics; *fetuses; food; health education; health maintenance organizations; informal social control; *mother fetus relationship; motivation; *nutrition; *patient compliance; *pregnant women; prenatal injuries; smoking; socioeconomic factors; survey; life style; *self care; California

Martone, Marilyn. Developing new models to ensure autonomy in home health care. *Linacre Quarterly.* 1997 Aug; 64(3): 29–37. 6 fn. BE59310.
*autonomy; *communication; *family members; *family relationship; females; *health personnel; *home care; patient compliance; patients; *professional autonomy; *professional family relationship; *professional patient relationship; psychological stress; technical expertise; terminal care; trust; dependency

Nelson, Judith E. Saving lives and saving deaths. *Annals of Internal Medicine.* 1999 May 4; 130(9): 776–777. BE61608.
attitudes to death; communication; *critically ill; *death; emotions; family members; *intensive care units; mortality; *palliative care; patient care; physician patient relationship; *physicians; professional family relationship; terminally ill

Nelson, Robert M. Ethics in the intensive care unit: creating an ethical environment. *Critical Care Clinics.* 1997 Jul; 13(3): 691–701. 28 refs. BE61557.
adults; advance directives; allowing to die; attitudes; attitudes to death; *communication; compassion; covenant; *critically ill; *decision making; dissent; informed consent; *institutional ethics; *intensive care units; interprofessional relations; newborns; nurses; parental consent; parents; *patient advocacy; *patient care; *patient care team; patient participation; pediatrics; *physician nurse relationship; physician patient relationship; physicians; professional autonomy; professional competence; professional family relationship; psychological stress; suffering; third party consent; trust; values; withholding treatment

Norrie, Peter. Ethical decision–making in intensive care: are nurses suitable patient advocates? *Intensive and Critical Care Nursing.* 1997 Jun; 13(3): 167–169. 22 refs. BE60481.
autonomy; decision making; institutional policies; *intensive care units; *nurse's role; *nurses; nursing ethics; paternalism;

BE = bioethics accession number   fn. = footnotes   refs. = references

*patient advocacy; *patient care; physician nurse relationship; professional competence; Great Britain

O'Connor, Bonnie B. Culture and the use of patient restraints. *HEC (HealthCare Ethics Committee) Forum.* 1998 Sep–Dec; 10(3–4): 263–275. 35 refs. BE61177.
> aged; alternatives; attitudes; *behavior control; comparative studies; cultural pluralism; economics; health personnel; historical aspects; hospitals; *international aspects; legal aspects; legal liability; nursing homes; *patient care; *physical restraint; professional patient relationship; risk; risks and benefits; standards; *values; *Great Britain; *United States

Orr, Robert D.; Genesen, Leigh B. Medicine, ethics and religion: rational or irrational? *Journal of Medical Ethics.* 1998 Dec; 24(6): 385–387. 10 fn. Commentary on J. Savulescu, p. 382–384. BE60787.
> cultural pluralism; decision making; futility; justice; *patient care; physicians; *prolongation of life; refusal to treat; *religion; resource allocation; social discrimination; suffering; values; atheists; rationality

Savulescu maintains that our paper, which encourages clinicians to honour requests for "inappropriate treatment" is prejudicial to his atheistic beliefs, and therefore wrong. In this paper we clarify and expand on our ideas, and respond to his assertion that medicine, ethics and atheism are objective, rational and true, while religion is irrational and false.

Pfettscher, Susan A. Making decisions about end-stage renal disease treatment: a review of theories and issues. *Advances in Renal Replacement Therapy.* 1997 Jan; 4(1): 81–88. 62 refs. BE60176.
> autonomy; communication; costs and benefits; *decision analysis; *decision making; family members; informed consent; *kidney diseases; *models, theoretical; organ transplantation; paternalism; *patient care; patient care team; *patient participation; patient satisfaction; *physician patient relationship; *physicians; professional autonomy; renal dialysis; treatment outcome; values; withholding treatment; United States

Pollock, Donald. Healing dilemmas. *Anthropological Quarterly.* 1996 Jul; 69(3): 149–157. 23 refs. 6 fn. BE61213.
> American Indians; *anthropology; attitudes; *cultural pluralism; developing countries; disease; drugs; ethical relativism; *international aspects; *non–Western World; paternalism; *patient care; *social dominance; *sociology of medicine; technical expertise; values; *Western World; *folk medicine; Brazil

Resnik, Robert. Cancer during pregnancy. [Editorial]. *New England Journal of Medicine.* 1999 Jul 8; 341(2): 120–121. 12 refs. BE62034.
> *cancer; drugs; fetal development; *fetuses; *patient care; *pregnant women; radiology; risks and benefits; surgery; time factors; treatment outcome

Richards, Tessa. Patients' priorities. [Editorial]. *BMJ (British Medical Journal).* 1999 Jan 30; 318(7179): 277. 11 refs. BE60579.
> decision making; *evaluation; information dissemination; international aspects; *patient care; *patient participation; patient satisfaction; primary health care; public participation; quality of health care; Europe; Great Britain

Richter, Gerd. Treatment of metastatic breast cancer — economic and ethical considerations. *Cancer Investigation.* 1997; 15(4): 335–341. 33 refs. BE59176.
> age factors; autonomy; bone marrow; *breast cancer; conflict of interest; *costs and benefits; *decision making; disclosure; drugs; *economics; evaluation; females; human

experimentation; informed consent; investigators; justice; *patient care; patients; physicians; practice guidelines; prognosis; *prolongation of life; quality adjusted life years; *quality of life; random selection; research design; *resource allocation; risks and benefits; *terminally ill; *therapeutic research; tissue transplantation; toxicity; *treatment outcome; values; vulnerable populations; chemotherapy; United States

Ristinen, Elaine; Mamtani, Ravinder. Ethics of transmission of hepatitis B virus by health–care workers. *Lancet.* 1998 Oct 24; 352(9137): 1381–1383. 17 refs. BE60798.
> confidentiality; counseling; employment; federal government; guidelines; *health personnel; *hepatitis; hospitals; *iatrogenic disease; immunization; informed consent; *institutional policies; mandatory testing; patient care; *public policy; *risk; Centers for Disease Control and Prevention; United States

Roberts, Laura Weiss; Battaglia, John; Smithpeter, Margaret, et al. An office on Main Street: health care dilemmas in small communities. *Hastings Center Report.* 1999 Jul–Aug; 29(4): 28–37. 35 fn. Includes inset article, "The problems of rural care: four new studies," p. 30–31. BE62467.
> *clinical ethics; community services; confidentiality; conflict of interest; cultural pluralism; *geographic factors; health; *health care delivery; mental health; *patient care; physician patient relationship; physicians; psychological stress; resource allocation; scarcity; social interaction; *socioeconomic factors; values; *rural population; United States

Rodriguez, Gonzalo Herranz. Contemporary ethical codes of professional conduct. *Dolentium Hominum: Church and Health in the World.* 1996; 31(11th Yr., No. 1): 33–36. BE61001.
> altruism; autonomy; beneficence; *Christian ethics; *codes of ethics; *emergency care; indigents; *international aspects; Jewish ethics; *medical ethics; misconduct; *moral obligations; nurses; *patient care; physician patient relationship; *physicians; professional ethics; sexuality; *social discrimination; value of life; values; vulnerable populations; war; dignity; Belgium; Ethical Principles of European Medicine; France; Geneva Declaration; *Good Samaritanism; Great Britain; Hippocratic Oath; International Code of Medical Ethics; Ireland; Italy; Portugal; Spain; United States; World Medical Association

Rosenczweig, Carolyn. Should relatives witness resuscitation? Ethical issues and practical considerations. *Canadian Medical Association Journal.* 1998 Mar 10; 158(5): 617–620. 9 refs. Second prize winning essay in the 1997 Dr. William Logie Medical Ethics Essay Contest for Canadian undergraduate medical students. BE60587.
> confidentiality; critically ill; *emergency care; *family members; *hospitals; *institutional policies; professional family relationship; psychological stress; *resuscitation; Canada

Rosner, Fred. The imperative to heal in traditional Judaism. *Mount Sinai Journal of Medicine.* 1997 Nov; 64(6): 413–416. 19 refs. BE59342.
> *AIDS; *communicable diseases; *Jewish ethics; moral obligations; occupational exposure; *patient care; patients; physician's role; *physicians; *refusal to treat; risk; value of life

Rosser, Walter W. Application of evidence from randomised controlled trials to general practice. *Lancet.* 1999 Feb 20; 353(9153): 661–664. 31 refs. BE61085.
> chronically ill; control groups; *costs and benefits; *decision

---

BE = bioethics accession number   fn. = footnotes   refs. = references

making; evaluation; *evidence-based medicine; *family practice; health insurance reimbursement; health promotion; *human experimentation; international aspects; *patient care; *patient participation; physician patient relationship; *physicians; preventive medicine; primary health care; quality of life; *random selection; research design; resource allocation; *risks and benefits; *socioeconomic factors; standards; *values

Savulescu, Julian. Two worlds apart: religion and ethics. *Journal of Medical Ethics.* 1998 Dec; 24(6): 382–384. 5 fn. Commentary on R.D. Orr and L.B. Genesen, "Requests for "inappropriate" treatment based on religious beliefs," *JME* 1997 Jun; 23(3): 142–147. BE60786.

allowing to die; Christian ethics; cultural pluralism; decision making; futility; justice; *patient care; physicians; *prolongation of life; refusal to treat; *religion; resource allocation; social discrimination; *values; atheists

In a recent article entitled, Requests "for inappropriate" treatment based on religious beliefs, Orr and Genesen claim that futile treatment should be provided to patients who request it if their request is based on a religious belief. I claim that this implies that we should also accede to requests for harmful or cost-ineffective treatments based on religious beliefs. This special treatment of religious requests is an example of special pleading on the part of theists and morally objectionable discrimination against atheists. It also provides an excellent illustration of how different the practices of religion and ethics are.

Schneck, Stuart A. "Doctoring" doctors and their families. *JAMA.* 1998 Dec 16; 280(23): 2039–2042. 74 refs. BE59582.

confidentiality; *family members; *guidelines; *interprofessional relations; married persons; *medical etiquette; *patient care; *patients; *physician patient relationship; physician's role; *physicians; privacy; professional family relationship; psychological stress; social dominance

Being selected to provide medical care to other physicians or their family members represents not only a gratifying professional recognition of competence by one's peers but also a challenge. Many personal and psychological factors may influence the medical care of physicians. Ill physicians may have difficulty with role reversal and "the VIP syndrome," while treating physicians may have to deal with their own anxiety and issues such as confidentiality, privacy, empathy, and intrusion by a physician-relative into the care of medical family members. Based on experience with more than 200 physician-patients and many adult family members of physicians, suggestions are offered for care of these patient groups.

Schneider, Carl E. Regulating doctors. *Hastings Center Report.* 1999 Jul–Aug; 29(4): 21–22. 5 refs. BE62465.

compensation; health care delivery; interprofessional relations; lawyers; legal aspects; *legal liability; *malpractice; managed care programs; medicine; *physicians; *professional autonomy; professional competence; self regulation; trust; physician's practice patterns; United States

Selwyn, Peter A.; Arnold, Robert. From fate to tragedy: the changing meanings of life, death, and AIDS. *Annals of Internal Medicine.* 1998 Dec 1; 129(11): 899–902. 29 refs. BE59327.

*AIDS; chronically ill; drugs; *HIV seropositivity; *palliative care; *patient care; physician patient relationship; *physician's role; psychological stress; *terminal care; terminally ill

The advent of highly active antiretroviral therapy (HAART) and quantitative viral load assays has revolutionized the care of HIV-infected patients. However, this paradigm shift has also had unexpected, sometimes adverse consequences that are not always obvious. Before antiretroviral therapy, physicians learned how to accompany patients through their illness; to bear witness to sickness and dying; and to help patients and their families with suffering, closure, and legacy. Since we have become better at treating the virus, a new temptation has emerged to dwell on quantitative aspects of HIV management and monitoring, although the skills that we learned earlier in the epidemic are no less necessary for providing good care. Our new-found therapeutic capabilities should not distract us from the sometimes more difficult and necessary task of simply "being there" for patients for whom HAART is no longer effective. The definition and practice of end-of-life care for patients with AIDS will continue to evolve as AIDS comes to resemble other chronic, treatable, but ultimately fatal illnesses, such as end-stage pulmonary disease and metastatic cancer, in which clinicians must continually readdress with their patients the balance of curative and palliative interventions as the disease process unfolds over time. The coming challenge in HIV care will be to encourage the maintenance of a "primary care" mentality-with attention to the larger psychosocial issues, end-of-life care, bereavement, and a focus on the patient as opposed to the illness-alongside our new antiretroviral paradigm. Otherwise, we run the risk of forgetting what we learned about healing, from a disease that we could not cure.

Shelton, Wayne. A broader look at medical futility. *Theoretical Medicine and Bioethics.* 1998 Aug; 19(4): 383–400. 18 refs. BE60160.

*allowing to die; case studies; *common good; cultural pluralism; *decision making; democracy; *dissent; economics; family members; *freedom; *futility; goals; health care; health care delivery; justice; managed care programs; medicine; models, theoretical; obligations to society; *patient care; patients; persistent vegetative state; physicians; *prolongation of life; public policy; quality of life; resource allocation; resuscitation orders; *rights; risks and benefits; standards; statistics; technical expertise; treatment outcome; uncertainty; *values; ventilators; *withholding treatment; United States

Siegal, Nina. Critics say inmates again are shackled in childbirth. [News]. *New York Times.* 1999 Apr 11: 33. BE62700.

*childbirth; hospitals; institutional policies; legal aspects; patient care; *physical restraint; *pregnant women; *prisoners; *Elmhurst Hospital Center (Queens, NY); New York; Rikers Island (NY)

Silvers, Anita; Wasserman, David; Mahowald, Mary B. Disability, Difference, Discrimination: Perspectives on Justice in Bioethics and Public Policy. Lanham, MD: Rowman and Littlefield; 1998. 343 p. (Point/counterpoint). Bibliography: p. 305–327. Afterword by L.C. Becker. ISBN 0-8476-9223-X. BE60751.

bioethical issues; *disabled; economics; education; employment; federal government; females; feminist ethics; government regulation; health; health care; home care; *justice; legal aspects; mentally disabled; models, theoretical; normality; physically disabled; prenatal diagnosis; resource allocation; self concept; *social discrimination; stigmatization; suffering; terminology; Americans with Disabilities Act 1990; United States

Sim, Julius. Respect for autonomy: issues in neurological

BE = bioethics accession number   fn. = footnotes   refs. = references

rehabilitation. *Clinical Rehabilitation.* 1998 Feb; 12(1): 3–10. 46 refs. BE61852.

*autonomy; beneficence; *central nervous system diseases; communication; competence; comprehension; decision making; family members; informed consent; mentally disabled; paternalism; *patient care; patient care team; patient participation; physically disabled; *rehabilitation

Skolnick, Andrew A. Critics denounce staffing jails and prisons with physicians convicted of misconduct. [News]. *JAMA.* 1998 Oct 28; 280(16): 1391–1392. BE60291.

*criminal law; *legal liability; *misconduct; patient care; *physicians; *prisoners; *professional competence; psychiatry; *quality of health care; *regulation; sex offenses; *licensing boards; *physician impairment; National Commission on Correctional Health Care; United States

Skolnick, Andrew A. Prison deaths spotlight how boards handle impaired, disciplined physicians. [News]. *JAMA.* 1998 Oct 28; 280(16): 1387–1390. Includes inset article, "Only the tip of the iceberg," by A.A. Skolnick, p. 1388–1389. BE60290.

*criminal law; fraud; *legal liability; *malpractice; mentally ill; *misconduct; negligence; patient care; *physicians; *prisoners; *professional competence; *quality of health care; *regulation; rehabilitation; *sex offenses; withholding treatment; *wrongful death; *licensing boards; *physician impairment; Correctional Medical Services; Mauney, Walter; United States; Williams, Gail

Sloan, R.P.; Bagiella, E.; Powell, T. Religion, spirituality, and medicine. *Lancet.* 1999 Feb 20; 353(9153): 664–667. 39 refs. BE61086.

alternative therapies; attitudes; *counseling; *empirical research; *health; health promotion; medical education; medicine; morbidity; mortality; pastoral care; *patient care; physician patient relationship; *physician's role; physicians; public opinion; quality of life; *religion; *research design; risks and benefits; treatment outcome

Söderberg, Anna; Gilje, Fredricka; Norberg, Astrid. Dignity in situations of ethical difficulty in intensive care. *Intensive and Critical Care Nursing.* 1997 Jun; 13(3): 135–144. 32 refs. BE60479.

allowing to die; caring; conscience; decision making; dehumanization; *intensive care units; *narrative ethics; nurse patient relationship; *nurses; *nursing ethics; *patient care; physician nurse relationship; psychological stress; terminal care; withholding treatment; *dignity; qualitative research; Sweden

Spike, Jeffrey. Brain death, pregnancy, and posthumous motherhood. [Case study]. *Journal of Clinical Ethics.* 1999 Spring; 10(1): 57–65. 9 fn. BE62707.

allowing to die; *brain death; *decision making; determination of death; dissent; ethics consultation; family members; fathers; feminist ethics; fetal development; *fetuses; health personnel; intensive care units; judicial action; moral policy; patient care; patient care team; posthumous reproduction; *pregnant women; *prolongation of life; quality of life; resource allocation; single persons; socioeconomic factors; third party consent; treatment outcome; ventilators; *withholding treatment

Spiro, Howard. The Power of Hope: A Doctor's Perspective. New Haven, CT: Yale University Press; 1998. 288 p. Bibliography: p.257–278. Prepared under the auspices of the Program for Humanities in Medicine, Yale University School of Medicine. Portions of this book previously appeared in *Doctors, Patients, and Placebos* (1986; Yale University Press). ISBN 0–300–07632–0. BE62582.

*alternative therapies; attitudes; autonomy; beneficence;

caring; communication; control groups; cultural pluralism; deception; diagnosis; disease; drugs; emotions; health; human experimentation; informed consent; intention; medical education; medicine; pain; paternalism; *patient care; patients; physician patient relationship; physician's role; physicians; *placebos; postmodernism; research subjects; risks and benefits; science; suffering; truth disclosure; uncertainty; hope; self care; United States

Stanberry, Ben. The legal and ethical aspects of telemedicine. 3: Telemedicine and malpractice. *Journal of Telemedicine and Telecare.* 1998; 4(2): 72–79. 31 fn. BE62406.

*computer communication networks; confidentiality; consent forms; emergency care; health personnel; *informed consent; *legal liability; *malpractice; negligence; *patient care; physician patient relationship; professional competence; *referral and consultation; *standards; treatment refusal; *telemedicine; Great Britain

Starr, Joann; Zawacki, Bruce E. Voices from the silent world of doctor and patient. *Cambridge Quarterly of Healthcare Ethics.* 1999 Spring; 8(2): 129–138. 12 fn. BE61230.

attitudes; *autonomy; *burns; *caring; clinical ethics committees; coercion; communication; compassion; competence; decision making; *emotions; empathy; ethicists; family members; hospitals; informed consent; intensive care units; *narrative ethics; nurse patient relationship; nurses; *pain; paternalism; *patient advocacy; *patient care; patient compliance; *patient participation; patients; *physician patient relationship; physician's role; physicians; professional family relationship; *psychological stress; psychology; *suffering; surgery; *treatment refusal; trust; vulnerable populations; empowerment

Sugarman, Jeremy; Burk, Larry. Physicians' ethical obligations regarding alternative medicine. *JAMA.* 1998 Nov 11; 280(18): 1623–1625. 24 refs. BE59653.

*alternative therapies; autonomy; beneficence; cultural pluralism; decision making; ethical relativism; evaluation; goals; health personnel; justice; *medicine; moral obligations; *patient care; patients; *physician's role; professional competence; referral and consultation; risks and benefits; values

Tiedje, Linda Beth. Ethical and legal issues in the care of substance-using women. *Journal of Obstetric, Gynecologic and Neonatal Nursing.* 1998 Jan–Feb; 27(1): 92–98. 46 refs. BE62060.

attitudes; autonomy; beneficence; child abuse; confidentiality; *drug abuse; federal government; *females; fetuses; government financing; guidelines; justice; legal aspects; mandatory testing; nurse patient relationship; nurses; *patient care; *pregnant women; *prenatal injuries; United States

Torrance, Caroline J.; Das, Robert; Allison, Miles C. Use of chaperones in clinics for genitourinary medicine: survey of consultants. *BMJ (British Medical Journal).* 1999 Jul 17; 319(7203): 159–160. 4 refs. BE62454.

adolescents; family members; *females; institutional policies; *knowledge, attitudes, practice; *males; nurses; *obstetrics and gynecology; organizational policies; *patient care; patients; *physician patient relationship; *physicians; *privacy; professional organizations; sexuality; survey; ambulatory care; *physical examination; General Medical Council (Great Britain); Great Britain; Royal College of Obstetricians and Gynaecologists

Vaught, Wayne; Lamdan, Ruth M. An ethics committee explores restraint use and practices. *HEC (HealthCare Ethics Committee) Forum.* 1998 Sep–Dec; 10(3–4): 306–316. 2 refs. BE61182.

aged; *behavior control; case studies; clinical ethics

BE = bioethics accession number   fn. = footnotes   refs. = references

committees; competence; emergency care; *hospitals; informed consent; injuries; institutional policies; intensive care units; mentally ill; *patient care; *physical restraint; Allegheny University Hospital (Philadelphia)

Veatch, Robert M. Ethical consensus formation in clinical cases. *In:* ten Have, Henk A.M.J.; Sass, Hans–Martin, eds. Consensus Formation in Healthcare Ethics. Boston, MA: Kluwer Academic; 1998: 17–34. 25 refs. ISBN 0-7923-4944-X. BE62585.
autonomy; *clinical ethics; *clinical ethics committees; competence; *consensus; contracts; covenant; cultural pluralism; *decision making; ethical theory; family members; health facilities; informed consent; legal guardians; moral policy; patient advocacy; *patient care; *patient care team; patient participation; *patients; peer review; *physicians; religious ethics; secularism; third party consent; values; absence of proxy

Wagner, James T.; Higdon, Tami L. Spiritual issues and bioethics in the intensive care unit: the role of the chaplain. *Critical Care Clinics.* 1996 Jan; 12(1): 15–27. 9 refs. BE59275.
adults; allowing to die; case studies; *clergy; clinical ethics committees; conflict of interest; counseling; critically ill; decision making; dissent; education; ethics consultation; family members; *hospitals; intensive care units; interprofessional relations; legal guardians; minors; organ donation; *pastoral care; *patient care; patient care team; patients; physicians; professional patient relationship; *professional role; referral and consultation; religion; required request; treatment refusal

Walters, D. Campbell. Just Take It Out! The Ethics and Economics of Cesarean Section and Hysterectomy. Mt. Vernon, IL: Topiary Publishing; 1998. 271 p. Bibliography: p. 267–271. ISBN 0-9667162-0-5. BE62741.
autonomy; brain pathology; *cesarean section; childbirth; congenital disorders; decision making; disclosure; economics; *females; fetuses; government financing; health insurance reimbursement; hospitals; informed consent; justice; legal liability; mortality; newborns; *obstetrics and gynecology; pain; paternalism; physician patient relationship; physicians; *pregnant women; public policy; *risks and benefits; standards; *surgery; treatment refusal; women's health services; *hysterectomy

Watson, Sidney Dean. In search of the story: physicians and charity care. *Saint Louis University Public Law Review.* 1996; 15(2): 353–369. 92 fn. BE59914.
*altruism; *bioethical issues; *bioethics; caring; case studies; economics; emergency care; ethicists; *health care delivery; hospitals; *indigents; literature; medical education; medical ethics; methods; minority groups; *moral obligations; *narrative ethics; obligations of society; *patient care; patient compliance; patient transfer; physician patient relationship; *physicians; *refusal to treat; remuneration; social problems; *socioeconomic factors; Medicaid; United States

Watts, Jonathan. Japanese victims of discrimination against lepers sue government. [News]. *Lancet.* 1998 Aug 22; 352(9128): 631. BE59639.
compensation; historical aspects; institutionalized persons; *legal aspects; legal rights; patient care; *public policy; *quarantine; residential facilities; social discrimination; *leprosy; *Japan; Twentieth Century

Wendell, Susan. Old women out of control: some thoughts on aging, ethics, and psychosomatic medicine. *In:* Walter, Margaret Urban, ed. Mother Time: Women, Aging, and Ethics. Lanham, MD: Rowman and Littlefield; 1999: 133–149. 24 refs. 4 fn. ISBN 0-8476-9260-4. BE61897.
adults; *age factors; aged; attitudes; chronically ill;

*diagnosis; disabled; *females; health; *medical errors; *mental health; morbidity; normality; patient care; physicians; *psychiatric diagnosis; *self concept; social discrimination; socioeconomic factors; sociology of medicine; stigmatization; *women's health; menopause; *psychosomatic medicine; North America

Wharton, Robert H. Pedestrian vs. train. *Hastings Center Report.* 1999 May–Jun; 29(3): 28–29. BE61411.
adolescents; attitudes; *communication; critically ill; *death; *decision making; *emergency care; *emotions; *family members; health personnel; injuries; *parents; personhood; *physician patient relationship; physicians; *professional family relationship; terminally ill; grief

Williamson, Charlotte. The rise of doctor–patient working groups. *BMJ (British Medical Journal).* 1998 Nov 14; 317(7169): 1374–1377. 31 refs. BE60838.
advisory committees; committee membership; communication; evaluation; patient advocacy; *patient care; *patient participation; *physician patient relationship; political activity; *quality of health care; standards; Great Britain

Wu, Albert W.; Cavanaugh, Thomas A.; McPhee, Stephen J., et al. To tell the truth: ethical and practical issues in disclosing medical mistakes to patients. *Journal of General Internal Medicine.* 1997 Dec; 12(12): 770–775. 31 refs. BE59534.
beneficence; communication; competence; deontological ethics; *disclosure; iatrogenic disease; injuries; interprofessional relations; legal liability; *medical errors; medical ethics; *moral obligations; *negligence; *patient care; patients; physician patient relationship; *physicians; *risks and benefits; teleological ethics; *truth disclosure; uncertainty; whistleblowing

Zusman, Jack. Restraint and Seclusion: Improving Practice and Conquering the JCAHO Standards. Marblehead, MA: Opus Communications; 1997. 198 p. Bibliography: p. 179–184. ISBN 1-885829-34-5. BE59869.
aged; alternatives; behavior control; communication; dangerousness; *health facilities; health personnel; injuries; institutional policies; institutionalized persons; mentally ill; patient care; *physical restraint; punishment; *regulation; risks and benefits; self regulation; *standards; terminology; *Joint Commission on Accreditation of Healthcare Organizations; United States

Zwitter, Matjaz; Nilstun, Tore; Knudsen, Lisbeth E., et al. Professional and public attitudes towards unsolicited medical intervention. *BMJ (British Medical Journal).* 1999 Jan 23; 318(7178): 251–253. 12 refs. BE60330.
altruism; *attitudes; autonomy; *beneficence; cancer; comparative studies; diagnosis; emergency care; genetic predisposition; health promotion; *international aspects; medical specialties; obligations to society; *paternalism; *patient care; physician patient relationship; *physicians; *privacy; *public opinion; risks and benefits; survey; traffic accidents; truth disclosure; incidental findings; *unsolicited intervention; Austria; Denmark; *Good Samaritanism; Slovenia; Sweden

PATIENT CARE/AGED

Altman, Lawrence K. Treating elderly's cancer is frustrating many experts. [News]. *New York Times.* 1998 May 20: A14. BE60469.
age factors; *aged; *cancer; drugs; *human experimentation; international aspects; *patient care; research subjects; risks and benefits; *selection of subjects; therapeutic research; Italy; United States

---

BE = bioethics accession number   fn. = footnotes   refs. = references

Antuono, Piero; Beyer, Jan. The burden of dementia: a medical and research perspective. *Theoretical Medicine and Bioethics.* 1999 Jan; 20(1): 3–13. 34 refs. BE62120.
*aged; autonomy; brain pathology; *dementia; diagnosis; drugs; economics; family members; genetic predisposition; home care; paternalism; *patient care; therapeutic research

Artnak, Kathryn E. Informed consent in the elderly: assessing decisional capacity. *Seminars in Perioperative Nursing.* 1997 Jan; 6(1): 59–64. 10 refs. BE59194.
*aged; attitudes; autonomy; beneficence; case studies; communication; *competence; comprehension; *decision making; disclosure; hospitals; *informed consent; moral obligations; *nurse's role; paternalism; *patient care; quality of life; risks and benefits; social discrimination; time factors; treatment refusal; values

Baker, Tina; Cooper, Colleen. What happens next? [Case study and commentaries]. *Hastings Center Report.* 1999 Mar–Apr; 29(2): 24–25. BE61657.
administrators; *aged; allied health personnel; *behavior control; behavior disorders; brain pathology; case studies; death; government regulation; health personnel; institutional policies; *nursing homes; *patient care; *physical restraint; cerebrovascular disorders

Barakat, Khalid; Wilkinson, Paul; Deaner, Andrew, et al. How should age affect management of acute myocardial infarction? A prospective cohort study. *Lancet.* 1999 Mar 20; 353(9157): 955–959. 23 refs. BE61462.
*age factors; *aged; drugs; evaluation studies; *heart diseases; hospitals; mortality; *patient care; *prognosis; *selection for treatment; social discrimination; treatment outcome; *myocardial infarction; prospective studies; thrombolytic therapy; Great Britain

Berghmans, Ron L.P. Ethical hazards of the substituted judgement test in decision making concerning the end of life of dementia patients. [Editorial]. *International Journal of Geriatric Psychiatry.* 1997 Mar; 12(3): 283–287. 23 refs. BE59429.
advance directives; *aged; *allowing to die; autonomy; competence; *decision making; *dementia; family members; *patient care; personhood; physicians; prolongation of life; quality of life; risks and benefits; *third party consent; time factors; treatment refusal; value of life; oral directives; personal identity

Binstock, Robert H. Old-age-based rationing: from rhetoric to risk? *Generations (American Society on Aging).* 1994 Winter; 18(4): 37–41. 41 refs. BE60550.
*age factors; *aged; *economics; federal government; government financing; *health care delivery; justice; *public policy; quality of life; *resource allocation; *selection for treatment; terminal care; wedge argument; withholding treatment; Medicare; *United States

Boyd, Kenneth. Old age, something to look forward to. *In:* Hanson, Mark J.; Callahan, Daniel, eds. The Goals of Medicine: The Forgotten Issue in Health Care Reform. Washington, DC: Georgetown University Press; 1999: 152–161. 21 fn. ISBN 0-87840-707-3. BE60523.
age factors; *aged; attitudes; economics; family members; *goals; health; *health care; health promotion; life extension; long-term care; *medicine; morbidity; patient care; resource allocation; selection for treatment; adult offspring; dependency; Great Britain

British Medical Association; Royal College of Nursing. The Older Person: Consent and Care: Report of the British Medical Association and the Royal College of

Nursing. London: British Medical Association; 1995 Apr. 63 p. 27 refs. ISBN 0-7279-0912-6. BE59169.
advance directives; *aged; autonomy; communication; competence; confidentiality; *decision making; disclosure; family members; health facilities; human experimentation; *informed consent; institutionalized persons; nurses; patient advocacy; *patient care; patient care team; patients' rights; physical restraint; physicians; *practice guidelines; professional organizations; resuscitation orders; third party consent; treatment refusal; elder abuse; *British Medical Association; *Great Britain; *Royal College of Nursing

Callahan, Daniel. Age, sex, and resource allocation. *In:* Walker, Margaret Urban, ed. Mother Time: Women, Aging, and Ethics. Lanham, MD: Rowman and Littlefield; 1999: 189–199. 9 fn. ISBN 0-8476-9260-4. BE61900.
age factors; *aged; biomedical technologies; chronically ill; disabled; disadvantaged; *economics; federal government; *females; *government financing; *health care; *health care reform; health promotion; home care; justice; long-term care; males; mortality; public policy; quality of life; rehabilitation; *resource allocation; social discrimination; *women's health; *women's health services; Medicare; *United States

Callahan, Daniel. Must the young and old struggle over health care resources? *Journal Of Long Term Home Health Care.* 1996 Fall; 15(4): 4–14. Edited version of the annual Iago Galdston Lecture, presented at the New York Academy of Medicine on 3 Jun 1996. BE60947.
*age factors; *aged; biomedical technologies; children; *economics; *health care; long-term care; moral obligations; obligations of society; public policy; *resource allocation; social impact; trends; withholding treatment; Medicare; United States

Cohen, Elias S.; Kruschwitz, Ann L. Restraint reduction: lessons from the asylum. *Journal of Ethics, Law, and Aging.* 1997 Spring-Summer; 3(1): 25–43. 72 fn. BE59202.
*aged; *behavior control; decision making; *dementia; education; federal government; government regulation; health personnel; historical aspects; *institutional policies; international aspects; legal aspects; *mental institutions; *mentally disabled; moral obligations; *nursing homes; patient advocacy; *patient care; *physical restraint; psychoactive drugs; quality of health care; state government; Eighteenth Century; Europe; Great Britain; Medicaid; Medicare; Nineteenth Century; Twentieth Century; *United States; Youngberg v. Romeo

Derse, Arthur R. Making decisions about life-sustaining medical treatment in patients with dementia: the problem of patient decision-making capacity. *Theoretical Medicine and Bioethics.* 1999 Jan; 20(1): 55–67. 42 refs. BE62124.
*aged; *allowing to die; assisted suicide; autonomy; beneficence; case studies; *compensation; comprehension; *decision making; *dementia; diagnosis; emergency care; heart diseases; human experimentation; *informed consent; patient care; patient participation; *prolongation of life; quality of life; recall; *resuscitation; standards; surgery; third party consent; *treatment refusal; truth disclosure; withholding treatment; rationality

DeSantis, Joe; Engberg, Sandra; Rogers, Joan. Geropsychiatric restraint use. *Journal of the American Geriatrics Society.* 1997 Dec; 45(12): 1515–1518. 25 refs. BE59692.
age factors; *aged; *behavior control; *behavior disorders; comparative studies; *dementia; hospitals; injuries; mental institutions; mentally ill; motivation; nurses; *patient care; *physical restraint; prospective studies

Fellows, Lesley K. Competency and consent in dementia. *Journal of the American Geriatrics Society.* 1998 Jul; 46(7):

BE = bioethics accession number   fn. = footnotes   refs. = references

922–926. 20 refs. BE62261.
    *advance directives; *aged; autonomy; beneficence;
coercion; communication; *competence; *decision making;
*dementia; family members; *informed consent; *patient
care; patient participation; personhood; physicians; *risks
and benefits; self concept; standards; terminal care; *third
party consent; time factors; values

Fisher, Carol; Gill, Denise. Limiting health care for the
elderly. *Plastic Surgical Nursing.* 1996 Summer; 16(2):
113–116. 20 refs. BE60198.
    *aged; beneficence; biomedical technologies; community
services; costs and benefits; ethical analysis; ethical theory;
government financing; *health care; hospitals; institutional
policies; intensive care units; justice; moral policy; nurses;
*resource allocation; selection for treatment; needs;
Medicaid; Medicare; United States

Frolik, Lawrence A., ed. Health care decision making.
In: his Aging and the Law: An Interdisciplinary Reader.
Philadelphia, PA: Temple University Press; 1999:
295–394. 14 refs. 296 fn. ISBN 1–56639–653–0. BE61059.
    advance care planning; advance directives; *aged; *allowing
to die; *assisted suicide; attitudes; *autonomy; chronically
ill; clinical ethics; coercion; communication; *competence;
critically ill; cultural pluralism; *decision making; disclosure;
family members; hospitals; *informed consent; judicial
action; *legal aspects; mentally disabled; minority groups;
nursing homes; patient advocacy; *patient care; patient care
team; patients; persistent vegetative state; physicians;
prolongation of life; resource allocation; resuscitation; *right
to die; standards; suffering; *terminal care; terminally ill;
*third party consent; treatment refusal; truth disclosure;
voluntary euthanasia; wedge argument; withholding
treatment; In re Fiori; In re Milton; Medicaid; Medicare;
Pocono Medical Center v. Harley; Study to Understand
Prognoses and Preferences for Outcomes and Risks of
Treatments (SUPPORT); Uniform Health Care Decisions
Act 1993; *United States

Goodwin, James S. Geriatrics and the limits of modern
medicine. *New England Journal of Medicine.* 1999 Apr
22; 340(16): 1283–1285. 11 refs. BE62027.
    *aged; compassion; diagnosis; hospices; iatrogenic disease;
managed care programs; *patient care; physician's role;
quality of life; suffering; values; geriatrics; United States

Gottlich, Vicki. Protection for nursing facility residents
under the ADA. *Generations (American Society on Aging).*
1994 Winter; 18(4): 43–47. 9 fn. BE60551.
    *aged; *disabled; federal government; *government
regulation; institutionalized persons; *legal aspects; *nursing
homes; patient admission; *patient care; patient discharge;
patient transfer; patients' rights; social discrimination;
*Americans with Disabilities Act 1990; *United States

**Hansen, Jennie Chin; Lynch, Marty; Estes, Carroll
L.** Is managed care good for older persons: Yes [and]
No. *In:* Scharlach, Andrew E.; Kaye, Lenard W., eds.
Controversial Issues in Aging. Boston, MA: Allyn and
Bacon; 1997: 114–124. 3 refs. ISBN 0–205–19381–1.
BE60964.
    *aged; community services; *costs and benefits; *economics;
*evaluation; gatekeeping; health care delivery; health
facilities; health maintenance organizations; home care;
incentives; indigents; long–term care; *managed care
programs; *patient care; patient care team; physicians;
preventive medicine; primary health care; program
descriptions; proprietary health facilities; *quality of health
care; referral and consultation; resource allocation;
withholding treatment; continuity of patient care; utilization
review; Medicaid; Medicare; Program of All–inclusive Care
for the Elderly (PACE); United States

Hardin, Steven B. VHA ethics rounds: [autonomy].

*NCCE News (Veterans Health Administration National
Center for Clinical Ethics).* 1994 Winter; 2(1): 4–5. 2 refs.
BE59848.
    *aged; *autonomy; beneficence; case studies; *decision
making; ethics consultation; hospitals; patient care team;
*patient discharge; risks and benefits; *terminally ill

Iglehart, John K. The American health care system:
Medicare. *New England Journal of Medicine.* 1999 Jan
28; 30(4): 327–332. 38 refs. BE60989.
    *aged; disabled; *economics; family practice; *federal
government; *government financing; *health care delivery;
health care reform; health insurance; managed care
programs; medical education; medical fees; medical
specialties; organization and administration; physicians;
political activity; politics; public opinion; statistics; *trends;
End Stage Renal Disease Program; Health Care Financing
Administration; *Medicare; *United States

Kane, Rosalie A.; Kane, Robert L.; Ladd, Richard C.
The Heart of Long–Term Care. New York, NY: Oxford
University Press; 1998. 328 p. Includes references. ISBN
0–19–512238–0. BE62732.
    accountability; *aged; allied health personnel; alternatives;
chronically ill; community services; disabled; family
members; federal government; goals; government financing;
health care delivery; health insurance; home care;
international aspects; *long–term care; managed care
programs; nursing homes; public policy; residential facilities;
state government; case managers; personal financing; quality
assurance; *United States

Kenyon, Georgina. Doctors refuse to operate on 80 year
old man. [News]. *BMJ (British Medical Journal).* 1998
Dec 5; 317(7172): 1548. BE60264.
    *aged; decision making; *heart diseases; *institutional
policies; patient care team; *public hospitals; *refusal to
treat; *resource allocation; *selection for treatment; social
discrimination; *surgery; *Australia; *Quinn, John

Kuczewski, Mark G. Ethics in long–term care: are the
principles different? *Theoretical Medicine and Bioethics.*
1999 Jan; 20(1): 15–29. 21 refs. 1 fn. BE62121.
    *aged; autonomy; beneficence; bioethics; case studies;
*casuistry; communication; communitarianism; competence;
deception; *decision making; ethical theory; family members;
*health personnel; informed consent; institutional ethics;
institutionalized persons; *long–term care; methods; *moral
obligations; *moral policy; narrative ethics; *nursing homes;
patient advocacy; *patient care; patients; physicians;
principle–based ethics; professional family relationship;
professional patient relationship; professional role; surgery;
third party consent; truth disclosure; values

Lantos, John D.; Mokalla, Mani; Meadow, William.
Resource allocation in neonatal and medical ICUs:
epidemiology and rationing at the extremes of life.
*American Journal of Respiratory and Critical Care
Medicine.* 1997 Jul; 156(1): 185–189. 12 refs. BE60028.
    age factors; *aged; comparative studies; costs and benefits;
*intensive care units; justice; *low birth weight; *mortality;
*newborns; patient discharge; prematurity; *resource
allocation; time factors; *treatment outcome; ventilators;
retrospective studies; University of Chicago Hospitals

Levinsky, Norman G. Can we afford medical care for
Alice C? *Lancet.* 1998 Dec 5; 352(9143): 1849–1851. 13
refs. BE60805.
    *age factors; *aged; allowing to die; biomedical
technologies; case studies; *economics; futility; government
financing; *health care; hospitals; intensive care units; justice;
mortality; patient admission; prolongation of life; *public
policy; quality of life; *resource allocation; social
discrimination; socioeconomic factors; Medicare; *United
States

BE = bioethics accession number   fn. = footnotes   refs. = references

Long, Ann; Slevin, Eamonn. Living with dementia: communicating with an older person and her family. *Nursing Ethics.* 1999 Jan; 6(1): 23–36. 54 refs. BE60152.
　　*aged; autonomy; beneficence; *caring; *communication; deception; dehumanization; *dementia; diagnosis; empathy; ethical analysis; family members; family relationship; humanism; *nurse patient relationship; *nurses; *nursing education; nursing research; paternalism; *patient care; *professional family relationship; psychological stress; psychology; social dominance; stigmatization; truth disclosure; adult offspring; University of Ulster (Northern Ireland)

Maly, Rose C.; Frank, Janet C.; Marshall, Grant N., et al. Perceived efficacy in patient-physician interactions (PEPPI): validation of an instrument in older persons. *Journal of the American Geriatrics Society.* 1998 Jul; 46(7): 889–894. 53 refs. BE62260.
　　*aged; *communication; comprehension; *evaluation; information dissemination; *patient care; *patient participation; *patient satisfaction; *physician patient relationship; *placebos; socioeconomic factors; *empowerment; physician's practice patterns; *questionnaires; self care; Los Angeles

Mattiasson, Anne-Cathrine; Hemberg, Maja. Intimacy -- meeting needs and respecting privacy in the care of elderly people: what is a good moral attitude on the part of the nurse/carer? *Nursing Ethics.* 1998 Nov; 5(6): 527–534. 27 refs. BE60813.
　　*aged; attitudes; *caring; communication; dementia; females; males; *nurse patient relationship; nurses; patient care; patients; *privacy; sexuality; trust

Mavretish, Barbara. Nursing home issues in restraint use. *HEC (HealthCare Ethics Committee) Forum.* 1998 Sep–Dec; 10(3–4): 300–305. 2 refs. BE61181.
　　*aged; behavior control; education; federal government; government regulation; health personnel; injuries; *institutional policies; *nursing homes; patient care; *physical restraint; statistics; *Frances Schervier Home and Hospital (New York City)

Meadow, William; Lantos, John D.; Mokalla, Mani, et al. Distributive justice across generations: epidemiology of ICU care for the very young and the very old. *Clinics in Perinatology.* 1996 Sep; 23(3): 597–608. 24 refs. BE60943.
　　adults; *age factors; *aged; comparative studies; *costs and benefits; economics; infants; *intensive care units; *justice; *low birth weight; medical records; *mortality; *newborns; patient care; patient discharge; prognosis; *resource allocation; selection for treatment; *treatment outcome; retrospective studies; survival; University of Chicago Medical Center

Miles, Steven H. Restraints: controlling a symptom or a symptom of control. *HEC (HealthCare Ethics Committee) Forum.* 1998 Sep–Dec; 10(3–4): 235–243. 18 refs. Paper presented at the 1990 Annual Meeting Convention of the American Geriatrics Society. BE61176.
　　*aged; *behavior control; consent forms; dehumanization; informed consent; injuries; institutional policies; legal aspects; *nursing homes; patient care; *physical restraint; risks and benefits; United States

Mold, James W.; Looney, Stephen W.; Viviani, Nancy J., et al. Predicting the health-related values and preferences of geriatric patients. *Journal of Family Practice.* 1994 Nov; 39(5): 461–467. 32 refs. BE60499.
　　*advance directives; *aged; *attitudes; competence; family relationship; health; patient care; *patients; persistent vegetative state; prolongation of life; *quality of life;

religion; resuscitation; socioeconomic factors; survey; terminal care; *value of life; *values; ventilators; *values histories; Oklahoma Health Sciences Center Geriatric Continuity Clinic

Moseley, Charles B. The impact of restraints on nursing home resident outcomes. *American Journal of Medical Quality.* 1997 Summer; 12(2): 94–102. 22 refs. BE59129.
　　*aged; comparative studies; evaluation studies; institutionalized persons; mentally disabled; *nursing homes; *patient care; *patients; *physical restraint; physically disabled; *treatment outcome; dependency; Virginia

O'Brien, James G., ed. Ethical and Legal Issues in Care of the Elderly. Proceedings of a Conference at Michigan State University, 14 Jun 1985. Issued by the Dept. of Family Practice, Michigan State University, East Lansing, MI; 1988. 119 p. BE62798.
　　advance care planning; *aged; autonomy; clinical ethics; competence; informed consent; institutionalized persons; long-term care; medical education; nursing homes; *patient care; social discrimination; third party consent; withholding treatment; elder abuse; geriatrics; United States

O'Connell, Laurence J. The role of religion in health-related decision making for elderly patients. *Generations (American Society on Aging).* 1994 Winter; 18(4): 27–30. 2 refs. BE60548.
　　*aged; bioethical issues; competence; *decision making; *patient care; *religion

Pascual, Julio; Liaño, Fernando; Madrid Acute Renal Failure Study Group. Causes and prognosis of acute renal failure in the very old. *Journal of the American Geriatrics Society.* 1998 Jun; 46(6): 721–725. 31 refs. BE62153.
　　*age factors; *aged; evaluation studies; intensive care units; *kidney diseases; *mortality; patient admission; *patient care; prevalence; *prognosis; quality of life; renal dialysis; resource allocation; *selection for treatment; social discrimination; withholding treatment; multicenter studies; prospective studies; *Madrid; Spain

Rakowski, Eric; Post, Stephen G. Should health care be rationed by age? Yes [and] No. *In:* Scharlach, Andrew E.; Kaye, Lenard W., eds. Controversial Issues in Aging. Boston, MA: Allyn and Bacon; 1997: 103–113. 9 refs. ISBN 0–205–19381–1. BE60963.
　　*age factors; *aged; autonomy; biomedical technologies; cultural pluralism; females; government financing; health care; justice; moral policy; prolongation of life; public policy; quality of life; *resource allocation; rights; *selection for treatment; social discrimination; value of life; values; needs; United States

Sachs, Greg A. Dementia and the goals of care. [Editorial]. *Journal of the American Geriatrics Society.* 1998 Jun; 46(6): 782–783. 5 refs. BE62256.
　　*advance care planning; *aged; *decision making; *dementia; family members; *goals; palliative care; *patient care; patient participation; physicians; preventive medicine; prolongation of life; rehabilitation; risks and benefits; values; withholding treatment; United States

Shaw, Allen B. Age as a basis for healthcare rationing: support for agist policies. *Drugs and Aging.* 1996 Dec; 9(6): 403–405. 21 refs. BE60379.
　　*age factors; *aged; *health care; justice; moral policy; public policy; *resource allocation; *selection for treatment; social discrimination; Great Britain

Smith, George P. Our hearts were once young and gay: health care rationing and the elderly. *University of Florida*

Journal of Law and Public Policy. 1996 Fall; 8(1): 1–23. 133 fn. BE59858.

age factors; *aged; decision making; economics; government financing; *health care delivery; justice; moral policy; obligations of society; obligations to society; paternalism; *public policy; *resource allocation; selection for treatment; social discrimination; value of life; withholding treatment; Medicaid; Medicare; United States

Sugarman, Jeremy; McCrory, Douglas C.; Hubal, Robert C. Getting meaningful informed consent from older adults: a structured literature review of empirical research. *Journal of the American Geriatrics Society.* 1998 Apr; 46(4): 517–524. 118 refs. BE60294.

age factors; *aged; competence; comprehension; consent forms; decision making; disclosure; education; *empirical research; evaluation studies; *human experimentation; *informed consent; literature; methods; *patient care; recall; research design; research subjects; selection of subjects; refusal to participate

Thomasma, David C. Stewardship of the aged: meeting the ethical challenge of ageism. *Cambridge Quarterly of Healthcare Ethics.* 1999 Spring; 8(2): 148–159. 38 fn. BE61232.

advance directives; *aged; allowing to die; autonomy; beneficence; biomedical technologies; case studies; casuistry; chronically ill; *clinical ethics; competence; covenant; *decision making; dissent; family members; health personnel; home care; hospitals; justice; legal guardians; long-term care; medicine; nursing homes; paternalism; *patient advocacy; *patient care; *patient participation; physical restraint; *physician patient relationship; prolongation of life; public policy; quality of life; resource allocation; right to die; risks and benefits; selection for treatment; social discrimination; terminal care; terminally ill; treatment refusal; *values; withholding treatment; elder abuse

Turner, N.J.; Haward, R.A.; Mulley, G.P., et al. Cancer in old age -- is it inadequately investigated and treated? *BMJ (British Medical Journal).* 1999 Jul 31; 319(7205): 309–312. 40 refs. BE62456.

*aged; *cancer; diagnosis; drugs; hormones; mass screening; palliative care; *patient care; quality of health care; radiology; *selection for treatment; social discrimination; surgery; treatment outcome; withholding treatment; *undertreatment; Great Britain

Varekamp, Inge; Meiland, Franka J.M.; Hoos, Aloysia M., et al. The meaning of urgency in the allocation of scarce health care resources; a comparison between renal transplantation and psychogeriatric nursing home care. *Health Policy.* 1998 May; 44(2): 135–148. 20 refs. 1 fn. BE59149.

*aged; critically ill; dementia; evaluation studies; family members; home care; *kidneys; nurses; *nursing homes; *organ transplantation; *patient admission; patient advocacy; patient compliance; physicians; *prognosis; psychological stress; *resource allocation; scarcity; *selection for treatment; *time factors; qualitative research; *Netherlands

Wasson, John H.; Bubolz, Thomas A.; Lynn, Joanne, et al. Can we afford comprehensive, supportive care for the very old? *Journal of the American Geriatrics Society.* 1998 Jul; 46(7): 829–832. 20 refs. BE62258.

*aged; *community services; *economics; government financing; health care; *health care delivery; health services research; *home care; *hospitals; managed care programs; mortality; patient admission; patient care; *resource allocation; *health services misuse; *Medicare; *United States

Weissman, David E.; Matson, Sandra. Pain assessment and management in the long-term care setting.

Theoretical Medicine and Bioethics. 1999 Jan; 20(1): 31–43. 53 refs. BE62122.

*aged; alternatives; attitudes; chronically ill; *dementia; diagnosis; education; health personnel; *institutional policies; *long-term care; *nursing homes; *opioid analgesics; *pain; *patient care; risks and benefits; technical expertise; toxicity; United States

Williams, Alan; Evans, J. Grimley. Rationing health care by age: the case for [and] The case against. *BMJ (British Medical Journal).* 1997 Mar 15; 314(7083): 820–825. BE60232.

*age factors; *aged; attitudes; common good; costs and benefits; goals; *health care; *justice; moral policy; patient care; quality adjusted life years; quality of life; *resource allocation; risks and benefits; *selection for treatment; social discrimination; social worth; treatment outcome; values; withholding treatment; needs; *Great Britain; *National Health Service

Wood, Erica; Karp, Naomi. Mediation: reframing care conflicts in nursing homes. *Generations (American Society on Aging).* 1994 Winter; 18(4): 54–57. 9 refs. BE60553.

*aged; bioethical issues; clinical ethics committees; decision making; dissent; family members; legal rights; long-term care; *mediation; *nursing homes; *patient care; patient care team; United States

Workman, Richard H.; Molinari, Victor; Rezabek, Pamela, et al. An ethical framework for understanding patients with antisocial personality disorder who develop dementia: diagnosing and managing disorders of autonomy. *Journal of Ethics, Law, and Aging.* 1997 Fall–Winter; 3(2): 79–90. 22 refs. BE60451.

accountability; *aged; aggression; *autonomy; *behavior disorders; case studies; *competence; comprehension; decision making; *dementia; diagnosis; evaluation; *hospitals; legal guardians; *paternalism; *patient care; patient care team; *patient compliance; *patient discharge; recall; standards; values

Zuccaro, Stefano Maria; Palleschi, Massimo; Italian Society of Hospital Geriatricians. Document on the rights of the sick elderly. *Dolentium Hominum: Church and Health in the World.* 1997; 36(12th Yr., No. 3): 32–35. 15 refs. BE60408.

*aged; autonomy; disclosure; freedom; *health care; health personnel; *organizational policies; patient care; *patients' rights; professional organizations; quality of health care; *rights; social worth; Europe; *Italian Society of Hospital Geriatricians

Zuckerman, Connie. Clinical ethics in geriatric care settings. *Generations (American Society on Aging).* 1994 Winter; 18(4): 9–12. 11 refs. BE60544.

*aged; autonomy; chronically ill; *clinical ethics; clinical ethics committees; *decision making; family members; home care; interdisciplinary communication; long-term care; mediation; nursing homes; *patient care; patient care team

PATIENT CARE/DRUGS

Abraham, John; Sheppard, Julie. Democracy, technocracy, and the secret state of medicines control: expert and nonexpert perspectives. *Science, Technology, and Human Values.* 1997 Spring; 22(2): 139–167. 38 refs. 2 fn. BE59854.

accountability; attitudes; committee membership; confidentiality; consensus; *decision making; drug abuse; *drug industry; *drugs; *government regulation; health personnel; investigators; mass media; patient care; physician's role; professional role; psychoactive drugs; public opinion; *public participation; public policy; risk; risks and benefits; science; survey; *technical expertise; trust; uncertainty; *values; questionnaires; Committee on the Safety of Medicines (Great Britain); *Great Britain; Medicines Commission (Great Britain)

Baleta, Adele. Huge percentage of women volunteer for zidovudine project. [News]. *Lancet.* 1999 Jan 16; 353(9148): 219. BE61564.
　　AIDS; *AIDS serodiagnosis; counseling; *drugs; economics; *HIV seropositivity; newborns; *patient care; *pregnant women; *preventive medicine; voluntary programs; *AZT; *South Africa; Western Cape

Beecham, Linda. UK issues guidance on prescribing Viagra. [News]. *BMJ (British Medical Journal).* 1999 Jan 30; 318(7179): 279. BE61556.
　　attitudes; diagnosis; dissent; drug industry; *drugs; *government financing; guidelines; *males; organizational policies; *patient care; *physicians; professional organizations; *public policy; *resource allocation; *selection for treatment; sexuality; social discrimination; *impotence; personal financing; British Medical Association; *Great Britain; *National Health Service; Royal College of Physicians; *Viagra

Beecham, Linda; Dorozynski, Alexander; Sheldon, Tony, et al. Viagra falls: the debate over rationing continues -- Britain, France, Netherlands, Italy, Switzerland, Spain, United States, Germany, Israel. *BMJ (British Medical Journal).* 1998 Sep 26; 317(7162): 836–838. BE59650.
　　*drugs; gatekeeping; *government financing; health care; *health insurance reimbursement; *international aspects; *males; national health insurance; *patient care; physicians; private sector; public policy; resource allocation; selection for treatment; sexuality; *impotence; personal financing; France; Germany; Great Britain; Israel; Italy; Netherlands; Spain; Switzerland; United States; *Viagra

Black, Douglas. Medicalised erections on demand? [Editorial]. *Journal of Medical Ethics.* 1999 Feb; 25(1): 5–7. 2 refs. BE61133.
　　decision making; drug industry; *drugs; *government financing; government regulation; health; health care; *health insurance reimbursement; international aspects; *males; *patient care; physicians; politics; public policy; quality of life; resource allocation; sexuality; *impotence; needs; personal financing; Great Britain; National Health Service; *Viagra

Blake, Robert L.; Early, Elizabeth K. Patients' attitudes about gifts to physicians from pharmaceutical companies. *Journal of the American Board of Family Practice.* 1995 Nov–Dec; 8(6): 457–464. 21 refs. BE61561.
　　advertising; *attitudes; *conflict of interest; continuing education; decision making; *drug industry; *drugs; economics; *financial support; *gifts; guidelines; incentives; *knowledge, attitudes, practice; *patient care; *patients; *physicians; professional organizations; survey; Missouri

Brooks, Alex. Viagra is licensed in Europe, but rationed in Britain. [News]. *BMJ (British Medical Journal).* 1998 Sep 19; 317(7161): 765. BE60827.
　　*drugs; *government financing; males; patient care; *public policy; *resource allocation; selection for treatment; sexuality; *impotence; *Great Britain; *National Health Service; *Viagra

Brown, Janet; Moore, Donna E.; Potter, David, et al. Placebos and the need for good communication: the case of George Hunter. [Case study and commentaries]. *Orthopaedic Nursing.* 1997 May–Jun; 16(3): 61–65. 2 refs. Reprinted from *Bioethics Bulletin,* 1994 Spring; 2(2): 1–7. BE61815.

aged; autonomy; beneficence; chronically ill; *deception; decision making; disclosure; drug abuse; drugs; informed consent; motivation; nurse patient relationship; nurses; *pain; paternalism; patient advocacy; *patient care; physician patient relationship; physicians; *placebos; risks and benefits; trust; opioids

Callahan, Joan C. Menopause: taking the cures or curing the takes? *In:* Walker, Margaret Urban, ed. Mother Time: Women, Aging, and Ethics. Lanham, MD: Rowman and Littlefield; 1999: 151–174. 48 fn. ISBN 0-8476-9260-4. BE61898.
　　adults; advertising; *age factors; cosmetic surgery; disclosure; drug industry; drugs; *females; *hormones; informed consent; *normality; *patient care; physicians; *risks and benefits; stigmatization; Western World; *women's health; *estrogen replacement therapy; *menopause; American Heart Association

Carnall, Douglas. American Medical Association moves to regulate prescribing on the Internet. [News]. *BMJ (British Medical Journal).* 1999 Jul 24; 319(7204): 213. BE62512.
　　*computer communication networks; *drugs; *patient care; physician patient relationship; *physicians; professional organizations; *regulation; risks and benefits; standards; *American Medical Association; *Internet; United States

Chase, Marilyn. Rationing scarce drugs has some questioning fairness and ethics. [News]. *Wall Street Journal.* 1998 Sep 28: B1. BE61125.
　　*breast cancer; *drug industry; females; *investigational drugs; patient care; *random selection; *resource allocation; *scarcity; *selection for treatment; selection of subjects; therapeutic research; *compassionate use; *Genentech Inc.; *Herceptin

Chisholm, John. Viagra: a botched test case for rationing. [Editorial]. *BMJ (British Medical Journal).* 1999 Jan 30; 318(7179): 273–274. 12 refs. BE60578.
　　*drugs; *government financing; *males; patient care; *public policy; *resource allocation; selection for treatment; sexuality; *impotence; *Great Britain; National Health Service; *Viagra

Collier, Joe. Patient-information leaflets and prescriber competence. *Lancet.* 1998 Nov 28; 352(9142): 1724. BE60800.
　　*drugs; government regulation; *information dissemination; international aspects; patient care; *patient education; *physicians; *professional competence; risks and benefits; standards; *European Union; *Great Britain; Medicines Control Agency (Great Britain)

DeLeon, Patrick H.; Bennett, Bruce E.; Bricklin, Patricia M. Ethics and public policy formulation: a case example related to prescription privileges. *Professional Psychology: Research and Practice.* 1997 Dec; 28(6): 518–525. 36 refs. BE59207.
　　*administrators; codes of ethics; conflict of interest; employment; *health personnel; interprofessional relations; patient care; physicians; politics; *professional autonomy; *professional ethics; professional organizations; psychiatry; *psychoactive drugs; *psychology; *public policy; technical expertise; American Psychological Association; United States

Elliott, Carl. The tyranny of happiness: ethics and cosmetic psychopharmacology. *In:* Parens, Erik, ed. Enhancing Human Traits: Ethical and Social Implications. Washington, DC: Georgetown University Press; 1998: 177–188. 11 fn. ISBN 0-87840-703-0. BE59752.
　　*behavior control; depressive disorder; *emotions;

BE = bioethics accession number　　　　　fn. = footnotes　　　　refs. = references

enhancement technologies; literature; *mental health; normality; psychiatry; *psychoactive drugs; psychological stress; *quality of life; *self concept; uncertainty; value of life; *values; Western World; authenticity; Listening to Prozac (Kramer, P.); Percy, Walker; Prozac; Twentieth Century; United States

Fieldston, Evan. AIDS, thalidomide and maternal–fetal rights in conflict. *Princeton Journal of Bioethics.* 1998 Spring; 1(1): 83–93. 9 refs. BE62495.
    *AIDS; autonomy; coercion; contraception; *drugs; *females; fetuses; *HIV seropositivity; iatrogenic disease; moral obligations; *patient care; preconception injuries; *pregnant women; *prenatal injuries; public health; quality of life; reproduction; selective abortion; *social control; toxicity; women's rights; *thalidomide

Freedman, Carol. Aspirin for the mind? Some ethical worries about psychopharmacology. *In:* Parens, Erik, ed. Enhancing Human Traits: Ethical and Social Implications. Washington, DC: Georgetown University Press; 1998: 135–150. 25 fn. ISBN 0–87840–703–0. BE59749.
    *emotions; enhancement technologies; mental health; moral policy; normality; pain; patient care; *psychoactive drugs; *psychological stress; psychotherapy; *self concept; suffering; Listening to Prozac (Kramer, P.)

Freudenheim, Milt. Psychiatric drugs are now promoted directly to patients. [News]. *New York Times.* 1998 Feb 17: D1, D3. BE59471.
    *advertising; computer communication networks; confidentiality; depressive disorder; *drug industry; economics; incentives; information dissemination; *mass media; *mentally ill; *patients; *psychoactive drugs; schizophrenia; Internet; United States

Glickman, Barry. Global challenges: ethical implications of the greening of modern Western medicine. *In:* Coward, Harold; Ratanakul, Pinit, eds. A Cross–Cultural Dialogue on Health Care Ethics. Waterloo, ON: Wilfrid Laurier University Press; 1999: 236–256. 45 refs. 1 fn. ISBN 0–88920–325–3. BE62796.
    *alternative therapies; drug industry; *ecology; economics; federal government; government regulation; internal medicine; medicine; folk medicine; vitamins; Canada; United States

Goldberg, Carey. Insurance for Viagra spurs coverage for birth control. [News]. *New York Times.* 1999 Jun 30: A1, A16. BE62445.
    *contraception; *drugs; *females; *government regulation; *health insurance reimbursement; *hormones; justice; *males; politics; state government; women's rights; United States; *Viagra

Grey, Matthew W. Medical use of marijuana: legal and ethical conflicts in the patient/physician relationship. [Comment]. *University of Richmond Law Review.* 1996 Jan; 30(1): 249–274. 66 fn. BE59862.
    AIDS; *autonomy; *beneficence; codes of ethics; federal government; government regulation; *legal aspects; *palliative care; patients; *physician patient relationship; physicians; professional organizations; *psychoactive drugs; terminally ill; compassionate use; *marijuana; American Medical Association; *United States

Griffith, David. Reasons for not seeing drug representatives: lightening workload, cutting costs, and improving quality. [Editorial]. *BMJ (British Medical Journal).* 1999 Jul 10; 319(7202): 69–70. 9 refs. BE62151.
    advertising; alternatives; communication; *conflict of interest; *drug industry; *drugs; *economics; information dissemination; motivation; *patient care; *physicians; quality

of health care; time factors; *physician's practice patterns; Great Britain

Haddox, J. David; Aronoff, Gerald M. Commentary: the potential for unintended consequences from public policy shifts in the treatment of pain. *Journal of Law, Medicine and Ethics.* 1998 Winter; 26(4): 350–352. 8 fn. BE61167.
    *chronically ill; drug abuse; *drugs; government regulation; misconduct; *opioid analgesics; *pain; *palliative care; *patient care; *physicians; politics; *practice guidelines; *public policy; *regulation; *risks and benefits; state government; *Federation of State Medical Boards; United States

Hassenfeld, Irwin N.; Hoge, Steven K. Consequences of involuntary treatment. [Letter and response]. *American Journal of Psychiatry.* 1998 Mar; 155(3): 450–451. 4 refs. BE59375.
    *autonomy; *coercion; decision making; empirical research; informed consent; involuntary commitment; judicial action; *mentally ill; *patient care; patient compliance; *patient participation; physician patient relationship; *psychoactive drugs; *treatment outcome; *treatment refusal; Massachusetts; New York; Virginia

Hoffmann, Diane E. Pain management and palliative care in the era of managed care: issues for health insurers. *Journal of Law, Medicine and Ethics.* 1998 Winter; 26(4): 267–289. 126 fn. BE61163.
    *administrators; aged; alternatives; anesthesia; attitudes; biomedical technologies; *chronically ill; *costs and benefits; diagnosis; drug abuse; *drugs; *economics; fraud; health facilities; *health insurance; *health insurance reimbursement; hospices; *managed care programs; medical devices; medical specialties; mental health; opioid analgesics; *organizational policies; *pain; *palliative care; *patient care; physicians; practice guidelines; public policy; *quality of health care; referral and consultation; resource allocation; surgery; survey; *terminal care; *terminally ill; therapeutic research; treatment outcome; acupuncture; biofeedback (psychology); *undertreatment; American Association of Health Plans; *Blue Cross–Blue Shield; Medicare; *United States

Hollon, Matthew F. Direct–to–consumer marketing of prescription drugs: creating consumer demand. *JAMA.* 1999 Jan 27; 281(4): 382–384. 32 refs. BE60238.
    *advertising; decision making; *drug industry; *drugs; economics; federal government; government regulation; information dissemination; *mass media; patient care; physician patient relationship; public health; *risks and benefits; Food and Drug Administration; United States

Holmer, Alan F. Direct–to–consumer prescription drug advertising builds bridges between patients and physicians. *JAMA.* 1999 Jan 27; 281(4): 380–382. 21 refs. BE60237.
    *advertising; *drug industry; *drugs; health education; information dissemination; *mass media; patient care; patient compliance; physician patient relationship; public health; *risks and benefits; social impact; United States

Jost, Timothy S. Public financing of pain management: leaky umbrellas and ragged safety nets. *Journal of Law, Medicine and Ethics.* 1998 Winter; 26(4): 290–307. 194 fn. BE61164.
    aged; alternatives; biomedical technologies; *chronically ill; costs and benefits; *drugs; economics; federal government; fraud; *government financing; hospices; hospitals; indigents; managed care programs; medical devices; nursing homes; opioid analgesics; *pain; *palliative care; *patient care; patients; quality of health care; state government; suffering; *terminal care; *terminally ill; time factors; utilization review; *Medicaid; *Medicare; *United States

---

Kolata, Gina; Eichenwald, Kurt. For the uninsured, drug trials are health care. [Stopgap medicine: a special report]. *New York Times.* 1999 Jun 22: A1, C12. BE62248.
    chronically ill; coercion; *conflict of interest; deception; drug industry; *human experimentation; *indigents; *investigational drugs; investigators; managed care programs; patient care; *patients; *physicians; placebos; quality of health care; research subjects; risks and benefits; patient abandonment; *private practice; United States

La Puma, John. Physician rewards for postmarketing surveillance (seeding studies) in the US. [Editorial]. *PharmacoEconomics.* 1995 Mar; 7(3): 187–190. 14 refs. BE59156.
    advertising; conflict of interest; *disclosure; *drug industry; *drugs; goals; *human experimentation; incentives; informed consent; *investigators; *physicians; *remuneration; *postmarketing research; United States

Lagnado, Lucette. Transplant patients ply an illicit market for vital medicines. [News]. *Wall Street Journal.* 1999 Jun 21: 1, A8. BE62450.
    *drugs; *economics; health insurance reimbursement; health personnel; hospitals; institutional policies; legal aspects: *misconduct; motivation; *organ transplantation; *patient care; patients; *transplant recipients; Medicaid; Medicare; United States

Long, Stephen P.; Medical Society of Virginia. Pain Management Subcommittee. MSV [Medical Society of Virginia] House of Delegates passes opioid guidelines. *Virginia Medical Quarterly.* 1998 Winter; 125(1): 8–11. BE60848.
    *chronically ill; *drugs; *guidelines; informed consent; medical records; *opioid analgesics; *pain; *palliative care; physicians; practice guidelines; professional organizations; *Medical Society of Virginia

McCaffery, Margo; Ferrell, Betty Rolling. Pain and placebos: ethical and professional issues. [Editorial]. *Orthopaedic Nursing.* 1997 Sep–Oct; 16(5): 8–11. 22 refs. Commentary on J. Brown et al., "Placebos and the need for good communication," *ON* 1997 Apr–May; 16(3): 61–65. BE60263.
    *attitudes; *deception; guideline adherence; health facilities; institutional policies; knowledge, attitudes, practice; misconduct; motivation; *nurses; *organizational policies; *pain; patient advocacy; *patient care; *placebos; practice guidelines; *professional organizations; risks and benefits; trust; analgesia

Margolis, Lewis H.; Rosner, Fred; Reynolds, Susan, et al. Personal use of drug samples by physicians and office staff. [Letters and responses]. *JAMA.* 1997 Nov 19; 278(19): 1567–1569. 13 refs. BE59340.
    *advertising; conflict of interest; *drug industry; *drugs; economics; family members; financial support; *gifts; medical ethics; *organizational policies; *patient care; *physicians; professional organizations; risks and benefits; *self care; American Medical Association

Mariner, Wendy K. Equitable access to biomedical advances: getting beyond the rights impasse. *Connecticut Law Review.* 1989 Spring; 21(3): 571–603. 103 fn. BE62127.
    abortion, induced; AIDS; *biomedical technologies; constitutional law; costs and benefits; drug industry; *drugs; federal government; government financing; *government regulation; *health care; *investigational drugs; justice; *legal aspects; *legal rights; *obligations of society; *organ transplantation; patient advocacy; patient care; patients; political activity; private sector; *public policy; public sector; *resource allocation; *unproven therapies; Food and

Drug Administration; *France; Roussel Uclaf; *RU–486; *United States

Martino, Ann M. In search of a new ethic for treating patients with chronic pain: what can medical boards do? *Journal of Law, Medicine and Ethics.* 1998 Winter; 26(4): 332–349. 83 fn. BE61166.
    accountability; *attitudes; *chronically ill; double effect; drug abuse; *drugs; empirical research; government regulation; health insurance reimbursement; institutional policies; legal liability; medical education; misconduct; *motivation; nurses; *opioid analgesics; *pain; *palliative care; patient advocacy; *patient care; peer review; pharmacists; *physicians; *practice guidelines; quality of health care; *regulation; religion; risk; sociology of medicine; standards; state government; stigmatization; suffering; survey; terminally ill; *values; withholding treatment; *undertreatment; Compassion in Dying; *United States

Nightingale, Stuart L.; Brown, Philip; Levin, Arthur Aaron, et al. Advertising prescription–only drugs. [Letters]. *Lancet.* 1998 May 23; 351(9115): 1582–1584. 9 refs. BE59248.
    *advertising; *drug industry; *drugs; economics; federal government; government regulation; *information dissemination; international aspects; *mass media; patient participation; patients; physician patient relationship; risks and benefits; Food and Drug Administration; United States

Post, Stephen G.; Whitehouse, Peter J. Emerging antidementia drugs: a preliminary ethical view. *Journal of the American Geriatrics Society.* 1998 Jun; 46(6): 784–787. 11 refs. BE62257.
    aged; beneficence; case studies; decision making; *dementia; *drugs; economics; family members; goals; justice; morbidity; nursing homes; patient admission; *patient care; patients; prolongation of life; psychological stress; *quality of life; *risks and benefits; *treatment outcome; *withholding treatment; Aricept

Rogers, Wendy A. Menopause: is this a disease and should we treat it? *In:* Donchin, Anne; Purdy, Laura M., eds. Embodying Bioethics: Recent Feminist Advances. Lanham, MD: Rowman and Littlefield; 1999: 203–219. 49 refs. 15 fn. ISBN 0–8476–8924–7. BE61022.
    age factors; aged; costs and benefits; *disease; drugs; *females; feminist ethics; *hormones; *normality; obstetrics and gynecology; patient care; risks and benefits; *women's health; *estrogen replacement therapy; *menopause; Australia

Rose, Steven P.R. Neurogenetic determinism and the new euphenics. *BMJ (British Medical Journal).* 1998 Dec 19–26; 317(7174): 1707–1708. 5 refs. BE60839.
    aggression; *behavior control; behavior disorders; *behavioral genetics; brain pathology; drug industry; *genetic determinism; genetic predisposition; hyperkinesis; *psychoactive drugs; social problems; trends

Rosenthal, Elisabeth. West's medicine is raising bills for China's sick. [News]. *New York Times.* 1998 Nov 19: A1, A12. BE61119.
    conflict of interest; *drug industry; *drugs; *economics; *health care; hospitals; *incentives; institutional policies; international aspects; misconduct; physicians; remuneration; Western World; *China

Roy, David J. The relief of pain and suffering: ethical principles and imperatives. [Editorial]. *Journal of Palliative Care.* 1998 Summer; 14(2): 3–5. 8 refs. BE61955.
    chronically ill; common good; communication; compassion; critically ill; *drugs; education; health care delivery; justice; *moral obligations; *moral policy; nurses; opioid analgesics; *pain; *palliative care; patient care; physicians; professional

---

BE = bioethics accession number   fn. = footnotes   refs. = references

competence; professional patient relationship; psychological stress; sedatives; *suffering; terminal care; terminally ill; dignity

Shapiro, Arthur K.; Shapiro, Elaine. The Powerful Placebo: From Ancient Priest to Modern Physician. Baltimore, MD: Johns Hopkins University Press; 1997. 280 p. Bibliography: p. 239–272. ISBN 0-8018-5569-1. BE62149.
alternative therapies; ancient history; attitudes; control groups; drugs; empirical research; ethicists; evaluation; fraud; *historical aspects; *human experimentation; international aspects; *patient care; patients; physicians; *placebos; psychoactive drugs; psychotherapy; random selection; *research design; review; risks and benefits; scientific misconduct; surgery; terminology; quackery; Eighteenth Century; Middle Ages; Nineteenth Century; Seventeenth Century; Twentieth Century

Smith, George P. Terminal sedation as palliative care: revalidating a right to a good death. *Cambridge Quarterly of Healthcare Ethics.* 1998 Fall; 7(4): 382–387. 37 fn. BE59139.
*drugs; legal aspects; pain; *palliative care; physicians; quality of health care; right to die; *sedatives; standards; suffering; *terminal care; terminally ill; United States

Smith, Richard. Viagra and rationing: let the sunlight in, let the people speak. [Editorial]. *BMJ (British Medical Journal).* 1998 Sep 19; 317(7161): 760–761. 6 refs. BE60826.
decision making; *drugs; government financing; males; public participation; *public policy; *resource allocation; sexuality; values; *impotence; *Great Britain; *National Health Service; Rationing Agenda Group (Great Britain); United States; *Viagra

Steinbrook, Robert. Caring for people with human immunodeficiency virus infection. [Editorial]. *New England Journal of Medicine.* 1998 Dec 24; 339(26): 1926–1928. 15 refs. BE60262.
adults; *AIDS; children; *disadvantaged; *drugs; *economics; federal government; *government financing; *health care delivery; *HIV seropositivity; mortality; *patient care; prevalence; *public policy; state government; statistics; Department of Veterans Affairs; Medicaid; Medicare; *United States

Stolberg, Sheryl Gay. Internet prescriptions boom in the "Wild West" of the Web: a special report. *New York Times.* 1999 Jun 27: 1, 14. BE62349.
advertising; *computer communication networks; deception; *drug industry; *drugs; economics; misconduct; patient care; pharmacists; *physicians; professional competence; regulation; standards; *Internet; United States; Viagra

VACO [VA Central Office] Bioethics Committee. Allocation of expensive medications. Report. *NCCE News (Veterans Health Administration National Center for Clinical Ethics).* 1995 Spring; 3(2, Suppl.): S1–S9. 4 refs. 1 fn. BE61470.
*costs and benefits; decision making; *drugs; *guidelines; military personnel; *patient care; practice guidelines; public hospitals; renal dialysis; *resource allocation; review committees; scarcity; pharmacy and therapeutics committees; erythropoietin; United States; *VACO (Veterans Affairs Central Office) Bioethics Committee

Veatch, Robert M.; Haddad, Amy. Case Studies in Pharmacy Ethics. New York, NY: Oxford University Press; 1999. 290 p. 165 fn. ISBN 0–19–513280–7. BE62740.
abortion, induced; autonomy; behavior control; beneficence; bioethical issues; capital punishment; *case studies;

competence; confidentiality; conflict of interest; conscience; contraception; decision making; drug industry; *drugs; economics; ethical analysis; futility; health insurance; human experimentation; justice; killing; misconduct; *moral obligations; pain; *patient care; patient education; *pharmacists; placebos; *professional ethics; professional patient relationship; terminal care; treatment refusal; truth disclosure; values; United States

Waldholz, Michael. AZT price cut for Third World mothers-to-be. [News]. *Wall Street Journal.* 1998 Mar 5: B1, B12. BE59369.
*developing countries; *drug industry; *drugs; *economics; *HIV seropositivity; human experimentation; newborns; patient care; placebos; *pregnant women; research design; *AZT; *Glaxo-Wellcome

Watts, Jonathan. When impotence leads contraception. [News]. *Lancet.* 1999 Mar 6; 353(9155): 819. BE61038.
*contraception; *drugs; *females; *government regulation; *hormones; *males; mass media; political activity; public policy; sexuality; social discrimination; *impotence; *Japan; *Viagra

Weissman, David E.; Matson, Sandra. Pain assessment and management in the long-term care setting. *Theoretical Medicine and Bioethics.* 1999 Jan; 20(1): 31–43. 53 refs. BE62122.
*aged; alternatives; attitudes; chronically ill; *dementia; diagnosis; *drugs; education; health personnel; *institutional policies; *long-term care; *nursing homes; *opioid analgesics; *pain; *patient care; risks and benefits; technical expertise; toxicity; United States

Wise, Jacqui. Aricept advertisement breached code. [News]. *BMJ (British Medical Journal).* 1998 Sep 19; 317(7161): 766. BE60952.
*advertising; *deception; *dementia; *drug industry; *drugs; misconduct; patient care; regulation; Great Britain; *Prescription Medicines Code of Practice Authority

Zuger, Abigail. Doctors' offices turn into salesrooms. [News]. *New York Times.* 1999 Mar 30: F1, F11. BE60875.
*alternative therapies; coercion; *conflict of interest; dissent; *drugs; *economics; *entrepreneurship; managed care programs; organizational policies; *patient care; *physicians; professional organizations; remuneration; American Medical Association; United States

Patients for hire, doctors for sale. [Editorial]. *New York Times.* 1999 May 22: A12. BE62247.
*conflict of interest; disclosure; *drug industry; fraud; *human experimentation; *incentives; indigents; *investigational drugs; medical ethics; misconduct; patient care; *physicians; *remuneration; research subjects; selection of subjects; *private practice; United States

World Medical Association adopts statements, etc., on miscellaneous matters. [Texts of statements and declarations]. *International Digest of Health Legislation.* 1997; 48(1): 92–97. Statements and declarations adopted by the 48th General Assembly of the World Medical Association, held in Somerset West, Republic of South Africa, Oct 1996; including the Declaration of Helsinki as amended Oct 1996. BE59591.
*bioethical issues; biomedical research; *contraception; *domestic violence; *drugs; *family planning; *guidelines; *human experimentation; informed consent; *international aspects; medical education; nontherapeutic research; *organizational policies; *patient care; *physicians; *professional competence; professional organizations; public policy; quality of health care; research ethics committees; self regulation; therapeutic research; third party consent; women's rights; *antibiotics; *Declaration of Helsinki;

BE = bioethics accession number   fn. = footnotes   refs. = references

*World Medical Association

PATIENT CARE/MENTALLY DISABLED

Adshead, Gwen. Ethics in psychiatric research and practice. *Current Opinion in Psychiatry.* 1996 Sep; 9(5): 348–351. 37 refs. BE60596.
  competence; confidentiality; *human experimentation; informed consent; *mentally ill; misconduct; *patient care; physician patient relationship; *psychiatry; research ethics committees; research subjects; social discrimination

Antuono, Piero; Beyer, Jan. The burden of dementia: a medical and research perspective. *Theoretical Medicine and Bioethics.* 1999 Jan; 20(1): 3–13. 34 refs. BE62120.
  *aged; autonomy; brain pathology; *dementia; diagnosis; drugs; economics; family members; genetic predisposition; home care; paternalism; *patient care; therapeutic research

Backlar, Patricia. Can we bridge the gap between the actual lives of persons with serious mental disorders and the therapeutic goals of their providers? *Community Mental Health Journal.* 1997 Dec; 33(6): 465–471. 22 refs. BE59382.
  *chronically ill; *community services; family members; friends; *mentally ill; *patient care; patient compliance; schizophrenia; social interaction

Bloch, Sidney; Harari, Edwin. Working with the family: the role of values. *American Journal of Psychotherapy.* 1996 Summer; 50(3): 274–284. 22 refs. BE62051.
  children; *family relationship; females; feminist ethics; informed consent; justice; males; minority groups; parents; *professional family relationship; *professional patient relationship; *psychotherapy; social discrimination; *values; *family therapy; relational ethics

Bursztajn, Harold J.; Pearlman, Theodore; Slovenko, Ralph, et al. Psychotherapist versus expert witness. [Letters and response]. *American Journal of Psychiatry.* 1998 Feb; 155(2): 307–308. 11 refs. BE59678.
  confidentiality; conflict of interest; disclosure; empathy; *expert testimony; *forensic psychiatry; legal aspects; physician's role; *psychotherapy

Callender, John S. Ethics and aims in psychotherapy: a contribution from Kant. *Journal of Medical Ethics.* 1998 Aug; 24(4): 274–278. 41 fn. BE61295.
  *autonomy; behavior control; deontological ethics; freedom; *goals; patients; philosophy; professional patient relationship; *psychotherapy; *self concept; suicide; rationality; *Kant, Immanuel
  Psychotherapy is an activity which takes many forms and which has many aims. The present paper argues that it can be viewed as a form of moral suasion. Kant's concepts of free will and ethics are described and these are then applied to the processes and outcome of psychotherapy. It is argued that his ideas, by linking rationality, free will and ethics into a single philosophical system, offer a valuable theoretical framework for thinking about aims and ethical issues in psychotherapy.

Chick, Jonathan. Treatment of alcoholic violent offenders: ethics and efficacy. *Alcohol and Alcoholism.* 1998 Jan–Feb; 33(1): 20–25. 38 refs. BE60680.
  *alcohol abuse; behavior disorders; *coercion; counseling; criminal law; dangerousness; employment; international aspects; law enforcement; legal aspects; *mandatory programs; outpatient commitment; *patient care; patient compliance; prisoners; psychoactive drugs; *treatment outcome; *violence; *voluntary programs

Chodoff, Paul. Ethical dimensions of psychotherapy: a personal perspective. *American Journal of Psychotherapy.* 1996 Summer; 50(3): 298–310. 20 refs. BE62053.
  child abuse; confidentiality; economics; health insurance reimbursement; health personnel; mentally ill; misconduct; *professional competence; *professional ethics; *professional patient relationship; *psychotherapy; recall; sex offenses; social dominance

Cohen, Elias S.; Kruschwitz, Ann L. Restraint reduction: lessons from the asylum. *Journal of Ethics, Law, and Aging.* 1997 Spring–Summer; 3(1): 25–43. 72 fn. BE59202.
  *aged; *behavior control; decision making; *dementia; education; federal government; government regulation; health personnel; historical aspects; *institutional policies; international aspects; legal aspects; *mental institutions; *mentally disabled; moral obligations; *nursing homes; patient advocacy; *patient care; *physical restraint; psychoactive drugs; quality of health care; state government; Eighteenth Century; Europe; Great Britain; Medicaid; Medicare; Nineteenth Century; Twentieth Century; *United States; Youngberg v. Romeo

Constantino, Rose E.; Boneysteele, Ginger; Gesmond, Sharyn A., et al. Restraining an aggressive suicidal, paraplegic patient: a look at the ethical and legal issues. *Dimensions of Critical Care Nursing.* 1997 May–Jun; 16(3): 144–151. 12 refs. BE59177.
  aggression; *behavior control; beneficence; case studies; decision making; freedom; hospitals; informed consent; *injuries; *intensive care units; legal liability; *nurses; nursing ethics; paralysis; *patient care; patient care team; *physical restraint; professional family relationship; referral and consultation; suicide; *violence

Dinwiddie, Stephen H.; Yutzy, Sean H. Ethical issues in psychiatric practice. *In:* Guze, Samuel B., ed. Adult Psychiatry. (Mosby's neurology psychiatry access series). St. Louis, MO: Mosby-Year Book; 1996: 445–453. 2 refs. ISBN 0-8151-3993-4. BE61058.
  alcohol abuse; assisted suicide; autonomy; beneficence; competence; confidentiality; conflict of interest; depressive disorder; human experimentation; informed consent; *medical ethics; *mentally ill; organ transplantation; paternalism; *patient care; physician patient relationship; *psychiatry; referral and consultation; risks and benefits; selection for treatment; treatment refusal

Downs, Murna. The emergence of the person in dementia research. *Ageing and Society.* 1997 Sep; 17(5): 597–607. 56 refs. BE59196.
  aged; autonomy; *behavioral research; communication; competence; *dementia; diagnosis; empirical research; family members; health services research; informed consent; *patient care; *patient participation; personhood; *research design; rights; risks and benefits; self concept; truth disclosure; support groups; United States

Dwyer, James; Shih, Anthony. The ethics of tailoring the patient's chart. *Psychiatric Services.* 1998 Oct; 49(10): 1309–1312. 16 refs. BE61447.
  beneficence; case studies; dangerousness; *deception; depressive disorder; health insurance reimbursement; involuntary commitment; legal liability; malpractice; managed care programs; *medical records; *mentally ill; *moral policy; *motivation; patient care; *physicians; *psychiatry; referral and consultation; resource allocation; schizophrenia; suicide; trust

Freudenheim, Milt. Psychiatric drugs are now promoted directly to patients. [News]. *New York Times.* 1998 Feb 17: D1, D3. BE59471.
  *advertising; computer communication networks; confidentiality; depressive disorder; *drug industry; economics; incentives; information dissemination; *mass

media; *mentally ill; *patients; *psychoactive drugs; schizophrenia; Internet; United States

Gigli, Gian Luigi. The unfinished project: ethical problems and strategies for action on mental retardation. *Dolentium Hominum: Church and Health in the World.* 1997; 34(12th Yr., No. 1): 64–76. 26 refs. BE60495.
  children; ecology; economics; education; family relationship; gene therapy; genetic counseling; genetic screening; health hazards; human rights; intelligence; mental institutions; mentally ill; *mentally retarded; obligations of society; *patient care; prenatal diagnosis; *preventive medicine; psychiatry; psychoactive drugs; public policy; selective abortion

Glover, Nicola. Community care -- same problems, different epithet? *Journal of Medical Ethics.* 1998 Oct; 24(5): 336–340. 9 refs. BE60256.
  coercion; *community services; dangerousness; *deinstitutionalized persons; evaluation; freedom; *legal aspects; legal guardians; *mentally ill; *outpatient commitment; paternalism; *patient care; patient compliance; psychoactive drugs; time factors; *Great Britain; *Mental Health (Patients in the Community) Act 1995
  A negative image of community care prevails. This method of care is perceived to be a relatively novel phenomenon and has received mixed media coverage. The negative image of community care has led to the growing belief that this care method has failed. This failure has largely been ascribed to the lack of powers available to control patients in the community and to the method's relative novelty. However, this paper contends that there are two flaws to the above assertion: first, community care is far from new, and second, the inherent problem is not the lack of powers available to control patients in the community, but, essentially, the absence of a secure and stable environment within the community.

Halasz, George. The rights of the child in psychotherapy. *American Journal of Psychotherapy.* 1996 Summer; 50(3): 285–297. 30 refs. BE62052.
  behavior disorders; case studies; *children; empathy; informed consent; managed care programs; parent child relationship; parental consent; patient compliance; professional patient relationship; *psychotherapy; rights

Hermann, Robert; Méhes, Károly. Physicians' attitudes regarding Down syndrome. *Journal of Child Neurology.* 1996 Jan; 11(1): 66–69. 15 refs. BE60189.
  active euthanasia; *allowing to die; *attitudes; children; clinical ethics committees; comparative studies; congenital disorders; *decision making; *Down syndrome; education; international aspects; medical specialties; mentally retarded; *newborns; nurses; parents; *patient care; pediatrics; *physicians; *prolongation of life; quality of life; selection for treatment; *surgery; survey; *withholding treatment; neurology; Canada; *Hungary

Hofland, Brian F. When capacity fades and autonomy is constricted: a client-centered approach to residential care. *Generations (American Society on Aging).* 1994 Winter; 18(4): 31–35. 22 refs. BE60549.
  advance directives; aged; *autonomy; beneficence; communication; *competence; decision making; *dementia; health personnel; *long-term care; nursing homes; *patient care; professional patient relationship; residential facilities

Holmes, Jeremy. Values in psychotherapy. *American Journal of Psychotherapy.* 1996 Summer; 50(3): 259–273. 31 refs. BE59882.
  health personnel; mentally ill; postmodernism; *professional ethics; professional patient relationship; *psychotherapy; religion; science; *values; Freud, Sigmund

Kjellin, Lars; Andersson, Kristina; Candefjord, Inga-Lill, et al. Ethical benefits and costs of coercion in short-term inpatient psychiatric care. *Psychiatric Services.* 1997 Dec; 48(12): 1567–1570. 12 refs. BE61624.
  *autonomy; beneficence; *coercion; comparative studies; evaluation studies; hospitals; *institutionalized persons; *involuntary commitment; mental health; mental institutions; *mentally ill; *patient care; patient discharge; patient satisfaction; risks and benefits; survey; *treatment outcome; *voluntary admission; *Sweden

Kjellin, Lars; Westrin, Claes-Göran. Involuntary admissions and coercive measures in psychiatric care: registered and reported. *International Journal of Law and Psychiatry.* 1998 Winter; 21(1): 31–42. 20 refs. BE59929.
  *coercion; comparative studies; family members; institutionalized persons; *involuntary commitment; medical records; mental institutions; *mentally ill; nurses; *patient admission; *patient care; patients; physical restraint; psychoactive drugs; standards; survey; time factors; *voluntary admission; *Sweden

Kullgren, G.; Jacobsson, L.; Lynöe, N., et al. Practices and attitudes among Swedish psychiatrists regarding the ethics of compulsory treatment. *Acta Psychiatrica Scandinavica.* 1996 May; 93(5): 389–396. 13 refs. BE61553.
  case studies; *coercion; dangerousness; decision making; electroconvulsive therapy; family members; *involuntary commitment; *knowledge, attitudes, practice; medical ethics; *mentally ill; misconduct; paternalism; *patient care; *physical restraint; physician patient relationship; *physicians; presumed consent; psychiatric diagnosis; *psychiatry; psychoactive drugs; sex offenses; sexuality; sterilization (sexual); therapeutic abortion; truth disclosure; *Sweden

Lamdan, Ruth M.; Ahmed, Ziauddin; Lee, Jean. General anesthesia: an extreme form of chemical and physical restraint. [Case analysis]. *HEC (HealthCare Ethics Committee) Forum.* 1998 Sep-Dec; 10(3-4): 317–322. BE61183.
  *anesthesia; *behavior control; case studies; competence; *critically ill; *mentally disabled; patient compliance; *physical restraint; *psychoactive drugs; renal dialysis; treatment refusal

Launer, John. A narrative approach to mental health in general practice: narrative based medicine. *BMJ (British Medical Journal).* 1999 Jan 9; 318(7176): 117–119. 21 refs. BE60844.
  behavior disorders; case studies; *communication; depressive disorder; diagnosis; drug abuse; family practice; *mentally disabled; narrative ethics; *patient care; physician patient relationship; socioeconomic factors; Great Britain

Lerner, Paul. Rationalizing the therapeutic arsenal: German neuropsychiatry in World War I. *In:* Berg, Manfred; Cocks, Geoffrey, eds. Medicine and Modernity: Public Health and Medical Care in Nineteenth- and Twentieth-Century Germany. New York, NY: Cambridge University Press; 1997: 121–148. 106 fn. ISBN 0-521-56411-5. BE59268.
  *attitudes; coercion; common good; deception; electroconvulsive therapy; *historical aspects; hypnosis; *mental health; *mentally ill; methods; *military personnel; misconduct; obligations to society; *patient care; physician patient relationship; physician's role; *physicians; psychiatric diagnosis; *psychiatry; psychotherapy; *public policy; rehabilitation; social control; social dominance; *war; post-traumatic stress disorders; *Germany; *Twentieth Century; *World War I

Long, Ann; Slevin, Eamonn. Living with dementia:

---

communicating with an older person and her family. *Nursing Ethics.* 1999 Jan; 6(1): 23–36. 54 refs. BE60152.
*aged; autonomy; beneficence; *caring; *communication; deception; dehumanization; *dementia; diagnosis; empathy; ethical analysis; family members; family relationship; humanism; *nurse patient relationship; *nurses; *nursing education; nursing research; paternalism; *patient care; *professional family relationship; psychological stress; psychology; social dominance; stigmatization; truth disclosure; adult offspring; University of Ulster (Northern Ireland)

Merskey, Harold. Ethical issues in the search for repressed memories. *American Journal of Psychotherapy.* 1996 Summer; 50(3): 323–335. 32 refs. BE62055.
*child abuse; health personnel; informed consent; knowledge, attitudes, practice; legal aspects; legislation; mandatory reporting; methods; organizational policies; professional organizations; *psychotherapy; *recall; sex offenses; Child Abuse Prevention and Treatment Act 1973; Great Britain; United States

Mester, Roberto; Mozes, Tamar; Blumensohn, Rachel, et al. The new Israeli psychiatric legislation for the minor (1995) and its relationship to the 1991 Law for the Treatment of the Mentally Ill. *International Journal of Law and Psychiatry.* 1998 Summer; 21(3): 281–289. 8 refs. BE61670.
adults; confidentiality; health personnel; involuntary commitment; *legal aspects; *legislation; *mentally ill; *minors; outpatient commitment; *patient care; professional competence; psychiatric diagnosis; psychiatry; psychology; *Israel; *Law for the Treatment of the Mentally Ill 1991 (Israel); *Youth (Care and Supervision) Law 1960 (1995 Amendments) (Israel)

Miller, Robert D. The continuum of coercion: constitutional and clinical considerations in the treatment of mentally disordered persons. *Denver University Law Review.* 1997; 74(4): 1169–1214. 244 fn. BE62219.
autonomy; cardiac death; child abuse; *coercion; competence; criminal law; dangerousness; deinstitutionalized persons; domestic violence; duty to warn; *informal social control; informed consent; institutionalized persons; involuntary commitment; judicial action; *legal aspects; managed care programs; mandatory reporting; mental institutions; *mentally ill; outpatient commitment; paternalism; patient advocacy; *patient care; physical restraint; physicians; prisoners; professional autonomy; psychiatric wills; psychiatry; psychoactive drugs; psychotherapy; right to treatment; sex offenses; *social control; stigmatization; treatment refusal; violence; voluntary admission; *United States

Murphy, Michael J.; DeBernardo, Caren R.; Shoemaker, Wendy E. Impact of managed care on independent practice and professional ethics: a survey of independent practitioners. *Professional Psychology: Research and Practice.* 1998 Feb; 29(1): 43–51. 18 refs. BE59209.
codes of ethics; confidentiality; deception; *decision making; disclosure; economics; health insurance reimbursement; *health personnel; incentives; *knowledge, attitudes, practice; *managed care programs; patient advocacy; patient care; professional autonomy; professional ethics; professional organizations; psychiatric diagnosis; psychoactive drugs; *psychology; *psychotherapy; *quality of health care; social impact; survey; utilization review; American Psychological Association; *United States

Olsen, Douglas P. Toward an ethical standard for coerced mental health treatment: least restrictive or most therapeutic? *Journal of Clinical Ethics.* 1998 Fall; 9(3): 235–246. 36 fn. BE61332.
alternative therapies; attitudes; autonomy; beneficence;

*coercion; common good; competence; dangerousness; freedom; guidelines; involuntary commitment; legal aspects; *mentally ill; minors; *patient care; physical restraint; psychoactive drugs; *standards; treatment refusal; voluntary admission; United States

Petrila, John. Ethics, money, and the problem of coercion in managed behavioral health care. *Saint Louis University Law Journal.* 1996 Spring; 40(2): 359–405. 145 fn. BE60063.
chronically ill; coercion; community services; *conflict of interest; dangerousness; *health care delivery; *health insurance reimbursement; incentives; involuntary commitment; *legal aspects; *legal liability; legal obligations; malpractice; *managed care programs; mental institutions; *mentally ill; moral obligations; *patient advocacy; *patient care; *patient discharge; physician patient relationship; *physicians; practice guidelines; private sector; public sector; quality of health care; remuneration; risk; standards; voluntary admission; withholding treatment; capitation fee; *continuity of patient care; Medicaid; United States

Post, Stephen G.; Whitehouse, Peter J. Emerging antidementia drugs: a preliminary ethical view. *Journal of the American Geriatrics Society.* 1998 Jun; 46(6): 784–787. 11 refs. BE62257.
aged; beneficence; case studies; decision making; *dementia; *drugs; economics; family members; goals; justice; morbidity; nursing homes; patient admission; *patient care; patients; prolongation of life; psychological stress; *quality of life; *risks and benefits; *treatment outcome; *withholding treatment; Aricept

Sachs, Greg A. Dementia and the goals of care. [Editorial]. *Journal of the American Geriatrics Society.* 1998 Jun; 46(6): 782–783. 5 refs. BE62256.
*advance care planning; *aged; *decision making; *dementia; family members; *goals; palliative care; *patient care; patient participation; physicians; preventive medicine; prolongation of life; rehabilitation; risks and benefits; values; withholding treatment; United States

Schiavone, Michele. Ethics and psychiatry. *Dolentium Hominum: Church and Health in the World.* 1997; 34(12th Yr., No. 1): 202–204. BE60497.
autonomy; beneficence; bioethics; freedom; *mentally ill; patient care; philosophy; physician patient relationship; *psychiatry

Schmiedebach, Heinz-Peter. The mentally ill patient caught between the state's demands and the professional interests of psychiatrists. *In:* Berg, Manfred; Cocks, Geoffrey, eds. Medicine and Modernity: Public Health and Medical Care in Nineteenth- and Twentieth-Century Germany. New York, NY: Cambridge University Press; 1997: 99–119. 61 fn. ISBN 0-521-56411-5. BE59267.
*attitudes; chronically ill; *dehumanization; eugenics; food; forensic psychiatry; health care delivery; *historical aspects; involuntary sterilization; medical specialties; *mental health; *mental institutions; *mentally ill; military personnel; mortality; patient care; *physicians; *psychiatry; public health; public policy; resource allocation; *social control; social problems; social worth; socioeconomic factors; *sociology of medicine; *stigmatization; war; prostitution; Darwinism; *Germany; *Nineteenth Century; *Twentieth Century; World War I

Sharkey, Joe. Bedlam: Greed, Profiteering, and Fraud in a Mental Health System Gone Crazy. New York, NY: St. Martin's Press; 1994. 294 p. ISBN 0-312-10421-9. BE62500.
adolescents; adults; advertising; alcohol abuse; behavior disorders; children; coercion; drug abuse; *fraud; *health insurance reimbursement; involuntary commitment; legal

---

BE = bioethics accession number   fn. = footnotes   refs. = references

aspects; mental health; *mental institutions; *misconduct; patient admission; *proprietary health facilities; psychiatric diagnosis; *referral and consultation; voluntary admission; *mental health services; National Medical Enterprises; Texas; *United States

Slomka, Jacquelyn; Agich, George J.; Stagno, Susan J., et al. Physical restraint elimination in the acute care setting: ethical considerations. *HEC (HealthCare Ethics Committee) Forum.* 1998 Sep-Dec; 10(3-4): 244-262. 35 refs. BE61178.
aged; autonomy; *behavior control; cultural pluralism; dangerousness; economics; family members; health care reform; health personnel; *hospitals; injuries; institutional policies; institutionalized persons; intention; international aspects; *mentally ill; paternalism; *patient care; patients; *physical restraint; physicians; psychiatry; psychological stress; risk; technical expertise; treatment refusal; values; United States

Snyder, Maryhelen. Ethical Issues in Feminist Family Therapy. New York, NY: Haworth Press; 1994. 83 p. Includes references. Published also as *Journal of Feminist Family Therapy*, 1994; 6(3). ISBN 1-56024-726-6. BE62150.
accountability; behavioral research; blacks; children; codes of ethics; cultural pluralism; education; *family relationship; females; *feminist ethics; health personnel; males; misconduct; patient advocacy; professional patient relationship; *psychotherapy; regulation; self regulation; social discrimination; whites; *family therapy; United States

Szmukler, George I.; Bloch, Sidney. Family involvement in the care of people with psychoses: an ethical argument. [Editorial]. *British Journal of Psychiatry.* 1997 Nov; 171: 401-405. 14 refs. BE60378.
confidentiality; disclosure; *family members; *family relationship; informed consent; *mentally ill; *patient care; professional family relationship; psychiatry; risks and benefits; third party consent; values

Watts, Jonathan. Patients not to be tied up in Japanese sanatoriums. [News]. *Lancet.* 1999 Jul 24; 354(9175): 316. BE62528.
aged; *behavior control; dementia; government regulation; *guidelines; *institutionalized persons; *mental institutions; *mentally ill; *physical restraint; public hospitals; *public policy; residential facilities; *Japan

Weissman, David E.; Matson, Sandra. Pain assessment and management in the long-term care setting. *Theoretical Medicine and Bioethics.* 1999 Jan; 20(1): 31-43. 53 refs. BE62122.
*aged; alternatives; attitudes; chronically ill; *dementia; diagnosis; *drugs; education; health personnel; *institutional policies; *long-term care; *nursing homes; *opioid analgesics; *pain; *patient care; risks and benefits; technical expertise; toxicity; United States

Winerip, Michael. Bedlam on the streets. *New York Times Magazine.* 1999 May 23: 42-49, 56, 65-66, 70. BE61010.
accountability; *community services; *dangerousness; *deinstitutionalized persons; *economics; government financing; *health care delivery; mental institutions; *mentally ill; mentally retarded; municipal government; outpatient commitment; patient compliance; patient discharge; patient transfer; psychoactive drugs; *public policy; residential facilities; schizophrenia; state government; *violence; voluntary admission; *homeless persons; New York City; *United States

Workman, Richard H.; Molinari, Victor; Rezabek, Pamela, et al. An ethical framework for understanding patients with antisocial personality disorder who develop

dementia: diagnosing and managing disorders of autonomy. *Journal of Ethics, Law, and Aging.* 1997 Fall-Winter; 3(2): 79-90. 22 refs. BE60451.
accountability; *aged; aggression; *autonomy; *behavior disorders; case studies; *competence; comprehension; decision making; *dementia; diagnosis; evaluation; *hospitals; legal guardians; *paternalism; *patient care; patient care team; *patient compliance; *patient discharge; recall; standards; values

PATIENT CARE/MINORS

Altman, Lawrence K. For surviving octuplets, progress comes in ounces. [News]. *New York Times.* 1998 Jan 17: 1, 20. BE59873.
biomedical technologies; critically ill; drugs; economics; hospitals; *infants; infertility; intensive care units; *multiple pregnancy; *newborns; *patient care; patient care team; *prematurity; prognosis; reproductive technologies; resource allocation; *Chukwu octuplets; Texas Children's Hospital (Houston)

Appleyard, James. The rights of children to health care. [Editorial]. *Journal of Medical Ethics.* 1998 Oct; 24(5): 293-294. 5 refs. BE60250.
*children; developing countries; *health care; health promotion; *human rights; *international aspects; nutrition; patients' rights; physicians; preventive medicine; professional organizations; quality of health care; rehabilitation; Convention on the Rights of the Child; *Declaration on the Rights of the Child to Health Care; United Nations; *World Medical Association

Bonati, Maurizio; Garattini, Silvio. Evidence- and ethical-based child health: update on therapeutic trials in children. *In:* Burgio, G. Roberto; Lantos, John D., eds. *Primum Non Nocere* Today. Second Edition. New York, NY: Elsevier; 1998: 101-106. 22 refs. ISBN 0-444-82923-7. BE60922.
*children; costs and benefits; drugs; *evidence-based medicine; *patient care; pediatrics; *practice guidelines; research design; risks and benefits; therapeutic research; treatment outcome; antibiotics; ear diseases

Borowski, A.; Schickendantz, S.; Mennicken, U., et al. Open heart interventions in premature, low- and very-low-birth-weight neonates: risk profile and ethical considerations. *Thoracic and Cardiovascular Surgeon.* 1997 Oct; 45(5): 238-241. 18 refs. BE60199.
brain pathology; case studies; *congenital disorders; *decision making; disclosure; *hearts; iatrogenic disease; *low birth weight; mentally retarded; morbidity; mortality; *newborns; parental consent; parents; patient care team; *prematurity; quality of life; risk; *risks and benefits; *surgery; therapeutic research; treatment outcome

Brinchmann, Berit Støre. When the home becomes a prison: living with a severely disabled child. *Nursing Ethics.* 1999 Mar; 6(2): 137-143. 14 refs. BE61933.
*attitudes; *children; *congenital disorders; decision making; *disabled; *emotions; family relationship; *home care; intensive care units; love; newborns; nursing research; *parent child relationship; *parents; prematurity; *prolongation of life; *psychological stress; quality of life; selective abortion; survey; qualitative research; Norway

Burgio, G. Roberto; Lantos, John D., eds. *Primum Non Nocere* Today. Second Edition. New York, NY: Elsevier; 1998. 171 p. (International congress series; no. 1171). Includes references. New edition of the proceedings of the international Symposium on Pediatric Bioethics, held in Pavia, Italy, 26-28 May 1994. ISBN 0-444-82923-7. BE60917.

BE = bioethics accession number   fn. = footnotes   refs. = references

active euthanasia; adolescents; allowing to die; anthropology; *beneficence; *bioethical issues; *bioethics; biomedical technologies; bone marrow; cancer; children; cord blood; decision making; directed donation; disease; drugs; ethical theory; evidence-based medicine; fetal research; fetal therapy; gene therapy; genetic predisposition; genetic screening; historical aspects; human experimentation; immunization; informed consent; international aspects; medical education; minors; moral policy; newborns; organ donation; palliative care; parental consent; *patient care; *pediatrics; practice guidelines; prenatal diagnosis; quality of life; risks and benefits; selective abortion; stem cells; tissue donation; ear diseases

Carson, Donna P. The socially complex family: new dilemmas for the neonatal social worker. *Clinics in Perinatology.* 1996 Sep; 23(3): 609-620. 5 refs. BE60944.
case studies; *critically ill; decision making; *family relationship; hospitals; intensive care units; low birth weight; *newborns; parents; *patient care; patient discharge; professional family relationship; *social problems; *social workers; values; Grady Memorial Hospital (Atlanta, GA)

Chase, Cheryl; Elliott, Carl. Intersexuality: waiting for change? [Letter and response]. *Hastings Center Report.* 1999 Mar-Apr; 29(2): 4. BE61651.
*children; congenital disorders; *cosmetic surgery; deception; females; *infants; *intersexuality; males; *normality; *sexuality

Chase, Cheryl. Surgical progress is not the answer to intersexuality. *Journal of Clinical Ethics.* 1998 Winter; 9(4): 385-392. 40 fn. BE60488.
adolescents; adults; attitudes; *children; circumcision; congenital disorders; *cosmetic surgery; females; homosexuals; *infants; informed consent; *intersexuality; males; normality; *patient care; patient satisfaction; patients; physicians; psychological stress; *risk; risks and benefits; *sexuality; suffering; *surgery; *treatment outcome

Clark, Graeme M.; Cowan, Robert S.C.; Dowell, Richard C. Ethical issues. *In:* Clark, Graeme M.; Cowan, Robert S.C.; Dowell, Richard C., eds. Cochlear Implantation for Infants and Children: Advances. San Diego, CA: Singular Publishing Group; 1997: 241-249. 9 refs. ISBN 1-56593-727-9. BE61114.
age factors; *children; congenital disorders; empirical research; *hearing disorders; infants; informed consent; international aspects; *medical devices; parental consent; *patient care; *physically disabled; *risks and benefits; *surgery; *therapeutic research; treatment outcome; *cochlear implants; Australia; United States

Clark, Reese H. The safe introduction of new technologies into neonatal medicine. *Clinics in Perinatology.* 1996 Sep; 23(3): 519-527. 28 refs. BE60939.
*biomedical technologies; *evaluation; health personnel; *human experimentation; mortality; *newborns; *patient care; research design; *risks and benefits; technical expertise; *technology assessment; *therapeutic research; treatment outcome; ventilators; extracorporeal membrane oxygenation; multicenter studies

Cooper, Ellen R. Caring for children with AIDS: new challenges for medicine and society. *Pediatrician.* 1990; 17(2): 118-123. 13 refs. BE59456.
adoption; AIDS; *children; confidentiality; disadvantaged; disclosure; family members; fetuses; *HIV seropositivity; informed consent; newborns; parental consent; patient care; *pediatrics; physicians; pregnant women; preventive medicine; research ethics committees; schools; stigmatization; therapeutic research; United States

Cooper, Rebecca; Koch, Kathryn A. Neonatal and pediatric critical care: ethical decision making. *Critical*

Care Clinics. 1996 Jan; 12(1): 149-164. 53 refs. BE59284.
*allowing to die; anencephaly; autonomy; *children; competence; congenital disorders; critically ill; *decision making; emergency care; futility; government regulation; *infants; informed consent; legal aspects; minors; *newborns; organ donation; organ donors; parental consent; *parents; paternalism; *patient care; physicians; *prolongation of life; quality of life; religion; risks and benefits; standards; suffering; surgery; treatment refusal; twins; values; conjoined twins; rationality; United States

Crouch, Robert A. Betwixt and between: the past and future of intersexuality. *Journal of Clinical Ethics.* 1998 Winter; 9(4): 372-384. 85 fn. BE60487.
adolescents; adults; anthropology; *attitudes; *children; congenital disorders; *cosmetic surgery; counseling; deception; *decision making; diagnosis; *females; *hormones; infants; *informal social control; *intersexuality; *males; medicine; motivation; *newborns; *normality; parents; paternalism; *patient care; *physicians; psychological stress; self concept; *sexuality; stigmatization; suffering; *surgery; treatment outcome; truth disclosure; uncertainty; *values

Diekema, Douglas S. Children first: the need to reform financing of health care services for children. [Editorial]. *Journal of Health Care for the Poor and Underserved.* 1996; 7(1): 3-14. 48 refs. BE60388.
adolescents; age factors; beneficence; *children; employment; *financial support; government financing; health care; *health care reform; health insurance; *indigents; justice; libertarianism; moral obligations; *obligations of society; resource allocation; socioeconomic factors; Medicaid; *United States

Dreger, Alice Domurat. A history of intersexuality: from the age of gonads to the age of consent. *Journal of Clinical Ethics.* 1998 Winter; 9(4): 345-355. 22 fn. BE60484.
adults; attitudes; autonomy; beneficence; *children; congenital disorders; *cosmetic surgery; *counseling; decision making; females; historical aspects; homosexuals; hormones; infants; informed consent; *intersexuality; males; normality; parental consent; parents; *patient care; patient participation; physicians; psychology; risks and benefits; *sexuality; sociology of medicine; *surgery; truth disclosure; Nineteenth Century; Twentieth Century

Elstein, D.; Steinberg, A.; Abrahamov, A., et al. Ethical guidelines for enzyme therapy in neuronopathic Gaucher disease. [Abstract]. *American Journal of Human Genetics.* 1997 Oct; 61(4): A354. BE59399.
*children; costs and benefits; decision making; drugs; *genetic disorders; *infants; *patient care; *practice guidelines; resource allocation; *risks and benefits; selection for treatment; suffering; *Gaucher's disease

Ferriman, Annabel. Trial by video: *Someone to watch over me,* ITV, 12 January. *BMJ (British Medical Journal).* 1999 Jan 23; 318(7178): 269. BE60347.
attitudes; *behavior disorders; *child abuse; children; *confidentiality; *deception; diagnosis; *forensic medicine; health personnel; hospitals; *mass media; *parents; risks and benefits; *covert monitoring; *Munchausen syndrome by proxy; *video recording; Great Britain

Fitzgerald, Wendy Anton. Engineering perfect offspring: devaluing children and childhood. *Hastings Constitutional Law Quarterly.* 1997 Summer; 24(4): 833-861. 183 fn. BE62163.
adults; *allowing to die; autonomy; behavior disorders; *children; *congenital disorders; *decision making; dehumanization; *disabled; Down syndrome; *eugenics; gene therapy; genetic counseling; *genetic determinism; *genetic disorders; genetic predisposition; genetic research;

BE = bioethics accession number   fn. = footnotes   refs. = references

hyperkinesis; *legal aspects; *newborns; *normality; *parents; *personhood; physicians; prognosis; *prolongation of life; psychiatric diagnosis; *quality of life; resource. allocation; social discrimination; social worth; *surgery; terminally ill; twins; *value of life; *values; *withholding treatment; *conjoined twins; dependency; seriously ill; Hensel twins; Holton twins; Lakeberg twins; Social Darwinism; United States

Fost, Norman. Decisions regarding treatment of seriously ill newborns. [Editorial]. *JAMA.* 1999 Jun 2; 281(21): 2041-2043. 18 refs. BE61905.
   adolescents; *allowing to die; attitudes; *congenital disorders; *decision making; disabled; empirical research; ethics consultation; intensive care units; *low birth weight; *newborns; nurses; parents; *patient care; physicians; prematurity; prognosis; *prolongation of life; *quality of life; resource allocation; *selection for treatment; *treatment outcome; trends; *uncertainty; withholding treatment; neonatology; United States

Fowlie, P.W.; Delahunty, C.; Tarnow-Mordi, W.O. What do doctors record in the medical notes following discussion with the parents of sick premature infants? *European Journal of Pediatrics.* 1998 Jan; 157(1): 63-65. 12 refs. BE62403.
   *communication; diagnosis; intensive care units; *low birth weight; *medical records; mortality; *newborns; *parents; *patient care; *physicians; *prematurity; *professional family relationship; prognosis; *records; statistics; survey; truth disclosure; withholding treatment; severity of illness index; Great Britain

Gallucci, Denise. Making decisions about premature infants. *American Journal of Nursing.* 1998 Jun; 98(6): 64, 66. 10 refs. BE61802.
   *allowing to die; communication; *decision making; intensive care units; *newborns; *nurse's role; parents; *patient care; patient care team; *prematurity; selection for treatment; treatment outcome; uncertainty

Gillett, Grant. The ethical challenge of sick children. *Pediatrician.* 1990; 17(2): 59-62. 1 ref. BE59450.
   active euthanasia; allowing to die; *children; congenital disorders; decision making; disabled; *newborns; parents; *patient care; pediatrics; personhood; quality of life; speciesism; value of life

Groveman, Sherri A. The Hanukkah bush: ethical implications in the clinical management of intersex. *Journal of Clinical Ethics.* 1998 Winter; 9(4): 356-359. BE60485.
   *adolescents; *children; congenital disorders; *counseling; *deception; diagnosis; females; *infants; *intersexuality; Jews; males; normality; parents; *patient care; physicians; *psychological stress; *sexuality; stigmatization; *surgery; *truth disclosure; support groups

Haimowitz, Stephan; Tucker, Bonnie. Deaf culture. [Letter and response]. *Hastings Center Report.* 1999 Mar-Apr; 29(2): 5. BE61653.
   *children; cultural pluralism; *hearing disorders; legal aspects; *medical devices; minority groups; normality; parents; *physically disabled; risks and benefits; social discrimination; *surgery; treatment refusal; *cochlear implants; Americans with Disabilities Act 1990; United States

Halasz, George. The rights of the child in psychotherapy. *American Journal of Psychotherapy.* 1996 Summer; 50(3): 285-297. 30 refs. BE62052.
   behavior disorders; case studies; *children; empathy; informed consent; managed care programs; parent child relationship; parental consent; patient compliance; professional patient relationship; *psychotherapy; rights

Haller, Karen B. When John became Joan. [Editorial]. *Journal of Obstetric, Gynecologic and Neonatal Nursing.* 1998 Jan-Feb; 27(1): 11. 2 refs. BE62056.
   case studies; decision making; females; guidelines; *infants; injuries; *intersexuality; *males; patient care; professional organizations; *sexuality; *surgery; treatment outcome; Intersex Society of North America

Harmon-Smith, Helena. 10 commandments. *Journal of Clinical Ethics.* 1998 Winter; 9(4): 371. BE60500.
   congenital disorders; *counseling; health personnel; *intersexuality; *newborns; *parents; *patient care; *sexuality; surgery

Hermann, Robert; Méhes, Károly. Physicians' attitudes regarding Down syndrome. *Journal of Child Neurology.* 1996 Jan; 11(1): 66-69. 15 refs. BE60189.
   active euthanasia; *allowing to die; *attitudes; children; clinical ethics committees; comparative studies; congenital disorders; *decision making; *Down syndrome; education; international aspects; medical specialties; mentally retarded; *newborns; nurses; parents; *patient care; pediatrics; *physicians; *prolongation of life; quality of life; selection for treatment; *surgery; survey; *withholding treatment; neurology; Canada; *Hungary

Howe, Edmund G. Intersexuality: what should careproviders do now? *Journal of Clinical Ethics.* 1998 Winter; 9(4): 337-344. 36 fn. BE60483.
   children; congenital disorders; *cosmetic surgery; *counseling; decision making; diagnosis; homosexuals; *infants; *intersexuality; normality; parents; *patient care; physicians; psychological stress; *risks and benefits; self concept; *sexuality; stigmatization; *surgery; truth disclosure

Howe, Edmund G. Treating infants who may die. *Journal of Clinical Ethics.* 1998 Fall; 9(3): 215-224. 25 fn. Commentary on C. Jones and J.M. Freeman, "Decision making in the nursery: an ethical dilemma," p. 314-322. BE61330.
   *allowing to die; attitudes; autonomy; case studies; coercion; communication; *critically ill; *decision making; disclosure; drug abuse; emotions; *health personnel; injuries; *newborns; *parents; paternalism; *patient care; professional family relationship; psychological stress; risks and benefits; socioeconomic factors; suffering; treatment refusal; analgesia; extracorporeal membrane oxygenation

Jones, Charlotte; Freeman, John M. Decision making in the nursery: an ethical dilemma. *Journal of Clinical Ethics.* 1998 Fall; 9(3): 314-322. 2 fn. Commented on by E.G. Howe, p. 215-224. BE61340.
   *allowing to die; autonomy; brain pathology; case studies; communication; *critically ill; *decision making; disabled; disclosure; drug abuse; intensive care units; *newborns; parental consent; *parents; patient advocacy; *patient care; *physicians; prognosis; resuscitation orders; risks and benefits; socioeconomic factors; treatment outcome; uncertainty; extracorporeal membrane oxygenation

Jonsen, Albert R. The ethics of pediatric medicine. *In:* Rudolph, Abraham M.; Hoffman, Julien I.E.; Rudolph, Colin D.; Sagan, Paul, eds. Rudolph's Pediatrics. Nineteenth Edition. Norwalk, CT: Appleton and Lange; 1991: 7-14. 8 refs. ISBN 0-8385-8488-8. BE61312.
   active euthanasia; *adolescents; allowing to die; case studies; *children; confidentiality; congenital disorders; *decision making; ethical analysis; futility; genetic screening; goals; human experimentation; immunization; *infants; medical ethics; organ donation; parental consent; parents; *patient care; patient participation; *pediatrics; physicians; quality of life; sterilization (sexual); terminally ill; treatment refusal; truth disclosure; withholding treatment

---

BE = bioethics accession number   fn. = footnotes   refs. = references

Kessler, Suzanne J. Lessons from the Intersexed. New Brunswick, NJ: Rutgers University Press; 1998. 193 p. Bibliography: p. 169–179. ISBN 0-8135-2530-6. BE62772.
adolescents; adults; attitudes; *children; communication; congenital disorders; *cosmetic surgery; *decision making; diagnosis; females; hormones; *infants; *intersexuality; males; normality; *parents; patient advocacy; *patient care; *physicians; self concept; *sexuality; *surgery; treatment outcome; values

Kipnis, Kenneth; Diamond, Milton. Pediatric ethics and the surgical assignment of sex. *Journal of Clinical Ethics.* 1998 Winter; 9(4): 398–410. 56 fn. BE60490.
adolescents; adults; age factors; attitudes; beneficence; case studies; congenital disorders; *cosmetic surgery; counseling; deception; diagnosis; empirical research; ethics consultation; females; hormones; *infants; *intersexuality; males; medical ethics; *newborns; *normality; organizational policies; parents; *patient care; patient satisfaction; patients; *pediatrics; *physicians; prevalence; professional organizations; psychological stress; psychology; *risks and benefits; selection for treatment; self concept; *sexuality; standards; *surgery; transsexualism; *treatment outcome; *truth disclosure; twins; uncertainty; values; support groups; American Academy of Pediatrics

Landman, Willem A.; Henley, Lesley D. Tensions in setting health care priorities for South Africa's children. *Journal of Medical Ethics.* 1998 Aug; 24(4): 268–273. 30 fn. BE61294.
beneficence; *children; chronically ill; costs and benefits; decision making; health; *health care; justice; legal aspects; long-term care; moral policy; preventive medicine; primary health care; public health; public participation; *public policy; quality of life; *resource allocation; standards; *health planning; needs; *South Africa

The new South African constitution commits the government to guarantee "basic health services" for every child under 18. Primary health care for pregnant women and children under six and elements of essential primary health care have received priority. At present, there is little analysis of the moral considerations involved in making choices about more advanced or costly health care which may, arguably, also be "basic". This paper illustrates some of the tensions in setting priorities for a just macro–allocation of children's health care, given the realities of need and scarce resources, and the commitment to equality of basic opportunities.

Lantos, John D.; Mokalla, Mani; Meadow, William. Resource allocation in neonatal and medical ICUs: epidemiology and rationing at the extremes of life. *American Journal of Respiratory and Critical Care Medicine.* 1997 Jul; 156(1): 185–189. 12 refs. BE60028.
age factors; *aged; comparative studies; costs and benefits; *intensive care units; justice; *low birth weight; *mortality; *newborns; patient discharge; prematurity; *resource allocation; time factors; *treatment outcome; ventilators; retrospective studies; University of Chicago Hospitals

Maher, John T.; Pask, Eleanor G. When truth hurts.... *In:* Adams, David W.; Deveau, Eleanor J., eds. Beyond the Innocence of Childhood: Helping Children and Adolescents Cope with Life-Threatening Illness and Dying. Amityville, NY: Baywood Publishing; 1995: 267–293. 38 refs. ISBN 0-89503-129-9. BE60658.
adolescents; age factors; autonomy; beneficence; cancer; *children; competence; comprehension; cultural pluralism; deception; decision making; diagnosis; futility; health personnel; HIV seropositivity; informed consent; parent child relationship; parents; patient participation; professional patient relationship; prognosis; psychological stress; quality of life; religion; rights; risks and benefits; suffering; terminal

care; *terminally ill; *truth disclosure

Matthews, Dennis J.; Meier, Robert H.; Bartholome, William. Ethical issues encountered in pediatric rehabilitation. *Pediatrician.* 1990; 17(2): 108–114. 7 refs. BE59454.
adolescents; allowing to die; autonomy; beneficence; *children; community services; congenital disorders; costs and benefits; decision making; *disabled; education; *goals; home care; injuries; justice; legal rights; newborns; normality; parents; *pediatrics; physicians; psychological stress; quality of life; *rehabilitation; *resource allocation; schools; selection for treatment; sexuality; uncertainty; withholding treatment

Meadow, William; Lantos, John D.; Mokalla, Mani, et al. Distributive justice across generations: epidemiology of ICU care for the very young and the very old. *Clinics in Perinatology.* 1996 Sep; 23(3): 597–608. 24 refs. BE60943.
adults; *age factors; *aged; comparative studies; *costs and benefits; economics; infants; *intensive care units; *justice; *low birth weight; medical records; *mortality; *newborns; patient care; patient discharge; prognosis; *resource allocation; selection for treatment; *treatment outcome; retrospective studies; survival; University of Chicago Medical Center

Mester, Roberto; Mozes, Tamar; Blumensohn, Rachel, et al. The new Israeli psychiatric legislation for the minor (1995) and its relationship to the 1991 Law for the Treatment of the Mentally Ill. *International Journal of Law and Psychiatry.* 1998 Summer; 21(3): 281–289. 8 refs. BE61670.
adults; confidentiality; health personnel; involuntary commitment; *legal aspects; *legislation; *mentally ill; *minors; outpatient commitment; *patient care; professional competence; psychiatric diagnosis; psychiatry; psychology; *Israel; *Law for the Treatment of the Mentally Ill 1991 (Israel); *Youth (Care and Supervision) Law 1960 (1995 Amendments) (Israel)

Muscari, Mary E. Rebels with a cause: when adolescents won't follow medical advice. *American Journal of Nursing.* 1998 Dec; 98(12): 26–31. 12 refs. Includes continuing education test, p. 31. BE61805.
*adolescents; autonomy; chronically ill; decision making; diabetes; females; motivation; nurse patient relationship; *nurses; *patient care; *patient compliance; patient participation; self concept

Oberfield, Sharon E. Growth hormone use in normal, short children -- a plea for reason. [Editorial]. *New England Journal of Medicine.* 1999 Feb 18; 340(7): 557–559. 11 refs. BE60336.
*children; decision making; enhancement technologies; *growth disorders; *hormones; *normality; *patient care; physicians; risks and benefits; *selection for treatment; self concept; treatment outcome; United States

Oppé, Thomas E. Ethical aspects of AIDS in childhood in England. *Pediatrician.* 1990; 17(2): 115–117. 5 refs. BE59455.
*AIDS; AIDS serodiagnosis; *children; confidentiality; disclosure; *HIV seropositivity; human experimentation; informed consent; parental consent; patient care; *pediatrics; physicians; *Great Britain

Preves, Sharon E. For the sake of the children: destigmatizing intersexuality. *Journal of Clinical Ethics.* 1998 Winter; 9(4): 411–420. 24 fn. BE60491.
*adolescents; *adults; *attitudes; *children; congenital disorders; *cosmetic surgery; deception; diagnosis; genetic counseling; hormones; *intersexuality; *newborns;

BE = bioethics accession number   fn. = footnotes   refs. = references

normality; parents; patient care; *patient satisfaction; *patients; physicians; *psychological stress; quality of life; *self concept; *sexuality; *stigmatization; *surgery; survey; transsexualism; *treatment outcome; *truth disclosure; empowerment; qualitative research; support groups; North America

Raffensperger, J. A philosophical approach to conjoined twins. *Pediatric Surgery International.* 1997 Apr; 12(4): 249-255. 29 refs. BE59192.
    *allowing to die; attitudes; case studies; *congenital disorders; decision making; diagnosis; double effect; futility; historical aspects; intention; killing; mass media; mental health; moral policy; mortality; organ donation; parents; physicians; privacy; prognosis; *quality of life; religious ethics; risks and benefits; *selection for treatment; *surgery; *treatment outcome; *twins; withholding treatment; *conjoined twins; Lakeberg twins; United States

Ramsay, Sarah. UK "Bristol case" inquiry formally opened. [News]. *Lancet.* 1999 Mar 20; 353(9157): 987. BE61957.
    children; heart diseases; hospitals; *misconduct; morbidity; mortality; patient care; *pediatrics; *physicians; *professional competence; quality of health care; self regulation; *surgery; technical expertise; Bristol; General Medical Council (Great Britain); *Great Britain; National Health Service

Ross, Lainie Friedman. Children, Families, and Health Care Decision Making. New York, NY: Clarendon Press; 1998. 197 p. (Issues in biomedical ethics). Bibliography: p. 177-190. ISBN 0-19-823763-4. BE61944.
    *adolescents; advisory committees; *autonomy; case studies; *children; *competence; *decision making; deontological ethics; directed donation; dissent; family members; *family relationship; federal government; futility; goals; government regulation; guidelines; *human experimentation; legal aspects; *minors; moral development; *moral obligations; nontherapeutic research; *organ donation; *parental consent; *parents; *patient care; pediatrics; personhood; physicians; prolongation of life; quality of life; refusal to treat; rights; risk; risks and benefits; sexuality; siblings; state interest; therapeutic research; *treatment refusal; utilitarianism; *values; liberalism; needs; National Commission for the Protection of Human Subjects; United States

Rylance, George. Privacy, dignity, and confidentiality: interview study with structured questionnaire. *BMJ (British Medical Journal).* 1999 Jan 30; 318(7179): 301. 4 refs. BE60580.
    *children; *confidentiality; disclosure; *hospitals; institutional policies; knowledge, attitudes, practice; *parents; *patient care; *privacy; survey; dignity; questionnaires; Great Britain

Saigal, Saroj; Stoskopf, Barbara L.; Feeny, David, et al. Differences in preferences for neonatal outcomes among health care professionals, parents, and adolescents. *JAMA.* 1999 Jun 2; 281(21): 1991-1997. 34 refs. BE62313.
    *adolescents; allowing to die; *attitudes; comparative studies; control groups; *decision making; disabled; *health; intensive care units; *low birth weight; *newborns; normality; *nurses; *parents; patient satisfaction; *physicians; *prolongation of life; *quality of life; survey; *treatment outcome; *value of life; neonatology; Canada
    CONTEXT: In neonatal intensive care, parents make important clinical management decisions in conjunction with health care professionals. Yet little information is available on whether preferences of health care professionals and parents for the resulting health outcomes differ. OBJECTIVE: To measure and compare preferences for selected health states from the perspectives of health care professionals (ie,

neonatologists and neonatal nurses), parents of extremely low-birth-weight (ELBW) or normal birth-weight infants, and adolescents who were either ELBW or normal birth-weight infants. DESIGN: Cross-sectional cohort study. SETTING AND PARTICIPANTS: A total of 742 participants were recruited and interviewed between 1993 and 1995, including 100 neonatologists from hospitals throughout Canada; 103 neonatal nurses from 3 regional neonatal intensive care units; 264 adolescents (aged 12-16 years), including 140 who were ELBW infants and 124 sociodemographically matched term controls; and 275 parents of the recruited adolescents. MAIN OUTCOME MEASURE: Preferences (utilities) for 4 to 5 hypothetical health states of children were obtained by direct interviews using the standard gamble method. RESULTS: Overall, neonatologists and nurses had similar preferences for the 5 health states, and a similar proportion rated some health states as worse than death (59% of neonatologists and 68% of nurses; P=.20). Health care professionals rated the health states lower than did parents of ELBW and term infants (P less than .001). Overall, 64% of health care professionals and 45% of parents rated 1 or more health states to be worse than death (P less than .001). Differences in mean utility scores between health care professionals and parents and adolescent respondents were most pronounced for the 2 most severely disabled health states (P less than .001). CONCLUSIONS: When asked to rate the health-related quality of life for the hypothetical conditions of children, health care professionals tend to provide lower utility scores than do adolescents and their parents. These findings have implications for decision making in the neonatal intensive care unit.

Schober, Justine Marut. A surgeon's response to the intersex controversy. *Journal of Clinical Ethics.* 1998 Winter; 9(4): 393-397. 12 fn. BE60489.
    adolescents; adults; age factors; attitudes; *children; congenital disorders; *cosmetic surgery; *counseling; diagnosis; females; *infants; informed consent; *intersexuality; males; parental consent; parents; *patient care; patient satisfaction; *physician's role; physicians; *risks and benefits; selection for treatment; *sexuality; surgery; treatment outcome; truth disclosure; support groups

Silverman, William A. Where's the Evidence? Controversies in Modern Medicine. New York, NY: Oxford University Press; 1998. 259 p. Bibliography: p. 225-247. A collection of essays and responses originally published in the journal *Paediatric and Perinatal Epidemiology* between 1987 and 1997. ISBN 0-19-262934-4. BE59723.
    active euthanasia; allowing to die; autonomy; *bioethical issues; biomedical technologies; conflict of interest; congenital disorders; control groups; *decision making; drug industry; *evidence-based medicine; futility; hearts; historical aspects; *human experimentation; informed consent; investigators; low birth weight; *newborns; organ transplantation; pain; parents; *patient care; physicians; *prematurity; prolongation of life; quality of life; *random selection; refusal to treat; *research design; research ethics committees; resource allocation; selection for treatment; social dominance; socioeconomic factors; therapeutic research; treatment outcome; withholding treatment; *neonatology; Great Britain; United States

Singh, Meharban. Ethical considerations in pediatric intensive care unit: Indian perspective. [Editorial]. *Indian Pediatrics.* 1996 Apr; 33(4): 271-278. 16 refs. BE60186.
    *allowing to die; artificial feeding; brain death; *children; communication; costs and benefits; critically ill; death; decision making; determination of death; futility; infants;

BE = bioethics accession number   fn. = footnotes   refs. = references

*intensive care units; newborns; organ donation; parents; *patient care; patient care team; pediatrics; persistent vegetative state; physician patient relationship; professional family relationship; resource allocation; resuscitation; trust; withholding treatment; *India

Soll, Roger. Consensus and controversy over resuscitation of the newborn infant. *Lancet.* 1999 Jul 3; 354(9172): 4–5. 13 refs. BE62407.
consensus; developing countries; emergency care; human experimentation; international aspects; mortality; *newborns; physicians; practice guidelines; professional organizations; prolongation of life; *resuscitation; selection for treatment; *International Liaison Committee on Resuscitation; World Health Organization

Van Haeringen, Alison R.; Dadds, Mark; Armstrong, Kenneth L. The child abuse lottery -- will the doctor suspect and report? Physician attitudes towards and reporting of suspected child abuse and neglect. *Child Abuse and Neglect.* 1998 Mar; 22(3): 159–169. 22 refs. BE61809.
*child abuse; comparative studies; confidentiality; decision making; diagnosis; injuries; *knowledge, attitudes, practice; legal aspects; *mandatory reporting; parents; pediatrics; *physicians; survey; Australia; *Queensland

Wharton, Robert H.; Levine, Karen R.; Buka, Stephen, et al. Advance care planning for children with special health care needs: a survey of parental attitudes. *Pediatrics.* 1996 May; 97(5): 682–687. 38 refs. BE60404.
*advance care planning; *advance directives; *attitudes; *children; *chronically ill; communication; comprehension; critically ill; *decision making; *disabled; knowledge, attitudes, practice; *parents; *patient care; physicians; *professional family relationship; prognosis; survey; truth disclosure; Massachusetts

Wilson, Bruce E.; Reiner, William G. Management of intersex: a shifting paradigm. *Journal of Clinical Ethics.* 1998 Winter; 9(4): 360–369. 32 fn. BE60486.
*adolescents; *children; congenital disorders; *cosmetic surgery; *counseling; *decision making; diagnosis; disclosure; empirical research; *hormones; *infants; informed consent; *intersexuality; *newborns; normality; *parents; *patient care; *patient care team; *patient participation; *physicians; psychological stress; *sexuality; *surgery; transsexualism; treatment outcome; trends; *truth disclosure

PATIENTS' RIGHTS

See also CONFIDENTIALITY, INFORMED CONSENT, TREATMENT REFUSAL, TRUTH DISCLOSURE

Baker, Robert. American independence and the right to emergency care. *JAMA.* 1999 Mar 3; 281(9): 859–860. 12 refs. BE60244.
administrators; codes of ethics; economics; *emergency care; historical aspects; *legal aspects; *legal rights; legislation; *managed care programs; *medical ethics; *moral obligations; patient advocacy; *patients' rights; physician patient relationship; *physicians; professional organizations; refusal to treat; *utilitarianism; *business ethics; *Patients' Bill of Rights; *United States

Bindless, Linda. The use of patients in health care education: the need for ethical justification. *Journal of Medical Ethics.* 1998 Oct; 24(5): 314–319. 27 fn. BE60252.
accountability; behavioral research; coercion; confidentiality; deception; disclosure; *education; *health personnel; human rights; informed consent; patient advocacy; patient care; *patients; *patients' rights; privacy; *professional ethics; professional patient relationship; research subjects; *students; vulnerable populations; Great Britain

This paper addresses ethical concerns emanating from the practice of using patients for health care education. It shows how some of the ways that patients are used in educational strategies to bridge theory–practice gaps can cause harm to patients and patient–practitioner relationships, thus failing to meet acceptable standards of professional practice. This will continue unless there is increased awareness of the need for protection of human rights in teaching situations. Unnecessary exposure of patients, failing to obtain explicit consent, causing harm to vulnerable or disadvantaged groups and inappropriate use of information, though normally regarded as unacceptable professional practices, may go unrecognised in meeting educational needs, widening rather than narrowing theory–practice gaps.

Buetow, Stephen. The scope for the involvement of patients in their consultations with health professionals: rights, responsibilities and preferences of patients. *Journal of Medical Ethics.* 1998 Aug; 24(4): 243–247. 53 refs. BE61289.
*accountability; common good; decision making; *health care delivery; *moral obligations; patient care; *patient participation; *patients; *patients' rights; *professional patient relationship; *Great Britain; National Health Service; Patient's Charter (Great Britain)

The degree and nature of patient involvement in consultations with health professionals influences problem and needs recognition and management, and public accountability. This paper suggests a framework for understanding the scope for patient involvement in such consultations. Patients are defined as co-producers of formal health services, whose potential for involvement in consultations depends on their personal rights, responsibilities and preferences. Patients' rights in consultations are poorly defined and, in the National Health Service (NHS), not legally enforceable. The responsibilities of patients are also undefined. I suggest that these are not to deny, of their own volition, the rights of others, which in consultations necessitate mutuality of involvement through information–exchange and shared decision–making. Preferences should be met insofar as they do not militate against responsibilities and rights.

Gecik, Karol. The need to protect patients' rights. *Medicine and Law.* 1993; 12(1–2): 109–112. 8 fn. BE60617.
health care; health personnel; *international aspects; legal aspects; *patients' rights; professional patient relationship; public policy; rights; *Europe; World Health Organization

Gross, Michael L. Autonomy and paternalism in communitarian society: patient rights in Israel. *Hastings Center Report.* 1999 Jul–Aug; 29(4): 13–20. 26 fn. BE62464.
*autonomy; clinical ethics committees; coercion; common good; *communitarianism; decision making; freedom; informed consent; Jewish ethics; legal aspects; legislation; *paternalism; *patients' rights; public policy; religion; rights; treatment refusal; value of life; values; *Israel; Patients' Rights Act 1996 (Israel); United States

The Israeli Patient Rights Act attempts to accommodate personal autonomy within an avowedly paternalist communitarian state. Although Israel is still groping toward a solution, the legislation begins to show the different form a communitarian version of autonomy must take.

BE = bioethics accession number   fn. = footnotes   refs. = references

Hill, Wan Ying; Fraser, Ian; Cotton, Philip. Patients' voices, rights and responsibilities: on implementing social audit in primary health care. *Journal of Business Ethics.* 1998 Oct; 17(13): 1481–1497. 59 refs. 23 fn. BE61217.
  *accountability; attitudes; decision making; economics; health care delivery; institutional ethics; legal rights; *organization and administration; *patient participation; *patient satisfaction; patients; *patients' rights; pharmacists; physician patient relationship; physicians; *primary health care; resource allocation; review committees; survey; trust; empowerment; Great Britain; *National Health Service; *Patients' Charter (Great Britain); *Scotland

Israel. The Patients' Rights Act, 1996. Dated 1 May 1996. (*Sefer Hakhukim,* 5756, 12 May 1996, p. 327). [Summary]. *International Digest of Health Legislation.* 1997; 48(2): 187–193. Summary derived from an unofficial English translation prepared in Israel. BE59594.
  administrators; clinical ethics committees; confidentiality; emergency care; health care; hospitals; informed consent; *legal rights; medical records; military personnel; patient access to records; patient care; *patients' rights; prisoners; quality of health care; review committees; treatment refusal; quality assurance; *Israel

Joint Commission on Accreditation of Healthcare Organizations. Ethical Issues and Patient Rights: Across the Continuum of Care. Oakbrook Terrace, IL: The Commission; 1998. 156 p. Includes references. ISBN 0-86688-591-9. BE62778.
  advance directives; allowing to die; bioethics; case studies; *clinical ethics; clinical ethics committees; competence; decision making; education; ethical analysis; ethical theory; ethics consultation; forms; guidelines; health care; health care delivery; *health facilities; home care; *institutional ethics; *institutional policies; organization and administration; patient care; *patients' rights; professional organizations; resuscitation orders; standards; terminal care; terminology; third party consent; values; withholding treatment; Joint Commission on Accreditation of Healthcare Organizations

Kahn, Charles N. Patients' rights proposals: the insurers' perspective. *JAMA.* 1999 Mar 3; 281(9): 858. 8 refs. BE60243.
  costs and benefits; economics; employment; federal government; *government regulation; *health insurance; *legal aspects; legislation; *managed care programs; *patients' rights; quality of health care; self regulation; state government; Patients' Bill of Rights; United States

Legemaate, Johan, ed.; Royal Dutch Medical Association. Patients' Rights in the Countries of the Toronto Group: The Results of a Survey Carried Out by the Royal Dutch Medical Association. Issued by the Association: Koninklijke Nederlandsche Maatschappij tot bevordering der Geneeskunst, P.O. Box 20051, 3502 LB, Utrecht, The Netherlands; 1992 Sep. 41 p. 16 refs. BE59259.
  adults; comparative studies; competence; confidentiality; disclosure; health care; informed consent; *international aspects; legal rights; medical records; minors; patient access to records; patient advocacy; patient care; patient compliance; *patients' rights; physician patient relationship; quality of health care; referral and consultation; survey; third party consent; Canada; Denmark; Finland; Great Britain; Iceland; Ireland; Jamaica; Netherlands; New Zealand; Norway; Sweden; *Toronto Group

Mariner, Wendy K. Going Hollywood with patient rights in managed care. *JAMA.* 1999 Mar 3; 281(9): 861. 5 refs. BE60245.
  accountability; *contracts; federal government;

*government regulation; *legal aspects; legislation; *managed care programs; mass media; *patients' rights; quality of health care; state government; Patients' Bill of Rights; *United States

Marx, Adina. The Society for Patient's Rights in Israel. *Nursing Ethics.* 1999 Mar; 6(2): 167–172. Includes principles of the Patients' Rights Law passed by the Knesset 1 May 1995. Paper presented at the 12th World Congress on Medical Law, Siófok, Hungary, 2–6 Aug 1998. BE61936.
  health care delivery; informed consent; *legal rights; legislation; *patient advocacy; *patients' rights; privacy; *Israel; *Patients' Rights Act 1996 (Israel)

Miller, Tracy E. Center stage on the patient protection agenda: grievance and appeal rights. *Journal of Law, Medicine and Ethics.* 1998 Summer; 26(2): 89–99. 77 fn. BE62676.
  disclosure; *due process; federal government; *government regulation; institutional policies; *legal rights; legislation; *managed care programs; *patient advocacy; *patients' rights; *physician's role; public policy; *quality of health care; self regulation; standards; state government; *withholding treatment; utilization review; Medicare; *United States

Shalala, Donna E. A Patients' Bill of Rights: the medical student's role. *JAMA.* 1999 Mar 3; 281(9): 857. 4 refs. BE60246.
  advisory committees; alternatives; disclosure; emergency care; federal government; government regulation; *health care delivery; incentives; insurance selection bias; *legal aspects; legislation; *managed care programs; medical education; *patients' rights; physicians; public policy; quality of health care; referral and consultation; students; withholding treatment; gag clauses; *Patients' Bill of Rights; *President's Advisory Commission on Consumer Protection and Quality in the Health Care Industry; *United States

Silva, Mary Cipriano. Ethics of consumer rights in managed care. *NursingConnections.* 1997 Summer; 10(2): 24–26. 3 refs. BE59189.
  disclosure; drugs; economics; gatekeeping; legal rights; legislation; *managed care programs; patient care; *patients' rights; quality of health care; referral and consultation; state government; withholding treatment; drug formularies; Managed Care Consumer Protection Act; United States

U.S. Congress. Senate. A bill to improve the access and choice of patients to quality, affordable health care [Patients' Bill of Rights Act of 1998]. S. 2330, 105th Cong., 2d Sess. Introduced by Trent Lott for Don Nickles, for himself, and others.; 1998 Jul 17 (first reading). 185 p. Read the second time and placed on the calendar 20 Jul 1998. BE59925.
  accountability; alternatives; biomedical research; confidentiality; *disclosure; emergency care; *health care delivery; *health insurance; health maintenance organizations; health services research; information dissemination; *legal aspects; legislation; medical records; patient access to records; patient care; *patients' rights; physicians; *quality of health care; referral and consultation; women's health; *women's health services; continuity of patient care; Centers for Disease Control and Prevention; Employee Retirement Income Security Act 1974 (ERISA); National Institutes of Health; Office of Research on Women's Health; *Patients' Bill of Rights Act (1998 bill); *United States

Weiss, Stefan C. Defining a "patients' bill of rights" for the next century. [Editorial]. *JAMA.* 1999 Mar 3; 281(9): 856. 4 refs. BE60242.
  *economics; *health care delivery; *legal aspects; *managed care programs; *patients' rights; physicians; public policy;

BE = bioethics accession number   fn. = footnotes   refs. = references

quality of health care; refusal to treat; *Patients' Bill of Rights; *United States

Zuccaro, Stefano Maria; Palleschi, Massimo; Italian Society of Hospital Geriatricians. Document on the rights of the sick elderly. *Dolentium Hominum: Church and Health in the World.* 1997; 36(12th Yr., No. 3): 32–35. 15 refs. BE60408.
  *aged; autonomy; disclosure; freedom; *health care; health personnel; *organizational policies; patient care; *patients' rights; professional organizations; quality of health care; *rights; social worth; Europe; *Italian Society of Hospital Geriatricians

PATIENTS' RIGHTS/MENTALLY DISABLED

Carmi, Amnon. The new Russian law on psychiatric care. *Dynamische Psychiatrie.* 1994; 27(3–4): 259–265. BE59756.
  aliens; coercion; competence; evaluation; institutionalized persons; involuntary commitment; *legal aspects; *legislation; *mentally ill; minors; patient care; *patients' rights; politics; psychiatric diagnosis; psychiatry; terminology; *Russia

Cohen, Pamela Schwartz. Psychiatric commitment in Japan: international concern and domestic reform. *UCLA Pacific Basin Law Journal.* 1995 Fall; 14(1): 28–74. 234 fn. BE59273.
  advisory committees; committee membership; community services; family members; health care reform; historical aspects; *human rights; *international aspects; *involuntary commitment; lawyers; *legal aspects; legal rights; mental institutions; *mentally ill; *non-Western World; paternalism; patient advocacy; patient care; *patient discharge; *patients' rights; physical restraint; physician patient relationship; *review committees; social discrimination; *standards; stigmatization; third party consent; values; voluntary admission; *International Commission of Jurists; *Japan; *Mental Health Act 1987 (Japan); Principles for the Protection of Persons with Mental Illness; *Psychiatric Review Boards (Japan); Twentieth Century; United Nations

Kellogg, Sarah C. The due process right to a safe and humane environment for patients in state custody: the voluntary/involuntary distinction. [Note]. *American Journal of Law and Medicine.* 1997; 23(2–3): 339–362. 219 fn. BE62504.
  constitutional law; *due process; equal protection; *institutionalized persons; *involuntary commitment; *legal aspects; *legal rights; *mental institutions; *mentally ill; *mentally retarded; *patients' rights; physical restraint; public hospitals; standards; Supreme Court decisions; *voluntary admission; *DeShaney v. Winnebago County Department of Social Services; *United States; *Youngberg v. Romeo

PERSONHOOD

Benjamin, Martin. Pragmatism and the determination of death. *In:* McGee, Glenn, ed. Pragmatic Bioethics. Nashville, TN: Vanderbilt University Press; 1999: 181–193, 280–281. 14 fn. ISBN 0-8265-1321-2. BE60671.
  advisory committees; *anencephaly; brain death; *determination of death; legal aspects; organ donation; *persistent vegetative state; *personhood; philosophy; standards; values; withholding treatment; pragmatism; Harvard Committee on Brain Death; Uniform Determination of Death Act

Benshoof, Janet; Knights of Columbus. Abortion and the "pro-life" v. "pro-choice" debate: should the human fetus be considered a person? *In:* Francoeur, Robert T., ed. Taking Sides: Clashing Views on Controversial

Issues in Human Sexuality. Fifth Edition. Guilford, CT: Dushkin Publishing Group/Brown and Benchmark; 1996: 120–133. 9 refs. Bibliography: p. 133. ISBN 0-697-31292-5. BE62044.
  *abortion, induced; *beginning of life; constitutional law; embryos; *fetuses; *legal aspects; legal liability; *legal rights; *personhood; *pregnant women; prenatal injuries; Supreme Court decisions; viability; wrongful death; Fourteenth Amendment; *Roe v. Wade; *United States; Webster v. Reproductive Health Services

Blustein, Jeffrey. Choosing for others as continuing a life story: the problem of personal identity revisited. *Journal of Law, Medicine and Ethics.* 1999 Spring; 27(1): 20–31. 37 fn. Commented on by M.G. Kuczewski, p. 32–36. BE61501.
  *advance directives; autonomy; communitarianism; competence; death; *decision making; dementia; *directive adherence; family members; friends; *moral policy; narrative ethics; patient care; persistent vegetative state; *personhood; philosophy; *self concept; standards; terminal care; *third party consent; time factors; Dresser, Rebecca; Robertson, John

Clarke, Liam. The person in abortion. *Nursing Ethics.* 1999 Jan; 6(1): 37–46. 28 refs. BE60153.
  *abortion, induced; *beginning of life; childbirth; children; emotions; *fetuses; infanticide; infants; moral development; *mother fetus relationship; *newborns; nurses; *personhood; pregnant women; speciesism; viability

Doyle, John P. Reflections on persons in petri dishes. *Linacre Quarterly.* 1997 Nov; 64(4): 62–76. 26 fn. BE61791.
  cloning; embryo disposition; embryo research; *embryos; human characteristics; in vitro fertilization; intelligence; morality; natural law; parent child relationship; *personhood; reproduction; self concept

Erde, Edmund L. Paradigms and personhood: a deepening of the dilemmas in ethics and medical ethics. *Theoretical Medicine and Bioethics.* 1999 Apr; 20(2): 141–160. 37 fn. BE62215.
  autonomy; bioethical issues; competence; deontological ethics; *ethical theory; freedom; law; medicine; *models, theoretical; paternalism; patient care; *personhood; *philosophy; psychology; rights; self concept; teleological ethics; treatment refusal

Fitzgerald, Wendy Anton. Engineering perfect offspring: devaluing children and childhood. *Hastings Constitutional Law Quarterly.* 1997 Summer; 24(4): 833–861. 183 fn. BE62163.
  adults; *allowing to die; autonomy; behavior disorders; *children; *congenital disorders; *decision making; dehumanization; *disabled; Down syndrome; *eugenics; gene therapy; genetic counseling; *genetic determinism; *genetic disorders; genetic predisposition; genetic research; hyperkinesis; *legal aspects; *newborns; *normality; *parents; *personhood; physicians; prognosis; *prolongation of life; psychiatric diagnosis; *quality of life; resource allocation; social discrimination; social worth; *surgery; terminally ill; twins; *value of life; *values; *withholding treatment; *conjoined twins; dependency; seriously ill; Hensel twins; Holton twins; Lakeberg twins; Social Darwinism; United States

Gould, Stephen Jay. Individuality: cloning and the discomfiting cases of Siamese twins. *Sciences.* 1997 Sep–Oct; 37(5): 14–16. BE61520.
  *cloning; evolution; normality; *personhood; *twins; *conjoined twins

Hunt, Geoffrey. Abortion: why bioethics can have no

BE = bioethics accession number   fn. = footnotes   refs. = references

answer -- a personal perspective. *Nursing Ethics.* 1999 Jan; 6(1): 47–57. 11 refs. BE60154.
  *abortion, induced; attitudes; *beginning of life; bioethics; *dissent; embryos; ethical analysis; ethicists; fetal development; *fetuses; *moral policy; *morality; newborns; *personhood; viability; *rationality

Jeffko, Walter G. Abortion, personhood, and community. *In: his* Contemporary Ethical Issues: A Personalistic Perspective. Amherst, NY: Humanity Books; 1999: 59–84. 42 fn. ISBN 1-57392-640-X. BE62245.
  *abortion, induced; *beginning of life; congenital disorders; drugs; embryos; *fetal development; *fetuses; infanticide; killing; legal aspects; methods; *moral policy; mother fetus relationship; newborns; *personhood; philosophy; population control; public policy; Roman Catholic ethics; selective abortion; sex offenses; therapeutic abortion; twinning; value of life; viability; RU–486

Jones, D. Gareth. The problematic symmetry between brain birth and brain death. *Journal of Medical Ethics.* 1998 Aug; 24(4): 237–242. 37 refs. BE61288.
  *beginning of life; *brain; *brain death; determination of death; *embryos; *fetal development; *fetuses; moral policy; *personhood; standards; terminology

The possible symmetry between the concepts of brain death and brain birth (life) is explored. Since the symmetry argument has tended to overlook the most appropriate definition of brain death, the fundamental concepts of whole brain death and higher brain death are assessed. In this way, a context is provided for a discussion of brain birth. Different writers have placed brain birth at numerous points: 25–40 days, eight weeks, 22–24 weeks, and 32–36 weeks gestation. For others, the concept itself is open to question. Apart from this, it needs to be asked whether a unitary concept is an oversimplification. The merits of defining two stages of brain birth, to parallel the two definitions of brain death, are discussed. An attempt is then made to map these various stages of brain birth and brain death onto a developmental continuum. Although the results hold biological interest, their ethical significance is less evident. Development and degeneration are not interchangeable, and definitions of death apply specifically to those who are dying, not those who are developing. I conclude that while a dual concept of brain death has proved helpful, a dual concept of brain birth still has problems, and the underlying concept of brain birth itself continues to be elusive.

Kischer, C. Ward. The big lie in human embryology: the case of the preembryo. *Linacre Quarterly.* 1997 Nov; 64(4): 53–61. 20 fn. BE61790.
  advisory committees; embryo research; *embryos; fetal development; moral obligations; *personhood; *terminology; twinning; American Fertility Society; Grobstein, Clifford; Human Embryo Research Panel; Warnock Committee

Koch, Tom; Rowell, Mary. Humanness, personhood, and a lamb named Dolly: response to "Cloning: technology, policy, and ethics" (*CQ* Vol. 7, No. 2). *Cambridge Quarterly of Healthcare Ethics.* 1999 Spring; 8(2): 241–245. 13 refs. BE61240.
  attitudes; *cloning; decision analysis; health personnel; human characteristics; *personhood; social interaction; *standards

Kuczewski, Mark G. Commentary: narrative views of personal identity and substituted judgment in surrogate decision making. *Journal of Law, Medicine and Ethics.* 1999 Spring; 27(1): 32–36. 19 fn. Commentary on J. Blustein, p. 20–31. BE61502.
  *advance directives; allowing to die; autonomy; competence; *decision making; dementia; *directive adherence; family members; friends; legal aspects; living wills; moral policy; narrative ethics; persistent vegetative state; *personhood; philosophy; physicians; prolongation of life; *self concept; standards; terminal care; *third party consent; time factors; withholding treatment; Dresser, Rebecca; Robertson, John

Lachs, John. Active euthanasia. *In: his* The Relevance of Philosophy to Life. Nashville, TN: Vanderbilt University Press; 1995: 181–187. 1 fn. ISBN 0-8265-1262-3. BE60863.
  *active euthanasia; adults; allowing to die; *anencephaly; *brain pathology; decision making; emotions; family members; health personnel; moral policy; newborns; *persistent vegetative state; *personhood; prolongation of life; public policy; quality of life; suffering

Leffel, Jim. Genetics and human rights in a postmodern age. *In:* Demy, Timothy J.; Stewart, Gary P., eds. Genetic Engineering: A Christian Response: Crucial Considerations in Shaping Life. Grand Rapids, MI: Kregel Publications; 1999: 126–138. 39 fn. ISBN 0-8254-2357-0. BE61364.
  autonomy; behavioral genetics; *Christian ethics; cloning; commodification; *cultural pluralism; dehumanization; embryo research; employment; *ethical relativism; eugenics; gene therapy; *genetic determinism; *genetic intervention; genetic materials; genetic research; genetic screening; health insurance; historical aspects; *human rights; humanism; patents; *personhood; *postmodernism; preimplantation diagnosis; prenatal diagnosis; property rights; secularism; selective abortion; sex determination; social discrimination; social problems; theology; transgenic organisms; *value of life; dignity; Social Darwinism; United States

Li, Hon–Lam. Abortion and degrees of personhood: understanding why the abortion problem (and the animal rights problem) are irresolvable. *Public Affairs Quarterly.* 1997 Jan; 11(1): 1–19. 26 fn. BE59161.
  *abortion, induced; age factors; animal rights; *beginning of life; fetal development; *fetuses; maternal health; moral policy; morality; *personhood; *pregnant women; speciesism; therapeutic abortion; *value of life

Linder, Douglas O. The other right–to–life debate: when does Fourteenth Amendment "life" end? *Arizona Law Review.* 1995; 37(4): 1183–1207. 138 fn. BE62218.
  *allowing to die; artificial feeding; bioethical issues; *brain death; brain pathology; coercion; constitutional law; *determination of death; due process; federal government; government financing; *legal aspects; legal rights; *persistent vegetative state; *personhood; *prolongation of life; *public policy; resource allocation; self concept; state government; Supreme Court decisions; *value of life; vulnerable populations; wedge argument; *withholding treatment; *Fourteenth Amendment; *United States

McMahan, Jeff. Brain death, cortical death and persistent vegetative state. *In:* Kuhse, Helga; Singer, Peter, eds. A Companion to Bioethics. Malden, MA: Blackwell; 1998: 250–260. 15 refs. ISBN 0-631-19737-0. BE59500.
  *brain; *brain death; *brain pathology; dementia; *determination of death; organ donation; *persistent vegetative state; *personhood; philosophy; self concept; uncertainty; withholding treatment; conjoined twins; locked-in syndrome

McMahan, Jeff. Cloning, killing, and identity. *Journal of Medical Ethics.* 1999 Apr; 25(2): 77–86. 8 fn. BE61907.
  *beginning of life; brain; *cloning; embryos; fetal development; fetuses; *killing; *moral policy; organ donation; *personhood; philosophy; self concept; tissue donation; twinning; twins; conjoined twins; nuclear transplantation; personal identity

---

BE = bioethics accession number   fn. = footnotes   refs. = references

One potentially valuable use of cloning is to provide a source of tissues or organs for transplantation. The most important objection to this use of cloning is that a human clone would be the sort of entity that it would be seriously wrong to kill. I argue that entities of the sort that you and I essentially are do not begin to exist until around the seventh month of fetal gestation. Therefore to kill a clone prior to that would not be to kill someone like you or me but would be only to prevent one of us from existing. And even after one of us begins to exist, the objections to killing it remain comparatively weak until its psychological capacities reach a certain level of maturation. These claims support the permissibility of killing a clone during the early stages of its development in order to use its organs for transplantation.

Morgan, Lynn M. Fetal relationality in feminist philosophy: an anthropological critique. *Hypatia.* 1996 Summer; 11(3): 47–70. 78 refs. 13 fn. BE61458.

> abortion, induced; anthropology; beginning of life; embryos; *feminist ethics; fetal development; *fetuses; infanticide; *mother fetus relationship; mothers; newborns; non–Western World; *personhood; philosophy; pregnant women; social interaction; value of life; Western World; relational ethics

Mori, Maurizio. On the concept of pre-embryo: the basis for a new "Copernican revolution" in the current view about human reproduction. *In:* Harris, John; Holm, Søren, eds. The Future of Human Reproduction: Ethics, Choice, and Regulation. New York, NY: Oxford University Press; 1998: 38–54. 15 fn. ISBN 0–19–823761–8. BE61261.

> abortion, induced; *beginning of life; biology; contraception; *embryos; *personhood; terminology; twinning; value of life

Pauer–Studer, Herlinde. Peter Singer on euthanasia. *Monist.* 1993 Apr; 76(2): 135–157. 22 refs. 42 fn. BE60218.

> abortion, induced; *active euthanasia; adults; *allowing to die; congenital disorders; death; *disabled; *dissent; ethical theory; eugenics; fetuses; infanticide; involuntary euthanasia; *killing; *moral policy; National Socialism; *newborns; pain; parental consent; *personhood; political activity; *quality of life; social worth; speciesism; *utilitarianism; value of life; voluntary euthanasia; wedge argument; withholding treatment; rationality; Austria; Germany; Rachels, James; *Singer, Peter

Scholl, Ann. Legally protecting fetuses: a study of the legal protections afforded organically united individuals. *Public Affairs Quarterly.* 1997 Apr; 11(2): 141–161. 17 refs. 26 fn. BE61896.

> abortion on demand; cesarean section; coercion; *fetuses; legal obligations; *legal rights; mother fetus relationship; *personhood; *pregnant women; therapeutic abortion; treatment refusal; twins; *women's rights; conjoined twins; Warren, Mary Anne

Shewmon, D. Alan. Recovery from "brain death": a neurologist's apologia. *Linacre Quarterly.* 1997 Feb; 64(1): 30–96. 268 refs. 9 fn. BE59309.

> adults; anencephaly; artificial feeding; *brain; *brain death; *brain pathology; cadavers; *cardiac death; childbirth; children; consensus; dementia; *determination of death; *dissent; historical aspects; infants; killing; legal aspects; organ donation; organizational policies; pain; *persistent vegetative state; *personhood; *philosophy; physicians; pregnant women; professional organizations; Roman Catholic ethics; standards; suffering; *uncertainty; utilitarianism; withholding treatment; Guillain-Barre syndrome; locked-in syndrome; neurology; American Academy of Neurology; American Medical Association; Aristotle; President's Commission for the Study of Ethical Problems; Thomas Aquinas; Twentieth Century

Sly, William S. When does human life begin? Does science provide the answer? *In:* Rainey, R. Randall; Magill, Gerard, eds. Abortion and Public Policy: An Interdisciplinary Investigation within the Catholic Tradition. Omaha, NE: Creighton University Press; 1996: 62–71. 23 fn. Paper presented at a conference held at Saint Louis University, 11–13 Mar 1993. ISBN 1–881871–18–5. BE61990.

> abortion, induced; *beginning of life; cryopreservation; embryo disposition; *embryos; *fetal development; legal aspects; *personhood; preimplantation diagnosis; public policy; *Roman Catholic ethics; science; United States

Tollefsen, Christopher. Advance directives and voluntary slavery: response to "Reassessing the reliability of advance directives," by Thomas May (*CQ* Vol. 6, No. 3). *Cambridge Quarterly of Healthcare Ethics.* 1998 Fall; 7(4): 405–413. 21 fn. BE59141.

> *advance directives; *autonomy; *competence; decision analysis; *decision making; *directive adherence; *evaluation; family members; informed consent; motivation; patient participation; *patients; *personhood; physicians; *self concept; third party consent; virtues; slavery

Tooley, Michael. Personhood. *In:* Kuhse, Helga; Singer, Peter, eds. A Companion to Bioethics. Malden, MA: Blackwell; 1998: 117–126. 17 refs. ISBN 0–631–19737–0. BE59488.

> animal rights; beginning of life; brain pathology; embryos; ethical theory; fetuses; killing; moral obligations; *moral policy; newborns; *personhood; philosophy; self concept; speciesism; standards; value of life

Vial Correa, Juan de Dios; Sgreccia, Elio, eds.; Pontificia Academia pro Vita. Identity and Statute [Status] of [the] Human Embryo: Proceedings of [the] Third Assembly of the Pontifical Academy for Life (Vatican City, February 14–16, 1997). Vatican City: Libreria Editrice Vaticana; 1998. 458 p. ISBN 88–209–2470–6. BE60114.

> abortion, induced; advisory committees; anthropology; *beginning of life; biology; embryo research; *embryos; fetal development; fetuses; historical aspects; human characteristics; human rights; international aspects; legal aspects; moral policy; morality; *personhood; philosophy; preimplantation diagnosis; prenatal diagnosis; public policy; reproductive technologies; *Roman Catholic ethics; *theology; *value of life; abortion, spontaneous; personal identity; United Nations; Universal Declaration of Human Rights

Wendler, Dave. Understanding the 'conservative' view on abortion. *Bioethics.* 1999 Jan; 13(1): 32–56. 16 fn. BE60887.

> *abortion, induced; cryopreservation; *embryos; *fetal development; fetal therapy; *fetuses; genetic determinism; genetic information; in vitro fertilization; moral obligations; *moral policy; morality; *personhood; policy analysis; abortion, spontaneous; potentiality

Wheale, Peter R. Moral and legal consequences for the fetus/unborn child of medical technologies derived from human genome research. *In:* Glasner, Peter; Rothman, Harry, eds. Genetic Imaginations: Ethical, Legal and Social Issues in Human Genome Research. Brookfield, VT: Ashgate; 1998: 83–96. 35 refs. Based on a paper presented at a workshop hosted by the Centre for Social and Economic Research at the University of the West of England; reprinted from *The Genetic Engineer and Biotechnologist*, 1995; 15(2–3). ISBN 1–84014–356–8. BE60020.

> abortion, induced; *beginning of life; coercion; *congenital disorders; deontological ethics; *embryo research; *embryos;

BE = bioethics accession number   fn. = footnotes   refs. = references

ethical analysis; fetal development; *fetuses; genetic disorders; genetic screening; genome mapping; government regulation; *legal aspects; legal liability; *moral obligations; *moral policy; negligence; *personhood; pregnant women; prenatal injuries; *public policy; *quality of life; rights; *selective abortion; social impact; treatment refusal; utilitarianism; *value of life; *wrongful life; *Great Britain

Court rules that fetuses are not "persons" entitled to be counted in the census: John Desmond Slattery v. William J. Clinton and William M. Daley, et al. (U.S. District Court, Southern District of New York, 1997). [News]. *Reporter on Human Reproduction and the Law.* 1997 Nov-Dec; No. 11-12: 62-63. BE60062.
federal government; *fetuses; *legal aspects; *personhood; statistics; *Slattery v. Clinton and Daley; *United States

PHYSICIAN PATIENT RELATIONSHIP *See* MEDICAL ETHICS, PROFESSIONAL PATIENT RELATIONSHIP

POPULATION CONTROL

See also CONTRACEPTION

Abrams, Paula. Reservations about women: population policy and reproductive rights. *Cornell International Law Journal.* 1996; 29(1): 1-41. 227 fn. BE59445.
*autonomy; *coercion; contraception; cultural pluralism; *decision making; developing countries; economics; family planning; *females; government regulation; *human rights; incentives; *international aspects; law; *legal rights; mandatory programs; non-Western World; *population control; *public policy; *reproduction; *social control; social discrimination; socioeconomic factors; sterilization (sexual); utilitarianism; voluntary programs; Western World; *women's rights; Convention on the Elimination of All Forms of Discrimination Against Women; United Nations International Conference on Population and Development; Universal Declaration of Human Rights

Baier, Kurt. Wrongful death and wrongful life. *In:* his Problems of Life and Death: A Humanist Perspective. Amherst, NY: Prometheus Books; 1997: 137-230. 74 fn. ISBN 1-57392-153-X. BE61848.
*allowing to die; *assisted suicide; capital punishment; contraception; disabled; disclosure; ethical theory; guidelines; *humanism; intention; *killing; law; legal aspects; legal liability; moral obligations; *moral policy; *morality; negligence; organ donation; physicians; *population control; prognosis; *prolongation of life; quality of life; suffering; suicide; value of life; values; *voluntary euthanasia; wrongful death; *wrongful life; rationality

Battin, Margaret Pabst. Population issues. *In:* Kuhse, Helga; Singer, Peter, eds. A Companion to Bioethics. Malden, MA: Blackwell; 1998: 149-162. 18 refs. ISBN 0-631-19737-0. BE59491.
contraception; family planning; feminist ethics; incentives; international aspects; mandatory programs; *population control; public policy; religious ethics; socioeconomic factors; voluntary programs

Gudorf, Christine E. Gender and culture in the globalization of bioethics. *Saint Louis University Public Law Review.* 1996; 15(2): 331-351. 122 fn. BE59913.
autonomy; beneficence; *bioethics; children; *circumcision; *coercion; *common good; contraception; *cultural pluralism; developing countries; ecology; *females; *feminist ethics; human rights; injuries; *international aspects; involuntary sterilization; justice; males; non-Western World; obligations to society; physicians; *population control; public policy; religion; reproduction; risks and benefits; sexuality;

social control; Western World; *women's health

Kligman, Gail. The Politics of Duplicity: Controlling Reproduction in Ceausecu's Romania. Berkeley, CA: University of California Press; 1998. 358 p. Bibliography: p. 331-346. ISBN 0-520-21075-1. BE60112.
*abortion, induced; adoption; coercion; communism; contraception; deception; dehumanization; dissent; economics; females; fraud; government regulation; historical aspects; *illegal abortion; incentives; information dissemination; international aspects; legal aspects; mass media; moral complicity; morbidity; mortality; paternalism; physicians; *political systems; politics; *population control; *public policy; *reproduction; *social control; social impact; socioeconomic factors; statistics; unwanted children; women's health; *Romania; *Twentieth Century

Robb, Carol S. Liberties, claims, entitlements, and trumps: reproductive rights and ecological responsibilities. *Journal of Religious Ethics.* 1998 Fall; 26(2): 283-294. 6 refs. 3 fn. BE61895.
Christian ethics; communitarianism; *ecology; freedom; *human rights; international aspects; justice; *moral obligations; natural law; *obligations to society; *population control; *reproduction; socioeconomic factors; speciesism; women's rights; International Covenant on Civil and Political Rights; International Covenant on Economic, Social and Cultural Rights

Sen, Amartya. Fertility and coercion. *University of Chicago Law Review.* 1996 Summer; 63(3): 1035-1061. 68 fn. BE60351.
autonomy; *coercion; decision making; *developing countries; *family planning; females; freedom; goals; historical aspects; international aspects; involuntary sterilization; justice; libertarianism; *population control; *public policy; reproduction; rights; *socioeconomic factors; utilitarianism; voluntary programs; women's rights; China; India

Tang, Julie. The United States' immigration laws: prospects for relief for foreign nationals seeking refuge from coercive sterilization or abortion practices in their homelands. *Saint Louis University Public Law Review.* 1996; 15(2): 371-401. 165 fn. BE59915.
*abortion, induced; *aliens; *coercion; federal government; *human rights; *international aspects; *involuntary sterilization; judicial action; *legal aspects; *mandatory programs; political systems; *population control; *public policy; reproduction; *emigration and immigration; *China; In re Chang; U.S. Congress; *United States

PRENATAL DIAGNOSIS

See also GENETIC COUNSELING, GENETIC SCREENING, SEX DETERMINATION

Anderson, Gwen. Nondirectiveness in prenatal genetics: patients read between the lines. *Nursing Ethics.* 1999 Mar; 6(2): 126-136. 33 refs. BE61932.
age factors; *attitudes; communication; congenital disorders; costs and benefits; decision making; *directive counseling; disclosure; fathers; females; *genetic counseling; genetic information; *genetic screening; genetic services; health personnel; males; marital relationship; married persons; moral obligations; narrative ethics; nurses; nursing research; *patients; *pregnant women; *prenatal diagnosis; professional patient relationship; quality of life; selective abortion; suffering; uncertainty; *values; qualitative research; right not to know

Andrews, Lori B. Prenatal screening and the culture of motherhood. *Hastings Law Journal.* 1996 Apr; 47(4):

967–1006. 185 fn. BE59844.
> autonomy; carriers; coercion; decision making; directive counseling; disabled; employment; family relationship; females; genetic disorders; genetic information; *genetic screening; genetic services; insurance selection bias; legal rights; mandatory testing; marital relationship; mass screening; *methods; mother fetus relationship; mothers; parent child relationship; policy analysis; *pregnant women; *prenatal diagnosis; privacy; psychological stress; *public policy; risks and benefits; selective abortion; self concept; social discrimination; *social impact; state interest; treatment refusal; ELSI-funded publication; Fourth Amendment; United States

Beech, Beverley A. Lawrence; Anderson, Gwen. 'We went through psychological hell': a case report of prenatal diagnosis. [Case study and commentaries]. *Nursing Ethics.* 1999 May; 6(3): 250–256. 12 refs. BE61769.
> age factors; amniocentesis; case studies; communication; congenital disorders; disclosure; Down syndrome; *genetic services; informed consent; interdisciplinary communication; interprofessional relations; *medical errors; patient advocacy; patient care team; *pregnant women; *prenatal diagnosis; professional patient relationship; *psychological stress; *quality of health care; risks and benefits; selective abortion; continuity of patient care; Australia

Boué, A. *Primum non nocere*: prenatal diagnosis and selective abortion. *In:* Burgio, G. Roberto; Lantos, John D., eds. *Primum Non Nocere* Today. Second Edition. New York, NY: Elsevier; 1998: 49–57. ISBN 0-444-82923-7. BE60920.
> *congenital disorders; *decision making; disabled; family relationship; fetal therapy; fetuses; genetic counseling; genetic disorders; information dissemination; legal aspects; mass media; maternal health; newborns; obstetrics and gynecology; *parents; patient care team; physicians; pregnant women; *prenatal diagnosis; prognosis; quality of life; risk; *selective abortion; surgery; uncertainty; ultrasonography; France

Bowes, Watson; Byrne, Paul; Cavanagh, Denis, et al. True integrity for the maternal–fetal medicine physician. *Linacre Quarterly.* 1997 Aug; 64(3): 77–86. 14 refs. Response to J. Blustein and A.R. Fleischman, "The pro-life maternal–fetal medicine physician: a problem of integrity," *Hastings Center Report*, 1995 Jan–Feb; 25(1): 22–26. BE59312.
> *abortion, induced; *attitudes; *beginning of life; children; *congenital disorders; *conscience; counseling; decision making; disclosure; Down syndrome; information dissemination; medical education; *moral complicity; *moral policy; morality; *obstetrics and gynecology; *physicians; pregnant women; *prenatal diagnosis; secularism; *selective abortion; *value of life; values; *integrity

Bowman, James E. To screen or not to screen: when should screening be offered? *Community Genetics.* 1998; 1(3): 145–147. 8 refs. BE62285.
> blacks; confidentiality; disadvantaged; disclosure; employment; genetic counseling; genetic information; *genetic screening; insurance; Jews; mass screening; phenylketonuria; *prenatal diagnosis; sickle cell anemia; single persons; social discrimination; Tay Sachs disease; United States

Campbell, Harry; Boyd, Kenneth. Screening and the new genetics: a public health perspective on the ethical debate. [Letter]. *Journal of Public Health Medicine.* 1996 Dec; 18(4): 485–486. 9 refs. BE60691.
> autonomy; costs and benefits; cystic fibrosis; eugenics; *genetic screening; mass screening; *prenatal diagnosis; public health; public policy

Choo, Vivien. Thin line between research and audit. *Lancet.* 1998 Aug 1; 352(9125): 337–338. 11 refs. Comment on R.J.M. Snijders et al., p. 343–346. BE60436.
> *Down syndrome; *editorial policies; *ethical review; *evaluation studies; human experimentation; informed consent; *methods; patient care; pregnant women; *prenatal diagnosis; *research ethics committees; *medical audit; Great Britain; Lancet

Cuckle, Howard. Rational Down syndrome screening policy. *American Journal of Public Health.* 1998 Apr; 88(4): 558–559. 13 refs. BE60129.
> age factors; chorionic villi sampling; costs and benefits; *decision analysis; *Down syndrome; fetal development; *mass screening; *methods; *pregnant women; *prenatal diagnosis; *public policy; risk; risks and benefits; values; ultrasonography

DauBach, Penelope P. Homegrown Eugenics: Socioeconomic Differentials in Utilization of Prenatal Testing. Ann Arbor, MI: University Microfilms International; 1997. 299 p. Bibliography: p. 269–299. Dissertation, Ph.D. in Anthropology, University of Kansas, 1997. UMI No. 9811292. BE60012.
> children; comparative studies; congenital disorders; costs and benefits; *decision making; *eugenics; females; genetic counseling; government financing; health insurance; indigents; *knowledge, attitudes, practice; minority groups; motivation; *pregnant women; *prenatal diagnosis; selective abortion; *socioeconomic factors; survey; whites; Medicaid; United States

Draper, Heather; Chadwick, Ruth. Beware! Preimplantation genetic diagnosis may solve some old problems but it also raises new ones. *Journal of Medical Ethics.* 1999 Apr; 25(2): 114–120. 6 fn. BE61913.
> abortion, induced; autonomy; beginning of life; case studies; children; *decision making; disabled; Down syndrome; *embryo transfer; *embryos; *genetic disorders; *genetic screening; hearing disorders; *in vitro fertilization; legal aspects; *moral obligations; *moral policy; motivation; *parents; *physicians; pregnant women; *preimplantation diagnosis; prenatal diagnosis; property rights; *quality of life; *reproduction; rights; risks and benefits; value of life

Preimplantation genetic diagnosis (PIGD) goes some way to meeting the clinical, psychological and ethical problems of antenatal testing. We should guard, however, against the assumption that PIGD is the answer to all our problems. It also presents some new problems and leaves some old problems untouched. This paper will provide an overview of how PIGD meets some of the old problems but will concentrate on two new challenges for ethics (and, indeed, law). First we look at whether we should always suppose that it is wrong for a clinician to implant a genetically abnormal zygote. The second concern is particularly important in the UK. The Human Fertilisation and Embryology Act (1990) gives clinicians a statutory obligation to consider the interests of the future children they help to create using in vitro fertilisation (IVF) techniques. Does this mean that because PIGD is based on IVF techniques the balance of power for determining the best interests of the future child shifts from the mother to the clinician?

Dunne, Cara; Warren, Catherine. Lethal autonomy: the malfunction of the informed consent mechanism within the context of prenatal diagnosis of genetic variants. *Issues in Law and Medicine.* 1998 Fall; 14(2): 165–202. 75 fn. BE62011.
> *autonomy; cancer; directive counseling; disclosure; Down syndrome; *eugenics; *genetic counseling; genetic disorders; genetic screening; genome mapping; health personnel;

BE = bioethics accession number   fn. = footnotes   refs. = references

historical aspects; *informed consent; killing; legal liability; mentally retarded; minority groups; National Socialism; physician's role; *prenatal diagnosis; quality of life; selective abortion; social discrimination; sterilization (sexual); wrongful life; Germany; Human Genome Project; Twentieth Century; United States

Eisenberg, Vered H.; Schenker, Joseph J. The moral aspects of prenatal diagnosis. *European Journal of Obstetrics, Gynecology, and Reproductive Biology.* 1997 Mar; 72(1): 35–45. 79 fn. BE60477.
attitudes; autonomy; chromosome abnormalities; congenital disorders; decision making; fetal development; fetal therapy; fetuses; genetic counseling; genetic disorders; guidelines; health personnel; legal aspects; methods; multiple pregnancy; obstetrics and gynecology; pregnant women; *prenatal diagnosis; privacy; professional organizations; religious ethics; risks and benefits; selective abortion; socioeconomic factors; International Federation of Gynecology and Obstetrics

Episcopal Diocese of Washington, D.C. Committee on Medical Ethics (Chair: Cynthia B. Cohen). Wrestling with the Future: Our Genes and Our Choices. Harrisburg, PA: Morehouse Publishing; 1998. 132 p. Bibliography: p. 125–127. ISBN 0-8192-1762-X. BE61310.
adolescents; adults; carriers; case studies; children; chromosome abnormalities; clergy; confidentiality; congenital disorders; decision making; disclosure; employment; family members; family relationship; genetic counseling; genetic disorders; genetic information; genetic intervention; genetic predisposition; *genetic screening; health insurance; health personnel; informed consent; late-onset disorders; morality; newborns; parents; pastoral care; preimplantation diagnosis; *prenatal diagnosis; privacy; *Protestant ethics; psychological stress; reproduction; *risks and benefits; *selective abortion; sex determination; social discrimination; stigmatization; theology; uncertainty; *Anglican Church; *Episcopal Church; United States

Evers-Kiebooms, Gerry. Adolescents' opinions about genetic risk and genetic testing. *In:* Sterckx, Sigrid, ed. Biotechnology, Patents and Morality. Proceedings of an International Workshop, "Biotechnology, Patents and Morality: Towards a Consensus," held in Ghent, Belgium, 17–19 Jan 1996. Brookfield, VT: Ashgate; 1997: 85–95. 8 refs. ISBN 1-84014-158-1. BE62237.
*adolescents; *attitudes; congenital disorders; genetic counseling; *genetic disorders; *genetic screening; *knowledge, attitudes, practice; mentally disabled; physically disabled; *prenatal diagnosis; *risk; risks and benefits; selective abortion; survey; Belgium

Freda, Margaret Comerford; DeVore, Nancy; Valentine-Adams, Nancy, et al. Informed consent for maternal serum alpha-fetoprotein screening in an inner city population: how informed is it? *Journal of Obstetric, Gynecologic and Neonatal Nursing.* 1998 Jan-Feb; 27(1): 99–106. 32 refs. BE62061.
*comprehension; congenital disorders; disadvantaged; disclosure; *informed consent; knowledge, attitudes, practice; *minority groups; nurse's role; *pregnant women; *prenatal diagnosis; survey; *alpha fetoproteins; prospective studies; qualitative research; *urban population; United States

Gillam, Lynn. Prenatal diagnosis and discrimination against the disabled. *Journal of Medical Ethics.* 1999 Apr; 25(2): 163–171. 34 fn. BE61921.
children; community services; *congenital disorders; *disabled; Down syndrome; fetuses; genetic disorders; genetic screening; genetic services; government financing; justice; killing; moral obligations; *moral policy; parents; personhood; pregnant women; *prenatal diagnosis;

prevalence; *quality of life; *selective abortion; *social discrimination; *social impact; social worth; stigmatization; value of life; values; *wedge argument
Two versions of the argument that prenatal diagnosis discriminates against the disabled are distinguished and analysed. Both are shown to be inadequate, but some valid concerns about the social effects of prenatal diagnosis are highlighted.

Golden, Frederic. Good eggs, bad eggs: the growing power of prenatal genetic tests is raising thorny new questions about ethics, fairness and privacy. *Time.* 1999 Jan 11; 153(1): 56–59. BE60309.
congenital disorders; decision making; disclosure; employment; family members; fetuses; genetic counseling; genetic disorders; *genetic information; genetic predisposition; *genetic screening; health insurance; late-onset disorders; parents; preimplantation diagnosis; *prenatal diagnosis; public opinion; selective abortion; *social discrimination; truth disclosure; United States

Goodey, Chris; Alderson, Priscilla; Appleby, John. The ethical implications of antenatal screening for Down's syndrome: Socratic inquiry; The good life?; [and] Calculating the costs and benefits. *Bulletin of Medical Ethics.* 1999 Apr; No. 147: 13–17. 14 refs. BE61823.
attitudes; behavioral research; costs and benefits; *Down syndrome; health personnel; mass screening; mentally retarded; motivation; parents; *prenatal diagnosis; quality of life; risks and benefits; stigmatization; suffering; Great Britain

Haddow, James E. Antenatal screening for Down's syndrome: where are we and where next? *Lancet.* 1998 Aug 1; 352(9125): 336–337. 10 refs. Commentary on R.J.M. Snijders et al., p. 343–346. BE60435.
*Down syndrome; evaluation; mass screening; *methods; *prenatal diagnosis; *risk; ultrasonography; Finland; Great Britain; United States

Hadley, Janet. Prenatal tests: blessings and burdens. *In:* Lee, Ellie, ed. Abortion Law and Politics Today. New York, NY: St. Martin's Press; 1998: 172–183. 27 fn. ISBN 0-312-21574-6. BE62337.
*congenital disorders; *decision making; directive counseling; *disabled; economics; *eugenics; genetic counseling; genetic disorders; genetic predisposition; genetic screening; international aspects; involuntary sterilization; late-onset disorders; parents; pregnant women; preimplantation diagnosis; *prenatal diagnosis; *public policy; rights; *selective abortion; *stigmatization; Great Britain

Harris, John. Doctors' orders, rationality and the good life: commentary on Savulescu. *Journal of Medical Ethics.* 1999 Apr; 25(2): 127–129. 7 fn. BE61915.
*autonomy; *beneficence; cloning; conscience; *decision making; *embryo transfer; freedom; in vitro fertilization; moral complicity; *moral obligations; moral policy; *motivation; parents; patients; *physicians; *preimplantation diagnosis; *reproduction; *reproductive technologies; *values; rationality

Hasadsri, Linda. The multi-faceted implications of preimplantation genetic testing. *Princeton Journal of Bioethics.* 1998 Spring; 1(1): 76–82. 8 refs. BE62494.
disabled; embryos; eugenics; genetic disorders; *genetic screening; late-onset disorders; moral obligations; normality; *preimplantation diagnosis; *risks and benefits; selective abortion; social discrimination

Heikkilä, Annaleena; Ryynänen, Markku; Kirkinen, Pertti, et al. Results and views of women in population-wide pregnancy screening for trisomy 21 in

East Finland. *Fetal Diagnosis and Therapy.* 1997 Mar-Apr; 12(2): 93-96. 22 refs. BE59230.
   age factors; *attitudes; *Down syndrome; *mass screening; *pregnant women; *prenatal diagnosis; survey; *Finland

Hoedemaekers, Rogeer; ten Have, Henk. Geneticization: the Cyprus paradigm. *Journal of Medicine and Philosophy.* 1998 Jun; 23(3): 274-287. 17 refs. BE59291.
   *attitudes; carriers; *coercion; decision making; *directive counseling; economics; eugenics; *genetic counseling; *genetic screening; genetic services; genetics; *goals; health education; *health personnel; international aspects; *mass screening; parents; paternalism; *prenatal diagnosis; prevalence; preventive medicine; public health; public opinion; quality of life; *selective abortion; social control; stigmatization; *thalassemia; *Cyprus; Great Britain; Quebec
Geneticization is a broad term referring to several related processes such as a spreading tendency to use a genetic model of disease explanation, a growing influence of genetics in medical practice, and the slow changing of individual and societal attitudes towards reproduction, prevention and control of disease. These processes can be demonstrated in medical literature on preventive genetic screening and counselling programs for beta-thalassaemia in Cyprus, the United Kingdom and Canada. The preventive possibilities of the new genetic and diagnostic technologies have been quickly understood and advocated by health professionals, and their educational strategies have created a web of social control, in marked contrast to the alleged voluntary decision-making process and free choice. Genetic diagnostic technologies have led to considerable changes in control and management of beta-thalassaemia, and have generated a number of unresolved incongruities.

Holm, Søren. Ethical issues in pre-implantation diagnosis. *In:* Harris, John; Holm, Søren, eds. The Future of Human Reproduction: Ethics, Choice, and Regulation. New York, NY: Oxford University Press; 1998: 176-190. 11 fn. ISBN 0-19-823761-8. BE61269.
   autonomy; communitarianism; decision making; disabled; eugenics; genetic disorders; genetic screening; government regulation; moral policy; parents; *preimplantation diagnosis; prenatal diagnosis; reproductive technologies; resource allocation; risks and benefits; sex preselection; standards

Kerr, Anne; Cunningham-Burley, Sarah; Amos, Amanda. Drawing the line: an analysis of lay people's discussions about the new genetics. *Public Understanding of Science.* 1998 Apr; 7(2): 113-133. 14 fn. BE60906.
   autonomy; behavioral genetics; children; cystic fibrosis; decision making; Down syndrome; eugenics; genetic counseling; genetic disorders; *genetic research; *genetic screening; *genetics; homosexuals; *knowledge, attitudes, practice; physicians; *prenatal diagnosis; *public opinion; *public participation; quality of life; selective abortion; socioeconomic factors; stigmatization; suffering; survey; focus groups; qualitative research; Scotland

King, David S. Preimplantation genetic diagnosis and the 'new' eugenics. *Journal of Medical Ethics.* 1999 Apr; 25(2): 176-182. 33 refs. BE61923.
   carriers; coercion; congenital disorders; decision making; directive counseling; disabled; embryo disposition; embryo transfer; embryos; *eugenics; gene pool; genetic counseling; genetic disorders; genetic predisposition; *genetic screening; goals; government regulation; health personnel; in vitro fertilization; informal social control; international aspects; knowledge, attitudes, practice; *moral policy; normality; parent child relationship; parents; physicians; *preimplantation diagnosis; prenatal diagnosis; public policy; selective abortion; social discrimination; *social impact;

socioeconomic factors; trends
Preimplantation genetic diagnosis (PID) is often seen as an improvement upon prenatal testing. I argue that PID may exacerbate the eugenic features of prenatal testing and make possible an expanded form of free-market eugenics. The current practice of prenatal testing is eugenic in that its aim is to reduce the numbers of people with genetic disorders. Due to social pressures and eugenic attitudes held by clinical geneticists in most countries, it results in eugenic outcomes even though no state coercion is involved. I argue that technological advances may soon make PID widely accessible. Because abortion is not involved, and multiple embryos are available, PID is radically more effective as a tool of genetic selection. It will also make possible selection on the basis of non-pathological characteristics, leading, potentially, to a full-blown free-market eugenics. For these reasons, I argue that PID should be strictly regulated.

Lafayette, DeeDee; Abuelo, Dianne; Passero, Mary Ann, et al. Attitudes toward cystic fibrosis carrier and prenatal testing and utilization of carrier testing among relatives of individuals with cystic fibrosis. *Journal of Genetic Counseling.* 1999 Feb; 8(1): 17-36. 57 refs. BE61642.
   *attitudes; *carriers; *cystic fibrosis; *family members; family planning; *genetic counseling; *genetic screening; *knowledge, attitudes, practice; *prenatal diagnosis; quality of life; *selective abortion; survey; Rhode Island

Lemonick, Michael D. Designer babies. *Time.* 1999 Jan 11; 153(1): 64-67. BE60312.
   eugenics; genetic disorders; *genetic enhancement; in vitro fertilization; methods; *preimplantation diagnosis; prenatal diagnosis; public opinion; selective abortion; *sex preselection; social impact; United States

McFadyen, Anne; Gledhill, Julia; Whitlow, Barry, et al. First trimester ultrasound screening carries ethical and psychological implications. [Editorial]. *BMJ (British Medical Journal).* 1998 Sep 12; 317(7160): 694-695. 11 refs. BE59883.
   chromosome abnormalities; congenital disorders; disclosure; fetal development; fetuses; genetic counseling; genetic disorders; *informed consent; mass screening; *pregnant women; *prenatal diagnosis; psychological stress; *risks and benefits; selective abortion; *time factors; treatment refusal; uncertainty; *ultrasonography

Mackler, Aaron L. An expanded partnership with God? In vitro fertilization in Jewish ethics. *Journal of Religious Ethics.* 1997 Fall; 25(2): 277-304. 76 refs. 16 fn. BE60304.
   cryopreservation; embryo disposition; embryo research; *embryo transfer; embryos; fetal development; fetuses; genetic screening; *in vitro fertilization; *Jewish ethics; *married persons; maternal health; mental health; mothers; multiple pregnancy; *ovum donors; parent child relationship; personhood; *preimplantation diagnosis; prenatal diagnosis; reproduction; *reproductive technologies; risks and benefits; selective abortion; *semen donors; *theology; therapeutic abortion

Mao, Xin. Chinese geneticists approach ethics. [Letter]. *Journal of Medical Ethics.* 1998 Jan; 35(1): 83. 14 refs. BE61126.
   *attitudes; confidentiality; developing countries; *directive counseling; disclosure; eugenics; *genetic counseling; genetic disorders; genetic predisposition; genetic research; *genetic screening; genetic services; genetics; guidelines; *health personnel; international aspects; investigators; *non-Western World; *prenatal diagnosis; *selective abortion; sex determination; survey; Western World; *China

Middleton, A.; Hewison, J.; Mueller, R.F. A pilot study of attitudes of deaf and hearing parents towards issues surrounding genetic testing for deafness. [Abstract]. *American Journal of Human Genetics.* 1997 Oct; 61(4): A190. BE59395.
    *attitudes; comparative studies; *genetic disorders; *genetic screening; *hearing disorders; *parents; *physically disabled; *prenatal diagnosis; *selective abortion; survey; Great Britain

Müller, H.J.; Deonna, Th.; Abbt, I., et al. Medical-ethical guidelines for genetic investigations in humans. *Schweizerische Medizinische Wochenschrift.* 1994 Jun 4; 124(22): 974-979. 5 refs. BE59774.
    confidentiality; disclosure; employment; *genetic counseling; genetic disorders; genetic predisposition; genetic research; *genetic screening; informed consent; insurance; physicians; *practice guidelines; *prenatal diagnosis; professional organizations; selective abortion; right not to know; *Swiss Academy of Medical Sciences

Nagy, Anne-Marie; De Man, Xavier; Ruibal, Nike, et al. Scientific and ethical issues of preimplantation diagnosis. [Editorial]. *Annals of Medicine.* 1998 Feb; 30(1): 1-6. 35 refs. BE62401.
    chromosome abnormalities; genetic disorders; genetic predisposition; *genetic screening; methods; *preimplantation diagnosis; sex preselection

Newell, Christopher. The social nature of disability, disease and genetics: a response to Gillam, Persson, Holtug, Draper and Chadwick. *Journal of Medical Ethics.* 1999 Apr; 25(2): 172-175. 13 fn. BE61922.
    bioethics; congenital disorders; decision making; *disabled; disease; embryo transfer; genetic disorders; genetic enhancement; genetic intervention; genetic screening; hearing disorders; normality; *preimplantation diagnosis; *prenatal diagnosis; quality of life; selective abortion; social control; *social discrimination; *social dominance; social worth; suffering; value of life; *values
The dominance of the biomedically informed view of disability, genetics, and diagnosis is explored. An understanding of the social nature of disability and genetics, especially in terms of oppression, adds a richer dimension to an understanding of ethical issues pertaining to genetics. This is much wider than the limited question of whether or not such technology discriminates. Instead, it is proposed that such technology will perpetuate the oppression and control of people with disability, especially if the knowledge of people with disability is not utilised in bioethical debates.

Paintin, David, ed. Ante-Natal Screening and Abortion for Fetal Abnormality. London: Birth Control Trust; 1997. 96 p. Includes references. Proceedings of a symposium held in London, 26 Sep 1996, at the Royal Society of Medicine. ISBN 0-906-233-37-2. BE59737.
    *congenital disorders; counseling; decision making; Down syndrome; economics; fetal development; methods; morality; nurse midwives; obstetrics and gynecology; parents; personhood; physicians; pregnant women; *prenatal diagnosis; preventive medicine; psychological stress; psychology; *selective abortion; needs; ultrasonography; Great Britain

Persson, Ingmar. Equality and selection for existence. *Journal of Medical Ethics.* 1999 Apr; 25(2): 130-136. 3 refs. BE61916.
    *beginning of life; congenital disorders; *disabled; embryo disposition; *embryo transfer; *embryos; genetic determinism; *genetic disorders; *genetic screening; germ cells; in vitro fertilization; *justice; *moral policy; personhood; *preimplantation diagnosis; public policy; *quality of life; rights; self concept; social interaction; *social worth; speciesism; *utilitarianism; *value of life
It is argued that the policy of excluding from further life some human gametes and pre-embryos as "unfit" for existence is not at odds with a defensible idea of human equality. Such an idea must be compatible with the obvious fact that the "functional" value of humans differs, that their "use" to themselves and others differs. A defensible idea of human equality is instead grounded in the fact that as this functional difference is genetically determined, it is nothing which makes humans deserve or be worthy of being better or worse off. Rather, nobody is worth a better life than anyone else. This idea of equality is, however, not applicable to gametes and pre-embryos, since they are not human beings, but something out of which human beings develop.

Rapp, Rayna. Refusing prenatal diagnosis: the meanings of bioscience in a multicultural world. *Science, Technology, and Human Values.* 1998 Winter; 23(1): 45-70. 19 refs. 5 fn. BE60419.
    aliens; *attitudes; blacks; *cultural pluralism; decision making; females; genetic counseling; genetic disorders; Hispanic Americans; indigents; Jews; males; *minority groups; *motivation; *pregnant women; *prenatal diagnosis; *religion; reproduction; risks and benefits; selective abortion; socioeconomic factors; treatment refusal; women's health services; ethnographic studies; *refusal to participate

Robinson, Paul. Prenatal screening, sex selection and cloning. *In:* Kuhse, Helga; Singer, Peter, eds. A Companion to Bioethics. Malden, MA: Blackwell; 1998: 173-185. 8 refs. ISBN 0-631-19737-0. BE59493.
    autonomy; *cloning; congenital disorders; costs and benefits; disabled; embryo disposition; embryos; fetuses; genetic counseling; genetic screening; killing; mass screening; moral obligations; *moral policy; pregnant women; preimplantation diagnosis; *prenatal diagnosis; psychological stress; risks and benefits; *selective abortion; sex determination; social impact; value of life

Saegusa, Asako. Japanese university approves genetic tests on in vitro embryos. [News]. *Nature.* 1999 Feb 11; 397(6719): 461. BE60397.
    Duchenne muscular dystrophy; ethical review; *genetic screening; guidelines; in vitro fertilization; physicians; political activity; *preimplantation diagnosis; professional organizations; research ethics committees; universities; *Japan; Japan Society of Obstetrics and Gynecology; Kagoshima University Medical School

Savulescu, Julian. Should doctors intentionally do less than the best? *Journal of Medical Ethics.* 1999 Apr; 25(2): 121-126. 11 fn. BE61914.
    artificial insemination; *autonomy; *beneficence; *cloning; *congenital disorders; conscience; *decision making; disabled; *embryo transfer; eugenics; freedom; *genetic disorders; *goals; in vitro fertilization; *medicine; mentally retarded; *moral complicity; *moral obligations; moral policy; *motivation; parent child relationship; *parents; *patients; *physicians; *preimplantation diagnosis; *quality of life; refusal to treat; *reproduction; *reproductive technologies; rights; selection for treatment; sex preselection; suffering; *values; rationality
The papers of Burley and Harris, and Draper and Chadwick, in this issue, raise a problem: what should doctors do when patients request an option which is not the best available? This commentary argues that doctors have a duty to offer that option which will result in the individual affected by that choice enjoying the highest level of wellbeing. Doctors can deviate from this duty and submaximise -- bring about an outcome that is less than the best -- only if there are good reasons to do so. The desire to have a child which is genetically

related provides little, if any, reason to submaximise. The implication for cloning, preimplantation diagnosis and embryo transfer is that doctors should only produce a clone or transfer embryos expected to enjoy a level of wellbeing which is less than that enjoyed by other children the couple could have, if there is a good reason to employ that technology. This paper sketches what might constitute a good reason to submaximise.

Schubert–Lehnhardt, Viola. Selective abortion after prenatal diagnosis. *Medicine and Law.* 1996; 15(1): 75–81. 11 fn. BE61204.

> attitudes; autonomy; *congenital disorders; *disabled; eugenics; *informal social control; mother fetus relationship; *prenatal diagnosis; quality of life; *selective abortion; *stigmatization; value of life; women's rights; *Germany

Serra–Prat, Mateu; Gallo, Pedro; Jovell, Albert J., et al. Trade-offs in prenatal detection of Down syndrome. *American Journal of Public Health.* 1998 Apr; 88(4): 551–557. 35 refs. BE60128.

> age factors; *alternatives; amniocentesis; comparative studies; costs and benefits; *decision analysis; decision making; *Down syndrome; *mass screening; *methods; *pregnant women; *prenatal diagnosis; *public policy; *risks and benefits; values; ultrasonography; Catalonia; Spain

OBJECTIVES: This paper presents the results of different screening policies for prenatal detection of Down syndrome that would allow decision makers to make informed choices. METHODS: A decision analysis model was built to compare 8 screening policies with regard to a selected set of outcome measures. Probabilities used in the analysis were obtained from official administrative data reports in Spain and Catalonia and from data published in the medical literature. Sensitivity analyses were carried out to test the robustness of screening policies' results to changes in uptake rates, diagnostic accuracy, and resources consumed. RESULTS: Selected screening policies posed major trades-offs regarding detection rates, false-positive results, fetal loss, and costs of the programs. All outcome measures considered were found quite robust to changes in uptake rates. Sensitivity and specificity rates of screening tests were shown to be the most influential factors in the outcome measures considered. CONCLUSIONS: The disclosed trade-offs emphasize the need to comprehensively inform decision makers about both positive and negative consequences of adopting one screening policy or another.

Sheiner, Eyal; Shoham–Vardi, Ilana; Weitzman, Dalia, et al. Decisions regarding pregnancy termination among Bedouin couples referred to third level ultrasound clinic. *European Journal of Obstetrics, Gynecology, and Reproductive Biology.* 1998 Feb; 76(2): 141–146. 14 refs. BE60478.

> *congenital disorders; *decision making; evaluation studies; fetal development; minority groups; parents; *pregnant women; *prenatal diagnosis; *selective abortion; ultrasonography; *Arabs; *Israel

Snijders, R.J.M.; Noble, P.; Sebire, N., et al. UK multicentre project on assessment of risk of trisomy 21 by maternal age and fetal nuchal–translucency thickness at 10–14 weeks of gestation. [For the Fetal Medicine Foundation First Trimester Screening Group (Great Britain)]. *Lancet.* 1998 Aug 1; 352(9125): 343–346. 20 refs. Commented on by J.E. Haddow, p. 336–337, and by V. Choo, p. 337–338. BE60437.

> age factors; chromosome abnormalities; *Down syndrome; evaluation studies; fetal development; *methods; pregnant women; *prenatal diagnosis; *risk; risks and benefits;

multicenter studies; ultrasonography; Great Britain

BACKGROUND: Prenatal diagnosis of trisomy 21 currently relies on assessment of risk followed by invasive testing in the 5% of pregnancies at the highest estimated risk. Selection of the high-risk group by a combination of maternal age and second-trimester maternal serum biochemistry gives a detection rate of about 60%. We investigated assessment of risk by a combination of maternal age and fetal nuchal–translucency thickness, measured by ultrasonography at 10–14 weeks of gestation. METHODS: The risk of trisomy 21 was estimated for 96127 women of median age 31 years (range 14–49) with singleton pregnancies. Ultrasonography was done by 306 appropriately trained sonographers in 22 centres. Risk of trisomy 21 was calculated from the maternal age and gestational-age-related prevalence, multiplied by a likelihood ratio depending on the deviation from normal in nuchal–translucency thickness for crown-rump length. The distribution of risks was investigated and the sensitivity of a cut-off risk of 1 in 300 was calculated. Phenotype was assessed by fetal karyotyping or clinical examination of liveborn infants. FINDINGS: The estimated trisomy–21 risk, from maternal age and fetal nuchal–translucency thickness, was 1 in 300 or higher in 7907 (8.3%) of 95476 normal pregnancies, 268 (82·2%) of 326 with trisomy 21, and 253 (77.9%) of 325 with other chromosomal defects. The 5% of the study population with the highest estimated risk included 77% of trisomy–21 cases. INTERPRETATION: Selection of the high-risk group for invasive testing by this method allows the detection of about 80% of affected pregnancies. However, even this method of risk assessment requires about 30 invasive tests for identification of one affected fetus.

Steinbock, Bonnie. Prenatal genetic testing for Alzheimer disease. *In:* Post, Stephen G.; Whitehouse, Peter J., eds. Genetic Testing for Alzheimer Disease: Ethical and Clinical Issues. Baltimore, MD: Johns Hopkins University Press; 1998: 140–151. 17 refs. ISBN 0-8018-5840-2. BE60721.

> autonomy; *dementia; disabled; genetic counseling; genetic disorders; *genetic screening; late-onset disorders; moral policy; parents; physicians; pregnant women; *prenatal diagnosis; selective abortion; sex determination

Stoller, David. Prenatal genetic screening: the enigma of selective abortion. *Journal of Law and Health.* 1997–98; 12(1): 121–140. 111 fn. BE61137.

> abortion, induced; congenital disorders; dehumanization; disabled; eugenics; federal government; fetuses; genetic counseling; genetic disorders; genetic enhancement; *genetic screening; genome mapping; government regulation; *legal aspects; *prenatal diagnosis; *selective abortion; sex determination; state government; state interest; stigmatization; Supreme Court decisions; viability; *United States

Trippitelli, Carol Lynn; Jamison, Kay R.; Folstein, Marshal F., et al. Pilot study on patients' and spouses' attitudes toward potential genetic testing for bipolar disorder. *American Journal of Psychiatry.* 1998 Jul; 155(7): 899–904. BE59826.

> adults; *attitudes; comparative studies; confidentiality; decision making; *depressive disorder; disclosure; *family members; genetic information; *genetic predisposition; *genetic screening; insurance; *married persons; *mentally ill; minors; motivation; *patients; *prenatal diagnosis; reproduction; risks and benefits; selective abortion; survey; Johns Hopkins University; Maryland

---

BE = bioethics accession number   fn. = footnotes   refs. = references

Walsh, Julia. Reproductive rights and the Human Genome Project. *Southern California Review of Law and Women's Studies.* 1994 Fall; 4(1): 145–181. 154 fn. BE62684.
autonomy; coercion; decision making; disclosure; eugenics; genetic information; *genetic screening; genome mapping; government financing; government regulation; health personnel; informed consent; legal rights; mandatory testing; mass screening; *pregnant women; *prenatal diagnosis; privacy; risks and benefits; selective abortion; social control; state government; voluntary programs; *women's rights; United States

Wertz, D.C. Is there a "women's ethic" in genetics? A survey of ASHG and NSGC. [Abstract]. *American Journal of Human Genetics.* 1996 Oct; 59(4): A340. BE60097.
adults; *attitudes; children; comparative studies; *directive counseling; *females; *genetic counseling; genetic disorders; *genetic screening; *health personnel; late-onset disorders; *males; *physicians; *prenatal diagnosis; selective abortion; sex determination; survey; United States

Wertz, Dorothy C. International perspectives on ethics and human genetics. *Suffolk University Law Review.* 1993 Winter; 27(4): 1411–1456. 102 fn. BE60738.
abortion, induced; *attitudes; autonomy; children; confidentiality; consensus; developing countries; directive counseling; disclosure; employment; family members; *genetic counseling; genetic disorders; genetic information; *genetic screening; genetic services; health personnel; informed consent; *international aspects; intersexuality; legal aspects; non-Western World; parent child relationship; *prenatal diagnosis; privacy; psychological stress; reproductive technologies; sex determination; survey; values; Western World; women's rights; United States

Wingerson, Lois. Unnatural Selection: The Promise and Power of Human Gene Research. New York, NY: Bantam Books; 1998. 399 p. Includes references. ISBN 0-553-09709-1. BE59741.
advisory committees; behavioral genetics; carriers; confidentiality; embryo research; eugenics; evolution; federal government; genes; genetic counseling; genetic disorders; genetic diversity; genetic predisposition; *genetic research; *genetic screening; *genetics; genome mapping; health insurance; informed consent; Jews; managed care programs; minority groups; preimplantation diagnosis; *prenatal diagnosis; property rights; public policy; risks and benefits; selective abortion; social discrimination; stigmatization; Human Embryo Research Panel; Human Genome Project; NCHGR Program on Ethical, Legal, and Social Implications (ELSI); United States

What price perfection? [Editorial]. *New Scientist.* 1997 Feb 22; 153(2070): 3. BE59711.
*eugenics; genetic predisposition; genetic research; *genetic screening; homosexuals; *prenatal diagnosis; selective abortion

PRENATAL INJURIES

See also FETUSES

Burns, Deborah L.; Catlin, Anita J. Positive toxicology screening in newborns: ethical issues in the decision to legally intervene. [Article and commentary]. *Pediatric Nursing.* 1997 Jan–Feb; 23(1): 73–78, 86. 43 refs. BE62417.
adoption; community services; costs and benefits; criminal law; *drug abuse; justice; *legal aspects; legal liability; newborns; nurses; parent child relationship; patient care; *pregnant women; *prenatal injuries; public policy; punishment; rehabilitation; resource allocation; women's health services; United States

Chavkin, David F. "For their own good": civil commitment of alcohol and drug-dependent pregnant women. *South Dakota Law Review.* 1992; 37(2): 224–288. 341 fn. BE61350.
*alcohol abuse; alternatives; *coercion; *drug abuse; due process; fetuses; goals; *involuntary commitment; *legal aspects; legal rights; *mandatory programs; outpatient commitment; *pregnant women; *prenatal injuries; social discrimination; standards; treatment refusal; voluntary programs; United States

De Ville, Kenneth A.; Kopelman, Loretta M. Moral and social issues regarding pregnant women who use and abuse drugs. *Obstetrics and Gynecology Clinics of North America.* 1998 Mar; 25(1): 237–254. 48 refs. BE60996.
alcohol abuse; blacks; coercion; criminal law; *drug abuse; females; fetuses; freedom; intention; involuntary commitment; justice; *legal aspects; legal liability; legislation; males; moral obligations; moral policy; *pregnant women; *prenatal injuries; *public policy; punishment; social discrimination; socioeconomic factors; state government; voluntary programs; United States

Farr, Kathryn Ann. Fetal abuse and the criminalization of behavior during pregnancy. *Crime and Delinquency.* 1995 Apr; 41(2): 235–245. 57 refs. BE59897.
child abuse; *criminal law; *drug abuse; fetuses; informed consent; legal aspects; *legal liability; minority groups; *pregnant women; *prenatal injuries; privacy; socioeconomic factors; state government; United States

Fieldston, Evan. AIDS, thalidomide and maternal-fetal rights in conflict. *Princeton Journal of Bioethics.* 1998 Spring; 1(1): 83–93. 9 refs. BE62495.
*AIDS; autonomy; coercion; contraception; *drugs; *females; fetuses; *HIV seropositivity; iatrogenic disease; moral obligations; *patient care; preconception injuries; *pregnant women; *prenatal injuries; public health; quality of life; reproduction; selective abortion; *social control; toxicity; women's rights; *thalidomide

Gómez, Laura E. Misconceiving Mothers: Legislators, Prosecutors, and the Politics of Prenatal Drug Exposure. Philadelphia, PA: Temple University Press; 1997. 207 p. (Gender, family, and the law). Bibliography: p. 153–197. ISBN 1-56639-558-5. BE60652.
abortion, induced; blacks; child abuse; criminal law; *drug abuse; empirical research; fetuses; government financing; health care; health education; Hispanic Americans; indigents; judicial action; law enforcement; *legal aspects; legal liability; *mass media; newborns; organizational policies; physicians; *political activity; *politics; *pregnant women; *prenatal injuries; prevalence; professional organizations; public health; public hospitals; public opinion; *public policy; punishment; rights; *social problems; *socioeconomic factors; state government; women's rights; *California; California Medical Association; Right to Life Movement; United States

Grubb, Andrew. Medical treatment (competent adult): pregnant woman and unborn child: Winnipeg Child and Family Services (Northwest Area) v. D.F.G. [Comment]. *Medical Law Review.* 1997 Spring; 5(1): 125–130. BE59765.
*coercion; competence; *drug abuse; fetuses; involuntary commitment; *legal aspects; legal rights; mentally ill; personhood; *pregnant women; *prenatal injuries; Canada; Great Britain; *Manitoba; Mental Health Act 1983 (Great Britain); Mental Health Act 1987 (MB); *Winnipeg Child and Family Services (Northwest Area) v. D.F.G.

Herbert, Bob. Pregnancy and addiction: South Carolina's misguided law. *New York Times.* 1998 Jun 11: A31.

BE = bioethics accession number   fn. = footnotes   refs. = references

BE59674.
   blacks; *child abuse; criminal law; *drug abuse; *fetuses; law enforcement; *legal liability; personhood; *pregnant women; *prenatal injuries; viability; Crawley, Malissa; *South Carolina

Hornstra, Deborah. A realistic approach to maternal–fetal conflict. *Hastings Center Report.* 1998 Sep–Oct; 28(5): 7–12. 18 fn. BE59547.
   abortion, induced; alcohol abuse; behavior control; cesarean section; coercion; disadvantaged; drug abuse; emotions; females; fetuses; legal aspects; *mother fetus relationship; *pregnant women; prenatal diagnosis; *prenatal injuries; rights; risk; smoking; *social control; social problems; treatment refusal; women's rights
We should not think of babies as having a right to be born healthy. We cannot say what such a right involves, and if we could, enforcing it would infringe on the mother's most basic rights. Most importantly, positing such a right casts the fetus and mother as adversaries, and so destroys the maternal–fetal relationship.

Kondro, Wayne. Canada upholds rights of pregnant women. [News]. *Lancet.* 1999 Jul 17; 354(9174): 232. BE62530.
   children; fetuses; *legal liability; *mothers; negligence; *pregnant women; *prenatal injuries; traffic accidents; *Canada

Markens, Susan; Browner, C.H.; Press, Nancy. Feeding the fetus: on interrogating the notion of maternal–fetal conflict. *Feminist Studies.* 1997 Summer; 23(2): 351–372. 46 fn. BE59795.
   attitudes; behavior control; feminist ethics; *fetuses; food; health education; health maintenance organizations; informal social control; *mother fetus relationship; motivation; *nutrition; *patient compliance; *pregnant women; prenatal injuries; smoking; socioeconomic factors; survey; life style; *self care; California

Mason, John Kenyon. Protection of the fetus. *In: his* Medico–Legal Aspects of Reproduction and Parenthood. Second Edition. Brookfield, VT: Ashgate; 1998: 143–186. 179 fn. ISBN 1–84104–065–8. BE61064.
   *aborted fetuses; abortion, induced; alcohol abuse; allowing to die; autonomy; beginning of life; brain death; cesarean section; coercion; compensation; competence; congenital disorders; criminal law; drug abuse; fetal development; *fetal therapy; *fetuses; genetic counseling; genetic disorders; infanticide; international aspects; *legal aspects; *legal liability; *legal rights; mentally ill; methods; negligence; personhood; physicians; *pregnant women; prenatal diagnosis; *prenatal injuries; prolongation of life; public policy; selective abortion; terminally ill; torts; treatment refusal; value of life; ventilators; viability; *wrongful death; *wrongful life; Abortion Act 1967 (Great Britain); Congenital Disabilities (Civil Liability) Act 1976 (Great Britain); *Great Britain; Infant Life (Preservation) Act 1929 (Great Britain); Scotland; United States

Millard, Dietra D. Toxicology testing in neonates: is it ethical, and what does it mean? *Clinics in Perinatology.* 1996 Sep; 23(3): 491–507. 84 refs. BE60937.
   confidentiality; congenital disorders; disclosure; *drug abuse; fetuses; intensive care units; *mass screening; morbidity; mortality; mothers; *newborns; parent child relationship; patient discharge; physicians; *pregnant women; *prenatal injuries; prevalence; prognosis; risks and benefits; social problems; social workers

Murphy, Sheigla; Rosenbaum, Marsha. Pregnant Women on Drugs: Combating Stereotypes and Stigma. New Brunswick, NJ: Rutgers University Press; 1999. 204 p. Bibliography: p. 185–198. ISBN 0–8135–2603–5.

BE62734.
   attitudes; child abuse; childbirth; criminal law; domestic violence; *drug abuse; family relationship; females; feminist ethics; fetuses; indigents; *motivation; parent child relationship; patient care; *pregnant women; *prenatal injuries; psychological stress; public policy; rehabilitation; social discrimination; *socioeconomic factors; *stigmatization; survey; harms; San Francisco

Panossian, André A.; Panossian, Vahé; Doumanian, Nancy P. Criminalization of perinatal HIV transmission. *Journal of Legal Medicine.* 1998 Jun; 19(2): 223–255. 155 fn. BE61249.
   child abuse; childbirth; *criminal law; drug abuse; females; *HIV seropositivity; infants; killing; *legal liability; males; mothers; *newborns; parent child relationship; patients; *pregnant women; *prenatal injuries; public policy; AZT; *United States

Parness, Jeffrey A. Arming the pregnancy police: more outlandish concoctions? *Louisiana Law Review.* 1992 Nov; 53(2): 427–448. 87 fn. BE61306.
   abortion, induced; child abuse; coercion; criminal law; drug abuse; economics; fetuses; *government regulation; historical aspects; killing; *legal aspects; legal liability; legal rights; *pregnant women; *prenatal injuries; public policy; social discrimination; state government; state interest; viability; Green, Melanie; *Illinois; Moore, Lee Ann

Selleck, Cynthia S.; Redding, Barbara A. Knowledge and attitudes of registered nurses toward perinatal substance abuse. *Journal of Obstetric, Gynecologic and Neonatal Nursing.* 1998 Jan–Feb; 27(1): 70–77. 11 refs. BE62057.
   *drug abuse; females; *knowledge, attitudes, practice; nurse patient relationship; *nurses; nursing education; *pregnant women; *prenatal injuries; socioeconomic factors; survey; Florida

Smith, George P. Procreative Liberty or Procreative Responsibility? Available from the author, Catholic University of America School of Law, 3600 John McCormack Rd., NE, Washington, DC 20064; 1998. 22 p. 120 fn. BE62199.
   alcohol abuse; autonomy; cesarean section; child abuse; coercion; contraception; disadvantaged; *drug abuse; *fetuses; freedom; government financing; hormones; involuntary sterilization; *legal liability; *pregnant women; *prenatal injuries; reproduction; smoking; surrogate mothers; treatment refusal; *Norplant; *United States

Steinbock, Bonnie. Mother–fetus conflict. *In:* Kuhse, Helga; Singer, Peter, eds. A Companion to Bioethics. Malden, MA: Blackwell; 1998: 135–146. 36 refs. ISBN 0–631–19737–0. BE59490.
   abortion, induced; alcohol abuse; *cesarean section; children; coercion; decision making; drug abuse; fetal development; fetal therapy; *fetuses; legal aspects; *moral obligations; moral policy; *mother fetus relationship; pain; physicians; *pregnant women; *prenatal injuries; public policy; surgery; *treatment refusal

Tiedje, Linda Beth. Ethical and legal issues in the care of substance–using women. *Journal of Obstetric, Gynecologic and Neonatal Nursing.* 1998 Jan–Feb; 27(1): 92–98. 46 refs. BE62060.
   attitudes; autonomy; beneficence; child abuse; confidentiality; *drug abuse; federal government; *females; fetuses; government financing; guidelines; justice; legal aspects; mandatory testing; nurse patient relationship; nurses; *patient care; *pregnant women; *prenatal injuries; United States

Tong, Rosemarie. Just caring about maternal–fetal

BE = bioethics accession number   fn. = footnotes   refs. = references

relations: the case of cocaine–using pregnant women. *In:* Donchin, Anne; Purdy, Laura M., eds. Embodying Bioethics: Recent Feminist Advances. Lanham, MD: Rowman and Littlefield; 1999: 33–43. 27 fn. ISBN 0-8476-8924-7. BE61013.
    bioethics; *caring; deontological ethics; *drug abuse; ethical theory; *feminist ethics; *justice; legal liability; *pregnant women; *prenatal injuries; public policy; punishment; rehabilitation; social discrimination; socioeconomic factors; utilitarianism; United States

PRIORITIES IN HEALTH CARE *See* RESOURCE ALLOCATION

PRIVILEGED COMMUNICATION *See* CONFIDENTIALITY

PROFESSIONAL ETHICS

See also BIOETHICS, FRAUD AND MISCONDUCT, MEDICAL ETHICS, NURSING ETHICS, PROFESSIONAL PATIENT RELATIONSHIP

Applebaum, Arthur Isak. Doctor, schmoctor: practice positivism and its complications. *In: his* Ethics for Adversaries: The Morality of Roles in Public and Professional Life. Princeton, NJ: Princeton University Press; 1999: 45–60. 9 fn. ISBN 0-691-00712-8. BE62129.
    conflict of interest; disclosure; duty to warn; gatekeeping; insurance; lawyers; legal obligations; managed care programs; *medical ethics; *moral obligations; mortality; occupational medicine; patient advocacy; physician patient relationship; *physician's role; professional competence; *professional ethics; *professional role; virtues

Berglund, Catherine Anne. Ethics for Health Care. New York, NY: Oxford University Press; 1998. 228 p. Bibliography: p. 211–224. Appendixes include medical and nursing codes of ethics from Australia and New Zealand. ISBN 0-19-554172-3. BE60704.
    abortion, induced; active euthanasia; assisted suicide; autonomy; beginning of life; *bioethical issues; biomedical research; caring; case studies; codes of ethics; competence; confidentiality; critically ill; drugs; economics; education; ethical theory; genome mapping; guidelines; health care; health care delivery; *health personnel; human experimentation; informed consent; institutional ethics; justice; patient care; patient care team; personhood; privacy; *professional ethics; professional organizations; professional patient relationship; public participation; quality of life; religious ethics; research ethics committees; risks and benefits; standards; trust; Australia; Australian Medical Association; Australian Nursing Council; National Health and Medical Research Council (Australia); New Zealand Medical Association

Bergsma, Jurrit; Mook, Bertha. Ethical considerations in psychotherapeutic systems. *Theoretical Medicine and Bioethics.* 1998 Aug; 19(4): 371–381. 21 fn. BE60159.
    autonomy; communication; disclosure; freedom; goals; health personnel; informed consent; methods; narrative ethics; professional autonomy; *professional ethics; *professional patient relationship; *psychotherapy; *social dominance; technical expertise; empowerment

Bishop, Laura Jane; Cherry, M. Nichelle; Darragh, Martina. Organizational ethics and health care: expanding bioethics to the institutional arena. [Bibliography]. *Kennedy Institute of Ethics Journal.* 1999 Jun; 9(2): 189–208. Also available, as Scope Note 36, from the National Reference Center for Bioethics

Literature, Kennedy Institute of Ethics, Georgetown University, Box 571212, Washington, DC 20057–1212, (202) 687–6806 or (800) MED-ETHX. BE62386.
    administrators; clinical ethics committees; codes of ethics; economics; health care delivery; *health facilities; *institutional ethics; professional ethics; *business ethics

Bouchard, Charles E. The virtuous manager. *Health Progress.* 1997 May–Jun; 78(3): 27–29. 6 refs. BE59686.
    *administrators; employment; health facilities; institutional ethics; justice; *professional ethics; Roman Catholic ethics; virtues; *business ethics; prudence

Cassidy, Judy. Calvary Hospital focuses on ethics: integrating clinical and organizational ethics meets needs of a changing healthcare system. *Health Progress.* 1998 Nov–Dec; 79(6): 48–50, 52. BE61480.
    clinical ethics; ethics committees; guidelines; health care delivery; *institutional ethics; institutional policies; managed care programs; palliative care; program descriptions; referral and consultation; *religious hospitals; *Roman Catholic ethics; values; *Calvary Hospital (Bronx, NY); Ethical and Religious Directives for Catholic Health Care Services

Chiodo, Gary T.; Tolle, Susan W. The ethical foundations of a duty to treat HIV–positive patients. *General Dentistry.* 1997 Jan–Feb; 45(1): 14, 16, 18, 20, 22. 35 refs. BE59426.
    autonomy; codes of ethics; *dentistry; *health personnel; *HIV seropositivity; *legal aspects; legislation; *occupational exposure; *patient care; privacy; *professional ethics; professional organizations; *refusal to treat; risk; social discrimination; *infection control; universal precautions; *American Dental Association; *Americans with Disabilities Act 1990; United States

Chodoff, Paul. Ethical dimensions of psychotherapy: a personal perspective. *American Journal of Psychotherapy.* 1996 Summer; 50(3): 298–310. 20 refs. BE62053.
    child abuse; confidentiality; economics; health insurance reimbursement; health personnel; mentally ill; misconduct; professional competence; *professional ethics; *professional patient relationship; *psychotherapy; recall; sex offenses; social dominance

Clark, Barbara J.; Abeles, Norman. Ethical issues and dilemmas in the mental health organization. *Administration and Policy in Mental Health.* 1994 Sep; 22(1): 7–17. 5 refs. BE59543.
    *administrators; advertising; confidentiality; conflict of interest; deception; disclosure; duty to warn; expert testimony; health care delivery; health insurance reimbursement; HIV seropositivity; institutional ethics; legal aspects; malpractice; mandatory reporting; mental health; *professional ethics; psychiatric diagnosis; *psychotherapy; quality of health care; records; resource allocation; suicide; quality assurance; United States

de Jong, Judith; Reatig, Natalie. SAMHSA philosophy and statement on ethical principles. *Ethics and Behavior.* 1998; 8(4): 339–343. BE60165.
    accountability; *alcohol abuse; autonomy; beneficence; codes of ethics; cultural pluralism; *drug abuse; federal government; health care delivery; *health promotion; *institutional ethics; justice; *mental health; *mentally ill; minority groups; preventive medicine; rehabilitation; resource allocation; social problems; trust; community consent; *community medicine; intervention studies; *Substance Abuse and Mental Health Services Administration; United States
    As the major federal agency responsible for improving the delivery and effectiveness of substance abuse and mental health services to the American public, the Substance Abuse and Mental Health Services

---

BE = bioethics accession number   fn. = footnotes   refs. = references

Administration (SAMHSA) is aware that its programs deal with especially sensitive issues. As a national leader in advancing effective services to persons with addictive and mental disorders, SAMHSA has stewardship over important interventions affecting personal, community, institutional, and social values. Inherent in SAMHSA's mission and goals is a commitment to protect and promote the human, civil, and legal rights and moral freedoms of those individuals and groups who participate in SAMHSA-funded activities and to demonstrate that Agency policies and procedures are congruent with publicly acceptable ethical principles and standards of conduct. A foundation of mutual trust between SAMHSA officials and participants as well as sensitivity to issues of public accountability will hasten and strengthen progress toward this shared vision.

DeLeon, Patrick H.; Bennett, Bruce E.; Bricklin, Patricia M. Ethics and public policy formulation: a case example related to prescription privileges. *Professional Psychology: Research and Practice.* 1997 Dec; 28(6): 518–525. 36 refs. BE59207.
　　*administrators; codes of ethics; conflict of interest; employment; *health personnel; interprofessional relations; patient care; physicians; politics; *professional autonomy; *professional ethics; professional organizations; psychiatry; *psychoactive drugs; *psychology; *public policy; technical expertise; American Psychological Association; United States

Guillen, Diego Gracia. The Hippocratic Oath in the development of medicine. *Dolentium Hominum: Church and Health in the World.* 1996; 31(11th Yr., No. 1): 22–28. BE60999.
　　ancient history; beneficence; clergy; *codes of ethics; compassion; confidentiality; *historical aspects; justice; legal obligations; love; *medical ethics; *medicine; *moral obligations; morality; obligations to society; physician patient relationship; *physician's role; *professional ethics; *religion; self regulation; technical expertise; *terminology; trust; *virtues; Western World; judges; Aristotle; *Hippocratic Oath; Socrates

Guilmette, Thomas J.; Hagan, Leigh D. Ethical considerations in forensic neuropsychological consultation. *Clinical Neuropsychologist.* 1997 Aug; 11(3): 287–290. 2 refs. BE60595.
　　brain pathology; case studies; *expert testimony; forensic psychiatry; *professional ethics; *psychology; *referral and consultation; *neuropsychology

Harris, John; Holm, Søren. Risk-taking and professional responsibility. *Journal of the Royal Society of Medicine.* 1997 Nov; 90(11): 625–629. 4 refs. BE62428.
　　AIDS; altruism; communicable diseases; contracts; emergency care; employment; HIV seropositivity; *medical ethics; *moral obligations; *occupational exposure; physicians; *professional ethics; *risk

Holmes, Jeremy. Values in psychotherapy. *American Journal of Psychotherapy.* 1996 Summer; 50(3): 259–273. 31 refs. BE59882.
　　health personnel; mentally ill; postmodernism; *professional ethics; professional patient relationship; *psychotherapy; religion; science; *values; Freud, Sigmund

Idziak, Janine M. Ethical Dilemmas in Allied Health. Dubuque, IA: Simon and Kolz; 2000. 288 p. Includes references. ISBN 0-9659350-3-5. BE61835.
　　aborted fetuses; abortion, induced; active euthanasia; advance directives; AIDS; *allied health personnel; allowing to die; artificial feeding; assisted suicide; *bioethical issues; case studies; clinical ethics committees; confidentiality;

congenital disorders; conscience; cultural pluralism; decision making; employment; ethical theory; health care; human experimentation; informed consent; moral policy; newborns; organ donation; palliative care; persistent vegetative state; prenatal diagnosis; *professional ethics; reproductive technologies; resource allocation; resuscitation orders; selective abortion; third party consent; truth disclosure; withholding treatment; United States

Koehn, Daryl. The Ground of Professional Ethics. New York, NY: Routledge; 1994. 224 p. (Professional ethics). Bibliography: p. 213–219. ISBN 0-415-11667-8. BE61841.
　　beneficence; *clergy; common good; confidentiality; conflict of interest; contracts; health; justice; law; *lawyers; *medical ethics; medicine; moral obligations; obligations to society; physician patient relationship; *physicians; *professional ethics; professional role; religion; self regulation; technical expertise; trust

Koocher, Gerald P.; Keith–Spiegel, Patricia. Ethics in Psychology: Professional Standards and Cases. Second Edition. New York, NY: Oxford University Press; 1998. 502 p. (Oxford textbooks in clinical psychology; v.3). Includes references. Appendices include the texts of the American Psychological Association's "Ethical Principles and Code of Conduct" (1992) and of its Ethics Committee's "Rules and Procedures" (1996). ISBN 0-19-509201-5. BE61942.
　　advertising; authorship; behavior control; case studies; codes of ethics; confidentiality; conflict of interest; dangerousness; deception; disclosure; duty to warn; expert testimony; HIV seropositivity; informed consent; interprofessional relations; law enforcement; legal liability; managed care programs; mass media; military personnel; misconduct; patient access to records; privacy; privileged communication; professional competence; *professional ethics; professional organizations; professional patient relationship; *psychology; psychotherapy; records; scientific misconduct; self regulation; sexuality; American Psychological Association

McCullough, Laurence B. Ethics in the management of health care organizations. *Physician Executive.* 1993 Nov–Dec; 19(6): 72–76. 4 refs. BE60638.
　　administrators; autonomy; beneficence; clinical ethics; *economics; ethics; *health care delivery; historical aspects; *hospitals; *institutional ethics; medical ethics; morality; organization and administration; patient advocacy; physicians; practice guidelines; *professional ethics; public policy; quality of health care; remuneration; resource allocation; trends; virtues; business ethics; preventive ethics; Eighteenth Century; Great Britain; Percival, Thomas; Twentieth Century; United States

O'Toole, Brian. Four ways people approach ethics: a practical guide to reaching consensus on moral problems. *Health Progress.* 1998 Nov–Dec; 79(6): 38–41, 43. BE61479.
　　*administrators; *decision making; ethical theory; *institutional ethics; morality; principle-based ethics; *professional ethics; standards; teleological ethics; values; virtues

Pentz, Rebecca D. Beyond case consultation: an expanded model for organizational ethics. *Journal of Clinical Ethics.* 1999 Spring; 10(1): 34–41. 31 fn. BE62704.
　　administrators; bioethics; bone marrow; clinical ethics; *clinical ethics committees; committee membership; conflict of interest; decision making; dissent; donors; *ethicists; *ethics consultation; evaluation; futility; hospitals; *institutional ethics; institutional policies; *models, theoretical; patient advocacy; physicians; professional competence; resource allocation; standards; tissue donation; withholding treatment; business ethics; preventive ethics; Core Competencies for Health Care Ethics Consultation

---

BE = bioethics accession number   fn. = footnotes   refs. = references

(SHHV-SBC Task Force); *M.D. Anderson Cancer Center

Perkins, David V.; Hudson, Brenda L.; Gray, Diana M., et al. Decisions and justifications by community mental health providers about hypothetical ethical dilemmas. *Psychiatric Services.* 1998 Oct; 49(10): 1317–1322. 23 refs. BE61448.
administrators; age factors; *community services; comparative studies; *confidentiality; *decision making; disclosure; education; *geographic factors; gifts; *health personnel; *mentally ill; nurses; *professional ethics; *professional patient relationship; psychology; *social interaction; social workers; survey; *case managers; *mental health services; rural population; urban population; Midwestern United States

Prilleltensky, Isaac. Values, assumptions, and practices: assessing the moral implications of psychological discourse and action. *American Psychologist.* 1997 May; 52(5): 517–535. 200 refs. BE59348.
autonomy; caring; *communitarianism; compassion; disadvantaged; postmodernism; *professional ethics; professional patient relationship; *psychology; psychotherapy; resource allocation; *values; vulnerable populations; empowerment

Pullman, Daryl. Role conflict and conflict of interest: a professional practice dilemma. *Journal of the American Optometric Association.* 1996 Feb; 67(2): 98–108. 19 refs. BE60295.
*conflict of interest; contracts; decision making; entrepreneurship; *health personnel; informed consent; interprofessional relations; medical devices; models, theoretical; *professional ethics; *professional patient relationship; *professional role; trust; *business ethics; *optometry

Resnik, David. Social epistemology and the ethics of research. *Studies in History and Philosophy of Science.* 1996 Dec; 27(4): 565–586. 39 fn. BE60462.
authorship; biomedical research; codes of ethics; deception; fraud; freedom; goals; information dissemination; interprofessional relations; investigators; moral obligations; moral policy; *philosophy; *professional ethics; *science; scientific misconduct; standards; values; knowledge; *research ethics

Resnik, David B. The Ethics of Science: An Introduction. New York, NY: Routledge; 1998. 221 p. (Philosophical issues in science). Bibliography: 206–216. ISBN 0-415-16698-5. BE61844.
animal experimentation; authorship; *biomedical research; case studies; conflict of interest; ecology; economics; education; ethical theory; expert testimony; faculty; fraud; goals; government financing; human experimentation; industry; information dissemination; interprofessional relations; *investigators; mass media; obligations to society; patents; peer review; *professional ethics; property rights; *science; *scientific misconduct; self regulation; standards; students; values; whistleblowing; publishing; *research ethics

Seedhouse, David. Ethics: The Heart of Health Care. Second Edition. New York, NY: Wiley; 1998. 232 p. Bibliography: p. 221–223. ISBN 0-471-97592-3. BE62100.
autonomy; case studies; codes of ethics; costs and benefits; deontological ethics; *ethical analysis; ethical relativism; ethical theory; *ethics; health; *health care; *health personnel; interprofessional relations; justice; law; methods; *moral policy; *morality; patient participation; personhood; principle-based ethics; *professional ethics; professional patient relationship; quality adjusted life years; resource allocation; teleological ethics; utilitarianism; values

Smith, Trevor. Ethics in Medical Research: A Handbook of Good Practice. New York, NY: Cambridge University Press; 1999. 403 p. Bibliography: p. 378–390. ISBN 0-521-62619-6. BE62737.
animal organs; children; compensation; confidentiality; critically ill; drug industry; drugs; epidemiology; ethical review; fetal research; forms; gene therapy; genetic materials; genetic research; *guidelines; *human experimentation; incentives; informed consent; injuries; international aspects; *investigators; medical records; mentally disabled; organ transplantation; *organization and administration; placebos; *professional ethics; *research design; *research ethics committees; research subjects; risks and benefits; selection of subjects; self regulation; volunteers; multicenter studies; questionnaires; Declaration of Helsinki; Great Britain; Internet

Swisher, Laura Lee; Krueger-Brophy, Carol. Legal and Ethical Issues in Physical Therapy. Boston, MA: Butterworth–Heinemann; 1998. 231 p. Includes references and glossary. ISBN 0-7506-9788-1. BE61846.
accountability; administrators; advance directives; advertising; *allied health personnel; assisted suicide; autonomy; caring; case studies; confidentiality; data banks; education; employment; ethical analysis; ethical theory; feminist ethics; fraud; human experimentation; informed consent; insurance; *legal aspects; legal liability; managed care programs; misconduct; negligence; patient care; physical restraint; *professional ethics; professional patient relationship; regulation; rehabilitation; resuscitation orders; sexuality; business ethics; elder abuse; *physical therapy; *United States

Thompson, Dennis F. The institutional turn in professional ethics. *Ethics and Behavior.* 1999; 9(2): 109–118. 10 refs. BE61783.
administrators; *assisted suicide; conflict of interest; *decision making; drugs; hospitals; *institutional ethics; *institutional policies; *lawyers; legal aspects; moral obligations; *physicians; professional autonomy; *professional ethics; *professional role; values; United States
The traditional ideal in which professionals alone or in small groups serve their patients and clients in accord with a public-spirited goal is giving way to practice in which professionals serve in organizations that value mainly their expertise and expect them to act in accord with the organization's goals. The study of professional ethics has not kept pace with this trend and, as a result, has neglected the institutional aspects of ethical problems. I focus attention on these aspects by considering a case that raises 2 problems that are particularly relevant in the context in which professionals now practice: the problem of representation (whom does the professional act for) and the problem of authority (who has the right to make the policy for the institution).

Veatch, Robert M.; Haddad, Amy. Case Studies in Pharmacy Ethics. New York, NY: Oxford University Press; 1999. 290 p. 165 fn. ISBN 0-19-513280-7. BE62740.
abortion, induced; autonomy; behavior control; beneficence; bioethical issues; capital punishment; *case studies; competence; confidentiality; conflict of interest; conscience; contraception; decision making; drug industry; *drugs; economics; ethical analysis; futility; health insurance; human experimentation; justice; killing; misconduct; *moral obligations; pain; *patient care; patient education; *pharmacists; placebos; *professional ethics; professional patient relationship; terminal care; treatment refusal; truth disclosure; values; United States

Weed, Douglas L. Preventing scientific misconduct. *American Journal of Public Health.* 1998 Jan; 88(1):

BE = bioethics accession number   fn. = footnotes   refs. = references

125–129. 50 refs. BE62601.
   biomedical research; due process; education; empirical research; *investigators; motivation; *professional ethics; regulation; science; *scientific misconduct; statistics; terminology; virtues; whistleblowing

Wells, Barron; Spinks, Nelda. The context of ethics in the health care industry. *Health Manpower Management.* 1996; 22(1): 21–29. 8 refs. BE59338.
   *administrators; *advertising; aged; disabled; drug industry; drugs; economics; *employment; females; *health care delivery; *health facilities; *institutional ethics; medical fees; minority groups; *misconduct; social discrimination; standards; *business ethics; quality assurance; United States

Wenger, Neil S.; Korenman, Stanley G.; Berk, Richard, et al. The ethics of scientific research: an analysis of focus groups of scientists and institutional representatives. *Journal of Investigative Medicine.* 1997 Aug; 45(6): 371–380. 20 refs. BE60389.
   accountability; *administrators; *attitudes; authorship; biomedical research; comparative studies; conflict of interest; education; financial support; fraud; information dissemination; interprofessional relations; *investigators; *professional ethics; punishment; *science; *scientific misconduct; self regulation; survey; universities; values; whistleblowing; *research ethics; United States

Ziman, John M. Why must scientists become more ethically sensitive than they used to be? *Science.* 1998 Dec 4; 282(5395): 1813–1814. 1 fn. BE59556.
   biomedical research; financial support; *industry; *investigators; *professional ethics; *science; *universities

PROFESSIONAL ETHICS/CODES OF ETHICS

American Health Information Management Association. AHIMA code of ethics and bylaws. *Journal of the American Health Information Management Association.* 1994 Jan; 65(1): 68–74. Bylaws amended Oct 1993; code of ethics amended 1991. BE60430.
   allied health personnel; *codes of ethics; *medical records; *professional ethics; professional organizations; *American Health Information Management Association; United States

Baumiller, Robert C.; Comley, Sarah; Cunningham, George, et al.; Council of Regional Networks [for Genetic Services] Committee on Ethics. Code of ethical principles for genetics professionals. *American Journal of Medical Genetics.* 1996 Oct 28; 65(3): 177–178. Accepted by the Council of Regional Networks Steering Committee 14 Apr 1994. BE59526.
   *codes of ethics; genetic counseling; genetic research; genetic screening; *genetic services; *health personnel; interprofessional relations; obligations to society; *professional ethics; professional organizations; professional patient relationship; *Council of Regional Networks for Genetic Services; United States

Baumiller, Robert C.; Cunningham, George; Fisher, Nancy, et al.; Council of Regional Networks [for Genetic Services] Committee on Ethics. Code of ethical principles for genetics professionals: an explication. *American Journal of Medical Genetics.* 1996 Oct 28; 65(3): 179–183. 4 refs. Approved by the Council of Regional Networks Executive Committee 9 Oct 1995. BE59527.
   autonomy; *codes of ethics; communication; confidentiality; directive counseling; genetic counseling; genetic research; genetic screening; *genetic services; *health personnel; information dissemination; interprofessional relations; laboratories; obligations to society; professional competence;

*professional ethics; professional organizations; professional patient relationship; standards; tissue banks; *Council of Regional Networks for Genetic Services; United States

Benatar, Solomon R.; Tavistock Group. Shared ethical principles for everybody in health care: a working draft from the Tavistock group. A shared statement of ethical principles for those who shape and give health care. *BMJ (British Medical Journal).* 1999 Jan 23; 318(7178): 249–251. Other members of the Tavistock Group are Donald M. Berwick, Maureen Bisognano, James Dalton, Frank Davidoff, Julio Frenk, Howard Hiatt, Brian Hurwitz, Penny Janeway, Margaret H. Marshall, Richard Norling, Mary Roch Rocklage, Hilary Scott, Amartya Sen, Richard Smith, and Ann Sommerville. BE60329.
   *codes of ethics; confidentiality; *consensus; economics; *guidelines; *health care; *health care delivery; health personnel; human rights; institutional ethics; *interdisciplinary communication; international aspects; obligations of society; patient advocacy; preventive medicine; *professional ethics; public health; quality of health care; resource allocation; Great Britain; Tavistock Group

Brodkin, C. Andrew; Frumkin, Howard; Kirkland, Katherine H., et al. AOEC position paper on the organizational code for ethical conduct. *Journal of Occupational and Environmental Medicine.* 1996 Sep; 38(9): 869–881. 14 refs. BE62426.
   *codes of ethics; comparative studies; confidentiality; conflict of interest; *health personnel; medical ethics; nursing ethics; *occupational medicine; *organizational policies; physicians; professional competence; *professional ethics; *professional organizations; social discrimination; *Association of Occupational and Environmental Clinics; Canada; *International Code of Ethics for Occupational Health Professionals; United States

Fisher, Celia B.; Younggren, Jeffrey N. The value and utility of the 1992 ethics code. *Professional Psychology: Research and Practice.* 1997 Dec; 28(6): 582–592. 60 refs. BE59208.
   behavioral research; *codes of ethics; education; evaluation; expert testimony; faculty; forensic psychiatry; goals; health personnel; informed consent; legal aspects; managed care programs; misconduct; *professional ethics; professional organizations; professional patient relationship; *psychology; psychotherapy; self regulation; sexuality; students; values; *American Psychological Association; *Ethical Principles of Psychologists and Code of Conduct

Gorlin, Rena A., ed. Health: allied health, chiropractic, dentistry, medicine, mental health, nursing, pharmacy, social work. *In: her* Codes of Professional Responsibility: Ethics Standards in Business, Health, and Law. Fourth Edition. Washington, DC: Bureau of National Affairs; 1999: 253–548. ISBN 1-57018-148-9. BE60740.
   administrators; allied health personnel; *codes of ethics; counseling; dentistry; *health personnel; hospitals; medical ethics; nurses; nursing ethics; pharmacists; physicians; *professional ethics; *professional organizations; psychiatry; psychology; social workers; *American Chiropractic Association; *American College of Healthcare Executives; *American College of Physicians; *American Counseling Association; *American Dental Association; *American Dental Hygenists' Association; *American Hospital Association; *American Medical Association; *American Nurses Association; *American Pharmaceutical Association; *American Psychiatric Association; *American Psychological Association; *American Society of Internal Medicine; *Clinical Social Work Federation; *National Association of Social Workers; United States

Hadjistavropoulos, Thomas; Malloy, David Cruise.

Ethical principles of the American Psychological Association: an argument for philosophical and practical ranking. *Ethics and Behavior.* 1999; 9(2): 127–140. 36 refs. BE61785.
 autonomy; caring; *codes of ethics; confidentiality; decision making; health personnel; models, theoretical; moral obligations; *moral policy; obligations to society; principle-based ethics; professional competence; *professional ethics; professional organizations; *psychology; rights; truth disclosure; values; virtues; dignity; integrity; *American Psychological Association; Canadian Psychological Association

Unlike the American Psychological Association (APA), the Canadian Psychological Association has adopted a code of ethics in which principles are organized in order of importance. The validity of this hierarchical organization has received some empirical and theoretical support. We conducted a theoretical analysis that revealed conceptual justification for a ranking of the 6 principles in the APA code. Such a ranking could assist psychologists in making more informed and consistent moral choices when confronted with ethical dilemmas that involve conflicts among principles.

Leach, Mark M.; Harbin, J. Judd. Psychological ethics codes: a comparison of twenty-four countries. *International Journal of Psychology.* 1997; 32(3): 181–192. 20 refs. BE59602.
 *codes of ethics; comparative studies; confidentiality; consensus; *cultural pluralism; education; ethical relativism; guidelines; health personnel; *international aspects; professional competence; *professional ethics; professional organizations; professional patient relationship; *psychology; psychotherapy; standards; survey; values; *American Psychological Association; Asia; Australia; Canada; Central America; Europe; Great Britain; Israel; New Zealand; Scandinavia; South Africa; South America; *United States

Limentani, Alexander E.; Miller, Saul; Neuberger, Julia, et al. An ethical code for everybody in health care. [Letters]. *BMJ (British Medical Journal).* 1998 May 9; 316(7142): 1458–1460. 7 refs. BE59227.
 *codes of ethics; health care; *health personnel; human rights; international aspects; medical ethics; patient participation; patients' rights; *professional ethics; Hippocratic Oath

Medical Library Association. Goals and Principles for Ethical Conduct. Chicago, IL: The Association (online). Downloaded from Internet Web site: http://www.mlanet.org.about.ethics.html on 11 Sep 1998; 1998 Sep 3. 2 p. BE62197.
 *codes of ethics; *professional ethics; professional organizations; *Medical Library Association

Robin, Eugene D.; McCauly, Robert F. A Hippocratic oath for our times. *Nurse Practitioner.* 1995 Jul; 20(7): 14–15. BE59388.
 *codes of ethics; health personnel; informed consent; interprofessional relations; nurses; patient access to records; patient care; *professional ethics; referral and consultation; truth disclosure; *Hippocratic Oath (updated version)

Smith, Richard; Hiatt, Howard; Berwick, Donald. A shared statement of ethical principles for those who shape and give health care: a working draft from the Tavistock Group. *Annals of Internal Medicine.* 1999 Jan 19; 130(2): 143–147. 1 ref. BE62602.
 administrators; *codes of ethics; *consensus; economics; goals; *guidelines; *health care; *health care delivery; health facilities; *health personnel; human rights; institutional ethics; *interdisciplinary communication; *international aspects; interprofessional relations; managed care programs; moral obligations; obligations to society; patient advocacy;

*professional ethics; public health; resource allocation; *Tavistock Group

Health care delivery in many countries has expanded over the past 150 years from a largely social service delivered by individual practitioners to an intricate network of services provided by teams of professionals. The problems of increasing resource consumption, financial constraints, complexity, and poor system design that have emerged as consequences of these changes have exacerbated many of the ethical tensions inherent in health care and have created new ones. Many groups of professionals that give and affect health care have established separate codes of ethics for their own disciplines, but no shared code exists that might bring all stakeholders in health care into a more consistent moral framework. A multidisciplinary group therefore recently met at Tavistock Square in London in an effort to prepare such a shared code. The result was not a code but a more basic and generic statement of ethical principles. The intent and hope is that it will offer clear guidance for tough calls in real world settings. It is presented here not as a finished work, but as a draft to elicit comment, critique, suggestions for revision, and, especially, ideas for implementation.

Smith, Richard; Hiatt, Howard; Berwick, Donald. Shared ethical principles for everybody in health care: a working draft from the Tavistock group. Introduction. *BMJ (British Medical Journal).* 1999 Jan 23; 318(7178): 248–249. 1 ref. BE60328.
 *codes of ethics; *consensus; *guidelines; *health care; health care delivery; health personnel; institutional ethics; *interdisciplinary communication; *international aspects; *professional ethics; Great Britain; Tavistock Group

PROFESSIONAL ETHICS/EDUCATION

Aroskar, Mila Ann. Teaching ethics in health care administration: a course profile. *Journal of Health Administration Education.* 1993 Fall; 11(4): 601–608. 6 refs. BE59776.
 *administrators; *curriculum; *education; ethical analysis; evaluation; faculty; goals; health facilities; *professional ethics; program descriptions; students; teaching methods; universities; University of Minnesota

Bindless, Linda. The use of patients in health care education: the need for ethical justification. *Journal of Medical Ethics.* 1998 Oct; 24(5): 314–319. 27 fn. BE60252.
 accountability; behavioral research; coercion; confidentiality; deception; disclosure; *education; *health personnel; human rights; informed consent; patient advocacy; patient care; *patients; *patients' rights; privacy; *professional ethics; professional patient relationship; research subjects; *students; vulnerable populations; Great Britain

This paper addresses ethical concerns emanating from the practice of using patients for health care education. It shows how some of the ways that patients are used in educational strategies to bridge theory-practice gaps can cause harm to patients and patient-practitioner relationships, thus failing to meet acceptable standards of professional practice. This will continue unless there is increased awareness of the need for protection of human rights in teaching situations. Unnecessary exposure of patients, failing to obtain explicit consent, causing harm to vulnerable or disadvantaged groups and inappropriate use of information, though normally regarded as unacceptable professional practices, may go unrecognised in meeting educational needs, widening rather than narrowing theory-practice gaps.

BE = bioethics accession number   fn. = footnotes   refs. = references

Gifford, Fred. Teaching scientific integrity. *Centennial Review.* 1994 Spring; 38(2): 297–314. 6 fn. BE59404.
*biomedical research; conflict of interest; curriculum; deception; *education; federal government; fraud; government regulation; interprofessional relations; *investigators; motivation; negligence; *professional ethics; science; *scientific misconduct; self regulation; *students; teaching methods; truth disclosure; *universities; Michigan State University; National Institutes of Health; United States

Glen, Sally. Educating for interprofessional collaboration: teaching about values. *Nursing Ethics.* 1999 May; 6(3): 202–213. 26 refs. BE61765.
cultural pluralism; *education; *health personnel; interdisciplinary communication; *interprofessional relations; moral development; nursing education; *patient care team; *professional ethics; social workers; *values

Glen, Sally. Health care education for dialogue and dialogic relationships. *Nursing Ethics.* 1999 Jan; 6(1): 3–11. 33 refs. BE60150.
autonomy; communication; cultural pluralism; democracy; *education; feminist ethics; *health personnel; *interprofessional relations; *moral development; narrative ethics; nursing education; postmodernism; professional ethics; self concept; *social interaction; teaching methods; Great Britain

Greene, David. The use of service learning in client environments to enhance ethical reasoning in students. *American Journal of Occupational Therapy.* 1997 Nov–Dec; 51(10): 844–852. 46 refs. BE61806.
aged; *allied health personnel; disabled; *education; evaluation studies; *moral development; *professional ethics; rehabilitation; teaching methods; *occupational therapy; United States

Wadeley, Alison. Ethics in Psychological Research and Practice. Leicester, England: British Psychological Association; 1991. 41 p. 29 refs. Open learning unit: models and methods in psychology. ISBN 1-85433-045-4. BE59462.
animal experimentation; animal testing alternatives; *behavioral research; *education; evaluation; guidelines; operant conditioning; *professional ethics; *psychology; teaching methods; British Psychological Society; Great Britain

PROFESSIONAL PATIENT RELATIONSHIP

See also PATIENT CARE, PROFESSIONAL ETHICS

American Academy of Ophthalmology. Ethics Committee. Patient–physician covenant. [Letter]. *Archives of Ophthalmology.* 1997 Jan; 115(1): 134. 1 ref. BE60078.
caring; conflict of interest; *covenant; economics; ethics committees; managed care programs; *patient advocacy; *physician patient relationship; *physicians; professional competence; professional organizations; trust; withholding treatment; American Academy of Ophthalmology

Arnow, Kathryn Smul. Medical technology transfer and physician–patient conversation. *International Journal of Technology Management.* 1996; 11(1–2): 70–88. 48 fn. BE59407.
*alternatives; autonomy; beneficence; *biomedical technologies; caring; *chronically ill; *communication; compassion; comprehension; *decision making; diagnosis; *disclosure; drugs; *emotions; *empathy; informed consent; malpractice; *medical devices; metaphor; narrative ethics; *patient care; *patient compliance; *patient participation; patients; *physician patient relationship; physicians;

prognosis; psychological stress; psychology; quality of life; *rehabilitation; *risks and benefits; self induced illness; *smoking; suffering; technical expertise; therapeutic research; treatment outcome; *trust; truth disclosure; *uncertainty; empowerment; *lung diseases; sick role; *technology transfer

Beaudoin, Claude; Maheux, Brigitte; Côté, Luc, et al. Clinical teachers as humanistic caregivers and educators: perceptions of senior clerks and second–year residents. *Canadian Medical Association Journal.* 1998 Oct 6; 159(7): 765–769. 19 refs. BE62356.
*attitudes; comparative studies; evaluation; *faculty; *humanism; *internship and residency; *interprofessional relations; *medical education; medical ethics; medical schools; *physician patient relationship; *physicians; *students; survey; *clinical clerkships; Laval University; Quebec; University of Montreal; University of Sherbrooke

Bergsma, Jurrit; Mook, Bertha. Ethical considerations in psychotherapeutic systems. *Theoretical Medicine and Bioethics.* 1998 Aug; 19(4): 371–381. 21 fn. BE60159.
autonomy; communication; disclosure; freedom; goals; health personnel; informed consent; methods; narrative ethics; professional autonomy; *professional ethics; *professional patient relationship; *psychotherapy; *social dominance; technical expertise; empowerment

Bignell, C.J. Chaperones for genital examination. [Editorial]. *BMJ (British Medical Journal).* 1999 Jul 17; 319(7203): 137–138. 7 refs. BE62453.
adolescents; adults; *females; institutional policies; knowledge, attitudes, practice; *males; nurses; obstetrics and gynecology; *patient care; patients; *physician patient relationship; physicians; *privacy; sexuality; ambulatory care; *physical examination; Great Britain

Bloch, Sidney; Harari, Edwin. Working with the family: the role of values. *American Journal of Psychotherapy.* 1996 Summer; 50(3): 274–284. 22 refs. BE62051.
children; *family relationship; females; feminist ethics; informed consent; justice; males; minority groups; parents; *professional family relationship; *professional patient relationship; *psychotherapy; social discrimination; *values; *family therapy; relational ethics

Bloche, M. Gregg. Clinical loyalties and the social purposes of medicine. *JAMA.* 1999 Jan 20; 281(3): 268–274. BE60693.
*beneficence; bioethics; capital punishment; clinical ethics; common good; *conflict of interest; disclosure; economics; forensic psychiatry; gatekeeping; goals; human rights; informed consent; injuries; law; legal aspects; managed care programs; mediation; *medical ethics; medicine; *obligations to society; patient advocacy; patient care; *physician patient relationship; *physician's role; *physicians; professional autonomy; public health; torture; trust; *loyalty; United States
Physicians increasingly face conflicts between the ethic of undivided loyalty to patients and pressure to use clinical methods and judgment for social purposes and on behalf of third parties. The principal legal and ethical paradigms by which these conflicts are managed are inadequate, because they either deny or unsuccessfully finesse the reality of contradiction between fidelity to patients and society's other expectations of medicine. This reality needs to be more squarely acknowledged. The challenge for ethics and law is not to resolve this tension -- an impossible task -- but to mediate it in myriad clinical circumstances in a way that preserves the primacy of keeping faith with patients while conceding the legitimacy of society's other expectations of medicine.

BE = bioethics accession number   fn. = footnotes   refs. = references

Branch, William T.; Pels, Richard J.; Hafler, Janet P. Medical students' empathic understanding of their patients. *Academic Medicine.* 1998 Apr; 73(4): 360–362. BE59876.
AIDS; compassion; domestic violence; drug abuse; *empathy; *medical education; medical ethics; *moral development; *physician patient relationship; *students; suffering; teaching methods

Brand, Donald A.; Kliger, Alan S. Planning for a kidney transplant: is my doctor listening? *JAMA.* 1999 Aug 18; 282(7): 691–694. 36 refs. BE62655.
case studies; *communication; *decision analysis; *decision making; kidney diseases; *kidneys; *organ transplantation; *patients; *physician patient relationship; physicians; quality of life; renal dialysis; *risks and benefits

Briant, Robin H.; St. George, Ian M.; White, Gillian. Sexual activity between doctors and patients. [Letter and response]. *New Zealand Medical Journal.* 1996 Apr 12; 109(1019): 127–128. 9 refs. BE60086.
attitudes; evaluation; family practice; *misconduct; morality; organizational policies; *physician patient relationship; *physicians; *sex offenses; standards; survey; Medical Council of New Zealand; *New Zealand

Budd, Susan; Sharma, Ursula, eds. The Healing Bond: The Patient–Practitioner Relationship and Therapeutic Responsibility. New York, NY: Routledge; 1994. 239 p. Includes references. ISBN 0–415–09052–0. BE59734.
accountability; *alternative therapies; anthropology; contraception; counseling; family planning; females; health personnel; interprofessional relations; lawyers; legal liability; males; malpractice; moral obligations; negligence; nurse midwives; *patient care; patient participation; *physician patient relationship; professional autonomy; *professional patient relationship; psychotherapy; referral and consultation; self regulation; sociology of medicine; trust; holistic medicine; quackery; self care; General Medical Council (Great Britain); Great Britain

Buetow, Stephen. The scope for the involvement of patients in their consultations with health professionals: rights, responsibilities and preferences of patients. *Journal of Medical Ethics.* 1998 Aug; 24(4): 243–247. 53 refs. BE61289.
*accountability; common good; decision making; *health care delivery; *moral obligations; patient care; *patient participation; *patients; *patients' rights; *professional patient relationship; *Great Britain; National Health Service; Patient's Charter (Great Britain)
The degree and nature of patient involvement in consultations with health professionals influences problem and needs recognition and management, and public accountability. This paper suggests a framework for understanding the scope for patient involvement in such consultations. Patients are defined as co–producers of formal health services, whose potential for involvement in consultations depends on their personal rights, responsibilities and preferences. Patients' rights in consultations are poorly defined and, in the National Health Service (NHS), not legally enforceable. The responsibilities of patients are also undefined. I suggest that these are not to deny, of their own volition, the rights of others, which in consultations necessitate mutuality of involvement through information–exchange and shared decision–making. Preferences should be met insofar as they do not militate against responsibilities and rights.

Bulger, Roger J. The Quest for Mercy: The Forgotten Ingredient in Health Care Reform. Charlottesville, VA: Carden Jennings; 1998. 117 p. Bibliography: p. 113–117.

ISBN 1–891524–01–1. BE61309.
attitudes to death; autonomy; caring; codes of ethics; common good; communication; compassion; disease; emotions; empathy; *health care reform; interprofessional relations; managed care programs; mass media; medical education; medical ethics; medicine; motivation; palliative care; patient care; patients; *physician patient relationship; physicians; placebos; *prolongation of life; psychology; public health; self concept; social impact; sociology of medicine; suffering; values; Hippocratic Oath; *United States

Carrillo, J. Emilio; Green, Alexander R.; Betancourt, Joseph R. Cross–cultural primary care: a patient–based approach. *Annals of Internal Medicine.* 1999 May 18; 130(10): 829–834. 44 refs. BE61610.
communication; *cultural pluralism; curriculum; *medical education; *minority groups; patient participation; *physician patient relationship; *primary health care; socioeconomic factors; United States
In today's multicultural society, assuring quality health care for all persons requires that physicians understand how each patient's sociocultural background affects his or her health beliefs and behaviors. Cross–cultural curricula have been developed to address these issues but are not widely used in medical education. Many curricula take a categorical and potentially stereotypic approach to "cultural competence" that weds patients of certain cultures to a set of specific, unifying characteristics. In addition, curricula frequently overlook the importance of social factors on the cross–cultural encounter. This paper discusses a patient–based cross–cultural curriculum for residents and medical students that teaches a framework for analysis of the individual patient's social context and cultural health beliefs and behaviors. The curriculum consists of five thematic units taught in four 2–hour sessions. The goal is to help physicians avoid cultural generalizations while improving their ability to understand, communicate with, and care for patients from diverse backgrounds.

Casarett, David J. Moral perception and the pursuit of medical philosophy. *Theoretical Medicine and Bioethics.* 1999 Apr; 20(2): 125–139. 58 fn. BE62214.
bioethics; clinical ethics; diagnosis; disease; health; *medical ethics; *medicine; moral development; *narrative ethics; patient care; patients; *philosophy; *physician patient relationship; *physicians; self concept; suffering; values; *phenomenology

Chodoff, Paul. Ethical dimensions of psychotherapy: a personal perspective. *American Journal of Psychotherapy.* 1996 Summer; 50(3): 298–310. 20 refs. BE62053.
child abuse; confidentiality; economics; health insurance reimbursement; health personnel; mentally ill; misconduct; professional competence; *professional ethics; *professional patient relationship; *psychotherapy; recall; sex offenses; social dominance

Connelly, Julia. Emotions, ethics, and decisions in primary care. *Journal of Clinical Ethics.* 1998 Fall; 9(3): 225–234. 36 fn. BE61331.
communication; *decision making; disclosure; *emotions; patient care; *physician patient relationship; physicians; *primary health care; psychological stress; risks and benefits; treatment refusal

Cooper–Patrick, Lisa; Gallo, Joseph J.; Gonzales, Junius J., et al. Race, gender, and partnership in the patient–physician relationship. *JAMA.* 1999 Aug 11; 282(6): 583–589. 53 refs. BE62667.
*attitudes; *blacks; communication; *decision making; evaluation studies; *females; *males; *minority groups; *patient participation; *patient satisfaction; *patients;

BE = bioethics accession number   fn. = footnotes   refs. = references

*physician patient relationship; *physicians; survey; *whites; *physician's practice patterns; District of Columbia; Maryland

CONTEXT: Many studies have documented race and gender differences in health care received by patients. However, few studies have related differences in the quality of interpersonal care to patient and physician race and gender. OBJECTIVE: To describe how the race/ethnicity and gender of patients and physicians are associated with physicians' participatory decision–making (PDM) styles. DESIGN, SETTING, AND PARTICIPANTS: Telephone survey conducted between November 1996 and June 1998 of 1816 adults aged 18 to 65 years (mean age, 41 years) who had recently attended 1 of 32 primary care practices associated with a large mixed–model managed care organization in an urban setting. Sixty–six percent of patients surveyed were female, 43% were white, and 45% were African American. The physician sample (n = 64) was 63% male, with 56% white, and 25% African American. MAIN OUTCOME MEASURE: Patients' ratings of their physicians' PDM style on a 100–point scale. RESULTS: African American patients rated their visits as significantly less participatory than whites in models adjusting for patient age, gender, education, marital status, health status, and length of the patient–physician relationship (mean [SE] PDM score, 58.0 [1.2] vs 60.6 [3.3]; P = .03). Ratings of minority and white physicians did not differ with respect to PDM style (adjusted mean [SE] PDM score for African Americans, 59.2 [1.7] vs whites, 61.7 [3.1]; P = .13). Patients in race–concordant relationships with their physicians rated their visits as significantly more participatory than patients in race–discordant relationships (difference [SE], 2.6 [1.1]; P = .02). Patients of female physicians had more participatory visits (adjusted mean [SE] PDM score for female, 62.4 [1.3] vs male, 59.5 [3.1]; P = .03), but gender concordance between physicians and patients was not significantly related to PDM score (unadjusted mean [SE] PDM score, 76.0 [1.0] for concordant vs 74.5 [0.9] for discordant; P = .12). Patient satisfaction was highly associated with PDM score within all race/ethnicity groups. CONCLUSIONS: Our data suggest that African American patients rate their visits with physicians as less participatory than whites. However, patients seeing physicians of their own race rate their physicians' decision–making styles as more participatory. Improving cross–cultural communication between primary care physicians and patients and providing patients with access to a diverse group of physicians may lead to more patient involvement in care, higher levels of patient satisfaction, and better health outcomes.

DesAutels, Peggy. Religious women, medical settings, and moral risk. *In:* Walker, Margaret Urban, ed. Mother Time: Women, Aging, and Ethics. Lanham, MD: Rowman and Littlefield; 1999: 175–187. 23 refs. 5 fn. ISBN 0-8476-9260-4. BE61899.
adults; age factors; aged; alternative therapies; attitudes; *bioethical issues; bioethics; Christian Scientists; clergy; clinical ethics committees; decision making; ethicists; *females; *feminist ethics; health; hospitals; palliative care; *paternalism; patient care; patient participation; *physician patient relationship; *religion; religious hospitals; Roman Catholics; *secularism; sociology of medicine; stigmatization; suffering; treatment refusal; *values; faith healing

Druzin, Paul; Shrier, Ian; Yacowar, Mayer, et al. Discrimination against gay, lesbian and bisexual family physicians by patients. *Canadian Medical Association Journal.* 1998 Mar 10; 158(5): 593–597. 13 refs. BE60585.
age factors; *attitudes; family practice; *females; *homosexuals; *males; *patients; *physician patient relationship; *physicians; *social discrimination; *stigmatization; survey; *urban population; *Quebec

Enbom, John A.; Thomas, Claire D. Evaluation of sexual misconduct complaints: the Oregon Board of Medical Examiners, 1991 to 1995. [Article and discussion]. *American Journal of Obstetrics and Gynecology.* 1997 Jun; 176(6): 1340–1348. 22 refs. BE59373.
age factors; comparative studies; emergency care; family practice; females; government regulation; internal medicine; males; medical specialties; *misconduct; obstetrics and gynecology; *physician patient relationship; *physicians; psychiatry; punishment; radiology; *sex offenses; *sexuality; sports medicine; state government; statistics; surgery; survey; *Oregon; *Oregon Board of Medical Examiners

Fahnestock, Deborah T. A piece of my mind: partnership for good dying. *JAMA.* 1999 Aug 18; 282(7): 615–616. BE62653.
*attitudes to death; caring; communication; *physician patient relationship; *terminal care; *terminally ill; continuity of patient care

Feldman, Debra S.; Novack, Dennis H.; Gracely, Edward. Effects of managed care on physician–patient relationships, quality of care, and the ethical practice of medicine. *Archives of Internal Medicine.* 1998 Aug 10–24; 158(15): 1626–1632. 54 refs. BE59173.
*attitudes; communication; confidentiality; *conflict of interest; decision making; disclosure; economics; females; gatekeeping; incentives; informed consent; males; *managed care programs; medical ethics; medical specialties; patient advocacy; patient care; patient participation; *physician patient relationship; *physicians; preventive medicine; *primary health care; professional autonomy; *quality of health care; referral and consultation; *social impact; survey; time factors; trust; continuity of patient care; Pennsylvania; United States

BACKGROUND: Survey studies have shown that physicians believe managed care is having significant impact on many of their professional obligations. METHODS: Primary care physicians were asked about the impact of managed care on: (1) physician–patient relationships, (2) the ability of physicians to carry out their professional ethical obligations, and (3) quality of patient care. In 1996 we surveyed 1011 primary care physicians in Pennsylvania. The survey group's responses were graded on a Likert scale. Space was provided for respondents to include written comments. The SPSS statistical software (SPSS Inc, Chicago, Ill) was used to analyze the data. RESULTS: The response rate was 55%. Most respondents indicated that under managed care physicians are less able to avoid conflicts of interest and less able to place the best interests of patients first. The majority responded that quality of health care is compromised by limitations in location of diagnostic tests, length of hospital stay, and choice of specialists. A significant minority (27%–49%) noted a decrease in the physician's ability to carry out ethical obligations, to respect patient autonomy, and to respect confidentiality in physician–patient communication. Most physicians expressed that managed care made no impact on ability to obtain informed consent or to provide information. There were small but statistically significant sex differences, with female physicians more negative toward managed care. CONCLUSIONS: Many physicians surveyed believe managed care has significant negative effects on the physician–patient relationship, the ability to carry out ethical obligations, and on quality of patient care. These results have implications for health

---

BE = bioethics accession number   fn. = footnotes   refs. = references

care system reform efforts.

Feldman, Miriam K. The doctor–patient bond: covenant or business contract? *Minnesota Medicine.* 1997 Sep; 80(9): 12–16. BE59932.
  *conflict of interest; decision making; disclosure; economics; gatekeeping; *managed care programs; *physician patient relationship; physicians; public opinion; *trust; withholding treatment; *Minnesota; United States

Fowlie, P.W.; Delahunty, C.; Tarnow–Mordi, W.O. What do doctors record in the medical notes following discussion with the parents of sick premature infants? *European Journal of Pediatrics.* 1998 Jan; 157(1): 63–65. 12 refs. BE62403.
  *communication; diagnosis; intensive care units; *low birth weight; *medical records; mortality; *newborns; *parents; *patient care; *physicians; *prematurity; *professional family relationship; prognosis; *records; statistics; survey; truth disclosure; withholding treatment; severity of illness index; Great Britain

Gabbard, Glen O. Lessons to be learned from the study of sexual boundary violations. *American Journal of Psychotherapy.* 1996 Summer; 50(3): 311–322. 17 refs. BE62054.
  health personnel; intention; love; *misconduct; privacy; *professional patient relationship; *psychotherapy; referral and consultation; self regulation; *sex offenses; sexuality

Gastmans, Chris; Dierckx de Casterle, Bernadette; Schotsmans, Paul. Nursing considered as moral practice: a philosophical–ethical interpretation of nursing. *Kennedy Institute of Ethics Journal.* 1998 Mar; 8(1): 43–69. 3 fn. Commented on by C.R. Taylor, p. 71–82. BE59354.
  altruism; beneficence; *caring; communication; emotions; goals; motivation; *nurse patient relationship; *nurse's role; nurses; *nursing ethics; patient admission; patient care; patient participation; patients; philosophy; professional competence; religion; technical expertise; trust; values; *virtues
Discussions of ethical approaches in nursing have been much enlivened in recent years, for instance by new developments in the theory of care. Nevertheless, many ethical concepts in nursing still need to be clarified. The purpose of this contribution is to develop a fundamental ethical view on nursing care considered as moral practice. Three main components are analyzed more deeply -- i.e., the caring relationship, caring behavior as the integration of virtue and expert activity, and "good care" as the ultimate goal of nursing practice. For the development of this philosophical–ethical interpretation of nursing, we have mainly drawn on the pioneering work of Anne Bishop and John Scudder, Alasdair MacIntyre, Lawrence Blum, and Louis Janssens. We will also show that the European philosophical background offers some original ideas for this endeavor.

Gaudiani, Vincent A. It's the patient. [Editorial]. *Pharos.* 1996 Fall; 59(4): 33. BE59699.
  biomedical research; health care delivery; historical aspects; international aspects; managed care programs; *misconduct; National Socialism; *physician patient relationship; *physicians; *scientific misconduct; *trends; Germany; Twentieth Century; United States

Gianakos, Dean. Conversations with Stella. *Annals of Internal Medicine.* 1999 Apr 20; 130(8): 698–699. BE61605.
  allowing to die; alternatives; chronically ill; *communication; critically ill; *patient care; *physician patient relationship; *treatment refusal; trust; uncertainty;

*ventilators; withholding treatment

Gilligan, Timothy; Raffin, Thomas A. End–of–life discussions with patients: timing and truth–telling. [Editorial]. *Chest.* 1996 Jan; 109(1): 11–12. 11 refs. BE60427.
  *advance care planning; advance directives; *allowing to die; chronically ill; communication; critically ill; *decision making; *patient participation; *physician patient relationship; *physicians; prognosis; terminally ill; *truth disclosure; ventilators

Greenhalgh, Trisha; Hurwitz, Brian. Why study narrative? Narrative based medicine. *BMJ (British Medical Journal).* 1999 Jan 2; 318(7175): 48–50. 18 refs. BE60841.
  attitudes; case studies; *communication; diagnosis; literature; medical education; narrative ethics; patient care; *physician patient relationship; physicians; *sick role

Grey, Matthew W. Medical use of marijuana: legal and ethical conflicts in the patient/physician relationship. [Comment]. *University of Richmond Law Review.* 1996 Jan; 30(1): 249–274. 66 fn. BE59862.
  AIDS; *autonomy; *beneficence; codes of ethics; federal government; government regulation; *legal aspects; *palliative care; patients; *physician patient relationship; physicians; professional organizations; *psychoactive drugs; terminally ill; compassionate use; *marijuana; American Medical Association; *United States

Hall, Judith A.; Epstein, Arnold M.; DeCiantis, Mary Lou, et al. Physician's liking for their patients: more evidence for the role of affect in medical care. *Health Psychology.* 1993; 12(2): 140–146. 52 refs. BE61829.
  aged; *attitudes; emotions; females; health; internal medicine; males; mental health; patient satisfaction; *physician patient relationship; *physicians; survey; Rhode Island

Hedges, Lawrence E.; Hilton, Robert; Hilton, Virginia Wink, et al. Therapists at Risk: Perils of the Intimacy of the Therapeutic Relationship. Northvale, NJ: Jason Aronson; 1997. 328 p. Bibliography: p. 305–318. Based on the proceedings of a conference held in Anaheim, CA, on 25 Apr 1994. ISBN 1–56821–827–3. BE61420.
  child abuse; health personnel; *legal aspects; legal liability; malpractice; mentally ill; methods; misconduct; professional competence; professional ethics; *professional patient relationship; *psychotherapy; *recall; sex offenses; *sexuality; time factors

Hellström, Olle. Symptoms or persons? A question for setting the goals of medicine. *In:* Hanson, Mark J.; Callahan, Daniel, eds. The Goals of Medicine: The Forgotten Issue in Health Care Reform. Washington, DC: Georgetown University Press; 1999: 118–136. 21 fn. Originally published as "Symptoms of the understanding of persons? A question of focus in relation to the setting of the goals of medicine," in Nordenfelt, L.; Tengland, P.A., eds., *The Goals and Limits of Medicine*, 1996; Stockholm: Almquist and Wiksell International. ISBN 0–87840–707–3. BE60521.
  communication; counseling; *goals; health; health care; health personnel; health promotion; *medicine; obligations to society; pain; patient advocacy; patient care; patient education; *physician patient relationship; *physician's role; public policy; quality of life; resource allocation; suffering; sick role

Herman, Joseph. The good old days. *Lancet.* 1998 Dec 12; 352(9144): 1930–1931. 13 refs. BE60391.
  altruism; biomedical technologies; caring; compassion; empathy; historical aspects; *physician patient relationship;

BE = bioethics accession number   fn. = footnotes   refs. = references

physicians; sociology of medicine; trends; Twentieth Century

Hester, D. Micah. Habits of healing. *In:* McGee, Glenn, ed. Pragmatic Bioethics. Nashville, TN: Vanderbilt University Press; 1999: 45-59, 261-264. 38 fn. ISBN 0-8265-1321-2. BE60662.
     attitudes; autonomy; common good; communication; human characteristics; humanism; intelligence; *medicine; *paternalism; patient care; *patient participation; philosophy; *physician patient relationship; physicians; social dominance; *social interaction; sociology of medicine; technical expertise; pragmatism; Dewey, John

Hester, D. Micah. The place of community in medical encounters. *Journal of Medicine and Philosophy.* 1998 Aug; 23(4): 369-383. 19 refs. 7 fn. BE60629.
     autonomy; chronically ill; *communication; communitarianism; disabled; *disease; *health; humanism; narrative ethics; paternalism; patient care; *patient participation; *physician patient relationship; physician's role; *self concept; social dominance; *social interaction
Disease and injury creates a break between the individual and the community which compromises the individual's status within the community as well as the integrity of the self as a "product" of social interaction. Our "everyday" activities are called into question since our ability to fulfill obligations and to achieve many of our ends is diminished through the weakening of our bodies. In light of this account of disease, healing is about restoring the individual to a state of vital functioning, and vital functioning entails communal participation. As John Dewey points out, health as "living healthily" can be understood only in context of each patient's pursuits which are always social and communal. But, if living in community with others is the end-in-view for medical encounters, it too must be implicated in the means to that end. A patient who is given the opportunity to participate as a member of the health care community has already begun within the medical encounter itself to live healthily. It follows, then, that we must work to promote new attitudes within health care towards aiding in the effective agency and participation of patients in their healing process -- i.e., we must see community as healing.

Hillman, Alan L. Mediators of patient trust. [Editorial]. *JAMA.* 1998 Nov 18; 280(19): 1703-1704. 4 refs. BE59654.
     attitudes; conflict of interest; incentives; knowledge, attitudes, practice; *managed care programs; patient advocacy; patients; *physician patient relationship; physicians; *remuneration; survey; *trust; capitation fee; United States

Honings, Bonifacio. The Charter for Health Care Workers: a synthesis of Hippocratic ethics and Christian morality. *Dolentium Hominum: Church and Health in the World.* 1996; 31(11th Yr., No. 1): 48-52. 41 fn. BE61002.
     abortion, induced; active euthanasia; allowing to die; beginning of life; beneficence; *Christian ethics; *codes of ethics; empathy; health personnel; marital relationship; *medical ethics; moral obligations; *morality; organ donation; patient education; *physician patient relationship; *physician's role; professional ethics; reproduction; reproductive technologies; *Roman Catholic ethics; suffering; terminal care; terminally ill; *theology; trust; *value of life; *Charter for Health Care Workers; Hippocrates; *Hippocratic Oath

Howe, Edmund G. Ethics consultants: could they do better? *Journal of Clinical Ethics.* 1999 Spring; 10(1): 13-25. 23 fn. BE62702.

case studies; *clinical ethics committees; communication; *conflict of interest; consensus; deception; decision making; dissent; emotions; *ethicist's role; *ethicists; *ethics consultation; evaluation; guidelines; interprofessional relations; patient advocacy; patient care team; professional competence; *professional family relationship; *professional patient relationship; psychology; social dominance; standards; *trust; Core Competencies for Health Care Ethics Consultation (SHHV-SBC Task Force)

Kao, Audiey C.; Green, Diane C.; Zaslavsky, Alan M., et al. The relationship between method of physician payment and patient trust. *JAMA.* 1998 Nov 18; 280(19): 1708-1714. 64 refs. BE59655.
     *attitudes; health insurance; health maintenance organizations; incentives; knowledge, attitudes, practice; *managed care programs; medical fees; *patients; *physician patient relationship; primary health care; *remuneration; social impact; survey; *trust; capitation fee; United States
CONTEXT: Trust is the cornerstone of the patient-physician relationship. Payment methods that place physicians at financial risk have raised concerns about patients' trust in physicians to act in patients' best interests. OBJECTIVE: To evaluate the extent to which methods of physician payment are related to patient trust. DESIGN: Cross-sectional telephone interview survey done between January and June 1997. SETTING: Health plans of a large national insurer in Atlanta, Ga, the Baltimore, Md-Washington, DC, area, and Orlando, Fla. PARTICIPANTS: A total of 2086 adult managed care and indemnity patients. MAIN OUTCOME MEASURE: A 10-item scale (alpha = .94) assessing patients' trust in physicians. RESULTS: More fee-for-service (FFS) indemnity patients (94%) completely or mostly trust their physicians to "put their health and well-being above keeping down the health plan's costs" than salary (77%), capitated (83%), or FFS managed care patients (85%) (P less than .001 for pairwise comparisons). In multivariate analyses that adjusted for potentially confounding factors, FFS indemnity patients also had higher scores on the 10-item trust scale than salary (P less than .001), capitated (P less than .001), or FFS managed care patients (P less than .01). The effects of payment method on patient trust were reduced when a measure based on patients' reports about physician behavior (eg, Does your physician take enough time to answer your questions?) was included in the regression analyses, but the differences remained statistically significant, except for the comparison between FFS managed care and FFS indemnity patients (P=.08). Patients' perceptions of how their physicians were paid were not independently associated with trust, but the 37.7% who said they did not know how their physicians were paid had higher levels of trust than other patients (P less than .01). A total of 30.2% of patients were incorrect about their physicians' method of payment. CONCLUSIONS: Most patients trusted their physicians, but FFS indemnity patients have higher levels of trust than salary, capitated, or FFS managed care patients. Patients' reports of physician behavior accounted for part of the variation in patients' trust in physicians who are paid differently. The impact of payment methods on patient trust may be mediated partly by physician behavior.

Lachs, John. Personal relations between physicians and patients. *In: his* The Relevance of Philosophy to Life. Nashville, TN: Vanderbilt University Press; 1995: 199-205. ISBN 0-8265-1262-3. BE60866.
     autonomy; decision making; informed consent; models, theoretical; paternalism; patient care; patient participation; *physician patient relationship; technical expertise

---

BE = bioethics accession number   fn. = footnotes   refs. = references

Levi, Banjamin H. Respecting Patient Autonomy. Urbana, IL: University of Illinois Press; 1999. 222 p. Bibliography: p. 205–217. ISBN 0–252–06749–5. BE62627.
 aged; *autonomy; bioethics; case studies; clinical ethics; communication; competence; decision making; freedom; health personnel; models, theoretical; nursing homes; paternalism; *patient care; *patient participation; physical restraint; *professional patient relationship; social interaction

Levine, Carol; Zuckerman, Connie. The trouble with families: toward an ethic of accommodation. *Annals of Internal Medicine.* 1999 Jan 19; 130(2): 148–152. 17 refs. BE62557.
 attitudes; communication; confidentiality; decision making; dissent; education; emotions; *family members; *family relationship; health personnel; hospitals; institutional policies; minority groups; patient advocacy; patient care; *professional family relationship; third party consent; truth disclosure; United States
Although some clinicians are extraordinarily sensitive to the legitimate roles of patients' families in medical crises, a persistent tendency to equate families with trouble is evident in both the literature and the practice of medicine. Some negative presumptions about families derive from western medicine's almost exclusive focus on the individual patient in codes of ethics, training, and practice. Modern bioethics has reinforced this individualistic approach. Physicians' primary responsibilities are unequivocally to their patients, but a complete understanding of the patient's personhood must include consideration of the significant persons who help define the patient's core identity. One source of tension between professionals and families lies in differing perceptions of the roles that family members should play and how they should play them. Members of a family may act as advocates, provide or manage care, serve as trusted companions on the journey through illness and death, and make decisions on behalf of an incompetent patient. Each role presents potential conflicts. Other sources of conflict include disagreement within a family; challenges to physician authority; fear of litigation; and differing religious, ethnic, or cultural traditions. An ethic of accommodation emphasizes the need to negotiate care plans that do not compromise patients' basic interests but that recognize the capacities and limitations of family members. Family caregivers want understandable and timely information, better training, compassionate recognition of their anxiety, guidance in defining their roles and responsibilities, and support for the setting of fair limits on their sacrifices. Health care professionals can better meet these needs through education and skills acquisition, the establishment of partnerships with families, and regular dialogue and communication.

Lo, Bernard; Quill, Timothy; Tulsky, James; American College of Physicians–American Society of Internal Medicine End-of-Life Care Consensus Panel. Discussing palliative care with patients. *Annals of Internal Medicine.* 1999 May 4; 130(9): 744–749. 27 refs. BE61607.
 advance care planning; aged; cancer; case studies; *communication; empathy; family members; heart diseases; home care; hospices; *palliative care; patient care; patient participation; *physician patient relationship; *physicians; religion; *terminal care; values

Long, Ann; Slevin, Eamonn. Living with dementia: communicating with an older person and her family. *Nursing Ethics.* 1999 Jan; 6(1): 23–36. 54 refs. BE60152.
 *aged; autonomy; beneficence; *caring; *communication;

deception; dehumanization; *dementia; diagnosis; empathy; ethical analysis; family members; family relationship; humanism; *nurse patient relationship; *nurses; *nursing education; nursing research; paternalism; *patient care; *professional family relationship; psychological stress; psychology; social dominance; stigmatization; truth disclosure; adult offspring; University of Ulster (Northern Ireland)

Lyckholm, Laurie J. Should physicians accept gifts from patients? *JAMA.* 1998 Dec 9; 280(22): 1944–1946. 14 refs. BE59580.
 conflict of interest; *gifts; guidelines; health facilities; incentives; medical ethics; misconduct; motivation; patient care; patients; *physician patient relationship

Macklin, Ruth. The doctor–patient relationship in different cultures. *In: her* Against Relativism: Cultural Diversity and the Search for Ethical Universals in Medicine. New York, NY: Oxford University Press; 1999: 85–107. 32 fn. ISBN 0–19–511632–1. BE62781.
 autonomy; beneficence; *cultural pluralism; *decision making; *ethical relativism; family members; freedom; historical aspects; informed consent; *international aspects; law; malpractice; medical ethics; misconduct; moral obligations; non-Western World; paternalism; patient participation; *physician patient relationship; professional family relationship; social control; trends; trust; truth disclosure; values; virtues; Western World; right not to know; China; Egypt; Europe; India; Japan; Mexico; Nigeria; Philippines; Twentieth Century; United States

McVaugh, Michael R. "Bedside manners in the Middle Ages." *Bulletin of the History of Medicine.* 1997 Summer; 71(2): 201–223. 50 fn. Revised version of the Fielding H. Garrison Lecture presented at the meeting of the American Association for the History of Medicine, 10 May 1996. BE60684.
 diagnosis; *historical aspects; medical education; medical etiquette; medical fees; *medicine; patient care; *physician patient relationship; physicians; prognosis; referral and consultation; social dominance; *sociology of medicine; surgery; trust; truth disclosure; uncertainty; Arnald of Villanova; Europe; *Middle Ages; Mondeville, Henry de; Sigerist, Henry; William of Saliceto; Zancariis, Albert de

Maly, Rose C.; Frank, Janet C.; Marshall, Grant N., et al. Perceived efficacy in patient–physician interactions (PEPPI): validation of an instrument in older persons. *Journal of the American Geriatrics Society.* 1998 Jul; 46(7): 889–894. 53 refs. BE62260.
 *aged; *communication; comprehension; *evaluation; information dissemination; *patient care; *patient participation; *patient satisfaction; *physician patient relationship; *placebos; socioeconomic factors; *empowerment; physician's practice patterns; *questionnaires; self care; Los Angeles

Mandl, Kenneth D.; Kohane, Isaac S.; Brandt, Allan M. Electronic patient–physician communication: problems and promise. *Annals of Internal Medicine.* 1998 Sep 15; 129(6): 495–500. 60 refs. BE59134.
 *communication; *computer communication networks; confidentiality; evaluation; health care delivery; legal aspects; patient care; patient participation; *physician patient relationship; risks and benefits; socioeconomic factors; standards; Internet; United States
A critical mass of Internet users will soon enable wide diffusion of electronic communication within medical practice. E-mail between physicians and patients offers important opportunities for better communication. Linking patients and physicians through e-mail may increase the involvement of patients in supervising and documenting their own health care, processes that may

activate patients and contribute to improved health. These new linkages may have profound implications for the patient–physician relationship. Although the federal government proposes regulation of telemedicine technologies and medical software, communications technologies are evolving under less scrutiny. Unless these technologies are implemented with substantial forethought, they may disturb delicate balances in the patient–physician relationship, widen social disparities in health outcomes, and create barriers to access to health care. This paper seeks to identify the promise and pitfalls of electronic patient–physician communication before such technology becomes widely distributed. A research agenda is proposed that would provide data that are useful for careful shaping of the communications infrastructure. The paper addresses the need to 1) define appropriate use of the various modes of patient–physician communication, 2) ensure the security and confidentiality of patient information, 3) create user interfaces that guide patients in effective use of the technology, 4) proactively assess medicolegal liability, and 5) ensure access to the technology by a multicultural, multilingual population with varying degrees of literacy.

Marta, Jan. Whose consent is it anyway? A poststructuralist framing of the person in medical decision-making. *Theoretical Medicine and Bioethics.* 1998 Aug; 19(4): 353–370. 33 fn. BE60158.
  *accountability; *autonomy; beneficence; communication; *competence; decision making; *emotions; *informed consent; mentally ill; *models, theoretical; patient participation; patients; personhood; *physician patient relationship; physician's role; physicians; *psychology; *psychotherapy; self concept; standards; *rationality; *poststructuralism

Martone, Marilyn. Developing new models to ensure autonomy in home health care. *Linacre Quarterly.* 1997 Aug; 64(3): 29–37. 6 fn. BE59310.
  *autonomy; *communication; *family members; *family relationship; females; *health personnel; *home care; patient compliance; patients; *professional autonomy; *professional family relationship; *professional patient relationship; psychological stress; technical expertise; terminal care; trust; dependency

Marvel, M. Kim; Epstein, Ronald M.; Flowers, Kristine, et al. Soliciting the patient's agenda: have we improved? *JAMA.* 1999 Jan 20; 281(3): 283–287. 14 refs. BE60381.
  *communication; family practice; patient participation; *physician patient relationship; physicians; survey; Canada; United States
CONTEXT: Previous research indicates physicians frequently choose a patient problem to explore before determining the patient's full spectrum of concerns. OBJECTIVE: To examine the extent to which experienced family physicians in various practice settings elicit the agenda of concerns patients bring to the office. DESIGN: A cross-sectional survey using linguistic analysis of a convenience sample of 264 patient–physician interviews. SETTING AND PARTICIPANTS: Primary care offices of 29 board-certified family physicians practicing in rural Washington (n = 1; 3%), semirural Colorado (n = 20; 69%), and urban settings in the United States and Canada (n = 8; 27%). Nine participants had fellowship training in communication skills and family counseling. MAIN OUTCOME MEASURES: Patient-physician verbal interactions, including physician solicitations of patient concerns, rate of completion of patient responses, length of time for patient responses, and frequency of late-arising patient

concerns. RESULTS: Physicians solicited patient concerns in 199 interviews (75.4%). Patients' initial statements of concerns were completed in 74 interviews (28.0%). Physicians redirected the patient's opening statement after a mean of 23.1 seconds. Patients allowed to complete their statement of concerns used only 6 seconds more on average than those who were redirected before completion of concerns. Late-arising concerns were more common when physicians did not solicit patient concerns during the interview (34.9% vs 14.9%). Fellowship-trained physicians were more likely to solicit patient concerns and allow patients to complete their initial statement of concerns (44% vs 22%). CONCLUSIONS: Physicians often redirect patients' initial descriptions of their concerns. Once redirected, the descriptions are rarely completed. Consequences of incomplete initial descriptions include late-arising concerns and missed opportunities to gather potentially important patient data. Soliciting the patient's agenda takes little time and can improve interview efficiency and yield increased data.

Mattiasson, Anne-Cathrine; Hemberg, Maja. Intimacy -- meeting needs and respecting privacy in the care of elderly people: what is a good moral attitude on the part of the nurse/carer? *Nursing Ethics.* 1998 Nov; 5(6): 527–534. 27 refs. BE60813.
  *aged; attitudes; *caring; communication; dementia; females; males; *nurse patient relationship; nurses; patient care; patients; *privacy; sexuality; trust

Mechanic, David. Public trust and initiatives for new health care partnerships. *Milbank Quarterly.* 1998; 76(2): 281–302. 54 refs. BE60057.
  audiovisual aids; autonomy; caring; chronically ill; *communication; computer communication networks; health care delivery; health education; health facilities; institutional ethics; managed care programs; *medical education; medical schools; paternalism; patient care; *patient education; patient participation; patient satisfaction; *physician patient relationship; physicians; professional competence; *sociology of medicine; teaching methods; trends; *trust; Internet

Mechanic, David. The functions and limitations of trust in the provision of medical care. *Journal of Health Politics, Policy and Law.* 1998 Aug; 23(4): 661–686. 53 refs. Commented on by S.D. Goold, p. 687–695. BE59782.
  communication; confidentiality; conflict of interest; decision making; *disclosure; *economics; evaluation; gatekeeping; health care delivery; incentives; informed consent; international aspects; *managed care programs; medical errors; negligence; organization and administration; patient advocacy; patient participation; patient satisfaction; *physician patient relationship; physician self-referral; *physicians; professional autonomy; professional competence; public opinion; quality of health care; referral and consultation; *regulation; resource allocation; standards; *trust; withholding treatment; gag clauses; quality assurance; Great Britain; United States
Trust, the expectation that institutions and professionals will act in one's interests, contributes to the effectiveness of medical care. With the rapid privatization of medical care and the growth of managed care, trust may be diminished. Five important aspects of trust are examined: technical and interpersonal competence, physician agency, physician control, confidentiality, and open communication and disclosure. In each case, changing health care arrangements increase the risks of trusting and encourage regulatory interventions that substitute for some aspects of trust. With the increased size and centralization of health care plans, inevitable errors are

attributed to health plans rather than to failures of individual judgment. Such generalized criticisms exacerbate distrust and encourage micromanagement of medical care processes.

Meinhardt, Robyn; Landis, Kenneth W. Bioethics update: the changing nature of the doctor/patient relationship. *Whittier Law Review.* 1995; 16(1): 177–186. 9 fn. BE59213.
   autonomy; conflict of interest; disclosure; economics; informed consent; legal aspects; *models (theoretical); paternalism; patient advocacy; patient participation; *physician patient relationship; physician's role; values

Michel, Vicki. Factoring ethnic and racial differences into bioethics decision making. *Generations (American Society on Aging).* 1994 Winter; 18(4): 23–26. 8 refs. BE60547.
   autonomy; coercion; communication; *cultural pluralism; *decision making; diagnosis; disclosure; *family members; family relationship; informed consent; *minority groups; physicians; privacy; professional family relationship; *professional patient relationship; prognosis; *truth disclosure; values; United States

Miller, Franklin G.; Rosenstein, Donald L.; DeRenzo, Evan G. Professional integrity in clinical research. *JAMA.* 1998 Oct 28; 280(16): 1449–1454. 30 refs. BE59636.
   beneficence; biomedical research; conflict of interest; drugs; financial support; *human experimentation; incentives; informed consent; *investigator subject relationship; *investigators; medical education; medical ethics; models, theoretical; *moral policy; nontherapeutic research; patients; physician patient relationship; *physicians; professional ethics; *professional role; regulation; research subjects; risks and benefits; teaching methods; therapeutic research; volunteers; withholding treatment; *integrity
In response to public concern over abuses in human medical experimentation, the dominant approach to the ethics of clinical research during the past 30 years has been regulation, particularly via institutional review board review and approval of scientific protocols and written consent forms. However, the effectiveness of regulatory mechanisms in ensuring the ethical conduct of clinical research is limited. Little attention has been devoted to the nature and role of professional integrity of physician investigators, a conscientious framework for guiding investigators in the socially important but morally complex activity of clinical research. Professional integrity is vital in forging an ethically sound relationship between investigators and patient volunteers, a relationship that differs in important ways from the patient–physician relationship in standard clinical practice. We examine critically 2 models of the moral identity of physician investigators, the investigator as clinician and the investigator as scientist; in neither of these 2 models can the physician investigator eliminate completely the moral conflicts posed by clinical research. The professional integrity of physician investigators depends on a coherent moral identity that is proper to the enterprise of clinical research. The roles of clinician and scientist must be integrated to manage conscientiously the ethical complexity, ambiguity, and tensions between the potentially competing loyalties of science and care of volunteer patients.

Morrison, Mary F. Obstacles to doctor–patient communication at the end of life. *In:* Steinberg, Maurice D.; Youngner, Stuart J., eds. End–of–Life Decisions: A Psychosocial Perspective. Washington, DC: American Psychiatric Press; 1998: 109–136. 63 fn. ISBN 0–88048–756–9. BE60121.

advance directives; age factors; aged; *allowing to die; attitudes; attitudes to death; chronically ill; *communication; cultural pluralism; *decision making; diagnosis; mentally ill; minority groups; patient participation; *patients; *physician patient relationship; *physicians; primary health care; professional family relationship; prognosis; prolongation of life; *psychiatry; referral and consultation; religion; resuscitation orders; socioeconomic factors; *terminal care; *terminally ill; time factors; truth disclosure; values; withholding treatment; United States

Nadelson, Carol C. Ethics and empathy in a changing health care system. *Pharos.* 1996 Fall; 59(4): 29–32. 16 refs. BE59698.
   accountability; compassion; confidentiality; *economics; *empathy; gatekeeping; *health care delivery; managed care programs; medical ethics; medical records; obligations of society; patient advocacy; patient compliance; *physician patient relationship; *physicians; resource allocation; sociology of medicine; *trends; trust; United States

Nessa, John; Malterud, Kirsti. Tell me what's wrong with me: a discourse analysis approach to the concept of patient autonomy. *Journal of Medical Ethics.* 1998 Dec; 24(6): 394–400. 29 fn. BE60789.
   *autonomy; case studies; *communication; competence; deception; decision making; depressive disorder; feminist ethics; informed consent; married persons; *patients; *physician patient relationship; rights; treatment refusal; qualitative research
BACKGROUND: Patient autonomy has gradually replaced physician paternalism as an ethical ideal. However, in a medical context, the principle of individual autonomy has different meanings. More knowledge is needed about what is and should be an appropriate understanding of the concept of patient autonomy in clinical practice. AIM: To challenge the traditional concept of patient autonomy by applying a discourse analysis to the issue. METHOD: A qualitative case study approach with material from one consultation. The discourse is interpreted according to pragmatic and text–linguistic principles and provides the basis of a theoretical discussion of different concepts of patient autonomy. RESULTS: The consultation transcript illustrates how the patient's wishes can be respected in real life. The patient, her husband and the doctor are all involved in the discourse dynamics, governed by the subject matter, namely her mental illness.
CONCLUSION: We suggest a dynamic and dialogue–based conception of autonomy as adequate for clinical purposes. These perspectives, based on mutual understanding, take communication between patient and doctor as their starting point. According to this approach, autonomy requires a genuine dialogue, an interpersonal mode of being which we choose to call "authentic interaction".

Neuberger, Julia; Tallis, Raymond. Do we need a new word for patients? [Article and commentary]. *BMJ (British Medical Journal).* 1999 Jun 26; 318(7200): 1756–1758. BE62306.
   alternatives; decision making; patient participation; *patients; *professional patient relationship; suffering; *terminology

Neufeld, Victor R. Physician as humanist: still an educational challenge. [Editorial]. *Canadian Medical Association Journal.* 1998 Oct 6; 159(7): 787–788. 7 refs. BE62358.
   attitudes; *communication; empirical research; *faculty; *humanism; internship and residency; interprofessional relations; *medical education; *physician patient relationship; *physicians; public opinion; students; Canada

---

BE = bioethics accession number   fn. = footnotes   refs. = references

O'Neill, Patrick. Negotiating Consent in Psychotherapy. New York, NY: New York University Press; 1998. 188 p. (Qualitative studies in psychology). Bibliography: p. 177–183. ISBN 0-8147-6195-X. BE61647.

adolescents; adults; alternatives; attitudes; behavior disorders; child abuse; coercion; *communication; confidentiality; dangerousness; disclosure; duty to warn; food; *health personnel; *informed consent; *knowledge, attitudes, practice; parental consent; patients; prisoners; *professional patient relationship; *psychology; *psychotherapy; sex offenses; survey; anorexia nervosa; bulimia; negotiation; qualitative research

Pang, Mei-che Samantha. Protective truthfulness: the Chinese way of safeguarding patients in informed treatment decisions. *Journal of Medical Ethics.* 1999 Jun; 25(3): 247–253. 42 refs. BE61859.

autonomy; *beneficence; competence; confidentiality; cultural pluralism; *decision making; diagnosis; disclosure; empirical research; evaluation studies; *family members; historical aspects; hospitals; *informed consent; *medical ethics; *moral obligations; non-Western World; *nurse patient relationship; *nurses; nursing ethics; nursing research; *paternalism; patient care; patients' rights; *physician patient relationship; physicians; privacy; professional competence; prognosis; psychological stress; survey; terminal care; *third party consent; trust; *truth disclosure; value of life; values; virtues; vulnerable populations; hope; *China

The first part of this paper examines the practice of informed treatment decisions in the protective medical system in China today. The second part examines how health care professionals in China perceive and carry out their responsibilities when relaying information to vulnerable patients, based on the findings of an empirical study that I had undertaken to examine the moral experience of nurses in practice situations. In the Chinese medical ethics tradition, refinement [jing] in skills and sincerity [cheng] in relating to patients are two cardinal virtues that health care professionals are required to possess. This notion of absolute sincerity carries a strong sense of parental protectiveness. The empirical findings reveal that most nurses are ambivalent about telling the truth to patients. Truth-telling would become an insincere act if a patient were to lose hope and confidence in life after learning of his or her disease. In this system of protective medical care, it is arguable as to whose interests are being protected: the patient, the family or the hospital. I would suggest that the interests of the hospital and the family members who legitimately represent the patient's interests are being honoured, but at the expense of the patient's right to know.

Pellissier, James M.; Venta, Enrique R. Introducing patient values into the decision making process for breast cancer screening. *Women and Health.* 1996; 24(4): 47–67. 40 refs. BE59442.

autonomy; *breast cancer; communication; *decision analysis; *decision making; evaluation; *females; *mass screening; models, theoretical; paternalism; *patient participation; *physician patient relationship; practice guidelines; risk; *values; United States

Perkins, David V.; Hudson, Brenda L.; Gray, Diana M., et al. Decisions and justifications by community mental health providers about hypothetical ethical dilemmas. *Psychiatric Services.* 1998 Oct; 49(10): 1317–1322. 23 refs. BE61448.

administrators; age factors; *community services; comparative studies; *confidentiality; *decision making; disclosure; education; *geographic factors; gifts; *health personnel; *mentally ill; nurses; *professional ethics; *professional patient relationship; psychology; *social interaction; social workers; survey; *case managers; *mental

health services; rural population; urban population; Midwestern United States

Perry, Clifton; Kuruc, Joan Wallman. Psychotherapists' sexual relationships with their patients. *Annals of Health Law.* 1993; 2: 35–54. 126 fn. BE59827.

compensation; criminal law; *health personnel; *legal aspects; legal liability; legislation; malpractice; mentally ill; *misconduct; *professional patient relationship; psychological stress; *psychotherapy; sex offenses; *sexuality; state government; torts; *United States

Pfettscher, Susan A. Making decisions about end-stage renal disease treatment: a review of theories and issues. *Advances in Renal Replacement Therapy.* 1997 Jan; 4(1): 81–88. 62 refs. BE60176.

autonomy; communication; costs and benefits; *decision analysis; *decision making; family members; informed consent; *kidney diseases; *models, theoretical; organ transplantation; paternalism; *patient care; patient care team; *patient participation; patient satisfaction; *physician patient relationship; *physicians; professional autonomy; renal dialysis; treatment outcome; values; withholding treatment; United States

Pullman, Daryl. Role conflict and conflict of interest: a professional practice dilemma. *Journal of the American Optometric Association.* 1996 Feb; 67(2): 98–108. 19 refs. BE60295.

*conflict of interest; contracts; decision making; entrepreneurship; *health personnel; informed consent; interprofessional relations; medical devices; models, theoretical; *professional ethics; *professional patient relationship; *professional role; trust; *business ethics; *optometry

Richards, Karlotta A.; Noblin, Charles D. Sanctions for ethics violations: does licensure of socioeconomic status matter? *Ethics and Behavior.* 1999; 9(2): 119–126. 10 refs. BE61784.

*attitudes; comparative studies; education; evaluation studies; *government regulation; guidelines; *health personnel; *misconduct; *patients; professional organizations; *professional patient relationship; *psychology; psychotherapy; *punishment; *sex offenses; *sexuality; *socioeconomic factors; state government; American Psychological Association; Mississippi

Although sexual relationships between therapists and their clients are unethical, such beahviors still occur. This study investigated whether psychologists with applied versus nonapplied training differed in the severity of sanctions advocated for psychologists charged with sexual ethical violations toward high- or low-socioeconomic status victims. Licensed and Nonlicensed psychologists (N=48) viewed a 15-min videotape simulating the adjudication process about an alleged sexual involvement between client and psychologist, then prescribed either: Dismissal of Charges, Educative Advisory, Educative Warning, Reprimand, Censure, Stipulated Resignation, Permitted Resignation, or Expulsion. The alleged victim was described as a college professor of home economics or a hairdresser. Licensed psychologists chose more severe sanctions ("Stipulated or Permitted Resignation") than did Nonlicensed psychologists ("Censure"). Socioeconomic status made no significant difference in sanctions. Apparently, applied therapy training results in more severe judgements toward those who violate American Psychological Association ethical guidelines than other types of psychology training.

Rosoff, Arnold J. Informed consent in the electronic age. *American Journal of Law and Medicine.* 1999; 25(2–3):

367–386. 73 fn. BE62505.
audiovisual aids; communication; comprehension; computer communication networks; *computers; disclosure; industry; information dissemination; *informed consent; legal liability; patient care; *patient education; *physician patient relationship; physician's role; risks and benefits; social impact; trends; *telemedicine; Internet

Saha, Somnath; Komaromy, Miriam; Koepsell, Thomas D., et al. Patient-physician racial concordance and the perceived quality and use of health care. *Archives of Internal Medicine.* 1999 May 10; 159(9): 997–1004. 42 refs. BE61389.
*attitudes; *blacks; comparative studies; cultural pluralism; evaluation; health care delivery; *Hispanic Americans; *minority groups; patient care; *patient satisfaction; *patients; *physician patient relationship; *physicians; preventive medicine; *quality of health care; socioeconomic factors; survey; *whites; *United States
BACKGROUND: Patients from racial and ethnic minority groups use fewer health care services and are less satisfied with their care than patients from the majority white population. These disparities may be attributable in part to racial or cultural differences between patients and their physicians. OBJECTIVE: To determine whether racial concordance between patients and physicians affects patients' satisfaction with and use of health care. METHODS: We analyzed data from the 1994 Commonwealth Fund's Minority Health Survey, a nationwide, telephone survey of noninstitutionalized adults. For the 2201 white, black, and Hispanic respondents who reported having a regular physician, we examined the association between patient-physician racial concordance and patients' ratings of their physicians, satisfaction with health care, reported receipt of preventive care, and reported receipt of needed medical care. RESULTS: Black respondents with black physicians were more likely than those with nonblack physicians to rate their physicians as excellent (adjusted odds ratio [OR], 2.40; 95% confidence interval [CI], 1.55–3.72) and to report receiving preventive care (adjusted OR, 1.74; 95% CI, 1.01–2.98) and all needed medical care (adjusted OR, 2.94; 95% CI, 1.10–7.87) during the previous year. Hispanics with Hispanic physicians were more likely than those with non–Hispanic physicians to be very satisfied with their health care overall (adjusted OR, 1.74; 95% CI, 1.01–2.99). CONCLUSIONS: Our findings confirm the importance of racial and cultural factors in the patient-physician relationship and reaffirm the role of black and Hispanic physicians in caring for black and Hispanic patients. Improving cultural competence among physicians may enhance the quality of health care for minority populations. In the meantime, by reducing the number of underrepresented minorities entering the US physician workforce, the reversal of affirmative action policies may adversely affect the delivery of health care to black and Hispanic Americans.

Schneck, Stuart A. "Doctoring" doctors and their families. *JAMA.* 1998 Dec 16; 280(23): 2039–2042. 74 refs. BE59582.
confidentiality; *family members; *guidelines; *interprofessional relations; married persons; *medical etiquette; *patient care; *patients; *physician patient relationship; physician's role; *physicians; privacy; professional family relationship; psychological stress; social dominance
Being selected to provide medical care to other physicians or their family members represents not only a gratifying professional recognition of competence by one's peers but also a challenge. Many personal and

psychological factors may influence the medical care of physicians. Ill physicians may have difficulty with role reversal and "the VIP syndrome," while treating physicians may have to deal with their own anxiety and issues such as confidentiality, privacy, empathy, and intrusion by a physician-relative into the care of medical family members. Based on experience with more than 200 physician-patients and many adult family members of physicians, suggestions are offered for care of these patient groups.

Schneider, Carl E. The Practice of Autonomy: Patients, Doctors, and Medical Decisions. New York, NY: Oxford University Press; 1998. 307 p. 1,224 fn. ISBN 0–19–511397–7. BE59665.
attitudes; *autonomy; bioethics; cancer; caring; chronically ill; *communication; compassion; comprehension; *decision making; disclosure; empirical research; family relationship; health care reform; *informed consent; law; literature; managed care programs; models, theoretical; narrative ethics; organization and administration; paternalism; *patient participation; *patients; *physician patient relationship; practice guidelines; professional autonomy; psychological stress; psychology; self concept; sociology of medicine; survey; terminally ill; time factors; truth disclosure; uncertainty; sick role; Great Britain; United States

Scott, P. Anne. Autonomy, power, and control in palliative care. *Cambridge Quarterly of Healthcare Ethics.* 1999 Spring; 8(2): 139–147. 35 fn. BE61231.
*autonomy; case studies; *communication; *hospices; institutionalized persons; *nurse patient relationship; nurse's role; nursing research; *palliative care; *patient advocacy; patient participation; physician patient relationship; professional family relationship; quality of health care; social dominance; *terminal care; terminally ill; dependency; *empowerment; sick role; Great Britain

Seedhouse, David. Death's moral sting. [Editorial]. *Health Care Analysis.* 1998 Dec; 6(4): 273–276. 12 fn. BE61585.
attitudes; attitudes to death; bioethics; *dehumanization; *economics; *health care delivery; incentives; informed consent; medical education; patient care; *physician patient relationship; physicians; privacy; prognosis; quality of life; social discrimination; *sociology of medicine; suffering; terminal care; truth disclosure; *values

Selby, Mary; Neuberger, Julia; Easmon, Charles, et al. Ethical dilemma: dealing with racist patients. [Article and commentaries]. *BMJ (British Medical Journal).* 1999 Apr 24; 318(7191): 1129–1131. 1 ref. BE62302.
attitudes; case studies; communication; dissent; hospitals; institutional policies; minority groups; moral complicity; nurses; *patients; physicians; *professional patient relationship; refusal to treat; *social discrimination

Setka, J. Relationship of medicine and physician toward patient at the advent of the 3rd millennium. *Sbornik Lekarsky.* 1997; 98(1): 11–19. 37 refs. BE62323.
biomedical technologies; historical aspects; international aspects; medical ethics; *medicine; *physician patient relationship; physician's role; *trends; values; Twenty-First Century

Smith, David H. Ethics in the doctor-patient relationship. *Critical Care Clinics.* 1996 Jan; 12(1): 179–197. 35 refs. BE59286.
advance directives; autonomy; bioethics; *communication; consent forms; decision making; disclosure; emotions; health care delivery; human experimentation; informed consent; legal aspects; living wills; patient care; *patient participation; patient satisfaction; *physician patient relationship; sociology of medicine; terminal care; *trends; trust; values; United States

---

BE = bioethics accession number   fn. = footnotes   refs. = references

Spielberg, Alissa R. On call and online: sociohistorical, legal, and ethical implications of e-mail for the patient–physician relationship. *JAMA.* 1998 Oct 21; 280(15): 1353–1359. 48 refs. BE60289.
*communication; *computer communication networks; *confidentiality; disclosure; government regulation; historical aspects; informed consent; *legal aspects; *medical records; patient care; *physician patient relationship; *physicians; privacy; referral and consultation; risks and benefits; sociology of medicine; *standards; state government; trends; computer security; *physician's practice patterns; American Medical Association; American Medical Informatics Association; Internet; United States
Increased use of e-mail by physicians, patients, and other health care organizations and staff has the potential to reshape the current boundaries of relationships in medical practice. By comparing reception of e-mail technology in medical practice with its historical analogue, reception of the telephone, this article suggests that new expectations, practice standards, and potential liabilities emerge with the introduction of this new communication technology. Physicians using e-mail should be aware of these considerations and construct their e-mail communications accordingly, recognizing that e-mail may be included in the patient's medical record. Likewise, physicians should discuss the ramifications of communicating electronically with patients and obtain documented informed consent before using e-mail. Physicians must keep patient information confidential, which will require taking precautions (including encryption to prevent interception) to preserve patient information, trust, and the integrity of the patient–physician relationship.

Spielberg, Alissa R. Online without a net: physician–patient communication by electronic mail. *American Journal of Law and Medicine.* 1999; 25(2–3): 267–295. 228 fn. BE62509.
*communication; *computer communication networks; *confidentiality; constitutional law; diagnosis; disclosure; federal government; health care delivery; health insurance reimbursement; informed consent; *legal aspects; legal liability; legal rights; malpractice; *medical records; *methods; *patient care; *physician patient relationship; *privacy; psychotherapy; public health; risks and benefits; standards; state government; Supreme Court decisions; *telemedicine; Internet; *United States

Starr, Joann; Zawacki, Bruce E. Voices from the silent world of doctor and patient. *Cambridge Quarterly of Healthcare Ethics.* 1999 Spring; 8(2): 129–138. 12 fn. BE61230.
attitudes; *autonomy; *burns; *caring; clinical ethics committees; coercion; communication; compassion; competence; decision making; *emotions; empathy; ethicists; family members; hospitals; informed consent; intensive care units; *narrative ethics; nurse patient relationship; nurses; *pain; paternalism; *patient advocacy; *patient care; patient compliance; *patient participation; patients; *physician patient relationship; physician's role; physicians; professional family relationship; *psychological stress; psychology; *suffering; surgery; *treatment refusal; trust; vulnerable populations; empowerment

Tauber, Alfred I. Confessions of a Medicine Man: An Essay in Popular Philosophy. Cambridge, MA: MIT Press; 1999. 159 p. Includes references. ISBN 0-262-20114-3. BE60753.
autonomy; biomedical research; biomedical technologies; decision making; economics; health care; medical education; *medical ethics; *medicine; patient advocacy; *philosophy; *physician patient relationship; physician's role; *physicians; postmodernism; resource allocation; self concept; Nietzsche, Friedrich; United States

Thom, David H.; Campbell, Bruce. Patient–physician trust: an exploratory study. *Journal of Family Practice.* 1997 Feb; 44(2): 169–176. 42 refs. BE60541.
*attitudes; blacks; caring; communication; family practice; Hispanic Americans; patient care; *patient satisfaction; *patients; *physician patient relationship; survey; *trust; qualitative research; California

Thomasma, David C. Stewardship of the aged: meeting the ethical challenge of ageism. *Cambridge Quarterly of Healthcare Ethics.* 1999 Spring; 8(2): 148–159. 38 fn. BE61232.
advance directives; *aged; allowing to die; autonomy; beneficence; biomedical technologies; case studies; casuistry; chronically ill; *clinical ethics; competence; covenant; *decision making; dissent; family members; health personnel; home care; hospitals; justice; legal guardians; long-term care; medicine; nursing homes; paternalism; *patient advocacy; *patient care; *patient participation; physical restraint; *physician patient relationship; prolongation of life; public policy; quality of life; resource allocation; right to die; risks and benefits; selection for treatment; social discrimination; terminal care; terminally ill; treatment refusal; *values; withholding treatment; elder abuse

Torrance, Caroline J.; Das, Robert; Allison, Miles C. Use of chaperones in clinics for genitourinary medicine: survey of consultants. *BMJ (British Medical Journal).* 1999 Jul 17; 319(7203): 159–160. 4 refs. BE62454.
adolescents; family members; *females; institutional policies; *knowledge, attitudes, practice; *males; nurses; *obstetrics and gynecology; organizational policies; *patient care; patients; *physician patient relationship; *physicians; *privacy; professional organizations; sexuality; survey; ambulatory care; *physical examination; General Medical Council (Great Britain); Great Britain; Royal College of Obstetricians and Gynaecologists

Trotter, C. Griffin. The medical covenant: a Roycean perspective. *In:* McGee, Glenn, ed. Pragmatic Bioethics. Nashville, TN: Vanderbilt University Press; 1999: 84–96, 266–269. 35 fn. ISBN 0-8265-1321-2. BE60665.
autonomy; beneficence; compassion; *covenant; economics; health care; mediation; *medical ethics; *medicine; *models, theoretical; obligations to society; patient care; *philosophy; *physician patient relationship; physician's role; regulation; standards; *virtues; *loyalty; *pragmatism; *Royce, Josiah

Verghese, Abraham. Showing doctors their biases. *New York Times.* 1999 Mar 1: A21. BE62697.
*blacks; diagnosis; females; heart diseases; humanism; literature; males; medical education; patient care; *physician patient relationship; *physicians; *social discrimination; stigmatization; *whites; United States

Verkerk, Marian. A care perspective on coercion and autonomy. *Bioethics.* 1999 Jul; 13(3–4): 358–368. 12 refs. BE61885.
*autonomy; beneficence; *caring; *coercion; feminist ethics; health personnel; paternalism; patient care; *professional patient relationship; psychiatry; self concept; Netherlands
In the Netherlands there is a growing debate over the possibility of introducing 'compassionate interference' as a form of good psychiatric care. Instead of respecting the autonomy of the patient by adopting an attitude of non-interference, professional carers should take a more active and committed role. There was a great deal of hostile reaction to this suggestion, the most commonly voiced criticism being that it smacked of 'modern paternalism.' Still, the current conception of care leaves us with a paradox. On the one hand patients are regarded as individuals who have a strong interest in (and a right to) freedom and non-interference; on the other hand many of them have a desperate need for flourishing,

---

BE = bioethics accession number   fn. = footnotes   refs. = references

viable relationships. In fact, part of their problem is that they cannot relate very well with other people. This creates a dichotomy, because respecting patients' autonomy often means that they cannot be given the help they so desperately need. In this respect current care practices do not answer the caring needs of these patients. The criticism on care practices is to be considered as important. It invites us to reexamine and reevaluate the current conception of caring relationships and its main values. In line with this reexamination an alternative perspective on care is introduced in this paper, a perspective in which 'compassionate interference' is not so much a threat to autonomy, but a means of attaining autonomy. For this we need a different definition of autonomy than that commonly used in current care practice.

Volkenandt, Matthias. Supportive care and euthanasia -- an ethical dilemma? *Supportive Care in Cancer.* 1998 Mar; 6(2): 114-119. 15 refs. Presented at the 9th International Symposium on Supportive Care in Cancer, held in St. Gallen, Switzerland, 26 Feb-1 Mar 1997. BE61573.
  *active euthanasia; allowing to die; *assisted suicide; autonomy; beneficence; *cancer; double effect; drugs; economics; intention; involuntary euthanasia; *moral obligations; moral policy; pain; *palliative care; *physician patient relationship; *physicians; resource allocation; social impact; suffering; *terminal care; *terminally ill; trust; voluntary euthanasia; wedge argument; withholding treatment; United States

Welie, Jos V.M. In the Face of Suffering: The Philosophical-Anthropological Foundations of Clinical Ethics. Omaha, NE: Creighton University Press; 1998. 304 p. Bibliography: p. 279-293. ISBN 1-881871-26-6. BE62440.
  anthropology; *autonomy; *beneficence; bioethics; caring; *clinical ethics; *compassion; cultural pluralism; *decision making; empathy; *ethical theory; freedom; human characteristics; paternalism; patients; personhood; *philosophy; *physician patient relationship; physicians; self concept; suffering; treatment refusal; trust; authenticity; patient abandonment; sick role; *sympathy; von Gebsattel, Viktor

Wharton, Robert H. Pedestrian vs. train. *Hastings Center Report.* 1999 May-Jun; 29(3): 28-29. BE61411.
  adolescents; attitudes; *communication; critically ill; *death; *decision making; *emergency care; *emotions; *family members; health personnel; injuries; *parents; personhood; *physician patient relationship; physicians; *professional family relationship; terminally ill; grief

Williamson, Charlotte. The rise of doctor-patient working groups. *BMJ (British Medical Journal).* 1998 Nov 14; 317(7169): 1374-1377. 31 refs. BE60838.
  advisory committees; committee membership; communication; evaluation; patient advocacy; *patient care; *patient participation; *physician patient relationship; political activity; *quality of health care; standards; Great Britain

Wincze, John P.; Richards, Jeff; Parsons, John, et al. A comparative survey of therapist sexual misconduct between an American state and an Australian state. *Professional Psychology: Research and Practice.* 1996 Jun; 27(3): 289-294. 25 refs. BE60223.
  comparative studies; disclosure; drug abuse; employment; females; fraud; health insurance reimbursement; *health personnel; international aspects; *knowledge, attitudes, practice; males; *misconduct; patients; *physicians; *professional patient relationship; *psychiatry; *psychology; *psychotherapy; *sexuality; social workers; statistics; survey; Australia; *Rhode Island; United States; *Western Australia

Zawacki, Bruce E. International bioethics at the bedside. [Editorial]. *Burns.* 1997 May; 23(3): iii-iv. 6 refs. BE62457.
  *allowing to die; burns; communication; *cultural pluralism; *decision making; family members; informed consent; international aspects; *minority groups; patient care; patients; *physician patient relationship; physicians; *professional family relationship; prognosis; third party consent; truth disclosure; Canada; United States

Zelas, Karen. Sex and the doctor-patient relationship. *New Zealand Medical Journal.* 1997 Feb 28; 110(1038): 60-62. 16 refs. BE60088.
  beneficence; continuing education; geographic factors; *misconduct; moral obligations; patients; *physician patient relationship; physicians; *sex offenses; *sexuality; social dominance; trust; dependency; physician impairment; New Zealand

PROLONGATION OF LIFE *See* ALLOWING TO DIE

PROXY DECISION MAKING *See* ADVANCE DIRECTIVES, ALLOWING TO DIE, INFORMED CONSENT, RESUSCITATION ORDERS

PSYCHOSURGERY

See also BEHAVIOR CONTROL

PUBLIC HEALTH

See also AIDS, HEALTH, HEALTH CARE, IMMUNIZATION, MASS SCREENING, OCCUPATIONAL HEALTH

Annas, George J. Human rights and health -- the Universal Declaration of Human Rights at 50. *New England Journal of Medicine.* 1998 Dec 10; 339(24): 1778-1781. 26 refs. BE60040.
  AIDS; capitalism; democracy; developing countries; economics; education; guidelines; *health; *health care; health promotion; historical aspects; *human rights; *international aspects; law; medical ethics; misconduct; natural law; obligations of society; obligations to society; physicians; political activity; prisoners; professional organizations; *public health; public policy; socialism; socioeconomic factors; torture; war; women's rights; Amnesty International; Consortium for Health and Human Rights; Global Lawyers and Physicians; Physicians for Social Responsibility; Physicians for the Prevention of Nuclear War; Physicians of the World; Twentieth Century Doctors without Borders; United Nations; *Universal Declaration of Human Rights

Bhopal, Raj; Donaldson, Liam. White, European, Western, Caucasian, or what? Inappropriate labeling in research on race, ethnicity, and health. *American Journal of Public Health.* 1998 Sep; 88(9): 1303-1307. 42 refs. BE62553.
  American Indians; blacks; comparative studies; control groups; cultural pluralism; editorial policies; epidemiology; health services research; international aspects; *minority groups; *public health; *research design; social discrimination; *socioeconomic factors; *terminology; *whites; United States
The request for scientifically appropriate terminology in research on race, ethnicity, and health has largely bypassed the term White. This and other words, such as Caucasian, are embedded in clinical and

epidemiological discourse, yet they are rarely defined. This commentary analyzes the issue from the perspective of the epidemiology of the health of minority ethnic and racial groups in Europe and the United States. Minority groups are usually compared with populations described as White, Caucasian, European, Europid, Western, Occidental, indigenous, native, and majority. Such populations are heterogeneous, the labels nonspecific, and the comparisons misleading. Terminology that reflects the research purpose – for example, reference, control, or comparison –– is better (unlike White, these terms imply no norm, allowing neither writers nor readers to make stereotyped assumptions about the comparison populations. This paper widens the debate on nomenclature for racial and ethnic groups. Many issues need exploration, including whether there is a shared understanding among the international research community of the terms discussed.

Buchanan, Robert J. Tuberculosis and HIV infection: utilization of public programs to fund treatment. *AIDS and Public Policy Journal.* 1997 Winter; 12(4): 122–136. 54 fn. Includes tables of states in which state or local health departments provide care or services to people with tuberculosis. BE59299.
    AIDS; communicable diseases; community services; drugs; *government financing; *health care delivery; HIV seropositivity; home care; indigents; municipal government; *patient care; prevalence; *public health; *public policy; *state government; survey; *tuberculosis; case managers; Medicaid; Medicare; Ryan White Comprehensive AIDS Resources Emergency Act; *United States

Campion, Edward W. Liberty and the control of tuberculosis. [Editorial]. *New England Journal of Medicine.* 1999 Feb 4; 340(5): 385–386. 8 refs. BE60991.
    coercion; *communicable diseases; drugs; freedom; hospitals; *legal aspects; patient care; patient compliance; patients; program descriptions; *public health; *public policy; quarantine; *tuberculosis; ambulatory care; New York City

Chapman, Simon. When outcomes threaten incomes: a case study of the obstruction of research to reduce teenage smoking. *Health Policy.* 1997 Jan; 39(1): 55–68. 54 refs. BE59796.
    *adolescents; advertising; *behavioral research; deception; economics; *ethical review; evidence-based medicine; *health promotion; *health services research; industry; *law enforcement; mass media; *public health; public policy; research design; *research ethics committees; risks and benefits; *smoking; state government; intervention studies; Australia; *New South Wales

Cheng, Leo H.H.; Whittington, Richard M. Natural deaths while driving: would screening for risk be ethically justified? *Journal of Medical Ethics.* 1998 Aug; 24(4): 248–251. 13 refs. BE61290.
    aged; autonomy; beneficence; confidentiality; *death; duty to warn; *heart diseases; mandatory programs; *mass screening; *mortality; paternalism; physicians; *preventive medicine; public health; public policy; *risk; survey; *traffic accidents; retrospective studies; Great Britain
OBJECTIVES: To determine the epidemiology and the underlying pathological conditions of natural deaths among motor vehicle drivers. Sudden death while driving may cause damage to properties, other vehicles or road users. Although the Medical Commission on Accident Prevention recommended restrictions to drivers at risk of sudden death due to their medical conditions, these restrictions are useless if they do not result in greater safety to the public. DESIGN: A retrospective study of natural deaths of motor vehicle drivers. SETTING: Natural deaths of motor vehicle

drivers reported to the coroner for Birmingham and Solihull. SUBJECTS: 86 consecutive natural deaths of motor vehicle drivers in a five-year period between 1984 and 1988. RESULTS: Of the 86 fatalities reviewed, 80 (93%) sudden deaths were caused by ischaemic heart disease. Fifty vehicles were involved in collision with 32 properties, 20 other vehicles and six pedestrians. Fifty-one out of 80 cardiac deaths had past cardiac history and three had reported chest pain prior to the sudden death. CONCLUSION: An applied normative ethical assessment based on the basic moral principles of autonomy, justice, beneficence and non-maleficence are discussed. We conclude that medical screening of drivers has little benefit for the drivers or other persons.

Coker, Richard. Public health, civil liberties, and tuberculosis. [Editorial]. *BMJ (British Medical Journal).* 1999 May 29; 318(7196): 1434–1435. 7 refs. BE62351.
    *coercion; communicable diseases; drugs; involuntary commitment; legal rights; *mandatory programs; *patient compliance; *public health; public policy; *tuberculosis; Great Britain

Crofts, Nick; Louie, Robyn; Loff, Bebe. The next plague: stigmatization and discrimination related to hepatitis C virus infection in Australia. *Health and Human Rights.* 1997; 2(2): 87–97. 7 refs. BE62088.
    attitudes; case studies; confidentiality; disclosure; drug abuse; employment; family members; health personnel; *hepatitis; hospitals; legislation; *public policy; *social discrimination; *stigmatization; infection control; *Australia

Darragh, Martina; McCarrick, Pat Milmoe. Public health ethics: health by the numbers. [Bibliography]. *Kennedy Institute of Ethics Journal.* 1998 Sep; 8(3): 339–358. Also available, as Scope Note 35, from the National Reference Center for Bioethics Literature, Kennedy Institute of Ethics, Georgetown University, Box 571212, Washington, DC 20057-1212, (202)687-6806 or (800)MED-ETHX. BE60171.
    epidemiology; genetic screening; health education; health promotion; *public health

de Jong, Judith; Reatig, Natalie. SAMHSA philosophy and statement on ethical principles. *Ethics and Behavior.* 1998; 8(4): 339–343. BE60165.
    accountability; *alcohol abuse; autonomy; beneficence; codes of ethics; cultural pluralism; *drug abuse; federal government; health care delivery; *health promotion; *institutional ethics; justice; *mental health; *mentally ill; minority groups; preventive medicine; rehabilitation; resource allocation; social problems; trust; community consent; *community medicine; intervention studies; *Substance Abuse and Mental Health Services Administration; United States
As the major federal agency responsible for improving the delivery and effectiveness of substance abuse and mental health services to the American public, the Substance Abuse and Mental Health Services Administration (SAMHSA) is aware that its programs deal with especially sensitive issues. As a national leader in advancing effective services to persons with addictive and mental disorders, SAMHSA has stewardship over important interventions affecting personal, community, institutional, and social values. Inherent in SAMHSA's mission and goals is a commitment to protect and promote the human, civil, and legal rights and moral freedoms of those individuals and groups who participate in SAMHSA-funded activities and to demonstrate that Agency policies and procedures are congruent with publicly acceptable ethical principles and standards of conduct. A foundation of mutual trust between

---

BE = bioethics accession number   fn. = footnotes   refs. = references

SAMHSA officials and participants as well as sensitivity to issues of public accountability will hasten and strengthen progress toward this shared vision.

Dute, Jos. Affected by the tooth of time: legislation on infectious diseases control in five European countries. *Medicine and Law.* 1993; 12(1-2): 101-108. 12 fn. BE60616.
    *communicable diseases; comparative studies; compensation; *government regulation; immunization; *international aspects; laboratories; legislation; mandatory programs; mandatory reporting; physicians; preventive medicine; *public health; *Germany; *Great Britain; *Netherlands; *Sweden; *Switzerland

Efferen, Linda S. In pursuit of tuberculosis control: civil liberty vs public health. [Editorial]. *Chest.* 1997 Jul; 112(1): 5-6. 10 refs. BE59836.
    coercion; *communicable diseases; involuntary commitment; legal aspects; *mandatory programs; *patient care; *patient compliance; *public health; public policy; *quarantine; standards; *tuberculosis; United States

Epstein, Andrew E. Lifestyle and ethical issues: driving and occupational aspects. *In:* Dunbar, Sandra B.; Ellenbogen, Kenneth A.; Epstein, A.E., eds. Sudden Cardiac Death: Past, Present, and Future. Armonk, NY: Futura; 1997: 321-334. 35 refs. ISBN 0-8799-3666-5. BE60021.
    age factors; alcohol abuse; behavior control; confidentiality; dangerousness; duty to warn; employment; government regulation; guidelines; *health; *heart diseases; insurance; morbidity; *mortality; physicians; professional organizations; public health; *risk; *traffic accidents; myocardial infarction; American Heart Association; North American Society of Pacing and Electrophysiology; United States

Fullilove, Mindy Thompson. Comment: abandoning "race" as a variable in public health research -- an idea whose time has come. *American Journal of Public Health.* 1998 Sep; 88(9): 1297-1298. 13 refs. BE62552.
    blacks; epidemiology; health; health services research; Hispanic Americans; human rights; *minority groups; *public health; *research design; *social discrimination; socioeconomic factors; *terminology; whites; United States

Gasner, M. Rose; Maw, Khin Lay; Feldman, Gabriel E., et al. The use of legal action in New York City to ensure treatment of tuberculosis. *New England Journal of Medicine.* 1999 Feb 4; 340(5): 359-366. 16 refs. BE60990.
    alcohol abuse; *coercion; *communicable diseases; comparative studies; drug abuse; drugs; evaluation studies; hospitals; incentives; *legal aspects; patient care; *patient compliance; patients; program descriptions; *public health; *public policy; quarantine; records; *tuberculosis; ambulatory care; homeless persons; retrospective studies; *New York City
BACKGROUND AND METHODS: After an increase in the number of cases of tuberculosis, New York City passed regulations to address the problem of nonadherence to treatment regimens. The commissioner of health can issue orders compelling a person to be examined for tuberculosis, to complete treatment, to receive treatment under direct observation, or to be detained for treatment. On the basis of a review of patients' records, we evaluated the use of these legal actions between April 1993 and April 1995. RESULTS: Among more than 8000 patients with tuberculosis, regulatory orders were issued for less than 4 percent. Among patients with a variety of social problems, only a minority required regulatory intervention: 10 percent of those with injection-drug use, 16 percent of those

with alcohol abuse, 17 percent of those who were homeless, 29 percent of those who used "crack" cocaine, and 38 percent of those with a history of incarceration. A total of 150 patients were ordered to undergo directly observed therapy, 139 patients to be detained during therapy, 12 patients to be examined for tuberculosis, and 3 patients to complete treatment. These 304 patients had a median of three prior hospitalizations related to tuberculosis and one episode of leaving the hospital against medical advice. Repeatedly noncompliant patients and those who left the hospital against medical advice were more likely than others to be detained. The median length of detention was 3 weeks for infectious patients and 28 weeks for noninfectious patients. As compared with patients ordered to receive directly observed therapy, the patients who were detained remained infectious longer, had left hospitals against medical advice more often, and were less likely to accept directly observed therapy voluntarily. Altogether, excluding those who died or moved, 96 percent of the patients completed treatment, and 2 percent continued to receive treatment for multidrug-resistant tuberculosis. CONCLUSIONS: For most patients with tuberculosis, even those with severe social problems, completion of treatment can usually be achieved without regulatory intervention. Patients were detained on the basis of their history of tuberculosis, rather than on the basis of their social characteristics, and the less restrictive measure of mandatory directly observed therapy was often effective.

Hoey, John. Human rights, ethics and the Krever inquiry. [Editorial]. *Canadian Medical Association Journal.* 1997 Nov 1; 157(9): 1231. 3 refs. BE59831.
    AIDS; AIDS serodiagnosis; *blood banks; blood donation; codes of ethics; *drug industry; *duty to warn; *hepatitis; *HIV seropositivity; human rights; legal aspects; misconduct; *public health; public policy; Supreme Court decisions; Baxter Corp.; *Canada; Canadian Red Cross; *Commission of Inquiry on the Blood System in Canada

Hoey, John. When the physician is the vector. [Editorial]. *Canadian Medical Association Journal.* 1998 Jul 14; 159(1): 45-46. 9 refs. BE62206.
    *communicable diseases; costs and benefits; dentistry; employment; *health personnel; *hepatitis; HIV seropositivity; *iatrogenic disease; immunization; insurance; international aspects; *mandatory testing; *patients; *physicians; *preventive medicine; privacy; *public policy; social discrimination; statistics; students; *Canada

Hurt, Richard D.; Robertson, Channing R. Prying open the door to the tobacco industry's secrets about nicotine: the Minnesota Tobacco Trial. *JAMA.* 1998 Oct 7; 280(13): 1173-1181. 96 refs. BE60287.
    *accountability; advertising; behavior control; biomedical research; cancer; *deception; *disclosure; drug abuse; *health hazards; *industry; investigators; *legal liability; moral complicity; *organizational policies; *public health; public policy; *records; *smoking; Minnesota
In 1994 the state of Minnesota filed suit against the tobacco industry. This trial is now history, but its legacy will carry on into the 21st century because of the revelations contained in the millions of pages of previously secret internal tobacco industry documents made public in the trial. In this article, we review representative documents relating to nicotine addiction, low-tar, low-nicotine cigarettes, and cigarette design and nicotine manipulation in cigarette manufacture. These documents reveal that for decades, the industry knew and internally acknowledged that nicotine is an addictive drug and cigarettes are the ultimate nicotine delivery device; that nicotine addiction can be

---

BE = bioethics accession number   fn. = footnotes   refs. = references

perpetuated and even enhanced through cigarette design alterations and manipulations; and that "health-conscious" smokers could be captured by low-tar, low-nicotine products, all the while ensuring the marketplace viability of their products. Appreciation of tobacco industry strategies over the past decades is essential to formulate an appropriate legislative and public policy response. We propose key elements for such legislation and urge no legal or financial immunity for the tobacco industry.

International Federation of Red Cross and Red Crescent Societies; François-Xavier Bagnoud Center for Health and Human Rights, Harvard School of Public Health. AIDS, Health and Human Rights: An Explanatory Model. Geneva: The Federation; Boston, MA: The Center; 1995. 162 p. Includes references. ISBN 92-9139-014-3. BE61599.
> *AIDS; AIDS serodiagnosis; confidentiality; counseling; females; guidelines; health; health care; health promotion; *HIV seropositivity; *human rights; *international aspects; patient care; preventive medicine; prisoners; *public health; public policy; social discrimination; voluntary programs; prostitution; Convention on the Elimination of All Forms of Discrimination Against Women; Convention on the Rights of the Child; Declaration of Alma-Ata; International Covenant on Civil and Political Rights; International Covenant on Economic, Social and Cultural Rights; United Nations; Universal Declaration of Human Rights

Kahn, Jeffrey. Bioethics and tobacco. *Bioethics Examiner.* 1997 Fall; 1(3): 1, 7. BE59792.
> *bioethics; economics; federal government; government regulation; industry; international aspects; *public health; *public policy; *smoking; United States

Krieger, Nancy; Birn, Anne-Emanuelle. A vision of social justice as the foundation of public health: commemorating 150 years of the spirit of 1848. *American Journal of Public Health.* 1998 Nov; 88(11): 1603-1606. 70 refs. BE59628.
> historical aspects; human rights; international aspects; *justice; *public health; social discrimination; socioeconomic factors; Nineteenth Century; Twentieth Century

Krieger, Nancy; Sidney, Stephen; Coakley, Eugenie. Racial discrimination and skin color in the CARDIA study: implications for public health research. *American Journal of Public Health.* 1998 Sep; 88(9): 1308-1313. 61 refs. BE62554.
> *attitudes; *blacks; *emotions; employment; females; *health; health care; Hispanic Americans; law enforcement; males; *minority groups; *public health; *research design; schools; self concept; *social discrimination; *socioeconomic factors; survey; whites; Coronary Artery Risk Development in Young Adults (CARDIA) Study; United States
OBJECTIVES: This study assessed whether skin color and ways of handling anger can serve as markers for experiences of racial discrimination and responses to unfair treatment in public health research. METHODS: Survey data on 1844 Black women and Black men (24 to 42 years old), collected in the year 5 (1990-1991) and year 7 (1992-1993) examinations of the Coronary Artery Risk Development in Young Adults (CARDIA) study, were examined. RESULTS: Skin color was not associated with self-reported experiences of racial discrimination in 5 of 7 specified situations (getting a job, at work, getting housing, getting medical care, in a public setting). Only moderate associations existed between darker skin color and being working class, having low income or low education, and being male (risk ratios under 2). Comparably moderate associations

existed between internalizing anger and typically responding to unfair treatment as a fact of life or keeping such treatment to oneself. CONCLUSIONS: Self-reported experiences of racial discrimination and responses to unfair treatment should be measured directly in public health research; data on skin color and ways of handling anger are not sufficient.

Lachmann, Peter J. Public health and bioethics. *Journal of Medicine and Philosophy.* 1998 Jun; 23(3): 297-302. 6 refs. BE59293.
> autonomy; bioethics; common good; *communicable diseases; drugs; genetic predisposition; genetic screening; HIV seropositivity; immunization; informed consent; international aspects; mandatory programs; morbidity; patients' rights; *public health; risks and benefits; trends; voluntary programs; antibiotics
Conduct that satisfies certain bioethical doctrines may come into conflict with the needs and ethics of public health. The growth of antibiotic resistance in bacteria and the spread of HIV both contribute to the difficulty of controlling infectious disease. These two sets of priorities need to be reconciled and this is likely to require a reassessment of prevailing ethical doctrines in the face of the needs of public health.

Lerner, Barron H.; Rothman, David J.; Tracy, Mark J., et al. Legal action to ensure treatment of tuberculosis. [Letters and response]. *New England Journal of Medicine.* 1999 Jul 8; 341(2): 130-131. 6 refs. BE62271.
> *coercion; communicable diseases; hospitals; legal aspects; mentally ill; patient care; *patient compliance; public health; *public policy; quarantine; self regulation; *tuberculosis; *New York City

Mann, Jonathan. Health and human rights: broadening the agenda for health professionals. [Editorial]. *Health and Human Rights.* 1996; 2(1): 1-5. 4 refs. BE62084.
> *health; health personnel; health promotion; *human rights; international aspects; misconduct; *public health; public policy

Mann, Jonathan, M.; Gruskin, Sofia; Grodin, Michael A., et al, eds. Health and Human Rights: A Reader. New York, NY: Routledge; 1999. 505 p. Includes references. ISBN 0-415-92102-3. BE62050.
> AIDS; circumcision; developing countries; family planning; females; genetic diversity; genetic research; *health; health care; HIV seropositivity; homosexuals; *human experimentation; *human rights; informed consent; *international aspects; killing; mass screening; medicine; minority groups; misconduct; National Socialism; newborns; patient advocacy; *physicians; *political activity; pregnant women; *public health; public policy; scientific misconduct; sexuality; social discrimination; *social impact; socioeconomic factors; tuberculosis; war; women's health; genocide; Doctors of the World; Doctors without Borders; International Covenant on Civil and Political Rights; International Covenant on Economic, Social and Cultural Rights; International Red Cross and Red Crescent Movement; Physicians for Human Rights; Universal Declaration of Human Rights

Nordin, Ingemar. The limits of medical practice. *Theoretical Medicine and Bioethics.* 1999 Apr; 20(2): 105-123. 16 fn. BE62213.
> cosmetic surgery; decision making; *goals; *health; *health care; *health personnel; health promotion; *medicine; models, theoretical; nurse's role; patient care; patient care team; patients; philosophy; physical restraint; *physician's role; physicians; politics; professional organizations; *professional role; *public health; resource allocation; social control; *social problems; technical expertise

---

BE = bioethics accession number   fn. = footnotes   refs. = references

Peng, Rui–cong. The goals of medicine and public health. *In:* Hanson, Mark J.; Callahan, Daniel, eds. The Goals of Medicine: The Forgotten Issue in Health Care Reform. Washington, DC: Georgetown University Press; 1999: 174–180. ISBN 0-87840-707-3. BE60525.
  costs and benefits; *goals; health care; health promotion; international aspects; *medicine; *preventive medicine; *public health; China

Pitkofsky, Rob. Race and tuberculosis: coincidence or correlation? *Princeton Journal of Bioethics.* 1998 Spring; 1(1): 32–41. 10 refs. BE62489.
  AIDS; aliens; communicable diseases; disadvantaged; geographic factors; *minority groups; patient care; patient compliance; prevalence; *public health; *socioeconomic factors; *tuberculosis; urban population; United States

Trickett, Edison J. Toward a framework for defining and resolving ethical issues in the protection of communities involved in primary prevention projects. *Ethics and Behavior.* 1998; 8(4): 321–337. 34 refs. BE60164.
  adolescents; *alcohol abuse; aliens; anthropology; behavior disorders; *behavioral research; children; cultural pluralism; disadvantaged; *drug abuse; ecology; education; health education; *health promotion; health services research; informed consent; injuries; investigator subject relationship; *mental health; mentally ill; metaphor; minority groups; patient education; *preventive medicine; professional ethics; psychology; public health; sexually transmitted diseases; social dominance; *social problems; trust; values; *community medicine; *intervention studies
Ethical issues flow from and are embedded in contexts of practice. *Contexts of practice* refer to the diverse social settings where interventions occur. Primary prevention activities require new professional roles in these diverse social settings. These new roles engage the professional in new activities, which in turn allow new ethical issues to arise. This article takes an ecological perspective on ethical issues arising from the enactment of new preventive roles intended to affect groups or communities. Within this perspective, the concepts of context and culture take on special conceptual significance. Four ecological assumptions about preventive interventions intended to affect groups or communities are offered as a means of framing ethical issues in such interventions. Finally, several approaches to developing ecological knowledge about the contexts of practice are presented as ways of furthering our ability to conceptualize and cope with ethical issues in preventive interventions intended to affect groups or communities.

Verweij, Marcel. Medicalization as a moral problem for preventative medicine. *Bioethics.* 1999 Apr; 13(2): 89–113. 35 fn. BE61671.
  autonomy; behavior control; beneficence; goals; *health; *health promotion; iatrogenic disease; mass screening; medicine; moral obligations; *moral policy; parents; patients; pregnant women; *preventive medicine; public health; *risks and benefits; self induced illness; social control; social impact; social problems; values
Preventive medicine is sometimes criticised as it contributes to medicalization of normal life. The concept 'medicalization' has been introduced by Zola to refer to processes in which the labels 'health' and 'ill' are made relevant for more and more aspects of human life. If preventive medicine contributes to medicalization, would that be morally problematic? My thesis is that such a contribution is indeed morally problematic. The concept is sometimes used to express moral intuitions regarding the practice of prevention and health promotion. Through analysis of these intuitions as well as some other moral concerns, I give an explication of the moral problems of medicalization within the context of preventive medicine.

Watts, Sheldon. Epidemics and History: Disease, Power and Imperialism. New Haven, CT: Yale University Press; 1997. 400 p. Bibliography: p. 368–384. ISBN 0-300-07015-2. BE60514.
  *communicable diseases; *developing countries; ecology; *epidemiology; *historical aspects; *international aspects; minority groups; morbidity; mortality; non-Western World; physicians; *political systems; public health; public opinion; *social dominance; social impact; *socioeconomic factors; *sociology of medicine; stigmatization; syphilis; Western World; slavery; *Africa; *Americas; *Asia; Eighteenth Century; *Europe; Middle Ages; Nineteenth Century; Seventeenth Century; Sixteenth Century; Twentieth Century

Witte, Kim. The manipulative nature of health communication research: ethical issues and guidelines. *American Behavioral Scientist.* 1994 Nov; 38(2): 285–293. 26 refs. BE61210.
  *behavior control; common good; *communication; decision making; goals; guidelines; *health education; health hazards; *health promotion; informal social control; information dissemination; preventive medicine; public participation; risk; standards

Wodak, Alex. Health, HIV infection, human rights, and injecting drug use. *Health and Human Rights.* 1998; 2(4): 24–41. 41 fn. BE61496.
  developing countries; *drug abuse; government regulation; hepatitis; *HIV seropositivity; *human rights; *international aspects; *law enforcement; *public health; *public policy; social discrimination; vulnerable populations; United Nations; Universal Declaration of Human Rights; World Health Organization

RANDOM SELECTION *See* HUMAN EXPERIMENTATION/RESEARCH DESIGN

RATIONING OF HEALTH CARE *See* RESOURCE ALLOCATION, SELECTION FOR TREATMENT

RECOMBINANT DNA RESEARCH

See also GENE THERAPY, GENETIC INTERVENTION, GENETIC RESEARCH, PATENTING LIFE FORMS

Anderson, J. Kerby. The ethics of genetic engineering and artificial reproduction. *In:* Demy, Timothy J.; Stewart, Gary P., eds. Genetic Engineering: A Christian Response: Crucial Considerations in Shaping Life. Grand Rapids, MI: Kregel Publications; 1999: 140–152. 20 fn. ISBN 0-8254-2357-0. BE61365.
  age factors; artificial insemination; *Christian ethics; *cloning; cryopreservation; embryo disposition; embryo research; embryo transfer; embryos; gamete intrafallopian transfer; gene therapy; in vitro fertilization; legal aspects; marital relationship; ovum donors; *parent child relationship; patents; pregnant women; *recombinant DNA research; *reproductive technologies; semen donors; sex preselection; social impact; surrogate mothers; theology; transgenic organisms; value of life; United States

Appleyard, Bryan. Brave New Worlds: Staying Human in the Genetic Future. New York, NY: Viking; 1998. 198 p. Bibliography: p. 183–186. ISBN 0-670-86989-9. BE60356.

---

*attitudes; behavioral genetics; biology; cloning; dehumanization; ecology; *eugenics; evolution; freedom; gene therapy; genetic counseling; genetic determinism; genetic disorders; *genetic intervention; genetic predisposition; genetic research; genetic screening; *genetics; genome mapping; historical aspects; humanism; investigators; life extension; minority groups; morality; National Socialism; normality; politics; preimplantation diagnosis; prenatal diagnosis; preventive medicine; public opinion; public policy; *recombinant DNA research; reproduction; *risks and benefits; *science; selective abortion; self regulation; social control; social discrimination; *social impact; transgenic organisms; value of life; *values; nature; Asilomar Conference

Fagan, John. Genetic Engineering: The Hazards -- Vedic Engineering: The Solutions. Fairfield, IA: Maharishi International University Press; 1995. 172 p. 50 refs. ISBN 0-923569-18-9. BE60504.
 *alternative therapies; *ecology; evolution; gene pool; gene therapy; *genetic intervention; genetic screening; germ cells; health; health hazards; preventive medicine; *recombinant DNA research; *risks and benefits; transgenic organisms; agriculture; *Ayurveda

Käppeli, Othmar; Auberson, Lillian. Biotech battlelines. [Letter]. *Nature.* 1998 Jul 2; 394(6688): 10. BE59934.
 attitudes; emotions; *genetic intervention; government regulation; *investigators; mass media; morality; *political activity; public opinion; *public participation; public policy; *recombinant DNA research; risks and benefits; transgenic organisms; *Switzerland

Lucassen, Emy. The ethics of genetic engineering. *Journal of Applied Philosophy.* 1996; 13(1): 51-61. 15 fn. BE59554.
 deontological ethics; ecology; ethical analysis; genetic diversity; *genetic intervention; *microbiology; *moral policy; *recombinant DNA research; risks and benefits; *transgenic organisms; agriculture; nature

Schatz, Gottfried. The Swiss vote on gene technology. *Science.* 1998 Sep 18; 281(5384): 1810-1811. 6 fn. BE59943.
 animal experimentation; *attitudes; cultural pluralism; ecology; *genetic intervention; humanities; interdisciplinary communication; investigators; males; mass media; patents; *political activity; public opinion; *public participation; public policy; *recombinant DNA research; *science; social dominance; transgenic animals; *transgenic organisms; *Gene Protection Initiative (Switzerland); *Switzerland

Schiermeier, Quirin. Germans mix support and scepticism for genetic engineering. [News]. *Nature.* 1998 May 28; 393(6683): 299. BE59886.
 *attitudes; eugenics; *genetic intervention; government regulation; industry; investigators; *public opinion; *recombinant DNA research; trust; *Germany

Turney, Jon. Frankenstein's Footsteps: Science, Genetics and Popular Culture. New Haven, CT: Yale University Press; 1998. 276 p. Bibliography: p. 249-270. ISBN 0-300-07417-4. BE61055.
 animal experimentation; *attitudes; bioethics; *biology; biomedical research; biomedical technologies; cloning; embryo research; eugenics; genes; *genetic intervention; *genetic research; genetics; genome mapping; *historical aspects; human body; in vitro fertilization; international aspects; investigators; *literature; mass media; nuclear warfare; *public opinion; *recombinant DNA research; regulation; reproductive technologies; risks and benefits; *science; social impact; knowledge; Brave New World (Huxley, A.); Dr. Jekyll and Mr. Hyde (Stevenson, R.L.); *Frankenstein (Shelley, M.); Great Britain; In His Image (Rorvik, D.); *Nineteenth Century; R.U.R. (Capek, K.); The Island of Dr. Moreau (Wells, H.G.); *Twentieth Century; United States

RECOMBINANT DNA RESEARCH/REGULATION

Berkeley (CA). City Manager's Report on Proposed Ordinance Regulating the Use of Hazardous Biological Research, Recombinant DNA Research or Use of DNA Technology in the City of Berkeley [and] Draft Ordinance No. 5010 Later Enacted into Law. Issued by the City of Berkeley, City Manager's office, 2180 Milvia St., Berkeley, CA; 1977 Sep 13 (date issued). 9 p. Ordinance effective 1997 Oct 21. BE59347.
 containment; *government regulation; municipal government; *recombinant DNA research; *Berkeley (CA); California

Glover, Eric. French panel calls for closer monitoring of genetic modification. [News]. *Nature.* 1998 Jul 2; 394(6688): 4. BE59888.
 *advisory committees; biomedical research; consensus; ecology; *genetic intervention; *public participation; public policy; public sector; *recombinant DNA research; *regulation; risks and benefits; *transgenic organisms; agriculture; *France

Malinowski, Michael J. Regulation of genetic modification of organisms: science or emotion? *Journal of Biolaw and Business.* 1998 Spring; 1(3): 3-7. 49 fn. BE62091.
 advisory committees; *cloning; drugs; federal government; food; *government regulation; human experimentation; international aspects; *public policy; *recombinant DNA research; *regulation; reproductive technologies; risks and benefits; *transgenic organisms; agriculture; Department of Agriculture; Environmental Protection Agency; European Union; Food and Drug Administration; National Bioethics Advisory Commission; *United States

Miller, Henry I. Policy Controversy in Biotechnology: An Insider's View. Austin, TX: R.G. Landes; 1997. 221 p. (Biotechnology intelligence unit). Includes references. ISBN 1-57059-408-2. BE62779.
 drugs; *federal government; food; gene therapy; genetic intervention; *government regulation; human experimentation; international aspects; microbiology; *politics; *public policy; *recombinant DNA research; risk; science; agriculture; *biotechnology; Department of Agriculture; Environmental Protection Agency; Food and Drug Administration; National Institutes of Health; *United States

Schiermeier, Quirin. Swiss reject curbs on genetic engineering. [News]. *Nature.* 1998 Jun 11; 393(6685): 507. BE59887.
 advisory committees; animal experimentation; ecology; *genetic intervention; *government regulation; industry; investigators; legal liability; mass media; *political activity; *public participation; public policy; *recombinant DNA research; research institutes; transgenic organisms; national ethics committees; *Switzerland

U.S. National Institutes of Health. Recombinant DNA research: actions under the guidelines; notice. *Federal Register.* 1995 Apr 27; 60(81): 20726-20737. BE59544.
 *advisory committees; confidentiality; containment; *ethical review; federal government; *gene therapy; *government regulation; guidelines; *human experimentation; informed consent; organization and administration; *recombinant DNA research; *Food and Drug Administration; *National Institutes of Health; *NIH Guidelines; Office of Recombinant DNA Activities; Points to Consider: Transfer of Recombinant DNA into Human Subjects; *Recombinant DNA Advisory Committee; *United States

---

BE = bioethics accession number   fn. = footnotes   refs. = references

REFUSAL OF TREATMENT *See* TREATMENT
    REFUSAL

REFUSAL TO TREAT *See* AIDS/HEALTH
    PERSONNEL, SELECTION FOR TREATMENT

REGULATION
    See under
        BEHAVIORAL RESEARCH/REGULATION
        HUMAN EXPERIMENTATION/REGULATION
        RECOMBINANT DNA
            RESEARCH/REGULATION

RELIGIOUS ASPECTS
    See under
        ABORTION/RELIGIOUS ASPECTS
        ALLOWING TO DIE/RELIGIOUS ASPECTS
        EUTHANASIA/RELIGIOUS ASPECTS

RENAL DIALYSIS *See* BIOMEDICAL
    TECHNOLOGIES, RESOURCE
    ALLOCATION/BIOMEDICAL
    TECHNOLOGIES

REPRODUCTION

    See also ABORTION, CONTRACEPTION,
        FETUSES, PRENATAL DIAGNOSIS,
        PRENATAL INJURIES, REPRODUCTIVE
        TECHNOLOGIES, STERILIZATION,
        WRONGFUL LIFE

Abrams, Paula. Reservations about women: population
policy and reproductive rights. *Cornell International Law
Journal.* 1996; 29(1): 1–41. 227 fn. BE59445.
    *autonomy; coercion; contraception; cultural pluralism;
    *decision making; developing countries; economics; family
    planning; *females; government regulation; *human rights;
    incentives; *international aspects; law; *legal rights;
    mandatory programs; non–Western World; *population
    control; *public policy; *reproduction; *social control; social
    discrimination; socioeconomic factors; sterilization (sexual);
    utilitarianism; voluntary programs; Western World;
    *women's rights; Convention on the Elimination of All
    Forms of Discrimination Against Women; United Nations
    International Conference on Population and Development;
    Universal Declaration of Human Rights

**American Society of Human Genetics. Board of
Directors.** Eugenics and the misuse of genetic
information to restrict reproductive freedom: ASHG
statement. *American Journal of Human Genetics.* 1999
Feb; 64(2): 335–338. 16 refs. BE62217.
    coercion; disabled; *eugenics; *freedom; genetic disorders;
    *genetic information; genetic screening; health personnel;
    historical aspects; incentives; *international aspects;
    investigators; involuntary sterilization; mentally retarded;
    National Socialism; *organizational policies; prenatal
    diagnosis; professional organizations; public policy;
    *reproduction; terminology; voluntary programs;
    *American Society of Human Genetics; China; Europe;
    Germany; Japan; United States

Andrews, Lori B. The sperminator. *New York Times
Magazine.* 1999 Mar 28: 62–65. BE60874.
    advance directives; cadavers; coercion; cryopreservation;
    decision making; directed donation; family members; family
    relationship; *informed consent; legal aspects; married
    persons; physicians; *posthumous reproduction; *semen
    donors; single persons; sperm; tissue donation; *coma; United

States

Benagiano, G. Reproductive health as an essential human
right. *Advances in Contraception.* 1996 Dec; 12(4):
243–250. 20 refs. BE60732.
    children; developing countries; education; *family planning;
    human rights; *international aspects; maternal health;
    *reproduction; *women's health; *women's rights

Brazier, Margaret. Reproductive rights: feminism or
patriarchy? *In:* Harris, John; Holm, Søren, eds. The
Future of Human Reproduction: Ethics, Choice, and
Regulation. New York, NY: Oxford University Press;
1998: 66–76. 28 fn. ISBN 0–19–823761–8. BE61263.
    aborted fetuses; embryo research; fathers; *females; feminist
    ethics; human rights; in vitro fertilization; legal aspects;
    *males; mentally retarded; ovum donors; parent child
    relationship; property rights; *reproduction; *reproductive
    technologies; rights; selection for treatment; single persons;
    *social discrimination; *social dominance; sterilization
    (sexual); *women's rights; Great Britain; Human Fertilisation
    and Embryology Act 1990

Clarke, Adele E. Disciplining Reproduction: Modernity,
American Life Sciences, and "the Problems of Sex."
Berkeley, CA: University of California Press; 1998. 421
p. Bibliography: p. 333–410. ISBN 0–520–20720–3.
BE60503.
    animal experimentation; *biology; *biomedical research;
    *contraception; eugenics; family planning; federal
    government; females; *financial support; genetics;
    government financing; historical aspects; infertility;
    interdisciplinary communication; investigators; males;
    medicine; morality; political activity; population control;
    private sector; *reproduction; reproductive technologies;
    *sexuality; *social control; social dominance; *sociology of
    medicine; universities; women's health; women's rights;
    agriculture; Ford Foundation; National Research Council;
    Rockefeller Foundation; *Twentieth Century; *United
    States

Dikötter, Frank. Imperfect Conceptions: Medical
Knowledge, Birth Defects and Eugenics in China. New
York, NY: Columbia University Press; 1998. 226 p.
Bibliography: p. 187–216. ISBN 0–231–11370–6.
BE60707.
    active euthanasia; *congenital disorders; *disabled; emotions;
    *eugenics; family relationship; genetic disorders;
    government regulation; *historical aspects; involuntary
    sterilization; medicine; political systems; pregnant women;
    *public policy; *reproduction; sexuality; *social control;
    value of life; values; *China; Eighteenth Century; Nineteenth
    Century; Seventeenth Century; Sixteenth Century;
    Twentieth Century

Draper, Heather; Chadwick, Ruth. Beware!
Preimplantation genetic diagnosis may solve some old
problems but it also raises new ones. *Journal of Medical
Ethics.* 1999 Apr; 25(2): 114–120. 6 fn. BE61913.
    abortion, induced; autonomy; beginning of life; case studies;
    children; *decision making; disabled; Down syndrome;
    *embryo transfer; *embryos; *genetic disorders; *genetic
    screening; hearing disorders; *in vitro fertilization; legal
    aspects; *moral obligations; *moral policy; motivation;
    *parents; *physicians; pregnant women; *preimplantation
    diagnosis; prenatal diagnosis; property rights; *quality of life;
    *reproduction; rights; risks and benefits; value of life
Preimplantation genetic diagnosis (PIGD) goes some
way to meeting the clinical, psychological and ethical
problems of antenatal testing. We should guard,
however, against the assumption that PIGD is the
answer to all our problems. It also presents some new
problems and leaves some old problems untouched. This
paper will provide an overview of how PIGD meets

BE = bioethics accession number   fn. = footnotes   refs. = references

some of the old problems but will concentrate on two new challenges for ethics (and, indeed, law). First we look at whether we should always suppose that it is wrong for a clinician to implant a genetically abnormal zygote. The second concern is particularly important in the UK. The Human Fertilisation and Embryology Act (1990) gives clinicians a statutory obligation to consider the interests of the future children they help to create using in vitro fertilisation (IVF) techniques. Does this mean that because PIGD is based on IVF techniques the balance of power for determining the best interests of the future child shifts from the mother to the clinician?

Fenwick, Lynda Beck. Private Choices, Public Consequences: Reproductive Technology and the New Ethics of Conception, Pregnancy, and Family. New York, NY: Dutton; 1998. 390 p. Bibliography: p. 377–380. ISBN 0-525-94263-7. BE62624.
    aborted fetuses; age factors; allowing to die; anencephaly; autonomy; brain death; cancer; cesarean section; cloning; congenital disorders; criminal law; *decision making; drug abuse; drugs; fetal therapy; fetal tissue donation; fetuses; genetic counseling; genetic disorders; genetic screening; government regulation; legal aspects; mass media; maternal health; multiple pregnancy; newborns; organ donation; parental consent; parents; posthumous reproduction; pregnant women; prenatal diagnosis; prenatal injuries; prolongation of life; public opinion; *reproduction; *reproductive technologies; rights; selection for treatment; siblings; single persons; surrogate mothers; survey; treatment refusal; questionnaires; United States

Galton, David J. Greek theories on eugenics. *Journal of Medical Ethics.* 1998 Aug; 24(4): 263–267. 21 refs. BE61293.
    *ancient history; carriers; children; disabled; *eugenics; females; *historical aspects; involuntary sterilization; legal aspects; males; mandatory programs; marital relationship; obligations to society; philosophy; population control; *reproduction; *social control; social discrimination; socioeconomic factors; *Aristotle; Athens; Europe; Galton, Francis; Great Britain; Greece; Nineteenth Century; *Plato; Twentieth Century; United States
With the recent developments in the Human Genome Mapping Project and the new technologies that are developing from it there is a renewal of concern about eugenic applications. Francis Galton (b1822, d1911), who developed the subject of eugenics, suggested that the ancient Greeks had contributed very little to social theories of eugenics. In fact the Greeks had a profound interest in methods of supplying their city states with the finest possible progeny. This paper therefore reviews the works of Plato (The Republic and Politics) and Aristotle (The Politics and The Athenian Constitution) which have a direct bearing on eugenic techniques and relates them to methods used in the present century.

Gibbons, John A. Who's your daddy?: a constitutional analysis of post–mortem insemination. [Comment]. *Journal of Contemporary Health Law and Policy.* 1997 Fall; 14(1): 187–210. 195 fn. BE60880.
    artificial insemination; children; *constitutional law; cryopreservation; embryo transfer; fathers; in vitro fertilization; *legal aspects; *legal rights; legislation; married persons; parent child relationship; *posthumous reproduction; privacy; public policy; *reproductive technologies; semen donors; single persons; sperm; surrogate mothers; *United States

Grubb, Andrew. Frozen embryos: rights of inheritance: In Re the Estate of the Late K. [Comment]. *Medical Law Review.* 1997 Spring; 5(1): 121–124. BE59764.

childbirth; *cryopreservation; embryo transfer; *embryos; fathers; fetuses; in vitro fertilization; *legal aspects; *legal rights; newborns; parent child relationship; personhood; *posthumous reproduction; property rights; *Australia; Great Britain; *In re Estate of the Late K; *Tasmania

Grubb, Andrew. Infertility treatment: posthumous use of sperm –– R. v. Human Fertilisation and Embryology Authority, ex parte D.B. [Comment]. *Medical Law Review.* 1996 Autumn; 4(3): 329–335. BE61517.
    *artificial insemination; *cryopreservation; death; informed consent; international aspects; *legal aspects; males; married persons; *posthumous reproduction; *sperm; coma; Belgium; *Great Britain; *R v. Human Fertilisation and Embryology Authority (ex parte Blood)

Harris, John. Doctors' orders, rationality and the good life: commentary on Savulescu. *Journal of Medical Ethics.* 1999 Apr; 25(2): 127–129. 7 fn. BE61915.
    *autonomy; *beneficence; cloning; conscience; *decision making; *embryo transfer; freedom; in vitro fertilization; moral complicity; *moral obligations; moral policy; *motivation; parents; patients; *physicians; *preimplantation diagnosis; *reproduction; *reproductive technologies; *values; rationality

Hartouni, Valerie. Cultural Conceptions: On Reproductive Technologies and the Remaking of Life. Minneapolis, MN: University of Minnesota Press; 1997. 175 p. Bibliography: p. 157–170. ISBN 0-8166-2623-5. BE62771.
    *abortion, induced; adoption; audiovisual aids; behavioral genetics; blacks; brain death; *cloning; disadvantaged; embryos; eugenics; *fetuses; genetic intervention; legal aspects; mass media; mothers; parent child relationship; personhood; political activity; posthumous reproduction; postmodernism; *pregnant women; prenatal diagnosis; prolongation of life; *reproduction; *reproductive technologies; social discrimination; *social impact; socioeconomic factors; Supreme Court decisions; *surrogate mothers; value of life; values; violence; women's rights; In re Baby M; Johnson v. Calvert; Right to Life Movement; S'Aline's Solution; The Bell Curve (Herrnstein, R.; Murray, C.); *United States

Jones, Nikki. Culture and reproductive health: challenges for feminist philanthrophy. *In:* Donchin, Anne; Purdy, Laura M., eds. Embodying Bioethics: Recent Feminist Advances. Lanham, MD: Rowman and Littlefield; 1999: 223–237. 46 fn. ISBN 0-8476-8924-7. BE61023.
    childbirth; circumcision; cultural pluralism; *developing countries; females; feminist ethics; human rights; injuries; international aspects; justice; morbidity; mortality; *reproduction; sexuality; social discrimination; values; *women's health; Nigeria; Philippines

Kligman, Gail. The Politics of Duplicity: Controlling Reproduction in Ceausescu's Romania. Berkeley, CA: University of California Press; 1998. 358 p. Bibliography: p. 331–346. ISBN 0-520-21075-1. BE60112.
    *abortion, induced; adoption; coercion; communism; contraception; deception; dehumanization; dissent; economics; females; fraud; government regulation; historical aspects; *illegal abortion; incentives; information dissemination; international aspects; legal aspects; mass media; moral complicity; morbidity; mortality; paternalism; physicians; *political systems; politics; *population control; *public policy; *reproduction; *social control; social impact; socioeconomic factors; statistics; unwanted children; women's health; *Romania; *Twentieth Century

Little, Margaret Olivia. Let me count the ways: feminism illuminating bioethics. [Book review essay]. *Medical Humanities Review.* 1997 Spring; 11(1): 76–81. BE59967.

---

abortion, induced; adoption; bioethical issues; *bioethics; drug abuse; employment; ethical theory; females; *feminist ethics; fetuses; HIV seropositivity; human experimentation; justice; males; parent child relationship; pregnant women; prenatal injuries; public policy; *reproduction; *reproductive technologies; rights; selection of subjects; social discrimination; *Feminism and Bioethics: Beyond Reproduction (Wolf, S.M., ed.); *Reproduction, Ethics, and the Law (Callahan, J.C., ed.)

Macklin, Ruth. International feminism and reproductive rights. *In: her* Against Relativism: Cultural Diversity and the Search for Ethical Universals in Medicine. New York, NY: Oxford University Press; 1999: 161–185. 30 fn. ISBN 0–19–511632–1. BE62783.
autonomy; *contraception; *cultural pluralism; decision making; *developing countries; *ethical relativism; females; *feminist ethics; freedom; *human rights; *international aspects; justice; legal aspects; males; methods; non–Western World; *paternalism; *political activity; postmodernism; pregnant women; public policy; *reproduction; reproductive technologies; Roman Catholic ethics; selective abortion; *sex determination; social control; social discrimination; values; Western World; *women's health; *women's rights; Brazil; China; Feminist International Network of Resistance to Reproductive and Genetic Engineering (FINRRAGE); India; International Conference on Population and Development (Cairo, 1994); Women's Global Network for Reproductive Rights

Marsiglio, William. Pathways to paternity and social fatherhood. *In: his* Procreative Man. New York, NY: New York University Press; 1998: 102–146, 213–222. 148 fn. ISBN 0–8147–5579–8. BE61950.
adoption; attitudes; confidentiality; DNA fingerprinting; emotions; *fathers; females; infertility; legal aspects; *males; married persons; motivation; *parent child relationship; pregnant women; *reproduction; *reproductive technologies; rights; semen donors; sexuality; single persons; tissue banks; trends; paternity; United States

Michie, Helena; Cahn, Naomi R. Confinements: Fertility and Infertility in Contemporary Culture. New Brunswick, NJ: Rutgers University Press; 1997. 187 p. Bibliography: p. 171–177. ISBN 0–8135–2433–4. BE62628.
autonomy; cesarean section; childbirth; coercion; criminal law; dehumanization; drug abuse; females; *feminist ethics; home care; hospitals; human body; indigents; *infertility; legal aspects; pain; parent child relationship; *pregnant women; prenatal diagnosis; prenatal injuries; *reproduction; *reproductive technologies; social control; *socioeconomic factors; United States

Mika, Karin; Hurst, Bonnie. One way to be born? Legislative inaction and the posthumous child. *Marquette Law Review.* 1996 Summer; 79(4): 993–1019. 223 fn. BE62221.
artificial insemination; children; *fathers; historical aspects; international aspects; *legal aspects; parent child relationship; *posthumous reproduction; privacy; reproduction; Supreme Court decisions; Davis v. Davis; France; Hecht v. Superior Court; Parpalaix v. CECOS; Twentieth Century; Uniform Parentage Act; Uniform Status of Children of Assisted Conception Act; *United States

Novaes, Simone Bateman; Salem, Tania. Embedding the embryo. *In:* Harris, John; Holm, Søren, eds. The Future of Human Reproduction: Ethics, Choice, and Regulation. New York, NY: Oxford University Press; 1998: 101–126. 30 fn. ISBN 0–19–823761–8. BE61265.
abortion, induced; autonomy; case studies; *cryopreservation; *decision making; *embryo disposition; *embryo transfer; *embryos; family relationship; hospitals; *in vitro fertilization; legal aspects; married persons; mother

fetus relationship; ovum donors; physicians; *posthumous reproduction; pregnant women; psychological stress; refusal to treat; *reproductive technologies; selection for treatment; semen donors; social sciences; *women's rights; France

Palmer, Eileen Alexa. Genetic Choice, Disability, and Regret. Ann Arbor, MI: UMI Dissertation Services; 1997. 159 p. Bibliography: p. 146–159. Dissertation, Ph.D. in philosophy, University of Wisconsin–Madison, 1997 May. UMI No. 9711004. BE61843.
children; congenital disorders; decision making; *disabled; *ethical analysis; *eugenics; *future generations; genetic disorders; genetic intervention; hearing disorders; intention; *moral obligations; *moral policy; *parents; philosophy; *quality of life; *reproduction; reproductive technologies; rights; teleological ethics; theology; time factors; value of life; harms; Adams, Robert; Heyd, David; Parfit, Derek; Woodward, James

Petchesky, Rosalind P.; Judd, Karen, eds.; International Reproductive Rights Research Action Group (IRRRAG). Negotiating Reproductive Rights: Women's Perspectives Across Countries and Cultures. New York, NY: Zed Books; 1998. 358 p. (Women's studies/health). Bibliography: p. 327–347. ISBN 1–85649–536–1. BE61113.
abortion, induced; autonomy; childbirth; circumcision; contraception; cultural pluralism; decision making; domestic violence; employment; family planning; females; human rights; indigents; *international aspects; legal rights; marital relationship; minority groups; political activity; religion; *reproduction; *sexuality; social discrimination; *socioeconomic factors; women's health; women's health services; *women's rights; *Brazil; *Egypt; International Reproductive Rights Research Action Group; *Malaysia; *Mexico; *Nigeria; *Philippines; *United States

Posner, Eric A.; Posner, Richard A. The demand for human cloning. *In:* Nussbaum, Martha C.; Sunstein, Cass R., eds. Clones and Clones: Facts and Fantasies About Human Cloning. New York, NY: Norton; 1998: 233–261. 33 fn. ISBN 0–393–04648–6. BE60364.
*cloning; eugenics; evolution; females; future generations; genetic diversity; government regulation; infertility; males; marital relationship; married persons; models, theoretical; *motivation; parent child relationship; public policy; *reproduction; reproductive technologies; risks and benefits; single persons; *social impact; socioeconomic factors

Robb, Carol S. Liberties, claims, entitlements, and trumps: reproductive rights and ecological responsibilities. *Journal of Religious Ethics.* 1998 Fall; 26(2): 283–294. 6 refs. 3 fn. BE61895.
Christian ethics; communitarianism; *ecology; freedom; *human rights; international aspects; justice; *moral obligations; natural law; *obligations to society; *population control; *reproduction; socioeconomic factors; speciesism; women's rights; International Covenant on Civil and Political Rights; International Covenant on Economic, Social and Cultural Rights

Roberts, Dorothy E. The genetic tie. *University of Chicago Law Review.* 1995 Winter; 62(1): 209–273. 277 fn. BE62436.
adoption; artificial insemination; *blacks; embryo transfer; family relationship; fathers; females; feminist ethics; *genetic identity; historical aspects; in vitro fertilization; *legal aspects; males; mothers; *parent child relationship; *reproduction; *reproductive technologies; semen donors; single persons; *social discrimination; *social worth; surrogate mothers; *whites; *personal identity; slavery; United States

Roberts, Melinda A. Child versus Childmaker: Future

BE = bioethics accession number   fn. = footnotes   refs. = references

Persons and Present Duties in Ethics and the Law. Lanham, MD: Rowman and Littlefield; 1998. 235 p. (Studies in social, political, and legal philosophy). Bibliography: p. 221–226. ISBN 0-8476-8901-8. BE59868.

children; *cloning; congenital disorders; constitutional law; embryos; freedom; *future generations; injuries; justice; legal aspects; *moral obligations; negligence; philosophy; privacy; quality of life; *reproduction; reproductive technologies; suffering; *teleological ethics; torts; value of life; *wrongful life; Broome, John; Fourteenth Amendment; United States

Roberts, Melinda A. Present duties and future persons: when are existence-inducing acts wrong? *Law and Philosophy.* 1995 Nov; 14(3–4): 297–327. 50 fn. BE59358.

adolescents; children; cloning; congenital disorders; contracts; embryo transfer; in vitro fertilization; injuries; judicial action; legal aspects; *moral policy; motivation; negligence; organ donation; parents; philosophy; physicians; quality of life; *reproduction; *reproductive technologies; surrogate mothers; value of life; *wrongful life

Robinson, John H.; Berry, Roberta M.; McDonnell, Kevin, eds. Reproduction. *In: their* A Health Law Reader: An Interdisciplinary Approach. Durham, NC: Carolina Academic Press; 1999: 73–180. 38 fn. ISBN 0-89089-907-X. BE62292.

*abortion, induced; attitudes; autonomy; children; cloning; *commodification; dehumanization; disabled; eugenics; family relationship; feminist ethics; fetuses; *freedom; gene therapy; *genetic intervention; genetic screening; government regulation; legal aspects; minority groups; *moral policy; morality; parent child relationship; personhood; prenatal diagnosis; *public policy; *reproduction; *reproductive technologies; rights; selective abortion; sex determination; sexuality; Supreme Court decisions; surrogate mothers; value of life; Roe v. Wade; United States

Savulescu, Julian. Should doctors intentionally do less than the best? *Journal of Medical Ethics.* 1999 Apr; 25(2): 121–126. 11 fn. BE61914.

artificial insemination; *autonomy; *beneficence; *cloning; *congenital disorders; conscience; *decision making; disabled; *embryo transfer; eugenics; freedom; *genetic disorders; *goals; in vitro fertilization; *medicine; mentally retarded; *moral complicity; *moral obligations; moral policy; *motivation; parent child relationship; *parents; *patients; *physicians; *preimplantation diagnosis; *quality of life; refusal to treat; *reproduction; *reproductive technologies; rights; selection for treatment; sex preselection; suffering; *values; rationality

The papers of Burley and Harris, and Draper and Chadwick, in this issue, raise a problem: what should doctors do when patients request an option which is not the best available? This commentary argues that doctors have a duty to offer that option which will result in the individual affected by that choice enjoying the highest level of wellbeing. Doctors can deviate from this duty and submaximise -- bring about an outcome that is less than the best -- only if there are good reasons to do so. The desire to have a child which is genetically related provides little, if any, reason to submaximise. The implication for cloning, preimplantation diagnosis and embryo transfer is that doctors should only produce a clone or transfer embryos expected to enjoy a level of wellbeing which is less than that enjoyed by other children the couple could have, if there is a good reason to employ that technology. This paper sketches what might constitute a good reason to submaximise.

Serour, Gamal I. Reproductive choice: a Muslim perspective. *In:* Harris, John; Holm, Søren, eds. The Future of Human Reproduction: Ethics, Choice, and

Regulation. New York, NY: Oxford University Press; 1998: 191–202. 37 fn. ISBN 0-19-823761-8. BE61270.

aborted fetuses; abortion, induced; age factors; contraception; *embryo research; females; *fetal research; fetal tissue donation; gene therapy; genetic counseling; genetic enhancement; *Islamic ethics; multiple pregnancy; *reproduction; *reproductive technologies; research embryo creation; selection for treatment; sex determination; sex preselection; *theology

Shah, Monica. Modern reproductive technologies: legal issues concerning cryopreservation and posthumous conception. *Journal of Legal Medicine.* 1996 Dec; 17(4): 547–571. 133 fn. BE61246.

children; *cryopreservation; *embryos; *germ cells; *legal aspects; legal rights; methods; ovum; parents; *posthumous reproduction; property rights; remuneration; *reproductive technologies; sperm; state government; wrongful death; *United States

Shanner, Laura. Abortion, Chernobyl, and unanswered genetic questions. *In:* Donchin, Anne; Purdy, Laura M., eds. Embodying Bioethics: Recent Feminist Advances. Lanham, MD: Rowman and Littlefield; 1999: 85–102. 18 refs. 1 fn. ISBN 0-8476-8924-7. BE61016.

childbirth; *decision making; *epidemiology; females; feminist ethics; fetuses; *genetic disorders; genetic screening; *health hazards; international aspects; methods; morbidity; nuclear energy; politics; pregnant women; prenatal diagnosis; psychological stress; public health; *radiation; *reproduction; research design; selective abortion; *social impact; socioeconomic factors; *uncertainty; *Chernobyl; Europe; Ukraine

Steinbock, Bonnie. A philosopher looks at assisted reproduction. *Journal of Assisted Reproduction and Genetics.* 1995 Sep; 12(8): 543–551. 45 fn. BE60568.

economics; embryo disposition; embryos; *freedom; HIV seropositivity; in vitro fertilization; moral obligations; *moral policy; ovum donors; parent child relationship; personhood; *religious ethics; remuneration; *reproduction; *reproductive technologies; *rights; *risks and benefits; Roman Catholic ethics; selection for treatment; semen donors; sexuality; social discrimination; surrogate mothers; values; women's health; *women's rights; Robertson, John

Steinbock, Bonnie. Sperm as property. *In:* Harris, John; Holm, Søren, eds. The Future of Human Reproduction: Ethics, Choice, and Regulation. New York, NY: Oxford University Press; 1998: 150–161. 39 fn. ISBN 0-19-823761-8. BE61267.

*artificial insemination; autonomy; body parts and fluids; commodification; *cryopreservation; decision making; dissent; *legal aspects; moral policy; *posthumous reproduction; *property rights; public policy; remuneration; reproduction; reproductive technologies; semen donors; *sperm; suicide; tissue banks; California; *Hecht v. Superior Court (Kane)

Thomson, Michael. Reproducing Narrative: Gender, Reproduction and Law. Brookfield, VT: Ashgate; 1998. 228 p. Includes references. ISBN 1-85521-929-8. BE62630.

*abortion, induced; attitudes; contraception; employment; *females; fetuses; health hazards; historical aspects; illegal abortion; international aspects; law; *legal aspects; legislation; males; narrative ethics; occupational exposure; physicians; political activity; politics; postmodernism; pregnant women; prenatal injuries; *reproduction; reproductive technologies; *social control; social discrimination; *sociology of medicine; women's health services; Abortion Act 1967 (Great Britain); Great Britain; Human Fertilisation and Embryology Act 1990 (Great Britain); Nineteenth Century; Twentieth Century; United States

---

BE = bioethics accession number   fn. = footnotes   refs. = references

Tong, Rosemarie. The way of feminist bioethics. [Book review essay]. *Medical Humanities Review.* 1997 Spring; 11(1): 72–75. BE59966.
    abortion on demand; abortion, induced; *bioethics; decision making; females; *feminist ethics; fetuses; moral obligations; pregnant women; *reproduction; reproductive technologies; *rights; risks and benefits; selective abortion; surrogate mothers; utilitarianism; *Reproducing Persons: Issues in Feminist Bioethics (Purdy, L.M.)

Weisman, Carol S.; Khoury, Amal J.; Cassirer, Christopher, et al. The implications of affiliations between Catholic and non–Catholic health care organizations for availability of reproductive health services. *Women's Health Issues.* 1999 May–Jun; 9(3): 121–134. 19 refs. BE62419.
    abortion, induced; contraception; *health facilities; obstetrics and gynecology; organization and administration; referral and consultation; *religious hospitals; *reproduction; reproductive technologies; Roman Catholic ethics; *Roman Catholics; sterilization (sexual); *women's health services; *health facility mergers; nonprofit organizations; United States

A birth spurs debate on using sperm after death. [Editorial]. *New York Times.* 1999 Mar 27: A11. BE60873.
    cadavers; cryopreservation; *informed consent; married persons; *posthumous reproduction; *semen donors; sperm; United States

REPRODUCTIVE TECHNOLOGIES

See also ARTIFICIAL INSEMINATION, BIOMEDICAL TECHNOLOGIES, CLONING, GENETIC INTERVENTION, IN VITRO FERTILIZATION, REPRODUCTION, SEX PRESELECTION, SURROGATE MOTHERS

Anderson, J. Kerby. Reproductive technologies. *In: his* Moral Dilemmas: Biblical Perspectives on Contemporary Ethical Issues. Nashville, TN: Word Publishing; 1998: 45–57, 230–231. 21 fn. ISBN 0–8499–1446–9. BE62394.
    artificial insemination; *Christian ethics; in vitro fertilization; marital relationship; *reproductive technologies; semen donors; sex preselection; surrogate mothers; United States

Anderson, J. Kerby. The ethics of genetic engineering and artificial reproduction. *In:* Demy, Timothy J.; Stewart, Gary P., eds. Genetic Engineering: A Christian Response: Crucial Considerations in Shaping Life. Grand Rapids, MI: Kregel Publications; 1999: 140–152. 20 fn. ISBN 0–8254–2357–0. BE61365.
    age factors; artificial insemination; *Christian ethics; *cloning; cryopreservation; embryo disposition; embryo research; embryo transfer; embryos; gamete intrafallopian transfer; gene therapy; in vitro fertilization; legal aspects; marital relationship; ovum donors; *parent child relationship; patents; pregnant women; *recombinant DNA research; *reproductive technologies; semen donors; sex preselection; social impact; surrogate mothers; theology; transgenic organisms; value of life; United States

Andrews, Lori B. The Clone Age: Adventures in the New World of Reproductive Technology. New York, NY: Henry Holt; 1999. 264 p. Notes on sources: p. 263–264. ISBN 0–8050–6080–4. BE61832.
    artificial insemination; cloning; cryopreservation; disclosure; economics; embryo transfer; eugenics; genetic disorders; genetic enhancement; genetic information; *genetic intervention; genetic research; genetic screening; genome mapping; health facilities; historical aspects; in vitro fertilization; *industry; infertility; international aspects; legal aspects; misconduct; motivation; multiple pregnancy; ovum

donors; parent child relationship; patents; physicians; posthumous reproduction; preimplantation diagnosis; prenatal diagnosis; regulation; remuneration; *reproductive technologies; risks and benefits; selective abortion; semen donors; social impact; surrogate mothers

Andrews, Lori B. The sperminator. *New York Times Magazine.* 1999 Mar 28: 62–65. BE60874.
    advance directives; cadavers; coercion; cryopreservation; decision making; directed donation; family members; family relationship; *informed consent; legal aspects; married persons; physicians; *posthumous reproduction; *semen donors; single persons; sperm; tissue donation; *coma; United States

Australia. Victoria. The Infertility Treatment Act 1995. No. 63 of 1995. Date of assent: 27 Jun 1995. [Summary]. *International Digest of Health Legislation.* 1997; 48(1): 24–33. BE59589.
    advisory committees; artificial insemination; counseling; donors; embryo disposition; *embryo research; embryo transfer; genetic intervention; *government regulation; in vitro fertilization; informed consent; *legal aspects; posthumous reproduction; records; *reproductive technologies; sex preselection; spousal consent; surrogate mothers; terminology; Australia; *Infertility Treatment Act 1995 (Victoria); Infertility Treatment Authority (Victoria); Standing Review and Advisory Committee on Infertility (Victoria); *Victoria

Bagness, Carmel. Genetics, the Fetus and Our Future. Hale, Cheshire, England: Hochland and Hochland; 1998. 105 p. Includes references. ISBN 1–898507–65–1. BE59721.
    aborted fetuses; cadavers; confidentiality; criminal law; disabled; embryo disposition; *embryo research; *embryos; eugenics; fetuses; gene therapy; genetic disorders; genetic enhancement; *genetic intervention; genetic materials; genome mapping; germ cells; legal aspects; moral obligations; multiple pregnancy; ovum donors; patents; personhood; preimplantation diagnosis; property rights; recombinant DNA research; regulation; remuneration; *reproductive technologies; research embryo creation; *risks and benefits; selective abortion; semen donors; social discrimination; social impact; torts; Great Britain; Human Genome Project

Bahnsen, Ulrich. Swiss to vote on ban on *in vitro* fertilization. [News]. *Nature.* 1998 Nov 12; 396(6707): 105. BE59659.
    embryo research; *government regulation; *in vitro fertilization; ovum donors; political activity; preimplantation diagnosis; *public participation; *reproductive technologies; stem cells; *Switzerland

Baird, Patricia. Proceed with care: new reproductive technologies and the need for boundaries. *Journal of Assisted Reproduction and Genetics.* 1995 Sep; 12(8): 491–498. 8 refs. BE60561.
    adoption; advisory committees; artificial insemination; drugs; embryo research; fetal research; fetal tissue donation; gene therapy; germ cells; government regulation; in vitro fertilization; infertility; prenatal diagnosis; public opinion; *public policy; *reproductive technologies; risks and benefits; semen donors; sex determination; sex preselection; surrogate mothers; *Canada; Proceed with Care: Final Report of the Royal Commission on New Reproductive Technologies (Canada); *Royal Commission on New Reproductive Technologies (Canada)

Bard, Jennifer S. When a woman doesn't need a man: legal issues regarding cloning as an infertility treatment. *Journal of Biolaw and Business.* 1998 Spring; 1(3): 56–58. 21 fn. BE62093.
    *cloning; cryopreservation; embryos; *legal aspects; marital

---

BE = bioethics accession number   fn. = footnotes   refs. = references

relationship; multiple pregnancy; parent child relationship; regulation; *reproductive technologies; risks and benefits; single persons

Barnhouse, Dorothy J. Birth of octuplets reignites fertilty debate. [News]. *New York Times.* 1999 Jan 5: F7. BE59874.
  drugs; health insurance; hormones; infertility; methods; *multiple pregnancy; patient care; physicians; *reproductive technologies

Berger, Joseph. Yale gene pool seen as route to better baby. *New York Times.* 1999 Jan 10: 19. BE60023.
  *advertising; *eugenics; intelligence; *ovum donors; parents; remuneration; students; universities; United States; *Yale University

Brazier, Margaret. Reproductive rights: feminism or patriarchy? *In:* Harris, John; Holm, Søren, eds. The Future of Human Reproduction: Ethics, Choice, and Regulation. New York, NY: Oxford University Press; 1998: 66–76. 28 fn. ISBN 0-19-823761-8. BE61263.
  aborted fetuses; embryo research; fathers; *females; feminist ethics; human rights; in vitro fertilization; legal aspects; *males; mentally retarded; ovum donors; parent child relationship; property rights; *reproduction; *reproductive technologies; rights; selection for treatment; single persons; *social discrimination; *social dominance; sterilization (sexual); *women's rights; Great Britain; Human Fertilisation and Embryology Act 1990

Brazil. Federal Medical Council. Federal Medical Council (CFM) of Brazil adopts resolutions on criteria for death and on medically assisted procreation. [Texts of Resolution CFM No. 1346/91, adopted 8 Aug 1991; and Resolution CFM No. 1358/92, adopted 11 Nov 1992]. *International Digest of Health Legislation.* 1994; 45(1): 100–102. BE62685.
  *brain death; confidentiality; cryopreservation; *determination of death; government regulation; *guidelines; health facilities; *legal aspects; multiple pregnancy; ovum donors; preimplantation diagnosis; records; *reproductive technologies; research embryo creation; selective abortion; sex preselection; standards; surrogate mothers; *Brazil; *Federal Medical Council (Brazil)

Burley, Justine C. The price of eggs: who should bear the costs of fertility treatments? *In:* Harris, John; Holm, Søren, eds. The Future of Human Reproduction: Ethics, Choice, and Regulation. New York, NY: Oxford University Press; 1998: 127–149. 51 fn. ISBN 0-19-823761-8. BE61266.
  biomedical technologies; *compensation; disabled; *government financing; health care; homosexuals; *infertility; *justice; *moral policy; multiple pregnancy; *obligations of society; philosophy; *public policy; reproduction; *reproductive technologies; *resource allocation; self induced illness; standards; values; voluntary sterilization; Dworkin, Ronald

Byers, Keith Alan. Infertility and in vitro fertilization: a growing need for consumer-oriented regulation of the in vitro fertilization industry. *Journal of Legal Medicine.* 1997 Sep; 18(3): 265–313. 304 fn. BE59838.
  advisory committees; AIDS serodiagnosis; communicable diseases; cryopreservation; economics; embryo disposition; embryo research; embryo transfer; federal government; genetic disorders; government financing; *government regulation; *health facilities; *in vitro fertilization; industry; *infertility; legal aspects; legislation; mandatory testing; misconduct; multiple pregnancy; ovum donors; physicians; psychological stress; public opinion; *public policy; quality of health care; remuneration; *reproductive technologies; standards; state government; statistics; treatment outcome; Ethics Advisory Board; Fertility Clinic Success Rate and

Certification Act 1992; Human Embryo Research Panel; *United States

Canada. Health Canada. Discussion Group on Embryo Research. Research on Human Embryos in Canada. Final Report of the Discussion Group on Embryo Research. Ottawa, ON: Health Canada; 1995 Nov 15. 33 p. 32 fn. BE59458.
  advisory committees; children; cloning; cultural pluralism; donors; embryo disposition; *embryo research; embryos; females; fetal development; genetic screening; germ cells; *government regulation; *guidelines; hybrids; incentives; industry; informed consent; moral obligations; moral policy; ovum donors; peer review; *preimplantation diagnosis; *public policy; remuneration; *reproductive technologies; research embryo creation; risk; risks and benefits; time factors; transgenic organisms; viability; women's health; *Canada; *Discussion Group on Embryo Research (Canada)

Canadian Nurses Association. The Role of the Nurse in Reproductive and Genetic Technologies. [Policy statement]. Issued by the Canadian Nurses Association, 50 Driveway, Ottawa, ON, Canada; 1996 Jun. 2 p. 4 refs. 2 fn. Approved by the CNA Board of Directors Jun 1996. BE62000.
  counseling; *genetic screening; *nurse's role; nurses; *organizational policies; professional organizations; *reproductive technologies; Canada; *Canadian Nurses Association

Capron, Alexander Morgan. Too many parents. *Hastings Center Report.* 1998 Sep–Oct; 28(5): 22–24. 10 refs. BE59550.
  accountability; artificial insemination; contracts; cryopreservation; embryo transfer; embryos; fathers; health facilities; *legal aspects; marital relationship; mothers; ovum donors; *parent child relationship; *reproductive technologies; semen donors; surrogate mothers; divorce; *Buzzanca v. Buzzanca; California; Connecticut; United States

Cataldo, Peter J. GIFT as assistance. *Ethics and Medics.* 1997 Dec; 22(12): 3–4. BE60411.
  *gamete intrafallopian transfer; marital relationship; methods; *Roman Catholic ethics

Catholic University of the Sacred Heart (Rome). On heterologous assisted fertilisation. *Bulletin of Medical Ethics.* 1997 Nov; 133: 10–11. BE59702.
  confidentiality; embryo disposition; ovum donors; *reproductive technologies; *Roman Catholic ethics; semen donors

Cooper, Susan Lewis; Glazer, Ellen Sarasohn. Choosing Assisted Reproduction: Social, Emotional and Ethical Considerations. Indianapolis, IN: Perspectives Press; 1998. 400 p. 91 fn. ISBN 0-944934-19-6. BE61044.
  adoption; age factors; artificial insemination; children; commodification; counseling; cryopreservation; deception; directed donation; disclosure; drugs; embryo disposition; embryo transfer; embryos; emotions; females; gamete intrafallopian transfer; genetic identity; health facilities; health insurance reimbursement; homosexuals; in vitro fertilization; infertility; legal aspects; males; moral policy; mother fetus relationship; multiple pregnancy; ovum donors; parent child relationship; preimplantation diagnosis; privacy; psychological stress; refusal to treat; remuneration; reproduction; *reproductive technologies; rights; risks and benefits; selective abortion; semen donors; single persons; surrogate mothers; abortion, spontaneous; grief; United States

Cutrer, William; Glahn, Sandra. Dealing with genetic reality: theological and clinical perspectives. *In:* Demy,

Timothy J.; Stewart, Gary P., eds. Genetic Engineering: A Christian Response: Crucial Considerations in Shaping Life. Grand Rapids, MI: Kregel Publications; 1999: 154-169. 11 fn. ISBN 0-8254-2357-0. BE61366.
  autonomy; beginning of life; beneficence; *Christian ethics; cloning; decision making; deontological ethics; *embryo research; embryos; ethical analysis; gene therapy; genetic disorders; genetic enhancement; genetic information; *genetic research; intention; justice; killing; moral complicity; moral policy; personhood; preimplantation diagnosis; *reproductive technologies; *risks and benefits; value of life; virtues; Human Embryo Research Panel; United States

de Beaufort, Inez. Letter from a post-menopausal mother. In: Harris, John; Holm, Søren, eds. The Future of Human Reproduction: Ethics, Choice, Regulation. New York, NY: Oxford University Press; 1998: 238-247. ISBN 0-19-823761-7. BE61273.
  *age factors; attitudes; children; fathers; females; morality; mothers; motivation; *parent child relationship; *reproductive technologies; risks and benefits; *selection for treatment

Deech, Ruth. Legal and ethical responsibilities of gamete banks. [Article and discussion]. Human Reproduction. 1998 May; 13(Suppl.): 80-89. BE61483.
  advertising; age factors; confidentiality; counseling; directed donation; disclosure; family members; *government regulation; *guidelines; informed consent; institutional ethics; international aspects; *legislation; *ovum; *ovum donors; registries; remuneration; reproductive technologies; *semen donors; *sperm; *tissue banks; tissue donation; *Great Britain; *Human Fertilisation and Embryology Act 1990; *Human Fertilisation and Embryology Authority

De Jonge, Christopher J.; Wolf, Don P. Embryo number for transfer should be regulated. [Editorial]. Fertility and Sterility. 1997 Nov; 68(5): 784-786. 10 refs. BE60335.
  economics; *embryo transfer; embryos; morbidity; *multiple pregnancy; *regulation; reproductive technologies; selective abortion; self regulation; *treatment outcome; United States

Demmer, K. Ethical aspects of reproductive medicine. In: Nieschlag, E.; Behre, H.M., eds. Andrology: Male Reproductive Health and Dysfunction. Berlin: Springer-Verlag; 1997: 409-417. 15 refs. Translated by T. Kopfensteiner. ISBN 3-540-61616-0. BE61325.
  artificial insemination; children; embryo research; embryos; genetic intervention; in vitro fertilization; infertility; males; marital relationship; methods; *reproductive technologies; *Roman Catholic ethics; semen donors; sperm; surrogate mothers; value of life; Evangelium Vitae; Instruction on Respect for Human Life

de Wert, Guido M.W.R. The post-menopause: playground for reproductive technology? Some ethical reflections. In: Harris, John; Holm, Søren, eds. The Future of Human Reproduction: Ethics, Choice, and Regulation. New York, NY: Oxford University Press; 1998: 221-237. 27 fn. ISBN 0-19-823761-8. BE61272.
  *age factors; autonomy; children; decision making; *females; government financing; guidelines; informed consent; international aspects; justice; males; maternal health; moral policy; multiple pregnancy; ovum donors; parent child relationship; physicians; *reproductive technologies; resource allocation; risk; scarcity; *selection for treatment; personal financing; Europe

Djerassi, Carl. Sex in an age of mechanical reproduction. Science. 1999 Jul 2; 285(5424): 53-54. BE62324.
  age factors; females; infertility; *literature; males; *methods; posthumous reproduction; *reproductive technologies;

*intracytoplasmic sperm injection; *An Immaculate Misconception (Djerassi, Carl)

Doerfler, John F. Is GIFT compatible with the teaching of Donum Vitae? Linacre Quarterly. 1997 Feb; 64(1): 16-29. 48 fn. BE59308.
  children; commodification; *gamete intrafallopian transfer; gifts; love; marital relationship; morality; reproduction; *Roman Catholic ethics; dignity; human body; *Instruction on Respect for Human Life

Donchin, Anne. Shaping reproductive technology policy: the search for consensus. In: ten Have, Henk A.M.J.; Sass, Hans-Martin, eds. Consensus Formation in Healthcare Ethics. Boston, MA: Kluwer Academic; 1998: 229-250. 36 refs. 28 fn. ISBN 0-7923-4944-X. BE62598.
  advisory committees; consensus; cultural pluralism; embryo research; government financing; *government regulation; international aspects; legislation; political activity; *politics; *public policy; *reproductive technologies; *Great Britain; Warnock Committee

Draper, Heather; Chadwick, Ruth. Beware! Preimplantation genetic diagnosis may solve some old problems but it also raises new ones. Journal of Medical Ethics. 1999 Apr; 25(2): 114-120. 6 fn. BE61913.
  abortion, induced; autonomy; beginning of life; case studies; children; *decision making; disabled; Down syndrome; *embryo transfer; *embryos; *genetic disorders; *genetic screening; hearing disorders; *in vitro fertilization; legal aspects; *moral obligations; *moral policy; motivation; *parents; *physicians; pregnant women; *preimplantation diagnosis; prenatal diagnosis; property rights; *quality of life; *reproduction; rights; risks and benefits; value of life
  Preimplantation genetic diagnosis (PIGD) goes some way to meeting the clinical, psychological and ethical problems of antenatal testing. We should guard, however, against the assumption that PIGD is the answer to all our problems. It also presents some new problems and leaves some old problems untouched. This paper will provide an overview of how PIGD meets some of the old problems but will concentrate on two new challenges for ethics (and, indeed, law). First we look at whether we should always suppose that it is wrong for a clinician to implant a genetically abnormal zygote. The second concern is particularly important in the UK. The Human Fertilisation and Embryology Act (1990) gives clinicians a statutory obligation to consider the interests of the future children they help to create using in vitro fertilisation (IVF) techniques. Does this mean that because PIGD is based on IVF techniques the balance of power for determining the best interests of the future child shifts from the mother to the clinician?

Easton, Megan. Infertility treatment: lack of consensus plagues an unregulated field. Canadian Medical Association Journal. 1998 May 19; 158(10): 1345-1348. BE59833.
  biomedical research; data banks; germ cells; *government regulation; health facilities; infertility; legislation; organizational policies; professional organizations; registries; remuneration; *reproductive technologies; self regulation; *Canada; Canadian Fertility and Andrology Society; Canadian Medical Association; Human Reproductive and Genetic Technologies Act (Bill C-47); Infertility Awareness Association (Canada); Society of Obstetricians and Gynaecologists of Canada

Eisenberg, V.H.; Schenker, J.G. Pre-embryo donation: ethical and legal aspects. International Journal of Gynaecology and Obstetrics. 1998 Jan; 60(1): 51-57. 39

BE = bioethics accession number   fn. = footnotes   refs. = references

refs. BE60695.

    age factors; confidentiality; cryopreservation; disclosure; *donors; *embryo transfer; *embryos; international aspects; legal aspects; medical records; *ovum donors; parent child relationship; property rights; registries; religion; remuneration; *reproductive technologies; selection for treatment; *semen donors; single persons; standards; tissue banks

Eisenberg, V.H.; Schenker, J.G. Pregnancy in the older woman: scientific and ethical aspects. *International Journal of Gynaecology and Obstetrics.* 1997 Feb; 56(2): 163–169. 41 refs. BE60689.

    adults; *age factors; females; human rights; international aspects; maternal health; morbidity; mortality; newborns; ovum donors; regulation; remuneration; reproduction; *reproductive technologies; resource allocation; risk; risks and benefits; *selection for treatment

Ellenson, David. Artificial fertilization (hafrayyah melakhutit) and procreative autonomy in light of two contemporary Israeli responsa. *In:* Jacob, Walter; Zemer, Moshe, eds. The Fetus and Fertility in Jewish Law: Essays and Responsa. Pittsburgh, PA: Rodef Shalom Press; Freehof Institute of Progressive Halakhah; 1995: 19–38. 23 fn. ISBN 0-929699-07-6. BE61837.

    artificial insemination; autonomy; children; drugs; embryo disposition; *embryo transfer; family relationship; genetic identity; genetic intervention; *in vitro fertilization; infertility; *Jewish ethics; married persons; multiple pregnancy; parent child relationship; reproduction; *reproductive technologies; risks and benefits; selective abortion; surrogate mothers; *theology; wedge argument; women's rights; Orthodox Judaism; Reform Judaism

Englert, Y. From medically assisted procreation to euthanasia: a modern way to deal with ethical dilemmas in modern medicine. *European Journal of Genetics in Society.* 1997; 3(2): 22–26. 3 refs. BE61454.

    assisted suicide; beginning of life; bioethics; embryo research; embryos; legal aspects; moral obligations; palliative care; personhood; physicians; *reproductive technologies; Roman Catholic ethics; suffering; terminal care; value of life; *voluntary euthanasia; wedge argument; Netherlands

Englert, Y.; Govaerts, I. Oocyte donation: particular technical and ethical aspects. *Human Reproduction.* 1998 May; 13(Suppl. 2): 90–97. 34 refs. BE61484.

    age factors; artificial insemination; attitudes; comparative studies; confidentiality; counseling; cryopreservation; directed donation; family members; females; in vitro fertilization; informed consent; methods; motivation; *ovum donors; remuneration; semen donors; socioeconomic factors; *tissue donation; Europe; United States

Farquhar, Dion. The Other Machine: Discourse and Reproductive Technologies. New York, NY: Routledge; 1996. 258 p. (Thinking gender). Bibliography: p. 235–246. ISBN 0-415-91279-2. BE62138.

    artificial insemination; commodification; economics; embryo transfer; family relationship; females; *feminist ethics; human body; in vitro fertilization; infertility; information dissemination; males; methods; minority groups; mother fetus relationship; mothers; multiple pregnancy; ovum donors; parent child relationship; philosophy; postmodernism; pregnant women; prenatal diagnosis; reproduction; *reproductive technologies; secularism; selective abortion; semen donors; sexuality; social dominance; *social impact; surrogate mothers

Fein, Esther B. Calling infertility a disease, couples battle with insurers. [News]. *New York Times.* 1998 Feb 22: 1, 34. BE59611.

    drugs; embryo transfer; *health insurance reimbursement; in vitro fertilization; *infertility; *reproductive technologies;

personal financing; United States

Feldmann, Linda. The ethics of putting eggs on ice. [News]. *Christian Science Monitor.* 1997 Oct 20: 1, 18. BE59607.

    age factors; *cryopreservation; *ovum; ovum donors; property rights; reproductive technologies; risks and benefits

Fenwick, Lynda Beck. Private Choices, Public Consequences: Reproductive Technology and the New Ethics of Conception, Pregnancy, and Family. New York, NY: Dutton; 1998. 390 p. Bibliography: p. 377–380. ISBN 0-525-94263-7. BE62624.

    aborted fetuses; age factors; allowing to die; anencephaly; autonomy; brain death; cancer; cesarean section; cloning; congenital disorders; criminal law; *decision making; drug abuse; drugs; fetal therapy; fetal tissue donation; fetuses; genetic counseling; genetic disorders; ·genetic screening; government regulation; legal aspects; mass media; maternal health; multiple pregnancy; newborns; organ donation; parental consent; parents; posthumous reproduction; pregnant women; prenatal diagnosis; prenatal injuries; prolongation of life; public opinion; *reproduction; *reproductive technologies; rights; selection for treatment; siblings; single persons; surrogate mothers; survey; treatment refusal; questionnaires; United States

Fine, Andrea. Fertility business hits Internet, weaving web of controversy. [News]. *Christian Science Monitor.* 1998 Sept 11: 3. BE60640.

    *advertising; commodification; *computer communication networks; females; *ovum donors; regulation; *remuneration; risk; *Internet

Fisher, Fleur; Sommerville, Ann. To everything there is a season? Are there medical grounds for refusing fertility treatment to older women? *In:* Harris, John; Holm, Søren, eds. The Future of Human Reproduction: Ethics, Choice, and Regulation. New York, NY: Oxford University Press; 1998: 203–220. 34 fn. ISBN 0-19-823761-8. BE61271.

    *age factors; attitudes; children; embryo transfer; *females; in vitro fertilization; infertility; legal aspects; maternal health; mortality; multiple pregnancy; ovum donors; *reproductive technologies; *selection for treatment; statistics; treatment outcome; life expectancy; Great Britain

Fisher, Ian. Bill would govern use of dead men's sperm. [News]. *New York Times.* 1998 Mar 7: B5. BE59612.

    advance directives; *cadavers; *government regulation; informed consent; legislation; *posthumous reproduction; *semen donors; state government; *New York

Fishman, Rachelle H.B. Infertility doctors use egg donors worldwide. [News]. *Lancet.* 1999 Feb 27; 353(9154): 736. BE61036.

    altruism; embryo transfer; *government regulation; in vitro fertilization; international aspects; legislation; *ovum donors; remuneration; scarcity; *Israel

Fishman, Rachelle H.B. Reproductive rights and risks in Israel. [News]. *Lancet.* 1998 Dec 19–26; 352(9145): 1998. BE60273.

    embryo transfer; government financing; guideline adherence; guidelines; low birth weight; morbidity; mortality; *multiple pregnancy; national health insurance; newborns; *reproductive technologies; risk; *Israel

Garcia, Sandra Anderson. Sociocultural and legal implications of creating and sustaining life through biomedical technology. *Journal of Legal Medicine.* 1996 Dec; 17(4): 469–525. 220 fn. BE61244.

    abortion, induced; allowing to die; bioethics; biomedical research; *biomedical technologies; cultural pluralism;

BE = bioethics accession number   fn. = footnotes   refs. = references

decision making; determination of death; disadvantaged; fetal research; futility; genetic counseling; *genetic intervention; genetic screening; genome mapping; intensive care units; international aspects; investigators; justice; law; legal aspects; minority groups; misconduct; newborns; physicians; political activity; prolongation of life; public policy; religion; reproduction; *reproductive technologies; resource allocation; rights; science; selection for treatment; socioeconomic factors; withholding treatment; United States

Gibbons, John A. Who's your daddy?: a constitutional analysis of post-mortem insemination. [Comment]. *Journal of Contemporary Health Law and Policy.* 1997 Fall; 14(1): 187–210. 195 fn. BE60880.
 artificial insemination; children; *constitutional law; cryopreservation; embryo transfer; fathers; in vitro fertilization; *legal aspects; *legal rights; legislation; married persons; parent child relationship; *posthumous reproduction; privacy; public policy; *reproductive technologies; semen donors; single persons; sperm; surrogate mothers; *United States

Gilbert, Bonny. Infertility and the ADA: health insurance coverage for infertility treatment. *Defense Council Journal.* 1996; 63(1): 42–57. 80 fn. BE59349.
 *disabled; drugs; economics; federal government; *health insurance reimbursement; *infertility; *legal aspects; legal rights; legislation; *patient care; *reproductive technologies; standards; state government; surgery; *Americans with Disabilities Act 1990; *United States

Golden, Frederic; Silver, Lee M. Boy? Girl? Up to you [and] A quandary that isn't. *Time.* 1998 Sep 21; 152(12): 82–83. BE60858.
 females; males; *reproductive technologies; *sex preselection; social impact; sperm

Golden, Frederic. The ice babies: long–lost frozen embryos are popping up all over. [News]. *Time.* 1998 Mar 2; 151(8): 65. BE59166.
 *cryopreservation; *embryo transfer; *embryos; in vitro fertilization; *time factors; United States

Gosden, Roger. Designing Babies: The Brave New World of Reproductive Technology. New York, NY: W.H. Freeman; 1999. 260 p. Bibliography: p. 247–254. ISBN 0–7167–3299–8. BE62625.
 age factors; attitudes; autonomy; cloning; congenital disorders; embryos; eugenics; evolution; family planning; females; gene therapy; genetic disorders; *genetic enhancement; *genetic intervention; genetic screening; genetics; germ cells; government regulation; historical aspects; males; methods; parent child relationship; preimplantation diagnosis; prenatal diagnosis; privacy; public policy; reproduction; *reproductive technologies; *risks and benefits; science; selective abortion; sex determination; sex preselection; social control; social impact; surrogate mothers

Great Britain. Human Fertilisation and Embryology Authority. Code of Practice. Fourth Edition. London: The Authority; 1998. 76 p. Revised Jul 1998. Includes references. BE60713.
 age factors; AIDS serodiagnosis; artificial insemination; cancer; competence; confidentiality; counseling; cryopreservation; disclosure; embryo disposition; embryo research; embryo transfer; embryos; forms; genetic counseling; genetic screening; germ cells; *government regulation; *guidelines; *health facilities; health personnel; informed consent; ovum donors; patient access to records; *practice guidelines; records; *reproductive technologies; selection for treatment; semen donors; *standards; surrogate mothers; *Great Britain; Human Fertilisation and Embryology Act 1990; *Human Fertilisation and Embryology Authority

Great Britain. Human Fertilisation and Embryology Authority. Sixth Annual Report [1995–1996]. London: The Authority; 1997. 45 p. Includes references. "This report covers the year beginning 1 Nov 1995 with a foreward look for the year beginning 1 Nov 1996." BE60714.
 age factors; artificial insemination; cloning; cryopreservation; *embryo research; embryos; genetic screening; *government regulation; guidelines; *health facilities; HIV seropositivity; *in vitro fertilization; information dissemination; informed consent; posthumous reproduction; preimplantation diagnosis; remuneration; *reproductive technologies; semen donors; sperm; *standards; statistics; *Great Britain; Human Fertilisation and Embryology Act 1990; *Human Fertilisation and Embryology Authority

Gross, Jane. The fight to cover infertility: suit says employer's refusal to pay is form of bias. [News]. *New York Times.* 1998 Dec 7: B1, B6. BE60367.
 *employment; *health insurance reimbursement; infertility; *legal aspects; *reproductive technologies; social discrimination; Equal Employment Opportunity Commission; New York; Saks, Rochelle; United States

Grubb, Andrew. Infertility treatment: access and judicial review -- R v. Sheffield Health Authority, ex parte Seale. [Comment]. *Medical Law Review.* 1996 Autumn; 4(3): 326–329. BE61516.
 *age factors; females; *government financing; *in vitro fertilization; *judicial action; *legal aspects; *public policy; refusal to treat; *reproductive technologies; *resource allocation; *selection for treatment; *Great Britain; National Health Service; *R v. Sheffield Health Authority, ex parte Seale

Grubb, Andrew. Use of fetal eggs and infertility treatment: Human Fertilisation and Embryology Act 1990, section 3A. [Comment]. *Medical Law Review.* 1995 Summer; 3(2): 203–204. BE59254.
 aborted fetuses; criminal law; embryo transfer; embryos; *fetal tissue donation; germ cells; *government regulation; in vitro fertilization; *legislation; *ovum; *reproductive technologies; *Great Britain; *Human Fertilisation and Embryology Act 1990

Gunning, Jennifer. Oocyte donation: the legislative framework in Western Europe. [Article and discussion]. *Human Reproduction.* 1998 May; 13(Suppl. 2): 98–104. 2 refs. BE61485.
 aborted fetuses; cadavers; confidentiality; cryopreservation; *government regulation; *international aspects; *legislation; married persons; *ovum donors; *reproductive technologies; single persons; *tissue donation; Austria; Denmark; *Europe; France; Germany; Great Britain; Human Fertilisation and Embryology Act 1990; Norway; Spain; Sweden; Switzerland

Handwerker, Lisa. Health commodification and the body politic: the example of female infertility in modern China. *In:* Donchin, Anne; Purdy, Laura M., eds. Embodying Bioethics: Recent Feminist Advances. Lanham, MD: Rowman and Littlefield; 1999: 141–157. 37 refs. 5 fn. ISBN 0–8476–8924–7. BE61019.
 *commodification; economics; eugenics; family planning; *females; feminist ethics; government regulation; health insurance reimbursement; indigents; *infertility; mandatory programs; physicians; population control; psychological stress; public policy; reproduction; *reproductive technologies; risks and benefits; social control; women's health; ethnographic studies; *China

Harris, John. Doctors' orders, rationality and the good life: commentary on Savulescu. *Journal of Medical Ethics.*

1999 Apr; 25(2): 127–129. 7 fn. BE61915.
*autonomy; *beneficence; cloning; conscience; *decision making; *embryo transfer; freedom; in vitro fertilization; moral complicity; *moral obligations; moral policy; *motivation; parents; patients; *physicians; *preimplantation diagnosis; *reproduction; *reproductive technologies; *values; rationality

Harris, John. Rights and reproductive choice. *In:* Harris, John; Holm, Søren, eds. The Future of Human Reproduction: Ethics, Choice, and Regulation. New York, NY: Oxford University Press; 1998: 5–37. 62 fn. ISBN 0-19-823761-8. BE61260.
aborted fetuses; age factors; *autonomy; cadavers; cloning; embryo transfer; embryos; eugenics; fetal tissue donation; freedom; genetic enhancement; genetic screening; government regulation; legal aspects; methods; minority groups; ovum donors; parental consent; posthumous reproduction; preimplantation diagnosis; prenatal diagnosis; *public policy; remuneration; *reproductive technologies; rights; selection for treatment; selective abortion; semen donors; sex determination; social control; tissue donation; embryo splitting; nuclear transplantation; ovaries; Great Britain

Harris, John; Holm, Søren, eds. The Future of Human Reproduction: Ethics, Choice, and Regulation. New York, NY: Oxford University Press; 1998. 254 p.. (Issues in biomedical ethics). Bibliography: p. 248–251 ISBN 0-19-823761-8. BE61259.
aborted fetuses; abortion, induced; age factors; autonomy; beginning of life; cadavers; cryopreservation; decision making; embryo disposition; embryo research; embryos; eugenics; fetal research; fetal tissue donation; informed consent; international aspects; Islamic ethics; justice; moral policy; National Socialism; obligations of society; ovum donors; personhood; posthumous reproduction; preimplantation diagnosis; property rights; public policy; reproduction; *reproductive technologies; resource allocation; selection for treatment; social control; sperm; women's rights

Hartouni, Valerie. Cultural Conceptions: On Reproductive Technologies and the Remaking of Life. Minneapolis, MN: University of Minnesota Press; 1997. 175 p. Bibliography: p. 157–170. ISBN 0-8166-2623-5. BE62771.
*abortion, induced; adoption; audiovisual aids; behavioral genetics; blacks; brain death; *cloning; disadvantaged; embryos; eugenics; *fetuses; genetic intervention; legal aspects; mass media; mothers; parent child relationship; personhood; political activity; posthumous reproduction; postmodernism; *pregnant women; prenatal diagnosis; prolongation of life; *reproduction; *reproductive technologies; social discrimination; *social impact; socioeconomic factors; Supreme Court decisions; *surrogate mothers; value of life; values; violence; women's rights; In re Baby M; Johnson v. Calvert; Right to Life Movement; S'Aline's Solution; The Bell Curve (Herrnstein, R.; Murray, C.); *United States

Hayes, Edward J.; Hayes, Paul J.; Kelly, Dorothy Ellen, et al. Principles relating to the origin of life. *In: their* Catholicism and Ethics. Norwood, MA: C.R. Publications; 1997: 79–119. Includes discussion questions and projects. References embedded in list at back of book. ISBN 0-9649087-7-8. BE61946.
abortion, induced; artificial insemination; clergy; cloning; *contraception; double effect; family planning; health personnel; historical aspects; in vitro fertilization; infertility; marital relationship; methods; prenatal diagnosis; reproduction; *reproductive technologies; *Roman Catholic ethics; sexuality; surrogate mothers; value of life

Hildt, Elisabeth; Mieth, Dietmar, eds. In Vitro

Fertilisation in the 1990s: Towards a Medical, Social and Ethical Evaluation. Brookfield, VT: Ashgate; 1998. 370 p. Includes references. This book is a collection of the lectures delivered at the symposium, "IVF in the 90s -- Methods, Contexts, Consequences," which was organized by the European Network for Biomedical Ethics and held in Stuttgart, Germany, 16–19 Jan 1997. ISBN 1-85972-685-2. BE61311.
alternatives; attitudes; autonomy; bioethics; counseling; cultural pluralism; decision making; directive counseling; embryo disposition; embryo research; *embryo transfer; embryos; evaluation; females; gene therapy; government regulation; historical aspects; *in vitro fertilization; infertility; males; moral obligations; multiple pregnancy; patients; preimplantation diagnosis; psychological stress; reproduction; *reproductive technologies; rights; selective abortion; statistics; treatment outcome; dignity; Europe

Hopkins, Patrick D., ed.; Tennessee. Supreme Court, at Knoxville. (Re)locating fetuses: technology and new body politics. *In: his* Sex/Machine: Readings in Culture, Gender, and Technology. Bloomington, IN: Indiana University Press; 1998: 171–235. 33 refs. 84 fn. ISBN 0-253-21230-8. BE62290.
*abortion, induced; alternatives; contracts; *cryopreservation; *embryo disposition; embryo transfer; *embryos; *females; feminist ethics; fetuses; human experimentation; *in vitro fertilization; infertility; intention; *legal aspects; *males; *methods; mother fetus relationship; parent child relationship; personhood; pregnant women; privacy; property rights; *reproductive technologies; *required request; *rights; *risks and benefits; social discrimination; social impact; viability; women's rights; divorce; *ectogenesis; *Davis v. Davis; Tennessee; United States

Jordan, Mary; Sullivan, Kevin. Japan takes dim view of fertility treatments. [News]. *Washington Post.* 1998 Jul 5: A13. BE59623.
artificial insemination; *attitudes; children; family relationship; in vitro fertilization; *infertility; informal social control; misconduct; organizational policies; ovum donors; physicians; professional organizations; religion; *reproductive technologies; semen donors; stigmatization; *Japan; Japan Society of Obstetrics and Gynecology; Netsu, Yahiro

Kakkar, Supriya. Unauthorized embryo transfer at the University of California, Irvine Center for Reproductive Health. [Note]. *Hastings Constitutional Law Quarterly.* 1997 Summer; 24(4): 1015–1033. 168 fn. BE62167.
children; constitutional law; contracts; cryopreservation; embryo disposition; *embryo transfer; embryos; genetic materials; health facilities; in vitro fertilization; industry; *legal aspects; *misconduct; *parent child relationship; physicians; privacy; property rights; *reproductive technologies; standards; *United States; *University of California, Irvine Center for Reproductive Health

Kennedy, Randy. U.S. agency says employer should pay for a woman's infertility treatments. [News]. *New York Times.* 1999 Apr 29: B3. BE61697.
*employment; federal government; *health insurance reimbursement; infertility; *legal aspects; *reproductive technologies; social discrimination; *Equal Employment Opportunity Commission; New York; Saks, Rochelle; *United States

Kerr, Susan M.; Caplan, Arthur; Polin, Glenn, et al. Postmortem sperm procurement. *Journal of Urology.* 1997 Jun; 157(6): 2154–2158. 9 refs. BE60194.
clinical ethics committees; *cryopreservation; decision making; *health facilities; institutional policies; *knowledge, attitudes, practice; married persons; methods; physicians; *posthumous reproduction; reproductive technologies;

BE = bioethics accession number   fn. = footnotes   refs. = references

*semen donors; *sperm; statistics; survey; time factors; questionnaires; Canada; United States

Kettner, Matthias; Schäfer, Dieter. Identifying moral perplexity in reproductive medicine: a discourse ethics rationale. *Human Reproduction and Genetic Ethics: An International Journal.* 1998; 4(1): 8–17. 46 refs. BE59799.
consensus; cryopreservation; cultural pluralism; embryo disposition; embryo research; embryos; goals; in vitro fertilization; moral obligations; *morality; parent child relationship; parents; physicians; preimplantation diagnosis; reproduction; *reproductive technologies; value of life

Khamsi, Firouz; Endman, Maxine W.; Lacanna, Iara C., et al. Some psychological aspects of oocyte donation from known donors on altruistic basis. *Fertility and Sterility.* 1997 Aug; 68(2): 323–327. 12 refs. BE60334.
*altruism; *attitudes; confidentiality; disclosure; emotions; females; gifts; *motivation; *ovum donors; *patients; psychology; social interaction; survey; Ontario

Kolata, Gina. Harrowing choices accompany advancements in fertility. [News]. *New York Times.* 1998 Mar 10: F3. BE59617.
*embryo transfer; government regulation; health facilities; in vitro fertilization; incentives; institutional policies; international aspects; *multiple pregnancy; physicians; *reproductive technologies; risks and benefits; selective abortion; statistics; twins; Australia; Europe; Great Britain; *United States

Kolata, Gina. Price soars for eggs, setting off a debate on a clinic's ethics. [News]. *New York Times.* 1998 Feb 25: A1, A16. BE59618.
health facilities; incentives; institutional policies; *ovum donors; *remuneration; risk; scarcity; St. Barnabas Medical Center (Livingston, NJ)

Kolata, Gina. $50,000 offered to tall, smart egg donor. [News]. *New York Times.* 1999 Mar 3: A10. BE62649.
*advertising; commodification; eugenics; incentives; *ovum donors; *patients; *remuneration; universities

Little, Margaret Olivia. Let me count the ways: feminism illuminating bioethics. [Book review essay]. *Medical Humanities Review.* 1997 Spring; 11(1): 76–81. BE59967.
abortion, induced; adoption; bioethical issues; *bioethics; drug abuse; employment; ethical theory; females; *feminist ethics; fetuses; HIV seropositivity; human experimentation; justice; males; parent child relationship; pregnant women; prenatal injuries; public policy; *reproduction; *reproductive technologies; rights; selection of subjects; social discrimination; *Feminism and Bioethics: Beyond Reproduction (Wolf, S.M., ed.); *Reproduction, Ethics, and the Law (Callahan, J.C., ed.)

Lyman, Rick. As octuplets remain in peril, ethics questions are raised. [News]. *New York Times.* 1998 Dec 22: A1, A22. BE60374.
drugs; morbidity; *multiple pregnancy; newborns; *reproductive technologies; risk; treatment outcome; Chukwu, Nkem; Texas

McDonnell, Orla. Ethical and social implications of technology in medicine: new possibilities and new dilemmas. *In:* Cleary, Anne; Treacy, Margaret P., eds. The Sociology of Health and Illness in Ireland. Dublin: University College of Dublin Press; 1997: 69–84. 13 refs. 4 fn. ISBN 1-900621-11-8. BE60509.
*allowing to die; artificial feeding; attitudes to death; autonomy; *biomedical technologies; decision making; determination of death; guidelines; infertility; killing; legal aspects; married persons; *mass media; patient advocacy; persistent vegetative state; physicians; privacy;

*prolongation of life; quality of life; *reproductive technologies; *right to die; selection for treatment; self regulation; *social impact; sociology of medicine; *values; withholding treatment; In re a Ward of Court; *Ireland

Mackler, Aaron L. An expanded partnership with God? In vitro fertilization in Jewish ethics. *Journal of Religious Ethics.* 1997 Fall; 25(2): 277–304. 76 refs. 16 fn. BE60304.
cryopreservation; embryo disposition; embryo research; *embryo transfer; embryos; fetal development; fetuses; genetic screening; *in vitro fertilization; *Jewish ethics; *married persons; maternal health; mental health; mothers; multiple pregnancy; *ovum donors; parent child relationship; personhood; *preimplantation diagnosis; prenatal diagnosis; reproduction; *reproductive technologies; risks and benefits; selective abortion; *semen donors; *theology; therapeutic abortion

Macklin, Ruth. Ethics, informed consent, and assisted reproduction. *Journal of Assisted Reproduction and Genetics.* 1995 Sep; 12(8): 484–490. 17 fn. BE60560.
autonomy; competence; comprehension; *contraception; cryopreservation; cultural pluralism; decision making; developing countries; *disclosure; embryo disposition; embryos; ethical relativism; females; in vitro fertilization; infertility; *informed consent; mentally retarded; multiple pregnancy; ovum donors; parent child relationship; physicians; professional competence; *reproductive technologies; risks and benefits; surrogate mothers; treatment outcome; values; Western World

Marsiglio, William. Pathways to paternity and social fatherhood. *In: his* Procreative Man. New York, NY: New York University Press; 1998: 102–146, 213–222. 148 fn. ISBN 0-8147-5579-8. BE61950.
adoption; attitudes; confidentiality; DNA fingerprinting; emotions; *fathers; females; infertility; legal aspects; *males; married persons; motivation; *parent child relationship; pregnant women; *reproduction; *reproductive technologies; rights; semen donors; sexuality; single persons; tissue banks; trends; paternity; United States

Mason, John Kenyon. The infertile woman. *In: his* Medico-Legal Aspects of Reproduction and Parenthood. Second Edition. Brookfield, VT: Ashgate; 1998: 227–250. 73 fn. ISBN 1-84104-065-8. BE61067.
aborted fetuses; advisory committees; age factors; costs and benefits; counseling; cryopreservation; embryo disposition; embryo research; embryo transfer; fathers; *females; gamete intrafallopian transfer; *government regulation; in vitro fertilization; *infertility; *legal aspects; moral policy; multiple pregnancy; organ donation; ovum donors; parent child relationship; parental consent; public policy; *reproductive technologies; research embryo creation; resource allocation; selection for treatment; selective abortion; semen donors; time factors; ovaries; *Great Britain; *Human Fertilisation and Embryology Act 1990; *Human Fertilisation and Embryology Authority; Human Tissue Act 1961 (Great Britain); National Health Service; Warnock Committee

Melo–Martín, Immaculada de. Making Babies: Biomedical Technologies, Reproductive Ethics, and Public Policy. Boston, MA: Kluwer Academic; 1998. 199 p. Includes references. ISBN 0-7923-5116-9. BE61842.
advisory committees; common good; disclosure; ethical theory; *evaluation; *in vitro fertilization; infertility; informed consent; *international aspects; legal aspects; methods; *public policy; *reproductive technologies; *risks and benefits; social impact; *technology assessment; treatment outcome; uncertainty; women's health; Australia; Canada; Europe; Great Britain; Spain; United States

Merchant, Jennifer. Confronting the consequences of

BE = bioethics accession number   fn. = footnotes   refs. = references

medical technology: policy frontiers in the United States and France. *In:* Githens, Marianne; Stetson, Dorothy McBride, eds. Abortion Politics: Public Policy in Cross–Cultural Perspective. New York, NY: Routledge; 1996: 189–209. 32 fn. ISBN 0-415-91225-3. BE60711.
   abortion, induced; advisory committees; comparative studies; cryopreservation; embryo disposition; *embryo research; eugenics; federal government; feminist ethics; *fetal research; fetuses; government financing; in vitro fertilization; infertility; international aspects; *legal aspects; legal liability; personhood; physicians; pregnant women; prenatal diagnosis; prenatal injuries; *public policy; *reproductive technologies; selective abortion; surrogate mothers; *women's rights; wrongful life; *France; *United States

Michaels, Meredith W. Other mothers: toward an ethic of postmaternal practice. *Hypatia.* 1996 Spring; 11(2): 49–70. 51 refs. 13 fn. BE61457.
   coercion; commodification; contracts; *females; *feminist ethics; *informal social control; males; mothers; *reproductive technologies; sexuality; social dominance; *surrogate mothers

Michie, Helena; Cahn, Naomi R. Confinements: Fertility and Infertility in Contemporary Culture. New Brunswick, NJ: Rutgers University Press; 1997. 187 p. Bibliography: p. 171–177. ISBN 0-8135-2433-4. BE62628.
   autonomy; cesarean section; childbirth; coercion; criminal law; dehumanization; drug abuse; females; *feminist ethics; home care; hospitals; human body; indigents; *infertility; legal aspects; pain; parent child relationship; *pregnant women; prenatal diagnosis; prenatal injuries; *reproduction; *reproductive technologies; social control; *socioeconomic factors; United States

Mika, Karin; Hurst, Bonnie. One way to be born? Legislative inaction and the posthumous child. *Marquette Law Review.* 1996 Summer; 79(4): 993–1019. 223 fn. BE62221.
   artificial insemination; children; *fathers; historical aspects; international aspects; *legal aspects; parent child relationship; *posthumous reproduction; privacy; reproduction; Supreme Court decisions; Davis v. Davis; France; Hecht v. Superior Court; Parpalaix v. CECOS; Twentieth Century; Uniform Parentage Act; Uniform Status of Children of Assisted Conception Act; *United States

Naessens, Katrien. Egg donor, or seller? *Christian Science Monitor.* 1999 Apr 9: 11. BE61006.
   commodification; decision making; females; motivation; *ovum donors; *remuneration

Novaes, Simone Bateman; Salem, Tania. Embedding the embryo. *In:* Harris, John; Holm, Søren, eds. The Future of Human Reproduction: Ethics, Choice, and Regulation. New York, NY: Oxford University Press; 1998: 101–126. 30 fn. ISBN 0-19-823761-8. BE61265.
   abortion, induced; autonomy; case studies; *cryopreservation; *decision making; *embryo disposition; *embryo transfer; *embryos; family relationship; hospitals; *in vitro fertilization; legal aspects; married persons; mother fetus relationship; ovum donors; physicians; *posthumous reproduction; pregnant women; psychological stress; refusal to treat; *reproductive technologies; selection for treatment; semen donors; social sciences; *women's rights; France

Pennings, Guido. Age and assisted reproduction. *International Journal of Medicine and Law.* 1995; 14(7/8): 531–541. 20 fn. BE61004.
   *age factors; *females; males; *moral obligations; motivation; parent child relationship; *parents; reproduction;

*reproductive technologies; risks and benefits; *selection for treatment; social discrimination; time factors

Purdy, Laura M. Assisted reproduction. *In:* Kuhse, Helga; Singer, Peter, eds. A Companion to Bioethics. Malden, MA: Blackwell; 1998: 163–172. 43 refs. ISBN 0-631-19737-0. BE59492.
   artificial insemination; coercion; cryopreservation; disadvantaged; embryo transfer; females; feminist ethics; genetic materials; in vitro fertilization; methods; moral policy; morality; ovum donors; remuneration; *reproductive technologies; resource allocation; risks and benefits; semen donors; surrogate mothers

Resnik, David B. The commodification of human reproductive materials. *Journal of Medical Ethics.* 1998 Dec; 24(6): 388–393. 21 refs. BE60788.
   autonomy; *body parts and fluids; *commodification; *embryos; *genes; *genetic materials; *germ cells; human body; moral policy; ovum donors; patents; personhood; property rights; regulation; *remuneration; reproductive technologies; semen donors; tissue donation; transgenic organisms
This essay develops a framework for thinking about the moral basis for the commodification of human reproductive materials. It argues that selling and buying gametes and genes is morally acceptable although there should not be a market for zygotes, embryos, or genomes. Also a market in gametes and genes should be regulated in order to address concerns about the adverse social consequences of commodification.

Roberts, Dorothy E. The genetic tie. *University of Chicago Law Review.* 1995 Winter; 62(1): 209–273. 277 fn. BE62436.
   adoption; artificial insemination; *blacks; embryo transfer; family relationship; fathers; females; feminist ethics; *genetic identity; historical aspects; in vitro fertilization; *legal aspects; males; mothers; *parent child relationship; *reproduction; *reproductive technologies; semen donors; single persons; *social discrimination; *social worth; surrogate mothers; *whites; *personal identity; slavery; United States

Roberts, Melinda A. Present duties and future persons: when are existence–inducing acts wrong? *Law and Philosophy.* 1995 Nov; 14(3–4): 297–327. 50 fn. BE59358.
   adolescents; children; cloning; congenital disorders; contracts; embryo transfer; in vitro fertilization; injuries; judicial action; legal aspects; *moral policy; motivation; negligence; organ donation; parents; philosophy; physicians; quality of life; *reproduction; *reproductive technologies; surrogate mothers; value of life; *wrongful life

Robinson, John H.; Berry, Roberta M.; McDonnell, Kevin, eds. Reproduction. *In: their* A Health Law Reader: An Interdisciplinary Approach. Durham, NC: Carolina Academic Press; 1999: 73–180. 38 fn. ISBN 0-89089-907-X. BE62292.
   *abortion, induced; attitudes; autonomy; children; cloning; *commodification; dehumanization; disabled; eugenics; family relationship; feminist ethics; fetuses; *freedom; gene therapy; *genetic intervention; genetic screening; government regulation; legal aspects; minority groups; *moral policy; morality; parent child relationship; personhood; prenatal diagnosis; *public policy; *reproduction; *reproductive technologies; rights; selective abortion; sex determination; sexuality; Supreme Court decisions; surrogate mothers; value of life; Roe v. Wade; United States

Rojanksy, Nathan; Schenker, Joseph G. Ethical aspects of assisted reproduction in AIDS patients. *Journal of Assisted Reproduction and Genetics.* 1995 Sep; 12(8):

537–542. 48 refs. BE60567.

*AIDS; AIDS serodiagnosis; artificial insemination; confidentiality; counseling; directive counseling; females; *HIV seropositivity; informed consent; ovum donors; physicians; privacy; refusal to treat; reproduction; *reproductive technologies; semen donors; partner notification

Savulescu, Julian. Should doctors intentionally do less than the best? *Journal of Medical Ethics.* 1999 Apr; 25(2): 121–126. 11 fn. BE61914.

artificial insemination; *autonomy; *beneficence; *cloning; *congenital disorders; conscience; *decision making; disabled; *embryo transfer; eugenics; freedom; *genetic disorders; *goals; in vitro fertilization; *medicine; mentally retarded; *moral complicity; *moral obligations; moral policy; *motivation; parent child relationship; *parents; *patients; *physicians; *preimplantation diagnosis; *quality of life; refusal to treat; *reproduction; *reproductive technologies; rights; selection for treatment; sex preselection; suffering; *values; rationality

The papers of Burley and Harris, and Draper and Chadwick, in this issue, raise a problem: what should doctors do when patients request an option which is not the best available? This commentary argues that doctors have a duty to offer that option which will result in the individual affected by that choice enjoying the highest level of wellbeing. Doctors can deviate from this duty and submaximise –– bring about an outcome that is less than the best –– only if there are good reasons to do so. The desire to have a child which is genetically related provides little, if any, reason to submaximise. The implication for cloning, preimplantation diagnosis and embryo transfer is that doctors should only produce a clone or transfer embryos expected to enjoy a level of wellbeing which is less than that enjoyed by other children the couple could have, if there is a good reason to employ that technology. This paper sketches what might constitute a good reason to submaximise.

Schenker, Joseph G. Sperm, oocyte, and pre-embryo donation. *Journal of Assisted Reproduction and Genetics.* 1995 Sep; 12(8): 499–508. 16 refs. BE60562.

aborted fetuses; age factors; artificial insemination; confidentiality; *donors; embryo transfer; *embryos; females; genetic materials; guidelines; in vitro fertilization; infertility; informed consent; males; medical records; ovum; *ovum donors; public policy; religious ethics; remuneration; *reproductive technologies; selection for treatment; *semen donors; single persons; sperm; tissue banks; tissue donation

Serour, Gamal I. Reproductive choice: a Muslim perspective. *In:* Harris, John; Holm, Søren, eds. The Future of Human Reproduction: Ethics, Choice, and Regulation. New York, NY: Oxford University Press; 1998: 191–202. 37 fn. ISBN 0-19-823761-8. BE61270.

aborted fetuses; abortion, induced; age factors; contraception; *embryo research; females; *fetal research; fetal tissue donation; gene therapy; genetic counseling; genetic enhancement; *Islamic ethics; multiple pregnancy; *reproduction; *reproductive technologies; research embryo creation; selection for treatment; sex determination; sex preselection; *theology

Shah, Monica. Modern reproductive technologies: legal issues concerning cryopreservation and posthumous conception. *Journal of Legal Medicine.* 1996 Dec; 17(4): 547–571. 133 fn. BE61246.

children; *cryopreservation; *embryos; *germ cells; *legal aspects; legal rights; methods; ovum; parents; *posthumous reproduction; property rights; remuneration; *reproductive technologies; sperm; state government; wrongful death; *United States

Shenfield, F. Current ethical dilemmas in assisted reproduction. *International Journal of Andrology.* 1997; 20 (Suppl. 3): 74–78. 42 refs. BE60482.

cryopreservation; embryo disposition; embryos; international aspects; legal aspects; methods; posthumous reproduction; preimplantation diagnosis; *reproductive technologies; semen donors; sex preselection; sperm; intracytoplasmic sperm injection; Great Britain

Sher, Geoffrey; Davis, Virginia Marriage; Stoess, Jean. Ethical implications of fertility technology. *In: their* In Vitro Fertilization: The A.R.T. of Making Babies. Updated Edition. New York, NY: Facts on File; 1998: 168–181. ISBN 0-8160-3827-9. BE62397.

cryopreservation; embryos; in vitro fertilization; methods; ovum; preimplantation diagnosis; regulation; *reproductive technologies; risks and benefits; sperm

Simini, Bruno. Italy moves on with in-vitro fertilisation legislation. [News]. *Lancet.* 1999 Jun 5; 353(9168): 1950. BE62681.

age factors; cloning; cryopreservation; donors; embryo disposition; embryos; females; germ cells; *government regulation; *in vitro fertilization; *legal aspects; legal liability; *legislation; physicians; *reproductive technologies; selection for treatment; *Italy

Smith, George P. Assisted reproductive technologies: artificial insemination, surrogation, and *in vitro* fertilization. *In: his* Family Values and the New Society: Dilemmas of the 21st Century. Westport, CT: Praeger; 1998: 95–140. 252 fn. ISBN 0-275-96221-0. BE62297.

abortion, induced; advisory committees; *artificial insemination; confidentiality; contracts; cryopreservation; disclosure; embryo disposition; embryo research; embryos; fathers; federal government; fetal research; government financing; *government regulation; guidelines; *in vitro fertilization; infertility; informed consent; *legal aspects; parent child relationship; personhood; professional organizations; public policy; remuneration; *reproductive technologies; risks and benefits; semen donors; state government; *surrogate mothers; divorce; American Fertility Society; Davis v. Davis; Human Embryo Research Panel; In re Baby M; In re Marriage of Moschetta; Johnson v. Calvert; *United States

Smith, George P. Testing the limits of procreational autonomy. *In: his* Family Values and the New Society: Dilemmas of the 21st Century. Westport, CT: Praeger; 1998: 69–92. 140 fn. ISBN 0-275-96221-0. BE62296.

abortion, induced; artificial insemination; autonomy; contraception; cryopreservation; cultural pluralism; embryo research; embryo transfer; embryos; family relationship; federal government; fetal research; government regulation; *in vitro fertilization; *legal aspects; married persons; privacy; public policy; religion; reproduction; *reproductive technologies; risks and benefits; Roman Catholic ethics; selection for treatment; single persons; state interest; surrogate mothers; value of life; values; United States

Smith, Orla. Theatre: a gamete gambol. *Science.* 1999 Jul 2; 285(5424): 56. BE62332.

*literature; methods; *reproductive technologies; *intracytoplasmic sperm injection; *An Immaculate Misconception (Djerassi, Carl)

Snyder, Rebecca S. Reproductive technology and stolen ova: who is the mother? [Note]. *Law and Inequality.* 1998 Winter; 16(1): 289–334. 305 fn. BE62432.

children; germ cells; health facilities; *legal rights; malpractice; misconduct; *mothers; ovum donors; *parent child relationship; physicians; property rights; reproduction; *reproductive technologies; *standards; *United States

---

BE = bioethics accession number   fn. = footnotes   refs. = references

Steinbock, Bonnie. A philosopher looks at assisted reproduction. *Journal of Assisted Reproduction and Genetics.* 1995 Sep; 12(8): 543–551. 45 fn. BE60568.

> economics; embryo disposition; embryos; *freedom; HIV seropositivity; in vitro fertilization; moral obligations; *moral policy; ovum donors; parent child relationship; personhood; *religious ethics; remuneration; *reproduction; *reproductive technologies; *rights; *risks and benefits; Roman Catholic ethics; selection for treatment; semen donors; sexuality; social discrimination; surrogate mothers; values; women's health; *women's rights; Robertson, John

Steinbock, Bonnie. Sperm as property. *In:* Harris, John; Holm, Søren, eds. The Future of Human Reproduction: Ethics; Choice, and Regulation. New York, NY: Oxford University Press; 1998: 150–161. 39 fn. ISBN 0-19-823761-8. BE61267.

> *artificial insemination; autonomy; body parts and fluids; commodification; *cryopreservation; decision making; dissent; *legal aspects; moral policy; *posthumous reproduction; *property rights; public policy; remuneration; reproduction; reproductive technologies; semen donors; *sperm; suicide; tissue banks; California; *Hecht v. Superior Court (Kane)

Stetson, Dorothy McBride. Feminist perspectives on abortion and reproductive technologies. *In:* Githens, Marianne; Stetson, Dorothy McBride, eds. Abortion Politics: Public Policy in Cross-Cultural Perspective. New York, NY: Routledge; 1996: 211–223. 25 refs. 1 fn. ISBN 0-415-91225-3. BE60712.

> *abortion, induced; autonomy; contraception; females; *feminist ethics; fetuses; freedom; international aspects; legal aspects; males; pregnant women; privacy; public policy; *reproductive technologies; rights; sexuality; social dominance; *women's rights; United States

Stewart, Gary P.; Cutrer, William R.; Demy, Timothy J., et al. Basic Questions on Sexuality and Reproductive Technology: When Is It Right to Intervene? Grand Rapids, MI: Kregel Publications; 1998. 77 p. (BioBasics series). 7 refs. 7 fn. ISBN 0-8254-3073-9. BE62738.

> adoption; artificial insemination; *Christian ethics; cloning; contraception; embryos; gamete intrafallopian transfer; in vitro fertilization; infertility; legal aspects; marital relationship; ovum donors; parent child relationship; preimplantation diagnosis; *reproductive technologies; semen donors; sexuality; surrogate mothers; intracytoplasmic sperm injection; zygote intrafallopian transfer

Sutcliffe, Alastair G.; Taylor, Brent; Grudzinskas, Gedis, et al. Children conceived by intracytoplasmic sperm injection. [Letter and response]. *Lancet.* 1998 Aug 15; 352(9127): 578–579. 7 refs. BE61081.

> *children; cryopreservation; evaluation studies; in vitro fertilization; infants; intelligence; *methods; *reproductive technologies; research design; risks and benefits; *sperm; *treatment outcome; *intracytoplasmic sperm injection

Swinn, Michael; Emberton, Mark; Ralph, David, et al. Retrieving semen from a dead patient: Utilitarianism in the absence of definitive guidelines; The patient was assaulted; Some ethical concerns were ignored; [and] An ethic of ambivalence. *BMJ (British Medical Journal).* 1998 Dec 5; 317(7172): 1583–1585. 7 refs. BE60233.

> advance directives; *brain death; *cadavers; case studies; competence; cryopreservation; family members; informed consent; married persons; physicians; *posthumous reproduction; *semen donors; sperm; third party consent; utilitarianism; Great Britain

Tizzard, Juliet. Reproductive technology: new ethical dilemmas and old moral prejudices. *In:* Lee, Ellie, ed.

Abortion Law and Politics Today. New York, NY: St. Martin's Press; 1998: 184–197. 12 refs. ISBN 0-312-21574-6. BE62338.

> advisory committees; beginning of life; clinical ethics committees; cryopreservation; decision making; embryo research; embryo transfer; embryos; fetal development; *government regulation; historical aspects; HIV seropositivity; in vitro fertilization; legal aspects; mass media; medical ethics; multiple pregnancy; posthumous reproduction; public participation; *public policy; *reproductive technologies; research ethics committees; selection for treatment; social impact; *Great Britain; Human Fertilisation and Embryology Act 1990 (Great Britain); *Human Fertilisation and Embryology Authority (Great Britain); Twentieth Century; *Warnock Committee

van Balen, Frank. Development of IVF children. *Developmental Review.* 1998 Mar; 18(1): 30–46. 42 refs. BE60348.

> attitudes; *children; congenital disorders; *empirical research; fathers; *in vitro fertilization; intelligence; international aspects; mothers; multiple pregnancy; *parent child relationship; psychology; *reproductive technologies; semen donors; *treatment outcome

Watts, Jonathan. In-vitro fertilisation guidelines fall behind the times. [News]. *Lancet.* 1999 Jan 23; 353(9149): 303. BE60392.

> *guideline adherence; *guidelines; *in vitro fertilization; married persons; obstetrics and gynecology; *organizational policies; ovum donors; physicians; professional organizations; regulation; *reproductive technologies; semen donors; *Japan; *Japan Society of Obstetrics and Gynecology

Weiss, Rick. Babies in limbo: law outpaced by fertility advances. [News]. *Washington Post.* 1998 Feb 8: A1, A16. BE59624.

> child abuse; children; counseling; cryopreservation; embryo transfer; *embryos; genetic disorders; *government regulation; health facilities; in vitro fertilization; informed consent; institutional ethics; *legal aspects; legal rights; mothers; ovum donors; *parent child relationship; parents; *posthumous reproduction; *property rights; records; *reproductive technologies; *risks and benefits; selection for treatment; semen donors; state government; surrogate mothers; *United States

Weiss, Rick. Fertility innovation or exploitation? *Washington Post.* 1998 Feb 9: A1, A12. BE59625.

> biomedical research; cancer; cryopreservation; disclosure; ethical review; females; government regulation; health facilities; *human experimentation; in vitro fertilization; *infertility; informed consent; laboratories; ovum; *private sector; *regulation; *reproductive technologies; research ethics committees; risks and benefits; *self regulation; standards; state government; ovaries; United States

Westergaard, Tine; Wohlfahrt, Jan; Aaby, Peter, et al. Population based study of rates of multiple pregnancies in Denmark, 1980–94. *BMJ (British Medical Journal).* 1997 Mar 15; 314(7083): 775–779. 27 refs. BE60231.

> age factors; childbirth; economics; low birth weight; morbidity; mortality; *multiple pregnancy; newborns; pregnant women; prematurity; *reproductive technologies; *social impact; statistics; *trends; twins; retrospective studies; *Denmark

OBJECTIVE: To study trends in multiple pregnancies not explained by changes in maternal age and parity patterns. DESIGN: Trends in population based figures for multiple pregnancies in Denmark studied from complete national records on parity history and vital status. POPULATION: 497,979 Danish women and 803,019 pregnancies, 1980–94. MAIN OUTCOME

BE = bioethics accession number   fn. = footnotes   refs. = references

MEASURES: National rates of multiple pregnancies, infant mortality, and stillbirths controlled for maternal age and parity. Special emphasis on primiparous women greater than or = 30 years of age, who are most likely to undergo fertility treatment. RESULTS: The national incidence of multiple pregnancies increased 1.7-fold during 1980–94, the increase primarily in 1989–94 and almost exclusively in primiparous women aged greater than or = 30 years, for whom the adjusted population based twinning rate increased 2.7-fold and the triplet rate 9.1-fold. During 1989–94, the adjusted yearly increase in multiple pregnancies for these women was 19% (95% confidence interval 16% to 21%) and in dizygotic twin pregnancies 25% (21% to 28%). The proportion of multiple births among infant deaths in primiparous women greater than or = 30 years increased from 11.5% to 26.9% during the study period. The total infant mortality, however, did not increase for these women because of a simultaneous significant decrease in infant mortality among singletons. CONCLUSIONS: A relatively small group of women has drastically changed the overall national rates of multiple pregnancies. The introduction of new treatments to enhance fertility has probably caused these changes and has also affected the otherwise decreasing trend in infant mortality. Consequently, the resources, both economical and otherwise, associated with these treatments go well beyond those invested in specific fertility enhancing treatments.

Wilder, Bruce L. Ethical issues related to the new reproductive technologies. *Current Opinion in Obstetrics and Gynecology.* 1995 Jun; 7(3): 199–202. 27 refs. BE62484.
  commodification; confidentiality; cryopreservation; embryos; eugenics; family relationship; fetal tissue donation; legal aspects; ovum donors; physician patient relationship; *reproductive technologies; selection for treatment; values

Wright, Robert; Gorney, Cynthia; Silver, Lee M., et al. Fertility for sale. *New York Times.* 1998 Mar 4: A21. BE59670.
  altruism; attitudes; drugs; females; health; incentives; *ovum donors; public policy; *remuneration; reproductive technologies; risk; risks and benefits; social discrimination; socioeconomic factors; surgery; United States

Yardley, Jim. Health officials investigating to determine how woman got the embryo of another. [News]. *New York Times.* 1999 Mar 31: B3. BE62698.
  blacks; cryopreservation; *embryo transfer; embryos; health facilities; in vitro fertilization; *negligence; physicians; whites; *Fasano, Donna; Nash, Lillian; New York; *Perry-Rogers, Deborah

A birth spurs debate on using sperm after death. [Editorial]. *New York Times.* 1999 Mar 27: All. BE60873.
  cadavers; cryopreservation; *informed consent; married persons; *posthumous reproduction; *semen donors; sperm; United States

Current European laws on gamete donation. *Human Reproduction.* 1998 May; 13(Suppl. 2): 105–134. BE61486.
  bone marrow; cadavers; cloning; confidentiality; cryopreservation; embryo research; embryo transfer; gene therapy; genetic counseling; genetic intervention; genetic screening; germ cells; *government regulation; health facilities; hybrids; informed consent; *international aspects; *legislation; organ donation; *ovum donors; posthumous reproduction; preimplantation diagnosis; prenatal diagnosis; *reproductive technologies; *semen donors; sex preselection; *tissue donation; Austria; Denmark; *Europe; France; Germany; Great Britain; Israel; Norway; Portugal; Spain;

Sweden; Switzerland

Fasten your seatbelts. [Editorial]. *New Scientist.* 1997 Dec 6; 156(2111): 3. BE60460.
  females; *posthumous reproduction; *reproductive technologies

Making Babies: A Frontline Television Program. [Videorecording]. Available from PBS Home Video, 1320 Braddock Pl., Alexandria, VA 22314; 1–800–328–PBS1; 1999. Videocassette; 58 min.; sd.; color; VHS. BE62650.
  age factors; cloning; cryopreservation; economics; embryo research; embryo transfer; eugenics; government regulation; homosexuals; in vitro fertilization; methods; motivation; multiple pregnancy; ovum donors; remuneration; *reproductive technologies; semen donors; single persons; sperm; tissue banks; treatment outcome; intracytoplasmic sperm injection

Too much of a good thing. [Editorial]. *New York Times.* 1998 Dec 23: A26. BE59775.
  drugs; economics; *multiple pregnancy; newborns; prematurity; *reproductive technologies; Chukwu octuplets

RESEARCH DESIGN
See under
  BEHAVIORAL RESEARCH/RESEARCH
    DESIGN
  HUMAN EXPERIMENTATION/RESEARCH
    DESIGN

RESEARCH ETHICS COMMITTEES *See* HUMAN EXPERIMENTATION/ETHICS COMMITTEES

RESOURCE ALLOCATION

See also SELECTION FOR TREATMENT

Binstock, Robert H. Old-age–based rationing: from rhetoric to risk? *Generations (American Society on Aging).* 1994 Winter; 18(4): 37–41. 41 refs. BE60550.
  *age factors; *aged; *economics; federal government; government financing; *health care delivery; justice; *public policy; quality of life; *resource allocation; *selection for treatment; terminal care; wedge argument; withholding treatment; Medicare; *United States

Bolan, Robert K.; Bessesen, Mary; McCollum, Marianne, et al. AIDS exceptionalism. [Letters and response]. *Annals of Internal Medicine.* 1999 Jan 5; 130(1): 79–80. 11 refs. BE61076.
  *AIDS; communicable diseases; drugs; *economics; federal government; government financing; health care; health insurance; HIV seropositivity; justice; medical education; patient care; political activity; public health; *public policy; *resource allocation; risks and benefits; *United States

Brown, Murray G. Rationing health care in Canada. *Annals of Health Law.* 1993; 2: 101–119. 22 fn. BE59829.
  compassion; costs and benefits; decision making; *economics; *government financing; *health care delivery; hospitals; justice; *national health insurance; organization and administration; physicians; private sector; *public policy; public sector; *resource allocation; treatment outcome; *values; needs; *Canada

Buchanan, Allen. Managed care: rationing without justice, but not unjustly. *Journal of Health Politics, Policy and Law.* 1998 Aug; 23(4): 617–634. 16 refs. Commented on by S.D. Goold, p. 687–695. BE59780.

BE = bioethics accession number   fn. = footnotes   refs. = references

contracts; costs and benefits; decision making; disadvantaged; disclosure; economics; ethical theory; gatekeeping; *health care; *health care delivery; health insurance; *institutional ethics; *justice; *managed care programs; *moral obligations; *moral policy; *physician's role; *private sector; proprietary health facilities; public participation; *public sector; *quality of health care; *resource allocation; *rights; *standards; terminology; *withholding treatment; *United States

Three ethical criticisms of managed care are often voiced: (1) by "skimming the cream" of the patient population, managed care organizations fail to discharge their obligations to improve access, or at least, to not worsen it; (2) managed care organizations engage in rationing, thereby depriving patients of care to which they are entitled; and (3) by pressuring physicians to ration care, managed care organizations interfere with physicians' fulfillment of their fiduciary obligations to provide the best care for each patient. This article argues that each of these criticisms is misconceived. The first rests on the false assumption that the health care system includes a workable division of responsibility regarding access that assigns obligations concerning access to managed care organizations. The second and third criticisms wrongly assume that we in the United States have taken the first step toward assuring equitable access to care for all, articulating a standard for what counts as an "adequate level of care" to which all are entitled. These three misguided criticisms obscure the most fundamental ethical flaw of managed care: the fact that it operates in an institutional setting within which no connection can be made between the activity of rationing and the basic requirements of justice.

Callahan, Daniel. Age, sex, and resource allocation. *In:* Walker, Margaret Urban, ed. Mother Time: Women, Aging, and Ethics. Lanham, MD: Rowman and Littlefield; 1999: 189–199. 9 fn. ISBN 0-8476-9260-4. BE61900.
> age factors; *aged; biomedical technologies; chronically ill; disabled; disadvantaged; *economics; federal government; *females; *government financing; *health care; *health care reform; health promotion; home care; justice; long–term care; males; mortality; public policy; quality of life; rehabilitation; *resource allocation; social discrimination; *women's health; *women's health services; Medicare; *United States

Callahan, Daniel. Must the young and old struggle over health care resources? *Journal Of Long Term Home Health Care.* 1996 Fall; 15(4): 4–14. Edited version of the annual Iago Galdston Lecture, presented at the New York Academy of Medicine on 3 Jun 1996. BE60947.
> *age factors; *aged; biomedical technologies; children; *economics; *health care; long–term care; moral obligations; obligations of society; public policy; *resource allocation; social impact; trends; withholding treatment; Medicare; United States

Cong, Yali. Ethical challenges in critical care medicine: a Chinese perspective. *Journal of Medicine and Philosophy.* 1998 Dec; 23(6): 581–600. 21 refs. 1 fn. BE62067.
> allowing to die; bioethics; *critically ill; decision making; *economics; family members; geographic factors; government financing; *health care delivery; hospitals; *intensive care units; justice; legal aspects; medical devices; non–Western World; patient admission; physician patient relationship; physicians; public policy; *resource allocation; values; personal financing; *China

The major ethical challenges for critical care medicine in China include the high cost of patient care in the ICU, the effect of payment mechanisms on access to critical care, the fact that much more money is spent on patients who die than on ones who live, the extent to which an attempt to rescue and save a patient is made, and the great geographical disparity in distribution of critical care. The ethical problems surrounding critical care medicine bear much relation to the culture, public policy and health care system in China. The essay concludes that China should allocate more resources to ordinary medical services rather than to critical care medicine.

Culpepper, Larry; Gilbert, Thomas T. Evidence and ethics. *Lancet.* 1999 Mar 6; 353(9155): 829–831. 10 refs. BE61220.
> biomedical technologies; chronically ill; costs and benefits; *decision making; diagnosis; *evidence–based medicine; *family practice; health care; health services research; human experimentation; iatrogenic disease; *medical specialties; medicine; patient advocacy; *patient care; patient participation; physician patient relationship; *physicians; practice guidelines; *primary health care; quality of life; random selection; research design; *resource allocation; *risks and benefits; treatment outcome; uncertainty; *values

de Beaufort, Inez. Individual responsibility for health. *In:* Bennett, Rebecca; Erin, Charles A., eds. HIV and AIDS: Testing, Screening, and Confidentiality. New York, NY: Oxford University Press; 1999: 107–124. 15 fn. ISBN 0-19-823801-0. BE62717.
> AIDS; alcohol abuse; autonomy; economics; *health; health care; health insurance; justice; *moral obligations; obligations of society; organ transplantation; physicians; *resource allocation; selection for treatment; *self induced illness; smoking; withholding treatment; personal financing; Netherlands

de Castro, Leonardo D.; Sy, Peter A. Critical care in the Philippines: the "Robin Hood principle" vs. *kagandahang loob. Journal of Medicine and Philosophy.* 1998 Dec; 23(6): 563–580. 14 refs. 2 fn. BE62066.
> allowing to die; attitudes; bioethical issues; biomedical technologies; *critically ill; decision making; developing countries; economics; emergency care; extraordinary treatment; *health care delivery; health maintenance organizations; hospitals; indigents; informed consent; international aspects; justice; legal aspects; newborns; non–Western World; nurses; obligations of society; organ donation; physicians; prolongation of life; public policy; religion; *resource allocation; *values; withholding treatment; *charity; technology transfer; *Philippines

Practical medical decisions are closely integrated with ethical and religious beliefs in the Philippines. This is shown in a survey of Filipino physicians' attitudes towards severely compromised neonates. This is also the reason why the ethical analysis of critical care practices must be situated within the context of local culture. Kagandahang loob and kusang loob are indigenous Filipino ethical concepts that provide a framework for the analysis of several critical care practices. The practice of taking-from-the-rich-to-give-to-the-poor in public hospitals is not compatible with these concepts. The legislated definition of death and other aspects of the Philippine Law on Organ Transplants also fail to be compatible with these concepts. Many ethical issues that arise in a critical care setting have their roots outside the seemingly isolated clinical setting. Critical care need not apply only to individuals in a serious clinical condition. Vulnerable populations require critical attention because potent threats to their lives exist in the water that they drink and the air that they breathe. We cannot ignore these threats even as we move inevitably towards a technologically dependent, highly commercialized approach to health management.

BE = bioethics accession number   fn. = footnotes   refs. = references

Dickens, Bernard M. Can doctors serve as double agents? [Editorial]. *Humane Health Care International.* 1997 Spring; 13(1): 8-9. 5 refs. BE59957.
*conflict of interest; *gatekeeping; legal aspects; *legal liability; negligence; patient advocacy; patient care; *physician's role; *physicians; *resource allocation; standards; Canada; Great Britain

Doyal, Len. Public participation and the moral quality of healthcare rationing. *Quality in Health Care.* 1998 Jun; 7(2): 98-102. 37 refs. BE62322.
*decision making; *democracy; futility; government financing; *health care delivery; health personnel; *justice; moral policy; patient participation; *public participation; *public policy; *resource allocation; rights; scarcity; needs; *Great Britain; *National Health Service

Fan, Ruiping. Critical care ethics in Asia: global or local? *Journal of Medicine and Philosophy.* 1998 Dec; 23(6): 549-562. 12 refs. 3 fn. BE62065.
autonomy; bioethical issues; bioethics; communitarianism; *critically ill; *cultural pluralism; decision making; developing countries; economics; ethical relativism; ethical theory; family members; *health care delivery; informed consent; intensive care units; *international aspects; *justice; libertarianism; morbidity; mortality; non-Western World; *quality of health care; *resource allocation; third party consent; utilitarianism; values; *Asia; China; Hong Kong; Japan; Philippines; Rawls, John; United States

Fears, Robin; Poste, George. Building population genetics resources using the U.K. NHS. *Science.* 1999 Apr 9; 284(5412): 267-268. 15 fn. BE61402.
confidentiality; *data banks; *DNA data banks; epidemiology; *genetic information; *genetic research; government financing; *health care delivery; *industry; informed consent; medical records; *population genetics; *private sector; *public policy; *public sector; regulation; research subjects; *resource allocation; tissue banks; pedigree studies; *Great Britain; *National Health Service

Finestone, Albert J.; Feldman, Debra; Beasley, John W., et al. Gatekeeping: good or bad, but never indifferent. [Letters and response]. *JAMA.* 1998 Mar 25; 279(12): 908-910. 6 refs. BE59233.
accountability; *attitudes; decision making; *economics; *gatekeeping; incentives; *managed care programs; organization and administration; patient advocacy; patient care; physician patient relationship; *physician's role; *physicians; preventive medicine; primary health care; professional autonomy; quality of health care; referral and consultation; remuneration; *resource allocation; *risks and benefits; trust; United States

Fisher, Carol; Gill, Denise. Limiting health care for the elderly. *Plastic Surgical Nursing.* 1996 Summer; 16(2): 113-116. 20 refs. BE60198.
*aged; beneficence; biomedical technologies; community services; costs and benefits; ethical analysis; ethical theory; government financing; *health care; hospitals; institutional policies; intensive care units; justice; moral policy; nurses; *resource allocation; selection for treatment; needs; Medicaid; Medicare; United States

Foster, Larry W.; McLellan, Linda J. Moral judgments in the rationing of health care resources: a comparative study of clinical health professionals. *Social Work in Health Care.* 1997; 25(4): 13-36. 56 refs. BE60341.
age factors; aged; *attitudes; comparative studies; costs and benefits; futility; health care; moral development; *nurses; *physicians; quality of life; *resource allocation; rights; selection for treatment; *social workers; social worth; survey; terminally ill; values; United States

Frazier, William D. Rationing of health care -- who determines who gets the cure, when, where, and why? *Annals of Health Law.* 1993; 2: 95-99. 9 fn. BE59828.
age factors; economics; health care; health care delivery; *resource allocation; *selection for treatment; social worth; United States

Fuchs, Victor R. Who Shall Live? Health, Economics, and Social Choice. Expanded Edition. River Edge, NJ: World Scientific; 1998. 278 p. (Economic ideas leading to the 21st century; v.3). Includes references. Six complementary papers dealing with national health insurance, poverty and health, and other policy issues, including Fuchs's 1996 presidential address to the American Economic Association, accompanying the original 1974 text. ISBN 981-02-3201-2. BE62770.
age factors; biomedical technologies; costs and benefits; *decision making; drug industry; drugs; *economics; employment; females; health; *health care delivery; *health care reform; health insurance; health maintenance organizations; historical aspects; hospitals; indigents; international aspects; males; morbidity; mortality; *national health insurance; organization and administration; physician's role; physicians; *public policy; *resource allocation; socioeconomic factors; values; *United States

Gross, Cary P.; Anderson, Gerard F.; Powe, Neil R. The relation between funding by the National Institutes of Health and the burden of disease. *New England Journal of Medicine.* 1999 Jun 17; 340(24): 1881-1887. 34 refs. BE62032.
age factors; AIDS; *biomedical research; breast cancer; comparative studies; decision making; dementia; depressive disorder; diabetes; diagnosis; disabled; *disease; federal government; financial support; *government financing; heart diseases; industry; morbidity; mortality; patient advocacy; political activity; prevalence; *resource allocation; schizophrenia; statistics; trends; values; *disability adjusted life years; *National Institutes of Health; *United States

BACKGROUND: The Institute of Medicine has proposed that the amount of disease-specific research funding provided by the National Institutes of Health (NIH) be systematically and consistently compared with the burden of disease for society. METHODS: We performed a cross-sectional study comparing estimates of disease-specific funding in 1996 with data on six measures of the burden of disease. The measures were total mortality, years of life lost, and number of hospital days in 1994 and incidence, prevalence, and disability-adjusted life-years (one disability-adjusted life-year is defined as the loss of one year of healthy life to disease) in 1990. With the use of these measures as explanatory variables in a regression analysis, predicted funding was calculated and compared with actual funding. RESULTS: There was no relation between the amount of NIH funding and the incidence, prevalence, or number of hospital days attributed to each condition or disease (P=0.82, P=0.23, and P=0.21, respectively). The numbers of deaths (r=0.40, P=0.03) and years of life lost (r=0.42, P=0.02) were weakly associated with funding, whereas the number of disability-adjusted life-years was strongly predictive of funding (r=0.62, P less than 0.001). When the latter three measures were used to predict expected funding, the conclusions about the appropriateness of funding for some diseases varied according to the measure used. However, the acquired immunodeficiency syndrome, breast cancer, diabetes mellitus, and dementia all received relatively generous funding, regardless of which measure was used as the basis for calculating support. Research on chronic obstructive pulmonary disease, perinatal conditions, and peptic ulcer was relatively

---

BE = bioethics accession number   fn. = footnotes   refs. = references

underfunded. CONCLUSIONS: The amount of NIH funding for research on a disease is associated with the burden of the disease; however, different measures of the burden of disease may yield different conclusions about the appropriateness of disease-specific funding levels.

Harris, John. Micro-allocation: deciding between patients. *In:* Kuhse, Helga; Singer, Peter, eds. A Companion to Bioethics. Malden, MA: Blackwell; 1998: 293–305. 12 refs. ISBN 0–631–19737–0. BE59504.
    *age factors; alcohol abuse; costs and benefits; decision making; disabled; health care; *justice; moral policy; obligations of society; quality adjusted life years; quality of life; *resource allocation; scarcity; *selection for treatment; *self induced illness; social discrimination; *social worth; needs

Holm, Søren. Goodbye to the simple solutions: the second phase of priority setting in health care. *BMJ (British Medical Journal).* 1998 Oct 10; 317(7164): 1000–1002. 6 refs. Presented at the Second International Conference on Priorities in Health Care held in London, 8–10 October 1998. BE60831.
    decision making; goals; government financing; *health care delivery; international aspects; *public policy; *resource allocation; severity of illness index; Denmark; Norway; *Scandinavia

Holm, Søren. Is society responsible for my health? *In:* Bennett, Rebecca; Erin, Charles A., eds. HIV and AIDS: Testing, Screening, and Confidentiality. New York, NY: Oxford University Press; 1999: 125–139. 23 fn. ISBN 0–19–823801–0. BE62718.
    AIDS; *health; *health care delivery; justice; moral obligations; *obligations of society; *resource allocation; self induced illness; state medicine; needs

Holmes, Colin A. QALYs: a nurse's view. *International Journal of Health Care Quality Assurance.* 1993; 6(5): 17–23. 28 refs. BE62253.
    age factors; chronically ill; commodification; costs and benefits; decision making; dehumanization; disabled; evaluation; health; health care; justice; nurses; politics; public policy; *quality adjusted life years; *quality of life; *resource allocation; social discrimination; socioeconomic factors; values; Great Britain

Jacobs, Lawrence; Marmor, Theodore; Oberlander, Jonathan. The Oregon Health Plan and the political paradox of rationing: what advocates and critics have claimed and what Oregon did. *Journal of Health Politics, Policy and Law.* 1999 Feb; 24(1): 161–180. 20 refs. 5 fn. BE61756.
    decision making; *economics; *evaluation; goals; *government financing; *health care delivery; *health reform; health insurance; *indigents; managed care programs; organ transplantation; policy analysis; political activity; *politics; public participation; *public policy; *resource allocation; standards; state government; withholding treatment; negotiation; universal coverage; *Oregon; *Oregon Health Plan; United States
The article proceeds in three sections. First, we very briefly review the original proposals and ensuing (and misleading) debate over rationing in Oregon. Next, we explore how the politics of rationing unfolded in Oregon from the enactment of OHP to its implementation. Finally, we consider the character of Oregon's innovation and the broader lessons that it holds for reform efforts elsewhere.

Joblin, Joseph. Health and the distribution of resources. *Dolentium Hominum: Church and Health in the World.*

1998; No. 37 [yr. 13(1)]: 63–68. 30 fn. BE61777.
    biomedical technologies; common good; developing countries; economics; *health; *health care; *human rights; indigents; international aspects; justice; morality; obligations of society; public policy; *resource allocation; *Roman Catholic ethics; socioeconomic factors; Western World

Jurevic, Amy. Disparate impact under Title VI: discrimination, by any other name, will still have the same impact. *Saint Louis University Public Law Review.* 1996; 15(2): 237–265. 260 fn. BE59909.
    *blacks; economics; federal government; females; *government financing; *government regulation; *health care delivery; hospitals; *indigents; institutional policies; *legal aspects; minority groups; morbidity; public policy; *resource allocation; selection for treatment; *social discrimination; *social impact; standards; state government; obesity; Civil Rights Act 1964; Department of Health and Human Services; *Medicaid; *Oregon; *Oregon Health Plan; *United States

Kapp, Marshall B. *De facto* health-care rationing by age: the law has no remedy. *Journal of Legal Medicine.* 1998 Sep; 19(3): 323–249. 152 fn. BE61250.
    *age factors; *aged; allowing to die; economics; future generations; government financing; health care; legal aspects; moral policy; *physicians; public policy; *resource allocation; *selection for treatment; *social discrimination; social impact; social worth; withholding treatment; duty to die; personal financing; Medicaid; Medicare; United States

Kegley, Jacquelyn Ann K. Community, autonomy, and managed care. *In:* McGee, Glenn, ed. Pragmatic Bioethics. Nashville, TN: Vanderbilt University Press; 1999: 204–227, 281–283. 31 fn. ISBN 0–8265–1321–2. BE60673.
    *autonomy; beneficence; biomedical technologies; caring; commodification; *common good; communication; cultural pluralism; decision making; disadvantaged; disease; *economics; freedom; health; *health care delivery; health education; informed consent; justice; *managed care programs; minority groups; paternalism; patient advocacy; patient care team; quality of health care; *resource allocation; social problems; trends; virtues; community consent; loyalty; quality assurance; *United States

Klein, Rudolf. Puzzling out priorities: why we must acknowledge that rationing is a political process. [Editorial]. *BMJ (British Medical Journal).* 1998 Oct 10; 317(7164): 959–960. 10 refs. BE60830.
    decision making; *health care delivery; international aspects; politics; *public policy; *resource allocation; *Great Britain; National Health Service

Kleinert, Sabine. Rationing of health care: how should it be done? [Commentary]. *Lancet.* 1998 Oct 17; 352(9136): 1244. 3 refs. Report on the Second International Conference on Priorities in Health Care held in London, 8–10 Oct 1998. BE60796.
    decision making; *evidence-based medicine; health care; *international aspects; public policy; *resource allocation; values

Kopelman, Loretta M. Help from Hume reconciling professionalism and managed care. *Journal of Medicine and Philosophy.* 1999 Aug; 24(4): 396–410. 28 refs. 8 fn. BE62616.
    age factors; beneficence; friends; *health care delivery; humanism; *justice; *managed care programs; medical ethics; minority groups; *moral obligations; moral policy; *obligations to society; *patient advocacy; philosophy; physician patient relationship; *physicians; *resource allocation; selection for treatment; social discrimination; socioeconomic factors; trust; *Hume, David; Rachels, James
Health care systems are widely criticized for limiting

BE = bioethics accession number   fn. = footnotes   refs. = references

doctors' roles as patient-advocates. Yet unrestricted advocacy can be unfairly partial, costly, and prejudicial. This essay considers three solutions to the problem of how to reconcile the demands of a just health care system for all patients, with the value of advocacy for some. Two views are considered and rejected, one supporting unlimited advocacy and another defending strict impartiality. A third view suggested by Hume's moral theory seeks to square the moral demands of professional advocacy and just health care systems. A moral basis for limited advocacy exists when it can be justified from a general or moral vantage. Consequently, ethical aspects of professionalism are not necessarily on a collision course with health care systems incorporating managed care. This solution is compatible with goals regarding the importance of humanistic education and professionalism to build patients' trust.

Kopelman, Loretta M.; Palumbo, Michael G. The U.S. health delivery system: inefficient and unfair to children. *American Journal of Law and Medicine.* 1997; 23(2-3): 319-337. 103 fn. BE62503.
>   age factors; biomedical technologies; *children; decision making; *economics; *ethical theory; *health care; *health care delivery; health insurance; immunization; indigents; infants; *justice; libertarianism; morbidity; mortality; obligations of society; parents; patient advocacy; physicians; preventive medicine; primary health care; public policy; *resource allocation; selection for treatment; standards; uncertainty; utilitarianism; egalitarianism; needs; *United States

Kosseff, Andrew L.; Gurewich, Victor; Moore, Michael R., et al. Managed care ethics. [Letters and response]. *Annals of Internal Medicine.* 1998 Oct 15; 129(8): 672-674. 3 refs. BE60076.
>   common good; conflict of interest; *decision making; *economics; *incentives; *managed care programs; medical ethics; *patient advocacy; physician patient relationship; *physicians; quality of health care; remuneration; *resource allocation; trust; withholding treatment; United States

Lamm, Richard D. Marginal medicine. *JAMA.* 1998 Sep 9; 280(10): 931-933. 14 refs. BE60284.
>   beneficence; *common good; disadvantaged; goals; *government financing; health; *health care delivery; health insurance; *managed care programs; medical ethics; moral obligations; obligations to society; patient advocacy; patient care; *physician's role; *public policy; *resource allocation; needs; United States

Lamm, Richard D. Redrawing the ethics map. *Hastings Center Report.* 1999 Mar-Apr; 29(2): 28-29. 5 refs. BE61659.
>   caring; *common good; *costs and benefits; economics; health; health care; *health care delivery; indigents; justice; medical ethics; patient advocacy; physicians; *public policy; *resource allocation; social problems; United States

Landman, Willem A.; Henley, Lesley D. Tensions in setting health care priorities for South Africa's children. *Journal of Medical Ethics.* 1998 Aug; 24(4): 268-273. 30 fn. BE61294.
>   beneficence; *children; chronically ill; costs and benefits; decision making; health; *health care; justice; legal aspects; long-term care; moral policy; preventive medicine; primary health care; public health; public participation; *public policy; quality of life; *resource allocation; standards; *health planning; needs; *South Africa

The new South African constitution commits the government to guarantee "basic health services" for every child under 18. Primary health care for pregnant women and children under six and elements of essential primary

health care have received priority. At present, there is little analysis of the moral considerations involved in making choices about more advanced or costly health care which may, arguably, also be "basic". This paper illustrates some of the tensions in setting priorities for a just macro-allocation of children's health care, given the realities of need and scarce resources, and the commitment to equality of basic opportunities.

Lears, Louise. The ethics and wisdom of collaboration. *Health Care Ethics USA.* 1998 Summer; 6(3): 6-7. 9 refs. BE60822.
>   economics; health care delivery; health maintenance organizations; health personnel; *interprofessional relations; medical specialties; *organization and administration; physicians; referral and consultation; *resource allocation

Lee, J.W.; Melgaard, Bjorn; Hull, Harry F., et al. Ethical dilemmas in polio eradication. *American Journal of Public Health.* 1998 Jan; 88(1): 130-132. 6 refs. BE62551.
>   *developing countries; economics; *immunization; *international aspects; *poliomyelitis; primary health care; public health; public policy; *resource allocation; World Health Organization

Leichter, Howard M. Oregon's bold experiment: whatever happened to rationing? *Journal of Health Politics, Policy and Law.* 1999 Feb; 24(1): 147-160. 17 refs. 18 fn. BE61755.
>   *evaluation; *government financing; *health care delivery; health care reform; *indigents; *managed care programs; *public policy; *resource allocation; standards; state government; withholding treatment; *Medicaid; *Oregon; *Oregon Health Plan

In 1994 Oregon began rationing health care for its Medicaid population, offering health policy makers and analysts around the country a view of one alternative future for health care delivery. The question now, four years after the experiment began, is what does that future look like? The short answer is that it does not look all that different from the present, but it looks different enough to offer important lessons to other states and the federal government. The Oregon experiment, including the prioritization of services and the aggressive use of managed care, has facilitated the expansion of health care coverage to over 100,000 additional Oregonians, helped decrease the percentage of the uninsured as well as reduce uncompensated care in hospitals, reduced the use of hospital emergency rooms, and reduced cost shifting. By most measures, the Oregon experiment appears to be a success.

Levinsky, Norman G. Can we afford medical care for Alice C? *Lancet.* 1998 Dec 5; 352(9143): 1849-1851. 13 refs. BE60805.
>   *age factors; *aged; allowing to die; biomedical technologies; case studies; *economics; futility; government financing; *health care; hospitals; intensive care units; justice; mortality; patient admission; prolongation of life; *public policy; quality of life; *resource allocation; social discrimination; socioeconomic factors; Medicare; *United States

MacLeod, Stuart M.; Bienenstock, John. Evidence-based rationing: Dutch pragmatism or government insensitivity? [Editorial]. *Canadian Medical Association Journal.* 1998 Jan 27; 158(2): 213-214. 5 refs. BE60582.
>   economics; *evidence-based medicine; *health care delivery; health services research; *public policy; quality of health care; *resource allocation; values; Canada; *Netherlands

---

McSherry, James; Dickie, Gordon L. Swords to ploughshares: gatekeepers turned advocates. [Editorial]. *Canadian Family Physician.* 1998 May; 44: 955–956. 5 refs. BE61851.
   costs and benefits; *economics; *gatekeeping; health care delivery; incentives; *patient advocacy; *physician's role; *physicians; *primary health care; *resource allocation; Canada

Malter, Alex; Sulmasy, Daniel P.; Schulman, Kevin A. Physician–assisted suicide. [Letter and response]. *Archives of Internal Medicine.* 1998 Dec 7–21; 158(22): 2513. 3 refs. BE61026.
   *assisted suicide; attitudes; economics; health care delivery; motivation; *physicians; public policy; *resource allocation; state government; suffering; terminally ill; rationality; Oregon; United States

Marchand, Sarah; Wikler, Daniel; Landesman, Bruce. Class, health and justice. *Milbank Quarterly.* 1998; 76(3): 449–467. 24 refs. BE59641.
   goals; *health; health care; health care delivery; indigents; international aspects; *justice; *moral policy; *obligations of society; *resource allocation; self induced illness; *socioeconomic factors; standards; egalitarianism
Class inequalities in health are intuitively unjust. Although the link between social class and health status has been fully documented, the precise nature of the injustice has not been made clear. Four alternative views are presented, corresponding to four goals: (1) maximizing the sum total of health; (2) equalizing the health status of higher and lower social classes; (3) maximizing the health status of the lowest social class; and (4) maximizing the health status of the sickest individuals in society. The nature of the injustice is further obscured by several theoretical and empirical questions, like the degree and significance of personal responsibility for illness and the relation of the degree of economic inequality to sum total of health.

Matthews, Dennis J.; Meier, Robert H.; Bartholome, William. Ethical issues encountered in pediatric rehabilitation. *Pediatrician.* 1990; 17(2): 108–114. 7 refs. BE59454.
   adolescents; allowing to die; autonomy; beneficence; *children; community services; congenital disorders; costs and benefits; decision making; *disabled; education; *goals; home care; injuries; justice; legal rights; newborns; normality; parents; *pediatrics; physicians; psychological stress; quality of life; *rehabilitation; *resource allocation; schools; selection for treatment; sexuality; uncertainty; withholding treatment

Mechanic, David. Muddling through elegantly: finding the proper balance in rationing. *Health Affairs.* 1997 Sep–Oct; 16(5): 83–92. 17 fn. BE59178.
   administrators; biomedical technologies; costs and benefits; cultural pluralism; decision making; *economics; evidence–based medicine; gatekeeping; government regulation; *health care delivery; international aspects; justice; managed care programs; *methods; national health insurance; physicians; political activity; politics; public opinion; *public policy; *resource allocation; socioeconomic factors; values; capitation fee; case managers; *Great Britain; Medicaid; National Health Service; Oregon Health Plan; *United States

Menzel, Paul; Gold, Marthe R.; Nord, Erik, et al. Toward a broader view of values in cost–effectiveness analysis of health. *Hastings Center Report.* 1999 May–Jun; 29(3): 7–15. 31 fn. BE61407.
   age factors; bioethics; chronically ill; *costs and benefits; critically ill; disabled; *economics; health; *health care;

justice; public participation; quality adjusted life years; quality of life; *resource allocation; selection for treatment; social discrimination; time factors; treatment outcome; utilitarianism; value of life; *values; hope; severity of illness index
By registering different health benefits on a common scale, CEA allows us to assess the relative social importance of different health care interventions and opens the way for the allocation decisions of health care policy. If it is really to be effective, however, CEA must be recalibrated so that it better reflects some of our widely held beliefs about the merits of different kinds of treatment.

Mooney, Gavin; Jan, Stephen. Vertical equity: weighing outcomes? or establishing procedures? *Health Policy.* 1997 Jan; 39(1): 79–87. 18 refs. BE59797.
   *communitarianism; decision making; economics; goals; health; *health care; *justice; *obligations of society; public participation; *resource allocation; rights; socioeconomic factors; treatment outcome; utilitarianism; values; Broome, John

Morris, Lynn; Martin, Desmond J.; Quinn, Thomas C., et al. The importance of doing HIV research in developing countries. *Nature Medicine.* 1998 Nov; 4(11): 1228–1229. 20 refs. BE62159.
   *AIDS; *biomedical research; *costs and benefits; *developing countries; drugs; economics; *HIV seropositivity; *human experimentation; newborns; patient care; pregnant women; preventive medicine; *resource allocation; *risks and benefits; sexually transmitted diseases; *Africa; AZT

Newdick, Christopher. Resource allocation in the National Health Service. *American Journal of Law and Medicine.* 1997; 23(2–3): 291–318. 196 fn. BE62502.
   aged; costs and benefits; *decision making; evidence–based medicine; futility; *health care delivery; health insurance reimbursement; judicial action; legal aspects; legal liability; long–term care; negligence; *organization and administration; physicians; refusal to treat; *resource allocation; risks and benefits; selection for treatment; self induced illness; social discrimination; state medicine; *Great Britain; *National Health Service

Orentlicher, David. Paying physicians more to do less: financial incentives to limit care. *University of Richmond Law Review.* 1996 Jan; 30(1): 155–197. 146 fn. BE59860.
   alternatives; biomedical technologies; costs and benefits; decision making; *economics; federal government; government regulation; health maintenance organizations; *incentives; *managed care programs; medical education; patient advocacy; patient care; patients; physician patient relationship; *physicians; practice guidelines; professional autonomy; quality of health care; referral and consultation; *remuneration; *resource allocation; risks and benefits; withholding treatment; capitation fee; utilization review; United States

Rai, Arti K. Reflective choice in health care: using information technology to present allocation options. *American Journal of Law and Medicine.* 1999; 25(2–3): 387–402. 122 fn. BE62510.
   autonomy; biomedical technologies; computer communication networks; *contracts; costs and benefits; counseling; decision making; *disclosure; evaluation; government regulation; *health insurance reimbursement; incentives; *information dissemination; *managed care programs; *patient participation; practice guidelines; quality adjusted life years; *resource allocation; personal financing; Internet; United States

Reay, Trish. Allocating scarce resources in a publicly

BE = bioethics accession number   fn. = footnotes   refs. = references

funded health system: ethical considerations of a Canadian managed care proposal. *Nursing Ethics.* 1999 May; 6(3): 240–249. 25 refs. BE61768.

conflict of interest; *decision making; federal government; *gatekeeping; government financing; health care delivery; *health care reform; incentives; justice; *managed care programs; moral obligations; patient advocacy; *physicians; public participation; *public policy; remuneration; *resource allocation; rights; capitation fee; *Alberta; *Canada

Richter, Gerd. Treatment of metastatic breast cancer -- economic and ethical considerations. *Cancer Investigation.* 1997; 15(4): 335–341. 33 refs. BE59176.

age factors; autonomy; bone marrow; *breast cancer; conflict of interest; *costs and benefits; *decision making; disclosure; drugs; *economics; evaluation; females; human experimentation; informed consent; investigators; justice; *patient care; patients; physicians; practice guidelines; prognosis; *prolongation of life; quality adjusted life years; *quality of life; random selection; research design; *resource allocation; risks and benefits; *terminally ill; *therapeutic research; tissue transplantation; toxicity; *treatment outcome; values; vulnerable populations; chemotherapy; United States

Rosenheck, Robert; Armstrong, Moe; Callahan, Daniel, et al. Obligation to the least well off in setting mental health service priorities: a consensus statement. *Psychiatric Services.* 1998 Oct; 49(10): 1273–1274, 1290. 13 refs. BE61446.

community services; consensus; *costs and benefits; decision making; *economics; federal government; *health care delivery; justice; mental health; *mentally ill; *obligations of society; psychiatry; *public policy; *resource allocation; schizophrenia; *selection for treatment; values; *mental health services; *seriously ill; United States; *Veterans Health Administration

Royal College of Physicians. Setting Priorities in the NHS: A Framework for Decision-Making. A Report of the Royal College of Physicians. London: Royal College of Physicians of London; 1995 Sep. 38 p. 50 refs. This report was approved by the Royal College of Physicians on 15 Jun 1995. ISBN 1-86016-020-4. BE59460.

administrators; advisory committees; biomedical research; common good; continuing education; costs and benefits; *decision making; *economics; education; evidence-based medicine; goals; *health care delivery; health promotion; health services research; justice; medical education; organization and administration; *organizational policies; patient care; patient care team; patient participation; *physician's role; physicians; preventive medicine; primary health care; private sector; professional organizations; *public participation; *public policy; *quality of health care; referral and consultation; *resource allocation; state medicine; time factors; treatment outcome; vulnerable populations; capitation fee; needs; *Great Britain; National Council for Health Care Priorities (Great Britain); *National Health Service; *Royal College of Physicians

Sabin, James E. Fairness as a problem of love and the heart: a clinician's perspective on priority setting. *BMJ (British Medical Journal).* 1998 Oct 10; 317(7164): 1002–1004. 11 refs. Presented at the Second International Conference on Priorities in Health Care held in London, 8-10 October 1998. BE60832.

communication; disclosure; *health care delivery; justice; managed care programs; mentally ill; obligations to society; patient advocacy; physician patient relationship; *physician's role; *physicians; public policy; *resource allocation; trust; *United States

Sackett, David. The Doctor's (Ethical and Economic) Dilemma: A Description of the Dilemmas Faced by a Physician Who Tries to Serve Both Individual Patients and Society. Office of Health Economics [OHE] Annual Lecture 1996. London: Office of Health Economics; 1996 Aug. 20 p. 9 refs. ISBN 0901-387-983. BE59419.

allowing to die; autonomy; beneficence; biomedical research; biomedical technologies; case studies; costs and benefits; *decision making; *economics; *evidence-based medicine; guideline adherence; guidelines; human experimentation; justice; *moral obligations; *obligations to society; *patient advocacy; patient care; *physicians; prolongation of life; quality of life; refusal to treat; *resource allocation; risks and benefits; selection for treatment; technical expertise; withholding treatment; *Great Britain; *National Health Service

Shaw, Allen B. Age as a basis for healthcare rationing: support for agist policies. *Drugs and Aging.* 1996 Dec; 9(6): 403–405. 21 refs. BE60379.

*age factors; *aged; *health care; justice; moral policy; public policy; *resource allocation; *selection for treatment; social discrimination; Great Britain

Smith, George P. Our hearts were once young and gay: health care rationing and the elderly. *University of Florida Journal of Law and Public Policy.* 1996 Fall; 8(1): 1–23. 133 fn. BE59858.

age factors; *aged; decision making; economics; government financing; *health care delivery; justice; moral policy; obligations of society; obligations to society; paternalism; *public policy; *resource allocation; selection for treatment; social discrimination; value of life; withholding treatment; Medicaid; Medicare; United States

ten Have, Henk A.M.J. Consensus formation and healthcare policy. *In:* ten Have, Henk A.M.J.; Sass, Hans-Martin, eds. Consensus Formation in Healthcare Ethics. Boston, MA: Kluwer Academic; 1998: 45–59. 13 refs. ISBN 0-7923-4944-X. BE62587.

advisory committees; attitudes; autonomy; biomedical technologies; *consensus; costs and benefits; *decision making; economics; health; *health care; *health care delivery; obligations of society; physicians; public opinion; public participation; *public policy; *resource allocation; rights; scarcity; standards; values; Dunning Committee; *Netherlands

Valdiserri, Ronald O.; Robinson, Carol; Lin, Lillian S., et al. Determining allocations for HIV-prevention interventions: assessing a change in federal funding policy. *AIDS and Public Policy Journal.* 1997 Winter; 12(4): 138–148. 31 fn. BE59300.

*AIDS; AIDS serodiagnosis; counseling; *federal government; *government financing; *HIV seropositivity; *municipal government; *preventive medicine; public health; *public policy; *resource allocation; *state government; health planning; *HIV Prevention Community Planning; *United States

Varekamp, Inge; Meiland, Franka J.M.; Hoos, Aloysia M., et al. The meaning of urgency in the allocation of scarce health care resources; a comparison between renal transplantation and psychogeriatric nursing home care. *Health Policy.* 1998 May; 44(2): 135–148. 20 refs. 1 fn. BE59149.

*aged; critically ill; dementia; evaluation studies; family members; home care; *kidneys; nurses; *nursing homes; *organ transplantation; *patient admission; patient advocacy; patient compliance; physicians; *prognosis; psychological stress; *resource allocation; scarcity; *selection for treatment; *time factors; qualitative research; *Netherlands

Varmus, Harold. Evaluating the burden of disease and spending the research dollars of the National Institutes of Health. [Editorial]. *New England Journal of Medicine.*

1999 Jun 17; 340(24): 1914–1915. 9 refs. BE62033.
*biomedical research; decision making; *disease; federal government; financial support; *government financing; industry; political activity; public participation; *resource allocation; trends; *disability adjusted life years; *National Institutes of Health; *United States

Veterans Affairs National Headquarters. Bioethics Committee. Ethical Considerations in Equitable Allocation and Distribution of Limited Health Care Resources: Report. Issued by the VA National Center for Clinical Ethics, White River Junction, VT 05009; 1996 Jan. 15 p. 43 refs. BE59264.
biomedical technologies; case studies; decision making; federal government; *guidelines; *health care; *institutional policies; justice; *public hospitals; rehabilitation; *resource allocation; selection for treatment; *standards; United States; *Veterans Health Administration

Vrbová, H.; Holmerová, I.; Hrubantová, L. Business ethics as a novel issue in health care economics. *Sbornik Lekarsky.* 1997; 98(3): 225–232. 6 refs. BE62418.
accountability; common good; community services; *economics; *health care delivery; health care reform; health insurance; patient participation; physician patient relationship; quality of health care; *resource allocation; trust; vulnerable populations; *Czech Republic

Wasson, John H.; Bubolz, Thomas A.; Lynn, Joanne, et al. Can we afford comprehensive, supportive care for the very old? *Journal of the American Geriatrics Society.* 1998 Jul; 46(7): 829–832. 20 refs. BE62258.
*aged; *community services; *economics; government financing; health care; *health care delivery; health services research; *home care; *hospitals; managed care programs; mortality; patient admission; patient care; *resource allocation; *health services misuse; *Medicare; *United States

Wikler, Daniel; Marchand, Sarah. Macro-allocation: dividing up the health care budget. *In:* Kuhse, Helga; Singer, Peter, eds. A Companion to Bioethics. Malden, MA: Blackwell; 1998: 306–315. 19 refs. ISBN 0-631-19737-0. BE59505.
costs and benefits; decision making; economics; health; *health care; justice; moral policy; public participation; public policy; quality adjusted life years; quality of life; *resource allocation; self induced illness

Williams, Alan. Intergenerational equity: an exploration of the 'fair innings' argument. *Health Economics.* 1997 Mar–Apr; 6(2): 117–132. 28 fn. BE59337.
*age factors; aged; health; *health care; international aspects; *justice; prolongation of life; *quality adjusted life years; quality of life; *resource allocation; selection for treatment; *socioeconomic factors; Great Britain

Williams, Alan; Evans, J. Grimley. Rationing health care by age: the case for [and] The case against. *BMJ (British Medical Journal).* 1997 Mar 15; 314(7083): 820–825. BE60232.
*age factors; *aged; attitudes; common good; costs and benefits; goals; *health care; *justice; moral policy; patient care; quality adjusted life years; quality of life; *resource allocation; risks and benefits; *selection for treatment; social discrimination; social worth; treatment outcome; values; withholding treatment; needs; *Great Britain; *National Health Service

Working Group on Prioritisation in Health Care (Finland). From Values to Choices: Report. Helsinki, Finland: National Research and Development Centre for Welfare and Health (STAKES); 1995. 78 p.

Bibliography: p. 72–77. ISBN 951-33-0035-8. BE62777.
advisory committees; age factors; aged; allowing to die; alternative therapies; biomedical technologies; decision making; developing countries; economics; genetic screening; government financing; health; health care; *health care delivery; health promotion; human rights; international aspects; justice; legislation; obligations of society; patient care; prenatal diagnosis; professional patient relationship; public participation; public policy; quality of life; *resource allocation; selection for treatment; self induced illness; terminal care; values; *Finland; *Working Group on Prioritisation in Health Care

Wright, Stephen G. The distribution of resources in health care. *Professional Nurse (London).* 1996 Jun; 11(9): 583–586. BE59988.
adolescents; deinstitutionalized persons; economics; *health care; infertility; low birth weight; mentally ill; newborns; pregnant women; public policy; refusal to treat; reproductive technologies; *resource allocation; selection for treatment; smoking; withholding treatment; *Great Britain; National Health Service

RESOURCE ALLOCATION/BIOMEDICAL TECHNOLOGIES

Alexander, G. Caleb; Sehgal, Ashwini R. Barriers to cadaveric renal transplantation among blacks, women, and the poor. *JAMA.* 1998 Oct 7; 280(13): 1148–1152. 21 refs. BE60285.
attitudes; blacks; cadavers; comparative studies; females; indigents; *kidneys; males; *organ transplantation; patients; prognosis; referral and consultation; renal dialysis; *resource allocation; *selection for treatment; *socioeconomic factors; *transplant recipients; whites; prospective studies; waiting lists; Indiana; Kentucky; Ohio
CONTEXT: Cadaveric renal transplantation rates differ greatly by race, sex, and income. Previous efforts to lessen these differences have focused on the transplant waiting list. However, the transplantation process involves a series of steps related to medical suitability, interest in transplantation, pretransplant workup, and movement up a waiting list to eventual transplantation. OBJECTIVE: To determine the relative importance of each step in explaining differences in cadaveric renal transplantation rates. DESIGN: Prospective cohort study. SETTING AND PATIENTS: A total of 7125 patients beginning long-term dialysis between January 1993 and December 1996 in Indiana, Kentucky, and Ohio. MAIN OUTCOME MEASURES: Completion of 4 separate steps during each patient-year of follow-up: (A) being medically suitable and possibly interested in transplantation; (B) being definitely interested in transplantation; (C) completing the pretransplant workup; and (D) moving up a waiting list and receiving a transplant. RESULTS: Compared with whites, blacks were less likely to complete steps B (odds ratio [OR], 0.68; 95% confidence interval [CI], 0.61–0.76), C (OR, 0.56; 95% CI, 0.48–0.65), and D (OR, 0.50; 95% CI, 0.40–0.62) after adjustment for age, sex, cause of renal failure, years receiving dialysis, and median income of patient ZIP code. Compared with men, women were less likely to complete each of the 4 steps, with ORs of 0.90, 0.89, 0.80, and 0.82, respectively. Poor individuals were less likely than wealthy individuals to complete steps A, B, and C, with ORs of 0.67, 0.78, and 0.77, respectively. CONCLUSIONS: Barriers at several steps are responsible for sociodemographic differences in access to cadaveric renal transplantation. Efforts to allocate kidneys equitably must address each step of the transplant process.

BE = bioethics accession number   fn. = footnotes   refs. = references

Ankeny, Rachel A. Recasting the debate on multiple listing for transplantation through consideration of both principles and practice. *Cambridge Quarterly of Healthcare Ethics.* 1999 Summer; 8(3): 330–339. 30 fn. BE62476.
  autonomy; body parts and fluids; *geographic factors; hospitals; institutional policies; justice; motivation; *organ transplantation; *patients; public policy; *resource allocation; scarcity; *selection for treatment; socioeconomic factors; standards; time factors; *transplant recipients; *waiting lists; United Network for Organ Sharing; United States

Asch, Steven; Frayne, Susan; Waitzkin, Howard. To discharge or not to discharge: ethics of care for an undocumented immigrant. *Journal of Health Care for the Poor and Underserved.* 1995; 6(1): 3–9. 27 refs. BE60569.
  *aliens; autonomy; beneficence; case studies; decision making; gatekeeping; government financing; health care delivery; hospitals; indigents; justice; *kidney diseases; legal aspects; *patient discharge; *physicians; public policy; *refusal to treat; *renal dialysis; *resource allocation; *selection for treatment; United States

Beecham, Linda. UK issues guidance on prescribing Viagra. [News]. *BMJ (British Medical Journal).* 1999 Jan 30; 318(7179): 279. BE61556.
  attitudes; diagnosis; dissent; drug industry; *drugs; *government financing; guidelines; *males; organizational policies; *patient care; *physicians; professional organizations; *public policy; *resource allocation; *selection for treatment; sexuality; social discrimination; *impotence; personal financing; British Medical Association; *Great Britain; *National Health Service; Royal College of Physicians; *Viagra

Bollinger, R. Randal. A UNOS [United Network for Organ Sharing] perspective on donor liver allocation. *Liver Transplantation and Surgery.* 1995 Jan; 1(1): 47–55. 6 refs. BE60881.
  dissent; federal government; geographic factors; goals; guidelines; health facilities; *livers; *organ transplantation; *organizational policies; physicians; prognosis; program descriptions; public policy; *resource allocation; scarcity; selection for treatment; standards; statistics; time factors; transplant recipients; voluntary programs; waiting lists; *United Network for Organ Sharing; *United States

Brooks, Alex. Viagra is licensed in Europe, but rationed in Britain. [News]. *BMJ (British Medical Journal).* 1998 Sep 19; 317(7161): 765. BE60827.
  *drugs; *government financing; males; patient care; *public policy; *resource allocation; selection for treatment; sexuality; *impotence; *Great Britain; *National Health Service; *Viagra

Burley, Justine C. The price of eggs: who should bear the costs of fertility treatments? *In:* Harris, John; Holm, Søren, eds. The Future of Human Reproduction: Ethics, Choice, and Regulation. New York, NY: Oxford University Press; 1998: 127–149. 51 fn. ISBN 0-19-823761-8. BE61266.
  biomedical technologies; *compensation; disabled; *government financing; health care; homosexuals; *infertility; *justice; *moral policy; multiple pregnancy; *obligations of society; philosophy; *public policy; reproduction; *reproductive technologies; *resource allocation; self induced illness; standards; values; voluntary sterilization; Dworkin, Ronald

Burrows, R. Removal of life support in intensive care units. *Medicine and Law.* 1994; 13(5–6): 489–500. 60 refs. BE60007.
  *allowing to die; autonomy; brain death; cardiac death; *decision making; deontological ethics; determination of death; economics; futility; informed consent; *intensive care units; legal aspects; patient admission; patient care; *physician's role; physicians; prognosis; *resource allocation; rights; *selection for treatment; third party consent; utilitarianism; withholding treatment; *South Africa

Caplan, Arthur L.; Coelho, Daniel H. The Ethics of Organ Transplants: The Current Debate. Amherst, NY: Prometheus Books; 1998. 350 p. Bibliography: p. 347–350. ISBN 1-57392-224-2. BE60916.
  aborted fetuses; abortion, induced; alcohol abuse; altruism; anencephaly; animal organs; blacks; brain death; cadavers; cardiac death; coercion; commodification; determination of death; directed donation; disadvantaged; donor cards; economics; family members; fetal tissue donation; health insurance reimbursement; incentives; international aspects; justice; kidneys; legal aspects; livers; *moral policy; *organ donation; organ donors; *organ transplantation; persistent vegetative state; presumed consent; primates; prognosis; *public policy; *remuneration; required request; *resource allocation; retreatment; *selection for treatment; *tissue transplantation; transplant recipients; mandated choice; refusal to donate; *unrelated donors; Medicaid; Medicare; Oregon; Uniform Anatomical Gift Act; United States

Chandna, Shahid M.; Schulz, Joerg; Lawrence, Christopher, et al. Is there a rationale for rationing chronic dialysis? A hospital based cohort study of factors affecting survival and morbidity. *BMJ (British Medical Journal).* 1999 Jan 23; 318(7178): 217–223. 25 refs. BE60327.
  age factors; diabetes; economics; evaluation studies; hospitals; kidney diseases; *morbidity; *mortality; *prognosis; *renal dialysis; *resource allocation; *selection for treatment; *treatment outcome; retrospective studies; Great Britain
  OBJECTIVES: To determine factors influencing survival and need for hospitalisation in patients needing dialysis, and to define the potential basis for rationing access to renal replacement therapy. DESIGN: Hospital based cohort study of all patients starting dialysis over a 4 year recruitment period (follow up 15–63 months). Groups were defined on the basis of age, comorbidity, functional status, and whether dialysis initiation was planned or unplanned. SETTING: Renal unit in a district general hospital, which acts as the main renal referral centre for four other such hospitals and serves a population of about 1.15 million people. SUBJECTS: 292 patients, mean age 61.3 years (18–92 years, SD 15.8), of whom 193 (66%) were male, and 59 (20%) were patients with diabetes. Dialysis initiation was planned in 163 (56%) patients and unplanned in 129 (44%). MAIN OUTCOME MEASURES: Overall survival, 1 year survival, and hospitalisation rate. RESULTS: Factors affecting survival in the Cox's proportional hazard model were Karnofsky performance score at presentation (hazard ratio 0.979, 95% confidence interval 0.972 to 0.986), comorbidity severity score (1.240, 1.131 to 1.340), age (1.036, 1.018 to 1.054), and myeloma (2.15, 1.140 to 4.042). The Karnofsky performance score used 3 months before presentation was significant (0.970, 0.956 to 0.981), as was unplanned presentation in this model (1.796, 1.233 to 2.617). Using these factors, a high risk group of 26 patients was defined, with 19.2% 1 year survival. Denying dialysis to this group would save 3.2% of the total cost of the chronic programme but would sacrifice five long term survivors. Less rigorous definition of the high risk group would save more money but lose more long term survivors. CONCLUSIONS: Severity of comorbid conditions and functional capacity are more important than age in predicting survival and morbidity of patients on dialysis. Late referral for dialysis

---

BE = bioethics accession number   fn. = footnotes   refs. = references

affects survival adversely. Denial of dialysis to patients in an extremely high risk group, defined by a new stratification based on logistic regression, would be of debatable benefit.

Chase, Marilyn. Rationing scarce drugs has some questioning fairness and ethics. [News]. *Wall Street Journal.* 1998 Sep 28: B1. BE61125.
>*breast cancer; *drug industry; females; *investigational drugs; patient care; *random selection; *resource allocation; *scarcity; *selection for treatment; selection of subjects; therapeutic research; *compassionate use; *Genentech Inc.; *Herceptin

Chisholm, John. Viagra: a botched test case for rationing. [Editorial]. *BMJ (British Medical Journal).* 1999 Jan 30; 318(7179): 273–274. 12 refs. BE60578.
>*drugs; *government financing; *males; patient care; *public policy; *resource allocation; selection for treatment; sexuality; *impotence; *Great Britain; National Health Service; *Viagra

Davis, Kathy. The rhetoric of cosmetic surgery: luxury or welfare? *In:* Parens, Erik, ed. Enhancing Human Traits: Ethical and Social Implications. Washington, DC: Georgetown University Press; 1998: 124–134. 13 fn. ISBN 0–87840–703–0. BE59748.
>*cosmetic surgery; decision making; enhancement technologies; females; feminist ethics; *government financing; guidelines; *health care; health care delivery; *health insurance reimbursement; national health insurance; normality; psychological stress; public participation; *public policy; *resource allocation; selection for treatment; state medicine; suffering; beauty; *Netherlands

Dossetor, John B. Economic, social, racial and age–related considerations in dialysis and transplantation. *Current Opinion in Nephrology and Hypertension.* 1995 Nov; 4(6): 498–501. 39 refs. BE59835.
>*age factors; aged; blacks; cadavers; developing countries; females; *international aspects; kidney diseases; *kidneys; males; *minority groups; organ donation; organ donors; *organ transplantation; remuneration; *renal dialysis; *resource allocation; selection for treatment; *socioeconomic factors; statistics; transplant recipients; treatment outcome; whites

Evans, Roger W. Liver transplantation in a managed care environment. *Liver Transplantation and Surgery.* 1995 Jan; 1(1): 61–75. 75 refs. BE60903.
>biomedical research; biomedical technologies; *costs and benefits; *economics; geographic factors; goals; health care; health care reform; health facilities; justice; *livers; *managed care programs; *organ transplantation; physicians; practice guidelines; prognosis; *resource allocation; risk; *selection for treatment; transplant recipients; treatment outcome; trends; *United States

Fleck, Leonard. Justice, rights, and Alzheimer disease genetics. *In:* Post, Stephen G.; Whitehouse, Peter J., eds. Genetic Testing for Alzheimer Disease: Ethical and Clinical Issues. Baltimore, MD: Johns Hopkins University Press; 1998: 190–208. 15 refs. ISBN 0–8018–5840–2. BE60724.
>age factors; artificial organs; beneficence; *biomedical technologies; breast cancer; costs and benefits; cystic fibrosis; decision making; *dementia; fetal therapy; gene therapy; genetic counseling; genetic disorders; genetic predisposition; *genetic screening; *genetic services; germ cells; *government financing; health care; hearts; *justice; late–onset disorders; *moral obligations; *moral policy; *obligations of society; organ transplantation; preimplantation diagnosis; prenatal diagnosis; public participation; *resource allocation; rights; risks and benefits;

selection for treatment; standards; therapeutic research

France. Order of 6 Nov 1996 approving the Rules for the distribution and allocation of transplants removed from deceased persons for the purpose of organ transplantation. (*Journal officiel de la Republique fran3aise, Lois et Decrets,* 10 Nov 1996, No. 263, pp. 16475–16476). *International Digest of Health Legislation.* 1997; 48(1): 15–18. BE59588.
>adults; *body parts and fluids; cadavers; children; *legal aspects; *organ transplantation; prognosis; *resource allocation; *selection for treatment; time factors; transplant recipients; *France

Grubb, Andrew. Infertility treatment: access and judicial review -- R v. Sheffield Health Authority, ex parte Seale. [Comment]. *Medical Law Review.* 1996 Autumn; 4(3): 326–329. BE61516.
>*age factors; females; *government financing; *in vitro fertilization; *judicial action; *legal aspects; *public policy; refusal to treat; *reproductive technologies; *resource allocation; *selection for treatment; *Great Britain; National Health Service; *R v. Sheffield Health Authority, ex parte Seale

Himma, Kenneth Einar. A critique of UNOS liver allocation policy. *Cambridge Quarterly of Healthcare Ethics.* 1999 Summer; 8(3): 311–320. 38 fn. Article followed by update on UNOS policy, p. 320. BE62474.
>chronically ill; critically ill; emergency care; ethical analysis; *justice; *livers; mortality; *organ transplantation; *organizational policies; *prognosis; *public policy; *resource allocation; scarcity; *selection for treatment; time factors; transplant recipients; treatment outcome; liver diseases; *needs; survival; waiting lists; *United Network for Organ Sharing; United States

Iqbal, Aamir; Holley, Jean L. Ethical issues in end–stage renal disease patients who use illicit intravenous drugs. *Seminars in Dialysis.* 1995 Jan–Feb; 8(1): 35–38. 30 refs. BE59922.
>case studies; *drug abuse; *kidney diseases; kidneys; methods; *organ transplantation; *patient compliance; *renal dialysis; *resource allocation; risks and benefits; *selection for treatment; self induced illness; social worth

Kenyon, Georgina. Doctors refuse to operate on 80 year old man. [News]. *BMJ (British Medical Journal).* 1998 Dec 5; 317(7172): 1548. BE60264.
>*aged; decision making; *heart diseases; *institutional policies; patient care team; *public hospitals; *refusal to treat; *resource allocation; *selection for treatment; social discrimination; *surgery; *Australia; *Quinn, John

Khauli, Raja B. Issues and controversies surrounding organ donation and transplantation: the need for laws that ensure equity and optimal utility of a scarce resource. *Suffolk University Law Review.* 1993 Winter; 27(4): 1225–1236. 37 fn. BE60734.
>accountability; body parts and fluids; cadavers; economics; family members; incentives; justice; kidneys; legal aspects; legislation; minority groups; *organ donation; *organ transplantation; patient compliance; presumed consent; prognosis; *public policy; remuneration; renal dialysis; required request; *resource allocation; retreatment; scarcity; selection for treatment; treatment outcome; National Organ Transplant Act 1984; Organ Procurement and Transplant Network; United Network for Organ Sharing; United States

Kjellstrand, Carl M. Duration and adequacy of dialysis -- overview: the science is easy, the ethic is difficult. *ASAIO Journal (American Society for Artificial Internal Organs).* 1997 May–Jun; 43(3): 220–224. 38 refs. BE60184.

BE = bioethics accession number   fn. = footnotes   refs. = references

chronically ill; comparative studies; international aspects; kidney diseases; mortality; *renal dialysis; *resource allocation; risks and benefits; selection for treatment; *time factors; treatment outcome; Japan; United States

Klintmalm, Goran B. Who should receive the liver allograft: the transplant center or the recipient? *Liver Transplantation and Surgery.* 1995 Jan; 1(1): 55–58. 2 refs. BE60882.
> geographic factors; health facilities; kidneys; *livers; *organ transplantation; prognosis; *resource allocation; scarcity; selection for treatment; time factors; transplant recipients; treatment outcome; waiting lists; United Network for Organ Sharing; *United States

Koch, Tom. The Limits of Principle: Deciding Who Lives and What Dies. Westport, CT: Praeger; 1998. 176 p. Bibliography: p. 159–168. ISBN 0-275-96407-8. BE60113.
> allowing to die; amyotrophic lateral sclerosis; *anencephaly; animal rights; *bioethical issues; bioethics; biomedical technologies; consensus; cultural pluralism; *decision making; disabled; Down syndrome; ethical analysis; eugenics; guidelines; historical aspects; intelligence; international aspects; legal aspects; methods; moral policy; newborns; organ donation; *organ transplantation; patient compliance; personhood; prognosis; prolongation of life; *quality of life; renal dialysis; *resource allocation; rights; scarcity; *selection for treatment; selective abortion; social worth; speciesism; transplant recipients; treatment outcome; *value of life; values

Landman, Willem A.; Henley, Lesley D. Equitable rationing of highly specialised health care services for children: a perspective from South Africa. *Journal of Medical Ethics.* 1999 Jun; 25(3): 224–229. 34 fn. BE61854.
> *biomedical technologies; *children; chronically ill; costs and benefits; cystic fibrosis; disabled; disease; futility; *government financing; *health care; *health care delivery; intensive care units; *justice; legal rights; leukemia; methods; moral policy; newborns; organ transplantation; palliative care; prevalence; primary health care; *prognosis; *public policy; quality of health care; *random selection; *resource allocation; scarcity; *selection for treatment; utilitarianism; needs; patient abandonment; *waiting lists; *South Africa
The principles of equality and equity, respectively in the Bill of Rights and the white paper on health, provide the moral and legal foundations for future health care for children in South Africa. However, given extreme health care need and scarce resources, the government faces formidable obstacles if it hopes to achieve a just allocation of public health care resources, especially among children in need of highly specialised health care. In this regard, there is a dearth of moral analysis which is practically useful in the South African situation. We offer a set of moral considerations to guide the macro–allocation of highly specialised public health care services among South Africa's children. We also mention moral considerations which should inform micro–allocation.

Lantos, John D.; Mokalla, Mani; Meadow, William. Resource allocation in neonatal and medical ICUs: epidemiology and rationing at the extremes of life. *American Journal of Respiratory and Critical Care Medicine.* 1997 Jul; 156(1): 185–189. 12 refs. BE60028.
> age factors; *aged; comparative studies; costs and benefits; *intensive care units; justice; *low birth weight; *mortality; *newborns; patient discharge; prematurity; *resource allocation; time factors; *treatment outcome; ventilators; retrospective studies; University of Chicago Hospitals

Layon, A. Joseph; D'Amico, Robert. Intensive care for patients with acquired immunodeficiency syndrome --

medicine versus ideology. *Critical Care Medicine.* 1990 Nov; 18(11): 1297–1299. 30 refs. BE60955.
> *AIDS; attitudes; economics; futility; HIV seropositivity; *intensive care units; patient admission; patients; prolongation of life; *resource allocation; self induced illness; social discrimination; terminally ill

McChesney, Lawrence P.; Braithwaite, Susan S. Expectations and outcomes in organ transplantation. *Cambridge Quarterly of Healthcare Ethics.* 1999 Summer; 8(3): 299–310. 18 fn. BE62473.
> allowing to die; committee membership; decision making; economics; hospitals; incentives; information dissemination; informed consent; morbidity; mortality; *organ transplantation; organization and administration; physician patient relationship; *physicians; prognosis; regulation; *resource allocation; risk; *selection for treatment; technical expertise; transplant recipients; *treatment outcome; treatment refusal; United States

McKenzie, John K.; Moss, Alvin H.; Feest, Terry G., et al. Dialysis decision making in Canada, the United Kingdom, and the United States. *American Journal of Kidney Diseases.* 1998 Jan; 31(1): 12–18. 23 refs. BE59626.
> age factors; allowing to die; comparative studies; *decision making; dementia; diabetes; diagnosis; drug abuse; Duchenne muscular dystrophy; economics; family members; *international aspects; *knowledge, attitudes, practice; malpractice; motivation; patient compliance; patients; persistent vegetative state; *physicians; prognosis; quality of life; *renal dialysis; *resource allocation; *selection for treatment; statistics; survey; treatment refusal; withholding treatment; *Canada; *Great Britain; *United States

Maiorca, Rosario. Ethical problems in dialysis: prospects for the year 2000. *Nephrology, Dialysis, Transplantation.* 1998; 13(Suppl. 1): 1–9. 46 refs. BE61570.
> advance directives; aged; allowing to die; autonomy; beneficence; decision making; economics; family members; health care delivery; international aspects; kidney diseases; medical ethics; moral development; *moral policy; patient participation; physicians; prognosis; public policy; quality of life; *renal dialysis; *resource allocation; risks and benefits; Roman Catholic ethics; *selection for treatment; social discrimination; suffering; theology; treatment refusal; value of life; *withholding treatment; Europe; Great Britain; Italy; National Health Service; United States

Mariner, Wendy K. Equitable access to biomedical advances: getting beyond the rights impasse. *Connecticut Law Review.* 1989 Spring; 21(3): 571–603. 103 fn. BE62127.
> abortion, induced; AIDS; *biomedical technologies; constitutional law; costs and benefits; drug industry; *drugs; federal government; government financing; *government regulation; *health care; *investigational drugs; justice; *legal aspects; *legal rights; *obligations of society; *organ transplantation; patient advocacy; patient care; patients; political activity; private sector; *public policy; public sector; *resource allocation; *unproven therapies; Food and Drug Administration; *France; Roussel Uclaf; *RU–486; *United States

Markovitz, Barry; May, Larry. Three patients, two hearts. [Case study and commentaries]. *Hastings Center Report.* 1998 Sep–Oct; 28(5): 20–21. BE59549.
> adolescents; adoption; advertising; *cadavers; case studies; critically ill; decision making; *directed donation; geographic factors; hearts; justice; *organ donation; *organ transplantation; parents; *resource allocation; scarcity; *selection for treatment; *transplant recipients

Meadow, William; Lantos, John D.; Mokalla, Mani, et al. Distributive justice across generations: epidemiology of ICU care for the very young and the

---

very old. *Clinics in Perinatology.* 1996 Sep; 23(3): 597–608. 24 refs. BE60943.

adults; *age factors; *aged; comparative studies; *costs and benefits; economics; infants; *intensive care units; *justice; *low birth weight; medical records; *mortality; *newborns; patient care; patient discharge; prognosis; *resource allocation; selection for treatment; *treatment outcome; retrospective studies; survival; University of Chicago Medical Center

Meester, Johan De. Eurotransplant allocation procedures: the basics, March 1996. *In:* Lachmann, Rolf; Meuter, Norbert, eds. Zur Gerechtigkeit der Organverteilung: Ein Problem der Transplantationsmedizin aus interdisziplinärer Sicht. Stuttgart, Germany: G. Fischer; 1997: 167–177. 2 refs. ISBN 3-437-21136-6. BE60742.

age factors; body parts and fluids; international aspects; kidneys; livers; *organ transplantation; program descriptions; *resource allocation; selection for treatment; time factors; transplant recipients; Europe; *Eurotransplant

Milford, Edgar L. Organ transplantation -- barriers, outcomes, and evolving policies. [Editorial]. *JAMA.* 1998 Oct 7; 280(13): 1184–1185. 11 refs. BE60288.

age factors; body parts and fluids; cadavers; critically ill; data banks; federal government; geographic factors; government financing; government regulation; kidneys; mortality; organ donation; *organ transplantation; prognosis; public policy; *resource allocation; *selection for treatment; *socioeconomic factors; time factors; transplant recipients; *treatment outcome; Department of Health and Human Services; End Stage Renal Disease Program; United Network for Organ Sharing; United States

Nakazato, Paul Z. Controversial aspects of the current liver donor allocation system for liver transplantation. *Academic Radiology.* 1995 Mar; 2(3): 244–248. 12 refs. BE62001.

geographic factors; hospitals; *livers; mortality; *organ transplantation; prognosis; *public policy; *resource allocation; retreatment; scarcity; selection for treatment; transplant recipients; treatment outcome; severity of illness index; waiting lists; United Network for Organ Sharing; United States

Neal, Bernard W. Ethical aspects in the care of very low birth weight infants. *Pediatrician.* 1990; 17(2): 92–99. 6 refs. BE59453.

active euthanasia; allowing to die; beneficence; *decision making; disabled; *intensive care units; justice; *low birth weight; moral obligations; *newborns; pediatrics; personhood; physicians; prognosis; quality of life; *resource allocation; *selection for treatment; suffering; value of life; Australia

Paterson, Ron. Rationing access to dialysis in New Zealand. *Ethics and Intellectual Disability.* 1999 Winter; 4(1): 5. BE62665.

allowing to die; *dementia; government financing; minority groups; *patient compliance; quality of life; *renal dialysis; *resource allocation; *selection for treatment; withholding treatment; Maoris; *New Zealand; Williams, Rau

Payne, William D. The rational development of liver allocation policy. *Liver Transplantation and Surgery.* 1995 Jan; 1(1): 58–61. 2 refs. BE60883.

federal government; geographic factors; health facilities; *livers; *organ transplantation; organizational policies; prognosis; public policy; *resource allocation; selection for treatment; transplant recipients; treatment outcome; waiting lists; United Network for Organ Sharing; *United States

Purtilo, Ruth B. What kind of a good is a donor liver anyway, and why should we care? *Liver Transplantation*

and Surgery. 1995 Jan; 1(1): 75–80. 8 refs. BE60884.

body parts and fluids; *common good; democracy; directed donation; *justice; *livers; *organ transplantation; patient advocacy; physicians; *public policy; *resource allocation; scarcity; selection for treatment; transplant recipients; values; United States

Rakowski, Eric; Post, Stephen G. Should health care be rationed by age? Yes [and] No. *In:* Scharlach, Andrew E.; Kaye, Lenard W., eds. Controversial Issues in Aging. Boston, MA: Allyn and Bacon; 1997: 103–113. 9 refs. ISBN 0-205-19381-1. BE60963.

*age factors; *aged; autonomy; biomedical technologies; cultural pluralism; females; government financing; health care; justice; moral policy; prolongation of life; public policy; quality of life; *resource allocation; rights; *selection for treatment; social discrimination; value of life; values; needs; United States

Russell, Paul S. Understanding resource use in liver transplantation. [Editorial]. *JAMA.* 1999 Apr 21; 281(15): 1431–1432. 9 refs. BE61903.

*economics; evaluation; hospitals; *livers; mortality; *organ transplantation; *public policy; *resource allocation; *scarcity; *selection for treatment; transplant recipients; treatment outcome; length of stay; severity of illness index; United States

Sass, Hans–Martin. Ethics of the allocation of highly advanced medical technologies. *Artificial Organs.* 1998 Mar; 22(3): 263–268. 14 refs. BE60080.

advisory committees; animal organs; artificial organs; *biomedical technologies; coercion; cultural pluralism; developing countries; economics; genetic predisposition; genetic screening; health education; health promotion; *incentives; international aspects; *justice; *organ donation; organ donors; *organ transplantation; preventive medicine; regulation; remuneration; *resource allocation; *socioeconomic factors

Savulescu, Julian. The cost of refusing treatment and equality of outcome. *Journal of Medical Ethics.* 1998 Aug; 24(4): 231–236. 23 fn. BE60728.

*alternatives; autonomy; *blood transfusions; *economics; *Jehovah's Witnesses; justice; legal aspects; obligations of society; *patient care; religion; *resource allocation; social discrimination; *treatment refusal; utilitarianism; values; Great Britain

Patients have a right to refuse medical treatment. But what should happen after a patient has refused recommended treatment? In many cases, patients receive alternative forms of treatment. These forms of care may be less cost-effective. Does respect for autonomy extend to providing these alternatives? How for does justice constrain autonomy? I begin by providing three arguments that such alternatives should not be offered to those who refuse treatment. I argue that the best argument which refusers can appeal to is based on the egalitarian principle of equality of outcome. However, this principle does not ultimately support a right to less cost-effective alternatives. I focus on Jehovah's Witnesses refusing blood and requesting alternative treatments. However, the point applies to many patients who refuse cost-effective medical care.

Scheinkestel, Carlos D. The evolution of the intensivist: from health care provider to economic rationalist and ethicist. *Medical Journal of Australia.* 1996 Mar 4; 164(5): 310–312. 14 refs. BE60196.

aged; critically ill; *decision making; health care delivery; hospitals; *intensive care units; patient admission; patient care; patient discharge; patient transfer; *physicians; prognosis; quality of life; *resource allocation; scarcity; *selection for treatment; treatment outcome; withholding

---

BE = bioethics accession number   fn. = footnotes   refs. = references

treatment; *Australia

Schmidt, Volker H. The politics of justice and the paradox of justification. *Social Justice Research.* 1998 Mar; 11(1): 3-19. 46 refs. BE59359.
    blacks; cultural pluralism; dissent; ethical analysis; ethical theory; *institutional policies; *justice; kidney diseases; kidneys; minority groups; organ donation; *organ transplantation; *public policy; *resource allocation; *selection for treatment; transplant recipients; treatment outcome; uncertainty; histocompatibility; rationality

Schwartz, William B. Life Without Disease: The Pursuit of Medical Utopia. Berkeley, CA: University of California Press; 1998. 178 p. Includes references. ISBN 0-520-21467-6. BE59738.
    anesthesia; biomedical research; *biomedical technologies; cloning; costs and benefits; drugs; *economics; fraud; gene therapy; genetic disorders; *genetic intervention; health care; *health care delivery; health insurance; health maintenance organizations; hospitals; international aspects; legal aspects; life extension; malpractice; *managed care programs; physicians; preventive medicine; *public policy; quality of health care; *resource allocation; *trends; Canada; Europe; Great Britain; *United States

Shaul, Randi Zlotnik; Mendelssohn, David C. Scarce resource allocation decisions: issues of physician conflict and liability. *Humane Health Care International.* 1997 Spring; 13(1): 25-28. 35 refs. BE59960.
    accountability; administrators; *conflict of interest; disclosure; *economics; *gatekeeping; informed consent; kidney diseases; *legal liability; negligence; patient advocacy; physician patient relationship; *physician's role; *physicians; public policy; *renal dialysis; *resource allocation; selection for treatment; social discrimination; standards; time factors; Canada; *Ontario

Showstack, Jonathan; Katz, Patricia P.; Lake, John R., et al.; National Institute of Diabetes and Digestive and Kidney Diseases. Liver Transplantation Database Group. Resource utilization in liver transplantation: effects of patient characteristics and clinical practice. *JAMA.* 1999 Apr 21; 281(15): 1381-1386. 29 refs. BE61901.
    adults; age factors; alcohol abuse; comparative studies; critically ill; *economics; *evaluation; *hospitals; intensive care units; *livers; *organ transplantation; *resource allocation; selection for treatment; *transplant recipients; length of stay; severity of illness index; *utilization review; California; *Mayo Clinic; Minnesota; Nebraska; *University of California, San Francisco; *University of Nebraska, Omaha
    CONTEXT: Liver transplantation is among the most costly of medical services, yet few studies have addressed the relationship between the resources utilized for this procedure and specific patient characteristics and clinical practices. OBJECTIVE: To assess the association of pretransplant patient characteristics and clinical practices with hospital resource utilization. DESIGN: Prospective cohort of patients who received liver transplants between January 1991 and July 1994. SETTING: University of California, San Francisco; Mayo Clinic, Rochester, Minn; and the University of Nebraska, Omaha. PATIENTS: Seven hundred eleven patients who received single-organ liver transplants, were at least 16 years old, and had nonfulminant liver disease. MAIN OUTCOME MEASURE: Standardized resource utilization derived from a database created by matching all services to a single price list. RESULTS: Higher adjusted resource utilization was associated with donor age of 60 years or older (28% [$53813] greater mean resource utilization; P=.005); recipient age of 60 years

or older (17% [$32795]; P=.01); alcoholic liver disease (26% [$49596]; P=.002); Child-Pugh class C (41% [$67 658]; P less than .001); care from the intensive care unit at time of transplant (42% [$77833]; P less than .001); death in the hospital (35% [$67 076]; P less than .001); and having multiple liver transplants during the index hospitalization (154% increase [$474 740 vs $186 726 for 1 transplant]; P less than .001). Adjusted length of stay and resource utilization also differed significantly among transplant centers. CONCLUSIONS: Clinical, economic, and ethical dilemmas in liver transplantation are highlighted by these findings. Recipients who were older, had alcoholic liver disease, or were severely ill were the most expensive to treat; this suggests that organ allocation criteria may affect transplant costs. Clinical practices and resource utilization varied considerably among transplant centers; methods to reduce variation in practice patterns, such as clinical guidelines, might lower costs while maintaining quality of care.

Silvers, Anita. A fatal attraction to normalizing: treating disabilities as deviations from "species-typical" functioning. *In:* Parens, Erik, ed. Enhancing Human Traits: Ethical and Social Implications. Washington, DC: Georgetown University Press; 1998: 95-123. 43 fn. ISBN 0-87840-703-0. BE59747.
    *biomedical technologies; community services; cosmetic surgery; costs and benefits; *disabled; disease; *enhancement technologies; genetic intervention; genetic predisposition; *health; *health care; hearing disorders; *justice; medicine; *normality; obligations of society; *physically disabled; public policy; *quality of life; *resource allocation; Daniels, Norman

Singer, Peter A.; Shaul, Randi Zlotnik. Resource allocation in coronary revascularization. *Canadian Journal of Cardiology.* 1997 Dec; 13(Suppl. D): 64D-66D. BE62105.
    constitutional law; costs and benefits; geographic factors; government regulation; guidelines; health care delivery; health facilities; *heart diseases; justice; organizational policies; physicians; professional organizations; *resource allocation; selection for treatment; social discrimination; standards; *surgery; needs; *Canada; Canada Health Act 1984; Canadian Cardiovascular Society; Canadian Charter of Rights and Freedoms; United Network for Organ Sharing

Smith, Richard. Viagra and rationing: let the sunlight in, let the people speak. [Editorial]. *BMJ (British Medical Journal).* 1998 Sep 19; 317(7161): 760-761. 6 refs. BE60826.
    decision making; *drugs; government financing; males; public participation; *public policy; *resource allocation; sexuality; values; *impotence; *Great Britain; *National Health Service; Rationing Agenda Group (Great Britain); United States; *Viagra

Stolberg, Sheryl Gay. Fight over organs shifts to states from Washington. [News]. *New York Times.* 1999 Mar 11: A1, A26. BE60870.
    *body parts and fluids; economics; *federal government; geographic factors; *government regulation; health facilities; organ donation; *organ transplantation; political activity; *resource allocation; scarcity; *state government; time factors; waiting lists; Department of Health and Human Services; *United States

Stolberg, Sheryl Gay. Health secretary urges donor priority for sickest patients. [News]. *New York Times.* 1998 Feb 27: A16. BE60466.
    critically ill; federal government; geographic factors; government regulation; livers; *organ transplantation; prognosis; *public policy; *resource allocation; *selection

---

BE = bioethics accession number   fn. = footnotes   refs. = references

for treatment; *transplant recipients; *Department of Health and Human Services; United Network for Organ Sharing; *United States

Stolberg, Sheryl Gay. Organ transplant panel urges a broad sharing of livers. [News]. *New York Times.* 1999 Jul 21: A14. BE62447.
  advisory committees; federal government; *geographic factors; *government regulation; *livers; *organ transplantation; *public policy; *resource allocation; scarcity; selection for treatment; waiting lists; Department of Health and Human Services; *Institute of Medicine; United Network for Organ Sharing; *United States

Thomasma, David C.; Micetich, Kenneth C.; Brems, John, et al. The ethics of competition in liver transplantation. *Cambridge Quarterly of Healthcare Ethics.* 1999 Summer; 8(3): 321–329. 28 fn. BE62475.
  beneficence; economics; federal government; *geographic factors; *government regulation; guidelines; hospitals; institutional policies; *justice; *livers; *misconduct; organ donation; organ donors; *organ transplantation; physicians; prisoners; public policy; *resource allocation; scarcity; *selection for treatment; standards; technical expertise; time factors; *transplant recipients; needs; *waiting lists; Department of Health and Human Services; United Network for Organ Sharing; *United States

Ubel, Peter A.; Caplan, Arthur L. Geographic favoritism in liver transplantation -- unfortunate or unfair? *New England Journal of Medicine.* 1998 Oct 29; 339(18): 1322–1325. 34 refs. BE60300.
  cadavers; critically ill; federal government; *geographic factors; *government regulation; hospitals; *justice; *livers; mortality; *organ transplantation; physicians; *prognosis; *public policy; *resource allocation; retreatment; *selection for treatment; self regulation; *standards; state government; time factors; *transplant recipients; treatment outcome; *seriously ill; United Network for Organ Sharing; *United States

Ubel, Peter A.; Baron, Jonathan; Asch, David A. Social responsibility, personal responsibility, and prognosis in public judgments about transplant allocation. *Bioethics.* 1999 Jan; 13(1): 57–68. 11 fn. BE60888.
  *drug abuse; *hearts; *nutrition; *organ transplantation; prognosis; *public opinion; *resource allocation; *selection for treatment; *self induced illness; *smoking; survey; transplant recipients; Pennsylvania

VACO [VA Central Office] Bioethics Committee. Allocation of expensive medications. Report. *NCCE News (Veterans Health Administration National Center for Clinical Ethics).* 1995 Spring; 3(2, Suppl.): S1–S9. 4 refs. 1 fn. BE61470.
  *costs and benefits; decision making; *drugs; *guidelines; military personnel; *patient care; practice guidelines; public hospitals; renal dialysis; *resource allocation; review committees; scarcity; pharmacy and therapeutics committees; erythropoietin; United States; *VACO (Veterans Affairs Central Office) Bioethics Committee

Veatch, Robert M. Egalitarian and maximin theories of justice: directed donation of organs for transplant. *Journal of Medicine and Philosophy.* 1998 Oct; 23(5): 456–476. 13 refs. 12 fn. Note: the journal issue cover shows a date of August 1998, which is incorrect. BE62113.
  beneficence; *directed donation; ethical analysis; *ethical theory; freedom; health; health care delivery; *justice; *moral policy; *organ donation; *organ transplantation; public policy; *resource allocation; rights; *selection for treatment; self concept; social discrimination; socioeconomic factors; transplant recipients; utilitarianism; whites; *egalitarianism; *Rawls, John; United Network for Organ

Sharing; United States
It is common to interpret Rawls's maximin theory of justice as egalitarian. Compared to utilitarian theories, this may be true. However, in special cases practices that distribute resources so as to benefit the worst off actually increase the inequality between the worst off and some who are better off. In these cases the Rawlsian maximin parts company with what is here called true egalitarianism. A policy question requiring a distinction between maximin and "true egalitarian" allocations has arisen in the arena of organ transplantation. This case is examined here as a venue for differentiating maximin and true egalitarian theories. Directed donation is the name given to donations of organs restricted to a particular social group. For example, the family of a member of the Ku Klux Klan donated his organs on the provision that they go only to members of the Caucasian race. While such donations appear to be discriminatory, if certain plausible assumptions are made, they satisfy the maximin criterion. They selectively advantage the recipient of the organs without harming anyone (assuming the organs would otherwise go unused). Moreover, everyone who is lower on the waiting list (who, thereby, could be considered worse off) is advantaged by moving up on the waiting list. This paper examines how maximin and more truly egalitarian theories handle this case arguing that, to the extent that directed donation in unethical, the best account of that conclusion is that an egalitarian principle of justice is to be preferred to the maximin.

Veterans Affairs National Headquarters. Bioethics Committee. Guidelines for the Allocation of Unproved Treatments: Report. Issued by the VA National Center for Clinical Ethics, White River Junction, VT 05009; 1996 Jan. 12 p. 11 fn. BE59265.
  *biomedical technologies; decision making; federal government; *guidelines; *institutional policies; *public hospitals; *resource allocation; *standards; *unproven therapies; United States; *Veterans Health Administration

Improving access to organs. [Editorial]. *New York Times.* 1999 Jul 26: A14. BE62448.
  federal government; *geographic factors; *government regulation; health facilities; justice; *organ transplantation; political activity; *resource allocation; time factors; Department of Health and Human Services; U.S. Congress; *United States

Misguided chauvinisim on organs. [Editorial]. *New York Times.* 1999 Mar 12: A22. BE60871.
  *body parts and fluids; *federal government; geographic factors; *government regulation; *organ transplantation; *resource allocation; scarcity; *state government; time factors; waiting lists; *United States

RESUSCITATION ORDERS

See also ALLOWING TO DIE

Alexandrov, Andrei V.; Pullicino, Patrick M.; Meslin, Eric M., et al. Agreement on disease-specific criteria for do-not-resuscitate orders in acute stroke. [For the members of the Canadian and Western New York Stroke Consortiums]. *Stroke.* 1996 Feb; 27(2): 232–237. 44 refs. BE61489.
  allowing to die; *brain pathology; consensus; critically ill; *decision making; family members; *futility; informed consent; morbidity; mortality; patients; physicians; *practice guidelines; *prognosis; *resuscitation; *resuscitation orders; selection for treatment; survey; terminally ill; time factors; ventilators; withholding treatment; *cerebrovascular

---

BE = bioethics accession number   fn. = footnotes   refs. = references

disorders; Canada; *Canadian Stroke Consortium; New York; United States; *Western New York Stroke Consortium

Bacon, Mike; Stewart, Kevin; Bowker, Lesley. CPR decision–making by elderly patients. [Letter]. *Journal of Medical Ethics.* 1998 Apr; 24(2): 134. 5 refs. BE59184.
*aged; competence; *decision making; futility; hospitals; morbidity; mortality; patient admission; *physicians; *resuscitation; *resuscitation orders; time factors; treatment outcome; London

Brown, Sharan E.; Valluzzi, Janet L. Do not resuscitate orders in early intervention settings: who should make the decision? *Infants and Young Children.* 1995 Jan; 7(3): 13–27. 69 fn. BE60498.
age factors; allowing to die; *children; community services; *decision making; directive adherence; *disabled; emergency care; faculty; federal government; government regulation; institutional policies; *legal aspects; *parents; patient care; *resuscitation orders; right to die; *schools; state government; *students; treatment refusal; withholding treatment; primary schools; Americans with Disabilities Act 1990; Education of the Handicapped Act Amendments 1986; Rehabilitation Act 1973; *United States

Carlsen, Mary S.; Pomeroy, Claire; Moldow, D. Gay. Optimizing discussions about resuscitation: development of a guide based on patients' recommendations. *Journal of Clinical Ethics.* 1998 Fall; 9(3): 263–272. 20 fn. BE61335.
*advance care planning; age factors; *attitudes; *communication; competence; comprehension; counseling; decision making; disclosure; evaluation studies; informed consent; nurses; *patient education; *patient participation; *patient satisfaction; *patients; physicians; recall; *resuscitation; *resuscitation orders; risk; social workers; statistics; survey; time factors; treatment outcome; United States

Carnevale, Franco A. The utility of futility: the construction of bioethical problems. *Nursing Ethics.* 1998 Nov; 5(6): 509–517. 29 refs. BE60885.
age factors; allowing to die; bioethical issues; *bioethics; communication; dissent; *futility; literature; patient discharge; philosophy; quality of life; *resuscitation; sociology of medicine; terminology; treatment outcome; trends; values; withholding treatment

Clemency, Mary V.; Thompson, Nancy J. Do not resuscitate orders in the perioperative period: patient perspectives. *Anesthesia and Analgesia.* 1997 Apr; 84(4): 859–864. 17 refs. BE60182.
AIDS; *anesthesia; *attitudes; cancer; communication; *decision making; disclosure; informed consent; intention; motivation; pain; palliative care; *patient participation; *patients; physicians; quality of life; *resuscitation; *resuscitation orders; risks and benefits; *surgery; survey; *terminally ill; treatment refusal; qualitative research; Atlanta; Georgia

Crelinsten, Gordon L.; Belik, Jacques; Bereza, Eugene, et al. CPR for patients in a persistent vegetative state? [Letters and response]. *Canadian Medical Association Journal.* 1998 Jul 14; 159(1): 18–19, 21. 8 refs. BE62204.
*allowing to die; *decision making; dissent; *family members; *futility; government financing; health facilities; institutional policies; *organizational policies; *persistent vegetative state; *physicians; professional organizations; *prolongation of life; refusal to treat; religious ethics; resource allocation; *resuscitation; *resuscitation orders; risks and benefits; value of life; values; withholding treatment; Canada; *Canadian Medical Association

Daly, Barbara J.; Gorecki, Julie; Sadowski, Alexis,

et al. Do-not-resuscitate practices in the chronically critically ill. *Heart and Lung.* 1996 Jul–Aug; 25(4): 310–317. 22 refs. BE59427.
chronically ill; comparative studies; competence; *critically ill; economics; evaluation studies; hospitals; *intensive care units; mortality; patient admission; patient discharge; *resuscitation orders; socioeconomic factors; University Hospitals of Cleveland

Flanigan, Rosemary. The most solemn moment of my living. [Editorial]. *Bioethics Forum.* 1998 Spring; 14(1): 3–4. 4 refs. BE59944.
*aged; attitudes; attitudes to death; *resuscitation; *resuscitation orders; statistics; treatment outcome; treatment refusal

Goldsmith, Jay P.; Ginsberg, Harley G.; McGettigan, Marie C. Ethical decisions in the delivery room. *Clinics in Perinatology.* 1996 Sep; 23(3): 529–550. 47 refs. BE60940.
active euthanasia; *allowing to die; attitudes; *congenital disorders; *decision making; deontological ethics; government regulation; health personnel; intensive care units; legal aspects; *low birth weight; moral policy; *newborns; parents; *physicians; *prematurity; prenatal injuries; *resuscitation; *selection for treatment; teleological ethics; values; viability; withholding treatment; United States

Heffner, John E.; Barbieri, Celia. Compliance with do–not–resuscitate orders for hospitalized patients transported to radiology departments. *Annals of Internal Medicine.* 1998 Nov 15; 129(10): 801–805. 20 refs. BE59323.
communication; *directive adherence; *hospitals; *institutional policies; medical records; *radiology; resuscitation; *resuscitation orders; survey; United States
BACKGROUND: Little is known about the effectiveness of do–not–resuscitate (DNR) orders during transport of hospitalized patients away from their rooms. OBJECTIVE: To determine compliance with DNR orders in radiology departments. DESIGN: Observational study. SETTING: 248 hospital-based radiology departments. PARTICIPANTS: 248 radiology department representatives. MEASUREMENTS: 10-item questionnaire examining the response of radiology personnel to patients with DNR orders who experience cardiopulmonary arrest. RESULTS: Written DNR protocols and structured procedures for communicating DNR status were used by 18.5% (CI, 13.7% to 23.4%) and 18.1% (CI, 13.3% to 23.0%) of departments, respectively. Medical chart review was the only source of information on DNR status for 41.5% (CI, 35.4% to 47.7%) of departments. It was found that 20.2% of respondents (CI, 15.2% to 25.2%) would resuscitate patients with DNR orders and that 38.3% (CI, 32.3% to 44.4%) had resuscitated patients with DNR orders in the past. CONCLUSIONS: Most radiology departments do not have formal procedures to prevent patients from undergoing unwanted or inappropriate resuscitative interventions, and DNR orders are frequently overruled.

Henderson, Shelley; Fins, Joseph J.; Moskowitz, Ellen H. Resuscitation in hospice. [Case study and commentaries]. *Hastings Center Report.* 1998 Nov–Dec; 28(6): 20–22. BE61280.
advance care planning; attitudes; autonomy; beneficence; case studies; *communication; *dissent; *family members; futility; goals; *home care; *hospices; informed consent; *palliative care; *patient care team; physician patient relationship; professional family relationship; *resuscitation orders; terminal care; *terminally ill; time factors

---

BE = bioethics accession number   fn. = footnotes   refs. = references

Hook, C. Christopher; Koch, Kathryn A. Ethics of resuscitation. *Critical Care Clinics.* 1996 Jan; 12(1): 135–148. 53 refs. BE59283.
> advance directives; allied health personnel; allowing to die; autonomy; beneficence; *decision making; disclosure; emergency care; family members; futility; guidelines; hospitals; informed consent; intensive care units; patient admission; patient discharge; patients; physicians; presumed consent; prolongation of life; resource allocation; *resuscitation; *resuscitation orders; right to die; time factors; treatment outcome; treatment refusal; withholding treatment; United States

Hosford, Ian; Brown, Edna; Duncan, Crawford. Formulating a "do not resuscitate" policy for a psychogeriatric service: need for consultation with Maori. *New Zealand Medical Journal.* 1995 Jun 14; 108(1001): 226–228. 20 refs. BE60058.
> *aged; communication; competence; *cultural pluralism; decision making; dementia; family members; *hospitals; *institutional policies; legal aspects; *mentally ill; *minority groups; patient care team; patient participation; *practice guidelines; resuscitation; *resuscitation orders; third party consent; hospital psychiatric units; *Maoris; *New Zealand; Porirua Hospital (NZ)

Illinois. Appellate Court, First District, Fourth Division. In re Estate of Austwick. *North Eastern Reporter, 2d Series.* 1995 Sep 7 (date of decision). 656: 773–779. BE59974.
> aged; competence; *decision making; institutionalized persons; *legal aspects; *legal guardians; nursing homes; patient care; psychoactive drugs; *resuscitation orders; *third party consent; Illinois; *In re Estate of Austwick
The Illinois Appellate Court for the First District held that a public guardian is not authorized to enter a do-not-resuscitate (DNR) order into a ward's medical chart when the ward has the decisional capacity to forgo life-sustaining treatment. Lucille Austwich, an 81-year-old woman in a nursing home, was adjudicated as disabled under the state's probate act and appointed a public guardian. The guardian entered a DNR order into Austwick's chart with her consent. Austwick petitioned the court one year later to have the order removed. The court here affirmed the trial court's order for removal of the DNR order because the guardian lacked authority to enter the order. Austwick had further argued that her public guardian should be removed for cause because he lacked legal authority when he consented to the DNR order and to psychotropic medication treatment. The court held that the public guardian's erroneous misinterpretation of the probate act was without bad faith and did not prejudice Austwick and, thus, did not warrant removal for cause. (KIE abstract)

Juhl, Marian Haglund. A tattoo in time: I want my last wish to be clearly visible so it will be honored by the doctor who treats me. *Newsweek.* 1997 Oct 13; 130(15): 19. BE60025.
> advance care planning; advance directives; aged; *communication; methods; registries; *resuscitation orders; treatment refusal; United States

Kane, Richard S.; Hammes, Bernard; Morgenweck, Cynthiane J., et al. Nursing home CPR policies. [Letter and response]. *Journal of the American Geriatrics Society.* 1998 Jan; 46(1): 116–117. 6 refs. BE59435.
> aged; autonomy; futility; *institutional policies; *nursing homes; prognosis; resource allocation; *resuscitation; *resuscitation orders; risks and benefits; selection for treatment; treatment outcome; withholding treatment

Kennedy, Ian. Adult: order concerning future non-treatment: Re R (Adult: Medical Treatment). [Comment]. *Medical Law Review.* 1997 Spring; 5(1): 104–108. BE59762.
> adults; allowing to die; *decision making; guidelines; *legal aspects; *mentally retarded; parents; *physically disabled; professional organizations; quality of life; *resuscitation orders; risks and benefits; third party consent; treatment outcome; withholding treatment; adult offspring; antibiotics; British Medical Association; *Great Britain; *Re R (Adult: Medical Treatment); Royal College of Nursing

Koenig, Kristi L.; Salvucci, Angelo A.; Goodwin, Peter A., et al. Out-of-hospital do-not-attempt-resuscitation in the suicidal patient: a special case [and] Death with dignity. [Letters and response]. *Academic Emergency Medicine.* 1997 Sep; 4(9): 926–928. 8 refs. BE59124.
> allied health personnel; *assisted suicide; attitudes; *emergency care; physicians; *resuscitation; *resuscitation orders; *suicide; terminally ill; California; Oregon

Kondro, Wayne. "Do-not-resuscitate" order lifted in Canada. [News]. *Lancet.* 1998 Nov 21; 352(9141): 1689. BE61103.
> aged; *decision making; *dissent; family members; hospitals; judicial action; *legal aspects; physicians; *resuscitation orders; third party consent; *Manitoba; *Sawatzky, Andrew

Lachs, John. Resuscitation. *In: his* The Relevance of Philosophy to Life. Nashville, TN: Vanderbilt University Press; 1995: 176–180. 1 fn. ISBN 0-8265-1262-3. BE60862.
> active euthanasia; allowing to die; intention; killing; moral policy; physicians; resuscitation; *resuscitation orders; *withholding treatment; dependency

Larkin, Marilynn. Resuscitation preferences for heart-failure patients likely to change. [News]. *Lancet.* 1998 Aug 28; 352(9129): 711. BE61101.
> *attitudes; *communication; *critically ill; empirical research; *heart diseases; *patients; physicians; *resuscitation; *seriously ill; *Study to Understand Prognoses and Preferences for Outcomes and Risks of Treatments (SUPPORT)

Lonchyna, Vassyl A. To resuscitate or not ... in the operating room: the need for hospital policies for surgeons regarding DNR orders. *Annals of Health Law.* 1997; 6: 209–227. 78 fn. BE59376.
> advance directives; allowing to die; anesthesia; autonomy; *decision making; directive adherence; futility; guidelines; *hospitals; iatrogenic disease; informed consent; *institutional policies; legal aspects; physicians; presumed consent; *resuscitation; *resuscitation orders; *surgery; treatment outcome; treatment refusal; withholding treatment; United States

McDermott, Vincent G. Resuscitation and the radiologist. [Editorial]. *Annals of Internal Medicine.* 1998 Nov 15; 129(10): 831–833. 15 refs. BE59324.
> communication; *directive adherence; *hospitals; *institutional policies; *radiology; resuscitation; *resuscitation orders

Marco, Catherine A.; Bessman, Edward S.; Schoenfeld, Charles N., et al. Ethical issues of cardiopulmonary resuscitation: current practice among emergency physicians. *Academic Emergency Medicine.* 1997 Sep; 4(9): 898–904. 53 refs. BE59123.
> advance directives; age factors; *decision making; directive adherence; *emergency care; evaluation studies; futility; guidelines; *knowledge, attitudes, practice; legal liability; *physicians; prognosis; *resuscitation; *resuscitation orders;

---

survey; treatment outcome; oral directives; *United States

Marik, Paul E.; Craft, Michele. An outcomes analysis of in-hospital cardiopulmonary resuscitation: the futility rationale for do not resuscitate orders. *Journal of Critical Care.* 1997 Sep; 12(3): 142–146. 27 refs. BE59432.
diagnosis; evaluation studies; *futility; *hospitals; institutional policies; mortality; patient discharge; *resuscitation; *resuscitation orders; selection for treatment; time factors; *treatment outcome; retrospective studies; St. Vincent Hospital (Worcester, MA)

Mason, Sue. The ethical dilemma of the do not resuscitate order. *British Journal of Nursing.* 1997 Jun 12–25; 6(11): 646–649. 27 refs. BE59424.
accountability; communication; decision making; living wills; *nurses; nursing ethics; patient advocacy; patient participation; physician nurse relationship; physicians; *resuscitation orders; Great Britain

Midwest Bioethics Center. Kansas City Area Ethics Committee Consortium. Honoring do-not-resuscitate (DNR) orders during invasive procedures. *Bioethics Forum.* 1998 Spring; 14(1): 23–26. 3 refs. This document was completed in 1994 and revised in 1997. BE59947.
communication; iatrogenic disease; informed consent; medical records; motivation; patient care team; patients; physicians; *practice guidelines; resuscitation; *resuscitation orders; risk; *surgery; third party consent; treatment outcome; treatment refusal; withholding treatment; *Kansas City Area Ethics Committee Consortium; Missouri

Mobeireek, Abdullah. The do-not-resuscitate order: indications on the current practice in Riyadh. *Annals of Saudi Medicine.* 1995 Jan; 15(1): 6–9. 29 refs. BE59197.
*attitudes; autonomy; *decision making; futility; hospitals; institutional policies; paternalism; patient participation; *physicians; resuscitation; *resuscitation orders; statistics; survey; treatment refusal; *Saudi Arabia

Mohr, M.; Kettler, D. Ethical aspects of prehospital CPR. *Acta Anaesthesiologica Scandinavica.* 1997; 41(Suppl. 111): 298–300. 20 refs. BE61551.
age factors; attitudes; critically ill; decision making; *emergency care; futility; guidelines; health personnel; patients; physicians; prognosis; *resuscitation; *resuscitation orders; terminally ill; time factors; treatment outcome; *withholding treatment; *ambulatory care

New York. Supreme Court, Albany County. In re Finn. *New York Supplement, 2d Series.* 1995 Feb 21 (date of decision). 625: 809–814. BE62193.
competence; constitutional law; *decision making; extraordinary treatment; futility; institutionalized persons; *legal aspects; legal guardians; *legislation; *mentally retarded; physicians; quality of life; *resuscitation orders; third party consent; treatment outcome; *In re Finn; *New York
The New York Supreme Court, Albany County, invalidated portions of New York's Do Not Resuscitate (DNR) law for vagueness and rescinded a DNR order written for a sixty-seven year old profoundly retarded man with many ailments, none life threatening. The New York DNR law permits orders to be written for the incompetent when two physicians concur that the order is in the patient's best interests and that to a reasonable degree of medical certainty, (1) the patient has a terminal condition, (2) the patient is permanently unconscious, (3) resuscitation would be medically futile, or (4) resuscitation would impose an extraordinary burden on the patient in light of the patient's medical condition and the expected outcome of resuscitation. The court held that the extraordinary burden prong of the test was

unconstitutionally vague, as the term was not legislatively defined and open to multiple interpretations. Additionally, the court found that the physician entering the DNR order had failed to make a written assessment of the patient's competence. (KIE abstract)

Pacheco, R.; Osuna, E.; Gómez–Zapata, M., et al. Medicolegal problems associated with do not resuscitate orders. *Medicine and Law.* 1994; 13(5–6): 461–466. 24 refs. BE60005.
autonomy; beneficence; critically ill; decision making; disclosure; emergency care; informed consent; *legal aspects; paternalism; patient participation; physicians; presumed consent; resuscitation; *resuscitation orders; treatment refusal; value of life; *Spain

Proulx, Amy J. Should you call a code? When a patient's condition is terminal, how do you handle a code? *American Journal of Nursing.* 1998 Jun; 98(6): 41. BE61816.
allowing to die; *decision making; family members; institutional policies; nurses; *nursing ethics; prolongation of life; *resuscitation orders; *terminally ill

Reynolds, Don F.; Garrett, Celia K. Avoiding resuscitation in non-hospital settings: *no consent* forms. *Bioethics Forum.* 1998 Spring; 14(1): 13–19. 11 refs. BE59946.
*advance directives; autonomy; compensation; consent forms; directive adherence; *emergency care; *forms; home care; hospices; *legal aspects; *legal liability; legal rights; legislation; nursing homes; physicians; prolongation of life; resuscitation; *resuscitation orders; terminally ill; third party consent; treatment refusal; withholding treatment; Kansas; Missouri; Murphy v. Wheeler; Younts v. St. Francis Hospital and School of Nursing

Sanders, Arthur B. Do we need a clinical decision rule for the discontinuation of cardiac arrest resuscitations? [Editorial]. *Archives of Internal Medicine.* 1999 Jan 25; 159(2): 119–121. 13 refs. BE60228.
adults; aged; critically ill; *decision making; *futility; *hospitals; morbidity; *mortality; *patient discharge; physicians; practice guidelines; *prognosis; resource allocation; *resuscitation; *selection for treatment; time factors; *treatment outcome; *withholding treatment

Sanders, Arthur B. When are resuscitation attempts futile? [Editorial]. *Academic Emergency Medicine.* 1997 Sep; 4(9): 852–853. 10 refs. BE59122.
age factors; consensus; *decision making; *emergency care; *futility; *goals; guidelines; hospitals; *physicians; *prognosis; quality of life; *resuscitation; resuscitation orders; treatment outcome; withholding treatment; ambulatory care; United States

Segal, Eran; Halamish–Shani, Talia; Rich, Harlin, et al. The slow code. [Letters and response]. *New England Journal of Medicine.* 1998 Jun 25; 338(26): 1921–1923. 8 refs. BE59239.
age factors; attitudes to death; communication; deception; decision making; dissent; family members; futility; *intention; methods; palliative care; paternalism; physician patient relationship; physicians; professional family relationship; prognosis; *resuscitation; *resuscitation orders; selection for treatment; terminal care; terminally ill; treatment outcome

Soll, Roger. Consensus and controversy over resuscitation of the newborn infant. *Lancet.* 1999 Jul 3; 354(9172): 4–5. 13 refs. BE62407.
consensus; developing countries; emergency care; human experimentation; international aspects; mortality; *newborns; physicians; practice guidelines; professional organizations; prolongation of life; *resuscitation; selection for treatment;

BE = bioethics accession number   fn. = footnotes   refs. = references

*International Liaison Committee on Resuscitation; World Health Organization

Sosna, Dennis. Advance directives for emergency medical service workers: the struggle continues. *Bioethics Forum.* 1998 Spring; 14(1): 33–36. BE59949.
*advance directives; *allied health personnel; directive adherence; education; *emergency care; *forms; *legal aspects; living wills; medical records; resuscitation; *resuscitation orders; *standards; withholding treatment; *Kansas; *Kansas City Area Ethics Committee Consortium; Midwest Bioethics Center

Square, David. Court verdict "splendid," ethics professor says. [News]. *Canadian Medical Association Journal.* 1998 Jan 27; 158(2): 159–160. BE60594.
child abuse; criminal law; *decision making; family members; *futility; infants; *legal aspects; legal liability; organizational policies; persistent vegetative state; *physicians; professional organizations; *resuscitation orders; *Manitoba; Manitoba Medical Association

Stoddard, Jim. A practical approach to DNR discussions. *Bioethics Forum.* 1998 Spring; 14(1): 27–32. 18 refs. BE59948.
advance directives; anesthesia; *communication; comprehension; decision making; family members; palliative care; patient care; *patients; *physicians; quality of life; *resuscitation; *resuscitation orders; risks and benefits; statistics; surgery; treatment outcome

Sullivan, M. C. The changing order of things [resuscitation]. *Bioethics Forum.* 1998 Spring; 14(1): 37–40. 3 refs. BE59950.
case studies; communication; decision making; physicians; resuscitation; *resuscitation orders; risks and benefits; terminal care

Teno, Joan M.; Branco, Kenneth J.; Mor, Vincent, et al. Changes in advance care planning in nursing homes before and after the Patient Self-Determination Act: report of a 10-state survey. *Journal of the American Geriatrics Society.* 1997 Aug; 45(8): 939–944. 43 refs. BE59434.
*advance care planning; *advance directives; aged; artificial feeding; comparative studies; evaluation studies; *geographic factors; hospitals; *institutional policies; institutionalized persons; legislation; living wills; medical records; *nursing homes; patient transfer; *resuscitation orders; *social impact; statistics; survey; third party consent; *time factors; treatment refusal; withholding treatment; *Patient Self-Determination Act 1990; *United States

van Walraven, Carl; Forster, Alan J.; Stiell, Ian G. Derivation of a clinical decision rule for the discontinuation of in-hospital cardiac arrest resuscitations. *Archives of Internal Medicine.* 1999 Jan 25; 159(2): 129–134. 30 refs. BE60229.
adults; age factors; aged; critically ill; *decision making; evaluation studies; *futility; *hospitals; morbidity; *mortality; *patient discharge; physicians; practice guidelines; *prognosis; resource allocation; *resuscitation; *selection for treatment; time factors; *treatment outcome; *withholding treatment; Ontario
BACKGROUND: Most patients undergoing in-hospital cardiac resuscitation will not survive to hospital discharge. OBJECTIVE: To derive a decision rule permitting the discontinuation of futile resuscitation attempts by identifying patients with no chance of surviving to hospital discharge. PATIENTS AND METHODS: Patient, arrest, and outcome data for 1077 adult patients undergoing in-hospital cardiac resuscitation was retrieved from 2 randomized clinical trials involving 5 teaching hospitals at 2 university

centers. Recursive partitioning was used to identify a decision rule using variables significantly associated with death in hospital. RESULTS: One hundred three patients (9.6%) survived to hospital discharge. Death in hospital was significantly more likely if patients were older than 75 years (P less than .001), the arrest was unwitnessed (P = .003), the resuscitation lasted longer than 10 minutes (P less than .001), and the initial cardiac rhythm was not ventricular tachycardia or fibrillation (P less than .001). All patients died if there was no pulse 10 minutes after the start of cardiopulmonary resuscitation, the initial cardiac rhythm was not ventricular tachycardia or fibrillation, and the arrest was not witnessed. As a resuscitation rule, these parameters identified all patients who survived to hospital discharge (sensitivity, 100%; 95% confidence interval, 97.1%–100%). Resuscitation could have been discontinued for 119 (12.1%) of 974 patients who did not survive, thereby avoiding 47 days of postresuscitative care. CONCLUSIONS: A practical and highly sensitive decision rule has been derived that identifies patients with no chance of surviving in-hospital cardiac arrest. Prospective validation of the rule is necessary before it can be used clinically.

Weijer, Charles. Cardiopulmonary resuscitation for patients in a persistent vegetative state: futile or acceptable? [Editorial]. *Canadian Medical Association Journal.* 1998 Feb 24; 158(4): 491–493. 19 refs. BE60584.
*allowing to die; case studies; *decision making; dissent; *family members; *futility; legal aspects; organizational policies; *persistent vegetative state; *physicians; professional organizations; *prolongation of life; refusal to treat; religious ethics; *resuscitation; *resuscitation orders; risks and benefits; value of life; withholding treatment; dignity; Canada; United States

Zweig, Steven C. An alternate policy for CPR in nursing homes. *Bioethics Forum.* 1998 Spring; 14(1): 5–11. 51 refs. BE59945.
advance directives; *aged; decision making; disclosure; family members; futility; health personnel; informed consent; *institutional policies; *nursing homes; palliative care; patients; *resuscitation; *resuscitation orders; risks and benefits; standards; treatment outcome; United States

Zweig, Steven C. Cardiopulmonary resuscitation and do-not-resuscitate orders in the nursing home. *Archives of Family Medicine.* 1997 Sep–Oct; 6(5): 424–429. 83 refs. BE61612.
advance care planning; advance directives; *aged; allowing to die; attitudes; autonomy; beneficence; blacks; chronically ill; costs and benefits; critically ill; decision making; directive adherence; disclosure; emergency care; family members; futility; *guidelines; hospitals; iatrogenic disease; informed consent; *institutional policies; medical records; mortality; *nursing homes; patient discharge; patient participation; patient transfer; physicians; prolongation of life; *resuscitation; *resuscitation orders; risks and benefits; selection for treatment; statistics; third party consent; *treatment outcome; whites; withholding treatment; United States

Do-not-resuscitate order; public school -- ABC School and DEF School v. Mr. and Mrs. M. *Mental and Physical Disability Law Reporter.* 1997 Nov–Dec; 21(6): 735. Synopsis of a 17 July 1997 ruling by a Massachusetts Superior Court. BE59846.
*children; *directive adherence; *disabled; *institutional policies; *legal aspects; legal rights; *parents; prolongation of life; *resuscitation orders; *schools; *students; *treatment refusal; *ABC School and DEF School v. Mr. and Mrs. M.; *Massachusetts

---

BE = bioethics accession number   fn. = footnotes   refs. = references

RIGHT TO DIE *See* ALLOWING TO DIE, EUTHANASIA, SUICIDE

RIGHTS
See under
HEALTH CARE/RIGHTS

SCIENTIFIC MISCONDUCT *See* FRAUD AND MISCONDUCT

SELECTION FOR TREATMENT

See also ALLOWING TO DIE, PATIENT CARE, RESOURCE ALLOCATION

Alexander, G. Caleb; Sehgal, Ashwini R. Barriers to cadaveric renal transplantation among blacks, women, and the poor. *JAMA.* 1998 Oct 7; 280(13): 1148–1152. 21 refs. BE60285.
    attitudes; blacks; cadavers; comparative studies; females; indigents; *kidneys; males; *organ transplantation; patients; prognosis; referral and consultation; renal dialysis; *resource allocation; *selection for treatment; *socioeconomic factors; *transplant recipients; whites; prospective studies; waiting lists; Indiana; Kentucky; Ohio
CONTEXT: Cadaveric renal transplantation rates differ greatly by race, sex, and income. Previous efforts to lessen these differences have focused on the transplant waiting list. However, the transplantation process involves a series of steps related to medical suitability, interest in transplantation, pretransplant workup, and movement up a waiting list to eventual transplantation. OBJECTIVE: To determine the relative importance of each step in explaining differences in cadaveric renal transplantation rates. DESIGN: Prospective cohort study. SETTING AND PATIENTS: A total of 7125 patients beginning long-term dialysis between January 1993 and December 1996 in Indiana, Kentucky, and Ohio. MAIN OUTCOME MEASURES: Completion of 4 separate steps during each patient-year of follow-up: (A) being medically suitable and possibly interested in transplantation; (B) being definitely interested in transplantation; (C) completing the pretransplant workup; and (D) moving up a waiting list and receiving a transplant. RESULTS: Compared with whites, blacks were less likely to complete steps B (odds ratio [OR], 0.68; 95% confidence interval [CI], 0.61–0.76), C (OR, 0.56; 95% CI, 0.48–0.65), and D (OR, 0.50; 95% CI, 0.40–0.62) after adjustment for age, sex, cause of renal failure, years receiving dialysis, and median income of patient ZIP code. Compared with men, women were less likely to complete each of the 4 steps, with ORs of 0.90, 0.89, 0.80, and 0.82, respectively. Poor individuals were less likely than wealthy individuals to complete steps A, B, and C, with ORs of 0.67, 0.78, and 0.77, respectively. CONCLUSIONS: Barriers at several steps are responsible for sociodemographic differences in access to cadaveric renal transplantation. Efforts to allocate kidneys equitably must address each step of the transplant process.

Ankeny, Rachel A. Recasting the debate on multiple listing for transplantation through consideration of both principles and practice. *Cambridge Quarterly of Healthcare Ethics.* 1999 Summer; 8(3): 330–339. 30 fn. BE62476.
    autonomy; body parts and fluids; *geographic factors; hospitals; institutional policies; justice; motivation; *organ transplantation; *patients; public policy; *resource

allocation; scarcity; *selection for treatment; socioeconomic factors; standards; time factors; *transplant recipients; *waiting lists; United Network for Organ Sharing; United States

Asch, Steven; Frayne, Susan; Waitzkin, Howard. To discharge or not to discharge: ethics of care for an undocumented immigrant. *Journal of Health Care for the Poor and Underserved.* 1995; 6(1): 3–9. 27 refs. BE60569.
    *aliens; autonomy; beneficence; case studies; decision making; gatekeeping; government financing; health care delivery; hospitals; indigents; justice; *kidney diseases; legal aspects; *patient discharge; *physicians; public policy; *refusal to treat; *renal dialysis; *resource allocation; *selection for treatment; United States

Baetens, P.; Ponjaert-Kristoffersen, I.; Devroey, P., et al. Artificial insemination by donor: an alternative for single women. *Human Reproduction.* 1995 Jun; 10(6): 1537–1542. 17 refs. BE60412.
    *artificial insemination; *counseling; *females; health facilities; institutional policies; mothers; motivation; parent child relationship; program descriptions; refusal to treat; *selection for treatment; semen donors; *single persons; socioeconomic factors; Belgium; Free University of Brussels

Barakat, Khalid; Wilkinson, Paul; Deaner, Andrew, et al. How should age affect management of acute myocardial infarction? A prospective cohort study. *Lancet.* 1999 Mar 20; 353(9157): 955–959. 23 refs. BE61462.
    *age factors; *aged; drugs; evaluation studies; *heart diseases; hospitals; mortality; *patient care; *prognosis; *selection for treatment; social discrimination; treatment outcome; *myocardial infarction; prospective studies; thrombolytic therapy; Great Britain

Barrow, Chelmer L.; Easley, Kirk A. The role of gender and race on the time delay for emergency department patients complaining of chest pain to be evaluated by a physician. *Saint Louis University Public Law Review.* 1996; 15(2): 267–277. 38 fn. Commented on by J. Barrow, p. 278–302. BE59910.
    *age factors; *blacks; comparative studies; *emergency care; *females; health care delivery; *heart diseases; *hospitals; institutional policies; *males; *quality of health care; *selection for treatment; social discrimination; *time factors; *whites; myocardial infarction; retrospective studies

Barrow, Jackie. Implications of the Emergency Medical Treatment and Active Labor Act (EMTALA) on differences based on race and gender in the treatment of patients presenting to a hospital emergency department with chest pain. *Saint Louis University Public Law Review.* 1996; 15(2): 278–302. 165 fn. Commentary on C.L. Barrow and K.A. Easley, p. 267–277. BE59911.
    age factors; blacks; *emergency care; federal government; females; *government regulation; heart diseases; *hospitals; indigents; institutional ethics; institutional policies; *legal aspects; legislation; males; minority groups; patient transfer; *quality of health care; *selection for treatment; social discrimination; *socioeconomic factors; standards; *Emergency Medical Treatment and Active Labor Act 1986; Medicare; *United States

Beecham, Linda. UK issues guidance on prescribing Viagra. [News]. *BMJ (British Medical Journal).* 1999 Jan 30; 318(7179): 279. BE61556.
    attitudes; diagnosis; dissent; drug industry; *drugs; *government financing; guidelines; *males; organizational policies; *patient care; *physicians; professional organizations; *public policy; *resource allocation; *selection for treatment; sexuality; social discrimination; *impotence; personal financing; British Medical Association;

BE = bioethics accession number   fn. = footnotes   refs. = references

*Great Britain; *National Health Service; Royal College of Physicians; *Viagra

Binstock, Robert H. Old-age-based rationing: from rhetoric to risk? *Generations (American Society on Aging)*. 1994 Winter; 18(4): 37-41. 41 refs. BE60550.
*age factors; *aged; *economics; federal government; government financing; *health care delivery; justice; *public policy; quality of life; *resource allocation; *selection for treatment; terminal care; wedge argument; withholding treatment; Medicare; *United States

Burrows, R. Removal of life support in intensive care units. *Medicine and Law*. 1994; 13(5-6): 489-500. 60 refs. BE60007.
*allowing to die; autonomy; brain death; cardiac death; *decision making; deontological ethics; determination of death; economics; futility; informed consent; *intensive care units; legal aspects; patient admission; patient care; *physician's role; physicians; prognosis; *resource allocation; rights; *selection for treatment; third party consent; utilitarianism; withholding treatment; *South Africa

Caplan, Arthur L.; Coelho, Daniel H. The Ethics of Organ Transplants: The Current Debate. Amherst, NY: Prometheus Books; 1998. 350 p. Bibliography: p. 347-350. ISBN 1-57392-224-2. BE60916.
aborted fetuses; abortion, induced; alcohol abuse; altruism; anencephaly; animal organs; blacks; brain death; cadavers; cardiac death; coercion; commodification; determination of death; directed donation; disadvantaged; donor cards; economics; family members; fetal tissue donation; health insurance reimbursement; incentives; international aspects; justice; kidneys; legal aspects; livers; *moral policy; *organ donation; organ donors; *organ transplantation; persistent vegetative state; presumed consent; primates; prognosis; *public policy; *remuneration; required request; *resource allocation; retreatment; *selection for treatment; *tissue transplantation; transplant recipients; mandated choice; refusal to donate; *unrelated donors; Medicaid; Medicare; Oregon; Uniform Anatomical Gift Act; United States

Chandna, Shahid M.; Schulz, Joerg; Lawrence, Christopher, et al. Is there a rationale for rationing chronic dialysis? A hospital based cohort study of factors affecting survival and morbidity. *BMJ (British Medical Journal)*. 1999 Jan 23; 318(7178): 217-223. 25 refs. BE60327.
age factors; diabetes; economics; evaluation studies; hospitals; kidney diseases; *morbidity; *mortality; *prognosis; *renal dialysis; *resource allocation; *selection for treatment; *treatment outcome; retrospective studies; Great Britain
OBJECTIVES: To determine factors influencing survival and need for hospitalisation in patients needing dialysis, and to define the potential basis for rationing access to renal replacement therapy. DESIGN: Hospital based cohort study of all patients starting dialysis over a 4 year recruitment period (follow up 15-63 months). Groups were defined on the basis of age, comorbidity, functional status, and whether dialysis initiation was planned or unplanned. SETTING: Renal unit in a district general hospital, which acts as the main renal referral centre for four other such hospitals and serves a population of about 1.15 million people. SUBJECTS: 292 patients, mean age 61.3 years (18-92 years, SD 15.8), of whom 193 (66%) were male, and 59 (20%) were patients with diabetes. Dialysis initiation was planned in 163 (56%) patients and unplanned in 129 (44%). MAIN OUTCOME MEASURES: Overall survival, 1 year survival, and hospitalisation rate. RESULTS: Factors affecting survival in the Cox's proportional hazard model were Karnofsky performance score at presentation (hazard ratio 0.979, 95% confidence interval

0.972 to 0.986), comorbidity severity score (1.240, 1.131 to 1.340), age (1.036, 1.018 to 1.054), and myeloma (2.15, 1.140 to 4.042). The Karnofsky performance score used 3 months before presentation was significant (0.970, 0.956 to 0.981), as was unplanned presentation in this model (1.796, 1.233 to 2.617). Using these factors, a high risk group of 26 patients was defined, with 19.2% 1 year survival. Denying dialysis to this group would save 3.2% of the total cost of the chronic programme but would sacrifice five long term survivors. Less rigorous definition of the high risk group would save more money but lose more long term survivors. CONCLUSIONS: Severity of comorbid conditions and functional capacity are more important than age in predicting survival and morbidity of patients on dialysis. Late referral for dialysis affects survival adversely. Denial of dialysis to patients in an extremely high risk group, defined by a new stratification based on logistic regression, would be of debatable benefit.

Chase, Marilyn. Rationing scarce drugs has some questioning fairness and ethics. [News]. *Wall Street Journal*. 1998 Sep 28: B1. BE61125.
*breast cancer; *drug industry; females; *investigational drugs; patient care; *random selection; *resource allocation; *scarcity; *selection for treatment; selection of subjects; therapeutic research; *compassionate use; *Genentech Inc.; *Herceptin

de Beaufort, Inez. Letter from a post-menopausal mother. *In:* Harris, John; Holm, Søren, eds. The Future of Human Reproduction: Ethics, Choice, Regulation. New York, NY: Oxford University Press; 1998: 238-247. ISBN 0-19-823761-7. BE61273.
*age factors; attitudes; children; fathers; females; morality; mothers; motivation; *parent child relationship; *reproductive technologies; risks and benefits; *selection for treatment

de Wert, Guido M.W.R. The post-menopause: playground for reproductive technology? Some ethical reflections. *In:* Harris, John; Holm, Søren, eds. The Future of Human Reproduction: Ethics, Choice, and Regulation. New York, NY: Oxford University Press; 1998: 221-237. 27 fn. ISBN 0-19-823761-8. BE61272.
*age factors; autonomy; children; decision making; *females; government financing; guidelines; informed consent; international aspects; justice; males; maternal health; moral policy; multiple pregnancy; ovum donors; parent child relationship; physicians; *reproductive technologies; resource allocation; risk; scarcity; *selection for treatment; personal financing; Europe

Eisenberg, V.H.; Schenker, J.G. Pregnancy in the older woman: scientific and ethical aspects. *International Journal of Gynaecology and Obstetrics*. 1997 Feb; 56(2): 163-169. 41 refs. BE60689.
adults; *age factors; females; human rights; international aspects; maternal health; morbidity; mortality; newborns; ovum donors; regulation; remuneration; reproduction; *reproductive technologies; resource allocation; risk; risks and benefits; *selection for treatment

Evans, Roger W. Liver transplantation in a managed care environment. *Liver Transplantation and Surgery*. 1995 Jan; 1(1): 61-75. 75 refs. BE60903.
biomedical research; biomedical technologies; *costs and benefits; *economics; geographic factors; goals; health care; health care reform; health facilities; justice; *livers; *managed care programs; *organ transplantation; physicians; practice guidelines; prognosis; *resource allocation; risk; *selection for treatment; transplant recipients; treatment outcome; trends; *United States

---

BE = bioethics accession number   fn. = footnotes   refs. = references

Fisher, Fleur; Sommerville, Ann. To everything there is a season? Are there medical grounds for refusing fertility treatment to older women? *In:* Harris, John; Holm, Søren, eds. The Future of Human Reproduction: Ethics, Choice, and Regulation. New York, NY: Oxford University Press; 1998: 203–220. 34 fn. ISBN 0-19-823761-8. BE61271.
*age factors; attitudes; children; embryo transfer; *females; in vitro fertilization; infertility; legal aspects; maternal health; mortality; multiple pregnancy; ovum donors; *reproductive technologies; *selection for treatment; statistics; treatment outcome; life expectancy; Great Britain

Fost, Norman. Decisions regarding treatment of seriously ill newborns. [Editorial]. *JAMA.* 1999 Jun 2; 281(21): 2041-2043. 18 refs. BE61905.
adolescents; *allowing to die; attitudes; *congenital disorders; *decision making; disabled; empirical research; ethics consultation; intensive care units; *low birth weight; *newborns; nurses; parents; *patient care; physicians; prematurity; prognosis; *prolongation of life; *quality of life; resource allocation; *selection for treatment; *treatment outcome; trends; *uncertainty; withholding treatment; neonatology; United States

France. Order of 6 Nov 1996 approving the Rules for the distribution and allocation of transplants removed from deceased persons for the purpose of organ transplantation. (*Journal officiel de la Republique fran3aise, Lois et Decrets*, 10 Nov 1996, No. 263, pp. 16475-16476). *International Digest of Health Legislation.* 1997; 48(1): 15-18. BE59588.
adults; *body parts and fluids; cadavers; children; *legal aspects; *organ transplantation; prognosis; *resource allocation; *selection for treatment; time factors; transplant recipients; *France

Frazier, William D. Rationing of health care -- who determines who gets the cure, when, where, and why? *Annals of Health Law.* 1993; 2: 95–99. 9 fn. BE59828.
age factors; economics; health care; health care delivery; *resource allocation; *selection for treatment; social worth; United States

Goldsmith, Jay P.; Ginsberg, Harley G.; McGettigan, Marie C. Ethical decisions in the delivery room. *Clinics in Perinatology.* 1996 Sep; 23(3): 529–550. 47 refs. BE60940.
active euthanasia; *allowing to die; attitudes; *congenital disorders; *decision making; deontological ethics; government regulation; health personnel; intensive care units; legal aspects; *low birth weight; moral policy; *newborns; parents; *physicians; *prematurity; prenatal injuries; *resuscitation; *selection for treatment; teleological ethics; values; viability; withholding treatment; United States

Grubb, Andrew. Infertility treatment: access and judicial review -- R v. Sheffield Health Authority, ex parte Seale. [Comment]. *Medical Law Review.* 1996 Autumn; 4(3): 326–329. BE61516.
*age factors; females; *government financing; *in vitro fertilization; *judicial action; *legal aspects; *public policy; refusal to treat; *reproductive technologies; *resource allocation; *selection for treatment; *Great Britain; National Health Service; *R v. Sheffield Health Authority, ex parte Seale

Hamel, Mary Beth; Teno, Joan M.; Goldman, Lee, et al. Patient age and decisions to withhold life-sustaining treatments from seriously ill, hospitalized adults. [For the SUPPORT Investigators]. *Annals of Internal Medicine.* 1999 Jan 19; 130(2): 116-125. 47 refs. BE62556.
*adults; *age factors; *aged; *allowing to die; attitudes; comparative studies; *decision making; dementia; evaluation studies; hospitals; medical records; patients; *physicians; *renal dialysis; resuscitation; *selection for treatment; *surgery; survey; *ventilators; *withholding treatment; seriously ill; Study to Understand Prognoses and Preferences for Outcomes and Risks of Treatments (SUPPORT); United States

BACKGROUND: Patient age may influence decisions to withhold life-sustaining treatments, independent of patients' preferences for or ability to benefit from such treatments. Controversy exists about the appropriateness of using age as a criterion for making treatment decisions. OBJECTIVE: To determine the effect of age on decisions to withhold life-sustaining therapies. DESIGN: Prospective cohort study. SETTING: Five medical centers participating in the Study to Understand Prognoses and Preferences for Outcomes and Risks of Treatments (SUPPORT). PATIENTS: 9105 hospitalized adults who had one of nine illnesses associated with an average 6-month mortality rate of 50%. MEASUREMENTS: Outcomes were the presence and timing of decisions to withhold ventilator support, surgery, and dialysis. Adjustment was made for sociodemographic characteristics, prognoses, baseline function, patients' preferences for life-extending care, and physicians' understanding of patients' preferences for life-extending care. RESULTS: The median patient age was 63 years; 44% of patients were women, and 53% survived to 180 days. In adjusted analyses, older age was associated with higher rates of withholding each of the three life–sustaining treatments studied. For ventilator support, the rate of decisions to withhold therapy increased 15% with each decade of age (hazard ratio, 1.15 [95% CI, 1.12 to 1.19]); for surgery, the increase per decade was 19% (hazard ratio, 1.19 [CI, 1.12 to 1.27]); and for dialysis, the increase per decade was 12% (hazard ratio, 1.12 [CI, 1.06 to 1.19]). Physicians underestimated older patients' preferences for life-extending care; adjustment for this underestimation resulted in an attenuation of the association between age and decisions to withhold treatments. CONCLUSION: Even after adjustment for differences in patients' prognoses and preferences, older age was associated with higher rates of decisions to withhold ventilator support, surgery, and dialysis.

Harris, John. Micro–allocation: deciding between patients. *In:* Kuhse, Helga; Singer, Peter, eds. A Companion to Bioethics. Malden, MA: Blackwell; 1998: 293–305. 12 refs. ISBN 0-631-19737-0. BE59504.
*age factors; alcohol abuse; costs and benefits; decision making; disabled; health care; *justice; moral policy; obligations of society; quality adjusted life years; quality of life; *resource allocation; scarcity; *selection for treatment; *self induced illness; social discrimination; *social worth; needs

Hefferman, Pam; Heilig, Steve. Giving "moral distress" a voice: ethical concerns among neonatal intensive care unit personnel. *Cambridge Quarterly of Healthcare Ethics.* 1999 Spring; 8(2): 173–178. 5 fn. BE61234.
allowing to die; *attitudes; biomedical technologies; *decision making; disabled; disclosure; futility; *intensive care units; *low birth weight; morbidity; mortality; *newborns; *nurses; parental consent; parents; patient care; physicians; practice guidelines; *prematurity; *prognosis; *prolongation of life; *psychological stress; *quality of life; *resuscitation; *selection for treatment; survey; *treatment outcome; ventilators; *viability; withholding treatment; neonatology; qualitative research; California; California Pacific Medical Center

---

BE = bioethics accession number   fn. = footnotes   refs. = references

Himma, Kenneth Einar. A critique of UNOS liver allocation policy. *Cambridge Quarterly of Healthcare Ethics.* 1999 Summer; 8(3): 311–320. 38 fn. Article followed by update on UNOS policy, p. 320. BE62474.
chronically ill; critically ill; emergency care; ethical analysis; *justice; *livers; mortality; *organ transplantation; *organizational policies; *prognosis; *public policy; *resource allocation; scarcity; *selection for treatment; time factors; transplant recipients; treatment outcome; liver diseases; *needs; survival; waiting lists; *United Network for Organ Sharing; United States

Iqbal, Aamir; Holley, Jean L. Ethical issues in end-stage renal disease patients who use illicit intravenous drugs. *Seminars in Dialysis.* 1995 Jan–Feb; 8(1): 35–38. 30 refs. BE59922.
case studies; *drug abuse; *kidney diseases; kidneys; methods; *organ transplantation; *patient compliance; *renal dialysis; *resource allocation; risks and benefits; *selection for treatment; self induced illness; social worth

Kapp, Marshall B. *De facto* health-care rationing by age: the law has no remedy. *Journal of Legal Medicine.* 1998 Sep; 19(3): 323–249. 152 fn. BE61250.
*age factors; *aged; allowing to die; economics; future generations; government financing; health care; legal aspects; moral policy; *physicians; public policy; *resource allocation; *selection for treatment; *social discrimination; social impact; social worth; withholding treatment; duty to die; personal financing; Medicaid; Medicare; United States

Kenyon, Georgina. Doctors refuse to operate on 80 year old man. [News]. *BMJ (British Medical Journal).* 1998 Dec 5; 317(7172): 1548. BE60264.
*aged; decision making; *heart diseases; *institutional policies; patient care team; *public hospitals; *refusal to treat; *resource allocation; *selection for treatment; social discrimination; *surgery; *Australia; *Quinn, John

Kinlaw, Kathy. The changing nature of neonatal ethics in practice. *Clinics in Perinatology.* 1996 Sep; 23(3): 417–428. 20 refs. BE60931.
*allowing to die; anencephaly; brain death; comprehension; *congenital disorders; *decision making; determination of death; disclosure; futility; government regulation; guidelines; informed consent; *intensive care units; *low birth weight; *newborns; parents; patient care; pediatrics; physicians; professional organizations; prognosis; prolongation of life; quality of life; risks and benefits; *selection for treatment; treatment outcome; uncertainty; withholding treatment; American Academy of Pediatrics; In re Baby K; United States

Kluge, Eike-Henner W. Severely disabled newborns. *In:* Kuhse, Helga; Singer, Peter, eds. A Companion to Bioethics. Malden, MA: Blackwell; 1998: 242–249. 29 refs. ISBN 0-631-19737-0. BE59499.
*active euthanasia; *allowing to die; *congenital disorders; decision making; disabled; moral policy; *newborns; parents; prolongation of life; *quality of life; *selection for treatment; suffering

Koch, Tom. The Limits of Principle: Deciding Who Lives and What Dies. Westport, CT: Praeger; 1998. 176 p. Bibliography: p. 159–168. ISBN 0-275-96407-8. BE60113.
allowing to die; amyotrophic lateral sclerosis; *anencephaly; animal rights; *bioethical issues; bioethics; biomedical technologies; consensus; cultural pluralism; *decision making; disabled; Down syndrome; ethical analysis; eugenics; guidelines; historical aspects; intelligence; international aspects; legal aspects; methods; moral policy; newborns; organ donation; *organ transplantation; patient compliance; personhood; prognosis; prolongation of life; *quality of life; renal dialysis; *resource allocation; rights;

scarcity; *selection for treatment; selective abortion; social worth; speciesism; transplant recipients; treatment outcome; *value of life; values

Kravitz, Richard L. Ethnic differences in use of cardiovascular procedures: new insights and new challenges. [Editorial]. *Annals of Internal Medicine.* 1999 Feb 2; 130(3): 231–233. 18 refs. BE60927.
*blacks; health insurance; *heart diseases; kidney diseases; *patient care; physician patient relationship; quality of health care; referral and consultation; *selection for treatment; *surgery; *whites; *angioplasty; continuity of patient care; *coronary artery bypass; undertreatment; Los Angeles; New York City; North Carolina

Kuczewski, Mark G.; Seiden, Dena J.; Frader, Joel, et al. Retransplantation and the "noncompliant" patient. [Case study and commentaries]. *Cambridge Quarterly of Healthcare Ethics.* 1999 Summer; 8(3): 375–381. BE62479.
adolescents; alternatives; case studies; communication; competence; counseling; depressive disorder; drugs; ethicists; justice; kidneys; *organ transplantation; *patient compliance; patient participation; professional patient relationship; refusal to treat; renal dialysis; resource allocation; *retreatment; *selection for treatment; socioeconomic factors; transplant recipients

Landman, Willem A.; Henley, Lesley D. Equitable rationing of highly specialised health care services for children: a perspective from South Africa. *Journal of Medical Ethics.* 1999 Jun; 25(3): 224–229. 34 fn. BE61854.
*biomedical technologies; *children; chronically ill; costs and benefits; cystic fibrosis; disabled; disease; futility; *government financing; *health care; *health care delivery; intensive care units; *justice; legal rights; leukemia; methods; moral policy; newborns; organ transplantation; palliative care; prevalence; primary health care; *prognosis; *public policy; quality of health care; *random selection; *resource allocation; scarcity; *selection for treatment; utilitarianism; needs; patient abandonment; *waiting lists; *South Africa
The principles of equality and equity, respectively in the Bill of Rights and the white paper on health, provide the moral and legal foundations for future health care for children in South Africa. However, given extreme health care need and scarce resources, the government faces formidable obstacles if it hopes to achieve a just allocation of public health care resources, especially among children in need of highly specialised health care. In this regard, there is a dearth of moral analysis which is practically useful in the South African situation. We offer a set of moral considerations to guide the macro-allocation of highly specialised public health care services among South Africa's children. We also mention moral considerations which should inform micro-allocation.

Leape, Lucian L.; Hilborne, Lee H.; Bell, Robert, et al. Underuse of cardiac procedures: do women, ethnic minorities, and the uninsured fail to receive needed revascularization? *Annals of Internal Medicine.* 1999 Feb 2; 130(3): 183–192. 38 refs. BE60926.
blacks; comparative studies; evaluation studies; *females; health insurance; *heart diseases; Hispanic Americans; hospitals; *indigents; *males; medical records; *minority groups; *patient care; proprietary hospitals; public hospitals; referral and consultation; *selection for treatment; *surgery; *angioplasty; *coronary artery bypass; retrospective studies; *undertreatment; Medicaid; Medicare; New York City
BACKGROUND: Women, ethnic minorities, and uninsured persons receive fewer cardiac procedures than affluent white male patients do, but rates of use are crude indicators of quality. The important question is, Do women, minorities, and the uninsured fail to receive

cardiac procedures when they need them? OBJECTIVE: To measure receipt of necessary coronary artery bypass graft (CABG) surgery and percutaneous transluminal coronary angioplasty (PTCA) overall; by patient sex, ethnicity, and payer status; and by availability of on-site revascularization. DESIGN: Retrospective, randomized medical record review. SETTING: 13 of the 24 hospitals in New York City that provide coronary angiography. PATIENTS: 631 patients who had coronary angiography in 1992 and met the RAND expert panel criteria for necessary revascularization. MEASUREMENTS: The percentage of patients who had CABG surgery or PTCA was measured, as were variations in use rates by sex, ethnic group, insurance status, and availability of on-site revascularization. Clinical and laboratory data were retrieved from medical records to identify patients who met the panel criteria for necessary revascularization. Receipt of revascularization was determined from state reports, medical records, and information provided by cardiologists. RESULTS: Overall, 74% (95% CI, 71% to 77%) of patients who met the panel criteria for necessary revascularization had CABG surgery or PTCA (underuse rate, 26%). No differences were found in use rates by patient sex, ethnic group, or payer status, but hospitals that provided on-site revascularization had higher use rates (76% [CI, 74% to 79%]) than hospitals that did not provide it (59% [CI, 56% to 65%]) (P less than 0.01). In hospitals that did not provide on-site revascularization, uninsured patients were less likely to have revascularization recommended to them (52% [CI, 32% to 78%]); rates of recommendation for patients with private insurance, Medicare, and Medicaid were 82%, 91%, and 75%, respectively (P = 0.026). CONCLUSIONS: Although revascularization procedures are substantially underused, no variations in rate of use by sex, ethnic group, or payer status were seen among patients treated in hospitals that provide CABG surgery and PTCA. However, underuse was significantly greater in hospitals that do not provide these procedures, particularly among uninsured persons.

McChesney, Lawrence P.; Braithwaite, Susan S. Expectations and outcomes in organ transplantation. *Cambridge Quarterly of Healthcare Ethics.* 1999 Summer; 8(3): 299–310. 18 fn. BE62473.
    allowing to die; committee membership; decision making; economics; hospitals; incentives; information dissemination; informed consent; morbidity; mortality; *organ transplantation; organization and administration; physician patient relationship; *physicians; prognosis; regulation; *resource allocation; risk; *selection for treatment; technical expertise; transplant recipients; *treatment outcome; treatment refusal; United States

MacKay, Karen; Moss, Alvin H. To dialyze or not to dialyze: an ethical and evidence-based approach to the patient with acute renal failure in the intensive care unit. *Advances in Renal Replacement Therapy.* 1997 Jul; 4(3): 288–296. 41 refs. BE62516.
    case studies; critically ill; *decision making; evidence-based medicine; family members; *intensive care units; *kidney diseases; mortality; patient care; patients; physicians; *prognosis; quality of life; *renal dialysis; *selection for treatment; time factors; *treatment outcome; withholding treatment

McKenzie, John K.; Moss, Alvin H.; Feest, Terry G., et al. Dialysis decision making in Canada, the United Kingdom, and the United States. *American Journal of Kidney Diseases.* 1998 Jan; 31(1): 12–18. 23 refs. BE59626.
    age factors; allowing to die; comparative studies; *decision

making; dementia; diabetes; diagnosis; drug abuse; Duchenne muscular dystrophy; economics; family members; *international aspects; *knowledge, attitudes, practice; malpractice; motivation; patient compliance; patients; persistent vegetative state; *physicians; prognosis; quality of life; *renal dialysis; *resource allocation; *selection for treatment; statistics; survey; treatment refusal; withholding treatment; *Canada; *Great Britain; *United States

Maiorca, Rosario. Ethical problems in dialysis: prospects for the year 2000. *Nephrology, Dialysis, Transplantation.* 1998; 13(Suppl. 1): 1–9. 46 refs. BE61570.
    advance directives; aged; allowing to die; autonomy; beneficence; decision making; economics; family members; health care delivery; international aspects; kidney diseases; medical ethics; moral development; *moral policy; patient participation; physicians; prognosis; public policy; quality of life; *renal dialysis; *resource allocation; risks and benefits; Roman Catholic ethics; *selection for treatment; social discrimination; suffering; theology; treatment refusal; value of life; *withholding treatment; Europe; Great Britain; Italy; National Health Service; United States

Markovitz, Barry; May, Larry. Three patients, two hearts. [Case study and commentaries]. *Hastings Center Report.* 1998 Sep–Oct; 28(5): 20–21. BE59549.
    adolescents; adoption; advertising; *cadavers; case studies; critically ill; decision making; *directed donation; geographic factors; hearts; justice; *organ donation; *organ transplantation; parents; *resource allocation; scarcity; *selection for treatment; *transplant recipients

Milford, Edgar L. Organ transplantation -- barriers, outcomes, and evolving policies. [Editorial]. *JAMA.* 1998 Oct 7; 280(13): 1184–1185. 11 refs. BE60288.
    age factors; body parts and fluids; cadavers; critically ill; data banks; federal government; geographic factors; government financing; government regulation; kidneys; mortality; organ donation; *organ transplantation; prognosis; public policy; *resource allocation; *selection for treatment; *socioeconomic factors; time factors; transplant recipients; *treatment outcome; Department of Health and Human Services; End Stage Renal Disease Program; United Network for Organ Sharing; United States

Morray, Barbara H. The lottery of life: should organ transplants be used to even the odds? *Dimensions of Critical Care Nursing.* 1995 Sep–Oct; 14(5): 266–272. 19 refs. BE60533.
    beneficence; case studies; *child abuse; clinical ethics committees; decision making; *infants; justice; legal guardians; *livers; mothers; nurses; *organ transplantation; parent child relationship; patient compliance; physicians; prognosis; quality of life; resource allocation; risks and benefits; *selection for treatment; *socioeconomic factors; utilitarianism

Muraskas, Jonathan; Marshall, Patricia A.; Tomich, Paul, et al. Neonatal viability in the 1990s: held hostage by technology. *Cambridge Quarterly of Healthcare Ethics.* 1999 Spring; 8(2): 160–172. 43 refs. BE61233.
    *allowing to die; *biomedical technologies; consensus; costs and benefits; critically ill; decision analysis; *decision making; disabled; extraordinary treatment; *futility; *intensive care units; *low birth weight; morbidity; mortality; *newborns; *parents; patient admission; patient care; *physicians; practice guidelines; *prematurity; professional family relationship; *prognosis; quality of life; resource allocation; *resuscitation; resuscitation orders; *selection for treatment; standards; *treatment outcome; treatment refusal; uncertainty; ventilators; *viability; *withholding treatment; neonatology; United States

Murphy, Donald J.; Barbour, Elizabeth. GUIDe (Guidelines for the Use of Intensive Care in Denver):

a community effort to define futile and inappropriate care. *New Horizons*. 1994 Aug; 2(3): 326–331. 36 refs. BE59890.
> adults; *allowing to die; artificial feeding; congenital disorders; *consensus; critically ill; decision making; dementia; economics; *futility; *guidelines; health facilities; hospitals; *intensive care units; *interdisciplinary communication; legal aspects; low birth weight; newborns; palliative care; persistent vegetative state; prognosis; *program descriptions; public participation; resource allocation; resuscitation; right to die; *selection for treatment; treatment outcome; withholding treatment; *Guidelines for the Use of Intensive Care in Denver (GUIDe)

Murphy, Julien S. Should lesbians count as infertile couples? Antilesbian discrimination in assisted reproduction. *In:* Donchin, Anne; Purdy, Laura M., eds. Embodying Bioethics: Recent Feminist Advances. Lanham, MD: Rowman and Littlefield; 1999: 103–120. 24 refs. 10 fn. ISBN 0-8476-8924-7. BE61017.
> *artificial insemination; *diagnosis; *females; *feminist ethics; health insurance reimbursement; *homosexuals; *infertility; legal rights; marital relationship; parent child relationship; physicians; refusal to treat; reproductive technologies; *selection for treatment; *social discrimination; United States

Murphy, Timothy F. Entitlement to cloning: response to "Cloning and infertilty" by Carson Strong (*CQ*, 1998 Summer; 7(3): 279–293). *Cambridge Quarterly of Healthcare Ethics*. 1999 Summer; 8(3): 364–368. 15 refs. BE62354.
> children; *cloning; females; *homosexuals; *infertility; injuries; males; methods; parent child relationship; reproduction; reproductive technologies; rights; *selection for treatment; harms; nuclear transplantation

Neal, Bernard W. Ethical aspects in the care of very low birth weight infants. *Pediatrician*. 1990; 17(2): 92–99. 6 refs. BE59453.
> active euthanasia; allowing to die; beneficence; *decision making; disabled; *intensive care units; justice; *low birth weight; moral obligations; *newborns; pediatrics; personhood; physicians; prognosis; quality of life; *resource allocation; *selection for treatment; suffering; value of life; Australia

Noble, Holcomb B. Of life, death and the rules of liver transplants. [News]. *New York Times*. 1999 Apr 6: F6. BE61072.
> economics; guidelines; health insurance reimbursement; *health maintenance organizations; *hepatitis; hospitals; *livers; *organ transplantation; prognosis; *refusal to treat; resource allocation; *selection for treatment; treatment outcome; personal financing; Florida

Oberfield, Sharon E. Growth hormone use in normal, short children -- a plea for reason. [Editorial]. *New England Journal of Medicine*. 1999 Feb 18; 340(7): 557–559. 11 refs. BE60336.
> *children; decision making; enhancement technologies; *growth disorders; *hormones; *normality; *patient care; physicians; risks and benefits; *selection for treatment; self concept; treatment outcome; United States

Pascual, Julio; Liaño, Fernando; Madrid Acute Renal Failure Study Group. Causes and prognosis of acute renal failure in the very old. *Journal of the American Geriatrics Society*. 1998 Jun; 46(6): 721–725. 31 refs. BE62153.
> *age factors; *aged; evaluation studies; intensive care units; *kidney diseases; *mortality; patient admission; *patient care; prevalence; *prognosis; quality of life; renal dialysis; resource allocation; *selection for treatment; social discrimination; withholding treatment; multicenter studies; prospective studies; *Madrid; Spain

Paterson, Ron. Rationing access to dialysis in New Zealand. *Ethics and Intellectual Disability*. 1999 Winter; 4(1): 5. BE62665.
> allowing to die; *dementia; government financing; minority groups; *patient compliance; quality of life; *renal dialysis; *resource allocation; *selection for treatment; withholding treatment; Maoris; *New Zealand; Williams, Rau

Peabody, Joyce L.; Martin, Gilbert I. From how small is too small to how much is too much: ethical issues at the limits of neonatal viability. *Clinics in Perinatology*. 1996 Sep; 23(3): 473–489. 75 refs. BE60936.
> *allowing to die; congenital disorders; *costs and benefits; *decision making; economics; *intensive care units; *low birth weight; morbidity; *newborns; parents; patient care; physicians; prognosis; public policy; quality of life; *selection for treatment; third party consent; treatment outcome; treatment refusal; value of life; *viability; withholding treatment; Americans with Disabilities Act 1990; United States

Pennings, Guido. Age and assisted reproduction. *International Journal of Medicine and Law*. 1995; 14(7/8): 531–541. 20 fn. BE61004.
> *age factors; *females; males; *moral obligations; motivation; parent child relationship; *parents; reproduction; *reproductive technologies; risks and benefits; *selection for treatment; social discrimination; time factors

Raffensperger, J. A philosophical approach to conjoined twins. *Pediatric Surgery International*. 1997 Apr; 12(4): 249–255. 29 refs. BE59192.
> *allowing to die; attitudes; case studies; *congenital disorders; decision making; diagnosis; double effect; futility; historical aspects; intention; killing; mass media; mental health; moral policy; mortality; organ donation; parents; physicians; privacy; prognosis; *quality of life; religious ethics; risks and benefits; *selection for treatment; *surgery; *treatment outcome; *twins; withholding treatment; *conjoined twins; Lakeberg twins; United States

Rakowski, Eric; Post, Stephen G. Should health care be rationed by age? Yes [and] No. *In:* Scharlach, Andrew E.; Kaye, Lenard W., eds. Controversial Issues in Aging. Boston, MA: Allyn and Bacon; 1997: 103–113. 9 refs. ISBN 0-205-19381-1. BE60963.
> *age factors; *aged; autonomy; biomedical technologies; cultural pluralism; females; government financing; health care; justice; moral policy; prolongation of life; public policy; quality of life; *resource allocation; rights; *selection for treatment; social discrimination; value of life; values; needs; United States

Rosenheck, Robert; Armstrong, Moe; Callahan, Daniel, et al. Obligation to the least well off in setting mental health service priorities: a consensus statement. *Psychiatric Services*. 1998 Oct; 49(10): 1273–1274, 1290. 13 refs. BE61446.
> community services; consensus; *costs and benefits; decision making; *economics; federal government; *health care delivery; justice; mental health; *mentally ill; *obligations of society; psychiatry; *public policy; *resource allocation; schizophrenia; *selection for treatment; values; *mental health services; *seriously ill; United States; *Veterans Health Administration

Russell, Paul S. Understanding resource use in liver transplantation. [Editorial]. *JAMA*. 1999 Apr 21; 281(15): 1431–1432. 9 refs. BE61903.
> *economics; evaluation; hospitals; *livers; mortality; *organ

---

BE = bioethics accession number   fn. = footnotes   refs. = references

transplantation; *public policy; *resource allocation; *scarcity; *selection for treatment; transplant recipients; treatment outcome; length of stay; severity of illness index; United States

Sanders, Arthur B. Do we need a clinical decision rule for the discontinuation of cardiac arrest resuscitations? [Editorial]. *Archives of Internal Medicine.* 1999 Jan 25; 159(2): 119–121. 13 refs. BE60228.
    adults; aged; critically ill; *decision making; *futility; *hospitals; morbidity; *mortality; *patient discharge; physicians; practice guidelines; *prognosis; resource allocation; *resuscitation; *selection for treatment; time factors; *treatment outcome; *withholding treatment

Scheinkestel, Carlos D. The evolution of the intensivist: from health care provider to economic rationalist and ethicist. *Medical Journal of Australia.* 1996 Mar 4; 164(5): 310–312. 14 refs. BE60196.
    aged; critically ill; *decision making; health care delivery; hospitals; *intensive care units; patient admission; patient care; patient discharge; patient transfer; *physicians; prognosis; quality of life; *resource allocation; scarcity; *selection for treatment; treatment outcome; withholding treatment; *Australia

Schmidt, Volker H. The politics of justice and the paradox of justification. *Social Justice Research.* 1998 Mar; 11(1): 3–19. 46 refs. BE59359.
    blacks; cultural pluralism; dissent; ethical analysis; ethical theory; *institutional policies; *justice; kidney diseases; kidneys; minority groups; organ donation; *organ transplantation; *public policy; *resource allocation; *selection for treatment; transplant recipients; treatment outcome; uncertainty; histocompatibility; rationality

Schulman, Kevin A.; Berlin, Jesse A.; Harless, William, et al. The effect of race and sex on physicians' recommendations for cardiac catheterization. *New England Journal of Medicine.* 1999 Feb 25; 340(8): 618–626. 40 refs. BE60948.
    age factors; audiovisual aids; *blacks; decision making; *diagnosis; *females; *heart diseases; *males; methods; *physicians; primary health care; *referral and consultation; *selection for treatment; survey; *whites; *heart catheterization; American Academy of Family Practice; American College of Physicians; United States
BACKGROUND: Epidemiologic studies have reported differences in the use of cardiovascular procedures according to the race and sex of the patient. Whether the differences stem from differences in the recommendations of physicians remains uncertain. METHODS: We developed a computerized survey instrument to assess physicians' recommendations for managing chest pain. Actors portrayed patients with particular characteristics in scripted interviews about their symptoms. A total of 720 physicians at two national meetings of organizations of primary care physicians participated in the survey. Each physician viewed a recorded interview and was given other data about a hypothetical patient. He or she then made recommendations about that patient's care. We used multivariate logistic-regression analysis to assess the effects of the race and sex of the patients on treatment recommendations, while controlling for the physicians' assessment of the probability of coronary artery disease as well as for the age of the patient, the level of coronary risk, the type of chest pain, and the results of an exercise stress test. RESULTS: The physicians' mean (+/-SD) estimates of the probability of coronary artery disease were lower for women (probability, 64.1+/-19.3 percent, vs. 69.2+/-18.2 percent for men; P less than 0.001), younger patients (63.8+/-19.5 percent for

patients who were 55 years old, vs. 69.5+/-17.9 percent for patients who were 70 years old; P less than 0.001), and patients with nonanginal pain (58.3+/-19.0 percent, vs. 64.4+/-18.3 percent for patients with possible angina and 77.1+/-14.0 percent for those with definite angina; P=0.001). Logistic-regression analysis indicated that women (odds ratio, 0.60; 95 percent confidence interval, 0.4 to 0.9; P=0.02) and blacks (odds ratio, 0.60; 95 percent confidence interval, 0.4 to 0.9; P=0.02) were less likely to be referred for cardiac catheterization than men and whites, respectively. Analysis of race–sex interactions showed that black women were significantly less likely to be referred for catheterization than white men (odds ratio, 0.4; 95 percent confidence interval, 0.2 to 0.7; P=0.004). CONCLUSIONS: Our findings suggest that the race and sex of a patient independently influence how physicians manage chest pain.

Shaw, Allen B. Age as a basis for healthcare rationing: support for agist policies. *Drugs and Aging.* 1996 Dec; 9(6): 403–405. 21 refs. BE60379.
    *age factors; *aged; *health care; justice; moral policy; public policy; *resource allocation; *selection for treatment; social discrimination; Great Britain

Stevenson, David K.; Goldworth, Amnon. Commentary: neonatal viability in the 1990s: held hostage by technology. *Cambridge Quarterly of Healthcare Ethics.* 1999 Spring; 8(2): 170–172. BE61253.
    advance care planning; *allowing to die; biomedical technologies; childbirth; *decision making; intensive care units; *low birth weight; *newborns; *parents; *physicians; *prematurity; prognosis; quality of life; *resuscitation; *selection for treatment; suffering; *treatment outcome; treatment refusal; uncertainty; *viability; *withholding treatment

Stolberg, Sheryl Gay. Health secretary urges donor priority for sickest patients. [News]. *New York Times.* 1998 Feb 27: A16. BE60466.
    critically ill; federal government; geographic factors; government regulation; livers; *organ transplantation; prognosis; *public policy; *resource allocation; *selection for treatment; *transplant recipients; *Department of Health and Human Services; United Network for Organ Sharing; *United States

Thomasma, David C.; Micetich, Kenneth C.; Brems, John, et al. The ethics of competition in liver transplantation. *Cambridge Quarterly of Healthcare Ethics.* 1999 Summer; 8(3): 321–329. 28 fn. BE62475.
    beneficence; economics; federal government; *geographic factors; *government regulation; guidelines; hospitals; institutional policies; *justice; *livers; *misconduct; organ donation; organ donors; *organ transplantation; physicians; prisoners; public policy; *resource allocation; scarcity; *selection for treatment; standards; technical expertise; time factors; *transplant recipients; needs; *waiting lists; Department of Health and Human Services; United Network for Organ Sharing; *United States

Turner, N.J.; Haward, R.A.; Mulley, G.P., et al. Cancer in old age -- is it inadequately investigated and treated? *BMJ (British Medical Journal).* 1999 Jul 31; 319(7205): 309–312. 40 refs. BE62456.
    *aged; *cancer; diagnosis; drugs; hormones; mass screening; palliative care; *patient care; quality of health care; radiology; *selection for treatment; social discrimination; surgery; treatment outcome; withholding treatment; *undertreatment; Great Britain

Ubel, Peter A.; Caplan, Arthur L. Geographic favoritism in liver transplantation -- unfortunate or unfair? *New*

England Journal of Medicine. 1998 Oct 29; 339(18): 1322–1325. 34 refs. BE60300.

cadavers; critically ill; federal government; *geographic factors; *government regulation; hospitals; *justice; *livers; mortality; *organ transplantation; physicians; *prognosis; *public policy; *resource allocation; retreatment; *selection for treatment; self regulation; *standards; state government; time factors; *transplant recipients; treatment outcome; *seriously ill; United Network for Organ Sharing; *United States

Ubel, Peter A.; Baron, Jonathan; Asch, David A. Social responsibility, personal responsibility, and prognosis in public judgments about transplant allocation. *Bioethics.* 1999 Jan; 13(1): 57–68. 11 fn. BE60888.

*drug abuse; *hearts; *nutrition; *organ transplantation; prognosis; *public opinion; *resource allocation; *selection for treatment; *self induced illness; *smoking; survey; transplant recipients; Pennsylvania

van Walraven, Carl; Forster, Alan J.; Stiell, Ian G. Derivation of a clinical decision rule for the discontinuation of in–hospital cardiac arrest resuscitations. *Archives of Internal Medicine.* 1999 Jan 25; 159(2): 129–134. 30 refs. BE60229.

adults; age factors; aged; critically ill; *decision making; evaluation studies; *futility; *hospitals; morbidity; *mortality; *patient discharge; physicians; practice guidelines; *prognosis; resource allocation; *resuscitation; *selection for treatment; time factors; *treatment outcome; *withholding treatment; Ontario

BACKGROUND: Most patients undergoing in–hospital cardiac resuscitation will not survive to hospital discharge. OBJECTIVE: To derive a decision rule permitting the discontinuation of futile resuscitation attempts by identifying patients with no chance of surviving to hospital discharge. PATIENTS AND METHODS: Patient, arrest, and outcome data for 1077 adult patients undergoing in–hospital cardiac resuscitation was retrieved from 2 randomized clinical trials involving 5 teaching hospitals at 2 university centers. Recursive partitioning was used to identify a decision rule using variables significantly associated with death in hospital. RESULTS: One hundred three patients (9.6%) survived to hospital discharge. Death in hospital was significantly more likely if patients were older than 75 years (P less than .001), the arrest was unwitnessed (P = .003), the resuscitation lasted longer than 10 minutes (P less than .001), and the initial cardiac rhythm was not ventricular tachycardia or fibrillation (P less than .001). All patients died if there was no pulse 10 minutes after the start of cardiopulmonary resuscitation, the initial cardiac rhythm was not ventricular tachycardia or fibrillation, and the arrest was not witnessed. As a resuscitation rule, these parameters identified all patients who survived to hospital discharge (sensitivity, 100%; 95% confidence interval, 97.1%–100%). Resuscitation could have been discontinued for 119 (12.1%) of 974 patients who did not survive, thereby avoiding 47 days of postresuscitative care. CONCLUSIONS: A practical and highly sensitive decision rule has been derived that identifies patients with no chance of surviving in–hospital cardiac arrest. Prospective validation of the rule is necessary before it can be used clinically.

Varekamp, Inge; Meiland, Franka J.M.; Hoos, Aloysia M., et al. The meaning of urgency in the allocation of scarce health care resources; a comparison between renal transplantation and psychogeriatric nursing home care. *Health Policy.* 1998 May; 44(2): 135–148. 20 refs. 1 fn. BE59149.

*aged; critically ill; dementia; evaluation studies; family members; home care; *kidneys; nurses; *nursing homes; *organ transplantation; *patient admission; patient advocacy; patient compliance; physicians; *prognosis; psychological stress; *resource allocation; scarcity; *selection for treatment; *time factors; qualitative research; *Netherlands

Veatch, Robert M. Egalitarian and maximin theories of justice: directed donation of organs for transplant. *Journal of Medicine and Philosophy.* 1998 Oct; 23(5): 456–476. 13 refs. 12 fn. Note: the journal issue cover shows a date of August 1998, which is incorrect. BE62113.

beneficence; *directed donation; ethical analysis; *ethical theory; freedom; health; health care delivery; *justice; *moral policy; *organ donation; *organ transplantation; public policy; *resource allocation; rights; *selection for treatment; self concept; social discrimination; socioeconomic factors; transplant recipients; utilitarianism; whites; *egalitarianism; *Rawls, John; United Network for Organ Sharing; United States

It is common to interpret Rawls's maximin theory of justice as egalitarian. Compared to utilitarian theories, this may be true. However, in special cases practices that distribute resources so as to benefit the worst off actually increase the inequality between the worst off and some who are better off. In these cases the Rawlsian maximin parts company with what is here called true egalitarianism. A policy question requiring a distinction between maximin and "true egalitarian" allocations has arisen in the arena of organ transplantation. This case is examined here as a venue for differentiating maximin and true egalitarian theories. Directed donation is the name given to donations of organs restricted to a particular social group. For example, the family of a member of the Ku Klux Klan donated his organs on the provision that they go only to members of the Caucasian race. While such donations appear to be discriminatory, if certain plausible assumptions are made, they satisfy the maximin criterion. They selectively advantage the recipient of the organs without harming anyone (assuming the organs would otherwise go unused). Moreover, everyone who is lower on the waiting list (who, thereby, could be considered worse off) is advantaged by moving up on the waiting list. This paper examines how maximin and more truly egalitarian theories handle this case arguing that, to the extent that directed donation in unethical, the best account of that conclusion is that an egalitarian principle of justice is to be preferred to the maximin.

Williams, Alan; Evans, J. Grimley. Rationing health care by age: the case for [and] The case against. *BMJ (British Medical Journal).* 1997 Mar 15; 314(7083): 820–825. BE60232.

*age factors; *aged; attitudes; common good; costs and benefits; goals; *health care; *justice; moral policy; patient care; quality adjusted life years; quality of life; *resource allocation; risks and benefits; *selection for treatment; social discrimination; social worth; treatment outcome; values; withholding treatment; needs; *Great Britain; *National Health Service

SEX DETERMINATION

See also PRENATAL DIAGNOSIS, SEX PRESELECTION

American College of Obstetricians and Gynecologists. Committee on Ethics. Sex selection. ACOG Committee Opinion No. 177. *ACOG Committee Opinions.* 1996 Nov.; No. 177: 4 p. 20 refs. BE61297.

BE = bioethics accession number   fn. = footnotes   refs. = references

conscience; disclosure; embryos; females; genetic disorders; in vitro fertilization; legal obligations; males; moral policy; motivation; *organizational policies; parents; *physicians; preimplantation diagnosis; prenatal diagnosis; professional organizations; risk; selective abortion; *sex determination; sex preselection; social discrimination; *American College of Obstetricians and Gynecologists; American Society for Reproductive Medicine; President's Commission for the Study of Ethical Problems; United Nations International Conference on Population and Development

Boetzkes, Elisabeth. Equality, autonomy, and feminist bioethics. *In:* Donchin, Anne; Purdy, Laura M., eds. Embodying Bioethics: Recent Feminist Advances. Lanham, MD: Rowman and Littlefield; 1999: 121–139. 36 refs. 8 fn. ISBN 0–8476–8924–7. BE61018.
abortion, induced; *autonomy; contracts; females; *feminist ethics; government regulation; legal rights; personhood; *pregnant women; reproduction; selective abortion; *self concept; *sex determination; *sex preselection; sexuality; social discrimination; *surrogate mothers; Canada

Hopkins, Patrick D., ed. (Mis?)conceptions: morality and gender politics in reproductive technology. *In: his* Sex/Machine: Readings in Culture, Gender, and Technology. Bloomington, IN: Indiana University Press; 1998: 95–170. 227 fn. ISBN 0–253–21230–8. BE62289.
abortion, induced; *artificial insemination; attitudes; children; developing countries; eugenics; family relationship; *fathers; *females; feminist ethics; genetic disorders; informed consent; international aspects; legal aspects; *males; methods; moral obligations; motivation; *parent child relationship; population control; pregnant women; public policy; remuneration; rights; *risks and benefits; selective abortion; *semen donors; *sex determination; *sex preselection; sexuality; single persons; social discrimination; social impact; socioeconomic factors; spousal notification; *surrogate mothers; wedge argument; women's rights; harms; United States

Macklin, Ruth. Death and birth. *In: her* Against Relativism: Cultural Diversity and the Search for Ethical Universals in Medicine. New York, NY: Oxford University Press; 1999: 136–160. 32 fn. ISBN 0–19–511632–1. BE62782.
*abortion, induced; autonomy; brain death; cardiac death; *cultural pluralism; *determination of death; *ethical relativism; family relationship; *females; feminist ethics; fetuses; infanticide; *international aspects; justice; morality; mortality; non-Western World; organ donation; organ transplantation; pregnant women; public policy; *selective abortion; *sex determination; *social discrimination; *social worth; value of life; values; women's rights; Cameroon; China; India; Japan; Philippines; United States

Macklin, Ruth. International feminism and reproductive rights. *In: her* Against Relativism: Cultural Diversity and the Search for Ethical Universals in Medicine. New York, NY: Oxford University Press; 1999: 161–185. 30 fn. ISBN 0–19–511632–1. BE62783.
autonomy; *contraception; *cultural pluralism; decision making; *developing countries; *ethical relativism; females; *feminist ethics; freedom; *human rights; *international aspects; justice; legal aspects; males; methods; non-Western World; *paternalism; *political activity; postmodernism; pregnant women; public policy; *reproduction; reproductive technologies; Roman Catholic ethics; selective abortion; *sex determination; social control; social discrimination; values; Western World; *women's health; *women's rights; Brazil; China; Feminist International Network of Resistance to Reproductive and Genetic Engineering (FINRRAGE); India; International Conference on Population and Development (Cairo, 1994); Women's Global Network for Reproductive Rights

Royal College of Obstetricians and Gynaecologists. Ethics Committee. Sex Selection. London: Royal College of Obstetricians and Gynaecologists Press; 1993. 16 p. 14 refs. ISBN 0–902331–60–4. BE59461.
counseling; cultural pluralism; disclosure; females; genetic disorders; goals; government regulation; infanticide; informed consent; international aspects; legal aspects; males; medicine; methods; physician's role; preimplantation diagnosis; prenatal diagnosis; *public policy; *risks and benefits; selective abortion; self regulation; *sex determination; *sex preselection; social discrimination; social worth; uncertainty; values; *Great Britain

Russell, Jeanie. "I'm the most hated physician in America." *Good Housekeeping.* 1998 May; 226(5): 108–111, 180. BE60210.
international aspects; methods; organizational policies; physicians; prenatal diagnosis; professional organizations; public opinion; public policy; selective abortion; *sex determination; sex preselection; stigmatization; ultrasonography; *Stephens, John

SEX PRESELECTION

See also REPRODUCTIVE TECHNOLOGIES, SEX DETERMINATION

Belkin, Lisa. Getting the girl. *New York Times Magazine.* 1999 Jul 25: 26–31, 38, 54–55. BE62249.
attitudes; females; human experimentation; international aspects; males; *methods; mothers; motivation; risks and benefits; sex determination; *sex preselection; social impact; Genetics and IVF Institute (Fairfax, VA); *Microsort; United States

Boetzkes, Elisabeth. Equality, autonomy, and feminist bioethics. *In:* Donchin, Anne; Purdy, Laura M., eds. Embodying Bioethics: Recent Feminist Advances. Lanham, MD: Rowman and Littlefield; 1999: 121–139. 36 refs. 8 fn. ISBN 0–8476–8924–7. BE61018.
abortion, induced; *autonomy; contracts; females; *feminist ethics; government regulation; legal rights; personhood; *pregnant women; reproduction; selective abortion; *self concept; *sex determination; *sex preselection; sexuality; social discrimination; *surrogate mothers; Canada

Danis, Jodi. Sexism and "the superfluous female": arguments for regulating pre-implantation sex selection. *Harvard Women's Law Journal.* 1995 Spring; 18: 219–264. 237 fn. BE59843.
attitudes; constitutional law; economics; equal protection; *females; feminist ethics; freedom; government regulation; international aspects; legal aspects; *males; methods; moral policy; physicians; privacy; *public policy; reproductive technologies; *risks and benefits; selective abortion; self regulation; sex determination; *sex preselection; social discrimination; social dominance; *social impact; teleological ethics; Canada; Great Britain; Human Embryo Research Panel; President's Commission for the Study of Ethical Problems; *United States

Golden, Frederic; Silver, Lee M. Boy? Girl? Up to you [and] A quandary that isn't. *Time.* 1998 Sep 21; 152(12): 82–83. BE60858.
females; males; *reproductive technologies; *sex preselection; social impact; sperm

Hopkins, Patrick D., ed. (Mis?)conceptions: morality and gender politics in reproductive technology. *In: his* Sex/Machine: Readings in Culture, Gender, and Technology. Bloomington, IN: Indiana University Press; 1998: 95–170. 227 fn. ISBN 0–253–21230–8. BE62289.

BE = bioethics accession number   fn. = footnotes   refs. = references

abortion, induced; *artificial insemination; attitudes; children; developing countries; eugenics; family relationship; *fathers; *females; feminist ethics; genetic disorders; informed consent; international aspects; legal aspects; *males; methods; moral obligations; motivation; *parent child relationship; population control; pregnant women; public policy; remuneration; rights; *risks and benefits; selective abortion; *semen donors; *sex determination; *sex preselection; sexuality; single persons; social discrimination; social impact; socioeconomic factors; spousal notification; *surrogate mothers; wedge argument; women's rights; harms; United States

Lemonick, Michael D. Designer babies. *Time.* 1999 Jan 11; 153(1): 64–67. BE60312.
  eugenics; genetic disorders; *genetic enhancement; in vitro fertilization; methods; *preimplantation diagnosis; prenatal diagnosis; public opinion; selective abortion; *sex preselection; social impact; United States

Royal College of Obstetricians and Gynaecologists. Ethics Committee. Sex Selection. London: Royal College of Obstetricians and Gynaecologists Press; 1993. 16 p. 14 refs. ISBN 0-902331-60-4. BE59461.
  counseling; cultural pluralism; disclosure; females; genetic disorders; goals; government regulation; infanticide; informed consent; international aspects; legal aspects; males; medicine; methods; physician's role; preimplantation diagnosis; prenatal diagnosis; *public policy; *risks and benefits; selective abortion; self regulation; *sex determination; *sex preselection; social discrimination; social worth; uncertainty; values; *Great Britain

Schiff, Daniel. Developing *halakhic* attitudes to sex preselection. *In:* Jacob, Walter; Zemer, Moshe, eds. The Fetus and Fertility in Jewish Law: Essays and Responsa. Pittsburgh, PA: Rodef Shalom Press; Freehof Institute of Progressive Halakhah; 1995: 91–117. 49 fn. ISBN 0-929699-07-6. BE61839.
  artificial insemination; embryos; females; historical aspects; in vitro fertilization; *Jewish ethics; males; marital relationship; married persons; *methods; preimplantation diagnosis; *sex preselection; social impact; sperm; Orthodox Judaism; Reform Judaism

Terry, Sara. The ethics of selecting child's sex. *Christian Science Monitor.* 1998 Sep 17: 1, 4. BE60965.
  children; commodification; parent child relationship; religion; reproductive technologies; *sex preselection; *social impact; social worth; values

SPECIAL POPULATIONS
See under
  BEHAVIORAL RESEARCH/SPECIAL
    POPULATIONS
  HUMAN EXPERIMENTATION/SPECIAL
    POPULATIONS

STERILIZATION

See also CONTRACEPTION

Bock, Gisela. Sterilization and "medical" massacres in National Socialist Germany: ethics, politics, and the law. *In:* Berg, Manfred; Cocks, Geoffrey, eds. Medicine and Modernity: Public Health and Medical Care in Nineteenth- and Twentieth-Century Germany. New York, NY: Cambridge University Press; 1997: 149–172. 85 fn. ISBN 0-521-56411-5. BE59269.
  aliens; chronically ill; *dehumanization; *disabled; *eugenics; genetic disorders; *historical aspects; *involuntary euthanasia; *involuntary sterilization; Jews; *killing; mentally disabled; minority groups; *National Socialism;

*physicians; *psychiatry; public health; *public policy; selective abortion; social control; social discrimination; *social worth; socioeconomic factors; *sociology of medicine; genocide; *Germany; *Twentieth Century

Cowdin, Daniel M.; Tuohey, John F. Sterilization, Catholic health care, and the legitimate autonomy of culture. *Christian Bioethics.* 1998 Apr; 4(1): 14–44. 57 refs. 48 fn. BE61979.
  beneficence; communication; cultural pluralism; decision making; dissent; double effect; ethical theory; goals; health; injuries; institutional policies; intention; interdisciplinary communication; maternal health; medicine; *morality; organ donation; *physicians; *professional autonomy; professional competence; religious hospitals; reproduction; *Roman Catholic ethics; science; *sterilization (sexual); surgery; theology; *voluntary sterilization; Aristotle; Gaudium et spes
Disagreement over the legitimacy of direct sterilization continues within Catholic moral debate, with painful and at times confusing ramifications for Catholic healthcare systems. This paper argues that the medical profession should be construed as a key *moral* authority in this debate, on two grounds. First, the recent revival of neo–Aristotelianism in moral philosophy as applied to medical ethics has brought out the inherently moral dimensions of the history and current practice of medicine. Second, this recognition can be linked to Catholic morality through Vatican II's affirmation of the legitimate autonomy of culture, including the sciences. A partial precedent for understanding the moral authority of medicine can be found in the recent history of Catholic medical morality, and we further argue that a full contemporary recognition of that authority would weigh against an absolute prohibition of direct sterilizations. Institutionally, we propose the allowance of direct sterilizations in cases where the clinically perceived biomedical good of the patient is at stake.

Crosby, John F. There is no moral authority in medicine: response to Cowdin and Tuohey. *Christian Bioethics.* 1998 Apr; 4(1): 63–82. 14 refs. 8 fn. Commentary on D.M. Cowdin and J.F. Tuohey, p. 14–44. BE61981.
  abortion, induced; contraception; *decision making; maternal health; medicine; moral development; *morality; *physicians; *professional autonomy; professional competence; *Roman Catholic ethics; *sterilization (sexual); theology; *voluntary sterilization
Central to the Cowdin-Tuohey paper is the concept of a moral authority proper to medical practitioners. Much as I agree with the authors in refusing to degrade doctors to the status of mere technicians, I argue that one does not succeed in retrieving the moral dimension of medical practice by investing doctors with moral authority. I show that none of the cases brought forth by Cowdin-Tuohey really amounts to a case of moral authority. Then I try to explain why no such cases can be found. Developing an insight that is common to all the major moral thinkers in the *philosophia perennis*, I show that doctors are professionally competent with respect only to a part of the human good; morally wise persons are competent with respect to that which makes man *good as man*. I try to show why it follows that a) professional expertise has no natural tendency to pass over into moral understanding, and that b) doctor and non-doctor alike start from the same point in developing their understanding of medical morality. It follows that the authors fail in their attempt to de–center the moral magisterium of the Church by setting up centers of moral authority outside of the Church.

Elton, Catherine. Peru's family planning became coerced sterilization. [News]. *Christian Science Monitor.* 1998 Feb

---

20: 1, 9. BE59562.
*coercion; deception; *family planning; *females; health personnel; *incentives; *indigents; *involuntary sterilization; minority groups; *public policy; remuneration; *sterilization (sexual); *Peru

Hodges, Jeffrey Alan. Euthenics, Eugenics and Compulsory Sterilization in Michigan: 1897–1960. Ann Arbor, MI: UMI Dissertation Services; 1995. 181 p. Bibliography: p. 176–181. Thesis, Master of Arts in History, Michigan State University, 1995. UMI No. 1378034. BE60650.
behavior control; blacks; *eugenics; females; *historical aspects; institutionalized persons; *involuntary sterilization; legislation; males; mentally ill; mentally retarded; National Socialism; prisoners; *public policy; sex offenses; social problems; socioeconomic factors; state government; whites; *Michigan; *Twentieth Century; United States

Keenan, James F.; O'Rourke, Kevin. Cooperation and "hard cases." Part 1: cooperation pro and con. [Article and response]. *Ethics and Medics.* 1998 Sep; 23(9): 3–4. BE61721.
administrators; *institutional ethics; institutional policies; intention; moral complicity; obstetrics and gynecology; physicians; *religious hospitals; *Roman Catholic ethics; *voluntary sterilization; women's health services; Ethical and Religious Directives for Catholic Health Care Services

Kumar, Sanjay. Health-care camps for the poor provide mass sterilisation quota. [News]. *Lancet.* 1999 Apr 10; 353(9160): 1251. BE61040.
deception; *females; incentives; *indigents; morbidity; *political activity; population control; *public policy; *sterilization (sexual); women's rights; Group Against Targeted Sterilisation (India); *India; Indian Population Project

Lustig, B. Andrew. Sexual ethics and communal judgments: on the pluralism of virtues, values, and practices. *Christian Bioethics.* 1998 Apr; 4(1): 3–13. 21 refs. Introduction to an article by D.M. Cowdin and J.F. Tuohey, p. 14–44; and to commentaries by J.E. Smith, p. 45–62; J.F. Crosby, p. 63–82; and G.P. McKenny, p. 100–109. BE61978.
*decision making; Eastern Orthodox ethics; marital relationship; *morality; natural law; personhood; *physicians; *professional autonomy; Protestant ethics; reproduction; *Roman Catholic ethics; *sexuality; *sterilization (sexual); theology; *voluntary sterilization
Different judgments by Christian communities on issues in sexual ethics involve different weightings of various sources of moral authority, different understandings of the normativity of the natural, and different assessments of the scope of freedom to be exercised in relation to the goods of marriage. These fundamental differences of interpretation can be exemplified by the ongoing Roman Catholic discussion of the legitimacy of voluntary sterilization in certain "hard cases." The contributors to this issue of *Christian Bioethics*, in their spirited exchange on that issue, exemplify the need for careful attention to the ways that differences of theological emphasis and moral method lead to different judgements in particular cases, both within and between particular Christian communities.

McKenny, Gerald P. A bad disease, a fatal cure: why sterilization is permissible and the autonomy of medicine is not. *Christian Bioethics.* 1998 Apr; 4(1): 100–109. 10 refs. 9 fn. Commentary on D.M. Cowdin and J.F. Tuohey, p. 14–44. BE61982.
contraception; married persons; medicine; *morality; *physicians; *professional autonomy; professional

competence; *Protestant ethics; *Roman Catholic ethics; sexuality; *sterilization (sexual); theology; *voluntary sterilization; nature
The debate in this issue regarding the Roman Catholic condemnation of the morality of sterilization is puzzling for Protestants. As I will argue the puzzlement arises on two grounds. First, why would anyone object to direct sterilization for the cure or prevention of disease? Second, if one wanted to challenge such an objection on moral grounds why would one turn to medicine to do so? For Christian ethics there is nothing wrong in principle with direct sterilization when there are good reasons for precluding the possibility of an additional pregnancy; and it is a serious theological mistake to treat medicine as an independent moral authority.

Mason, John Kenyon. Sterilisation. *In: his* Medico-Legal Aspects of Reproduction and Parenthood. Second Edition. Brookfield, VT: Ashgate; 1998: 67–106. 149 fn. ISBN 1-84104-065-8. BE61062.
adults; autonomy; compensation; competence; decision making; eugenics; females; historical aspects; human rights; informed consent; international aspects; *involuntary sterilization; judicial action; *legal aspects; legal liability; legal rights; males; mentally disabled; minors; National Socialism; parental consent; paternalism; physicians; punishment; reproduction; risks and benefits; sex offenses; spousal consent; state interest; *sterilization (sexual); Supreme Court decisions; third party consent; *voluntary sterilization; *wrongful life; Australia; Canada; Declaration of Tokyo; European Convention for the Protection of Human Rights; Germany; *Great Britain; Twentieth Century; United States

Rosenthal, Elisabeth. Scientists debate China's law on sterilizing the carriers of genetic defects. [News]. *New York Times.* 1998 Aug 16: 14. BE59567.
attitudes; *eugenics; genetic counseling; *genetic disorders; informed consent; *international aspects; investigators; *involuntary sterilization; legislation; *public policy; sterilization (sexual); *China; International Congress on Genetics; Law on Maternal and Infant Health Care (China)

Schoen, Johanna. "A Great Thing for Poor Folks": Birth Control, Sterilization, and Abortion in Public Health and Welfare in the Twentieth Century. Ann Arbor, MI: UMI Dissertation Services; 1996. 267 p. Bibliography: p. 240–267. Dissertation, Ph.D. in History, University of North Carolina, 1995. Order No. 9631980. BE62797.
*abortion, induced; blacks; *coercion; *contraception; eugenics; *females; government regulation; historical aspects; *indigents; *involuntary sterilization; legal aspects; males; mentally retarded; motivation; public health; *public policy; sexuality; *social control; social discrimination; state government; whites; *North Carolina; Twentieth Century; United States

Sims, Calvin. Using gifts as bait, Peru sterilizes poor women. [News]. *New York Times.* 1998 Feb 15: 1, 12. BE59568.
*coercion; *family planning; *females; *gifts; health personnel; *incentives; *indigents; *involuntary sterilization; *public policy; *sterilization (sexual); *Peru

Smith, Janet E. Sterilizations reconsidered? *Christian Bioethics.* 1998 Apr; 4(1): 45–62. 19 refs. 16 fn. Commentary on D.M. Cowdin and J.F. Tuohey, p. 14–44. BE61980.
contraception; *decision making; double effect; historical aspects; intention; maternal health; medicine; moral development; *morality; natural law; organ donation; *physicians; *professional autonomy; *Roman Catholic ethics; science; sexuality; *sterilization (sexual); theology; *voluntary sterilization; rationality

---

BE = bioethics accession number   fn. = footnotes   refs. = references

Cowdin and Tuohey argue for a rethinking of Catholic bioethical principles and the Church's moral authority. Citing the Second Vatican Council for support, they argue that if the Church were to respect the proper autonomy of medicine, it would allow sterilizations. In this essay I argue against Cowdin and Tuohey's understanding that the Church has derived its moral laws independent of consultation with medicine and that it treats medicine simply as a source of technical expertise. I also argue that they misunderstand that nature of autonomy as well as the Church's position regarding the type of autonomy they request for medicine. I will especially argue against their understanding of the principles of totality and double effect as "dispensations" from the moral order. I conclude that they have provided no grounds to cause the Church to reconsider its condemnation of all sterilizations.

Tang, Julie. The United States' immigration laws: prospects for relief for foreign nationals seeking refuge from coercive sterilization or abortion practices in their homelands. *Saint Louis University Public Law Review.* 1996; 15(2): 371–401. 165 fn. BE59915.
> *abortion, induced; *aliens; *coercion; federal government; *human rights; *international aspects; *involuntary sterilization; judicial action; *legal aspects; *mandatory programs; political systems; *population control; *public policy; reproduction; *emigration and immigration; *China; In re Chang; U.S. Congress; *United States

Telling, Douglas Cushman. Science in Politics: Eugenics, Sterilization, and Genetic Screening. Ann Arbor, MI: UMI Dissertation Services; 1988. 264 p. Bibliography: p. 251–264. Dissertation, Ph.D. in Political Science, University of Massachusetts, 1988. Order No. 8906337. BE61053.
> bioethical issues; carriers; coercion; employment; *eugenics; fetuses; *genetic screening; government regulation; health hazards; historical aspects; industry; involuntary sterilization; legal aspects; legal liability; newborns; normality; *politics; prenatal diagnosis; *public policy; reproduction; reproductive technologies; science; selective abortion; *social control; social discrimination; socioeconomic factors; state government; *sterilization (sexual); trends; wrongful life; Galton, Francis; Muller, Hermann; Osborn, Frederick; Sanger, Margaret; Twentieth Century; *United States

Tsuchiya, Takashi. Eugenic sterilizations in Japan and recent demands for an apology: a report. *Ethics and Intellectual Disability.* 1997 Fall; 3(1): 1–4. BE59951.
> compensation; *disabled; *eugenics; females; historical aspects; *involuntary sterilization; *legal aspects; *mandatory programs; *mentally disabled; physically disabled; political activity; public policy; voluntary sterilization; *Eugenic Protection Law (Japan); *Japan; Twentieth Century

Sweden plans to pay sterilization victims. [News]. *New York Times.* 1999 Jan 27: A8. BE60971.
> *compensation; eugenics; females; historical aspects; *involuntary sterilization; minors; *public policy; socioeconomic factors; *Sweden; Twentieth Century

STERILIZATION/MENTALLY DISABLED

Cica, Natasha. Sterilising the intellectually disabled: the approach of the High Court of Australia in Department of Health v. J.W.B. and S.M.B. [Comment]. *Medical Law Review.* 1993 Summer; 1(2): 186–231. 252 fn. BE60601.
> eugenics; females; human rights; informed consent; *judicial action; *legal aspects; *mentally retarded; motivation; parents; *risks and benefits; *sterilization (sexual); third party consent; *Australia; *Department of Health v. J.W.B. and

S.M.B.; Northwest Territories

Denekens, Joke P.M.; Nys, Herman; Stuer, Hugo. Sterilisation of incompetent mentally handicapped persons: a model for decision making. *Journal of Medical Ethics.* 1999 Jun; 25(3): 237–241. 22 refs. BE61856.
> age factors; competence; comprehension; contraception; *decision making; *family members; family relationship; financial support; genetic disorders; guidelines; informed consent; intelligence; legal aspects; *mentally retarded; parent child relationship; *patient care team; patient education; *patient participation; physicians; reproduction; *risks and benefits; sexuality; *sterilization (sexual); third party consent

Doctors are regularly confronted with requests for sterilisation of mentally handicapped people who cannot give consent for themselves. They ought to act in a medical vacuum because there doesn't exist a consensus about a model for decision making on this matter. In this article a model for decision making is proposed, based on a review of the literature and our own research data. We have attempted to select and classify certain factors which could enable us to arrive at an ethically justifiable method of making a medical decision. In doing so we distinguish two major criteria: heredity and parenting competence, and six minor criteria: conception risk, IQ, age, personality, medical aspects and prognosis and finally support and guidance for the mentally handicapped person. The major criteria give rise to a "situation of necessity". In this situation the physician is confronted with a conflict of values and interests. The minor criteria are of an entirely different ethical order. They can only be considered once the major criteria have created a "situation of necessity". Ultimately it comes down to deciding whether the benefits of sterilisation outweigh the drawbacks and whether the means are appropriate to the end, where efficient contraception is the end and irreversible sterilisation is the means.

Great Britain. England. High Court of Justice, Family Division. Re D (A Minor) (Wardship:Sterilisation). *All England Law Reports.* 1975 Sep 17. 1976: 326–336. BE59972.
> females; *legal aspects; legal guardians; legal rights; *mentally retarded; *minors; parental consent; risks and benefits; *sterilization (sexual); *Great Britain; *Re D (A Minor) (Wardship: Sterilisation)

The Family Division of England's High Court of Justice decided to continue wardship of a mentally retarded minor and refused to consent to her sterilization. D, age 11, suffered from Sotos syndrome and was mentally retarded. A year earlier, she had reached puberty and her mother and pediatrician sought her sterilization for reproductive and eugenic reasons. There was professional testimony that by age 18, D would understand the implications of a hysterectomy and be able to give informed consent. The court found that the proposed hysterectomy for nontherapeutic purposes was neither medically indicated nor necessary and refused to consent to D's sterilization. (KIE abstract)

Johnson, Linda. Expanding eugenics or improving health care in China: commentary on the Provisions of the Standing Committee of the Gansu People's Congress concerning the prohibition of reproduction by intellectually impaired persons. *Journal of Law and Society.* 1997 Jun; 24(2): 199–234. 126 fn. BE62168.
> abortion, induced; coercion; *eugenics; females; *intelligence; *involuntary sterilization; *legal aspects; legislation; *mandatory programs; married persons; *mentally retarded; normality; population control; pregnant

---

women; *public policy; reproduction; *China; *Gansu Province; Law on Maternal and Infant Health Care 1994 (China)

Kennedy, Ian. Minor: consent; sterilisation; best interests -- L and G.M. v. M.M.: The Director-General, Department of Family Services and Aboriginal and Islander Affairs. [Comment]. *Medical Law Review.* 1995 Spring; 3(1): 94–97. BE60000.
  females; *legal aspects; legal rights; *mentally retarded; *minors; parents; risks and benefits; *sterilization (sexual); third party consent; *Australia; *L and G.M. v. M.M.

Kennedy, Ian. Treatment without consent (sterilisation): adult -- Re W (A Patient). [Comment]. *Medical Law Review.* 1993 Summer; 1(2): 234–236. BE59996.
  *adults; decision making; females; judicial action; *legal aspects; *mentally retarded; physicians; risks and benefits; *sterilization (sexual); third party consent; *Great Britain; *Re W (A Patient)

Keown, Rebecca M. A case–based approach to sterilization of mentally incompetent women. *Princeton Journal of Bioethics.* 1998 Spring; 1(1): 94–113. 15 refs. 10 fn. BE62496.
  adults; contraception; eugenics; *females; health; international aspects; involuntary sterilization; judicial action; *legal aspects; *legal rights; *mentally retarded; minors; motivation; parental consent; *risks and benefits; *standards; state interest; *sterilization (sexual); Australia; Canada; Great Britain; *Re B (A Minor) (Wardship: Sterilisation); *Re Eve; *Re Marion

Larson, Edward J. Confronting scientific authority with religious values: eugenics in American history. *In:* Demy, Timothy J.; Stewart, Gary P., eds. Genetic Engineering: A Christian Response: Crucial Considerations in Shaping Life. Grand Rapids, MI: Kregel Publications; 1999: 104–124. 80 fn. ISBN 0-8254-2357-0. BE61363.
  clergy; contraception; disadvantaged; *eugenics; gene therapy; genetic determinism; genetic information; genetic screening; genome mapping; *historical aspects; human rights; institutionalized persons; *involuntary sterilization; justice; *legislation; mass media; *mentally ill; *mentally retarded; organizational policies; patient discharge; physicians; *political activity; *politics; prisoners; privacy; *religion; Roman Catholic ethics; *Roman Catholics; sex offenses; state government; Supreme Court decisions; value of life; *Alabama; Buck v. Bell; *Christian Fundamentalists; *Louisiana; Medical Association of Alabama; Twentieth Century; United States

Thomson, Mathew. Sterilization, segregation and community care: ideology and solutions to the problem of mental deficiency in inter–war Britain. *History of Psychiatry.* 1992 Dec; 3(12): 473–498. 119 fn. BE61498.
  attitudes; deinstitutionalized persons; *eugenics; family relationship; females; *historical aspects; indigents; involuntary sterilization; males; mental institutions; *mentally retarded; motivation; paternalism; physicians; political systems; psychiatry; public policy; residential facilities; sexuality; *social control; social discrimination; social problems; social workers; socioeconomic factors; sociology of medicine; *voluntary sterilization; *Great Britain; *Nineteenth Century; *Twentieth Century

Thomson, Mathew. The Problem of Mental Deficiency: Eugenics, Democracy, and Social Policy in Britain c. 1870–1959. New York, NY: Oxford University Press; 1998. 351 p. Bibliography: p. 307–342. ISBN 0-19-820692-5. BE60511.
  attitudes; community services; democracy; *eugenics; females; *historical aspects; legal aspects; males; mental institutions; *mentally retarded; organization and administration; physicians; politics; psychiatry; *public

policy; social discrimination; socioeconomic factors; *sterilization (sexual); Board of Control (Great Britain); *Great Britain; Mental Deficiency Act 1913 (Great Britain); *Nineteenth Century; Royal Commission on Care and Control of the Feeble-Minded; *Twentieth Century

Alberta to compensate victims of sterilization. [News]. *New York Times.* 1998 Jun 6: A6. BE59360.
  *compensation; eugenics; females; institutionalized persons; *involuntary sterilization; *mentally retarded; physically disabled; *public policy; *Alberta; Sexual Sterilization Act 1927 (AB)

The Lynchburg Story: Eugenic Sterilization in America. [Videorecording].New York, NY: Filmakers Library; 1994. 1 videocassette; 55 min.; sd.; color; VHS. Director: Stephen Trombley; producer: Bruce Eadie. A Worldview Pictures Production. Certificate of Merit, San Francisco International Film Festival, 1994. BE59872.
  adolescents; attitudes; children; *disabled; *eugenics; females; *historical aspects; *indigents; institutionalized persons; investigators; *involuntary sterilization; legal aspects; males; mass media; *mentally retarded; National Socialism; nurses; physically disabled; physicians; public hospitals; public opinion; *public policy; state government; Supreme Court decisions; *whites; Buck v. Bell; Germany; Laughlin, Harry; *Lynchburg Colony for the Epileptic and Feebleminded; Priddy, Albert; *Twentieth Century; *United States; Virginia

SUICIDE

See also EUTHANASIA

Annas, George J. The "right to die" in America: sloganeering from Quinlan and Cruzan to Quill and Kevorkian. *Duquesne Law Review.* 1996 Summer; 34(4): 875–897. 37 fn. BE62533.
  *allowing to die; anencephaly; artificial feeding; *assisted suicide; brain death; competence; congenital disorders; *decision making; determination of death; Down syndrome; family members; futility; informed consent; *legal aspects; *legal rights; newborns; paternalism; patients; persistent vegetative state; physicians; resuscitation orders; *right to die; risks and benefits; social discrimination; standards; state government; terminally ill; third party consent; treatment refusal; ventilators; withholding treatment; Cruzan v. Director, Missouri Department of Health; In re Quinlan; *United States

Australia. Euthanasia Laws Act 1997. *Acts of the Australian Parliament.* 1997 Mar 27 (date effective). 7 p. Nov 17, 1997, passed by the Senate and the House of Representatives, assented to by the Governor–General, 27 Mar 1997. BE59924.
  *active euthanasia; allowing to die; *assisted suicide; federal government; intention; killing; *legal aspects; *legislation; palliative care; state government; suicide; third party consent; withholding treatment; *Australia; *Euthanasia Laws Act 1997 (Australia); Rights of the Terminally Ill Act 1995 (Northern Territory)

Back, Anthony; Ganzini, Linda; Sullivan, Mark, et al. Responding to patient requests for physician–assisted suicide. [Letters and response]. *JAMA.* 1999 Jan 20; 281(3): 227–229. 12 refs. BE61619.
  *assisted suicide; communication; competence; conscience; decision analysis; depressive disorder; drugs; moral obligations; palliative care; physician patient relationship; *physicians; practice guidelines; sedatives; suffering; *terminal care; coma

Baggett, David J. On the legality and morality of

BE = bioethics accession number   fn. = footnotes   refs. = references

physician–assisted suicide. *Asbury Theological Journal.*
1995 Spring; 50(1): 51–66. 13 fn. BE61347.
> allowing to die; *assisted suicide; attitudes; *Christian ethics;
> compassion; cultural pluralism; involuntary euthanasia;
> moral policy; *morality; pain; *physicians; public opinion;
> *public policy; quality of life; *religion; *right to die; rights;
> suffering; suicide; utilitarianism; value of life; voluntary
> euthanasia; *wedge argument; Kevorkian, Jack; United
> States

Baier, Kurt. Wrongful death and wrongful life. *In: his*
Problems of Life and Death: A Humanist Perspective.
Amherst, NY: Prometheus Books; 1997: 137–230. 74 fn.
ISBN 1–57392–153–X. BE61848.
> *allowing to die; *assisted suicide; capital punishment;
> contraception; disabled; disclosure; ethical theory;
> guidelines; *humanism; intention; *killing; law; legal aspects;
> legal liability; moral obligations; *moral policy; *morality;
> negligence; organ donation; physicians; *population control;
> prognosis; *prolongation of life; quality of life; suffering;
> suicide; value of life; values; *voluntary euthanasia; wrongful
> death; *wrongful life; rationality

Battin, Margaret Pabst; Snyder, Lois. Should older
persons have the right to commit suicide? Yes [and] No.
In: Scharlach, Andrew E.; Kaye, Lenard W., eds.
Controversial Issues in Aging. Boston, MA: Allyn and
Bacon; 1997: 92–102. 8 refs. ISBN 0–205–19381–1.
BE60962.
> active euthanasia; *aged; allowing to die; *assisted suicide;
> autonomy; coercion; constitutional law; depressive disorder;
> economics; *human rights; legal aspects; *legal rights;
> motivation; physicians; *right to die; state government;
> *suicide; treatment refusal; value of life; duty to die; Death
> with Dignity Act (OR); Oregon; United States

Beckett, Alexandra. End–of–life decisions in AIDS. *In:*
Steinberg, Maurice D.; Youngner, Stuart J., eds.
End–of–Life Decisions: A Psychosocial Perspective.
Washington, DC: American Psychiatric Press; 1998:
179–203. 68 fn. ISBN 0–88048–756–9. BE60119.
> *AIDS; alcohol abuse; *allowing to die; *assisted suicide;
> autonomy; case studies; competence; decision making;
> dementia; depressive disorder; drug abuse; drugs; futility;
> patient care; patients; *physicians; prognosis; psychiatric
> diagnosis; psychiatry; quality of life; referral and
> consultation; risks and benefits; *suicide; treatment refusal;
> withholding treatment; United States

Belluck, Pam. Kevorkian seen as 'distraction' on suicide
aid. [News]. *New York Times.* 1999 Mar 30: A1, A17.
BE60911.
> *active euthanasia; *assisted suicide; chronically ill; *legal
> aspects; legal liability; palliative care; *physicians; public
> opinion; public policy; right to die; terminally ill; wedge
> argument; *Kevorkian, Jack; United States; Youk, Thomas

Bottum, J. Debriefing the philosophers. *First Things.* 1997
Jun–Jul; No. 74: 26–30. BE60101.
> *assisted suicide; attitudes; coercion; disadvantaged;
> *ethicists; indigents; *philosophy; physicians; professional
> competence; public policy; regulation; *right to die; social
> impact; *Supreme Court decisions; value of life; wedge
> argument; liberalism; Dworkin, Ronald; Nagel, Thomas;
> Nozick, Robert; Rawls, John; Scanlon, Thomas; Thomson,
> Judith Jarvis; United States; Vacco v. Quill; Washington
> v. Glucksberg

Bresnahan, James F. Palliative care or assisted suicide?
America. 1998 Mar 14; 178(8): 16–21. BE59701.
> allowing to die; *assisted suicide; compassion; government
> regulation; *hospices; killing; *legal aspects; *palliative care;
> physicians; right to die; Roman Catholic ethics; state
> government; suffering; Supreme Court decisions; *terminal
> care; terminally ill; Oregon; *United States; *Vacco v. Quill;

*Washington v. Glucksberg

**British Columbia. Special Advisory Committee on
Ethical Issues in Health Care.** Euthanasia and
Physician–Assisted Suicide. Victoria, BC: British
Columbia Ministry of Health and Ministry Responsible
for Seniors; 1994 Feb. 43 p. 52 fn. ISBN 0–7726–2137–3.
BE59216.
> *active euthanasia; advance directives; advisory committees;
> *allowing to die; artificial feeding; *assisted suicide;
> autonomy; *beneficence; coercion; compassion; competence;
> double effect; drugs; intention; justice; killing; legal aspects;
> *moral policy; pain; palliative care; persistent vegetative
> state; *physicians; public policy; quality of life; right to die;
> suffering; Supreme Court decisions; terminally ill; third party
> consent; treatment refusal; value of life; *voluntary
> euthanasia; vulnerable populations; wedge argument;
> withholding treatment; dignity; duty to die; *British
> Columbia; *Canada; Canadian Charter of Rights and
> Freedoms; Criminal Code of Canada; Law Reform
> Commission of Canada; Rodriguez v. British Columbia
> (Attorney–General); *Special Advisory Committee on
> Ethical Issues in Health Care (BC)

Brodie, Gilbert E. Assisted suicide: an analysis of the legal
(i.e., moral) arguments in judgments of the Supreme
Court of Canada in the Sue Rodriguez case. *In:* Morgan,
John D., ed. Readings in Thanatology. Amityville, NY:
Baywood Publishing; 1997: 439–473. 2 refs. 17 fn. ISBN
0–89503–149–3. BE62334.
> active euthanasia; allowing to die; amyotrophic lateral
> sclerosis; *assisted suicide; *autonomy; constitutional law;
> criminal law; double effect; drugs; *ethical analysis;
> extraordinary treatment; *freedom; intention; justice;
> *killing; *law; *legal aspects; legal rights; *morality;
> motivation; pain; palliative care; physically disabled; right
> to die; risks and benefits; self concept; state interest;
> *Supreme Court decisions; treatment refusal; *value of life;
> values; withholding treatment; analgesia; dignity; *Canada;
> Canadian Charter of Rights and Freedoms; Criminal Code
> of Canada; *Rodriguez v. British Columbia
> (Attorney–General)

Brody, Howard. Physician–assisted suicide should be
legalized. *Archives of Neurology.* 1996 Nov; 53(11):
1182–1183. 12 refs. BE60528.
> *assisted suicide; guidelines; palliative care; physicians;
> *public policy; quality of health care; referral and
> consultation; resource allocation; terminal care; United
> States

Brovins, Joan; Oehmke, Thomas. Dr. Death: Dr. Jack
Kevorkian's Rx: Death. Hollywood, FL: Lifetime
Books; 1993. 256 p. 59 fn. ISBN 0–8119–0782–1.
BE62799.
> *assisted suicide; case studies; killing; legal liability; patients;
> physicians; right to die; *Kevorkian, Jack; Michigan; United
> States

Brushwood, David B.; Allen, William L. Constitutional
right to pharmaceutically assisted death. *American
Journal of Health–System Pharmacy.* 1996 Aug 1; 53(15):
1797–1799. 2 refs. BE59422.
> *assisted suicide; attitudes; conscience; *drugs; *legal
> aspects; *pharmacists; physicians; *right to die; *terminally
> ill; *Compassion in Dying v. State of Washington; United
> States; Washington

Callahan, Daniel. Physician–assisted suicide: moral
questions. *In:* Steinberg, Maurice D.; Youngner, Stuart
J., eds. End–of–Life Decisions: A Psychosocial
Perspective. Washington, DC: American Psychiatric
Press; 1998: 283–297. ISBN 0–88048–756–9. BE60116.
> *assisted suicide; autonomy; compassion; empathy;

BE = bioethics accession number   fn. = footnotes   refs. = references

involuntary euthanasia; killing; *moral obligations; obligations of society; pain; physician's role; *physicians; psychological stress; suffering; terminally ill; value of life; voluntary euthanasia; wedge argument; United States

Callahan, Jay. Assisted suicide, community, and the common good. [Editorial]. *Health and Social Work.* 1997 Nov; 22(4): 243-245. 23 refs. BE59231.

    *assisted suicide; *autonomy; *common good; freedom; legal rights; organizational policies; professional organizations; *social workers; National Association of Social Workers; *United States

Candilis, Philip J.; Appelbaum, Kenneth L. Physician-assisted suicide and the Supreme Court: the Washington and Vacco verdicts. *Journal of the American Academy of Psychiatry and the Law.* 1997; 25(4): 595-606. 22 refs. BE59152.

    advisory committees; allowing to die; *assisted suicide; *constitutional law; drugs; due process; equal protection; government regulation; intention; involuntary euthanasia; *legal aspects; legal rights; palliative care; physician's role; *physicians; public policy; *right to die; state government; state interest; *Supreme Court decisions; terminally ill; treatment refusal; value of life; vulnerable populations; withholding treatment; Fourteenth Amendment; New York State Task Force on Life and the Law; *United States; *Vacco v. Quill; *Washington v. Glucksberg

Catholic Health Association of the United States. CHA amicus curiae brief on physician-assisted suicide. *Health Progress.* 1997 May-Jun; 78(3): 36-43, 47. 10 fn. BE59687.

    allowing to die; *assisted suicide; clergy; constitutional law; double effect; due process; equal protection; killing; *legal aspects; legal rights; managed care programs; moral policy; physicians; public policy; right to die; *Roman Catholic ethics; state interest; suicide; Supreme Court decisions; terminal care; withholding treatment; Bernardin, Joseph; *Catholic Health Association; National Conference of Catholic Bishops; *United States; Vacco v. Quill; Washington v. Glucksberg

Cavanaugh, Thomas A. Currently accepted practices that are known to lead to death, and PAS: is there an ethically relevant difference? *Cambridge Quarterly of Healthcare Ethics.* 1998 Fall; 7(4): 375-381. 8 fn. BE59138.

    *allowing to die; *assisted suicide; drugs; *ethical analysis; *intention; killing; *moral policy; pain; *palliative care; physicians; *sedatives; *terminal care; treatment refusal; withholding treatment

Chesterman, Simon. Last rights: euthanasia, the sanctity of life, and the law in the Netherlands and the Northern Territory of Australia. *International and Comparative Law Quarterly.* 1998 Apr; 47(2): 362-393. 201 fn. BE61460.

    *active euthanasia; adults; allowing to die; *assisted suicide; attitudes; autonomy; comparative studies; depressive disorder; double effect; drugs; government regulation; guidelines; intention; international aspects; involuntary euthanasia; judicial action; killing; *legal aspects; legal liability; legislation; moral policy; newborns; pain; palliative care; physicians; political activity; public policy; statistics; suffering; terminally ill; *value of life; *voluntary euthanasia; *wedge argument; Australia; Euthanasia Laws Act 1997 (Australia); *Netherlands; Nitschke, Philip; *Northern Territory; Rights of the Terminally Ill Act 1995 (NT)

Chin, Arthur E.; Hedberg, Katrina; Higginson, Grant K., et al. Legalized physician-assisted suicide in Oregon -- the first year's experience. *New England Journal of Medicine.* 1999 Feb 18; 340(7): 577-583. 24 refs. BE60994.

    *assisted suicide; attitudes; autonomy; comparative studies; control groups; diagnosis; disabled; *drugs; emotions; evaluation studies; guideline adherence; guidelines;

legislation; *mortality; motivation; pain; *physicians; public policy; refusal to treat; social impact; socioeconomic factors; statistics; survey; *terminally ill; *Death with Dignity Act (OR); *Oregon

BACKGROUND AND METHODS: On October 27, 1997, Oregon legalized physician-assisted suicide. We collected data on all terminally ill Oregon residents who received prescriptions for lethal medications under the Oregon Death with Dignity Act and who died in 1998. The data were obtained from physicians' reports, death certificates, and interviews with physicians. We compared persons who took lethal medications prescribed under the act with those who died from similar illnesses but did not receive prescriptions for lethal medications. RESULTS: Information on 23 persons who received prescriptions for lethal medications was reported to the Oregon Health Division; 15 died after taking the lethal medications, 6 died from underlying illnesses, and 2 were alive as of January 1, 1999. The median age of the 15 patients who died after taking lethal medications was 69 years; 8 were male, and all 15 were white. Thirteen of the 15 patients had cancer. The case patients and controls were similar with regard to sex, race, urban or rural residence, level of education, health insurance coverage, and hospice enrollment. No case patients or controls expressed concern about the financial impact of their illness. One case patient and 15 controls expressed concern about inadequate control of pain (P=0.10). The case patients were more likely than the controls to have never married (P=0.04) and were more likely to be concerned about loss of autonomy due to illness (P=0.01) and loss of control of bodily functions (P=0.02). At death, 21 percent of the case patients and 84 percent of the controls were completely disabled (P less than 0.001). CONCLUSIONS: During the first year of legalized physician-assisted suicide in Oregon, the decision to request and use a prescription for lethal medication was associated with concern about loss of autonomy or control of bodily functions, not with fear of intractable pain or concern about financial loss. In addition, we found that the choice of physician-assisted suicide was not associated with level of education or health insurance coverage.

Cicirelli, Victor G. Elders' end-of-life decisions: implications for hospice care. *Hospice Journal.* 1997; 12(1): 57-72. 26 refs. BE59180.

    *aged; *allowing to die; *assisted suicide; *attitudes; chronically ill; *comparative studies; *decision making; dementia; family members; hospices; *patient participation; physicians; *prolongation of life; *quality of life; socioeconomic factors; *suicide; survey; terminal care; terminally ill; *voluntary euthanasia; withholding treatment; Indiana

Cohen, Lewis M. Suicide, hastening death, and psychiatry. *Archives of Internal Medicine.* 1998 Oct 12; 158(18): 1973-1976. 49 refs. BE59576.

    *allowing to die; *assisted suicide; competence; drugs; historical aspects; legal aspects; palliative care; physician's role; *psychiatry; quality of life; referral and consultation; religion; renal dialysis; sedatives; *suicide; terminal care; terminally ill; treatment refusal; withholding treatment; United States

Coleman, Gerald. Basic issues in the debate over dying. *Origins.* 1998 Mar 19; 27(39): 663-668. 56 fn. Address delivered to the annual Archbishop John R. Quinn Colloquim on Catholic Social Teaching, University of San Francisco, 28 Feb 1998. BE59812.

    *active euthanasia; allowing to die; artificial feeding;

---

*assisted suicide; autonomy; extraordinary treatment; killing; persistent vegetative state; quality of life; right to die; *Roman Catholic ethics; suffering; terminal care; value of life; United States

Connelly, R.J. Death with dignity: fifty years of soul-searching. *Journal of Religion and Health.* 1998 Fall; 37(3): 195–213. 58 fn. BE61218.
*active euthanasia; advance directives; aged; *allowing to die; artificial feeding; *assisted suicide; *attitudes; consensus; depressive disorder; dissent; extraordinary treatment; health personnel; hospices; legal aspects; pain; palliative care; physicians; public opinion; public policy; *right to die; Roman Catholic ethics; Supreme Court decisions; *terminal care; *trends; ventilators; voluntary euthanasia; withholding treatment; Compassion in Dying; Cruzan v. Director, Missouri Department of Health; Death with Dignity Act (OR); Hemlock Society; In re Quinlan; *United States; Vacco v. Quill; Washington v. Glucksberg

Conner, Paul. Is there a secular answer to euthanasia, American style? *Angelicum.* 1996; 73: 381–400. 24 fn. BE60098.
*active euthanasia; allowing to die; *assisted suicide; attitudes; autonomy; compassion; criminal law; ethicists; intention; killing; moral policy; *morality; motivation; palliative care; physicians; public policy; quality of life; Roman Catholic ethics; suffering; terminally ill; *voluntary euthanasia; withholding treatment; Brock, Dan; Kevorkian, Jack; United States

Cuperus–Bosma, Jacqueline M.; van der Wal, Gerrit; Looman, Caspar W.N., et al. Assessment of physician–assisted death by members of the public prosecution in the Netherlands. *Journal of Medical Ethics.* 1999 Feb; 25(1): 8–15. 7 fn. BE61188.
*active euthanasia; advance directives; *assisted suicide; cancer; case studies; *decision making; drugs; evaluation studies; family members; guideline adherence; guidelines; involuntary euthanasia; knowledge, attitudes, practice; *law enforcement; lawyers; legal liability; mandatory reporting; pain; *physicians; prognosis; referral and consultation; standards; suffering; *survey; terminally ill; third party consent; voluntary euthanasia; dignity; life expectancy; *prosecutors; *Netherlands
OBJECTIVES: To identify the factors that influence the assessment of reported cases of physician–assisted death by members of the public prosecution. DESIGN/SETTING: At the beginning of 1996, during verbal interviews, 12 short case-descriptions were presented to a representative group of 47 members of the public prosecution in the Netherlands. RESULTS: Assessment varied considerably between respondents. Some respondents made more "lenient" assessments than others. Characteristics of the respondents, such as function, personal-life philosophy and age, were not related to the assessment. Case characteristics, i.e. the presence of an explicit request, life expectancy and the type of suffering, strongly influenced the assessment. Of these characteristics, the presence or absence of an explicit request was the most important determinant of the decision whether or not to hold an inquest. CONCLUSIONS: Although the presence of an explicit request, life expectancy and the type of suffering each influenced the assessment, each individual assessment was dependent on the assessor. The resulting danger of legal inequality and legal uncertainty, particularly in complicated cases, should be kept to a minimum by the introduction of some form of protocol and consultation in doubtful or boundary cases. The notification procedure already promotes a certain degree of uniformity in the prosecution policy.

Curran, Patrick. Regulating death: Oregon's Death with Dignity Act and the legalization of physician–assisted suicide. [Note]. *Georgetown Law Journal.* 1998 Jan; 86(3): 725–749. 165 fn. BE61257.
*assisted suicide; autonomy; coercion; compensation; drugs; *evaluation; *government regulation; legal aspects; palliative care; patients; physicians; prognosis; right to die; socioeconomic factors; state government; terminally ill; terminology; time factors; voluntary euthanasia; dignity; *Death with Dignity Act (OR); *Oregon

De Leo, Diego; Marietta, Paola. Suicide: determinism or freedom? *Dolentium Hominum: Church and Health in the World.* 1997; 34(12th Yr., No. 1): 148–154. 44 refs. BE60496.
active euthanasia; allowing to die; *assisted suicide; attitudes; decision making; *freedom; health personnel; historical aspects; legal aspects; physicians; preventive medicine; psychiatry; public opinion; quality of life; right to die; risk; *suicide; value of life; rationality; Germany; Italy; Netherlands; United States

Delury, George E. But What If She Wants to Die? A Husband's Diary. New York, NY: Carol Publishing Group; 1997. 224 p. ISBN 1–55972–411–0. BE61475.
active euthanasia; *assisted suicide; attitudes to death; central nervous system diseases; coercion; criminal law; decision making; depressive disorder; *family members; legal liability; *married persons; mass media; *motivation; psychological stress; public policy; right to die; suffering; uncertainty; *multiple sclerosis; *Delury, George; *Lebov, Myrna; New York City

Demy, Timothy J.; Stewart, Gary P. Suicide: A Christian Response: Crucial Considerations for Choosing Life. Grand Rapids, MI: Kregel Publications; 1998. 490 p. Includes references. Foreword by Carl F.H. Henry. ISBN 0–8254–2355–4. BE61352.
*active euthanasia; adolescents; advance directives; allowing to die; *assisted suicide; autonomy; beneficence; cancer; *Christian ethics; disabled; killing; legal aspects; morality; pain; palliative care; paternalism; physicians; Protestant ethics; public policy; quality of life; right to die; social discrimination; suffering; *suicide; terminally ill; *theology; treatment refusal; value of life; *voluntary euthanasia; wedge argument; withholding treatment; *Evangelical Christians; United States

Devlin, Maureen M. Compassion in Dying v. State of Washington. [Note]. *Issues in Law and Medicine.* 1996 Summer; 12(1): 59–63. BE61148.
abortion, induced; adults; allowing to die; *assisted suicide; coercion; competence; *constitutional law; *drugs; *due process; government regulation; *legal aspects; *legal rights; *physicians; *right to die; state government; *state interest; *terminally ill; treatment refusal; *Compassion in Dying v. State of Washington; Fourteenth Amendment; *Washington

Devlin, Maureen M. Quill v. Vacco. [Note]. *Issues in Law and Medicine.* 1996 Summer; 12(1): 65–67. BE61149.
adults; allowing to die; *assisted suicide; competence; *constitutional law; *drugs; due process; *equal protection; government regulation; *legal aspects; *legal rights; *physicians; *right to die; state government; state interest; *terminally ill; treatment refusal; withholding treatment; Fourteenth Amendment; *New York; *Quill v. Vacco

Dickinson, George E.; Lancaster, Carol J.; Sumner, Edward D., et al. Attitudes toward assisted suicide and euthanasia among physicians in South Carolina and Washington. *Omega: A Journal of Death and Dying.* 1997–1998; 36(3): 201–218. 17 refs. BE61223.
*active euthanasia; *assisted suicide; *attitudes; clinical ethics committees; comparative studies; competence;

decision making; family members; guidelines; medical specialties; morality; pain; physician patient relationship; *physicians; public opinion; public policy; quality of life; referral and consultation; right to die; survey; terminally ill; *voluntary euthanasia; *South Carolina; United States; *Washington

Dixon, Nicholas. On the difference between physician–assisted suicide and active euthanasia. *Hastings Center Report.* 1998 Sep–Oct; 28(5): 25–29. 12 fn. BE59551.
   *active euthanasia; *assisted suicide; coercion; *killing; *moral policy; *physician's role; *public policy; socioeconomic factors; *voluntary euthanasia; wedge argument; United States

Those who defend physician–assisted suicide often seek to distinguish it from active euthanasia, but in fact, the two acts face the same objections. Both can lead to abuse, both implicate the physician in the death of a patient, and both violate whatever objections there are to killing. Their moral similarity derives from the similar roles of the physician.

Doerflinger, Richard M. An uncertain future for assisted suicide. [News]. *Hastings Center Report.* 1999 Jan–Feb; 29(1): 52. BE61640.
   *assisted suicide; federal government; *legal aspects; legislation; palliative care; political activity; public opinion; *public policy; right to die; *state government; Michigan; Oregon; *United States

Doukas, David J.; Gorenflo, Daniel W.; Supanich, Barbara. Primary care physician attitudes and values toward end–of–life care and physician–assisted death. *Ethics and Behavior.* 1999; 9(3): 219–230. 12 refs. BE62083.
   *active euthanasia; advance directives; *allowing to die; *assisted suicide; *attitudes; family practice; internal medicine; *physicians; *primary health care; survey; *values; Michigan

This study explores how primary care physician attitudes toward physician–assisted death (PAD) are related to their personal values toward end–of–life care and PAD. A group of 810 Michigan family physicians, internists, and general practitioners, divided into 4 typology groups by their intention toward participating in PAD, rated their attitudes toward PAD, along with their values and preferences for their own end–of–life care. Respondents who most objected to PAD were less likely to have executed an advance directive and more likely to have values promoting continued life-sustaining treatment in their own terminal care. Furthermore, a significant number of physicians, who had strong values against their own withdrawal of treatment in terminal care, were opposed to the withdrawing or withholding of life-sustaining treatment in patient care. Considerations of personal physician values are relevant in the discussion of PAD and the withdrawal of treatment in terminal care.

Downie, Jocelyn; Sherwin, Susan. A feminist exploration of issues around assisted death. *Saint Louis University Public Law Review.* 1996; 15(2): 303–330. 78 fn. BE59912.
   abortion, induced; *active euthanasia; allowing to die; *assisted suicide; *autonomy; coercion; competence; decision making; *females; *feminist ethics; guidelines; home care; involuntary euthanasia; killing; *legal aspects; palliative care; *public policy; right to die; *social discrimination; *social impact; terminal care; treatment refusal; *voluntary euthanasia; wedge argument; Canada; United States

Dworkin, Gerald; Frey, R.G.; Bok, Sissela. Euthanasia and Physician–Assisted Suicide: For and Against. New York, NY: Cambridge University Press; 1998. 139 p. Includes references. ISBN 0–521–58789–1. BE60708.
   *active euthanasia; allowing to die; artificial feeding; *assisted suicide; autonomy; Christian ethics; double effect; intention; *killing; legal rights; medical ethics; medicine; *moral policy; natural law; palliative care; physician patient relationship; *physician's role; *physicians; *public policy; quality of life; risks and benefits; suffering; terminal care; terminally ill; treatment refusal; *voluntary euthanasia; *wedge argument; withholding treatment; United States

Engelhardt, H. Tristram. Physician–assisted death: doctrinal develoment vs. Christian tradition. [Introduction to five articles]. *Christian Bioethics.* 1998 Aug; 4(2): 115–121. 7 refs. 3 fn. Introduction to a set of articles by D.C. Thomasma, H.T. Engelhardt, A. Young, C. Kaczor, and W.E. Stempsey. BE61157.
   *active euthanasia; *assisted suicide; attitudes to death; *Christian ethics; Eastern Orthodox ethics; historical aspects; intention; killing; physicians; Roman Catholic ethics; suicide; theology; *voluntary euthanasia

Physician–assisted suicide offers a moral and theological Rorschach test. Foundational commitments regarding morality and theology are disclosed by how the issue is perceived and by what moral problems it is seen to present. One of the cardinal differences disclosed is that between Western and Orthodox Christian approaches to theology in general, and the theology of dying and suicide in particular. Confrontation with the issue of suicide is likely to bring further doctrinal development in many of the Western Christian religions, so as to be able to accept physician–assisted suicide and euthanasia.

Engelhardt, H. Tristram. Physician–assisted suicide reconsidered: dying as a Christian in a post–Christian age. *Christian Bioethics.* 1998 Aug; 4(2): 143–167. 41 refs. 31 fn. Commented on by C. Kaczor, p. 183–201. BE61159.
   *active euthanasia; *assisted suicide; attitudes to death; autonomy; *Christian ethics; Eastern Orthodox ethics; freedom; legal aspects; morality; physicians; *postmodernism; right to die; *secularism; suffering; suicide; *theology; trends; *values; *voluntary euthanasia; dignity; United States

The traditional Christian focus concerning dying is on repentance, not dignity. The goal of a traditional Christian death is not a pleasing, final chapter to life, but union with God: holiness. The pursuit of holiness requires putting on Christ and accepting His cross. In contrast, post–traditional Christian and secular concerns with self–determination, control, dignity, and self–esteem make physician–assisted suicide and voluntary active euthanasia plausible moral choices. Such is not the case within the context of the traditional Christian experience of God, which throughout its 2000 years has sternly condemned suicide and assisted suicide. The wrongness of such actions cannot adequately be appreciated outside the experience of that Christian life. Traditional Christian appreciations of death involve an epistemology and metaphysics of values in discordance with those of secular morality. This difference in the appreciation of the meaning of dying and death, as well as in the appreciation of the moral significance of suicide, discloses a new battle in the culture wars separating traditional Christian morality from that of the surrounding society.

Filene, Peter G. In the Arms of Others: A Cultural History of the Right–to–Die in America. Chicago, IL: Ivan R. Dee; 1998. 282 p. 637 fn. ISBN 1–56663–188–2. BE60014.
   *active euthanasia; *allowing to die; artificial feeding;

BE = bioethics accession number   fn. = footnotes   refs. = references

*assisted suicide; attitudes; attitudes to death; autonomy; competence; congenital disorders; decision making; determination of death; ethicists; extraordinary treatment; government regulation; *historical aspects; judicial action; legal aspects; living wills; mass media; newborns; persistent vegetative state; physicians; political activity; politics; privacy; public opinion; *right to die; state government; suffering; *terminal care; terminally ill; treatment refusal; *trends; withholding treatment; Cruzan v. Director, Missouri Department of Health; Cruzan v. Harmon; In re Conroy; In re Quinlan; Netherlands; Nineteenth Century; Superintendent v. Saikewicz; *Twentieth Century; *United States

Flanders, Steven; Shelanski, Vivien B.; Ickes, Cynthia, et al. Physician–assisted suicide: potential impact of recent court decisions. *Journal of Long Term Home Health Care.* 1997 Winter; 16(1): 4–13. 14 refs. Proceedings of PRIDE Institute's symposium held at Saint Vincent's Hospital and Medical Center of New York City, 16 Jul 1996. BE62110.
aged; *assisted suicide; autonomy; constitutional law; due process; *equal protection; freedom; government regulation; *legal aspects; opioid analgesics; pain; palliative care; physician's role; physicians; prognosis; right to die; state government; state interest; suffering; *terminally ill; vulnerable populations; Fourteenth Amendment; *New York; *Quill v. Vacco; Washington

Fletcher, John C. Deciding about death:
physician–assisted suicide and the courts -- a panel discussion. *Pharos.* 1998 Winter; 61(1): 2–7. 5 refs. Program participants: Timothy E. Quill, John Arras, Richard J. Bonnie, and John C. Fletcher. BE59986.
allowing to die; *assisted suicide; autonomy; coercion; competence; decision making; depressive disorder; equal protection; hospices; *legal aspects; legal rights; moral policy; pain; *palliative care; *physicians; privacy; public policy; sedatives; suffering; *terminal care; terminally ill; third party consent; vulnerable populations; wedge argument; withholding treatment; *United States

Foley, Kathleen; Hendin, Herbert. The Oregon report: don't ask, don't tell. *Hastings Center Report.* 1999 May–Jun; 29(3): 37–42. 22 refs. BE61413.
*assisted suicide; competence; depressive disorder; diagnosis; economics; empirical research; *evaluation; *legislation; motivation; pain; palliative care; patients; physicians; professional competence; prognosis; psychiatry; *public policy; quality of health care; referral and consultation; state government; statistics; *Death with Dignity Act (OR); *Oregon; *Oregon Health Division
The Oregon Health Division's report on assisted suicide under the state's new legislation does not provide enough data to support its reassuring conclusions. Especially glaring is the lack of data on the palliative care offered to patients who requested assisted suicide, on their financial situation, and on their emotional state.

Frankel, Sherman. The dementia dilemma. *Perspectives in Biology and Medicine.* 1999 Winter; 42(2): 174–178. A longer draft version of this article appears at Internet Website
http://www.physics.upenn.edu/facultyinfo/frankel.html. BE62119.
*advance directives; aged; *assisted suicide; competence; *dementia; diagnosis; *directive adherence; patient advocacy; *right to die; voluntary euthanasia; Society for an Assisted Graceful Exit (SAGE); United States

Frey, R.G. Hume on suicide. *Journal of Medicine and Philosophy.* 1999 Aug; 24(4): 336–351. 17 refs. 2 fn. BE62612.
autonomy; Christian ethics; historical aspects; morality;

obligations to society; philosophy; *suicide; theology; Eighteenth Century; *Hume, David
Anyone interested in the morality of suicide reads David Hume's essay on the subject even today. There are numerous reasons for this, but the central one is that it sets up the starting point for contemporary debate about the morality of suicide, namely, the debate about whether some condition of life could present one with a morally acceptable reason for autonomously deciding to end one's life. We shall only be able to have this debate if we think that at least some acts of suicide can be moral, and we shall only be able to think this if we give up the blanket condemnation of suicide that theology has put in place. I look at this strategy of argument in the context of the wider eighteenth–century attempt to develop a non–theologically based ethic. The result in Hume's case is a very modern tract on suicide, with voluntariness and autonomy to the fore and with reflection on the condition of one's life and one's desire to carry on living a life in that condition the motivating circumstance.

Frolik, Lawrence A., ed. Health care decision making. *In: his* Aging and the Law: An Interdisciplinary Reader. Philadelphia, PA: Temple University Press; 1999: 295–394. 14 refs. 296 fn. ISBN 1–56639–653–0. BE61059.
advance care planning; advance directives; *aged; *allowing to die; *assisted suicide; attitudes; *autonomy; chronically ill; clinical ethics; coercion; communication; *competence; critically ill; cultural pluralism; *decision making; disclosure; family members; hospitals; *informed consent; judicial action; *legal aspects; mentally disabled; minority groups; nursing homes; patient advocacy; *patient care; patient care team; patients; persistent vegetative state; physicians; prolongation of life; resource allocation; resuscitation; *right to die; standards; suffering; *terminal care; terminally ill; *third party consent; treatment refusal; truth disclosure; voluntary euthanasia; wedge argument; withholding treatment; In re Fiori; In re Milton; Medicaid; Medicare; Pocono Medical Center v. Harley; Study to Understand Prognoses and Preferences for Outcomes and Risks of Treatments (SUPPORT); Uniform Health Care Decisions Act 1993; *United States

Ganzini, Linda; Johnston, Wendy S.; McFarland, Bentson H., et al. Attitudes of patients with amyotrophic lateral sclerosis and their care givers toward assisted suicide. *New England Journal of Medicine.* 1998 Oct 1; 339(14): 967–973. 30 refs. BE60035.
*amyotrophic lateral sclerosis; *assisted suicide; *attitudes; drugs; *family members; home care; males; motivation; *patients; physicians; prolongation of life; psychological stress; quality of life; religion; socioeconomic factors; survey; terminal care; treatment refusal; *Oregon; *Washington
BACKGROUND AND METHODS: Amyotrophic lateral sclerosis (ALS) is a neuromuscular disease that causes gradual paralysis, respiratory failure, and death, usually within three to five years after it has been diagnosed. Between 1995 and 1997, we surveyed patients with this disease in Oregon and Washington, as well as their family care givers, in order to determine their attitudes toward assisted suicide. Patients were considered to be willing to contemplate assisted suicide if they agreed with the statement, "Under some circumstances I would consider taking a prescription for a medicine whose sole purpose was to end my life," and disagreed with the statement, "I would never request or take a prescription for a medication whose sole purpose was to end my life." The Oregon Death with Dignity Act, which legalized physician–assisted suicide, was approved by Oregon voters in 1994 but did not go into effect until October 1997, after data collection for this study had been completed. RESULTS: Of 140

BE = bioethics accession number   fn. = footnotes   refs. = references

eligible persons with ALS, 100 (71 percent) agreed to participate in the study, as did 91 family care givers. The mean age of the patients with ALS was 54 years; the mean duration of illness since the diagnosis was 2.8 years. Fifty-six patients (56 percent) said they would consider assisted suicide, and 44 of the 56 agreed with the statement, "If physician-assisted suicide were legal, I would request a lethal prescription from a physician." One patient would have taken the medication immediately, and 36 would have kept it for future use. As compared with the patients who were opposed to assisted suicide, those who would consider it were more likely to be men, had a higher level of education, were less likely to be religious, had higher scores for hopelessness, and rated their quality of life as lower. In 66 of 91 instances (73 percent), care givers and patients had the same attitude toward assisted suicide. CONCLUSIONS: In Oregon and Washington, a majority of persons with ALS whom we surveyed would consider assisted suicide. Many would request a prescription for a lethal dose of medication well before they intended to use it.

Garrison, Jayne. Rushing heaven's door: assisted suicide -- do we really know what we want? *Health.* 1997 May/Jun; 11(4): 123-124, 126, 128-130. BE60450.
   active euthanasia; aged; allowing to die; *assisted suicide; attitudes; coercion; competence; decision making; family members; family relationship; hospices; quality of life; *terminal care; treatment refusal; adult offspring

Gilham, Charles; Leibold, Peter. A voice against physician-assisted suicide. [Cardinal Bernardin's letter; excerpts]. *Health Progress.* 1997 May-Jun; 78(3): 44-47. 10 fn. BE59688.
   *assisted suicide; clergy; *legal aspects; physician patient relationship; physicians; public policy; right to die; Roman Catholic ethics; Supreme Court decisions; value of life; wedge argument; Bernardin, Joseph; United States; Vacco v. Quill; Washington v. Glucksberg

Gillon, Raanan. Euthanasia in the Netherlands -- down the slippery slope? [Editorial]. *Journal of Medical Ethics.* 1999 Feb; 25(1): 3-4. 3 refs. BE61187.
   *active euthanasia; adults; allowing to die; *assisted suicide; autonomy; coercion; decision making; drugs; *empirical research; *guideline adherence; guidelines; infants; intention; *involuntary euthanasia; legal liability; palliative care; *physicians; *public policy; referral and consultation; right to die; statistics; suffering; treatment refusal; *voluntary euthanasia; *wedge argument; withholding treatment; *Netherlands

Glick, Shimon M. Euthanasia: an unbiased decision? *American Journal of Medicine.* 1997 Mar; 102(3): 294-296. 21 refs. BE62007.
   *active euthanasia; aged; *assisted suicide; autonomy; chronically ill; coercion; communication; conflict of interest; guideline adherence; involuntary euthanasia; managed care programs; patient advocacy; patients; physician patient relationship; physicians; suffering; suicide; terminally ill; trust; vulnerable populations; wedge argument; *duty to die

Grant, Sharon. Physician-assisted suicide: a chaplain's perspective. *Humane Health Care International.* 1997 Spring; 13(1): 21-24. 17 refs. BE59959.
   *assisted suicide; attitudes to death; autonomy; chronically ill; coercion; competence; guidelines; pastoral care; physician patient relationship; physicians; public policy; *religious ethics; terminally ill; theology; value of life; values; dignity; Quill, Timothy

Green, Gill. AIDS and euthanasia. *AIDS Care.* 1995; 7(Suppl. 2): S169-S173. 6 refs. BE60344.
   *active euthanasia; *AIDS; *assisted suicide; *attitudes; communication; family members; friends; health personnel; *HIV seropositivity; legal aspects; *patients; quality of life; suicide; survey; Scotland

Green, Michael J.; Fost, Norman. Seven reasons for Wisconsin physicians to oppose proposed legislation to legalize physician-assisted suicide. *Wisconsin Medical Journal.* 1995 Dec; 94(12): 693-695. 14 refs. BE61576.
   *assisted suicide; chronically ill; economics; health care; involuntary euthanasia; legal liability; *legislation; pain; palliative care; physician patient relationship; *physicians; political activity; right to die; rights; state government; suffering; terminally ill; wedge argument; duty to die; Netherlands; *Wisconsin

Griffiths, Pauline. Physician-assisted suicide and voluntary euthanasia: is it time the UK law caught up? *Nursing Ethics.* 1999 Mar; 6(2): 107-117. 35 refs. BE61930.
   allowing to die; *assisted suicide; congenital disorders; criminal law; double effect; guidelines; international aspects; involuntary euthanasia; killing; knowledge, attitudes, practice; *legal aspects; *legal liability; newborns; *nurses; opioid analgesics; pain; palliative care; *physicians; public policy; *right to die; treatment refusal; *voluntary euthanasia; wedge argument; withholding treatment; Australia; *Great Britain; Netherlands; Suicide Act 1961 (Great Britain); United States

Grubb, Andrew. Assisting suicide: Sue Rodriguez v. Attorney General of Canada and Others. [Comment]. *Medical Law Review.* 1994 Spring; 2(1): 119-126. BE59998.
   *amyotrophic lateral sclerosis; *assisted suicide; autonomy; coercion; constitutional law; criminal law; drugs; equal protection; freedom; justice; *legal aspects; legal rights; *physically disabled; physicians; state interest; Supreme Court decisions; terminally ill; value of life; vulnerable populations; *Canada; Canadian Charter of Rights and Freedoms; Criminal Code of Canada; European Convention on Human Rights; *Rodriguez v. British Columbia (Attorney-General)

Hall, Alison C. To die with dignity: comparing physician assisted suicide in the United States, Japan, and the Netherlands. [Note]. *Washington University Law Quarterly.* 1996 Fall; 74(3): 803-840. 236 fn. BE60111.
   adults; allowing to die; alternatives; *assisted suicide; autonomy; competence; constitutional law; depressive disorder; disclosure; drugs; due process; equal protection; freedom; *guidelines; international aspects; judicial action; *legal aspects; legal rights; legislation; pain; *physicians; privacy; psychiatric diagnosis; public policy; quality of life; referral and consultation; *right to die; state government; *suffering; *terminally ill; treatment refusal; voluntary euthanasia; withholding treatment; rationality; Compassion in Dying v. State of Washington; *Japan; Japan Society for Dying with Dignity; *Netherlands; New York; Quill v. Vacco; Royal Dutch Medical Association; *United States

Hassan, T.B.; MacNamara, A.F.; Davy, A., et al. Managing patients with deliberate self harm who refuse treatment in the accident and emergency department. *BMJ (British Medical Journal).* 1999 Jul 10; 319(7202): 107-109. 10 refs. BE61751.
   case studies; coercion; *competence; critically ill; decision making; *emergency care; evaluation; hospitals; *knowledge, attitudes, practice; *legal aspects; legal liability; *patient care; *physicians; psychiatric diagnosis; referral and consultation; *suicide; survey; *treatment refusal; Great Britain

Haverkate, Ilinka; van der Wal, Gerrit; van der Maas,

BE = bioethics accession number   fn. = footnotes   refs. = references

Paul J., et al. Guidelines on euthanasia and pain alleviation: compliance and opinions of physicians. *Health Policy.* 1998 Apr; 44(1): 45–55. 13 refs. BE59927.
*active euthanasia; administrators; *assisted suicide; double effect; family practice; *guideline adherence; *guidelines; hospitals; *institutional policies; *knowledge, attitudes, practice; medical specialties; nursing homes; *palliative care; *physicians; referral and consultation; suffering; survey; *Netherlands

Hendin, Herbert. Seduced by Death: Doctors, Patients, and Assisted Suicide. Revised and Updated. New York, NY: W.W. Norton; 1998. 304 p. 359 fn. ISBN 0–393–31791–9. BE59170.
*active euthanasia; allowing to die; *assisted suicide; attitudes to death; autonomy; chronically ill; coercion; competence; *decision making; depressive disorder; futility; guidelines; intention; involuntary euthanasia; judicial action; legal aspects; legal liability; mass media; palliative care; physician patient relationship; *physician's role; *physicians; political activity; politics; professional organizations; psychiatry; psychological stress; *public policy; referral and consultation; right to die; self regulation; statistics; suffering; suicide; Supreme Court decisions; terminally ill; treatment refusal; voluntary euthanasia; wedge argument; withholding treatment; Chabot, Boudewijn; Cohen, Herbert; Compassion in Dying; Dutch Voluntary Euthanasia Society; Hemlock Society; Kevorkian, Jack; Mulder-Meiss, Wine; *Netherlands; Quill, Timothy; Remmelink Commission; Royal Dutch Medical Association; *United States

Hendlin, Herbert. Physician-assisted suicide: what next? *Responsive Community.* 1997 Fall; 7(4): 21–34. BE59718.
*active euthanasia; *assisted suicide; autonomy; coercion; competence; depressive disorder; drugs; government regulation; guideline adherence; guidelines; involuntary euthanasia; motivation; pain; palliative care; physicians; public policy; quality of health care; right to die; suffering; suicide; *terminal care; terminally ill; treatment refusal; *voluntary euthanasia; vulnerable populations; wedge argument; Netherlands; United States

Hester, D. Micah. Significance at the end of life. *In:* McGee, Glenn, ed. Pragmatic Bioethics. Nashville, TN: Vanderbilt University Press; 1999: 113–128, 271–274. 31 fn. ISBN 0–8265–1321–2. BE60667.
*assisted suicide; attitudes to death; autonomy; family members; friends; health personnel; killing; *moral obligations; right to die; rights; suicide; terminal care; *terminally ill; *voluntary euthanasia; dignity; James, William

Humphry, Derek; Clement, Mary. Freedom to Die: People, Politics, and the Right-to-Die Movement. New York, NY: St. Martin's Press; 1998. 388 p. 523 fn. Appendixes include "A twentieth-century chronology of voluntary euthanasia and physician-assisted suicide," "Laws on physician-assisted suicide in the United States," and "The Oregon Death with Dignity Act." ISBN 0–312–19415–3. BE62300.
advance directives; AIDS; allowing to die; *assisted suicide; *attitudes; biomedical technologies; federal government; government regulation; historical aspects; international aspects; *legal aspects; palliative care; patient advocacy; patients' rights; physician patient relationship; physicians; political activity; politics; public opinion; *public policy; religion; resource allocation; *right to die; rights; state government; terminal care; *trends; *voluntary euthanasia; Australia; Hemlock Society; In re Quinlan; Kevorkian, Jack; Netherlands; Oregon; Quill, Timothy; Twentieth Century; *United States

Jacobson, Jay A. Preaching to the choir: new voices in the end of life discussion. [Editorial]. *Journal of Clinical Oncology.* 1997 Feb; 15(2): 413–415. 5 refs. BE59533.
*active euthanasia; allowing to die; *assisted suicide; *attitudes; cancer; empirical research; food; patients; physicians; public opinion; terminally ill; treatment refusal; trends; voluntary euthanasia; oncology; United States

Jamison, Stephen. Assisted Suicide: A Decision-Making Guide for Health Professionals. San Francisco, CA: Jossey-Bass; 1997. 248 p. Bibliography: p. 223–242 ISBN 0–7879–0873–8. BE62139.
active euthanasia; allowing to die; *alternatives; *assisted suicide; autonomy; chronically ill; coercion; *communication; compassion; competence; confidentiality; *decision making; depressive disorder; dissent; double effect; drugs; economics; family members; hospices; killing; legal aspects; motivation; opioid analgesics; pain; palliative care; patients; physician patient relationship; *physician's role; physicians; professional family relationship; *professional role; psychotherapy; quality of life; right to die; sedatives; suffering; Supreme Court decisions; *terminal care; terminally ill; trust; vulnerable populations; wedge argument; withholding treatment; rationality; United States; Vacco v. Quill; Washington v. Glucksberg

Jochemsen, Henk; Keown, John. Voluntary euthanasia under control? Further empirical evidence from the Netherlands. *Journal of Medical Ethics.* 1999 Feb; 25(1): 16–21. 46 fn. BE61189.
*active euthanasia; adults; *allowing to die; *assisted suicide; competence; decision making; depressive disorder; drugs; *empirical research; *guideline adherence; *guidelines; intention; *involuntary euthanasia; *knowledge, attitudes, practice; law enforcement; mandatory reporting; newborns; pain; palliative care; parental consent; *physicians; psychiatry; quality of life; referral and consultation; *regulation; *social control; statistics; suffering; terminal care; *voluntary euthanasia; *wedge argument; withholding treatment; *Netherlands
Nineteen ninety-six saw the publication of a major Dutch survey into euthanasia in the Netherlands. This paper outlines the main statistical findings of this survey and considers whether it shows that voluntary euthanasia is under effective control in the Netherlands. The paper concludes that although there has been some improvement in compliance with procedural requirements, the practice of voluntary euthanasia remains beyond effective control.

Jonsen, Albert R. Physician-assisted suicide. *Seattle University Law Review.* 1995 Spring; 18(3): 459–471. 45 fn. BE59817.
active euthanasia; *assisted suicide; autonomy; beneficence; government regulation; knowledge, attitudes, practice; *legal aspects; legal rights; *physicians; public policy; state government; treatment refusal; vulnerable populations; wedge argument; Ballot Measure 16 (OR); Compassion in Dying v. State of Washington; Initiative 119 (WA); *Oregon; *Washington

Kaczor, Christopher. Faith and reason and physician-assisted suicide. *Christian Bioethics.* 1998 Aug; 4(2): 183–201. 33 refs. 9 fn. Commentary on D.C. Thomasma, p. 122–142, and on H.T. Engelhardt, p. 143–167. BE61161.
*assisted suicide; attitudes to death; *Christian ethics; Eastern Orthodox ethics; historical aspects; intention; philosophy; Roman Catholic ethics; secularism; suicide; *theology; Jesus; Thomas Aquinas
Aquinas's conception of the relationship of faith and reason calls into question the arguments and some of the conclusions advanced in contributions to the debate on physician-assisted suicide by David Thomasma and H. Tristram Engelhardt. An understanding of the nature of theology as based on revelation calls into question Thomasma's theological argument in favor of

---

physician-assisted suicide based on the example of Christ and the martyrs. On the other hand, unaided reason calls into question his assumptions about the nature of death as in some cases a good for the human person. Finally, if Aquinas is right about the relationship of faith and reason, Engelhardt's sharp contrast between "Christian" and "secular" approaches to physician-assisted suicide needs reconsideration, although his conclusions about physician-assisted suicide would find support.

Kamisar, Yale. No constitutional right to physician-assisted suicide. *Health Law News.* 1997 Sep; 11(1): 2-3. BE60856.
     artificial feeding; *assisted suicide; *constitutional law; double effect; drugs; due process; *legal aspects; *legal rights; palliative care; physicians; *right to die; state government; Supreme Court decisions; terminal care; treatment refusal; withholding treatment; *United States; *Vacco v. Quill; *Washington v. Glucksberg

Kaplan, Kalman J. The case of Dr. Kevorkian and Mr. Gale: a brief historical note. *Omega: A Journal of Death and Dying.* 1997-1998; 36(2): 169-176. 9 refs. 1 fn. BE59773.
     *assisted suicide; coercion; *legal liability; physically disabled; physicians; *Gale, Hugh; *Kevorkian, Jack; Michigan

Kapp, Marshall B. Annotated bibliography on physician-assisted suicide. *Journal of Ethics, Law, and Aging.* 1997 Spring-Summer; 3(1): 45-51. BE59203.
     *assisted suicide; euthanasia; *physicians

Kapp, Marshall B. The physician-assisted suicide debate: which side is "gerontologically correct"? [Editorial]. *Journal of Ethics, Law, and Aging.* 1997 Spring-Summer; 3(1): 3-4. 3 refs. BE59204.
     *aged; *assisted suicide; autonomy; competence; palliative care; patient advocacy; patient care; *physicians; public policy

Keenan, James F. The case for physician-assisted suicide? *America.* 1998 Nov 14; 179(15): 14-19. BE61208.
     active euthanasia; aged; *assisted suicide; blacks; chronically ill; depressive disorder; females; indigents; involuntary euthanasia; motivation; pain; palliative care; *physicians; public opinion; public policy; quality of health care; Roman Catholic ethics; *vulnerable populations; wedge argument; whites; Netherlands; United States

Kelly, Brian; Varghese, Francis T. Euthanasia legislation. [Letter]. *Lancet.* 1998 Dec 5; 352(9143): 1863-1864. 5 refs. BE61707.
     *assisted suicide; communication; depressive disorder; emotions; motivation; patients; physician patient relationship; physician's role; psychiatry; referral and consultation; terminally ill; voluntary euthanasia; Australia

Kirk, Kathy. How Oregon's Death with Dignity Act affects practice. *American Journal of Nursing.* 1998 Aug; 98(8): 54-55. 4 refs. BE61803.
     accountability; active euthanasia; *assisted suicide; conscience; government regulation; *nurse's role; physician's role; state government; terminal care; Death with Dignity Act (OR); *Oregon

Kitchener, Betty; Jorm, Anthony F. Conditions required for a law on active voluntary euthanasia: a survey of nurses' opinions in the Australian Capital Territory. *Journal of Medical Ethics.* 1999 Feb; 25(1): 25-30. 27 refs. BE61191.
     advance directives; age factors; AIDS; *assisted suicide; *attitudes; cancer; case studies; competence; counseling; dementia; depressive disorder; drugs; family members; government regulation; *guidelines; informed consent; legal aspects; legislation; *nurses; pain; palliative care; paralysis; physicians; public opinion; *public policy; quality of life; referral and consultation; statistics; suffering; survey; terminally ill; *voluntary euthanasia; Australia; *Australian Capital Territory
     OBJECTIVES: To ascertain which conditions nurses believe should be in a law allowing active voluntary euthanasia (AVE). DESIGN: Survey questionnaire posted to registered nurses (RNs). SETTING: Australian Capital Territory (ACT) at the end of 1996, when active voluntary euthanasia was legal in the Northern Territory. SURVEY SAMPLE: A random sample of 2,000 RNs, representing 54 per cent of the RN population in the ACT. MAIN MEASURES: Two methods were used to look at nurses' opinions. The first involved four vignettes which varied in terms of critical characteristics of each patient who was requesting help to die. The respondents were asked if the law should be changed to allow any of these requests. There was also a checklist of conditions, most of which have commonly been included in Australian proposed laws on AVE. The respondents chose those which they believed should apply in a law on AVE. RESULTS: The response rate was 61%. Support for a change in the law to allow AVE was 38% for a young man with AIDS, 39% for an elderly man with early stage Alzheimer's disease, 44% for a young woman who had become quadriplegic and 71% for a middle-aged woman with metastases from breast cancer. The conditions most strongly supported in any future AVE law were: "second doctor's opinion," "cooling off period," "unbearable protracted suffering," "patient fully informed about illness and treatment" and "terminally ill." There was only minority support for "not suffering from treatable depression," "administer the fatal dose themselves" and "over a certain age." CONCLUSION: Given the lack of support for some conditions included in proposed AVE laws, there needs to be further debate about the conditions required in any future AVE bills.

Knobel, Peter. Suicide, assisted suicide, active euthanasia: a *Halakhic* inquiry. *In:* Jacob, Walter; Zemer, Moshe, eds. Death and Euthanasia in Jewish Law: Essays and Responsa. Pittsburgh, PA: Freehof Institute of Progressive Halakhah; Rodef Shalom Press; 1995: 27-59. 68 fn. ISBN 0-929699-06-8. BE60072.
     advance directives; *assisted suicide; autonomy; compassion; competence; *covenant; decision making; guidelines; informed consent; *Jewish ethics; justice; killing; methods; pain; quality of life; suffering; *suicide; terminally ill; theology; value of life; virtues; *voluntary euthanasia; dignity; *Reform Judaism

Koch, Tom; Heilig, Steve. On the subject(s) of Jack Kevorkian, M.D.: a retrospective analysis. [Article and commentary]. *Cambridge Quarterly of Healthcare Ethics.* 1998 Fall; 7(4): 436-442. 7 refs. BE59147.
     amyotrophic lateral sclerosis; *assisted suicide; autonomy; autopsies; cancer; central nervous system diseases; *chronically ill; depressive disorder; *diagnosis; family members; *motivation; pain; palliative care; *patients; physicians; prognosis; quality of life; treatment refusal; *voluntary euthanasia; dependency; multiple sclerosis; *Kevorkian, Jack

Koenig, Kristi L.; Salvucci, Angelo A.; Goodwin, Peter A., et al. Out-of-hospital do-not-attempt-resuscitation in the suicidal patient: a special case [and] Death with dignity. [Letters and response]. *Academic Emergency Medicine.* 1997 Sep; 4(9): 926-928. 8 refs. BE59124.

BE = bioethics accession number   fn. = footnotes   refs. = references

allied health personnel; *assisted suicide; attitudes; *emergency care; physicians; *resuscitation; *resuscitation orders; *suicide; terminally ill; California; Oregon

Kreimer, Seth F. The second time as tragedy: the assisted suicide cases and the heritage of *Roe v. Wade*. *Hastings Constitutional Law Quarterly*. 1997 Summer; 24(4): 863–901. 179 fn. BE62164.
   abortion, induced; *assisted suicide; *constitutional law; drugs; *due process; government regulation; *legal aspects; legal rights; pain; palliative care; pregnant women; *right to die; sedatives; state government; state interest; suffering; *Supreme Court decisions; terminal care; terminally ill; Planned Parenthood of Southeastern Pennsylvania v. Casey; Roe v. Wade; *United States; *Washington v. Glucksberg

Kuczewski, Mark G. Physician–assisted death: can philosophical bioethics aid social policy? *Cambridge Quarterly of Healthcare Ethics*. 1998 Fall; 7(4): 339–347. 19 fn. BE59135.
   *allowing to die; *assisted suicide; autonomy; bioethics; *casuistry; *communitarianism; drugs; *ethical analysis; ethical theory; *intention; killing; legal rights; *moral policy; palliative care; physicians; public policy; treatment refusal; United States

Laane, Henk–Maarten. Euthanasia, assisted suicide and AIDS. *AIDS Care*. 1995; 7(Suppl. 2): S163–S167. 13 refs. BE60343.
   *AIDS; *assisted suicide; criminal law; drugs; economics; empirical research; knowledge, attitudes, practice; legal aspects; mortality; physicians; statistics; suffering; *voluntary euthanasia; *Netherlands

Lachs, John. Dying old as a social problem. *In:* McGee, Glenn, ed. Pragmatic Bioethics. Nashville, TN: Vanderbilt University Press; 1999: 194–203, 281. 5 fn. ISBN 0–8265–1321–2. BE60672.
   *aged; assisted suicide; *autonomy; caring; depressive disorder; quality of life; *right to die; suffering; *suicide; *terminal care; terminally ill; value of life; voluntary euthanasia; rationality

Lachs, John. When abstract moralizing runs amok. *In: his* The Relevance of Philosophy to Life. Nashville, TN: Vanderbilt University Press; 1995: 188–194. 7 fn. ISBN 0–8265–1262–3. BE60864.
   *active euthanasia; *assisted suicide; *autonomy; drugs; moral policy; physicians; public policy; quality of life; *right to die; rights; suffering; voluntary euthanasia; wedge argument; *Callahan, Daniel

Larkin, Marilynn. Psychologists grapple with patient requests to hasten death. [News]. *Lancet*. 1999 Jun 19; 353(9170): 2133. BE62682.
   *assisted suicide; attitudes; *competence; depressive disorder; empirical research; *evaluation; *health personnel; mentally ill; physicians; professional competence; *psychiatric diagnosis; *psychology; referral and consultation; terminally ill; Oregon

Larson, Edward J. Seeking compassion in dying: the Washington State law against assisted suicide. *Seattle University Law Review*. 1995 Spring; 18(3): 509–519. 55 fn. BE59820.
   aged; allowing to die; *assisted suicide; coercion; constitutional law; drugs; *equal protection; *freedom; *government regulation; *legal aspects; *legal rights; physicians; right to die; state government; state interest; *terminally ill; treatment refusal; vulnerable populations; *Compassion in Dying v. State of Washington; Cruzan v. Director, Missouri Department of Health; Fourteenth Amendment; *Washington

Leone, Daniel A., ed. The Ethics of Euthanasia. San Diego, CA: Greenhaven Press; 1999. 88 p. (At issue: an opposing viewpoints series). Bibliography: p. 83–85. ISBN 0–7377–0004–1. BE61047.
   abortion, induced; *active euthanasia; *allowing to die; *assisted suicide; autonomy; Christian ethics; historical aspects; involuntary euthanasia; killing; legal aspects; moral policy; motivation; National Socialism; physicians; public policy; right to die; suffering; terminally ill; value of life; wedge argument; Germany; Netherlands; United States

Letvak, Richard; Pochard, Frédéric; Grassin, Marc, et al. Palliative options at the end of life. [Letters and response]. *JAMA*. 1998 Apr 8; 279(14): 1065–1067. 9 refs. BE59234.
   *allowing to die; artificial feeding; *assisted suicide; autonomy; beneficence; competence; conscience; cultural pluralism; double effect; *drugs; family members; food; informed consent; intention; pain; *palliative care; physicians; public policy; *sedatives; suffering; *terminal care; terminally ill; treatment refusal; *voluntary euthanasia; withholding treatment; coma; United States

Lewis, Neil A. Reno lifts barrier to Oregon's law on aided suicide. [News]. *New York Times*. 1998 Jun 6: A1, A7. BE60472.
   *assisted suicide; *drugs; federal government; *legal aspects; legal liability; *physicians; public policy; state government; terminally ill; *Death with Dignity Act (OR); Department of Justice; Drug Enforcement Agency; *Oregon; United States

Lindsay, Ronald Alan. Self-Determination, Suicide and Euthanasia: The Implications of Autonomy for the Morality and Legality of Assisted Suicide and Voluntary Active Euthanasia. Ann Arbor, MI: UMI Dissertation Services; 1996. 592 p. Bibliography: p. 572–592. Dissertation, Ph.D. in Philosophy, Georgetown University, August 1996. UMI No. 9713205. BE61112.
   active euthanasia; *assisted suicide; *autonomy; beneficence; coercion; competence; government regulation; guidelines; involuntary euthanasia; legal aspects; medical fees; model legislation; *moral policy; palliative care; paternalism; philosophy; physically disabled; physician patient relationship; physician's role; physicians; *public policy; *right to die; suffering; suicide; terminally ill; treatment refusal; trust; value of life; *voluntary euthanasia; vulnerable populations; wedge argument; Engelhardt, H. Tristram; Feinberg, Joel; Rachels, James

Lund, Nelson. Two precipices, one chasm: the economics of physician–assisted suicide and euthanasia. *Hastings Constitutional Law Quarterly*. 1997 Summer; 24(4): 903–946. 119 fn. BE62165.
   abortion, induced; active euthanasia; allowing to die; artificial feeding; *assisted suicide; biomedical research; codes of ethics; coercion; decision making; dehumanization; *economics; family members; government financing; government regulation; guideline adherence; guidelines; *health care delivery; health insurance; incentives; involuntary euthanasia; *legal aspects; managed care programs; medical ethics; persistent vegetative state; physician patient relationship; *physicians; politics; *public policy; quality of life; resource allocation; right to die; social impact; state government; *Supreme Court decisions; trust; voluntary euthanasia; vulnerable populations; *wedge argument; withholding treatment; *duty to die; *Hippocratic Oath; Netherlands; Roe v. Wade; *United States; Vacco v. Quill; Washington v. Glucksberg

McCormick, Richard A. Vive la différence! Killing and allowing to die. *America*. 1997 Dec 6; 177(18): 6–12. BE59444.
   active euthanasia; *allowing to die; *assisted suicide; autonomy; ethicists; *killing; legal aspects; moral policy;

BE = bioethics accession number   fn. = footnotes   refs. = references

physician's role; Supreme Court decisions; treatment refusal; withholding treatment; Beauchamp, Tom; Brock, Dan; Rachels, James; United States; Vacco v. Quill; Washington v. Glucksberg

McGough, Peter M. Medical concerns about physician–assisted suicide. *Seattle University Law Review.* 1995 Spring; 18(3): 521–530. 26 fn. BE59821.
    active euthanasia; allowing to die; *assisted suicide; attitudes; attitudes to death; beneficence; decision making; depressive disorder; double effect; drugs; guidelines; intention; legal rights; pain; palliative care; *physicians; public policy; right to die; social impact; terminal care; terminally ill; treatment refusal; trust; vulnerable populations; withholding treatment; Netherlands; United States

McIlwain, James T. Comments on "Euthanasia." *Rhode Island Medicine.* 1993 Dec; 76(12): 602. Commentary on D.W. Brock, "Euthanasia," p. 585–589. BE59415.
    *assisted suicide; attitudes to death; autonomy; *euthanasia; medical ethics; physician's role; *public policy; value of life; values; voluntary euthanasia; wedge argument; United States

McKhann, Charles F. A Time to Die: The Place for Physician Assistance. New Haven, CT: Yale University Press; 1999. 268 p. 240 fn. ISBN 0-300-07631-2. BE62341.
    *active euthanasia; advance directives; allowing to die; *assisted suicide; autonomy; chronically ill; competence; dementia; depressive disorder; double effect; economics; family members; guidelines; hospices; killing; legal aspects; medical ethics; organizational policies; palliative care; physician's role; *physicians; professional organizations; public opinion; *public policy; religious ethics; suffering; suicide; terminal care; terminally ill; treatment refusal; *voluntary euthanasia; wedge argument; rationality; Netherlands; *United States

McQuillen, Michael P.; Menken, Matthew; Hachinski, Vladimir. Managed care and managed death: peas from the same pod? [Article and commentaries]. *Archives of Neurology.* 1997 Mar; 54(3): 326–330. 45 refs. BE60326.
    active euthanasia; allowing to die; *assisted suicide; autonomy; economics; empirical research; intention; killing; legal aspects; *managed care programs; palliative care; physician's role; physicians; public opinion; resource allocation; right to die; terminology; treatment outcome; utilitarianism; neurology; United States

Malter, Alex; Sulmasy, Daniel P.; Schulman, Kevin A. Physician–assisted suicide. [Letter and response]. *Archives of Internal Medicine.* 1998 Dec 7–21; 158(22): 2513. 3 refs. BE61026.
    *assisted suicide; attitudes; economics; health care delivery; motivation; *physicians; public policy; *resource allocation; state government; suffering; terminally ill; rationality; Oregon; United States

Maltsberger, John T.; American Association of Suicidology. Committee on Physician–Assisted Death. Report of the Committee on Physician–Assisted Suicide and Euthanasia. *Suicide and Life–Threatening Behavior.* 1996; 26(Suppl.): 1–19. 36 fn. BE61572.
    *active euthanasia; aged; allowing to die; *assisted suicide; attitudes; autonomy; chronically ill; depressive disorder; disadvantaged; double effect; drugs; economics; females; intention; involuntary euthanasia; managed care programs; nurses; *organizational policies; pain; *palliative care; physician patient relationship; *physicians; public policy; right to die; suffering; *suicide; terminal care; terminally ill; voluntary euthanasia; withholding treatment; duty to die; *American Association of Suicidology; Netherlands; United States

Mannan, Haripriya M. Death as defined by Hinduism. *Saint Louis University Public Law Review.* 1996; 15(2): 423–432. 85 fn. BE59918.
    allowing to die; *attitudes to death; *Hindu ethics; legal aspects; right to die; *suicide; *India

Manning, Michael. Euthanasia and Physician–Assisted Suicide: Killing or Caring? New York, NY: Paulist Press; 1998. 120 p. Bibliography: p.108–120. ISBN 0-8091-3804-2. BE61048.
    *active euthanasia; allowing to die; artificial feeding; *assisted suicide; autonomy; common good; compassion; double effect; drugs; historical aspects; involuntary euthanasia; *killing; legal aspects; medical ethics; National Socialism; physician patient relationship; physicians; right to die; *Roman Catholic ethics; socioeconomic factors; theology; trust; wedge argument; withholding treatment; Germany; Netherlands; United States

Marlin, George J. Assisted suicide and euthanasia. *In: his* The Politician's Guide to Assisted Suicide, Cloning, and Other Current Controversies. Washington, DC: Morley Books; 1998: 63–124, 205–211. 172 fn. ISBN 0-9660597-1-9. BE62395.
    *active euthanasia; allowing to die; artificial feeding; *assisted suicide; Christian ethics; government regulation; historical aspects; human rights; killing; *legal aspects; legal rights; National Socialism; physician's role; physicians; politics; public policy; right to die; social impact; social worth; Supreme Court decisions; wedge argument; Germany; Kevorkian, Jack; Netherlands; United States

Martyn, Susan R.; Bourguignon, Henry J. Physician–assisted suicide: the lethal flaws of the Ninth and Second Circuit decisions. *California Law Review.* 1997 Mar; 85(2): 371–426. 265 fn. BE59896.
    abortion, induced; allowing to die; *assisted suicide; coercion; competence; *constitutional law; due process; economics; equal protection; freedom; guidelines; incentives; international aspects; involuntary euthanasia; killing; *legal aspects; *legal rights; legislation; palliative care; *physicians; *right to die; state government; state interest; suffering; *terminally ill; treatment refusal; voluntary euthanasia; *Compassion in Dying v. State of Washington; Cruzan v. Director, Missouri Department of Health; *Fourteenth Amendment; Netherlands; *New York; Planned Parenthood of Southeastern Pennsylvania v. Casey; *Quill v. Vacco; *Washington

Matzo, Marianne LaPorte. The search to end suffering: a historical perspective. *Journal of Gerontological Nursing.* 1997 Mar; 23(3): 11–17. 29 refs. BE60383.
    *active euthanasia; *allowing to die; artificial feeding; *assisted suicide; *attitudes; autonomy; historical aspects; international aspects; *nurse's role; *nurses; physicians; public policy; quality of life; religion; right to die; suffering; *suicide; terminal care; terminally ill; trends; voluntary euthanasia; withholding treatment

Mayo, David. Termination-of-treatment decisions: ethical underpinnings. *In:* Steinberg, Maurice D.; Youngner, Stuart J., eds. End-of-Life Decisions: A Psychosocial Perspective. Washington, DC: American Psychiatric Press; 1998: 259–281. 47 fn. ISBN 0-88048-756-9. BE60117.
    advance directives; advisory committees; *allowing to die; *assisted suicide; autonomy; competence; death; *decision making; *disclosure; *double effect; drugs; historical aspects; human rights; informed consent; *intention; *killing; legal rights; palliative care; paternalism; patients; physician patient relationship; *physicians; psychiatric diagnosis; psychiatry; referral and consultation; right to die; suffering; *terminally ill; treatment refusal; values; withholding treatment; Patient Self-Determination Act 1990; President's Commission for the Study of Ethical Problems; United States

---

BE = bioethics accession number   fn. = footnotes   refs. = references

Meisel, Alan; Jernigan, Jan C.; Youngner, Stuart J. Prosecutors and end-of-life decision making. *Archives of Internal Medicine.* 1999 May 24; 159(10): 1089–1095. 22 refs. BE61391.

active euthanasia; *allowing to die; artificial feeding; *assisted suicide; *attitudes; *criminal law; decision making; drugs; hospitals; killing; *knowledge, attitudes, practice; law enforcement; *lawyers; *legal liability; morality; *opioid analgesics; *palliative care; persistent vegetative state; *physicians; prolongation of life; right to die; survey; *terminal care; terminally ill; third party consent; ventilators; withholding treatment; *prosecutors; *United States

OBJECTIVE: To examine personal beliefs and professional behavior of state criminal prosecutors toward end-of-life decisions. DESIGN: Mail survey. SETTING: District attorney offices nationwide. PARTICIPANTS: All prosecuting attorneys who are members of the National District Attorneys Association. A total of 2844 surveys were mailed with 2 follow-up mailings at 6-week intervals; 761 surveys were returned for a response rate of 26.8%. The majority of respondents were white men, Protestant, and served in rural areas. INTERVENTIONS: None. MAIN OUTCOME MEASURES: On the basis of 4 case scenarios, (1) professional behavior as determined by respondents' willingness to prosecute and what criminal charges they would seek; and (2) personal beliefs as determined by whether prosecutors believed the physicians' actions were morally wrong and whether they would want the same action taken if they were in the patient's condition. RESULTS: Most respondents would not seek prosecution in 3 of the 4 cases. In the fourth case, involving physician-assisted suicide, only about one third of the respondents said that they definitely would prosecute. Those who would prosecute would most often seek a charge of criminal homicide. A majority of respondents believed that the physicians' actions were morally correct in each of the 4 cases and would want the same action taken if they were in the patient's position. There was a strong correlation between personal beliefs and professional behaviors. CONCLUSIONS: A large majority of responding prosecutors were unwilling to prosecute physicians in cases that clearly fall within currently accepted legal and professional boundaries. In the case of physician-assisted suicide, results reflected a surprisingly large professional unwillingness to prosecute and an even greater personal acceptance of physician-assisted suicide.

Michigan Catholic Conference. Living and dying according to the voice of faith. *Origins.* 1997 Oct 23; 27(19): 317, 319–322. BE60461.

allowing to die; *assisted suicide; *attitudes to death; compassion; economics; pain; palliative care; *Roman Catholic ethics; suffering; suicide; *terminal care; terminally ill; treatment refusal; value of life; voluntary euthanasia

Miller, Bradley W. A time to kill: Ronald Dworkin and the ethics of euthanasia. *Res Publica.* 1996; 2(1): 31–61. 105 fn. BE59210.

abortion, induced; advance directives; *assisted suicide; *autonomy; competence; intention; involuntary euthanasia; justice; killing; law; mentally disabled; moral policy; morality; *natural law; persistent vegetative state; personhood; physicians; *public policy; quality of life; state interest; utilitarianism; *value of life; *voluntary euthanasia; wedge argument; dignity; *Dworkin, Ronald

Monahan, Emmy S. An analysis of the mandatory notification procedure pertaining to termination of life in the Netherlands and recent developments. *Saint Louis University Public Law Review.* 1996; 15(2): 411–422. 77

fn. BE59917.

*active euthanasia; adults; *assisted suicide; competence; criminal law; depressive disorder; guidelines; *legal aspects; legal liability; *mandatory reporting; mentally ill; newborns; nurses; physician patient relationship; physicians; psychiatry; public policy; referral and consultation; suffering; *Netherlands

Morrison, R. Sean; Meier, Diane E. Physician-assisted dying: fashioning public policy with an absence of data. *Generations (American Society on Aging).* 1994 Winter; 18(4): 48–53. 21 refs. BE60552.

*assisted suicide; autonomy; *empirical research; hospices; international aspects; involuntary euthanasia; knowledge, attitudes, practice; legal aspects; motivation; pain; palliative care; physicians; public opinion; *public policy; risks and benefits; suffering; terminally ill; *voluntary euthanasia; wedge argument; Netherlands; *United States

Moyers, Peter. A Rawlsian case for physician-assisted suicide. *Princeton Journal of Bioethics.* 1998 Spring; 1(1): 23–31. 4 refs. BE62488.

*assisted suicide; competence; ethical theory; freedom; *justice; legal aspects; *morality; physicians; *public policy; quality of life; rights; *terminally ill; values; Devlin, Patrick; *Rawls, John; United States; Vacco v. Quill; Washington v. Glucksberg

New York State Task Force on Life and the Law. When Death Is Sought: Assisted Suicide and Euthanasia in the Medical Context; Supplement to Report. New York, NY: The Task Force; 1997 Apr. 18 p. 70 fn. ISBN 1-881268-02-0. BE62735.

*active euthanasia; advisory committees; *allowing to die; *assisted suicide; competence; double effect; due process; equal protection; government regulation; *guidelines; judicial action; *legal aspects; legal rights; opioid analgesics; pain; *palliative care; physicians; *public policy; right to die; risks and benefits; state government; suffering; terminally ill; treatment refusal; vulnerable populations; withholding treatment; *New York; *New York State Task Force on Life and the Law; United States; *Vacco v. Quill; Washington; *Washington v. Glucksberg

Ogden, Russel. AIDS, euthanasia and nursing. *Nursing Standard.* 1996 May 29; 10(36): 49–51. 12 refs. BE60401.

*AIDS; *assisted suicide; attitudes; conscience; drugs; friends; *nurse's role; nursing ethics; physicians; suicide; terminally ill; *voluntary euthanasia; British Columbia

Onwuteaka-Philipsen, Bregje D.; Muller, Martien T.; van der Wal, Gerrit. Euthanatics: implementation of a protocol to standardise euthanatics among pharmacists and GPs. *Patient Education and Counseling.* 1997 Jun; 31(2): 131–137. 9 refs. BE59389.

*active euthanasia; *assisted suicide; *drugs; knowledge, attitudes, practice; *methods; *pharmacists; *physicians; *practice guidelines; *standards; survey; *Netherlands

Orentlicher, David. The Supreme Court and terminal sedation: rejecting assisted suicide, embracing euthanasia. *Hastings Constitutional Law Quarterly.* 1997 Summer; 24(4): 947–968. 100 fn. BE62166.

*allowing to die; *artificial feeding; *assisted suicide; competence; double effect; drugs; *euthanasia; government regulation; *intention; involuntary euthanasia; *legal aspects; moral policy; pain; *palliative care; *physicians; right to die; *sedatives; suffering; *Supreme Court decisions; terminally ill; vulnerable populations; wedge argument; *withholding treatment; *United States; *Vacco v. Quill; *Washington v. Glucksberg

O'Rourke, Kevin D. Physician assisted suicide, a religious perspective. *Saint Louis University Public Law Review.*

1996; 15(2): 433–446. 72 fn. BE59919.
*assisted suicide; autonomy; compassion; historical aspects; motivation; physicians; *Roman Catholic ethics; suffering; suicide; theology; value of life

Peck, M. Scott. Denial of the Soul: Spiritual and Medical Perspectives on Euthanasia and Mortality. New York, NY: Harmony Books; 1997. 242 p. Includes references. ISBN 0-517-70865-5. BE61600.
allowing to die; *assisted suicide; *attitudes to death; chronically ill; competence; decision making; dementia; depressive disorder; *drugs; electroconvulsive therapy; empathy; euthanasia; extraordinary treatment; family members; futility; hospices; hospitals; killing; mentally ill; opioid analgesics; *pain; *palliative care; pastoral care; patient care; physicians; prolongation of life; psychiatric diagnosis; psychiatry; psychoactive drugs; *psychological stress; psychotherapy; public policy; quality of life; *religion; right to die; schizophrenia; secularism; *suffering; *suicide; terminal care; terminally ill; treatment refusal; withholding treatment; *opioids

Pfettscher, Susan. Nephrology nurses, euthanasia, and assisted suicide. *ANNA Journal (American Nephrology Nurses' Association).* 1996 Oct; 23(5): 524–525. 3 refs. BE62101.
*allowing to die; *assisted suicide; *attitudes; case studies; *nurses; patients; *renal dialysis; suffering; treatment refusal; voluntary euthanasia; withholding treatment

Place, Michael D. How faith and public policy intersect. *Health Progress.* 1999 Jan–Feb; 80(1): 10–13. BE61618.
*assisted suicide; communication; democracy; health care; morality; political activity; *public policy; *religion; *Roman Catholic ethics; secularism; theology; value of life; United States

Poenisch, Carol. Merian Frederick's story. *New England Journal of Medicine.* 1998 Oct 1; 339(14): 996–998. 1 ref. BE60036.
*amyotrophic lateral sclerosis; *assisted suicide; *attitudes; autonomy; case studies; clergy; decision making; drugs; emotions; *family members; hospices; motivation; parent child relationship; *patients; physically disabled; physicians; public policy; suffering; terminal care; adult offspring; dependency; *Kevorkian, Jack; Michigan

Prado, C.G.; Taylor, S.J. Assisted Suicide: Theory and Practice in Elective Death. Amherst, NY: Humanity Books; 1999. 223 p. Bibliography: p. 185–217. ISBN 1-57392-633-7. BE62736.
active euthanasia; *assisted suicide; autonomy; competence; *decision making; economics; ethical theory; *evaluation; informed consent; legal aspects; managed care programs; *moral policy; motivation; physician's role; prolongation of life; public policy; social impact; standards; suffering; suicide; *terminal care; third party consent; values; voluntary euthanasia; wedge argument; rationality; United States

Preston, Thomas A. Physician involvement in life–ending practices. *Seattle University Law Review.* 1995 Spring; 18(3): 531–544. 28 fn. BE59822.
active euthanasia; *allowing to die; *assisted suicide; attitudes to death; double effect; drugs; iatrogenic disease; intention; *killing; *knowledge, attitudes, practice; palliative care; persistent vegetative state; *physician's role; *physicians; prolongation of life; resuscitation orders; suffering; *terminal care; terminally ill; withholding treatment

Price, David P.T. Assisted suicide and refusing medical treatment: linguistics, morals and legal contortions. *Medical Law Review.* 1996 Autumn; 4(3): 270–299. 141 fn. BE61513.
active euthanasia; allowing to die; *assisted suicide; double

effect; *intention; international aspects; *legal aspects; moral policy; physicians; right to die; *suicide; *treatment refusal; Canada; Great Britain; New Zealand; United States

Reagan, Peter. Helen. *Lancet.* 1999 Apr 10; 353(9160): 1265–1267. BE61201.
aged; *assisted suicide; attitudes; breast cancer; case studies; drugs; *emotions; legislation; physician patient relationship; *physicians; professional family relationship; right to die; *terminally ill; Death with Dignity Act (OR); *Oregon

Reiling, Jennifer, ed. *JAMA* 100 years ago: the right to die. [Reprint]. *JAMA.* 1999 Sep 22–29; 282(12): 1112b. BE62668.
*assisted suicide; *attitudes; *historical aspects; *physicians; *right to die; *voluntary euthanasia; *Nineteenth Century

Robinson, John H.; Berry, Roberta M.; McDonnell, Kevin, eds. Death and dying. *In: their* A Health Law Reader: An Interdisciplinary Approach. Durham, NC: Carolina Academic Press; 1999: 339–426. 64 fn. ISBN 0-89089-907-X. BE62295.
*active euthanasia; *advance directives; *allowing to die; artificial feeding; *assisted suicide; brain death; competence; decision making; determination of death; directive adherence; *disabled; economics; freedom; intention; *legal aspects; legal liability; legal rights; living wills; moral policy; physician's role; physicians; public policy; quality of life; *right to die; risks and benefits; standards; state government; state interest; third party consent; treatment refusal; value of life; withholding treatment; wrongful life; Patient Self-Determination Act 1990; *United States

Rowland, Lewis P. Assisted suicide and alternatives in amyotrophic lateral sclerosis. [Editorial]. *New England Journal of Medicine.* 1998 Oct 1; 339(14): 987–989. 20 refs. BE60037.
advance care planning; *alternatives; *amyotrophic lateral sclerosis; artificial feeding; *assisted suicide; attitudes; double effect; drugs; hospices; legal aspects; *palliative care; patients; physically disabled; physicians; prognosis; prolongation of life; psychological stress; sedatives; *terminal care; time factors; truth disclosure; voluntary euthanasia; Death with Dignity Act (OR); Oregon

Ryan, Christopher James. Pulling up the runaway: the effect of new evidence on euthanasia's slippery slope. *Journal of Medical Ethics.* 1998 Oct; 24(5): 341–344. 29 refs. BE60257.
*assisted suicide; empirical research; *involuntary euthanasia; legal aspects; physician patient relationship; physicians; *public policy; *social impact; statistics; *voluntary euthanasia; *wedge argument; *Australia; *Netherlands; Remmelink Commission

The slippery slope argument has been the mainstay of many of those opposed to the legalisation of physician–assisted suicide and euthanasia. In this paper I re-examine the slippery slope in the light of two recent studies that examined the prevalence of medical decisions concerning the end of life in the Netherlands and in Australia. I argue that these two studies have robbed the slippery slope of the source of its power -- its intuitive obviousness. Finally I propose that, contrary to the warnings of the slippery slope, the available evidence suggests that the legalisation of physician–assisted suicide might actually decrease the prevalence of non–voluntary and involuntary euthanasia.

Sachs, Susan. Man accused of assisting wife's suicide. [News]. *New York Times.* 1999 Aug 7: B1, B3. BE62544.
*assisted suicide; *family members; *legal liability; married persons; Florio, Ann; *Florio, Peter; New York City

---

Sage, William M.; Jõe, Linda; Emanuel, Ezekiel J., et al. Potential cost savings from legalizing physician–assisted suicide. [Letters and response]. *New England Journal of Medicine.* 1998 Dec 10; 339(24): 1789–1790. 5 refs. BE60984.
*assisted suicide; costs and benefits; decision making; *economics; government financing; health care; long–term care; physicians; public policy; resource allocation; *terminal care; value of life; personal financing

Salem, Tania. Physician–assisted suicide: promoting autonomy — or medicalizing suicide? *Hastings Center Report.* 1999 May-Jun; 29(3): 30–36. 30 fn. BE61412.
*assisted suicide; attitudes to death; *autonomy; competence; *decision making; evaluation; government regulation; medicine; paternalism; *physician's role; *social control; *social dominance; *suicide; United States
Assisted suicide, many argue, honors self-determination in returning control of their dying to patients themselves. But physician assistance and measures proposed to safeguard patients from coercion in fact return ultimate authority over this "private and deeply personal" decision to medicine and society.

Scanlon, Colleen; Rushton, Cindy Hylton. Assisted suicide: clinical realities and ethical challenges. *American Journal of Critical Care.* 1996 Nov; 5(6): 397–405. 25 refs. Includes a continuing education quiz, p. 404–405. BE60527.
*assisted suicide; autonomy; beneficence; codes of ethics; communication; conscience; informed consent; nurse patient relationship; *nurse's role; *nurses; nursing ethics; organizational policies; professional organizations; public policy; social impact; terminal care; American Nurses Association; United States

Scherer, Jennifer M.; Simon, Rita J. Euthanasia and the Right to Die: A Comparative View. Lanham, MD: Rowman and Littlefield; 1999. 151 p. 270 fn. Includes tables of "Status of Right–to–Die Legislation in the U.S., by State, July 1997," and "Social Indicators, Euthanasia and Right–to–Die Regulations, Twenty Countries." ISBN 0-8476-9167-5. BE61316.
*active euthanasia; advance directives; *allowing to die; *assisted suicide; attitudes to death; autonomy; beneficence; coercion; comparative studies; compassion; *cultural pluralism; disabled; economics; eugenics; goals; health care delivery; historical aspects; *international aspects; involuntary euthanasia; knowledge, attitudes, practice; *legal aspects; medicine; National Socialism; pain; palliative care; persistent vegetative state; physicians; political activity; *public opinion; *public policy; quality of life; religious ethics; *right to die; standards; *state government; suffering; suicide; terminal care; terminally ill; treatment refusal; value of life; *voluntary euthanasia; wedge argument; withholding treatment; Australia; Canada; China; Colombia; France; Germany; Great Britain; India; Iran; Israel; Japan; Netherlands; South Africa; Spain; Switzerland; United States

Schoenholtz, Jack C.; Freedman, Alfred M.; Halpern, Abraham L. The "legal" abuse of physicians in deaths in the United States: the erosion of ethics and morality in medicine. *Wayne Law Review.* 1996 Spring; 42(3): 1505–1601. 306 fn. BE62178.
active euthanasia; allowing to die; *assisted suicide; *capital punishment; competence; economics; forensic medicine; forensic psychiatry; health care delivery; *killing; *legal aspects; medical ethics; moral obligations; organizational policies; patient care; *physicians; prisoners; professional organizations; psychiatric diagnosis; psychiatry; quality of life; wedge argument; American Medical Association; American Psychiatric Association; United States

Scofield, Giles R. Exposing some myths about

physician–assisted suicide. *Seattle University Law Review.* 1995 Spring; 18(3): 473–493. 37 fn. BE59818.
allowing to die; *assisted suicide; autonomy; beneficence; competence; disabled; disadvantaged; health care; health care delivery; justice; *legal aspects; legal rights; pain; patients; *physicians; *public policy; *right to die; social dominance; terminally ill; third party consent; treatment refusal; value of life; withholding treatment; Netherlands; *United States

Shah, Nisha; Warner, James; Blizard, Bob, et al. National survey of UK psychiatrists' attitudes to euthanasia. [Letter]. *Lancet.* 1998 Oct 24; 352(9137): 1360. 5 refs. BE60797.
active euthanasia; *allowing to die; *assisted suicide; *attitudes; *physicians; psychiatric diagnosis; *psychiatry; survey; *voluntary euthanasia; *Great Britain

Sheldon, Tony. Euthanasia endorsed in Dutch patient with dementia. [News]. *BMJ (British Medical Journal).* 1999 Jul 10; 319(7202): 75. BE61976.
*assisted suicide; *competence; *dementia; informed consent; organizational policies; physicians; psychiatry; referral and consultation; *Netherlands; Royal Dutch Medical Association

Siegel, Mark C. Lethal pity: the Oregon Death with Dignity Act, its implications for the disabled, and the struggle for equality in an able–bodied world. *Law and Inequality.* 1998 Winter; 16(1): 259–288. 225 fn. BE62431.
*assisted suicide; *disabled; equal protection; government regulation; *legal aspects; legal rights; public policy; quality of life; *social impact; social worth; socioeconomic factors; state government; terminally ill; *Death with Dignity Act (OR); *Oregon; United States

Simpson, William G. A different kind of Holocaust: from euthanasia to tyranny. *Linacre Quarterly.* 1997 Aug; 64(3): 87–92. BE59313.
abortion on demand; *abortion, induced; *active euthanasia; aged; *assisted suicide; chronically ill; disabled; eugenics; historical aspects; involuntary sterilization; *killing; National Socialism; public policy; right to die; social discrimination; *social worth; terminally ill; *value of life; genocide; Darwinism; Germany; Netherlands; Twentieth Century; United States

Smith, George P. Death. In: his Family Values and the New Society: Dilemmas of the 21st Century. Westport, CT: Praeger; 1998: 217–246. 192 fn. ISBN 0-275-96221-0. BE62298.
*active euthanasia; *allowing to die; artificial feeding; *assisted suicide; attitudes to death; beneficence; double effect; extraordinary treatment; futility; government regulation; *legal aspects; legal liability; moral policy; physicians; quality of life; *right to die; Roman Catholic ethics; standards; state government; terminal care; terminology; treatment refusal; *withholding treatment; *United States

Smith, Wesley J. Assisted suicide comes to Oregon. *Human Life Review.* 1995 Spring; 21(2): 25–40. 34 fn. BE61348.
active euthanasia; *assisted suicide; compassion; competence; counseling; depressive disorder; drugs; international aspects; involuntary euthanasia; legal aspects; *physicians; *political activity; quality of life; *right to die; Roman Catholics; suffering; terminally ill; value of life; voluntary euthanasia; vulnerable populations; wedge argument; *Ballot Measure 16 (OR); *Death with Dignity Act (OR); Initiative 119 (WA); Netherlands; *Oregon; Proposition 161 (CA); United States

Smith, Wesley J. Forced Exit: The Slippery Slope from Assisted Suicide to Legalized Murder. New York, NY:

BE = bioethics accession number   fn. = footnotes   refs. = references

Times Books; 1997. 291 p. 657 fn. ISBN 0–8129–2790–7. BE59666.

allowing to die; artificial feeding; *assisted suicide; coercion; compassion; disabled; economics; *euthanasia; guideline adherence; guidelines; hospices; *involuntary euthanasia; killing; legal aspects; managed care programs; pain; palliative care; *public policy; quality of life; resource allocation; right to die; terminal care; value of life; values; vulnerable populations; wedge argument; withholding treatment; Netherlands; United States

Somerville, Margaret A. Euthanasia in the media: jounalists' values, media ethics and "public square" messages. *Humane Health Care International.* 1997 Spring; 13(1): 17–20. 17 fn. BE59958.

*active euthanasia; *attitudes to death; autonomy; chronically ill; compassion; disabled; journalism; *mass media; professional ethics; right to die; suffering; terminally ill; *values; Australia; Canada; Netherlands; United States

Spencer, Donald E. Practical implications for health care providers in a physician–assisted suicide environment. *Seattle University Law Review.* 1995 Spring; 18(3): 545–556. 14 fn. BE59823.

alternatives; *assisted suicide; coercion; competence; counseling; decision making; depressive disorder; guidelines; health care reform; health personnel; home care; hospices; informed consent; lawyers; *legal aspects; palliative care; patient education; patients; *physicians; public opinion; *public policy; referral and consultation; *terminal care; terminally ill; continuity of patient care; United States

Spike, Jeffrey. Physicians' responsibilities in the care of suicidal patients: three case studies. *Journal of Clinical Ethics.* 1998 Fall; 9(3): 306–313. 5 fn. BE61339.

adults; advance directives; aged; *allowing to die; assisted suicide; autonomy; case studies; chronically ill; decision making; directive adherence; ethics consultation; family relationship; futility; patient care; *physician's role; physicians; *prolongation of life; resuscitation orders; right to die; *suicide; terminally ill; treatment refusal; withholding treatment

Sprung, Charles L.; Oppenheim, Arieh. End–of–life decisions in critical care medicine –– where are we headed? [Editorial]. *Critical Care Medicine.* 1998 Feb; 26(2): 200–202. 39 refs. BE62109.

*active euthanasia; *allowing to die; *assisted suicide; attitudes; autonomy; *critically ill; decision making; economics; hospitals; intensive care units; intention; international aspects; legal aspects; physician's role; physicians; right to die; suffering; terminally ill; treatment refusal; vulnerable populations; wedge argument; withholding treatment; Australia; Netherlands; United States

Starace, F.; Ogden, R.D. Suicidal behaviours and euthanasia. *AIDS Care.* 1997 Feb; 9(1): 106–108. Report on the XIth International Conference on AIDS, Vancouver, BC, Canada. BE62004.

*AIDS; *assisted suicide; attitudes; *HIV seropositivity; nurses; patients; physicians; statistics; *suicide; *voluntary euthanasia; British Columbia; California; Canada; Great Britain; Netherlands

Stead, William W.; Miller, Douglas P.; Lewis, Gregory L., et al. Terminal dehydration as an alternative to physician–assisted suicide. [Letters and responses]. *Annals of Internal Medicine.* 1998 Dec 15; 129(12): 1080–1082. 18 refs. BE60227.

allowing to die; *alternatives; *artificial feeding; *assisted suicide; competence; drugs; *food; intention; *palliative care; physicians; sedatives; suffering; suicide; *terminal care; terminally ill; terminology; *treatment refusal; *withholding treatment; *dehydration

Steinberg, Maurice D.; Youngner, Stuart J., eds. End–of–Life Decisions: A Psychosocial Perspective. Washington, DC: American Psychiatric Press; 1998. 322 p. (Issues in psychiatry). 686 fn. ISBN 0–88048–756–9. BE60115.

adults; age factors; AIDS; *allowing to die; *assisted suicide; autonomy; children; *communication; competence; *decision making; depressive disorder; dissent; emotions; family members; family relationship; legal aspects; morality; patient care team; physician patient relationship; *physician's role; physicians; psychiatric diagnosis; *psychiatry; psychological stress; referral and consultation; *terminally ill; third party consent; treatment refusal; values; withholding treatment; rationality; United States

Stempsey, William E. Laying down one's life for oneself. *Christian Bioethics.* 1998 Aug; 4(2): 202–224. 37 refs. 11 fn. BE61162.

altruism; *assisted suicide; double effect; *historical aspects; intention; motivation; physicians; *Roman Catholic ethics; *suicide; theology

Roman Catholicism has long opposed suicide. Although Scripture neither condones nor condemns suicide explicitly, cases in the Bible that are purported to be suicides fall into several different categories, and the Roman Catholic tradition can show why some of these should be considered morally wrong and some should not. While Christian martyrdom is praised, it is not correct to argue that this Christian outlook invites suicide, or that it recommends physician–assisted suicide for altruistic motives. Church Tradition, from its earliest days, has clearly distinguished martyrdom from suicide. The principles of double effect and cooperation, mainstays in Roman Catholic moral theology, enable one to see the moral difference between martyrdom and suicide, and to appreciate why physician–assisted suicide is wrong for both patient and physician.

Stephany, Theresa. Assisted suicide for the terminally ill: why we must have the choice. *Home Care Provider.* 1997 Oct; 2(5): 212–213. BE59428.

*assisted suicide; autonomy; conscience; health personnel; nurses; psychological stress; quality of life; *suffering; terminal care; *terminally ill

Stewart, Barbara. Grand jury refuses to indict in an assisted suicide. [News]. *New York Times.* 1999 Jul 17: B1, B4. BE62545.

*assisted suicide; friends; *legal liability; terminally ill; *Beigel, Cara; New York City; *Zancope, Marco

Stoffell, Brian. Voluntary euthanasia, suicide and physician–assisted suicide. *In:* Kuhse, Helga; Singer, Peter, eds. A Companion to Bioethics. Malden, MA: Blackwell; 1998: 272–279. 14 refs. ISBN 0–631–19737–0. BE59502.

*assisted suicide; autonomy; cultural pluralism; historical aspects; justice; killing; *moral policy; morality; physicians; *public policy; right to die; suffering; *suicide; *voluntary euthanasia; rationality

Stolberg, Sheryl Gay. Assisted suicides are rare, survey of doctors finds. [News]. *New York Times.* 1998 Apr 23: A1, A21. BE60323.

*active euthanasia; *assisted suicide; double effect; drugs; *knowledge, attitudes, practice; legal aspects; motivation; *physicians; suffering; terminally ill; United States

Stolberg, Sheryl Gay. In death, the goal is no questions asked. [News]. *New York Times.* 1998 Apr 26: WK 3. BE60471.

*assisted suicide; attitudes; *death; drugs; family members; legal liability; physicians; *records; Oregon; United States

---

BE = bioethics accession number   fn. = footnotes   refs. = references

Sullivan, Mark; Ormel, Johan; Kempen, G.I.J.M., et al. Beliefs concerning death, dying, and hastening death among older, functionally impaired Dutch adults: a one-year longitudinal study. *Journal of the American Geriatrics Society.* 1998 Oct; 46(10): 1251-1257. 26 refs. BE62265.

*active euthanasia; age factors; *aged; *allowing to die; *assisted suicide; *attitudes; *attitudes to death; chronically ill; decision making; dementia; health; involuntary euthanasia; mental health; mentally ill; *persistent vegetative state; *physically disabled; psychological stress; religion; socioeconomic factors; suffering; survey; time factors; withholding treatment; dependency; *Netherlands

Sunstein, Cass R. The right to die. *Yale Law Journal.* 1997 Jan; 106(4): 1123-1163. 169 fn. BE59662.

abortion, induced; active euthanasia; allowing to die; *assisted suicide; autonomy; coercion; competence; *constitutional law; contraception; *decision making; democracy; depressive disorder; *due process; *equal protection; family members; federal government; *government regulation; judicial action; *legal aspects; *legal rights; *physicians; privacy; prognosis; public policy; *right to die; social impact; state government; *state interest; suffering; *Supreme Court decisions; terminally ill; treatment refusal; value of life; wedge argument; Compassion in Dying v. State of Washington; Quill v. Vacco; *United States

Thomasma, David C.; Kimbrough-Kushner, Thomasine; Kimsma, Gerrit K., et al, eds. Asking to Die: Inside the Dutch Debate About Euthanasia. Boston, MA: Kluwer Academic; 1998. 584 p. Includes reference. ISBN 0-7923-5185-1. BE61054.

accountability; *active euthanasia; advisory committees; allowing to die; alternatives; *assisted suicide; case studies; Christian ethics; competence; continuing education; criminal law; disclosure; double effect; drugs; empirical research; ethical analysis; guidelines; hospices; hospitals; informed consent; institutional policies; international aspects; involuntary euthanasia; judicial action; killing; legal aspects; legislation; mandatory reporting; *moral policy; motivation; organizational policies; palliative care; patients; physicians; professional organizations; psychiatry; public opinion; *public policy; referral and consultation; review; *standards; suffering; *voluntary euthanasia; wedge argument; dignity; Free University of Amsterdam Academic Hospital; Medical Center of Alkmaar (Netherlands); *Netherlands; Remmelink Commission; Royal Dutch Medical Association; United States

Thomasma, David C. Assessing the arguments for and against euthanasia and assisted suicide: part two. *Cambridge Quarterly of Healthcare Ethics.* 1998 Fall; 7(4): 388-401. 37 fn. BE59140.

*active euthanasia; advance directives; aged; allowing to die; *assisted suicide; autonomy; compassion; economics; ethical analysis; eugenics; *intention; killing; mentally disabled; moral obligations; *moral policy; *motivation; National Socialism; physician's role; public policy; quality of life; right to die; social worth; suffering; values; *voluntary euthanasia; withholding treatment; Germany; Kevorkian, Jack; United States

Thomasma, David C. Assisted death and martyrdom. *Christian Bioethics.* 1998 Aug; 4(2): 122-142. 53 refs. 15 fn. Commented on by C. Kaczor, p. 183-201. BE61158.

*active euthanasia; *assisted suicide; attitudes to death; capital punishment; *historical aspects; *intention; *killing; love; *Roman Catholic ethics; theology; value of life; violence; *voluntary euthanasia; war; Jesus
Against the backdrop of ancient, mediaeval and modern Catholic teaching prohibiting killing (the rule against killing), the question of assisted suicide and euthanasia is examined. In the past the Church has modified its initial repugnance for killing by developing specific

guidelines for permitting killing under strict conditions. This took place with respect to capital punishment and a just war, for example. One wonders why in the least objectionable instance, when a person is already dying, suffering, and repeatedly requesting assistance in dying, there is still such widespread condemnation of assisted suicide and euthanasia. In a *Gedankexperiment*, I suggest that certain stories of martyrdom in the history of the Christian Church shed some light on the role of taking one's life, or putting one's life in danger out of love. I further suggest that requesting assisted suicide and/or euthanasia from the motive of love of one's family or care givers might possibly qualify as one instance of justifiable euthanasia, although I acknowledge that the Church will not be making changes in its stance any time soon.

Thompson, Dennis F. The institutional turn in professional ethics. *Ethics and Behavior.* 1999; 9(2): 109-118. 10 refs. BE61783.

administrators; *assisted suicide; conflict of interest; *decision making; drugs; hospitals; *institutional ethics; *institutional policies; *lawyers; legal aspects; moral obligations; *physicians; professional autonomy; *professional ethics; *professional role; values; United States
The traditional ideal in which professionals alone or in small groups serve their patients and clients in accord with a public-spirited goal is giving way to practice in which professionals serve in organizations that value mainly their expertise and expect them to act in accord with the organization's goals. The study of professional ethics has not kept pace with this trend and, as a result, has neglected the institutional aspects of ethical problems. I focus attention on these aspects by considering a case that raises 2 problems that are particularly relevant in the context in which professionals now practice: the problem of representation (whom does the professional act for) and the problem of authority (who has the right to make the policy for the institution).

Tucker, Kathryn L.; Burman, David J. Physician aid in dying: a humane option, a constitutionally protected choice. *Seattle University Law Review.* 1995 Spring; 18(3): 495-508. 59 fn. BE59819.

abortion, induced; allowing to die; *assisted suicide; competence; *constitutional law; drugs; due process; equal protection; freedom; government regulation; *legal aspects; *legal rights; *physicians; *right to die; state government; state interest; terminally ill; treatment refusal; Compassion in Dying v. State of Washington; Cruzan v. Director, Missouri Department of Health; *Fourteenth Amendment; Planned Parenthood of Southeastern Pennsylvania v. Casey; *United States; Washington

U.S. District Court, D. Oregon. In the United States District Court for the District of Oregon: Lee v. State of Oregon, Order, Civil No. 94-6467-HO, 9 May 1996. *Issues in Law and Medicine.* 1996 Summer; 12(1): 79-92. 18 fn. BE61150.

*assisted suicide; competence; constitutional law; criminal law; depressive disorder; due process; equal protection; *legal aspects; legal rights; *physicians; professional competence; psychiatric diagnosis; referral and consultation; right to die; social discrimination; standards; state government; terminally ill; *Ballot Measure 16 (OR); *Compassion in Dying v. State of Washington; *Lee v. State of Oregon; *Oregon

U.S. District Court, D. Oregon. Lee v. State of Oregon. *Federal Supplement.* 1995 Aug 3 (date of decision). 891: 1429-1439. BE62390.

*assisted suicide; competence; constitutional law; decision

BE = bioethics accession number   fn. = footnotes   refs. = references

making; drugs; equal protection; informed consent; *legal aspects; legal rights; legislation; *physicians; state interest; *terminally ill; rationality; *Death with Dignity Act (OR); Fourteenth Amendment; *Lee v. State of Oregon; *Oregon The U.S. District Court for the District of Oregon found unconstitutional the Oregon Death with Dignity Act, which allows a terminally ill patient to obtain a doctor's prescription for a fatal drug dosage in order to commit suicide. The court held that the state law, which classified competent terminally ill patients as a group and established procedures for them to opt for assisted suicide, was not rationally related to any legitimate state interest for purposes of the equal protection clause of the Fourteenth Ammendment. The law did not ensure rational and voluntary decision making by the terminally ill. (KIE abstract)

Underwood, James L. The Supreme Court's assisted suicide opinions in international perspective: avoiding a bureaucracy of death. *North Dakota Law Review.* 1997; 73(4): 641–684. 296 fn. BE62434.
 *active euthanasia; allowing to die; *assisted suicide; autonomy; depressive disorder; due process; equal protection; freedom; government regulation; guideline adherence; guidelines; historical aspects; *international aspects; *legal aspects; legal liability; legal rights; mentally ill; pain; physically disabled; physicians; privacy; *right to die; state government; suffering; Supreme Court decisions; terminally ill; value of life; vulnerable populations; *Australia; *Canada; Chabot, Boudewijn; *Colombia; *Netherlands; Northern Territory; Rodriguez v. British Columbia (Attorney-General); *United States; Vacco v. Quill; Washington v. Glucksberg

Urofsky, Melvin I. Leaving the door ajar: the Supreme Court and assisted suicide. *University of Richmond Law Review.* 1998 Mar; 32(2): 313–405. 421 fn. BE61523.
 advance directives; allowing to die; *assisted suicide; autonomy; constitutional law; due process; *equal protection; freedom; government regulation; historical aspects; international aspects; *legal aspects; legal rights; persistent vegetative state; physicians; public opinion; public policy; *right to die; state government; state interest; suffering; suicide; *Supreme Court decisions; terminally ill; treatment refusal; voluntary euthanasia; wedge argument; Compassion in Dying v. State of Washington; Cruzan v. Director, Missouri Department of Health; In re Quinlan; Kevorkian, Jack; Nineteenth Century; Quill, Timothy; Twentieth Century; *United States; *Vacco v. Quill; *Washington v. Glucksberg

Verhovek, Sam Howe. Legal suicide has killed 8, Oregeon says. [News]. *New York Times.* 1998 Aug 19: A16. BE60324.
 adults; *assisted suicide; competence; death; drugs; legal aspects; *physicians; *statistics; terminally ill; *Death with Dignity Act (OR); *Oregon

Verhovek, Sam Howe. Oregon reporting 15 deaths in 1998 under suicide law. [News]. *New York Times.* 1999 Feb 18: A1, A17. BE60868.
 *assisted suicide; death; drugs; evaluation; government regulation; legislation; motivation; physicians; social impact; state government; statistics; terminally ill; Health Division (Oregon); *Oregon

Vlaardingerbroek, W.F.C., comp.; Netherlands. Ministry of Health, Welfare and Sport. Documentation and Library Department. Euthanasia and Physician–Assisted Suicide in the Netherlands: Bibliography 1984–1995. Rijswijk, Netherlands: Ministry of Health, Welfare and Sport; 1995 Feb. 20 p. BE59475.
 *active euthanasia; *assisted suicide; physicians; *Netherlands; Remmelink Commission

Volkenandt, Matthias. Supportive care and euthanasia -- an ethical dilemma? *Supportive Care in Cancer.* 1998 Mar; 6(2): 114–119. 15 refs. Presented at the 9th International Symposium on Supportive Care in Cancer, held in St. Gallen, Switzerland, 26 Feb–1 Mar 1997. BE61573.
 *active euthanasia; allowing to die; *assisted suicide; autonomy; beneficence; *cancer; double effect; drugs; economics; intention; involuntary euthanasia; *moral obligations; moral policy; pain; *palliative care; *physician patient relationship; *physicians; resource allocation; social impact; suffering; *terminal care; *terminally ill; trust; voluntary euthanasia; wedge argument; withholding treatment; United States

Wagner, Bertil K.J.; Christian Pharmacists Fellowship International. Pharmacists should not participate in abortion or assisted suicide. [Position paper]. *Annals of Pharmacotherapy.* 1996 Oct; 30(10): 1192–1196. 56 refs. 1 fn. BE60183.
 *abortion, induced; active euthanasia; alternatives; *assisted suicide; beneficence; *Christian ethics; *conscience; counseling; depressive disorder; *drugs; mortality; motivation; *organizational policies; palliative care; *pharmacists; pregnant women; professional ethics; psychological stress; theology; value of life; *Christian Pharmacists Fellowship International; United States

Wehrwein, Peter. US physicians confused about end–of–life care. [News]. *Lancet.* 1998 Aug 15; 352(9127): 549. BE59656.
 *active euthanasia; allowing to die; *assisted suicide; cancer; empirical research; *euthanasia; guideline adherence; *knowledge, attitudes, practice; *physicians; *terminally ill; withholding treatment; United States

Werth, James L.; Gordon, Judith R.; Sullivan, Mark D., et al. Gatekeepers. [Letter and response]. *Hastings Center Report.* 1999 May–Jun; 29(3): 4. BE61404.
 abortion, induced; *assisted suicide; competence; decision making; *gatekeeping; health personnel; *mandatory programs; mental health; patient care team; *physician's role; professional role; psychiatric diagnosis; *psychiatry; quality of health care; *referral and consultation; terminal care; treatment refusal; United States

Werth, James L. Mental health professionals and assisted death: perceived ethical obligations and proposed guidelines for practice. *Ethics and Behavior.* 1999; 9(2): 159–183. 42 refs. BE61787.
 *assisted suicide; attitudes; codes of ethics; competence; confidentiality; *counseling; dangerousness; disclosure; duty to warn; *guidelines; *health personnel; informed consent; legal obligations; legislation; mental health; *organizational policies; palliative care; *practice guidelines; professional ethics; professional organizations; *professional role; psychiatric diagnosis; psychiatry; psychology; *psychotherapy; quality of life; *referral and consultation; social workers; state government; suicide; terminally ill; *American Counseling Association; *American Psychiatric Association; *American Psychological Association; Bellah v. Greenson; *National Association of Social Workers; Tarasoff v. Regents of the University of California; United States
I have three purposes in this article: (a) to briefly review the legal obligations a mental health professional has when working with a client who is talking about taking some action that could lead to his or her death, (b) to clarify the positions of the 4 major national mental health organizations regarding the acceptable roles of their members with clients who are discussing the possibility of receiving assisted death, and (c) to propose a set of guidelines for practice for mental health professionals working with clients who are considering assisted death that comport with the various laws and codes of ethics.

BE = bioethics accession number   fn. = footnotes   refs. = references

Werth, James L. When is a mental health professional competent to assess a person's decision to hasten death? *Ethics and Behavior.* 1999; 9(2): 141-157. 39 refs. BE61786.
　*assisted suicide; attitudes to death; coercion; communication; competence; continuing education; *counseling; decision making; education; *evaluation; *health personnel; legal aspects; *mental health; *professional competence; professional organizations; professional role; *psychotherapy; quality of life; *referral and consultation; *standards; terminally ill; American Association of Suicidology; Association for Death Education and Counseling; United States

As the country continues to debate the legality of aid-in-dying, it appears inevitable that at some point there will be a need for mental health professionals to be involved in assessments of individuals asking for a hastened death. I designed this article to provide a set of guidelines that will allow both mental health professionals and potential consultees to determine if a professional has the training and expertise necessary to be a competent consultant.

Wineberg, Howard. Oregon's Death with Dignity Act: ten months later. [Letter]. *Annals of Internal Medicine.* 1999 Mar 16; 130(6): 538. 3 refs. BE62560.
　*assisted suicide; drugs; legislation; physicians; social impact; statistics; *Oregon

Wooddell, Victor; Kaplan, Kalman J. An expanded typology of suicide, assisted suicide, and euthanasia. *Omega: A Journal of Death and Dying.* 1997-1998; 36(3): 219-226. 15 refs. BE61224.
　*active euthanasia; *allowing to die; *assisted suicide; coercion; *euthanasia; health personnel; *involuntary euthanasia; legal aspects; physician patient relationship; *physician's role; *physicians; *suicide; terminology; third party consent; treatment refusal; voluntary euthanasia; United States

Young, Alexey. Natural death and the work of perfection. *Christian Bioethics.* 1998 Aug; 4(2): 168-182. 20 refs. 10 fn. BE61160.
　active euthanasia; *assisted suicide; attitudes to death; clergy; *Eastern Orthodox ethics; love; pain; *suffering; suicide; *theology; voluntary euthanasia; Russia

The historic or traditional Christian view of pain (suffering) and death, especially as preserved by the Christians East (i.e., the Orthodox), is radically opposed to the modern secular obsession with avoidance of pain. Everything about this life has its goal or aim in a mystical reality, the Kingdom of Heaven, for which earthly life is a preparation. While neither illness nor health are seen as ends in themselves, both are viewed as proceeding from the will of God for our benefit and have no ultimate meaning or purpose outside of eternal life. Death may be a relief or an ending of suffering, but in itself it is not "good" but evil. Because they are the embodiment of lived theology, saints' lives can be a sure guide to understanding how to die as a traditional Christian. To illustrate this, I have chosen some examples from the lives of relatively recent saints. I myself am from the Russian Orthodox spiritual tradition, so all but one of my examples come from pre-Revolutionary Russia. The question is not so much whether or not a traditional Christian can countenance physician-assisted suicide, but rather, what is the meaning or purpose of pain and suffering in general. Is it part of the "work of perfection" required of those who wish to enter the Kingdom of Heaven and therefore not to be completely denied?

Zwier, Paul J. Looking for a nonlegal process:

physician-assisted suicide and the care perspective. *University of Richmond Law Review.* 1996 Jan; 30(1): 199-248. 173 fn. BE59861.
　abortion, induced; adults; allowing to die; alternatives; *assisted suicide; autonomy; *caring; communication; consensus; constitutional law; criminal law; decision making; due process; equal protection; family members; freedom; health personnel; killing; *legal aspects; legal rights; newborns; patients; *physicians; privacy; public policy; *right to die; suffering; terminally ill; treatment refusal; values; wedge argument; withholding treatment; Compassion in Dying v. State of Washington; Cruzan v. Director, Missouri Department of Health; Death with Dignity Act (OR); Planned Parenthood of Southeastern Pennsylvania v. Casey; *United States

A better death in Oregon. [Editorial]. *New York Times.* 1998 Mar 28: A14. BE60470.
　*assisted suicide; drugs; guidelines; legal aspects; *physicians; *public policy; state government; *Death with Dignity Act (OR); *Oregon

A suicide tape on TV inflames the issue in Spain. [News]. *New York Times.* 1998 Mar 9: A9. BE60322.
　*assisted suicide; *mass media; paralysis; *physically disabled; *Sampedro, Ramón; *Spain

Assisted suicide, at state discretion. [Editorial]. *New York Times.* 1998 Jun 8: A20. BE60475.
　*assisted suicide; *drugs; federal government; *legal aspects; legal liability; legislation; *physicians; public opinion; public policy; right to die; state government; Supreme Court decisions; terminally ill; *Death with Dignity Act (OR); Department of Justice; Drug Enforcement Agency; *Oregon; United States

Assisted suicide, in practice. [Editorial]. *New York Times.* 1999 Feb 27: A14. BE60869.
　*assisted suicide; evaluation; government regulation; legislation; social impact; state government; statistics; Netherlands; *Oregon

Euthanasia study challenged. *American Nurses Association Center for Ethics and Human Rights Communique.* 1996 Spring; 5(1): 6. *nurses BE60406.
　*active euthanasia; *assisted suicide; intensive care units; palliative care; *research design; terminal care

Guidelines issued on assisted suicide. [News]. *New York Times.* 1998 Mar 4: A15. BE60467.
　*assisted suicide; *guidelines; legal aspects; *physicians; state government; *Death with Dignity Act (OR); *Oregon

Kevorkian offers organs in assisted-suicide case. [News]. *New York Times.* 1998 Jun 8: A18. BE60474.
　*assisted suicide; cadavers; hospitals; *kidneys; *organ donation; patients; physicians; standards; *Kevorkian, Jack; Michigan

Oregon lets state pay for suicides. [News]. *New York Times.* 1998 Feb 27: A10. BE60320.
　*assisted suicide; *drugs; *government financing; *indigents; legal aspects; physicians; *public policy; state government; *terminally ill; *Oregon

The euthanasia war: last rights -- human beings do not start their own life; do they have the right to invite a doctor to end it? The pros and cons of doctor-assisted suicide. *Economist.* 1997 Jun 21; 343(8022): 21-24. BE60898.
　*active euthanasia; allowing to die; *assisted suicide; chronically ill; double effect; futility; international aspects; involuntary euthanasia; legal aspects; pain; palliative care; physicians; regulation; *right to die; suicide; terminally ill; *voluntary euthanasia; vulnerable populations; wedge

BE = bioethics accession number　　fn. = footnotes　　refs. = references

argument; withholding treatment; Australia; Colombia; Netherlands; United States

The right to choose to die. [Editorial]. *Economist.* 1997 Jun 21; 343(8022): 15-16. BE60897.
*assisted suicide; autonomy; health personnel; intention; killing; *legal aspects; palliative care; *right to die; *United States

United Kingdom Government publishes response to House of Lords report on medical ethics. [Summary of *Government Response to the Report of the Select Committee on Medical Ethics*, presented to Parliament by command of Her Majesty, May 1994]. *International Digest of Health Legislation.* 1995; 46(4): 570-572. BE62686.
*active euthanasia; advance directives; advisory committees; *allowing to die; *assisted suicide; decision making; drugs; guidelines; legal aspects; palliative care; persistent vegetative state; *public policy; resource allocation; *terminal care; terminally ill; treatment refusal; *Great Britain; *House of Lords Select Committee on Medical Ethics

SURROGATE DECISION MAKING *See*
ALLOWING TO DIE, INFORMED CONSENT, RESUSCITATION ORDERS

SURROGATE MOTHERS

See also REPRODUCTIVE TECHNOLOGIES

Boetzkes, Elisabeth. Equality, autonomy, and feminist bioethics. *In:* Donchin, Anne; Purdy, Laura M., eds. Embodying Bioethics: Recent Feminist Advances. Lanham, MD: Rowman and Littlefield; 1999: 121-139. 36 refs. 8 fn. ISBN 0-8476-8924-7. BE61018.
abortion, induced; *autonomy; contracts; females; *feminist ethics; government regulation; legal rights; personhood; *pregnant women; reproduction; selective abortion; *self concept; *sex determination; *sex preselection; sexuality; social discrimination; *surrogate mothers; Canada

British Medical Association. Changing Conceptions of Motherhood: The Practice of Surrogacy in Britain. London: The Association; 1996. 74 p. 34 fn. ISBN 0-7279-1006-X. BE59733.
children; coercion; confidentiality; counseling; decision making; depressive disorder; disclosure; economics; fathers; government regulation; guidelines; health facilities; infertility; legal aspects; legal liability; maternal health; moral obligations; mother fetus relationship; mothers; motivation; organizational policies; parent child relationship; physicians; professional organizations; risks and benefits; *surrogate mothers; British Medical Association; *Great Britain; Human Fertilisation and Embryology Act 1990; Human Fertilisation and Embryology Authority; Surrogacy Arrangements Act 1985 (Great Britain)

Bromham, David R. Surrogacy: ethical, legal and social aspects. *Journal of Assisted Reproduction and Genetics.* 1995 Sep; 12(8): 509-516. 31 refs. BE60563.
altruism; artificial feeding; children; coercion; commodification; embryo transfer; family members; females; government regulation; in vitro fertilization; legal aspects; motivation; parent child relationship; remuneration; risks and benefits; *surrogate mothers; prostitution; Family Law Reform Act 1987 (Great Britain); Great Britain; Human Fertilisation and Embryology Act 1990; Surrogacy Arrangements Act 1985 (Great Britain)

Freilicher, Liza; Scheu, Jennifer; Wetanson, Suzanne. Conceiving Luc: A Family Story. New York, NY: William Morrow; 1999. 302 p. ISBN 0-688-15986-9.

BE62099.
embryo transfer; *family members; *family relationship; in vitro fertilization; *surrogate mothers; United States

Grubb, Andrew. Surrogate arrangements and parental orders: the Parental Orders (Human Fertilisation and Embryology) Regulations 1994 (S.I. 1994 No. 2767). [Comment]. *Medical Law Review.* 1995 Summer; 3(2): 204-208. BE59257.
government regulation; *legal aspects; legislation; ovum donors; *parent child relationship; semen donors; *surrogate mothers; *Great Britain; Human Fertilisation and Embryology Act 1990

Grubb, Andrew. Surrogate contract: parentage -- In Re Marriage of Moschetta. [Comment]. *Medical Law Review.* 1995 Summer; 3(2): 219-221. BE60001.
artificial insemination; contracts; fathers; *legal aspects; marital relationship; *mothers; *parent child relationship; semen donors; *surrogate mothers; divorce; California; Great Britain; *In re Marriage of Moschetta; Uniform Parentage Act

Hartouni, Valerie. Cultural Conceptions: On Reproductive Technologies and the Remaking of Life. Minneapolis, MN: University of Minnesota Press; 1997. 175 p. Bibliography: p. 157-170. ISBN 0-8166-2623-5. BE62771.
*abortion, induced; adoption; audiovisual aids; behavioral genetics; blacks; brain death; *cloning; disadvantaged; embryos; eugenics; *fetuses; genetic intervention; legal aspects; mass media; mothers; parent child relationship; personhood; political activity; posthumous reproduction; postmodernism; *pregnant women; prenatal diagnosis; prolongation of life; *reproduction; *reproductive technologies; social discrimination; *social impact; socioeconomic factors; Supreme Court decisions; *surrogate mothers; value of life; values; violence; women's rights; In re Baby M; Johnson v. Calvert; Right to Life Movement; S'Aline's Solution; The Bell Curve (Herrnstein, R.; Murray, C.); *United States

Hopkins, Patrick D., ed. (Mis?)conceptions: morality and gender politics in reproductive technology. *In:* his Sex/Machine: Readings in Culture, Gender, and Technology. Bloomington, IN: Indiana University Press; 1998: 95-170. 227 fn. ISBN 0-253-21230-8. BE62289.
abortion, induced; *artificial insemination; attitudes; children; developing countries; eugenics; family relationship; *fathers; *females; feminist ethics; genetic disorders; informed consent; international aspects; legal aspects; *males; methods; moral obligations; motivation; *parent child relationship; population control; pregnant women; public policy; remuneration; rights; *risks and benefits; selective abortion; *semen donors; *sex determination; *sex preselection; sexuality; single persons; social discrimination; social impact; socioeconomic factors; spousal notification; *surrogate mothers; wedge argument; women's rights; harms; United States

Marshall, Adam. Choices for a child: an ethical and legal analysis of a failed surrogate birth contract. [Comment]. *University of Richmond Law Review.* 1996 Jan; 30(1): 275-302. 139 fn. BE59863.
*allowing to die; beneficence; child abuse; *congenital disorders; contracts; *decision making; *dissent; Down syndrome; *legal aspects; mother fetus relationship; *newborns; parent child relationship; *parents; standards; surgery; *surrogate mothers; withholding treatment; Americans with Disabilities Act 1990; Baby Jane Doe; Child Abuse Amendments 1984; In re Baby M; In re Conroy; Johnson v. Calvert; Superintendent v. Saikewicz; *United States

---

Mason, John Kenyon. A third party to marriage. *In: his* Medico–Legal Aspects of Reproduction and Parenthood. Second Edition. Brookfield, VT: Ashgate; 1998: 251–279. 99 fn. ISBN 1–84104–065–8. BE61068.
adoption; advisory committees; altruism; artificial insemination; children; contracts; embryo transfer; fathers; in vitro fertilization; industry; international aspects; judicial action; *legal aspects; model legislation; morality; mother fetus relationship; mothers; motivation; ovum donors; parent child relationship; *public policy; remuneration; semen donors; *surrogate mothers; *Great Britain; Human Fertilisation and Embryology Act 1990; Human Fertilisation and Embryology Authority; Israel; Surrogacy Arrangements Act 1985 (Great Britain); United States; Warnock Committee

Michaels, Meredith W. Other mothers: toward an ethic of postmaternal practice. *Hypatia.* 1996 Spring; 11(2): 49–70. 51 refs. 13 fn. BE61457.
coercion; commodification; contracts; *females; *feminist ethics; *informal social control; males; mothers; *reproductive technologies; sexuality; social dominance; *surrogate mothers

Neuhaus, Richard John; Morris, Monica B. Should surrogate motherhood be outlawed? *In:* Francoeur, Robert T., ed. Taking Sides: Clashing Views on Controversial Issues in Human Sexuality. Fifth Edition. Guilford, CT: Dushkin Publishing Group/Brown and Benchmark; 1996: 144–159. 5 refs. ISBN 0–697–31292–5. BE62046.
commodification; contracts; *government regulation; legal aspects; parent child relationship; remuneration; socioeconomic factors; *surrogate mothers

Warden, John. Surrogate mothers should be paid expenses only. [News]. *BMJ (British Medical Journal).* 1998 Oct 24; 317(7166): 1104. BE60853.
advisory committees; attitudes; physicians; *public policy; *remuneration; *surrogate mothers; *Great Britain

TECHNOLOGIES, BIOMEDICAL *See* BIOMEDICAL TECHNOLOGIES

TERMINAL CARE

See also ALLOWING TO DIE, PATIENT CARE, RESUSCITATION ORDERS

Alpers, Ann. Criminal act or palliative care? Prosecutions involving the care of the dying. *Journal of Law, Medicine and Ethics.* 1998 Winter; 26(4): 308–331. 200 fn. BE61165.
allowing to die; case studies; *criminal law; double effect; *drugs; intention; killing; law enforcement; *legal liability; negligence; *nurses; *opioid analgesics; *pain; *palliative care; *physicians; practice guidelines; suffering; *terminal care; *terminally ill; withholding treatment; *United States

Back, Anthony; Ganzini, Linda; Sullivan, Mark, et al. Responding to patient requests for physician–assisted suicide. [Letters and response]. *JAMA.* 1999 Jan 20; 281(3): 227–229. 12 refs. BE61619.
*assisted suicide; communication; competence; conscience; decision analysis; depressive disorder; drugs; moral obligations; palliative care; physician patient relationship; *physicians; practice guidelines; sedatives; suffering; *terminal care; coma

Begley, Anne Marie; Farsides, Bobby. Response to the National Council for Hospice and Specialist Palliative Care Services — voluntary euthanasia: the Council's view, by Ann Marie Begley, with reply by Bobby Farsides on behalf of the National Council for Hospice and Specialist Palliative Care Services. *Nursing Ethics.* 1999 Mar; 6(2): 157–161. 11 refs. BE61935.
autonomy; double effect; drugs; health personnel; hospices; *organizational policies; pain; *palliative care; paternalism; public policy; right to die; *terminal care; terminally ill; values; *voluntary euthanasia; wedge argument; analgesia; Great Britain; *National Council for Hospice and Specialist Palliative Care Services (Great Britain)

Bleich, J. David. On "The ethics of pain management." [Editorial]. *Cancer Investigation.* 1994; 12(3): 362–363. 3 refs. Commentary on J.J. Mitchell, "Administering mercy: the ethics of pain management," p. 343–349. BE60100.
double effect; opioid analgesics; *pain; *palliative care; physicians; professional competence; risks and benefits; *terminal care

Block, Susan; Billings, J. Andrew. Nurturing humanism through teaching palliative care. *Academic Medicine.* 1998 Jul; 73(7): 763–765. 12 refs. BE59880.
cultural pluralism; curriculum; hospices; *humanism; interprofessional relations; *medical education; medical ethics; medical schools; *palliative care; patient care team; physician patient relationship; professional family relationship; students; *terminal care; teaching hospitals

Bradley, Elizabeth H.; Peiris, Vasum; Wetle, Terrie. Discussions about end-of-life care in nursing homes. *Journal of the American Geriatrics Society.* 1998 Oct; 46(10): 1235–1241. 44 refs. BE62263.
*advance care planning; advance directives; aged; artificial feeding; *communication; competence; decision making; *family members; institutionalized persons; legislation; medical records; *nursing homes; *patient participation; *patients; *physicians; resuscitation; statistics; survey; *terminal care; third party consent; time factors; ventilators; retrospective studies; Connecticut; Patient Self-Determination Act 1990

Brown, Norman K.; Thompson, Donovan J.; Prentice, Ross L. Nontreatment and aggressive narcotic therapy among hospitalized pancreatic cancer patients. *Journal of the American Geriatrics Society.* 1998 Jul; 46(7): 839–848. 30 refs. BE62259.
active euthanasia; advance directives; *allowing to die; blood transfusions; *cancer; comparative studies; *decision making; drugs; evaluation studies; family members; futility; *intention; knowledge, attitudes, practice; medical records; medical specialties; nurses; *opioid analgesics; physicians; primary health care; prognosis; religious hospitals; resuscitation orders; Roman Catholics; *sedatives; selection for treatment; statistics; surgery; *terminal care; *terminally ill; time factors; *withholding treatment; antibiotics; *coma; fluid therapy; King County (WA); Washington

Bruera, Eduardo; Lawlor, Peter. Defining palliative care interventions. *Journal of Palliative Care.* 1998 Summer; 14(2): 23–24. 9 refs. BE61956.
biomedical technologies; decision making; family members; *palliative care; patient participation; physicians; risks and benefits; selection for treatment; *terminal care; needs

Burgess, Michael; Stephenson, Peter; Ratanakul, Pinit, et al. End-of-life decisions: clinical decisions about dying and perspectives on life and death. *In:* Coward, Harold; Ratanakul, Pinit, eds. A Cross-Cultural Dialogue on Health Care Ethics. Waterloo, ON: Wilfrid Laurier University Press; 1999: 190–206. 23 refs. 2 fn. ISBN 0–88920–325–3. BE62794.
advance directives; allowing to die; assisted suicide; attitudes to death; autonomy; *Buddhist ethics; compassion; *cultural pluralism; decision making; economics; family members;

gatekeeping; justice; minority groups; physicians; prolongation of life; religion; religious ethics; secularism; *terminal care; terminally ill; treatment refusal; *values; Canada; Hutterites; Thailand

Burnside, Gordon. New paths in end-of-life care. *Health Progress.* 1998 May-Jun; 79(3): 18-20. 5 fn. Report on the Innovators in End-of-Life Care National Conference held in Washington, DC, in Mar 1998. BE61614.
  attitudes to death; health insurance; health personnel; hospices; pain; palliative care; pastoral care; quality of health care; religion; *terminal care; Medicare; MediCaring; United States

Buss, Mary K.; Marx, Eric S.; Sulmasy, Daniel P. The preparedness of students to discuss end-of-life issues with patients. *Academic Medicine.* 1998 Apr; 73(4): 418-422. 16 refs. BE59878.
  *advance care planning; *advance directives; age factors; allowing to die; assisted suicide; communication; ethics consultation; *knowledge, attitudes, practice; *medical education; medical schools; physician patient relationship; *students; survey; *terminal care; *Georgetown University School of Medicine; Mayo Medical School

Byrne, Paul A.; Colliton, William F.; Evers, Joseph C., et al. Life, life support, and death principles, guidelines, policies and procedures for making decisions that respect life. [Booklet, third edition; published by the American Life League; 1996]. *Linacre Quarterly.* 1997 Nov; 64(4): 3-31. 11 fn. BE61788.
  allowing to die; artificial feeding; brain death; *Christian ethics; determination of death; euthanasia; extraordinary treatment; *guidelines; health personnel; intention; moral obligations; opioid analgesics; organ donation; pain; persistent vegetative state; quality of life; resuscitation orders; *terminal care; third party consent; *value of life; ventilators; withholding treatment

Califano, Joseph A. Physician-assisted living. *America.* 1998 Nov 14; 179(15): 10-12. BE61207.
  assisted suicide; palliative care; *physician's role; *terminal care; dignity

Campbell, Margaret L. Forgoing Life - Sustaining Therapy: How to Care for the Patient Who Is Near Death. Aliso Viejo, CA: AACN Critical Care; 1998. 140 p. 322 refs. ISBN 0-945812-77-9. BE60066.
  advance care planning; advance directives; *allowing to die; *artificial feeding; attitudes to death; autonomy; case studies; communication; compassion; competence; cultural pluralism; decision making; diagnosis; double effect; *drugs; family members; hospitals; informed consent; intention; legal aspects; minority groups; nurse patient relationship; nurses; *palliative care; persistent vegetative state; *practice guidelines; professional family relationship; prognosis; psychological stress; quality of life; *renal dialysis; resuscitation orders; right to die; sedatives; suffering; *terminal care; terminally ill; third party consent; treatment refusal; truth disclosure; *ventilators; *withholding treatment; analgesia; grief; United States

Carrick, Paul. Environmental ethics and medical ethics: some implications for end-of-life care, Part I. *Cambridge Quarterly of Healthcare Ethics.* 1999 Winter; 8(1): 107-117. 32 fn. BE60532.
  *aged; assisted suicide; case studies; dementia; *ecology; future generations; *moral obligations; moral policy; obligations to society; population control; public policy; quality of life; resource allocation; *speciesism; teleological ethics; *terminal care; *terminally ill; theology; *value of life; voluntary euthanasia; duty to die; nature

Carrick, Paul. Environmental ethics and medical ethics:

some implications for end-of-life care, part II. *Cambridge Quarterly of Healthcare Ethics.* 1999 Spring; 8(2): 250-256. 15 fn. BE61241.
  aged; allowing to die; assisted suicide; autonomy; behavior control; beneficence; biomedical technologies; chronically ill; dementia; developing countries; *ecology; freedom; *future generations; justice; *moral obligations; moral policy; palliative care; *paternalism; population control; public policy; *quality of life; resource allocation; smoking; social worth; *speciesism; *terminal care; terminally ill; *value of life; values; voluntary euthanasia; vulnerable populations; withholding treatment; duty to die; nature

Carron, Annette T.; Lynn, Joanne; Keaney, Patrick. End-of-life care in medical textbooks. *Annals of Internal Medicine.* 1999 Jan 5; 130(1): 82-86. 26 refs. BE59333.
  advance care planning; comparative studies; decision making; diagnosis; epidemiology; evaluation; *literature; medical education; *medicine; palliative care; prognosis; *terminal care
Improvement in end-of-life care has become a demand of the public and a priority for health care professionals. Medical textbooks could support this improvement by functioning as educational resources and as reference material. In this paper, four widely used general medical textbooks are assessed for their coverage of nine content domains for 12 illnesses that often cause death; each domain in each disease and in each text was graded for presence and helpfulness of advice. Helpful information was rare, and only prognostication and medical treatments to alter the course of the disease were usually mentioned. Harrison's Textbook of Medicine, The Merck Manual, and Scientific American Medicine often mentioned at least a few of the domains in each disease, although not often in a way that would guide a clinician. Manual of Medical Therapeutics (The Washington Manual) includes little information about end-of-life care. Improvement seems possible. Short additions of information on end-of-life care would probably be effective. Many chapters discussed at length certain topics that are clearly optional; other textbooks addressed these topics only briefly. When dealing with end-of-life care, physicians should seek guidance from other sources and textbook authors and editors should improve the utility and completeness of their texts.

Cavanaugh, Thomas A. Currently accepted practices that are known to lead to death, and PAS: is there an ethically relevant difference? *Cambridge Quarterly of Healthcare Ethics.* 1998 Fall; 7(4): 375-381. 8 fn. BE59138.
  *allowing to die; *assisted suicide; drugs; *ethical analysis; *intention; killing; *moral policy; pain; *palliative care; physicians; *sedatives; *terminal care; treatment refusal; withholding treatment

Cavanaugh, Thomas A. The ethics of death-hastening or death-causing palliative analgesic administration to the terminally ill. *Journal of Pain and Symptom Management.* 1996 Oct; 12(4): 248-254. 18 refs. BE60192.
  accountability; death; *double effect; *drugs; *ethical analysis; ethical theory; intention; moral obligations; pain; *palliative care; suffering; *terminal care; *terminally ill; *analgesia

Chochinov, Harvey Max; Tataryn, Douglas; Clinch, Jennifer J., et al. Will to live in the terminally ill. *Lancet.* 1999 Sep 4; 354(9181): 816-819. 17 refs. BE62519.
  aged; assisted suicide; *attitudes to death; *cancer; depressive disorder; hospitals; pain; *palliative care; *psychology; survey; terminal care; *terminally ill; *time factors; voluntary euthanasia; Manitoba
BACKGROUND: Complex biomedical and psychosocial considerations figure prominently in the

debate about euthanasia and assisted suicide. No study to date, however, has examined the extent to which a dying patient's will to live fluctuates as death approaches. METHODS: This study examined patients with cancer in palliative care. Will to live was measured twice daily throughout the hospital stay on a self-report 100 mm visual analogue scale. This scale was incorporated into the Edmonton symptom assessment system, a series of visual analogue scales measuring pain, nausea, shortness of breath, appetite, drowsiness, depression, sense of well-being, anxiety, and activity. Maximum and median fluctuations in will-to-live ratings, separated by 12 h, 24 h, 7 days, and 30 days, were calculated for each patient. FINDINGS: Of 585 patients admitted to palliative care during the study period (November, 1993, to May, 1995), 168 (29%; aged 31–89 years) met criteria of cognitive and physical fitness and agreed to take part. The pattern of median changes in will-to-live score suggested that will to live was stable (median changes less than 10 mm on 100 mm scale for all time intervals). By contrast, the average maximum changes in will-to-live score were substantial (12 h 33.1 mm, 24 h 35.8 mm, 7 days 48.8 mm, 30 days 68.0 mm). In a series of stepwise regression models carried out at 12 h, 24 h, and 1–4 weeks after admission, the four main predictor variables of will to live were depression, anxiety, shortness of breath, and sense of well-being, with the prominence of these variables changing over time. INTERPRETATION: Among dying patients, will to live shows substantial fluctuation, with the explanation for these changes shifting as death approaches.

Colebunders, Robert; Schrooten, W.; Singer, Peter A., et al. Euthanasia and end-of-life care. [Letter and response]. *JAMA.* 1999 Apr 28; 281(16): 1488. 2 refs. BE62564.
> *active euthanasia; *attitudes; HIV seropositivity; legal aspects; pain; *patients; quality of life; *terminal care; *terminally ill; *voluntary euthanasia; Belgium; Ontario

Connelly, R.J. Death with dignity: fifty years of soul-searching. *Journal of Religion and Health.* 1998 Fall; 37(3): 195–213. 58 fn. BE61218.
> *active euthanasia; advance directives; aged; *allowing to die; artificial feeding; *assisted suicide; *attitudes; consensus; depressive disorder; dissent; extraordinary treatment; health personnel; hospices; legal aspects; pain; palliative care; physicians; public opinion; public policy; *right to die; Roman Catholic ethics; Supreme Court decisions; *terminal care; *trends; ventilators; voluntary euthanasia; withholding treatment; Compassion in Dying; Cruzan v. Director, Missouri Department of Health; Death with Dignity Act (OR); Hemlock Society; In re Quinlan; *United States; Vacco v. Quill; Washington v. Glucksberg

Cooper-Mahkorn, Déirdre. Guidelines on assisted deaths criticised. [News]. *BMJ (British Medical Journal).* 1998 Oct 3; 317(7163): 904. BE60851.
> active euthanasia; *allowing to die; autonomy; *guidelines; newborns; physicians; politics; prematurity; professional organizations; rights; *terminal care; *terminally ill; third party consent; withholding treatment; coma; *German Medical Council; *Germany

Costantini-Ferrando, Maria F.; Foley, Kathleen M.; Rapkin, Bruce D., et al. Communicating with patients about advanced cancer. [Letters and responses]. *JAMA.* 1998 Oct 28; 280(16): 1403–1404. 5 refs. BE60083.
> advance care planning; advance directives; *cancer; *communication; comparative studies; *comprehension; *decision making; mortality; *palliative care; *patients; *physicians; *prognosis; *prolongation of life; risk; suffering; survey; *terminal care; *terminally ill; *truth disclosure;

Memorial Sloan-Kettering Cancer Center (NYC)

Danis, Marion. Improving end-of-life care in the intensive care unit: what's to be learned from outcomes research? *New Horizons.* 1998 Feb; 6(1): 110–118. 52 refs. BE61814.
> *advance care planning; advance directives; allowing to die; communication; critically ill; death; decision making; *empirical research; health services research; hospitals; *intensive care units; *palliative care; patient satisfaction; prognosis; prolongation of life; *quality of health care; resuscitation orders; *terminal care; terminally ill; treatment outcome; uncertainty; withholding treatment; continuity of patient care; Study to Understand Prognoses and Preferences for Outcomes and Risks of Treatments (SUPPORT); United States

de Bousingen, Denis Durand. Euthanasia and pain relief discussed in Europe. [News]. *Lancet.* 1998 Oct 3; 352(9134): 1129. BE60453.
> assisted suicide; euthanasia; health care delivery; hospices; information dissemination; organizational policies; pain; *palliative care; physicians; professional organizations; *public policy; *terminal care; Austria; Council of Europe; *Europe; France; Germany

Dickinson, George E.; Mermann, Alan C. Death education in U.S. medical schools, 1975–1995. *Academic Medicine.* 1996 Dec; 71(12): 1348–1349. 5 refs. BE61381.
> *curriculum; *death; *medical education; *medical schools; survey; teaching methods; *terminal care; trends; *United States

Dubler, Nancy Neveloff. The collision of confinement and care: end-of-life care in prisons and jails. *Journal of Law, Medicine and Ethics.* 1998 Summer; 26(2): 149–156. 42 fn. BE62677.
> advance directives; aged; AIDS; alternatives; drugs; institutional policies; institutionalized persons; legal rights; palliative care; patient transfer; physical restraint; *prisoners; public policy; *quality of health care; resuscitation orders; socioeconomic factors; *terminal care; *terminally ill; treatment refusal; trust; vulnerable populations; withholding treatment; *United States

Fahnestock, Deborah T. A piece of my mind: partnership for good dying. *JAMA.* 1999 Aug 18; 282(7): 615–616. BE62653.
> *attitudes to death; caring; communication; *physician patient relationship; *terminal care; *terminally ill; continuity of patient care

Farriman, Annabel. Surgeons carry out too many operations on dying patients. [News]. *BMJ (British Medical Journal).* 1998 Nov 7; 317(7168): 1269. BE60854.
> futility; *mortality; prognosis; *surgery; terminal care; *terminally ill; *treatment outcome; *health services misuse; Great Britain

Filene, Peter G. In the Arms of Others: A Cultural History of the Right-to-Die in America. Chicago, IL: Ivan R. Dee; 1998. 282 p. 637 fn. ISBN 1-56663-188-2. BE60014.
> *active euthanasia; *allowing to die; artificial feeding; *assisted suicide; attitudes; attitudes to death; autonomy; competence; congenital disorders; decision making; determination of death; ethicists; extraordinary treatment; government regulation; *historical aspects; judicial action; legal aspects; living wills; mass media; newborns; persistent vegetative state; physicians; political activity; politics; privacy; public opinion; *right to die; state government; suffering; *terminal care; terminally ill; treatment refusal; *trends; withholding treatment; Cruzan v. Director, Missouri Department of Health; Cruzan v. Harmon; In re Conroy; In re Quinlan; Netherlands; Nineteenth Century; Superintendent v. Saikewicz; *Twentieth Century; *United

---

BE = bioethics accession number   fn. = footnotes   refs. = references

States

Fimbrez, Karen Jean. Life-Sustaining Treatment: The Family Decision-Making Process. Ann Arbor, MI: UMI Dissertation Services; 1995. 90 p. Bibliography: p. 87-90. Thesis, Master of Social Work, California State University, Long Beach, Jun 1995. Order No. 1362278. BE60067.

*advance care planning; advance directives; age factors; aged; *allowing to die; artificial feeding; attitudes; communication; costs and benefits; cultural pluralism; *decision making; *emotions; *family members; *family relationship; minority groups; nursing homes; patient care team; patient participation; prognosis; *prolongation of life; quality of life; religion; resuscitation; social workers; survey; *terminal care; third party consent; ventilators; withholding treatment; adult offspring; antibiotics; qualitative research; United States

Fitzgerald, Faith T. Dying in America. *Pharos.* 1997 Spring; 60(2): 29-31. BE60338.

allowing to die; *assisted suicide; *attitudes to death; euthanasia; futility; prolongation of life; quality of life; resuscitation; resuscitation orders; right to die; *terminal care; terminally ill; treatment outcome; withholding treatment; United States

Fletcher, John C. Deciding about death: physician-assisted suicide and the courts -- a panel discussion. *Pharos.* 1998 Winter; 61(1): 2-7. 5 refs. Program participants: Timothy E. Quill, John Arras, Richard J. Bonnie, and John C. Fletcher. BE59986.

allowing to die; *assisted suicide; autonomy; coercion; competence; decision making; depressive disorder; equal protection; hospices; *legal aspects; legal rights; moral policy; pain; *palliative care; *physicians; privacy; public policy; sedatives; suffering; *terminal care; terminally ill; third party consent; vulnerable populations; wedge argument; withholding treatment; *United States

Foley, Kathleen. A 44-year-old woman with severe pain at the end of life. *JAMA.* 1999 May 26; 281(20): 1937-1945. 51 refs. BE62311.

*attitudes; *attitudes to death; *cancer; case studies; communication; compassion; comprehension; diagnosis; drugs; family members; medical education; *opioid analgesics; *pain; *palliative care; patient care team; *patients; physician patient relationship; *physicians; professional competence; prognosis; psychological stress; quality of health care; quality of life; radiology; risks and benefits; *terminal care; *terminally ill; truth disclosure

Frolik, Lawrence A., ed. Health care decision making. *In: his* Aging and the Law: An Interdisciplinary Reader. Philadelphia, PA: Temple University Press; 1999: 295-394. 14 refs. 296 fn. ISBN 1-56639-653-0. BE61059.

advance care planning; advance directives; *aged; *allowing to die; *assisted suicide; attitudes; *autonomy; chronically ill; clinical ethics; coercion; communication; *competence; critically ill; cultural pluralism; *decision making; disclosure; family members; hospitals; *informed consent; judicial action; *legal aspects; mentally disabled; minority groups; nursing homes; patient advocacy; *patient care; patient care team; patients; persistent vegetative state; physicians; prolongation of life; resource allocation; resuscitation; *right to die; standards; suffering; *terminal care; terminally ill; *third party consent; treatment refusal; truth disclosure; voluntary euthanasia; wedge argument; withholding treatment; In re Fiori; In re Milton; Medicaid; Medicare; Pocono Medical Center v. Harley; Study to Understand Prognoses and Preferences for Outcomes and Risks of Treatments (SUPPORT); Uniform Health Care Decisions Act 1993; *United States

Garrison, Jayne. Rushing heaven's door: assisted suicide

-- do we really know what we want? *Health.* 1997 May/Jun; 11(4): 123-124, 126, 128-130. BE60450.

active euthanasia; aged; allowing to die; *assisted suicide; attitudes; coercion; competence; decision making; family members; family relationship; hospices; quality of life; *terminal care; treatment refusal; adult offspring

Gavin, William J. On "tame" and "untamed" death: Jamesian reflections. *In:* McGee, Glenn, ed. Pragmatic Bioethics. Nashville, TN: Vanderbilt University Press; 1999: 97-112, 269-271. 56 fn. ISBN 0-8265-1321-2. BE60666.

*attitudes to death; cultural pluralism; *death; *determination of death; emotions; historical aspects; narrative ethics; philosophy; psychology; public policy; *terminal care; *terminally ill; dignity; pragmatism; James, William

Goetschius, Suzanne K. Families and end-of-life care: how do we meet their needs? *Journal of Gerontological Nursing.* 1997 Mar; 23(3): 43-49. 1 ref. BE60387.

advance directives; allowing to die; communication; emotions; *family members; *nurses; *professional family relationship; *terminal care

Goff, Robert. A matter of life and death. *Medical Law Review.* 1995 Spring; 3(1): 1-21. 19 fn. Text of the Cassel Lecture at the University of Stockholm, 4 June 1993. BE59255.

*active euthanasia; advisory committees; *allowing to die; artificial feeding; assisted suicide; competence; criminal law; decision making; drugs; guidelines; hospices; international aspects; involuntary euthanasia; killing; *legal aspects; *legal liability; pain; palliative care; persistent vegetative state; *physicians; public opinion; public policy; right to die; suffering; *terminal care; treatment refusal; *voluntary euthanasia; wedge argument; withholding treatment; *Airedale NHS Trust v. Bland; *Great Britain; House of Lords Select Committee on Medical Ethics; Netherlands; *R v. Cox; Sweden

Gramelspacher, Gregory P.; Zhou, Xiao-Hua; Hanna, Mark P., et al. Preferences of physicians and their patients for end-of-life care. *Journal of General Internal Medicine.* 1997 Jun; 12(6): 346-351. 33 refs. BE60248.

advance directives; aged; *allowing to die; artificial feeding; *attitudes; chronically ill; communication; comparative studies; intensive care units; internal medicine; *patients; *physicians; primary health care; *prolongation of life; resuscitation; socioeconomic factors; surgery; survey; *terminal care; terminally ill; ventilators; withholding treatment; Indiana

Haisfield-Wolfe, Mary Ellen. End-of-life care: evolution of the nurse's role. *Oncology Nursing Forum.* 1996 Jul; 23(6): 931-935. 28 refs. BE60197.

advance directives; attitudes to death; biomedical technologies; cancer; communication; *decision making; nurse patient relationship; *nurse's role; pain; palliative care; patient advocacy; patient care team; resuscitation orders; *terminal care; terminally ill; empowerment

Hanson, Laura C.; Earp, Jo Anne; Garrett, Joanne, et al. Community physicians who provide terminal care. *Archives of Internal Medicine.* 1999 May 24; 159(10): 1133-1138. 25 refs. BE61392.

advance care planning; *aged; *allowing to die; blacks; cancer; chronically ill; communication; death; *decision making; diagnosis; family members; family relationship; home care; hospices; hospitals; living wills; morbidity; palliative care; physician patient relationship; *physicians; *primary health care; professional family relationship; *prolongation of life; resuscitation; selection for treatment; survey; *terminal care; terminally ill; ventilators; whites; withholding treatment; community hospitals; *physician's

practice patterns; retrospective studies; North Carolina
BACKGROUND: Most dying patients are treated by physicians in community practice, yet studies of terminal care rarely include these physicians. OBJECTIVE: To examine the frequency of life–sustaining treatment use and describe what factors influence physicians' treatment decisions in community–based practices. METHODS: Family members and treating physicians for decedents 65 years and older who died of cancer, congestive heart failure, chronic lung disease, cirrhosis, or stroke completed interviews about end–of–life care in community settings. RESULTS: Eighty percent of eligible family and 68.8% of eligible physicians participated (N = 165). Most physicians were trained in primary care and 85.4% were primary care physicians for the decedents. Physicians typically knew the decedent a year or more (68.9%), and 93.3% treated them for at least 1 month before death. In their last month of life, 2.4% of decedents received cardiopulmonary resuscitation, 5.5% received ventilatory support, and 34.1% received hospice care. Family recalled a discussion of treatment options in 78.2% of deaths. Most discussions (72.1%) took place a month or more before death. Place of death, cancer, and having a living will were independent predictors of less aggressive treatment before death. Physicians believed that advanced planning and good relationships were the major determinants of good decision making. CONCLUSIONS: Community physicians use few life–sustaining treatments for dying patients. Treatment decisions are made in the context of long–term primary care relationships, and living wills influence treatment decisions. The choice to remain in community settings with a familiar physician may influence the dying experience.

Harrold, Joan K.; Lynn, Joanne, eds. A Good Dying: Shaping Health Care for the Last Months of Life. New York, NY: Haworth Press; 1998. 188 p. Includes references. Co–published simultaneously as *The Hospice Journal*, 1998; 13(1/2). ISBN 0–7890–0502–6. BE60653.
aged; cancer; chronically ill; evaluation; family members; government financing; health care delivery; health insurance reimbursement; health personnel; home care; *hospices; humanities; managed care programs; mortality; pain; *palliative care; professional organizations; prognosis; quality of health care; referral and consultation; standards; suffering; *terminal care; terminally ill; Medicare; National Hospice Organization; United States

Haverkate, Ilinka; van der Wal, Gerrit; van der Maas, Paul J., et al. Guidelines on euthanasia and pain alleviation: compliance and opinions of physicians. *Health Policy.* 1998 Apr; 44(1): 45–55. 13 refs. BE59927.
*active euthanasia; administrators; *assisted suicide; double effect; family practice; *guideline adherence; *guidelines; hospitals; *institutional policies; *knowledge, attitudes, practice; medical specialties; nursing homes; *palliative care; *physicians; referral and consultation; suffering; survey; *Netherlands

Hendlin, Herbert. Physician–assisted suicide: what next? *Responsive Community.* 1997 Fall; 7(4): 21–34. BE59718.
*active euthanasia; *assisted suicide; autonomy; coercion; competence; depressive disorder; drugs; government regulation; guideline adherence; guidelines; involuntary euthanasia; motivation; pain; palliative care; physicians; public policy; quality of health care; right to die; suffering; suicide; *terminal care; terminally ill; treatment refusal; *voluntary euthanasia; vulnerable populations; wedge argument; Netherlands; United States

Hines, Stephen C.; Glover, Jacqueline J.; Holley, Jean

L., et al. Dialysis patients' preferences for family–based advance care planning. *Annals of Internal Medicine.* 1999 May 18; 130(10): 825–828. 20 refs. BE61609.
*advance care planning; *advance directives; *attitudes; *chronically ill; communication; decision making; *family members; family relationship; legal aspects; *patients; physician patient relationship; *physician's role; renal dialysis; state government; survey; *terminal care; third party consent; trust; New York; Pennsylvania; Rochester (NY); West Virginia
BACKGROUND: Most patients do not participate in advance care planning with physicians. OBJECTIVE: To examine patients' preferences for involving their physicians and families in advance care planning. DESIGN: Face–to–face interviews with randomly selected patients. SETTING: Community–based dialysis units in one rural and one urban region. PARTICIPANTS: 400 hemodialysis patients. MEASUREMENTS: Questions about whom patients involve in advance care planning, whom patients would like to include in this planning, and patients' reactions to state legislation on surrogate decision makers in end–of–life care. RESULTS: Patients more frequently discussed preferences for end–of–life care with family members than with physicians (50% compared with 6%; P less than 0.001). More patients wanted to include family members in future discussions of advance care planning than wanted to include physicians (91% compared with 36%; P less than 0.001). Patients were most comfortable with legislation that granted their family end–of–life decision–making authority in the event of their own incapacity (P less than 0.001). CONCLUSION: Most patients want to include their families more than their physicians in advance care planning.

Hoffmann, Diane E. Pain management and palliative care in the era of managed care: issues for health insurers. *Journal of Law, Medicine and Ethics.* 1998 Winter; 26(4): 267–289. 126 fn. BE61163.
*administrators; aged; alternatives; anesthesia; attitudes; biomedical technologies; *chronically ill; *costs and benefits; diagnosis; drug abuse; *drugs; *economics; fraud; health facilities; *health insurance; *health insurance reimbursement; hospices; *managed care programs; medical devices; medical specialties; mental health; opioid analgesics; *organizational policies; *pain; *palliative care; *patient care; physicians; practice guidelines; public policy; *quality of health care; referral and consultation; resource allocation; surgery; survey; *terminal care; *terminally ill; therapeutic research; treatment outcome; acupuncture; biofeedback (psychology); *undertreatment; American Association of Health Plans; *Blue Cross–Blue Shield; Medicare; *United States

Huser, Frank A. Palliative Care and Euthanasia. Edinburgh: Campion Press; 1995. 69 p. 61 refs. Papers presented at a symposium entitled, "Palliative Care and Euthanasia," held in London, Fall 1993. ISBN 1–873732–16–3. BE60506.
allowing to die; artificial feeding; cancer; caring; competence; criminal law; ethics; guidelines; hospices; informed consent; killing; legal aspects; nurses; *palliative care; persistent vegetative state; philosophy; politics; principle–based ethics; *public policy; quality of life; resource allocation; suffering; *terminal care; terminally ill; treatment refusal; *voluntary euthanasia; withholding treatment; *Great Britain; *Netherlands

Jamison, Stephen. Assisted Suicide: A Decision–Making Guide for Health Professionals. San Francisco, CA: Jossey–Bass; 1997. 248 p. Bibliography: p. 223–242 ISBN 0–7879–0873–8. BE62139.

BE = bioethics accession number   fn. = footnotes   refs. = references

active euthanasia; allowing to die; *alternatives; *assisted suicide; autonomy; chronically ill; coercion; *communication; compassion; competence; confidentiality; *decision making; depressive disorder; dissent; double effect; drugs; economics; family members; hospices; killing; legal aspects; motivation; opioid analgesics; pain; palliative care; patients; physician patient relationship; *physician's role; physicians; professional family relationship; *professional role; psychotherapy; quality of life; right to die; sedatives; suffering; Supreme Court decisions; *terminal care; terminally ill; trust; vulnerable populations; wedge argument; withholding treatment; rationality; United States; Vacco v. Quill; Washington v. Glucksberg

Johnson, Philip R.S. An analysis of "dignity". *Theoretical Medicine and Bioethics.* 1998 Aug; 19(4): 337–352. 35 refs. BE60157.
    allowing to die; *attitudes to death; autonomy; *communication; family members; hospices; hospitals; humanism; palliative care; patient care team; persistent vegetative state; professional patient relationship; quality of life; *terminal care; *terminally ill; terminology; value of life; *dignity

Jost, Timothy S. Public financing of pain management: leaky umbrellas and ragged safety nets. *Journal of Law, Medicine and Ethics.* 1998 Winter; 26(4): 290–307. 194 fn. BE61164.
    aged; alternatives; biomedical technologies; *chronically ill; costs and benefits; *drugs; economics; federal government; fraud; *government financing; hospices; hospitals; indigents; managed care programs; medical devices; nursing homes; opioid analgesics; *pain; *palliative care; *patient care; patients; quality of health care; state government; suffering; *terminal care; *terminally ill; time factors; utilization review; *Medicaid; *Medicare; *United States

Kaldjian, Lauris C.; Jekel, James F.; Friedland, Gerald. End-of-life decisions in HIV-positive patients: the role of spiritual beliefs. *AIDS.* 1998 Jan 1; 12(1): 103–107. 13 refs. BE60526.
    *advance care planning; advance directives; assisted suicide; *attitudes to death; *decision making; disadvantaged; emotions; *HIV seropositivity; living wills; pastoral care; *patients; physician patient relationship; *religion; resuscitation; suicide; survey; *terminal care; urban population; Yale-New Haven Hospital

Karlawish, Jason H.T.; Quill, Timothy; Meier, Diane E.; American College of Physicians–American Society of Internal Medicine End-of-Life Care Consensus Panel. A consensus-based approach to providing palliative care to patients who lack decision-making capacity. *Annals of Internal Medicine.* 1999 May 18; 130(10): 835–840. 26 refs. BE61611.
    advance care planning; aged; allowing to die; artificial feeding; case studies; *communication; consensus; counseling; *decision making; *dementia; drugs; *family members; food; goals; institutionalized persons; nursing homes; *palliative care; patient care; patient care team; *physician nurse relationship; *physician's role; *physicians; quality of life; terminal care; terminally ill; third party consent; values; withholding treatment; antibiotics
Making palliative care decisions for a patient who lacks decision-making capacity presents several challenges. Other people, such as family and caregivers, must choose for the patient. The goals and values of these decision makers may conflict with those of each other and with those of the patient, who now lacks the capacity to participate in the decision. This paper presents a case study of a patient with severe Alzheimer disease who has two common clinical problems: neurogenic dysphagia and aspiration pneumonia. The case study describes a consensus-based decision-making strategy

that keeps what is known about the patient's wishes and values in the foreground but also expects guidance from the physician and elicits input from family members and other people who care for and have knowledge about the patient. The steps of this process, including key clinical prompts and potential transition statements, are outlined and described. The overall goal of the case commentary is to demonstrate that physicians can guide a highly emotional and personal process in a structured manner that has meaning for the patient, family, physician, and other caregivers.

Kazanowski, Mary. A commitment to palliative care: could it impact assisted suicide? *Journal of Gerontological Nursing.* 1997 Mar; 23(3): 36–42. 29 refs. BE60386.
    aged; assisted suicide; cancer; health insurance reimbursement; hospices; nurses; *pain; *palliative care; prognosis; quality of health care; referral and consultation; suffering; *terminal care; United States

Knudsen, Nancy S.; Pisetsky, David S. Doing everything. [Letter and response]. *Annals of Internal Medicine.* 1999 Jan 19; 130(2): 165–166. 5 refs. BE62558.
    palliative care; *physician's role; *terminal care

Koch, Kathryn A. The language of death: euthanatos et mors -- the science of uncertainty. *Critical Care Clinics.* 1996 Jan; 12(1): 1–14. 35 refs. BE59274.
    *allowing to die; assisted suicide; attitudes to death; competence; *decision making; determination of death; double effect; drugs; emotions; euthanasia; family members; futility; legal aspects; pain; palliative care; patient participation; *physicians; prognosis; *terminal care; terminally ill; third party consent; *uncertainty; withholding treatment; United States

Kopfensteiner, Thomas R. Death with dignity: a Roman Catholic perspective. *Linacre Quarterly.* 1996 Nov; 63(4): 64–75. 23 fn. BE59306.
    *allowing to die; artificial feeding; *attitudes to death; biomedical technologies; caring; compassion; double effect; drugs; extraordinary treatment; metaphor; pain; palliative care; persistent vegetative state; physician patient relationship; *Roman Catholic ethics; suffering; *terminal care; terminally ill; theology; treatment refusal; truth disclosure; value of life; withholding treatment; analgesia; dignity; patient abandonment

Kow, Jim. Autonomy and the person in the dying patient. *In:* Morgan, John D., ed. Readings in Thanatology. Amityville, NY: Baywood Publishing; 1997: 423–438. 57 refs. ISBN 0-89503-149-3. BE62333.
    advance directives; allowing to die; assisted suicide; *autonomy; caring; common good; compassion; competence; comprehension; death; decision making; dementia; determination of death; disclosure; empathy; family relationship; freedom; informed consent; moral obligations; pain; palliative care; paternalism; persistent vegetative state; personhood; physician patient relationship; physicians; privacy; quality of life; right to die; rights; social interaction; standards; suffering; *terminal care; *terminally ill; third party consent; treatment refusal; value of life; voluntary euthanasia; dependency

Kuczewski, Mark G.; DeVita, Michael. Managed care and end-of-life decisions: learning to live ungagged. *Archives of Internal Medicine.* 1998 Dec 7–21; 158(22): 2424–2428. 13 refs. BE61277.
    allowing to die; case studies; *communication; decision making; *disclosure; economics; ethicists; *family members; *health insurance reimbursement; hospices; informed consent; *managed care programs; medical records; *patient care team; patient transfer; *physician's role; professional family relationship; *professional role; social workers;

technical expertise; *terminal care; time factors; *case managers

Lachs, John. Dying old as a social problem. *In:* McGee, Glenn, ed. Pragmatic Bioethics. Nashville, TN: Vanderbilt University Press; 1999: 194–203, 281. 5 fn. ISBN 0-8265-1321-2. BE60672.
    *aged; assisted suicide; *autonomy; caring; depressive disorder; quality of life; *right to die; suffering; *suicide; *terminal care; terminally ill; value of life; voluntary euthanasia; rationality

Lascaratos, John; Poulakou–Rebelakou, Effie; Marketos, Spyros. Abandonment of terminally ill patients in the Byzantine era: an ancient tradition? *Journal of Medical Ethics.* 1999 Jun; 25(3): 254–258. 36 fn. BE61860.
    *ancient history; *attitudes to death; Christian ethics; famous persons; futility; goals; *historical aspects; *medical ethics; medicine; physician patient relationship; physician's role; *physicians; *refusal to treat; *terminal care; *terminally ill; *patient abandonment; *rituals; *Byzantium; *Middle Ages
Our research on the texts of the Byzantine historians and chroniclers revealed an apparently curious phenomenon, namely, the abandonment of terminally ill emperors by their physicians when the latter realised that they could not offer any further treatment. This attitude tallies with the mentality of the ancient Greek physicians, who even in Hippocratic times thought the treatment and care of the terminally ill to be a challenge to nature and hubris to the gods. Nevertheless, it is a very curious attitude in the light of the concepts of the Christian Byzantine physicians who, according to the doctrines of the Christian religion, should have been imbued with the spirit of philanthropy and love for their fellowmen. The meticulous analysis of three examples of abandonment of Byzantine emperors, and especially that of Alexius I Comnenus, by their physicians reveals that this custom, following ancient pagan ethics, in those times took on a ritualised form without any significant or real content.

Latimer, Elizabeth J. Ethical care at the end of life. *Canadian Medical Association Journal.* 1998 Jun 30; 158(13): 1741–1747. 30 refs. BE62203.
    allowing to die; autonomy; beneficence; case studies; communication; compassion; cultural pluralism; decision making; double effect; drugs; family members; *goals; informed consent; intention; interprofessional relations; medical records; pain; palliative care; patient care team; *physician's role; professional family relationship; professional patient relationship; prognosis; prolongation of life; psychological stress; quality of life; resuscitation orders; suffering; *terminal care; terminally ill; treatment refusal; trust; truth disclosure; values

Lesage, Pauline; Latimer, Elizabeth. An approach to ethical issues. *In:* MacDonald, Neil, ed. Palliative Medicine: A Case–Based Manual. New York, NY: Oxford University Press; 1998: 253–277. 25 fn. ISBN 0-19-262657-4. BE59171.
    active euthanasia; alternatives; assisted suicide; autonomy; beneficence; case studies; communication; competence; confidentiality; decision making; diagnosis; disclosure; double effect; drugs; emotions; family members; futility; goals; informed consent; intention; pain; *palliative care; patient care team; patient participation; physicians; prognosis; quality of life; resource allocation; right to die; risks and benefits; sedatives; suffering; *terminal care; terminally ill; treatment refusal; truth disclosure; uncertainty; values; wedge argument; withholding treatment; analgesia

Letvak, Richard; Pochard, Frédéric; Grassin, Marc,

et al. Palliative options at the end of life. [Letters and response]. *JAMA.* 1998 Apr 8; 279(14): 1065–1067. 9 refs. BE59234.
    *allowing to die; artificial feeding; *assisted suicide; autonomy; beneficence; competence; conscience; cultural pluralism; double effect; *drugs; family members; food; informed consent; intention; pain; *palliative care; physicians; public policy; *sedatives; suffering; *terminal care; terminally ill; treatment refusal; *voluntary euthanasia; withholding treatment; coma; United States

Lo, Bernard; Snyder, Lois. Care at the end of life: guiding practice where there are no easy answers. [Editorial]. *Annals of Internal Medicine.* 1999 May 4; 130(9): 772–774. 16 refs. BE61606.
    *communication; decision making; pain; *palliative care; patient care; patient participation; *physicians; professional competence; professional organizations; psychological stress; quality of life; suffering; *terminal care; terminally ill; time factors; American College of Physicians; American Society of Internal Medicine

Lo, Bernard; Quill, Timothy; Tulsky, James; American College of Physicians–American Society of Internal Medicine End–of–Life Care Consensus Panel. Discussing palliative care with patients. *Annals of Internal Medicine.* 1999 May 4; 130(9): 744–749. 27 refs. BE61607.
    advance care planning; aged; cancer; case studies; *communication; empathy; family members; heart diseases; home care; hospices; *palliative care; patient care; patient participation; *physician patient relationship; *physicians; religion; *terminal care; values

MacDonald, Neil. A march of folly. [Editorial]. *Canadian Medical Association Journal.* 1998 Jun 30; 158(13): 1699–1701. 20 refs. BE62202.
    active euthanasia; attitudes; biomedical research; *cancer; communication; economics; family members; *home care; medical education; *palliative care; physician patient relationship; physicians; professional family relationship; *terminal care; terminally ill; Canada

Maltsberger, John T.; American Association of Suicidology. Committee on Physician–Assisted Death. Report of the Committee on Physician–Assisted Suicide and Euthanasia. *Suicide and Life–Threatening Behavior.* 1996; 26(Suppl.): 1–19. 36 fn. BE61572.
    *active euthanasia; aged; allowing to die; *assisted suicide; attitudes; autonomy; chronically ill; depressive disorder; disadvantaged; double effect; drugs; economics; females; intention; involuntary euthanasia; managed care programs; nurses; *organizational policies; pain; *palliative care; physician patient relationship; *physicians; public policy; right to die; suffering; *suicide; terminal care; terminally ill; voluntary euthanasia; withholding treatment; duty to die; *American Association of Suicidology; Netherlands; United States

Matthews, Hugh. Better palliative care could cut euthanasia. [News]. *BMJ (British Medical Journal).* 1998 Dec 12; 317(7173): 1613. BE60733.
    *active euthanasia; attitudes; guidelines; involuntary euthanasia; killing; *palliative care; physicians; quality of health care; suffering; *terminal care; *Netherlands

Meisel, Alan; Jernigan, Jan C.; Youngner, Stuart J. Prosecutors and end–of–life decision making. *Archives of Internal Medicine.* 1999 May 24; 159(10): 1089–1095. 22 refs. BE61391.
    active euthanasia; *allowing to die; artificial feeding; *assisted suicide; *attitudes; *criminal law; decision making; drugs; hospitals; killing; *knowledge, attitudes, practice; law enforcement; *lawyers; *legal liability; morality; *opioid

analgesics; *palliative care; persistent vegetative state; *physicians; prolongation of life; right to die; survey; *terminal care; terminally ill; third party consent; ventilators; withholding treatment; *prosecutors; *United States

OBJECTIVE: To examine personal beliefs and professional behavior of state criminal prosecutors toward end-of-life decisions. DESIGN: Mail survey. SETTING: District attorney offices nationwide. PARTICIPANTS: All prosecuting attorneys who are members of the National District Attorneys Association. A total of 2844 surveys were mailed with 2 follow-up mailings at 6-week intervals; 761 surveys were returned for a response rate of 26.8%. The majority of respondents were white men, Protestant, and served in rural areas. INTERVENTIONS: None. MAIN OUTCOME MEASURES: On the basis of 4 case scenarios, (1) professional behavior as determined by respondents' willingness to prosecute and what criminal charges they would seek; and (2) personal beliefs as determined by whether prosecutors believed the physicians' actions were morally wrong and whether they would want the same action taken if they were in the patient's condition. RESULTS: Most respondents would not seek prosecution in 3 of the 4 cases. In the fourth case, involving physician-assisted suicide, only about one third of the respondents said that they definitely would prosecute. Those who would prosecute would most often seek a charge of criminal homicide. A majority of respondents believed that the physicians' actions were morally correct in each of the 4 cases and would want the same action taken if they were in the patient's position. There was a strong correlation between personal beliefs and professional behaviors. CONCLUSIONS: A large majority of responding prosecutors were unwilling to prosecute physicians in cases that clearly fall within currently accepted legal and professional boundaries. In the case of physician-assisted suicide, results reflected a surprisingly large professional unwillingness to prosecute and an even greater personal acceptance of physician-assisted suicide.

Meyer, Charles. A Good Death: Challenges, Choices, and Care Options. Mystic, CT: Twenty-Third Publications; 1998. 57 p. ISBN 0-89622-923-8. BE59474.
advance care planning; allowing to die; alternative therapies; artificial feeding; assisted suicide; biomedical technologies; clinical ethics committees; economics; euthanasia; health care delivery; home care; hospitals; pain; palliative care; pastoral care; paternalism; physicians; prolongation of life; quality of life; resuscitation orders; *terminal care

Michigan Catholic Conference. Living and dying according to the voice of faith. *Origins.* 1997 Oct 23; 27(19): 317, 319-322. BE60461.
allowing to die; *assisted suicide; *attitudes to death; compassion; economics; pain; palliative care; *Roman Catholic ethics; suffering; suicide; *terminal care; terminally ill; treatment refusal; value of life; voluntary euthanasia

Mitchell, John J. Administering mercy: the ethics of pain management. *Cancer Investigation.* 1994; 12(3): 343-349. 33 refs. Commented on by J. David Bleich, p. 362-363. BE60099.
double effect; drugs; hospitals; institutional policies; legal liability; *pain; *palliative care; patient participation; patients; physician patient relationship; physicians; professional competence; religion; rights; risks and benefits; Roman Catholic ethics; suffering; teleological ethics; *terminal care

Morgan, John, ed. An Easeful Death? Perspectives on Death, Dying and Euthanasia. Sydney, NSW, Australia:

Federation Press; 1996. 218 p. 276 fn. ISBN 1-86287-222-8. BE62733.
*active euthanasia; allowing to die; assisted suicide; *attitudes to death; autonomy; biomedical technologies; caring; determination of death; emotions; historical aspects; hospices; involuntary euthanasia; killing; legal aspects; legislation; nurses; palliative care; physicians; prolongation of life; quality of life; resource allocation; right to die; suffering; suicide; *terminal care; terminally ill; value of life; *values; voluntary euthanasia; withholding treatment; *Australia; Netherlands; Northern Territory; South Australia; Victoria

Morrison, Mary F. Obstacles to doctor-patient communication at the end of life. *In:* Steinberg, Maurice D.; Youngner, Stuart J., eds. End-of-Life Decisions: A Psychosocial Perspective. Washington, DC: American Psychiatric Press; 1998: 109-136. 63 fn. ISBN 0-88048-756-9. BE60121.
advance directives; age factors; aged; *allowing to die; attitudes; attitudes to death; chronically ill; *communication; cultural pluralism; *decision making; diagnosis; mentally ill; minority groups; patient participation; *patients; *physician patient relationship; *physicians; primary health care; professional family relationship; prognosis; prolongation of life; *psychiatry; referral and consultation; religion; resuscitation orders; socioeconomic factors; *terminal care; *terminally ill; time factors; truth disclosure; values; withholding treatment; United States

Murphy, Donald; Buchanan, Susan Fox. Community guidelines for end-of-life care: incremental change or significant reform? *Bioethics Forum.* 1998 Summer; 14(2): 19-24. 4 refs. BE61581.
advance directives; *allowing to die; artificial feeding; congenital disorders; *decision making; dementia; dissent; ethics consultation; futility; *guidelines; *hospitals; *institutional policies; long-term care; newborns; nursing homes; palliative care; persistent vegetative state; prognosis; *public participation; *public policy; renal dialysis; resource allocation; resuscitation; *terminal care; treatment outcome; withholding treatment; *community policies; *Colorado; *Colorado Collective for Medical Decisions

Nelson, Judith E. Saving lives and saving deaths. *Annals of Internal Medicine.* 1999 May 4; 130(9): 776-777. BE61608.
attitudes to death; communication; *critically ill; *death; emotions; family members; *intensive care units; mortality; *palliative care; patient care; physician patient relationship; *physicians; professional family relationship; terminally ill

O'Neill, J. A peaceful death. [Personal view]. *BMJ (British Medical Journal).* 1999 Jul 31; 319(7205): 327. BE62469.
communication; drugs; family members; hospitals; institutional policies; medical education; pain; *palliative care; *physicians; *terminal care; terminally ill; Great Britain

Parry, Richard D. Death, dignity and morality. *America.* 1998 Nov 14; 179(15): 20-21. BE61209.
aged; assisted suicide; dementia; motivation; parent child relationship; physicians; *terminal care; adult offspring; dependency; dignity

Payne, S. A.; Langley-Evans, A.; Hillier, R. Perceptions of a "good" death: a comparative study of the views of hospice staff and patients. *Palliative Medicine.* 1996 Oct; 10(4): 307-312. 14 refs. BE60042.
*attitudes to death; comparative studies; *health personnel; *hospices; pain; *palliative care; *patients; psychological stress; suffering; survey; *terminal care; *terminally ill; dignity; qualitative research; Great Britain

Perrin, Kathleen Ouimet. Giving voice to the wishes of elders for end-of-life care. *Journal of Gerontological*

Nursing. 1997 Mar; 23(3): 18–27. 25 refs. BE60384.
　　*advance care planning; *advance directives; *aged; allowing to die; communication; competence; *decision making; directive adherence; family members; informed consent; living wills; *nurse's role; patient advocacy; patient education; physician patient relationship; standards; *terminal care; third party consent; treatment refusal

Porta, Miguel; Busquet, Xavier; Jariod, Manuel. Attitudes and views of physicians and nurses towards cancer patients dying at home. *Palliative Medicine.* 1997 Mar; 11(2): 116–126. 37 refs. BE60043.
　　age factors; *attitudes; *cancer; diagnosis; drugs; evaluation studies; females; *home care; males; *nurses; pain; palliative care; *physicians; primary health care; professional family relationship; professional patient relationship; psychological stress; quality of health care; survey; *terminal care; *terminally ill; truth disclosure; Spain

Potter, Robert Lyman. Treatment redirection: moving from curative to palliative care. *Bioethics Forum.* 1998 Summer; 14(2): 3–9. 18 refs. BE61579.
　　attitudes; *communication; *decision making; family members; goals; informed consent; *palliative care; patient care; *patient care team; patients; physicians; prognosis; terminal care; time factors; withholding treatment

Prado, C.G.; Taylor, S.J. Assisted Suicide: Theory and Practice in Elective Death. Amherst, NY: Humanity Books; 1999. 223 p. Bibliography: p. 185–217. ISBN 1-57392-633-7. BE62736.
　　active euthanasia; *assisted suicide; autonomy; competence; *decision making; economics; ethical theory; *evaluation; informed consent; legal aspects; managed care programs; *moral policy; motivation; physician's role; prolongation of life; public policy; social impact; standards; suffering; suicide; *terminal care; third party consent; values; voluntary euthanasia; wedge argument; rationality; United States

Preston, Thomas A. Physician involvement in life-ending practices. *Seattle University Law Review.* 1995 Spring; 18(3): 531–544. 28 fn. BE59822.
　　active euthanasia; *allowing to die; *assisted suicide; attitudes to death; double effect; drugs; iatrogenic disease; intention; *killing; *knowledge, attitudes, practice; palliative care; persistent vegetative state; *physician's role; *physicians; prolongation of life; resuscitation orders; suffering; *terminal care; terminally ill; withholding treatment

Preston, Thomas A.; Patterson, James R.; Hodges, Marian O., et al. The rule of double effect. [Letters and response]. *New England Journal of Medicine.* 1998 May 7; 338(19): 1389–1390. 6 refs. BE59240.
　　assisted suicide; autonomy; decision making; *double effect; drugs; informed consent; *intention; opioid analgesics; *palliative care; physicians; sedatives; suffering; *terminal care; terminally ill

Pritchard, Robert S.; Fisher, Elliott S.; Teno, Joan M., et al. Influence of patient preferences and local health system characteristics on the place of death. [For the SUPPORT Investigators]. *Journal of the American Geriatrics Society.* 1998 Oct; 46(10): 1242–1250. 40 refs. BE62264.
　　aged; death; decision making; economics; evaluation studies; geographic factors; health care delivery; home care; hospices; *hospitals; *mortality; nursing homes; patient participation; prognosis; socioeconomic factors; statistics; *terminal care; terminally ill; physician's practice patterns; Medicare; Study to Understand Prognoses and Preferences for Outcomes and Risks of Treatments (SUPPORT); *United States

Renal Physicians Association; American Society of Nephrology. RPA/ASN position on quality of care at the end of life. [Position paper]. *Dialysis and Transplantation.* 1997 Nov; 26(11): 776, 778–780, 782–783. 16 refs. BE60956.
　　*advance care planning; advance directives; *allowing to die; assisted suicide; competence; family members; guidelines; hospices; informed consent; *kidney diseases; *organizational policies; palliative care; patient care team; *physicians; professional organizations; quality of health care; *renal dialysis; resuscitation orders; *terminal care; third party consent; treatment refusal; withholding treatment; *nephrology; *American Society of Nephrology; *Renal Physicians Association

Robb, Yvonne A. Ethical considerations relating to terminal weaning in intensive care. *Intensive and Critical Care Nursing.* 1997 Jun; 13(3): 156–162. 26 refs. BE60480.
　　*allowing to die; autonomy; beneficence; case studies; decision making; disclosure; dissent; family members; futility; informed consent; intensive care units; nurses; pain; patient advocacy; persistent vegetative state; physicians; prolongation of life; quality of life; suffering; *terminal care; terminally ill; third party consent; treatment refusal; *ventilators; *withholding treatment

Robinson, Walter M.; Ravilly, Sophie; Berde, Charles, et al. End-of-life care in cystic fibrosis. *Pediatrics.* 1997 Aug; 100(2, Pt. 1): 205–209. 29 refs. BE61296.
　　adolescents; adults; cancer; *children; comparative studies; *cystic fibrosis; drugs; hospitals; opioid analgesics; pain; *palliative care; prognosis; prolongation of life; resuscitation orders; *terminal care; terminally ill; uncertainty; antibiotics; retrospective studies; Children's Hospital (Boston)

Rowland, Lewis P. Assisted suicide and alternatives in amyotrophic lateral sclerosis. [Editorial]. *New England Journal of Medicine.* 1998 Oct 1; 339(14): 987–989. 20 refs. BE60037.
　　advance care planning; *alternatives; *amyotrophic lateral sclerosis; artificial feeding; *assisted suicide; attitudes; double effect; drugs; hospices; legal aspects; *palliative care; patients; physically disabled; physicians; prognosis; prolongation of life; psychological stress; sedatives; *terminal care; time factors; truth disclosure; voluntary euthanasia; Death with Dignity Act (OR); Oregon

Roy, David J. The relief of pain and suffering: ethical principles and imperatives. [Editorial]. *Journal of Palliative Care.* 1998 Summer; 14(2): 3–5. 8 refs. BE61955.
　　chronically ill; common good; communication; compassion; critically ill; *drugs; education; health care delivery; justice; *moral obligations; *moral policy; nurses; opioid analgesics; *pain; *palliative care; patient care; physicians; professional competence; professional patient relationship; psychological stress; sedatives; *suffering; terminal care; terminally ill; dignity

Sachs, Greg A. Improving care of the the dying. *Generations (American Society on Aging).* 1994 Winter; 18(4): 19–22. 6 refs. BE60546.
　　aged; allowing to die; attitudes to death; autonomy; education; government financing; guidelines; health insurance reimbursement; hospices; organizational policies; pain; *palliative care; patient care team; professional organizations; *terminal care; terminally ill; truth disclosure; American Geriatrics Society; Medicare; The Troubled Dream of Life (Callahan, D.); United States

Sage, William M.; Jōe, Linda; Emanuel, Ezekiel J., et al. Potential cost savings from legalizing physician-assisted suicide. [Letters and response]. *New England Journal of Medicine.* 1998 Dec 10; 339(24): 1789–1790. 5 refs. BE60984.

BE = bioethics accession number　　　fn. = footnotes　　　refs. = references

*assisted suicide; costs and benefits; decision making; *economics; government financing; health care; long–term care; physicians; public policy; resource allocation; *terminal care; value of life; personal financing

Schneiderman, Lawrence J. The family physician and end–of–life care. *Journal of Family Practice.* 1997 Sep; 45(3): 259–262. 38 refs. BE59341.
advance care planning; *advance directives; *allowing to die; competence; economics; family practice; hospices; palliative care; physicians; resource allocation; resuscitation orders; *terminal care; withholding treatment; United States

Selwyn, Peter A.; Arnold, Robert. From fate to tragedy: the changing meanings of life, death, and AIDS. *Annals of Internal Medicine.* 1998 Dec 1; 129(11): 899–902. 29 refs. BE59327.
*AIDS; chronically ill; drugs; *HIV seropositivity; *palliative care; *patient care; physician patient relationship; *physician's role; psychological stress; *terminal care; terminally ill
The advent of highly active antiretroviral therapy (HAART) and quantitative viral load assays has revolutionized the care of HIV–infected patients. However, this paradigm shift has also had unexpected, sometimes adverse consequences that are not always obvious. Before antiretroviral therapy, physicians learned how to accompany patients through their illness; to bear witness to sickness and dying; and to help patients and their families with suffering, closure, and legacy. Since we have become better at treating the virus, a new temptation has emerged to dwell on quantitative aspects of HIV management and monitoring, although the skills that we learned earlier in the epidemic are no less necessary for providing good care. Our new–found therapeutic capabilities should not distract us from the sometimes more difficult and necessary task of simply "being there" for patients for whom HAART is no longer effective. The definition and practice of end–of–life care for patients with AIDS will continue to evolve as AIDS comes to resemble other chronic, treatable, but ultimately fatal illnesses, such as end–stage pulmonary disease and metastatic cancer, in which clinicians must continually readdress with their patients the balance of curative and palliative interventions as the disease process unfolds over time. The coming challenge in HIV care will be to encourage the maintenance of a "primary care" mentality–with attention to the larger psychosocial issues, end–of–life care, bereavement, and a focus on the patient as opposed to the illness–alongside our new antiretroviral paradigm. Otherwise, we run the risk of forgetting what we learned about healing, from a disease that we could not cure.

Singer, Peter A.; MacDonald, Neil. Bioethics for clinicians: 15. Quality end–of–life care. *Canadian Medical Association Journal.* 1998 Jul 28; 159(2): 159–162. 29 refs. Includes a list of "Resources for physicians providing end–of–life care" (textbook, manuals, professional standards and policy statements, journal, and web sites). BE59834.
active euthanasia; advance care planning; assisted suicide; communication; decision making; family members; legal aspects; pain; *palliative care; physicians; quality of health care; suffering; *terminal care; terminally ill; withholding treatment

Singer, Peter A.; Martin, Douglas K.; Kelner, Merrijoy. Quality end–of–life care: patients' perspectives. *JAMA.* 1999 Jan 13; 281(2): 163–168. 31 refs. BE60236.
adults; advance care planning; advance directives; aged; allowing to die; *attitudes; chronically ill; decision making; family relationship; HIV seropositivity; long–term care; pain; palliative care; patient participation; *patient satisfaction; patients; *quality of health care; *quality of life; renal dialysis; suffering; survey; *terminal care; terminally ill; withholding treatment; qualitative research; Ontario; Toronto

CONTEXT: Quality end–of–life care is increasingly recognized as an ethical obligation of health care providers, both clinicians and organizations. However, this concept has not been examined from the perspective of patients. OBJECTIVE: To identify and describe elements of quality end–of–life care from the patient's perspective. DESIGN: Qualitative study using in–depth, open–ended, face–to–face interviews and content analysis. SETTING: Toronto, Ontario. PARTICIPANTS: A total of 126 participants from 3 patient groups: dialysis patients (n = 48), people with human immunodeficiency virus infection (n = 40), and residents of a long–term care facility (n = 38). OUTCOME MEASURES: Participants' views on end–of–life issues. RESULTS: Participants identified 5 domains of quality end–of–life care: receiving adequate pain and symptom management, avoiding inappropriate prolongation of dying, achieving a sense of control, relieving burden, and strengthening relationships with loved ones. CONCLUSION: These domains, which characterize patients' perspectives on end–of–life care, can serve as focal points for improving the quality of end–of–life care.

Smith, George P. Terminal sedation as palliative care: revalidating a right to a good death. *Cambridge Quarterly of Healthcare Ethics.* 1998 Fall; 7(4): 382–387. 37 fn. BE59139.
*drugs; legal aspects; pain; *palliative care; physicians; quality of health care; right to die; *sedatives; standards; suffering; *terminal care; terminally ill; United States

Spencer, Donald E. Practical implications for health care providers in a physician–assisted suicide environment. *Seattle University Law Review.* 1995 Spring; 18(3): 545–556. 14 fn. BE59823.
alternatives; *assisted suicide; coercion; competence; counseling; decision making; depressive disorder; guidelines; health care reform; health personnel; home care; hospices; informed consent; lawyers; *legal aspects; palliative care; patient education; patients; *physicians; public opinion; *public policy; referral and consultation; *terminal care; terminally ill; continuity of patient care; United States

Stead, William W.; Miller, Douglas P.; Lewis, Gregory L., et al. Terminal dehydration as an alternative to physician–assisted suicide. [Letters and responses]. *Annals of Internal Medicine.* 1998 Dec 15; 129(12): 1080–1082. 18 refs. BE60227.
allowing to die; *alternatives; *artificial feeding; *assisted suicide; competence; drugs; *food; intention; *palliative care; physicians; sedatives; suffering; suicide; *terminal care; terminally ill; terminology; *treatment refusal; *withholding treatment; *dehydration

Stingl, Michael; Burgess, Michael M.; Hubert, John, et al. Euthanasia and health reform in Canada. [Article and commentaries]. *Cambridge Quarterly of Healthcare Ethics.* 1998 Fall; 7(4): 348–370. 46 fn. BE59136.
*active euthanasia; aged; caring; chronically ill; community services; competence; economics; goals; *health care delivery; *health care reform; home care; involuntary euthanasia; *justice; obligations of society; organization and administration; palliative care; primary health care; *public policy; *quality of health care; quality of life; socioeconomic factors; suffering; *terminal care; terminally ill; *voluntary

euthanasia; *Canada; Netherlands

Sulmasy, Daniel P.; Pellegrino, Edmund D. The rule of double effect: clearing up the double talk. *Archives of Internal Medicine.* 1999 Mar 22; 159(6): 545–550. 44 refs. BE62605.

active euthanasia; allowing to die; assisted suicide; autonomy; conscience; *double effect; *drugs; *intention; law; moral complicity; morality; *opioid analgesics; *pain; *palliative care; physicians; public policy; religion; *sedatives; *terminal care; withholding treatment

Tolle, Susan W.; Rosenfeld, Anne G.; Tilden, Virginia P., et al. Oregon's low in–hospital death rates: what determines where people die and satisfaction with decisions on place of death? *Annals of Internal Medicine.* 1999 Apr 20; 130(8): 681–685. 24 refs. BE61602.

*advance care planning; allowing to die; *alternatives; *death; evaluation studies; family members; *geographic factors; home care; hospices; *hospitals; managed care programs; mortality; nursing homes; palliative care; patient admission; patient discharge; patient transfer; resource allocation; resuscitation orders; statistics; *terminal care; terminally ill; patient satisfaction; *Oregon; United States

Where Americans die is much more influenced by what part of the country they live in than by what their preferences are for location of death. Although most Americans report a preference for death at home, a majority still die in acute care hospitals. We describe the experiences of patients who died in Oregon (the state that currently has the lowest in–hospital death rate in the United States -- 31%) and the views of their families. We examine the factors influencing respect for dying patients' preferred location of death. Data from Oregon studies confirm that decisions to avoid hospital admission are far more common than discharge of the actively dying. Do–not–resuscitate orders were reported for 91% of nursing home residents in one study and living wills were reported for 67% of a random sample of adult Oregon decedents in a second study. In the second study, decisions not to start treatment were far more common than decisions to stop treatment (79% compared with 21%). Only 2.4% of families reported that "too little" treatment was given. Throughout the United States, use and availability of beds in acute care hospitals have been confirmed to be the principal determining factors in location of death. Within that constraint, however, the availability of other resources and services both facilitates the process of arranging for patients to die outside the hospital and improves satisfaction with the quality of terminal care.

Tonelli, Mark R.; Lynn, Joanne; Orentlicher, David. Terminal sedation. [Letters and response]. *New England Journal of Medicine.* 1998 Apr 23; 338(17): 1230–1231. 5 refs. BE59238.

*active euthanasia; artificial feeding; assisted suicide; double effect; *drugs; *intention; pain; physicians; *sedatives; suffering; *terminal care; *terminally ill; time factors; withholding treatment; coma

Vaux, Kenneth L.; Vaux, Sara A. Dying Well. Nashville, TN: Abingdon Press; 1996. 147 p. (Challenges in ethics). 97 fn. Edited by Kenneth L. Vaux. ISBN 0–687–10933–7. BE61358.

aged; allowing to die; assisted suicide; attitudes to death; autonomy; biomedical technologies; cancer; case studies; common good; economics; home care; hospices; hospitals; humanism; intensive care units; legal aspects; medical education; nursing homes; palliative care; pastoral care; patient advocacy; physicians; prognosis; prolongation of life; Protestant ethics; psychological stress; quality of life; *religious ethics; resource allocation; right to die; suffering;

*terminal care; terminally ill; theology; values; United States

Volkenandt, Matthias. Supportive care and euthanasia -- an ethical dilemma? *Supportive Care in Cancer.* 1998 Mar; 6(2): 114–119. 15 refs. Presented at the 9th International Symposium on Supportive Care in Cancer, held in St. Gallen, Switzerland, 26 Feb–1 Mar 1997. BE61573.

*active euthanasia; allowing to die; *assisted suicide; autonomy; beneficence; *cancer; double effect; drugs; economics; intention; involuntary euthanasia; *moral obligations; moral policy; pain; *palliative care; *physician patient relationship; *physicians; resource allocation; social impact; suffering; *terminal care; *terminally ill; trust; voluntary euthanasia; wedge argument; withholding treatment; United States

Webb, Marilyn. The Good Death: The New American Search to Reshape the End of Life. New York, NY: Bantam Books; 1997. 479 p. 396 fn. Foreward by Timothy E. Quill; introduction by Joanne Lynn. ISBN 0–553–09555–2. BE60515.

advance directives; AIDS; *allowing to die; amyotrophic lateral sclerosis; artificial feeding; assisted suicide; *attitudes to death; cancer; case studies; cultural pluralism; *death; decision making; dementia; drugs; family members; family relationship; government regulation; hospices; legal aspects; opioid analgesics; *pain; *palliative care; persistent vegetative state; physicians; psychological stress; quality of health care; regulation; right to die; standards; *terminal care; *terminally ill; treatment refusal; trends; withholding treatment; United States

Wronska, Irena; Gozdek, Nina. Aims and ethics of palliative care: the views of a selected group of Polish nursing students. *Scandinavian Journal of Caring Sciences.* 1994; 8(1): 25–27. 4 refs. BE61590.

aged; *attitudes; communication; goals; nurse patient relationship; nurse's role; *nurses; nursing education; pain; *palliative care; patient care team; professional competence; quality of life; *students; suffering; survey; *terminal care; *terminally ill; dignity; *Poland

Zalcberg, John R.; Buchanan, John D. Clinical issues in euthanasia. [Editorial]. *Medical Journal of Australia.* 1997 Feb 3; 166(3): 150–152. 16 refs. BE60195.

allowing to die; cancer; communication; depressive disorder; family members; palliative care; physicians; professional competence; public policy; suffering; *terminal care; terminally ill; *voluntary euthanasia; vulnerable populations; withholding treatment; Australia

United Kingdom Government publishes response to House of Lords report on medical ethics. [Summary of *Government Response to the Report of the Select Committee on Medical Ethics*, presented to Parliament by command of Her Majesty, May 1994]. *International Digest of Health Legislation.* 1995; 46(4): 570–572. BE62686.

*active euthanasia; advance directives; advisory committees; *allowing to die; *assisted suicide; decision making; drugs; guidelines; legal aspects; palliative care; persistent vegetative state; *public policy; resource allocation; *terminal care; terminally ill; treatment refusal; *Great Britain; *House of Lords Select Committee on Medical Ethics

TERMINAL CARE/HOSPICES

Bresnahan, James F. Palliative care or assisted suicide? *America.* 1998 Mar 14; 178(8): 16–21. BE59701.

allowing to die; *assisted suicide; compassion; government regulation; *hospices; killing; *legal aspects; *palliative care; physicians; right to die; Roman Catholic ethics; state government; suffering; Supreme Court decisions; *terminal care; terminally ill; Oregon; *United States; *Vacco v. Quill;

*Washington v. Glucksberg

Fish, Peter. A harder better death. [Personal narrative]. *Health.* 1997 Nov–Dec; 11(8): 108–114. BE59200.
assisted suicide; cancer; drugs; family members; government financing; health insurance; home care; *hospices; organizational policies; pain; palliative care; patient care team; quality of health care; suffering; *terminal care; terminally ill; withholding treatment; Medicare; National Hospice Organization; United States

Harrold, Joan K.; Lynn, Joanne, eds. A Good Dying: Shaping Health Care for the Last Months of Life. New York, NY: Haworth Press; 1998. 188 p. Includes references. Co-published simultaneously as *The Hospice Journal*, 1998; 13(1/2). ISBN 0–7890–0502–6. BE60653.
aged; cancer; chronically ill; evaluation; family members; government financing; health care delivery; health insurance reimbursement; health personnel; home care; *hospices; humanities; managed care programs; mortality; pain; *palliative care; professional organizations; prognosis; quality of health care; referral and consultation; standards; suffering; *terminal care; terminally ill; Medicare; National Hospice Organization; United States

Henderson, Shelley; Fins, Joseph J.; Moskowitz, Ellen H. Resuscitation in hospice. [Case study and commentaries]. *Hastings Center Report.* 1998 Nov–Dec; 28(6): 20–22. BE61280.
advance care planning; attitudes; autonomy; beneficence; case studies; *communication; *dissent; *family members; futility; goals; *home care; *hospices; informed consent; *palliative care; *patient care team; physician patient relationship; professional family relationship; *resuscitation orders; terminal care; *terminally ill; time factors

McGrath, Pam. Autonomy, discourse, and power: a postmodern reflection on principlism and bioethics. *Journal of Medicine and Philosophy.* 1998 Oct; 23(5): 516–532. 75 refs. 2 fn. Note: the journal issue cover shows a date of August 1998, which is incorrect. BE62116.
alternatives; *autonomy; *bioethics; biomedical technologies; Buddhist ethics; decision making; ethicists; *home care; *hospices; hospitals; philosophy; physicians; *postmodernism; *principle-based ethics; *social discrimination; *sociology of medicine; *terminal care; terminally ill; empowerment; Foucault, Michel; Karuna Hospice Service (Brisbane, QLD)
In recent years there has been an increasing critique of the philosophy based reasoning in bioethics which is known as principlism. This article seeks to make a postmodern contribution to this emerging debate by using notions of power and discourse to highlight the limits and superficiality of this abstract, rationalistic mode of reflection. The focus of the discussion will be on the principle of autonomy. Recent doctoral research on a hospice organization (Karuna Hospice Service) will be used to contextualize the debate to end–of–life ethical dilemmas. The conclusion will be reached that the discursive richness of this organization's notion of autonomy or choice, which incorporates a holistic respect for the individual and the active creation of alternatives, can provide important insights to our understanding of autonomy in bioethics. The concern is raised that if autonomy is reified as a principle outside of the context of discourse, it may only complement the hegemonic power of biomedicine.

Mak, June Mui Hing; Clinton, Michael. Promoting a good death: an agenda for outcomes research -- a review of the literature. *Nursing Ethics.* 1999 Mar; 6(2): 97–106. 55 refs. BE61929.

*attitudes to death; autonomy; cultural pluralism; goals; *hospices; non–Western World; nurses; nursing research; pain; palliative care; patient participation; patient satisfaction; quality of health care; *terminal care; terminally ill; *treatment outcome; Western World; hope

Reitman, James S.; Calhoun, Byron C.; Hoeldtke, Nathan J. Perinatal hospice: a response to early termination for severe congenital anomalies. *In:* Demy, Timothy J.; Stewart, Gary P., eds. Genetic Engineering: A Christian Response: Crucial Considerations in Shaping Life. Grand Rapids, MI: Kregel Publications; 1999: 196–211. 63 fn. ISBN 0–8254–2357–0. BE61368.
alternatives; autonomy; *Christian ethics; *congenital disorders; conscience; females; fetal development; fetuses; *hospices; *newborns; personhood; pregnant women; psychological stress; risks and benefits; *selective abortion; suffering; *terminal care; terminally ill; theology; viability; grief; United States

Scott, P. Anne. Autonomy, power, and control in palliative care. *Cambridge Quarterly of Healthcare Ethics.* 1999 Spring; 8(2): 139–147. 35 fn. BE61231.
*autonomy; case studies; *communication; *hospices; institutionalized persons; *nurse patient relationship; nurse's role; nursing research; *palliative care; *patient advocacy; patient participation; physician patient relationship; professional family relationship; quality of health care; social dominance; *terminal care; terminally ill; dependency; *empowerment; sick role; Great Britain

Stolberg, Sheryl Gay. As life ebbs, so does time to elect comforts of hospice. *New York Times.* 1998 Mar 4: A1, A18. BE60321.
attitudes; biomedical technologies; family members; home care; *hospices; hospitals; palliative care; physicians; prolongation of life; referral and consultation; suffering; *terminal care; *terminally ill; Medicare; United States

TEST TUBE FERTILIZATION *See* IN VITRO FERTILIZATION

TESTING AND SCREENING

See also GENETIC SCREENING, MASS SCREENING
See under
AIDS/TESTING AND SCREENING

THERAPEUTIC RESEARCH *See* HUMAN EXPERIMENTATION

THIRD PARTY CONSENT *See* ALLOWING TO DIE, INFORMED CONSENT, RESUSCITATION ORDERS

TISSUE DONATION *See* ORGAN AND TISSUE DONATION

TORTURE

Charatan, Fred. Brazil challenges doctors accused of torture. [News]. *BMJ (British Medical Journal).* 1999 Mar 20; 318(7186): 757. BE62511.
human rights; military personnel; *misconduct; *physicians; prisoners; professional organizations; self regulation; *torture; *Brazil

Rohter, Larry. Brazil rights group hopes to bar doctors

BE = bioethics accession number   fn. = footnotes   refs. = references

linked to torture. [News]. *New York Times.* 1999 Mar 11: A15. BE61550.
  moral complicity; *physicians; prisoners; *professional organizations; *punishment; self regulation; *torture; *Brazil

Welsh, James; van Es, Adriaan. Health and human rights: an international minefield. *Lancet.* 1998 Dec 19-26; 352 (Suppl. 4): 14. 5 refs. BE60807.
  capital punishment; circumcision; females; *human rights; *international aspects; *misconduct; *physicians; political activity; public health; *torture; war

Welsh, James. Truth and reconciliation ... and justice. *Lancet.* 1998 Dec 5; 352(9143): 1852-1853. 5 refs. BE60806.
  accountability; blacks; *human rights; justice; *misconduct; *physicians; prisoners; social discrimination; *torture; *Chile; *South Africa

TRANSGENIC ANIMALS *See* GENETIC INTERVENTION, PATENTING LIFE FORMS, RECOMBINANT DNA RESEARCH

TRANSPLANTATION *See* ORGAN AND TISSUE TRANSPLANTATION

TREATMENT REFUSAL

See also ALLOWING TO DIE, ADVANCE DIRECTIVES, INFORMED CONSENT, PATIENTS' RIGHTS

Andersen, David; Cavalier, Robert; Covey, Preston K. A Right to Die? The Dax Cowart Case. [CD-ROM computer file]. New York, NY: Routledge; 1996 Jun. 1 computer laser optical disc; sd., col.; 4 - 3/4 in. + user guide and teacher's guide.. Interactive; contains scenes of medical treatment which some may find distressing. Versions available for Windows or Macintosh (single user ISBN 0-415-91753-0, multiple user pack ISBN 0-415-91754-9); contact Routledge (e-mail: info.dax@routledge.com; http://www.routledge.com/routledge.html). BE59871.
  *allowing to die; assisted suicide; *autonomy; beneficence; *burns; case studies; coercion; decision making; dissent; moral obligations; *pain; paternalism; *patient care; patient care team; physically disabled; physician patient relationship; physicians; *prolongation of life; quality of life; rehabilitation; *right to die; *suffering; suicide; teaching methods; treatment outcome; *treatment refusal; *Cowart, Dax

Banja, John D.; Adler, Richard K.; Stringer, Anthony Y. Ethical dimensions of caring for defiant patients: a case study. *Journal of Head Trauma Rehabilitation.* 1996 Dec; 11(6): 93-97. 1 ref. BE60501.
  alcohol abuse; autonomy; *behavior disorders; *brain pathology; case studies; coercion; *competence; dissent; injuries; involuntary commitment; parents; paternalism; *patient compliance; patient discharge; rehabilitation; *treatment refusal; adult offspring; neuropsychology

Branigin, William. Sect's transfusion ban puts believer at risk. [News]. *Washington Post.* 1999 Jan 21: A2. BE60024.
  advance directives; *blood transfusions; competence; critically ill; decision making; dissent; family members; *Jehovah's Witnesses; married persons; *treatment refusal; Los Angeles; *Villagomez, Rosario Rios

Bridgeman, Jo. Medical treatment: the mother's rights. *Family Law.* 1993 Sep; 23: 534-535. BE61825.
  *cesarean section; competence; *fetuses; judicial action; *legal aspects; legal rights; *pregnant women; *treatment refusal; *Great Britain; *Re S (An Adult: Surgical Treatment)

Brown, Lowell C.; Paine, Shirley J. Thunder from California: the *Thor* decision and the ever-expanding right to die. *HealthSpan.* 1993 Oct; 10(9): 13-17. 56 fn. BE61559.
  *allowing to die; *artificial feeding; autonomy; competence; food; force feeding; *legal aspects; legal liability; legal obligations; *legal rights; paralysis; patients; *physically disabled; physicians; *prisoners; quality of life; *right to die; state interest; suicide; surgery; *treatment refusal; value of life; withholding treatment; quadriplegia; *California; California Medical Association; *Thor v. Superior Court (Andrews)

Cale, Gita S. Risk-related standards of competence: continuing the debate over risk-related standards of competence. *Bioethics.* 1999 Apr; 13(2): 131-148. 28 fn. Commentary on I. Wilks, "The debate over risk-related standards of competence," *Bioethics,* 1997 Oct; 11(5): 413-426. BE61673.
  *autonomy; beneficence; *competence; *decision making; evaluation; *informed consent; *moral policy; patient care; patients; *risk; *risks and benefits; *standards; *treatment refusal

This discussion paper addresses Ian Wilks' defence of the risk-related standard of competence that appears in *Bioethics 11.* Wilks there argues that the puzzle posed by Mark Wicclair in *Bioethics 5* against Dan Brock's argument in favour of a risk-related standard of competence -- namely that Brock's argument allows for situations of asymmetrical competence -- is not a genuine problem for a risk-related standard of competence. To show this, Wilks presents what he believes to be two examples of real situations in which asymmetrical competence arises. I argue that insofar as Wilks equivocates two senses of competence in his examples -- namely, competence to perform a task and competence in performing a task -- Wilks is unable to illustrate the existence of real situations of asymmetrical competence. By examining the way in which Wilks equivocates two senses of competence in his examples, and by applying the results of this examination to the problem of patient competency within the medical field, I argue that not only does Wilks fail to show that situations of asymmetrical competence exist, but he is also unable to provide a foundation for understanding how the risk-related standard of competence can strike a balance between an individual's autonomy and benevolent intervention. I thus conclude that insofar as Wilks fails to answer the objections raised by Wicclair and others against the risk-related standard of competence, the risk-related standard of competence continues to be undermined by the problem of asymmetrical competence.

Gianakos, Dean. Conversations with Stella. *Annals of Internal Medicine.* 1999 Apr 20; 130(8): 698-699. BE61605.
  allowing to die; alternatives; chronically ill; *communication; critically ill; *patient care; *physician patient relationship; *treatment refusal; trust; uncertainty; *ventilators; withholding treatment

Grubb, Andrew. Treatment without consent (anorexia nervosa): adult -- Riverside Mental Health Trust v. Fox. [Comment]. *Medical Law Review.* 1994 Spring; 2(1): 95-99. BE59904.
  artificial feeding; *behavior disorders; females; *food; *force feeding; judicial action; *legal aspects; mentally ill;

BE = bioethics accession number   fn. = footnotes   refs. = references

*treatment refusal; *anorexia nervosa; *Great Britain; *Riverside Mental Health NHS Trust v. Fox

Hassan, T.B.; MacNamara, A.F.; Davy, A., et al. Managing patients with deliberate self harm who refuse treatment in the accident and emergency department. *BMJ (British Medical Journal).* 1999 Jul 10; 319(7202): 107–109. 10 refs. BE61751.
case studies; coercion; *competence; critically ill; decision making; *emergency care; evaluation; hospitals; *knowledge, attitudes, practice; *legal aspects; legal liability; *patient care; *physicians; psychiatric diagnosis; referral and consultation; *suicide; survey; *treatment refusal; Great Britain

Hurwitz, Brian. Pressuring Mrs Thomas to accept treatment: a case history. *Journal of Medical Ethics.* 1998 Oct; 24(5): 320–321. BE60253.
aged; *cancer; case studies; *coercion; home care; hospitals; *paternalism; patient admission; *patient care; physician's role; *radiology; resource allocation; *treatment refusal
A general practitioner (GP) recounts events which unfolded after visiting a patient at home. She was found to be suffering from an entirely curable clinical condition which was worsening as a result of refusal to accept effective medical treatment. The effects upon a grown-up son of the patient's refusal, and the increasing burden of care falling upon local district nursing services, were factors which influenced the GP's thinking and decision making.

Illinois. Appellate Court, First District, Fifth Division. In re Brown. *North Eastern Reporter, 2d Series.* 1997 Dec 31 (date of decision). 689: 397–406. BE60046.
autonomy; *blood transfusions; coercion; *fetuses; *Jehovah's Witnesses; *legal aspects; legal guardians; legal rights; *pregnant women; religion; state interest; third party consent; *treatment refusal; value of life; viability; *Illinois; *In re Brown
The Appellate Court of Illinois, First District, held that a competent pregnant woman's right to refuse medical treatment overrides the state's substantial interest in the welfare of a viable fetus. Darlene Brown entered a hospital for a cystoscopy and removal of a urethral mass. She lost 1,500 cubic centimeters of blood and refused blood transfusions because of her beliefs as a Jehovah's Witness. In her physician's opinion, Brown's chances of survival, as well as those of the fetus, were only 5%. The trial court appointed a guardian *ad litem* pursuant to the state's request to protect the interest of the fetus. The guardian ordered Brown to undergo transfusions and she gave birth to a healthy child. The court here held that the trial court abused its discretion in appointing the guardian and forcing Brown to undergo treatment, reasoning that the state's interest in preserving the life of the mother and of the fetus cannot override a pregnant woman's competent refusal of recommended invasive medical procedures. (KIE abstract)

Kennedy, Ian. Treatment without consent (adult): force feeding of detainee -- Department of Immigration v. Mok and Another. [Comment]. *Medical Law Review.* 1994 Spring; 2(1): 102–105. BE59905.
adults; *aliens; emergency care; *force feeding; law enforcement; *legal aspects; *prisoners; *treatment refusal; emigration and immigration; *Australia; *Department of Immigration v. Mok

Leggat, John E.; Swartz, Richard D.; Port, Friedrich K. Withdrawal from dialysis: a review with an emphasis on the black experience. *Advances in Renal Replacement Therapy.* 1997 Jan; 4(1): 22–29. 44 refs. BE60177.
advance directives; age factors; aged; *allowing to die; attitudes to death; *blacks; communication; comparative studies; cultural pluralism; decision making; diabetes; family relationship; kidney diseases; *knowledge, attitudes, practice; morbidity; physician patient relationship; prolongation of life; quality of life; religion; *renal dialysis; social interaction; social worth; *socioeconomic factors; statistics; suicide; *treatment refusal; trust; *whites; *withholding treatment; United States

Levi, Joel. Refusal of life-sustaining treatment recognized by court of law. *Medicine and Law.* 1993; 12(1–2): 191–192. BE60621.
*allowing to die; amyotrophic lateral sclerosis; decision making; Jewish ethics; *legal aspects; physicians; *right to die; terminally ill; *treatment refusal; ventilators; withholding treatment; *Israel

Malyon, David. Transfusion-free treatment of Jehovah's Witnesses: respecting the autonomous patient's motives. *Journal of Medical Ethics.* 1998 Dec; 24(6): 376–381. 31 fn. BE60731.
alternatives; *blood transfusions; children; coercion; computer communication networks; conscience; decision making; freedom; *Jehovah's Witnesses; motivation; parents; physicians; *religion; risks and benefits; surgery; *treatment refusal
What makes Jehovah's Witnesses tick? What motivates practitioners of medicine? How is benevolent human behaviour to be interpreted? The explanation that fear of censure, mind-control techniques or enlightened self-interest are the real motivators of human conduct is questioned. Those who believe that man was created in "God's image", hold that humanity has the potential to rise above selfishly driven attitudes and actions, and reflect the qualities of love, kindness and justice that separate us from the beasts. A comparison of general medical ethics and disciplines, and those of the Jehovah's Witness community, is made in this context. The easy charge that frequent deaths result from refusal of blood transfusions is examined. The central source of antipathy towards Jehovah's Witnesses, namely the alleged imposition of extreme and even harmful refusal of blood therapy on our children is addressed. Of course, "... few dilemmas are likely to be resolved wisely or satisfactorily by a blinkered adherence to abstract principles alone. Solutions to most cases will be dictated by a combination of factors. The support of medical ethics by Jehovah's Witnesses, and their willingness to share in reasoned and ethical debate, while at the same time holding firm to their religious and conscientious principles are emphasised.

Malyon, David. Transfusion-free treatment of Jehovah's Witnesses: respecting the autonomous patient's rights. *Journal of Medical Ethics.* 1998 Oct; 24(5): 302–307. 28 fn. BE60730.
advance directives; alternatives; *autonomy; *blood transfusions; children; coercion; competence; confidentiality; *decision making; dissent; *Jehovah's Witnesses; parents; patient care; physician patient relationship; physicians; *religion; surgery; *treatment refusal; rationality
Do six million Jehovah's Witnesses mean what they say? Muramoto's not-so-subtle proposition is that they don't, because of a system of control akin to the Orwellian "thought police". My response is that the fast developing cooperative relationship between our worldwide community and the medical profession as a whole, and the proven record of that community's steadfast integrity in relation to their Christian principles is the evidence that we do! I seek to highlight the inaccuracy of information, which Muramoto admits came largely from dis-enchanted ex-members, by quoting "established"

---

medical ethical opinion that refusal of blood transfusions must be respected as evidence of patient autonomy. Personal experience of my work on hospital liaison committees for Jehovah's Witnesses is reviewed and I endeavour to prove that our view of blood, and its association with life, goes to the very core of the human psyche. Lastly I suggest that faith transcends rationality. Human beings are more than just minds! Our deep moral sense and consciousness that our dignity is diminished by living our lives solely on the "self interest" principle, lies at the heart of true personal autonomy. Maybe it's a case of "two men looking through the same bars: one seeing mud, the other stars."

Muramoto, Osamu. Bioethics of the refusal of blood by Jehovah's Witnesses: Part 1. Should bioethical deliberation consider dissidents' views? *Journal of Medical Ethics.* 1998 Aug; 24(4): 223–230. 40 refs. BE60727.
  attitudes; autonomy; *blood transfusions; coercion; computer communication networks; confidentiality; decision making; *dissent; guidelines; health personnel; *Jehovah's Witnesses; patient care; *physicians; *religion; *treatment refusal; Internet

Jehovah's Witnesses' (JWs) refusal of blood transfusions has recently gained support in the medical community because of the growing popularity of "no-blood" treatment. Many physicians, particularly so-called "sympathetic doctors", are establishing a close relationship with this religious organization. On the other hand, it is little known that this blood doctrine is being strongly criticized by reform-minded current and former JWs who have expressed conscientious dissent from the organization. Their arguments reveal religious practices that conflict with many physicians' moral standards. They also suggest that a certain segment of "regular" or orthodox JWs may have different attitudes towards the blood doctrine. The author considers these viewpoints and argues that there are ethical flaws in the blood doctrine, and that the medical community should reconsider its supportive position. The usual physician assumption that JWs are acting autonomously and uniformly in refusing blood is seriously questioned.

Muramoto, Osamu. Bioethics of the refusal of blood by Jehovah's Witnesses: Part 2. A novel approach based on rational non-interventional paternalism. *Journal of Medical Ethics.* 1998 Oct; 24(5): 295–301. 32 fn. BE60729.
  autonomy; *blood transfusions; coercion; *communication; counseling; *decision making; disclosure; dissent; emergency care; *informed consent; *Jehovah's Witnesses; *paternalism; patient care; physician patient relationship; *physicians; *treatment refusal

Most physicians dealing with Jehovah's Witnesses (JWs) who refuse blood-based treatment are uncertain as to any obligation to educate patients where it concerns the JW blood doctrine itself. They often feel they must unquestioningly comply when demands are framed as religiously based. Recent discussion by dissidents and reformers of morally questionable policies by the JW organisation raise ethical dilemmas about "passive" support of this doctrine by some concerned physicians. In this paper, Part 2, I propose that physicians discuss the misinformation and irrationality behind the blood doctrine with the JW patient by raising questions that provide new perspectives. A meeting should be held non-coercively and in strict confidence, and the patient's decision after the meeting should be fully honoured (non-interventional). A rational deliberation based on new information and a new perspective would enable a certain segment of JW patients to make truly informed,

autonomous and rational decisions.

Muramoto, Osamu. Jehovah's Witnesses and blood transfusions. [Letter]. *Lancet.* 1998 Sep 5; 352(9130): 824. 1 ref. BE61082.
  *blood transfusions; *dissent; human rights; *Jehovah's Witnesses; *organizational policies; patient compliance; punishment; *treatment refusal; European Commission on Human Rights

Oliver, Jo. Anorexia and the refusal of medical treatment. *Victoria University of Wellington Law Review.* 1997 Dec; 27(4): 621–647. 105 fn. BE61524.
  artificial feeding; autonomy; behavior disorders; *competence; females; food; *force feeding; *legal aspects; mentally ill; mothers; paternalism; *treatment refusal; *anorexia nervosa; *New Zealand; *Re C MC

Price, David P.T. Assisted suicide and refusing medical treatment: linguistics, morals and legal contortions. *Medical Law Review.* 1996 Autumn; 4(3): 270–299. 141 fn. BE61513.
  active euthanasia; allowing to die; *assisted suicide; double effect; *intention; international aspects; *legal aspects; moral policy; physicians; right to die; *suicide; *treatment refusal; Canada; Great Britain; New Zealand; United States

Rowan, Cathy. Court-ordered caesareans -- choice or control? *Nursing Ethics.* 1998 Nov; 5(6): 542–544. 10 refs. BE60815.
  *cesarean section; *coercion; competence; *fetuses; *judicial action; *legal aspects; nurse midwives; *pregnant women; *treatment refusal; *Great Britain

Savulescu, Julian. The cost of refusing treatment and equality of outcome. *Journal of Medical Ethics.* 1998 Aug; 24(4): 231–236. 23 fn. BE60728.
  *alternatives; autonomy; *blood transfusions; *economics; *Jehovah's Witnesses; justice; legal aspects; obligations of society; *patient care; religion; *resource allocation; social discrimination; *treatment refusal; utilitarianism; values; Great Britain

Patients have a right to refuse medical treatment. But what should happen after a patient has refused recommended treatment? In many cases, patients receive alternative forms of treatment. These forms of care may be less cost-effective. Does respect for autonomy extend to providing these alternatives? How for does justice constrain autonomy? I begin by providing three arguments that such alternatives should not be offered to those who refuse treatment. I argue that the best argument which refusers can appeal to is based on the egalitarian principle of equality of outcome. However, this principle does not ultimately support a right to less cost-effective alternatives. I focus on Jehovah's Witnesses refusing blood and requesting alternative treatments. However, the point applies to many patients who refuse cost-effective medical care.

Smith, Martin L. Ethical perspectives on Jehovah's Witnesses' refusal of blood. *Cleveland Clinic Journal of Medicine.* 1997 Oct; 64(9): 475–481. 25 refs. BE59229.
  *adolescents; *adults; *autonomy; *beneficence; *blood transfusions; casuistry; *children; competence; conscience; *decision making; ethical analysis; informed consent; *Jehovah's Witnesses; justice; legal aspects; mentally retarded; *moral obligations; *parents; patient care; *physicians; referral and consultation; resource allocation; risks and benefits; *state interest; *treatment refusal

Starr, Joann; Zawacki, Bruce E. Voices from the silent world of doctor and patient. *Cambridge Quarterly of Healthcare Ethics.* 1999 Spring; 8(2): 129–138. 12 fn.

BE = bioethics accession number   fn. = footnotes   refs. = references

BE61230.
 attitudes; *autonomy; *burns; *caring; clinical ethics committees; coercion; communication; compassion; competence; decision making; *emotions; empathy; ethicists; family members; hospitals; informed consent; intensive care units; *narrative ethics; nurse patient relationship; nurses; *pain; paternalism; *patient advocacy; *patient care; patient compliance; *patient participation; patients; *physician patient relationship; physician's role; physicians; professional family relationship; *psychological stress; psychology; *suffering; surgery; *treatment refusal; trust; vulnerable populations; empowerment

Stead, William W.; Miller, Douglas P.; Lewis, Gregory L., et al. Terminal dehydration as an alternative to physician–assisted suicide. [Letters and responses]. *Annals of Internal Medicine.* 1998 Dec 15; 129(12): 1080–1082. 18 refs. BE60227.
 allowing to die; *alternatives; *artificial feeding; *assisted suicide; competence; drugs; *food; intention; *palliative care; physicians; sedatives; suffering; suicide; *terminal care; terminally ill; terminology; *treatment refusal; *withholding treatment; *dehydration

Steinbock, Bonnie. Mother–fetus conflict. *In:* Kuhse, Helga; Singer, Peter, eds. A Companion to Bioethics. Malden, MA: Blackwell; 1998: 135–146. 36 refs. ISBN 0–631–19737–0. BE59490.
 abortion, induced; alcohol abuse; *cesarean section; children; coercion; decision making; drug abuse; fetal development; fetal therapy; *fetuses; legal aspects; *moral obligations; moral policy; *mother fetus relationship; pain; physicians; *pregnant women; *prenatal injuries; public policy; surgery; *treatment refusal

Swartz, Richard D.; Perry, Erica; Schneider, Carl, et al. The option to withdraw from chronic dialysis treatment. *Advances in Renal Replacement Therapy.* 1994 Oct; 1(3): 264–273. 84 refs. BE62003.
 *allowing to die; autonomy; case studies; *chronically ill; communication; competence; *decision making; depressive disorder; family members; interdisciplinary communication; legal aspects; patient care team; patients; professional patient relationship; prognosis; psychiatric diagnosis; quality of life; religious ethics; *renal dialysis; suffering; *treatment refusal

Tomlin, P.J. A memorable incident: when a spade is not a spade. *BMJ (British Medical Journal).* 1999 Jan 23; 318(7178): 256. BE60346.
 *blood transfusions; case studies; decision making; emergency care; family members; *Jehovah's Witnesses; paternalism; physicians; surgery; *treatment refusal

Walsh, Marcia K. Difficult decisions in health care: one woman's journey. [Personal narrative]. *Bioethics Forum.* 1997 Summer; 13(2): 35–37. 13 refs. 2 fn. BE59401.
 *advance directives; *allowing to die; artificial feeding; attitudes; dementia; *patients; persistent vegetative state; *quality of life; terminally ill; *treatment refusal; withholding treatment

Wicclair, Mark R. The continuing debate over risk–related standards of competence. *Bioethics.* 1999 Apr; 13(2): 149–153. 10 fn. Commentary on I. Wilks, "The debate over risk–related standards of competence," *Bioethics,* 1997 Oct; 11(5): 413–426. BE61674.
 *competence; *decision making; *informed consent; *moral policy; paternalism; patient care; patients; *risk; *risks and benefits; *standards; *treatment refusal

Wilks, Ian. Asymmetrical competence. *Bioethics.* 1999 Apr; 13(2): 154–159. 4 fn. BE61675.
 *competence; *decision making; *informed consent; *moral policy; patient care; patients; *risk; *risks and benefits;

 *standards; *treatment refusal

Youngner, Stuart J. Competence to refuse life–sustaining treatment. *In:* Steinberg, Maurice D.; Youngner, Stuart J., eds. End–of–Life Decisions: A Psychosocial Perspective. Washington, DC: American Psychiatric Press; 1998: 19–54. 60 fn. ISBN 0–88048–756–9. BE60122.
 *allowing to die; alternatives; assisted suicide; autonomy; beneficence; communication; *competence; comprehension; *decision making; dementia; disclosure; informed consent; legal aspects; mentally ill; paternalism; *patients; physician patient relationship; *physician's role; *psychiatry; referral and consultation; risks and benefits; standards; terminally ill; *treatment refusal; values; withholding treatment; rationality; United States

TREATMENT REFUSAL/MENTALLY DISABLED

Allan, Alfred; Allan, Marietjie. The right of mentally ill patients in South Africa to refuse treatment. *South African Law Journal.* 1997; 114(Pt. 4): 724–737. 77 fn. BE61472.
 competence; electroconvulsive therapy; informed consent; *institutionalized persons; involuntary commitment; involuntary sterilization; *legal aspects; legal rights; legislation; mental institutions; *mentally ill; patient advocacy; patient care; patient discharge; psychoactive drugs; psychosurgery; review committees; third party consent; *treatment refusal; voluntary admission; mental health services; Mental Health Act (South Africa); *South Africa

Boronow, John; Stoline, Anne; Sharfstein, Steven S. Refusal of ECT by a patient with recurrent depression, psychosis, and catatonia. *American Journal of Psychiatry.* 1997 Sep; 154(9): 1285–1291. 19 refs. BE60201.
 beneficence; case studies; chronically ill; communication; competence; *decision making; *depressive disorder; economics; *electroconvulsive therapy; *family members; family relationship; food; government financing; hospitals; institutionalized persons; judicial action; justice; *mentally ill; paternalism; *patient care; patient care team; professional family relationship; professional patient relationship; psychiatric diagnosis; *psychoactive drugs; *schizophrenia; *treatment refusal; *catatonia; Medicare; United States

Brakman, Sarah–Vaughan; Amari–Vaught, Eileen. Resistance and refusal. [Case study and commentaries]. *Hastings Center Report.* 1999 Jan–Feb; 29(1): 22–23. BE61632.
 anesthesia; autonomy; beneficence; case studies; competence; decision making; dissent; females; health personnel; legal aspects; legal guardians; *mentally retarded; obstetrics and gynecology; preventive medicine; residential facilities; risks and benefits; *third party consent; *treatment refusal

Cichon, Dennis E. The right to "just say no": a history and analysis of the right to refuse antipsychotic drugs. *Louisiana Law Review.* 1992 Nov; 53(2): 283–426. 934 fn. BE61305.
 competence; constitutional law; dangerousness; due process; historical aspects; institutionalized persons; *legal aspects; *legal rights; *mentally ill; prisoners; psychiatry; *psychoactive drugs; review; risks and benefits; standards; *state interest; Supreme Court decisions; *treatment refusal; *United States; Washington v. Harper

Derse, Arthur R. Making decisions about life–sustaining medical treatment in patients with dementia: the problem of patient decision–making capacity. *Theoretical Medicine and Bioethics.* 1999 Jan; 20(1): 55–67. 42 refs. BE62124.
 *aged; *allowing to die; assisted suicide; autonomy; beneficence; case studies; *compensation; comprehension;

---

*decision making; *dementia; diagnosis; emergency care; heart diseases; human experimentation; *informed consent; patient care; patient participation; *prolongation of life; quality of life; recall; *resuscitation; standards; surgery; third party consent; *treatment refusal; truth disclosure; withholding treatment; rationality

Douglas, Gillian. Re C (Refusal of Medical Treatment). [Comment]. *Family Law.* 1994 Mar; 24: 131–132. BE61827.
*advance directives; autonomy; *competence; critically ill; directive adherence; informed consent; institutionalized persons; *legal aspects; mental institutions; *mentally ill; schizophrenia; *surgery; *treatment refusal; *amputation; *Great Britain; *Re C (Refusal of Medical Treatment)

Eilers, Robert. Hospitalized psychiatric patients' resistance to routine medical care. *Administration and Policy in Mental Health.* 1994 May; 21(5): 407–415. 27 refs. BE62125.
autonomy; coercion; competence; continuing education; decision making; health personnel; informed consent; institutionalized persons; involuntary commitment; legal aspects; mental institutions; *mentally ill; paternalism; patient care; physical restraint; risks and benefits; sedatives; third party consent; *treatment refusal

Great Britain. England. High Court of Justice, Family Division. Re K, W and H (Minors) (Medical Treatment). *Family Law Reports.* 1992 Sep 10 (date of decision). 1993: 854–859. BE59973.
adolescents; behavior disorders; competence; emergency care; *informed consent; *legal aspects; mental institutions; *mentally ill; *minors; *parental consent; *treatment refusal; Children Act 1989 (Great Britain); *Great Britain; Mental Health Act 1983 (Great Britain); *Re K, W and H (Minors) (Medical Treatment); Re R (A Minor) (Wardship: Medical Treatment)

The Family Division of the High Court of Justice of England's Supreme Court of Judicature refused to rule on a mental hospital's application for clarification of the law regarding consent of minors to receive emergency medication under the Mental Health Act and the Children Act. Three girls, all about 15 years of age, had been admitted for psychiatric care at St. Andrew's Hospital and, prior to their admission, consent for use of medication in emergency situations had been obtained from their parents. After complaints had been received from the girls that they had not consented to receive medication and about other matters, a committee investigation and report followed. The committee recommended that a court ruling be obtained on the issue. The court found the hospital's application "misconceived and unnecessary." Following the Court of Appeal in *Re R (A Minor) (Wardship: Medical Treatment)*, the court held that "a child with *Gillick* competence can consent to treatment, but if he or she declines to do so, consent can be given by someone else *who has parental rights or responsibilities.? In this case, none of the patients were Gillick* competent, and even if that was not the case, any refusal of treatment would not put the hospital or doctors at risk for liability because the requisite parental consent had been obtained. (KIE abstract)

Grubb, Andrew. Competent adult: refusal of treatment (renal dialysis) -- Re J.T. (Adult: Refusal of Treatment). [Comment]. *Medical Law Review.* 1998 Spring; 6(1): 105–107. BE61831.
allowing to die; *competence; *legal aspects; *mentally disabled; *renal dialysis; *treatment refusal; *Great Britain; *Re J.T. (Adult: Refusal of Treatment)

Grubb, Andrew. Refusal of treatment (incompetent patient): best interests and practicality -- Re D (Medical Treatment: Mentally Disabled Patient). [Comment]. *Medical Law Review.* 1998 Spring; 6(1): 103–105. BE61830.
allowing to die; coercion; competence; *legal aspects; *mentally ill; *renal dialysis; *treatment refusal; *Great Britain; *Re D (Medical Treatment: Mentally Disabled Patient)

Grubb, Andrew. Treatment without consent: adult -- Re C (Refusal of Medical Treatment). [Comment]. *Medical Law Review.* 1994 Spring; 2(1): 92–95. BE59903.
adults; advance directives; *competence; institutionalized persons; *legal aspects; legal rights; *mentally ill; schizophrenia; *surgery; *treatment refusal; amputation; *Great Britain; Re C (Adult: Refusal of Medical Treatment)

Hassenfeld, Irwin N.; Hoge, Steven K. Consequences of involuntary treatment. [Letter and response]. *American Journal of Psychiatry.* 1998 Mar; 155(3): 450–451. 4 refs. BE59375.
*autonomy; *coercion; decision making; empirical research; informed consent; involuntary commitment; judicial action; *mentally ill; *patient care; patient compliance; *patient participation; physician patient relationship; *psychoactive drugs; *treatment outcome; *treatment refusal; Massachusetts; New York; Virginia

Inwald, A.C.; Hippisley-Cox, Julia; Hippisley-Cox, Stephen, et al. Competency, consent, and the duty of care: ethical dilemma. [Case study and commentaries]. *BMJ (British Medical Journal).* 1998 Sep 19; 317(7161): 809–810. 4 refs. BE60849.
case studies; *competence; decision making; informed consent; legal aspects; *mentally ill; moral obligations; physicians; *schizophrenia; social workers; *surgery; *treatment refusal; Great Britain

Kennedy, Ian. Treatment without consent (diagnostic procedure): adult -- Re H (Mental Patient). [Comment]. *Medical Law Review.* 1993 Summer; 1(2): 236–238. BE60603.
diagnosis; informed consent; judicial action; *legal aspects; *mentally ill; *patient care; *schizophrenia; sterilization (sexual); *treatment refusal; *Great Britain; *Re H (Mental Patient)

McHale, J.V. Mental incapacity: some proposals for legislative reform. *Journal of Medical Ethics.* 1998 Oct; 24(5): 322–327. 67 fn. BE60254.
adults; advance directives; advisory committees; allowing to die; blood transfusions; *competence; *decision making; evaluation; family members; *informed consent; *judicial action; *legal aspects; *legislation; *mentally disabled; nontherapeutic research; patient care; persistent vegetative state; practice guidelines; *public policy; risks and benefits; *standards; sterilization (sexual); *third party consent; tissue donation; *treatment refusal; withholding treatment; *Who Decides? Making Decisions on Behalf of Mentally Incompetent Patients; Airedale NHS Trust v. Bland; *Great Britain; House of Lords Select Committee on Medical Ethics; *Law Commission (Great Britain); Re C (Adult: Refusal of Treatment); Re F (Mental Patient: Sterilisation); Re T (Adult: Refusal of Medical Treatment)

While the decision of the House of Lords in Re F in [1990] clarified somewhat the law concerning the treatment of the mentally incapacitated adult, many uncertainties remained. This paper explores proposals discussed in a recent government green paper for reform of the law in an area involving many difficult ethical dilemmas.

Moldow, D. Gay. VHA ethics rounds: [refusal to eat].

BE = bioethics accession number   fn. = footnotes   refs. = references

NCCE News (Veterans Health Administration National Center for Clinical Ethics). 1994 Fall; 2(4): 4–5. 10 refs. BE59847.
  aged; allowing to die; *artificial feeding; beneficence; case studies; clinical ethics committees; coercion; competence; decision making; *dementia; *depressive disorder; electroconvulsive therapy; ethics consultation; *food; force feeding; hospitals; nursing homes; *patient care; patient care team; quality of life; risks and benefits; *treatment refusal

Purtell, Dennis J.; Brakman, Sarah–Vaughan. Autonomy and the mentally disabled. [Letter and response]. *Hastings Center Report.* 1999 Jul–Aug; 29(4): 5. BE62461.
  autonomy; beneficence; institutionalized persons; legal guardians; *mentally retarded; obstetrics and gynecology; preventive medicine; risks and benefits; *third party consent; *treatment refusal

Singer, Beth J. Mental illness: rights, competence, and communication. *In:* McGee, Glenn, ed. Pragmatic Bioethics. Nashville, TN: Vanderbilt University Press; 1999: 141–151, 275–278. 31 fn. ISBN 0–8265–1321–2. BE60668.
  autonomy; beneficence; *communication; *competence; comprehension; decision making; disclosure; health personnel; informed consent; legal aspects; *mentally ill; paternalism; patient advocacy; patient care; patient participation; *psychoactive drugs; rights; standards; *treatment refusal; empowerment; pragmatism; United States

Szasz, Thomas. Parity for mental illness, disparity for the mental patient. *Lancet.* 1998 Oct 10; 352(9135): 1213–1215. 12 refs. BE60794.
  *advance directives; autonomy; brain pathology; competence; dangerousness; government regulation; health insurance; involuntary commitment; *legal aspects; mental institutions; *mentally ill; *psychiatric wills; *treatment refusal; Patient Self-Determination Act 1990; United States

TREATMENT REFUSAL/MINORS

Burgess, Michael; Rodney, Patricia; Coward, Harold, et al. Pediatric care: judgments about best interests at the onset of life. *In:* Coward, Harold; Ratanaku, Pinit, eds. A Cross–Cultural Dialogue on Health Care Ethics. Waterloo, ON: Wilfrid Laurier University Press; 1999: 160–175. 18 refs. 2 fn. ISBN 0–88920–325–3. BE62792.
  allowing to die; *American Indians; autonomy; *Buddhist ethics; children; compassion; *cultural pluralism; *decision making; dissent; economics; family relationship; females; *Hindu ethics; *infants; international aspects; legal aspects; males; organ transplantation; *parents; physicians; prognosis; quality of life; risks and benefits; treatment outcome; *treatment refusal; *values;' Canada; India; Thailand

Canada. Supreme Court. B. v. Children's Aid Society of Metropolitan Toronto. *Dominion Law Reports, 4th Series.* 1995 Jan 27 (date of decision). 122: 1–92. BE59472.
  autonomy; *blood transfusions; congenital disorders; constitutional law; decision making; freedom; *infants; *Jehovah's Witnesses; *legal aspects; *legal rights; parent child relationship; *parents; quality of life; religion; *state interest; Supreme Court decisions; *treatment refusal; value of life; *B. v. Children's Aid Society of Metropolitan Toronto; *Canada; *Canadian Charter of Rights and Freedoms

The Canadian Supreme Court held that the right of parents to choose or refuse medical treatment for their children based on religious beliefs is not a liberty included in the Canadian Charter of Rights and Freedoms. The parents of S.B., a premature infant, consented to all medical treatment except blood transfusions, to which they objected as Jehovah's Witnesses. Because of a potentially life-threatening condition and a projected later surgery, S.B. was made a temporary ward of the Children's Aid Society of Metropolitan Toronto in order to administer the blood. Section 7 of the Charter proclaims that "[e]veryone has the right to life, liberty and security of the person and the right not to be deprived thereof except in accordance with the principles of fundamental justice." The Chief Justice viewed parental autonomy as outside the concept of "liberty", because liberty had a physical connection or dimension specific to criminal justice. Four other judges, however, interpreted "liberty" not to mean unconstrained freedom, not mere freedom from physical restraint, and consequently under their view the state can intervene where parental decision making threatens a child's autonomy or health. (KIE abstract)

Clark, Frank I. Making sense of State v. Messenger. *Pediatrics.* 1996 Apr; 97(4): 579–583. 20 refs. BE59983.
  *allowing to die; *communication; decision making; *dissent; fathers; institutional policies; intensive care units; killing; *legal aspects; morbidity; *newborns; parental consent; *parents; physicians; prematurity; professional family relationship; prognosis; resuscitation; standards; *treatment refusal; uncertainty; ventilators; Messinger, Gregory; Michigan; *State v. Messenger

Coney, Sandra. Chemotherapy in children -- where to draw the line? [News]. *Lancet.* 1999 Mar 6; 353(9155): 819. BE61037.
  alternative therapies; *cancer; *children; *drugs; legal aspects; mass media; *parents; public opinion; *treatment refusal; *New Zealand

Cretney, Stephen. Re S (A Minor) (Blood Transfusion: Adoption Order Condition). [Comment]. *Family Law.* 1994 Nov; 24: 608–610. BE61828.
  *adoption; *blood transfusions; *Jehovah's Witnesses; judicial action; *legal aspects; *minors; *parents; *treatment refusal; *Great Britain; *Re S (A Minor)(Blood Transfusion: Adoption Order Condition)

Dickenson, Donna L.; Nicholson, Richard. Children's rights. [Letter and response]. *Hastings Center Report.* 1999 Jan–Feb; 29(1): 5. BE61628.
  children; competence; *decision making; *informed consent; international aspects; legal aspects; *minors; parental consent; *treatment refusal; Great Britain; United States

Dyer, Clare. Parents can choose child's treatment. [News]. *BMJ (British Medical Journal).* 1998 Oct 24; 317(7166): 1102. BE62644.
  *decision making; *legal aspects; *minors; *parents; *treatment refusal; chronic fatigue syndrome; *Great Britain

Great Britain. England. High Court of Justice, Family Division. Re K, W and H (Minors) (Medical Treatment). *Family Law Reports.* 1992 Sep 10 (date of decision). 1993: 854–859. BE59973.
  adolescents; behavior disorders; competence; emergency care; *informed consent; *legal aspects; mental institutions; *mentally ill; *minors; *parental consent; *treatment refusal; Children Act 1989 (Great Britain); *Great Britain; Mental Health Act 1983 (Great Britain); *Re K, W and H (Minors) (Medical Treatment); Re R (A Minor) (Wardship: Medical Treatment)

The Family Division of the High Court of Justice of England's Supreme Court of Judicature refused to rule on a mental hospital's application for clarification of the law regarding consent of minors to receive emergency

---

medication under the Mental Health Act and the Children Act. Three girls, all about 15 years of age, had been admitted for psychiatric care at St. Andrew's Hospital and, prior to their admission, consent for use of medication in emergency situations had been obtained from their parents. After complaints had been received from the girls that they had not consented to receive medication and about other matters, a committee investigation and report followed. The committee recommended that a court ruling be obtained on the issue. The court found the hospital's application "misconceived and unnecessary." Following the Court of Appeal in *Re R (A Minor) (Wardship: Medical Treatment)*, the court held that "a child with *Gillick* competence can consent to treatment, but if he or she declines to do so, consent can be given by someone else who has parental rights or responsibilities." In this case, none of the patients were *Gillick* competent, and even if that was not the case, any refusal of treatment would not put the hospital or doctors at risk for liability because the requisite parental consent had been obtained. (KIE abstract)

Grubb, Andrew. Medical treatment (child): parental refusal and role of the court -- Re T (A Minor) (Wardship: Medical Treatment). [Comment]. *Medical Law Review.* 1996 Autumn; 4(3): 315–319. BE61515.
   allowing to die; *children; congenital disorders; *decision making; *infants; judicial action; *legal aspects; livers; mothers; *organ transplantation; *parents; surgery; *treatment refusal; *Great Britain; *Re T (A Minor) (Wardship: Medical Treatment)

Kennedy, Ian. Treatment of incompetent child: parental wishes and Charter of Rights and Freedoms -- B. v. Children's Aid Society of Metropolitan Toronto. [Comment]. *Medical Law Review.* 1996 Spring; 4(1): 117–122. BE60002.
   *blood transfusions; constitutional law; freedom; *infants; *Jehovah's Witnesses; *legal aspects; *legal rights; moral obligations; *parents; religion; Supreme Court decisions; *treatment refusal; value of life; *B. v. Children's Aid Society of Metropolitan Toronto; *Canada; Canadian Charter of Rights and Freedoms

Kondro, Wayne. Boy refuses cancer treatment in favour of prayer. [News]. *Lancet.* 1999 Mar 27; 353(9158): 1078. BE61986.
   *adolescents; alternative therapies; cancer; competence; legal aspects; parents; *religion; *treatment refusal; *Christian Fundamentalists; *Dueck, Tyrell; Saskatchewan

Lawry, Kathleen; Slomka, Jacquelyn; Goldfarb, Johanna. What went wrong: multiple perspectives on an adolescent's decision to refuse blood transfusions. *Clinical Pediatrics.* 1996 Jun; 35(6): 317–321. 6 refs. BE62107.
   *adolescents; autonomy; beneficence; *blood transfusions; case studies; communication; competence; *decision making; disadvantaged; dissent; *Jehovah's Witnesses; patient care; patient care team; physician patient relationship; physicians; professional family relationship; religion; socioeconomic factors; *treatment refusal; trust; uncertainty; values

Maine. Supreme Judicial Court. In re Nikolas E. *Atlantic Reporter, 2d Series.* 1998 Nov 19 (date of decision). 720: 562–568. BE62344.
   *children; *HIV seropositivity; *investigational drugs; *legal aspects; minors; *mothers; parents; patient care; *risks and benefits; state interest; *therapeutic research; *treatment refusal; *In re Nikolas E.; Maine
   The Supreme Judicial Court of Maine upheld a lower court decision allowing a mother who had been charged

with parental neglect to retain custody of her HIV-positive four-year-old son, whose recommended, but highly aggressive and experimental antiviral drug treatment, she had delayed. Both of the child's divorced parents are HIV positive, and his older sister died at age 4 from AIDS complications after receiving the drug therapy. The court found that there was insufficient proof of likely benefit and lack of significant harm from the drug regimen. Furthermore the court was unable to determine the likely effects of treatment on the child. Consequently the court decided that the mother's decision to delay new and experimental treatment was not serious parental neglect. (KIE abstract)

Mason, John Kenyon. Consent to treatment and research in children. *In: his* Medico-Legal Aspects of Reproduction and Parenthood. Second Edition. Brookfield, VT: Ashgate; 1998: 319–339. 83 fn. ISBN 1-84104-065-8. BE61070.
   adolescents; *alternative therapies; animal organs; blood transfusions; *competence; comprehension; decision making; donors; *human experimentation; *informed consent; international aspects; Jehovah's Witnesses; judicial action; *legal aspects; *minors; nontherapeutic research; *organ donation; organ donors; organ transplantation; *parental consent; *parents; *patient care; religion; research subjects; risks and benefits; siblings; state interest; therapeutic research; *tissue donation; *treatment refusal; *Great Britain; United States

Neild, Patricia. Irreconcilable differences: a parent's right to refuse to consent to the medical treatment of a child. *Family and Conciliation Courts Review.* 1995 Jul; 33(3): 342–360. 46 fn. BE59199.
   allowing to die; autonomy; *children; congenital disorders; disabled; drugs; fetuses; *judicial action; *legal aspects; legal rights; leukemia; mentally retarded; newborns; *parents; personhood; pregnant women; prenatal injuries; privacy; prolongation of life; quality of life; state interest; surgery; terminally ill; *treatment refusal; value of life; withholding treatment; chemotherapy; *Canada; Freeman, Craig; Nova Scotia

Nicholls, Michael. Keyholders and flak jackets: consent to medical treatment for children. *Family Law.* 1994 Feb; 24: 81–85. BE61826.
   adolescents; age factors; competence; decision making; emergency care; *informed consent; judicial action; *legal aspects; *minors; parental consent; parents; patient care; *treatment refusal; *Great Britain

Otten, Marc. Parents refuse to allow life-saving treatment for newborn: our moral obligation. *Princeton Journal of Bioethics.* 1998 Spring; 1(1): 61–64. 2 refs. BE62492.
   *allowing to die; *congenital disorders; decision making; killing; moral obligations; *newborns; *parents; physicians; rights; selection for treatment; *treatment refusal; wedge argument; withholding treatment

Paris, John J.; Schreiber, Michael D. Parental discretion in refusal of treatment for newborns: a real but limited right. *Clinics in Perinatology.* 1996 Sep; 23(3): 573–581. 21 refs. BE60942.
   *allowing to die; *congenital disorders; *decision making; dissent; Down syndrome; legal aspects; *low birth weight; morbidity; mortality; *newborns; *parents; physicians; prognosis; resuscitation; rights; risks and benefits; selection for treatment; treatment outcome; *treatment refusal; uncertainty; values; withholding treatment; State v. Messenger; United States

Robinson, John H.; Berry, Roberta M.; McDonnell, Kevin, eds. Neonates and children. *In: their* A Health

---

Law Reader: An Interdisciplinary Approach. Durham, NC: Carolina Academic Press; 1999: 181–238. 46 fn. ISBN 0-89089-907-X. BE62293.
  *allowing to die; *anencephaly; *children; Christian Scientists; *congenital disorders; cultural pluralism; *decision making; determination of death; *disabled; futility; human experimentation; informed consent; *legal aspects; legal liability; legal rights; *newborns; nontherapeutic research; *organ donation; *parents; patient care; personhood; prolongation of life; quality of life; religion; *rights; risks and benefits; social discrimination; standards; therapeutic research; third party consent; *treatment refusal; *value of life; wedge argument; withholding treatment; Americans with Disabilities Act 1990; United States

Ross, Lainie Friedman. Children, Families, and Health Care Decision Making. New York, NY: Clarendon Press; 1998. 197 p. (Issues in biomedical ethics). Bibliography: p. 177–190. ISBN 0-19-823763-4. BE61944.
  *adolescents; advisory committees; *autonomy; case studies; *children; *competence; *decision making; deontological ethics; directed donation; dissent; family members; *family relationship; federal government; futility; goals; government regulation; guidelines; *human experimentation; legal aspects; *minors; moral development; *moral obligations; nontherapeutic research; *organ donation; *parental consent; *parents; *patient care; pediatrics; personhood; physicians; prolongation of life; quality of life; refusal to treat; rights; risk; risks and benefits; sexuality; siblings; state interest; therapeutic research; *treatment refusal; utilitarianism; *values; liberalism; needs; National Commission for the Protection of Human Subjects; United States

Schmidt, Kelli. "Who are you to say what my best interest is?" Minors' due process rights when admitted by parents for inpatient mental health treatment. [Comment]. *Washington Law Review.* 1996 Oct; 71(4): 1187–1217. 202 fn. BE59417.
  behavior disorders; constitutional law; *due process; freedom; *involuntary commitment; *judicial action; *legal aspects; *legal rights; mental institutions; *mentally ill; *minors; parental consent; privacy; proprietary health facilities; psychiatric diagnosis; Supreme Court decisions; *treatment refusal; voluntary admission; Parham v. J.R.; *State ex rel. T.B. v. CPC Fairfax Hospital; United States; *Washington

Schneider, Carl E. Justification by faith. *Hastings Center Report.* 1999 Jan–Feb; 29(1): 24–25. 4 refs. BE61633.
  child abuse; death; *legal aspects; *legal liability; legal rights; *minors; *parents; *religion; state government; *treatment refusal; faith healing; Child Protective Services Act (PA); *Pennsylvania; *Pennsylvania v. Nixon

Smith, Martin L. Ethical perspectives on Jehovah's Witnesses' refusal of blood. *Cleveland Clinic Journal of Medicine.* 1997 Oct; 64(9): 475–481. 25 refs. BE59229.
  *adolescents; *adults; *autonomy; *beneficence; *blood transfusions; casuistry; *children; competence; conscience; *decision making; ethical analysis; informed consent; *Jehovah's Witnesses; justice; legal aspects; mentally retarded; *moral obligations; *parents; patient care; *physicians; referral and consultation; resource allocation; risks and benefits; *state interest; *treatment refusal

Smith, Stacey. Parents refuse to allow life-saving treatment for newborn: the right to choose. *Princeton Journal of Bioethics.* 1998 Spring; 1(1): 58–60. 4 refs. BE62491.
  *allowing to die; case studies; *congenital disorders; decision making; *newborns; *parents; physicians; prognosis; risks and benefits; standards; state interest; surgery; *treatment refusal; withholding treatment

Teicher, Stacy A. When minors refuse medical treatment.

[News]. *Christian Science Monitor.* 1999 Feb 9: 3. BE60966.
  *adolescents; autonomy; *blood transfusions; competence; decision making; *Jehovah's Witnesses; *legal aspects; *minors; parents; religion; *treatment refusal; value of life; Demos, Alexis; Massachusetts

Williams, L.; Harris, A.; Thompson, M., et al. Consent to treatment by minors attending accident and emergency departments: guidelines. *Journal of Accident and Emergency Medicine.* 1997 Sep; 14(5): 286–289. 2 refs. BE59430.
  adolescents; children; competence; critically ill; decision analysis; *emergency care; *guidelines; hospitals; *informed consent; judicial action; *legal aspects; *minors; *parental consent; *parents; physical restraint; *physicians; referral and consultation; third party consent; *treatment refusal; Children Act 1989 (Great Britain); Family Law Reform Act 1969 (Great Britain); *Great Britain

Court says mother has right to stop HIV drugs for son. *AIDS Policy and Law.* 1998 Oct 2; 13(18): 1, 4–5. 1 ref. BE61300.
  child abuse; *children; decision making; *drugs; *HIV seropositivity; *legal aspects; *legal rights; mothers; *parents; *risks and benefits; state interest; *treatment refusal; uncertainty; *In re Nikolas Emerson; Maine

Do-not-resuscitate order; public school — ABC School and DEF School v. Mr. and Mrs. M. *Mental and Physical Disability Law Reporter.* 1997 Nov–Dec; 21(6): 735. Synopsis of a 17 July 1997 ruling by a Massachusetts Superior Court. BE59846.
  *children; *directive adherence; *disabled; *institutional policies; *legal aspects; legal rights; *parents; prolongation of life; *resuscitation orders; *schools; *students; *treatment refusal; *ABC School and DEF School v. Mr. and Mrs. M.; *Massachusetts

TRIAGE *See* SELECTION FOR TREATMENT

TRUTH DISCLOSURE

Berger, Jeffrey T. Culture and ethnicity in clinical care. *Archives of Internal Medicine.* 1998 Oct 26; 158(19): 2085–2090. 110 refs. BE59577.
  *advance directives; *alternative therapies; American Indians; Asian Americans; *attitudes; autopsies; blacks; cancer; *cultural pluralism; family relationship; health; Hispanic Americans; knowledge, attitudes, practice; living wills; *minority groups; nutrition; *organ donation; *patient care; physicians; preventive medicine; prolongation of life; socioeconomic factors; *truth disclosure; whites; withholding treatment; United States

Caulfield, Timothy; Dossetor, John; Boshkov, Lynn, et al. Notifying patients exposed to blood products associated with Creutzfeldt-Jakob disease: integrating science, legal duties and ethical mandates. *Canadian Medical Association Journal.* 1997 Nov 15; 157(10): 1389–1392. 41 refs. BE59682.
  autonomy; beneficence; *blood transfusions; brain pathology; central nervous system diseases; *disclosure; *duty to warn; health personnel; hemophilia; iatrogenic disease; *information dissemination; informed consent; *legal obligations; *moral obligations; *moral policy; patients; *public policy; resource allocation; *risk; risks and benefits; *truth disclosure; *Creutzfeldt-Jakob syndrome; recontact; Canada

Chadwick, Ruth. The philosophy of the right to know and the right not to know. *In:* Chadwick, Ruth; Levitt, Mairi; Shickle, Darren, eds. The Right to Know and

the Right Not to Know. Brookfield, VT: Ashgate; 1997: 13–22. 13 refs. ISBN 1-85972-424-8. BE62184.
autonomy; communitarianism; confidentiality; disclosure; *ethical analysis; family members; genetic counseling; genetic disorders; *genetic information; genetic predisposition; *genetic screening; insurance; mass screening; moral obligations; patients; privacy; reproduction; *rights; teleological ethics; *truth disclosure; utilitarianism; duty to know; *right not to know

Charlton, Rodger; Simone, Charles B.; Simone, Nicole L., et al. Do we always need to tell patients the truth? [Letters]. *Lancet.* 1998 Nov 28; 352(9142): 1787. 11 refs. BE61028.
*attitudes; *cancer; cultural pluralism; diagnosis; disclosure; informed consent; *international aspects; legal aspects; mortality; *patients; physicians; *prognosis; *public opinion; quality of life; risks and benefits; survey; terminally ill; *truth disclosure; Arato v. Avedon; Australia; Denmark; Italy; *Japan; United Arab Emirates; *United States

Costantini-Ferrando, Maria F.; Foley, Kathleen M.; Rapkin, Bruce D., et al. Communicating with patients about advanced cancer. [Letters and responses]. *JAMA.* 1998 Oct 28; 280(16): 1403–1404. 5 refs. BE60083.
advance care planning; advance directives; *cancer; *communication; comparative studies; *comprehension; *decision making; mortality; *palliative care; *patients; *physicians; *prognosis; *prolongation of life; risk; suffering; survey; *terminal care; *terminally ill; *truth disclosure; Memorial Sloan-Kettering Cancer Center (NYC)

Dickerson, Denise Ann. A doctor's duty to disclose life expectancy information to terminally ill patients. [Note]. *Cleveland State Law Review.* 1995; 43(2): 319–350. 293 fn. BE59241.
cancer; decision making; disclosure; family members; informed consent; *legal aspects; legal obligations; physicians; *prognosis; standards; terminal care; *terminally ill; *truth disclosure; *life expectancy; *Arato v. Avedon; California

Gilligan, Timothy; Raffin, Thomas A. End-of-life discussions with patients: timing and truth-telling. [Editorial]. *Chest.* 1996 Jan; 109(1): 11–12. 11 refs. BE60427.
*advance care planning; advance directives; *allowing to die; chronically ill; communication; critically ill; *decision making; *patient participation; *physician patient relationship; *physicians; prognosis; terminally ill; *truth disclosure; ventilators

Groveman, Sherri A. The Hanukkah bush: ethical implications in the clinical management of intersex. *Journal of Clinical Ethics.* 1998 Winter; 9(4): 356–359. BE60485.
*adolescents; *children; congenital disorders; *counseling; *deception; diagnosis; females; *infants; *intersexuality; Jews; males; normality; parents; *patient care; physicians; *psychological stress; *sexuality; stigmatization; *surgery; *truth disclosure; support groups

Hamajima, Nobuyuki; Tajima, Kazuo; Morishita, Mayumi, et al. Patients' expectations of information provided at cancer hospitals in Japan. *Japanese Journal of Clinical Oncology.* 1996 Oct; 26(5): 362–367. 15 refs. BE60187.
age factors; alternatives; *attitudes; *cancer; *diagnosis; drugs; females; hospitals; males; patient care; *patients; prognosis; survey; *truth disclosure; *Aichi Cancer Center Hospital; *Japan

Hassn, A.M.F.; Hassan, A. Do we always need to tell patients the truth? [Letter]. *Lancet.* 1998 Oct 3;

352(9134): 1153. 2 refs. BE60085.
cancer; death; diagnosis; mentally ill; paternalism; physicians; prognosis; *psychological stress; risks and benefits; terminally ill; *truth disclosure

Higgs, Roger. Truth-telling. *In:* Kuhse, Helga; Singer, Peter, eds. A Companion to Bioethics. Malden, MA: Blackwell; 1998: 432–440. 30 refs. ISBN 0-631-19737-0. BE59516.
autonomy; beneficence; communication; cultural pluralism; deception; diagnosis; moral policy; paternalism; physician patient relationship; prognosis; risks and benefits; *truth disclosure; uncertainty

Hingorani, Melanie; Wong, Tina; Vafidis, Gilli. Patients' and doctors' attitudes to amount of information given after unintended injury during treatment: cross sectional, questionnaire survey. *BMJ (British Medical Journal).* 1999 Mar 6; 318(7184): 640–641. 5 refs. BE61701.
*attitudes; *disclosure; *iatrogenic disease; injuries; *medical errors; ophthalmology; *patients; *physicians; prognosis; self regulation; surgery; survey; *truth disclosure; General Medical Council (Great Britain); Great Britain

King, Susan M.; Watson, Heather; Heurter, Helen, et al. Notifying patients exposed to blood products associated with Creutzfeldt-Jakob disease: theoretical risk for real people. *Canadian Medical Association Journal.* 1998 Oct 6; 159(7): 771–774. 23 refs. BE62357.
adolescents; *attitudes; *blood transfusions; central nervous system diseases; children; communication; *disclosure; duty to warn; iatrogenic disease; parental notification; *parents; *patients; psychological stress; *risk; risks and benefits; survey; *truth disclosure; *Creutzfeldt-Jakob syndrome; recontact; Canada; Hospital for Sick Children (Toronto); Ontario

Kipnis, Kenneth; Diamond, Milton. Pediatric ethics and the surgical assignment of sex. *Journal of Clinical Ethics.* 1998 Winter; 9(4): 398–410. 56 fn. BE60490.
adolescents; adults; age factors; attitudes; beneficence; case studies; congenital disorders; *cosmetic surgery; counseling; deception; diagnosis; empirical research; ethics consultation; females; hormones; *infants; *intersexuality; males; medical ethics; *newborns; *normality; organizational policies; parents; *patient care; patient satisfaction; patients; *pediatrics; *physicians; prevalence; professional organizations; psychological stress; psychology; *risks and benefits; selection for treatment; self concept; *sexuality; standards; *surgery; transsexualism; *treatment outcome; *truth disclosure; twins; uncertainty; values; support groups; American Academy of Pediatrics

Larke, Bryce. The quandary of Creutzfeldt-Jakob disease. [Editorial]. *Canadian Medical Association Journal.* 1998 Oct 6; 159(7): 789–792. 22 refs. BE62359.
attitudes; blood donation; *blood transfusions; brain pathology; central nervous system diseases; *disclosure; *duty to warn; iatrogenic disease; industry; patients; physicians; public policy; *risk; risks and benefits; *truth disclosure; uncertainty; *Creutzfeldt-Jakob syndrome; recontact; Canada

Levitt, Mairi. Sociological perspectives on the right to know and the right not to know. *In:* Chadwick, Ruth; Levitt, Mairi; Shickle, Darren, eds. The Right to Know and the Right Not to Know. Brookfield, VT: Ashgate; 1997: 29–36. 16 refs. 3 fn. ISBN 1-85972-424-8. BE62186.
autonomy; disadvantaged; genetic counseling; *genetic information; *genetic screening; health promotion; mass screening; paternalism; rights; *risks and benefits; self induced illness; social sciences; *socioeconomic factors;

BE = bioethics accession number   fn. = footnotes   refs. = references

*truth disclosure; right not to know; Great Britain

Maher, John T.; Pask, Eleanor G. When truth hurts.... *In:* Adams, David W.; Deveau, Eleanor J., eds. Beyond the Innocence of Childhood: Helping Children and Adolescents Cope with Life–Threatening Illness and Dying. Amityville, NY: Baywood Publishing; 1995: 267–293. 38 refs. ISBN 0–89503–129–9. BE60658.
    adolescents; age factors; autonomy; beneficence; cancer; *children; competence; comprehension; cultural pluralism; deception; decision making; diagnosis; futility; health personnel; HIV seropositivity; informed consent; parent child relationship; parents; patient participation; professional patient relationship; prognosis; psychological stress; quality of life; religion; rights; risks and benefits; suffering; terminal care; *terminally ill; *truth disclosure

Michel, Vicki. Factoring ethnic and racial differences into bioethics decision making. *Generations (American Society on Aging).* 1994 Winter; 18(4): 23–26. 8 refs. BE60547.
    autonomy; coercion; communication; *cultural pluralism; *decision making; diagnosis; disclosure; *family members; family relationship; informed consent; *minority groups; physicians; privacy; professional family relationship; *professional patient relationship; prognosis; *truth disclosure; values; United States

Okamura, Hitoshi; Uchitomi, Yosuke; Sasako, Mitsuru, et al. Guidelines for telling the truth to cancer patients. *Japanese Journal of Clinical Oncology.* 1998 Jan; 28(1): 1–4. 8 refs. BE60188.
    *cancer; communication; comprehension; *diagnosis; family members; *guidelines; hospitals; institutional policies; nurse's role; patients; physicians; privacy; psychiatry; psychological stress; referral and consultation; *truth disclosure; continuity of patient care; *Japan; National Cancer Center Hospital (Tokyo)

Pang, Mei–che Samantha. Protective truthfulness: the Chinese way of safeguarding patients in informed treatment decisions. *Journal of Medical Ethics.* 1999 Jun; 25(3): 247–253. 42 refs. BE61859.
    autonomy; *beneficence; competence; confidentiality; cultural pluralism; *decision making; diagnosis; disclosure; empirical research; evaluation studies; *family members; historical aspects; hospitals; *informed consent; *medical ethics; *moral obligations; non–Western World; *nurse patient relationship; *nurses; nursing ethics; nursing research; *paternalism; patient care; patients' rights; *physician patient relationship; physicians; privacy; professional competence; prognosis; psychological stress; survey; terminal care; *third party consent; trust; *truth disclosure; value of life; values; virtues; vulnerable populations; hope; *China
The first part of this paper examines the practice of informed treatment decisions in the protective medical system in China today. The second part examines how health care professionals in China perceive and carry out their responsibilities when relaying information to vulnerable patients, based on the findings of an empirical study that I had undertaken to examine the moral experience of nurses in practice situations. In the Chinese medical ethics tradition, refinement [jing] in skills and sincerity [cheng] in relating to patients are two cardinal virtues that health care professionals are required to possess. This notion of absolute sincerity carries a strong sense of parental protectiveness. The empirical findings reveal that most nurses are ambivalent about telling the truth to patients. Truth–telling would become an insincere act if a patient were to lose hope and confidence in life after learning of his or her disease. In this system of protective medical care, it is arguable as to whose interests are being protected: the patient, the family or the hospital. I would suggest that the interests of the hospital and the family members who legitimately

represent the patient's interests are being honoured, but at the expense of the patient's right to know.

Phillips, Ben; Reagan, James E. VHA ethics rounds: [truth–telling]. *NCCE News (Veterans Health Administration National Center for Clinical Ethics).* 1998 Winter; 6(1): 4–5. 1 fn. BE59849.
    case studies; deception; diagnosis; family members; patients; physician patient relationship; prognosis; trust; *truth disclosure

Preves, Sharon E. For the sake of the children: destigmatizing intersexuality. *Journal of Clinical Ethics.* 1998 Winter; 9(4): 411–420. 24 fn. BE60491.
    *adolescents; *adults; *attitudes; *children; congenital disorders; *cosmetic surgery; deception; diagnosis; genetic counseling; hormones; *intersexuality; *newborns; normality; parents; patient care; *patient satisfaction; *patients; physicians; *psychological stress; quality of life; *self concept; *sexuality; *stigmatization; *surgery; survey; transsexualism; *treatment outcome; *truth disclosure; empowerment; qualitative research; support groups; North America

Ruddick, William. Hope and deception. *Bioethics.* 1999 Jul; 13(3–4): 343–357. 16 fn. BE61884.
    allowing to die; autonomy; beneficence; children; *deception; emotions; family members; futility; motivation; parents; patients; physician patient relationship; physicians; placebos; principle–based ethics; professional family relationship; prognosis; *risks and benefits; terminally ill; trust; *truth disclosure; *hope
Convinced of hope's therapeutic benefits, physicians routinely support patients' false hopes, often with family collusion and vague, euphemistic diagnoses and prognoses, if not overt lies. Bioethicists charge them with paternalistic violations of Patient Autonomy. There are, I think, too many morally significant exceptions to accept the physician's rationales, or the bioethicist's criticisms, stated sweepingly. Physicians need to take account of the harms caused by loss of hopes, especially false hopes due to deception, as well as of the harms of successfully maintained deceptive hopes. As for autonomy, hopes –– even if based on deception –– can protect and enhance autonomy, understood broadly as the capacity to lead a chosen or embraced life. Deception aside, patients' hopes often rest on beliefs about *possible* rather than *probable* outcomes –– beliefs themselves supported by optimism, 'denial', or self-deception. Such 'possibility-hopes' may conflict with physicians' often more fact-sensitive 'probability hopes.' To resolve such conflicts physicians may try to 'down-shift' patients' or parents' hopes to lesser, more realistic hopes. Alternatively, physicians may alter or enlarge their own professional hopes to include the 'vital hopes' that define the lives of patients or parents, as well as 'survival hopes' needed to face and bear the loss of loved ones, especially children. A principle of Hope-giving might help guide such sympathetic hope-accommodations. More generally, it would give Hope a distinct place among Beneficence, Autonomy, and the other moral factors already highlighted by canonical principles of Medical Ethics. To formulate such a principle, however, we will need a collective Project Hope to pursue deeper philosophical and psychological studies.

Sibbald, Barbara. Blood recipients and CJD: to notify or not to notify, that is the question. *Canadian Medical Association Journal.* 1998 Oct 6; 159(7): 829–831. BE62361.
    *attitudes; blood donation; *blood transfusions; central nervous system diseases; *disclosure; *duty to warn;

BE = bioethics accession number   fn. = footnotes   refs. = references

iatrogenic disease; parents; *patients; public policy; *risk; risks and benefits; *truth disclosure; *Creutzfeldt-Jakob syndrome; recontact; Canada

Silverman, Ralph. Informing the cancer patient. *Missouri Medicine.* 1997 Jul; 94(7): 317–318. 3 refs. BE61444.
    *cancer; decision making; diagnosis; physicians; prognosis; *truth disclosure

Spinsanti, Sandro. Obtaining consent from the family: a horizon for clinical ethics. *In:* ten Have, Henk A.M.J.; Sass, Hans–Martin, eds. Consensus Formation in Healthcare Ethics. Boston, MA: Kluwer Academic; 1998: 209–217. 5 refs. 3 fn. ISBN 0–7923–4944–X. BE62596.
    allowing to die; autonomy; beneficence; cancer; caring; case studies; consensus; *decision making; diagnosis; *family members; family relationship; paternalism; patient advocacy; *physician's role; physicians; *professional family relationship; prognosis; prolongation of life; terminal care; terminally ill; *third party consent; *truth disclosure; withholding treatment; *Italy

Takala, Tuija. The right to genetic ignorance confirmed. *Bioethics.* 1999 Jul; 13(3–4): 288–293. 15 fn. BE61879.
    *autonomy; children; decision making; family members; genetic disorders; *genetic information; *genetic screening; *moral obligations; *moral policy; reproduction; *rights; suffering; *truth disclosure; harms; *right not to know
One of the much debated issues around the evolving human genetics is the question of the right to know versus the right not to know. The core question of this theme is whether an *individual* has the right to know about her own genetic constitution and further, does she also have the right to remain in ignorance. Within liberal traditions it is usually held that people, if they so wish, have the right to all the knowledge available about themselves. This right is based on the value of autonomy or on the right of self–determination, and it is sometimes partly justified as a countermeasure to the authorities' control over people. I do not wish to deny the right to genetic knowledge (about oneself). I think that its existence is self–evident. The argument I want to put forth in this paper is that in liberal societies we should acknowledge people's right to remain in ignorance as well. The only reason for not doing this would be that grave harm to others would follow if people were allowed to make these seemingly self–regarding decisions. Arguments presented against the right to ignorance are two–fold. First there are those arguing against the right to ignorance on the grounds of harm to others, that is, philosophers who do not deny people's right to ignorance in self–related matters but wish to state that genetic ignorance causes harm to others, and this is one of the most commonly accepted reasons for restricting people's freedom. The other line of argument flows from the Kantian view that not even merely self–regarding foolishness (in the eyes of others) should be allowed.

Vassilas, C.A.; Donaldson, J. Few GPs tell patients of their diagnosis of Alzheimer's disease. [Letter]. *BMJ (British Medical Journal).* 1999 Feb 20; 318(7182): 536. 2 refs. BE62251.
    cancer; *dementia; *diagnosis; *family practice; *knowledge, attitudes, practice; *physicians; survey; terminally ill; *truth disclosure; Great Britain

Whitney, Simon N.; Spiegel, David. The patient, the physician, and the truth. [Case study and commentaries]. *Hastings Center Report.* 1999 May–Jun; 29(3): 24–25. BE61409.

autonomy; *cancer; case studies; communication; competence; diagnosis; moral obligations; paternalism; physician patient relationship; physicians; prognosis; *truth disclosure; *right not to know

Wilson, Bruce E.; Reiner, William G. Management of intersex: a shifting paradigm. *Journal of Clinical Ethics.* 1998 Winter; 9(4): 360–369. 32 fn. BE60486.
    *adolescents; *children; congenital disorders; *cosmetic surgery; *counseling; *decision making; diagnosis; disclosure; empirical research; *hormones; *infants; informed consent; *intersexuality; *newborns; normality; *parents; *patient care; *patient care team; *patient participation; *physicians; psychological stress; *sexuality; *surgery; transsexualism; treatment outcome; trends; *truth disclosure

Wu, Albert W.; Cavanaugh, Thomas A.; McPhee, Stephen J., et al. To tell the truth: ethical and practical issues in disclosing medical mistakes to patients. *Journal of General Internal Medicine.* 1997 Dec; 12(12): 770–775. 31 refs. BE59534.
    beneficence; communication; competence; deontological ethics; *disclosure; iatrogenic disease; injuries; interprofessional relations; legal liability; *medical errors; medical ethics; *moral obligations; *negligence; *patient care; patients; physician patient relationship; *physicians; *risks and benefits; teleological ethics; *truth disclosure; uncertainty; whistleblowing

WAR

Barnaby, Wendy. Biological weapons and genetic engineering. *GenEthics News.* 1997 Jun–Jul; No. 18: 4–5. BE60819.
    *biological warfare; *genetic intervention; genetic research; international aspects; microbiology; minority groups; United States

Blumenthal, Ralph; Miller, Judith. Japanese germ–war atrocities: a half–century of stonewalling the world. *New York Times.* 1999 Mar 4: A12. BE60974.
    *biological warfare; dehumanization; disclosure; federal government; historical aspects; *human experimentation; investigators; military personnel; *misconduct; moral complicity; *prisoners; *public policy; records; *scientific misconduct; torture; China; *Japan; Twentieth Century; United States; *World War II

Lerner, Paul. Rationalizing the therapeutic arsenal: German neuropsychiatry in World War I. *In:* Berg, Manfred; Cocks, Geoffrey, eds. Medicine and Modernity: Public Health and Medical Care in Nineteenth– and Twentieth–Century Germany. New York, NY: Cambridge University Press; 1997: 121–148. 106 fn. ISBN 0–521–56411–5. BE59268.
    *attitudes; coercion; common good; deception; electroconvulsive therapy; *historical aspects; hypnosis; *mental health; *mentally ill; methods; *military personnel; misconduct; obligations to society; *patient care; physician patient relationship; physician's role; *physicians; psychiatric diagnosis; *psychiatry; psychotherapy; *public policy; rehabilitation; social control; social dominance; *war; post–traumatic stress disorders; *Germany; *Twentieth Century; *World War I

Maddocks, Ian. Evolution of the physicians' peace movement: a historical perspective. *Health and Human Rights.* 1996; 2(1): 89–109. 36 fn. BE62086.
    developing countries; ecology; *historical aspects; human rights; international aspects; lawyers; nuclear warfare; organizational policies; *physician's role; *physicians; *political activity; professional organizations; public health; *war; Africa; Europe; Great Britain; *International

---

BE = bioethics accession number   fn. = footnotes   refs. = references

Physicians for the Prevention of Nuclear War; Medical Association for the Prevention of War; Medical Campaign Against Nuclear Weapons; Physicians for Social Responsibility; Twentieth Century; United States

Morris, Kelly. US military face punishment for refusing anthrax vaccine. [News]. *Lancet.* 1999 Jan 9; 353(9147): 130. BE60981.
  *biological warfare; *immunization; mandatory programs; *military personnel; *punishment; *risks and benefits; voluntary programs; *refusal to participate; *Canada; Great Britain; *United States

Myers, Steven Lee. Airman discharged for refusal to take anthrax vaccine as rebellion grows. [News]. *New York Times.* 1999 Mar 11: A24. BE60908.
  *biological warfare; *immunization; *military personnel; *punishment; *refusal to participate; Bettendorf, Jeffrey; United States

O'Rourke, Dennis. Half Life: A Parable for the Nuclear Age. [Videorecording]. Available from Direct Cinema Ltd., P.O. Box 69799, Los Angeles, CA, 90069, (213)396-4774; 1986. Videocassette; 86 min.; sd., color; VHS. ISBN 1-55974-135-X. Written, directed, and produced by Dennis O'Rourke. BE62227.
  cancer; deception; developing countries; federal government; genetic disorders; health hazards; *human experimentation; injuries; *morbidity; *nontherapeutic research; *nuclear warfare; *public policy; *radiation; *scientific misconduct; Atomic Energy Commission; Department of Energy; *Micronesia; *United States

Pearson, Graham S. How to make microbes safer. *Nature.* 1998 Jul 16; 394(6690): 217-218. BE59154.
  *biological warfare; ecology; genetic intervention; guidelines; health hazards; *international aspects; *microbiology; recombinant DNA research; *regulation; risks and benefits; *transgenic organisms

Richey, Warren. A vaccination war erupts in military. [News]. *Christian Science Monitor.* 1999 Jan 28: 2. BE61007.
  *biological warfare; *immunization; mandatory programs; *military personnel; punishment; *risks and benefits; voluntary programs; *refusal to participate; Great Britain; *United States

Schofer, Joel Martin. Violations of informed consent during war. *JAMA.* 1999 May 5; 281(17): 1657. 8 refs. BE62310.
  *biological warfare; decision making; *drugs; federal government; government regulation; human experimentation; *immunization; *informed consent; *investigational drugs; mandatory programs; *military personnel; *preventive medicine; research subjects; risks and benefits; therapeutic research; voluntary programs; *war; chemical warfare; Department of Defense; Food and Drug Administration; *Persian Gulf War; United States

Tanaka, Yuki. Japanese biological warfare plans and experiments on POWs. *In: his* Hidden Horrors: Japanese War Crimes in World War II. Boulder, CO: Westview Press; 1996: 135-165, 238-242. 72 fn. ISBN 0-8133-2718-0. BE60510.
  *biological warfare; communicable diseases; *dehumanization; *historical aspects; *human experimentation; international aspects; *investigators; killing; military personnel; misconduct; National Socialism; nutrition; *physicians; *prisoners; psychology; public policy; *scientific misconduct; China; *Japan; Manchuria; Rabaul; *Twentieth Century; World War II

Tokuda, Yasuharu; Kadlec, Robert F.; Zelicoff, Alan

P. Physicians and biological warfare agents. [Letter and response]. *JAMA.* 1998 Jan 28; 279(4): 273-274. 8 refs. BE59183.
  *biological warfare; international aspects; investigators; microbiology; misconduct; *physicians; Biological and Toxin Weapons Convention 1972; Japan; United States; World War II

U.S. Food and Drug Administration. Accessibility to new drugs for use in military and civilian exigencies when traditional human efficacy studies are not feasible; determination under the interim rule that informed consent is not feasible for military exigencies; request for comments. *Federal Register.* 1997 Jul 31; 62(147): 40996-41001. BE59405.
  *biological warfare; federal government; *government regulation; *human experimentation; *informed consent; *investigational drugs; *military personnel; public policy; toxicity; volunteers; *war; Department of Defense; *Food and Drug Administration; *Persian Gulf War; United States

WITHHOLDING TREATMENT *See* ALLOWING TO DIE, RESUSCITATION ORDERS

WOMEN'S HEALTH *See* HEALTH

WRONGFUL BIRTH *See* WRONGFUL LIFE

WRONGFUL LIFE

Baier, Kurt. Wrongful death and wrongful life. *In: his* Problems of Life and Death: A Humanist Perspective. Amherst, NY: Prometheus Books; 1997: 137-230. 74 fn. ISBN 1-57392-153-X. BE61848.
  *allowing to die; *assisted suicide; capital punishment; contraception; disabled; disclosure; ethical theory; guidelines; *humanism; intention; *killing; law; legal aspects; legal liability; moral obligations; *moral policy; *morality; negligence; organ donation; physicians; *population control; prognosis; *prolongation of life; quality of life; suffering; suicide; value of life; values; *voluntary euthanasia; wrongful death; *wrongful life; rationality

Gillon, Raanan. 'Wrongful life' claims. [Editorial]. *Journal of Medical Ethics.* 1998 Dec; 24(6): 363-364. 1 ref. BE60784.
  abortion, induced; children; contraception; *disabled; *genetic counseling; health personnel; *legal liability; *negligence; wedge argument; *wrongful life

Mason, John Kenyon. Protection of the fetus. *In: his* Medico-Legal Aspects of Reproduction and Parenthood. Second Edition. Brookfield, VT: Ashgate; 1998: 143-186. 179 fn. ISBN 1-84104-065-8. BE61064.
  *aborted fetuses; abortion, induced; alcohol abuse; allowing to die; autonomy; beginning of life; brain death; cesarean section; coercion; compensation; competence; congenital disorders; criminal law; drug abuse; fetal development; *fetal therapy; *fetuses; genetic counseling; genetic disorders; infanticide; international aspects; *legal aspects; *legal liability; *legal rights; mentally ill; methods; negligence; personhood; physicians; *pregnant women; prenatal diagnosis; *prenatal injuries; prolongation of life; public policy; selective abortion; terminally ill; torts; treatment refusal; value of life; ventilators; viability; *wrongful death; *wrongful life; Abortion Act 1967 (Great Britain); Congenital Disabilities (Civil Liability) Act 1976 (Great Britain); *Great Britain; Infant Life (Preservation) Act 1929 (Great Britain); Scotland; United States

Mason, John Kenyon. Sterilisation. *In: his* Medico-Legal

BE = bioethics accession number   fn. = footnotes   refs. = references

Aspects of Reproduction and Parenthood. Second Edition. Brookfield, VT: Ashgate; 1998: 67-106. 149 fn. ISBN 1-84104-065-8. BE61062.

  adults; autonomy; compensation; competence; decision making; eugenics; females; historical aspects; human rights; informed consent; international aspects; *involuntary sterilization; judicial action; *legal aspects; legal liability; legal rights; males; mentally disabled; minors; National Socialism; parental consent; paternalism; physicians; punishment; reproduction; risks and benefits; sex offenses; spousal consent; state interest; *sterilization (sexual); Supreme Court decisions; third party consent; *voluntary sterilization; *wrongful life; Australia; Canada; Declaration of Tokyo; European Convention for the Protection of Human Rights; Germany; *Great Britain; Twentieth Century; United States

Perry, Clifton. Children's suits for suffering life. *Pediatrician.* 1990; 17(2): 79-86. 20 fn. BE59451.

  allowing to die; compensation; congenital disorders; disclosure; federal government; *legal liability; legal rights; negligence; *newborns; parents; physicians; prenatal diagnosis; risk; selective abortion; state government; *torts; *wrongful life; *United States

Roberts, Melinda A. Child versus Childmaker: Future Persons and Present Duties in Ethics and the Law. Lanham, MD: Rowman and Littlefield; 1998. 235 p. (Studies in social, political, and legal philosophy). Bibliography: p. 221-226. ISBN 0-8476-8901-8. BE59868.

  children; *cloning; congenital disorders; constitutional law; embryos; freedom; *future generations; injuries; justice; legal aspects; *moral obligations; negligence; philosophy; privacy; quality of life; *reproduction; reproductive technologies; suffering; *teleological ethics; torts; value of life; *wrongful life; Broome, John; Fourteenth Amendment; United States

Roberts, Melinda A. Present duties and future persons: when are existence-inducing acts wrong? *Law and Philosophy.* 1995 Nov; 14(3-4): 297-327. 50 fn. BE59358.

  adolescents; children; cloning; congenital disorders; contracts; embryo transfer; in vitro fertilization; injuries; judicial action; legal aspects; *moral policy; motivation; negligence; organ donation; parents; philosophy; physicians; quality of life; *reproduction; *reproductive technologies; surrogate mothers; value of life; *wrongful life

Shapira, Amos. 'Wrongful life' lawsuits for faulty genetic counselling: should the impaired newborn be entitled to sue? *Journal of Medical Ethics.* 1998 Dec; 24(6): 369-375. 4 fn. BE60785.

  compensation; congenital disorders; *disabled; disclosure; *genetic counseling; genetic screening; health personnel; *legal aspects; *legal liability; *negligence; *newborns; parents; prenatal diagnosis; public health; public policy; right to die; selective abortion; value of life; wedge argument; *wrongful life; *Israel

A "wrongful life" suit is based on the purported tortious liability of a genetic counsellor towards an infant with hereditary defects, with the latter asserting that he or she would not have been born at all if not for the counsellor's negligence. This negligence allegedly lies in the failure on the part of the defendant adequately to advice the parents or to conduct properly the relevant testing and thereby prevent the child's conception or birth (where unimpaired life was not possible). This paper will offer support for the thesis that it would be both feasible and desirable to endorse "wrongful life" compensation actions. The genetic counsellor owed a duty of due professional care to the impaired newborn who now claims that but for the counsellor's negligence, he or she would not have been born at all. The plaintiff's defective life (where healthy life was never an option)

constitutes a compensable injury. A sufficient causal link may exist between the plaintiff's injury and the defendant's breach of duty of due professional care and an appropriate measure of damages can be allocated to the disabled newborn. Sanctioning a "wrongful life" cause of action does not necessarily entail abandoning valuable constraints with regard to abortion and euthanasia. Nor does it inevitably lead to an uncontrolled slide down a "slippery slope".

Wheale, Peter R. Moral and legal consequences for the fetus/unborn child of medical technologies derived from human genome research. *In:* Glasner, Peter; Rothman, Harry, eds. Genetic Imaginations: Ethical, Legal and Social Issues in Human Genome Research. Brookfield, VT: Ashgate; 1998: 83-96. 35 refs. Based on a paper presented at a workshop hosted by the Centre for Social and Economic Research at the University of the West of England; reprinted from *The Genetic Engineer and Biotechnologist*, 1995; 15(2-3). ISBN 1-84014-356-8. BE60020.

  abortion, induced; *beginning of life; coercion; *congenital disorders; deontological ethics; *embryo research; *embryos; ethical analysis; fetal development; *fetuses; genetic disorders; genetic screening; genome mapping; government regulation; *legal aspects; legal liability; *moral obligations; *moral policy; negligence; *personhood; pregnant women; prenatal injuries; *public policy; *quality of life; rights; *selective abortion; social impact; treatment refusal; utilitarianism; *value of life; *wrongful life; *Great Britain

---

BE = bioethics accession number   fn. = footnotes   refs. = references

AUTHOR INDEX

AUTHOR INDEX

A

Aaby, Peter see **Westergaard, Tine**

Aakvaag, Asbjørn see **Nylenna, Magne**

Aarons, D. Medical ethics: a sensitization to some important issues. *West Indian Medical Journal.* 1996 Sep; 45(3): 74–77.
(MEDICAL ETHICS)

Aarons, Derrick E. Medicine and its alternatives: health care priorities in the Caribbean. *Hastings Center Report.* 1999 Jul–Aug; 29(4): 23–27.
(HEALTH CARE/FOREIGN COUNTRIES)

Abbaszadegan, Mohammad R. see **Lerman, Caryn**

Abbott, Alison. 'Don't try to change embryo research law.' [News]. *Nature.* 1999 Mar 25; 398(6725): 275.
(EMBRYO AND FETAL RESEARCH)

Abbott, Alison. German scientists may escape fraud trial. [News]. *Nature.* 1998 Oct 8; 395(6702): 532–533.
(BIOMEDICAL RESEARCH; FRAUD AND MISCONDUCT)

Abbott, Alison. Science comes to terms with the lessons of fraud. [News]. *Nature.* 1999 Mar 4; 398(6722): 13–17.
(BIOMEDICAL RESEARCH; FRAUD AND MISCONDUCT)

Abbt, I. see **Müller, H.J.**

Abeles, Norman see **Clark, Barbara J.**

Abraham, John; Sheppard, Julie. Democracy, technocracy, and the secret state of medicines control: expert and nonexpert perspectives. *Science, Technology, and Human Values.* 1997 Spring; 22(2): 139–167.
(HEALTH CARE/FOREIGN COUNTRIES; PATIENT CARE/DRUGS)

Abrahamov, A. see **Elstein, D.**

Abrams, Judith Z.; Abrams, Steven A. The use of animals in medical research -- the health of the fetus and the newborn: a liberal halakhic perspective. *In:* Jacob, Walter; Zemer, Moshe, eds. The Fetus and Fertility in Jewish Law: Essays and Responsa. Pittsburgh, PA: Rodef Shalom Press; Freehof Institute of Progressive Halakhah; 1995: 119–130.
(ANIMAL EXPERIMENTATION)

Abrams, Judith Z. see **Freeman, David L.**

Abrams, Paula. Reservations about women: population policy and reproductive rights. *Cornell International Law Journal.* 1996; 29(1): 1–41.
(POPULATION CONTROL; REPRODUCTION)

Abrams, Steven A. see **Abrams, Judith Z.**

Abuelo, Dianne see **Lafayette, DeeDee**

Ach, Johann S. see **Boshammer, Susanne**

Achille, Marie A.; Ogloff, James R.P. When is a request for assisted suicide legitimate? Factors influencing public attitudes toward euthanasia. *Canadian Journal of Behavioural Science.* 1997 Jan; 29(1): 19–27.
(ALLOWING TO DIE/ATTITUDES; EUTHANASIA/ATTITUDES)

Achilles, Jennifer S. see **Croyle, Robert T.**

Achrekar, Abinash; Gupta, Rajesh; Pichayangkura, Chart; Chokevivat, Vichai; Limpakarnjanarat, Khanchit; Chuachoowong, Rutt; Bhadrakom, Chaiporn; Siriwasin, Wimol; Chearskul, Sanay; Chotpitayasunondh, Tawee; Shaffer, Nathan. Informed consent for a clinical trial in Thailand. [Letter and responses]. *New England Journal of Medicine.* 1998 Oct 29; 339(18): 1331–1332.
(AIDS/HUMAN EXPERIMENTATION; HUMAN EXPERIMENTATION/FOREIGN COUNTRIES; HUMAN EXPERIMENTATION/INFORMED CONSENT; HUMAN EXPERIMENTATION/RESEARCH DESIGN; HUMAN EXPERIMENTATION/SPECIAL POPULATIONS)

Ackerman, Elise see **Waldman, Steven**

Ad Hoc Committee on Health Care Issues and the Church. The non–profit nature of Catholic health care ministry. *Dolentium Hominum: Church and Health in the World.* 1997; 36(12th Yr., No. 3): 44.
(HEALTH CARE/ECONOMICS)

Adam, S. see **Wiggins, S.**

Adams, Betsy see **Slovenko, Ralph**

Adams, Betsy see **Sugarman, Jeremy**

Adams, Eleanor see **McKee, Katherine**

Adams, James; Society for Academic Emergency Medicine. Ethics Committee. Virtue in emergency medicine. *Academic Emergency Medicine.* 1996 Oct; 3(10): 961–966.
(MEDICAL ETHICS)

Addington, Whitney see **McCally, Michael**

Adler, N.E. see **Weiss, A.H.**

Adler, Richard K. see **Banja, John D.**

Admiraal, Pieter; Ardila, Ruben; Berlin, Isaiah, et al.;

Humanist Laureates of the International Academy of Humanism. Declaration in defense of cloning and the integrity of scientific research. *Free Inquiry.* 1997 Summer; 17(3): 11-12.
(CLONING)

Adshead, Gwen. Ethics in psychiatric research and practice. *Current Opinion in Psychiatry.* 1996 Sep; 9(5): 348-351.
(HUMAN EXPERIMENTATION/SPECIAL POPULATIONS; PATIENT CARE/MENTALLY DISABLED)

Al-Adwani, Andrew see **Joy, Mark**

Agar, Nicholas. Liberal eugenics. *Public Affairs Quarterly.* 1998 Apr; 12(2): 137-155.
(EUGENICS; GENETIC INTERVENTION)

Agarwal, Manoj R.; Ferran, Jose; Ost, Katherine; Wilson, Kenneth C.M. Ethics of 'informed consent' in dementia research -- the debate continues. *International Journal of Geriatric Psychiatry.* 1996 Sep; 11(9): 801-806.
(HUMAN EXPERIMENTATION/INFORMED CONSENT; HUMAN EXPERIMENTATION/SPECIAL POPULATIONS)

Aggoune, Michéle see **Lot, Florence**

Agich, George J. From Pittsburgh to Cleveland: NHBD [non-heart-beating donor] controversies and bioethics. *Cambridge Quarterly of Healthcare Ethics.* 1999 Summer; 8(3): 269-274.
(ETHICISTS AND ETHICS COMMITTEES; ORGAN AND TISSUE DONATION)

Agich, George J. see **Slomka, Jacquelyn**

Ahmed, Ziauddin see **Lamdan, Ruth M.**

Ahr, Willfried see **Sponholz, Gerlinde**

Aikman, Peter J.; Thiel, Elaine C.; Martin, Douglas K.; Singer, Peter A. Proxy, health, and personal care preferences: implications for end-of-life care. *Cambridge Quarterly of Healthcare Ethics.* 1999 Spring; 8(2): 200-210.
(ADVANCE DIRECTIVES; AIDS)

Akabayashi, Akira. Transplantation from a brain dead donor in Japan. [News]. *Hastings Center Report.* 1999 May-Jun; 29(3): 48.
(DETERMINATION OF DEATH/BRAIN DEATH; ORGAN AND TISSUE DONATION)

Akveld, Hans see **Price, David**

Alaska. Supreme Court. Valley Hospital Association, Inc. v. Mat-Su Coalition for Choice. *Pacific Reporter, 2d Series.* 1997 Nov 21 (date of decision). 948: 963-973.
(ABORTION/LEGAL ASPECTS)

Albert, Steven M.; Frank, Lori; Kleinman, Leah; Leidy, Nancy Kline; Legro, Marcia; Shikiar, Rich; Revicki, Dennis; Murri, Rita; Fantoni, Massimo; Antinori, Andrea; Ortona, Luigi; Hyland, Michael E.; Apolone, Giovanni; Leplége, Alain; Hunt, Sonja. Defining and measuring quality of life in medicine. [Letters and response]. *JAMA.* 1998 Feb 11; 279(6): 429-431.
(HEALTH)

Alberta Law Reform Institute. Advance Directives and Substitute Decision-Making in Personal Healthcare: A Joint Report of the Alberta Law Reform Institute and the Health Law Institute. Edmonton, AB: The Institute; 1993 Mar. 60 p.
(ADVANCE DIRECTIVES; INFORMED CONSENT)

Alberts, Bruce see **Burris, John**

Alcantara, Oscar L. see **Waller, Adele A.**

Alderson, Priscilla. Childhood, genetics, ethics and the social context. *In:* Clarke, Angus, ed. The Genetic Testing of Children. Washington, DC: BIOS Scientific Publishers; 1998: 223-235.
(EUGENICS)

Alderson, Priscilla; Goodey, Christopher. Theories of consent. *BMJ (British Medical Journal).* 1998 Nov 7; 317(7168): 1313-1315.
(INFORMED CONSENT)

Alderson, Priscilla see **Goodey, Chris**

Alderson, Priscilla see **Pfeffer, Naomi**

Aldhous, Peter. The fears of a clone. *New Scientist.* 1998 Feb 21; 157(2122): 8.
(CLONING)

Alexander, Elizabeth; Brody, Howard. Ethics by the numbers: monitoring physicians' integrity in managed care. *Journal of Clinical Ethics.* 1998 Fall; 9(3): 297-305.
(HEALTH CARE/ECONOMICS)

Alexander, G. Caleb; Sehgal, Ashwini R. Barriers to cadaveric renal transplantation among blacks, women, and the poor. *JAMA.* 1998 Oct 7; 280(13): 1148-1152.
(ORGAN AND TISSUE TRANSPLANTATION; RESOURCE ALLOCATION/BIOMEDICAL TECHNOLOGIES; SELECTION FOR TREATMENT)

Alexandrov, Andrei V.; Pullicino, Patrick M.; Meslin, Eric M.; Norris, John W. Agreement on disease-specific criteria for do-not-resuscitate orders in acute stroke. [For the members of the Canadian and Western New York Stroke Consortiums]. *Stroke.* 1996 Feb; 27(2): 232-237.
(RESUSCITATION ORDERS)

Ali, S.M. see **Swinburn, J.M.A.**

Alkas, Peri H.; Shandera, Wayne X. HIV and AIDS in Africa: African policies in response to AIDS in relation to various national legal traditions. *Journal of Legal Medicine.* 1996 Dec; 17(4): 527-546.
(AIDS)

Allan, Alfred; Allan, Marietjie. The right of mentally ill patients in South Africa to refuse treatment. *South African Law Journal.* 1997; 114(Pt. 4): 724-737.
(TREATMENT REFUSAL/MENTALLY DISABLED)

Allan, Marietjie see **Allan, Alfred**

Allanson, J. see **Cappelli, M.**

Allebeck, Peter. Forensic psychiatric studies and research ethical considerations. *Nordic Journal of Psychiatry.* 1997; 51(Suppl. 39): 53-56.
(HUMAN EXPERIMENTATION/SPECIAL POPULATIONS)

Allen, Arthur. Exposed: why doctor–patient confidentiality isn't what it used to be. *Washington Post Magazine.* 1998 Feb 8: 11–15, 27–32.
(CONFIDENTIALITY)

Allen, Arthur see **Redenbaugh, Russell**

Allen, Katrina; Williamson, Robert. Should we genetically test everyone for haemochromatosis? *Journal of Medical Ethics.* 1999 Apr; 25(2): 209–214.
(GENETIC SCREENING; MASS SCREENING)

Allen, Keith D.; Hodges, Eric D.; Knudsen, Sharon K. Comparing four methods to inform parents about child behavior management: how to inform for consent. *Pediatric Dentistry.* 1995 May–Jun; 17(3): 180–186.
(BEHAVIOR CONTROL; INFORMED CONSENT/MINORS)

Allen, William L. see **Brushwood, David B.**

Allert, Gebhard; Sponholz, Gerlinde; Baitsch, Helmut; Kautenburger, Monika. Consensus formation in genetic counseling: a complex process. *In:* ten Have, Henk A.M.J.; Sass, Hans–Martin, eds. Consensus Formation in Healthcare Ethics. Boston, MA: Kluwer Academic; 1998: 193–207.
(GENETIC COUNSELING)

Allert, Gebhard see **Sponholz, Gerlinde**

Allison, Miles C. see **Torrance, Caroline J.**

Almario, Donna A. see **Stoto, Michael A.**

Almeder, Robert F. see **Humber, James M.**

Alper, Joseph. A man in a hurry: stem cells. [Profile of Michael West]. *Science.* 1999 Mar 5; 283(5407): 1434–1435.
(BIOMEDICAL RESEARCH; GENETIC RESEARCH)

Alpers, Ann. Criminal act or palliative care? Prosecutions involving the care of the dying. *Journal of Law, Medicine and Ethics.* 1998 Winter; 26(4): 308–331.
(TERMINAL CARE)

Alpers, Ann; Lo, Bernard. Avoiding family feuds: responding to surrogate demands for life-sustaining interventions. *Journal of Law, Medicine and Ethics.* 1999 Spring; 27(1): 74–80.
(ADVANCE DIRECTIVES; ALLOWING TO DIE; INFORMED CONSENT)

Altman, Dennis. HIV, homophobia, and human rights. *Health and Human Rights.* 1998; 2(4): 15–22.
(AIDS)

Altman, Ellen; Hernon, Peter, eds. Research Misconduct: Issues, Implications, and Strategies. Greenwich, CT: Ablex; 1997. 206 p.
(BIOMEDICAL RESEARCH; FRAUD AND MISCONDUCT)

Altman, Lawrence K. British cast spotlight on misconduct in scientific research. [News]. *New York Times.* 1998 Jun 9: F3.
(BIOMEDICAL RESEARCH; FRAUD AND MISCONDUCT)

Altman, Lawrence K. Ethics panel urges easing of curbs on AIDS vaccine tests. [News]. *New York Times.* 1998 Jun 28: 6.
(AIDS/HUMAN EXPERIMENTATION; HUMAN EXPERIMENTATION/FOREIGN COUNTRIES; IMMUNIZATION)

Altman, Lawrence K. F.D.A. authorizes first full testing for H.I.V. vaccine. [News]. *New York Times.* 1998 Jun 4: A1, A23.
(AIDS/HUMAN EXPERIMENTATION; IMMUNIZATION)

Altman, Lawrence K. For surviving octuplets, progress comes in ounces. [News]. *New York Times.* 1998 Jan 17: 1, 20.
(PATIENT CARE/MINORS)

Altman, Lawrence K. New direction for transplants raises hopes and questions. [Rebuilding the body: a special report]. *New York Times.* 1999 May 2: 1, 46–47.
(HUMAN EXPERIMENTATION; ORGAN AND TISSUE TRANSPLANTATION)

Altman, Lawrence K. 'Role model' with a past clouds medical triumph. [News]. *New York Times.* 1999 Apr 27: F6.
(ORGAN AND TISSUE TRANSPLANTATION)

Altman, Lawrence K. Treating elderly's cancer is frustrating many experts. [News]. *New York Times.* 1998 May 20: A14.
(HUMAN EXPERIMENTATION/SPECIAL POPULATIONS; PATIENT CARE/AGED)

Altman, Lawrence K. Who Goes First? The Story of Self-Experimentation in Medicine. With a New Preface. Berkeley, CA: University of California Press; 1998. 430 p.
(HUMAN EXPERIMENTATION/SPECIAL POPULATIONS)

Alvarez, Lizette. Senate, 54–42, rejects Republican bill to ban human cloning. [News]. *New York Times.* 1998 Feb 12: A10.
(CLONING)

Alves, Wayne A.; Macciocchi, Stephen N. Ethical considerations in clinical neuroscience: current concepts in neuroclinical trials. *Stroke.* 1996 Oct; 27(10): 1903–1909.
(HUMAN EXPERIMENTATION/INFORMED CONSENT; HUMAN EXPERIMENTATION/RESEARCH DESIGN)

Amari–Vaught, Eileen see **Brakman, Sarah–Vaughan**

Amer, Mona S. Breaking the mold: human embryo cloning and its implications for a right to individuality. [Comment]. *UCLA Law Review.* 1996 Jun; 43(5): 1659–1688.
(CLONING)

American Academy of Ophthalmology. Ethics Committee. Patient–physician covenant. [Letter]. *Archives of Ophthalmology.* 1997 Jan; 115(1): 134.
(PROFESSIONAL PATIENT RELATIONSHIP)

American Association of Occupational Health Nurses; American College of Occupational and Environmental Medicine. AAOHN and ACOEM consensus statement for confidentiality of employee health information. *AAOHN Journal (American Association of Occupational Health Nurses).* 1997 Nov; 45(11): 613.
(CONFIDENTIALITY; OCCUPATIONAL HEALTH)

American Association of Suicidology. Committee on Physician–Assisted Death see **Maltsberger, John T.**

American Civil Liberties Union see **Crawford, Colin**

American College of Healthcare Executives. Health information confidentiality: ethical policy statement, November 1997. *Journal of the American Health Information Management Association.* 1998 Mar; 69(3): 27.
(CONFIDENTIALITY)

American College of Obstetricians and Gynecologists. Committee on Ethics. Ethical considerations in research involving pregnant women. ACOG Committee Opinon No. 213, Nov 1998. *Women's Health Issues.* 1999 Jul–Aug; 9(4): 194–198.
(HUMAN EXPERIMENTATION/SPECIAL POPULATIONS)

American College of Obstetricians and Gynecologists. Committee on Ethics. Obstetrician-gynecologists' ethical responsibilities, concerns, and risks pertaining to adoption. ACOG Committee Opinion No. 194. *ACOG Committee Opinions.* 1997 Nov; No. 194: 4 p.
(PATIENT CARE)

American College of Obstetricians and Gynecologists. Committee on Ethics. Sex selection. ACOG Committee Opinion No. 177. *ACOG Committee Opinions.* 1996 Nov.; No. 177: 4 p.
(SEX DETERMINATION)

American College of Obstetricians and Gynecologists. Committee on Health Care for Underserved Women. Mandatory reporting of domestic violence. ACOG Committee Opinion No. 200. *ACOG Committee Opinions.* 1998 Mar; No. 200: 3 p.
(CONFIDENTIALITY/LEGAL ASPECTS)

American College of Obstetricians and Gynecologists. Committee on Obstetrics: Maternal and Fetal Medicine. Current status of cystic fibrosis carrier screening. ACOG Committee Opinion No. 101. *ACOG Committee Opinions.* 1991 Nov; No. 101: 2 p.
(GENETIC SCREENING)

American College of Occupational and Environmental Medicine see **American Association of Occupational Health Nurses**

American College of Physicians–American Society of Internal Medicine End-of-Life Care Consensus Panel see **Karlawish, Jason H.T.**

American College of Physicians–American Society of Internal Medicine End-of-Life Care Consensus Panel see **Lo, Bernard**

American Geriatrics Society. Ethics Committee. Informed consent for research on human subjects with dementia. [Position statement]. *Journal of the American Geriatrics Society.* 1998 Oct; 46(10): 1308–1310.
(HUMAN EXPERIMENTATION/INFORMED CONSENT; INFORMED CONSENT/MENTALLY DISABLED)

American Health Information Management Association. AHIMA code of ethics and bylaws. *Journal of the American Health Information Management Association.* 1994 Jan; 65(1): 68–74.
(PROFESSIONAL ETHICS/CODES OF ETHICS)

American Hospital Association. AIDS/HIV Infection: Recommendations for Health Care Practices and Public Policy. Chicago, IL: The Association; 1992. 19 p.
(AIDS)

American Medical Association. Council on Ethical and Judicial Affairs. Code of Medical Ethics: Current Opinions with Annotations, 1998–1999 Edition. Chicago, IL: American Medical Association; 1998. 228 p.
(BIOETHICS/CODES OF ETHICS; MEDICAL ETHICS/CODES OF ETHICS)

American Medical Association. Council on Ethical and Judicial Affairs. Medical futility in end-of-life care: report of the Council on Ethical and Judicial Affairs. *JAMA.* 1999 Mar 10; 281(10): 937–941.
(ALLOWING TO DIE)

American Medical Association. Council on Ethical and Judicial Affairs. Subject selection for clinical trials. *IRB: A Review of Human Subjects Research.* 1998 Mar–Jun; 20(2–3): 12–15.
(HUMAN EXPERIMENTATION)

American Psychiatric Association. Committee on Confidentiality; American Psychiatric Association. Council on Psychiatry and Law. American Psychiatric Association resource document on preserving patient confidentiality in the era of information technology. *Journal of the American Academy of Psychiatry and the Law.* 1997; 25(4): 551–559.
(CONFIDENTIALITY/MENTAL HEALTH)

American Psychiatric Association. Council on Psychiatry and Law see **American Psychiatric Association. Committee on Confidentiality**

American Society for Reproductive Medicine. Ethics Committee. Informed consent and the use of gametes and embryos for research. *Fertility and Sterility.* 1997 Nov; 68(5): 780–781.
(EMBRYO AND FETAL RESEARCH; INFORMED CONSENT; ORGAN AND TISSUE DONATION)

American Society of Human Genetics. Board of Directors. Eugenics and the misuse of genetic information to restrict reproductive freedom: ASHG statement. *American Journal of Human Genetics.* 1999 Feb; 64(2): 335–338.
(EUGENICS; REPRODUCTION)

American Society of Nephrology see **Renal Physicians Association**

Ammann, Arthur see **Wilfert, Catherine M.**

Amnesty International. Danish Working Group for Children see **Fasting, Ulla**

Amos, Amanda see **Kerr, Anne**

Andalman, Robert see **Baram, Michael**

Andersen, Bogi. Icelandic health records. [Letter]. *Science.* 1998 Dec 11; 282(5396): 1993.
(GENETIC RESEARCH)

Andersen, Bogi; Arnason, Einar. Iceland's database is ethically questionable. *BMJ (British Medical Journal).* 1999 Jun 5; 318(7197): 1565.
(GENETIC RESEARCH)

Andersen, Daniel see **Nylenna, Magne**

Andersen, David; Cavalier, Robert; Covey, Preston K.
A Right to Die? The Dax Cowart Case. [CD-ROM computer file]. New York, NY: Routledge; 1996 Jun. 1 computer laser optical disc; sd., col.; 4 – 3/4 in. + user guide and teacher's guide..
(ALLOWING TO DIE; PATIENT CARE; TREATMENT REFUSAL)

Anderson, Donna G.; Vojir, Carol; Johnson, MeriLou.
Three medical schools' responses to the HIV/AIDS epidemic and the effect on students' knowledge and attitudes. *Academic Medicine.* 1997 Feb; 72(2): 144–146.
(AIDS/HEALTH PERSONNEL)

Anderson, Gerard F. see **Gross, Cary P.**

Anderson, Gwen. Nondirectiveness in prenatal genetics: patients read between the lines. *Nursing Ethics.* 1999 Mar; 6(2): 126–136.
(GENETIC COUNSELING; GENETIC SCREENING; PRENATAL DIAGNOSIS)

Anderson, Gwen see **Beech, Beverley A. Lawrence**

Anderson, J. Kerby. Abortion. *In: his* Moral Dilemmas: Biblical Perspectives on Contemporary Ethical Issues. Nashville, TN: Word Publishing; 1998: 1–15, 227–228.
(ABORTION/RELIGIOUS ASPECTS)

Anderson, J. Kerby. Euthanasia. *In: his* Moral Dilemmas: Biblical Perspectives on Contemporary Ethical Issues. Nashville, TN: Word Publishing; 1998: 17–31, 228–229.
(EUTHANASIA/RELIGIOUS ASPECTS)

Anderson, J. Kerby. Genetic engineering. *In: his* Moral Dilemmas: Biblical Perspectives on Contemporary Ethical Issues. Nashville, TN: Word Publishing; 1998: 33–43, 229–230.
(GENETIC INTERVENTION)

Anderson, J. Kerby. Reproductive technologies. *In: his* Moral Dilemmas: Biblical Perspectives on Contemporary Ethical Issues. Nashville, TN: Word Publishing; 1998: 45–57, 230–231.
(REPRODUCTIVE TECHNOLOGIES)

Anderson, J. Kerby. The ethics of genetic engineering and artificial reproduction. *In:* Demy, Timothy J.; Stewart, Gary P., eds. Genetic Engineering: A Christian Response: Crucial Considerations in Shaping Life. Grand Rapids, MI: Kregel Publications; 1999: 140–152.
(CLONING; RECOMBINANT DNA RESEARCH; REPRODUCTIVE TECHNOLOGIES)

Anderson, Jeremy. A prayer from the dying: [an advertisement sponsored by the Voluntary Euthanasia Society of New South Wales]. *BMJ (British Medical Journal).* 1999 Apr 17; 318(7190): 1084.
(EUTHANASIA)

Anderson, Warwick P.; Perry, Michael A. Australian animal ethics committees: we have come a long way. *Cambridge Quarterly of Healthcare Ethics.* 1999 Winter; 8(1): 80–86.
(ANIMAL EXPERIMENTATION)

Andersson, Kristina see **Kjellin, Lars**

Andre, Judith; Fleck, Leonard; Tomlinson, Tom.
Improving our aim. [Bioethics and the press]. *Journal of Medicine and Philosophy.* 1999 Apr; 24(2): 130–147.
(BIOETHICS; ETHICISTS AND ETHICS COMMITTEES)

Andrews, Edmund L. German company to leave China over sales of organs. [News]. *New York Times.* 1998 Mar 7: A5.
(ORGAN AND TISSUE DONATION)

Andrews, Lori; Elster, Nanette. International regulation of human embryo research: embryo research in the US. *Human Reproduction.* 1998 Jan; 13(1): 1–4.
(EMBRYO AND FETAL RESEARCH)

Andrews, Lori see **Nelkin, Dorothy**

Andrews, Lori B. Genetic privacy: from the laboratory to the legislature. *Genome Research.* 1995 Oct; 5(3): 209–213.
(CONFIDENTIALITY/LEGAL ASPECTS; GENETIC SCREENING)

Andrews, Lori B. Prenatal screening and the culture of motherhood. *Hastings Law Journal.* 1996 Apr; 47(4): 967–1006.
(GENETIC SCREENING; PRENATAL DIAGNOSIS)

Andrews, Lori B. The Clone Age: Adventures in the New World of Reproductive Technology. New York, NY: Henry Holt; 1999. 264 p.
(GENETIC INTERVENTION; REPRODUCTIVE TECHNOLOGIES)

Andrews, Lori B. The sperminator. *New York Times Magazine.* 1999 Mar 28: 62–65.
(INFORMED CONSENT; REPRODUCTION; REPRODUCTIVE TECHNOLOGIES)

Andrulis, Dennis P. Access to care is the centerpiece in the elimination of socioeconomic disparities in health. *Annals of Internal Medicine.* 1998 Sep 1; 129(5): 412–416.
(HEALTH; HEALTH CARE)

Andrykowski, Michael A.; Lightner, Robin; Studts, Jamie L.; Munn, Rita K. Hereditary cancer risk notification and testing: how interested is the general population? *Journal of Clinical Oncology.* 1997 May; 15(5): 2139–2148.
(GENETIC SCREENING)

Anfang, Stuart A.; Appelbaum, Paul S. Twenty years after *Tarasoff*: reviewing the duty to protect. *Harvard Review of Psychiatry.* 1996 Jul–Aug; 4(2): 67–76.
(CONFIDENTIALITY/LEGAL ASPECTS; CONFIDENTIALITY/MENTAL HEALTH)

Angelides, Kimon; Pianelli, James V. It will take more than notebooks to stop fraud. [Letter]. *Nature.* 1998 Dec 3; 396(6710): 404.
(BIOMEDICAL RESEARCH; FRAUD AND MISCONDUCT)

Angell, Marcia see **Desvarieux, Moïse**

Ankeny, Rachel A. Recasting the debate on multiple listing for transplantation through consideration of both principles and practice. *Cambridge Quarterly of Healthcare Ethics.* 1999 Summer; 8(3): 330–339.
(ORGAN AND TISSUE TRANSPLANTATION; RESOURCE ALLOCATION/BIOMEDICAL TECHNOLOGIES; SELECTION FOR TREATMENT)

Annas, George J. Burden of proof: judging science and

protecting public health in (and out of) the courtroom. *American Journal of Public Health*. 1999 Apr; 89(4): 490–493.
(BIOMEDICAL RESEARCH; BIOMEDICAL TECHNOLOGIES)

Annas, George J. Genetic prophecy and genetic privacy. *Trial*. 1996 Jan; 32(1): 18–20, 22–25.
(GENETIC SCREENING)

Annas, George J. Human rights and health -- the Universal Declaration of Human Rights at 50. *New England Journal of Medicine*. 1998 Dec 10; 339(24): 1778–1781.
(HEALTH; HEALTH CARE/RIGHTS; PUBLIC HEALTH)

Annas, George J. Protecting patients from discrimination -- the Americans with Disabilities Act and HIV infection. *New England Journal of Medicine*. 1998 Oct 22; 339(17): 1255–1259.
(AIDS/HEALTH PERSONNEL)

Annas, George J. Some Choice: Law, Medicine, and the Market. New York, NY: Oxford University Press; 1998. 303 p.
(BIOETHICS)

Annas, George J. The prospect of human cloning: an opportunity for national and international cooperation in bioethics. *In:* Humber, James M.; Almeder, Robert F., eds. Human Cloning. Totowa, NJ: Humana Press; 1998: 51–63.
(CLONING)

Annas, George J. The "right to die" in America: sloganeering from Quinlan and Cruzan to Quill and Kevorkian. *Duquesne Law Review*. 1996 Summer; 34(4): 875–897.
(ALLOWING TO DIE/LEGAL ASPECTS; SUICIDE)

Annas, George J. Waste and longing -- the legal status of placental-blood banking. *New England Journal of Medicine*. 1999 May 13; 340(19): 1521–1524.
(BLOOD DONATION)

Annas, George J.; Grodin, Michael A. Human rights and maternal-fetal HIV transmission prevention trials in Africa. *American Journal of Public Health*. 1998 Apr; 88(4): 560–563.
(AIDS/HUMAN EXPERIMENTATION; HUMAN EXPERIMENTATION/FOREIGN COUNTRIES; HUMAN EXPERIMENTATION/RESEARCH DESIGN; HUMAN EXPERIMENTATION/SPECIAL POPULATIONS)

Annas, George J.; Grodin, Michael A. Reflections on the fiftieth anniversary of the Doctors' Trial. *Health and Human Rights*. 1996; 2(1): 7–21.
(FRAUD AND MISCONDUCT; HUMAN EXPERIMENTATION)

Annas, George J. see **Bopp, James**

Annas, George J. see **Glantz, Leonard H.**

Annas, George J. see **Limentani, Alexander E.**

Annas, George J. see **Mann, Jonathan, M.**

Annas, George J. see **Pence, Gregory E.**

Annas, George J. see **Roche, Patricia**

Annas, George J. see **Tessman, Irwin**

Antinori, Andrea see **Albert, Steven M.**

Antle, Beverley J.; Carlin, Kathleen. Enhancing patient participation in team decision making. *Humane Health Care International*. 1997 Spring; 13(1): 32–35.
(PATIENT CARE)

Antuono, Piero; Beyer, Jan. The burden of dementia: a medical and research perspective. *Theoretical Medicine and Bioethics*. 1999 Jan; 20(1): 3–13.
(PATIENT CARE/AGED; PATIENT CARE/MENTALLY DISABLED)

Aoki, Eiko; Watanabe, Toru. Patients' concerns about clinical trials in Japan. [Letter and response]. *Lancet*. 1999 Mar 20; 353(9157): 1019–1020.
(HUMAN EXPERIMENTATION/FOREIGN COUNTRIES; HUMAN EXPERIMENTATION/INFORMED CONSENT; HUMAN EXPERIMENTATION/RESEARCH DESIGN)

Apolone, Giovanni see **Albert, Steven M.**

Appelbaum, Binyamin C.; Appelbaum, Paul S.; Grisso, Thomas. Competence to consent to voluntary psychiatric hospitalization: a test of a standard proposed by APA. *Psychiatric Services*. 1998 Sep; 49(9): 1193–1196.
(INFORMED CONSENT/MENTALLY DISABLED)

Appelbaum, Kenneth L. see **Candilis, Philip J.**

Appelbaum, Paul S. Child abuse reporting laws: time for reform? *Psychiatric Services*. 1999 Jan; 50(1): 27–29.
(CONFIDENTIALITY/LEGAL ASPECTS; CONFIDENTIALITY/MENTAL HEALTH)

Appelbaum, Paul S. Jaffee v. Redmond: psychotherapist-patient privilege in the federal courts. *Psychiatric Services*. 1996 Oct; 47(10): 1033–1034, 1052.
(CONFIDENTIALITY/LEGAL ASPECTS; CONFIDENTIALITY/MENTAL HEALTH)

Appelbaum, Paul S. Ought we to require emotional capacity as part of decisional competence? *Kennedy Institute of Ethics Journal*. 1998 Dec; 8(4): 377–387.
(INFORMED CONSENT)

Appelbaum, Paul S.; Grisso, Thomas. Capacities of hospitalized, medically ill patients to consent to treatment. *Psychosomatics*. 1997 Mar-Apr; 38(2): 119–125.
(INFORMED CONSENT)

Appelbaum, Paul S. see **Anfang, Stuart A.**

Appelbaum, Paul S. see **Appelbaum, Binyamin C.**

Appelbaum, Paul S. see **Halpern, Abraham L.**

Applebaum, Arthur Isak. Doctor, schmoctor: practice positivism and its complications. *In: his* Ethics for Adversaries: The Morality of Roles in Public and Professional Life. Princeton, NJ: Princeton University Press; 1999: 45–60.
(MEDICAL ETHICS; PROFESSIONAL ETHICS)

Appleby, Brenda Margaret. Responsible Parenthood: Decriminalizing Contraception in Canada. Toronto, ON: University of Toronto Press; 1999. 301 p.
(CONTRACEPTION)

Appleby, John see **Goodey, Chris**

Appleyard, Bryan. Brave New Worlds: Staying Human in the Genetic Future. New York, NY: Viking; 1998. 198 p.
(EUGENICS; GENETIC INTERVENTION; RECOMBINANT DNA RESEARCH)

Appleyard, James. The rights of children to health care. [Editorial]. *Journal of Medical Ethics.* 1998 Oct; 24(5): 293–294.
(HEALTH CARE/RIGHTS; PATIENT CARE/MINORS)

Appleyard, James. Withdrawal of treatment in children. [Letter]. *Journal of Medical Ethics.* 1998 Oct; 24(5): 350.
(ALLOWING TO DIE/INFANTS)

Arboleda-Flórez, Julio; Weisstub, David N. Ethical research with the mentally disordered. *Canadian Journal of Psychiatry.* 1997 Jun; 42(5): 485–491.
(HUMAN EXPERIMENTATION/FOREIGN COUNTRIES; HUMAN EXPERIMENTATION/INFORMED CONSENT; HUMAN EXPERIMENTATION/SPECIAL POPULATIONS)

Arboleda-Flórez, Julio see **Weisstub, David N.**

Ardila, Ruben see **Admiraal, Pieter**

Argentina. Law No. 24193 of 24 Mar 1993 on the transplantation of organs and anatomical materials. (*Boletin Oficial de la Repdblica Argentina*, 26 Apr 1993, Section 1, No. 27625, p. 1–5). [Summary]. *International Digest of Health Legislation.* 1994. 45(1). 35–36.
(ORGAN AND TISSUE DONATION)

Arican, Nadir see **Frank, Martina W.**

Arluke, Arnold. Moral elevation in medical research. *Advances in Medical Sociology.* 1990; 1: 189–204.
(ANIMAL EXPERIMENTATION)

Arluke, Arnold; Groves, Julian. Pushing the boundaries: scientists in the public arena. *In:* Hart, Lynette A., ed. Responsible Conduct with Animals in Research. New York, NY: Oxford University Press; 1998: 145–164.
(ANIMAL EXPERIMENTATION)

Armstrong, John D. see **Crausman, Robert S.**

Armstrong, Kenneth L. see **Van Haeringen, Alison R.**

Armstrong, Moe see **Rosenheck, Robert**

Arnason, Einar see **Andersen, Bogi**

Arnold, L. Eugene; Stoff, David M.; Cook, Edwin; Wright, Clinton; Cohen, Donald J.; Kruesi, Markus; Hattab, Jocelyn; Graham, Philip; Zametkin, Alan; Castellanos, F. Xavier; McMahon, William; Leckman, James F. Biologic procedures: ethical issues in research with children and adolescents. *In:* Hoagwood, Kimberly; Jensen, Peter S.; Fisher, Celia B., eds. Ethical Issues in Mental Health Research with Children and Adolescents. Mahwah, NJ: Lawrence Erlbaum Associates; 1996: 89–111.
(HUMAN EXPERIMENTATION/MINORS; HUMAN EXPERIMENTATION/SPECIAL POPULATIONS)

Arnold, Lori see **Wright, Robert**

Arnold, Robert see **Selwyn, Peter A.**

Arnold, Robert see **Siminoff, Laura A.**

Arnold, Robert M.; Siminoff, Laura A.; Frader, Joel E. Ethical issues in organ procurement: a review for intensivists. *Critical Care Clinics.* 1996 Jan; 12(1): 29–48.
(ORGAN AND TISSUE DONATION)

Arnold, Robert M. see **Aulisio, Mark P.**

Arnold, Robert M. see **Tulsky, James A.**

Arnold, Robert M. see **Youngner, Stuart J.**

Arnow, Kathryn Smul. Medical technology transfer and physician–patient conversation. *International Journal of Technology Management.* 1996; 11(1–2): 70–88.
(BIOMEDICAL TECHNOLOGIES; PROFESSIONAL PATIENT RELATIONSHIP)

Aronoff, Gerald M. see **Haddox, J. David**

Aroskar, Mila Ann. Teaching ethics in health care administration: a course profile. *Journal of Health Administration Education.* 1993 Fall; 11(4): 601–608.
(PROFESSIONAL ETHICS/EDUCATION)

Arras, John D. A case approach. *In:* Kuhse, Helga; Singer, Peter, eds. A Companion to Bioethics. Malden, MA: Blackwell; 1998: 106–114.
(BIOETHICS)

Arras, John D. see **Crouch, Robert A.**

Arrow, Kenneth J. see **Lanza, Robert P.**

Artal, Raul see **Oldenettel, Debra**

Arthur, John, ed. Abortion. *In:* Arthur, John, ed. Morality and Moral Controversies. Fifth Edition. Upper Saddle River, NJ: Prentice Hall; 1999: 166–210.
(ABORTION; FETUSES)

Arthur, John, ed. Euthanasia. *In:* Arthur, John, ed. Morality and Moral Controversies. Fifth Edition. Upper Saddle River, NJ: Prentice Hall; 1999: 211–235.
(ALLOWING TO DIE; EUTHANASIA)

Artnak, Kathryn E. Informed consent in the elderly: assessing decisional capacity. *Seminars in Perioperative Nursing.* 1997 Jan; 6(1): 59–64.
(INFORMED CONSENT; PATIENT CARE/AGED)

Asch, David A. see **Ubel, Peter A.**

Asch, Steven; Frayne, Susan; Waitzkin, Howard. To discharge or not to discharge: ethics of care for an undocumented immigrant. *Journal of Health Care for the Poor and Underserved.* 1995; 6(1): 3–9.
(HEALTH CARE/ECONOMICS; RESOURCE ALLOCATION/BIOMEDICAL TECHNOLOGIES; SELECTION FOR TREATMENT)

Ashcroft, Richard. Equipoise, knowledge and ethics in clinical research and practice. *Bioethics.* 1999 Jul; 13(3–4): 314–326.
(HUMAN EXPERIMENTATION/RESEARCH DESIGN)

Ashraf, Haroon. BMA address the issue of withholding and withdrawing treatment. [News]. *Lancet.* 1999 Jun 26; 353(9171): 2220.
(ALLOWING TO DIE)

Asian Society of Transplantation. Declaration of Seoul

on brain death. *International Digest of Health Legislation.* 1997; 48(2): 229.
(DETERMINATION OF DEATH/BRAIN DEATH)

Aspen Health Law and Compliance Center see **Roach, William H.**

Association of Canadian Universities for Northern Studies. Board Committee on Revising the Ethical Principles see **Graham, Amanda**

Association of the British Pharmaceutical Industry. Clinical Trial Compensation Guidelines. Issued by the Association of the British Pharmaceutical Industry, 12 Whitehall, London SW1A 2DY, England; 1991 Jan. 2 p.
(HUMAN EXPERIMENTATION/FOREIGN COUNTRIES)

Astagneau, Pascal see **Lot, Florence**

Astrow, Alan B. see **Dietz, Sarah M.**

Astrue, Michael J. see **Stoddard, Joan C.**

Atkinson, Jeffrey see **van der Valk, Jan**

Attkisson, C. Clifford; Rosenblatt, Abram; Hoagwood, Kimberly. Research ethics and human subjects protection in child mental health services research and community studies. *In:* Hoagwood, Kimberly; Jensen, Peter S.; Fisher, Celia B., eds. Ethical Issues in Mental Health Research with Children and Adolescents. Mahwah, NJ: Lawrence Erlbaum Associates; 1996: 43–57.
(HUMAN EXPERIMENTATION/MINORS; HUMAN EXPERIMENTATION/SPECIAL POPULATIONS)

Auberson, Lillian see **Käppeli, Othmar**

Aulisio, Mark P. The foundations of bioethics: contingency and relevance. *Journal of Medicine and Philosophy.* 1998 Aug; 23(4): 428–438.
(BIOETHICS)

Aulisio, Mark P.; Arnold, Robert M.; Youngner, Stuart J. An ongoing conversation: the Task Force report and bioethics consultation. [Introduction to a set of articles by E.D. Pellegrino, E.G. Howe, J.W. Ross, R. Pentz, A.H. Moss, and the authors]. *Journal of Clinical Ethics.* 1999 Spring; 10(1): 3–4.
(ETHICISTS AND ETHICS COMMITTEES)

Aulisio, Mark P.; Arnold, Robert M.; Youngner, Stuart J. Moving the conversation forward. *Journal of Clinical Ethics.* 1999 Spring; 10(1): 49–56.
(ETHICISTS AND ETHICS COMMITTEES)

Ault, Alicia. Drug industry hopes to moderate genetic privacy laws. [News]. *Nature Medicine.* 1998 Jan; 4(1): 6.
(CONFIDENTIALITY/LEGAL ASPECTS; GENETIC RESEARCH)

Aurran, Y. see **Julian-Reyneir, C.**

Austad, Torleiv. The right not to know -- worthy of preservation any longer? An ethical perspective. *Clinical Genetics.* 1996 Aug; 50(2): 85–88.
(GENETIC SCREENING)

Australia. Euthanasia Laws Act 1997. *Acts of the Australian Parliament.* 1997 Mar 27 (date effective). 7 p.
(EUTHANASIA/LEGAL ASPECTS; SUICIDE)

Australia. Victoria. The Infertility Treatment Act 1995. No. 63 of 1995. Date of assent: 27 Jun 1995. [Summary]. *International Digest of Health Legislation.* 1997; 48(1): 24–33.
(EMBRYO AND FETAL RESEARCH; REPRODUCTIVE TECHNOLOGIES)

Australie, K. see **Malkin, D.**

Avallone, Fran; Focus on the Family; Family Research Council. Do parental notification laws benefit minors seeking abortions? *In:* Francoeur, Robert T., ed. Taking Sides: Clashing Views on Controversial Issues in Human Sexuality. Fifth Edition. Guilford, CT: Dushkin Publishing Group/Brown and Benchmark; 1996: 174–191.
(ABORTION/LEGAL ASPECTS; ABORTION/MINORS)

Averhoff, Francisco M. see **Gordon, Todd E.**

Avins, Andrew L. Can unequal be more fair? Ethics, subject allocation, and randomised clinical trials. *Journal of Medical Ethics.* 1998 Dec; 24(6): 401–408.
(HUMAN EXPERIMENTATION/RESEARCH DESIGN)

Avise, John C. The Genetic Gods: Evolution and Belief in Human Affairs. Cambridge, MA: Harvard University Press; 1998. 279 p.
(GENETIC RESEARCH)

Awong, Linda; Miles, Al. Asking patients about revising advance directives. *American Journal of Nursing.* 1998 Apr; 98(4): 71.
(ADVANCE DIRECTIVES)

Axelrod, Julius see **Lanza, Robert P.**

Ayd, Frank J. Human cloning and the rights of human beings. *Medical–Moral Newsletter.* 1998 May–Jun; 35(5–6): 17–23.
(CLONING; EMBRYO AND FETAL RESEARCH)

Ayd, Frank J. Research on the decisionally impaired: overview and commentary. *Medical–Moral Newsletter.* 1998 Jan–Feb; 35(1–2): 1–8.
(HUMAN EXPERIMENTATION/INFORMED CONSENT; HUMAN EXPERIMENTATION/SPECIAL POPULATIONS)

Aydin, A.E. see **Sever, M.S.**

Aymerich, Marta see **Serra–Prat, Mateu**

B

Babrow, Austin S. see **Hines, Stephen C.**

Bacchetta, Matthew D. see **Fins, Joseph J.**

Bacchetta, Matthew D. see **Richter, Gerd**

Bach, Fritz H. see **Sachs, David H.**

Bachmann, C. see **Müller, H.J.**

Back, Anthony; Ganzini, Linda; Sullivan, Mark; Menzel, Paul; Rieger, Dean; Emanuel, Linda. Responding to patient requests for physician–assisted

suicide. [Letters and response]. *JAMA.* 1999 Jan 20; 281(3): 227–229.
(SUICIDE; TERMINAL CARE)

Back, G. see **Houghton, D.J.**

Backlar, Patricia. Can we bridge the gap between the actual lives of persons with serious mental disorders and the therapeutic goals of their providers? *Community Mental Health Journal.* 1997 Dec; 33(6): 465–471.
(PATIENT CARE/MENTALLY DISABLED)

Bacon, Mike; Stewart, Kevin; Bowker, Lesley. CPR decision–making by elderly patients. [Letter]. *Journal of Medical Ethics.* 1998 Apr; 24(2): 134.
(RESUSCITATION ORDERS)

Badzek, Laurie A. see **Hines, Stephen C.**

Baergen, Carolyn see **Baergen, Ralph**

Baergen, Ralph; Baergen, Carolyn. Paternalism, risk and patient choice. *Journal of the American Dental Association.* 1997 Apr; 128(4): 481–484.
(PATIENT CARE)

Baetens, P.; Ponjaert-Kristoffersen, I.; Devroey, P.; Van Steirteghem, A.C. Artificial insemination by donor: an alternative for single women. *Human Reproduction.* 1995 Jun; 10(6): 1537–1542.
(ARTIFICIAL INSEMINATION; SELECTION FOR TREATMENT)

Baggaley, Rachel see **Edi-Osagie, E.C.O.**

Baggaley, Rachel see **Godfrey-Faussett, Peter**

Baggett, David J. On the legality and morality of physician–assisted suicide. *Asbury Theological Journal.* 1995 Spring; 50(1): 51–66.
(SUICIDE)

Bagiella, E. see **Sloan, R.P.**

Bagla, Pallava. Animal experimentation: strict rules rile Indian scientists. [News]. *Science.* 1998 Sep 18; 281(5384): 1777–1778.
(ANIMAL EXPERIMENTATION)

Bagla, Pallava. Animal research: 50 monkeys taken from Indian lab. [News]. *Science.* 1999 Aug 13; 285(5430): 997.
(ANIMAL EXPERIMENTATION)

Bagla, Pallava. India backs off on central control. [News]. *Science.* 1998 Dec 11; 282(5396): 1967.
(ANIMAL EXPERIMENTATION)

Bagla, Pallava. New Indian rules disrupt research. [News]. *Science.* 1999 Jul 9; 285(5425): 180–181.
(ANIMAL EXPERIMENTATION)

Bagness, Carmel. Genetics, the Fetus and Our Future. Hale, Cheshire, England: Hochland and Hochland; 1998. 105 p.
(EMBRYO AND FETAL RESEARCH; GENETIC INTERVENTION; REPRODUCTIVE TECHNOLOGIES)

Bahnsen, Ulrich. Swiss to vote on ban on *in vitro* fertilization. [News]. *Nature.* 1998 Nov 12; 396(6707): 105.
(IN VITRO FERTILIZATION; REPRODUCTIVE

TECHNOLOGIES)

Bahnsen, Ulrich. Switzerland adopts transplant guidelines. [News]. *Nature.* 1999 Feb 18; 397(6720): 553.
(ORGAN AND TISSUE DONATION; ORGAN AND TISSUE TRANSPLANTATION)

Baier, Kurt. Wrongful death and wrongful life. *In: his* Problems of Life and Death: A Humanist Perspective. Amherst, NY: Prometheus Books; 1997: 137–230.
(ALLOWING TO DIE; EUTHANASIA; POPULATION CONTROL; SUICIDE; WRONGFUL LIFE)

Bailey, Lisa see **MacKay, Charles**

Bailey, Susan see **Wincze, John P.**

Baird, Karen L. The new NIH and FDA medical research policies: targeting gender, promoting justice. *Journal of Health Politics, Policy and Law.* 1999 Jun; 24(3): 531–565.
(HUMAN EXPERIMENTATION/REGULATION; HUMAN EXPERIMENTATION/SPECIAL POPULATIONS)

Baird, Patricia. Human embryo research in Canada: legal and policy aspects. *Human Reproduction.* 1997 Nov; 12(11): 2343–2345.
(EMBRYO AND FETAL RESEARCH)

Baird, Patricia. Patenting and human genes. *Perspectives in Biology and Medicine.* 1998 Spring; 41(3): 391–408.
(PATENTING LIFE FORMS)

Baird, Patricia. Proceed with care: new reproductive technologies and the need for boundaries. *Journal of Assisted Reproduction and Genetics.* 1995 Sep; 12(8): 491–498.
(REPRODUCTIVE TECHNOLOGIES)

Baitsch, Helmut see **Allert, Gebhard**

Baitsch, Helmut see **Sponholz, Gerlinde**

Baker, A. Cornelius see **Solomon, Liza**

Baker, Debra. Positively truthful: appeal asks whether doctors have duty to disclose HIV status to patients. *ABA Journal: The Lawyer's Magazine.* 1998 Aug; 84: 38–40.
(AIDS/CONFIDENTIALITY; AIDS/HEALTH PERSONNEL)

Baker, Michael. Korean report sparks anger and inquiry. [News]. *Science.* 1999 Jan 1; 283(5398): 16–17.
(CLONING)

Baker, Michael. Report casts doubt on Korean experiment. [News]. *Science.* 1999 Jan 29; 283(5402): 617, 619.
(CLONING)

Baker, Robert. A theory of international bioethics: multiculturalism, postmodernism, and the bankruptcy of fundamentalism. *Kennedy Institute of Ethics Journal.* 1998 Sep; 8(3): 201–231.
(BIOETHICS; FRAUD AND MISCONDUCT; HUMAN EXPERIMENTATION/REGULATION)

Baker, Robert. A theory of international bioethics: the negotiable and the non–negotiable. *Kennedy Institute of Ethics Journal.* 1998 Sep; 8(3): 233–273.
(BIOETHICS; HUMAN EXPERIMENTATION)

Baker, Robert. American independence and the right to

emergency care. *JAMA.* 1999 Mar 3; 281(9): 859–860.
(HEALTH CARE/ECONOMICS; HEALTH CARE/RIGHTS; MEDICAL ETHICS; PATIENTS' RIGHTS)

Baker, Robert. Negotiating international bioethics: a response to Tom Beauchamp and Ruth Macklin. *Kennedy Institute of Ethics Journal.* 1998 Dec; 8(4): 423–453.
(BIOETHICS; HUMAN EXPERIMENTATION)

Baker, Tina; Cooper, Colleen. What happens next? [Case study and commentaries]. *Hastings Center Report.* 1999 Mar–Apr; 29(2): 24–25.
(BEHAVIOR CONTROL; PATIENT CARE/AGED)

Bakke, O.M. see **García–Alonso, F.**

Bakran, A. see **Engelhart, Karlheinz**

Balano, Kirsten; Beckerman, Karen; Ng, Valerie; Minkoff, Howard; O'Sullivan, Mary Jo. Rapid HIV screening during labor. [Letter and response]. *JAMA.* 1998 Nov 18; 280(19): 1664.
(AIDS/TESTING AND SCREENING)

Balcombe, Jonathan see **van der Valk, Jan**

Baleta, Adele. Huge percentage of women volunteer for zidovudine project. [News]. *Lancet.* 1999 Jan 16; 353(9148): 219.
(AIDS/TESTING AND SCREENING; PATIENT CARE/DRUGS)

Ball, Eric see **Slovenko, Ralph**

Ball, Eric see **Sugarman, Jeremy**

Balls, M. see **van Zutphen, L.F.M.**

Balls, Michael. Reducing animal testing: tests matter more than what is tested. [Editorial]. *ATLA: Alternatives to Laboratory Animals.* 1997 Nov–Dec; 25(6): 613–617.
(ANIMAL EXPERIMENTATION)

Balls, Michael. The precautionary principle should be used with caution -- and should be applied to animal experimentation and genetic manipulation, not merely to protection of the environment. [Editorial]. *ATLA: Alternatives to Laboratory Animals.* 1999 Jan–Feb; 27(1): 1–5.
(ANIMAL EXPERIMENTATION; GENETIC INTERVENTION)

Balls, Michael. The production of genetically modified animals and humans: an inescapable moral challenge to scientists and laypeople alike. [Editorial]. *ATLA: Alternatives to Laboratory Animals.* 1998 Jan–Feb; 26(1): 1–2.
(CLONING; GENETIC INTERVENTION)

Balls, Michael. The Three Rs concept of alternatives to animal experimentation. *In:* van Zutphen, L.F.M.; Balls, M., eds. Animal Alternatives, Welfare and Ethics. New York, NY: Elsevier; 1997: 27–41.
(ANIMAL EXPERIMENTATION)

Balls, Michael see **Mepham, T. Ben**

Balter, Michael. French AIDS research pioneers to testify in trial of ministers. [News]. *Science.* 1999 Feb 12; 283(5404): 910–911.
(AIDS/TESTING AND SCREENING; FRAUD AND MISCONDUCT)

Bande–Knops, Jacqueline see **Welkenhuysen, Myriam**

Banerjee, D.J. see **Swinburn, J.M.A.**

Banja, John D.; Adler, Richard K.; Stringer, Anthony Y. Ethical dimensions of caring for defiant patients: a case study. *Journal of Head Trauma Rehabilitation.* 1996 Dec; 11(6): 93–97.
(TREATMENT REFUSAL)

Bar El, Yair Carlos; Durst, Rimona; Rabinowitz, Jonathan; Kalian, Moshe; Teitelbaum, Alexander; Shlafman, Michael. Implementation of order of compulsory ambulatory treatment in Jerusalem. *International Journal of Law and Psychiatry.* 1998 Winter; 21(1): 65–71.
(INVOLUNTARY COMMITMENT/FOREIGN COUNTRIES)

Bär, W. see **Müller, H.J.**

Barakamfitiye, D. see **Lee, J.W.**

Barakat, Khalid; Wilkinson, Paul; Deaner, Andrew; Fluck, David; Ranjadayalan, Kulasegaram; Timmis, Adam. How should age affect management of acute myocardial infarction? A prospective cohort study. *Lancet.* 1999 Mar 20; 353(9157): 955–959.
(PATIENT CARE/AGED; SELECTION FOR TREATMENT)

Baram, Michael; Proctor, Susan; Andalman, Robert; van Eyl, Diderico. Human gene therapy research: technological temptations and social control. *Genetic Resource.* 1993; 7(2): 10–15.
(GENE THERAPY)

Baraza, Richard see **Edi–Osagie, E.C.O.**

Barbasch, Avi see **Garber, Judy E.**

Barber, John C.K. "Code of practice and guidance on human genetic testing services supplied direct to the public": Advisory Committee on Genetic Testing. *Journal of Medical Genetics.* 1998 Jun; 35(6): 443–445.
(GENETIC SCREENING; GENETIC SERVICES)

Barbieri, Celia see **Heffner, John E.**

Barbieri, Ottavia see **Mepham, T. Ben**

Barbour, Elizabeth see **Murphy, Donald J.**

Barchard, Chris see **Thomas, Sandy**

Bard, Jennifer S. When a woman doesn't need a man: legal issues regarding cloning as an infertility treatment. *Journal of Biolaw and Business.* 1998 Spring; 1(3): 56–58.
(CLONING; REPRODUCTIVE TECHNOLOGIES)

Barkun, Harvey see **Ferris, Lorraine E.**

Barnaby, Wendy. Biological weapons and genetic engineering. *GenEthics News.* 1997 Jun–Jul; No. 18: 4–5.
(GENETIC INTERVENTION; WAR)

Barnard, Kate. Basingstoke LREC revisited. [Letter and editorial comment]. *Bulletin of Medical Ethics.* 1997 Aug; No. 130: 13–17.
(HUMAN EXPERIMENTATION/ETHICS COMMITTEES; HUMAN EXPERIMENTATION/FOREIGN COUNTRIES)

Barnett, Michael L. The assessment of new biotechnologies: would the world be different if Napoleon had received recombinant growth hormone? [Editorial]. *Journal of Dental Research.* 1995 Dec; 74(12): 1820–1821.
(BIOMEDICAL TECHNOLOGIES)

Barnhouse, Dorothy J. Birth of octuplets reignites fertilty debate. [News]. *New York Times.* 1999 Jan 5: F7.
(REPRODUCTIVE TECHNOLOGIES)

Barns, Ian. The Human Genome Project and the self. *Soundings.* 1994 Spring–Summer; 77(1–2): 99–128.
(GENOME MAPPING)

Baron, Jonathan see **Ubel, Peter A.**

Barondess, Jeremiah A. Care of the medical ethos: reflections on Social Darwinism, racial hygiene, and the Holocaust. *Annals of Internal Medicine.* 1998 Dec 1; 129(11): 891–898.
(EUGENICS; FRAUD AND MISCONDUCT; MEDICAL ETHICS)

Barr, Bernadine Courtright. Spare Children, 1900–1945: Inmates of Orphanages as Subjects of Research in Medicine and in the Social Sciences in America. Ann Arbor, MI: University Microfilms International; 1992. 341 p.
(BEHAVIORAL RESEARCH/MINORS; HUMAN EXPERIMENTATION/MINORS)

Barr, Patricia see **Garber, Judy E.**

Barragan, Javier Lozano. The demands of health and morality: the health paradigm in WHO. *Dolentium Hominum: Church and Health in the World.* 1997; 36(12th Yr., No. 3): 36–42.
(HEALTH)

Barrera, M. see **Malkin, D.**

Barrett, J. Carl see **Sharp, Richard R.**

Barrow, Chelmer L.; Easley, Kirk A. The role of gender and race on the time delay for emergency department patients complaining of chest pain to be evaluated by a physician. *Saint Louis University Public Law Review.* 1996; 15(2): 267–277.
(HEALTH CARE; PATIENT CARE; SELECTION FOR TREATMENT)

Barrow, Jackie. Implications of the Emergency Medical Treatment and Active Labor Act (EMTALA) on differences based on race and gender in the treatment of patients presenting to a hospital emergency department with chest pain. *Saint Louis University Public Law Review.* 1996; 15(2): 278–302.
(HEALTH CARE; PATIENT CARE; SELECTION FOR TREATMENT)

Bartels, Dianne; Youngner, Stuart; Levine, June. HealthCare Ethics Forum '94: ethics committees: living up to your potential. *AACN Clinical Issues in Critical Care Nursing.* 1994 Aug; 5(3): 313–323.
(ETHICISTS AND ETHICS COMMITTEES)

Bartholet, Elizabeth see **Wright, Robert**

Bartholome, William see **Matthews, Dennis J.**

Bartko, John J. see **Trippitelli, Carol Lynn**

Bartlett, Rachel. The ethics of xenotransplantation. [Letter]. *Journal of Medical Ethics.* 1998 Dec; 24(6): 414–415.
(ORGAN AND TISSUE TRANSPLANTATION)

Bartlett, Rachel see **Thomas, Sandy**

Barton, C. Dennis; Mallik, Harminder S.; Orr, William B.; Janofsky, Jeffrey S. Clinicians' judgment of capacity of nursing home patients to give informed consent. *Psychiatric Services.* 1996 Sep; 47(9): 956–960.
(INFORMED CONSENT)

Barton, John; Crandon, John; Kennedy, Donald; Miller, Henry. A model protocol to assess the risks of agricultural introductions: a risk–based approach to rationalizing field trial regulations. *Nature Biotechnology.* 1997 Sep; 15(9): 845–848.
(GENETIC INTERVENTION)

Baskin, Shari A. see **Morrison, R. Sean**

Basu, Sandip K.; Rath, Satyajit. Animal experimentation rules in India. [Letter]. *Science.* 1998 Oct 16; 282(5388): 415.
(ANIMAL EXPERIMENTATION)

Bates, Carol K. see **Covinsky, Kenneth E.**

Battaglia, John see **Roberts, Laura Weiss**

Battin, Margaret P. see **Sage, William M.**

Battin, Margaret Pabst. Population issues. *In:* Kuhse, Helga; Singer, Peter, eds. A Companion to Bioethics. Malden, MA: Blackwell; 1998: 149–162.
(POPULATION CONTROL)

Battin, Margaret Pabst; Snyder, Lois. Should older persons have the right to commit suicide? Yes [and] No. *In:* Scharlach, Andrew E.; Kaye, Lenard W., eds. Controversial Issues in Aging. Boston, MA: Allyn and Bacon; 1997: 92–102.
(SUICIDE)

Battistini, Michelle see **Grisso, Jeane Ann**

Batzel, Alice M. The HIM professional's role on the ethics committee. *Journal of the American Health Information Management Association.* 1996 Nov–Dec; 67(10): 58–60.
(ETHICISTS AND ETHICS COMMITTEES)

Bauer, Heidi M. see **Frank, Martina W.**

Baume, Peter see **Yuan, Zong F.**

Baumiller, Robert C.; Comley, Sarah; Cunningham, George; Fisher, Nancy; Fox, Lynda; Henderson, Merrill; Lebel, Robert; McGrath, Geraldine; Pelias, Mary Z.; Porter, Ian; Roper Willson, Nancy; Council of Regional Networks [for Genetic Services] Committee on Ethics. Code of ethical principles for genetics professionals. *American Journal of Medical Genetics.* 1996 Oct 28; 65(3): 177–178.
(GENETIC SERVICES; PROFESSIONAL ETHICS/CODES OF ETHICS)

Baumiller, Robert C.; Cunningham, George; Fisher, Nancy; Fox, Lynda; Henderson, Merrill; Lebel, Robert; McGrath, Geraldine; Pelias, Mary Z.;

Porter, Ian; Seydel, Frank; Roper Willson, Nancy; Council of Regional Networks [for Genetic Services] Committee on Ethics. Code of ethical principles for genetics professionals: an explication. *American Journal of Medical Genetics.* 1996 Oct 28; 65(3): 179–183.
(GENETIC SERVICES; PROFESSIONAL ETHICS/CODES OF ETHICS)

Bayer, Ronald. Clinical progress and the future of HIV exceptionalism. *Archives of Internal Medicine.* 1999 May 24; 159(10): 1042–1048.
(AIDS/CONFIDENTIALITY; AIDS/TESTING AND SCREENING)

Bayer, Ronald. Responsibility and intimacy in the AIDS epidemic. *Responsive Community.* 1997 Fall; 7(4): 45–55.
(AIDS/CONFIDENTIALITY)

Bayer, Ronald. Science, justice, and breast implants. [Editorial]. *American Journal of Public Health.* 1999 Apr; 89(4): 483.
(BIOMEDICAL RESEARCH; BIOMEDICAL TECHNOLOGIES)

Bayer, Ronald. The debate over maternal–fetal HIV transmission prevention trials in Africa, Asia, and the Caribbean: racist exploitation or exploitation of racism? *American Journal of Public Health.* 1998 Apr; 88(4): 567–570.
(AIDS/HUMAN EXPERIMENTATION; HUMAN EXPERIMENTATION/FOREIGN COUNTRIES; HUMAN EXPERIMENTATION/RESEARCH DESIGN; HUMAN EXPERIMENTATION/SPECIAL POPULATIONS)

Bayer, Ronald see **Fairchild, Amy L.**

Bayer, Ronald see **Feldman, Eric A.**

Bayer, Ronald see **Wilfert, Catherine M.**

Bayertz, Kurt. What's special about molecular genetic diagnostics? *Journal of Medicine and Philosophy.* 1998 Jun; 23(3): 247–254.
(GENETIC SCREENING; MASS SCREENING)

Baylis, Françoise; Downie, Jocelyn; Sherwin, Susan. Women and health research: from theory, to practice, to policy. *In:* Donchin, Anne; Purdy, Laura M., eds. Embodying Bioethics: Recent Feminist Advances. Lanham, MD: Rowman and Littlefield; 1999: 253–268.
(HUMAN EXPERIMENTATION/FOREIGN COUNTRIES; HUMAN EXPERIMENTATION/SPECIAL POPULATIONS)

Beasley, John W. Primary care research and protection for human subjects. [Letter]. *JAMA.* 1999 May 12; 281(18): 1697–1698.
(HUMAN EXPERIMENTATION/ETHICS COMMITTEES)

Beasley, John W. see **Finestone, Albert J.**

Beauchamp, Thomas L. see **Potts, John T.**

Beauchamp, Tom L. Hume on the nonhuman animal. *Journal of Medicine and Philosophy.* 1999 Aug; 24(4): 322–335.
(ANIMAL EXPERIMENTATION)

Beauchamp, Tom L. The mettle of moral fundamentalism: a reply to Robert Baker. *Kennedy Institute of Ethics Journal.* 1998 Dec.; 8(4): 389–401.
(BIOETHICS; HUMAN EXPERIMENTATION)

Beauchamp, Tom L.; Walters, LeRoy, eds.

Contemporary Issues in Bioethics. Fifth Edition. Belmont, CA: Wadsworth; 1999. 786 p.
(BIOETHICS)

Beauchamp, Tom L. see **Herdman, Roger**

Beaudoin, Claude; Maheux, Brigitte; Côté, Luc; Des Marchais, Jacques E.; Jean, Pierre; Berkson, Laeora. Clinical teachers as humanistic caregivers and educators: perceptions of senior clerks and second–year residents. *Canadian Medical Association Journal.* 1998 Oct 6; 159(7): 765–769.
(MEDICAL ETHICS/EDUCATION; PROFESSIONAL PATIENT RELATIONSHIP)

Beck, James C. Psychiatry and the death penalty. *Harvard Review of Psychiatry.* 1996 Nov–Dec; 4(4): 225–229.
(CAPITAL PUNISHMENT)

Beckel, Jean. Resolving ethical problems in long–term care. *Journal of Gerontological Nursing.* 1996 Jan; 22(1): 20–26.
(ALLOWING TO DIE)

Becker, Carl. Money talks, money kills -- the economics of transplantation in Japan and China. *Bioethics.* 1999 Jul; 13(3–4): 236–243.
(CAPITAL PUNISHMENT; DETERMINATION OF DEATH/BRAIN DEATH; ORGAN AND TISSUE DONATION; ORGAN AND TISSUE TRANSPLANTATION)

Becker, Gay see **Nachtigall, Robert D.**

Beckerman, Karen see **Balano, Kirsten**

Beckett, Alexandra. End–of–life decisions in AIDS. *In:* Steinberg, Maurice D.; Youngner, Stuart J., eds. End–of–Life Decisions: A Psychosocial Perspective. Washington, DC: American Psychiatric Press; 1998: 179–203.
(AIDS; ALLOWING TO DIE; SUICIDE)

Beckett, William S. see **Merrill, William W.**

Beckman, Howard B. see **Marvel, M. Kim**

Beckman, Linda J.; Harvey, S. Marie, eds. The New Civil War: The Psychology, Culture, and Politics of Abortion. Washington, DC: American Psychological Association; 1998. 406 p.
(ABORTION)

Beckwith, Jon. The responsibility of scientists in the genetics and race controversies. *In:* Smith, Edward; Sapp, Walter, eds. Plain Talk about the the Human Genome Project: A Tuskegee University Conference on Its Promise and Perils ... and Matters of Race. Tuskegee, AL: Tuskegee University Press; 1997: 83–94.
(BEHAVIORAL GENETICS)

Beech, Beverley A. Lawrence; Anderson, Gwen. 'We went through psychological hell': a case report of prenatal diagnosis. [Case study and commentaries]. *Nursing Ethics.* 1999 May; 6(3): 250–256.
(GENETIC SERVICES; PRENATAL DIAGNOSIS)

Beecham, Linda. GMC advises doctors on seeking consent. [News]. *BMJ (British Medical Journal).* 1999 Feb 27; 318(7183): 553.
(INFORMED CONSENT)

Beecham, Linda. UK issues guidance on prescribing Viagra. [News]. *BMJ (British Medical Journal).* 1999 Jan 30; 318(7179): 279.
(PATIENT CARE/DRUGS; RESOURCE ALLOCATION/BIOMEDICAL TECHNOLOGIES; SELECTION FOR TREATMENT)

Beecham, Linda; Dorozynski, Alexander; Sheldon, Tony; Turone, Fabio; Mach, Adrea; Bosch, Xavier; Charatan, Fred B.; Mahkorn, Déirdre Tilmann; Siegel–Itzkovich, Judy. Viagra falls: the debate over rationing continues -- Britain, France, Netherlands, Italy, Switzerland, Spain, United States, Germany, Israel. *BMJ (British Medical Journal).* 1998 Sep 26; 317(7162): 836–838.
(HEALTH CARE/ECONOMICS; PATIENT CARE/DRUGS)

Begley, Anne Marie; Farsides, Bobby. Response to the National Council for Hospice and Specialist Palliative Care Services -- voluntary euthanasia: the Council's view, by Ann Marie Begley, with reply by Bobby Farsides on behalf of the National Council for Hospice and Specialist Palliative Care Services. *Nursing Ethics.* 1999 Mar; 6(2): 157–161.
(EUTHANASIA; TERMINAL CARE)

Begum, Hasna. Health care, ethics and nursing in Bangladesh: a personal perspective. *Nursing Ethics.* 1998 Nov; 5(6): 535–541.
(HEALTH CARE/FOREIGN COUNTRIES)

Belgium. Agreement on cooperation establishing a Consultative Committee on Bioethics, done at Brussels on 15 Jan 1993 between the State, the Flemish Community, the French Community, the German–Speaking Community, and the Joint Inter–Community Commission. (*Moniteur Belge*, 12 May 1993, No. 93, p. 10824–10828). [Summary]. *International Digest of Health Legislation.* 1994. 45(1). 47–48.
(BIOETHICS; ETHICISTS AND ETHICS COMMITTEES)

Belik, Jacques see **Crelinsten, Gordon L.**

Belkin, Lisa. Getting the girl. *New York Times Magazine.* 1999 Jul 25: 26–31, 38, 54–55.
(SEX PRESELECTION)

Belkin, Lisa. Splice Einstein and Sammy Glick, add a little Magellan: banking on genes. *New York Times Magazine.* 1998 Aug 23: 26–31, 56, 58, 60–61.
(GENOME MAPPING)

Bell, Elmerine Allen Whitfield. Testimony of Elmerine Allen Whitfield Bell [concerning human experimentation with plutonium]. *Accountability in Research.* 1998 Jan; 6(1–2): 167–181.
(FRAUD AND MISCONDUCT; HUMAN EXPERIMENTATION)

Bell, P.R.F. see **Lloyd, A.J.**

Bell, Robert see **Leape, Lucian L.**

Belle, Steven see **Showstack, Jonathan**

Beller, Fritz K.; Zlatnik, Gail P. The beginning of human life. *Journal of Assisted Reproduction and Genetics.* 1995 Sep; 12(8): 477–483.
(FETUSES)

Belluck, Pam. Dr. Kevorkian is a murderer, the jury finds. [News]. *New York Times.* 1999 Mar 27: A1, A9.

(EUTHANASIA/LEGAL ASPECTS)

Belluck, Pam. For Kevorkian, a fifth but very different, trial. [News]. *New York Times.* 1999 Mar 20: A1, A11.
(EUTHANASIA/LEGAL ASPECTS)

Belluck, Pam. Kevorkian seen as 'distraction' on suicide aid. [News]. *New York Times.* 1999 Mar 30: A1, A17.
(EUTHANASIA/LEGAL ASPECTS; SUICIDE)

Beloqui, Jorge; Chokevivat, Vichai; Collins, Chris. HIV vaccine research and human rights: examples from three countries planning efficacy trials. *Health and Human Rights.* 1998; 3(1): 38–58.
(AIDS/HUMAN EXPERIMENTATION; IMMUNIZATION)

Benach, Marta O. see **McGovern, Margaret M.**

Benagiano, G. Reproductive health as an essential human right. *Advances in Contraception.* 1996 Dec; 12(4): 243–250.
(CONTRACEPTION; REPRODUCTION)

Benagiano, G.; Cottingham, J. Contraceptive methods: potential for abuse. *International Journal of Gynaecology and Obstetrics.* 1997 Jan; 56(1): 39–46.
(CONTRACEPTION)

Benatar, Solomon R. Global disparities in health and human rights: a critical commentary. *American Journal of Public Health.* 1998 Feb; 88(2): 295–300.
(HEALTH)

Benatar, Solomon R. Imperialism, research ethics, and global health. [Editorial]. *Journal of Medical Ethics.* 1998 Aug; 24(4): 221–222.
(HUMAN EXPERIMENTATION/FOREIGN COUNTRIES; HUMAN EXPERIMENTATION/RESEARCH DESIGN)

Benatar, Solomon R.; Tavistock Group. Shared ethical principles for everybody in health care: a working draft from the Tavistock group. A shared statement of ethical principles for those who shape and give health care. *BMJ (British Medical Journal).* 1999 Jan 23; 318(7178): 249–251.
(HEALTH CARE; PROFESSIONAL ETHICS/CODES OF ETHICS)

Benedict, James. The use of fetal tissue: a cautious approval. *Christian Century.* 1998 Feb 18; 115(5): 164–165.
(FETUSES; ORGAN AND TISSUE DONATION)

Benjamin, Georges see **Solomon, Liza**

Benjamin, Martin. Pragmatism and the determination of death. *In:* McGee, Glenn, ed. Pragmatic Bioethics. Nashville, TN: Vanderbilt University Press; 1999: 181–193, 280–281.
(DETERMINATION OF DEATH; PERSONHOOD)

Bennett, Bruce E. see **DeLeon, Patrick H.**

Bennett, Gerry see **White, D.M.D.**

Bennett, J.D. see **Houghton, D.J.**

Bennett, Nancy see **Pokorski, Robert J.**

Bennett, Rebecca. Should we routinely test pregnant women for HIV? *In:* Bennett, Rebecca; Erin, Charles

A., eds. HIV and AIDS: Testing, Screening, and Confidentiality. New York, NY: Oxford University Press; 1999: 228–239.
(AIDS/TESTING AND SCREENING)

Bennett, Rebecca; Erin, Charles A., eds. HIV and AIDS: Testing, Screening, and Confidentiality. New York, NY: Oxford University Press; 1999. 285 p.
(AIDS/CONFIDENTIALITY; AIDS/TESTING AND SCREENING)

Benshoof, Janet; Knights of Columbus. Abortion and the "pro–life" *v.* "pro–choice" debate: should the human fetus be considered a person? *In:* Francoeur, Robert T., ed. Taking Sides: Clashing Views on Controversial Issues in Human Sexuality. Fifth Edition. Guilford, CT: Dushkin Publishing Group/Brown and Benchmark; 1996: 120–133.
(ABORTION/LEGAL ASPECTS; FETUSES; PERSONHOOD)

Bentley, Margaret E. see **de Zoysa, Isabelle**

Benzi, Guido see **Gbolade, Babatunde A.**

Beran, Roy Gary. Professional privilege, driving and epilepsy, the doctor's responsibility. *Epilepsy Research.* 1997 Mar; 26(3): 415–421.
(CONFIDENTIALITY/LEGAL ASPECTS)

Berde, Charles see **Robinson, Walter M.**

Berenson, Robert A. see **Kosseff, Andrew L.**

Berenson, Robert A. see **Menendez, Roger**

Bereza, Eugene see **Crelinsten, Gordon L.**

Berg, Kåre see **Wertz, Dorothy C.**

Berg, Paul; Singer, Maxine. Regulating human cloning. [Editorial]. *Science.* 1998 Oct 16; 282(5388): 413.
(CLONING)

Berger, Abi. Private company wins rights to Icelandic gene database. [News]. *BMJ (British Medical Journal).* 1999 Jan 2; 318(7175): 11.
(GENETIC RESEARCH)

Berger, Jeffrey T. Culture and ethnicity in clinical care. *Archives of Internal Medicine.* 1998 Oct 26; 158(19): 2085–2090.
(ADVANCE DIRECTIVES; ORGAN AND TISSUE DONATION; PATIENT CARE; TRUTH DISCLOSURE)

Berger, Joseph. Yale gene pool seen as route to better baby. *New York Times.* 1999 Jan 10: 19.
(EUGENICS; REPRODUCTIVE TECHNOLOGIES)

Berghmans, Ron L.P. Ethical hazards of the substituted judgement test in decision making concerning the end of life of dementia patients. [Editorial]. *International Journal of Geriatric Psychiatry.* 1997 Mar; 12(3): 283–287.
(ALLOWING TO DIE; INFORMED CONSENT/MENTALLY DISABLED; PATIENT CARE/AGED)

Berglund, Catherine Anne. Bioethics: a balancing of concerns in context. *Australian Health Review.* 1997; 20(1): 43–52.
(BIOETHICS)

Berglund, Catherine Anne. Ethics for Health Care. New

York, NY: Oxford University Press; 1998. 228 p.
(BIOETHICS; PROFESSIONAL ETHICS)

Bergsma, Jan H. Dutch Union of Medical Ethics Committees. *Bulletin of Medical Ethics.* 1999 Feb; No. 145: 19–20.
(HUMAN EXPERIMENTATION/ETHICS COMMITTEES; HUMAN EXPERIMENTATION/FOREIGN COUNTRIES)

Bergsma, Jurrit; Mook, Bertha. Ethical considerations in psychotherapeutic systems. *Theoretical Medicine and Bioethics.* 1998 Aug; 19(4): 371–381.
(PROFESSIONAL ETHICS; PROFESSIONAL PATIENT RELATIONSHIP)

Berk, Richard see **Wenger, Neil S.**

Berkeley (CA). City Manager's Report on Proposed Ordinance Regulating the Use of Hazardous Biological Research, Recombinant DNA Research or Use of DNA Technology in the City of Berkeley [and] Draft Ordinance No. 5010 Later Enacted into Law. Issued by the City of Berkeley, City Manager's office, 2180 Milvia St., Berkeley, CA; 1977 Sep 13 (date issued). 9 p.
(RECOMBINANT DNA RESEARCH/REGULATION)

Berkeley (CA). Use of electric shock treatment prohibited. *Berkeley Municipal Code.* 1982 Dec 30 (date effective). Sect. 12.26.010 to 12.26.050. 2 p.
(ELECTROCONVULSIVE THERAPY)

Berkson, Laeora see **Beaudoin, Claude**

Berlin, Isaiah see **Admiraal, Pieter**

Berlin, Jesse A. see **Schulman, Kevin A.**

Bernard, David B.; Shulkin, David J. The media vs managed health care: are we seeing a full court press? *Archives of Internal Medicine.* 1998 Oct 26; 158(19): 2109–2111.
(HEALTH CARE/ECONOMICS)

Bernard, Lynn E.; McGillivray, Barbara; Van Allen, Margot I.; Friedman, J.M.; Langlois, Sylvie. Duty to re–contact: a study of families at risk for Fragile X. *Journal of Genetic Counseling.* 1999 Feb; 8(1): 3–15.
(GENETIC COUNSELING; GENETIC SCREENING)

Bernat, James L. Refinements in the definition and criterion of death. *In:* Youngner, Stuart J.; Arnold, Robert M.; Schapiro, Renie, eds. The Definition of Death: Contemporary Controversies. Baltimore, MD: Johns Hopkins University Press; 1999: 83–92.
(DETERMINATION OF DEATH/BRAIN DEATH)

Bernat, James L. VHA ethics rounds: [ethics committee role]. *NCCE News (Veterans Health Administration National Center for Clinical Ethics).* 1995 Spring; 3(2): 4–5.
(ALLOWING TO DIE; ETHICISTS AND ETHICS COMMITTEES)

Bernat, James L. see **Lizza, John B.**

Bernhardt, B. see **Schoonmaker, M.**

Bernhardt, B.A. see **James, C.A.**

Bernheim, Jan L. How to get serious answers to the serious question: "How have you been?": subjective quality of life (QOL) as an individual experiential

emergent construct. *Bioethics.* 1999 Jul; 13(3–4): 272–287.
(HEALTH)

Bernstein, Nina. For subjects in Haiti study, free AIDS care has a price: a special report. *New York Times.* 1999 Jun 6: A1, A10.
(AIDS/HUMAN EXPERIMENTATION; HUMAN EXPERIMENTATION/FOREIGN COUNTRIES)

Bero, Lisa A. see **Hsu, John**

Berry, Roberta M. The Human Genome Project and the end of insurance. *University of Florida Journal of Law and Public Policy.* 1996 Spring; 7(2): 205–256.
(GENETIC SCREENING; GENOME MAPPING)

Berry, Roberta M. see **Robinson, John H.**

Berry, Sandy see **Wenger, Neil S.**

Berwick, Donald see **Smith, Richard**

Bessesen, Mary see **Bolan, Robert K.**

Bessman, Edward S. see **Marco, Catherine A.**

Betancourt, Joseph R. see **Carrillo, J. Emilio**

Bettman, Jerome W. Ethics and the American Academy of Ophthalmology in historical perspective. *Ophthalmology.* 1996 Aug; 103(8, Suppl.): S29–S39.
(MEDICAL ETHICS)

Bevington, Linda K. see **Stewart, Gary P.**

Bewley, Susan see **Swinn, Michael**

Beyer, Jan see **Antuono, Piero**

Bhadrakom, Chaiporn see **Achrekar, Abinash**

Bhopal, Raj; Donaldson, Liam. White, European, Western, Caucasian, or what? Inappropriate labeling in research on race, ethnicity, and health. *American Journal of Public Health.* 1998 Sep; 88(9): 1303–1307.
(PUBLIC HEALTH)

Biagioli, Mario. Publication and promotion: long live the deans! *Lancet.* 1998 Sep 12; 352(9131): 899–900.
(BIOMEDICAL RESEARCH; FRAUD AND MISCONDUCT)

Bickel, Janet. Proceedings of the AAMC Conference on Students' and Residents' Ethical and Professional Development: introduction. *Academic Medicine.* 1996 Jun; 71(6): 622–623.
(MEDICAL ETHICS/EDUCATION)

Bickel, Janet. Summaries of break-out sessions [AAMC Conference on Students' and Residents' Ethical and Professional Development, 27–28 Oct 1995]. *Academic Medicine.* 1996 Jun; 71(6): 634–640.
(MEDICAL ETHICS/EDUCATION)

Biederman, Joseph see **Leonard, Henrietta**

Bienenstock, John see **MacLeod, Stuart M.**

Biesecker, Leslie G. see **DeRenzo, Evan G.**

Bignell, C.J. Chaperones for genital examination.

[Editorial]. *BMJ (British Medical Journal).* 1999 Jul 17; 319(7203): 137–138.
(PATIENT CARE; PROFESSIONAL PATIENT RELATIONSHIP)

Bilger, Burkhard. Cell block: moral relativism and news of practical benefits are nudging human cloning toward public acceptance, even as the first laws are written to ban it. *Sciences.* 1997 Sep–Oct; 37(5): 17–19.
(CLONING)

Billauer, Barbara Pfeffer. On Judaism and genes: a response to Paul Root Wolpe. *Kennedy Institute of Ethics Journal.* 1999 Jun; 9(2): 159–165.
(BEHAVIORAL GENETICS)

Billings, J. Andrew see **Block, Susan**

Billings, J. Andrew see **Stead, William W.**

Billings, Paul see **Handelin, Barbara**

Billings, Paul R.; Newman, Stuart A. Crossing the germline. *GeneWATCH.* 1999 Jan; 11(5–6): 1, 3–4.
(EMBRYO AND FETAL RESEARCH; GENE THERAPY)

Billings, Paul R.; Schneider, Holm; Coutelle, Charles. In utero gene therapy: the case against [and] the case for. *Nature Medicine.* 1999 Mar; 5(3): 255–257.
(EMBRYO AND FETAL RESEARCH; GENE THERAPY)

Billings, Paul R. see **Stoddard, Joan C.**

Bin Saeed, Khalid Saad. How physician executives and clinicians perceive ethical issues in Saudi Arabian hospitals. *Journal of Medical Ethics.* 1999 Feb; 25(1): 51–56.
(BIOETHICS; MEDICAL ETHICS)

Binder, Renée L. see **McNiel, Dale E.**

Bindless, Linda. The use of patients in health care education: the need for ethical justification. *Journal of Medical Ethics.* 1998 Oct; 24(5): 314–319.
(PATIENTS' RIGHTS; PROFESSIONAL ETHICS/EDUCATION)

Bindman, Andrew B.; Osmond, Dennis; Hecht, Frederick M.; Lehman, J. Stan; Vranizan, Karen; Keane, Dennis; Reingold, Arthur. Multistate evaluation of anonymous HIV testing and access to medical care. [For the Multistate Evaluation of Surveillance of HIV (MESH) Study Group]. *JAMA.* 1998 Oct 28; 280(16): 1416–1420.
(AIDS/TESTING AND SCREENING)

Bindman, Andrew B. see **Colfax, Grant Nash**

Bindman, Andrew B. see **Grumbach, Kevin**

Bindman, Andrew B. see **Saha, Somnath**

Binedell, Julia. Adolescent requests for predictive genetic testing. *In:* Clarke, Angus, ed. The Genetic Testing of Children. Washington, DC: BIOS Scientific Publishers; 1998: 123–132.
(GENETIC SCREENING)

Bing, A. see **Hassan, T.B.**

Binstock, Robert H. Old-age-based rationing: from rhetoric to risk? *Generations (American Society on Aging).*

1994 Winter; 18(4): 37–41.
(HEALTH CARE/ECONOMICS; PATIENT CARE/AGED; RESOURCE ALLOCATION; SELECTION FOR TREATMENT)

Binstock, Robert H.; Murray, Thomas H. Genetics and long–term–care insurance: ethical and policy issues. *In:* Post, Stephen G.; Whitehouse, Peter J., eds. Genetic Testing for Alzheimer Disease: Ethical and Clinical Issues. Baltimore, MD: Johns Hopkins University Press; 1998: 155–176.
(GENETIC SCREENING; HEALTH CARE/ECONOMICS)

Birchard, Karen. Irish doctors concerned by information access. [News]. *Lancet.* 1998 Oct 24; 352(9137): 1368.
(CONFIDENTIALITY/LEGAL ASPECTS; PATIENT ACCESS TO RECORDS)

Birchard, Karen. New ethical guidelines on abortion released in Ireland. [News]. *Lancet.* 1998 Dec 5; 352(9143): 1840.
(ABORTION/FOREIGN COUNTRIES)

Birleson, Peter. Legal rights and responsibilities of adolescents and staff in Victorian Child and Adolescent Mental Health Services. *Australian and New Zealand Journal of Psychiatry.* 1996 Dec; 30(6): 805–812.
(INFORMED CONSENT/MENTALLY DISABLED; INFORMED CONSENT/MINORS)

Birmingham, Karen. UK leads on science and technology bioethics. [News]. *Nature Medicine.* 1998 Jun; 4(6): 651–652.
(BIOETHICS; DNA FINGERPRINTING; GENETIC INTERVENTION)

Birmingham, Karen; Cimons, Marlene. Government report highlights the lack of clinical trial protection in the US. [News]. *Nature Medicine.* 1998 Jul; 4(7): 749.
(HUMAN EXPERIMENTATION/ETHICS COMMITTEES; HUMAN EXPERIMENTATION/REGULATION)

Birn, Anne–Emanuelle see **Krieger, Nancy**

Biros, Michelle H. Institutional review board approval: when and why? *Academic Emergency Medicine.* 1998 Feb; 5(2): 91–92.
(HUMAN EXPERIMENTATION/ETHICS COMMITTEES)

Bishop, Laura Jane; Cherry, M. Nichelle; Darragh, Martina. Organizational ethics and health care: expanding bioethics to the institutional arena. [Bibliography]. *Kennedy Institute of Ethics Journal.* 1999 Jun; 9(2): 189–208.
(PROFESSIONAL ETHICS)

Bito, Seiji see **Wenger, Neil**

Biven, Miranda. Administrative developments: NIH backs federal funding for stem cell research. *Journal of Law, Medicine and Ethics.* 1999 Spring; 27(1): 95–99.
(EMBRYO AND FETAL RESEARCH)

Bjørn, Else; Rossel, Peter; Holm, Søren. Can the written information to research subjects be improved? -- an empirical study. *Journal of Medical Ethics.* 1999 Jun; 25(3): 263–267.
(HUMAN EXPERIMENTATION/INFORMED CONSENT)

Black, Douglas. Medicalised erections on demand? [Editorial]. *Journal of Medical Ethics.* 1999 Feb; 25(1): 5–7.
(HEALTH CARE/ECONOMICS; PATIENT CARE/DRUGS)

Black, Peter. Managed care and the patient: surgical, ethical and legal considerations. *Journal of Clinical Neuroscience.* 1997 Apr; 4(2): 149–151.
(HEALTH CARE/ECONOMICS)

Black, Robert E. see **Edi–Osagie, E.C.O.**

Blackwell, Barry see **Menendez, Roger**

Blair, Jayson see **Pérez–Peña, Richard**

Blair, P.S. see **West, Charles**

Blake, Robert L.; Early, Elizabeth K. Patients' attitudes about gifts to physicians from pharmaceutical companies. *Journal of the American Board of Family Practice.* 1995 Nov–Dec; 8(6): 457–464.
(HEALTH CARE/ECONOMICS; PATIENT CARE/DRUGS)

Blanche, Stéphane see **Merson, Michael H.**

Blank, Robert H. Brain Policy: How the New Neuroscience Will Change Our Lives and Our Politics. Washington, DC: Georgetown University Press; 1999. 199 p.
(BIOMEDICAL RESEARCH; BIOMEDICAL TECHNOLOGIES)

Blechner, Barbara see **Walker, Leslie**

Bleich, J. David. Bioethical Dilemmas: A Jewish Perspective. Hoboken, NJ: Ktav; 1998. 375 p.
(BIOETHICS)

Bleich, J. David. Moral debate and semantic sleight of hand. *Suffolk University Law Review.* 1993 Winter; 27(4): 1173–1193.
(DETERMINATION OF DEATH/BRAIN DEATH; FETUSES; ORGAN AND TISSUE DONATION)

Bleich, J. David. On "The ethics of pain management." [Editorial]. *Cancer Investigation.* 1994; 12(3): 362–363.
(TERMINAL CARE)

Bleich, J. David; Caplan, Arthur L.; Murray, Joseph E.; Lafferty, Kevin J.; Robertson, John A. Defining the limits of organ and tissue research and transplantation. [Proceedings of the International Symposium on Law and Science at the Crossroads: Biomedical Technology, Ethics, Public Policy, and the Law; panel discussion]. *Suffolk University Law Review.* 1993 Winter; 27(4): 1457–1476.
(DETERMINATION OF DEATH/BRAIN DEATH; FETUSES; ORGAN AND TISSUE DONATION)

Bliss, Laura E. see **Cook, Rebecca J.**

Blizard, Bob see **Shah, Nisha**

Bloch, Alexia see **Siminoff, Laura A.**

Bloch, Sidney; Harari, Edwin. Working with the family: the role of values. *American Journal of Psychotherapy.* 1996 Summer; 50(3): 274–284.
(PATIENT CARE/MENTALLY DISABLED; PROFESSIONAL PATIENT RELATIONSHIP)

Bloch, Sidney see **Pargiter, Russell**

Bloch, Sidney see **Szmukler, George I.**

Bloche, M. Gregg. Clinical loyalties and the social

purposes of medicine. *JAMA.* 1999 Jan 20; 281(3): 268–274.
(MEDICAL ETHICS; PROFESSIONAL PATIENT RELATIONSHIP)

Block, Susan; Billings, J. Andrew. Nurturing humanism through teaching palliative care. *Academic Medicine.* 1998 Jul; 73(7): 763–765.
(MEDICAL ETHICS/EDUCATION; TERMINAL CARE)

Block, Susan D. see **Simon, Steven R.**

Block, Susan D. see **Stead, William W.**

Blokhuis, Harry J. see **Mepham, T. Ben**

Blondeau, Danielle; Valois, Pierre; Keyserlingk, Edward W.; Hébert, Martin; Lavoie, Mireille. Comparison of patients' and health care professionals' attitudes towards advance directives. *Journal of Medical Ethics.* 1998 Oct; 24(5): 328–335.
(ADVANCE DIRECTIVES)

Bloom, Barry R. see **Mann, Jonathan M.**

Bloom, Floyd E. see **Miller, Linda J.**

Blue, Arthur; Keyserlingk, Edward; Rodney, Patricia; Starzomski, Rosalie. A critical view of North American health policy. *In:* Coward, Harold; Ratanakul, Pinit, eds. A Cross-Cultural Dialogue on Health Care Ethics. Waterloo, ON: Wilfrid Laurier University Press; 1999: 215–225.
(HEALTH CARE)

Blumensohn, Rachel see **Mester, Roberto**

Blumenthal, David. Ethics issues in academic-industry relationships in the life sciences: the continuing debate. *Academic Medicine.* 1996 Dec; 71(12): 1291–1296.
(BIOMEDICAL RESEARCH)

Blumenthal, David see **Finestone, Albert J.**

Blumenthal, David see **Hsu, John**

Blumenthal, Ralph; Miller, Judith. Japanese germ-war atrocities: a half-century of stonewalling the world. *New York Times.* 1999 Mar 4: A12.
(FRAUD AND MISCONDUCT; HUMAN EXPERIMENTATION/FOREIGN COUNTRIES; HUMAN EXPERIMENTATION/SPECIAL POPULATIONS; WAR)

Blustein, Jeffrey. Choosing for others as continuing a life story: the problem of personal identity revisited. *Journal of Law, Medicine and Ethics.* 1999 Spring; 27(1): 20–31.
(ADVANCE DIRECTIVES; INFORMED CONSENT; PERSONHOOD)

Blustein, Jeffrey see **Post, Linda Farber**

Bock, Gisela. Sterilization and "medical" massacres in National Socialist Germany: ethics, politics, and the law. *In:* Berg, Manfred; Cocks, Geoffrey, eds. Medicine and Modernity: Public Health and Medical Care in Nineteenth- and Twentieth-Century Germany. New York, NY: Cambridge University Press; 1997: 149–172.
(EUGENICS; EUTHANASIA; STERILIZATION)

Bodenheimer, Thomas. Disease management -- promises and pitfalls. *New England Journal of Medicine.* 1999 Apr

15; 340(15): 1202–1205.
(HEALTH CARE/ECONOMICS; PATIENT CARE)

Bodenheimer, Thomas. The American health care system: physicians and the changing medical marketplace. *New England Journal of Medicine.* 1999 Feb 18; 340(7): 584–588.
(HEALTH CARE/ECONOMICS)

Bodiwala, G.G. see **Hassan, T.B.**

Boettcher, Brian. Fatal episodes in medical history. [Personal view]. *BMJ (British Medical Journal).* 1998 Dec 5; 317(7172): 1603.
(FRAUD AND MISCONDUCT; PATIENT CARE)

Boetzkes, Elisabeth. Equality, autonomy, and feminist bioethics. *In:* Donchin, Anne; Purdy, Laura M., eds. Embodying Bioethics: Recent Feminist Advances. Lanham, MD: Rowman and Littlefield; 1999: 121–139.
(SEX DETERMINATION; SEX PRESELECTION; SURROGATE MOTHERS)

Boetzkes, Elisabeth. Genetic knowledge and third-party interests. *Cambridge Quarterly of Healthcare Ethics.* 1999 Summer; 8(3): 386–392.
(CONFIDENTIALITY; GENETIC SCREENING)

Bogardus, Sidney T.; Holmboe, Eric; Jekel, James F. Perils, pitfalls, and possibilities in talking about medical risk. *JAMA.* 1999 Mar 17; 281(11): 1037–1041.
(INFORMED CONSENT)

Bohlin, Raymond G. The possibilities and ethics of human cloning. *In:* Demy, Timothy J.; Stewart, Gary P., eds. Genetic Engineering: A Christian Response: Crucial Considerations in Shaping Life. Grand Rapids, MI: Kregel Publications; 1999: 260–277.
(CLONING)

Boisvert, D.P.J. Editorial policies and animal welfare. *In:* van Zutphen, L.F.M.; Balls, M., eds. Animal Alternatives, Welfare and Ethics. New York, NY: Elsevier; 1997: 399–404.
(ANIMAL EXPERIMENTATION)

Bok, Sissela see **Dworkin, Gerald**

Bolan, Robert K.; Bessesen, Mary; McCollum, Marianne; Frothingham, Richard; Casarett, David; Lantos, John. AIDS exceptionalism. [Letters and response]. *Annals of Internal Medicine.* 1999 Jan 5; 130(1): 79–80.
(AIDS; RESOURCE ALLOCATION)

Bollinger, R. Randal. A UNOS [United Network for Organ Sharing] perspective on donor liver allocation. *Liver Transplantation and Surgery.* 1995 Jan; 1(1): 47–55.
(ORGAN AND TISSUE TRANSPLANTATION; RESOURCE ALLOCATION/BIOMEDICAL TECHNOLOGIES)

Bombard, Allan see **Freda, Margaret Comerford**

Bonati, Maurizio; Garattini, Silvio. Evidence- and ethical-based child health: update on therapeutic trials in children. *In:* Burgio, G. Roberto; Lantos, John D., eds. *Primum Non Nocere* Today. Second Edition. New York, NY: Elsevier; 1998: 101–106.
(PATIENT CARE/MINORS)

Bonecutter, Faith J. see **Gorelick, Philip B.**

Bonetta, Laura. Inquiry into clinical trial scandal at Canadian research hospital. [News]. *Nature Medicine.* 1998 Oct; 4(10): 1095.
(BIOMEDICAL RESEARCH; HUMAN EXPERIMENTATION/FOREIGN COUNTRIES)

Boneysteele, Ginger see **Constantino, Rose E.**

Bonney, Aba see **Lerman, Caryn**

Bonnicksen, Andrea L. Procreation by cloning: crafting anticipatory guidelines. *Journal of Law, Medicine and Ethics.* 1997 Winter; 25(4): 273–282.
(CLONING; EMBRYO AND FETAL RESEARCH)

Bonnie, Richard J. Research with cognitively impaired subjects: unfinished business in the regulation of human research. *Archives of General Psychiatry.* 1997 Feb; 54(2): 105–111.
(HUMAN EXPERIMENTATION/REGULATION; HUMAN EXPERIMENTATION/SPECIAL POPULATIONS)

Bood, Alex see **Griffiths, John**

Boogaerts, Andrea see **Decruyenaere, Marleen**

Bopp, James; Cook, Curtis R. Partial–birth abortion: the final frontier of abortion jurisprudence. *Issues in Law and Medicine.* 1998 Summer; 14(1): 3–57.
(ABORTION/LEGAL ASPECTS)

Bopp, James; Cook, Curtis R.; Heilig, Steve; Annas, George J. Partial–birth abortion. [Letters and response]. *New England Journal of Medicine.* 1998 Dec 3; 339(23): 1716–1717.
(ABORTION/LEGAL ASPECTS)

Bordo, Susan. *Braveheart, Babe,* and the contemporary body. *In:* Parens, Erik, ed. Enhancing Human Traits: Ethical and Social Implications. Washington, DC: Georgetown University Press; 1998: 189–221.
(BIOMEDICAL TECHNOLOGIES; HEALTH)

Boronow, John; Stoline, Anne; Sharfstein, Steven S. Refusal of ECT by a patient with recurrent depression, psychosis, and catatonia. *American Journal of Psychiatry.* 1997 Sep; 154(9): 1285–1291.
(ELECTROCONVULSIVE THERAPY; TREATMENT REFUSAL/MENTALLY DISABLED)

Borowski, A.; Schickendantz, S.; Mennicken, U.; Korb, H. Open heart interventions in premature, low- and very–low–birth–weight neonates: risk profile and ethical considerations. *Thoracic and Cardiovascular Surgeon.* 1997 Oct; 45(5): 238–241.
(PATIENT CARE/MINORS)

Borrmans, Maurice. Health, illness, and healing in the great religions: IV. Islam. *Dolentium Hominum: Church and Health in the World.* 1998; No. 37 [yr. 13(1)]: 118–120.
(HEALTH; HEALTH CARE)

Borzi, Phyllis see **Rosenbaum, Sara**

Bosch, Xavier. Commission set up to deal with HIV infected doctors in Spain. [News]. *BMJ (British Medical Journal).* 1998 Oct 10; 317(7164): 970.
(AIDS/HEALTH PERSONNEL)

Bosch, Xavier. Confidential Spanish registry of HIV–infected individuals. [News]. *JAMA.* 1999 Mar 17; 281(11): 977.
(AIDS/CONFIDENTIALITY)

Bosch, Xavier. Eating disorders may warrant compulsory hospital admission. [News]. *Lancet.* 1999 Mar 20; 353(9157): 993.
(INVOLUNTARY COMMITMENT/FOREIGN COUNTRIES)

Bosch, Xavier. European body to oversee tissue banks. [News]. *Nature Medicine.* 1998 Sep; 4(9): 988.
(ORGAN AND TISSUE DONATION)

Bosch, Xavier. Geneticists discuss ethics of human genome project. [News]. *Lancet.* 1998 Oct 31; 352(9138): 1448.
(GENOME MAPPING)

Bosch, Xavier. Spain brings forward mifepristone approval. [News]. *Lancet.* 1998 Oct 17; 352(9136): 1293.
(ABORTION/FOREIGN COUNTRIES)

Bosch, Xavier. Spain fails to extend its criteria for legal abortions. [News]. *Lancet.* 1998 Oct 3; 352(9134): 1130.
(ABORTION/FOREIGN COUNTRIES)

Bosch, Xavier. Spain leads world in organ donation and transplantation. [News]. *JAMA.* 1999 Jul 7; 282(1): 17–18.
(ORGAN AND TISSUE DONATION; ORGAN AND TISSUE TRANSPLANTATION)

Bosch, Xavier. Spain releases xenotransplantation guidelines. [News]. *Nature Medicine.* 1998 Aug; 4(8): 876.
(ORGAN AND TISSUE TRANSPLANTATION)

Bosch, Xavier. Spanish patients' access to records boosted. [News]. *Lancet.* 1999 Jul 17; 354(9174): 232.
(PATIENT ACCESS TO RECORDS)

Bosch, Xavier. Spanish watchdog sees way ahead for stem–cell research. [News]. *Nature.* 1999 Apr 22; 398(6729): 645.
(CLONING)

Bosch, Xavier see **Beecham, Linda**

Boshammer, Susanne; Kayss, Matthias; Runtenberg, Christa; Ach, Johann S. Discussing HUGO: the German debate on the ethical implications of the Human Genome Project. *Journal of Medicine and Philosophy.* 1998 Jun; 23(3): 324–333.
(GENOME MAPPING)

Boshkov, Lynn see **Caulfield, Timothy**

Bostrom, Barry A. Evans v. Kelley. [Note]. *Issues in Law and Medicine.* 1998 Summer; 14(1): 103–106.
(ABORTION/LEGAL ASPECTS)

Bostrom, Barry A. In the matter of the guardianship and protective placement of Edna M.F. [Note]. *Issues in Law and Medicine.* 1998 Fall; 14(2): 205–207.
(ALLOWING TO DIE/LEGAL ASPECTS)

Bostrom, Barry A. Planned Parenthood of Wisconsin v. Doyle. [Note]. *Issues in Law and Medicine.* 1998 Fall; 14(2): 209–214.
(ABORTION/LEGAL ASPECTS)

Botkin, Jeffrey R. see **Schrock, Charles R.**

Botstein, David. Of genes and genomes. *In:* Smith, Edward; Sapp, Walter, eds. Plain Talk about the Human

Genome Project: A Tuskegee University Conference on Its Promise and Perils ... and Matters of Race. Tuskegee, AL: Tuskegee University Press; 1997: 207–214.
(GENOME MAPPING)

Bottum, J. Debriefing the philosophers. *First Things*. 1997 Jun–Jul; No. 74: 26–30.
(ETHICISTS AND ETHICS COMMITTEES; SUICIDE)

Bouchard, Charles E. The virtuous manager. *Health Progress*. 1997 May–Jun; 78(3): 27–29.
(PROFESSIONAL ETHICS)

Boué, A. *Primum non nocere*: prenatal diagnosis and selective abortion. *In:* Burgio, G. Roberto; Lantos, John D., eds. *Primum Non Nocere* Today. Second Edition. New York, NY: Elsevier; 1998: 49–57.
(ABORTION; PRENATAL DIAGNOSIS)

Boulyjenkov, Victor see **Wertz, Dorothy C.**

Bourguignon, Henry J. see **Martyn, Susan R.**

Bourke, Brian. Decisions, decisions. *Healthcare Alabama*. 1997 Mar; 10(1): 12–15, 20.
(ETHICISTS AND ETHICS COMMITTEES)

Bova, Ben. The impact of immortality. *In: his* Immortality: How Science Is Extending Your Life Span -- and Changing the World. New York, NY: Avon Books; 1998: 183–251.
(LIFE EXTENSION)

Bowen, Jennifer R. see **Sutcliffe, Alastair G.**

Bower, Bruce. Psychology's tangled web: deceptive methods may backfire on behavioral researchers. *Science News*. 1998 Jun 20; 153(25): 394–395.
(BEHAVIORAL RESEARCH/RESEARCH DESIGN)

Bowes, Watson; Byrne, Paul; Cavanagh, Denis; Colliton, William; Foye, Gerard; Klaus, Hanna; Pellegrino, Edmund. True integrity for the maternal–fetal medicine physician. *Linacre Quarterly*. 1997 Aug; 64(3): 77–86.
(ABORTION/ATTITUDES; PRENATAL DIAGNOSIS)

Bowker, Lesley see **Bacon, Mike**

Bowman, James E. Minority health issues and genetics. *Community Genetics*. 1998; 1(3): 142–144.
(GENETIC SCREENING)

Bowman, James E. To screen or not to screen: when should screening be offered? *Community Genetics*. 1998; 1(3): 145–147.
(GENETIC SCREENING; PRENATAL DIAGNOSIS)

Boyce, Nell. Psychiatric guinea pigs are left in limbo. [News]. *New Scientist*. 1998 Nov 28; 160(2162): 21.
(HUMAN EXPERIMENTATION/SPECIAL POPULATIONS)

Boyd, Jeff see **MacKay, Charles**

Boyd, Kenneth. Bringing both sides together. *Cambridge Quarterly of Healthcare Ethics*. 1999 Winter; 8(1): 43–45.
(ANIMAL EXPERIMENTATION)

Boyd, Kenneth. Old age, something to look forward to.

In: Hanson, Mark J.; Callahan, Daniel, eds. The Goals of Medicine: The Forgotten Issue in Health Care Reform. Washington, DC: Georgetown University Press; 1999: 152–161.
(HEALTH CARE; PATIENT CARE/AGED)

Boyd, Kenneth see **Campbell, Harry**

Boyd, Kenneth see **Cash, John**

Boyes, Edward see **Hill, Ruaraidh**

Boyle, J.M. see **Jaeger, A.S.**

Boyle, Joseph. An absolute rule approach. *In:* Kuhse, Helga; Singer, Peter, eds. A Companion to Bioethics. Malden, MA: Blackwell; 1998: 72–79.
(BIOETHICS)

Boyle, Philip see **O'Rourke, Kevin D.**

Bradley, Elizabeth see **Walker, Leslie**

Bradley, Elizabeth H.; Peiris, Vasum; Wetle, Terrie. Discussions about end-of-life care in nursing homes. *Journal of the American Geriatrics Society*. 1998 Oct; 46(10): 1235–1241.
(ADVANCE DIRECTIVES; TERMINAL CARE)

Bradley, Elizabeth H.; Rizzo, John A. Public information and private search: evaluating the Patient Self–Determination Act. *Journal of Health Politics, Policy and Law*. 1999 Apr; 24(2): 239–273.
(ADVANCE DIRECTIVES)

Bradley, Elizabeth H.; Wetle, Terrie; Horwitz, Sarah. The Patient Self–Determination Act and advance directive completion in nursing homes. *Archives of Family Medicine*. 1998 Sep–Oct; 7(5): 417–423.
(ADVANCE DIRECTIVES)

Bradley, J. Andrew see **Nicholson, Michael L.**

Bragg, Rick. A family shooting and a twist like no other. [News]. *New York Times*. 1999 May 19: A1, A16.
(ALLOWING TO DIE/LEGAL ASPECTS)

Bragg, Rick. Woman avoids murder charge over daughter. [News]. *New York Times*. 1999 May 26: A26.
(ALLOWING TO DIE/LEGAL ASPECTS)

Brahmachari, Samir K. see **Chatterji, Somnath**

Braithwaite, Susan S. see **McChesney, Lawrence P.**

Brakman, Sarah–Vaughan; Amari–Vaught, Eileen. Resistance and refusal. [Case study and commentaries]. *Hastings Center Report*. 1999 Jan–Feb; 29(1): 22–23.
(INFORMED CONSENT/MENTALLY DISABLED; TREATMENT REFUSAL/MENTALLY DISABLED)

Brakman, Sarah–Vaughan see **Dietz, Sarah M.**

Brakman, Sarah–Vaughan see **Purtell, Dennis J.**

Branch, William T.; Pels, Richard J.; Hafler, Janet P. Medical students' empathic understanding of their patients. *Academic Medicine*. 1998 Apr; 73(4): 360–362.
(MEDICAL ETHICS/EDUCATION; PROFESSIONAL PATIENT RELATIONSHIP)

Branco, Kenneth J. see **Teno, Joan M.**

Brand, Donald A.; Kliger, Alan S. Planning for a kidney transplant: is my doctor listening? *JAMA.* 1999 Aug 18; 282(7): 691–694.
(ORGAN AND TISSUE TRANSPLANTATION; PROFESSIONAL PATIENT RELATIONSHIP)

Brandt, Allan M. see **Mandl, Kenneth D.**

Branigin, William. Sect's transfusion ban puts believer at risk. [News]. *Washington Post.* 1999 Jan 21: A2.
(TREATMENT REFUSAL)

Bratton, Letitia B.; Griffin, Linner Ward. A kidney donor's dilemma: the sibling who can donate -- but doesn't. *Social Work in Health Care.* 1994; 20(2): 75–96.
(ORGAN AND TISSUE DONATION)

Braun, Hans see **van der Valk, Jan**

Braunholtz, David A. see **Edwards, Sarah J.L.**

Brayshaw, A. see **Williams, L.**

Brazell, Nancy E. The significance and application of informed consent. *AORN Journal (Association of Operating Room Nurses).* 1997 Feb; 65(2): 377, 379–380, 382, 385–386.
(INFORMED CONSENT)

Brazier, Margaret. Reproductive rights: feminism or patriarchy? *In:* Harris, John; Holm, Søren, eds. The Future of Human Reproduction: Ethics, Choice, and Regulation. New York, NY: Oxford University Press; 1998: 66–76.
(REPRODUCTION; REPRODUCTIVE TECHNOLOGIES)

Brazier, Margaret; Lobjoit, Mary. Fiduciary relationship: an ethical approach and a legal concept? *In:* Bennett, Rebecca; Erin, Charles A., eds. HIV and AIDS: Testing, Screening, and Confidentiality. New York, NY: Oxford University Press; 1999: 179–199.
(AIDS/CONFIDENTIALITY; AIDS/HEALTH PERSONNEL; AIDS/TESTING AND SCREENING)

Brazil. Federal Medical Council. Federal Medical Council (CFM) of Brazil adopts resolutions on criteria for death and on medically assisted procreation. [Texts of Resolution CFM No. 1346/91, adopted 8 Aug 1991; and Resolution CFM No. 1358/92, adopted 11 Nov 1992]. *International Digest of Health Legislation.* 1994; 45(1): 100–102.
(DETERMINATION OF DEATH/BRAIN DEATH; REPRODUCTIVE TECHNOLOGIES)

Breen, Kerry J.; Plueckhahn, Vernon D.; Cordner, Stephen M. Ethics, Law and Medical Practice. St. Leonards, NSW, Australia: Allen and Unwin; 1997. 367 p.
(HEALTH CARE/FOREIGN COUNTRIES; MEDICAL ETHICS; PATIENT CARE)

Breier, Alan see **Pinals, Debra A.**

Breimer, Lars; Brown, Laura; Skinner, Andrew; Gani, Akif; Hillman, Harold; Rymer, Janice. Fraud. [Letters]. *BMJ (British Medical Journal).* 1998 Dec 5; 317(7172): 1590–1591.
(BIOMEDICAL RESEARCH; FRAUD AND MISCONDUCT)

Bremberg, Stefan see **Zwitter, Matjaz**

Brems, John see **Thomasma, David C.**

Brennan, Andrew. Ethics, codes and animal research. *In:* van Zutphen, L.F.M.; Balls, M., eds. Animal Alternatives, Welfare and Ethics. New York, NY: Elsevier; 1997: 43–54.
(ANIMAL EXPERIMENTATION)

Brenner, Zara R.; Duffy-Durnin, Karen. Toward restraint-free care. *American Journal of Nursing.* 1998 Dec; 98(12): 16F, 16H–16I.
(PATIENT CARE)

Bresnahan, James F. Palliative care or assisted suicide? *America.* 1998 Mar 14; 178(8): 16–21.
(SUICIDE; TERMINAL CARE/HOSPICES)

Brewster, M.F. see **Godfrey-Faussett, Peter**

Brewster, M.F. see **Limentani, Alexander E.**

Briant, Robin H.; St. George, Ian M.; White, Gillian. Sexual activity between doctors and patients. [Letter and response]. *New Zealand Medical Journal.* 1996 Apr 12; 109(1019): 127–128.
(FRAUD AND MISCONDUCT; PROFESSIONAL PATIENT RELATIONSHIP)

Bricklin, Patricia M. see **DeLeon, Patrick H.**

Bridgeman, Jo. Declared innocent? *Medical Law Review.* 1995 Summer; 3(2): 117–141.
(ALLOWING TO DIE/LEGAL ASPECTS)

Bridgeman, Jo. Medical treatment: the mother's rights. *Family Law.* 1993 Sep; 23: 534–535.
(FETUSES; TREATMENT REFUSAL)

Brinchmann, Berit Støre. When the home becomes a prison: living with a severely disabled child. *Nursing Ethics.* 1999 Mar; 6(2): 137–143.
(PATIENT CARE/MINORS)

Brindle, Lucy. Exploring the approach of psychology as a discipline to the childhood testing debate: issues of theory, empiricism and power. *In:* Clarke, Angus, ed. The Genetic Testing of Children. Washington, DC: BIOS Scientific Publishers; 1998: 183–193.
(GENETIC SCREENING)

British Association for Tissue Banks see **Institute of Biology (Great Britain)**

British Columbia. Special Advisory Committee on Ethical Issues in Health Care. Euthanasia and Physician-Assisted Suicide. Victoria, BC: British Columbia Ministry of Health and Ministry Responsible for Seniors; 1994 Feb. 43 p.
(ALLOWING TO DIE; EUTHANASIA; SUICIDE)

British Diabetic Association. Ethical issues in research into prevention of insulin-dependent diabetes mellitus (IDDM). [Editorial]. *Diabetic Medicine.* 1996 May; 13(5): 399–400.
(GENETIC RESEARCH)

British Electrophoresis Society see **Institute of Biology (Great Britain)**

British Medical Association. Changing Conceptions of Motherhood: The Practice of Surrogacy in Britain. London: The Association; 1996. 74 p.
(SURROGATE MOTHERS)

British Medical Association. Human Genetics: Choice and Responsibility. New York, NY: Oxford University Press; 1998. 236 p.
(GENETIC COUNSELING; GENETIC SCREENING; GENETIC SERVICES)

British Medical Association; Royal College of Nursing. The Older Person: Consent and Care: Report of the British Medical Association and the Royal College of Nursing. London: British Medical Association; 1995 Apr. 63 p.
(INFORMED CONSENT; PATIENT CARE/AGED)

Broadhead, Caren. Challenging the regulatory authorities to justify their requirements. *ATLA: Alternatives to Laboratory Animals.* 1998 Jan–Feb; 26(1): 69–70.
(ANIMAL EXPERIMENTATION)

Broadhead, Caren. The ethical review process. [Meeting report]. *ATLA: Alternatives to Laboratory Animals.* 1998 Jan–Feb; 26(1): 71–72.
(ANIMAL EXPERIMENTATION)

Brock, Dan W. Cloning human beings: an assessment of the ethical issues pro and con. *In:* Nussbaum, Martha C.; Sunstein, Cass R., eds. Clones and Clones: Facts and Fantasies About Human Cloning. New York, NY: Norton; 1998: 141–164.
(CLONING)

Brock, Dan W. Enhancements of human function: some distinctions for policymakers. *In:* Parens, Erik, ed. Enhancing Human Traits: Ethical and Social Implications. Washington, DC: Georgetown University Press; 1998: 48–69.
(BIOMEDICAL TECHNOLOGIES)

Brock, Dan W. Euthanasia. *Rhode Island Medicine.* 1993 Dec; 76(12): 585–589.
(EUTHANASIA)

Brock, Dan W. Medical decisions at the end of life. *In:* Kuhse, Helga; Singer, Peter, eds. A Companion to Bioethics. Malden, MA: Blackwell; 1998: 231–241.
(ALLOWING TO DIE)

Brock, Dan W. The role of the public in public policy on the definition of death. *In:* Youngner, Stuart J., Arnold, Robert M.; Schapiro, Renie, eds. The Definition of Death: Contemporary Controversies. Baltimore, MD: Johns Hopkins University Press; 1999: 293–307.
(DETERMINATION OF DEATH)

Brock, Dan W. see **Letvak, Richard**

Brock, Dan W. see **Preston, Thomas A.**

Brodie, Gilbert E. Assisted suicide: an analysis of the legal (i.e., moral) arguments in judgments of the Supreme Court of Canada in the Sue Rodriguez case. *In:* Morgan, John D., ed. Readings in Thanatology. Amityville, NY: Baywood Publishing; 1997: 439–473.
(SUICIDE)

Brodkin, C. Andrew; Frumkin, Howard; Kirkland, Katherine H.; Orris, Peter; Schenk, Maryjean. AOEC position paper on the organizational code for ethical conduct. *Journal of Occupational and Environmental Medicine.* 1996 Sep; 38(9): 869–881.
(PROFESSIONAL ETHICS/CODES OF ETHICS)

Brodsky, Archie see **Bursztajn, Harold J.**

Brody, Baruch. Religion and bioethics. *In:* Kuhse, Helga; Singer, Peter, eds. A Companion to Bioethics. Malden, MA: Blackwell; 1998: 41–48.
(BIOETHICS)

Brody, Baruch A. How much of the brain must be dead? *In:* Youngner, Stuart J.; Arnold, Robert M.; Schapiro, Renie, eds. The Definition of Death: Contemporary Controversies. Baltimore, MD: Johns Hopkins University Press; 1999: 71–82.
(DETERMINATION OF DEATH/BRAIN DEATH)

Brody, Baruch A. see **Halevy, Amir**

Brody, Howard. Ethics in managed care: a matter of focus, a matter of integrity. *Michigan Medicine.* 1998 Dec; 97(12): 28–32.
(HEALTH CARE/ECONOMICS)

Brody, Howard. Physician–assisted suicide should be legalized. *Archives of Neurology.* 1996 Nov; 53(11): 1182–1183.
(SUICIDE)

Brody, Howard; Miller, Franklin G. The internal morality of medicine: explication and application to managed care. *Journal of Medicine and Philosophy.* 1998 Aug; 23(4): 384–410.
(HEALTH CARE/ECONOMICS; MEDICAL ETHICS)

Brody, Howard see **Alexander, Elizabeth**

Brody, Howard see **Menendez, Roger**

Bromham, David R. Surrogacy: ethical, legal and social aspects. *Journal of Assisted Reproduction and Genetics.* 1995 Sep; 12(8): 509–516.
(SURROGATE MOTHERS)

Brook, Robert H. see **Leape, Lucian L.**

Brooks, Alex. Mentally ill patients need protection from inappropriate genetic testing. [News]. *BMJ (British Medical Journal).* 1998 Oct 3; 317(7163): 903.
(GENETIC SCREENING)

Brooks, Alex. Viagra is licensed in Europe, but rationed in Britain. [News]. *BMJ (British Medical Journal).* 1998 Sep 19; 317(7161): 765.
(HEALTH CARE/FOREIGN COUNTRIES; PATIENT CARE/DRUGS; RESOURCE ALLOCATION/BIOMEDICAL TECHNOLOGIES)

Broumand, B. Living donors: the Iran experience. *Nephrology, Dialysis, Transplantation.* 1997 Sep; 12(9): 1830–1831.
(ORGAN AND TISSUE DONATION)

Brovins, Joan; Oehmke, Thomas. Dr. Death: Dr. Jack Kevorkian's Rx: Death. Hollywood, FL: Lifetime Books; 1993. 256 p.
(SUICIDE)

Brower, Vicki. Bioethics commission "constituted for

consensus." [News]. *Nature Biotechnology.* 1996 Sep; 14(9): 1069.
(ETHICISTS AND ETHICS COMMITTEES)

Brower, Vicki. Boston meeting blasts IRBs. [News]. *Nature Medicine.* 1998 Jan; 4(1): 9.
(HUMAN EXPERIMENTATION/ETHICS COMMITTEES)

Brower, Vicki. Experts criticize NBAC cloning report's defensive posture. [News]. *Nature Biotechnology.* 1997 Aug; 15(8): 705.
(CLONING)

Brower, Vicki. Insurers keep genetic test options open. [News]. *Nature Biotechnology.* 1997 Aug; 15(8): 708–709.
(GENETIC SCREENING)

Brower, Vicki. Lawyers, physicians seek genomics rules. [News]. *Nature Biotechnology.* 1997 Jan; 15(1): 10.
(GENETIC SCREENING)

Brown, Barry. Genetic testing, access to genetic data and discrimination: conceptual legislative models. *Suffolk University Law Review.* 1993 Winter; 27(4): 1573–1592.
(CONFIDENTIALITY/LEGAL ASPECTS; GENETIC SCREENING)

Brown, Craig K. see **Limentani, Alexander E.**

Brown, Edna see **Hosford, Ian**

Brown, Harold O.J.; Budziszewski, J.; Chaput, Charles J.; Chevlen, Eric; Hinlicky, Sarah E.; Meilaender, Gilbert; Turner, Philip; Mohler, R. Albert; Mosier, Alicia; Smith, Janet E. Contraception: a symposium. *First Things.* 1998 Dec; No. 88: 17–29.
(CONTRACEPTION)

Brown, Janet; Moore, Donna E.; Potter, David; Stewart, Robert. Placebos and the need for good communication: the case of George Hunter. [Case study and commentaries]. *Orthopaedic Nursing.* 1997 May–Jun; 16(3): 61–65.
(PATIENT CARE/DRUGS)

Brown, Laura see **Breimer, Lars**

Brown, Lowell C.; Paine, Shirley J. Thunder from California: the *Thor* decision and the ever-expanding right to die. *HealthSpan.* 1993 Oct; 10(9): 13–17.
(ALLOWING TO DIE/LEGAL ASPECTS; TREATMENT REFUSAL)

Brown, Murray G. Rationing health care in Canada. *Annals of Health Law.* 1993; 2: 101–119.
(HEALTH CARE/ECONOMICS; HEALTH CARE/FOREIGN COUNTRIES; RESOURCE ALLOCATION)

Brown, Norman K.; Thompson, Donovan J.; Prentice, Ross L. Nontreatment and aggressive narcotic therapy among hospitalized pancreatic cancer patients. *Journal of the American Geriatrics Society.* 1998 Jul; 46(7): 839–848.
(ALLOWING TO DIE; TERMINAL CARE)

Brown, Philip see **Nightingale, Stuart L.**

Brown, Phyllida. WHO urges "coverage for all, not coverage of everything." [News]. *BMJ (British Medical Journal).* 1999 May 15; 318(7194): 1305.
(HEALTH CARE/FOREIGN COUNTRIES)

Brown, Robert S. see **Showstack, Jonathan**

Brown, Sharan E.; Valluzzi, Janet L. Do not resuscitate orders in early intervention settings: who should make the decision? *Infants and Young Children.* 1995 Jan; 7(3): 13–27.
(RESUSCITATION ORDERS)

Browner, C.H. see **Markens, Susan**

Bruce, Donald M. Cloning –– a step too far? An article on the ethical aspects of cloning in animals and humans. *Human Reproduction and Genetic Ethics: An International Journal.* 1998; 4(2): 34–38.
(CLONING)

Brücker, Gilles see **Lot, Florence**

Brückner, Ch. see **Müller, H.J.**

Bruera, Eduardo; Lawlor, Peter. Defining palliative care interventions. *Journal of Palliative Care.* 1998 Summer; 14(2): 23–24.
(TERMINAL CARE)

Brunner, Eric. Gene tests survey: results. *Splice of Life.* 1996 Dec; 3(3): 7–8.
(GENETIC SCREENING)

Brushwood, David B.; Allen, William L. Constitutional right to pharmaceutically assisted death. *American Journal of Health–System Pharmacy.* 1996 Aug 1; 53(15): 1797–1799.
(SUICIDE)

Bubolz, Thomas A. see **Wasson, John H.**

Buchanan, Allen. Choosing who will be disabled: genetic intervention and the morality of inclusion. *In:* Paul, Ellen Frankel; Miller, Fred D.; Paul, Jeffrey, eds. Scientific Innovation, Philosophy, and Public Policy. New York, NY: Cambridge University Press; 1996: 18–46.
(GENETIC INTERVENTION)

Buchanan, Allen. Managed care: rationing without justice, but not unjustly. *Journal of Health Politics, Policy and Law.* 1998 Aug; 23(4): 617–634.
(HEALTH CARE/ECONOMICS; HEALTH CARE/RIGHTS; RESOURCE ALLOCATION)

Buchanan, John D. see **Zalcberg, John R.**

Buchanan, Robert J. Tuberculosis and HIV infection: utilization of public programs to fund treatment. *AIDS and Public Policy Journal.* 1997 Winter; 12(4): 122–136.
(HEALTH CARE/ECONOMICS; PUBLIC HEALTH)

Buchanan, Susan Fox see **Murphy, Donald**

Buck, Catherine see **Perry, Erica**

Buckley, Jonathan see **Kodish, Eric D.**

Budai, Pamela. Mandatory reporting of child abuse: is it in the best interests of the child? *Australian and New Zealand Journal of Psychiatry.* 1996 Dec; 30(6): 794–804.
(CONFIDENTIALITY/LEGAL ASPECTS; CONFIDENTIALITY/MENTAL HEALTH)

Budd, Susan; Sharma, Ursula, eds. The Healing Bond: The Patient–Practitioner Relationship and Therapeutic

Responsibility. New York, NY: Routledge; 1994. 239 p.
(PATIENT CARE; PROFESSIONAL PATIENT RELATIONSHIP)

Budziszewski, J. see **Brown, Harold O.J.**

Buetow, Stephen. The scope for the involvement of patients in their consultations with health professionals: rights, responsibilities and preferences of patients. *Journal of Medical Ethics.* 1998 Aug; 24(4): 243–247.
(HEALTH CARE/FOREIGN COUNTRIES; PATIENTS' RIGHTS; PROFESSIONAL PATIENT RELATIONSHIP)

Bühler, E. see **Müller, H.J.**

Buka, Stephen see **Wharton, Robert H.**

Bulger, Roger J. The Quest for Mercy: The Forgotten Ingredient in Health Care Reform. Charlottesville, VA: Carden Jennings; 1998. 117 p.
(HEALTH CARE; PROFESSIONAL PATIENT RELATIONSHIP)

Burack, Robert see **Butler, Dennis J.**

Burdette, Tom see **Swartz, Richard D.**

Burdon, Justin see **Edi-Osagie, E.C.O.**

Burgess, Michael; Rodney, Patricia; Coward, Harold; Ratanakul, Pinit; Suwonnakote, Khannika. Pediatric care: judgments about best interests at the onset of life. *In:* Coward, Harold; Ratanaku, Pinit, eds. A Cross-Cultural Dialogue on Health Care Ethics. Waterloo, ON: Wilfrid Laurier University Press; 1999: 160–175.
(TREATMENT REFUSAL/MINORS)

Burgess, Michael; Stephenson, Peter; Ratanakul, Pinit; Suwonnakote, Khannika. End-of-life decisions: clinical decisions about dying and perspectives on life and death. *In:* Coward, Harold; Ratanakul, Pinit, eds. A Cross-Cultural Dialogue on Health Care Ethics. Waterloo, ON: Wilfrid Laurier University Press; 1999: 190–206.
(TERMINAL CARE)

Burgess, Michael M.; Laberge, Claude M.; Knoppers, Bartha Maria. Bioethics for clinicians: 14. Ethics and genetics in medicine. *Canadian Medical Association Journal.* 1998 May 19; 158(10): 1309–1313.
(GENETIC COUNSELING; GENETIC SCREENING)

Burgess, Michael M. see **Stingl, Michael**

Burgio, G. Roberto; Lantos, John D., eds. *Primum Non Nocere* Today. Second Edition. New York, NY: Elsevier; 1998. 171 p.
(BIOETHICS; PATIENT CARE/MINORS)

Burgio, G. Roberto; Locatelli, F.; Nespoli, L. Hematopoietic stem cell transplantation in pediatric practice: a bioethical reassessment. *In:* Burgio, G. Roberto; Lantos, John D., eds. *Primum Non Nocere* Today. Second Edition. New York, NY: Elsevier; 1998: 85–99.
(BLOOD DONATION; ORGAN AND TISSUE DONATION)

Burk, Dan L.; Hess, Jennifer A. Genetic privacy: constitutional considerations in forensic DNA testing. *George Mason University Civil Rights Law Journal.* 1994 Winter; 5(1): 1–53.

(DNA FINGERPRINTING)

Burk, Larry see **Sugarman, Jeremy**

Burke, J. Daniel. A comment on Dan Brock's essay, "Euthanasia." *Rhode Island Medicine.* 1993 Dec; 76(12): 603–604.
(EUTHANASIA/RELIGIOUS ASPECTS)

Burke, Jennifer E. see **Schulman, Kevin A.**

Burke, W. see **Eisinger, F.**

Burke, Wylie see **MacKay, Charles**

Burke, Wylie see **Welch, H. Gilbert**

Burley, Justine; Harris, John. Human cloning and child welfare. *Journal of Medical Ethics.* 1999 Apr; 25(2): 108–113.
(CLONING)

Burley, Justine C. The price of eggs: who should bear the costs of fertility treatments? *In:* Harris, John; Holm, Søren, eds. The Future of Human Reproduction: Ethics, Choice, and Regulation. New York, NY: Oxford University Press; 1998: 127–149.
(REPRODUCTIVE TECHNOLOGIES; RESOURCE ALLOCATION/BIOMEDICAL TECHNOLOGIES)

Burman, David J. see **Tucker, Kathryn L.**

Burmeister, Leon F. see **Shavers-Hornaday, Vickie L.**

Burnett, Barbara see **Gorelick, Philip B.**

Burns, Deborah L.; Catlin, Anita J. Positive toxicology screening in newborns: ethical issues in the decision to legally intervene. [Article and commentary]. *Pediatric Nursing.* 1997 Jan–Feb; 23(1): 73–78, 86.
(PRENATAL INJURIES)

Burnside, Gordon. New paths in end-of-life care. *Health Progress.* 1998 May–Jun; 79(3): 18–20.
(TERMINAL CARE)

Burris, John; Cook-Deegan, Robert; Alberts, Bruce. The Human Genome Project after a decade: policy issues. *Nature Genetics.* 1998 Dec; 20(4): 333–335.
(GENOME MAPPING)

Burrows, Elizabeth see **Saigal, Saroj**

Burrows, R. Removal of life support in intensive care units. *Medicine and Law.* 1994; 13(5–6): 489–500.
(ALLOWING TO DIE; RESOURCE ALLOCATION/BIOMEDICAL TECHNOLOGIES; SELECTION FOR TREATMENT)

Bursztajn, Harold J.; Pearlman, Theodore; Slovenko, Ralph; Strasburger, Larry H.; Gutheil, Thomas G.; Brodsky, Archie. Psychotherapist versus expert witness. [Letters and response]. *American Journal of Psychiatry.* 1998 Feb; 155(2): 307–308.
(PATIENT CARE/MENTALLY DISABLED)

Burt, Robert A. Where do we go from here? *In:* Youngner, Stuart J.; Arnold, Robert M.; Schapiro, Renie, eds. The Definition of Death: Contemporary Controversies. Baltimore, MD: Johns Hopkins University Press; 1999: 332–339.

(DETERMINATION OF DEATH)

Burton, Laurel Arthur; Tarlos–Benka, Judy. Grief–driven ethical decision–making. *Journal of Religion and Health.* 1997 Winter; 36(4): 333–343.
(ALLOWING TO DIE/INFANTS)

Burton, Thomas M. A prostate researcher tested firm's product -- and sat on its board. [News]. *Wall Street Journal.* 1998 Mar 19: A1, A8.
(BIOMEDICAL RESEARCH; FRAUD AND MISCONDUCT; HEALTH CARE/ECONOMICS; HUMAN EXPERIMENTATION)

Burton, William B. see **Zelenik, Jomarie**

Busquet, Xavier see **Porta, Miguel**

Buss, Mary K.; Marx, Eric S.; Sulmasy, Daniel P. The preparedness of students to discuss end–of–life issues with patients. *Academic Medicine.* 1998 Apr; 73(4): 418–422.
(ADVANCE DIRECTIVES; MEDICAL ETHICS/EDUCATION; TERMINAL CARE)

Butler, Declan. Breakthrough stirs US embryo debate ... while Europe contemplates funding ban. [News]. *Nature.* 1998 Nov 12; 396(6707): 104–105.
(EMBRYO AND FETAL RESEARCH)

Butler, Declan. Europe is urged to hold back on xenotransplant clinical trials. [News]. *Nature.* 1999 Jan 28; 397(6717): 281–282.
(HUMAN EXPERIMENTATION/REGULATION; ORGAN AND TISSUE TRANSPLANTATION)

Butler, Declan. FDA warns on primate xenotransplants. [News]. *Nature.* 1999 Apr 15; 398(6728): 549.
(HUMAN EXPERIMENTATION/REGULATION; ORGAN AND TISSUE TRANSPLANTATION)

Butler, Declan. Fraud squad files report to prosecutor in INSERM case. [News]. *Nature.* 1998 Jul 23; 394(6691): 308.
(BIOMEDICAL RESEARCH; FRAUD AND MISCONDUCT)

Butler, Declan. Human genome declaration looks set for United Nations approval. [News]. *Nature.* 1998 Nov 26; 396(6709): 297.
(GENETIC INTERVENTION; GENOME MAPPING)

Butler, Declan. Pressure grows for relaxation of French embryo research laws. [News]. *Nature.* 1998 Oct 8; 395(6702): 532–533.
(EMBRYO AND FETAL RESEARCH)

Butler, Declan. Transplant panel to play 'honest broker.' [News]. *Nature.* 1999 Apr 22; 398(6729): 643.
(ORGAN AND TISSUE TRANSPLANTATION)

Butler, Declan. WHO's bioethics code likely to stir debate. [News]. *Nature.* 1999 Mar 18; 398(6724): 179.
(GENETIC RESEARCH)

Butler, Declan; Reichhardt, Tony. Long–term effect of GM crops serves up food for thought. *Nature.* 1999 Apr 22; 398(6729): 651–656.
(GENETIC INTERVENTION)

Butler, Dennis J.; Edwards, Ann; Tzelepis, Angela; Klingbeil, Carol; Melgar, Thomas; Speece, Mark; Schubiner, Howard; Burack, Robert. Informed consent for videotaping. [Letter and response]. *Academic*

Medicine. 1996 Dec; 71(12): 1276–1277.
(CONFIDENTIALITY; INFORMED CONSENT)

Butzow, James J. see **Murphy, Edmond A.**

Byers, Keith Alan. Infertility and in vitro fertilization: a growing need for consumer–oriented regulation of the in vitro fertilization industry. *Journal of Legal Medicine.* 1997 Sep; 18(3): 265–313.
(IN VITRO FERTILIZATION; REPRODUCTIVE TECHNOLOGIES)

Byk, Christian. A map to a new treasure island: the human genome and the concept of common heritage. *Journal of Medicine and Philosophy.* 1998 Jun; 23(3): 234–246.
(GENETIC INTERVENTION; GENETIC RESEARCH)

Byk, Christian. International Association for Law, Ethics and Science organizes third international meeting (Paris, 23–24 Sep 1994). *International Digest of Health Legislation.* 1995; 46(4): 572–574.
(BEHAVIOR CONTROL; BEHAVIORAL RESEARCH/SPECIAL POPULATIONS)

Byk, Christian. International colloquy, "From Ethics to Law, from Law to Ethics" (Lausanne, 17–18 Oct 1996). [Meeting report]. *International Digest of Health Legislation.* 1997; 48(2): 252–254.
(BIOETHICS)

Byk, Christian. Reply to Lebech or the ontological humility of the lawyer faced with philosophical consistency. *Journal of Medical Ethics.* 1998 Oct; 24(5): 348–349.
(EMBRYO AND FETAL RESEARCH)

Byrne, Paul see **Bowes, Watson**

Byrne, Paul A.; Colliton, William F.; Evers, Joseph C.; Fangman, Timothy R.; L'Ecuyer, Jerome; Simon, Frank G.; Nilges, Richard G.; Shen, Jerome T.Y.; Kramper, Ralph J.; Sadick, Mary H. Life, life support, and death principles, guidelines, policies and procedures for making decisions that respect life. [Booklet, third edition; published by the American Life League; 1996]. *Linacre Quarterly.* 1997 Nov; 64(4): 3–31.
(TERMINAL CARE)

Byrnes, Margot see **van Hooft, Stan**

C

Caelleigh, Addeane S. The guillotine. *Academic Medicine.* 1997 Mar; 72(3): 166.
(CAPITAL PUNISHMENT)

Cahill, Jo. Patient participation -- a review of the literature. *Journal of Clinical Nursing.* 1998 Mar; 7(2): 119–128.
(PATIENT CARE)

Cahill, Lisa Sowle. Catholic commitment and public responsibility. *In:* Rainey, R. Randall; Magill, Gerard, eds. Abortion and Public Policy: An Interdisciplinary Investigation within the Catholic Tradition. Omaha, NE: Creighton University Press; 1996: 131–162.
(ABORTION/LEGAL ASPECTS; ABORTION/RELIGIOUS ASPECTS)

Cahill, Lisa Sowle. The new biotech world order. [Symposium: human primordial stem cells]. *Hastings*

Center Report. 1999 Mar–Apr; 29(2): 45–48.
(BIOMEDICAL RESEARCH; EMBRYO AND FETAL RESEARCH; GENETIC RESEARCH)

Cahn, Naomi R. see **Michie, Helena**

Calangu, S. see **Sever, M.S.**

Caldicott, Fiona see **Thomas, Sandy**

Cale, Gita S. Risk–related standards of competence: continuing the debate over risk–related standards of competence. *Bioethics.* 1999 Apr; 13(2): 131–148.
(INFORMED CONSENT; TREATMENT REFUSAL)

Calhoun, Byron C. see **Reitman, James S.**

Califano, Joseph A. Physician–assisted living. *America.* 1998 Nov 14; 179(15): 10–12.
(TERMINAL CARE)

Callahan, Daniel. Age, sex, and resource allocation. *In:* Walker, Margaret Urban, ed. Mother Time: Women, Aging, and Ethics. Lanham, MD: Rowman and Littlefield; 1999: 189–199.
(HEALTH; HEALTH CARE/ECONOMICS; PATIENT CARE/AGED; RESOURCE ALLOCATION)

Callahan, Daniel. Calling scientific ideology to account. *Society.* 1996 May–Jun; 33(4): 14–19.
(BIOETHICS; BIOMEDICAL RESEARCH)

Callahan, Daniel. Must the young and old struggle over health care resources? *Journal Of Long Term Home Health Care.* 1996 Fall; 15(4): 4–14.
(HEALTH CARE/ECONOMICS; PATIENT CARE/AGED; RESOURCE ALLOCATION)

Callahan, Daniel. Physician–assisted suicide: moral questions. *In:* Steinberg, Maurice D.; Youngner, Stuart J., eds. End–of–Life Decisions: A Psychosocial Perspective. Washington, DC: American Psychiatric Press; 1998: 283–297.
(SUICIDE)

Callahan, Daniel. The Hastings Center and the early years of bioethics. *Kennedy Institute of Ethics Journal.* 1999 Mar; 9(1): 53–71.
(BIOETHICS)

Callahan, Daniel see **Hanson, Mark J.**

Callahan, Daniel see **Rosenheck, Robert**

Callahan, Daniel see **Steinfels, Peter**

Callahan, Jay. Assisted suicide, community, and the common good. [Editorial]. *Health and Social Work.* 1997 Nov; 22(4): 243–245.
(SUICIDE)

Callahan, Joan C. Menopause: taking the cures or curing the takes? *In:* Walker, Margaret Urban, ed. Mother Time: Women, Aging, and Ethics. Lanham, MD: Rowman and Littlefield; 1999: 151–174.
(HEALTH; PATIENT CARE/DRUGS)

Callahan, Leigh F. see **Pincus, Theodore**

Callari Galli, M. Viewing bioethics from an anthropological viewpoint. *In:* Burgio, G. Roberto;

Lantos, John D., eds. *Primum Non Nocere* Today. Second Edition. New York, NY: Elsevier; 1998: 23–26.
(BIOETHICS)

Callender, John S. Ethics and aims in psychotherapy: a contribution from Kant. *Journal of Medical Ethics.* 1998 Aug; 24(4): 274–278.
(PATIENT CARE/MENTALLY DISABLED)

Callens, Stefaan H. The automatic processing of medical data in Belgium: is the individual protected? *Medicine and Law.* 1993; 12(1–2): 55–59.
(CONFIDENTIALITY/LEGAL ASPECTS)

Callum, Janet; Chalker, Rebecca; Raymond, Janice; Klein, Renate; Dumble, Lynette. Should RU486 be legalized? *In:* Francoeur, Robert T., ed. Taking Sides: Clashing Views on Controversial Issues in Human Sexuality. Fifth Edition. Guilford, CT: Dushkin Publishing Group/Brown and Benchmark; 1996: 134–143.
(ABORTION)

Campbell, Alastair V. Presidential address: Global bioethics –– dream or nightmare? *Bioethics.* 1999 Jul; 13(3–4): 183–190.
(BIOETHICS)

Campbell, Bruce see **Thom, David H.**

Campbell, Courtney S. Can what you don't know hurt you?: the case of genetic screening for breast cancer. *In:* Smith, Edward; Sapp, Walter, eds. Plain Talk about the Human Genome Project: A Tuskegee University Conference on Its Promise and Perils ... and Matters of Race. Tuskegee, AL: Tuskegee University Press; 1997: 117–122.
(GENETIC SCREENING)

Campbell, Courtney S. Fundamentals of life and death: Christian fundamentalism and medical science. *In:* Youngner, Stuart J.; Arnold, Robert M.; Schapiro, Renie, eds. The Definition of Death: Contemporary Controversies. Baltimore, MD: Johns Hopkins University Press; 1999: 194–209.
(DETERMINATION OF DEATH/BRAIN DEATH)

Campbell, Courtney S. Religion and the body in medical research. *Kennedy Institute of Ethics Journal.* 1998 Sep; 8(3): 275–305.
(BIOMEDICAL RESEARCH; GENETIC RESEARCH; HUMAN EXPERIMENTATION; ORGAN AND TISSUE DONATION)

Campbell, Courtney S.; Woolfrey, Joan. Norms and narratives: religious reflections on the human cloning controversy. *Journal of Biolaw and Business.* 1998 Spring; 1(3): 8–20.
(CLONING)

Campbell, Eric G. see **Hsu, John**

Campbell, Harry; Boyd, Kenneth. Screening and the new genetics: a public health perspective on the ethical debate. [Letter]. *Journal of Public Health Medicine.* 1996 Dec; 18(4): 485–486.
(GENETIC SCREENING; MASS SCREENING; PRENATAL DIAGNOSIS)

Campbell, Harry see **Pfeffer, Naomi**

Campbell, Keith. Look on the bright side of cloning.

Nature Medicine. 1998 May; 4(5): 557–558.
(CLONING)

Campbell, Margaret L. Forgoing Life – Sustaining Therapy: How to Care for the Patient Who Is Near Death. Aliso Viejo, CA: AACN Critical Care; 1998. 140 p.
(ALLOWING TO DIE; TERMINAL CARE)

Campbell, Neil. A problem for the idea of voluntary euthanasia. *Journal of Medical Ethics.* 1999 Jun; 25(3): 242–244.
(ADVANCE DIRECTIVES; EUTHANASIA)

Campion, Edward W. Liberty and the control of tuberculosis. [Editorial]. *New England Journal of Medicine.* 1999 Feb 4; 340(5): 385–386.
(PUBLIC HEALTH)

Canada. Alberta. Personal Directives Act [Chapter P–4.03]. Alberta, Canada: The Queen's Printer for Alberta; 1996 May 24 (date of enactment). 21 p.
(ADVANCE DIRECTIVES)

Canada. Health Canada. Discussion Group on Embryo Research. Research on Human Embryos in Canada. Final Report of the Discussion Group on Embryo Research. Ottawa, ON: Health Canada; 1995 Nov 15. 33 p.
(EMBRYO AND FETAL RESEARCH; REPRODUCTIVE TECHNOLOGIES)

Canada. Supreme Court. B. v. Children's Aid Society of Metropolitan Toronto. *Dominion Law Reports, 4th Series.* 1995 Jan 27 (date of decision). 122: 1–92.
(TREATMENT REFUSAL/MINORS)

Canadian Home Care Association see **Canadian Nurses Association**

Canadian Hospital Association see **Canadian Nurses Association**

Canadian Long Term Care Association see **Canadian Nurses Association**

Canadian Nurses Association. The Role of the Nurse in Reproductive and Genetic Technologies. [Policy statement]. Issued by the Canadian Nurses Association, 50 Driveway, Ottawa, ON, Canada; 1996 Jun. 2 p.
(GENETIC SCREENING; REPRODUCTIVE TECHNOLOGIES)

Canadian Nurses Association; Canadian Home Care Association; Canadian Hospital Association; et al. Joint Statement on Advance Directives. [Policy statement]. Ottawa, ON: Issued by the Canadian Nurses Association, 50 Driveway, Ottawa, ON K2P 1E2, Canada; 1994 Sep. 4 p.
(ADVANCE DIRECTIVES)

Candefjord, Inga–Lill see **Kjellin, Lars**

Candilis, Philip J.; Appelbaum, Kenneth L. Physician–assisted suicide and the Supreme Court: the Washington and Vacco verdicts. *Journal of the American Academy of Psychiatry and the Law.* 1997; 25(4): 595–606.
(SUICIDE)

Candotti, Fabio; Notarangelo, Luigi D.; Ugazio, Alberto G. Gene therapy: current status, perspectives

and problematic issues. *In:* Burgio, G. Roberto; Lantos, John D., eds. *Primum Non Nocere* Today. Second Edition. New York, NY: Elsevier; 1998: 133–145.
(GENE THERAPY)

Cannold, Leslie. "There is no evidence to suggest...": changing the way we judge information for disclosure in the informed consent process. *Hypatia.* 1997 Spring; 12(2): 165–184.
(HUMAN EXPERIMENTATION/FOREIGN COUNTRIES; HUMAN EXPERIMENTATION/INFORMED CONSENT; HUMAN EXPERIMENTATION/SPECIAL POPULATIONS)

Cantor, Charles R. How will the Human Genome Project improve our quality of life? *Nature Biotechnology.* 1998 Mar; 16(3): 212–213.
(GENOME MAPPING)

Cantor, Norman L. The real ethic of death and dying. [Book review essay]. *Michigan Law Review.* 1996 May; 94(6): 1718–1738.
(ALLOWING TO DIE; EUTHANASIA)

Cantor, Scott B. see **Chavey, William E.**

Capen, Karen. There's more to Krever's report than the blood issue -- much more. *Canadian Medical Association Journal.* 1998 Jan 13; 158(1): 92–94.
(INFORMED CONSENT)

Caplan, Arthur. Bioethics: *The Birth of Bioethics* by Albert R. Jonsen. [Book review essay]. *JAMA.* 1999 Mar 3; 281(9): 849–850.
(BIOETHICS)

Caplan, Arthur. Due Consideration: Controversy in the Age of Medical Miracles. New York, NY: Wiley; 1998. 282 p.
(BIOETHICS)

Caplan, Arthur see **Kerr, Susan M.**

Caplan, Arthur see **Lebacqz, Karen**

Caplan, Arthur see **McGee, Glenn**

Caplan, Arthur L. Am I my brother's keeper? *Suffolk University Law Review.* 1993 Winter; 27(4): 1195–1208.
(ORGAN AND TISSUE DONATION)

Caplan, Arthur L. Wearing your organ transplant on your sleeve. *Hastings Center Report.* 1999 Mar–Apr; 29(2): 52.
(ORGAN AND TISSUE TRANSPLANTATION)

Caplan, Arthur L. What's so special about the human genome? *Cambridge Quarterly of Healthcare Ethics.* 1998 Fall; 7(4): 422–424.
(GENOME MAPPING)

Caplan, Arthur L. Why the rush to ban cloning? *New York Times.* 1998 Jan 28: A25.
(CLONING)

Caplan, Arthur L.; Coelho, Daniel H. The Ethics of Organ Transplants: The Current Debate. Amherst, NY: Prometheus Books; 1998. 350 p.
(ORGAN AND TISSUE DONATION; ORGAN AND TISSUE TRANSPLANTATION; RESOURCE ALLOCATION/BIOMEDICAL TECHNOLOGIES; SELECTION FOR TREATMENT)

Caplan, Arthur L. see **Bleich, J. David**

Caplan, Arthur L. see **Coelho, Daniel H.**

Caplan, Arthur L. see **McGee, Glenn**

Caplan, Arthur L. see **Moreno, Jonathan**

Caplan, Arthur L. see **Ubel, Peter A.**

Cappelli, M.; Surh, L.; Verma, S.; Ryan, W.; Logan, D.; Korneluk, Y.; Feeny, D.; Hunter, A.; Allanson, J. Canadian women's attitudes towards breast cancer gene testing. [Abstract]. *American Journal of Human Genetics.* 1997 Oct; 61(4): A187.
(GENETIC SCREENING)

Capron, Alexander Morgan. Advance directives. *In:* Kuhse, Helga; Singer, Peter, eds. A Companion to Bioethics. Malden, MA: Blackwell; 1998: 261–271.
(ADVANCE DIRECTIVES)

Capron, Alexander Morgan. Ethical and human–rights issues in research on mental disorders that may affect decision–making capacity. *New England Journal of Medicine.* 1999 May 6; 340(18): 1430–1434.
(HUMAN EXPERIMENTATION/REGULATION; HUMAN EXPERIMENTATION/SPECIAL POPULATIONS)

Capron, Alexander Morgan. Good intentions. *Hastings Center Report.* 1999 Mar–Apr; 29(2): 26–27.
(EMBRYO AND FETAL RESEARCH)

Capron, Alexander Morgan. The bifurcated legal standard for determining death: does it work? *In:* Youngner, Stuart J.; Arnold, Robert M.; Schapiro, Renie, eds. The Definition of Death: Contemporary Controversies. Baltimore, MD: Johns Hopkins University Press; 1999: 117–136.
(DETERMINATION OF DEATH; DETERMINATION OF DEATH/BRAIN DEATH)

Capron, Alexander Morgan. Too many parents. *Hastings Center Report.* 1998 Sep–Oct; 28(5): 22–24.
(REPRODUCTIVE TECHNOLOGIES)

Carin, M. see **Sever, M.S.**

Carlberg, Axel. The Moral Rubicon: A Study of the Principles of Sanctity of Life and Quality of Life in Bioethics. Lund, Sweden: Lund University Press; 1998. 208 p.
(BIOETHICS)

Carlin, Kathleen see **Antle, Beverley J.**

Carlisle, John see **Ferris, Lorraine E.**

Carlsen, Mary S.; Pomeroy, Claire; Moldow, D. Gay. Optimizing discussions about resuscitation: development of a guide based on patients' recommendations. *Journal of Clinical Ethics.* 1998 Fall; 9(3): 263–272.
(RESUSCITATION ORDERS)

Carlsson, Hans–Erik see **Hagelin, Joakim**

Carmi, Amnon. The new Russian law on psychiatric care. *Dynamische Psychiatrie.* 1994; 27(3–4): 259–265.
(PATIENTS' RIGHTS/MENTALLY DISABLED)

Carmi, Rivka see **Sheiner, Eyal**

Carnall, Douglas. American Medical Association moves to regulate prescribing on the Internet. [News]. *BMJ (British Medical Journal).* 1999 Jul 24; 319(7204): 213.
(PATIENT CARE/DRUGS)

Carné, X. see **García–Alonso, F.**

Carnevale, Franco A. The utility of futility: the construction of bioethical problems. *Nursing Ethics.* 1998 Nov; 5(6): 509–517.
(BIOETHICS; RESUSCITATION ORDERS)

Carr, T.R. see **Virgo, Katherine S.**

Carrick, Paul. Environmental ethics and medical ethics: some implications for end-of-life care, Part I. *Cambridge Quarterly of Healthcare Ethics.* 1999 Winter; 8(1): 107–117.
(TERMINAL CARE)

Carrick, Paul. Environmental ethics and medical ethics: some implications for end-of-life care, part II. *Cambridge Quarterly of Healthcare Ethics.* 1999 Spring; 8(2): 250–256.
(TERMINAL CARE)

Carrillo, J. Emilio; Green, Alexander R.; Betancourt, Joseph R. Cross-cultural primary care: a patient-based approach. *Annals of Internal Medicine.* 1999 May 18; 130(10): 829–834.
(PATIENT CARE; PROFESSIONAL PATIENT RELATIONSHIP)

Carroll, Alex see **Doyle, Kathy**

Carron, Annette T.; Lynn, Joanne; Keaney, Patrick. End-of-life care in medical textbooks. *Annals of Internal Medicine.* 1999 Jan 5; 130(1): 82–86.
(TERMINAL CARE)

Carse, Alisa L. Facing up to moral perils: the virtues of care in bioethics. *In:* Gordon, Suzanne; Benner, Patricia; Noddings, Nel, eds. Caregiving: Readings in Knowledge, Practice, Ethics, and Politics. Philadelphia, PA: University of Pennsylvania Press; 1996: 83–110.
(BIOETHICS)

Carson, Donna P. The socially complex family: new dilemmas for the neonatal social worker. *Clinics in Perinatology.* 1996 Sep; 23(3): 609–620.
(PATIENT CARE/MINORS)

Carter, Thomas H. see **Foster, Morris W.**

Cartwright, Will. The pig, the transplant surgeon and the Nuffield Council. *Medical Law Review.* 1996 Autumn; 4(3): 250–269.
(ETHICISTS AND ETHICS COMMITTEES; ORGAN AND TISSUE TRANSPLANTATION)

Casarett, David see **Bolan, Robert K.**

Casarett, David J. Moral perception and the pursuit of medical philosophy. *Theoretical Medicine and Bioethics.* 1999 Apr; 20(2): 125–139.
(MEDICAL ETHICS; PROFESSIONAL PATIENT RELATIONSHIP)

Casarett, David J.; Daskal, Frona; Lantos, John. Experts in ethics? The authority of the clinical ethicist. *Hastings Center Report.* 1998 Nov–Dec; 28(6): 6–11.
(BIOETHICS; ETHICISTS AND ETHICS COMMITTEES)

Cascardi, Michele; Poythress, Norman G. Correlates of perceived coercion during psychiatric hospital admission. *International Journal of Law and Psychiatry.* 1997 Fall; 20(4): 445-458.
(INVOLUNTARY COMMITMENT)

Cash, John; Boyd, Kenneth. Blood transfusion: Bayer's initiative. *Lancet.* 1999 Feb 27; 353(9154): 691-692.
(BLOOD DONATION; ETHICISTS AND ETHICS COMMITTEES)

Casper, Monica J. Working on and around human fetuses: the contested domain of fetal surgery. *In:* Berg, Marc; Mol, Annemarie, eds. Differences in Medicine: Unraveling Practices, Techniques, and Bodies. Durham, NC: Duke University Press; 1998: 28-52.
(FETUSES; PATIENT CARE)

Cassel, Christine K. see **McCally, Michael**

Cassell, Cynthia see **Slovenko, Ralph**

Cassell, Cynthia see **Sugarman, Jeremy**

Cassell, Eric J. Pain, suffering, and the goals of medicine. *In:* Hanson, Mark J.; Callahan, Daniel, eds. The Goals of Medicine: The Forgotten Issue in Health Care Reform. Washington, DC: Georgetown University Press; 1999: 101-117.
(HEALTH CARE)

Cassidy, Judy. Calvary Hospital focuses on ethics: integrating clinical and organizational ethics meets needs of a changing healthcare system. *Health Progress.* 1998 Nov-Dec; 79(6): 48-50, 52.
(HEALTH CARE; PROFESSIONAL ETHICS)

Cassiman, Jean-Jacques see **Decruyenaere, Marleen**

Cassirer, Christopher see **Weisman, Carol S.**

Castellanos, F. Xavier see **Arnold, L. Eugene**

Castle, Nicholas G. Advance directives in nursing homes: resident and facility characteristics. *Omega: A Journal of Death and Dying.* 1996-1997; 34(4): 321-332.
(ADVANCE DIRECTIVES)

Catalano, Joseph T. The ethics of cadaver experimentation. *Critical Care Nurse.* 1994 Dec; 14(6): 82-85.
(HUMAN EXPERIMENTATION/SPECIAL POPULATIONS; NURSING ETHICS/EDUCATION)

Cataldo, Peter J. GIFT as assistance. *Ethics and Medics.* 1997 Dec; 22(12): 3-4.
(REPRODUCTIVE TECHNOLOGIES)

Catholic Health Association of the United States. CHA amicus curiae brief on physician-assisted suicide. *Health Progress.* 1997 May-Jun; 78(3): 36-43, 47.
(SUICIDE)

Catholic University of the Sacred Heart (Rome). On heterologous assisted fertilisation. *Bulletin of Medical Ethics.* 1997 Nov; 133: 10-11.
(REPRODUCTIVE TECHNOLOGIES)

Catlin, Anita J. see **Burns, Deborah L.**

Caudill, O. Brandt see **Hedges, Lawrence E.**

Caulfield, Timothy. The commercialization of human genetics: profits and problems. *Molecular Medicine Today.* 1998 Apr; 4(4): 148-150.
(GENETIC RESEARCH)

Caulfield, Timothy; Dossetor, John; Boshkov, Lynn; Hannon, Judith; Sawyer, Douglas; Robertson, Gerald. Notifying patients exposed to blood products associated with Creutzfeldt-Jakob disease: integrating science, legal duties and ethical mandates. *Canadian Medical Association Journal.* 1997 Nov 15; 157(10): 1389-1392.
(BLOOD DONATION; TRUTH DISCLOSURE)

Causino, Nancyanne see **Finestone, Albert J.**

Cavalier, Robert see **Andersen, David**

Cavanagh, Denis see **Bowes, Watson**

Cavanaugh, Thomas A. Currently accepted practices that are known to lead to death, and PAS: is there an ethically relevant difference? *Cambridge Quarterly of Healthcare Ethics.* 1998 Fall; 7(4): 375-381.
(ALLOWING TO DIE; SUICIDE; TERMINAL CARE)

Cavanaugh, Thomas A. The ethics of death-hastening or death-causing palliative analgesic administration to the terminally ill. *Journal of Pain and Symptom Management.* 1996 Oct; 12(4): 248-254.
(TERMINAL CARE)

Cavanaugh, Thomas A. see **Wu, Albert W.**

Cavanna, J.S. see **Galton, D.J.**

CBS Video. 60 Minutes: Choosing Life (A.L.S.). [Videorecording]. Produced by 60 Minutes, 524 West 57th St., New York, NY 10019; 1999. 1 videocassette; 14 min.; sd.; color; VHS..
(EUTHANASIA/ATTITUDES)

CBS Video. 60 Minutes: Death by Doctor. [Videorecording]. Produced by 60 Minutes, 524 West 57th St., New York, NY 10019; 1998. 1 videocassette; 14 min.; sd.; color; VHS.
(EUTHANASIA)

Chabal, F. see **Julian-Reyneir, C.**

Chadwick, Ruth. Dimensions of quality in genetic services -- an ethical comment. *European Journal of Human Genetics.* 1997; 5(Suppl. 2): 22-24.
(GENETIC COUNSELING; GENETIC SERVICES)

Chadwick, Ruth. Gene therapy. *In:* Kuhse, Helga; Singer, Peter, eds. A Companion to Bioethics. Malden, MA: Blackwell; 1998: 189-197.
(GENE THERAPY)

Chadwick, Ruth. The philosophy of the right to know and the right not to know. *In:* Chadwick, Ruth; Levitt, Mairi; Shickle, Darren, eds. The Right to Know and the Right Not to Know. Brookfield, VT: Ashgate; 1997: 13-22.
(GENETIC SCREENING; TRUTH DISCLOSURE)

Chadwick, Ruth; Levitt, Mairi. Mass media and public discussion in bioethics. *In:* Chadwick, Ruth; Levitt, Mairi; Shickle, Darren, eds. The Right to Know and

the Right Not to Know. Brookfield, VT: Ashgate; 1997: 79–86.
(GENETIC SCREENING)

Chadwick, Ruth; Levitt, Mairi; Shickle, Darren, eds. The Right to Know and the Right Not to Know. Brookfield, VT: Ashgate; 1997. 101 p.
(GENETIC SCREENING)

Chadwick, Ruth; ten Have, Henk; Husted, Jörgen; Levitt, Mairi; McGleenan, Tony; Shickle, Darren; Wiesing, Urban. Genetic screening and ethics: European perspectives. *Journal of Medicine and Philosophy.* 1998 Jun; 23(3): 255–273.
(GENETIC SCREENING)

Chadwick, Ruth see **Draper, Heather**

Chaisson, Richard E. see **Morris, Lynn**

Chakravarti, Aravinda see **Collins, Francis S.**

Chalker, Rebecca see **Callum, Janet**

Chally, Pamela S.; Loriz, Lillia. Ethics in the trenches: decision making in practice -- a practical model for resolving the types of ethical dilemmas you face daily. *American Journal of Nursing.* 1998 Jun; 98(6): 17–20.
(NURSING ETHICS)

Chalmers, Don; Schwartz, Robert. Rogers v. Whitaker and informed consent in Australia: a fair dinkum duty of disclosure. *Medical Law Review.* 1993 Summer; 1(2): 139–159.
(INFORMED CONSENT)

Chalmers, Iain. Publication and promotion: the public interest. *Lancet.* 1998 Sep 12; 352(9131): 893–894.
(BIOMEDICAL RESEARCH)

Chambers, Tod. Retrodiction and the histories of bioethics. *Medical Humanities Review.* 1998 Spring; 12(1): 9–22.
(BIOETHICS)

Chambers, Tod. The Fiction of Bioethics: Cases as Literary Text. New York, NY: Routledge; 1999. 207 p.
(BIOETHICS)

Chandna, Shahid M.; Schulz, Joerg; Lawrence, Christopher; Greenwood, Roger N.; Farrington, Ken. Is there a rationale for rationing chronic dialysis? A hospital based cohort study of factors affecting survival and morbidity. *BMJ (British Medical Journal).* 1999 Jan 23; 318(7178): 217–223.
(RESOURCE ALLOCATION/BIOMEDICAL TECHNOLOGIES; SELECTION FOR TREATMENT)

Chapman, I.H. Informed consent: survey of Auckland, N.Z. anaesthetists' practice and attitudes. *Anaesthesia and Intensive Care.* 1997 Dec; 25(6): 671–674.
(INFORMED CONSENT)

Chapman, Simon. When outcomes threaten incomes: a case study of the obstruction of research to reduce teenage smoking. *Health Policy.* 1997 Jan; 39(1): 55–68.
(BEHAVIORAL RESEARCH/ETHICS COMMITTEES; PUBLIC HEALTH)

Chaput, Charles J. see **Brown, Harold O.J.**

Charatan, Fred. AMA issues guidelines on end of life care. [News]. *BMJ (British Medical Journal).* 1999 Mar 13; 318(7185): 690.
(ALLOWING TO DIE)

Charatan, Fred. Brazil challenges doctors accused of torture. [News]. *BMJ (British Medical Journal).* 1999 Mar 20; 318(7186): 757.
(FRAUD AND MISCONDUCT; TORTURE)

Charatan, Fred. Pennsylvania plans to reward organ donation. [News]. *BMJ (British Medical Journal).* 1999 May 22; 318(7195): 1371.
(ORGAN AND TISSUE DONATION)

Charatan, Fred B. see **Beecham, Linda**

Charland, Louis C. Appreciation and emotion: theoretical reflections on the MacArthur Treatment Competence Study. *Kennedy Institute of Ethics Journal.* 1998 Dec; 8(4): 359–376.
(INFORMED CONSENT)

Charles, J. Daryl. Blame it on the beta–boosters: genetics, self–determination, and moral accountability. *In:* Demy, Timothy J.; Stewart, Gary P., eds. Genetic Engineering: A Christian Response: Crucial Considerations in Shaping Life. Grand Rapids, MI: Kregel Publications; 1999: 240–258.
(BEHAVIORAL GENETICS)

Charlesworth, Max see **Skene, Loane**

Charlton, Rodger; Simone, Charles B.; Simone, Nicole L.; Simone, Charles B., II; Tanida, Noritoshi. Do we always need to tell patients the truth? [Letters]. *Lancet.* 1998 Nov 28; 352(9142): 1787.
(TRUTH DISCLOSURE)

Charo, R. Alta. Dusk, dawn, and defining death: legal classifications and biological categories. *In:* Youngner, Stuart J., Arnold, Robert M., Schapiro, Renie, eds. The Definition of Death: Contemporary Controversies. Baltimore, MD: Johns Hopkins University Press; 1999: 277–292.
(DETERMINATION OF DEATH)

Charo, R. Alta. Update on the National Bioethics Advisory Commission. *Protecting Human Subjects.* 1997 Fall: 10–11.
(ETHICISTS AND ETHICS COMMITTEES)

Charrow, Robert P. Wheat, guns, and science: human research subjects and the commerce clause. *Journal of NIH Research.* 1997 Nov; 9(11): 55–57.
(HUMAN EXPERIMENTATION/REGULATION)

Chase, Cheryl. Surgical progress is not the answer to intersexuality. *Journal of Clinical Ethics.* 1998 Winter; 9(4): 385–392.
(PATIENT CARE/MINORS)

Chase, Cheryl; Elliott, Carl. Intersexuality: waiting for change? [Letter and response]. *Hastings Center Report.* 1999 Mar–Apr; 29(2): 4.
(PATIENT CARE/MINORS)

Chase, Marilyn. Rationing scarce drugs has some questioning fairness and ethics. [News]. *Wall Street Journal.* 1998 Sep 28: B1.
(PATIENT CARE/DRUGS; RESOURCE

ALLOCATION/BIOMEDICAL TECHNOLOGIES; SELECTION FOR TREATMENT)

Chastain, Garvin; Landrum, R. Eric, eds. Protecting Human Subjects: Departmental Subject Pools and Institutional Review Boards. Washington, DC: American Psychological Association; 1999. 228 p.
(BEHAVIORAL RESEARCH; BEHAVIORAL RESEARCH/ETHICS COMMITTEES)

Chatterjee, Anjan see **Marson, Daniel C.**

Chatterji, Somnath; Jain, Sanjeev; Brahmachari, Samir K.; Majumder, Partha; Reich, Theodore. International collaboration in genetics research. [Letter]. *Nature Genetics.* 1997 Feb; 15(2): 124.
(GENETIC RESEARCH)

Chavey, William E.; Cantor, Scott B.; Clover, Richard D.; Reinarz, James A.; Spann, Stephen J. Cost-effectiveness analysis of screening health care workers for HIV. *Journal of Family Practice.* 1994 Mar; 38(3): 249–257.
(AIDS/HEALTH PERSONNEL; AIDS/TESTING AND SCREENING)

Chavkin, David F. "For their own good": civil commitment of alcohol and drug-dependent pregnant women. *South Dakota Law Review.* 1992; 37(2): 224–288.
(INVOLUNTARY COMMITMENT; PRENATAL INJURIES)

Chavkin, Wendy. Unwanted pregnancy in Armenia -- the larger context. [Editorial]. *American Journal of Public Health.* 1998 May; 88(5): 732–733.
(ABORTION/FOREIGN COUNTRIES; CONTRACEPTION)

Chearskul, Sanay see **Achrekar, Abinash**

Cheng, F.; Ip, Mary; Wong, K.K.; Yan, W.W. Critical care ethics in Hong Kong: cross-cultural conflicts as East meets West. *Journal of Medicine and Philosophy.* 1998 Dec; 23(6): 616–627.
(ALLOWING TO DIE; HEALTH CARE/FOREIGN COUNTRIES)

Cheng, Leo H.H.; Whittington, Richard M. Natural deaths while driving: would screening for risk be ethically justified? *Journal of Medical Ethics.* 1998 Aug; 24(4): 248–251.
(MASS SCREENING; PUBLIC HEALTH)

Cheron, Mireille see **Lot, Florence**

Cherry, M. Nichelle see **Bishop, Laura Jane**

Chervenak, Frank A.; McCullough, Laurence B. Ethical considerations in research involving pregnant women. *Women's Health Issues.* 1999 Jul–Aug; 9(4): 206–207.
(HUMAN EXPERIMENTATION/SPECIAL POPULATIONS)

Chervenak, Frank A.; McCullough, Laurence B.; Wapner, Ronald. Three ethically justified indications for selective termination in multifetal pregnancy: a practical and comprehensive management strategy. *Journal of Assisted Reproduction and Genetics.* 1995 Sep; 12(8): 531–536.
(ABORTION)

Chervenak, Frank A. see **Perone, Nicola**

Chesterman, Simon. Last rights: euthanasia, the sanctity

of life, and the law in the Netherlands and the Northern Territory of Australia. *International and Comparative Law Quarterly.* 1998 Apr; 47(2): 362–393.
(EUTHANASIA/LEGAL ASPECTS; SUICIDE)

Chevlen, Eric see **Brown, Harold O.J.**

Chez, Ronald A. see **Perone, Nicola**

Chick, Jonathan. Treatment of alcoholic violent offenders: ethics and efficacy. *Alcohol and Alcoholism.* 1998 Jan–Feb; 33(1): 20–25.
(PATIENT CARE/MENTALLY DISABLED)

Children's Defense Fund see **Redenbaugh, Russell**

Childress, James F. A principle-based approach. *In:* Kuhse, Helga; Singer, Peter, eds. A Companion to Bioethics. Malden, MA: Blackwell; 1998: 61–71.
(BIOETHICS)

Childress, James F. The gift of life: ethical issues in organ transplantation. *Bulletin of the American College of Surgeons.* 1996 Mar; 81(3): 8–22.
(ORGAN AND TISSUE DONATION)

Chin, Arthur E.; Hedberg, Katrina; Higginson, Grant K.; Fleming, David W. Legalized physician-assisted suicide in Oregon -- the first year's experience. *New England Journal of Medicine.* 1999 Feb 18; 340(7): 577–583.
(SUICIDE)

Chin, Marshall H. Health outcomes and managed care: discussing the hidden issues. *American Journal Of Managed Care.* 1997 May; 3(5): 756–762.
(HEALTH CARE/ECONOMICS)

Chiodo, Gary T.; Tolle, Susan W. The ethical foundations of a duty to treat HIV-positive patients. *General Dentistry.* 1997 Jan–Feb; 45(1): 14, 16, 18, 20, 22.
(AIDS/HEALTH PERSONNEL; PROFESSIONAL ETHICS)

Chisholm, John. Viagra: a botched test case for rationing. [Editorial]. *BMJ (British Medical Journal).* 1999 Jan 30; 318(7179): 273–274.
(HEALTH CARE/ECONOMICS; PATIENT CARE/DRUGS; RESOURCE ALLOCATION/BIOMEDICAL TECHNOLOGIES)

Chiu, John T. see **Margolis, Lewis H.**

Cho, Mildred K. see **Merz, Jon F.**

Chochinov, Harvey Max; Tataryn, Douglas; Clinch, Jennifer J.; Dudgeon, Deborah. Will to live in the terminally ill. *Lancet.* 1999 Sep 4; 354(9181): 816–819.
(TERMINAL CARE)

Chodoff, Paul. Ethical dimensions of psychotherapy: a personal perspective. *American Journal of Psychotherapy.* 1996 Summer; 50(3): 298–310.
(PATIENT CARE/MENTALLY DISABLED; PROFESSIONAL ETHICS; PROFESSIONAL PATIENT RELATIONSHIP)

Choi, Hae Won. Koreans honor dead lab animals (who knows -- they may return). [News]. *Wall Street Journal.* 1998 Nov 10: B1.
(ANIMAL EXPERIMENTATION)

Chokevivat, Vichai see **Achrekar, Abinash**

Chokevivat, Vichai see **Beloqui, Jorge**

Chokevivat, Vichai see **Schüklenk, Udo**

Choo, Vivien. Thin line between research and audit. *Lancet.* 1998 Aug 1; 352(9125): 337–338.
(HUMAN EXPERIMENTATION/ETHICS COMMITTEES; PRENATAL DIAGNOSIS)

Chotpitayasunondh, Tawee see **Achrekar, Abinash**

Christakis, Dimitri see **Hundert, Edward M.**

Christensen, Jan see **Fasting, Ulla**

Christian Pharmacists Fellowship International see **Wagner, Bertil K.J.**

Christianson, David J. Insurance concerns: are the fears exaggerated? *In:* Smith, Edward; Sapp, Walter, eds. Plain Talk about the Human Genome Project: A Tuskegee University Conference on its Promise and Perils ... and Matters of Race. Tuskegee, AL: Tuskegee University Press; 1997: 169–177.
(GENETIC SCREENING)

Chuachoowong, Rutt see **Achrekar, Abinash**

Chugh, Kirpal S.; Jha, Vivekanand. Commerce in transplantation in Third World countries. *Kidney International.* 1996 May; 49(5): 1181–1186.
(ORGAN AND TISSUE DONATION; ORGAN AND TISSUE TRANSPLANTATION)

Churchill, Larry R. Looking to Hume for justice: on the utility of Hume's view of justice for American health care reform. *Journal of Medicine and Philosophy.* 1999 Aug; 24(4): 352–364.
(HEALTH CARE)

Churchill, Larry R. Mapping the ethical terrain of managed care. *NCCE News (Veterans Health Administration National Center for Clinical Ethics).* 1998 Winter; 6(1): 1–2, 10–11.
(HEALTH CARE/ECONOMICS)

Cica, Natasha. Sterilising the intellectually disabled: the approach of the High Court of Australia in Department of Health v. J.W.B. and S.M.B. [Comment]. *Medical Law Review.* 1993 Summer; 1(2): 186–231.
(STERILIZATION/MENTALLY DISABLED)

Cichon, Dennis E. The right to "just say no": a history and analysis of the right to refuse antipsychotic drugs. *Louisiana Law Review.* 1992 Nov; 53(2): 283–426.
(TREATMENT REFUSAL/MENTALLY DISABLED)

Cicirelli, Victor G. Elders' end-of-life decisions: implications for hospice care. *Hospice Journal.* 1997; 12(1): 57–72.
(ALLOWING TO DIE/ATTITUDES; EUTHANASIA/ATTITUDES; SUICIDE)

Ciesielski–Carlucci, Chris see **Thomasma, David C.**

Ciliberti, Rosella. Biotechnological patents and ethical aspects. *Cancer Detection and Prevention.* 1993; 17(2): 313–315.
(PATENTING LIFE FORMS)

Ciment, James. Most deaths related to abortion occur in the developing world. [News]. *BMJ (British Medical Journal).* 1999 Jun 5; 318(7197): 1509.
(ABORTION/FOREIGN COUNTRIES)

Cimons, Marlene see **Birmingham, Karen**

Claes, Tom. Cultural background of the ethical and social debate about biotechnology. *In:* Sterckx, Sigrid, ed. Biotechnology, Patents and Morality. Proceedings of an International Workshop, "Biotechnology, Patents and Morality: Towards a Consensus," held in Ghent, Belgium, 17–19 Jan 1996. Brookfield, VT: Ashgate; 1997: 121–127.
(GENETIC INTERVENTION)

Clark, Barbara J.; Abeles, Norman. Ethical issues and dilemmas in the mental health organization. *Administration and Policy in Mental Health.* 1994 Sep; 22(1): 7–17.
(PROFESSIONAL ETHICS)

Clark–Chiarelli, Nancy see **Simon, Steven R.**

Clark, Frank I. Making sense of State v. Messenger. *Pediatrics.* 1996 Apr; 97(4): 579–583.
(ALLOWING TO DIE/INFANTS; ALLOWING TO DIE/LEGAL ASPECTS; TREATMENT REFUSAL/MINORS)

Clark, Graeme M.; Cowan, Robert S.C.; Dowell, Richard C. Ethical issues. *In:* Clark, Graeme M.; Cowan, Robert S.C.; Dowell, Richard C., eds. Cochlear Implantation for Infants and Children: Advances. San Diego, CA: Singular Publishing Group; 1997: 241–249.
(HUMAN EXPERIMENTATION/MINORS; HUMAN EXPERIMENTATION/SPECIAL POPULATIONS; PATIENT CARE/MINORS)

Clark, Peter A. A legacy of mistrust: African–Americans, the medical profession, and AIDS. *Linacre Quarterly.* 1998 Feb; 65(1): 66–88.
(AIDS)

Clark, Reese H. The safe introduction of new technologies into neonatal medicine. *Clinics in Perinatology.* 1996 Sep; 23(3): 519–527.
(BIOMEDICAL TECHNOLOGIES; HUMAN EXPERIMENTATION/MINORS; PATIENT CARE/MINORS)

Clark, Richard E. Bone-marrow donation by mentally incapable adults. *Lancet.* 1998 Dec 5; 352(9143): 1847–1848.
(ORGAN AND TISSUE DONATION)

Clark, William R. The ethics of molecular medicine. *In: his:* The New Healers: The Promise and Problems of Molecular Medicine in the Twenty–First Century. New York, NY: Oxford University Press; 1997: 207–231, 236.
(DNA FINGERPRINTING; GENE THERAPY; GENETIC SCREENING)

Clarke, Adele E. Disciplining Reproduction: Modernity, American Life Sciences, and "the Problems of Sex." Berkeley, CA: University of California Press; 1998. 421 p.
(BIOMEDICAL RESEARCH; CONTRACEPTION; REPRODUCTION)

Clarke, Angus. Genetic screening and counselling. *In:* Kuhse, Helga; Singer, Peter, eds. A Companion to Bioethics. Malden, MA: Blackwell; 1998: 215–228.
(GENETIC COUNSELING; GENETIC SCREENING)

Clarke, Angus, ed. The Genetic Testing of Children. Washington, DC: BIOS Scientific Publishers; 1998. 334 p.
(GENETIC SCREENING)

Clarke, Angus; Michie, Susan. Parents' responses to predictive genetic testing in their children. [Letter and response]. *Journal of Medical Genetics*. 1997 Feb; 34(2): 174–175.
(GENETIC SCREENING)

Clarke, Liam. The person in abortion. *Nursing Ethics*. 1999 Jan; 6(1): 37–46.
(ABORTION; FETUSES; PERSONHOOD)

Clarke, M.P. There are ethical issues in ophthalmology. *BMJ (British Medical Journal)*. 1999 Apr 24; 318(7191): 1153.
(GENETIC SCREENING)

Clayton, Ellen Wright. Issues in state newborn screening programs. *Pediatrics*. 1992 Oct; 90(4): 641–646.
(GENETIC SCREENING; MASS SCREENING)

Clayton, Paul D. Improving the privacy and security of electronic health information. *Academic Medicine*. 1997 Jun; 72(6): 522–523.
(CONFIDENTIALITY)

Cleary, Paul D. see **Kao, Audiey C.**

Clemency, Mary V.; Thompson, Nancy J. Do not resuscitate orders in the perioperative period: patient perspectives. *Anesthesia and Analgesia*. 1997 Apr; 84(4): 859–864.
(RESUSCITATION ORDERS)

Clement, Mary see **Humphry, Derek**

Clever, Linda Hawes see **Kirsch, Michael**

Clinch, Jennifer J. see **Chochinov, Harvey Max**

Clinton, Michael see **Mak, June Mui Hing**

Cloostermans, Trees see **Decruyenaere, Marleen**

Clouser, K. Danner; Hufford, David J.; Morrison, Catherine J. What's in a word? *Alternative Therapies in Health and Medicine*. 1995 Jul; 1(3): 78–79.
(PATIENT CARE)

Clover, Richard D. see **Chavey, William E.**

Cloyd, J. Timothy see **Elshtain, Jean Bethke**

Coakley, Eugenie see **Krieger, Nancy**

Coburn, Tom; Senak, Mark S.; Stein, Robert E.; Wilcox, W. Bradford; Krauthammer, Charles; Shepherd, H.R. What can be done to curtail the AIDS epidemic? *In:* Dudley, William, ed. Epidemics: Opposing Viewpoints. San Diego, CA: Greenhaven Press; 1999: 53–85, 173.
(AIDS)

Coburn, Tom A. see **Solomon, Liza**

Cocks, Geoffrey. The old as new: the Nuremberg Doctors' Trial and medicine in modern Germany. *In:* Berg, Manfred; Cocks, Geoffrey, eds. Medicine and Modernity: Public Health and Medical Care in Nineteenth- and Twentieth-Century Germany. New York, NY: Cambridge University Press; 1997: 173–191.
(FRAUD AND MISCONDUCT; HUMAN EXPERIMENTATION/FOREIGN COUNTRIES)

Cocks, Geoffrey. The old as new: the Nuremberg Doctors' Trial and medicine in modern Germany. *In: his* Treating Mind and Body: Essays in the History of Science, Professions, and Society Under Extreme Conditions. New Brunswick, NJ: Transaction Publishers; 1998: 193–213.
(FRAUD AND MISCONDUCT; HUMAN EXPERIMENTATION/FOREIGN COUNTRIES)

Coelho, Daniel H.; Caplan, Arthur L. The unclaimed cadaver. *Academic Medicine*. 1997 Sep; 72(9): 741–743.
(ORGAN AND TISSUE DONATION)

Coelho, Daniel H. see **Caplan, Arthur L.**

Coghlan, Andy. Named and shamed: genetic engineers who flouted the rules are brought to book. [News]. *New Scientist*. 1998 Apr 4; 158(2128): 4.
(FRAUD AND MISCONDUCT; GENETIC INTERVENTION)

Coghlan, Andy. Perfect People's Republic. [News]. *New Scientist*. 1998 Oct 24; 160(2157): 18.
(EUGENICS)

Coghlan, Andy. Selling the family secrets. [News]. *New Scientist*. 1998 Dec 5; 160(2163): 20–21.
(GENETIC RESEARCH)

Coghlan, Andy. The price of profit. [News]. *New Scientist*. 1998 May 16; 158(2134): 20–21.
(GENETIC RESEARCH; GENOME MAPPING)

Cohen, Adam. Showdown for Doctor Death. *Time*. 1998 Dec 7; 152(23): 46–47.
(EUTHANASIA)

Cohen, Cynthia B. Moving away from the Huntington's disease paradigm in the predictive genetic testing of children. *In:* Clarke, Angus, ed. The Genetic Testing of Children. Washington, DC: BIOS Scientific Publishers; 1998: 133–143.
(GENETIC SCREENING)

Cohen, Donald J. see **Arnold, L. Eugene**

Cohen, Elias S.; Kruschwitz, Ann L. Restraint reduction: lessons from the asylum. *Journal of Ethics, Law, and Aging*. 1997 Spring–Summer; 3(1): 25–43.
(BEHAVIOR CONTROL; PATIENT CARE/AGED; PATIENT CARE/MENTALLY DISABLED)

Cohen–Haguenauer, Odile. Gene therapy: regulatory issues and international approaches to regulation. *Current Opinion In Biotechnology*. 1997 Jun; 8(3): 361–369.
(GENE THERAPY)

Cohen, Jon. No consensus on rules for AIDS vaccine trials. [News]. *Science*. 1998 Jul 3; 281(5373): 22–23.
(AIDS/HUMAN EXPERIMENTATION; IMMUNIZATION)

Cohen, Jon. Research shutdown roils Los Angeles VA. [News]. *Science*. 1999 Apr 2; 284(5411): 18–19, 21.
(FRAUD AND MISCONDUCT; HUMAN EXPERIMENTATION/REGULATION)

Cohen, Jon. Researchers urged not to inject virulent HIV strain into chimps. [News]. *Science.* 1999 Feb 19; 283(5405): 1090–1091.
(AIDS; ANIMAL EXPERIMENTATION)

Cohen, Jon; Ivinson, Adrian J. Clarifying AIDS vaccine trial guidelines. [Letter and response]. *Nature Medicine.* 1998 Oct; 4(10): 1091.
(AIDS/HUMAN EXPERIMENTATION; HUMAN EXPERIMENTATION/FOREIGN COUNTRIES; IMMUNIZATION)

Cohen, Jonathan R. In God's garden: creation and cloning in Jewish thought. *Hastings Center Report.* 1999 Jul–Aug; 29(4): 7–12.
(CLONING)

Cohen, Jonathan S. see **Dickinson, George E.**

Cohen, Lewis M. Suicide, hastening death, and psychiatry. *Archives of Internal Medicine.* 1998 Oct 12; 158(18): 1973–1976.
(ALLOWING TO DIE; SUICIDE)

Cohen, Lynne. Jewish and secular medical ethics share themes but diverge on issues such as heroic measures. *Canadian Medical Association Journal.* 1997 Nov 15; 157(10): 1415–1416.
(ALLOWING TO DIE/RELIGIOUS ASPECTS; EUTHANASIA/RELIGIOUS ASPECTS)

Cohen, Pamela Schwartz. Psychiatric commitment in Japan: international concern and domestic reform. *UCLA Pacific Basin Law Journal.* 1995 Fall; 14(1): 28–74.
(INVOLUNTARY COMMITMENT/FOREIGN COUNTRIES; PATIENTS' RIGHTS/MENTALLY DISABLED)

Cohen, Peter J. The placebo is not dead: three historical vignettes. *IRB: A Review of Human Subjects Research.* 1998 Mar–Jun; 20(2–3): 6–8.
(HUMAN EXPERIMENTATION/RESEARCH DESIGN)

Cohen, Philip. Totems and taboos: an Apache tribe has signed a historic deal with geneticists. [News]. *New Scientist.* 1998 Aug 29; 159(2149): 5.
(GENETIC RESEARCH)

Cohen, Simon see **Winter, Bob**

Cohen, Sophie see **Julvez, Jean**

Coker, Richard. Public health, civil liberties, and tuberculosis. [Editorial]. *BMJ (British Medical Journal).* 1999 May 29; 318(7196): 1434–1435.
(PUBLIC HEALTH)

Cole–Turner, Ronald. Do means matter? *In:* Parens, Erik, ed. Enhancing Human Traits: Ethical and Social Implications. Washington, DC: Georgetown University Press; 1998: 151–161.
(BIOMEDICAL TECHNOLOGIES)

Colebunders, Robert; Schrooten, W.; Singer, Peter A.; Martin, Douglas K.; Kelner, Merrijoy. Euthanasia and end–of–life care. [Letter and response]. *JAMA.* 1999 Apr 28; 281(16): 1488.
(EUTHANASIA; TERMINAL CARE)

Coleman, Gerald. Basic issues in the debate over dying. *Origins.* 1998 Mar 19; 27(39): 663–668.
(EUTHANASIA/RELIGIOUS ASPECTS; SUICIDE)

Coles, Robert see **Wright, Robert**

Colfax, Grant Nash; Bindman, Andrew B. Health benefits and risks of reporting HIV–infected individuals by name. [Comment]. *American Journal of Public Health.* 1998 Jun; 88(6): 876–879.
(AIDS/CONFIDENTIALITY)

Collier, Joe. Patient–information leaflets and prescriber competence. *Lancet.* 1998 Nov 28; 352(9142): 1724.
(PATIENT CARE/DRUGS)

Collins, Chris see **Beloqui, Jorge**

Collins, Francis S. Shattuck Lecture –– medical and societal consequences of the Human Genome Project. *New England Journal of Medicine.* 1999 Jul 1; 341(1): 28–37.
(GENOME MAPPING)

Collins, Francis S.; Patrinos, Ari; Jordan, Elke; Chakravarti, Aravinda; Gesteland, Raymond; Walters, LeRoy. New goals for the U.S. Human Genome Project: 1998–2003. *Science.* 1998 Oct 23; 282(5389): 682–689.
(GENOME MAPPING)

Collins, Francis S. see **Karanjawala, Zarir E.**

Collins, Harry; Pinch, Trevor. ACTing UP: AIDS cures and lay expertise. *In: their* The Golem at Large: What You Should Know About Technology. New York, NY: Cambridge University Press; 1998: 126–150.
(AIDS/HUMAN EXPERIMENTATION; HUMAN EXPERIMENTATION/RESEARCH DESIGN)

Collins, Michael F. The role of Catholic hospitals in the new millennium. *Dolentium Hominum: Church and Health in the World.* 1998; No. 37 [yr. 13(1)]: 85–89.
(HEALTH CARE)

Colliton, William see **Bowes, Watson**

Colliton, William F. see **Byrne, Paul A.**

Collopy, Bart J. The moral underpinning of the proxy–provider relationship: issues of trust and distrust. *Journal of Law, Medicine and Ethics.* 1999 Spring; 27(1): 37–45.
(ADVANCE DIRECTIVES; INFORMED CONSENT)

Colvin, Robert B. see **Sachs, David H.**

Combes, Robert D. see **Mepham, T. Ben**

Comley, Sarah see **Baumiller, Robert C.**

Concar, David. Their learned friends: was a scientific society really a front for one of the world's biggest tobacco firms? [News]. *New Scientist.* 1998 May 16; 158(2134): 5.
(BIOMEDICAL RESEARCH)

Coney, Sandra. Chemotherapy in children –– where to draw the line? [News]. *Lancet.* 1999 Mar 6; 353(9155): 819.
(TREATMENT REFUSAL/MINORS)

Cong, Yali. Ethical challenges in critical care medicine: a Chinese perspective. *Journal of Medicine and*

Philosophy. 1998 Dec; 23(6): 581–600.
(HEALTH CARE/ECONOMICS; HEALTH CARE/FOREIGN COUNTRIES; RESOURCE ALLOCATION)

Conn, P. Michael; Parker, James. Animal rights: reaching the public. [Editorial]. *Science.* 1998 Nov 20; 282(5393): 1417.
(ANIMAL EXPERIMENTATION)

Connelly, Julia. Emotions, ethics, and decisions in primary care. *Journal of Clinical Ethics.* 1998 Fall; 9(3): 225–234.
(PROFESSIONAL PATIENT RELATIONSHIP)

Connelly, Maureen T. see **Simon, Steven R.**

Connelly, R.J. Death with dignity: fifty years of soul-searching. *Journal of Religion and Health.* 1998 Fall; 37(3): 195–213.
(ALLOWING TO DIE/ATTITUDES; EUTHANASIA/ATTITUDES; SUICIDE; TERMINAL CARE)

Conner, Paul. Euthanasia -- why not? *Rhode Island Medicine.* 1993 Dec; 76(12): 595–599.
(ALLOWING TO DIE/RELIGIOUS ASPECTS; EUTHANASIA/RELIGIOUS ASPECTS)

Conner, Paul. Is there a secular answer to euthanasia, American style? *Angelicum.* 1996; 73: 381–400.
(EUTHANASIA; SUICIDE)

Connor, Susan Scholle; Fuenzalida-Puelma, Hernán L., eds. Bioethics: Issues and Perspectives. Washington, DC: Pan American Health Organization; 1990. 239 p.
(BIOETHICS)

Connors, Alfred F. see **Hamel, Mary Beth**

Constantino, Rose E.; Boneysteele, Ginger; Gesmond, Sharyn A.; Nelson, Beverly. Restraining an aggressive suicidal, paraplegic patient: a look at the ethical and legal issues. *Dimensions of Critical Care Nursing.* 1997 May–Jun; 16(3): 144–151.
(BEHAVIOR CONTROL; PATIENT CARE/MENTALLY DISABLED)

Cook, Curtis R. see **Bopp, James**

Cook-Deegan, Robert see **Burris, John**

Cook-Deegan, Robert Mullan. Finding a voice for bioethics in public policy: federal initiatives in the United States, 1974–1991. *In:* ten Have, Henk A.M.J.; Sass, Hans-Martin, eds. Consensus Formation in Healthcare Ethics. Boston, MA: Kluwer Academic; 1998: 107–140.
(BIOETHICS; ETHICISTS AND ETHICS COMMITTEES)

Cook, E. David. Genetics and the British insurance industry. *Journal of Medical Ethics.* 1999 Apr; 25(2): 157–162.
(GENETIC SCREENING)

Cook, Edwin see **Arnold, L. Eugene**

Cook, Rebecca J.; Dickens, Bernard M.; Bliss, Laura E. International developments in abortion law from 1988 to 1998. *American Journal of Public Health.* 1999 Apr; 89(4): 579–586.
(ABORTION/FOREIGN COUNTRIES; ABORTION/LEGAL ASPECTS)

Cook, Robin. Chromosome 6. [Fiction]. New York, NY: Berkley Books; 1997. 460 p.
(GENETIC INTERVENTION)

Cook, William see **Crelinsten, Gordon L.**

Cooper, Colleen see **Baker, Tina**

Cooper, Ellen R. Caring for children with AIDS: new challenges for medicine and society. *Pediatrician.* 1990; 17(2): 118–123.
(AIDS; PATIENT CARE/MINORS)

Cooper, J.A. see **Welton, A.J.**

Cooper-Mahkorn, Déirdre. Guidelines on assisted deaths criticised. [News]. *BMJ (British Medical Journal).* 1998 Oct 3; 317(7163): 904.
(ALLOWING TO DIE; TERMINAL CARE)

Cooper-Patrick, Lisa; Gallo, Joseph J.; Gonzales, Junius J.; Vu, Hong Thi; Powe, Neil R.; Nelson, Christine; Ford, Daniel E. Race, gender, and partnership in the patient-physician relationship. *JAMA.* 1999 Aug 11; 282(6): 583–589.
(PROFESSIONAL PATIENT RELATIONSHIP)

Cooper, Rebecca; Koch, Kathryn A. Neonatal and pediatric critical care: ethical decision making. *Critical Care Clinics.* 1996 Jan; 12(1): 149–164.
(ALLOWING TO DIE/INFANTS; PATIENT CARE/MINORS)

Cooper, Susan Lewis; Glazer, Ellen Sarasohn. Choosing Assisted Reproduction: Social, Emotional and Ethical Considerations. Indianapolis, IN: Perspectives Press; 1998. 400 p.
(REPRODUCTIVE TECHNOLOGIES)

Coovadia, Hoosen M. see **Karim, Quarraisha Abdool**

Cordner, Stephen see **Loff, Bebe**

Cordner, Stephen M. see **Breen, Kerry J.**

Cornell, Morna see **Heywood, Mark**

Cosimi, A. Benedict see **Sachs, David H.**

Costa, Patrizia see **Mepham, T. Ben**

Costa, T. see **Fitzpatrick, J.**

Costa, T. see **Huggins, M.**

Costantini-Ferrando, Maria F.; Foley, Kathleen M.; Rapkin, Bruce D.; Kennedy, B.J.; Weeks, Jane C.; Smith, Thomas J. Communicating with patients about advanced cancer. [Letters and responses]. *JAMA.* 1998 Oct 28; 280(16): 1403–1404.
(TERMINAL CARE; TRUTH DISCLOSURE)

Costanza, Mary see **Pokorski, Robert J.**

Côté, Luc see **Beaudoin, Claude**

Cottingham, J. see **Benagiano, G.**

Cotton, Philip see **Hill, Wan Ying**

Coulter, Angela; Entwistle, Vikki; Gilbert, David. Sharing decisions with patients: is the information good

enough? *BMJ (British Medical Journal)*. 1999 Jan 30; 318(7179): 318–322.
(PATIENT CARE)

Council of Regional Networks [for Genetic Services] Committee on Ethics see **Baumiller, Robert C.**

Courvoisier, B. see **Müller, H.J.**

Coutelle, Charles see **Billings, Paul R.**

Couzin, Jennifer. RAC confronts in utero gene therapy proposals. [News]. *Science*. 1998 Oct 2; 282(5386): 27.
(EMBRYO AND FETAL RESEARCH; GENE THERAPY)

Covey, Preston K. see **Andersen, David**

Covinsky, Kenneth E.; Bates, Carol K.; Davis, Roger B.; Delbanco, Thomas L. Physicians' attitudes toward using patient reports to assess quality of care. *Academic Medicine*. 1996 Dec; 71(12): 1353–1356.
(PATIENT CARE)

Cowan, Robert S.C. see **Clark, Graeme M.**

Coward, Harold; Ratanakul, Pinit, eds. A Cross–Cultural Dialogue on Health Care Ethics. Waterloo, ON: Wilfrid Laurier University Press; 1999. 274 p.
(BIOETHICS; HEALTH; HEALTH CARE)

Coward, Harold see **Burgess, Michael**

Cowdin, Daniel M.; Tuohey, John F. Sterilization, Catholic health care, and the legitimate autonomy of culture. *Christian Bioethics*. 1998 Apr; 4(1): 14–44.
(STERILIZATION)

Cowell, Alan. Obeying pope, German bishops end role in abortion system. [News]. *New York Times*. 1998 Jan 28: A3.
(ABORTION/FOREIGN COUNTRIES; ABORTION/RELIGIOUS ASPECTS)

Cowen, Robert C. Academics face abuse of rules designed to protect research. *Christian Science Monitor*. 1998 Mar 25: 13.
(BIOMEDICAL RESEARCH; FRAUD AND MISCONDUCT)

Cox, Paul M. see **Rae, Scott B.**

Craddock, Nick see **Jones, Ian**

Craft, Michele see **Marik, Paul E.**

Crandon, John see **Barton, John**

Cranford, Ronald see **Lynn, Joanne**

Cranford, Ronald E. Discontinuation of ventilation after brain stem death: policy should be balanced with concern for the family. *BMJ (British Medical Journal)*. 1999 Jun 26; 318(7200): 1754–1755.
(DETERMINATION OF DEATH/BRAIN DEATH)

Crausman, Robert S.; Armstrong, John D. Ethically based medical decision making in the intensive care unit: residency teaching strategies. *Critical Care Clinics*. 1996 Jan; 12(1): 71–84.
(BIOETHICS/EDUCATION; MEDICAL ETHICS/EDUCATION)

Crausman, Robert S. see **Merrill, William W.**

Crawford, Colin; American Civil Liberties Union. Should HIV testing be required for all pregnant women? *In:* Francoeur, Robert T., ed. Taking Sides: Clashing Views on Controversial Issues in Human Sexuality. Fifth Edition. Guilford, CT: Dushkin Publishing Group/Brown and Benchmark; 1996: 192–207.
(AIDS/TESTING AND SCREENING)

Crawshaw, Ralph. Cautionary note on reforming medical oaths. *Bulletin of Medical Ethics*. 1997 Nov; No. 133: 13–14.
(MEDICAL ETHICS/CODES OF ETHICS)

Crelinsten, Gordon L.; Belik, Jacques; Bereza, Eugene; Cook, William; McCarthy, Martha; Zawadowski, Andrew; Turnbull, John; Jespersen, Bruce W.; Walker, Paul; Gutowski, William D.; Weijer, Charles. CPR for patients in a persistent vegetative state? [Letters and response]. *Canadian Medical Association Journal*. 1998 Jul 14; 159(1): 18–19, 21.
(ALLOWING TO DIE; RESUSCITATION ORDERS)

Creskoff, Katharine. Scientific imperialism or service to humanity? The complexities of the Human Genome Diversity Project. *Princeton Journal of Bioethics*. 1998 Spring; 1(1): 6–22.
(GENETIC RESEARCH; GENOME MAPPING)

Cretney, Stephen. Re S (A Minor) (Blood Transfusion: Adoption Order Condition). [Comment]. *Family Law*. 1994 Nov; 24: 608–610.
(TREATMENT REFUSAL/MINORS)

Crigger, Bette–Jane. The battle over babies: international research in perinatal HIV transmission. *IRB: A Review of Human Subjects Research*. 1998 Jul–Aug; 20(4): 13–15.
(AIDS/HUMAN EXPERIMENTATION; HUMAN EXPERIMENTATION/FOREIGN COUNTRIES; HUMAN EXPERIMENTATION/RESEARCH DESIGN; HUMAN EXPERIMENTATION/SPECIAL POPULATIONS)

Crigger, Bette–Jane. Xenotransplantation [title supplied]. *Hastings Center Report*. 1999 Jan–Feb; 29(1): 50.
(ORGAN AND TISSUE TRANSPLANTATION)

Crilly, R.E. see **Mepham, T.B.**

Crilly, Robert E. see **Mepham, T. Ben**

Critser, John K. Current status of semen banking in the USA. [Article and discussion]. *Human Reproduction*. 1998 May; 13(Suppl. 2): 55–69.
(ARTIFICIAL INSEMINATION)

Crofts, Nick; Louie, Robyn; Loff, Bebe. The next plague: stigmatization and discrimination related to hepatitis C virus infection in Australia. *Health and Human Rights*. 1997; 2(2): 87–97.
(PUBLIC HEALTH)

Crosby, John F. There is no moral authority in medicine: response to Cowdin and Tuohey. *Christian Bioethics*. 1998 Apr; 4(1): 63–82.
(STERILIZATION)

Crossland, Nigel see **Evans, Donald**

Crosson, Francis J. see **Menendez, Roger**

Crosthwaite, Jan. Gender and bioethics. *In:* Kuhse, Helga; Singer, Peter, eds. A Companion to Bioethics. Malden, MA: Blackwell; 1998: 32–40.
(BIOETHICS)

Crouch, Robert A. Betwixt and between: the past and future of intersexuality. *Journal of Clinical Ethics.* 1998 Winter; 9(4): 372–384.
(PATIENT CARE/MINORS)

Crouch, Robert A.; Arras, John D. AZT trials and tribulations. *Hastings Center Report.* 1998 Nov–Dec; 28(6): 26–34.
(AIDS/HUMAN EXPERIMENTATION; HUMAN EXPERIMENTATION/FOREIGN COUNTRIES; HUMAN EXPERIMENTATION/RESEARCH DESIGN; HUMAN EXPERIMENTATION/SPECIAL POPULATIONS)

Crouch, Robert A.; Elliott, Carl. Moral agency and the family: the case of living related organ transplantation. *Cambridge Quarterly of Healthcare Ethics.* 1999 Summer; 8(3): 275–287.
(ORGAN AND TISSUE DONATION)

Croyle, Robert T.; Achilles, Jennifer S.; Lerman, Caryn. Psychologic aspects of cancer genetic testing: a research update for clinicians. *Cancer.* 1997 Aug 1; 80(3, Suppl.): 569–575.
(GENETIC SCREENING)

Csillag, Claudio. Brazil abolishes "presumed consent" in organ donation. [News]. *Lancet.* 1998 Oct 24; 352(9137): 1367.
(INFORMED CONSENT; ORGAN AND TISSUE DONATION)

Cuckle, Howard. Rational Down syndrome screening policy. *American Journal of Public Health.* 1998 Apr; 88(4): 558–559.
(MASS SCREENING; PRENATAL DIAGNOSIS)

Cuckle, Howard see **Moss, Sue**

Culpepper, Larry; Gilbert, Thomas T. Evidence and ethics. *Lancet.* 1999 Mar 6; 353(9155): 829–831.
(HEALTH CARE; PATIENT CARE; RESOURCE ALLOCATION)

Cunningham–Burley, Sarah see **Kerr, Anne**

Cunningham, George see **Baumiller, Robert C.**

Cunningham, Paige C. see **Stewart, Gary P.**

Cunningham, Peter J.; Grossman, Joy M.; St. Peter, Robert F.; Lesser, Cara S. Managed care and physicians' provision of charity care. *JAMA.* 1999 Mar 24–31; 281(12): 1087–1092.
(HEALTH CARE/ECONOMICS)

Cuperus–Bosma, Jacqueline M.; van der Wal, Gerrit; Looman, Caspar W.N.; van der Maas, Paul J. Assessment of physician–assisted death by members of the public prosecution in the Netherlands. *Journal of Medical Ethics.* 1999 Feb; 25(1): 8–15.
(EUTHANASIA; SUICIDE)

Curran, James W. see **Wilfert, Catherine M.**

Curran, Patrick. Regulating death: Oregon's Death with Dignity Act and the legalization of physician–assisted suicide. [Note]. *Georgetown Law Journal.* 1998 Jan; 86(3): 725–749.

(SUICIDE)

Currie, Rebecca. MRC funds large–scale human genetic database. [News]. *Nature Medicine.* 1998 Dec; 4(12): 1346.
(GENETIC RESEARCH)

Currie, Rebecca. UK moves ahead on the xenotransplantation issue. [News]. *Nature Medicine.* 1998 Sep; 4(9): 988.
(ORGAN AND TISSUE TRANSPLANTATION)

Curtis, George see **Swartz, Richard D.**

Cust, Kenneth F.T. Justice and rights to health care. *Reason Papers.* 1993 Fall; 18: 153–168.
(HEALTH CARE/RIGHTS)

Cusveller, Bart; Jochemsen, Henk. Life–terminating actions with severely demented patients: critical assessment of a report of the Royal Dutch Society of Medicine. *Issues in Law and Medicine.* 1996 Summer; 12(1): 31–45.
(ALLOWING TO DIE; EUTHANASIA)

Cutrer, William; Glahn, Sandra. Dealing with genetic reality: theological and clinical perspectives. *In:* Demy, Timothy J.; Stewart, Gary P., eds. Genetic Engineering: A Christian Response: Crucial Considerations in Shaping Life. Grand Rapids, MI: Kregel Publications; 1999: 154–169.
(EMBRYO AND FETAL RESEARCH; GENETIC RESEARCH; REPRODUCTIVE TECHNOLOGIES)

Cutrer, William R. see **Stewart, Gary P.**

Cutter, Mary Ann G.; Drexler, Edward; McCullough, Laurence B.; McInerney, Joseph D.; Murray, Jeffrey C.; Rossiter, Belinda; Zola, John. Mapping and Sequencing the Human Genome: Science, Ethics, and Public Policy. Colorado Springs, CO: BSCS, the Colorado College; Chicago, IL: American Medical Association; 1992. 94 p.
(GENOME MAPPING)

Cutter, William. Rabbi Judah's handmaid: narrative influence on life's important decisions. *In:* Jacob, Walter; Zemer, Moshe, eds. Death and Euthanasia in Jewish Law: Essays and Responsa. Pittsburgh, PA: Freehof Institute of Progressive Halakhah; Rodef Shalom Press; 1995: 61–87.
(ALLOWING TO DIE/RELIGIOUS ASPECTS)

Cutting, Keith see **Rix, Gary**

D

Daar, A.S. Paid organ donation -- the Grey Basket concept. [Editorial]. *Journal of Medical Ethics.* 1998 Dec; 24(6): 365–368.
(ORGAN AND TISSUE DONATION)

Daar, Judith F. Informed consent: defining limits through therapeutic parameters. *Whittier Law Review.* 1995; 16(1): 187–209.
(INFORMED CONSENT)

Dadds, Mark see **Van Haeringen, Alison R.**

D'Agostino, Francesco. The person and the right to health. *Dolentium Hominum: Church and Health in the*

World. 1998; No. 37 [yr. 13(1)]: 29–30.
(HEALTH)

Dahlquist, Gisela see **Nylenna, Magne**

Daily, O. Patrick see **Lin, Hung–Mo**

Dal–Ré, Rafael; Espada, Julián; Ortega, Rafael. Performance of research ethics committees in Spain: a prospective study of 100 applications for clinical trial protocols on medicines. *Journal of Medical Ethics.* 1999 Jun; 25(3): 268–273.
(HUMAN EXPERIMENTATION/ETHICS COMMITTEES; HUMAN EXPERIMENTATION/FOREIGN COUNTRIES)

Dalby, Shirley. Commercial testing. *In:* Clarke, Angus, ed. The Genetic Testing of Children. Washington, DC: BIOS Scientific Publishers; 1998: 265–270.
(GENETIC SCREENING; GENETIC SERVICES)

Dalton, Rex. Arizona professor files lawsuit after being fired for misconduct. [News]. *Nature.* 1998 Aug 27; 394(6696): 817.
(BIOMEDICAL RESEARCH; FRAUD AND MISCONDUCT)

Dalton, Rex. Federal panel endorses Baylor fraud claim. [News]. *Nature.* 1999 Feb 18; 397(6720): 549.
(BIOMEDICAL RESEARCH; FRAUD AND MISCONDUCT)

Dalton, Rex. Salk Institute investigated after claims of inhumane research. [News]. *Nature.* 1998 Aug 20; 394(6695): 709.
(ANIMAL EXPERIMENTATION; FRAUD AND MISCONDUCT)

Daly, Barbara J.; Gorecki, Julie; Sadowski, Alexis; Rudy, Ellen B.; Montenegro, Hugo D.; Song, Rhayun; Dyer, Mary Ann. Do–not–resuscitate practices in the chronically critically ill. *Heart and Lung.* 1996 Jul–Aug; 25(4): 310–317.
(RESUSCITATION ORDERS)

Dalyell, Tam. More comment from Westminster [research ethics committees]. [News]. *New Scientist.* 1998 Oct 3; 160(2154): 55.
(HUMAN EXPERIMENTATION/ETHICS COMMITTEES; HUMAN EXPERIMENTATION/FOREIGN COUNTRIES)

Damberg, Cheryl see **Grumbach, Kevin**

D'Amico, Robert see **Layon, A. Joseph**

Dan, Zhang; Lei, Xiong. Chinese center sues over study coverage. [News]. *Science.* 1999 Mar 26; 283(5410): 1990–1992.
(GENETIC RESEARCH)

Daniel, C. Ralph; Elewski, Boni E.; Scher, Richard K. Proposed guidelines for speakers discussing medications and other products. *Cutis.* 1997 May; 59(5): 271–272.
(HEALTH CARE/ECONOMICS)

Daniels, Norman. Is there a right to health care and, if so, what does it encompass? *In:* Kuhse, Helga; Singer, Peter, eds. A Companion to Bioethics. Malden, MA: Blackwell; 1998: 316–325.
(HEALTH CARE/RIGHTS)

Daniels, Norman see **Sachs, David H.**

Danis, Jodi. Sexism and "the superfluous female":

arguments for regulating pre–implantation sex selection. *Harvard Women's Law Journal.* 1995 Spring; 18: 219–264.
(SEX PRESELECTION)

Danis, Marion. Improving end–of–life care in the intensive care unit: what's to be learned from outcomes research? *New Horizons.* 1998 Feb; 6(1): 110–118.
(TERMINAL CARE)

Danis, Marion see **Hanson, Laura C.**

Danoff, Deborah see **Swick, Herbert M.**

Darragh, Martina. BIOETHICSLINE on ·the World Wide Web. [News]. *Kennedy Institute of Ethics Journal.* 1998 Dec; 8(4): 467–468.
(BIOETHICS)

Darragh, Martina; McCarrick, Pat Milmoe. Public health ethics: health by the numbers. [Bibliography]. *Kennedy Institute of Ethics Journal.* 1998 Sep; 8(3): 339–358.
(PUBLIC HEALTH)

Darragh, Martina see **Bishop, Laura Jane**

Das, Robert see **Torrance, Caroline J.**

Daskal, Frona see **Casarett, David J.**

Date, Jan see **Jones, Steve**

DauBach, Penelope P. Homegrown Eugenics: Socioeconomic Differentials in Utilization of Prenatal Testing. Ann Arbor, MI: University Microfilms International; 1997. 299 p.
(EUGENICS; PRENATAL DIAGNOSIS)

Daube, Jasper R. Searching for cures: the necessity of animal research. [Editorial]. *Minnesota Medicine.* 1997 Sep; 80(9): 27–29.
(ANIMAL EXPERIMENTATION)

David, Edward E. Non–starters and no brainers: an outside perspective. *Accountability in Research.* 1997; 5(4): 255–263.
(BIOMEDICAL RESEARCH; FRAUD AND MISCONDUCT)

Davidoff, Frank. Publication and promotion: intelligence work. *Lancet.* 1998 Sep 12; 352(9131): 895–896.
(BIOMEDICAL RESEARCH)

Davidoff, Frank. Weighing the alternatives: lessons from the paradoxes of alternative medicine. [Editorial]. *Annals of Internal Medicine.* 1998 Dec 15; 129(12): 1068–1070.
(PATIENT CARE)

Davidoff, Frank; Reinecke, Robert D. The 28th Amendment. [Editorial]. *Annals of Internal Medicine.* 1999 Apr 20; 130(8): 692–694.
(HEALTH CARE/RIGHTS)

Davidson, Sylvia. New European clinical trial regulations are "unacceptable" to industry. [News]. *Nature Biotechnology.* 1998 Feb; 16(2): 127.
(HUMAN EXPERIMENTATION/FOREIGN COUNTRIES; HUMAN EXPERIMENTATION/REGULATION)

Davies, Darcy B. see **Lin, Hung–Mo**

Davies, Huw T.O.; Rennie, Drummond. Independence,

governance, and trust: redefining the relationship between JAMA and the AMA. [Editorial]. *JAMA*. 1999 Jun 23–30; 281(24): 2344–2346.
(BIOMEDICAL RESEARCH)

Davis, Anne J. Global influence of American nursing: some ethical issues. *Nursing Ethics*. 1999 Mar; 6(2): 118–125.
(NURSING ETHICS)

Davis, Dena S. Medical research with college athletes: some ethical issues. *IRB: A Review of Human Subjects Research*. 1998 Jul–Aug; 20(4): 10–11.
(HUMAN EXPERIMENTATION/SPECIAL POPULATIONS)

Davis, Dena S.; Forster, Heidi P. Legal trends in bioethics. *Journal of Clinical Ethics*. 1998 Fall; 9(3): 323–332.
(BIOETHICS)

Davis, Kathy. The rhetoric of cosmetic surgery: luxury or welfare? *In:* Parens, Erik, ed. Enhancing Human Traits: Ethical and Social Implications. Washington, DC: Georgetown University Press; 1998: 124–134.
(HEALTH CARE/FOREIGN COUNTRIES; RESOURCE ALLOCATION/BIOMEDICAL TECHNOLOGIES)

Davis, Roger B. see **Covinsky, Kenneth E.**

Davis, Roger B. see **Hamel, Mary Beth**

Davis, Virginia Marriage see **Sher, Geoffrey**

Davison, Alex M. Commercialization in organ donation. [Editorial]. *Nephrology, Dialysis, Transplantation*. 1994; 9(4): 348–349.
(ORGAN AND TISSUE DONATION; ORGAN AND TISSUE TRANSPLANTATION)

Davy, A. see **Hassan, T.B.**

Dawkins, Richard. Thinking clearly about clones: how dogma and ignorance get in the way. *Free Inquiry*. 1997 Summer; 17(3): 13–14.
(CLONING)

Day, Michael. How the West gets well. *New Scientist*. 1997 May 17; 154(2082): 14–15.
(HUMAN EXPERIMENTATION/FOREIGN COUNTRIES)

Day, Michael. This won't hurt ... have we fully investigated the risks associated with immunisation. [News]. *New Scientist*. 1998 Mar 7; 157(2124): 4.
(IMMUNIZATION)

Dayer, P. see **Müller, H.J.**

Dea, Robin see **Rosenheck, Robert**

Deaner, Andrew see **Barakat, Khalid**

DeBakey, Lois see **Greenfield, Barak**

DeBakey, Selma see **Greenfield, Barak**

de Beaufort, Inez. Individual responsibility for health. *In:* Bennett, Rebecca; Erin, Charles A., eds. HIV and AIDS: Testing, Screening, and Confidentiality. New York, NY: Oxford University Press; 1999: 107–124.
(HEALTH; RESOURCE ALLOCATION)

de Beaufort, Inez. Letter from a post–menopausal mother. *In:* Harris, John; Holm, Søren, eds. The Future of Human Reproduction: Ethics, Choice, Regulation. New York, NY: Oxford University Press; 1998: 238–247.
(REPRODUCTIVE TECHNOLOGIES; SELECTION FOR TREATMENT)

DeBernardo, Caren R. see **Murphy, Michael J.**

Debono, M. see **Lui, S.C.**

de Bousingen, Denis Durand. Euthanasia and pain relief discussed in Europe. [News]. *Lancet*. 1998 Oct 3; 352(9134): 1129.
(EUTHANASIA; TERMINAL CARE)

de Castro, Leonardo D. Ethical issues in human experimentation. *In:* Kuhse, Helga; Singer, Peter, eds. A Companion to Bioethics. Malden, MA: Blackwell; 1998: 379–389.
(HUMAN EXPERIMENTATION)

de Castro, Leonardo D. Is there an Asian bioethics? *Bioethics*. 1999 Jul; 13(3–4): 227–235.
(BIOETHICS)

de Castro, Leonardo D.; Sy, Peter A. Critical care in the Philippines: the "Robin Hood principle" vs. *kagandahang loob*. *Journal of Medicine and Philosophy*. 1998 Dec; 23(6): 563–580.
(HEALTH CARE/FOREIGN COUNTRIES; RESOURCE ALLOCATION)

DeCew, Judith Wagner. In Pursuit of Privacy: Law, Ethics, and the Rise of Technology. Ithaca, NY: Cornell University Press; 1997. 199 p.
(CONFIDENTIALITY/LEGAL ASPECTS)

DeCiantis, Mary Lou see **Hall, Judith A.**

de Cock Buning, Tjard. Training members of ethics committees. *In:* van Zutphen, L.F.M.; Balls, M., eds. Animal Alternatives, Welfare and Ethics. New York, NY: Elsevier; 1997: 379–383.
(ANIMAL EXPERIMENTATION)

de Cock Buning, Tjard see **Mepham, T. Ben**

Decruyenaere, Marleen; Evers-Kiebooms, Gerry; Boogaerts, Andrea; Cloostermans, Trees; Cassiman, Jean-Jacques; Demyttenaere, Koen; Dom, René; Fryns, Jean-Pierre; Van den Berghe, Herman. Non-participation in predictive testing for Huntington's disease: individual decision-making, personality and avoidant behaviour in the family. *European Journal of Human Genetics*. 1997 Nov–Dec; 5(6): 351–363.
(GENETIC SCREENING)

Decruyenaere, Marleen see **Welkenhuysen, Myriam**

Decter, Sheila R. see **Roberts, John**

Deech, Ruth. Legal and ethical responsibilities of gamete banks. [Article and discussion]. *Human Reproduction*. 1998 May; 13(Suppl. 2): 80–89.
(ORGAN AND TISSUE DONATION; REPRODUCTIVE TECHNOLOGIES)

Deftos, L.J. Genomic torts: the law of the future -- the duty of physicians to disclose the presence of a genetic disease to the relatives of their patients with the disease.

University of San Francisco Law Review. 1997 Fall; 32(1): 105–137.
(GENETIC COUNSELING)

DeGrazia, David. Biology, consciousness, and the definition of death. *Philosophy and Public Policy.* 1998 Winter–Spring; 18(1–2): 18–22.
(DETERMINATION OF DEATH/BRAIN DEATH)

DeGrazia, David. The ethics of animal research: what are the prospects for agreement? *Cambridge Quarterly of Healthcare Ethics.* 1999 Winter; 8(1): 23–34.
(ANIMAL EXPERIMENTATION)

de Haes, Johanna C.J.M. see **Varekamp, Inge**

de Jong, Judith; Reatig, Natalie. SAMHSA philosophy and statement on ethical principles. *Ethics and Behavior.* 1998; 8(4): 339–343.
(MENTAL HEALTH; PROFESSIONAL ETHICS; PUBLIC HEALTH)

De Jonge, Christopher J.; Wolf, Don P. Embryo number for transfer should be regulated. [Editorial]. *Fertility and Sterility.* 1997 Nov; 68(5): 784–786.
(REPRODUCTIVE TECHNOLOGIES)

Dekkers, Wim J.M.; ten Have, Henk A.M.J. Biomedical research with human body "parts". *In:* ten Have, Henk A.M.J.; Welie, Jos V.M., eds. Ownership of the Human Body: Philosophical Considerations on the Use of the Human Body and Its Parts in Health Care. Boston, MA: Kluwer Academic; 1998: 49–63.
(BIOMEDICAL RESEARCH; ORGAN AND TISSUE DONATION)

de Klerk, Anton. The right of patients to have access to their medical records: the position in South African law. *Medicine and Law.* 1993; 12(1–2): 77–83.
(PATIENT ACCESS TO RECORDS)

Delahunty, C. see **Fowlie, P.W.**

Delbanco, Thomas L. see **Covinsky, Kenneth E.**

De Leo, Diego; Marietta, Paola. Suicide: determinism or freedom? *Dolentium Hominum: Church and Health in the World.* 1997; 34(12th Yr., No. 1): 148–154.
(SUICIDE)

DeLeon, Patrick H.; Bennett, Bruce E.; Bricklin, Patricia M. Ethics and public policy formulation: a case example related to prescription privileges. *Professional Psychology: Research and Practice.* 1997 Dec; 28(6): 518–525.
(PATIENT CARE/DRUGS; PROFESSIONAL ETHICS)

Delpire, Véronique C. see **Mepham, T. Ben**

del Rio, Carlos. Is ethical research feasible in developed and developing countries? *Bioethics.* 1998 Oct; 12(4): 328–330.
(AIDS/HUMAN EXPERIMENTATION; HUMAN EXPERIMENTATION/FOREIGN COUNTRIES; HUMAN EXPERIMENTATION/RESEARCH DESIGN)

Del Rio, Carlos see **Schüklenk, Udo**

del Rio, Carlos see **Wilfert, Catherine M.**

Delury, George E. But What If She Wants to Die? A Husband's Diary. New York, NY: Carol Publishing Group; 1997. 224 p.
(SUICIDE)

Del Vecchio, Paolo see **Rosenheck, Robert**

De Man, Xavier see **Nagy, Anne–Marie**

Demmer, K. Ethical aspects of reproductive medicine. *In:* Nieschlag, E.; Behre, H.M., eds. Andrology: Male Reproductive Health and Dysfunction. Berlin: Springer–Verlag; 1997: 409–417.
(REPRODUCTIVE TECHNOLOGIES)

Demy, Timothy J.; Stewart, Gary P., eds. Genetic Engineering: A Christian Response: Crucial Considerations in Shaping Life. Grand Rapids, MI: Kregel Publications; 1999. 320 p.
(GENETIC INTERVENTION)

Demy, Timothy J.; Stewart, Gary P. Suicide: A Christian Response: Crucial Considerations for Choosing Life. Grand Rapids, MI: Kregel Publications; 1998. 490 p.
(EUTHANASIA/RELIGIOUS ASPECTS; SUICIDE)

Demy, Timothy J. see **Stewart, Gary P.**

Demyttenaere, Koen see **Decruyenaere, Marleen**

den Hartogh, Govert. The slippery slope argument. *In:* Kuhse, Helga; Singer, Peter, eds. A Companion to Bioethics. Malden, MA: Blackwell; 1998: 280–290.
(BIOETHICS)

Denekens, Joke P.M.; Nys, Herman; Stuer, Hugo. Sterilisation of incompetent mentally handicapped persons: a model for decision making. *Journal of Medical Ethics.* 1999 Jun; 25(3): 237–241.
(STERILIZATION/MENTALLY DISABLED)

Denley, Ian; Smith, Simon Weston; Gardner, Martin; O'Conor, Rory. Privacy in clinical information systems in secondary care. [Article and commentaries]. *BMJ (British Medical Journal).* 1999 May 15; 318(7194): 1328–1331.
(CONFIDENTIALITY)

Dennison, David K. see **Levine, Robert J.**

Deonna, Th. see **Müller, H.J.**

DePaulo, J. Raymond see **Trippitelli, Carol Lynn**

de Pomerai, David. Dolly mixtures: retrospect and prospects for animal and human cloning. *Human Reproduction and Genetic Ethics: An International Journal.* 1998; 4(2): 39–48.
(CLONING)

de Pomerai, David I. Are there limits to animal transgenesis? *European Journal of Genetics in Society.* 1997; 3(1): 4–12.
(GENETIC INTERVENTION)

de Raeve, Louise. Maintaining integrity through clinical supervision. *Nursing Ethics.* 1998 Nov; 5(6): 486–496.
(NURSING ETHICS)

Derbyshire, Stuart W.G. Locating the beginnings of pain. *Bioethics.* 1999 Jan; 13(1): 1–31.

(FETUSES)

DeRenzo, Evan G. A bioethicist's perspective. *In:* Hoagwood, Kimberly; Jensen, Peter S.; Fisher, Celia B., eds. Ethical Issues in Mental Health Research with Children and Adolescents. Mahwah, NJ: Lawrence Erlbaum Associates; 1996: 269–286.
(HUMAN EXPERIMENTATION/MINORS; HUMAN EXPERIMENTATION/SPECIAL POPULATIONS)

DeRenzo, Evan G. Ethical considerations in dysphagia treatment and research: secular and sacred. *In:* Sonies, Barbara C., ed. Dysphagia: A Continuum of Care. Gaithersburg, MD: Aspen Publishing; 1997: 91–106.
(PATIENT CARE)

DeRenzo, Evan G.; Biesecker, Leslie G.; Meltzer, Noah. Genetics and the dead: implications for genetics research with samples from deceased persons. *American Journal of Medical Genetics.* 1997 Mar 31; 69(3): 332–334.
(GENETIC RESEARCH; HUMAN EXPERIMENTATION/ETHICS COMMITTEES)

DeRenzo, Evan G. see **Miller, Franklin G.**

Derickson, Alan. Black Lung: Anatomy of a Public Health Disaster. Ithaca, NY: Cornell University Press; 1998. 237 p.
(OCCUPATIONAL HEALTH)

Derse, Arthur R. Making decisions about life–sustaining medical treatment in patients with dementia: the problem of patient decision–making capacity. *Theoretical Medicine and Bioethics.* 1999 Jan; 20(1): 55–67.
(ALLOWING TO DIE; INFORMED CONSENT/MENTALLY DISABLED; PATIENT CARE/AGED; TREATMENT REFUSAL/MENTALLY DISABLED)

Derse, Arthur R. see **Larkin, Gregory Luke**

Des Jarlais, Don C.; Vanischseni, Suphak; Marmor, Michael; Kitayaporn, Dwip; Kalebic, Thea; Mbidde, Edward K. HIV vaccine trials. [Letters and response]. *Science.* 1998 Mar 6; 279(5356): 1433–1436.
(AIDS/HUMAN EXPERIMENTATION; HUMAN EXPERIMENTATION/FOREIGN COUNTRIES)

Des Marchais, Jacques E. see **Beaudoin, Claude**

DeSantis, Joe; Engberg, Sandra; Rogers, Joan. Geropsychiatric restraint use. *Journal of the American Geriatrics Society.* 1997 Dec; 45(12): 1515–1518.
(BEHAVIOR CONTROL; PATIENT CARE/AGED)

DesAutels, Peggy. Religious women, medical settings, and moral risk. *In:* Walker, Margaret Urban, ed. Mother Time: Women, Aging, and Ethics. Lanham, MD: Rowman and Littlefield; 1999: 175–187.
(BIOETHICS; PROFESSIONAL PATIENT RELATIONSHIP)

Desbiens, Norman see **Hamel, Mary Beth**

Deschoolmeester, G. see **Roels, L.**

Desenclos, Jean–Claude see **Lot, Florence**

Desnick, Robert J. see **McGovern, Margaret M.**

Desvarieux, Moïse; Turner, Marie T.; Whalen, Christopher C.; Johnson, John L.; Mugerwa, Roy D.; Ellner, Jerrold J.; Msamanga, Gernard; Angell, **Marcia.** Questions about a placebo–controlled trial of preventive therapy for tuberculosis in HIV–infected Ugandans. [Letters and responses]. *New England Journal of Medicine.* 1998 Mar 19; 338(12): 841–843.
(AIDS/HUMAN EXPERIMENTATION; HUMAN EXPERIMENTATION/FOREIGN COUNTRIES; HUMAN EXPERIMENTATION/RESEARCH DESIGN)

De Tavernier, Johan. Biotechnology policy and ethics. *In:* Sterckx, Sigrid, ed. Biotechnology, Patents and Morality. Proceedings of an International Workshop, "Biotechnology, Patents and Morality: Towards a Consensus," held in Ghent, Belgium, 17–19 Jan 1996. Brookfield, VT: Ashgate; 1997: 114–120.
(GENETIC INTERVENTION)

Deutsch, Lisa B. Medicaid payment for organ transplants: the extent of mandated coverage. *Columbia Journal of Law and Social Problems.* 1997 Winter; 30(2): 185–213.
(HEALTH CARE/ECONOMICS; ORGAN AND TISSUE TRANSPLANTATION)

De Ville, Kenneth. Act first and look up the law afterward?: medical malpractice and the ethics of defensive medicine. *Theoretical Medicine and Bioethics.* 1998 Dec; 19(6): 569–589.
(PATIENT CARE)

De Ville, Kenneth A.; Kopelman, Loretta M. Moral and social issues regarding pregnant women who use and abuse drugs. *Obstetrics and Gynecology Clinics of North America.* 1998 Mar; 25(1): 237–254.
(PRENATAL INJURIES)

DeVita, Michael see **Kuczewski, Mark G.**

Devlin, Maureen M. Compassion in Dying v. State of Washington. [Note]. *Issues in Law and Medicine.* 1996 Summer; 12(1): 59–63.
(SUICIDE)

Devlin, Maureen M. Quill v. Vacco. [Note]. *Issues in Law and Medicine.* 1996 Summer; 12(1): 65–67.
(SUICIDE)

DeVore, Nancy see **Freda, Margaret Comerford**

Devroey, P. see **Baetens, P.**

de Wachter, Maurice A.M. Sociology and bioethics in the U.S.A. [Book review essay]. *Hastings Center Report.* 1998 Sep–Oct; 28(5): 40–42.
(BIOETHICS)

DeWalt, Darren A. see **Pincus, Theodore**

de Wert, Guido M.W.R. The post–menopause: playground for reproductive technology? Some ethical reflections. *In:* Harris, John; Holm, Søren, eds. The Future of Human Reproduction: Ethics, Choice, and Regulation. New York, NY: Oxford University Press; 1998: 221–237.
(REPRODUCTIVE TECHNOLOGIES; SELECTION FOR TREATMENT)

Dewhurst, David see **van der Valk, Jan**

Dewsbury, Donald A. Is the fox guarding the henhouse? A historical study of the dual role of the Committee on Animal Research and Ethics. *In:* Hart, Lynette A., ed. Responsible Conduct with Animals in Research. New York, NY: Oxford University Press; 1998: 18–29.

(ANIMAL EXPERIMENTATION)

de Zoysa, Isabelle; Elias, Christopher J.; Bentley, Margaret E. Ethical challenges in efficacy trials of vaginal microbicides for HIV prevention. *American Journal of Public Health.* 1998 Apr; 88(4): 571–575.
(AIDS/HUMAN EXPERIMENTATION; HUMAN EXPERIMENTATION/RESEARCH DESIGN; HUMAN EXPERIMENTATION/SPECIAL POPULATIONS)

de Zulueta, Paquita see **Gbolade, Babatunde A.**

Dhavamoni, Mariasusai. Health, illness, and healing in the great religions: II. Hinduism. *Dolentium Hominum: Church and Health in the World.* 1998; No. 37 [yr. 13(1)]: 112–115.
(HEALTH)

Diamond, Milton see **Kipnis, Kenneth**

Dicke, Arnold A. see **Pokorski, Robert J.**

Dickens, Bernard M. Can doctors serve as double agents? [Editorial]. *Humane Health Care International.* 1997 Spring; 13(1): 8–9.
(RESOURCE ALLOCATION)

Dickens, Bernard M. see **Cook, Rebecca J.**

Dickens, Bernard M. see **Weijer, Charles**

Dickenson, Donna see **Pattison, Stephen**

Dickenson, Donna L. Cross-cultural issues in European bioethics. *Bioethics.* 1999 Jul; 13(3–4): 249–255.
(BIOETHICS)

Dickenson, Donna L.; Geller, Gail. Can children and young people consent to be tested for adult onset genetic disorders? [and] Weighing burdens and benefits rather than competence. [Article and commentary]. *BMJ (British Medical Journal).* 1999 Apr 17; 318(7190): 1063–1066.
(GENETIC SCREENING; INFORMED CONSENT/MINORS)

Dickenson, Donna L.; Nicholson, Richard. Children's rights. [Letter and response]. *Hastings Center Report.* 1999 Jan–Feb; 29(1): 5.
(INFORMED CONSENT/MINORS; TREATMENT REFUSAL/MINORS)

Dickerson, Denise Ann. A doctor's duty to disclose life expectancy information to terminally ill patients. [Note]. *Cleveland State Law Review.* 1995; 43(2): 319–350.
(TRUTH DISCLOSURE)

Dickert, Neal; Grady, Christine. What's the price of a research subject? Approaches to payment for research participation. *New England Journal of Medicine.* 1999 Jul 15; 341(3): 198–203.
(HUMAN EXPERIMENTATION)

Dickie, Gordon L. see **McSherry, James**

Dickinson, George E.; Lancaster, Carol J.; Sumner, Edward D.; Cohen, Jonathan S. Attitudes toward assisted suicide and euthanasia among physicians in South Carolina and Washington. *Omega: A Journal of Death and Dying.* 1997–1998; 36(3): 201–218.
(EUTHANASIA/ATTITUDES; SUICIDE)

Dickinson, George E.; Mermann, Alan C. Death education in U.S. medical schools, 1975–1995. *Academic Medicine.* 1996 Dec; 71(12): 1348–1349.
(TERMINAL CARE)

Dickson, David. Back on track: the rebirth of human genetics in China. [News]. *Nature.* 1998 Nov 26; 396(6709): 303–306.
(GENETIC RESEARCH; GENOME MAPPING)

Dickson, David. British MRC reprimanded over clinical test record. [News]. *Nature Medicine.* 1998 Jul; 4(7): 752.
(HUMAN EXPERIMENTATION/FOREIGN COUNTRIES; HUMAN EXPERIMENTATION/INFORMED CONSENT)

Dickson, David. China brings in regulations to put a stop to 'genetic piracy'. [News]. *Nature.* 1998 Sep 3; 395(6697): 5.
(GENETIC RESEARCH)

Dickson, David. Congress grabs eugenics common ground. [News]. *Nature.* 1998 Aug 20; 394(6695): 711.
(EUGENICS)

Dickson, David. Panel urges caution on genetic testing for mental disorders. [News]. *Nature.* 1998 Sep 24; 395(6700): 309.
(GENETIC SCREENING)

Dickson, David. Proceed with caution, says UK report on ethics of GM foods. [News]. *Nature.* 1999 Jun 3; 399(6735): 396.
(GENETIC INTERVENTION)

Dickson, David. Survey: some countries side with China on genetic issues. [News]. *Nature Medicine.* 1998 Oct; 4(10): 1096.
(EUGENICS)

Dickson, David. Wellcome Trust funds new "Medicine in Society" program. [News]. *Nature Medicine.* 1998 May; 4(5): 542.
(BIOETHICS)

Diekema, Douglas S. Children first: the need to reform financing of health care services for children. [Editorial]. *Journal of Health Care for the Poor and Underserved.* 1996; 7(1): 3–14.
(HEALTH CARE/ECONOMICS; PATIENT CARE/MINORS)

Dierckx de Casterle, Bernadette see **Gastmans, Chris**

Dietz, Sarah M.; Brakman, Sarah-Vaughan; Dresser, Rebecca; Astrow, Alan B. The incompetent self: metamorphosis of a person? [Letters and responses]. *Hastings Center Report.* 1998 Sep–Oct; 28(5): 4–5.
(ADVANCE DIRECTIVES; ALLOWING TO DIE)

Dijon, Xavier. Abortion and genetic manipulation: breaking with reasoning founded on disrespect for life and human dignity. *Medicine and Law.* 1993; 12(1–2): 85–92.
(ABORTION; EMBRYO AND FETAL RESEARCH)

Dikötter, Frank. Imperfect Conceptions: Medical Knowledge, Birth Defects and Eugenics in China. New York, NY: Columbia University Press; 1998. 226 p.
(EUGENICS; REPRODUCTION)

Dimand, R.J. see **Weiss, A.H.**

DiMatteo, M. Robin see Maly, Rose C.

Diniz, Debora; Guilhem, Dirce Bellezi; Garrafa, Volnei. Biothics in Brazil. *Bioethics.* 1999 Jul; 13(3–4): 244–248.
(BIOETHICS)

Dinwiddie, Stephen H.; Yutzy, Sean H. Ethical issues in psychiatric practice. *In:* Guze, Samuel B., ed. Adult Pyschiatry. (Mosby's neurology psychiatry access series). St. Louis, MO: Mosby-Year Book; 1996: 445–453.
(MEDICAL ETHICS; PATIENT CARE/MENTALLY DISABLED)

Dixon, Nicholas. On the difference between physician–assisted suicide and active euthanasia. *Hastings Center Report.* 1998 Sep–Oct; 28(5): 25–29.
(EUTHANASIA; SUICIDE)

Dixon, Nicholas. The morality of anti–abortion civil disobedience. *Public Affairs Quarterly.* 1997 Jan; 11(1): 21–38.
(ABORTION/LEGAL ASPECTS)

Djerassi, Carl. Sex in an age of mechanical reproduction. *Science.* 1999 Jul 2; 285(5424): 53–54.
(REPRODUCTIVE TECHNOLOGIES)

Djerassi, Carl. Who will mentor the mentors? *Nature.* 1999 Jan 28; 397(6717): 291.
(BIOMEDICAL RESEARCH; FRAUD AND MISCONDUCT)

Dodson, Michael; Williamson, Robert. Indigenous peoples and the morality of the Human Genome Diversity Project. *Journal of Medical Ethics.* 1999 Apr; 25(2): 204–208.
(GENETIC RESEARCH; GENOME MAPPING)

Doerfler, John F. Is GIFT compatible with the teaching of *Donum Vitae*? *Linacre Quarterly.* 1997 Feb; 64(1): 16–29.
(REPRODUCTIVE TECHNOLOGIES)

Doerflinger, Richard M. An uncertain future for assisted suicide. [News]. *Hastings Center Report.* 1999 Jan–Feb; 29(1): 52.
(SUICIDE)

Doerflinger, Richard M. The ethics of funding embryonic stem cell research: a Catholic viewpoint. *Kennedy Institute of Ethics Journal.* 1999 Jun; 9(2): 137–150.
(EMBRYO AND FETAL RESEARCH)

Doksum, T. see James, C.A.

Dolian, Gayane; Lüdicke, Frank; Katchatrian, Naira; Morabia, Alfredo. Contraception and induced abortion in Armenia: a critical need for family planning programs in Eastern Europe. *American Journal of Public Health.* 1998 May; 88(5): 803–805.
(ABORTION/FOREIGN COUNTRIES; CONTRACEPTION)

Dom, René see Decruyenaere, Marleen

Donaldson, J. see Vassilas, C.A.

Donaldson, Liam see Bhopal, Raj

Donchin, Anne. Shaping reproductive technology policy: the search for consensus. *In:* ten Have, Henk A.M.J.; Sass, Hans-Martin, eds. Consensus Formation in Healthcare Ethics. Boston, MA: Kluwer Academic; 1998: 229–250.
(REPRODUCTIVE TECHNOLOGIES)

Donchin, Anne; Purdy, Laura M., eds. Embodying Bioethics: Recent Feminist Advances. Lanham, MD: Rowman and Littlefield; 1999. 286 p.
(BIOETHICS)

Dondero, Timothy J. see Merson, Michael H.

Donnellan, Craig, ed. Animal experiments. *In:* Donnellan, Craig, ed. Do Animals Have Rights? Cambridge, England: Independence Educational Publishers; 1995: 1–21.
(ANIMAL EXPERIMENTATION)

Donovan, Jenny L. see Featherstone, Katie

Donovan, Patricia. Hospital mergers and reproductive health care. *Family Planning Perspectives.* 1996 Nov–Dec; 28(6): 281–284.
(ABORTION/RELIGIOUS ASPECTS; CONTRACEPTION; HEALTH CARE)

Dooha, Susan M. see Halkitis, Perry N.

Dorff, Elliot N. Matters of Life and Death: A Jewish Approach to Modern Medical Ethics. Philadelphia, PA: Jewish Publication Society; 1998. 456 p.
(BIOETHICS)

Dorff, Elliot N. The Jewish Tradition: Religious Beliefs and Health Care Decisions. [Booklet]. Chicago, IL: Park Ridge Center for the Study of Health, Faith, and Ethics; 1996. 23 p.
(BIOETHICS)

Dorozynski, Alexander see Beecham, Linda

Dósa, Agnes. Bioethics and health law in Hungary. *Saint Louis University Public Law Review.* 1996; 15(2): 403–409.
(BIOETHICS; HEALTH CARE/FOREIGN COUNTRIES)

Dossetor, John see Caulfield, Timothy

Dossetor, John B. Economic, social, racial and age–related considerations in dialysis and transplantation. *Current Opinion in Nephrology and Hypertension.* 1995 Nov; 4(6): 498–501.
(ORGAN AND TISSUE TRANSPLANTATION; RESOURCE ALLOCATION/BIOMEDICAL TECHNOLOGIES)

Douglas, Gillian. Re C (Refusal of Medical Treatment). [Comment]. *Family Law.* 1994 Mar; 24: 131–132.
(ADVANCE DIRECTIVES; TREATMENT REFUSAL/MENTALLY DISABLED)

Doukas, David J.; Gorenflo, Daniel W.; Supanich, Barbara. Primary care physician attitudes and values toward end–of–life care and physician–assisted death. *Ethics and Behavior.* 1999; 9(3): 219–230.
(ALLOWING TO DIE/ATTITUDES; EUTHANASIA/ATTITUDES; SUICIDE)

Doukas, David J. see Nease, Donald E.

Doumanian, Nancy P. see Panossian, André A.

Dove, Alan. Genetics research on the town hall agenda, courtesy of ELSI. [News]. *Nature Medicine.* 1998 May;

4(5): 541.
(GENETIC RESEARCH)

Dove, Alan. No-consent trials raise concern. [News]. *Nature Medicine.* 1999 Mar; 5(3): 250–251.
(HUMAN EXPERIMENTATION/INFORMED CONSENT)

Dowell, Richard C. see **Clark, Graeme M.**

Downie, Jocelyn; Sherwin, Susan. A feminist exploration of issues around assisted death. *Saint Louis University Public Law Review.* 1996; 15(2): 303–330.
(EUTHANASIA; SUICIDE)

Downie, Jocelyn see **Baylis, Françoise**

Downs, Murna. The emergence of the person in dementia research. *Ageing and Society.* 1997 Sep; 17(5): 597–607.
(BEHAVIORAL RESEARCH/SPECIAL POPULATIONS; PATIENT CARE/MENTALLY DISABLED)

Doxiadis, Spyros A. Why medical ethics? *Pediatrician.* 1990; 17(2): 56–58.
(MEDICAL ETHICS)

Doyal, L. see **Galton, D.J.**

Doyal, Len. Human need and the right of patients to privacy. *Journal of Contemporary Health Law and Policy.* 1997 Fall; 14(1): 1–21.
(CONFIDENTIALITY)

Doyal, Len. Moral quality entails a high standard of informed consent. [Editorial]. *Quality in Health Care.* 1998 Jun; 7(2): 63–64.
(INFORMED CONSENT)

Doyal, Len. Public participation and the moral quality of healthcare rationing. *Quality in Health Care.* 1998 Jun; 7(2): 98–102.
(HEALTH CARE/FOREIGN COUNTRIES; RESOURCE ALLOCATION)

Doyle, John P. Reflections on persons in petri dishes. *Linacre Quarterly.* 1997 Nov; 64(4): 62–76.
(FETUSES; PERSONHOOD)

Doyle, Kathy; Carroll, Alex. The slippery slope [comparison of treatment withdrawal in English and Irish law]. *New Law Journal.* 1996 May 24; 146(6745): 759–761.
(ALLOWING TO DIE/LEGAL ASPECTS)

Drane, James F. Decisionmaking and consensus formation in clinical ethics. *In:* ten Have, Henk A.M.J.; Sass, Hans-Martin, eds. Consensus Formation in Healthcare Ethics. Boston, MA: Kluwer Academic; 1998: 143–157.
(BIOETHICS; MEDICAL ETHICS)

Draper, Heather; Chadwick, Ruth. Beware! Preimplantation genetic diagnosis may solve some old problems but it also raises new ones. *Journal of Medical Ethics.* 1999 Apr; 25(2): 114–120.
(GENETIC SCREENING; PRENATAL DIAGNOSIS; REPRODUCTION; REPRODUCTIVE TECHNOLOGIES)

Draper, Heather see **Sorell, Tom**

Dreger, Alice Domurat. A history of intersexuality: from the age of gonads to the age of consent. *Journal of Clinical Ethics.* 1998 Winter; 9(4): 345–355.

(PATIENT CARE/MINORS)

Dreger, Alice Domurat. Hemaphrodites and the Medical Invention of Sex. Cambridge, MA: Harvard University Press; 1998. 268 p.
(PATIENT CARE)

Dresser, Rebecca. Science in the courtroom: a new approach. *Hastings Center Report.* 1999 May–Jun; 29(3): 26–27.
(BIOMEDICAL TECHNOLOGIES)

Dresser, Rebecca. Time for new rules on human subjects research? *Hastings Center Report.* 1998 Nov–Dec; 28(6): 23–24.
(HUMAN EXPERIMENTATION/ETHICS COMMITTEES; HUMAN EXPERIMENTATION/REGULATION)

Dresser, Rebecca see **Dietz, Sarah M.**

Dresser, Rebecca see **Preston, Thomas A.**

Drew, Christopher. U.S. says 2 Chinese offered organs from the executed. [News]. *New York Times.* 1998 Feb 24: A1, B5.
(ORGAN AND TISSUE DONATION)

Drexler, Edward see **Cutter, Mary Ann G.**

Dronamraju, Krishna R. Biological and Social Issues in Biotechnology Sharing. Brookfield, VT: Ashgate; 1998. 165 p.
(GENETIC INTERVENTION; GENETIC RESEARCH)

Drucker, Jacques see **Lot, Florence**

Drukker, Alfred see **Velasco, N.**

Drummey, James J. see **Hayes, Edward J.**

Drutchas, Geoffrey G. Is Life Sacred? Cleveland, OH: Pilgrim Press; 1998. 209 p.
(BIOETHICS)

Druzin, Paul; Shrier, Ian; Yacowar, Mayer; Rossignol, Michel. Discrimination against gay, lesbian and bisexual family physicians by patients. *Canadian Medical Association Journal.* 1998 Mar 10; 158(5): 593–597.
(PROFESSIONAL PATIENT RELATIONSHIP)

Dubé, Ross see **Schulman, Kevin A.**

Dubler, Nancy Neveloff. Current ethical issues in aging: introduction. *Generations (American Society on Aging).* 1994 Winter; 18(4): 5–8.
(BIOETHICS)

Dubler, Nancy Neveloff. The collision of confinement and care: end-of-life care in prisons and jails. *Journal of Law, Medicine and Ethics.* 1998 Summer; 26(2): 149–156.
(TERMINAL CARE)

Dubler, Nancy Neveloff see **Fleischman, Alan R.**

Dubler, Nancy Neveloff see **Post, Linda Farber**

Dubler, Nancy Neveloff see **Zelenik, Jomarie**

DuBois, James M. Recent attacks on brain death: do they merit a reconsideration of our current policies? *Health*

Care Ethics USA. 1998 Summer; 6(3): 4–5.
(DETERMINATION OF DEATH/BRAIN DEATH)

DuBose, Edwin R., ed. The Jehovah's Witness Tradition: Religious Beliefs and Health Care Decisions. [Booklet]. Chicago, IL: Park Ridge Center for the Study of Health, Faith, and Ethics; 1995. 10 p.
(BIOETHICS)

DuBose, Edwin R., ed. The Seventh–Day Adventist Tradition: Religious Beliefs and Health Care Decisions. [Booklet]. Chicago, IL: Park Ridge Center for the Study of Health, Faith, and Ethics; 1996. 7 p.
(BIOETHICS)

Dubow, Saul. Scientific Racism in Modern South Africa. New York, NY: Cambridge University Press; 1995. 320 p.
(EUGENICS)

Dudgeon, Deborah see **Chochinov, Harvey Max**

Dudley, R. Adams see **Showstack, Jonathan**

Duffield, Patricia. Advance directives in primary care. *American Journal of Nursing.* 1998 Apr; 98(4): 16CCC–16DDD.
(ADVANCE DIRECTIVES)

Duffy–Durnin, Karen see **Brenner, Zara R.**

Dumble, Lynette see **Callum, Janet**

Duncan, Crawford see **Hosford, Ian**

Duncan, Nigel. World Medical Association opposes Icelandic gene database. [News]. *BMJ (British Medical Journal).* 1999 Apr 24; 318(7191): 1096.
(GENETIC RESEARCH)

Dunn, Debra Geller. Bioethics and nursing. *NursingConnections.* 1994 Fall; 7(3): 43–51.
(NURSING ETHICS)

Dunne, Cara; Warren, Catherine. Lethal autonomy: the malfunction of the informed consent mechanism within the context of prenatal diagnosis of genetic variants. *Issues in Law and Medicine.* 1998 Fall; 14(2): 165–202.
(EUGENICS; GENETIC COUNSELING; INFORMED CONSENT; PRENATAL DIAGNOSIS)

Dunphy, Kilian. Death on request: euthanasia revisited. [Editorial]. *British Journal of Nursing.* 1995 Apr 13–26; 4(7): 365–366.
(EUTHANASIA)

Dunstan, G.R. Pre-embryo research. *Journal of Assisted Reproduction and Genetics.* 1995 Sep; 12(8): 517–523.
(EMBRYO AND FETAL RESEARCH)

Dunstan, G.R. The ethics of organ donation. *British Medical Bulletin.* 1997; 53(4): 921–939.
(ORGAN AND TISSUE DONATION)

Durán, Deborah Guadalupe. Lack of Hispanics' involvement in research –– is it Hispanics or scientists? *Community Genetics.* 1998; 1(3): 183–189.
(BIOMEDICAL RESEARCH; GENETIC RESEARCH)

Durand, Kate T.H. see **Kern, David G.**

Durfy, S.J. see **Ulrich, C.M.**

Durlabhji, Subhash see **Fusilier, Marcelline R.**

Durnan, Richard J.; Lomax, Karen J. Ethics consultation: the need for continuing education and outcome evaluation, not credentialing. [Article and commentary]. *NCCE News (Veterans Health Administration National Center for Clinical Ethics).* 1995 Spring; 3(2): 1–2, 5, 9, 11.
(ETHICISTS AND ETHICS COMMITTEES)

Durst, Rimona see **Bar El, Yair Carlos**

Duster, Troy. Molecular halos and behavioral glows. *In:* Smith, Edward; Sapp, Walter, eds. Plain Talk about the Human Genome Project: A Tuskegee University Conference on Its Promise and Perils ... and Matters of Race. Tuskegee, AL: Tuskegee University Press; 1997: 215–222.
(BEHAVIORAL GENETICS)

Dute, Jos. Affected by the tooth of time: legislation on infectious diseases control in five European countries. *Medicine and Law.* 1993; 12(1–2): 101–108.
(PUBLIC HEALTH)

Dworkin, Gerald; Frey, R.G.; Bok, Sissela. Euthanasia and Physician–Assisted Suicide: For and Against. New York, NY: Cambridge University Press; 1998. 139 p.
(EUTHANASIA; SUICIDE)

Dworkin, Gerald; Kennedy, Ian. Human tissue: rights in the body and its parts. *Medical Law Review.* 1993 Autumn; 1(3): 291–319.
(BIOMEDICAL RESEARCH; ORGAN AND TISSUE DONATION)

Dworkin, Mark; Young, Melissa. Gene Blues: Dilemmas of DNA Testing. [Videorecording]. Oley, PA: Bullfrog Films; 1997. 1 videocassette; 30 min.; sd.; color; VHS.
(GENETIC SCREENING)

Dworkin, Roger B. see **Smith, David H.**

Dwyer, James; Shih, Anthony. The ethics of tailoring the patient's chart. *Psychiatric Services.* 1998 Oct; 49(10): 1309–1312.
(FRAUD AND MISCONDUCT; PATIENT CARE/MENTALLY DISABLED)

Dye, Timothy D. see **Oldenettel, Debra**

Dyer, Clare. British GP cleared of murder charge. [News]. *BMJ (British Medical Journal).* 1999 May 15; 318(7194): 1306.
(EUTHANASIA/LEGAL ASPECTS)

Dyer, Clare. Parents can choose child's treatment. [News]. *BMJ (British Medical Journal).* 1998 Oct 24; 317(7166): 1102.
(TREATMENT REFUSAL/MINORS)

Dyer, Clare. Power of attorney change in England and Wales. [News]. *BMJ (British Medical Journal).* 1999 Jul 24; 319(7204): 211.
(ADVANCE DIRECTIVES)

Dyer, Clare. Sale of prescription data breaches confidentiality. [News]. *BMJ (British Medical Journal).* 1999 Jun 5; 318(7197): 1505.
(CONFIDENTIALITY/LEGAL ASPECTS)

Dyer, Clare. Transsexuals win case for NHS funded surgery. [News]. *BMJ (British Medical Journal).* 1999 Jan 9; 318(7176): 75.
(HEALTH CARE/ECONOMICS; HEALTH CARE/FOREIGN COUNTRIES; HEALTH CARE/RIGHTS)

Dyer, Clare. UK Human Rights Act will allow challenges to treatment refusals. [News]. *BMJ (British Medical Journal).* 1998 Nov 14; 317(7169): 1339.
(HEALTH CARE/FOREIGN COUNTRIES; HEALTH CARE/RIGHTS)

Dyer, Mary Ann see **Daly, Barbara J.**

Dyer, Owen. GP found guilty of forging trial consent forms. [News]. *BMJ (British Medical Journal).* 1998 Nov 28; 317(7171): 1475.
(FRAUD AND MISCONDUCT; HUMAN EXPERIMENTATION/FOREIGN COUNTRIES; HUMAN EXPERIMENTATION/INFORMED CONSENT)

E

Early, Elizabeth K. see **Blake, Robert L.**

Earp, Jo Anne see **Hanson, Laura C.**

Easley, Kirk A. see **Barrow, Chelmer L.**

Easmon, Charles see **Selby, Mary**

Easterbrook, Gregg. Medical evolution: will *Homo sapiens* become obsolete? *New Republic.* 1999 Mar 1; 220(9): 20–25.
(EMBRYO AND FETAL RESEARCH)

Eastman, Nigel. Public health psychiatry or crime prevention? [Editorial]. *BMJ (British Medical Journal).* 1999 Feb 27; 318(7183): 549–551.
(INVOLUNTARY COMMITMENT/FOREIGN COUNTRIES)

Easton, Megan. Infertility treatment: lack of consensus plagues an unregulated field. *Canadian Medical Association Journal.* 1998 May 19; 158(10): 1345–1348.
(REPRODUCTIVE TECHNOLOGIES)

Eaton, Thomas A. see **Larson, Edward J.**

Ebbers, Andrea see **Hall, Mark A.**

Ecder, T. see **Sever, M.S.**

Eckenwiler, Lisa Ann. Women and the Ethics of Clinical Research: Broadening Conceptions of Justice. Ann Arbor, MI: UMI Dissertation Services; 1997. 237 p.
(HUMAN EXPERIMENTATION/SPECIAL POPULATIONS)

Eckholm, Erik. Arrests put focus on human organs from China. [News]. *New York Times.* 1998 Feb 25: B4.
(ORGAN AND TISSUE DONATION)

Eckholm, Erik. Hoping to control spread of AIDS, China bans the sale of blood. [News]. *New York Times.* 1998 Oct 1: A7.
(BLOOD DONATION)

Economides, Demetrios see **McFadyen, Anne**

Eddy, Timothy J. see **Gallup, Gordon G.**

Edi-Osagie, E.C.O.; Edi-Osagie, N.E.; Lurie, Peter;

Wolfe, Sidney M.; Burdon, Justin; Baraza, Richard; Landray, Martin J.; Halsey, Neal A.; Sommer, Alfred; Black, Robert E.; Godfrey-Faussett, Peter; Mwinga, Alwyn; Hosp, Maria; Baggaley, Rachel; Quigley, Maria; Porter, John. Ethics and international research. [Letters and response]. *BMJ (British Medical Journal).* 1998 Feb 21; 316(7131): 625–628.
(AIDS/HUMAN EXPERIMENTATION; HUMAN EXPERIMENTATION/RESEARCH DESIGN; HUMAN EXPERIMENTATION/SPECIAL POPULATIONS)

Edi-Osagie, N.E. see **Edi-Osagie, E.C.O.**

Edwards, Ann see **Butler, Dennis J.**

Edwards, Erick B. see **Lin, Hung-Mo**

Edwards, Sarah J.L.; Braunholtz, David A.; Lilford, Richard J.; Stevens, Andrew J. Ethical issues in the design and conduct of cluster randomised controlled trials. *BMJ (British Medical Journal).* 1999 May 22; 318(7195): 1407–1409.
(HUMAN EXPERIMENTATION/INFORMED CONSENT; HUMAN EXPERIMENTATION/RESEARCH DESIGN)

Edwards, Sarah J.L.; Lilford, R.J.; Hewison, J. The ethics of randomised controlled trials from the perspectives of patients, the public, and healthcare professionals. *BMJ (British Medical Journal).* 1998 Oct 31; 317(7167): 1209–1212.
(HUMAN EXPERIMENTATION/INFORMED CONSENT; HUMAN EXPERIMENTATION/RESEARCH DESIGN)

Efferen, Linda S. In pursuit of tuberculosis control: civil liberty vs public health. [Editorial]. *Chest.* 1997 Jul; 112(1): 5–6.
(PUBLIC HEALTH)

Effros, Richard M. see **Pence, Gregory E.**

Egilman, David; Wallace, Wes; Hom, Candace. Corporate corruption of medical literature: asbestos studies concealed by W.R. Grace & Co. *Accountability in Research.* 1998 Jan; 6(1–2): 127–147.
(BIOMEDICAL RESEARCH; FRAUD AND MISCONDUCT; OCCUPATIONAL HEALTH)

Egilman, David; Wallace, Wes; Stubbs, Cassandra; Mora-Corrasco, Fernando. A little too much of the Buchenwald touch? Military radiation research at the University of Cincinnati, 1960–1972. *Accountability in Research.* 1998 Jan; 6(1–2): 63–102.
(FRAUD AND MISCONDUCT; HUMAN EXPERIMENTATION)

Egilman, David; Wallace, Wes; Stubbs, Cassandra; Mora-Corrasco, Fernando. Ethical aerobics: ACHRE's flight from responsibility. *Accountability in Research.* 1998 Jan; 6(1–2): 15–61.
(FRAUD AND MISCONDUCT; HUMAN EXPERIMENTATION/ETHICS COMMITTEES; HUMAN EXPERIMENTATION/INFORMED CONSENT)

Eguchi, Kenji see **Okamura, Hitoshi**

Eichenwald, Kurt. Monitoring of drug tests is faulted. [News]. *New York Times.* 1998 Jun 12: A14.
(HUMAN EXPERIMENTATION/ETHICS COMMITTEES; HUMAN EXPERIMENTATION/REGULATION)

Eichenwald, Kurt; Kolata, Gina. A doctor's drug studies turn into fraud. [Research for hire: second of two

articles]. *New York Times.* 1999 May 17: A1, A16.
(FRAUD AND MISCONDUCT; HUMAN EXPERIMENTATION)

Eichenwald, Kurt; Kolata, Gina. Drug trials hide conflicts for doctors. [Research for hire: first of two articles]. *New York Times.* 1999 May 16: 1, 34.
(FRAUD AND MISCONDUCT; HUMAN EXPERIMENTATION)

Eichenwald, Kurt see **Kolata, Gina**

Eidelman, Arthur I. see **Hammerman, Cathy**

Eidelman, Leonid A. see **Nyman, Deborah J.**

Eijk, W.J. Ethical models for health management. *Dolentium Hominum: Church and Health in the World.* 1998; No. 37 [yr. 13(1)]: 58–62.
(HEALTH CARE)

Eilers, Robert. Hospitalized psychiatric patients' resistance to routine medical care. *Administration and Policy in Mental Health.* 1994 May; 21(5): 407–415.
(TREATMENT REFUSAL/MENTALLY DISABLED)

Eisemann, Martin; Richter, Jörg. Relationships between various attitudes towards self–determination in health care with special reference to an advance directive. *Journal of Medical Ethics.* 1999 Feb; 25(1): 37–41.
(ADVANCE DIRECTIVES)

Eisenberg, John M. see **Schulman, Kevin A.**

Eisenberg, Leon. Would cloned humans really be like sheep? *New England Journal of Medicine.* 1999 Feb 11; 340(6): 471–475.
(CLONING)

Eisenberg, V.H.; Schenker, J.G. Pre–embryo donation: ethical and legal aspects. *International Journal of Gynaecology and Obstetrics.* 1998 Jan; 60(1): 51–57.
(ORGAN AND TISSUE DONATION; REPRODUCTIVE TECHNOLOGIES)

Eisenberg, V.H.; Schenker, J.G. Pregnancy in the older woman: scientific and ethical aspects. *International Journal of Gynaecology and Obstetrics.* 1997 Feb; 56(2): 163–169.
(REPRODUCTIVE TECHNOLOGIES; SELECTION FOR TREATMENT)

Eisenberg, Vered H.; Schenker, Joseph G. Genetic engineering: moral aspects and control of practice. *Journal of Assisted Reproduction and Genetics.* 1997 Jul; 14(6): 297–316.
(GENE THERAPY; GENETIC INTERVENTION)

Eisenberg, Vered H.; Schenker, Joseph J. The moral aspects of prenatal diagnosis. *European Journal of Obstetrics, Gynecology, and Reproductive Biology.* 1997 Mar; 72(1): 35–45.
(PRENATAL DIAGNOSIS)

Eisenbraun, Ann J. see **Foster, Morris W.**

Eiser, Arnold R.; Seiden, Dena J. Discontinuing dialysis in persistent vegetative state: the roles of autonomy, community, and professional moral agency. *American Journal of Kidney Diseases.* 1997 Aug; 30(2): 291–296.
(ALLOWING TO DIE)

Eisinger, F.; Geller, G.; Burke, W.; Holtzman, N.A. Cultural basis for differences between US and French clinical recommendations for women at increased risk of breast and ovarian cancer. *Lancet.* 1999 Mar 13; 353(9156): 919–920.
(PATIENT CARE)

Eisinger, F. see **Julian–Reyneir, C.**

Eldegez, U. see **Sever, M.S.**

Elewski, Boni E. see **Daniel, C. Ralph**

Elias, Christopher J. see **de Zoysa, Isabelle**

Elizalde, Jose. The patentability of human genes: an ethical debate in the European Community. *Journal of Medicine and Philosophy.* 1998 Jun; 23(3): 318–323.
(PATENTING LIFE FORMS)

Ellenson, David. Artificial fertilization (hafrayyah melakhutit) and procreative autonomy in light of two contemporary Israeli responsa. *In:* Jacob, Walter; Zemer, Moshe, eds. The Fetus and Fertility in Jewish Law: Essays and Responsa. Pittsburgh, PA: Rodef Shalom Press; Freehof Institute of Progressive Halakhah; 1995: 19–38.
(IN VITRO FERTILIZATION; REPRODUCTIVE TECHNOLOGIES)

Elliott, Carl. A Philosophical Disease: Bioethics, Culture and Identity. New York, NY: Routledge; 1999. 188 p.
(BIOETHICS)

Elliott, Carl. Bioethics as commodity: does the exchange of money alter the nature of an ethics consultation? *Bioethics Examiner.* 1997 Fall; 1(3): 1–2.
(ETHICISTS AND ETHICS COMMITTEES)

Elliott, Carl. Patients doubtfully capable or incapable of consent. *In:* Kuhse, Helga; Singer, Peter, eds. A Companion to Bioethics. Malden, MA: Blackwell; 1998: 452–462.
(INFORMED CONSENT)

Elliott, Carl. The tyranny of happiness: ethics and cosmetic psychopharmacology. *In:* Parens, Erik, ed. Enhancing Human Traits: Ethical and Social Implications. Washington, DC: Georgetown University Press; 1998: 177–188.
(BEHAVIOR CONTROL; MENTAL HEALTH; PATIENT CARE/DRUGS)

Elliott, Carl see **Chase, Cheryl**

Elliott, Carl see **Crouch, Robert A.**

Ellner, Jerrold J. see **Desvarieux, Moïse**

Elsaadany, Susie see **King, Susan M.**

Elshtain, Jean Bethke. The hard questions: our bodies, our clones. *New Republic.* 1997 Aug 4; 217(5): 25.
(CLONING)

Elshtain, Jean Bethke. To clone or not to clone. *In:* Nussbaum, Martha C.; Sunstein, Cass R., eds. Clones and Clones: Facts and Fantasies About Human Cloning. New York, NY: Norton; 1998: 181–189.
(CLONING)

Elshtain, Jean Bethke; Cloyd, J. Timothy, eds. Politics

and the Human Body: Assault on Dignity. Nashville, TN: Vanderbilt University Press; 1995. 323 p.
(BIOETHICS)

Elstein, D.; Steinberg, A.; Abrahamov, A.; Zimran, A. Ethical guidelines for enzyme therapy in neuronopathic Gaucher disease. [Abstract]. *American Journal of Human Genetics.* 1997 Oct; 61(4): A354.
(PATIENT CARE/MINORS)

Elster, Nanette see **Andrews, Lori**

Elton, Catherine. Peru's family planning became coerced sterilization. [News]. *Christian Science Monitor.* 1998 Feb 20: 1, 9.
(STERILIZATION)

Emanuel, Ezekiel J. A world of research subjects. [Introduction to a set of articles by R.A. Crouch and J.D. Arras; by C. Grady; by L.H. Glantz, G.J. Annas, M.A. Grodin, and W.K. Mariner; and by C. Levine]. *Hastings Center Report.* 1998 Nov–Dec; 28(6): 25.
(HUMAN EXPERIMENTATION/FOREIGN COUNTRIES)

Emanuel, Ezekiel J. The blossoming of bioethics at NIH. *Kennedy Institute of Ethics Journal.* 1998 Dec; 8(4): 455–466.
(BIOETHICS)

Emanuel, Ezekiel J.; Goldman, Lee. Protecting patient welfare in managed care: six safeguards. *Journal of Health Politics, Policy and Law.* 1998 Aug; 23(4): 635–659.
(HEALTH CARE/ECONOMICS)

Emanuel, Ezekiel J. see **Sage, William M.**

Emanuel, Linda see **Back, Anthony**

Emanuel, Linda see **Greenfield, Barak**

Emanuel, Linda see **Wharton, Robert H.**

Emberton, Mark see **Swinn, Michael**

Emmott, Helen see **Potter, Robert**

Enbom, John A.; Thomas, Claire D. Evaluation of sexual misconduct complaints: the Oregon Board of Medical Examiners, 1991 to 1995. [Article and discussion]. *American Journal of Obstetrics and Gynecology.* 1997 Jun; 176(6): 1340–1348.
(FRAUD AND MISCONDUCT; PROFESSIONAL PATIENT RELATIONSHIP)

Endman, Maxine W. see **Khamsi, Firouz**

Engberg, Sandra see **DeSantis, Joe**

Engelhardt, Dietrich V. The ethics of pediatrics and the ill child in history. *In:* Burgio, G. Roberto; Lantos, John D., eds. *Primum Non Nocere* Today. Second Edition. New York, NY: Elsevier; 1998: 11–21.
(MEDICAL ETHICS)

Engelhardt, H. Tristram. Critical care: why there is no global bioethics. *Journal of Medicine and Philosophy.* 1998 Dec; 23(6): 643–651.
(BIOETHICS; HEALTH CARE/FOREIGN COUNTRIES)

Engelhardt, H. Tristram. Germ–line genetic engineering and moral diversity: moral controversies in a post–Christian world. *In:* Paul, Ellen Frankel; Miller, Fred D.; Paul, Jeffrey, eds. Scientific Innovation, Philosophy, and Public Policy. New York, NY: Cambridge University Press; 1996: 47–62.
(GENE THERAPY; GENETIC INTERVENTION)

Engelhardt, H. Tristram. Physician–assisted death: doctrinal develoment vs. Christian tradition. [Introduction to five articles]. *Christian Bioethics.* 1998 Aug; 4(2): 115–121.
(EUTHANASIA/RELIGIOUS ASPECTS; SUICIDE)

Engelhardt, H. Tristram. Physician–assisted suicide reconsidered: dying as a Christian in a post–Christian age. *Christian Bioethics.* 1998 Aug; 4(2): 143–167.
(EUTHANASIA/RELIGIOUS ASPECTS; SUICIDE)

Engelhardt, H. Tristram. Redefining death: the mirage of consensus. *In:* Youngner, Stuart J.; Arnold, Robert M.; Schapiro, Renie, eds. The Definition of Death: Contemporary Controversies. Baltimore, MD: Johns Hopkins University Press; 1999: 319–331.
(DETERMINATION OF DEATH)

Engelhart, Karlheinz; King, T.T.; Bakran, A.; Evans, David W.; Treloar, Adrian; Hoffenberg, Raymond. Organ donation and permanent vegetative state. [Letters and response]. *Lancet.* 1998 Jan 17; 351(9097): 211–213.
(DETERMINATION OF DEATH; ORGAN AND TISSUE DONATION)

Englert, Y. From medically assisted procreation to euthanasia: a modern way to deal with ethical dilemmas in modern medicine. *European Journal of Genetics in Society.* 1997; 3(2): 22–26.
(EUTHANASIA; REPRODUCTIVE TECHNOLOGIES)

Englert, Y.; Govaerts, I. Oocyte donation: particular technical and ethical aspects. *Human Reproduction.* 1998 May; 13(Suppl. 2): 90–97.
(ORGAN AND TISSUE DONATION; REPRODUCTIVE TECHNOLOGIES)

English, Veronica see **Sommerville, Ann**

Enserink, Martin. Iceland OKs private health databank. [News]. *Science.* 1999 Jan 1; 283(5398): 13.
(GENETIC RESEARCH)

Enserink, Martin. Opponents criticize Iceland's database. [News]. *Science.* 1998 Oct 30; 282(5390): 859.
(GENETIC RESEARCH)

Entwistle, Vikki see **Coulter, Angela**

Episcopal Diocese of Washington, D.C. Committee on Medical Ethics (Chair: Cynthia B. Cohen). Wrestling with the Future: Our Genes and Our Choices. Harrisburg, PA: Morehouse Publishing; 1998. 132 p.
(ABORTION/RELIGIOUS ASPECTS; GENETIC SCREENING; PRENATAL DIAGNOSIS)

Epstein, Andrew E. Lifestyle and ethical issues: driving and occupational aspects. *In:* Dunbar, Sandra B.; Ellenbogen, Kenneth A.; Epstein, A.E., eds. Sudden Cardiac Death: Past, Present, and Future. Armonk, NY: Futura; 1997: 321–334.
(HEALTH; PUBLIC HEALTH)

Epstein, Arnold M. see **Hall, Judith A.**

Epstein, Richard A. A rush to caution: cloning human beings. *In:* Nussbaum, Martha C.; Sunstein, Cass R. eds. Clones and Clones: Facts and Fantasies About Human Cloning. New York, NY: Norton; 1998: 262–279.
(CLONING)

Epstein, Richard A.; Lindsay, Donald G.; Lally, James F.; Reinhardt, Uwe E. Articulating a social ethic for health care. [Letters and response]. *JAMA.* 1998 Mar 11; 279(10): 745–746.
(HEALTH CARE/ECONOMICS)

Epstein, Richard S. see Roberts, Laura Weiss

Epstein, Ronald M. Mindful practice. *JAMA.* 1999 Sep 1; 282(9): 833–839.
(PATIENT CARE)

Epstein, Ronald M. see Marvel, M. Kim

Eraksoy, H. see Sever, M.S.

Erde, Edmund L. Paradigms and personhood: a deepening of the dilemmas in ethics and medical ethics. *Theoretical Medicine and Bioethics.* 1999 Apr; 20(2): 141–160.
(PERSONHOOD)

Erin, Charles A. Is there a right to remain in ignorance of HIV status? *In:* Bennett, Rebecca; Erin, Charles A., eds. HIV and AIDS: Testing, Screening, and Confidentiality. New York, NY: Oxford University Press; 1999: 251–266.
(AIDS/TESTING AND SCREENING)

Erin, Charles A. Some comments on the ethics of consent to the use of ovarian tissue from aborted fetuses and dead women. *In:* Harris, John; Holm, Søren, eds. The Future of Human Reproduction: Ethics, Choice, and Regulation. New York, NY: Oxford University Press; 1998: 162–175.
(FETUSES; INFORMED CONSENT; ORGAN AND TISSUE DONATION)

Erin, Charles A. see Bennett, Rebecca

Ernst, E. Towards a risk–benefit evaluation of placebos. *Wiener Medizinische Wochenschrift.* 1998; 148(20): 461–463.
(HUMAN EXPERIMENTATION/RESEARCH DESIGN; PATIENT CARE)

Escarce, José J. see Schulman, Kevin A.

Esch, Julie Funesti see Frank, Stacy

Espada, Julián see Dal–Ré, Rafael

Essex, Ben see Gbolade, Babatunde A.

Essex, Max see Merson, Michael H.

Estes, Carroll L. see Hansen, Jennie Chin

Esther, Robert see Pincus, Theodore

Estrada, M. Dolors see Serra–Prat, Mateu

Etzioni, Amitai. HIV testing of infants: privacy and public health. *Health Affairs.* 1998 Jul–Aug; 17(4): 170–183.
(AIDS/CONFIDENTIALITY; AIDS/TESTING AND SCREENING)

Etzioni, Amitai. HIV testing of infants: should public health override privacy? *In: his* The Limits of Privacy. New York, NY: Basic Books; 1999: 17–42, 220–226.
(AIDS/CONFIDENTIALITY; AIDS/TESTING AND SCREENING)

Etzioni, Amitai. Medical records: big brother versus big bucks. *In: his* The Limits of Privacy. New York, NY: Basic Books; 1999: 139–182, 248–258.
(CONFIDENTIALITY)

Etzioni, Amitai. Medical records: enhancing privacy, preserving the common good. *Hastings Center Report.* 1999 Mar–Apr; 29(2): 14–23.
(CONFIDENTIALITY)

European Commission. Group of Advisers to the European Commission on the Ethical Implications of Biotechnology. Luxembourg: Office for Official Publications of the European Communities; 1996. 24 p.
(ETHICISTS AND ETHICS COMMITTEES; GENETIC INTERVENTION)

European Commission. Proposal for a good clinical practice directive. [Official statement]. *Bulletin of Medical Ethics.* 1998 Feb; No. 135: 6–11.
(HUMAN EXPERIMENTATION/FOREIGN COUNTRIES)

European Commission. Group of Advisers on the Ethical Implications of Biotechnology. Ethical aspects of patenting inventions involving elements of human origin. *European Journal of Genetics in Society.* 1997; 3(1): 1–3.
(PATENTING LIFE FORMS)

European Federation of Scientific Networks. European Scientific Co–operation Network: "Medicine and Human Rights". The Human Rights, Ethical and Moral Dimensions of Health Care. Strasbourg, France: Council of Europe Publishing; 1998 Mar. 485 p.
(BIOETHICS)

European Parliament. Scientific and Technological Options Assessment (STOA) Programme Contractor. Bioethics in Europe. Final Report, July 1992. Luxembourg: European Parliament, Directorate General for Research; 1992 Sep 8. 257 p.
(BIOETHICS; BIOMEDICAL TECHNOLOGIES; GENETIC INTERVENTION)

Evans, David W. see Engelhart, Karlheinz

Evans, Donald; Crossland, Nigel; Graham, I.M.F.; Preece, Alan. Issues for research ethics committees: third installment. [Letters]. *Bulletin of Medical Ethics.* 1998 Feb; No. 135: 13–16.
(HUMAN EXPERIMENTATION/ETHICS COMMITTEES; HUMAN EXPERIMENTATION/FOREIGN COUNTRIES)

Evans, J. Grimley see Williams, Alan

Evans, Mark I.; Johnson, Mark Paul; Quintero, Ruben A.; Fletcher, John C. Ethical issues surrounding multifetal pregnancy reduction and selective termination. *Clinics in Perinatology.* 1996 Sep; 23(3): 437–451.
(ABORTION)

Evans, Martyn. Bioethics and the newspapers. *Journal of Medicine and Philosophy.* 1999 Apr; 24(2): 164–180.
(BIOETHICS)

Evans, Martyn. The utility of the body. *In:* ten Have, Henk A.M.J.; Welie, Jos V.M., eds. Ownership of the Human Body: Philosophical Considerations on the Use of the Human Body and Its Parts in Healthcare. Boston, MA: Kluwer Academic; 1998: 207–226. (BIOETHICS)

Evans, Roger W. Liver transplantation in a managed care environment. *Liver Transplantation and Surgery.* 1995 Jan; 1(1): 61–75. (HEALTH CARE/ECONOMICS; ORGAN AND TISSUE TRANSPLANTATION; RESOURCE ALLOCATION/BIOMEDICAL TECHNOLOGIES; SELECTION FOR TREATMENT)

Everhart, James see **Showstack, Jonathan**

Evers, Joseph C. see **Byrne, Paul A.**

Evers-Kiebooms, Gerry. Adolescents' opinions about genetic risk and genetic testing. *In:* Sterckx, Sigrid, ed. Biotechnology, Patents and Morality. Proceedings of an International Workshop, "Biotechnology, Patents and Morality: Towards a Consensus," held in Ghent, Belgium, 17–19 Jan 1996. Brookfield, VT: Ashgate; 1997: 85–95. (GENETIC SCREENING; PRENATAL DIAGNOSIS)

Evers-Kiebooms, Gerry see **Decruyenaere, Marleen**

Evers-Kiebooms, Gerry see **Welkenhuysen, Myriam**

Eyre, Harmon see **Pokorski, Robert J.**

F

Faden, Ruth; Guttman, Dan. In response: speaking truth to historiography. *Medical Humanities Review.* 1997 Fall; 11(2): 37–43. (ETHICISTS AND ETHICS COMMITTEES; FRAUD AND MISCONDUCT; HUMAN EXPERIMENTATION)

Faden, Ruth; Kass, Nancy. HIV research, ethics, and the developing world. [Editorial]. *American Journal of Public Health.* 1998 Apr; 88(4): 548–550. (AIDS/HUMAN EXPERIMENTATION; HUMAN EXPERIMENTATION/FOREIGN COUNTRIES; HUMAN EXPERIMENTATION/INFORMED CONSENT; HUMAN EXPERIMENTATION/RESEARCH DESIGN; HUMAN EXPERIMENTATION/SPECIAL POPULATIONS)

Faden, Ruth R. see **Sugarman, Jeremy**

Faden, Ruth R. see **Wilfert, Catherine M.**

Fagan, John. Genetic Engineering: The Hazards -- Vedic Engineering: The Solutions. Fairfield, IA: Maharish: International University Press; 1995. 172 p. (GENETIC INTERVENTION; RECOMBINANT DNA RESEARCH)

Fagot-Largeault, Anne. Ownership of the human body: judicial and legislative responses in France. *In:* ten Have, Henk A.M.J.; Welie, Jos V.M., eds. Ownership of the Human Body: Philosophical Considerations on the Use of the Human Body and Its Parts in Healthcare. Boston, MA: Kluwer Academic; 1998: 115–140. (BIOETHICS; ORGAN AND TISSUE DONATION)

Fahnestock, Deborah T. A piece of my mind: partnership for good dying. *JAMA.* 1999 Aug 18; 282(7): 615–616. (PROFESSIONAL PATIENT RELATIONSHIP; TERMINAL CARE)

Fahy, Bonnie see **Heffner, John E.**

Fahy, Tom see **Howard, Louise**

Fairchild, Amy L.; Bayer, Ronald. Uses and abuses of Tuskegee. *Science.* 1999 May 7; 284(5416): 919–921. (AIDS/HUMAN EXPERIMENTATION; HUMAN EXPERIMENTATION/RESEARCH DESIGN; HUMAN EXPERIMENTATION/SPECIAL POPULATIONS)

Fairman, Julie; Happ, Mary Beth. For their own good? A historical examination of restraint use. *HEC (HealthCare Ethics Committee) Forum.* 1998 Sep–Dec; 10(3–4): 290–299. (BEHAVIOR CONTROL; PATIENT CARE)

Family Research Council see **Focus on the Family**

Fan, Ruiping. Critical care ethics in Asia: global or local? *Journal of Medicine and Philosophy.* 1998 Dec; 23(6): 549–562. (HEALTH CARE/FOREIGN COUNTRIES; RESOURCE ALLOCATION)

Fangman, Timothy R. see **Byrne, Paul A.**

Fano, Alix. Lethal Laws: Animal Testing, Human Health and Environmental Policy. New York, NY: Zed Books; 1997. 242 p. (ANIMAL EXPERIMENTATION)

Fanos, Joanna H. Developmental tasks of childhood and adolescence: implications for genetic testing. *American Journal of Medical Genetics.* 1997 Jul 11; 71(1): 22–28. (GENETIC SCREENING)

Fantoni, Massimo see **Albert, Steven M.**

Faraone, Stephen V.; Gottesman, Irving I.; Tsuang, Ming T. Fifty years of the Nuremberg Code: a time for retrospection and introspection. [Editorial]. *American Journal of Medical Genetics.* 1997 Jul 25; 74(4): 345–347. (FRAUD AND MISCONDUCT; GENETIC RESEARCH; HUMAN EXPERIMENTATION)

Farlow, Martin see **Koepp, Robert**

Farquhar, Dion. The Other Machine: Discourse and Reproductive Technologies. New York, NY: Routledge; 1996. 258 p. (REPRODUCTIVE TECHNOLOGIES)

Farr, Kathryn Ann. Fetal abuse and the criminalization of behavior during pregnancy. *Crime and Delinquency.* 1995 Apr; 41(2): 235–245. (PRENATAL INJURIES)

Farriman, Annabel. Surgeons carry out too many operations on dying patients. [News]. *BMJ (British Medical Journal).* 1998 Nov 7; 317(7168): 1269. (TERMINAL CARE)

Farrington, Ken see **Chandna, Shahid M.**

Farsides, Bobby see **Begley, Anne Marie**

Farsides, Calliope C.S. HIV infection and the health care worker: the case for limited disclosure. *In:* Bennett, Rebecca; Erin, Charles A., eds. HIV and AIDS: Testing, Screening, and Confidentiality. New York, NY: Oxford University Press; 1999: 166–178.

(AIDS/CONFIDENTIALITY; AIDS/HEALTH PERSONNEL)

Farthing, Michael J.G. Fraud in medicine: coping with fraud. *Lancet*. 1998 Dec 19-26; 352 (Suppl. 4): 11.
(BIOMEDICAL RESEARCH; FRAUD AND MISCONDUCT)

Fasting, Ulla; Christensen, Jan; Glending, Susanne; Amnesty International. Danish Working Group for Children. Children sold for transplants: medical and legal aspects. *Nursing Ethics*. 1998 Nov; 5(6): 518-526.
(ORGAN AND TISSUE DONATION)

Fazel, Seena; Hope, Tony; Jacoby, Robin. Assessment of competence to complete advance directives: validation of a patient centred approach. *BMJ (British Medical Journal)*. 1999 Feb 20; 318(7182): 493-497.
(ADVANCE DIRECTIVES)

Fazel, Seena; Hope, Tony; Jacoby, Robin. Dementia, intelligence, and the competence to complete advance directives. [Research letter]. *Lancet*. 1999 Jul 3; 354(9172): 48.
(ADVANCE DIRECTIVES)

Fazel, Seena; Hope, Tony; Jacoby, Robin. Ways of assessing capacity to complete an advance directive should be developed. [Letter]. *BMJ (British Medical Journal)*. 1998 Apr 25; 316(7140): 1321-1322.
(ADVANCE DIRECTIVES)

Fears, Robin; Poste, George. Building population genetics resources using the U.K. NHS. *Science*. 1999 Apr 9; 284(5412): 267-268.
(GENETIC RESEARCH; HEALTH CARE/FOREIGN COUNTRIES; RESOURCE ALLOCATION)

Featherstone, Katie; Donovan, Jenny L. Random allocation or allocation at random? Patients' perspectives of participation in a randomised controlled trial. *BMJ (British Medical Journal)*. 1998 Oct 31; 317(7167): 1177-1180.
(HUMAN EXPERIMENTATION/INFORMED CONSENT; HUMAN EXPERIMENTATION/RESEARCH DESIGN)

Federman, Daniel D. Protecting the future of medicine -- from themselves. [Editorial]. *Annals of Internal Medicine*. 1999 Jan 5; 130(1): 66-67.
(AIDS/HEALTH PERSONNEL; MEDICAL ETHICS/EDUCATION)

Feeny, D. see **Cappelli, M.**

Feeny, David see **Saigal, Saroj**

Feest, Terry G. see **McKenzie, John K.**

Fégueux, Sophie see **Lot, Florence**

Fein, Esther B. Calling infertility a disease, couples battle with insurers. [News]. *New York Times*. 1998 Feb 22: 1, 34.
(HEALTH CARE/ECONOMICS; REPRODUCTIVE TECHNOLOGIES)

Fein, Oliver see **McCally, Michael**

Feinberg, Mark B. see **Wilfert, Catherine M.**

Feldblum, Chai see **Gostin, Lawrence O.**

Feldman, David M. Birth Control in Jewish Law: Marital Relations, Contraception, and Abortion as Set Forth in the Classic Texts of Jewish Law. First Jason Aronson Edition. Northvale, NJ: Jason Aronson; 1998. 349 p.
(ABORTION/RELIGIOUS ASPECTS; CONTRACEPTION)

Feldman, Debra see **Finestone, Albert J.**

Feldman, Debra S.; Novack, Dennis H.; Gracely, Edward. Effects of managed care on physician-patient relationships, quality of care, and the ethical practice of medicine. *Archives of Internal Medicine*. 1998 Aug 10-24; 158(15): 1626-1632.
(HEALTH CARE/ECONOMICS; PROFESSIONAL PATIENT RELATIONSHIP)

Feldman, Eric A. Testing the force: HIV and discrimination in the Australian military. *AIDS and Public Policy Journal*. 1998 Summer; 13(2): 85-90.
(AIDS/TESTING AND SCREENING)

Feldman, Eric A.; Bayer, Ronald, eds. Blood Feuds: AIDS, Blood, and the Politics of Medical Disaster. New York, NY: Oxford University Press; 1999. 375 p.
(AIDS; BLOOD DONATION)

Feldman, Gabriel E. see **Gasner, M. Rose**

Feldman, Miriam K. The doctor-patient bond: covenant or business contract? *Minnesota Medicine*. 1997 Sep; 80(9): 12-16.
(HEALTH CARE/ECONOMICS; PROFESSIONAL PATIENT RELATIONSHIP)

Feldmann, Linda. The ethics of putting eggs on ice. [News]. *Christian Science Monitor*. 1997 Oct 20: 1, 18.
(REPRODUCTIVE TECHNOLOGIES)

Fellows, Lesley K. Competency and consent in dementia. *Journal of the American Geriatrics Society*. 1998 Jul; 46(7): 922-926.
(ADVANCE DIRECTIVES; INFORMED CONSENT/MENTALLY DISABLED; PATIENT CARE/AGED)

Felsman, Janine P. Eliminating parental consent and notification for adolescent HIV testing: a legitimate statutory response to the AIDS epidemic. [Note]. *Journal of Law and Policy*. 1996; 5(1): 339-383.
(AIDS/TESTING AND SCREENING; CONFIDENTIALITY/LEGAL ASPECTS; INFORMED CONSENT/MINORS)

Fenn, Darien S. see **Lee, Melinda A.**

Fennell, Phil. Statutory authority to treat, relatives and treatment proxies. *Medical Law Review*. 1994 Spring; 2(1): 30-56.
(INFORMED CONSENT/MENTALLY DISABLED)

Fentiman, Linda C. Organ donation as national service: a proposed federal organ donation law. *Suffolk University Law Review*. 1993 Winter; 27(4): 1593-1612.
(ORGAN AND TISSUE DONATION)

Fenwick, Lynda Beck. Private Choices, Public Consequences: Reproductive Technology and the New Ethics of Conception, Pregnancy, and Family. New York, NY: Dutton; 1998. 390 p.
(REPRODUCTION; REPRODUCTIVE TECHNOLOGIES)

Ferenz, Leonard. Ethical considerations of federal guidelines and models of moral responsibility governing neuropharmacologic research. *In:* Hertzman, Marc;

Feltner, Douglas, E., eds. The Handbook of Psychopharmacology Trials: An Overview of Scientific, Political, and Ethical Concerns. New York, NY: New York University Press; 1997: 23–45.
(HUMAN EXPERIMENTATION/REGULATION)

Ferguson, P.R. Causing death or allowing to die? A rejoinder to Randall's comments. [Letter]. *Journal of Medical Ethics.* 1998 Aug; 24(4): 281–282.
(ALLOWING TO DIE/LEGAL ASPECTS; EUTHANASIA/LEGAL ASPECTS)

Fernandes, Praveen see Sugarman, Jeremy

Fernando, M. Daniel see Solomon, Liza

Ferran, Jose see Agarwal, Manoj R.

Ferrell, Betty R. Pain management: a moral imperative. *American Nurses Association Center for Ethics and Human Rights Communique.* 1996–1997 Winter; 5(2): 4–5.
(PATIENT CARE)

Ferrell, Betty Rolling see McCaffery, Margo

Ferriman, Annabel. Trial by video: *Someone to watch over me,* ITV, 12 January. *BMJ (British Medical Journal).* 1999 Jan 23; 318(7178): 269.
(CONFIDENTIALITY/MENTAL HEALTH; PATIENT CARE/MINORS)

Ferris, Lorraine E.; Barkun, Harvey; Carlisle, John; Hoffman, Brian; Katz, Cheryl; Silverman, Marvin. Defining the physician's duty to warn: consensus statement of Ontario's Medical Expert Panel on Duty to Inform. *Canadian Medical Association Journal.* 1998 Jun 2; 158(11): 1473–1479.
(CONFIDENTIALITY/LEGAL ASPECTS; CONFIDENTIALITY/MENTAL HEALTH)

Ferris, Sandy see Pincus, Harold Alan

Festing, M.F.W.; van Zutphen, L.F.M. Guidelines for reviewing manuscripts on studies involving live animals: synopsis of the workshop. *In:* van Zutphen, L.F.M.; Balls, M., eds. Animal Alternatives, Welfare and Ethics. New York, NY: Elsevier; 1997: 405–410.
(ANIMAL EXPERIMENTATION)

Fiddler, Morris; Pergament, Eugene. Germline gene therapy: its time is near. *Molecular Human Reproduction.* 1996 Feb; 2(2): 75–76.
(GENE THERAPY)

Field, Julie Kunce see Scarnecchia, Suellyn

Fielding, Helen A. Body measures: phenomenological considerations of corporeal ethics. *Journal of Medicine and Philosophy.* 1998 Oct; 23(5): 533–545.
(BIOETHICS; ORGAN AND TISSUE DONATION)

Fieldston, Evan. AIDS, thalidomide and maternal–fetal rights in conflict. *Princeton Journal of Bioethics.* 1998 Spring; 1(1): 83–93.
(AIDS; PATIENT CARE/DRUGS; PRENATAL INJURIES)

Filene, Peter G. In the Arms of Others: A Cultural History of the Right-to-Die in America. Chicago, IL: Ivan R. Dee; 1998. 282 p.
(ALLOWING TO DIE; EUTHANASIA; SUICIDE; TERMINAL CARE)

Fimbrez, Karen Jean. Life-Sustaining Treatment: The Family Decision-Making Process. Ann Arbor, MI: UMI Dissertation Services; 1995. 90 p.
(ALLOWING TO DIE; TERMINAL CARE)

Fincanci, Sebnem Korur see Frank, Martina W.

Finder, Stuart G.; Fox, Mark D.; Frist, William H.; Zaner, Richard M. The ethicist's role on the transplant team: a study of heart, lung, and liver transplantation programs in the United States. *Clinical Transplantation.* 1993 Dec; 7(6): 559–564.
(ETHICISTS AND ETHICS COMMITTEES; ORGAN AND TISSUE TRANSPLANTATION)

Fine, Andrea. Fertility business hits Internet, weaving web of controversy. [News]. *Christian Science Monitor.* 1998 Sept 11: 3.
(ORGAN AND TISSUE DONATION; REPRODUCTIVE TECHNOLOGIES)

Fineberg, Harvey V. see Sachs, David H.

Finestone, Albert J.; Feldman, Debra; Beasley, John W.; Volpintesta, Edward; Zarin, Deborah A.; Pincus, Harold Alan; Halm, Ethan A.; Blumenthal, David; Causino, Nancyanne. Gatekeeping: good or bad, but never indifferent. [Letters and response]. *JAMA.* 1998 Mar 25; 279(12): 908–910.
(HEALTH CARE/ECONOMICS; RESOURCE ALLOCATION)

Fink, Diane see Garber, Judy E.

Finn, Lisa. It's for (y)our own good: an analysis of the discourses surrounding mandatory, unblinded HIV testing of newborns. *Journal of Medical Humanities.* 1998 Summer; 19(2–3): 133–162.
(AIDS/TESTING AND SCREENING)

Fins, Joseph J. Commentary: from contract to covenant in advance care planning. *Journal of Law, Medicine and Ethics.* 1999 Spring; 27(1): 46–51.
(ADVANCE DIRECTIVES; INFORMED CONSENT)

Fins, Joseph J.; Miller, Franklin G.; Bacchetta, Matthew D. Clinical pragmatism: bridging theory and practice. *Kennedy Institute of Ethics Journal.* 1998 Mar; 8(1): 37–42.
(BIOETHICS)

Fins, Joseph J. see Henderson, Shelley

Finucane, Thomas E. see Kane, Richard S.

Firn, David. Roslin Institute upset by human cloning suggestions. [News]. *Nature Medicine.* 1999 Mar; 5(3): 253.
(CLONING)

First, M. Roy. Controversies in organ donation: minority donation and living unrelated renal donors. *Transplantation Proceedings.* 1997 Feb–Mar; 29(1–2): 67–69.
(ORGAN AND TISSUE DONATION)

Fischer, Gary S. see Tulsky, James A.

Fish, Peter. A harder better death. [Personal narrative]. *Health.* 1997 Nov–Dec; 11(8): 108–114.
(TERMINAL CARE/HOSPICES)

Fisher, Barbara Loe see **Redenbaugh, Russell**

Fisher, Carol; Gill, Denise. Limiting health care for the elderly. *Plastic Surgical Nursing.* 1996 Summer; 16(2): 113–116.
(PATIENT CARE/AGED; RESOURCE ALLOCATION)

Fisher, Celia B.; Hoagwood, Kimberly; Jensen, Peter S. Casebook on ethical issues in research with children and adolescents with mental disorders. *In:* Hoagwood, Kimberly; Jensen, Peter S.; Fisher, Celia B., eds. Ethical Issues in Mental Health Research with Children and Adolescents. Mahwah, NJ: Lawrence Erlbaum Associates; 1996: 135–266.
(BEHAVIORAL RESEARCH/MINORS; BEHAVIORAL RESEARCH/SPECIAL POPULATIONS; HUMAN EXPERIMENTATION/MINORS; HUMAN EXPERIMENTATION/SPECIAL POPULATIONS)

Fisher, Celia B.; Younggren, Jeffrey N. The value and utility of the 1992 ethics code. *Professional Psychology: Research and Practice.* 1997 Dec; 28(6): 582–592.
(PROFESSIONAL ETHICS/CODES OF ETHICS)

Fisher, Celia B. see **Hoagwood, Kimberly**

Fisher, Elliott S.; Welch, H. Gilbert. Avoiding the unintended consequences of growth in medical care: how might more be worse? *JAMA.* 1999 Feb 3; 281(5): 446–453.
(BIOMEDICAL TECHNOLOGIES; HEALTH CARE; PATIENT CARE)

Fisher, Elliott S. see **Pritchard, Robert S.**

Fisher, Fleur; Sommerville, Ann. To everything there is a season? Are there medical grounds for refusing fertility treatment to older women? *In:* Harris, John; Holm, Søren, eds. The Future of Human Reproduction: Ethics, Choice, and Regulation. New York, NY: Oxford University Press; 1998: 203–220.
(REPRODUCTIVE TECHNOLOGIES; SELECTION FOR TREATMENT)

Fisher, Ian. Bill would govern use of dead men's sperm. [News]. *New York Times.* 1998 Mar 7: B5.
(REPRODUCTIVE TECHNOLOGIES)

Fisher, Ian. Families providing complex medical care, tubes and all. *New York Times.* 1998 Jun 7: 1, 30.
(BIOMEDICAL TECHNOLOGIES; PATIENT CARE)

Fisher, Nancy see **Baumiller, Robert C.**

Fishman, Jay A. see **Sachs, David H.**

Fishman, Rachelle H.B. Infertility doctors use egg donors worldwide. [News]. *Lancet.* 1999 Feb 27; 353(9154): 736.
(REPRODUCTIVE TECHNOLOGIES)

Fishman, Rachelle H.B. Israeli cloning ban endorsed by scientists. [News]. *Lancet.* 1999 Jan 16; 353(9148): 218.
(CLONING)

Fishman, Rachelle H.B. Reproductive rights and risks in Israel. [News]. *Lancet.* 1998 Dec 19–26; 352(9145): 1998.
(REPRODUCTIVE TECHNOLOGIES)

Fister, Susan see **Schlomann, Pamela**

Fitzgerald, Faith T. Dying in America. *Pharos.* 1997

Spring; 60(2): 29–31.
(TERMINAL CARE)

Fitzgerald, Jennifer. Geneticizing disability: the Human Genome Project and the commodification of self. *Issues in Law and Medicine.* 1998 Fall; 14(2): 147–163.
(GENOME MAPPING)

Fitzgerald, Wendy Anton. Engineering perfect offspring: devaluing children and childhood. *Hastings Constitutional Law Quarterly.* 1997 Summer; 24(4): 833–861.
(ALLOWING TO DIE/INFANTS; EUGENICS; PATIENT CARE/MINORS; PERSONHOOD)

Fitzpatrick, J.; Hahn, C.; Costa, T.; Huggins, M. The duty to recontact: attitudes of genetics service providers. [Abstract]. *American Journal of Human Genetics.* 1997 Oct; 61(4): A57.
(GENETIC COUNSELING; GENETIC SERVICES)

Flanders, Steven; Shelanski, Vivien B.; Ickes, Cynthia; Salinas, Jean–Louis; Sierra, Silvia. Physician–assisted suicide: potential impact of recent court decisions. *Journal of Long Term Home Health Care.* 1997 Winter; 16(1): 4–13.
(SUICIDE)

Flanigan, Rosemary. The most solemn moment of my living. [Editorial]. *Bioethics Forum.* 1998 Spring; 14(1): 3–4.
(RESUSCITATION ORDERS)

Fleck, Leonard. Justice, rights, and Alzheimer disease genetics. *In:* Post, Stephen G.; Whitehouse, Peter J., eds. Genetic Testing for Alzheimer Disease: Ethical and Clinical Issues. Baltimore, MD: Johns Hopkins University Press; 1998: 190–208.
(GENETIC SCREENING; GENETIC SERVICES; RESOURCE ALLOCATION/BIOMEDICAL TECHNOLOGIES)

Fleck, Leonard see **Andre, Judith**

Fleetwood, Janet. Editor's introduction [to a set of nine articles on the use of restraints in healthcare]. *HEC (HealthCare Ethics Committee) Forum.* 1998 Sep–Dec; 10(3–4): 231–234.
(BEHAVIOR CONTROL; PATIENT CARE)

Flegel, Kenneth M. Physicians, finder's fees and free, informed consent. [Editorial]. *Canadian Medical Association Journal.* 1997 Nov 15; 157(10): 1373–1374.
(HUMAN EXPERIMENTATION)

Flegel, Kenneth M. Society's interest in protection for the fetus. [Editorial]. *Canadian Medical Association Journal.* 1998 Apr 7; 158(7): 895–896.
(ABORTION/FOREIGN COUNTRIES)

Flegel, Kenneth M.; Lant, Mary. Sound privacy for patients. [Editorial]. *Canadian Medical Association Journal.* 1998 Mar 10; 158(5): 613–614.
(CONFIDENTIALITY)

Fleischman, Alan R.; Post, Linda Farber; Dubler, Nancy Neveloff. Mandatory newborn screening for human immunodeficiency virus. *Bulletin of the New York Academy of Medicine.* 1994 Summer; 71(1): 4–17.
(AIDS/TESTING AND SCREENING)

Fleissner, Erwin. Race and the human genome. [Book

review essay]. *Hastings Center Report.* 1999 Jul–Aug; 29(4): 40–42.
(GENOME MAPPING)

Fleming, David W. see Chin, Arthur E.

Fleming, P.J. see West, Charles

Fleming, Patricia L. see Nakashima, Allyn K.

Fletcher, J.C.; Wertz, D.C. Refusal of employment or insurance. [Abstract]. *American Journal of Human Genetics.* 1997 Oct; 61(4): A56.
(GENETIC SCREENING)

Fletcher, John C. Deciding about death: physician–assisted suicide and the courts –– a panel discussion. *Pharos.* 1998 Winter; 61(1): 2–7.
(SUICIDE; TERMINAL CARE)

Fletcher, John C.; Richter, Gerd. Ethical issues of perinatal human gene therapy. *Journal of Maternal–Fetal Medicine.* 1996 Sep–Oct; 5(5): 232–244.
(EMBRYO AND FETAL RESEARCH; GENE THERAPY; HUMAN EXPERIMENTATION/MINORS)

Fletcher, John C. see Evans, Mark I.

Fletcher, John C. see Wertz, Dorothy C.

Flew, Antony. Advance directives are the solution to Dr. Campbell's problem for voluntary euthanasia. *Journal of Medical Ethics.* 1999 Jun; 25(3): 245–246.
(ADVANCE DIRECTIVES; EUTHANASIA)

Flowers, Kristine see Marvel, M. Kim

Fluck, David see Barakat, Khalid

Fluhr, Haya see Mester, Roberto

Flynn, Eileen P. Issues in Medical Ethics. Kansas City, MO: Sheed and Ward; 1997. 384 p.
(BIOETHICS)

Flynn, Laurie see Rosenheck, Robert

Focus on the Family see Avallone, Fran

Foley, Elizabeth see Gbolade, Babatunde A.

Foley, Kathleen. A 44–year–old woman with severe pain at the end of life. *JAMA.* 1999 May 26; 281(20): 1937–1945.
(TERMINAL CARE)

Foley, Kathleen; Hendin, Herbert. The Oregon report: don't ask, don't tell. *Hastings Center Report.* 1999 May–Jun; 29(3): 37–42.
(SUICIDE)

Foley, Kathleen M. see Costantini–Ferrando, Maria F.

Folstein, Marshal F. see Holzer, Jacob C.

Folstein, Marshal F. see Trippitelli, Carol Lynn

Ford, Daniel E. see Cooper–Patrick, Lisa

Forder, Caroline J. Abortion: a constitutional problem in European perspective. *Maastricht Journal of European and Comparative Law.* 1994; 1: 56–100.
(ABORTION/FOREIGN COUNTRIES; ABORTION/LEGAL ASPECTS)

Forret, Patricia; McGuire, Beverly. Ethical guidelines for managed care contract negotiations. *Journal of Health Care Finance.* 1996 Winter; 23(2): 38–45.
(HEALTH CARE/ECONOMICS)

Forrow, Lachlan see Sachs, David H.

Forster, Alan J. see van Walraven, Carl

Forster, Heidi P. Legal trends in bioethics. *Journal of Clinical Ethics.* 1998 Winter; 9(4): 421–430.
(BIOETHICS)

Forster, Heidi P. Legal trends in bioethics. *Journal of Clinical Ethics.* 1999 Spring; 10(1): 66–75.
(BIOETHICS)

Forster, Heidi P.; Robertson, John. Frozen embryo disposition. [Letter and response]. *Hastings Center Report.* 1999 Mar–Apr; 29(2): 4–5.
(FETUSES; IN VITRO FERTILIZATION)

Forster, Heidi P. see Davis, Dena S.

Fortinsky, R.H. see Weiss, A.H.

Fost, Norman. Decisions regarding treatment of seriously ill newborns. [Editorial]. *JAMA.* 1999 Jun 2; 281(21): 2041–2043.
(ALLOWING TO DIE/INFANTS; PATIENT CARE/MINORS; SELECTION FOR TREATMENT)

Fost, Norman. The unimportance of death. *In:* Youngner, Stuart J.; Arnold, Robert M.; Schapiro, Renie, eds. The Definition of Death: Contemporary Controversies. Baltimore, MD: Johns Hopkins University Press; 1999: 161–178.
(DETERMINATION OF DEATH/BRAIN DEATH; ORGAN AND TISSUE DONATION)

Fost, Norman see Green, Michael J.

Fost, Norman C. see Love, Richard R.

Foster, Claire; Holley, Sandra. Ethical review of multi–centre research: a survey of multi–centre researchers in the South Thames region. *Journal of the Royal College of Physicians of London.* 1998 May–Jun; 32(3): 242–245.
(HUMAN EXPERIMENTATION/ETHICS COMMITTEES; HUMAN EXPERIMENTATION/FOREIGN COUNTRIES)

Foster, Claire see Holley, Sandra

Foster, Larry W.; McLellan, Linda J. Moral judgments in the rationing of health care resources: a comparative study of clinical health professionals. *Social Work in Health Care.* 1997; 25(4): 13–36.
(RESOURCE ALLOCATION)

Foster, Morris W.; Eisenbraun, Ann J.; Carter, Thomas H. Communal discourse as a supplement to informed consent for genetic research. *Nature Genetics.* 1997 Nov; 17(3): 277–279.
(GENETIC RESEARCH; HUMAN EXPERIMENTATION/INFORMED CONSENT)

Foster, Peggy; Hudson, Stephanie. From compliance to concordance: a challenge for contraceptive prescribers. *Health Care Analysis.* 1998 Jun; 6(2): 123–130.
(CONTRACEPTION)

Fowlie, P.W.; Delahunty, C.; Tarnow–Mordi, W.O. What do doctors record in the medical notes following discussion with the parents of sick premature infants? *European Journal of Pediatrics.* 1998 Jan; 157(1): 63–65.
(PATIENT CARE/MINORS; PROFESSIONAL PATIENT RELATIONSHIP)

Fowlie, Peter W. see **McHaffie, Hazel E.**

Fox, Daniel M. Comment: epidemiology and the new political economy of medicine. *American Journal of Public Health.* 1999 Apr; 89(4): 493–496.
(BIOMEDICAL RESEARCH; BIOMEDICAL TECHNOLOGIES)

Fox–Genovese, Elizabeth. Abortion and morality revisited. *Human Life Review.* 1997 Summer; 23(3): 50–59.
(ABORTION)

Fox, Jeffrey L. Forget Washington: state laws threaten to restrict genetic research, too. [News]. *Journal of NIH Research.* 1997 Nov; 9(11): 19–20.
(GENETIC RESEARCH; GENETIC SCREENING)

Fox, Jeffrey L. Future tense for in utero gene therapy. [News]. *Nature Biotechnology.* 1998 Nov; 16(11): 1002–1003.
(EMBRYO AND FETAL RESEARCH; GENE THERAPY)

Fox, Jeffrey L. Gene therapy experts ponder readiness for enhancements. [News]. *Nature Biotechnology.* 1997 Nov; 15(12): 1236–1237.
(GENE THERAPY)

Fox, Jeffrey L. Germline gene therapy contemplated. [News]. *Nature Biotechnology.* 1998 May; 16(5): 407.
(GENE THERAPY; HUMAN EXPERIMENTATION)

Fox, Jeffrey L. U.S. Bioethics Commission meets, outlines agenda. [News]. *Nature Biotechnology.* 1996 Nov; 14(11): 1533.
(BIOETHICS; ETHICISTS AND ETHICS COMMITTEES)

Fox, Jeffrey L. US bioethicists say continue human cloning moratorium. [News]. *Nature Biotechnology.* 1997 Jul; 15(7): 609.
(CLONING)

Fox, Lynda see **Baumiller, Robert C.**

Fox, Marie. A woman's right to choose? A feminist critique. *In:* Harris, John; Holm, Søren, eds. The Future of Human Reproduction: Ethics, Choice, and Regulation. New York, NY: Oxford University Press; 1998: 77–100.
(ABORTION)

Fox, Marie. Abortion decision–making: taking men's needs seriously. *In:* Lee, Ellie, ed. Abortion Law and Politics Today. New York, NY: St. Martin's Press; 1998: 198–215.
(ABORTION/FOREIGN COUNTRIES; ABORTION/LEGAL ASPECTS)

Fox, Marie; McHale, Jean. Xenotransplantation: the ethical and legal ramifications. *Medical Law Review.* 1998

Spring; 6(1): 42–61.
(HUMAN EXPERIMENTATION/REGULATION; ORGAN AND TISSUE TRANSPLANTATION)

Fox, Mark D. see **Finder, Stuart G.**

Fox, Michael W. Concepts in Ethology: Animal Behavior and Bioethics. Second Edition. Malabar, FL: Krieger; 1998. 163 p.
(ANIMAL EXPERIMENTATION; BEHAVIORAL RESEARCH)

Fox, Renée C. see **Rosenheck, Robert**

Foye, Gerard see **Bowes, Watson**

Frader, Joel see **Kuczewski, Mark G.**

Frader, Joel E. see **Arnold, Robert M.**

France. Decree No. 96–1041 of 2 Dec 1996 on the determination of death prior to the removal of organs, tissues, and cells for therapeutic or scientific purposes, and amending the Public Health Code (Second Part: decrees made after consulting the *Conseil d'Etat*). (*Journal officiel de la Republique fran3aise, Lois et Decrets*, 4 Dec 1996, No. 282, p. 17615). *International Digest of Health Legislation.* 1997; 48(2): 197–198.
(DETERMINATION OF DEATH; ORGAN AND TISSUE DONATION)

France. Order of 6 Nov 1996 approving the Rules for the distribution and allocation of transplants removed from deceased persons for the purpose of organ transplantation. (*Journal officiel de la Republique fran3aise, Lois et Decrets*, 10 Nov 1996, No. 263, pp. 16475–16476). *International Digest of Health Legislation.* 1997; 48(1): 15–18.
(ORGAN AND TISSUE TRANSPLANTATION; RESOURCE ALLOCATION/BIOMEDICAL TECHNOLOGIES; SELECTION FOR TREATMENT)

Francis, Donald P. see **Merson, Michael H.**

François–Xavier Bagnoud Center for Health and Human Rights, Harvard School of Public Health see **International Federation of Red Cross and Red Crescent Societies**

Francome, Colin. Attitudes of general practitioners in Northern Ireland toward abortion and family planning. *Family Planning Perspectives.* 1997 Sep–Oct; 29(5): 234–236.
(ABORTION/ATTITUDES; ABORTION/FOREIGN COUNTRIES; CONTRACEPTION)

Frank, Janet C. see **Maly, Rose C.**

Frank, Lori see **Albert, Steven M.**

Frank, Martina W.; Bauer, Heidi M.; Arican, Nadir; Fincanci, Sebnem Korur; Iacopino, Vincent. Virginity examinations in Turkey: role of forensic physicians in controlling female sexuality. *JAMA.* 1999 Aug 4; 282(5): 485–490.
(BEHAVIOR CONTROL)

Frank, Stacy; Esch, Julie Funesti; Margeson, Nancy E. Mandatory HIV testing of newborns: the impact on women. *American Journal of Nursing.* 1998 Oct; 98(10): 49–51.
(AIDS/TESTING AND SCREENING; MASS SCREENING)

Frankel, Mark S. Perception, reality, and the political context of conflict of interest in university–industry relationships. *Academic Medicine.* 1996 Dec; 71(12): 1297–1304.
(BIOMEDICAL RESEARCH)

Frankel, Sherman. The dementia dilemma. *Perspectives in Biology and Medicine.* 1999 Winter; 42(2): 174–178.
(ADVANCE DIRECTIVES; SUICIDE)

Frankford, David M. The treatment/enhancement distinction as an armament in the policy wars. *In:* Parens, Erik, ed. Enhancing Human Traits: Ethical and Social Implications. Washington, DC: Georgetown University Press; 1998: 70–94.
(BIOMEDICAL TECHNOLOGIES)

Frankford, David M. see **Rosenbaum, Sara**

Franklin, Barbara A. see **Lerman, Caryn**

Fraser, Ian see **Hill, Wan Ying**

Frayne, Susan see **Asch, Steven**

Frazier, William D. Rationing of health care -- who determines who gets the cure, when, where, and why? *Annals of Health Law.* 1993; 2: 95–99.
(RESOURCE ALLOCATION; SELECTION FOR TREATMENT)

Freda, Margaret Comerford; DeVore, Nancy; Valentine–Adams, Nancy; Bombard, Allan; Merkatz, Irwin R. Informed consent for maternal serum alpha–fetoprotein screening in an inner city population: how informed is it? *Journal of Obstetric, Gynecologic and Neonatal Nursing.* 1998 Jan–Feb; 27(1): 99–106.
(INFORMED CONSENT; PRENATAL DIAGNOSIS)

Freedman, Alfred M. see **Halpern, Abraham L.**

Freedman, Alfred M. see **Schoenholtz, Jack C.**

Freedman, Benjamin. Duty and Healing: Foundations of a Jewish Bioethic. New York, NY: Routledge; 1999. 344 p.
(BIOETHICS; ETHICISTS AND ETHICS COMMITTEES; INFORMED CONSENT)

Freedman, Carol. Aspirin for the mind? Some ethical worries about psychopharmacology. *In:* Parens, Erik, ed. Enhancing Human Traits: Ethical and Social Implications. Washington, DC: Georgetown University Press; 1998: 135–150.
(PATIENT CARE/DRUGS)

Freeman, Daniel M. see **Zweig, Franklin M.**

Freeman, David L.; Abrams, Judith Z., eds. Illness and Health in the Jewish Tradition: Writings from the Bible to Today. Philadelphia, PA: Jewish Publication Society; 1999. 291 p.
(HEALTH)

Freeman, John M. see **Jones, Charlotte**

Freeman, Michael. Deciding for the intellectually impaired. *Medical Law Review.* 1994 Spring; 2(1): 77–91.
(INFORMED CONSENT/MENTALLY DISABLED)

Freiberg, Nancy. The ethos of ethics [Edmund D. Pellegrino]. *Georgetown Magazine.* 1996 Fall; 28(2–3–4): 14–18.
(ETHICISTS AND ETHICS COMMITTEES)

Freilicher, Liza; Scheu, Jennifer; Wetanson, Suzanne. Conceiving Luc: A Family Story. New York, NY: William Morrow; 1999. 302 p.
(SURROGATE MOTHERS)

Frenk, Julio. Medical care and health improvement: the critical link. [Editorial]. *Annals of Internal Medicine.* 1998 Sep 1; 129(5): 419–420.
(HEALTH; HEALTH CARE)

Frentz, Gerda see **Zwitter, Matjaz**

Fretz, Leo. Biotechnology and the public debate: some philosophical reflections. *In:* Sterckx, Sigrid, ed. Biotechnology, Patents and Morality. Proceedings of an International Workshop, "Biotechnology, Patents and Morality: Towards a Consensus," held in Ghent, Belgium, 17–19 Jan 1996. Brookfield, VT: Ashgate; 1997: 257–265.
(GENETIC INTERVENTION)

Freudenheim, Milt. Medicine at the click of a mouse: on-line health files are convenient; are they private? [News]. *New York Times.* 1998 Aug 12: Business 1,8.
(CONFIDENTIALITY)

Freudenheim, Milt. Psychiatric drugs are now promoted directly to patients. [News]. *New York Times.* 1998 Feb 17: D1, D3.
(PATIENT CARE/DRUGS; PATIENT CARE/MENTALLY DISABLED)

Freudenthal, Gad, ed. AIDS in Jewish Thought and Law. Hoboken, NJ: Ktav; 1998. 175 p.
(AIDS)

Frey, R.G. Hume on suicide. *Journal of Medicine and Philosophy.* 1999 Aug; 24(4): 336–351.
(SUICIDE)

Frey, R.G. Medicine, animal experimentation, and the moral problem of unfortunate humans. *In:* Paul, Ellen Frankel; Miller, Fred D.; Paul, Jeffrey, eds. Scientific Innovation, Philosophy, and Public Policy. New York, NY: Cambridge University Press; 1996: 181–211.
(ANIMAL EXPERIMENTATION)

Frey, R.G. see **Dworkin, Gerald**

Frey, Robert L. see **Nakashima, Allyn K.**

Fried, Terri R. see **Segal, Eran**

Frieden, Thomas R. see **Gasner, M. Rose**

Frieden, Thomas R. see **Lerner, Barron H.**

Friedland, Gerald see **Kaldjian, Lauris C.**

Friedland, Steven I. The criminal law implications of the Human Genome Project: reimagining a genetically oriented criminal justice system. *Kentucky Law Journal.* 1997–1998; 86(2): 303–366.
(BEHAVIORAL GENETICS)

Friedman, J.M. see **Bernard, Lynn E.**

Fries, Brant E. see **Teno, Joan M.**

Frist, William H. see **Finder, Stuart G.**

Frolik, Lawrence A., ed. Health care decision making. *In: his* Aging and the Law: An Interdisciplinary Reader. Philadelphia, PA: Temple University Press; 1999: 295–394.
(ALLOWING TO DIE/LEGAL ASPECTS; INFORMED CONSENT; PATIENT CARE/AGED; SUICIDE; TERMINAL CARE)

Frothingham, Richard see **Bolan, Robert K.**

Frumkin, Howard see **Brodkin, C. Andrew**

Fryns, Jean-Pierre see **Decruyenaere, Marleen**

Fuchs, E. see **Müller, H.J.**

Fuchs, Victor; Iglehart, John K. Physicians as agents of social control: the thoughts of Victor Fuchs. [Interview]. *Health Affairs.* 1998 Jan–Feb; 17(1): 90–96.
(HEALTH CARE/ECONOMICS)

Fuchs, Victor R. Who Shall Live? Health, Economics, and Social Choice. Expanded Edition. River Edge, NJ: World Scientific; 1998. 278 p.
(HEALTH CARE/ECONOMICS; RESOURCE ALLOCATION)

Fuenzalida-Puelma, Hernán L. see **Connor, Susan Scholle**

Fujiwara, Paula I. see **Gasner, M. Rose**

Fujiwara, Paula I. see **Lerner, Barron H.**

Fukushima, Masanori. Clinical trials in Japan. *Nature Medicine.* 1995 Jan; 1(1): 12–13.
(HUMAN EXPERIMENTATION/FOREIGN COUNTRIES; HUMAN EXPERIMENTATION/REGULATION)

Fulford, K.W.M. Dissent and dissensus: the limits of consensus formation in psychiatry. *In:* ten Have, Henk A.M.J.; Sass, Hans-Martin, eds. Consensus Formation in Healthcare Ethics. Boston, MA: Kluwer Academic; 1998: 175–192.
(MENTAL HEALTH)

Fulford, K.W.M. see **Hope, R.A.**

Fullilove, Mindy Thompson. Comment: abandoning "race" as a variable in public health research -- an idea whose time has come. *American Journal of Public Health.* 1998 Sep; 88(9): 1297–1298.
(PUBLIC HEALTH)

Fulton, Forrest M. see **McNiel, Dale E.**

Furedi, Ann. Wrong but the right thing to do: public opinion and abortion. *In:* Lee, Ellie, ed. Abortion Law and Politics Today. New York, NY: St. Martin's Press; 1998: 159–171.
(ABORTION/ATTITUDES; ABORTION/FOREIGN COUNTRIES)

Furer, Julie J. see **Lafferty, Kevin J.**

Furlong, William see **Saigal, Saroj**

Fusilier, Marcelline; Manning, Michael R.; Villar, Armando J. Santini; Rodriguez, Daniel Torres. AIDS knowledge and attitudes of health-care workers in Mexico. *Journal of Social Psychology.* 1998 Apr; 138(2): 203–210.
(AIDS/HEALTH PERSONNEL)

Fusilier, Marcelline R.; Durlabhji, Subhash. Health care workers' AIDS attitudes and willingness to provide care -- India. *Journal of Health and Human Services Administration.* 1997 Fall; 20(2): 145–158.
(AIDS/HEALTH PERSONNEL)

Fuss, Michael. Health, illness, and healing in the great religions: I. Buddhism. *Dolentium Hominum: Church and Health in the World.* 1998; No. 37 [yr. 13(1)]: 108–111.
(HEALTH)

G

Gabbard, Glen O. Lessons to be learned from the study of sexual boundary violations. *American Journal of Psychotherapy.* 1996 Summer; 50(3): 311–322.
(FRAUD AND MISCONDUCT; PROFESSIONAL PATIENT RELATIONSHIP)

Gabrielson, Karin see **van der Valk, Jan**

Gadow, Sally. Whose body? Whose story? The question about narrative in women's health care. *Soundings.* 1994 Fall–Winter; 77(3–4): 295–307.
(HEALTH)

Galanos, Anthony N. see **Hamel, Mary Beth**

Gallo, Joseph J. see **Cooper-Patrick, Lisa**

Gallo, Pedro see **Serra-Prat, Mateu**

Galloway, John. Dogged by controversy [review of *The Brown Dog Affair*, by Peter Mason; and of *Lethal Laws: Animal Testing, Human Health, and Environmental Policy*, by Alix Fano]. [Book review essay]. *Nature.* 1998 Aug 13; 394(6694): 635–636.
(ANIMAL EXPERIMENTATION)

Gallucci, Denise. Making decisions about premature infants. *American Journal of Nursing.* 1998 Jun; 98(6): 64, 66.
(ALLOWING TO DIE/INFANTS; PATIENT CARE/MINORS)

Gallup, Gordon G.; Eddy, Timothy J. Animal facilities survey. *American Psychologist.* 1990 Mar; 45(3): 400–401.
(ANIMAL EXPERIMENTATION)

Galton, D.J.; Doyal, L. "Goodbye Dolly?" The ethics of human cloning. [Letter]. *Journal of Medical Ethics.* 1998 Aug; 24(4): 279.
(CLONING)

Galton, D.J.; Kay, A.; Cavanna, J.S. Human cloning: safety is the issue. [Letter]. *Nature Medicine.* 1998 Jun; 4(6): 644.
(CLONING)

Galton, David J. Greek theories on eugenics. *Journal of Medical Ethics.* 1998 Aug; 24(4): 263–267.
(EUGENICS; REPRODUCTION)

Gani, Akif see **Breimer, Lars**

Gans Epner, Janet E.; Jonas, Harry S.; Seckinger, Daniel L. Late-term abortion. *JAMA.* 1998 Aug 26;

280(8): 724–729.
(ABORTION)

Gansler, David A. see **Holzer, Jacob C.**

Ganz, Peter R. see **Tackaberry, Eilleen**

Ganzini, Linda; Johnston, Wendy S.; McFarland, Bentson H.; Tolle, Susan W.; Lee, Melinda A. Attitudes of patients with amyotrophic lateral sclerosis and their care givers toward assisted suicide. *New England Journal of Medicine.* 1998 Oct 1; 339(14): 967–973.
(SUICIDE)

Ganzini, Linda see **Back, Anthony**

Ganzini, Linda see **Lee, Melinda A.**

Ganzini, Linda see **Werth, James L.**

Garattini, Silvio. Alternatives to animal experiments: expectations and limitations. *In:* van Zutphen, L.F.M.; Balls, M., eds. Animal Alternatives, Welfare and Ethics. New York, NY: Elsevier; 1997: 55–66.
(ANIMAL EXPERIMENTATION)

Garattini, Silvio see **Bonati, Maurizio**

Garber, Judy E.; Offit, Kenneth; Olopade, O.I. (Funmi); Fink, Diane; Barbasch, Avi; Barr, Patricia; Gleeson, Robert K.; Le Stage, Barbara. The American Society of Clinical Oncology position on genetic testing: implications for health care providers: workshop no. 4. *Cancer.* 1997 Aug 1; 80(3, Suppl.): 632–634.
(GENETIC SCREENING)

García–Alonso, F.; Guallar, E.; Bakke, O.M.; Carné, X. Use and abuse of placebo in phase III trials. *European Journal Of Clinical Pharmacology.* 1998 Apr; 54(2): 101–105.
(HUMAN EXPERIMENTATION/RESEARCH DESIGN)

Garcia, Sandra Anderson. Sociocultural and legal implications of creating and sustaining life through biomedical technology. *Journal of Legal Medicine.* 1996 Dec; 17(4): 469–525.
(BIOMEDICAL TECHNOLOGIES; GENETIC INTERVENTION; REPRODUCTIVE TECHNOLOGIES)

Gardner, Martin see **Denley, Ian**

Garner, Robert. Animal research and pluralist politics: the British and American experience. *In:* van Zutphen, L.F.M.; Balls, M., eds. Animal Alternatives, Welfare and Ethics. New York, NY: Elsevier; 1997: 67–79.
(ANIMAL EXPERIMENTATION)

Garrafa, Volnei see **Diniz, Debora**

Garrett, Celia K. see **Reynolds, Don F.**

Garrett, Joanne see **Hanson, Laura C.**

Garrison, Jayne. Rushing heaven's door: assisted suicide -- do we really know what we want? *Health.* 1997 May/Jun; 11(4): 123–124, 126, 128–130.
(SUICIDE; TERMINAL CARE)

Garver, Kenneth L.; Santorum, Rick. Eugenics and Catholic medicine. *Ethics and Medics.* 1998 Jul; 23(7): 1–2.
(EUGENICS)

Gasner, M. Rose; Maw, Khin Lay; Feldman, Gabriel E.; Fujiwara, Paula I.; Frieden, Thomas R. The use of legal action in New York City to ensure treatment of tuberculosis. *New England Journal of Medicine.* 1999 Feb 4; 340(5): 359–366.
(PUBLIC HEALTH)

Gasner, M. Rose see **Lerner, Barron H.**

Gastmans, Chris. Care as a moral attitude in nursing. *Nursing Ethics.* 1999 May; 6(3): 214–223.
(NURSING ETHICS)

Gastmans, Chris. The significance of the Convention on Human Rights and Biomedicine of the Council of Europe for healthcare ethics committees. *HEC (HealthCare Ethics Committee) Forum.* 1998 Sep–Dec; 10(3–4): 350–358.
(BIOETHICS; ETHICISTS AND ETHICS COMMITTEES)

Gastmans, Chris; Dierckx de Casterle, Bernadette; Schotsmans, Paul. Nursing considered as moral practice: a philosophical–ethical interpretation of nursing. *Kennedy Institute of Ethics Journal.* 1998 Mar; 8(1): 43–69.
(NURSING ETHICS; PROFESSIONAL PATIENT RELATIONSHIP)

Gates, Elena. Two challenges for research ethics: innovative treatment and fetal therapy. *Women's Health Issues.* 1999 Jul–Aug; 9(4): 208–210.
(EMBRYO AND FETAL RESEARCH; HUMAN EXPERIMENTATION/SPECIAL POPULATIONS)

Gates, Elena see **Kim, H. Nina**

Gates, Elena A. New surgical procedures: can our patients benefit while we learn? [Article and discussion]. *American Journal of Obstetrics and Gynecology.* 1997 Jun; 176(6): 1293–1299.
(PATIENT CARE)

Gatter, Robert. Communicative ethics for bioethics. *Bioethics Examiner.* 1997 Fall; 1(3): 4–5.
(BIOETHICS)

Gatter, Robert see **Kuczewski, Mark G.**

Gaudiani, Vincent A. It's the patient. [Editorial]. *Pharos.* 1996 Fall; 59(4): 33.
(FRAUD AND MISCONDUCT; PROFESSIONAL PATIENT RELATIONSHIP)

Gavaghan, Helen. Embryo research tests NIH's mettle. [News]. *Nature Medicine.* 1995 Jan; 1(1): 5–6.
(EMBRYO AND FETAL RESEARCH)

Gavin, William J. On "tame" and "untamed" death: Jamesian reflections. *In:* McGee, Glenn, ed. Pragmatic Bioethics. Nashville, TN: Vanderbilt Univesity Press; 1999: 97–112, 269–271.
(DETERMINATION OF DEATH; TERMINAL CARE)

Gay, David see **Lynxwiler, John**

Gazelle, Gail see **Segal, Eran**

Gbadegesin, Segun. Bioethics and cultural diversity. *In:* Kuhse, Helga; Singer, Peter, eds. A Companion to Bioethics. Malden, MA: Blackwell; 1998: 24–31.
(BIOETHICS)

Gbadegesin, Segun see **Schüklenk, Udo**

Gbolade, Babatunde A.; Tan, K.H.; Teo, K.P.; Essex, Ben; Waldron, Mary A.; Foley, Elizabeth; Harindra, V.; Goodman, Meg; Olaitan, Adeola; Madge, Sara; Jones, Melvyn; Johnson, Margaret; Parazzini, Fabio; Ricci, Elena; Grasso, Paola; Surace, Matteo; Benzi, Guido; de Zulueta, Paquita. Reducing the vertical transmission of HIV. [Letters]. *BMJ (British Medical Journal).* 1998 Jun 20; 316(7148): 1899–1901.
(AIDS/TESTING AND SCREENING)

Gearhart, John. New potential for human embryonic stem cells. *Science.* 1998 Nov 6; 282(5391): 1061–1062.
(EMBRYO AND FETAL RESEARCH)

Gecik, Karol. The need to protect patients' rights. *Medicine and Law.* 1993; 12(1–2): 109–112.
(PATIENTS' RIGHTS)

Geller, G. see **Eisinger, F.**

Geller, G. see **James, C.A.**

Geller, Gail see **Dickenson, Donna L.**

Geltman, Paul L.; Meyers, Alan F. Immigration reporting laws: ethical dilemmas in pediatric practice. *American Journal of Public Health.* 1998 Jun; 88(6): 967–968.
(CONFIDENTIALITY/LEGAL ASPECTS)

Gelzer, J. see **Müller, H.J.**

Gemelli, Agostino. Against experimentation on human embryos. *European Journal of Genetics in Society.* 1997; 3(1): 13–15.
(EMBRYO AND FETAL RESEARCH)

General Conference of Seventh–Day Adventists. Christian View of Human Life Committee. The Seventh–Day Adventist Church Focuses on Ethical Issues. Washington, DC: General Conference of Seventh–Day Adventists; 1996 Jul. 39 p.
(BIOETHICS)

Genesen, Leigh B. see **Orr, Robert D.**

Genetics Forum (London). Public oppose insurers' genetic test policy. *Splice of Life.* 1997 Apr; 3(5): 10–11.
(GENETIC RESEARCH; GENETIC SCREENING)

Genetics Forum (London). The Case Against Patents in Genetic Engineering: A Special Report from the Genetics Forum. London: Genetics Forum; 1996 Apr. 28 p.
(GENETIC INTERVENTION; PATENTING LIFE FORMS)

Gerberding, Julie. Provider–to–patient HIV transmission: how to keep it exceedingly rare. [Editorial]. *Annals of Internal Medicine.* 1999 Jan 5; 130(1): 64–65.
(AIDS/HEALTH PERSONNEL)

Gersh, Bernard J. see **Schulman, Kevin A.**

Gervais, Karen G.; Priester, Reinhard; Vawter, Dorothy E.; Otte, Kimberly K.; Solberg, Mary M., eds. Ethical Challenges in Managed Care: A Casebook. Washington, DC: Georgetown University Press; 1999. 372 p.
(HEALTH CARE/ECONOMICS)

Gesmond, Sharyn A. see **Constantino, Rose E.**

Gesteland, Raymond see **Collins, Francis S.**

Gevers, Sjef. Population screening: the role of the law. *European Journal of Health Law.* 1998 Mar; 5(1): 7–18.
(GENETIC SCREENING; MASS SCREENING)

Gevers, Sjef. Third trimester abortion for fetal abnormality. *Bioethics.* 1999 Jul; 13(3–4): 306–313.
(ABORTION/FOREIGN COUNTRIES; ABORTION/LEGAL ASPECTS)

Gianakos, Dean. Conversations with Stella. *Annals of Internal Medicine.* 1999 Apr 20; 130(8): 698–699.
(PROFESSIONAL PATIENT RELATIONSHIP; TREATMENT REFUSAL)

Gianopoulos, John G. see **Muraskas, Jonathan**

Gibbons, John A. Who's your daddy?: a constitutional analysis of post–mortem insemination. [Comment]. *Journal of Contemporary Health Law and Policy.* 1997 Fall; 14(1): 187–210.
(REPRODUCTION; REPRODUCTIVE TECHNOLOGIES)

Gibeau, Anne M. Female genital mutilation: when a cultural practice generates clinical and ethical dilemmas. *Journal of Obstetric, Gynecologic and Neonatal Nursing.* 1998 Jan–Feb; 27(1): 85–91.
(HEALTH)

Gibson, Joan McIver. Mediation for ethics committees: a promising process. *Generations (American Society on Aging).* 1994 Winter; 18(4): 58–60.
(ETHICISTS AND ETHICS COMMITTEES)

Giesen, Dieter. Civil liability of physicians for new methods of treatment and experimentation: a comparative examination. *Medical Law Review.* 1995 Spring; 3(1): 22–52.
(HUMAN EXPERIMENTATION)

Giesen, Dieter. Compensation and consent: a brief comparative examination of liability for HIV–infected blood. *In:* Bennett, Rebecca; Erin, Charles A., eds. HIV and AIDS: Testing, Screening, and Confidentiality. New York, NY: Oxford University Press; 1999: 91–106.
(AIDS; BLOOD DONATION)

Gifford, Fred. Teaching scientific integrity. *Centennial Review.* 1994 Spring; 38(2): 297–314.
(BIOMEDICAL RESEARCH; FRAUD AND MISCONDUCT; PROFESSIONAL ETHICS/EDUCATION)

Gigli, Gian Luigi. The unfinished project: ethical problems and strategies for action on mental retardation. *Dolentium Hominum: Church and Health in the World.* 1997; 34(12th Yr., No. 1): 64–76.
(PATIENT CARE/MENTALLY DISABLED)

Gilbert, Bonny. Infertility and the ADA: health insurance coverage for infertility treatment. *Defense Council Journal.* 1996; 63(1): 42–57.

(PATIENT CARE; REPRODUCTIVE TECHNOLOGIES)

Gilbert, David see **Coulter, Angela**

Gilbert, Scott F. see **Pence, Gregory E.**

Gilbert, Thomas T. see **Culpepper, Larry**

Gilham, Charles; Leibold, Peter. A voice against physician–assisted suicide. [Cardinal Bernardin's letter; excerpts]. *Health Progress.* 1997 May–Jun; 78(3): 44–47.
(SUICIDE)

Gilham, Charles S. see **Leibold, Peter**

Gilhooly, Mary L.M.; Smith, Alexander McCall; Nichols, David, eds.; Scottish Action on Dementia. Rights and Legal Protection Sub–Committee. Dementia: Consent to Treatment, Volume 1 [and] Dementia: Consent to Research, Volume 2. Two Discussion Papers. Edinburgh, Scotland: Scottish Action on Dementia; 1992 Mar. 52 p.
(HUMAN EXPERIMENTATION/FOREIGN COUNTRIES; HUMAN EXPERIMENTATION/INFORMED CONSENT; HUMAN EXPERIMENTATION/SPECIAL POPULATIONS; INFORMED CONSENT/MENTALLY DISABLED)

Gilje, Fredricka see **Söderberg, Anna**

Gill, Denise see **Fisher, Carol**

Gill, Satvir see **Toth, Ellen L.**

Gillam, Lynn. Prenatal diagnosis and discrimination against the disabled. *Journal of Medical Ethics.* 1999 Apr; 25(2): 163–171.
(ABORTION; PRENATAL DIAGNOSIS)

Gillam, Lynn. The 'more–abortions' objection to fetal tissue transplantation. *Journal of Medicine and Philosophy.* 1998 Aug; 23(4): 411–427.
(ABORTION; FETUSES; ORGAN AND TISSUE DONATION)

Gillam, Lynn see **van Hooft, Stan**

Gillespie, Rosemary. Women, the body and brand extension in medicine: cosmetic surgery and the paradox of choice. *Women and Health.* 1996; 24(4): 69–85.
(HEALTH; PATIENT CARE)

Gillett, Grant. The ethical challenge of sick children. *Pediatrician.* 1990; 17(2): 59–62.
(PATIENT CARE/MINORS)

Gilligan, Mary Ann; Jensen, Norman. Use of advance directives: a survey in three clinics. *Wisconsin Medical Journal.* 1995; 94(5): 239–243.
(ADVANCE DIRECTIVES)

Gilligan, Timothy; Raffin, Thomas A. End-of-life discussions with patients: timing and truth–telling. [Editorial]. *Chest.* 1996 Jan; 109(1): 11–12.
(ALLOWING TO DIE; PROFESSIONAL PATIENT RELATIONSHIP; TRUTH DISCLOSURE)

Gillon, Raanan. Confidentiality. *In:* Kuhse, Helga; Singer, Peter, eds. A Companion to Bioethics. Malden, MA: Blackwell; 1998: 425–431.
(CONFIDENTIALITY)

Gillon, Raanan. Ethical issues. *In:* Weber, Walter;

Mulvihill, John J.; Narod, Steven A., eds. Familial Cancer Management. Boca Raton, FL: CRC Press; 1996: 142–158.
(GENETIC INTERVENTION; GENETIC SCREENING; PATIENT CARE)

Gillon, Raanan. Eugenics, contraception, abortion and ethics. [Editorial]. *Journal of Medical Ethics.* 1998 Aug; 24(4): 219–220.
(ABORTION; CONTRACEPTION; EUGENICS)

Gillon, Raanan. Euthanasia in the Netherlands -- down the slippery slope? [Editorial]. *Journal of Medical Ethics.* 1999 Feb; 25(1): 3–4.
(EUTHANASIA; SUICIDE)

Gillon, Raanan. 'Wrongful life' claims. [Editorial]. *Journal of Medical Ethics.* 1998 Dec; 24(6): 363–364.
(GENETIC COUNSELING; WRONGFUL LIFE)

Gillott, John. Childhood testing for carrier status: the perspectives of the Genetic Interest Group. *In:* Clarke, Angus, ed. The Genetic Testing of Children. Washington, DC: BIOS Scientific Publishers; 1998: 97–102.
(GENETIC SCREENING)

Gilman, Sander L. Making the Body Beautiful: A Cultural History of Aesthetic Surgery. Princeton, NJ: Princeton University Press; 1999. 396 p.
(PATIENT CARE)

Gin, Brian R. Genetic discrimination: Huntington's disease and the Americans with Disabilities Act. [Note]. *Columbia Law Review.* 1997 Jun; 97(5): 1406–1434.
(GENETIC SCREENING)

Ginsberg, Harley G. see **Goldsmith, Jay P.**

Ginzberg, Eli. The uncertain future of managed care. *New England Journal of Medicine.* 1999 Jan 14; 340(2): 144–146.
(HEALTH CARE/ECONOMICS)

Ginzberg, Eli. US health system reform in the early 21st century. *JAMA.* 1998 Nov 4; 280(17): 1539.
(HEALTH CARE/ECONOMICS)

Githens, Marianne; Stetson, Dorothy McBride, eds. Abortion Politics: Public Policy in Cross-Cultural Perspective. New York, NY: Routledge; 1996. 234 p.
(ABORTION/FOREIGN COUNTRIES; ABORTION/LEGAL ASPECTS)

Glahn, Sandra see **Cutrer, William**

Glannon, Walter. The ethics of human cloning. *Public Affairs Quarterly.* 1998 Jul; 12(3): 287–305.
(CLONING)

Glantz, Leonard H.; Annas, George J.; Grodin, Michael A.; Mariner, Wendy K. Research in developing countries: taking "benefit" seriously. *Hastings Center Report.* 1998 Nov–Dec; 28(6): 38–42.
(HEALTH CARE/ECONOMICS; HEALTH CARE/FOREIGN COUNTRIES; HUMAN EXPERIMENTATION/FOREIGN COUNTRIES)

Glantz, Leonard H. see **Merson, Michael H.**

Glantz, Leonard H. see **Roche, Patricia**

Glasner, Peter; Rothman, Harry, eds. Genetic Imaginations: Ethical, Legal and Social Issues in Human Genome Research. Brookfield, VT: Ashgate; 1998. 140 p.
(GENOME MAPPING)

Glass, Kathleen Cranley; Weijer, Charles; Lemmens, Trudo; Palmour, Roberta M.; Shapiro, Stanley H. Structuring the review of human genetics protocols, Part II: diagnostic and screening studies. *IRB: A Review of Human Subjects Research.* 1997 May–Aug; 19(3–4): 1–13.
(GENETIC RESEARCH; GENETIC SCREENING; HUMAN EXPERIMENTATION/ETHICS COMMITTEES)

Glasser, Ronald J. The doctor is not in: on the managed failure of managed health care. *Harper's Magazine.* 1998 Mar; 296(1774): 35–41.
(HEALTH CARE/ECONOMICS)

Glazer, Ellen Sarasohn see **Cooper, Susan Lewis**

Gledhill, Julia see **McFadyen, Anne**

Gleeson, Robert K. see **Garber, Judy E.**

Gleeson, Robert K. see **MacKay, Charles**

Glen, Sally. Educating for interprofessional collaboration: teaching about values. *Nursing Ethics.* 1999 May; 6(3): 202–213.
(PROFESSIONAL ETHICS/EDUCATION)

Glen, Sally. Health care education for dialogue and dialogic relationships. *Nursing Ethics.* 1999 Jan; 6(1): 3–11.
(PROFESSIONAL ETHICS/EDUCATION)

Glending, Susanne see **Fasting, Ulla**

Glendon, Mary Ann; Treene, Eric W. The legacy of Justice William Brennan. *Human Life Review.* 1998 Winter; 24(1): 65–76.
(ABORTION/LEGAL ASPECTS)

Glick, Shimon. Ethical aspects of organ transplantation. *Jewish Medical Ethics.* 1997 Jan; 3(1): 11–13.
(ORGAN AND TISSUE DONATION; ORGAN AND TISSUE TRANSPLANTATION)

Glick, Shimon M. Euthanasia: an unbiased decision? *American Journal of Medicine.* 1997 Mar; 102(3): 294–296.
(EUTHANASIA; SUICIDE)

Glick, Shimon M. see **Yakir, Avi**

Glickman, Barry. Global challenges: ethical implications of the greening of modern Western medicine. *In:* Coward, Harold; Ratanakul, Pinit, eds. A Cross–Cultural Dialogue on Health Care Ethics. Waterloo, ON: Wilfrid Laurier University Press; 1999: 236–256.
(PATIENT CARE/DRUGS)

Glover, Eric. French panel calls for closer monitoring of genetic modification. [News]. *Nature.* 1998 Jul 2; 394(6688): 4.
(GENETIC INTERVENTION; RECOMBINANT DNA RESEARCH/REGULATION)

Glover, Jacqueline J. see **Hines, Stephen C.**

Glover, Jonathan. Eugenics: some lessons from the Nazi experience. *In:* Harris, John; Holm, Søren, eds. The Future of Human Reproduction: Ethics, Choice, and Regulation. New York, NY: Oxford University Press; 1998: 55–65.
(EUGENICS)

Glover, Nicola. Community care -- same problems, different epithet? *Journal of Medical Ethics.* 1998 Oct; 24(5): 336–340.
(INVOLUNTARY COMMITMENT/FOREIGN COUNTRIES; PATIENT CARE/MENTALLY DISABLED)

Gluck, John P. Change during a life in animal research: the loss and regaining of ambivalence. *In:* Hart, Lynette A., ed. Responsible Conduct with Animals in Research. New York, NY: Oxford University Press; 1998: 30–48.
(ANIMAL EXPERIMENTATION)

Godfrey–Faussett, Peter; Baggaley, Rachel; Brewster, M.F. Exceptionalism in HIV. [Letters]. *BMJ (British Medical Journal).* 1998 Jun 13; 316(7147): 1826.
(AIDS/TESTING AND SCREENING)

Godfrey–Faussett, Peter see **Edi–Osagie, E.C.O.**

Godkin, Diane see **Toth, Ellen L.**

Goerl, Hans S. Who's that fish on my line? The dangers of electronic distribution of genetic information. *In:* Smith, Edward; Sapp, Walter, eds. Plain Talk about the Human Genome Project: A Tuskegee University Conference on Its Promise and Perils ... and Matters of Race. Tuskegee, AL: Tuskegee University Press; 1997: 201–203.
(GENETIC SERVICES)

Goetschius, Suzanne K. Families and end–of–life care: how do we meet their needs? *Journal of Gerontological Nursing.* 1997 Mar; 23(3): 43–49.
(TERMINAL CARE)

Goff, Robert. A matter of life and death. *Medical Law Review.* 1995 Spring; 3(1): 1–21.
(ALLOWING TO DIE/LEGAL ASPECTS; EUTHANASIA/LEGAL ASPECTS; TERMINAL CARE)

Gohar, Josef see **Sheiner, Eyal**

Gold, Marthe R. see **Menzel, Paul**

Gold, Rachel Benson; Richards, Cory L. Managed care and unintended pregnancy. *Women's Health Issues.* 1998 May–Jun; 8(3): 134–147.
(CONTRACEPTION; HEALTH CARE/ECONOMICS)

Gold, Richard. Owning our bodies: an examination of property law and biotechnology. *San Diego Law Review.* 1995; 32(4): 1167–1247.
(BIOMEDICAL RESEARCH; ORGAN AND TISSUE DONATION)

Goldbeck–Wood, Sandra. Bavaria forced to lift abortion restrictions. [News]. *BMJ (British Medical Journal).* 1998 Nov 7; 317(7168): 1272.
(ABORTION/FOREIGN COUNTRIES)

Goldberg, Alan M. see **Zurlo, Joanne**

Goldberg, Carey. DNA databanks giving police a powerful weapon, and critics. [News]. *New York Times.* 1998 Feb 19: A1, A12.
(DNA FINGERPRINTING)

Goldberg, Carey. Insurance for Viagra spurs coverage for birth control. [News]. *New York Times.* 1999 Jun 30: A1, A16.
(CONTRACEPTION; PATIENT CARE/DRUGS)

Goldberg, David J. see **Simpson, Wendy M.**

Goldberg, Susan L. Legal aspects of restraint use in hospitals and nursing homes. *HEC (HealthCare Ethics Committee) Forum.* 1998 Sep–Dec; 10(3–4): 276–289.
(BEHAVIOR CONTROL; PATIENT CARE)

Golden, Frederic. Good eggs, bad eggs: the growing power of prenatal genetic tests is raising thorny new questions about ethics, fairness and privacy. *Time.* 1999 Jan 11; 153(1): 56–59.
(GENETIC SCREENING; PRENATAL DIAGNOSIS)

Golden, Frederic. The ice babies: long-lost frozen embryos are popping up all over. [News]. *Time.* 1998 Mar 2; 151(8): 65.
(FETUSES; REPRODUCTIVE TECHNOLOGIES)

Golden, Frederic; Silver, Lee M. Boy? Girl? Up to you [and] A quandary that isn't. *Time.* 1998 Sep 21; 152(12): 82–83.
(REPRODUCTIVE TECHNOLOGIES; SEX PRESELECTION)

Goldenberg, Robert L. see **Stringer, Jeffrey S.A.**

Goldfarb, Johanna see **Lawry, Kathleen**

Golding, J. see **West, Charles**

Goldman, Howard H. see **Rosenheck, Robert**

Goldman, Lee see **Emanuel, Ezekiel J.**

Goldman, Lee see **Hamel, Mary Beth**

Goldman, Marina. Physical restraints. [Bibliography]. *HEC (HealthCare Ethics Committee) Forum.* 1998 Sep–Dec; 10(3–4): 323–337.
(BEHAVIOR CONTROL; PATIENT CARE)

Goldsmith, Jay P.; Ginsberg, Harley G.; McGettigan, Marie C. Ethical decisions in the delivery room. *Clinics in Perinatology.* 1996 Sep; 23(3): 529–550.
(ALLOWING TO DIE/INFANTS; RESUSCITATION ORDERS; SELECTION FOR TREATMENT)

Goldstein, Doris Mueller, comp. Bibliography of resources by and about André Hellegers. *Kennedy Institute of Ethics Journal.* 1999 Mar; 9(1): 89–107.
(BIOETHICS)

Goldstein, Mark R. see **Nightingale, Stuart L.**

Goldworth, Amnon. Informed consent in the genetic age. *Cambridge Quarterly of Healthcare Ethics.* 1999 Summer; 8(3): 393–400.
(CONFIDENTIALITY; GENETIC SCREENING; INFORMED CONSENT)

Goldworth, Amnon see **Stevenson, David K.**

Golub, Edward S. Finding a vocabulary for the extrascientific significance of technology. *Nature Biotechnology.* 1997 May; 15(5): 394.
(CLONING; GENETIC INTERVENTION)

Golway, Terry. Life in the 90's. [Peter Singer]. *America.* 1998 Sep 12; 179(6): 4.
(ETHICISTS AND ETHICS COMMITTEES)

Gómez, Laura E. Misconceiving Mothers: Legislators, Prosecutors, and the Politics of Prenatal Drug Exposure. Philadelphia, PA: Temple University Press; 1997. 207 p.
(PRENATAL INJURIES)

Gómez–Zapata, M. see **Pacheco, R.**

Gonen, Julianna S. Managed care and unintended pregnancy: testing the limits of prevention. *Women's Health Issues.* 1999 Mar–Apr; 9(2, Suppl.): 26S–35S.
(CONTRACEPTION; CONTRACEPTION/MINORS; HEALTH CARE/ECONOMICS)

Gonzales, Junius J. see **Cooper–Patrick, Lisa**

Goode, E.L. see **Jaeger, A.S.**

Goodey, Chris; Alderson, Priscilla; Appleby, John. The ethical implications of antenatal screening for Down's syndrome: Socratic inquiry; The good life?; [and] Calculating the costs and benefits. *Bulletin of Medical Ethics.* 1999 Apr; No. 147: 13–17.
(PRENATAL DIAGNOSIS)

Goodey, Christopher see **Alderson, Priscilla**

Goodman, Kenneth W. A DiMaggio rule on medical privacy. *New York Times.* 1998 Dec 30: A17.
(CONFIDENTIALITY; HEALTH)

Goodman, Kenneth W. Critical care computing: outcomes, confidentiality, and appropriate use. *Critical Care Clinics.* 1996 Jan; 12(1): 109–122.
(CONFIDENTIALITY; PATIENT CARE)

Goodman, Kenneth W. Philosophy as news: bioethics, journalism and public policy. *Journal of Medicine and Philosophy.* 1999 Apr; 24(2): 181–200.
(BIOETHICS; ETHICISTS AND ETHICS COMMITTEES)

Goodman, Meg see **Gbolade, Babatunde A.**

Goodman, Steven N. see **Sugarman, Jeremy**

Goodwin, James S. Geriatrics and the limits of modern medicine. *New England Journal of Medicine.* 1999 Apr 22; 340(16): 1283–1285.
(PATIENT CARE/AGED)

Goodwin, Peter A. see **Koenig, Kristi L.**

Goold, Susan Dorr. Money and trust: relationships between patients, physicians, and health plans. *Journal of Health Politics, Policy and Law.* 1998 Aug; 23(4): 687–695.
(HEALTH CARE/ECONOMICS)

Gordon, Bruce see **Prentice, Ernest D.**

Gordon, Jon W. Genetic enhancement in humans. *Science.* 1999 Mar 26; 283(5410): 2023–2024.
(GENETIC INTERVENTION)

Gordon, Judith R. see **Werth, James L.**

Gordon, Lisa B. see **Tishler, L. Carl**

Gordon, Meg. Space monkeys 'were put at risk.' [News]. *New Scientist.* 1997 May 3; 154(2080): 6.
(ANIMAL EXPERIMENTATION)

Gordon, Nancy P.; Shade, Starley P. Advance directives are more likely among seniors asked about end–of–life care preferences. *Archives of Internal Medicine.* 1999 Apr 12; 159(7): 701–704.
(ADVANCE DIRECTIVES)

Gordon, Todd E.; Zook, Eric G.; Averhoff, Francisco M.; Williams, Walter W. Consent for adolescent vaccination: issues and current practices. *Journal of School Health.* 1997 Sep; 67(7): 259–264.
(IMMUNIZATION; INFORMED CONSENT/MINORS)

Gorecki, Julie see **Daly, Barbara J.**

Gorelick, Philip B.; Harris, Yvonne; Burnett, Barbara; Bonecutter, Faith J. The recruitment triangle: reasons why African Americans enroll, refuse to enroll, or voluntarily withdraw from a clinical trial: an interim report from the African–American Antiplatelet Stroke Prevention Study (AAASPS). *Journal of the National Medical Association.* 1998 Mar; 90(3): 141–145.
(HUMAN EXPERIMENTATION/SPECIAL POPULATIONS)

Gorenflo, Daniel W. see **Doukas, David J.**

Gorlin, Rena A., ed. Health: allied health, chiropractic, dentistry, medicine, mental health, nursing, pharmacy, social work. *In: her* Codes of Professional Responsibility: Ethics Standards in Business, Health, and Law. Fourth Edition. Washington, DC: Bureau of National Affairs; 1999: 253–548.
(PROFESSIONAL ETHICS/CODES OF ETHICS)

Gormley, Siobhan M. see **Simpson, Wendy M.**

Gorney, Cynthia. Articles of Faith: A Frontline History of the Abortion Wars. New York, NY: Simon and Schuster; 1998. 575 p.
(ABORTION)

Gorney, Cynthia see **Wright, Robert**

Gosden, Roger. Designing Babies: The Brave New World of Reproductive Technology. New York, NY: W.H. Freeman; 1999. 260 p.
(GENETIC INTERVENTION; REPRODUCTIVE TECHNOLOGIES)

Gostin, Lawrence O.; Feldblum, Chai; Webber, David W. Disability discrimination in America: HIV/AIDS and other health conditions. *JAMA.* 1999 Feb 24; 281(8): 745–752.
(AIDS; HEALTH)

Gostin, Lawrence O.; Hadley, Jack. Health services research: public benefits, personal privacy, and proprietary interests. [Editorial]. *Annals of Internal Medicine.* 1998 Nov 15; 129(10): 833–835.
(CONFIDENTIALITY; HEALTH CARE)

Gostin, Lawrence O.; Webber, David W. The AIDS Litigation Project: HIV/AIDS in the courts in the 1990s, part 1. *AIDS and Public Policy Journal.* 1997 Winter; 12(4): 105–121.
(AIDS)

Gostin, Lawrence O.; Webber, David W. The AIDS Litigation Project: HIV/AIDS in the courts in the 1990s, part 2. *AIDS and Public Policy Journal.* 1998 Spring; 13(1): 3–19.
(AIDS; AIDS/CONFIDENTIALITY)

Gostin, Lawrence O. see **Solomon, Liza**

Goto, Takahisa see **Nakata, Yoshinori**

Gottesman, Irving I. see **Faraone, Stephen V.**

Gottlich, Vicki. Protection for nursing facility residents under the ADA. *Generations (American Society on Aging).* 1994 Winter; 18(4): 43–47.
(PATIENT CARE/AGED)

Gottlieb, Scott. NCI defends research involving minority groups. [News]. *Nature Medicine.* 1999 Mar; 5(3): 254.
(BIOMEDICAL RESEARCH; HUMAN EXPERIMENTATION/SPECIAL POPULATIONS)

Gough, Pippa see **Selby, Mary**

Gould, Randi see **MacKay, Charles**

Gould, Stephen Jay. Individuality: cloning and the discomfiting cases of Siamese twins. *Sciences.* 1997 Sep–Oct; 37(5): 14–16.
(CLONING; PERSONHOOD)

Govaerts, I. see **Englert, Y.**

Gozdek, Nina see **Wronska, Irena**

Graber, Glenn C. see **Walsh, Marie E.**

Grabois, Ellen W. The liability of psychotherapists for breach of confidentiality. *Journal of Law and Health.* 1997–98; 12(1): 39–84.
(CONFIDENTIALITY/LEGAL ASPECTS; CONFIDENTIALITY/MENTAL HEALTH)

Gracely, Edward see **Feldman, Debra S.**

Gracia, Diego. What kind of values? A historical perspective on the ends of medicine. *In:* Hanson, Mark J.; Callahan, Daniel, eds. The Goals of Medicine: The Forgotten Issue in Health Care Reform. Washington, DC: Georgetown University Press; 1999: 88–100.
(HEALTH)

Grady, Christine. Science in the service of healing. *Hastings Center Report.* 1998 Nov–Dec; 28(6): 34–38.
(AIDS/HUMAN EXPERIMENTATION; HUMAN EXPERIMENTATION/FOREIGN COUNTRIES; HUMAN EXPERIMENTATION/RESEARCH DESIGN; HUMAN EXPERIMENTATION/SPECIAL POPULATIONS)

Grady, Christine see **Dickert, Neal**

Grady, Denise. Fraud found in analyzing breast cancer. [News]. *New York Times.* 1999 Feb 6: A13.
(FRAUD AND MISCONDUCT; HUMAN EXPERIMENTATION/REGULATION)

Grady, Denise. Live donors revolutionize liver care. [News]. *New York Times.* 1999 Aug 2: A1, A12.
(ORGAN AND TISSUE DONATION)

Grady, Denise. Patient or guinea pig? Dilemma of clinical trials. [News]. *New York Times.* 1999 Jan 5: F1, F4.

(HUMAN EXPERIMENTATION/INFORMED CONSENT)

Graff, Sylvester see **Rigali, Justin**

Graham, Amanda; McDonald, Jim; Association of Canadian Universities for Northern Studies. Board Committee on Revising the Ethical Principles. Ethical Principles for the Conduct of Research in the North. Ottawa, ON: Association of Canadian Universities for Northern Studies; 1998. 28 p.
(HUMAN EXPERIMENTATION/FOREIGN COUNTRIES; HUMAN EXPERIMENTATION/SPECIAL POPULATIONS)

Graham, I.M.F. see **Evans, Donald**

Graham, John Remington. Natural law, our constitutions, and the unborn. *Revue Generale de Droit.* 1996; 27(1): 21–53.
(ABORTION/FOREIGN COUNTRIES; ABORTION/LEGAL ASPECTS)

Graham, Peter E.; Miller, Norman M.; Harel–Raviv, Mili. The law and ethics in relation to dentists treating HIV–positive patients: two recent court cases. *Journal of the Canadian Dental Association.* 1995 Jun; 61(6): 487–491.
(AIDS/HEALTH PERSONNEL)

Graham, Philip see **Arnold, L. Eugene**

Graham, Wendy J.; Newell, Marie–Louise. Seizing the opportunity: collaborative initiatives to reduce HIV and maternal mortality. *Lancet.* 1999 Mar 6; 353(9155): 836–839.
(AIDS; HEALTH; HEALTH CARE/FOREIGN COUNTRIES)

Gramelspacher, Gregory P.; Zhou, Xiao–Hua; Hanna, Mark P.; Tierney, William M. Preferences of physicians and their patients for end–of–life care. *Journal of General Internal Medicine.* 1997 Jun; 12(6): 346–351.
(ALLOWING TO DIE/ATTITUDES; TERMINAL CARE)

Gramelspacher, Gregory P. see **Smith, David H.**

Granbois, Judith A. see **Smith, David H.**

Grant, Sharon. Physician–assisted suicide: a chaplain's perspective. *Humane Health Care International.* 1997 Spring; 13(1): 21–24.
(SUICIDE)

Grassin, Marc see **Letvak, Richard**

Grasso, Paola see **Gbolade, Babatunde A.**

Gray, Diana M. see **Perkins, David V.**

Gray, Gwen. Access to medical care under strain: new pressures in Canada and Australia. *Journal of Health Politics, Policy and Law.* 1998 Dec; 23(6): 905–947.
(HEALTH CARE/ECONOMICS; HEALTH CARE/FOREIGN COUNTRIES)

Gray, Paul. Cursed by eugenics. *Time.* 1999 Jan 11; 153(1): 84–85.
(EUGENICS)

Great Britain. Advisory Committee on Genetic Testing. Genetic research and ethics. *Bulletin of Medical Ethics.* 1999 Feb; No. 145: 21–24.
(GENETIC RESEARCH; GENETIC SCREENING)

Great Britain. England. High Court of Justice, Family Division. Re D (A Minor) (Wardship:Sterilisation). *All England Law Reports.* 1975 Sep 17. 1976: 326–336.
(STERILIZATION/MENTALLY DISABLED)

Great Britain. England. High Court of Justice. Family Division. Re H (Mental Patients: Diagnosis). *Family Law Reports.* 1992 Jul 1 (date of decision). [1993] 1: 28–33.
(INFORMED CONSENT/MENTALLY DISABLED)

Great Britain. England. High Court of Justice, Family Division. Re K, W and H (Minors) (Medical Treatment). *Family Law Reports.* 1992 Sep 10 (date of decision). 1993: 854–859.
(INFORMED CONSENT/MENTALLY DISABLED; INFORMED CONSENT/MINORS; TREATMENT REFUSAL/MENTALLY DISABLED; TREATMENT REFUSAL/MINORS)

Great Britain. Health Departments of the United Kingdom. Advisory Committee on Genetic Testing. Code of practice on human genetic testing services supplied direct to the public. *Community Genetics.* 1998; 1(1): 48.
(GENETIC SCREENING; GENETIC SERVICES)

Great Britain. Human Fertilisation and Embryology Authority. Code of Practice. Fourth Edition. London: The Authority; 1998. 76 p.
(REPRODUCTIVE TECHNOLOGIES)

Great Britain. Human Fertilisation and Embryology Authority. Sixth Annual Report [1995–1996]. London: The Authority; 1997. 45 p.
(EMBRYO AND FETAL RESEARCH; IN VITRO FERTILIZATION; REPRODUCTIVE TECHNOLOGIES)

Great Britain. Human Fertilisation and Embryology Authority see **Human Genetics Advisory Commission (Great Britain)**

Great Britain. Parliament. House of Commons. Science and Technology Committee. Association of British Insurers' Policy Statement on Life Insurance and Genetics. Second Report. London: The Stationery Office; 1997 Feb 19. 7 p.
(GENETIC SCREENING)

Greece. Circular No. 4548 of 13 Jun 1990 on indications and deontological principles in respect of laboratory tests for the detection of antibodies to the human immunodeficiency virus (HIV). [Summary]. *International Digest of Health Legislation.* 1994. 45(4). 501–502.
(AIDS/TESTING AND SCREENING)

Greely, H.T. see **McConnell, L.M.**

Greely, Henry T. Genomics research and human subjects. [Editorial]. *Science.* 1998 Oct 23; 282(5389): 625.
(GENETIC RESEARCH; HUMAN EXPERIMENTATION)

Greely, Henry T. see **Koenig, Barbara A.**

Greely, Henry T. see **Tessman, Irwin**

Green, Alexander R. see **Carrillo, J. Emilio**

Green, Diane C. see **Kao, Audiey C.**

Green, Gill. AIDS and euthanasia. *AIDS Care.* 1995;

7(Suppl. 2): S169–S173.
(AIDS; EUTHANASIA/ATTITUDES; SUICIDE)

Green, Michael J.; Fost, Norman. Seven reasons for Wisconsin physicians to oppose proposed legislation to legalize physician–assisted suicide. *Wisconsin Medical Journal.* 1995 Dec; 94(12): 693–695.
(SUICIDE)

Green, T. see **Wiggins, S.**

Greenberg, Daniel S. DNA in the mortuary. *Washington Post.* 1999 Jan 1: A25.
(DNA FINGERPRINTING)

Greenberg, Daniel S. When institutional review boards fail the system. [News]. *Lancet.* 1999 May 22; 353(9166): 1773.
(HUMAN EXPERIMENTATION/ETHICS COMMITTEES)

Greene, David. The use of service learning in client environments to enhance ethical reasoning in students. *American Journal of Occupational Therapy.* 1997 Nov–Dec; 51(10): 844–852.
(PROFESSIONAL ETHICS/EDUCATION)

Greene, Kathryn; Serovich, Julianne M. Appropriateness of disclosure of HIV testing information: the perspective of the PLWAs [people living with HIV/AIDS]. *Journal of Applied Communication Research.* 1996 Feb; 24(1): 50–65.
(AIDS/CONFIDENTIALITY)

Greenfield, Barak; Kaufman, Jeffrey L.; Hueston, William J.; Mainous, Arch G.; DeBakey, Lois; DeBakey, Selma; Rennie, Drummond; Yank, Veronica; Emanuel, Linda. Authors vs contributors: accuracy, accountability, and responsibility. [Letters and response]. *JAMA.* 1998 Feb 4; 279(5): 356–357.
(BIOMEDICAL RESEARCH; FRAUD AND MISCONDUCT)

Greenfield, L. John see **Segal, Eran**

Greenhalgh, Trisha; Hurwitz, Brian. Why study narrative? Narrative based medicine. *BMJ (British Medical Journal).* 1999 Jan 2; 318(7175): 48–50.
(PROFESSIONAL PATIENT RELATIONSHIP)

Greenwood, Roger N. see **Chandna, Shahid M.**

Greer, Margaret see **Sprague, Joey**

Grey, Matthew W. Medical use of marijuana: legal and ethical conflicts in the patient/physician relationship. [Comment]. *University of Richmond Law Review.* 1996 Jan; 30(1): 249–274.
(PATIENT CARE/DRUGS; PROFESSIONAL PATIENT RELATIONSHIP)

Griffin, Linner Ward see **Bratton, Letitia B.**

Griffith, David. Reasons for not seeing drug representatives: lightening workload, cutting costs, and improving quality. [Editorial]. *BMJ (British Medical Journal).* 1999 Jul 10; 319(7202): 69–70.
(HEALTH CARE/ECONOMICS; PATIENT CARE/DRUGS)

Griffith, Ezra E.H. Ethics in forensic psychiatry: a cultural response to Stone and Appelbaum. *Journal of the American Academy of Psychiatry and the Law.* 1998; 26(2): 171–184.

(MEDICAL ETHICS)

Griffiths, John; Bood, Alex; Weyers, Heleen. Euthanasia and Law in the Netherlands. Amsterdam: Amsterdam University Press; 1998. 382 p.
(EUTHANASIA/LEGAL ASPECTS)

Griffiths, John R. Consent –– Scots law and the patient's right to know. *Medicine and Law.* 1996; 15(1): 1–6.
(INFORMED CONSENT)

Griffiths, Pauline. Physician–assisted suicide and voluntary euthanasia: is it time the UK law caught up? *Nursing Ethics.* 1999 Mar; 6(2): 107–117.
(EUTHANASIA/LEGAL ASPECTS; SUICIDE)

Grimes, David A. A 26–year–old woman seeking an abortion. *JAMA.* 1999 Sep 22–29; 282(12): 1169–1175.
(ABORTION)

Grimes, David A. The continuing need for late abortions. *JAMA.* 1998 Aug 26; 280(8): 747–750.
(ABORTION)

Grisez, Germain. About health care issues. *In: his* The Way of the Lord Jesus. Volume 3: Difficult Moral Questions. Chicago, IL: Franciscan Herald Press; 1997: 203–419.
(BIOETHICS)

Grisolía, Santiago. Ethical and social aspects of the Human Genome Project. [Meeting report]. *Impact of Science on Society.* 1991; 41[1(161)]: 37–43.
(GENOME MAPPING)

Grisso, Jeane Ann; Battistini, Michelle; Ryan, Lesley. Women's health textbooks: codifying science and calling for change. *Annals of Internal Medicine.* 1998 Dec 1; 129(11): 916–918.
(HEALTH; HEALTH CARE)

Grisso, Thomas see **Appelbaum, Binyamin C.**

Grisso, Thomas see **Appelbaum, Paul S.**

Grodin, Michael A. see **Annas, George J.**

Grodin, Michael A. see **Glantz, Leonard H.**

Grodin, Michael A. see **Limentani, Alexander E.**

Grodin, Michael A. see **Mann, Jonathan, M.**

Grodin, Michael A. see **Merson, Michael H.**

Grodin, Michael A. see **Roche, Patricia A.**

Grody, Wayne W.; Pyeritz, Reed E. Report card on molecular genetic testing: room for improvement? [Editorial]. *JAMA.* 1999 Mar 3; 281(9): 845–847.
(GENETIC SCREENING; GENETIC SERVICES)

Groopman, Jerome. The moral way to pay for human organs. *New York Times.* 1999 May 7: A27.
(ORGAN AND TISSUE DONATION)

Gross, Cary P.; Anderson, Gerard F.; Powe, Neil R. The relation between funding by the National Institutes of Health and the burden of disease. *New England Journal of Medicine.* 1999 Jun 17; 340(24): 1881–1887.
(BIOMEDICAL RESEARCH; RESOURCE ALLOCATION)

Gross, Jane. The fight to cover infertility: suit says employer's refusal to pay is form of bias. [News]. *New York Times.* 1998 Dec 7: B1, B6.
(HEALTH CARE/ECONOMICS; REPRODUCTIVE TECHNOLOGIES)

Gross, Michael L. Autonomy and paternalism in communitarian society: patient rights in Israel. *Hastings Center Report.* 1999 Jul–Aug; 29(4): 13–20.
(PATIENTS' RIGHTS)

Grossman, Joy M. see **Cunningham, Peter J.**

Grossman, Linda S. see **Klamen, Debra L.**

Grossmann, Atina. The debate that will not end: the politics of abortion in Germany from Weimar to National Socialism and the postwar period. *In:* Berg, Manfred; Cocks, Geoffrey, eds. Medicine and Modernity: Public Health and Medical Care in Nineteenth- and Twentieth-Century Germany. New York, NY: Cambridge University Press; 1997: 193–211.
(ABORTION/FOREIGN COUNTRIES; ABORTION/LEGAL ASPECTS)

Groveman, Sherri A. The Hanukkah bush: ethical implications in the clinical management of intersex. *Journal of Clinical Ethics.* 1998 Winter; 9(4): 356–359.
(PATIENT CARE/MINORS; TRUTH DISCLOSURE)

Groves, Julian see **Arluke, Arnold**

Grubb, Andrew. Access to medical records — Breen v. Williams. [Comment]. *Medical Law Review.* 1995 Spring; 3(1): 102–107.
(PATIENT ACCESS TO RECORDS)

Grubb, Andrew. Assisting suicide: Sue Rodriguez v. Attorney General of Canada and Others. [Comment]. *Medical Law Review.* 1994 Spring; 2(1): 119–126.
(SUICIDE)

Grubb, Andrew. Attempted murder of terminally ill patient: R. v. Cox. [Comment]. *Medical Law Review.* 1993 Summer; 1(2): 232–234.
(EUTHANASIA/LEGAL ASPECTS)

Grubb, Andrew. Competent adult: refusal of treatment (renal dialysis) — Re J.T. (Adult: Refusal of Treatment). [Comment]. *Medical Law Review.* 1998 Spring; 6(1): 105–107.
(TREATMENT REFUSAL/MENTALLY DISABLED)

Grubb, Andrew. Frozen embryos: rights of inheritance: In Re the Estate of the Late K. [Comment]. *Medical Law Review.* 1997 Spring; 5(1): 121–124.
(FETUSES; IN VITRO FERTILIZATION; REPRODUCTION)

Grubb, Andrew. Incompetent patient in PVS: views of relatives and "best interests": Re G. [Comment]. *Medical Law Review.* 1995 Spring; 3(1): 80–84.
(ALLOWING TO DIE/LEGAL ASPECTS)

Grubb, Andrew. Incompetent patient (PVS): withdrawal of feeding (Scotland) — Law Hospital N.H.S. Trust v. The Lord Advocate. [Comment]. *Medical Law Review.* 1996 Autumn; 4(3): 300–311.
(ALLOWING TO DIE/LEGAL ASPECTS)

Grubb, Andrew. Infertility treatment: access and judicial review — R v. Sheffield Health Authority, ex parte Seale. [Comment]. *Medical Law Review.* 1996 Autumn; 4(3): 326–329.
(REPRODUCTIVE TECHNOLOGIES; RESOURCE ALLOCATION/BIOMEDICAL TECHNOLOGIES; SELECTION FOR TREATMENT)

Grubb, Andrew. Infertility treatment: posthumous use of sperm -- R. v. Human Fertilisation and Embryology Authority, ex parte D.B. [Comment]. *Medical Law Review.* 1996 Autumn; 4(3): 329–335.
(ARTIFICIAL INSEMINATION; REPRODUCTION)

Grubb, Andrew. Medical treatment (child): parental refusal and role of the court -- Re T (A Minor) (Wardship: Medical Treatment). [Comment]. *Medical Law Review.* 1996 Autumn; 4(3): 315–319.
(ORGAN AND TISSUE TRANSPLANTATION; TREATMENT REFUSAL/MINORS)

Grubb, Andrew. Medical treatment (competent adult): pregnant woman and unborn child: Winnipeg Child and Family Services (Northwest Area) v. D.F.G. [Comment]. *Medical Law Review.* 1997 Spring; 5(1): 125–130.
(PRENATAL INJURIES)

Grubb, Andrew. PVS patient: disclosure after death: Re C (Adult Patient: Restriction of Publicity After Death). [Comment]. *Medical Law Review.* 1997 Spring; 5(1): 108–110.
(CONFIDENTIALITY/LEGAL ASPECTS)

Grubb, Andrew. Refusal of treatment (incompetent patient): best interests and practicality -- Re D (Medical Treatment: Mentally Disabled Patient). [Comment]. *Medical Law Review.* 1998 Spring; 6(1): 103–105.
(TREATMENT REFUSAL/MENTALLY DISABLED)

Grubb, Andrew. Surrogate arrangements and parental orders: the Parental Orders (Human Fertilisation and Embryology) Regulations 1994 (S.I. 1994 No. 2767). [Comment]. *Medical Law Review.* 1995 Summer; 3(2): 204–208.
(SURROGATE MOTHERS)

Grubb, Andrew. Surrogate contract: parentage -- In Re Marriage of Moschetta. [Comment]. *Medical Law Review.* 1995 Summer; 3(2): 219–221.
(SURROGATE MOTHERS)

Grubb, Andrew. Treatment without consent: adult -- Re C (Refusal of Medical Treatment). [Comment]. *Medical Law Review.* 1994 Spring; 2(1): 92–95.
(TREATMENT REFUSAL/MENTALLY DISABLED)

Grubb, Andrew. Treatment without consent (anorexia nervosa): adult -- Riverside Mental Health Trust v. Fox. [Comment]. *Medical Law Review.* 1994 Spring; 2(1): 95–99.
(FORCE FEEDING; TREATMENT REFUSAL)

Grubb, Andrew. Use of fetal eggs and infertility treatment: Human Fertilisation and Embryology Act 1990, section 3A. [Comment]. *Medical Law Review.* 1995 Summer; 3(2): 203–204.
(FETUSES; ORGAN AND TISSUE DONATION; REPRODUCTIVE TECHNOLOGIES)

Grubb, Andrew; Walsh, Pat; Lambe, Neil. Reporting on the persistent vegetative state in Europe. *Medical Law Review.* 1999 Summer; 6(2): 161–219.
(ALLOWING TO DIE/ATTITUDES; ALLOWING TO

DIE/LEGAL ASPECTS)

Gruber, Franz see **van der Valk, Jan**

Gruber, Franz P.; Kolar, Roman. Animal test advisory commissions: ethics committees in Germany. *In:* van Zutphen, L.F.M.; Balls, M., eds. Animal Alternatives, Welfare and Ethics. New York, NY: Elsevier; 1997: 373–376.
(ANIMAL EXPERIMENTATION)

Grudzinskas, Gedis see **Sutcliffe, Alastair G.**

Gruman, Cynthia see **Walker, Leslie**

Grumbach, Kevin; Osmond, Dennis; Vranizan, Karen; Jaffe, Deborah; Bindman, Andrew B. Primary care physicians' experience of financial incentives in managed–care systems. *New England Journal of Medicine.* 1998 Nov 19; 339(21): 1516–1521.
(HEALTH CARE/ECONOMICS)

Grumbach, Kevin; Selby, Joe V.; Damberg, Cheryl; Bindman, Andrew B.; Quesenberry, Charles; Truman, Alison; Uratsu, Connie. Resolving the gatekeeper conundrum: what patients value in primary care and referrals to specialists. *JAMA.* 1999 Jul 21; 282(3): 261–266.
(HEALTH CARE/ECONOMICS)

Gruskin, Sofia. The highest priority: making use of UN conference documents to remind governments of their commitments to HIV/AIDS. *Health and Human Rights.* 1998; 3(1): 107–142.
(AIDS)

Gruskin, Sofia; Mann, Jonathan; Tarantola, Daniel. Past, present, and future: AIDS and human rights. [Editorial]. *Health and Human Rights.* 1998; 2(4): 1–3.
(AIDS)

Gruskin, Sofia see **Mann, Jonathan, M.**

Gruskin, Sofia see **Tarantola, Daniel**

Guallar, E. see **García–Alonso, F.**

Gudorf, Christine E. Gender and culture in the globalization of bioethics. *Saint Louis University Public Law Review.* 1996; 15(2): 331–351.
(BIOETHICS; HEALTH; POPULATION CONTROL)

Guenin, Louis M. The logical geography of concepts and shared responsibilities concerning research misconduct. *Academic Medicine.* 1996 Jun; 71(6): 595–603.
(BIOMEDICAL RESEARCH; FRAUD AND MISCONDUCT)

Guernsey, Thomas F. see **Loftus, Elizabeth F.**

Guido, Ginny Wacker. Ethics. *In: her* Legal Issues in Nursing. Second Edition. Stamford, CT: Appleton and Lange; 1997: 355–366.
(NURSING ETHICS)

Guilhem, Dirce Bellezi see **Diniz, Debora**

Guillen, Diego Gracia. The Hippocratic Oath in the development of medicine. *Dolentium Hominum: Church and Health in the World.* 1996; 31(11th Yr., No. 1): 22–28.
(MEDICAL ETHICS/CODES OF ETHICS; PROFESSIONAL ETHICS)

Guillod, O. see **Müller, H.J.**

Guilmette, Thomas J.; Hagan, Leigh D. Ethical considerations in forensic neuropsychological consultation. *Clinical Neuropsychologist.* 1997 Aug; 11(3): 287–290.
(PROFESSIONAL ETHICS)

Guither, Harold D. The debate over animals in research, testing, and teaching. *In: his* Animal Rights: History and Scope of a Radical Social Movement. Carbondale, IL: Southern Illinois University Press; 1998: 73–85, 240–241.
(ANIMAL EXPERIMENTATION)

Gunn, Michael. The meaning of incapacity. *Medical Law Review.* 1994 Spring; 2(1): 8–29.
(INFORMED CONSENT/MENTALLY DISABLED)

Gunning, Jennifer. Oocyte donation: the legislative framework in Western Europe. [Article and discussion]. *Human Reproduction.* 1998 May; 13(Suppl. 2): 98–104.
(ORGAN AND TISSUE DONATION; REPRODUCTIVE TECHNOLOGIES)

Gupta, Rajesh see **Achrekar, Abinash**

Gurewich, Victor see **Kosseff, Andrew L.**

Guston, David H. The demise of the social contract for science: misconduct in science and the nonmodern world. *Centennial Review.* 1994 Spring; 38(2): 215–248.
(BIOMEDICAL RESEARCH; FRAUD AND MISCONDUCT)

Gutheil, Thomas G. see **Bursztajn, Harold J.**

Gutowski, William D. see **Crelinsten, Gordon L.**

Guttman, Dan. Disclosure and consent: through the Cold War prism. *Accountability in Research.* 1998 Jan; 6(1–2): 1–14.
(HUMAN EXPERIMENTATION/INFORMED CONSENT)

Guttman, Dan see **Faden, Ruth**

Guttmann, Ronald D. see **Wu, John**

Gutzwiller, F. see **Müller, H.J.**

Guyatt, Gordon. Determining an ethical stance: pharmaceutical industry involvement and family medicine residency training. [Editorial]. *Canadian Family Physician.* 1997 Nov; 43: 1898–1900, 1905–1907.
(HEALTH CARE/ECONOMICS)

Gwyther, Lisa P. see **Martin, Richard J.**

H

Haber, Edgar. Industry and the university. *Nature Biotechnology.* 1996 Apr; 14(4): 441–442.
(BIOMEDICAL RESEARCH)

Hachinski, Vladimir see **McQuillen, Michael P.**

Hackler, Chris. Consensus and futility of treatment: some policy suggestions. *In:* ten Have, Henk A.M.J.; Sass, Hans-Martin, eds. Consensus Formation in Healthcare Ethics. Boston, MA: Kluwer Academic; 1998: 219–228.
(ALLOWING TO DIE)

Haddad, Amy see **Veatch, Robert M.**

Haddow, James E. Antenatal screening for Down's syndrome: where are we and where next? *Lancet.* 1998 Aug 1; 352(9125): 336–337.
(PRENATAL DIAGNOSIS)

Haddox, J. David; Aronoff, Gerald M. Commentary: the potential for unintended consequences from public policy shifts in the treatment of pain. *Journal of Law, Medicine and Ethics.* 1998 Winter; 26(4): 350–352.
(PATIENT CARE/DRUGS)

Hadfield, Peter. Cloning's maverick goes east. [News]. *New Scientist.* 1998 Dec 12; 160(2164): 26.
(CLONING)

Hadjistavropoulos, Thomas; Malloy, David Cruise. Ethical principles of the American Psychological Association: an argument for philosophical and practical ranking. *Ethics and Behavior.* 1999; 9(2): 127–140.
(PROFESSIONAL ETHICS/CODES OF ETHICS)

Hadley, Jack see Gostin, Lawrence O.

Hadley, Janet. Prenatal tests: blessings and burdens. *In:* Lee, Ellie, ed. Abortion Law and Politics Today. New York, NY: St. Martin's Press; 1998: 172–183.
(ABORTION; EUGENICS; PRENATAL DIAGNOSIS)

Hafferty, Fred see Hundert, Edward M.

Hafler, Janet P. see Branch, William T.

Hagan, Leigh D. see Guilmette, Thomas J.

Hagelin, Joakim; Carlsson, Hans-Erik; Hau, Jann. The use of animals in biomedical research. [Letter]. *Nursing Ethics.* 1999 Mar; 6(2): 173.
(ANIMAL EXPERIMENTATION)

Häggman–Laitila, Arja. The authenticity and ethics of phenomenological research: how to overcome the researcher's own views. *Nursing Ethics.* 1999 Jan; 6(1): 12–22.
(BEHAVIORAL RESEARCH/RESEARCH DESIGN; HEALTH)

Haglund, Keith. Research coalition promises no human cloning by members. [News]. *Journal of NIH Research.* 1997 Nov; 9(11): 20–21.
(CLONING)

Hahn, C. see Fitzpatrick, J.

Hahn, C. see Huggins, M.

Haiken, Elizabeth. Venus Envy: A History of Cosmetic Surgery. Baltimore, MD: Johns Hopkins University Press; 1997. 370 p.
(BIOMEDICAL TECHNOLOGIES; PATIENT CARE)

Haimowitz, Stephan; Tucker, Bonnie. Deaf culture. [Letter and response]. *Hastings Center Report.* 1999 Mar–Apr; 29(2): 5.
(PATIENT CARE/MINORS)

Haines, Andrew see McCally, Michael

Haisfield–Wolfe, Mary Ellen. End-of-life care: evolution of the nurse's role. *Oncology Nursing Forum.* 1996 Jul; 23(6): 931–935.
(TERMINAL CARE)

Halamish–Shani, Talia see Segal, Eran

Halasz, George. The rights of the child in psychotherapy. *American Journal of Psychotherapy.* 1996 Summer; 50(3): 285–297.
(PATIENT CARE/MENTALLY DISABLED; PATIENT CARE/MINORS)

Haldane, John see Thomas, Sandy

Halevy, Amir; Brody, Baruch A. The Houston process-based approach to medical futility. *Bioethics Forum.* 1998 Summer; 14(2): 10–17.
(ALLOWING TO DIE)

Halkitis, Perry N.; Dooha, Susan M. The perceptions and experiences of managed care by HIV–positive individuals in New York City. *AIDS and Public Policy Journal.* 1998 Summer; 13(2): 75–84.
(AIDS; HEALTH CARE/ECONOMICS)

Hall, Alison C. To die with dignity: comparing physician assisted suicide in the United States, Japan, and the Netherlands. [Note]. *Washington University Law Quarterly.* 1996 Fall; 74(3): 803–840.
(SUICIDE)

Hall, Judith A.; Epstein, Arnold M.; DeCiantis, Mary Lou; McNeil, Barbara J. Physician's liking for their patients: more evidence for the role of affect in medical care. *Health Psychology.* 1993; 12(2): 140–146.
(PROFESSIONAL PATIENT RELATIONSHIP)

Hall, Mark A.; Smith, Teresa Rust; Naughton, Michelle; Ebbers, Andrea. Judicial protection of managed care consumers: an empirical study of insurance coverage disputes. *Seton Hall Law Review.* 1996; 26: 1055–1068.
(HEALTH CARE/ECONOMICS)

Hall, Mark A. see Kosseff, Andrew L.

Hall, Mark A. see Menendez, Roger

Hall, Phyllis H. see Pokorski, Robert J.

Haller, Karen B. When John became Joan. [Editorial]. *Journal of Obstetric, Gynecologic and Neonatal Nursing.* 1998 Jan–Feb; 27(1): 11.
(PATIENT CARE/MINORS)

Hallowell, Christopher. Playing the odds: health insurers want to know what's in your DNA. *Time.* 1999 Jan 11; 153(1): 60.
(GENETIC SCREENING)

Halm, Ethan A. see Finestone, Albert J.

Halpern, Abraham L.; Freedman, Alfred M.; Schoenholtz, Jack C.; Appelbaum, Paul S. Ethics in forensic psychiatry. [Letter and response]. *American Journal of Psychiatry.* 1998 Apr; 155(4): 575–577.
(CAPITAL PUNISHMENT; MEDICAL ETHICS)

Halpern, Abraham L. see Schoenholtz, Jack C.

Halsey, Neal A. see Edi–Osagie, E.C.O.

Hamajima, Nobuyuki; Tajima, Kazuo. Patients' views on reference to clinical data. *Journal of Epidemiology.*

1997 Mar; 7(1): 17–19.
(BIOMEDICAL RESEARCH; HEALTH CARE)

Hamajima, Nobuyuki; Tajima, Kazuo; Morishita, Mayumi; Hyodo, Chigusa; Sakakibara, Noriko; Kawai, Chisato; Moritaka, Shigeko. Patients' expectations of information provided at cancer hospitals in Japan. *Japanese Journal of Clinical Oncology.* 1996 Oct; 26(5): 362–367.
(TRUTH DISCLOSURE)

Hamel, Mary Beth; Teno, Joan M.; Goldman, Lee; Lynn, Joanne; Davis, Roger B.; Galanos, Anthony N.; Desbiens, Norman; Connors, Alfred F.; Wenger, Neil; Phillips, Russell S. Patient age and decisions to withhold life–sustaining treatments from seriously ill, hospitalized adults. [For the SUPPORT Investigators]. *Annals of Internal Medicine.* 1999 Jan 19; 130(2): 116–125.
(ALLOWING TO DIE; SELECTION FOR TREATMENT)

Hamel, Ron. A question of value. *Health Progress.* 1997 May–Jun; 78(3): 24–26, 32.
(HEALTH CARE)

Hamilton, Peter. Fatal accident inquiry: death during research. *Bulletin of Medical Ethics.* 1997 Aug; No. 130: 22–24.
(HUMAN EXPERIMENTATION/FOREIGN COUNTRIES; HUMAN EXPERIMENTATION/INFORMED CONSENT)

Hammer, Scott see **Merson, Michael H.**

Hammerman, Cathy; Lavie, Ofer; Kornbluth, Eti; Rabinson, Jakob; Schimmel, Michael S.; Eidelman, Arthur I. Does pregnancy affect medical ethical decision making? *Journal of Medical Ethics.* 1998 Dec; 24(6): 409–413.
(ALLOWING TO DIE/ATTITUDES; ALLOWING TO DIE/INFANTS)

Hammerman, Cathy see **Kottow, Michael H.**

Hammerschmidt, Dale E. "There is no substantive due process right to conduct human–subject research": the saga of the Minnesota Gamma Hydroxybutyrate Study. *IRB: A Review of Human Subjects Research.* 1997 May–Aug; 19(3–4): 13–15.
(FRAUD AND MISCONDUCT; HUMAN EXPERIMENTATION/ETHICS COMMITTEES)

Hammes, Bernard see **Kane, Richard S.**

Hamolsky, Milton W. Some reflections on Brock's "Euthanasia." *Rhode Island Medicine.* 1993 Dec; 76(12): 590–591.
(EUTHANASIA)

Handelin, Barbara; Wachbroit, Robert; Billings, Paul; Scheck, Barry; Reilly, Philip; Milunsky, Aubrey. Genetic testing and individual rights. [Proceedings of the International Symposium on Law and Science at the Crossroads: Biomedical Technology, Ethics, Public Policy, and the Law; panel discussion]. *Suffolk University Law Review.* 1993 Winter; 27(4): 1477–1497.
(GENETIC SCREENING)

Handwerker, Lisa. Health commodification and the body politic: the example of female infertility in modern China. *In:* Donchin, Anne; Purdy, Laura M., eds. Embodying Bioethics: Recent Feminist Advances. Lanham, MD: Rowman and Littlefield; 1999: 141–157.

(REPRODUCTIVE TECHNOLOGIES)

Hanford, Jack T. Mental health and managed care. *Journal of Religion and Health.* 1998 Summer; 37(2): 159–165.
(HEALTH CARE/ECONOMICS; MENTAL HEALTH)

Hanigsberg, Julia E. Homologizing pregnancy and motherhood: a consideration of abortion. *Michigan Law Review.* 1995 Nov; 94(2): 371–418.
(ABORTION/LEGAL ASPECTS)

Hanna, Mark P. see **Gramelspacher, Gregory P.**

Hannay, Timo. Japan on verge of first gene therapy trial. [News]. *Nature Medicine.* 1995 Jan; 1(1): 9.
(GENE THERAPY; HUMAN EXPERIMENTATION/FOREIGN COUNTRIES; HUMAN EXPERIMENTATION/REGULATION)

Hannibal, Kari; Lawrence, Robert S. The health professional as human rights promoter: ten years of Physicians for Human Rights (USA). *Health and Human Rights.* 1996; 2(1): 111–127.
(FRAUD AND MISCONDUCT)

Hannon, Judith see **Caulfield, Timothy**

Hansen, Jennie Chin; Lynch, Marty; Estes, Carroll L. Is managed care good for older persons: Yes [and] No. *In:* Scharlach, Andrew E.; Kaye, Lenard W., eds. Controversial Issues in Aging. Boston, MA: Allyn and Bacon; 1997: 114–124.
(HEALTH CARE/ECONOMICS; PATIENT CARE/AGED)

Hanson, Kristina W. Public opinion and the mental health parity debate: lessons from the survey literature. *Psychiatric Services.* 1998 Aug; 49(8): 1059–1066.
(HEALTH CARE/ECONOMICS; MENTAL HEALTH)

Hanson, Laura C.; Earp, Jo Anne; Garrett, Joanne; Menon, Manoj; Danis, Marion. Community physicians who provide terminal care. *Archives of Internal Medicine.* 1999 May 24; 159(10): 1133–1138.
(ALLOWING TO DIE; TERMINAL CARE)

Hanson, Mark J. The idea of progress and the goals of medicine. *In:* Hanson, Mark J.; Callahan, Daniel, eds. The Goals of Medicine: The Forgotten Issue in Health Care Reform. Washington, DC: Georgetown University Press; 1999: 137–151.
(BIOMEDICAL TECHNOLOGIES)

Hanson, Mark J.; Callahan, Daniel, eds. The Goals of Medicine: The Forgotten Issue in Health Care Reform. Washington, DC: Georgetown University Press; 1999. 239 p.
(HEALTH CARE)

Happ, Mary Beth see **Fairman, Julie**

Harari, Edwin see **Bloch, Sidney**

Harbin, J. Judd see **Leach, Mark M.**

Hardin, Steven B. VHA ethics rounds: [autonomy]. *NCCE News (Veterans Health Administration National Center for Clinical Ethics).* 1994 Winter; 2(1): 4–5.
(PATIENT CARE/AGED)

Hardon, Anita; Hayes, Elizabeth, eds. Reproductive Rights in Practice: A Feminist Report on Quality of

Care. New York, NY: Zed Books; 1997. 235 p.
(CONTRACEPTION)

Hare, R.M. A utilitarian approach. *In:* Kuhse, Helga; Singer, Peter, eds. A Companion to Bioethics. Malden, MA: Blackwell; 1998: 80–85.
(BIOETHICS)

Harel–Raviv, Mili see **Graham, Peter E.**

Harindra, V. see **Gbolade, Babatunde A.**

Harless, William see **Schulman, Kevin A.**

Harmon–Smith, Helena. 10 commandments. *Journal of Clinical Ethics.* 1998 Winter; 9(4): 371.
(PATIENT CARE/MINORS)

Harper, Max see **White, D.M.D.**

Harper, Peter S. What do we mean by genetic testing? *Journal of Medical Genetics.* 1997 Sep; 34(9): 749–752.
(GENETIC SCREENING)

Harper, William. Judging who should live: Schneiderman and Jecker on the duty not to treat. *Journal of Medicine and Philosophy.* 1998 Oct; 23(5): 500–515.
(ALLOWING TO DIE)

Harper, William. The role of futility judgments in improperly limiting the scope of clinical research. *Journal of Medical Ethics.* 1998 Oct; 24(5): 308–313.
(BIOMEDICAL RESEARCH; HUMAN EXPERIMENTATION/RESEARCH DESIGN)

Harr, Helmut see **Sponholz, Gerlinde**

Harrell, Lindy E. see **Marson, Daniel C.**

Harris, A. see **Williams, L.**

Harris–Abbott, Deborah, ed. The Latter-Day Saints Tradition: Religious Beliefs and Health Care Decisions. [Booklet]. Chicago, IL: Park Ridge Center for the Study of Health, Faith, and Ethics; 1995. 19 p.
(BIOETHICS)

Harris, John. Doctors' orders, rationality and the good life: commentary on Savulescu. *Journal of Medical Ethics.* 1999 Apr; 25(2): 127–129.
(PRENATAL DIAGNOSIS; REPRODUCTION; REPRODUCTIVE TECHNOLOGIES)

Harris, John. Micro–allocation: deciding between patients. *In:* Kuhse, Helga; Singer, Peter, eds. A Companion to Bioethics. Malden, MA: Blackwell; 1998: 293–305.
(RESOURCE ALLOCATION; SELECTION FOR TREATMENT)

Harris, John. Rights and reproductive choice. *In:* Harris, John; Holm, Søren, eds. The Future of Human Reproduction: Ethics, Choice, and Regulation. New York, NY: Oxford University Press; 1998: 5–37.
(REPRODUCTIVE TECHNOLOGIES)

Harris, John; Holm, Søren. Risk–taking and professional responsibility. *Journal of the Royal Society of Medicine.* 1997 Nov; 90(11): 625–629.
(MEDICAL ETHICS; PROFESSIONAL ETHICS)

Harris, John; Holm, Søren, eds. The Future of Human Reproduction: Ethics, Choice, and Regulation. New

York, NY: Oxford University Press; 1998. 254 p..
(REPRODUCTIVE TECHNOLOGIES)

Harris, John see **Burley, Justine**

Harris, Yvonne see **Gorelick, Philip B.**

Harrold, Joan K.; Lynn, Joanne, eds. A Good Dying: Shaping Health Care for the Last Months of Life. New York, NY: Haworth Press; 1998. 188 p.
(TERMINAL CARE; TERMINAL CARE/HOSPICES)

Hart, David see **Limentani, Alexander E.**

Hart, Graham J. see **Simpson, Wendy M.**

Hart, Lynette A. Responsible animal care and use: moving toward a less–troubled middle ground. *In:* Hart, Lynette A., ed. Responsible Conduct with Animals in Research. New York, NY: Oxford University Press; 1998: 3–17.
(ANIMAL EXPERIMENTATION)

Hart, Lynette A., ed. Responsible Conduct with Animals in Research. New York, NY: Oxford University Press; 1998. 193 p.
(ANIMAL EXPERIMENTATION)

Hartouni, Valerie. Cultural Conceptions: On Reproductive Technologies and the Remaking of Life. Minneapolis, MN: University of Minnesota Press; 1997. 175 p.
(ABORTION; CLONING; FETUSES; REPRODUCTION; REPRODUCTIVE TECHNOLOGIES; SURROGATE MOTHERS)

Hartshorne, J.E. Principles of valid informed consent to treatment in dentistry. *Journal of the Dental Association of South Africa.* 1993 Aug; 48(8): 465–468.
(INFORMED CONSENT)

Harty, Anne E. see **Lerman, Caryn**

Harvey, John Collins. Doctors, ethics, and managed care. *Linacre Quarterly.* 1996 Nov; 63(4): 84–93.
(HEALTH CARE/ECONOMICS)

Harvey, S. Marie see **Beckman, Linda J.**

Hasadsri, Linda. The multi–faceted implications of preimplantation genetic testing. *Princeton Journal of Bioethics.* 1998 Spring; 1(1): 76–82.
(GENETIC SCREENING; PRENATAL DIAGNOSIS)

Hasian, Marouf Arif. The Uses of "Necessity" in Anglo–American Discourse: An Ideographic Analysis of the Eugenics Movement, 1900–1940. Ann Arbor, MI: UMI Dissertation Services; 1993. 447 p.
(EUGENICS)

Hass, Janis. Storage of cord blood attracts private–sector interest. *Canadian Medical Association Journal.* 1999 Feb 23; 160(4): 551–552.
(BLOOD DONATION)

Hassan, A. see **Hassn, A.M.F.**

Hassan, Riaz see **Stevens, Christine A.**

Hassan, T.B.; MacNamara, A.F.; Davy, A.; Bing, A.; Bodiwala, G.G. Managing patients with deliberate self harm who refuse treatment in the accident and emergency department. *BMJ (British Medical Journal).*

1999 Jul 10; 319(7202): 107–109.
(SUICIDE; TREATMENT REFUSAL)

Hassenfeld, Irwin N.; Hoge, Steven K. Consequences of involuntary treatment. [Letter and response]. *American Journal of Psychiatry.* 1998 Mar; 155(3): 450–451.
(PATIENT CARE/DRUGS; TREATMENT REFUSAL/MENTALLY DISABLED)

Hassn, A.M.F.; Hassan, A. Do we always need to tell patients the truth? [Letter]. *Lancet.* 1998 Oct 3; 352(9134): 1153.
(TRUTH DISCLOSURE)

Hattab, Jocelyn see **Arnold, L. Eugene**

Hau, Jann see **Hagelin, Joakim**

Hausman, Shawn see **Pokorski, Robert J.**

Haverkate, Ilinka; van der Wal, Gerrit; van der Maas, Paul J.; Onwuteaka–Philipsen, Bregje D.; Kostense, Piet J. Guidelines on euthanasia and pain alleviation: compliance and opinions of physicians. *Health Policy.* 1998 Apr; 44(1): 45–55.
(EUTHANASIA/ATTITUDES; SUICIDE; TERMINAL CARE)

Haward, R.A. see **Turner, N.J.**

Hawes, Catherine see **Teno, Joan M.**

Hay, D.M. see **Lui, S.C.**

Hayden, M.R. see **Wiggins, S.**

Hayes, Edward J.; Hayes, Paul J.; Kelly, Dorothy Ellen; Drummey, James J. Principles relating to the origin of life. *In:* their Catholicism and Ethics. Norwood, MA: C.R. Publications; 1997: 79–119.
(CONTRACEPTION; REPRODUCTIVE TECHNOLOGIES)

Hayes, Edward J.; Hayes, Paul J.; Kelly, Dorothy Ellen; Drummey, James J. Principles relating to the preservation of life. *In:* their Catholicism and Ethics. Norwood, MA: C.R. Publications; 1997: 153–175.
(BIOETHICS)

Hayes, Edward J.; Hayes, Paul J.; Kelly, Dorothy Ellen; Drummey, James J. Principles relating to the taking of life. *In:* their Catholicism and Ethics. Norwood, MA: C.R. Publications; 1997: 121–151.
(ABORTION/RELIGIOUS ASPECTS; EUTHANASIA/RELIGIOUS ASPECTS)

Hayes, Elizabeth see **Hardon, Anita**

Hayes, P.D. see **Lloyd, A.J.**

Hayes, Paul J. see **Hayes, Edward J.**

Haynor, Patricia M. Meeting the challenge of advance directives. *American Journal of Nursing.* 1998 Mar; 98(3): 26–33.
(ADVANCE DIRECTIVES)

Häyry, Heta. Who should know about my HIV positivity and why? *In:* Bennett, Rebecca; Erin, Charles A., eds. HIV and AIDS: Testing, Screening, and Confidentiality. New York, NY: Oxford University Press; 1999: 240–250.

(AIDS/CONFIDENTIALITY; AIDS/TESTING AND SCREENING)

Hayter, Mark. Confidentiality and the acquired immune deficiency syndrome (AIDS): an analysis of the legal and professional issues. *Journal of Advanced Nursing.* 1997 Jun; 25(6): 1162–1166.
(AIDS/CONFIDENTIALITY; CONFIDENTIALITY/LEGAL ASPECTS)

Headings, V.E. Revisiting foundations of autonomy and beneficence in genetic counseling. *Genetic Counseling.* 1997; 8(4): 291–294.
(GENETIC COUNSELING)

Healy, Bernadine. Hippocrates vs. Big Brother. *New York Times.* 1998 Jul 24: A25.
(CONFIDENTIALITY)

Hebel, J. Richard see **Muncie, Herbert L.**

Hebel, Richard see **Lynn, Joanne**

Hébert, Martin see **Blondeau, Danielle**

Hecht, Frederick M. see **Bindman, Andrew B.**

Hedberg, Katrina see **Chin, Arthur E.**

Hedges, Lawrence E.; Hilton, Robert; Hilton, Virginia Wink; Caudill, O. Brandt. Therapists at Risk: Perils of the Intimacy of the Therapeutic Relationship. Northvale, NJ: Jason Aronson; 1997. 328 p.
(PROFESSIONAL PATIENT RELATIONSHIP)

Hefferman, Pam; Heilig, Steve. Giving "moral distress" a voice: ethical concerns among neonatal intensive care unit personnel. *Cambridge Quarterly of Healthcare Ethics.* 1999 Spring; 8(2): 173–178.
(ALLOWING TO DIE/ATTITUDES; ALLOWING TO DIE/INFANTS; SELECTION FOR TREATMENT)

Heffner, John E.; Barbieri, Celia. Compliance with do–not–resuscitate orders for hospitalized patients transported to radiology departments. *Annals of Internal Medicine.* 1998 Nov 15; 129(10): 801–805.
(RESUSCITATION ORDERS)

Heffner, John E.; Fahy, Bonnie; Hilling, Lana; Barbieri, Celia. Outcomes of advance directive education of pulmonary rehabilitation patients. *American Journal of Respiratory and Critical Care Medicine.* 1997 Mar; 155(3): 1055–1059.
(ADVANCE DIRECTIVES)

Heguesh, Roni see **Mester, Roberto**

Hehir, J. Bryan. The Church and abortion in the 1990s: the role of institutional leadership. *In:* Rainey, R. Randall; Magill, Gerard, eds. Abortion and Public Policy: An Interdisciplinary Investigation within the Catholic Tradition. Omaha, NE: Creighton University Press; 1996: 203–228.
(ABORTION/RELIGIOUS ASPECTS)

Heierli, C. see **Müller, H.J.**

Heikkilä, Annaleena; Ryynänen, Markku; Kirkinen, Pertti; Saarikoski, Seppo. Results and views of women in population–wide pregnancy screening for trisomy 21 in East Finland. *Fetal Diagnosis and Therapy.* 1997

Mar–Apr; 12(2): 93–96.
(MASS SCREENING; PRENATAL DIAGNOSIS)

Heilig, Steve see **Bopp, James**

Heilig, Steve see **Hefferman, Pam**

Heilig, Steve see **Koch, Tom**

Heller, Jan C. Religiously based objections to human cloning: are they sustainable? *In:* Humber, James M.; Almeder, Robert F.,eds. Human Cloning. Totowa, NJ: Humana Press; 1998: 153–176.
(CLONING)

Heller, Tom see **Pattison, Stephen**

Hellman, Deborah. Trial and error: can good science be bad medicine? *New Republic.* 1998 Apr 27; 218(17): 14, 16–17.
(AIDS/HUMAN EXPERIMENTATION; HUMAN EXPERIMENTATION/FOREIGN COUNTRIES; HUMAN EXPERIMENTATION/RESEARCH DESIGN; HUMAN EXPERIMENTATION/SPECIAL POPULATIONS)

Hellman, Deborah. Trials on trial. *Philosophy and Public Policy.* 1998 Winter–Spring; 18(1–2): 13–18.
(AIDS/HUMAN EXPERIMENTATION; HUMAN EXPERIMENTATION/FOREIGN COUNTRIES; HUMAN EXPERIMENTATION/RESEARCH DESIGN; HUMAN EXPERIMENTATION/SPECIAL POPULATIONS)

Hellström, Olle. Symptoms or persons? A question for setting the goals of medicine. *In:* Hanson, Mark J.; Callahan, Daniel, eds. The Goals of Medicine: The Forgotten Issue in Health Care Reform. Washington, DC: Georgetown University Press; 1999: 118–136.
(PROFESSIONAL PATIENT RELATIONSHIP)

Hemberg, Maja see **Mattiasson, Anne–Cathrine**

Hemmings, Gwynneth see **Joy, Mark**

Henderson, Merrill see **Baumiller, Robert C.**

Henderson, Shelley; Fins, Joseph J.; Moskowitz, Ellen H. Resuscitation in hospice. [Case study and commentaries]. *Hastings Center Report.* 1998 Nov–Dec; 28(6): 20–22.
(RESUSCITATION ORDERS; TERMINAL CARE/HOSPICES)

Hendin, Herbert. Seduced by Death: Doctors, Patients, and Assisted Suicide. Revised and Updated. New York, NY: W.W. Norton; 1998. 304 p.
(EUTHANASIA; SUICIDE)

Hendin, Herbert see **Foley, Kathleen**

Hendlin, Herbert. Physician–assisted suicide: what next? *Responsive Community.* 1997 Fall; 7(4): 21–34.
(EUTHANASIA; SUICIDE; TERMINAL CARE)

Henley, Lesley D. see **Landman, Willem A.**

Henn, Wolfram. Genetic screening with the DNA chip: a new Pandora's box? *Journal of Medical Ethics.* 1999 Apr; 25(2): 200–203.
(GENETIC SCREENING)

Herbert, Bob. Pregnancy and addiction: South Carolina's misguided law. *New York Times.* 1998 Jun 11: A31.
(PRENATAL INJURIES)

Herdman, Roger; Beauchamp, Tom L.; Potts, John T. The Institute of Medicine's report on non–heart–beating organ transplantation. *Kennedy Institute of Ethics Journal.* 1998 Mar; 8(1): 89–90.
(ORGAN AND TISSUE DONATION)

Herdman, Roger C. see **Potts, John T.**

Herman, Joan. Genetic testing and insurance: a question of balance. *In:* Smith, Edward; Sapp; Walter, eds. Plain Talk about the Human Genome Project: A Tuskegee University Conference on Its Promise and Perils ... and Matters of Race. Tuskegee, AL: Tuskegee University Press; 1997: 179–185.
(GENETIC SCREENING)

Herman, Joseph. The good old days. *Lancet.* 1998 Dec 12; 352(9144): 1930–1931.
(PROFESSIONAL PATIENT RELATIONSHIP)

Hermann, Robert; Méhes, Károly. Physicians' attitudes regarding Down syndrome. *Journal of Child Neurology.* 1996 Jan; 11(1): 66–69.
(ALLOWING TO DIE/ATTITUDES; ALLOWING TO DIE/INFANTS; PATIENT CARE/MENTALLY DISABLED; PATIENT CARE/MINORS)

Hernández–Arriaga, Jorge; Navarrete de Olivares, Victoria; Iserson, Kenneth V. The development of bioethics in Mexico. *Cambridge Quarterly of Healthcare Ethics.* 1999 Summer; 8(3): 382–385.
(BIOETHICS)

Hernon, Peter see **Altman, Ellen**

Herrera, C.D. Research ethics at the empirical side: Research Ethics: A Psychological Approach, edited by Barbara Stanley, Joan Sieber, and Gary Melton; Illusions of Reality: A History of Deception in Social Psychology, by James Korn. [Book review essay]. *Theoretical Medicine and Bioethics.* 1999 April; 20(2): 191–200.
(BEHAVIORAL RESEARCH)

Herrington, David see **Merson, Michael H.**

Hervé, Christian see **Letvak, Richard**

Herz, Susan E. Two steps to three choices: a new approach to mandated choice. *Cambridge Quarterly of Healthcare Ethics.* 1999 Summer; 8(3): 340–347.
(ORGAN AND TISSUE DONATION)

Herzog, Harold A. Understanding animal activism. *In:* Hart, Lynette A., ed. Responsible Conduct with Animals in Research. New York, NY: Oxford University Press; 1998: 165–183.
(ANIMAL EXPERIMENTATION)

Hess, Jennifer A. see **Burk, Dan L.**

Hesse, Manfred see **Peters, Malte**

Hester, D. Micah. Habits of healing. *In:* McGee, Glenn, ed. Pragmatic Bioethics. Nashville, TN: Vanderbilt University Press; 1999: 45–59, 261–264.
(PROFESSIONAL PATIENT RELATIONSHIP)

Hester, D. Micah. Significance at the end of life. *In:* McGee, Glenn, ed. Pragmatic Bioethics. Nashville, TN: Vanderbilt University Press; 1999: 113–128, 271–274.
(EUTHANASIA; SUICIDE)

Hester, D. Micah. The place of community in medical encounters. *Journal of Medicine and Philosophy.* 1998 Aug; 23(4): 369–383.
(HEALTH; PROFESSIONAL PATIENT RELATIONSHIP)

Heurter, Helen see **King, Susan M.**

Hewison, J. see **Edwards, Sarah J.L.**

Hewison, J. see **Middleton, A.**

Heywood, Mark; Cornell, Morna. Human rights and AIDS in South Africa: from right margin to left margin. *Health and Human Rights.* 1998; 2(4): 60–82.
(AIDS)

Hiatt, Howard see **Smith, Richard**

Hibbs, Euthymia D.; Krener, Penelope. Ethical issues in psychosocial treatment research with children and adolescents. *In:* Hoagwood, Kimberly; Jensen, Peter S.; Fisher, Celia B., eds. Ethical Issues in Mental Health Research with Children and Adolescents. Mahwah, NJ: Lawrence Erlbaum Associates; 1996: 59–71.
(BEHAVIORAL RESEARCH/MINORS; BEHAVIORAL RESEARCH/SPECIAL POPULATIONS)

Hicks, Stephen C. The regulation of fetal tissue transplantation: different legislative models for different purposes. *Suffolk University Law Review.* 1993 Winter; 27(4): 1613–1629.
(EMBRYO AND FETAL RESEARCH; FETUSES; ORGAN AND TISSUE DONATION)

Higdon, Tami L. see **Wagner, James T.**

Higgins, Julian see **Koepp, Robert**

Higginson, Grant K. see **Chin, Arthur E.**

Higgs, Roger. Do studies of the nature of cases mislead about the reality of cases? A response to Pattison *et al. Journal of Medical Ethics.* 1999 Feb; 25(1): 47–50.
(BIOETHICS/EDUCATION; MEDICAL ETHICS/EDUCATION)

Higgs, Roger. Truth-telling. *In:* Kuhse, Helga; Singer, Peter, eds. A Companion to Bioethics. Malden, MA: Blackwell; 1998: 432–440.
(TRUTH DISCLOSURE)

Hilborne, Lee H. see **Leape, Lucian L.**

Hildt, Elisabeth; Mieth, Dietmar, eds. In Vitro Fertilisation in the 1990s: Towards a Medical, Social and Ethical Evaluation. Brookfield, VT: Ashgate; 1998. 370 p.
(IN VITRO FERTILIZATION; REPRODUCTIVE TECHNOLOGIES)

Hile, Allison see **Virgo, Katherine S.**

Hilhorst, Medard T. Can health care workers care for their patients and be advocates of third-party interests? *In:* Bennett, Rebecca; Erin, Charles A., eds. HIV and AIDS: Testing, Screening, and Confidentiality. New York, NY: Oxford University Press; 1999: 149–165.
(AIDS/CONFIDENTIALITY; AIDS/HEALTH PERSONNEL)

Hill, Richard N.; Stokes, William S. Validation and regulatory acceptance of alternatives. *Cambridge Quarterly of Healthcare Ethics.* 1999 Winter; 8(1): 73–79.
(ANIMAL EXPERIMENTATION)

Hill, Ruaraidh; Stanisstreet, Martin; Boyes, Edward; O'Sullivan, Helen. Animal experimentation needs dissection. [Letter]. *Nature.* 1998 Jan 8; 391(6663): 117.
(ANIMAL EXPERIMENTATION; GENETIC INTERVENTION)

Hill-Smith, Ian see **Inwald, A.C.**

Hill, Wan Ying; Fraser, Ian; Cotton, Philip. Patients' voices, rights and responsibilities: on implementing social audit in primary health care. *Journal of Business Ethics.* 1998 Oct; 17(13): 1481–1497.
(HEALTH CARE/FOREIGN COUNTRIES; PATIENTS' RIGHTS)

Hillam, Jonathan see **White, D.M.D.**

Hillier, R. see **Payne, S. A.**

Hilling, Lana see **Heffner, John E.**

Hillman, Alan L. Mediators of patient trust. [Editorial]. *JAMA.* 1998 Nov 18; 280(19): 1703–1704.
(HEALTH CARE/ECONOMICS; PROFESSIONAL PATIENT RELATIONSHIP)

Hillman, Alan L. see **Ramsey, Scott D.**

Hillman, Harold see **Breimer, Lars**

Hilton, Robert see **Hedges, Lawrence E.**

Hilton, Virginia Wink see **Hedges, Lawrence E.**

Hilts, Philip J. Duke's plan ends the ban on research. [News]. *New York Times.* 1999 May 15: A10.
(FRAUD AND MISCONDUCT; HUMAN EXPERIMENTATION/REGULATION)

Hilts, Philip J. Psychiatric researchers under fire. [News]. *New York Times.* 1998 May 19: F1, F5.
(HUMAN EXPERIMENTATION/INFORMED CONSENT; HUMAN EXPERIMENTATION/SPECIAL POPULATIONS)

Hilts, Philip J. Psychiatric unit's ethics faulted. [News]. *New York Times.* 1998 May 28: A26.
(FRAUD AND MISCONDUCT; HUMAN EXPERIMENTATION/SPECIAL POPULATIONS)

Hilts, Philip J. Study or human experiment? Face-lift project stirs ethical concerns. [News]. *New York Times.* 1998 Jun 21: 25–26.
(HUMAN EXPERIMENTATION/INFORMED CONSENT)

Hilts, Philip J. V.A. hospital is told to halt all research. [News]. *New York Times.* 1999 Mar 25: A25.
(FRAUD AND MISCONDUCT; HUMAN EXPERIMENTATION/REGULATION; HUMAN EXPERIMENTATION/SPECIAL POPULATIONS)

Hilts, Philip J.; Stolberg, Sheryl Gay. Ethics lapses at Duke halt dozens of human experiments. [News]. *New York Times.* 1999 May 13: A26.
(FRAUD AND MISCONDUCT; HUMAN EXPERIMENTATION/REGULATION)

Hilzenrath, David S. Healing vs. honesty? For doctors, managed care's cost controls pose moral dilemma. [News]. *Washington Post.* 1998 Mar 15: H1, H6–H7.
(HEALTH CARE/ECONOMICS)

Himma, Kenneth Einar. A critique of UNOS liver

allocation policy. *Cambridge Quarterly of Healthcare Ethics.* 1999 Summer; 8(3): 311–320.
(ORGAN AND TISSUE TRANSPLANTATION; RESOURCE ALLOCATION/BIOMEDICAL TECHNOLOGIES; SELECTION FOR TREATMENT)

Himmelstein, David U.; Woolhandler, Steffie. The silence of the doctors: fifty years after Nuremberg. [Editorial]. *Journal of General Internal Medicine.* 1998 Jun; 13(6): 422–423.
(HEALTH CARE/ECONOMICS)

Hinds, Di see **Jones, Steve**

Hines, Stephen C.; Glover, Jacqueline J.; Holley, Jean L.; Babrow, Austin S.; Badzek, Laurie A.; Moss, Alvin H. Dialysis patients' preferences for family-based advance care planning. *Annals of Internal Medicine.* 1999 May 18; 130(10): 825–828.
(ADVANCE DIRECTIVES; TERMINAL CARE)

Hingorani, Melanie; Wong, Tina; Vafidis, Gilli. Patients' and doctors' attitudes to amount of information given after unintended injury during treatment: cross sectional, questionnaire survey. *BMJ (British Medical Journal).* 1999 Mar 6; 318(7184): 640–641.
(TRUTH DISCLOSURE)

Hinlicky, Sarah E. see **Brown, Harold O.J.**

Hippisley-Cox, Julia see **Inwald, A.C.**

Hippisley-Cox, Stephen see **Inwald, A.C.**

Hitzig, W. see **Müller, H.J.**

Hoagwood, Kimberly; Jensen, Peter S.; Fisher, Celia B., eds. Ethical Issues in Mental Health Research with Children and Adolescents. Mahwah, NJ: Lawrence Erlbaum Associates; 1996. 313 p.
(HUMAN EXPERIMENTATION/MINORS; HUMAN EXPERIMENTATION/SPECIAL POPULATIONS)

Hoagwood, Kimberly see **Attkisson, C. Clifford**

Hoagwood, Kimberly see **Fisher, Celia B.**

Hobsons Publishing PLC. Genes, Diseases and Dilemmas: A Resource Book for A-Level General Studies and 16–19 Entitlement Curriculum. [Teachers' notes and student booklet; sponsored by the Association of the British Pharmaceutical Industry (ABPI)]. Cambridge, England: Hobsons Scientific Publishing; 1993. 27 p.
(GENETIC INTERVENTION)

Hodge, James G. Privacy and antidiscrimination issues: genetics legislation in the United States. *Community Genetics.* 1998; 1(3): 169–174.
(CONFIDENTIALITY/LEGAL ASPECTS; GENETIC SCREENING)

Hodge, Susan E. Paternalistic and protective? [Letter]. *Journal of Genetic Counseling.* 1995 Dec; 4(4): 351–352.
(GENETIC COUNSELING; GENETIC SCREENING)

Hodges, Eric D. see **Allen, Keith D.**

Hodges, Jeffrey Alan. Euthenics, Eugenics and Compulsory Sterilization in Michigan: 1897–1960. Ann Arbor, MI: UMI Dissertation Services; 1995. 181 p.
(EUGENICS; STERILIZATION)

Hodges, Marian O. see **Preston, Thomas A.**

Hodgson, John. A genetic heritage betrayed or empowered? *Nature Biotechnology.* 1998 Nov; 16(11): 1017–1021.
(GENETIC RESEARCH)

Hodgson, John. New "deCODE bill" restarts controversy. [News]. *Nature Biotechnology.* 1998 Sep; 16(9): 816.
(GENETIC RESEARCH)

Hoedemaekers, Rogeer. Predictive genetic screening and the concept of risk. *In:* Clarke, Angus, ed. The Genetic Testing of Children. Washington, DC: BIOS Scientific Publishers; 1998: 245–264.
(GENETIC COUNSELING; GENETIC SCREENING)

Hoedemaekers, Rogeer; ten Have, Henk. Geneticization: the Cyprus paradigm. *Journal of Medicine and Philosophy.* 1998 Jun; 23(3): 274–287.
(ABORTION/ATTITUDES; ABORTION/FOREIGN COUNTRIES; GENETIC COUNSELING; GENETIC SCREENING; MASS SCREENING; PRENATAL DIAGNOSIS)

Hoefler, James M. see **Stead, William W.**

Hoeldtke, Nathan J. see **Reitman, James S.**

Hoey, John. Human rights, ethics and the Krever inquiry. [Editorial]. *Canadian Medical Association Journal.* 1997 Nov 1; 157(9): 1231.
(AIDS; PUBLIC HEALTH)

Hoey, John. When the physician is the vector. [Editorial]. *Canadian Medical Association Journal.* 1998 Jul 14; 159(1): 45–46.
(PUBLIC HEALTH)

Hoffenberg, Raymond see **Engelhart, Karlheinz**

Hoffman, Brian see **Ferris, Lorraine E.**

Hoffmann, Diane E. Pain management and palliative care in the era of managed care: issues for health insurers. *Journal of Law, Medicine and Ethics.* 1998 Winter; 26(4): 267–289.
(HEALTH CARE/ECONOMICS; PATIENT CARE/DRUGS; TERMINAL CARE)

Hoffmann, Diane E.; Zimmerman, Sheryl Itkin; Tompkins, Catherine. How close is enough? Family relationships and attitudes toward advance directives and life-sustaining treatments. *Journal of Ethics, Law, and Aging.* 1997 Spring–Summer; 3(1): 5–24.
(ADVANCE DIRECTIVES; ALLOWING TO DIE/ATTITUDES)

Hoffmaster, Barry. Part II, conclusion. *In:* Coward, Harold; Ratanakul, Pinit, eds. A Cross-Cultural Dialogue on Health Care Ethics. Waterloo, ON: Wilfrid Laurier University Press; 1999: 146–153.
(BIOETHICS)

Hoffmaster, Barry. Secular health care ethics. *In:* Coward, Harold; Ratanakul, Pinit, eds. A Cross-Cultural Dialogue on Health Care Ethics. Waterloo, ON: Wilfrid Laurier University Press; 1999: 139–145.
(BIOETHICS)

Hofland, Brian F. When capacity fades and autonomy

is constricted: a client–centered approach to residential care. *Generations (American Society on Aging).* 1994 Winter; 18(4): 31–35.
(PATIENT CARE/MENTALLY DISABLED)

Hoge, Steven K. see **Hassenfeld, Irwin N.**

Hoge, Warren. British researchers on animal rights death list. [News]. *New York Times.* 1999 Jan 10: 10.
(ANIMAL EXPERIMENTATION)

Holden, Constance, ed. Clone rangers. [News]. *Science.* 1999 Jun 25; 284(5423): 2083.
(CLONING)

Holland, Anthony J.; Wong, Josephine. Genetically determined obesity in Prader–Willi syndrome: the ethics and legality of treatment. *Journal of Medical Ethics.* 1999 Jun; 25(3): 230–236.
(BEHAVIOR CONTROL)

Holland, Julie. Should parents be permitted to authorize genetic testing for their children? *Family Law Quarterly.* 1997 Summer; 31(2): 321–353.
(GENETIC SCREENING; INFORMED CONSENT/MINORS)

Holley, Jean L. see **Hines, Stephen C.**

Holley, Jean L. see **Iqbal, Aamir**

Holley, Sandra; Foster, Claire. Ethical review of multi–centre research: a survey of local research ethics committees in the South Thames region. *Journal of the Royal College of Physicians of London.* 1998 May–Jun; 32(3): 238–241.
(HUMAN EXPERIMENTATION/ETHICS COMMITTEES; HUMAN EXPERIMENTATION/FOREIGN COUNTRIES)

Holley, Sandra see **Foster, Claire**

Hollinger, Dennis P. A theology of healing and genetic engineering. *In:* Demy, Timothy J.; Stewart, Gary P., eds. Genetic Engineering: A Christian Response: Crucial Considerations in Shaping Life. Grand Rapids, MI: Kregel Publications; 1999: 294–303.
(GENE THERAPY; GENETIC INTERVENTION)

Hollon, Matthew F. Direct–to–consumer marketing of prescription drugs: creating consumer demand. *JAMA.* 1999 Jan 27; 281(4): 382–384.
(PATIENT CARE/DRUGS)

Holm, Søren. Ethical issues in pre–implantation diagnosis. *In:* Harris, John; Holm, Søren, eds. The Future of Human Reproduction: Ethics, Choice, and Regulation. New York, NY: Oxford University Press; 1998: 176–190.
(PRENATAL DIAGNOSIS)

Holm, Søren. Goodbye to the simple solutions: the second phase of priority setting in health care. *BMJ (British Medical Journal).* 1998 Oct 10; 317(7164): 1000–1002.
(HEALTH CARE/FOREIGN COUNTRIES; RESOURCE ALLOCATION)

Holm, Søren. Is society responsible for my health? *In:* Bennett, Rebecca; Erin, Charles A., eds. HIV and AIDS: Testing, Screening, and Confidentiality. New York, NY: Oxford University Press; 1999: 125–139.
(HEALTH; HEALTH CARE; RESOURCE ALLOCATION)

Holm, Søren; Rossel, Peter. Ethical aspects of the use

of 'sensitive information' in health care research. *In:* Bennett, Rebecca; Erin, Charles A., eds. HIV and AIDS: Testing, Screening, and Confidentiality. New York, NY: Oxford University Press; 1999: 200–215.
(BIOMEDICAL RESEARCH; CONFIDENTIALITY)

Holm, Søren see **Bjørn, Else**

Holm, Søren see **Harris, John**

Holm, Søren see **Rossel, Peter**

Holmboe, Eric see **Bogardus, Sidney T.**

Holmer, Alan F. Direct–to–consumer prescription drug advertising builds bridges between patients and physicians. *JAMA.* 1999 Jan 27; 281(4): 380–382.
(PATIENT CARE/DRUGS)

Holmerová, I. see **Vrbová, H.**

Holmes, Colin A. QALYs: a nurse's view. *International Journal of Health Care Quality Assurance.* 1993; 6(5): 17–23.
(RESOURCE ALLOCATION)

Holmes, Helen Bequaert. Closing the gaps: an imperative for feminist bioethics. *In:* Donchin, Anne; Purdy, Laura M., eds. Embodying Bioethics: Recent Feminist Advances. Lanham, MD: Rowman and Littlefield; 1999: 45–63.
(BIOETHICS; HEALTH CARE/ECONOMICS)

Holmes, Jeremy. Values in psychotherapy. *American Journal of Psychotherapy.* 1996 Summer; 50(3): 259–273.
(PATIENT CARE/MENTALLY DISABLED; PROFESSIONAL ETHICS)

Holmes, Steven A. Right to abortion quietly advances in state courts. [News]. *New York Times.* 1998 Dec 6: 1, 25.
(ABORTION/LEGAL ASPECTS)

Holt, Natalie. The business of medicine: the professionalization/commercialization boundary in nineteenth–century medical practice. *Pharos.* 1998 Winter; 61(1): 32–37.
(HEALTH CARE/ECONOMICS)

Holtgrave, David R. see **Valdiserri, Ronald O.**

Holtug, Nils. Creating and patenting new life forms. *In:* Kuhse, Helga; Singer, Peter, eds. A Companion to Bioethics. Malden, MA: Blackwell; 1998: 206–214.
(GENETIC INTERVENTION; PATENTING LIFE FORMS)

Holtug, Nils. Does justice require genetic enhancements? *Journal of Medical Ethics.* 1999 Apr; 25(2): 137–143.
(GENE THERAPY; GENETIC INTERVENTION)

Holtzman, N.A. see **Eisinger, F.**

Holtzman, N.A. see **James, C.A.**

Holtzman, N.A. see **Schoonmaker, M.**

Holtzman, Neil A. The UK's policy on genetic testing services supplied direct to the public –– two spheres and two tiers. *Community Genetics.* 1998; 1(1): 49–52.
(GENETIC SCREENING; GENETIC SERVICES)

Holzer, Jacob C.; Gansler, David A.; Moczynski, Nancy P.; Folstein, Marshal F. Cognitive functions in the informed consent evaluation process: a pilot study. *Journal of the American Academy of Psychiatry and the Law.* 1997; 25(4): 531–540.
(INFORMED CONSENT)

Hölzer, Michael see Sponholz, Gerlinde

Hom, Candace see Egilman, David

Honings, Bonifacio. The Charter for Health Care Workers: a synthesis of Hippocratic ethics and Christian morality. *Dolentium Hominum: Church and Health in the World.* 1996; 31(11th Yr., No. 1): 48–52.
(MEDICAL ETHICS/CODES OF ETHICS; PROFESSIONAL PATIENT RELATIONSHIP)

Hook, C. Christopher; Koch, Kathryn A. Ethics of resuscitation. *Critical Care Clinics.* 1996 Jan; 12(1): 135–148.
(RESUSCITATION ORDERS)

Hoos, Aloysia M. see Varekamp, Inge

Hope, R.A.; Fulford, K.W.M.; Yates, Anne. The Oxford Practice Skills Course: Ethics, Law, and Communication Skills in Health Care Education. [Instructor's Manual]. New York, NY: Oxford University Press; 1996. 181 p.
(MEDICAL ETHICS/EDUCATION)

Hope, Tony. Empirical medical ethics. [Editorial]. *Journal of Medical Ethics.* 1999 Jun; 25(3): 219–220.
(BIOETHICS)

Hope, Tony. Medical research needs lay involvement. [Editorial]. *Journal of Medical Ethics.* 1998 Oct; 24(5): 291–292.
(BIOMEDICAL RESEARCH; HUMAN EXPERIMENTATION/RESEARCH DESIGN)

Hope, Tony see Fazel, Seena

Hopkins, Patrick D., ed. (Mis?)conceptions: morality and gender politics in reproductive technology. *In: his* Sex/Machine: Readings in Culture, Gender, and Technology. Bloomington, IN: Indiana University Press; 1998: 95–170.
(ARTIFICIAL INSEMINATION; SEX DETERMINATION; SEX PRESELECTION; SURROGATE MOTHERS)

Hopkins, Patrick D., ed.; Tennessee. Supreme Court, at Knoxville. (Re)locating fetuses: technology and new body politics. *In: his* Sex/Machine: Readings in Culture, Gender, and Technology. Bloomington, IN: Indiana University Press; 1998: 171–235.
(ABORTION; FETUSES; REPRODUCTIVE TECHNOLOGIES)

Horn, David. Unnatural acts: procreation and the genealogy of artifice. *In:* Terry, Jennifer; Calvert, Melodie, eds. Processed Lives: Gender and Technology in Everyday Life. New York, NY: Routledge; 1997: 145–154.
(ARTIFICIAL INSEMINATION; EUGENICS)

Hornby, Sonia see Thomas, Sandy

Hornstra, Deborah. A realistic approach to maternal–fetal conflict. *Hastings Center Report.* 1998 Sep–Oct; 28(5): 7–12.
(PRENATAL INJURIES)

Horsley, Rosemarie see Nakashima, Allyn K.

Horst, J. see Nippert, I.

Horton, Richard. Publication and promotion: a fair reward. *Lancet.* 1998 Sep 12; 352(9131): 892.
(BIOMEDICAL RESEARCH)

Horton, Richard. Scientific misconduct: exaggerated fear but still real and requiring a proportionate response. *Lancet.* 1999 Jul 3; 354(9172): 7–8.
(BIOMEDICAL RESEARCH; FRAUD AND MISCONDUCT)

Horvath, Thomas see Rosenheck, Robert

Horwitz, Sarah see Bradley, Elizabeth H.

Hosford, Ian; Brown, Edna; Duncan, Crawford. Formulating a "do not resuscitate" policy for a psychogeriatric service: need for consultation with Maori. *New Zealand Medical Journal.* 1995 Jun 14; 108(1001): 226–228.
(RESUSCITATION ORDERS)

Hosp, Maria see Edi–Osagie, E.C.O.

Houdebine, Louis–Marie see Mepham, T. Ben

Hough, M. Catherine. Ethical dilemmas faced by critical care nurses in clinical practice: walking the line. *Critical Care Clinics.* 1996 Jan; 12(1): 123–133.
(NURSING ETHICS; PATIENT CARE)

Houghton, D.J.; Williams, S.; Bennett, J.D.; Back, G.; Jones, A.S. Informed consent: patients' and junior doctors' perceptions of the consent procedure. *Clinical Otolaryngology.* 1997 Dec; 22(6): 515–518.
(INFORMED CONSENT)

Hoult, Lorraine see Saigal, Saroj

Howard, Louise; Fahy, Tom. Liver transplantation for alcoholic liver disease. [Editorial]. *British Journal of Psychiatry.* 1997 Dec; 171: 497–500.
(ORGAN AND TISSUE TRANSPLANTATION)

Howe, Edmund G. Ethics consultants: could they do better? *Journal of Clinical Ethics.* 1999 Spring; 10(1): 13–25.
(ETHICISTS AND ETHICS COMMITTEES; PROFESSIONAL PATIENT RELATIONSHIP)

Howe, Edmund G. Intersexuality: what should careproviders do now? *Journal of Clinical Ethics.* 1998 Winter; 9(4): 337–344.
(PATIENT CARE/MINORS)

Howe, Edmund G. Treating infants who may die. *Journal of Clinical Ethics.* 1998 Fall; 9(3): 215–224.
(ALLOWING TO DIE/INFANTS; PATIENT CARE/MINORS)

Howe, Edmund G. see Shamoo, Adil E.

Howsepian, A.A. The 1994 Multi–Society Task Force consensus statement on the persistent vegetative state: a critical analysis. *Issues in Law and Medicine.* 1996 Summer; 12(1): 3–29.
(ALLOWING TO DIE)

Howsepian, A.A. see **Letvak, Richard**

Hoyle, Russ. Clinton's cloning ban may threaten genetic research. *Nature Biotechnology.* 1997 Jul; 15(7): 600.
(CLONING)

Hoyle, Russ. Forensics: the FBI's national DNA database. *Nature Biotechnology.* 1998 Nov; 16(11): 987.
(DNA FINGERPRINTING)

Hoyle, Russ. US national bioethics commission: politics as usual? *Nature Biotechnology.* 1996 Aug; 14(8): 927.
(BIOETHICS; ETHICISTS AND ETHICS COMMITTEES)

Hoyt, John W. see **Kelly, David F.**

Hrubantová, L. see **Vrbová, H.**

Hsu, John; Trevett, Kenneth P.; Campbell, Eric G.; Blumenthal, David; Louis, Karen Seashore; Bero, Lisa A. Corporate gifts to academic researchers. [Letters and responses]. *JAMA.* 1998 Sep 9; 280(10): 883–884.
(BIOMEDICAL RESEARCH)

Hu, Peicheng. The acceptability of active euthanasia in China. *Medicine and Law.* 1993; 12(1–2): 47–53.
(EUTHANASIA/ATTITUDES)

Hubal, Robert C. see **Sugarman, Jeremy**

Hubbard, Ruth. Predictive genetics and the construction of the healthy ill. *Suffolk University Law Review.* 1993 Winter; 27(4): 1209–1224.
(GENETIC SCREENING)

Huber, Ch. see **Waibel, U.G.**

Hubert, John see **Stingl, Michael**

Huddleston, John F. see **Webb, Gilbert W.**

Hudson, Brenda L. see **Perkins, David V.**

Hudson, C.N.; Sherr, Lorraine. Antenatal HIV testing in Europe. [Letter]. *Lancet.* 1997 Dec 13; 350(9093): 1783.
(AIDS/TESTING AND SCREENING)

Hudson, Stephanie see **Foster, Peggy**

Hueston, William J. see **Greenfield, Barak**

Hufford, David J. see **Clouser, K. Danner**

Huggins, M.; Hahn, C.; Costa, T. Staying informed and recontacting patients about research advances: a study of patient attitudes. [Abstract]. *American Journal of Human Genetics.* 1996 Oct; 59(4): A335.
(GENETIC COUNSELING; GENETIC RESEARCH)

Huggins, M. see **Fitzpatrick, J.**

Hughes, Chanita see **Lerman, Caryn**

Hughes, Ian see **van der Valk, Jan**

Hui, Edwin. Chinese health care ethics. *In:* Coward, Harold; Ratanakul, Pinit, eds. A Cross-Cultural Dialogue on Health Care Ethics. Waterloo, ON: Wilfrid Laurier University Press; 1999: 128–138.
(BIOETHICS)

Hull, Harry F. see **Lee, J.W.**

Hull, Richard T. No fear: how a humanist faces science's new creation. *Free Inquiry.* 1997 Summer; 17(3): 18–20.
(CLONING)

Human Genetics Advisory Commission (Great Britain). Cloning Issues in Reproduction, Science and Medicine. [Consultation paper]. London: The Commission [online]. Internet Web site: http://www.dti.gov.uk/hgac/papers/papers—c.htm [1998 December 7]; 1998 Jan. 23 p.
(CLONING)

Human Genetics Advisory Commission (Great Britain). The Implications of Genetic Testing for Insurance. [Report]. London: The Commission [online]. Internet Web site: http://www.dti.gov.uk/hgac/papers/papers—b.htm [1998 December 7]; 1997 Dec. 32 p.
(GENETIC SCREENING)

Human Genetics Advisory Commission (Great Britain). The Implications of Genetic Testing for Life Insurance. [Paper; request for responses]. London: The Commission [online]. Internet Web site: http://www.dti.gov.uk/hgac/papers/papers—a.htm [1998 December 7]; 1997 Jul 9. 9 p.
(GENETIC SCREENING)

Human Genetics Advisory Commission (Great Britain); Great Britain. Human Fertilisation and Embryology Authority. Cloning Issues in Reproduction, Science and Medicine. [Report]. London: The Commission [online]. Web site: http://www.dti.gov.uk/hgac/papers/papers—d.htm [1998 December 9]; 1998 Dec. 39 p.
(CLONING)

Human Genome Education [HuGEM] Project. The HuGEM Project: I. An Overview of the Human Genome Project and Its Ethical, Legal and Social Issues (19 min.); II. Opportunities and Challenges of the Human Genome Project (24 min.); III. Issues of Genetic Privacy and Discrimination (45 min.); IV. Genetic Testing Across the Lifespan (30 min.); V. Working Together to Improve Genetic Services (28 min.). Available from the Georgetown University Child Development Center, 3307 M St., NW, Suite 401, Washington, DC 20007; (202) 687–8803; 1996. 5 videocassettes; 146 min. total (19–45 min. each); sd., color; VHS.
(GENETIC SCREENING; GENETIC SERVICES; GENOME MAPPING)

Humanist Laureates of the International Academy of Humanism see **Admiraal, Pieter**

Humber, James M.; Almeder, Robert F., eds. Human Cloning. Totowa, NJ: Humana Press; 1998. 214 p.
(CLONING)

Humphry, Derek; Clement, Mary. Freedom to Die: People, Politics, and the Right-to-Die Movement. New York, NY: St. Martin's Press; 1998. 388 p.
(EUTHANASIA/ATTITUDES; EUTHANASIA/LEGAL ASPECTS; SUICIDE)

Hundert, Edward M.; Hafferty, Fred; Christakis,

Dimitri. Characteristics of the informal curriculum and trainees' ethical choices. *Academic Medicine.* 1996 Jun; 71(6): 624–633.
(MEDICAL ETHICS/EDUCATION)

Hunsicker, Lawrence G. see **Lin, Hung–Mo**

Hunt, Geoffrey. Abortion: why bioethics can have no answer -- a personal perspective. *Nursing Ethics.* 1999 Jan; 6(1): 47–57.
(ABORTION; FETUSES; PERSONHOOD)

Hunt, Geoffrey see **Tschudin, Verena**

Hunt, J.R. see **Ulrich, C.M.**

Hunt, Jean; Joffe, Carole. Problems and prospects of contemporary abortion provision. *In:* Dan, Alice J., ed. Reframing Women's Health: Multidisciplinary Research and Practice. Thousand Oaks, CA: Sage Publications; 1994: 163–174.
(ABORTION)

Hunt, John. Abortion and Nazism: is there really a connection? *Linacre Quarterly.* 1996 Nov; 63(4): 53–63.
(ABORTION)

Hunt, Sonja see **Albert, Steven M.**

Hunter, A. see **Cappelli, M.**

Hurst, Bonnie see **Mika, Karin**

Hurt, Richard D.; Robertson, Channing R. Prying open the door to the tobacco industry's secrets about nicotine: the Minnesota Tobacco Trial. *JAMA.* 1998 Oct 7; 280(13): 1173–1181.
(PUBLIC HEALTH)

Hurwitz, Brian. Pressuring Mrs Thomas to accept treatment: a case history. *Journal of Medical Ethics.* 1998 Oct; 24(5): 320–321.
(TREATMENT REFUSAL)

Hurwitz, Brian see **Greenhalgh, Trisha**

Huser, Frank A. Palliative Care and Euthanasia. Edinburgh: Campion Press; 1995. 69 p.
(EUTHANASIA; TERMINAL CARE)

Husted, Jørgen. Autonomy and a right not to know. *In:* Chadwick, Ruth; Levitt, Mairi; Shickle, Darren, eds. The Right to Know and the Right Not to Know. Brookfield, VT: Ashgate; 1997: 55–68.
(GENETIC SCREENING)

Husted, Jörgen see **Chadwick, Ruth**

Hutcheon, R. Gordon; Mitchell, John J.; Schmerler, Susan. The Pediatric Ethics Forum: exploring the ethical dimensions of pediatric care. [Case analysis]. *HEC (HealthCare Ethics Committee) Forum.* 1998 Sep–Dec; 10(3–4): 338–349.
(ALLOWING TO DIE; ETHICISTS AND ETHICS COMMITTEES)

Hyer, Steven see **Limentani, Alexander E.**

Hyland, Michael E. see **Albert, Steven M.**

Hyodo, Chigusa see **Hamajima, Nobuyuki**

I

Iacopino, Vincent see **Frank, Martina W.**

Ickes, Cynthia see **Flanders, Steven**

Idziak, Janine M. Ethical Dilemmas in Allied Health. Dubuque, IA: Simon and Kolz; 2000. 288 p.
(BIOETHICS; PROFESSIONAL ETHICS)

Iglehart, John K. The American health care system: Medicaid. *New England Journal of Medicine.* 1999 Feb 4; 340(5): 403–408.
(HEALTH CARE/ECONOMICS)

Iglehart, John K. The American health care system: Medicare. *New England Journal of Medicine.* 1999 Jan 28; 30(4): 327–332.
(HEALTH CARE/ECONOMICS; PATIENT CARE/AGED)

Iglehart, John K. see **Fuchs, Victor**

IJsselmuiden, Carel B. see **Merson, Michael H.**

Ikels, Charlotte. Ethical issues in organ procurement in Chinese societies. *China Journal.* 1997 Jul; No. 38: 95–119.
(ORGAN AND TISSUE DONATION; ORGAN AND TISSUE TRANSPLANTATION)

Ikemoto, Lisa C. When a hospital becomes Catholic. *Mercer Law Review.* 1996 Summer; 47(4): 1087–1134.
(HEALTH CARE/ECONOMICS)

Ilani, Zvi; Weinberger, Yaakov, comps. The obligation to heal and medical malpractice. *Jewish Medical Ethics.* 1997 Jan; 3(1): 18–29.
(PATIENT CARE)

Iles, Alastair T. The Human Genome Project: a challenge to the human rights framework. *Harvard Human Rights Journal.* 1996 Spring; 9: 27–60.
(GENOME MAPPING)

Illhardt, Franz J. Ownership of the human body: deontological approaches. *In:* ten Have, Henk A.M.J.; Welie, Jos V.M., eds. Ownership of the Human Body: Philosophical Considerations on the Use of the Human Body and Its Parts in Healthcare. Boston, MA: Kluwer Academic; 1998: 187–206.
(ORGAN AND TISSUE DONATION)

Illinois. Appellate Court, First District, Fifth Division. In re Brown. *North Eastern Reporter, 2d Series.* 1997 Dec 31 (date of decision). 689: 397–406.
(FETUSES; TREATMENT REFUSAL)

Illinois. Appellate Court, First District, Fourth Division. In re Estate of Austwick. *North Eastern Reporter, 2d Series.* 1995 Sep 7 (date of decision). 656: 773–779.
(INFORMED CONSENT; RESUSCITATION ORDERS)

Indiana. Supreme Court. A Woman's Choice–East Side Women's Clinic v. Newman. *North Eastern Reporter, 2d Series.* 1996 Aug 7 (date of decision). 671: 104–113.
(ABORTION/LEGAL ASPECTS)

Ingram, Kellie K. see **Marson, Daniel C.**

Inlander, Charles B. see **Nightingale, Stuart L.**

Institute of Biology (Great Britain). Institute of Biology Response to the Advisory Group on the Ethics of Xenotransplantation, made to the Department of Health. [Consultation response]. London: Institute of Biology [online]. Downloaded from Internet Web site: http://www.primex.co.uk/iob/d13.html on 16 Jan 1998; 1996 Apr 1. 5 p.
(ORGAN AND TISSUE TRANSPLANTATION)

Institute of Biology (Great Britain); British Electrophoresis Society; British Association for Tissue Banks; et al. Xenotransplantation -- Reply to the Government's Response from the Institute of Biology and British Electrophoresis Society (with additional comments from the British Association of Tissue Banks and the Society for Low Temperature Biology). [Consultations]. London: Institute of Biology [online]. Downloaded from Web site: http://www.thomson.com/iob/xenotrans2.html on 16 Jan 1998; 1997 May 6. 2 p.
(ORGAN AND TISSUE TRANSPLANTATION)

Institute of Medicine. Committee on Perinatal Transmission of HIV see **Stoto, Michael A.**

International Committee of Medical Journal Editors. Statement on project-specific industry support for research. [Editorial]. *Canadian Medical Association Journal.* 1998 Mar 10; 158(5): 615–616.
(BIOMEDICAL RESEARCH)

International Federation of Red Cross and Red Crescent Societies; François-Xavier Bagnoud Center for Health and Human Rights, Harvard School of Public Health. AIDS, Health and Human Rights: An Explanatory Model. Geneva: The Federation; Boston, MA: The Center; 1995. 162 p.
(AIDS; PUBLIC HEALTH)

International Reproductive Rights Research Action Group (IRRRAG) see **Petchesky, Rosalind P.**

Inui, Thomas S. see **Simon, Steven R.**

Inwald, A.C.; Hippisley-Cox, Julia; Hippisley-Cox, Stephen; Hill-Smith, Ian. Competency, consent, and the duty of care: ethical dilemma. [Case study and commentaries]. *BMJ (British Medical Journal).* 1998 Sep 19; 317(7161): 809–810.
(TREATMENT REFUSAL/MENTALLY DISABLED)

Iozzio, M.J. Science, ethics, and cloning technologies. *Linacre Quarterly.* 1997 Nov; 64(4): 46–52.
(CLONING)

Ip, Mary see **Cheng, F.**

Iqbal, Aamir; Holley, Jean L. Ethical issues in end-stage renal disease patients who use illicit intravenous drugs. *Seminars in Dialysis.* 1995 Jan–Feb; 8(1): 35–38.
(ORGAN AND TISSUE TRANSPLANTATION; RESOURCE ALLOCATION/BIOMEDICAL TECHNOLOGIES; SELECTION FOR TREATMENT)

Ireland. An act (No. 5 of 1995) to prescribe the conditions subject to which certain information relating to services lawfully available outside the state for termination of pregnancies and to persons who provide such services may be given to individual women or the general public, and other matters. Dated 12 May 1995. (The Regulation of Information (Services Outside the State for Termination of Pregnancies) Act, 1995). [Summary]. *International Digest of Health Legislation.* 1995. 46(4). 481–482.
(ABORTION/FOREIGN COUNTRIES; ABORTION/LEGAL ASPECTS)

Iserson, Kenneth V. see **Hernández–Arriaga, Jorge**

Ish, Christopher see **Segal, Eran**

Isoniemi, H. Living kidney donation: a surgeon's opinion. *Nephrology, Dialysis, Transplantation.* 1997 Sep; 12(9): 1828–1829.
(ORGAN AND TISSUE DONATION)

Israel. The Patients' Rights Act, 1996. Dated 1 May 1996. (*Sefer Hakhukim*, 5756, 12 May 1996, p. 327). [Summary]. *International Digest of Health Legislation.* 1997; 48(2): 187–193.
(PATIENTS' RIGHTS)

Israeli, Saul. Organ transplants: responsa. *Jewish Medical Ethics.* 1997 Jan; 3(1): 14–17.
(ORGAN AND TISSUE DONATION)

Italian Society of Hospital Geriatricians see **Zuccaro, Stefano Maria**

Ivinson, Adrian J. Hard-won consensus on AIDS vaccine trial guidelines. [News]. *Nature Medicine.* 1998 Aug; 4(8): 874.
(AIDS/HUMAN EXPERIMENTATION; HUMAN EXPERIMENTATION/FOREIGN COUNTRIES; IMMUNIZATION)

Ivinson, Adrian J. see **Cohen, Jon**

J

Jackson, Fatimah. Assessing the Human Genome Project: an African–American and bioanthropological critique. *In:* Smith, Edward; Sapp, Walter, eds. Plain Talk about the Human Genome Project: A Tuskegee University Conference on Its Promise and Perils ... and Matters of Race. Tuskegee, AL: Tuskegee University Press; 1997: 95–103.
(GENETIC RESEARCH; GENOME MAPPING)

Jackson, Jean E. Hippocrates in the bush. *Anthropological Quarterly.* 1996 Jul; 69(3): 120–122.
(PATIENT CARE)

Jacob, Walter. End-stage euthanasia: some other considerations. *In:* Jacob, Walter; Zemer, Moshe, eds. Death and Euthanasia in Jewish Law: Essays and Responsa. Pittsburgh, PA: Freehof Institute of Progressive Halakhah; Rodef Shalom Press; 1995: 89–103.
(ALLOWING TO DIE/RELIGIOUS ASPECTS)

Jacob, Walter; Zemer, Moshe, eds. Death and Euthanasia in Jewish Law: Essays and Responsa. Pittsburgh, PA: Freehof Institute of Progressive Halakhah: Rodef Shalom Press; 1995. 204 p.
(ALLOWING TO DIE/RELIGIOUS ASPECTS; EUTHANASIA/RELIGIOUS ASPECTS)

Jacob, Walter; Zemer, Moshe, eds. The Fetus and Fertility in Jewish Law: Essays and Responsa. Pittsburgh, PA: Rodef Shalom Press; Freehof Institute of Progressive Halakhah; 1995. 224 p.
(BIOETHICS)

Jacobs, Laurie G. see Zelenik, Jomarie

Jacobs, Lawrence; Marmor, Theodore; Oberlander, Jonathan. The Oregon Health Plan and the political paradox of rationing: what advocates and critics have claimed and what Oregon did. *Journal of Health Politics, Policy and Law.* 1999 Feb; 24(1): 161–180.
(HEALTH CARE/ECONOMICS; RESOURCE ALLOCATION)

Jacobson, Jay A. Preaching to the choir: new voices in the end of life discussion. [Editorial]. *Journal of Clinical Oncology.* 1997 Feb; 15(2): 413–415.
(EUTHANASIA/ATTITUDES; SUICIDE)

Jacobson, Nora. The socially constructed breast: breast implants and the medical construction of need. *American Journal of Public Health.* 1998 Aug; 88(8): 1254–1261.
(BIOMEDICAL TECHNOLOGIES; PATIENT CARE)

Jacobsson, L. see Kullgren, G.

Jacoby, Kerry N. Souls, Bodies, Spirits: The Drive to Abolish Abortion Since 1973. Westport, CT: Praeger; 1998. 230 p.
(ABORTION)

Jacoby, Robin see Fazel, Seena

Jaeger, A.S.; Goode, E.L.; Boyle, J.M. Attitudes and opinions towards genetic testing among US Hispanics. [Abstract]. *American Journal of Human Genetics.* 1997 Oct; 61(4): A221.
(GENETIC SCREENING)

Jaffe, Deborah see Grumbach, Kevin

Jain, Renu; Thomasma, David C.; Ragas, Rasa. Ethical challenges in the treatment of infants of drug-abusing mothers. *Cambridge Quarterly of Healthcare Ethics.* 1999 Spring; 8(2): 179–188.
(ALLOWING TO DIE/INFANTS)

Jain, Sanjeev see Chatterji, Somnath

Jakobsen, A. Living renal transplantation -- the Oslo experience. *Nephrology, Dialysis, Transplantation.* 1997 Sep; 12(9): 1825–1827.
(ORGAN AND TISSUE DONATION; ORGAN AND TISSUE TRANSPLANTATION)

James, C.A.; Bernhardt, B.A.; Doksum, T.; Holtzman, N.A.; Geller, G. Attitudes toward BRCA1 testing among physicians and medical students. [Abstract]. *American Journal of Human Genetics.* 1996 Oct; 59(4): A7.
(GENETIC SCREENING)

James, Caryn. '60 Minutes,' Kevorkian and a death for the cameras. *New York Times.* 1998 Nov 23: A12.
(EUTHANASIA)

James, P.B. see West, Charles

James, Trudi; Platzer, Hazel. Ethical considerations in qualitative research with vulnerable groups: exploring lesbians' and gay men's experiences of health care -- a personal perspective. *Nursing Ethics.* 1999 Jan; 6(1): 73–81.
(BEHAVIORAL RESEARCH/SPECIAL POPULATIONS)

Jamison, Kay R. see Trippitelli, Carol Lynn

Jamison, Stephen. Assisted Suicide: A Decision–Making Guide for Health Professionals. San Francisco, CA: Jossey–Bass; 1997. 248 p.
(SUICIDE; TERMINAL CARE)

Jan, Stephen see Mooney, Gavin

Janofsky, Jeffrey S. see Barton, C. Dennis

Janofsky, Michael. Judge backs Virginia limit on abortions. [News]. *New York Times.* 1998 Jul 2: A12.
(ABORTION/LEGAL ASPECTS)

Jansen, Lynn A. Assessing clinical pragmatism. *Kennedy Institute of Ethics Journal.* 1998 Mar; 8(1): 23–36.
(BIOETHICS)

Janson, C.G. Thoughts on medical ethics and education. *Pharos.* 1997 Fall; 60(4): 31–34.
(MEDICAL ETHICS/EDUCATION)

Jariod, Manuel see Porta, Miguel

Jaroff, Leon. Fixing the genes. *Time.* 1999 Jan 11; 153(1): 68–70, 73.
(GENE THERAPY)

Jaroff, Leon. Success stories: the verdict on the pioneering children of gene therapy -- so far, so good. *Time.* 1999 Jan 11; 153(1): 72–73.
(GENE THERAPY)

Jaworowski, Solomon; Nachmias, Solomon; Zabow, Aubrey. Enforced psychiatric treatment of minors in Israel: the interface between the Mental Health Act and the Youth Law. *Israel Journal of Psychiatry and Related Sciences.* 1995; 32(2): 114–119.
(INVOLUNTARY COMMITMENT/FOREIGN COUNTRIES; INVOLUNTARY COMMITMENT/MINORS)

Jayaraman, K.S. Ban on sale may cause Indian blood shortage. [News]. *Nature Medicine.* 1998 Feb; 4(2): 139.
(BLOOD DONATION)

Jayaraman, K.S. Indian state plans compulsory HIV testing, segregation and branding. [News]. *Nature Medicine.* 1998 Apr; 4(4): 378.
(AIDS/TESTING AND SCREENING)

Jayaraman, K.S. Row in India over rules on animal experiments. [News]. *Nature.* 1998 Sep 10; 395(6698): 108.
(ANIMAL EXPERIMENTATION)

Jayaraman, K.S. Will new guidelines protect or expose the Indian gene pool? [News]. *Nature Medicine.* 1998 Jun; 4(6): 653.
(GENETIC RESEARCH)

Jean, Pierre see Beaudoin, Claude

Jeffko, Walter G. Abortion, personhood, and community. *In: his* Contemporary Ethical Issues: A Personalistic Perspective. Amherst, NY: Humanity Books; 1999: 59–84.
(ABORTION; FETUSES; PERSONHOOD)

Jeffko, Walter G. Euthanasia: a reinterpretation. *In: his* Contemporary Ethical Issues: A Personalistic Perspective. Amherst, NY: Humanity Books; 1999: 85–105.

(ALLOWING TO DIE; EUTHANASIA)

Jekel, James F. see **Bogardus, Sidney T.**

Jekel, James F. see **Kaldjian, Lauris C.**

Jellinek, Michael S. see **Van der Feen, Julie R.**

Jennett, Bryan. Discontinuation of ventilation after brain stem death: brain stem death defines death in law. *BMJ (British Medical Journal).* 1999 Jun 26; 318(7200): 1755.
(DETERMINATION OF DEATH/BRAIN DEATH)

Jensen, Norman see **Gilligan, Mary Ann**

Jensen, Peter S. see **Fisher, Celia B.**

Jensen, Peter S. see **Hoagwood, Kimberly**

Jensen, Peter S. see **Leonard, Henrietta**

Jernigan, Jan C. see **Meisel, Alan**

Jespersen, Bruce W. see **Crelinsten, Gordon L.**

Jha, Vivekanand see **Chugh, Kirpal S.**

Joblin, Joseph. Health and the distribution of resources. *Dolentium Hominum: Church and Health in the World.* 1998; No. 37 [yr. 13(1)]: 63–68.
(HEALTH; HEALTH CARE/RIGHTS; RESOURCE ALLOCATION)

Jochemsen, Henk; Keown, John. Voluntary euthanasia under control? Further empirical evidence from the Netherlands. *Journal of Medical Ethics.* 1999 Feb; 25(1): 16–21.
(ALLOWING TO DIE; EUTHANASIA; SUICIDE)

Jochemsen, Henk see **Cusveller, Bart**

Jõe, Linda see **Sage, William M.**

Joffe, Carole see **Hunt, Jean**

Johannes, Laura. Sham surgery is used to test effectiveness of novel operations. [News]. *Wall Street Journal.* 1998 Dec 11: A1.
(HUMAN EXPERIMENTATION/RESEARCH DESIGN)

Johnson, Dirk. Kevorkian faces a murder charge in death of man. [News]. *New York Times.* 1998 Nov 26: A1, A18.
(EUTHANASIA/LEGAL ASPECTS)

Johnson, Dirk. Kevorkian sentenced to 10 to 25 years in prison. [News]. *New York Times.* 1999 Apr 14: A1, A23.
(EUTHANASIA/LEGAL ASPECTS)

Johnson, John L. see **Desvarieux, Moïse**

Johnson, Linda. Expanding eugenics or improving health care in China: commentary on the Provisions of the Standing Committee of the Gansu People's Congress concerning the prohibition of reproduction by intellectually impaired persons. *Journal of Law and Society.* 1997 Jun; 24(2): 199–234.
(EUGENICS; STERILIZATION/MENTALLY DISABLED)

Johnson, Margaret see **Gbolade, Babatunde A.**

Johnson, Mark Paul see **Evans, Mark I.**

Johnson, MeriLou see **Anderson, Donna G.**

Johnson, N.E.; Rusche, B. Ethics committees: how do they contribute to the Three Rs? Synopsis of the workshop. *In:* van Zutphen, L.F.M.; Balls, M., eds. Animal Alternatives, Welfare and Ethics. New York, NY: Elsevier; 1997: 391–395.
(ANIMAL EXPERIMENTATION)

Johnson, Paul see **West, Charles**

Johnson, Philip R.S. An analysis of "dignity". *Theoretical Medicine and Bioethics.* 1998 Aug; 19(4): 337–352.
(TERMINAL CARE)

Johnson, T.R. see **Rosner, Mary**

Johnston, Wendy S. see **Ganzini, Linda**

Johnstone, Frank D. see **Simpson, Wendy M.**

Joint Commission on Accreditation of Healthcare Organizations. Ethical Issues and Patient Rights: Across the Continuum of Care. Oakbrook Terrace, IL: The Commission; 1998. 156 p.
(BIOETHICS; PATIENTS' RIGHTS)

Joint Commission on Accreditation of Healthcare Organizations. Standards for restraint and seclusion. *Joint Commission Perspectives.* 1996 Jan–Feb; 16(1): RS1–RS8.
(BEHAVIOR CONTROL)

Jonas, Harry S. see **Gans Epner, Janet E.**

Jones, A.S. see **Houghton, D.J.**

Jones, Anne Hudson. Narrative based medicine: narrative in medical ethics. *BMJ (British Medical Journal).* 1999 Jan 23; 318(7178): 253–256.
(MEDICAL ETHICS)

Jones, Anne Hudson. Publication and promotion: is the system really broken? *Lancet.* 1998 Sep 12; 352(9131): 894–895.
(BIOMEDICAL RESEARCH)

Jones, Charlotte; Freeman, John M. Decision making in the nursery: an ethical dilemma. *Journal of Clinical Ethics.* 1998 Fall; 9(3): 314–322.
(ALLOWING TO DIE/INFANTS; PATIENT CARE/MINORS)

Jones, D. Gareth. The problematic symmetry between brain birth and brain death. *Journal of Medical Ethics.* 1998 Aug; 24(4): 237–242.
(DETERMINATION OF DEATH/BRAIN DEATH; FETUSES; PERSONHOOD)

Jones, Gary E. Do the 'Baby Doe' rules discriminate against infants? *Pediatrician.* 1990; 17(2): 87–91.
(ALLOWING TO DIE/INFANTS)

Jones, Ian; Craddock, Nick. Ethical issues in genetics of mental disorders. [Letter]. *Lancet.* 1998 Nov 28; 352(9142): 1788.
(GENETIC SCREENING)

Jones, Judy. Government sets up inquiry into ventilation

trial. [News]. *BMJ (British Medical Journal).* 1999 Feb 27; 318(7183): 553.
(HUMAN EXPERIMENTATION/FOREIGN COUNTRIES; HUMAN EXPERIMENTATION/INFORMED CONSENT; HUMAN EXPERIMENTATION/MINORS)

Jones, Melvyn see **Gbolade, Babatunde A.**

Jones, Nikki. Culture and reproductive health: challenges for feminist philanthrophy. *In:* Donchin, Anne; Purdy, Laura M., eds. Embodying Bioethics: Recent Feminist Advances. Lanham, MD: Rowman and Littlefield; 1999: 223–237.
(HEALTH; REPRODUCTION)

Jones, Steve; Oswald, Nigel; Date, Jan; Hinds, Di. Attitudes of patients to medical student participation: general practice consultations on the Cambridge Community-Based Clinical Course. *Medical Education.* 1996 Jan; 30(1): 14–17.
(PATIENT CARE)

Jones, Valerie A. In the same boat. *JAMA.* 1998 Nov 4; 280(17): 1537–1538.
(GENETIC SCREENING)

Jonsen, Albert R. Physician-assisted suicide. *Seattle University Law Review.* 1995 Spring; 18(3): 459–471.
(SUICIDE)

Jonsen, Albert R. The birth of bioethics: the origins and evolution of a demi-discipline. *Medical Humanities Review.* 1997 Spring; 11(1): 9–21.
(BIOETHICS)

Jonsen, Albert R. The ethics of pediatric medicine. *In:* Rudolph, Abraham M.; Hoffman, Julien I.E.; Rudolph, Colin D.; Sagan, Paul, eds. Rudolph's Pediatrics. Nineteenth Edition. Norwalk, CT: Appleton and Lange; 1991: 7–14.
(PATIENT CARE/MINORS)

Jonsson, Lena. The Swedish transplantation law. *International Digest of Health Legislation.* 1997; 48(2): 237–239.
(FETUSES; ORGAN AND TISSUE DONATION)

Jordan, Elke see **Collins, Francis S.**

Jordan, Mary; Sullivan, Kevin. Japan takes dim view of fertility treatments. [News]. *Washington Post.* 1998 Jul 5: A13.
(REPRODUCTIVE TECHNOLOGIES)

Jorm, Anthony F. see **Kitchener, Betty**

Josefson, Deborah. Prisoner wants to donate his second kidney. [News]. *BMJ (British Medical Journal).* 1999 Jan 2; 318(7175): 7.
(ORGAN AND TISSUE DONATION)

Josefson, Deborah. U.S. doctors want no part in executions. [News]. *BMJ (British Medical Journal).* 1998 Sep 12; 317(7160): 702.
(CAPITAL PUNISHMENT)

Jost, Timothy S. Public financing of pain management: leaky umbrellas and ragged safety nets. *Journal of Law, Medicine and Ethics.* 1998 Winter; 26(4): 290–307.
(HEALTH CARE/ECONOMICS; PATIENT CARE/DRUGS; TERMINAL CARE)

Jourdin, Gonzague see **Merson, Michael H.**

Jovell, Albert J. see **Serra-Prat, Mateu**

Joy, Mark; Hemmings, Gwynneth; Al-Adwani, Andrew; Szasz, Thomas. Parity of mental illness, disparity for the mental patient. [Letters and response]. *Lancet.* 1999 Jan 2; 353(9146): 73–74.
(BEHAVIOR CONTROL; MENTAL HEALTH)

Judd, Karen see **Petchesky, Rosalind P.**

Juengst, Eric T. Self-critical federal science? The ethics experiment within the U.S. Human Genome Project. *In:* Paul, Ellen Frankel; Miller, Fred D.; Paul, Jeffrey, eds. Scientific Innovation, Philosophy, and Public Policy. New York, NY: Cambridge University Press; 1996: 63–95.
(GENOME MAPPING)

Juengst, Eric T. The ethical implications of Alzheimer disease risk testing for other clinical uses of APOE genotyping. *In:* Post, Stephen G.; Whitehouse, Peter J., eds. Genetic Testing for Alzheimer Disease: Ethical and Clinical Issues. Baltimore, MD: Johns Hopkins University Press; 1998: 177–189.
(GENETIC SCREENING)

Juengst, Eric T. What does *enhancement* mean? *In:* Parens, Erik, ed. Enhancing Human Traits: Ethical and Social Implications. Washington, DC: Georgetown University Press; 1998: 29–47.
(BIOMEDICAL TECHNOLOGIES; HEALTH; HEALTH CARE)

Juhl, Marian Haglund. A tattoo in time: I want my last wish to be clearly visible so it will be honored by the doctor who treats me. *Newsweek.* 1997 Oct 13; 130(15): 19.
(RESUSCITATION ORDERS)

Julian-Reyneir, C.; Eisinger, F.; Aurran, Y.; Chabal, F.; Sobol, H. Attitudes about breast cancer genetics and preventive strategies: a national survey of French medical and surgical gynecologists. [Abstract]. *American Journal of Human Genetics.* 1997 Oct; 61(4): A222.
(GENETIC SCREENING)

Julvez, Jean; Tuppin, Phillippe; Cohen, Sophie. Survey in France of response to xenotransplantation. [Research letter]. *Lancet.* 1999 Feb 27; 353(9154): 726.
(ORGAN AND TISSUE DONATION; ORGAN AND TISSUE TRANSPLANTATION)

Jurevic, Amy. Disparate impact under Title VI: discrimination, by any other name, will still have the same impact. *Saint Louis University Public Law Review.* 1996; 15(2): 237–265.
(HEALTH CARE/ECONOMICS; RESOURCE ALLOCATION)

K

Kaczor, Christopher. Faith and reason and physician-assisted suicide. *Christian Bioethics.* 1998 Aug; 4(2): 183–201.
(SUICIDE)

Kadlec, Robert F. see **Tokuda, Yasuharu**

Kagawa-Singer, Marjorie see **Wenger, Neil**

Kahn, Charles N. Patients' rights proposals: the insurers'

perspective. *JAMA.* 1999 Mar 3; 281(9): 858.
(HEALTH CARE/ECONOMICS; PATIENTS' RIGHTS)

Kahn, Jeffrey. Bioethics and tobacco. *Bioethics Examiner.* 1997 Fall; 1(3): 1, 7.
(BIOETHICS; PUBLIC HEALTH)

Kahn, Jeffrey. Ethical issues in genetic testing for Alzheimer's disease. *Geriatrics.* 1997 Sep; 52(Suppl. 2): S30–S32.
(GENETIC SCREENING)

Kahn, Katherine see **Wenger, Neil**

Kahn, Tamar Joy see **Walters, LeRoy**

Kaikati, Jack G. see **Virgo, Katherine S.**

Kaiser, Jocelyn. Activists ransack Minnesota labs. [News]. *Science.* 1999 Apr 16; 284(5413): 410–411.
(ANIMAL EXPERIMENTATION)

Kaiser, Jocelyn. Baylor saga comes to an end. [News]. *Science.* 1999 Feb 19; 283(5405): 1091.
(BIOMEDICAL RESEARCH; FRAUD AND MISCONDUCT)

Kaiser, Jocelyn. EPA ponders pesticide tests in humans. [News]. *Science.* 1999 Jan 1; 283(5398): 18–19.
(HUMAN EXPERIMENTATION)

Kaiser, Jocelyn, ed. Ethics of studying cybernauts. [News]. *Science.* 1999 Jun 25; 284(5423): 2051.
(BEHAVIORAL RESEARCH)

Kaiser, Jocelyn. ORI report tracks gun-shy feds. [News]. *Science.* 1999 May 7; 284(5416): 901.
(BIOMEDICAL RESEARCH; FRAUD AND MISCONDUCT)

Kaiser, Jocelyn. Tulane inquiry clears lead researcher. [News]. *Science.* 1999 Jun 18; 284(5422): 1905.
(BIOMEDICAL RESEARCH; FRAUD AND MISCONDUCT)

Kaiser, Jocelyn, ed. Weighing in on bioethics. [News]. *Science.* 1999 Apr 23; 284(5414): 551.
(BIOETHICS)

Kakizoe, Tadao see **Okamura, Hitoshi**

Kakkar, Supriya. Unauthorized embryo transfer at the University of California, Irvine Center for Reproductive Health. [Note]. *Hastings Constitutional Law Quarterly.* 1997 Summer; 24(4): 1015–1033.
(FRAUD AND MISCONDUCT; REPRODUCTIVE TECHNOLOGIES)

Kalb, Paul E. Health care fraud and abuse. *JAMA.* 1999 Sep 22–29; 282(12): 1163–1168.
(FRAUD AND MISCONDUCT; HEALTH CARE/ECONOMICS)

Kaldjian, Lauris C.; Jekel, James F.; Friedland, Gerald. End-of-life decisions in HIV-positive patients: the role of spiritual beliefs. *AIDS.* 1998 Jan 1; 12(1): 103–107.
(AIDS; TERMINAL CARE)

Kalebic, Thea see **Des Jarlais, Don C.**

Kalian, Moshe see **Bar El, Yair Carlos**

Kalian, Moshe see **Mester, Roberto**

Kaltiala–Heino, Riittakerttu; Laippala, Pekka; Salokangas, Raimo K.R. Impact of coercion on treatment outcome. *International Journal of Law and Psychiatry.* 1997 Summer; 20(3): 311–322.
(INVOLUNTARY COMMITMENT/FOREIGN COUNTRIES)

Kamberg, Caren see **Leape, Lucian L.**

Kamisar, Yale. No constitutional right to physician–assisted suicide. *Health Law News.* 1997 Sep; 11(1): 2–3.
(SUICIDE)

Kane, Richard S.; Hammes, Bernard; Morgenweck, Cynthiane J.; Finucane, Thomas E.; Leal–Mora, David. Nursing home CPR policies. [Letter and response]. *Journal of the American Geriatrics Society.* 1998 Jan; 46(1): 116–117.
(RESUSCITATION ORDERS)

Kane, Robert L. see **Kane, Rosalie A.**

Kane, Rosalie A.; Kane, Robert L.; Ladd, Richard C. The Heart of Long-Term Care. New York, NY: Oxford University Press; 1998. 328 p.
(HEALTH CARE; PATIENT CARE/AGED)

Kantor, Jay E. Ethics consultations in psychiatric private practice. *SBC Newsletter (Society for Bioethics Consultation).* 1996 Spring: 10–12.
(ETHICISTS AND ETHICS COMMITTEES)

Kao, Audiey C.; Green, Diane C.; Zaslavsky, Alan M.; Koplan, Jeffrey P.; Cleary, Paul D. The relationship between method of physician payment and patient trust. *JAMA.* 1998 Nov 18; 280(19): 1708–1714.
(HEALTH CARE/ECONOMICS; PROFESSIONAL PATIENT RELATIONSHIP)

Kaplan, Kalman J. The case of Dr. Kevorkian and Mr. Gale: a brief historical note. *Omega: A Journal of Death and Dying.* 1997–1998; 36(2): 169–176.
(SUICIDE)

Kaplan, Kalman J. see **Wooddell, Victor**

Kaplan, Laura. The Story of Jane: The Legendary Underground Feminist Abortion Service. Chicago, IL: University of Chicago Press; 1995. 314 p.
(ABORTION)

Kaplan, Starr (Esther) Rose. Germ–line genetic engineering revisited. *Pharos.* 1997 Fall; 60(4): 21–25.
(GENE THERAPY)

Kapp, Marshall B. Annotated bibliography on physician–assisted suicide. *Journal of Ethics, Law, and Aging.* 1997 Spring-Summer; 3(1): 45–51.
(SUICIDE)

Kapp, Marshall B. Can managed care be managed? *Pharos.* 1998 Spring; 61(2): 15–17.
(HEALTH CARE/ECONOMICS)

Kapp, Marshall B. Commentary: anxieties as a legal impediment to the doctor-proxy relationship. *Journal of Law, Medicine and Ethics.* 1999 Spring; 27(1): 69–73.
(ADVANCE DIRECTIVES; ALLOWING TO DIE/LEGAL ASPECTS; INFORMED CONSENT)

Kapp, Marshall B. *De facto* health–care rationing by age:

the law has no remedy. *Journal of Legal Medicine.* 1998 Sep; 19(3): 323–249.
(RESOURCE ALLOCATION; SELECTION FOR TREATMENT)

Kapp, Marshall B. The physician–assisted suicide debate: which side is "gerontologically correct"? [Editorial]. *Journal of Ethics, Law, and Aging.* 1997 Spring–Summer; 3(1): 3–4.
(SUICIDE)

Käppeli, Othmar; Auberson, Lillian. Biotech battlelines. [Letter]. *Nature.* 1998 Jul 2; 394(6688): 10.
(GENETIC INTERVENTION; RECOMBINANT DNA RESEARCH)

Karanjawala, Zarir E.; Collins, Francis S. Genetics in the context of medical practice. *JAMA.* 1998 Nov 4; 280(17): 1533–1534.
(GENETIC SCREENING)

Karim, Quarraisha Abdool; Karim, Salim S. Abdool; Coovadia, Hoosen M.; Susser, Mervyn. Informed consent for HIV testing in a South African hospital: is it truly informed and truly voluntary? *American Journal of Public Health.* 1998 Apr; 88(4): 637–640.
(AIDS/HUMAN EXPERIMENTATION; AIDS/TESTING AND SCREENING; HUMAN EXPERIMENTATION/FOREIGN COUNTRIES; HUMAN EXPERIMENTATION/INFORMED CONSENT)

Karim, Salim S. Abdool. Placebo controls in HIV perinatal transmission trials: a South African's viewpoint. *American Journal of Public Health.* 1998 Apr; 88(4): 564–566.
(AIDS/HUMAN EXPERIMENTATION; HUMAN EXPERIMENTATION/FOREIGN COUNTRIES; HUMAN EXPERIMENTATION/RESEARCH DESIGN)

Karim, Salim S. Abdool see **Karim, Quarraisha Abdool**

Karlawish, Jason H.T. Shared decision making in critical care: a clinical reality and an ethical necessity. *American Journal of Critical Care.* 1996 Nov; 5(6): 391–396.
(INFORMED CONSENT)

Karlawish, Jason H.T.; Quill, Timothy; Meier, Diane E.; American College of Physicians–American Society of Internal Medicine End–of–Life Care Consensus Panel. A consensus–based approach to providing palliative care to patients who lack decision–making capacity. *Annals of Internal Medicine.* 1999 May 18; 130(10): 835–840.
(TERMINAL CARE)

Karli, Pierre. Conceptual and ethical problems raised by the study of brain–behavior relationships underlying aggression. *In:* Feshbach, Seymour; Zagrodzka, Jolanta, eds. Aggression: Biological, Developmental, and Social Perspectives. New York, NY: Plenum Press; 1997: 3–14.
(BEHAVIORAL RESEARCH)

Karlin, Patricia Devine see **Wilfert, Catherine M.**

Karlinsky, Harry. Genetic testing and counseling for early–onset autosomal–dominant Alzheimer disease. *In:* Post, Stephen G.; Whitehouse, Peter J., eds. Genetic Testing for Alzheimer Disease: Ethical and Clinical Issues. Baltimore, MD: Johns Hopkins University Press; 1998: 103–117.
(GENETIC COUNSELING; GENETIC SCREENING)

Karp, Naomi see **Wood, Erica**

Karro, Helle. Abortion in the framework of family planning in Estonia. *Acta Obstetricia et Gynecologica Scandinavica.* 1997; 76(Suppl. 164): 46–50.
(ABORTION/FOREIGN COUNTRIES)

Kash, Kathryn M. Psychosocial and ethical implications of defining genetic risk for cancers. *Annals of the New York Academy of Sciences.* 1995 Sep 30; 768: 41–52.
(GENETIC COUNSELING; GENETIC SCREENING)

Kass, Leon R.; Wilson, James Q. The Ethics of Human Cloning. Washington, DC: AEI Press; 1998. 101 p.
(CLONING)

Kass, Nancy see **Faden, Ruth**

Kass, Nancy E. see **Sugarman, Jeremy**

Kassirer, Jerome P. see **Menendez, Roger**

Katchatrian, Naira see **Dolian, Gayane**

Kater, Michael H. The Sewering scandal of 1993 and the German medical establishment. *In:* Berg, Manfred; Cocks, Geoffrey, eds. Medicine and Modernity: Public Health and Medical Care in Nineteenth– and Twentieth–Century Germany. New York, NY: Cambridge University Press; 1997: 213–234.
(EUTHANASIA; FRAUD AND MISCONDUCT)

Katz, Cheryl see **Ferris, Lorraine E.**

Katz, Patricia P. see **Showstack, Jonathan**

Katzoff, Michael see **Kosseff, Andrew L.**

Kauffman, H. Myron see **Lin, Hung–Mo**

Kaufman, Jeffrey L. see **Greenfield, Barak**

Kautenburger, Monika see **Allert, Gebhard**

Kavanaugh, John F. Ethical commitments in health care systems. *America.* 1998 Nov 7; 179(14): 20.
(ABORTION/RELIGIOUS ASPECTS; CONTRACEPTION; HEALTH CARE)

Kawai, Chisato see **Hamajima, Nobuyuki**

Kawakami, Ikuko see **Kitamura, Fusako**

Kay, A. see **Galton, D.J.**

Kaye, Howard L. Anxiety and genetic manipulation: a sociological view. *Perspectives in Biology and Medicine.* 1998 Summer; 41(4): 483–490.
(CLONING; GENETIC INTERVENTION)

Kayss, Matthias see **Boshammer, Susanne**

Kazanowski, Mary. A commitment to palliative care: could it impact assisted suicide? *Journal of Gerontological Nursing.* 1997 Mar; 23(3): 36–42.
(TERMINAL CARE)

Keane, Dennis see **Bindman, Andrew B.**

Keaney, Patrick see **Carron, Annette T.**

Keenan, James F. Institutional cooperation and the ethical

and religious directives. *Linacre Quarterly*. 1997 Aug; 64(3): 53–76.
(HEALTH CARE)

Keenan, James F. The case for physician–assisted suicide? *America*. 1998 Nov 14; 179(15): 14–19.
(SUICIDE)

Keenan, James F.; O'Rourke, Kevin. Cooperation and "hard cases." Part 1: cooperation pro and con. [Article and response]. *Ethics and Medics*. 1998 Sep; 23(9): 3–4.
(STERILIZATION)

Keenlyside, Richard see **McGovern, Margaret M.**

Keeth, Merrill Beth see **Webb, Cynthia M.**

Kefalides, Paul. Solid organ transplantation. 1: Many problems, new solutions. *Annals of Internal Medicine*. 1998 Dec 15; 129(12): 1093–1095.
(ORGAN AND TISSUE DONATION)

Kefalides, Paul. Solid organ transplantation. 2: Ethical considerations. *Annals of Internal Medicine*. 1999 Jan 19; 130(2): 169–170.
(ORGAN AND TISSUE DONATION; ORGAN AND TISSUE TRANSPLANTATION)

Keffer, M. Jan. Ethical decisions with limited resources: how is that possible? *Nursing Case Management*. 1997 Sep–Oct; 2(5): 196–202.
(HEALTH CARE/ECONOMICS)

Kegley, Jacquelyn Ann K. Community, autonomy, and managed care. *In:* McGee, Glenn, ed. Pragmatic Bioethics. Nashville, TN: Vanderbilt University Press; 1999: 204–227, 281–283.
(HEALTH CARE/ECONOMICS; RESOURCE ALLOCATION)

Keith–Spiegel, Patricia see **Koocher, Gerald P.**

Kelen, Gabor D. see **Marco, Catherine A.**

Keller, Frieder see **Sponholz, Gerlinde**

Kellogg, Sarah C. The due process right to a safe and humane environment for patients in state custody: the voluntary/involuntary distinction. [Note]. *American Journal of Law and Medicine*. 1997; 23(2–3): 339–362.
(INVOLUNTARY COMMITMENT; PATIENTS' RIGHTS/MENTALLY DISABLED)

Kellough, Gail. Aborting Law: An Exploration of the Politics of Motherhood and Medicine. Buffalo, NY: University of Toronto Press; 1996. 340 p.
(ABORTION/FOREIGN COUNTRIES; ABORTION/LEGAL ASPECTS)

Kelly, Brian; Varghese, Francis T. Euthanasia legislation. [Letter]. *Lancet*. 1998 Dec 5; 352(9143): 1863–1864.
(SUICIDE)

Kelly, David F.; Hoyt, John W. Ethics consultation. *Critical Care Clinics*. 1996 Jan; 12(1): 49–70.
(ETHICISTS AND ETHICS COMMITTEES)

Kelly, Dorothy Ellen see **Hayes, Edward J.**

Kelly, Robert. On human cloning. *Nature Biotechnology*. 1998 Sep; 16(9): 798.

(CLONING)

Kelner, Merrijoy see **Colebunders, Robert**

Kelner, Merrijoy see **Singer, Peter A.**

Kempen, G.I.J.M. see **Sullivan, Mark**

Kempf, Judith. Collecting medical specimens in South America: a dilemma in medical ethics. *Anthropological Quarterly*. 1996 Jul; 69(3): 142–148.
(HUMAN EXPERIMENTATION/FOREIGN COUNTRIES; HUMAN EXPERIMENTATION/RESEARCH DESIGN)

Kennedy, B.J. see **Costantini–Ferrando, Maria F.**

Kennedy, Donald see **Barton, John**

Kennedy, Ian. Adult: order concerning future non–treatment: Re R (Adult: Medical Treatment). [Comment]. *Medical Law Review*. 1997 Spring; 5(1): 104–108.
(RESUSCITATION ORDERS)

Kennedy, Ian. Child: discontinuation of treatment: Re C (A Baby). [Comment]. *Medical Law Review*. 1997 Spring; 5(1): 102–104.
(ALLOWING TO DIE/INFANTS; ALLOWING TO DIE/LEGAL ASPECTS)

Kennedy, Ian. Child: terminal illness; withdrawal of treatment -- Re C (A Minor) (Medical Treatment). [Comment]. *Medical Law Review*. 1998 Spring; 6(1): 99–103.
(ALLOWING TO DIE/INFANTS; ALLOWING TO DIE/LEGAL ASPECTS)

Kennedy, Ian. Illness and treatment: meaning for purposes of insurance contract: Katskee v. Blue Cross/Blue Shield. [Comment]. *Medical Law Review*. 1995 Summer; 3(2): 224–227.
(GENETIC SCREENING)

Kennedy, Ian. Minor: consent; sterilisation; best interests -- L and G.M. v. M.M.: The Director–General, Department of Family Services and Aboriginal and Islander Affairs. [Comment]. *Medical Law Review*. 1995 Spring; 3(1): 94–97.
(STERILIZATION/MENTALLY DISABLED)

Kennedy, Ian. Physicians' duty of confidentiality : Saur v. Probes. [Comment]. *Medical Law Review*. 1993 Summer; 1(2): 254–256.
(CONFIDENTIALITY/LEGAL ASPECTS; CONFIDENTIALITY/MENTAL HEALTH)

Kennedy, Ian. Treatment of incompetent child: parental wishes and Charter of Rights and Freedoms -- B. v. Children's Aid Society of Metropolitan Toronto. [Comment]. *Medical Law Review*. 1996 Spring; 4(1): 117–122.
(TREATMENT REFUSAL/MINORS)

Kennedy, Ian. Treatment without consent (adult): force feeding of detainee -- Department of Immigration v. Mok and Another. [Comment]. *Medical Law Review*. 1994 Spring; 2(1): 102–105.
(FORCE FEEDING; TREATMENT REFUSAL)

Kennedy, Ian. Treatment without consent (diagnostic procedure): adult -- Re H (Mental Patient). [Comment]. *Medical Law Review*. 1993 Summer; 1(2): 236–238.

(TREATMENT REFUSAL/MENTALLY DISABLED)

Kennedy, Ian. Treatment without consent (sterilisation): adult -- Re W (A Patient). [Comment]. *Medical Law Review.* 1993 Summer; 1(2): 234–236.
(STERILIZATION/MENTALLY DISABLED)

Kennedy, Ian; Sewell, Herb. Xenotransplantation moratorium. [Letter]. *Nature Biotechnology.* 1998 Feb; 16(2): 120.
(HUMAN EXPERIMENTATION/FOREIGN COUNTRIES; HUMAN EXPERIMENTATION/REGULATION; ORGAN AND TISSUE TRANSPLANTATION)

Kennedy, Ian see **Dworkin, Gerald**

Kennedy Institute of Ethics (Georgetown University). Bioethics Information Retrieval Project. Bioethics Thesaurus. 1999 Edition. Washington, DC: The Institute; 1999. 92 p.
(BIOETHICS)

Kennedy, Randy. U.S. agency says employer should pay for a woman's infertility treatments. [News]. *New York Times.* 1999 Apr 29: B3.
(HEALTH CARE/ECONOMICS; REPRODUCTIVE TECHNOLOGIES)

Kent, Gerry. Responses by four local research ethics committees to submitted proposals. *Journal of Medical Ethics.* 1999 Jun; 25(3): 274–277.
(HUMAN EXPERIMENTATION/ETHICS COMMITTEES; HUMAN EXPERIMENTATION/FOREIGN COUNTRIES)

Kenyon, Georgina. Australian army infected troops and internees in Second World War. [News]. *BMJ (British Medical Journal).* 1999 May 8; 318(7193): 1233.
(FRAUD AND MISCONDUCT; HUMAN EXPERIMENTATION/FOREIGN COUNTRIES)

Kenyon, Georgina. Doctors refuse to operate on 80 year old man. [News]. *BMJ (British Medical Journal).* 1998 Dec 5; 317(7172): 1548.
(PATIENT CARE/AGED; RESOURCE ALLOCATION/BIOMEDICAL TECHNOLOGIES; SELECTION FOR TREATMENT)

Keown, John. A reply to McLachlan. *Journal of Medical Ethics.* 1998 Aug; 24(4): 255–256.
(BLOOD DONATION)

Keown, John see **Jochemsen, Henk**

Keown, Rebecca M. A case–based approach to sterilization of mentally incompetent women. *Princeton Journal of Bioethics.* 1998 Spring; 1(1): 94–113.
(STERILIZATION/MENTALLY DISABLED)

Kerby, Christina see **Pierce, Jessica**

Kerin, Jacinta. Double standards: principled or arbitrary? [Editorial]. *Bioethics.* 1998 Oct; 12(4): iii–vii.
(BIOETHICS)

Kern, David G.; Kern, Robin K.; Durand, Kate T.H.; Shuchman, Miriam. Secrecy in science: the flock worker's lung investigation. [Letter and response]. *Annals of Internal Medicine.* 1999 Apr 6; 130(7): 616.
(BIOMEDICAL RESEARCH; OCCUPATIONAL HEALTH)

Kern, David G. see **Merrill, William W.**

Kern, Robin K. see **Kern, David G.**

Kerner, Jon F. see **Schulman, Kevin A.**

Kerr, Anne; Cunningham-Burley, Sarah; Amos, Amanda. Drawing the line: an analysis of lay people's discussions about the new genetics. *Public Understanding of Science.* 1998 Apr; 7(2): 113–133.
(GENETIC RESEARCH; GENETIC SCREENING; PRENATAL DIAGNOSIS)

Kerr, Anne; Cunningham-Burley, Sarah; Amos, Amanda. The new genetics and health: mobilizing lay expertise. *Public Understanding of Science.* 1998 Jan; 7(1): 41–60.
(GENETIC RESEARCH; GENETIC SCREENING)

Kerr, Susan M.; Caplan, Arthur; Polin, Glenn; Smugar, Steve; O'Neill, Kathryn; Urowitz, Sara. Postmortem sperm procurement. *Journal of Urology.* 1997 Jun; 157(6): 2154–2158.
(ORGAN AND TISSUE DONATION; REPRODUCTIVE TECHNOLOGIES)

Kessler, Seymour. Genetic counseling is directive? Look again. [Letter]. *American Journal of Human Genetics.* 1997 Aug; 61(2): 466–467.
(GENETIC COUNSELING)

Kessler, Suzanne J. Lessons from the Intersexed. New Brunswick, NJ: Rutgers University Press; 1998. 193 p.
(PATIENT CARE/MINORS)

Kettelberger, Denise M. see **Smith, G. Kenneth**

Kettler, D. see **Mohr, M.**

Kettner, Matthias; Schäfer, Dieter. Identifying moral perplexity in reproductive medicine: a discourse ethics rationale. *Human Reproduction and Genetic Ethics: An International Journal.* 1998; 4(1): 8–17.
(REPRODUCTIVE TECHNOLOGIES)

Kevles, Daniel J. Star chambers will result in injustice. [Letter]. *Nature.* 1998 Sep 24; 395(6700): 317.
(BIOMEDICAL RESEARCH; FRAUD AND MISCONDUCT)

Kevles, Daniel J. The Baltimore Case: A Trial of Politics, Science, and Character. New York, NY: Norton; 1998. 509 p.
(BIOMEDICAL RESEARCH; FRAUD AND MISCONDUCT)

Keyserlingk, Edward. Comparing the participation of Native North American and Euro–North American patients in health care decisions. *In:* Coward, Harold; Ratanakul, Pinit, eds. A Cross–Cultural Dialogue on Health Care Ethics. Waterloo, ON: Wilfrid Laurier University Press; 1999: 176–189.
(PATIENT CARE)

Keyserlingk, Edward see **Blue, Arthur**

Keyserlingk, Edward W. see **Blondeau, Danielle**

Khaïat, Lucette. The law and AIDS: issues and objectives (a comparative approach). *Medicine and Law.* 1993; 12(1–2): 3–10.
(AIDS)

Khalsa, Devi Kirin see **Workman, Richard H.**

Khamsi, Firouz; Endman, Maxine W.; Lacanna, Iara C.; Wong, Jeremy. Some psychological aspects of oocyte donation from known donors on altruistic basis. *Fertility and Sterility.* 1997 Aug; 68(2): 323–327.
(ORGAN AND TISSUE DONATION; REPRODUCTIVE TECHNOLOGIES)

Khan, Izhar H. see **Velasco, N.**

Khan, Z.P. see **Swinburn, J.M.A.**

Khanna, Vikram; Silverman, Henry; Schwartz, Jack. Disclosure of operating practices by managed–care organizations to consumers of healthcare: obligations of informed consent. *Journal of Clinical Ethics.* 1998 Fall; 9(3): 291–296.
(HEALTH CARE/ECONOMICS; INFORMED CONSENT)

Al–Khannan, M. see **Shah, V.S.**

Khauli, Raja B. Issues and controversies surrounding organ donation and transplantation: the need for laws that ensure equity and optimal utility of a scarce resource. *Suffolk University Law Review.* 1993 Winter; 27(4): 1225–1236.
(ORGAN AND TISSUE DONATION; ORGAN AND TISSUE TRANSPLANTATION; RESOURCE ALLOCATION/BIOMEDICAL TECHNOLOGIES)

Khoury, Amal J. see **Weisman, Carol S.**

Kilborn, Peter T. Definition of abortion is found to vary abroad. [News]. *New York Times.* 1999 Nov 24: A18.
(ABORTION/FINANCIAL SUPPORT; ABORTION/FOREIGN COUNTRIES; CONTRACEPTION)

Kilborn, Peter T. Pressure growing to cover the cost of birth control. [News]. *New York Times.* 1998 Aug 2: 1, 30.
(CONTRACEPTION; HEALTH CARE/ECONOMICS)

Kiliçaslan, I. see **Sever, M.S.**

Killick, S.R. see **Lui, S.C.**

Kilner, John F.; Orr, Robert D.; Shelly, Judith Allen, eds. The Changing Face of Health Care: A Christian Appraisal of Managed Care, Resource Allocation, and Patient–Caregiver Relationships. Grand Rapids, MI: Eerdmans, Paternoster Press; 1998. 314 p.
(HEALTH CARE/ECONOMICS)

Kilner, John F. see **Neerhof, Mark G.**

Kilner, John F. see **Stewart, Gary P.**

Kim, H. Nina; Gates, Elena; Lo, Bernard. What hysterectomy patients want to know about the roles of residents and medical students in their care. *Academic Medicine.* 1998 Mar; 73(3): 339–341.
(PATIENT CARE)

Kim, Hyang Nina. Prescription for prophecy: confronting the ambiguity of susceptibility testing. *JAMA.* 1998 Nov 4; 280(17): 1535–1536.
(GENETIC SCREENING)

Kim, Roy J. see **Merson, Michael H.**

Kimbrough–Kushner, Thomasine see **Thomasma, David C.**

Kimsma, Gerrit K. see **Thomasma, David C.**

Kin, Curtis A. Coming soon to the "genetic supermarket" near you. [Note]. *Stanford Law Review.* 1996 Jul; 48(6): 1573–1604.
(BIOMEDICAL TECHNOLOGIES; GENETIC INTERVENTION)

King, David. Led by the nose. *GenEthics News.* 1997 Jan–Mar; No. 16: 7.
(CLONING)

King, David. The persistence of eugenics. *GenEthics News.* 1998 Feb–Mar; No. 22: 6–8.
(EUGENICS; GENETIC COUNSELING)

King, David S. Preimplantation genetic diagnosis and the 'new' eugenics. *Journal of Medical Ethics.* 1999 Apr; 25(2): 176–182.
(EUGENICS; GENETIC SCREENING; PRENATAL DIAGNOSIS)

King, Michael see **Shah, Nisha**

King, Patricia. The dilemma of difference. *In:* Smith, Edward; Sapp, Walter, eds. Plain Talk about the Human Genome Project: A Tuskegee University Conference on Its Promise and Perils ... and Matters of Race. Tuskegee, AL: Tuskegee University Press; 1997: 75–81.
(GENOME MAPPING)

King, Ralph T. The pill U.S. drug companies dare not market. [News]. *Wall Street Journal.* 1998 Jun 26: B1, B6.
(CONTRACEPTION)

King, Susan M.; Watson, Heather; Heurter, Helen; Ricketts, Maura; Elsaadany, Susie. Notifying patients exposed to blood products associated with Creutzfeldt–Jakob disease: theoretical risk for real people. *Canadian Medical Association Journal.* 1998 Oct 6; 159(7): 771–774.
(BLOOD DONATION; TRUTH DISCLOSURE)

King, Suzanne see **Low, Lawrence**

King, T.T. see **Engelhart, Karlheinz**

Kinghorn, Warren. Indecision. [Excerpt]. *JAMA.* 1998 Nov 4; 280(17): 1538.
(GENETIC SCREENING)

Kinlaw, Kathy. The changing nature of neonatal ethics in practice. *Clinics in Perinatology.* 1996 Sep; 23(3): 417–428.
(ALLOWING TO DIE/INFANTS; SELECTION FOR TREATMENT)

Kipnis, Kenneth; Diamond, Milton. Pediatric ethics and the surgical assignment of sex. *Journal of Clinical Ethics.* 1998 Winter; 9(4): 398–410.
(PATIENT CARE/MINORS; TRUTH DISCLOSURE)

Kirberger, Elizabeth see **Moore, Kirsten**

Kirk, Kathy. How Oregon's Death with Dignity Act affects practice. *American Journal of Nursing.* 1998 Aug; 98(8): 54–55.
(SUICIDE)

Kirkinen, Pertti see **Heikkilä, Annaleena**

Kirkland, Katherine H. see **Brodkin, C. Andrew**

Kirklin, James see **Lin, Hung–Mo**

Kirp, David L. Blood, sweat, and tears: the Tuskegee experiment and the era of AIDS. *Tikkun.* 1995 May–Jun; 10(3): 50–54.
(AIDS; FRAUD AND MISCONDUCT; HUMAN EXPERIMENTATION/SPECIAL POPULATIONS)

Kirsch, Michael; Rothschild, Bruce M.; Ridzon, Renée; Onorato, Ida; Snider, Dixie E.; Clever, Linda Hawes. Patient consent for publication. [Letters and responses]. *JAMA.* 1997 Dec 24–31; 278(24): 2139–2141.
(BIOMEDICAL RESEARCH; CONFIDENTIALITY; HUMAN EXPERIMENTATION/INFORMED CONSENT)

Kirschbaum, Mark Stephen. Deciding to Authorize, Forego, or Withdraw Life Support: The Meaning for Parents. Ann Arbor, MI: UMI Dissertation Services; 1994. 172 p.
(ALLOWING TO DIE)

Kirschner, Melvin H. see **Letvak, Richard**

Kischer, C. Ward. The big lie in human embryology: the case of the preembryo. *Linacre Quarterly.* 1997 Nov; 64(4): 53–61.
(FETUSES; PERSONHOOD)

Kishore, R.R. Organ donation consanguinity or universality. *Medicine and Law.* 1996; 15(1): 93–104.
(ORGAN AND TISSUE DONATION)

Kissane, David W.; Street, Annette; Nitschke, Philip. Seven deaths in Darwin: case studies under the Rights of the Terminally Ill Act, Northern Territory, Australia. *Lancet.* 1998 Oct 3; 352(9134): 1097–1102.
(EUTHANASIA)

Kissell, Judith Lee. Complicity in thought and language: toleration of wrong. *Journal of Medical Humanities.* 1999 Spring; 20(1): 49–60.
(FRAUD AND MISCONDUCT)

Kitamura, Fusako; Tomoda, Atsuko; Tsukada, Kazumi; Tanaka, Makoto; Kawakami, Ikuko; Mishima, Shuuichi; Kitamura, Toshinori. Method for assessment of competency to consent in the mentally ill: rationale, development, and comparison with the medically ill. *International Journal of Law and Psychiatry.* 1998 Summer; 21(3): 223–244.
(INFORMED CONSENT/MENTALLY DISABLED)

Kitamura, Toshinori see **Kitamura, Fusako**

Kitayaporn, Dwip see **Des Jarlais, Don C.**

Kitchener, Betty; Jorm, Anthony F. Conditions required for a law on active voluntary euthanasia: a survey of nurses' opinions in the Australian Capital Territory. *Journal of Medical Ethics.* 1999 Feb; 25(1): 25–30.
(EUTHANASIA; SUICIDE)

Kitcher, Philip. Whose self is it, anyway? *Sciences.* 1997 Sep–Oct; 37(5): 58–62.
(CLONING)

Kittay, Eva Feder; Kittay, Leo. On the expressivity and ethics of selective abortion for disability: conversations with my son. *In:* Haber, Joram G.; Halfon, Mark S., eds. Norms and Values: Essays on the Work of Virginia Held. Lanham, MD: Rowman and Littlefield; 1998: 173–203.
(ABORTION)

Kittay, Leo see **Kittay, Eva Feder**

Kjellin, Lars; Andersson, Kristina; Candefjord, Inga–Lill; Palmstierna, Tom; Wallsten, Tuula. Ethical benefits and costs of coercion in short–term inpatient psychiatric care. *Psychiatric Services.* 1997 Dec; 48(12): 1567–1570.
(INVOLUNTARY COMMITMENT/FOREIGN COUNTRIES; PATIENT CARE/MENTALLY DISABLED)

Kjellin, Lars; Westrin, Claes–Göran. Involuntary admissions and coercive measures in psychiatric care: registered and reported. *International Journal of Law and Psychiatry.* 1998 Winter; 21(1): 31–42.
(INVOLUNTARY COMMITMENT/FOREIGN COUNTRIES; PATIENT CARE/MENTALLY DISABLED)

Kjellstrand, Carl M. Duration and adequacy of dialysis -- overview: the science is easy, the ethic is difficult. *ASAIO Journal (American Society for Artificial Internal Organs).* 1997 May–Jun; 43(3): 220–224.
(RESOURCE ALLOCATION/BIOMEDICAL TECHNOLOGIES)

Klaffke, Oliver. The sacred and the profane: Swiss attitudes to genetic engineering have deep cultural roots. [News]. *New Scientist.* 1998 Jun 6; 158(2137): 61.
(GENETIC INTERVENTION)

Klamen, Debra L.; Grossman, Linda S.; Kopacz, David R. Attitudes about abortion among second–year medical students. *Medical Teacher.* 1996 Dec; 18(4): 345–346.
(ABORTION/ATTITUDES)

Klaus, Hanna see **Bowes, Watson**

Klein, Renate see **Callum, Janet**

Klein, Rudolf. Puzzling out priorities: why we must acknowledge that rationing is a political process. [Editorial]. *BMJ (British Medical Journal).* 1998 Oct 10; 317(7164): 959–960.
(HEALTH CARE/FOREIGN COUNTRIES; RESOURCE ALLOCATION)

Kleinert, Sabine. Rationing of health care: how should it be done? [Commentary]. *Lancet.* 1998 Oct 17; 352(9136): 1244.
(RESOURCE ALLOCATION)

Kleinert, Sabine. Validation of genetic tests for insurance in UK. [News]. *Lancet.* 1998 Nov 14; 352(9140): 1608.
(GENETIC SCREENING)

Kleinman, Leah see **Albert, Steven M.**

Klen, Rudolf. Aborted embryos -- law and ethics. *Bulletin of Medical Ethics.* 1998 Feb; No. 135: 22–23.
(FETUSES; ORGAN AND TISSUE DONATION)

Kliger, Alan S. see **Brand, Donald A.**

Kligman, Gail. The Politics of Duplicity: Controlling Reproduction in Ceausescu's Romania. Berkeley, CA: University of California Press; 1998. 358 p.
(ABORTION/FOREIGN COUNTRIES; POPULATION CONTROL; REPRODUCTION)

Klingbeil, Carol see **Butler, Dennis J.**

Klintmalm, Goran B. Who should receive the liver allograft: the transplant center or the recipient? *Liver Transplantation and Surgery.* 1995 Jan; 1(1): 55–58.
(ORGAN AND TISSUE TRANSPLANTATION; RESOURCE ALLOCATION/BIOMEDICAL TECHNOLOGIES)

Klocker, Johann see **Zwitter, Matjaz**

Klocker–Kaiser, Ursula see **Zwitter, Matjaz**

Klotzko, Arlene Judith. Immortal longings. *New Scientist.* 1998 Dec 5; 160(2163): 49.
(EMBRYO AND FETAL RESEARCH; LIFE EXTENSION)

Kluge, Eike–Henner W. Severely disabled newborns. *In:* Kuhse, Helga; Singer, Peter, eds. A Companion to Bioethics. Malden, MA: Blackwell; 1998: 242–249.
(ALLOWING TO DIE/INFANTS; EUTHANASIA; SELECTION FOR TREATMENT)

Kluger, Jeffrey. DNA detectives. *Time.* 1999 Jan 11; 153(1): 62–63.
(DNA FINGERPRINTING)

Kluger, Jeffrey. Who owns our genes? *Time.* 1999 Jan 11; 153(1): 51.
(GENOME MAPPING)

Klugman, Craig M.; Murray, Thomas H. Cloning, historical ethics, and NBAC. *In:* Humber, James M.; Almeder, Robert F.,eds. Human Cloning. Totowa, NJ: Humana Press; 1998: 1–50.
(CLONING)

Knaus, William A. see **Pritchard, Robert S.**

Knights of Columbus see **Benshoof, Janet**

Knobel, Peter. Suicide, assisted suicide, active euthanasia: a *Halakhic* inquiry. *In:* Jacob, Walter; Zemer, Moshe, eds. Death and Euthanasia in Jewish Law: Essays and Responsa. Pittsburgh, PA: Freehof Institute of Progressive Halakhah; Rodef Shalom Press; 1995: 27–59.
(EUTHANASIA/RELIGIOUS ASPECTS; SUICIDE)

Knoppers, Bartha Maria see **Burgess, Michael M.**

Knowles, Lori P. Property, progeny, and patents. [Symposium: human primordial stem cells]. *Hastings Center Report.* 1999 Mar–Apr; 29(2): 38–40.
(BIOMEDICAL RESEARCH; EMBRYO AND FETAL RESEARCH)

Knudsen, Lisbeth E. see **Zwitter, Matjaz**

Knudsen, Nancy S.; Pisetsky, David S. Doing everything. [Letter and response]. *Annals of Internal Medicine.* 1999 Jan 19; 130(2): 165–166.
(TERMINAL CARE)

Knudsen, Sharon K. see **Allen, Keith D.**

Koch, Kathryn A. The language of death: euthanatos et mors — the science of uncertainty. *Critical Care Clinics.* 1996 Jan; 12(1): 1–14.
(ALLOWING TO DIE; TERMINAL CARE)

Koch, Kathryn A. see **Cooper, Rebecca**

Koch, Kathryn A. see **Hook, C. Christopher**

Koch, Tom. The Limits of Principle: Deciding Who Lives and What Dies. Westport, CT: Praeger; 1998. 176 p.
(BIOETHICS; ORGAN AND TISSUE TRANSPLANTATION; RESOURCE ALLOCATION/BIOMEDICAL TECHNOLOGIES; SELECTION FOR TREATMENT)

Koch, Tom; Heilig, Steve. On the subject(s) of Jack Kevorkian, M.D.: a retrospective analysis. [Article and commentary]. *Cambridge Quarterly of Healthcare Ethics.* 1998 Fall; 7(4): 436–442.
(EUTHANASIA; SUICIDE)

Koch, Tom; Rowell, Mary. Humanness, personhood, and a lamb named Dolly: response to "Cloning: technology, policy, and ethics" (*CQ* Vol. 7, No. 2). *Cambridge Quarterly of Healthcare Ethics.* 1999 Spring; 8(2): 241–245.
(CLONING; PERSONHOOD)

Kocieniewski, David. Ban on a type of abortion is struck down. [News]. *New York Times.* 1998 Dec 9: B1, B4.
(ABORTION/LEGAL ASPECTS)

Kodish, Eric. Commentary: risks and benefits, testing and screening, cancer, genes and dollars. *Journal of Law, Medicine and Ethics.* 1997 Winter; 25(4): 252–255.
(GENETIC SCREENING)

Kodish, Eric; Murray, Thomas; Whitehouse, Peter. Conflict of interest in university–industry research relationships: realities, politics, and values. *Academic Medicine.* 1996 Dec; 71(12): 1287–1290.
(BIOMEDICAL RESEARCH)

Kodish, Eric D.; Pentz, Rebecca D.; Noll, Robert B.; Ruccione, Kathy; Buckley, Jonathan; Lange, Beverly J. Informed consent in the Childrens Cancer Group: results of preliminary research. [For the Children's Cancer Group]. *Cancer.* 1998 Jun 15; 82(12): 2467–2481.
(HUMAN EXPERIMENTATION/INFORMED CONSENT; HUMAN EXPERIMENTATION/MINORS)

Koehn, Daryl. The Ground of Professional Ethics. New York, NY: Routledge; 1994. 224 p.
(MEDICAL ETHICS; PROFESSIONAL ETHICS)

Koenig, B.A. see **McConnell, L.M.**

Koenig, Barbara A.; Greely, Henry T.; McConnell, Laura M.; Silverberg, Heather L.; Raffin, Thomas A. Genetic testing for BRCA1 and BRCA2: recommendations of the Stanford Program in Genomics, Ethics, and Society. *Journal of Women's Health.* 1998 Jun; 7(5): 531–545.
(GENETIC SCREENING)

Koenig, Kristi L.; Salvucci, Angelo A.; Goodwin, Peter A.; Schmidt, Terri A.; Zechnich, Andrew D. Out–of–hospital do–not–attempt–resuscitation in the suicidal patient: a special case [and] Death with dignity. [Letters and response]. *Academic Emergency Medicine.* 1997 Sep; 4(9): 926–928.
(RESUSCITATION ORDERS; SUICIDE)

Koenig, Robert. European researchers grapple with animal rights. [News]. *Science.* 1999 Jun 4; 284(5420): 1604–1606.
(ANIMAL EXPERIMENTATION)

Koepp, Robert; Miles, Stephen H.; Qizilbash, Nawab; Schneider, Lon; Farlow, Martin; Whitehead, Anne;

644

Higgins, Julian. Meta–analysis of tacrine for Alzheimer disease: the influence of industry sponsors. [Letter and response]. *JAMA.* 1999 Jun 23–30; 281(24): 2287–2288.
(BIOMEDICAL RESEARCH; HUMAN EXPERIMENTATION/RESEARCH DESIGN)

Koepsell, Thomas D. see **Saha, Somnath**

Kohane, Isaac S. see **Mandl, Kenneth D.**

Kohane, Isaac S. see **Roberts, John**

Kohn, R. see **Kullgren, G.**

Kokkonen, Paula. Coercion and legal protection in psychiatric care in Finland. *Medicine and Law.* 1993; 12(1–2): 113–124.
(INVOLUNTARY COMMITMENT/FOREIGN COUNTRIES)

Kolar, Roman see **Gruber, Franz P.**

Kolata, Gina. Harrowing choices accompany advancements in fertility. [News]. *New York Times.* 1998 Mar 10: F3.
(REPRODUCTIVE TECHNOLOGIES)

Kolata, Gina. In big advance in cloning, biologists create 50 mice. [News]. *New York Times.* 1998 Jul 23: A1, A20.
(CLONING)

Kolata, Gina. In the game of cloning, women hold all the cards. [News]. *New York Times.* 1998 Feb 22: 6.
(CLONING)

Kolata, Gina. Price soars for eggs, setting off a debate on a clinic's ethics. [News]. *New York Times.* 1998 Feb 25: A1, A16.
(REPRODUCTIVE TECHNOLOGIES)

Kolata, Gina. Scientists brace for changes in path of human evolution. [News]. *New York Times.* 1998 Mar 21: A1, A12.
(GENE THERAPY)

Kolata, Gina. When a cell does an embryo's work, a debate is born. *New York Times.* 1999 Feb 9: F2.
(EMBRYO AND FETAL RESEARCH)

Kolata, Gina. Where marketing and medicine meet. [News]. *New York Times.* 1998 Feb 10: A14.
(BIOMEDICAL TECHNOLOGIES; HEALTH CARE/ECONOMICS)

Kolata, Gina. $50,000 offered to tall, smart egg donor. [News]. *New York Times.* 1999 Mar 3: A10.
(REPRODUCTIVE TECHNOLOGIES)

Kolata, Gina; Eichenwald, Kurt. For the uninsured, drug trials are health care. [Stopgap medicine: a special report]. *New York Times.* 1999 Jun 22: A1, C12.
(HUMAN EXPERIMENTATION/SPECIAL POPULATIONS; PATIENT CARE/DRUGS)

Kolata, Gina see **Eichenwald, Kurt**

Kolehmainen, Sophia. CRG brings ethics into NIH prenatal gene therapy debate. *GeneWATCH.* 1999 Feb; 12(1): 15–16.
(EMBRYO AND FETAL RESEARCH; GENE THERAPY)

Kolehmainen, Sophia. Iceland's genetic $ell-out.

GeneWATCH. 1999 Feb; 12(1): 12–13.
(GENETIC RESEARCH)

Komaromy, Miriam see **Saha, Somnath**

Kondro, Wayne. Boy refuses cancer treatment in favour of prayer. [News]. *Lancet.* 1999 Mar 27; 353(9158): 1078.
(TREATMENT REFUSAL/MINORS)

Kondro, Wayne. Canada upholds rights of pregnant women. [News]. *Lancet.* 1999 Jul 17; 354(9174): 232.
(PRENATAL INJURIES)

Kondro, Wayne. Canadian government will revisit human–cloning legislation. [News]. *Lancet.* 1999 May 8; 353(9164): 1599.
(CLONING)

Kondro, Wayne. Canadian panel calls for review of drug–trial confidentiality agreements. [News]. *Lancet.* 1998 Dec 19–26; 352(9145): 1996.
(BIOMEDICAL RESEARCH; HUMAN EXPERIMENTATION/FOREIGN COUNTRIES)

Kondro, Wayne. "Do-not-resuscitate" order lifted in Canada. [News]. *Lancet.* 1998 Nov 21; 352(9141): 1689.
(RESUSCITATION ORDERS)

Kondro, Wayne. Voluntary blood tests for Canadian doctors? [News]. *Lancet.* 1998 Oct 10; 352(9135): 1205.
(AIDS/HEALTH PERSONNEL; AIDS/TESTING AND SCREENING)

Koocher, Gerald P.; Keith–Spiegel, Patricia. Ethics in Psychology: Professional Standards and Cases. Second Edition. New York, NY: Oxford University Press; 1998. 502 p.
(PROFESSIONAL ETHICS)

Kopacz, David R. see **Klamen, Debra L.**

Kopelman, Loretta M. Bioethics and humanities: what makes us one field? *Journal of Medicine and Philosophy.* 1998 Aug; 23(4): 356–368.
(BIOETHICS)

Kopelman, Loretta M. Help from Hume reconciling professionalism and managed care. *Journal of Medicine and Philosophy.* 1999 Aug; 24(4): 396–410.
(HEALTH CARE/ECONOMICS; RESOURCE ALLOCATION)

Kopelman, Loretta M.; McCullough, Laurence B. Hume, bioethics, and philosophy of medicine. [Introduction to a set of articles by T.L. Beauchamp, R.G. Frey, L.R. Churchill, K.F. Schaffner, L.B. McCullough, and L.M. Kopelman]. *Journal of Medicine and Philosophy.* 1999 Aug; 24(4): 315–321.
(BIOETHICS)

Kopelman, Loretta M.; Palumbo, Michael G. The U.S. health delivery system: inefficient and unfair to children. *American Journal of Law and Medicine.* 1997; 23(2–3): 319–337.
(HEALTH CARE; HEALTH CARE/ECONOMICS; RESOURCE ALLOCATION)

Kopelman, Loretta M. see **De Ville, Kenneth A.**

Kopfensteiner, Thomas R. Death with dignity: a Roman Catholic perspective. *Linacre Quarterly.* 1996 Nov; 63(4): 64–75.

(ALLOWING TO DIE/RELIGIOUS ASPECTS; TERMINAL CARE)

Koplan, Jeffrey P. see **Kao, Audiey C.**

Korb, H. see **Borowski, A.**

Korenman, Stanley G. see **Wenger, Neil S.**

Korn, James H. Illusions of Reality: A History of Deception in Social Psychology. Albany, NY: State University of New York Press; 1997. 204 p.
(BEHAVIORAL RESEARCH)

Kornbluth, Eti see **Hammerman, Cathy**

Kornbluth, Eti see **Kottow, Michael H.**

Korneluk, Y. see **Cappelli, M.**

Kornetsky, Susan. Questions and answers regarding clinical research: an educational brochure. *IRB: A Review of Human Subjects Research.* 1998 Jul–Aug; 20(4): 12–13.
(HUMAN EXPERIMENTATION; HUMAN EXPERIMENTATION/MINORS)

Korszniak, N. A review of the use of radio-isotopes in medicine and medical research in Australia (1947–73). *Australasian Radiology.* 1997 May; 41(2): 211–219.
(HUMAN EXPERIMENTATION/FOREIGN COUNTRIES; HUMAN EXPERIMENTATION/REGULATION)

Korzick, Karen A.; Terry, Peter B. Cadaveric organ donation: rethinking SPRT [Selection of Potential Recipients of Transplants]. [Editorial]. *Archives of Internal Medicine.* 1999 Mar 8; 159(5): 427–428.
(ORGAN AND TISSUE DONATION)

Kosseff, Andrew L.; Gurewich, Victor; Moore, Michael R.; Temianka, Daniel; Volpintesta, Edward J.; Prechter, Gary C.; Katzoff, Michael; Hall, Mark A.; Berenson, Robert A. Managed care ethics. [Letters and response]. *Annals of Internal Medicine.* 1998 Oct 15; 129(8): 672–674.
(HEALTH CARE/ECONOMICS; RESOURCE ALLOCATION)

Kostense, Piet J. see **Haverkate, Ilinka**

Kottow, Michael H.; Hammerman, Cathy; Kornbluth, Eti. Decision making in the critically ill neonate. [Letter and response]. *Journal of Medical Ethics.* 1998 Aug; 24(4): 280–281.
(BEHAVIORAL RESEARCH/SPECIAL POPULATIONS)

Koval, John J. see **McCarthy, Gillian M.**

Kow, Jim. Autonomy and the person in the dying patient. *In:* Morgan, John D., ed. Readings in Thanatology. Amityville, NY: Baywood Publishing; 1997: 423–438.
(TERMINAL CARE)

Kozma, C. see **Lapham, E.V.**

Kozma, C. see **Weiss, J.O.**

Krainacker, David A.; Mondragon, Delfi. Ethical responsibilities in a managed care system. *Nebraska Medical Journal.* 1995 Oct; 80(10): 306–308.
(HEALTH CARE/ECONOMICS)

Krakauer, Eric L. Prescriptions: autonomy, humanism and

the purpose of health technology. *Theoretical Medicine and Bioethics.* 1998 Dec; 19(6): 525–545.
(BIOETHICS; BIOMEDICAL TECHNOLOGIES)

Kramper, Ralph J. see **Byrne, Paul A.**

Krasny, Alex see **Slovenko, Ralph**

Krasny, Alex see **Sugarman, Jeremy**

Krause, Robert G. see **Segal, Eran**

Krauthammer, Charles. Of headless mice...and men: the ultimate cloning horror: human organ farms. *Time.* 1998 Jan 19; 151(2): 76.
(CLONING; ORGAN AND TISSUE DONATION)

Krauthammer, Charles. Yes, let's pay for organs. *Time.* 1999 May 17; 153(19): 100.
(ORGAN AND TISSUE DONATION)

Krauthammer, Charles see **Coburn, Tom**

Kravitz, Leonard. Euthanasia. *In:* Jacob, Walter; Zemer, Moshe, eds. Death and Euthanasia in Jewish Law: Essays and Responsa. Pittsburgh, PA: Freehof Institute of Progressive Halakhah; Rodef Shalom Press; 1995: 11–25.
(ALLOWING TO DIE/RELIGIOUS ASPECTS; EUTHANASIA/RELIGIOUS ASPECTS)

Kravitz, Richard L. Ethnic differences in use of cardiovascular procedures: new insights and new challenges. [Editorial]. *Annals of Internal Medicine.* 1999 Feb 2; 130(3): 231–233.
(PATIENT CARE; SELECTION FOR TREATMENT)

Kreimer, Seth F. The second time as tragedy: the assisted suicide cases and the heritage of *Roe v. Wade.* Hastings Constitutional Law Quarterly. 1997 Summer; 24(4): 863–901.
(SUICIDE)

Krener, Penelope see **Hibbs, Euthymia D.**

Krieger, Nancy; Birn, Anne-Emanuelle. A vision of social justice as the foundation of public health: commemorating 150 years of the spirit of 1848. *American Journal of Public Health.* 1998 Nov; 88(11): 1603–1606.
(PUBLIC HEALTH)

Krieger, Nancy; Sidney, Stephen; Coakley, Eugenie. Racial discrimination and skin color in the CARDIA study: implications for public health research. *American Journal of Public Health.* 1998 Sep; 88(9): 1308–1313.
(HEALTH; PUBLIC HEALTH)

Kristal, A.R. see **Ulrich, C.M.**

Kristjanson, Linda see **McAlpine, Heather**

Krizek, Thomas J. see **Phipps, Etienne**

Krol, Leendert J. see **Varekamp, Inge**

Krueger-Brophy, Carol see **Swisher, Laura Lee**

Kruesi, Markus see **Arnold, L. Eugene**

Kruschwitz, Ann L. see **Cohen, Elias S.**

Kuczewski, Mark. Casuistry and principlism: the convergence of method in biomedical ethics. *Theoretical Medicine and Bioethics.* 1998 Dec; 19(6): 509–524.
(BIOETHICS)

Kuczewski, Mark G. Commentary: narrative views of personal identity and substituted judgment in surrogate decision making. *Journal of Law, Medicine and Ethics.* 1999 Spring; 27(1): 32–36.
(ADVANCE DIRECTIVES; INFORMED CONSENT; PERSONHOOD)

Kuczewski, Mark G. Ethics in long-term care: are the principles different? *Theoretical Medicine and Bioethics.* 1999 Jan; 20(1): 15–29.
(PATIENT CARE/AGED)

Kuczewski, Mark G. Physician-assisted death: can philosophical bioethics aid social policy? *Cambridge Quarterly of Healthcare Ethics.* 1998 Fall; 7(4): 339–347.
(ALLOWING TO DIE; SUICIDE)

Kuczewski, Mark G.; DeVita, Michael. Managed care and end-of-life decisions: learning to live ungagged. *Archives of Internal Medicine.* 1998 Dec 7–21; 158(22): 2424–2428.
(HEALTH CARE/ECONOMICS; TERMINAL CARE)

Kuczewski, Mark G.; Pinkus, Rosa Lynn B. An Ethics Casebook for Hospitals: Practical Approaches to Everyday Cases. Washington, DC: Georgetown University Press; 1999. 219 p.
(BIOETHICS)

Kuczewski, Mark G.; Seiden, Dena J.; Frader, Joel; Gatter, Robert; Rhodes, Rosamond. Retransplantation and the "noncompliant" patient. [Case study and commentaries]. *Cambridge Quarterly of Healthcare Ethics.* 1999 Summer; 8(3): 375–381.
(ORGAN AND TISSUE TRANSPLANTATION; SELECTION FOR TREATMENT)

Kuhn, Charles see **Merrill, William W.**

Kuhse, Helga. Critical notice: why killing is not always worse -- and is sometimes better -- than letting die. *Cambridge Quarterly of Healthcare Ethics.* 1998 Fall; 7(4): 371–374.
(ALLOWING TO DIE; EUTHANASIA)

Kuhse, Helga; Singer, Peter, eds. A Companion to Bioethics. Malden, MA: Blackwell; 1998. 512 p.
(BIOETHICS)

Kuhse, Helga; Singer, Peter. Still no academic freedom in Germany. [Editorial]. *Bioethics.* 1999 Apr; 13(2): iii–vi.
(EUTHANASIA)

Kuhse, Helga see **Singer, Peter**

Kulczychi, Andrzej. The Abortion Debate in the World Arena. New York, NY: Routledge; 1999. 246 p.
(ABORTION/FOREIGN COUNTRIES)

Kullgren, G.; Jacobsson, L.; Lynöe, N.; Kohn, R.; Levav, I. Practices and attitudes among Swedish psychiatrists regarding the ethics of compulsory treatment. *Acta Psychiatrica Scandinavica.* 1996 May; 93(5): 389–396.
(INVOLUNTARY COMMITMENT/FOREIGN COUNTRIES; PATIENT CARE/MENTALLY DISABLED)

Kumar, Sanjay. Health-care camps for the poor provide mass sterilisation quota. [News]. *Lancet.* 1999 Apr 10; 353(9160): 1251.
(STERILIZATION)

Kumar, Sanjay. Medical confidentiality broken to stop marriage of man infected with HIV. [News]. *Lancet.* 1998 Nov 28; 352(9142): 1764.
(AIDS/CONFIDENTIALITY; CONFIDENTIALITY/LEGAL ASPECTS)

Kumar, Sanjay. New medical council to create code of ethics for Delhi's doctors. [News]. *Lancet.* 1998 Oct 31; 352(9138): 1453.
(MEDICAL ETHICS/CODES OF ETHICS)

Kumar, Sanjay. Research into anti-fertility vaccine continues despite protests. [News]. *Lancet.* 1998 Nov 7; 352(9139): 1528.
(CONTRACEPTION; HUMAN EXPERIMENTATION/SPECIAL POPULATIONS)

Kunene, Sibusiso Sixtus; Zungu, Busie Maya. An investigation into the attitude of professional nurses towards euthanasia. *Curationis.* 1996 Dec; 19(4): 26–30.
(ALLOWING TO DIE/ATTITUDES; EUTHANASIA/ATTITUDES)

Kunik, Mark E. see **Workman, Richard H.**

Kurm, Margus see **Sootak, Jaan**

Kurtz, Zarrina. Appropriate paternalism and the best interests of the child. *In:* Clarke, Angus, ed. The Genetic Testing of Children. Washington, DC: BIOS Scientific Publishers; 1998: 237–243.
(GENETIC SCREENING)

Kuruc, Joan Wallman see **Perry, Clifton**

Kuttner, Robert. The American health care system: employer-sponsored health coverage. *New England Journal of Medicine.* 1999 Jan 21; 340(3): 248–252.
(HEALTH CARE/ECONOMICS)

Kuttner, Robert. The American health care system: health insurance coverage. *New England Journal of Medicine.* 1999 Jan 14; 340(2): 163–168.
(HEALTH CARE/ECONOMICS)

Kuttner, Robert. The American health care system: Wall Street and health care. *New England Journal of Medicine.* 1999 Feb 25; 340(8): 664–668.
(HEALTH CARE/ECONOMICS)

Kylmä, Jari; Vehviläinen-Julkunen, Katri; Lähdevirta, Juhani. Ethical considerations in a grounded theory study on the dynamics of hope in HIV-positive adults and their significant others. *Nursing Ethics.* 1999 May; 6(3): 224–239.
(AIDS/HUMAN EXPERIMENTATION; BEHAVIORAL RESEARCH/SPECIAL POPULATIONS)

L

La Puma, John. Physician rewards for postmarketing surveillance (seeding studies) in the US. [Editorial]. *PharmacoEconomics.* 1995 Mar; 7(3): 187–190.
(HUMAN EXPERIMENTATION; PATIENT CARE/DRUGS)

La Puma, John. Satisfying managed care patients through ethics consultation. *SBC Newsletter (Society for Bioethics*

Consultation). 1996 Spring: 12–13.
(ETHICISTS AND ETHICS COMMITTEES; HEALTH
CARE/ECONOMICS)

Laane, Henk–Maarten. Euthanasia, assisted suicide and
AIDS. *AIDS Care.* 1995; 7(Suppl. 2): S163–S167.
(AIDS; EUTHANASIA; SUICIDE)

Laberge, Claude M. see **Burgess, Michael M.**

Lacanna, Iara C. see **Khamsi, Firouz**

Lachmann, Peter J. Public health and bioethics. *Journal
of Medicine and Philosophy.* 1998 Jun; 23(3): 297–302.
(PUBLIC HEALTH)

Lachs, John. Active euthanasia. *In: his* The Relevance
of Philosophy to Life. Nashville, TN: Vanderbilt
University Press; 1995: 181–187.
(EUTHANASIA; PERSONHOOD)

Lachs, John. Dying old as a social problem. *In:* McGee,
Glenn, ed. Pragmatic Bioethics. Nashville, TN:
Vanderbilt University Press; 1999: 194–203, 281.
(SUICIDE; TERMINAL CARE)

Lachs, John. On selling organs. *In: his* The Relevance
of Philosophy to Life. Nashville, TN: Vanderbilt
University Press; 1995: 195–198.
(ORGAN AND TISSUE DONATION)

Lachs, John. Personal relations between physicians and
patients. *In: his* The Relevance of Philosophy to Life.
Nashville, TN: Vanderbilt University Press; 1995:
199–205.
(PROFESSIONAL PATIENT RELATIONSHIP)

Lachs, John. Resuscitation. *In: his* The Relevance of
Philosophy to Life. Nashville, TN: Vanderbilt
University Press; 1995: 176–180.
(RESUSCITATION ORDERS)

Lachs, John. The element of choice in criteria of death.
In: his The Relevance of Philosophy to Life. Nashville,
TN: Vanderbilt University Press; 1995: 209–227.
(DETERMINATION OF DEATH; DETERMINATION OF
DEATH/BRAIN DEATH)

Lachs, John. When abstract moralizing runs amok. *In: his*
The Relevance of Philosophy to Life. Nashville, TN:
Vanderbilt University Press; 1995: 188–194.
(EUTHANASIA; SUICIDE)

Ladd, Richard C. see **Kane, Rosalie A.**

Ladimer, Irving. Self–determination for life and death.
Medicine and Law. 1996; 15(1): 83–92.
(ADVANCE DIRECTIVES; ALLOWING TO DIE)

**Lafayette, DeeDee; Abuelo, Dianne; Passero, Mary
Ann; Tantravahi, Umadevi.** Attitudes toward cystic
fibrosis carrier and prenatal testing and utilization of
carrier testing among relatives of individuals with cystic
fibrosis. *Journal of Genetic Counseling.* 1999 Feb; 8(1):
17–36.
(ABORTION/ATTITUDES; GENETIC COUNSELING; GENETIC
SCREENING; PRENATAL DIAGNOSIS)

Lafferty, Kevin J.; Furer, Julie J. Legal and medical
implications of fetal tissue transplantation. *Suffolk
University Law Review.* 1993 Winter; 27(4): 1237–1248.

(EMBRYO AND FETAL RESEARCH; FETUSES; ORGAN AND
TISSUE DONATION; ORGAN AND TISSUE
TRANSPLANTATION)

Lafferty, Kevin J. see **Bleich, J. David**

Lagay, Faith L. Science, rhetoric, and public discourse
in genetic research. *Cambridge Quarterly of Healthcare
Ethics.* 1999 Spring; 8(2): 226–237.
(GENE THERAPY; GENETIC INTERVENTION; GENETIC
RESEARCH)

Lagnado, Lucette. Their role growing, Catholic hospitals
juggle doctrine and medicine. *Wall Street Journal.* 1999
Feb 4: A1, A8.
(ETHICISTS AND ETHICS COMMITTEES; HEALTH CARE)

Lagnado, Lucette. Transplant patients ply an illicit market
for vital medicines. [News]. *Wall Street Journal.* 1999
Jun 21: 1, A8.
(FRAUD AND MISCONDUCT; HEALTH CARE/ECONOMICS;
ORGAN AND TISSUE TRANSPLANTATION; PATIENT
CARE/DRUGS)

Lähdevirta, Juhani see **Kylmä, Jari**

Laippala, Pekka see **Kaltiala–Heino, Riittakerttu**

Lake, John R. see **Showstack, Jonathan**

Lallemant, Marc see **Merson, Michael H.**

Lally, James F. see **Epstein, Richard A.**

Lamb, David. Organ transplants, death, and policies for
procurement. *Monist.* 1993 Apr; 76(2): 203–221.
(DETERMINATION OF DEATH/BRAIN DEATH; ORGAN AND
TISSUE DONATION)

Lambe, Neil see **Grubb, Andrew**

Lamberg, Lynne. Researchers urged to tell public how
animal studies benefit human health. [News]. *JAMA.* 1999
Aug 18; 282(7): 619–621.
(ANIMAL EXPERIMENTATION)

Lambert, Bruce. Giuliani backs DNA testing of newborns
for identification. [News]. *New York Times.* 1998 Dec
17: B4.
(DNA FINGERPRINTING)

Lamdan, Ruth M.; Ahmed, Ziauddin; Lee, Jean.
General anesthesia: an extreme form of chemical and
physical restraint. [Case analysis]. *HEC (HealthCare
Ethics Committee) Forum.* 1998 Sep–Dec; 10(3–4):
317–322.
(BEHAVIOR CONTROL; PATIENT CARE/MENTALLY
DISABLED)

Lamdan, Ruth M. see **Vaught, Wayne**

Lamm, Richard D. Marginal medicine. *JAMA.* 1998 Sep
9; 280(10): 931–933.
(HEALTH CARE/ECONOMICS; RESOURCE ALLOCATION)

Lamm, Richard D. Redrawing the ethics map. *Hastings
Center Report.* 1999 Mar–Apr; 29(2): 28–29.
(HEALTH CARE/ECONOMICS; RESOURCE ALLOCATION)

Lampman, Jane. Cloning's double trouble. [News].
Christian Science Monitor. 1998 Aug 13: B1, B3–B4.
(CLONING)

Lancaster, Carol J. see **Dickinson, George E.**

Landesman, Bruce see **Marchand, Sarah**

Landis, Kenneth W. see **Meinhardt, Robyn**

Landman, Willem A.; Henley, Lesley D. Equitable rationing of highly specialised health care services for children: a perspective from South Africa. *Journal of Medical Ethics.* 1999 Jun; 25(3): 224–229.
(HEALTH CARE/FOREIGN COUNTRIES; RESOURCE ALLOCATION/BIOMEDICAL TECHNOLOGIES; SELECTION FOR TREATMENT)

Landman, Willem A.; Henley, Lesley D. Tensions in setting health care priorities for South Africa's children. *Journal of Medical Ethics.* 1998 Aug; 24(4): 268–273.
(HEALTH CARE/FOREIGN COUNTRIES; PATIENT CARE/MINORS; RESOURCE ALLOCATION)

Landray, Martin J. see **Edi-Osagie, E.C.O.**

Landrum, R. Eric see **Chastain, Garvin**

Landsverk, John see **Putnam, Frank W.**

Lange, Beverly J. see **Kodish, Eric D.**

Langer, Pamela J. see **Resnik, David B.**

Langley-Evans, A. see **Payne, S. A.**

Langley, Gill. Animal tests and alternatives: an animal protection viewpoint. *In:* van Zutphen, L.F.M.; Balls, M., eds. Animal Alternatives, Welfare and Ethics. New York, NY: Elsevier; 1997: 347–354.
(ANIMAL EXPERIMENTATION)

Langlois, Sylvie see **Bernard, Lynn E.**

Lant, Mary see **Flegel, Kenneth M.**

Lantos, John see **Bolan, Robert K.**

Lantos, John see **Casarett, David J.**

Lantos, John D.; Mokalla, Mani; Meadow, William. Resource allocation in neonatal and medical ICUs: epidemiology and rationing at the extremes of life. *American Journal of Respiratory and Critical Care Medicine.* 1997 Jul; 156(1): 185–189.
(PATIENT CARE/AGED; PATIENT CARE/MINORS; RESOURCE ALLOCATION/BIOMEDICAL TECHNOLOGIES)

Lantos, John D. see **Burgio, G. Roberto**

Lantos, John D. see **Meadow, William**

Lanza, Robert P.; Arrow, Kenneth J.; Axelrod, Julius, et al. Science over politics. [Letter]. *Science.* 1999 Mar 19; 283(5409): 1849–1850.
(EMBRYO AND FETAL RESEARCH)

Lapham, E.V.; Kozma, C.; Weiss, J.O. Consumer experience in genetic research. [Abstract]. *American Journal of Human Genetics.* 1997 Oct; 61(4): A189.
(GENETIC RESEARCH)

Lapham, E.V. see **Weiss, J.O.**

Lapierre, Yvon D.; Weijer, Charles. Placebo: pro and con. *NCEHR Communique (National Council on Ethics in Human Research).* 1997–1998 Winter–Spring; 8(2): 11–15.
(HUMAN EXPERIMENTATION/ETHICS COMMITTEES; HUMAN EXPERIMENTATION/RESEARCH DESIGN; HUMAN EXPERIMENTATION/SPECIAL POPULATIONS)

Larimore, Walter L.; Orr, Robert D. Medical abortion is not just a medical issue. [Editorial]. *Today's Christian Doctor.* 1997 Winter; 28(4): 4–6.
(ABORTION)

Larke, Bryce. The quandary of Creutzfeldt–Jakob disease. [Editorial]. *Canadian Medical Association Journal.* 1998 Oct 6; 159(7): 789–792.
(BLOOD DONATION; TRUTH DISCLOSURE)

Larkin, Gregory Luke; Weber, James E.; Derse, Arthur R. Universal emergency access under managed care: universal doubt or mission impossible? *Cambridge Quarterly of Healthcare Ethics.* 1999 Spring; 8(2): 213–225.
(HEALTH CARE/ECONOMICS)

Larkin, Marilynn. Psychologists grapple with patient requests to hasten death. [News]. *Lancet.* 1999 Jun 19; 353(9170): 2133.
(SUICIDE)

Larkin, Marilynn. Resuscitation preferences for heart-failure patients likely to change. [News]. *Lancet.* 1998 Aug 28; 352(9129): 711.
(RESUSCITATION ORDERS)

Larkin, Marilynn. Whose article is it anyway? *Lancet.* 1999 Jul 10; 354(9173): 136.
(BIOMEDICAL RESEARCH; FRAUD AND MISCONDUCT)

Larkins, Richard G. Victorian orphans and clinical research. [Editorial]. *Medical Journal of Australia.* 1997 Jul 21; 167(2): 60–61.
(HUMAN EXPERIMENTATION/FOREIGN COUNTRIES)

Larson, Edward J. Confronting scientific authority with religious values: eugenics in American history. *In:* Demy, Timothy J.; Stewart, Gary P., eds. Genetic Engineering: A Christian Response: Crucial Considerations in Shaping Life. Grand Rapids, MI: Kregel Publications; 1999: 104–124.
(EUGENICS; STERILIZATION/MENTALLY DISABLED)

Larson, Edward J. Seeking compassion in dying: the Washington State law against assisted suicide. *Seattle University Law Review.* 1995 Spring; 18(3): 509–519.
(SUICIDE)

Larson, Edward J.; Eaton, Thomas A. The limits of advance directives: a history and assessment of the Patient Self-Determination Act. *Wake Forest Law Review.* 1997 Summer; 32(2): 249–293.
(ADVANCE DIRECTIVES)

Lasby, Clarence G. Eisenhower's Heart Attack: How Ike Beat Heart Disease and Held on to the Presidency. Lawrence, KS: University Press of Kansas; 1997. 384 p.
(CONFIDENTIALITY; HEALTH)

Lascaratos, John; Poulakou-Rebelakou, Effie; Marketos, Spyros. Abandonment of terminally ill patients in the Byzantine era: an ancient tradition?

Journal of Medical Ethics. 1999 Jun; 25(3): 254–258.
(MEDICAL ETHICS; TERMINAL CARE)

Lasley, Elizabeth Norton. Research lab to surrender chimps. [News]. *Science.* 1999 Sep 10; 285(5434): 1649–1650.
(ANIMAL EXPERIMENTATION)

Latimer, Elizabeth see **Lesage, Pauline**

Latimer, Elizabeth J. Ethical care at the end of life. *Canadian Medical Association Journal.* 1998 Jun 30; 158(13): 1741–1747.
(TERMINAL CARE)

Laughlin, J. see **Weiss, A.H.**

Launer, John. A narrative approach to mental health in general practice: narrative based medicine. *BMJ (British Medical Journal).* 1999 Jan 9; 318(7176): 117–119.
(PATIENT CARE/MENTALLY DISABLED)

Lavelle, Marianne. When abortions come late in pregnancy: though rare, most aren't for medical reasons. [News]. *U.S. News and World Report.* 1998 Jan 19; 124(2): 31–32.
(ABORTION)

Lavie, Ofer see **Hammerman, Cathy**

Lavoie, Mireille see **Blondeau, Danielle**

Law, Bernard see **Rigali, Justin**

Law, Sylvia A. Silent no more: physicians' legal and ethical obligations to patients seeking abortions. *New York University Review of Law and Social Change.* 1994–1995; 21(2): 279–321.
(ABORTION/LEGAL ASPECTS)

Lawlor, Peter see **Bruera, Eduardo**

Lawrence, Christopher see **Chandna, Shahid M.**

Lawrence, Robert S. see **Hannibal, Kari**

Lawrence, Robert S. see **McCally, Michael**

Lawry, Kathleen; Slomka, Jacquelyn; Goldfarb, Johanna. What went wrong: multiple perspectives on an adolescent's decision to refuse blood transfusions. *Clinical Pediatrics.* 1996 Jun; 35(6): 317–321.
(TREATMENT REFUSAL/MINORS)

Layon, A. Joseph; D'Amico, Robert. Intensive care for patients with acquired immunodeficiency syndrome -- medicine versus ideology. *Critical Care Medicine.* 1990 Nov; 18(11): 1297–1299.
(AIDS; RESOURCE ALLOCATION/BIOMEDICAL TECHNOLOGIES)

Le Coeur, Sophie see **Merson, Michael H.**

Le Stage, Barbara see **Garber, Judy E.**

Leach, C.E.A. see **West, Charles**

Leach, Mark M.; Harbin, J. Judd. Psychological ethics codes: a comparison of twenty-four countries. *International Journal of Psychology.* 1997; 32(3): 181–192.

(PROFESSIONAL ETHICS/CODES OF ETHICS)

Leal–Mora, David see **Kane, Richard S.**

Leape, Lucian L.; Hilborne, Lee H.; Bell, Robert; Kamberg, Caren; Brook, Robert H. Underuse of cardiac procedures: do women, ethnic minorities, and the uninsured fail to receive needed revascularization? *Annals of Internal Medicine.* 1999 Feb 2; 130(3): 183–192.
(PATIENT CARE; SELECTION FOR TREATMENT)

Lears, Louise. Research in the emergency department. *Health Care Ethics USA.* 1997 Spring; 5(2): 4–5.
(HUMAN EXPERIMENTATION/INFORMED CONSENT; HUMAN EXPERIMENTATION/REGULATION)

Lears, Louise. The ethics and wisdom of collaboration. *Health Care Ethics USA.* 1998 Summer; 6(3): 6–7.
(RESOURCE ALLOCATION)

Lebacqz, Karen. Research with human embryonic stem cells: ethical considerations. [Symposium: human primordial stem cells]. *Hastings Center Report.* 1999 Mar–Apr; 29(2): 31–36.
(EMBRYO AND FETAL RESEARCH)

Lebacqz, Karen; Tauer, Carol; McGee, Glenn; Caplan, Arthur. Stem cells. [Letter and responses]. *Hastings Center Report.* 1999 Jul–Aug; 29(4): 4–5.
(EMBRYO AND FETAL RESEARCH)

Lebech, Anne Mette Maria. Principles, compromise and human embryos in Europe. *Bulletin of Medical Ethics.* 1997 Aug; No. 130: 18–21.
(FETUSES)

Lebech, Mette Maria. Comment on a proposed draft protocol for the European Convention on Biomedicine relating to research on the human embryo and fetus. *Journal of Medical Ethics.* 1998 Oct; 24(5): 345–347.
(EMBRYO AND FETAL RESEARCH)

Lebel, R.R. see **Swiglo, B.A.**

Lebel, Robert see **Baumiller, Robert C.**

Leckman, James F. see **Arnold, L. Eugene**

L'Ecuyer, Jerome see **Byrne, Paul A.**

Lederberg, Marguerite S. Making a situational diagnosis: psychiatrists at the interface of psychiatry and ethics in the consultation–liaison setting. *Psychosomatics.* 1997 Jul–Aug; 38(4): 327–338.
(ETHICISTS AND ETHICS COMMITTEES)

Lee, Ellie, ed. Abortion Law and Politics Today. New York, NY: St. Martin's Press; 1998. 233 p.
(ABORTION/FOREIGN COUNTRIES; ABORTION/LEGAL ASPECTS)

Lee, J.W.; Melgaard, Bjorn; Hull, Harry F.; Barakamfitiye, D.; Okwo–Bele, J.M. Ethical dilemmas in polio eradication. *American Journal of Public Health.* 1998 Jan; 88(1): 130–132.
(IMMUNIZATION; RESOURCE ALLOCATION)

Lee, Jean see **Lamdan, Ruth M.**

Lee, Kwoc–Choy see **Toth, Ellen L.**

Lee, Melinda A.; Smith, David M.; Fenn, Darien S.; Ganzini, Linda. Do patients' treatment decisions match advance statements of their preferences? *Journal of Clinical Ethics.* 1998 Fall; 9(3): 258–262.
(ADVANCE DIRECTIVES; ALLOWING TO DIE/ATTITUDES)

Lee, Melinda A. see **Ganzini, Linda**

Lee, Tun–Hou see **Merson, Michael H.**

Leffel, Jim. Genetics and human rights in a postmodern age. *In:* Demy, Timothy J.; Stewart, Gary P., eds. Genetic Engineering: A Christian Response: Crucial Considerations in Shaping Life. Grand Rapids, MI: Kregel Publications; 1999: 126–138.
(GENETIC INTERVENTION; PERSONHOOD)

Legemaate, Johan, ed.; Royal Dutch Medical Association. Patients' Rights in the Countries of the Toronto Group: The Results of a Survey Carried Out by the Royal Dutch Medical Association. Issued by the Association: Koninklijke Nederlandsche Maatschappij tot bevordering der Geneeskunst, P.O. Box 20051, 3502 LB, Utrecht, The Netherlands; 1992 Sep. 41 p.
(PATIENTS' RIGHTS)

Leggat, John E.; Swartz, Richard D.; Port, Friedrich K. Withdrawal from dialysis: a review with an emphasis on the black experience. *Advances in Renal Replacement Therapy.* 1997 Jan; 4(1): 22–29.
(ALLOWING TO DIE/ATTITUDES; TREATMENT REFUSAL)

Legro, Marcia see **Albert, Steven M.**

Lehman, J. Stan see **Bindman, Andrew B.**

Lehrman, Nathaniel S. The ethics of harmful psychiatric research: a faulty effort to defend them. *Accountability in Research.* 1997; 5(4): 283–288.
(HUMAN EXPERIMENTATION/SPECIAL POPULATIONS)

Lehrman, Sally. Prisoner's DNA database ruled unlawful. [News]. *Nature.* 1998 Aug 27; 394(6696): 818.
(DNA FINGERPRINTING)

Lehrman, Sally. Virus treatment questioned after gene therapy death. [News]. *Nature.* 1999 Oct 7; 401(6753): 517–518.
(GENE THERAPY; HUMAN EXPERIMENTATION)

Lei, Xiong see **Dan, Zhang**

Leibold, Peter; Gilham, Charles S. When physicians perform abortions outside the Catholic hospital. *Health Progress.* 1998 Mar–Apr; 79(2): 12–14.
(ABORTION/LEGAL ASPECTS; ABORTION/RELIGIOUS ASPECTS)

Leibold, Peter see **Gilham, Charles**

Leichter, Howard M. Oregon's bold experiment: whatever happened to rationing? *Journal of Health Politics, Policy and Law.* 1999 Feb; 24(1): 147–160.
(HEALTH CARE/ECONOMICS; RESOURCE ALLOCATION)

Leidy, Nancy Kline see **Albert, Steven M.**

Leigh, Wilhelmina A. Participant protection with the use of records: ethical issues and recommendations. *Ethics and Behavior.* 1998; 8(4): 305–319.

(BEHAVIORAL RESEARCH/REGULATION; CONFIDENTIALITY/MENTAL HEALTH)

Lemkow, Louis. Public Attitudes to Genetic Engineering: Some European Perspectives. Shankill, Ireland: European Foundation for the Improvement of Living and Working Conditions; 1993. 44 p.
(GENETIC INTERVENTION)

Lemmens, Trudo see **Glass, Kathleen Cranley**

Lemonick, Michael D. Designer babies. *Time.* 1999 Jan 11; 153(1): 64–67.
(GENETIC INTERVENTION; PRENATAL DIAGNOSIS; SEX PRESELECTION)

Lemonick, Michael D. Good news at a price : a study finds that AIDS drugs can help poor kids -- but was it ethical? *Time.* 1999 Feb 15; 153(6): 64.
(AIDS/HUMAN EXPERIMENTATION; HUMAN EXPERIMENTATION/FOREIGN COUNTRIES; HUMAN EXPERIMENTATION/SPECIAL POPULATIONS)

Lemonick, Michael D. The biological mother lode. [News]. *Time.* 1998 Nov 16; 152(20): 96–97.
(EMBRYO AND FETAL RESEARCH)

Lemonick, Michael D.; Thompson, Dick. Racing to map our DNA. [News]. *Time.* 1999 Jan 11; 153(1): 44–51.
(GENOME MAPPING)

Leng, Ter Kah; Sy, Susanna Leong Huey. Advance medical directives in Singapore. *Medical Law Review.* 1997 Spring; 5(1): 63–101.
(ADVANCE DIRECTIVES; ALLOWING TO DIE/LEGAL ASPECTS)

Leonard, Debra G.B. see **Merz, Jon F.**

Leonard, Henrietta; Jensen, Peter S.; Vitiello, Benedetto; Ryan, Neal; March, John; Riddle, Mark; Biederman, Joseph. Ethical issues in psychopharmacological treatment research with children and adolescents. *In:* Hoagwood, Kimberly; Jensen, Peter S.; Fisher, Celia B., eds. Ethical Issues in Mental Health Research with Children and Adolescents. Mahwah, NJ: Lawrence Erlbaum Associates; 1996: 73–88.
(HUMAN EXPERIMENTATION/MINORS; HUMAN EXPERIMENTATION/SPECIAL POPULATIONS)

Leone, Daniel A., ed. The Ethics of Euthanasia. San Diego, CA: Greenhaven Press; 1999. 88 p.
(ALLOWING TO DIE; EUTHANASIA; SUICIDE)

Leonir, Noëlle. French, European, and international legislation on bioethics. *Suffolk University Law Review.* 1993 Winter; 27(4): 1249–1270.
(BIOETHICS)

Leplége, Alain see **Albert, Steven M.**

Lerman, Caryn; Hughes, Chanita; Trock, Bruce J.; Myers, Ronald E.; Main, David; Bonney, Aba; Abbaszadegan, Mohammad R.; Harty, Anne E.; Franklin, Barbara A.; Lynch, Jane F.; Lynch, Henry T. Genetic testing in families with hereditary nonpolyposis colon cancer. *JAMA.* 1999 May 5; 281(17): 1618–1622.
(GENETIC SCREENING)

Lerman, Caryn see **Croyle, Robert T.**

Lerman, Caryn see Peshkin, Beth N.

Lerman, Caryn see Wilfond, Benjamin S.

Lerner, Barron H.; Rothman, David J.; Tracy, Mark J.; Gasner, M. Rose; Frieden, Thomas R.; Fujiwara, Paula I. Legal action to ensure treatment of tuberculosis. [Letters and response]. *New England Journal of Medicine.* 1999 Jul 8; 341(2): 130–131.
(PUBLIC HEALTH)

Lerner, Paul. Rationalizing the therapeutic arsenal: German neuropsychiatry in World War I. *In:* Berg, Manfred; Cocks, Geoffrey, eds. Medicine and Modernity: Public Health and Medical Care in Nineteenth– and Twentieth–Century Germany. New York, NY: Cambridge University Press; 1997: 121–148.
(HEALTH CARE/FOREIGN COUNTRIES; MENTAL HEALTH; PATIENT CARE/MENTALLY DISABLED; WAR)

Lesage, Pauline; Latimer, Elizabeth. An approach to ethical issues. *In:* MacDonald, Neil, ed. Palliative Medicine: A Case-Based Manual. New York, NY: Oxford University Press; 1998: 253–277.
(TERMINAL CARE)

Lessard, Hester. The construction of health care and the ideology of the private in Canadian constitutional law. *Annals of Health Law.* 1993; 2: 121–159.
(ABORTION/FOREIGN COUNTRIES; ABORTION/LEGAL ASPECTS; HEALTH CARE/FOREIGN COUNTRIES; HEALTH CARE/RIGHTS)

Lesser, Cara S. see Cunningham, Peter J.

Letvak, Richard; Pochard, Frédéric; Grassin, Marc; Hervé, Christian; Kirschner, Melvin H.; Howsepian, A.A.; Quill, Timothy E.; Lo, Bernard; Brock, Dan W. Palliative options at the end of life. [Letters and response]. *JAMA.* 1998 Apr 8; 279(14): 1065–1067.
(ALLOWING TO DIE; EUTHANASIA; SUICIDE; TERMINAL CARE)

Levav, I. see Kullgren, G.

Levi, Banjamin H. Respecting Patient Autonomy. Urbana, IL: University of Illinois Press; 1999. 222 p.
(PROFESSIONAL PATIENT RELATIONSHIP)

Levi, Jeffrey. Can access to care for people living with HIV be expanded? *AIDS and Public Policy Journal.* 1998 Summer; 13(2): 56–74.
(AIDS; HEALTH CARE/ECONOMICS)

Levi, Joel. Refusal of life-sustaining treatment recognized by court of law. *Medicine and Law.* 1993; 12(1–2): 191–192.
(ALLOWING TO DIE/LEGAL ASPECTS; TREATMENT REFUSAL)

Levin, Arthur Aaron see Nightingale, Stuart L.

Levine, Carol. Placebos and HIV: lessons learned. *Hastings Center Report.* 1998 Nov–Dec; 28(6): 43–48.
(AIDS/HUMAN EXPERIMENTATION; HUMAN EXPERIMENTATION/FOREIGN COUNTRIES; HUMAN EXPERIMENTATION/RESEARCH DESIGN; HUMAN EXPERIMENTATION/SPECIAL POPULATIONS)

Levine, Carol, ed. Taking Sides: Clashing Views on Controversial Bioethical Issues. Eighth Edition. Guilford, CT: Dushkin Publishing Group; 1999. 355 p.
(BIOETHICS)

Levine, Carol. The loneliness of the long-term care giver. [Personal narrative]. *New England Journal of Medicine.* 1999 May 20; 340(20): 1587–1590.
(HEALTH CARE/ECONOMICS; PATIENT CARE)

Levine, Carol; Zuckerman, Connie. The trouble with families: toward an ethic of accommodation. *Annals of Internal Medicine.* 1999 Jan 19; 130(2): 148–152.
(PROFESSIONAL PATIENT RELATIONSHIP)

Levine, June see Bartels, Dianne

Levine, Karen R. see Wharton, Robert H.

Levine, Myron M. see Matz, Robert

Levine, Noga Morag. Abortion in Israel: community, rights, and the context of compromise. *Law and Social Inquiry.* 1994 Spring; 19(2): 313–335.
(ABORTION/FOREIGN COUNTRIES)

Levine, Richard S. Avoiding conflicts of interest in surrogate decision making: why ethics committees should assign surrogacy to a separate committee. *Journal of Clinical Ethics.* 1998 Fall; 9(3): 273–290.
(ETHICISTS AND ETHICS COMMITTEES)

Levine, Robert A.; Lieberson, Alan. Physicians' perceptions of managed care. *American Journal Of Managed Care.* 1998 Feb; 4(2): 171–180.
(HEALTH CARE/ECONOMICS)

Levine, Robert J.; Dennison, David K. Randomized clinical trials in periodontology: ethical considerations. *Annals of Periodontology.* 1997 Mar; 2(1): 83–94.
(HUMAN EXPERIMENTATION/RESEARCH DESIGN)

Levine, Robert J. see Wilfert, Catherine M.

Levinsky, Norman G. Can we afford medical care for Alice C? *Lancet.* 1998 Dec 5; 352(9143): 1849–1851.
(HEALTH CARE/ECONOMICS; PATIENT CARE/AGED; RESOURCE ALLOCATION)

Levitt, Mairi. A sociological perspective on genetic screening. *European Journal of Genetics in Society.* 1997; 3(2): 19–21.
(GENETIC SCREENING)

Levitt, Mairi. Sociological perspectives on the right to know and the right not to know. *In:* Chadwick, Ruth; Levitt, Mairi; Shickle, Darren, eds. The Right to Know and the Right Not to Know. Brookfield, VT: Ashgate; 1997: 29–36.
(GENETIC SCREENING; TRUTH DISCLOSURE)

Levitt, Mairi see Chadwick, Ruth

Lewin, Tamar. A prisoner is the focus of an abortion debate. [News]. *New York Times.* 1999 Jan 10: 12.
(ABORTION/FINANCIAL SUPPORT; ABORTION/LEGAL ASPECTS)

Lewin, Tamar. Study on late term abortion finds procedure is little used. [News]. *New York Times.* 1998 Dec 11: A12.
(ABORTION)

Lewin, Tamar. Wisconsin abortion clinics shut down, citing new law. [News]. *New York Times.* 1998 May 15: A27.
(ABORTION/LEGAL ASPECTS)

Lewis, Gregory L. see **Stead, William W.**

Lewis, Neil A. Reno lifts barrier to Oregon's law on aided suicide. [News]. *New York Times.* 1998 Jun 6: A1, A7.
(SUICIDE)

Lewontin, R.C. People are not commodities. *New York Times.* 1999 Jan 23: A19.
(GENETIC RESEARCH)

Li, Hon-Lam. Abortion and degrees of personhood: understanding why the abortion problem (and the animal rights problem) are irresolvable. *Public Affairs Quarterly.* 1997 Jan; 11(1): 1–19.
(ABORTION; FETUSES; PERSONHOOD)

Liaño, Fernando see **Pascual, Julio**

Lichterman, Boleslav see **Swinn, Michael**

Lie, Reidar K. Ethics of placebo-controlled trials in developing countries. *Bioethics.* 1998 Oct; 12(4): 307–311.
(AIDS/HUMAN EXPERIMENTATION; HUMAN EXPERIMENTATION/FOREIGN COUNTRIES; HUMAN EXPERIMENTATION/RESEARCH DESIGN; HUMAN EXPERIMENTATION/SPECIAL POPULATIONS)

Lieberman, Brian see **Sutcliffe, Alastair G.**

Lieberman, Jeffrey A. see **Pincus, Harold Alan**

Lieberson, Alan see **Levine, Robert A.**

Light, Donald. Saving John Worthy. [Letter]. *Hastings Center Report.* 1999 May–Jun; 29(3): 5.
(HEALTH CARE/ECONOMICS)

Light, Donald W. Good managed care needs universal health insurance. *Annals of Internal Medicine.* 1999 Apr 20; 130(8): 686–689.
(HEALTH CARE/ECONOMICS)

Lightner, Robin see **Andrykowski, Michael A.**

Lii, Jane H. Suit over adopted boy's H.I.V. seen as a first. [News]. *New York Times.* 1998 Feb 8: 35.
(AIDS)

Lilford, R.J. see **Edwards, Sarah J.L.**

Lilford, Richard J. see **Edwards, Sarah J.L.**

Limaye, Ajit P. see **Margolis, Lewis H.**

Limentani, Alexander E.; Miller, Saul; Neuberger, Julia; Annas, George J.; Grodin, Michael A.; Brewster, M.F.; Hyer, Steven; Wilcox, Hervey; Brown, Craig K.; Philipp, Robin; Hart, David. An ethical code for everybody in health care. [Letters]. *BMJ (British Medical Journal).* 1998 May 9; 316(7142): 1458–1460.
(PROFESSIONAL ETHICS/CODES OF ETHICS)

Limpakarnjanarat, Khanchit see **Achrekar, Abinash**

Lin-Fu, Jane S. Advances in genetics: issues for US racial and ethnic minorities: an Asian American and Pacific Islander perspective. *Community Genetics.* 1998; 1(3): 124–129.
(GENETIC RESEARCH; GENETIC SERVICES)

Lin, Hung-Mo; Kauffman, H. Myron; McBride, Maureen A.; Davies, Darcy B.; Rosendale, John D.; Smith, Carol M.; Edwards, Erick B.; Daily, O. Patrick; Kirklin, James; Shield, Charles F.; Hunsicker, Lawrence G. Center-specific graft and patient survival rates: 1997 United Network for Organ Sharing (UNOS) report. *JAMA.* 1998 Oct 7; 280(13): 1153–1160.
(ORGAN AND TISSUE TRANSPLANTATION)

Lin, Jonathan H. Divining and altering the future: implications from the Human Genome Project. [Editorial]. *JAMA.* 1998 Nov 4; 280(17): 1532.
(GENETIC SCREENING)

Lin, Lillian S. see **Valdiserri, Ronald O.**

Linburn, Geoffrey E. *Donaldson* revisited: is dangerousness a constitutional requirement for civil commitment? *Journal of the American Academy of Psychiatry and the Law.* 1998; 26(3): 343–351.
(INVOLUNTARY COMMITMENT)

Linder, Douglas O. The other right-to-life debate: when does Fourteenth Amendment "life" end? *Arizona Law Review.* 1995; 37(4): 1183–1207.
(ALLOWING TO DIE/LEGAL ASPECTS; DETERMINATION OF DEATH/BRAIN DEATH; PERSONHOOD)

Lindsay, Donald G. see **Epstein, Richard A.**

Lindsay, Michael K. Routine voluntary antepartum HIV antibody counseling and testing: a sound public health prevention strategy. *Clinical Obstetrics and Gynecology.* 1996 Jun; 39(2): 305–315.
(AIDS/TESTING AND SCREENING)

Lindsay, Ronald A. Taboos without a clue: sizing up religious objections to cloning. *Free Inquiry.* 1997 Summer; 17(3): 15–17.
(CLONING)

Lindsay, Ronald Alan. Self-Determination, Suicide and Euthanasia: The Implications of Autonomy for the Morality and Legality of Assisted Suicide and Voluntary Active Euthanasia. Ann Arbor, MI: UMI Dissertation Services; 1996. 592 p.
(EUTHANASIA; SUICIDE)

Lints, Frédéric A. see **Nagy, Anne-Marie**

Lipschutz, Joshua H. To clone or not to clone -- a Jewish perspective. *Journal of Medical Ethics.* 1999 Apr; 25(2): 105–107.
(CLONING)

Lisko, Elaine A. Genetic information and long-term care insurance. *Health Law News.* 1998 Sep; 12(1): 3, 12–13.
(GENETIC SCREENING)

Liss, Marsha B. see **Putnam, Frank W.**

Little, Margaret Olivia. Cosmetic surgery, suspect norms, and the ethics of complicity. *In:* Parens, Erik, ed. Enhancing Human Traits: Ethical and Social

Implications. Washington, DC: Georgetown University Press; 1998: 162–176.
(BIOMEDICAL TECHNOLOGIES)

Little, Margaret Olivia. Let me count the ways: feminism illuminating bioethics. [Book review essay]. *Medical Humanities Review.* 1997 Spring; 11(1): 76–81.
(BIOETHICS; REPRODUCTION; REPRODUCTIVE TECHNOLOGIES)

Little, Miles. Research, ethics and conflicts of interest. *Journal of Medical Ethics.* 1999 Jun; 25(3): 259–262.
(HUMAN EXPERIMENTATION/ETHICS COMMITTEES)

Liu, Honghu see **Wenger, Neil**

Livolsi, Virginia see **Merz, Jon F.**

Lizza, John B.; Truog, Robert D.; Robertson, John A.; Bernat, James L. Death: merely biological? [Letters and response]. *Hastings Center Report.* 1999 Jan–Feb; 29(1): 4–5.
(DETERMINATION OF DEATH/BRAIN DEATH)

Lloyd, A.J.; Hayes, P.D.; London, N.J.M.; Bell, P.R.F.; Naylor, A.R. Patients' ability to recall risk associated with treatment options. [Research letter]. *Lancet.* 1999 Feb 20; 353(9153): 645.
(INFORMED CONSENT)

Lloyd, Geoffrey see **Thorns, Andrew**

Lo, B. see **Weiss, A.H.**

Lo, Bernard; Quill, Timothy; Tulsky, James; American College of Physicians–American Society of Internal Medicine End–of–Life Care Consensus Panel. Discussing palliative care with patients. *Annals of Internal Medicine.* 1999 May 4; 130(9): 744–749.
(PROFESSIONAL PATIENT RELATIONSHIP; TERMINAL CARE)

Lo, Bernard; Snyder, Lois. Care at the end of life: guiding practice where there are no easy answers. [Editorial]. *Annals of Internal Medicine.* 1999 May 4; 130(9): 772–774.
(TERMINAL CARE)

Lo, Bernard see **Alpers, Ann**

Lo, Bernard see **Kim, H. Nina**

Lo, Bernard see **Letvak, Richard**

Lo, Bernard see **Wu, Albert W.**

Lobjoit, Mary see **Brazier, Margaret**

Locatelli, F. see **Burgio, G. Roberto**

Lock, Margaret. The problem of brain death: Japanese disputes about bodies and modernity. *In:* Youngner, Stuart J., Arnold, Robert M., Schapiro, Renie, eds. The Definition of Death: Contemporary Controversies. Baltimore, MD: Johns Hopkins University Press; 1999: 239–256.
(DETERMINATION OF DEATH/BRAIN DEATH; ORGAN AND TISSUE DONATION)

Loder, Natasha. Allow cloning in embryo research, says UK report. [News]. *Nature.* 1998 Dec 10; 396(6711): 503.
(CLONING; EMBRYO AND FETAL RESEARCH)

Loehle, Craig. Untainted by money. *New Scientist.* 1997 Aug 16; 155(2095): 44.
(BIOMEDICAL RESEARCH)

Loewy, Erich H. Curiosity, imagination, compassion, science and ethics: do curiosity and imagination serve a central function? *Health Care Analysis.* 1998 Dec; 6(4): 286–294.
(BIOETHICS)

Loewy, Erich H.; Loewy, Roberta Springer. Ethics and managed care: reconstructing a system and refashioning a society. [Editorial]. *Archives of Internal Medicine.* 1998 Dec 7–21; 158(22): 2419–2422.
(HEALTH CARE/ECONOMICS)

Loewy, Roberta Springer see **Loewy, Erich H.**

Loff, Bebe; Cordner, Stephen. Aboriginal people trade land claim for dialysis. [News]. *Lancet.* 1998 Oct 31; 352(9138): 1451.
(BIOMEDICAL TECHNOLOGIES; HEALTH CARE/FOREIGN COUNTRIES)

Loff, Bebe; Cordner, Stephen. Australian doctor reveals details of assisted suicides. [News]. *Lancet.* 1998 Dec 5; 352(9143): 1838.
(EUTHANASIA)

Loff, Bebe; Cordner, Stephen. Confusion over use of cadaver gametes for assisted fertilisation. [News]. *Lancet.* 1998 Aug 1; 352(9125): 382.
(ARTIFICIAL INSEMINATION)

Loff, Bebe; Cordner, Stephen. Learning a culture of respect for human rights. [Commentary]. *Lancet.* 1998 Dec 5; 352(9143): 1800.
(FRAUD AND MISCONDUCT; HEALTH CARE/FOREIGN COUNTRIES)

Loff, Bebe; Cordner, Stephen. World War II malaria trials revisited. [News]. *Lancet.* 1999 May 8; 353(9164): 1597.
(FRAUD AND MISCONDUCT; HUMAN EXPERIMENTATION/FOREIGN COUNTRIES)

Loff, Bebe see **Crofts, Nick**

Loftus, Elizabeth F.; Paddock, John R.; Guernsey, Thomas F. Patient–psychotherapist privilege: access to clinical records in the tangled web of repressed memory litigation. *University of Richmond Law Review.* 1996 Jan; 30(1): 109–154.
(CONFIDENTIALITY/LEGAL ASPECTS; CONFIDENTIALITY/MENTAL HEALTH)

Logan, D. see **Cappelli, M.**

Lomax, Karen J. see **Durnan, Richard J.**

Lonchyna, Vassyl A. To resuscitate or not ... in the operating room: the need for hospital policies for surgeons regarding DNR orders. *Annals of Health Law.* 1997; 6: 209–227.
(RESUSCITATION ORDERS)

London, Leslie; McCarthy, G. Teaching medical students on the ethical dimensions of human rights: meeting the challenge in South Africa. *Journal of Medical Ethics.* 1998 Aug; 24(4): 257–262.
(MEDICAL ETHICS/EDUCATION)

London, N.J.M. see **Lloyd, A.J.**

London, Stephanie J. see **Wilcox, Allen J.**

Long, Ann; Slevin, Eamonn. Living with dementia: communicating with an older person and her family. *Nursing Ethics.* 1999 Jan; 6(1): 23–36.
(NURSING ETHICS/EDUCATION; PATIENT CARE/AGED; PATIENT CARE/MENTALLY DISABLED; PROFESSIONAL PATIENT RELATIONSHIP)

Long, Stephen P.; Medical Society of Virginia. Pain Management Subcommittee. MSV [Medical Society of Virginia] House of Delegates passes opioid guidelines. *Virginia Medical Quarterly.* 1998 Winter; 125(1): 8–11.
(PATIENT CARE/DRUGS)

Longenecker, J. Craig see **Wong, Jeffrey G.**

Looman, Caspar W.N. see **Cuperus-Bosma, Jacqueline M.**

Looney, Stephen W. see **Mold, James W.**

Loriz, Lillia see **Chally, Pamela S.**

Lot, Florence; Séguier, Jean–Christophe; Fégueux, Sophie; Astagneau, Pascal; Simon, Philippe; Aggoune, Michéle; van Amerongen, Patrice; Ruch, Martine; Cheron, Mireille; Brücker, Gilles; Desenclos, Jean–Claude; Drucker, Jacques. Probable transmission of HIV from an orthopedic surgeon to a patient in France. *Annals of Internal Medicine.* 1999 Jan 5; 130(1): 1–6.
(AIDS/HEALTH PERSONNEL)

Louie, Robyn see **Crofts, Nick**

Louis, Karen Seashore see **Hsu, John**

Love, Richard R.; Fost, Norman C. Ethical and regulatory challenges in a randomized control trial of adjuvant treatment for breast cancer in Vietnam. *Journal of Investigative Medicine.* 1997 Oct; 45(8): 423–431.
(HUMAN EXPERIMENTATION/ETHICS COMMITTEES; HUMAN EXPERIMENTATION/FOREIGN COUNTRIES; HUMAN EXPERIMENTATION/INFORMED CONSENT; HUMAN EXPERIMENTATION/RESEARCH DESIGN)

Low, Lawrence; King, Suzanne; Wilkie, Tom. Genetic discrimination in life insurance: empirical evidence from a cross sectional survey of genetic support groups in the United Kingdom. *BMJ (British Medical Journal).* 1998 Dec 12; 317(7173): 1632–1635.
(GENETIC SCREENING)

Lowy, Cathy. What is 'ethics'? [Comment]. *Australian and New Zealand Journal of Psychiatry.* 1997 Feb; 31(1): 83–84.
(ETHICISTS AND ETHICS COMMITTEES; MEDICAL ETHICS)

Lu, Leonard. Commerce in organ transplantation. *Pharos.* 1998 Spring; 61(2): 2–5.
(ORGAN AND TISSUE DONATION)

Lucassen, Anneke. Ethical issues in genetics of mental disorders. *Lancet.* 1998 Sep 26; 352(9133): 1004–1005.
(GENETIC COUNSELING; GENETIC SCREENING)

Lucassen, Emy. The ethics of genetic engineering. *Journal of Applied Philosophy.* 1996; 13(1): 51–61.

(GENETIC INTERVENTION; RECOMBINANT DNA RESEARCH)

Lüdicke, Frank see **Dolian, Gayane**

Ludmerer, Kenneth M. Instilling professionalism in medical education. [Editorial]. *JAMA.* 1999 Sep 1; 282(9): 881–882.
(MEDICAL ETHICS/EDUCATION)

Lui, S.C.; Weaver, S.M.; Robinson, J.; Debono, M.; Nieland, M.; Killick, S.R.; Hay, D.M. A survey of semen donor attitudes. *Human Reproduction.* 1995 Jan; 10(1): 234–238.
(ARTIFICIAL INSEMINATION)

Luna, A. see **Pacheco, R.**

Luna, Florencia. Corruption and research. *Bioethics.* 1999 Jul; 13(3–4): 262–271.
(BIOMEDICAL RESEARCH; FRAUD AND MISCONDUCT; HUMAN EXPERIMENTATION)

Lund, Nelson. Two precipices, one chasm: the economics of physician–assisted suicide and euthanasia. *Hastings Constitutional Law Quarterly.* 1997 Summer; 24(4): 903–946.
(HEALTH CARE/ECONOMICS; SUICIDE)

Lundberg, George D. JAMA, abortion, and editorial responsibility. [Editorial]. *JAMA.* 1998 Aug 26; 280(8): 740.
(ABORTION)

Lundberg, George D. Publication and promotion: writing is all. *Lancet.* 1998 Sep 12; 352(9131): 898.
(BIOMEDICAL RESEARCH)

Luo, Chewe see **Wilfert, Catherine M.**

Lupton, M.L. Behaviour modification by genetic intervention –– the law's response. *Medicine and Law.* 1994; 13(5–6): 417–431.
(GENE THERAPY)

Lurie, Peter; Wolfe, Sidney M. Ethics of HIV trials. [Letter]. *Lancet.* 1998 Jan 17; 351(9097): 220.
(AIDS/HUMAN EXPERIMENTATION; HUMAN EXPERIMENTATION/FOREIGN COUNTRIES; HUMAN EXPERIMENTATION/RESEARCH DESIGN; HUMAN EXPERIMENTATION/SPECIAL POPULATIONS)

Lurie, Peter see **Edi–Osagie, E.C.O.**

Lurie, Peter see **Merson, Michael H.**

Lustig, B. Andrew. Concepts and methods in recent bioethics: critical responses. [Introduction to articles by R.M. Veatch, B.C. White and J. Zimbelman, W. Harper, P. McGrath, and H. Fielding]. *Journal of Medicine and Philosophy.* 1998 Oct; 23(5): 445–455.
(BIOETHICS)

Lustig, B. Andrew. Sexual ethics and communal judgments: on the pluralism of virtues, values, and practices. *Christian Bioethics.* 1998 Apr; 4(1): 3–13.
(STERILIZATION)

Luttrell, Steven. Withdrawing or withholding life prolonging treatment: a new BMA report fills an ethical vacuum. [Editorial]. *BMJ (British Medical Journal).* 1999 Jun 26; 318(7200): 1709–1710.

(ALLOWING TO DIE/LEGAL ASPECTS)

Lyall, Sarah. A country unveils its gene pool and debate flares. [News]. *New York Times.* 1999 Feb 16: F1, F4.
(GENETIC RESEARCH)

Lyckholm, Laurie J. Should physicians accept gifts from patients? *JAMA.* 1998 Dec 9; 280(22): 1944–1946.
(PROFESSIONAL PATIENT RELATIONSHIP)

Lyman, Rick. As octuplets remain in peril, ethics questions are raised. [News]. *New York Times.* 1998 Dec 22: A1, A22.
(REPRODUCTIVE TECHNOLOGIES)

Lynch, Charles F. see **Shavers–Hornaday, Vickie L.**

Lynch, Eugene C. see **Stoddard, Joan C.**

Lynch, Henry T. see **Lerman, Caryn**

Lynch, Jane see **Pokorski, Robert J.**

Lynch, Jane F. see **Lerman, Caryn**

Lynch, Marty see **Hansen, Jennie Chin**

Lynn, David J.; Vaillant, George E. Anonymity, neutrality, and confidentiality in the actual methods of Sigmund Freud: a review of 43 cases, 1907–1939. *American Journal of Psychiatry.* 1998 Feb; 155(2): 163–171.
(CONFIDENTIALITY/MENTAL HEALTH)

Lynn, Joanne; Cranford, Ronald. The persisting perplexities in the determination of death. *In:* Youngner, Stuart J.; Arnold, Robert M.; Schapiro, Renie, eds. The Definition of Death: Contemporary Controversies. Baltimore, MD: Johns Hopkins University Press; 1999: 101–114.
(DETERMINATION OF DEATH)

Lynn, Joanne; Muncie, Herbert L.; Magaziner, Jay; Hebel, Richard; Warren, John W. Ethical concerns about research on incompetent persons. [Letter and response]. *Journal of the American Geriatrics Society.* 1998 May; 46(5): 660.
(HUMAN EXPERIMENTATION/INFORMED CONSENT; HUMAN EXPERIMENTATION/SPECIAL POPULATIONS)

Lynn, Joanne see **Carron, Annette T.**

Lynn, Joanne see **Hamel, Mary Beth**

Lynn, Joanne see **Harrold, Joan K.**

Lynn, Joanne see **Pritchard, Robert S.**

Lynn, Joanne see **Tonelli, Mark R.**

Lynn, Joanne see **Wasson, John H.**

Lynn, Lorna A. AIDS clinical trials: is there access for all? [Editorial]. *Journal of General Internal Medicine.* 1997 Mar; 12(3): 198–199.
(AIDS/HUMAN EXPERIMENTATION)

Lynöe, N. see **Kullgren, G.**

Lynxwiler, John; Gay, David. The abortion attitudes of black women: 1972–1991. *Journal of Black Studies.* 1996 Nov; 27(2): 260–277.
(ABORTION/ATTITUDES)

Lyon, Sue see **Velasco, N.**

Lysaker, John T.; Sullivan, Michael. Untying the gag: reason in the world of health care reform. *In:* McGee, Glenn, ed. Pragmatic Bioethics. Nashville, TN: Vanderbilt University Press; 1999: 228–245, 283–287.
(HEALTH CARE/ECONOMICS)

M

McAlpine, Heather; Kristjanson, Linda; Poroch, Davina. Development and testing of the ethical reasoning tool (ERT): an instrument to measure the ethical reasoning of nurses. *Journal of Advanced Nursing.* 1997 Jun; 25(6): 1151–1161.
(NURSING ETHICS)

McBride, Maureen A. see **Lin, Hung–Mo**

McCabe, Jennifer see **Margolis, Lewis H.**

McCaffery, Margo; Ferrell, Betty Rolling. Pain and placebos: ethical and professional issues. [Editorial]. *Orthopaedic Nursing.* 1997 Sep–Oct; 16(5): 8–11.
(FRAUD AND MISCONDUCT; PATIENT CARE/DRUGS)

McCally, Michael; Haines, Andrew; Fein, Oliver; Addington, Whitney; Lawrence, Robert S.; Cassel, Christine K. Poverty and ill health: physicians can, and should, make a difference. *Annals of Internal Medicine.* 1998 Nov 1; 129(9): 726–733.
(HEALTH)

McCarrick, Pat Milmoe see **Darragh, Martina**

McCarthy, David. Persons and their copies. *Journal of Medical Ethics.* 1999 Apr; 25(2): 98–104.
(CLONING)

McCarthy, G. see **London, Leslie**

McCarthy, Gillian M.; Koval, John J.; MacDonald, John K. Factors associated with refusal to treat HIV–infected patients: the results of a national survey of dentists in Canada. *American Journal of Public Health.* 1999 Apr; 89(4): 541–545.
(AIDS/HEALTH PERSONNEL)

McCarthy, James. Placebo in research on schizophrenia. [Letter]. *Psychiatric Services.* 1998 May; 49(5): 699.
(HUMAN EXPERIMENTATION/RESEARCH DESIGN; HUMAN EXPERIMENTATION/SPECIAL POPULATIONS)

McCarthy, Martha see **Crelinsten, Gordon L.**

McCauly, Robert F. see **Robin, Eugene D.**

McChesney, Lawrence P.; Braithwaite, Susan S. Expectations and outcomes in organ transplantation. *Cambridge Quarterly of Healthcare Ethics.* 1999 Summer; 8(3): 299–310.
(ORGAN AND TISSUE TRANSPLANTATION; RESOURCE ALLOCATION/BIOMEDICAL TECHNOLOGIES; SELECTION FOR TREATMENT)

Macciocchi, Stephen N. see **Alves, Wayne A.**

McCollum, Marianne see **Bolan, Robert K.**

McConnell, L.M.; Koenig, B.A.; Greely, H.T.; Raffin, T.A.; Stanford Program in Genomics, Ethics and Society. Alzheimer Disease Working Group. Genetic testing and Alzheimer disease: has the time come? *Nature Medicine.* 1998 Jul; 4(7): 757–759.
(GENETIC SCREENING)

McConnell, Laura M. see **Koenig, Barbara A.**

McCormick, Marie C. see **Stoto, Michael A.**

McCormick, Richard A. Vive la différence! Killing and allowing to die. *America.* 1997 Dec 6; 177(18): 6–12.
(ALLOWING TO DIE; SUICIDE)

McCorvey, Norma. I Am Roe: My Life, *Roe v. Wade,* and Freedom of Choice. New York, NY: HarperPerennial; 1994. 216 p.
(ABORTION/LEGAL ASPECTS)

McCorvey, Norma. Won by Love: Norma McCorvey, Jane Roe of Roe v. Wade, Speaks Out for the Unborn as She Shares Her New Conviction for Life. Nashville, TN: Thomas Nelson; 1997. 244 p.
(ABORTION)

McCrory, Douglas C. see **Slovenko, Ralph**

McCrory, Douglas C. see **Sugarman, Jeremy**

McCubbin, Michael; Weisstub, David N. Toward a pure best interests model of proxy decision making for incompetent psychiatric patients. *International Journal of Law and Psychiatry.* 1998 Winter; 21(1): 1–30.
(INFORMED CONSENT/MENTALLY DISABLED)

McCullough, Laurence B. A transcultural, preventive ethics approach to critical–care medicine: restoring the critical care physician's power and authority. *Journal of Medicine and Philosophy.* 1998 Dec; 23(6): 628–642.
(ALLOWING TO DIE; HEALTH CARE/FOREIGN COUNTRIES)

McCullough, Laurence B. Ethics in the management of health care organizations. *Physician Executive.* 1993 Nov–Dec; 19(6): 72–76.
(HEALTH CARE/ECONOMICS; PROFESSIONAL ETHICS)

McCullough, Laurence B. Hume's influence on John Gregory and the history of medical ethics. *Journal of Medicine and Philosophy.* 1999 Aug; 24(4): 376–395.
(MEDICAL ETHICS)

McCullough, Laurence B. John Gregory and the Invention of Professional Medical Ethics and the Profession of Medicine. Boston, MA: Kluwer Academic; 1998. 347 p.
(MEDICAL ETHICS)

McCullough, Laurence B. John Gregory's Writings on Medical Ethics and Philosophy of Medicine. Boston, MA: Kluwer Academic; 1998. 254 p.
(MEDICAL ETHICS)

McCullough, Laurence B. Laying medicine open: understanding major turning points in the history of medical ethics. *Kennedy Institute of Ethics Journal.* 1999 Mar; 9(1): 7–23.
(BIOETHICS; MEDICAL ETHICS)

McCullough, Laurence B.; Reich, Warren Thomas. Laying medicine open: innovative interaction between medicine and the humanities. [Introduction to articles by L.B. McCullough, W.T. Reich, D. Callahan, and E.D. Pellegrino, and to a bibliography of resources by and about A.E. Hellegers compiled by D.M. Goldstein]. *Kennedy Institute of Ethics Journal.* 1999 Mar; 9(1): 1–5.
(BIOETHICS)

McCullough, Laurence B. see **Chervenak, Frank A.**

McCullough, Laurence B. see **Cutter, Mary Ann G.**

McCullough, Laurence B. see **Kopelman, Loretta M.**

McCullough, Laurence B. see **Perone, Nicola**

McCullough, Laurence B. see **Workman, Richard H.**

McDaniels, Andrea. Brazil mandates organ 'donation' for transplants. [News]. *Christian Science Monitor.* 1998 Jan 16: 1, 9.
(ORGAN AND TISSUE DONATION)

McDermott, Vincent G. Resuscitation and the radiologist. [Editorial]. *Annals of Internal Medicine.* 1998 Nov 15; 129(10): 831–833.
(RESUSCITATION ORDERS)

McDonald, Jim see **Graham, Amanda**

MacDonald, John K. see **McCarthy, Gillian M.**

McDonald, Michael. Health, health care, and culture: diverse meanings, shared agendas. *In:* Coward, Harold; Ratanakul, Pinit, eds. A Cross–Cultural Dialogue on Health Care Ethics. Waterloo, ON: Wilfrid Laurier University Press; 1999: 92–112.
(HEALTH; HEALTH CARE)

MacDonald, Neil. A march of folly. [Editorial]. *Canadian Medical Association Journal.* 1998 Jun 30; 158(13): 1699–1701.
(TERMINAL CARE)

MacDonald, Neil see **Singer, Peter A.**

McDonnell, Kevin see **Robinson, John H.**

McDonnell, Orla. Ethical and social implications of technology in medicine: new possibilities and new dilemmas. *In:* Cleary, Anne; Treacy, Margaret P., eds. The Sociology of Health and Illness in Ireland. Dublin: University College of Dublin Press; 1997: 69–84.
(ALLOWING TO DIE; BIOMEDICAL TECHNOLOGIES; REPRODUCTIVE TECHNOLOGIES)

McDonough, Paul G. The ethics of somatic and germline gene therapy. *Annals of the New York Academy of Sciences.* 1997 Jun 17; 816: 378–382.
(GENE THERAPY)

Macer, Darryl R.J. Bioethics Is Love of Life: An Alternative Textbook. Christchurch, NZ: Eubios Ethics Institute; 1998. 158 p.
(BIOETHICS)

McFadyen, Anne; Gledhill, Julia; Whitlow, Barry; Economides, Demetrios. First trimester ultrasound screening carries ethical and psychological implications. [Editorial]. *BMJ (British Medical Journal).* 1998 Sep 12;

317(7160): 694–695.
(INFORMED CONSENT; PRENATAL DIAGNOSIS)

McFarland, Bentson H. see **Ganzini, Linda**

MacFarquhar, Neil. In Islam, brain death ends life support. *New York Times.* 1999 Feb 6: A6.
(ALLOWING TO DIE/RELIGIOUS ASPECTS; DETERMINATION OF DEATH/BRAIN DEATH)

MacFie, J. Ethical implications of recognizing nutritional support as a medical therapy. *British Journal of Surgery.* 1996 Nov; 83(11): 1567–1568.
(PATIENT CARE)

McGee, Ellen M. see **Maguire, G.Q.**

McGee, Glenn. Breaking bioethics: an introduction and mission. *Cambridge Quarterly of Healthcare Ethics.* 1998 Fall; 7(4): 414–416.
(BIOETHICS; ETHICISTS AND ETHICS COMMITTEES)

McGee, Glenn. Ethics and the future of genetic testing. *In:* Smith, Edward; Sapp, Walter, eds. Plain Talk about the Human Genome Project: A Tuskegee University Conference on Its Promise and Perils ... and Matters of Race. Tuskegee, AL: Tuskegee University Press; 1997: 151–158.
(GENETIC INTERVENTION)

McGee, Glenn. Gene patents can be ethical. *Cambridge Quarterly of Healthcare Ethics.* 1998 Fall; 7(4): 417–421.
(GENOME MAPPING)

McGee, Glenn. Genetic enhancement of families. *In:* McGee, Glenn, ed. Pragmatic Bioethics. Nashville, TN: Vanderbilt University Press; 1999: 168–180, 279–280.
(GENETIC INTERVENTION)

McGee, Glenn. Paper shields: why advance directives still don't work. *Princeton Journal of Bioethics.* 1998 Spring; 1(1): 42–57.
(ADVANCE DIRECTIVES)

McGee, Glenn, ed. Pragmatic Bioethics. Nashville, TN: Vanderbilt University Press; 1999. 302 p.
(BIOETHICS)

McGee, Glenn. Pragmatic method and bioethics. *In:* McGee, Glenn, ed. Pragmatic Bioethics. Nashville, TN: Vanderbilt University Press; 1999: 18–29, 258–260.
(BIOETHICS)

McGee, Glenn; Caplan, Arthur. The ethics and politics of small sacrifices in stem cell research. *Kennedy Institute of Ethics Journal.* 1999 June; 9(2): 151–158.
(EMBRYO AND FETAL RESEARCH)

McGee, Glenn; Caplan, Arthur L. What's in the dish? [Symposium: human primordial stem cells]. *Hastings Center Report.* 1999 Mar–Apr; 29(2): 36–38.
(EMBRYO AND FETAL RESEARCH)

McGee, Glenn see **Lebacqz, Karen**

McGettigan, Marie C. see **Goldsmith, Jay P.**

McGillivray, Barbara see **Bernard, Lynn E.**

McGleenan, Tony. Rights to know and not to know: is there a need for a genetic privacy law? *In:* Chadwick,

Ruth; Levitt, Mairi; Shickle, Darren, eds. The Right to Know and the Right Not to Know. Brookfield, VT: Ashgate; 1997: 43–54.
(CONFIDENTIALITY/LEGAL ASPECTS; GENETIC SCREENING)

McGleenan, Tony see **Chadwick, Ruth**

McGough, Peter M. Medical concerns about physician–assisted suicide. *Seattle University Law Review.* 1995 Spring; 18(3): 521–530.
(SUICIDE)

McGovern, Margaret M.; Benach, Marta O.; Wallenstein, Sylvan; Desnick, Robert J.; Keenlyside, Richard. Quality assurance in molecular genetic testing laboratories. *JAMA.* 1999 Mar 3; 281(9): 835–840.
(GENETIC SCREENING; GENETIC SERVICES)

McGovern, Thomas F. Vulnerability: reflection on its ethical implications for the protection of participants in SAMHSA programs. *Ethics and Behavior.* 1998; 8(4): 293–304.
(BEHAVIORAL RESEARCH/SPECIAL POPULATIONS)

McGowan, Ruth. Beyond the disorder: one parent's reflection on genetic counselling. *Journal of Medical Ethics.* 1999 Apr; 25(2): 195–199.
(GENETIC COUNSELING)

McGrath, Geraldine see **Baumiller, Robert C.**

McGrath, Pam. Autonomy, discourse, and power: a postmodern reflection on principlism and bioethics. *Journal of Medicine and Philosophy.* 1998 Oct; 23(5): 516–532.
(BIOETHICS; TERMINAL CARE/HOSPICES)

McGregor, Christopher G.A. see **Sachs, David H.**

MacGregor, Scott N. see **Neerhof, Mark G.**

McGuffin, Peter see **Thomas, Sandy**

McGuire, Beverly see **Forret, Patricia**

Mach, Adrea see **Beecham, Linda**

Machado, Nora. Using the Bodies of the Dead: Legal, Ethical and Organisational Dimensions of Organ Transplantation. Brookfield, VT: Ashgate/Dartmouth; 1998. 262 p.
(ORGAN AND TISSUE DONATION; ORGAN AND TISSUE TRANSPLANTATION)

McHaffie, Hazel E.; Fowlie, Peter W. Life, Death and Decisions: Doctors and Nurses Reflect on Neonatal Practice. Hale, Cheshire, England: Hochland and Hochland; 1996. 294 p.
(ALLOWING TO DIE/ATTITUDES; ALLOWING TO DIE/INFANTS)

McHale, J.V. Guidelines for medical research -- some ethical and legal problems. *Medical Law Review.* 1993 Summer; 1(2): 160–185.
(HUMAN EXPERIMENTATION/ETHICS COMMITTEES; HUMAN EXPERIMENTATION/FOREIGN COUNTRIES)

McHale, J.V. Mental incapacity: some proposals for legislative reform. *Journal of Medical Ethics.* 1998 Oct; 24(5): 322–327.

(INFORMED CONSENT/MENTALLY DISABLED; TREATMENT REFUSAL/MENTALLY DISABLED)

McHale, Jean see **Fox, Marie**

Macilwain, Colin. Proposed restrictions relaxed on research on mentally disabled. [News]. *Nature.* 1998 Oct 22; 395(6704): 731.
(HUMAN EXPERIMENTATION/REGULATION; HUMAN EXPERIMENTATION/SPECIAL POPULATIONS)

McIlwain, James T. Comments on "Euthanasia." *Rhode Island Medicine.* 1993 Dec; 76(12): 602.
(EUTHANASIA; SUICIDE)

McInerney, Joseph D. see **Cutter, Mary Ann G.**

McIntosh, Kenneth. Short (and shorter) courses of zidovudine. [Editorial]. *New England Journal of Medicine.* 1998 Nov 12; 339(20): 1467–1468.
(AIDS/HUMAN EXPERIMENTATION; HUMAN EXPERIMENTATION/SPECIAL POPULATIONS)

McIntosh, Kenneth see **Merson, Michael H.**

MacKay, Charles; Murphy, Patricia D.; Smith, Robert A.; Bailey, Lisa; Boyd, Jeff; Burke, Wylie; Gleeson, Robert K.; Gould, Randi; Moore, Michael L.; Steinberg, Karen; Worsham, G. Fred. Industry, ethics, and general medicine: workshop no. 5. *Cancer.* 1997 Aug 1; 80(3, Suppl.): 635.
(GENETIC SCREENING)

MacKay, Karen; Moss, Alvin H. To dialyze or not to dialyze: an ethical and evidence–based approach to the patient with acute renal failure in the intensive care unit. *Advances in Renal Replacement Therapy.* 1997 Jul; 4(3): 288–296.
(BIOMEDICAL TECHNOLOGIES; SELECTION FOR TREATMENT)

McKee, Katherine; Adams, Eleanor. Nurse midwives' attitudes toward abortion performance and related procedures. *Journal of Nurse–Midwifery.* 1994 Sep–Oct; 39(5): 300–311.
(ABORTION/ATTITUDES)

McKenna, Juliet J. Where ignorance is not bliss: a proposal for mandatory HIV testing of pregnant women. *Stanford Law and Policy Review.* 1996 Summer; 7(2): 133–157.
(AIDS/TESTING AND SCREENING)

McKenny, Gerald P. A bad disease, a fatal cure: why sterilization is permissible and the autonomy of medicine is not. *Christian Bioethics.* 1998 Apr; 4(1): 100–109.
(STERILIZATION)

McKenny, Gerald P. Enhancements and the ethical significance of vulnerability. *In:* Parens, Erik, ed. Enhancing Human Traits: Ethical and Social Implications. Washington, DC: Georgetown University Press; 1998: 222–237.
(BIOMEDICAL TECHNOLOGIES; HEALTH)

McKenzie, John K.; Moss, Alvin H.; Feest, Terry G.; Stocking, Carol B.; Siegler, Mark. Dialysis decision making in Canada, the United Kingdom, and the United States. *American Journal of Kidney Diseases.* 1998 Jan; 31(1): 12–18.
(RESOURCE ALLOCATION/BIOMEDICAL TECHNOLOGIES; SELECTION FOR TREATMENT)

McKhann, Charles F. A Time to Die: The Place for Physician Assistance. New Haven, CT: Yale University Press; 1999. 268 p.
(EUTHANASIA; SUICIDE)

Mackler, Aaron L. An expanded partnership with God? In vitro fertilization in Jewish ethics. *Journal of Religious Ethics.* 1997 Fall; 25(2): 277–304.
(IN VITRO FERTILIZATION; PRENATAL DIAGNOSIS; REPRODUCTIVE TECHNOLOGIES)

Macklin, Ruth. A defense of fundamental principles and human rights: a reply to Robert Baker. *Kennedy Institute of Ethics Journal.* 1998 Dec; 8(4): 403–422.
(BIOETHICS; FRAUD AND MISCONDUCT; HUMAN EXPERIMENTATION)

Macklin, Ruth. Against Relativism: Cultural Diversity and the Search for Ethical Universals in Medicine. New York, NY: Oxford University Press; 1999. 290 p.
(BIOETHICS)

Macklin, Ruth. Death and birth. *In:* her Against Relativism: Cultural Diversity and the Search for Ethical Universals in Medicine. New York, NY: Oxford University Press; 1999: 136–160.
(ABORTION/FOREIGN COUNTRIES; DETERMINATION OF DEATH; SEX DETERMINATION)

Macklin, Ruth. Ethical relativism in a multicultural society. *Kennedy Institute of Ethics Journal.* 1998 Mar; 8(1): 1–22.
(PATIENT CARE)

Macklin, Ruth. Ethics, epidemiology, and law: the case of silicone breast implants. *American Journal of Public Health.* 1999 Apr; 89(4): 487–489.
(BIOMEDICAL RESEARCH; BIOMEDICAL TECHNOLOGIES)

Macklin, Ruth. Ethics, informed consent, and assisted reproduction. *Journal of Assisted Reproduction and Genetics.* 1995 Sep; 12(8): 484–490.
(INFORMED CONSENT; REPRODUCTIVE TECHNOLOGIES)

Macklin, Ruth. International feminism and reproductive rights. *In:* her Against Relativism: Cultural Diversity and the Search for Ethical Universals in Medicine. New York, NY: Oxford University Press; 1999: 161–185.
(ABORTION/FOREIGN COUNTRIES; CONTRACEPTION; REPRODUCTION; SEX DETERMINATION)

Macklin, Ruth. International research and ethical imperialism. *In:* her Against Relativism: Cultural Diversity and the Search for Ethical Universals in Medicine. New York, NY: Oxford University Press; 1999: 187–217.
(HUMAN EXPERIMENTATION/FOREIGN COUNTRIES; HUMAN EXPERIMENTATION/INFORMED CONSENT; HUMAN EXPERIMENTATION/SPECIAL POPULATIONS)

Macklin, Ruth. The doctor–patient relationship in different cultures. *In:* her Against Relativism: Cultural Diversity and the Search for Ethical Universals in Medicine. New York, NY: Oxford University Press; 1999: 85–107.
(PROFESSIONAL PATIENT RELATIONSHIP)

McLachlan, Hugh V. The unpaid donation of blood and altruism: a comment on Keown. *Journal of Medical Ethics.* 1998 Aug; 24(4): 252–254.
(BLOOD DONATION)

McLean, Margaret R. When what we know outstrips what we can do. *Issues in Ethics (Markkula Center for Applied Ethics).* 1998 Spring–Summer; 9(2): 6–10. (GENETIC INTERVENTION; GENETIC SCREENING)

Maclean, Norman. Transgenic animals in perspective. *In:* Maclean, Norman, ed. Animals with Novel Genes. New York, NY: Cambridge University Press; 1994: 1–20. (GENETIC INTERVENTION)

McLean, Sheila A.M. The genetic testing of children: some legal and ethical concerns. *In:* Clarke, Angus, ed. The Genetic Testing of Children. Washington, DC: BIOS Scientific Publishers; 1998: 17–26. (GENETIC SCREENING)

McLellan, Linda J. see **Foster, Larry W.**

MacLeod, Stuart M.; Bienenstock, John. Evidence-based rationing: Dutch pragmatism or government insensitivity? [Editorial]. *Canadian Medical Association Journal.* 1998 Jan 27; 158(2): 213–214. (HEALTH CARE/FOREIGN COUNTRIES; RESOURCE ALLOCATION)

McMahan, Jeff. Brain death, cortical death and persistent vegetative state. *In:* Kuhse, Helga; Singer, Peter, eds. A Companion to Bioethics. Malden, MA: Blackwell; 1998: 250–260. (DETERMINATION OF DEATH/BRAIN DEATH; PERSONHOOD)

McMahan, Jeff. Cloning, killing, and identity. *Journal of Medical Ethics.* 1999 Apr; 25(2): 77–86. (CLONING; PERSONHOOD)

McMahon, William see **Arnold, L. Eugene**

McMahon, William M. see **Schrock, Charles R.**

McNally, Ruth. Eugenics here and now. *In:* Glasner, Peter; Rothman, Harry; eds. Genetic Imaginations: Ethical, Legal and Social Issues in Human Genome Research. Brookfield, VT: Ashgate; 1998: 69–82. (ABORTION/FOREIGN COUNTRIES; EUGENICS; GENETIC SERVICES)

MacNamara, A.F. see **Hassan, T.B.**

McNeil, Barbara J. see **Hall, Judith A.**

McNeill, Paul M. Experimentation on human beings. *In:* Kuhse, Helga; Singer, Peter, eds. A Companion to Bioethics. Malden, MA: Blackwell; 1998: 369–378. (HUMAN EXPERIMENTATION/REGULATION)

McNiel, Dale E.; Binder, Renée L.; Fulton, Forrest M. Management of threats of violence under California's duty–to–protect statute. *American Journal of Psychiatry.* 1998 Aug; 155(8): 1097–1101. (CONFIDENTIALITY/LEGAL ASPECTS; CONFIDENTIALITY/MENTAL HEALTH)

McPhee, Stephen J. see **Wu, Albert W.**

Macpherson, Cheryl Cox. Research ethics committees: a regional approach. *Theoretical Medicine and Bioethics.* 1999 Apr; 20(2): 161–179. (HUMAN EXPERIMENTATION/ETHICS COMMITTEES; HUMAN EXPERIMENTATION/FOREIGN COUNTRIES)

Macpherson, Cheryl Cox see **Mann, Jonathan M.**

McQuay, Henry J. see **Tramèr, Martin R.**

McQuillen, Michael P.; Menken, Matthew; Hachinski, Vladimir. Managed care and managed death: peas from the same pod? [Article and commentaries]. *Archives of Neurology.* 1997 Mar; 54(3): 326–330. (HEALTH CARE/ECONOMICS; SUICIDE)

McSherry, James; Dickie, Gordon L. Swords to ploughshares: gatekeepers turned advocates. [Editorial]. *Canadian Family Physician.* 1998 May; 44: 955–956. (HEALTH CARE/ECONOMICS; RESOURCE ALLOCATION)

McVaugh, Michael R. "Bedside manners in the Middle Ages." *Bulletin of the History of Medicine.* 1997 Summer; 71(2): 201–223. (PROFESSIONAL PATIENT RELATIONSHIP)

Maddocks, Ian. Evolution of the physicians' peace movement: a historical perspective. *Health and Human Rights.* 1996; 2(1): 89–109. (WAR)

Madge, Sara see **Gbolade, Babatunde A.**

Madigan, Timothy J. Cloning and human dignity. [Editorial]. *Free Inquiry.* 1998 Spring; 18(2): 57–58. (CLONING)

Madison, Melinda. Tragic life or tragic death: mandatory testing of newborns for HIV -- mothers' rights versus children's health. *Journal of Legal Medicine.* 1997 Sep; 18(3): 361–386. (AIDS/TESTING AND SCREENING)

Madrid Acute Renal Failure Study Group see **Pascual, Julio**

Magaziner, Jay see **Lynn, Joanne**

Magaziner, Jay see **Muncie, Herbert L.**

Magill, Gerard see **Rainey, R. Randall**

Magis, Carlos see **Schüklenk, Udo**

Magnus, David. Disease gene patenting: the clinician's dilemma. *Cambridge Quarterly of Healthcare Ethics.* 1998 Fall; 7(4): 433–435. (GENETIC SCREENING; GENOME MAPPING)

Maguire, G.Q.; McGee, Ellen M. Implantable brain chips? Time for debate. *Hastings Center Report.* 1999 Jan–Feb; 29(1): 7–13. (BIOMEDICAL TECHNOLOGIES)

Maher, Daniel P. The moral triangle. *Ethics and Medics.* 1997 May; 22(5): 1–2. (CONTRACEPTION)

Maher, Effat A. Ethical and intellectual property in the biological sciences. *Cellular and Molecular Biology.* 1997 May; 43(3): 263–267. (PATENTING LIFE FORMS)

Maher, John T.; Pask, Eleanor G. When truth hurts.... *In:* Adams, David W.; Deveau, Eleanor J., eds. Beyond the Innocence of Childhood: Helping Children and Adolescents Cope with Life–Threatening Illness and Dying. Amityville, NY: Baywood Publishing; 1995:

267–293.
(PATIENT CARE/MINORS; TRUTH DISCLOSURE)

Maheux, Brigitte see **Beaudoin, Claude**

Mahkorn, Déirdre Tilmann see **Beecham, Linda**

Mahony, Roger see **Rigali, Justin**

Mahowald, Mary B. Collaboration and casuistry. *In:* McGee, Glenn, ed. Pragmatic Bioethics. Nashville, TN: Vanderbilt University Press; 1999: 73–83, 265–266.
(BIOETHICS)

Mahowald, Mary B. see **Silvers, Anita**

Main, David see **Lerman, Caryn**

Maine. Supreme Judicial Court. In re Nikolas E. *Atlantic Reporter, 2d Series.* 1998 Nov 19 (date of decision). 720: 562–568.
(AIDS/HUMAN EXPERIMENTATION; TREATMENT REFUSAL/MINORS)

Mainous, Arch G. see **Greenfield, Barak**

Maiorca, Rosario. Ethical problems in dialysis: prospects for the year 2000. *Nephrology, Dialysis, Transplantation.* 1998; 13(Suppl. 1): 1–9.
(RESOURCE ALLOCATION/BIOMEDICAL TECHNOLOGIES; SELECTION FOR TREATMENT)

Majumder, Partha see **Chatterji, Somnath**

Mak, June Mui Hing; Clinton, Michael. Promoting a good death: an agenda for outcomes research -- a review of the literature. *Nursing Ethics.* 1999 Mar; 6(2): 97–106.
(TERMINAL CARE/HOSPICES)

Makover, Michael E. Mismanaged Care: How Corporate Medicine Jeopardizes Your Health. Amherst, NY: Prometheus Books; 1998. 300 p.
(HEALTH CARE/ECONOMICS)

Malakoff, David. Alternatives to animals urged for producing antibodies. [News]. *Science.* 1999 Apr 9; 284(5412): 230.
(ANIMAL EXPERIMENTATION)

Malakoff, David. Groups sue to tighten oversight of rodents. [News]. *Science.* 1999 Feb 5; 283(5403): 767, 769.
(ANIMAL EXPERIMENTATION)

Maldonato, A. Ethical aspects in the prediction of Type I diabetes. *Diabetes, Nutrition and Metabolism.* 1996 Dec; 9(6): 325–329.
(GENETIC SCREENING)

Malhotra, Anil K. see **Pinals, Debra A.**

Malinowski, Michael J. Regulation of genetic modification of organisms: science or emotion? *Journal of Biolaw and Business.* 1998 Spring; 1(3): 3–7.
(CLONING; RECOMBINANT DNA RESEARCH/REGULATION)

Malkin, D.; Australie, K.; Shuman, C.; Barrera, M.; Weksberg, R. Parental attitudes to genetic counseling and predictive testing for childhood cancer. [Abstract]. *American Journal of Human Genetics.* 1996 Oct; 59(4): A7.
(GENETIC COUNSELING; GENETIC SCREENING)

Mallik, Harminder S. see **Barton, C. Dennis**

Malloy, David Cruise see **Hadjistavropoulos, Thomas**

Malloy, David Cruise see **Ross, Saul**

Malm, H.M. Medical screening and the value of early detection: when unwarranted faith leads to unethical recommendations. *Hastings Center Report.* 1999 Jan–Feb; 29(1): 26–37.
(MASS SCREENING)

Malone, Ruth E. Policy as product: morality and metaphor in health policy discourse. *Hastings Center Report.* 1999 May–Jun; 29(3): 16–22.
(HEALTH CARE/ECONOMICS)

Maloney, Dennis M. Federal agency proposal will lead to more children serving as research subjects. *Human Research Report.* 1997 Oct; 12(10): 1–2.
(HUMAN EXPERIMENTATION/MINORS; HUMAN EXPERIMENTATION/REGULATION)

Maloney, Dennis M. Federal investigation concludes that institutional review boards are in trouble. *Human Research Report.* 1998 Aug; 13(8): 1–2.
(HUMAN EXPERIMENTATION/ETHICS COMMITTEES; HUMAN EXPERIMENTATION/REGULATION)

Maloney, Dennis M. First federal agency to now require treatment for injured research subjects. [News]. *Human Research Report.* 1998 Apr; 13(4): 1–2.
(HUMAN EXPERIMENTATION/REGULATION)

Maloney, Dennis M. New federal commission proposed on bioethics. *Human Research Report.* 1998 Mar; 13(3): 6.
(BIOETHICS; ETHICISTS AND ETHICS COMMITTEES)

Maloney, Dennis M. New human subject regulations would change certain IRB reviews. [News]. *Human Research Report.* 1998 Jul; 13(7): 1–2.
(HUMAN EXPERIMENTATION/REGULATION; HUMAN EXPERIMENTATION/SPECIAL POPULATIONS)

Maloney, Dennis M. New policy on research with children is part of trend toward including more research subjects. *Human Research Report.* 1998 May; 13(5): 1–2.
(HUMAN EXPERIMENTATION/MINORS; HUMAN EXPERIMENTATION/REGULATION)

Maloney, Dennis M. Proposal on waiver of informed consent poses major issues for research ethics. *Human Research Report.* 1997 Sep; 12(9): 1–3.
(HUMAN EXPERIMENTATION/INFORMED CONSENT; HUMAN EXPERIMENTATION/REGULATION; HUMAN EXPERIMENTATION/SPECIAL POPULATIONS)

Maloney, Dennis M. Report says institutional review boards are conducting inadequate reviews. *Human Research Report.* 1998 Sep; 13(9): 1–2.
(HUMAN EXPERIMENTATION/ETHICS COMMITTEES; HUMAN EXPERIMENTATION/REGULATION)

Maloney, Dennis M. Researchers and the privacy act: Fisher v. National Institutes of Health (Part I). *Human Research Report.* 1998 Sep; 13(9): 4–5.
(CONFIDENTIALITY/LEGAL ASPECTS; FRAUD AND MISCONDUCT)

Malter, Alex; Sulmasy, Daniel P.; Schulman, Kevin A. Physician–assisted suicide. [Letter and response].

Archives of Internal Medicine. 1998 Dec 7–21; 158(22): 2513.
(RESOURCE ALLOCATION; SUICIDE)

Malterud, Kirsti see **Nessa, John**

Maltsberger, John T.; American Association of Suicidology. Committee on Physician–Assisted Death. Report of the Committee on Physician–Assisted Suicide and Euthanasia. *Suicide and Life–Threatening Behavior.* 1996; 26(Suppl.): 1–19.
(EUTHANASIA; SUICIDE; TERMINAL CARE)

Maly, Rose C.; Frank, Janet C.; Marshall, Grant N.; DiMatteo, M. Robin; Reuben, David B. Perceived efficacy in patient–physician interactions (PEPPI): validation of an instrument in older persons. *Journal of the American Geriatrics Society.* 1998 Jul; 46(7): 889–894.
(PATIENT CARE/AGED; PROFESSIONAL PATIENT RELATIONSHIP)

Malyon, David. Transfusion–free treatment of Jehovah's Witnesses: respecting the autonomous patient's motives. *Journal of Medical Ethics.* 1998 Dec; 24(6): 376–381.
(TREATMENT REFUSAL)

Malyon, David. Transfusion–free treatment of Jehovah's Witnesses: respecting the autonomous patient's rights. *Journal of Medical Ethics.* 1998 Oct; 24(5): 302–307.
(TREATMENT REFUSAL)

Mamtani, Ravinder see **Ristinen, Elaine**

Man, Rae. Will Israel be the first to allow organ sales? [News]. *Nature Medicine.* 1998 Apr; 4(4): 376.
(ORGAN AND TISSUE DONATION)

Mandl, Kenneth D.; Kohane, Isaac S.; Brandt, Allan M. Electronic patient–physician communication: problems and promise. *Annals of Internal Medicine.* 1998 Sep 15; 129(6): 495–500.
(PROFESSIONAL PATIENT RELATIONSHIP)

Manfredi, Paolo L. see **Preston, Thomas A.**

Mann, Jonathan. Health and human rights: broadening the agenda for health professionals. [Editorial]. *Health and Human Rights.* 1996; 2(1): 1–5.
(HEALTH; PUBLIC HEALTH)

Mann, Jonathan see **Gruskin, Sofia**

Mann, Jonathan M. AIDS and human rights: where do we go from here? *Health and Human Rights.* 1998; 3(1): 143–149.
(AIDS)

Mann, Jonathan, M.; Gruskin, Sofia; Grodin, Michael A.; Annas, George J., eds. Health and Human Rights: A Reader. New York, NY: Routledge; 1999. 505 p.
(HEALTH; HUMAN EXPERIMENTATION; PUBLIC HEALTH)

Mann, Jonathan M.; Zion, Deborah; Macpherson, Cheryl Cox; Bloom, Barry R. The ethics of AIDS vaccine trials. [Letters and response]. *Science.* 1998 May 29; 280(5368): 1327, 1329–1331.
(AIDS/HUMAN EXPERIMENTATION; HUMAN EXPERIMENTATION/FOREIGN COUNTRIES; IMMUNIZATION)

Mannan, Haripriya M. Death as defined by Hinduism.

Saint Louis University Public Law Review. 1996; 15(2): 423–432.
(SUICIDE)

Manning, Michael. Euthanasia and Physician–Assisted Suicide: Killing or Caring? New York, NY: Paulist Press; 1998. 120 p.
(EUTHANASIA/RELIGIOUS ASPECTS; SUICIDE)

Manning, Michael R. see **Fusilier, Marcelline**

Manning, Rita C. A care approach. *In:* Kuhse, Helga; Singer, Peter, eds. A Companion to Bioethics. Malden, MA: Blackwell; 1998: 98–105.
(BIOETHICS)

Manuel, Catherine. HIV screening: benefits and harms for the individual and the community. *In:* Bennett, Rebecca; Erin, Charles A., eds. HIV and AIDS: Testing, Screening, and Confidentiality. New York, NY: Oxford University Press; 1999: 61–74.
(AIDS/TESTING AND SCREENING)

Mao, Xin. Chinese geneticists approach ethics. [Letter]. *Journal of Medical Ethics.* 1998 Jan; 35(1): 83.
(ABORTION/ATTITUDES; ABORTION/FOREIGN COUNTRIES; GENETIC COUNSELING; GENETIC SCREENING; PRENATAL DIAGNOSIS)

Mao, Xin. Ethics and genetics in China: an inside story. [Letter]. *Nature Genetics.* 1997 Sep; 17(1): 20.
(EUGENICS; GENETIC COUNSELING; GENETIC RESEARCH)

March, John see **Leonard, Henrietta**

Marchand, Sarah; Wikler, Daniel; Landesman, Bruce. Class, health and justice. *Milbank Quarterly.* 1998; 76(3): 449–467.
(HEALTH; RESOURCE ALLOCATION)

Marchand, Sarah see **Wikler, Daniel**

Marco, Catherine A.; Bessman, Edward S.; Schoenfeld, Charles N.; Kelen, Gabor D. Ethical issues of cardiopulmonary resuscitation: current practice among emergency physicians. *Academic Emergency Medicine.* 1997 Sep; 4(9): 898–904.
(RESUSCITATION ORDERS)

Margeson, Nancy E. see **Frank, Stacy**

Margolis, Lewis H.; Rosner, Fred; Reynolds, Susan; Chiu, John T.; Mehta, Hemendra J.; Tenery, Robert M.; Limaye, Ajit P.; Paauw, Douglas S.; Westfall, John M.; McCabe, Jennifer; Nicholas, Richard A. Personal use of drug samples by physicians and office staff. [Letters and responses]. *JAMA.* 1997 Nov 19; 278(19): 1567–1569.
(HEALTH CARE/ECONOMICS; PATIENT CARE/DRUGS)

Marietta, Paola see **De Leo, Diego**

Marik, Paul E.; Craft, Michele. An outcomes analysis of in–hospital cardiopulmonary resuscitation: the futility rationale for do not resuscitate orders. *Journal of Critical Care.* 1997 Sep; 12(3): 142–146.
(RESUSCITATION ORDERS)

Mariner, Wendy K. Equitable access to biomedical advances: getting beyond the rights impasse. *Connecticut Law Review.* 1989 Spring; 21(3): 571–603.

(HEALTH CARE/RIGHTS; PATIENT CARE/DRUGS; RESOURCE ALLOCATION/BIOMEDICAL TECHNOLOGIES)

Mariner, Wendy K. Going Hollywood with patient rights in managed care. *JAMA.* 1999 Mar 3; 281(9): 861.
(HEALTH CARE/ECONOMICS; PATIENTS' RIGHTS)

Mariner, Wendy K. see **Glantz, Leonard H.**

Marjan, R.S.R.; Ruminjo, J.K. Attitudes to prenatal testing and notification for HIV infection in Nairobi, Kenya. *East African Medical Journal.* 1996 Oct; 73(10): 665–669.
(AIDS/TESTING AND SCREENING)

Markens, Susan; Browner, C.H.; Press, Nancy. Feeding the fetus: on interrogating the notion of maternal–fetal conflict. *Feminist Studies.* 1997 Summer; 23(2): 351–372.
(FETUSES; PATIENT CARE; PRENATAL INJURIES)

Marketos, Spyros see **Lascaratos, John**

Markman, Maurie. Ethical issues in clinical trials in oncology. *Cleveland Clinic Journal of Medicine.* 1997 May; 64(5): 275–277.
(HUMAN EXPERIMENTATION/RESEARCH DESIGN)

Markovitz, Barry; May, Larry. Three patients, two hearts. [Case study and commentaries]. *Hastings Center Report.* 1998 Sep–Oct; 28(5): 20–21.
(ORGAN AND TISSUE DONATION; ORGAN AND TISSUE TRANSPLANTATION; RESOURCE ALLOCATION/BIOMEDICAL TECHNOLOGIES; SELECTION FOR TREATMENT)

Marks, Beverly L. see **Webb, Cynthia M.**

Marlier, Eric. Opinions of Europeans on Biotechnology in 1991: Report Undertaken on Behalf of the Directorate–General for Science, Research and Development of the Commission of the European Communities. Brussels, Belgium: INRA (Europe). European Coordination Office; 1991. 98 p.
(GENETIC INTERVENTION)

Marlin, George J. Assisted suicide and euthanasia. *In: his* The Politician's Guide to Assisted Suicide, Cloning, and Other Current Controversies. Washington, DC: Morley Books; 1998: 63–124, 205–211.
(EUTHANASIA/LEGAL ASPECTS; SUICIDE)

Marlin, George J. Eugenics and cloning. *In: his* The Politician's Guide to Assisted Suicide, Cloning, and Other Current Controversies. Washington, DC: Morley Books; 1998: 125–168, 212–216.
(CLONING; EUGENICS)

Marmor, Michael see **Des Jarlais, Don C.**

Marmor, Theodore see **Jacobs, Lawrence**

Marquis, Don. How to resolve an ethical dilemma concerning randomized clinical trials. *New England Journal of Medicine.* 1999 Aug 26; 341(9): 691–693.
(HUMAN EXPERIMENTATION/INFORMED CONSENT; HUMAN EXPERIMENTATION/RESEARCH DESIGN)

Marshall, Adam. Choices for a child: an ethical and legal analysis of a failed surrogate birth contract. [Comment]. *University of Richmond Law Review.* 1996 Jan; 30(1): 275–302.

(ALLOWING TO DIE/INFANTS; SURROGATE MOTHERS)

Marshall, Andrew. Genetic tests forge ahead, despite scientific concerns. [News]. *Nature Biotechnology.* 1996 Dec; 14(13): 1642–1643.
(GENETIC SCREENING)

Marshall, Eliot. A second private genome project. [News]. *Science.* 1998 Aug 21; 281(5380): 1121.
(GENOME MAPPING)

Marshall, Eliot. A versatile cell line raises scientific hopes, legal questions. [News]. *Science.* 1998 Nov 6; 282(5391): 1014–1015.
(EMBRYO AND FETAL RESEARCH)

Marshall, Eliot. Beryllium screening raises ethical issues. [News]. *Science.* 1999 Jul 9; 285(5425): 178–179.
(GENETIC SCREENING; OCCUPATIONAL HEALTH)

Marshall, Eliot. Britain urged to expand embryo studies. [News]. *Science.* 1998 Dec 18; 282(5397): 2167–2168.
(EMBRYO AND FETAL RESEARCH)

Marshall, Eliot. Claim of human–cow embryo greeted with skepticism. [News]. *Science.* 1998 Nov 20; 282(5393): 1390–1391.
(GENETIC RESEARCH)

Marshall, Eliot. DNA studies challenge the meaning of race. [News]. *Science.* 1998 Oct 23; 282(5389): 654–655.
(GENETIC RESEARCH; GENOME MAPPING)

Marshall, Eliot. Drug firms to create public database of genetic mutations. [News]. *Science.* 1999 Apr 16; 284(5413): 406–407.
(GENOME MAPPING)

Marshall, Eliot. Ethicists back stem cell research, White House treads cautiously. [News]. *Science.* 1999 Jul 23; 285(5427): 502.
(EMBRYO AND FETAL RESEARCH)

Marshall, Eliot. Investigations on trial in a Texas court. [News]. *Science.* 1999 Feb 12; 283(5404): 913–914.
(BIOMEDICAL RESEARCH; FRAUD AND MISCONDUCT)

Marshall, Eliot. Legal fight over patents on life. [News]. *Science.* 1999 Jun 25; 284(5423): 2067, 2069.
(PATENTING LIFE FORMS)

Marshall, Eliot. NIMH to screen studies for science and human risks. [News]. *Science.* 1999 Jan 22; 283(5401): 464–465.
(HUMAN EXPERIMENTATION/SPECIAL POPULATIONS)

Marshall, Eliot. Panel proposes tighter rules for tissue studies. [News]. *Science.* 1998 Dec 18; 282(5397): 2165–6.
(GENETIC RESEARCH; HUMAN EXPERIMENTATION/INFORMED CONSENT; ORGAN AND TISSUE DONATION)

Marshall, Eliot. Panel pulls back report after NIH critique. [News]. *Science.* 1998 Oct 30; 282(5390): 857,859.
(HUMAN EXPERIMENTATION/REGULATION; HUMAN EXPERIMENTATION/SPECIAL POPULATIONS)

Marshall, Eliot. Panel tightens rules on mental disorders. [News]. *Science.* 1998 Nov 27; 282(5394): 1617.
(HUMAN EXPERIMENTATION/REGULATION; HUMAN EXPERIMENTATION/SPECIAL POPULATIONS)

Marshall, Eliot. Ruling may free NIH to fund stem cell studies. [News]. *Science.* 1999 Jan 22; 283(5401): 465, 467.
(EMBRYO AND FETAL RESEARCH)

Marshall, Eliot. Shutdown of research at Duke sends a message. [News]. *Science.* 1999 May 21; 284(5418): 1246.
(FRAUD AND MISCONDUCT; HUMAN EXPERIMENTATION/REGULATION)

Marshall, Eliot. Stem cell research: NIH plans ethics review of proposals. [News]. *Science.* 1999 Apr 16; 284(5413): 413, 415.
(EMBRYO AND FETAL RESEARCH)

Marshall, Eliot. Use of stem cells still legally murky, but hearing offers hope. [News]. *Science.* 1998 Dec 11; 282(5396): 1962–1963.
(EMBRYO AND FETAL RESEARCH)

Marshall, Grant N. see **Maly, Rose C.**

Marshall, Patricia A. see **Muraskas, Jonathan**

Marsiglio, William. Abortion and gender politics. *In: his* Procreative Man. New York, NY: New York University Press; 1998: 86–101, 211–213.
(ABORTION/ATTITUDES)

Marsiglio, William. Pathways to paternity and social fatherhood. *In: his* Procreative Man. New York, NY: New York University Press; 1998: 102–146, 213–222.
(REPRODUCTION; REPRODUCTIVE TECHNOLOGIES)

Marson, Daniel C.; Chatterjee, Anjan; Ingram, Kellie K.; Harrell, Lindy E. Toward a neurologic model of competency: cognitive predictors of capacity to consent in Alzheimer's disease using three different legal standards. *Neurology.* 1996 Mar; 46(3): 666–672.
(INFORMED CONSENT/MENTALLY DISABLED)

Marta, Jan. Whose consent is it anyway? A poststructuralist framing of the person in medical decision-making. *Theoretical Medicine and Bioethics.* 1998 Aug; 19(4): 353–370.
(INFORMED CONSENT; PROFESSIONAL PATIENT RELATIONSHIP)

Marteau, T.M. see **Welton, A.J.**

Martensen, Robert. If only it were so: medical physics, U.S. human radiation experiments, and the *Final Report* of the President's Advisory Committee (ACHRE). *Medical Humanities Review.* 1997 Fall; 11(2): 21–36.
(BIOMEDICAL RESEARCH; ETHICISTS AND ETHICS COMMITTEES; FRAUD AND MISCONDUCT; HUMAN EXPERIMENTATION)

Martin, Desmond J. see **Morris, Lynn**

Martin, Douglas K.; Thiel, Elaine C.; Singer, Peter A. A new model of advance care planning: observations from people with HIV. *Archives of Internal Medicine.* 1999 Jan 11; 159(1): 86–92.
(ADVANCE DIRECTIVES; AIDS)

Martin, Douglas K. see **Aikman, Peter J.**

Martin, Douglas K. see **Colebunders, Robert**

Martin, Douglas K. see **Singer, Peter A.**

Martin, Gilbert I. see **Peabody, Joyce L.**

Martin, Jeanett. Contraception and the under–16s: the legal issues. *Nursing Standard.* 1996 Jun 12; 10(38): 46–48.
(CONTRACEPTION/MINORS)

Martin, Richard J.; Gwyther, Lisa P.; Whitehouse, Peter J. Special care unit research: ethical issues. *Alzheimer Disease and Associated Disorders.* 1994; 8(Suppl. 1): S360–S367.
(BEHAVIORAL RESEARCH/SPECIAL POPULATIONS)

Martinez, William. Genetic testing of children and adolescents: ethical, legal and psychosocial implications. *Princeton Journal of Bioethics.* 1998 Spring; 1(1): 65–75.
(GENETIC SCREENING)

Martino, Ann M. In search of a new ethic for treating patients with chronic pain: what can medical boards do? *Journal of Law, Medicine and Ethics.* 1998 Winter; 26(4): 332–349.
(PATIENT CARE/DRUGS)

Martone, Marilyn. Developing new models to ensure autonomy in home health care. *Linacre Quarterly.* 1997 Aug; 64(3): 29–37.
(PATIENT CARE; PROFESSIONAL PATIENT RELATIONSHIP)

Martyn, Susan R.; Bourguignon, Henry J. Physician-assisted suicide: the lethal flaws of the Ninth and Second Circuit decisions. *California Law Review.* 1997 Mar; 85(2): 371–426.
(SUICIDE)

Marvel, M. Kim; Epstein, Ronald M.; Flowers, Kristine; Beckman, Howard B. Soliciting the patient's agenda: have we improved? *JAMA.* 1999 Jan 20; 281(3): 283–287.
(PROFESSIONAL PATIENT RELATIONSHIP)

Marwick, Charles. Funding stem cell research. [News]. *JAMA.* 1999 Feb 24; 281(8): 692–693.
(EMBRYO AND FETAL RESEARCH)

Marwick, Charles. IOM committee gazes into new vaccine future. [News]. *JAMA.* 1999 Apr 21; 281(15): 1366–1367.
(IMMUNIZATION)

Marwick, Charles. Protecting subjects of clinical research. [News]. *JAMA.* 1999 Aug 11; 282(6): 516–517.
(HUMAN EXPERIMENTATION/REGULATION)

Marx, Adina. The Society for Patient's Rights in Israel. *Nursing Ethics.* 1999 Mar; 6(2): 167–172.
(PATIENTS' RIGHTS)

Marx, Eric S. see **Buss, Mary K.**

Maryland. Health Care Decisions Act. *Maryland (Health-General) Code Annotated (Michie).* 1993 (date approved). Sects. 5–601 to 5–618. 102–119.
(ADVANCE DIRECTIVES)

Mason, John Kenyon. A third party to marriage. *In: his* Medico-Legal Aspects of Reproduction and Parenthood. Second Edition. Brookfield, VT: Ashgate; 1998: 251–279.
(SURROGATE MOTHERS)

Mason, John Kenyon. Abortion. *In: his* Medico-Legal Aspects of Reproduction and Parenthood. Second Edition. Brookfield, VT: Ashgate; 1998: 107–141.
(ABORTION/FOREIGN COUNTRIES; ABORTION/LEGAL ASPECTS)

Mason, John Kenyon. Consent to treatment and research in children. *In: his* Medico-Legal Aspects of Reproduction and Parenthood. Second Edition. Brookfield, VT: Ashgate; 1998: 319–339.
(HUMAN EXPERIMENTATION/MINORS; INFORMED CONSENT/MINORS; ORGAN AND TISSUE DONATION; TREATMENT REFUSAL/MINORS)

Mason, John Kenyon. Contraception. *In: his* Medico-Legal Aspects of Reproduction and Parenthood. Second Edition. Brookfield, VT: Ashgate; 1998: 41–65.
(CONTRACEPTION)

Mason, John Kenyon. Defective neonates and infants. *In: his* Medico-Legal Aspects of Reproduction and Parenthood. Second Edition. Brookfield, VT: Ashgate; 1998: 281–318.
(ALLOWING TO DIE/INFANTS)

Mason, John Kenyon. Fetal experimentation. *In: his* Medico-Legal Aspects of Reproduction and Parenthood. Second Edition. Brookfield, VT: Ashgate; 1998: 187–206.
(EMBRYO AND FETAL RESEARCH; ORGAN AND TISSUE DONATION)

Mason, John Kenyon. Protection of the fetus. *In: his* Medico-Legal Aspects of Reproduction and Parenthood. Second Edition. Brookfield, VT: Ashgate; 1998: 143–186.
(FETUSES; PRENATAL INJURIES; WRONGFUL LIFE)

Mason, John Kenyon. Sterilisation. *In: his* Medico-Legal Aspects of Reproduction and Parenthood. Second Edition. Brookfield, VT: Ashgate; 1998: 67–106.
(STERILIZATION; WRONGFUL LIFE)

Mason, John Kenyon. The infertile man. *In: his* Medico-Legal Aspects of Reproduction and Parenthood. Second Edition. Brookfield, VT: Ashgate; 1998: 207–226.
(ARTIFICIAL INSEMINATION)

Mason, John Kenyon. The infertile woman. *In: his* Medico-Legal Aspects of Reproduction and Parenthood. Second Edition. Brookfield, VT: Ashgate; 1998: 227–250.
(REPRODUCTIVE TECHNOLOGIES)

Mason, Sue. The ethical dilemma of the do not resuscitate order. *British Journal of Nursing.* 1997 Jun 12–25; 6(11): 646–649.
(RESUSCITATION ORDERS)

Masood, Ehsan. Britain opens biotech regulation to greater public involvement. [News]. *Nature.* 1999 May 27; 399(6734): 287–288.
(GENETIC INTERVENTION)

Masood, Ehsan. Iceland poised to sell exclusive rights to national health data. [News]. *Nature.* 1998 Dec 3; 396(6710): 395.
(GENETIC RESEARCH)

Massachusetts. Supreme Judicial Court. Planned Parenthood League of Massachusetts v. Attorney General. *North Eastern Reporter, 2d Series.* 1997 Mar 18 (date of decision). 677: 101–114.
(ABORTION/LEGAL ASPECTS; ABORTION/MINORS)

Massachusetts. Trial Court, Probate and Family Department, Suffolk County. AZ v. BZ. Unpublished redacted copy; 1996. 31 p.
(FETUSES; IN VITRO FERTILIZATION)

Masters, Brooke A. Family's life-and-death battle plays out in court. [News]. *Washington Post.* 1998 Sep 9: A1, A14.
(ALLOWING TO DIE/LEGAL ASPECTS)

Mathews, Steve. Protection of personal data -- the European view. *Journal of the American Health Information Management Association.* 1998 Mar; 69(3): 42–44.
(CONFIDENTIALITY)

Matson, Sandra see **Weissman, David E.**

Matthews, Dennis J.; Meier, Robert H.; Bartholome, William. Ethical issues encountered in pediatric rehabilitation. *Pediatrician.* 1990; 17(2): 108–114.
(PATIENT CARE/MINORS; RESOURCE ALLOCATION)

Matthews, Hugh. Better palliative care could cut euthanasia. [News]. *BMJ (British Medical Journal).* 1998 Dec 12; 317(7173): 1613.
(EUTHANASIA; TERMINAL CARE)

Matthews, Hugh. British public opposes human cloning. [News]. *BMJ (British Medical Journal).* 1998 Dec 12; 317(7173): 1613.
(CLONING)

Mattiasson, Anne-Cathrine; Hemberg, Maja. Intimacy -- meeting needs and respecting privacy in the care of elderly people: what is a good moral attitude on the part of the nurse/carer? *Nursing Ethics.* 1998 Nov; 5(6): 527–534.
(PATIENT CARE/AGED; PROFESSIONAL PATIENT RELATIONSHIP)

Matz, Robert; Levine, Myron M.; Tacket, Carol O.; Rabinovich, Regina. Recruiting volunteers for a typhoid vaccine. [Letter and response]. *JAMA.* 1998 Nov 4; 280(17): 1480–1481.
(HUMAN EXPERIMENTATION; IMMUNIZATION)

Matzo, Marianne LaPorte. The search to end suffering: a historical perspective. *Journal of Gerontological Nursing.* 1997 Mar; 23(3): 11–17.
(ALLOWING TO DIE/ATTITUDES; EUTHANASIA/ATTITUDES; SUICIDE)

Matzo, Marianne LaPorte see **Webb, Cynthia M.**

Mavretish, Barbara. Nursing home issues in restraint use. *HEC (HealthCare Ethics Committee) Forum.* 1998 Sep-Dec; 10(3–4): 300–305.
(PATIENT CARE/AGED)

Maw, Khin Lay see **Gasner, M. Rose**

Mawer, Simon. Iceland, the nation of clones. *New York Times.* 1999 Jan 23: A19.
(GENETIC RESEARCH; GENOME MAPPING)

May, Larry see **Markovitz, Barry**

May, Thomas. Assessing competency without judging merit. *Journal of Clinical Ethics.* 1998 Fall; 9(3): 247–257.
(INFORMED CONSENT)

May, Thomas. Slavery, commitment, and choice: do advance directives reflect autonomy? Response to "Advance directives and voluntary slavery" by Christopher Tollefsen (*CQ*, 1998 Fall; 7(4):405–413). *Cambridge Quarterly of Healthcare Ethics.* 1999 Summer; 8(3): 358–363.
(ADVANCE DIRECTIVES)

May, William E. Bioethics and human life. *In:* Forte, David F., ed. Natural Law and Contemporary Public Policy. Washington, DC: Georgetown University Press; 1998: 41–54.
(BIOETHICS)

May, William E. Making health care decisions for others. *Ethics and Medics.* 1997 Jun; 22(6): 1–3.
(ADVANCE DIRECTIVES; INFORMED CONSENT)

Mayo, David. Termination–of–treatment decisions: ethical underpinnings. *In:* Steinberg, Maurice D.; Youngner, Stuart J., eds. End–of–Life Decisions: A Psychosocial Perspective. Washington, DC: American Psychiatric Press; 1998: 259–281.
(ALLOWING TO DIE; SUICIDE)

Mayor, Susan. UK authorities recommend human cloning for therapeutic research. [News]. *BMJ (British Medical Journal).* 1998 Dec 12; 317(7173): 1613.
(CLONING; EMBRYO AND FETAL RESEARCH)

Mazur, Dennis J. Medical Risk and the Right to an Informed Consent in Clinical Care and Clinical Research. Tampa, FL: American College of Physician Executives; 1998. 183 p.
(HUMAN EXPERIMENTATION/INFORMED CONSENT; INFORMED CONSENT)

Mbidde, Edward K. see **Des Jarlais, Don C.**

Mbidde, Edward K. see **Merson, Michael H.**

Meade, Harry M. Dairy gene. *Sciences.* 1997 Sep–Oct; 37(5): 20–25.
(CLONING; GENETIC INTERVENTION)

Meade, T.W. see **Welton, A.J.**

Meadow, William; Lantos, John D.; Mokalla, Mani; Reimshisel, Tyler. Distributive justice across generations: epidemiology of ICU care for the very young and the very old. *Clinics in Perinatology.* 1996 Sep; 23(3): 597–608.
(PATIENT CARE/AGED; PATIENT CARE/MINORS; RESOURCE ALLOCATION/BIOMEDICAL TECHNOLOGIES)

Meadow, William see **Lantos, John D.**

Mechanic, David. Muddling through elegantly: finding the proper balance in rationing. *Health Affairs.* 1997 Sep–Oct; 16(5): 83–92.
(HEALTH CARE/ECONOMICS; HEALTH CARE/FOREIGN COUNTRIES; RESOURCE ALLOCATION)

Mechanic, David. Public trust and initiatives for new health care partnerships. *Milbank Quarterly.* 1998; 76(2): 281–302.
(PROFESSIONAL PATIENT RELATIONSHIP)

Mechanic, David. The functions and limitations of trust in the provision of medical care. *Journal of Health Politics, Policy and Law.* 1998 Aug; 23(4): 661–686.
(HEALTH CARE/ECONOMICS; PROFESSIONAL PATIENT RELATIONSHIP)

Mecsas–Faxon, S.; Tishler, S.; Pauker, S.P. Cancer genetics program within an HMO: a model of confidential service. [Abstract]. *American Journal of Human Genetics.* 1997 Oct; 61(4): A224.
(GENETIC SCREENING; GENETIC SERVICES)

Medawar, Charles see **Nightingale, Stuart L.**

Medical Library Association. Goals and Principles for Ethical Conduct. Chicago, IL: The Association (online). Downloaded from Internet Web site: http://www.mlanet.org.about.ethics.html on 11 Sep 1998; 1998 Sep 3. 2 p.
(PROFESSIONAL ETHICS/CODES OF ETHICS)

Medical Research Council (Great Britain). Responsibility in Investigations on Human Participants and Material and on Personal Information. [Guidance]. London: The Council; 1992 Nov. 15 p.
(HUMAN EXPERIMENTATION/FOREIGN COUNTRIES)

Medical Research Council (Great Britain). Responsibility in the Use of Animals in Medical Research: Guidance Issued by the Medical Research Council. [Pamphlet]. London: The Council; 1993 Jul. 13 p.
(ANIMAL EXPERIMENTATION)

Medical Society of Virginia. Pain Management Subcommittee see **Long, Stephen P.**

Meester, Johan De. Eurotransplant allocation procedures: the basics, March 1996. *In:* Lachmann, Rolf; Meuter, Norbert, eds. Zur Gerechtigkeit der Organverteilung: Ein Problem der Transplantationsmedizin aus interdisziplinärer Sicht. Stuttgart, Germany: G. Fischer; 1997: 167–177.
(ORGAN AND TISSUE TRANSPLANTATION; RESOURCE ALLOCATION/BIOMEDICAL TECHNOLOGIES)

Meguid, Michael M. Editors' responsibility in defeating fraud. [Letter]. *Nature.* 1999 May 6; 399(6731): 13.
(BIOMEDICAL RESEARCH; FRAUD AND MISCONDUCT)

Méhes, Károly see **Hermann, Robert**

Mehta, Hemendra J. see **Margolis, Lewis H.**

Meier–Allmendinger, Diana see **Sponholz, Gerlinde**

Meier, Diane E. see **Karlawish, Jason H.T.**

Meier, Diane E. see **Morrison, R. Sean**

Meier, Diane E. see **Preston, Thomas A.**

Meier, Diane E. see **Stead, William W.**

Meier, Robert H. see **Matthews, Dennis J.**

Meilaender, Gilbert. Begetting and cloning. *First Things.* 1997 Jun–Jul; No. 74: 41–43.

(CLONING)

Meilaender, Gilbert see Brown, Harold O.J.

Meiland, Franka J.M. see Varekamp, Inge

Meinert, Curtis L. IRBs and randomized clinical trials. *IRB: A Review of Human Subjects Research.* 1998 Mar–Jun; 20(2–3): 9–12.
(HUMAN EXPERIMENTATION/ETHICS COMMITTEES)

Meinhardt, Robyn; Landis, Kenneth W. Bioethics update: the changing nature of the doctor/patient relationship. *Whittier Law Review.* 1995; 16(1): 177–186.
(PROFESSIONAL PATIENT RELATIONSHIP)

Meisel, Alan. Legal aspects of end–of–life decision making. *In:* Steinberg, Maurice D.; Youngner, Stuart J., eds. End–of–Life Decisions: A Psychosocial Perspective. Washington, DC: American Psychiatric Press; 1998: 235–257.
(ALLOWING TO DIE/LEGAL ASPECTS)

Meisel, Alan; Jernigan, Jan C.; Youngner, Stuart J. Prosecutors and end–of–life decision making. *Archives of Internal Medicine.* 1999 May 24; 159(10): 1089–1095.
(ALLOWING TO DIE/ATTITUDES; SUICIDE; TERMINAL CARE)

Melbye, Mads see Westergaard, Tine

Meldrum, Marcia. "A calculated risk": the Salk polio vaccine field trials of 1954. *BMJ (British Medical Journal).* 1998 Oct 31; 317(7167): 1233–1236.
(HUMAN EXPERIMENTATION/RESEARCH DESIGN; IMMUNIZATION)

Melgaard, Bjorn see Lee, J.W.

Melgar, Thomas see Butler, Dennis J.

Melnick, Vijaya L. The brave new world of DNA: transcendence or transgression? *In:* Smith, Edward; Sapp, Walter, eds. Plain Talk about the Human Genome Project: A Tuskegee University Conference on Its Promise and Perils ... and Matters of Race. Tuskegee, AL: Tuskegee University Press; 1997: 197–200.
(GENETIC INTERVENTION; HEALTH)

Melo–Martín, Immaculada de. Making Babies: Biomedical Technologies, Reproductive Ethics, and Public Policy. Boston, MA: Kluwer Academic; 1998. 199 p.
(IN VITRO FERTILIZATION; REPRODUCTIVE TECHNOLOGIES)

Meltzer, Noah see DeRenzo, Evan G.

Mendelssohn, David C. see Shaul, Randi Zlotnik

Menendez, Roger; Zwelling–Aamot, Marcy L.; White, T. Michael; Blackwell, Barry; Shelman, Keith; Brody, Howard; Hall, Mark A.; Berenson, Robert A.; Crosson, Francis J.; Rubin, Herbert; Kassirer, Jerome P. A new ethic for medicine? [Letters and response]. *New England Journal of Medicine.* 1998 Oct 29; 339(18): 1326–1328.
(HEALTH CARE/ECONOMICS)

Menikoff, Jerry. Doubts about death: the silence of the Institute of Medicine. *Journal of Law, Medicine and Ethics.* 1998 Summer; 26(2): 157–165.
(DETERMINATION OF DEATH; ORGAN AND TISSUE DONATION)

Menken, Matthew see McQuillen, Michael P.

Mennicken, U. see Borowski, A.

Menon, Manoj see Hanson, Laura C.

Menzel, Paul; Gold, Marthe R.; Nord, Erik; Pinto–Prades, Jose–Louis; Richardson, Jeff; Ubel, Peter. Toward a broader view of values in cost–effectiveness analysis of health. *Hastings Center Report.* 1999 May–Jun; 29(3): 7–15.
(HEALTH CARE/ECONOMICS; RESOURCE ALLOCATION)

Menzel, Paul see Back, Anthony

Mepham, T.B.; Crilly, R.E. Transgenic xenotransplantation: utilitarian and deontological caveats. *In:* van Zutphen, L.F.M.; Balls, M., eds. Animal Alternatives, Welfare and Ethics. New York, NY: Elsevier; 1997: 355–360.
(ORGAN AND TISSUE TRANSPLANTATION)

Mepham, T. Ben; Combes, Robert D.; Balls, Michael; Barbieri, Ottavia; Blokhuis, Harry J.; Costa, Patrizia; Crilly, Robert E.; de Cock Buning, Tjard; Delpire, Véronique C.; O'Hare, Michael J.; Houdebine, Louis–Marie; van Kreijl, Coen F.; van der Meer, Miriam; Reinhardt, Christoph A.; Wolf, Eckhard; van Zeller, Anne–Marie. The Use of Transgenic Animals in the European Union: The Report and Recommendations of ECVAM [European Centre for the Validation of Alternative Methods] Workshop 28. *ATLA: Alternatives to Laboratory Animals.* 1998 Jan–Feb; 26(1): 21–43.
(ANIMAL EXPERIMENTATION; GENETIC INTERVENTION)

Merchant, Jennifer. Confronting the consequences of medical technology: policy frontiers in the United States and France. *In:* Githens, Marianne; Stetson, Dorothy McBride, eds. Abortion Politics: Public Policy in Cross–Cultural Perspective. New York, NY: Routledge; 1996: 189–209.
(EMBRYO AND FETAL RESEARCH; REPRODUCTIVE TECHNOLOGIES)

Merkatz, Irwin R. see Freda, Margaret Comerford

Merkatz, Ruth B. Inclusion of women in clinical trials: a historical overview of scientific, ethical, and legal issues. *Journal of Obstetric, Gynecologic and Neonatal Nursing.* 1998 Jan–Feb; 27(1): 78–84.
(HUMAN EXPERIMENTATION/SPECIAL POPULATIONS)

Merlino, Joseph P. The hospital ethics committee: a role for the contemporary psychoanalyst. *Journal of the American Academy of Psychoanalysis.* 1997 Summer; 25(2): 295–305.
(ALLOWING TO DIE; ETHICISTS AND ETHICS COMMITTEES)

Mermann, Alan C. see Dickinson, George E.

Merrill, Sonya. Genetic screening: suffering and sovereignty. *In:* Demy, Timothy J.; Stewart, Gary P., eds. Genetic Engineering: A Christian Response: Crucial Considerations in Shaping Life. Grand Rapids, MI: Kregel Publications; 1999: 304–313.
(BIOMEDICAL TECHNOLOGIES; GENETIC SCREENING)

Merrill, William W.; Beckett, William S.; Raymond, Lawrence W.; Kern, David G.; Crausman, Robert S.; Kuhn, Charles. Flock worker's lung. [Letters and response]. *Annals of Internal Medicine.* 1999 Apr 6; 130(7): 615–616.
(OCCUPATIONAL HEALTH)

Merskey, Harold. Ethical issues in the search for repressed memories. *American Journal of Psychotherapy.* 1996 Summer; 50(3): 323–335.
(PATIENT CARE/MENTALLY DISABLED)

Merson, Michael H.; Simonds, R.J.; Rogers, Martha F.; Dondero, Timothy J.; Francis, Donald P.; Mbidde, Edward K.; Blanche, Stéphane; Kim, Roy J.; Sharif, Shahnaaz K.; Tafesse, Eskinder; Murphy, Timothy F.; IJsselmuiden, Carel B.; Herrington, David; Piot, Peter; Glantz, Leonard H.; Grodin, Michael A.; Lallemant, Marc; McIntosh, Kenneth; Jourdin, Gonzague; Le Coeur, Sophie; Vithayasai, Vicharn; Lee, Tun-Hou; Hammer, Scott; Prescott, Nicholas; Essex, Max; Lurie, Peter; Wolfe, Sidney M. Ethics of placebo-controlled trials of zidovudine to prevent the perinatal transmission of HIV in the Third World. [Letters and response; editor's note]. *New England Journal of Medicine.* 1998 Mar 19; 338(12): 836–841.
(AIDS/HUMAN EXPERIMENTATION; HUMAN EXPERIMENTATION/FOREIGN COUNTRIES; HUMAN EXPERIMENTATION/RESEARCH DESIGN; HUMAN EXPERIMENTATION/SPECIAL POPULATIONS)

Merz, Jon F.; Cho, Mildred K. Disease genes are not patentable: a rebuttal of McGee. *Cambridge Quarterly of Healthcare Ethics.* 1998 Fall; 7(4): 425–428.
(GENOME MAPPING)

Merz, Jon F.; Leonard, Debra G.B.; Miller, Elizabeth R. IRB review and consent in human tissue research. *Science.* 1999 Mar 12; 283(5408): 1647–1648.
(GENETIC RESEARCH; HUMAN EXPERIMENTATION/ETHICS COMMITTEES; HUMAN EXPERIMENTATION/INFORMED CONSENT; ORGAN AND TISSUE DONATION)

Merz, Jon F.; Sankar, Pamela; Taube, Sheila E.; Livolsi, Virginia. Use of human tissues in research: clarifying clinician and researcher roles and information flows. *Journal of Investigative Medicine.* 1997 Jun; 45(5): 252–257.
(GENETIC RESEARCH; HUMAN EXPERIMENTATION/INFORMED CONSENT; ORGAN AND TISSUE DONATION)

Meslin, Eric M. see Alexandrov, Andrei V.

Mester, Roberto; Mozes, Tamar; Blumensohn, Rachel; Fluhr, Haya; Spivak, Baruch; Heguesh, Roni; Kalian, Moshe. The new Israeli psychiatric legislation for the minor (1995) and its relationship to the 1991 Law for the Treatment of the Mentally Ill. *International Journal of Law and Psychiatry.* 1998 Summer; 21(3): 281–289.
(PATIENT CARE/MENTALLY DISABLED; PATIENT CARE/MINORS)

Meyer, Charles. A Good Death: Challenges, Choices, and Care Options. Mystic, CT: Twenty-Third Publications; 1998. 57 p.
(TERMINAL CARE)

Meyer, G. Rex, ed. Bioethics in Education. Münster, Germany: Lit; 1991. 190 p.
(BIOETHICS/EDUCATION)

Meyer, Roberta B. Justification for permitting life insurers to continue to underwrite on the basis of genetic information and genetic test results. *Suffolk University Law Review.* 1993 Winter; 27(4): 1271–1305.
(GENETIC SCREENING)

Meyer, Roberta B. see Pokorski, Robert J.

Meyers, Alan F. see Geltman, Paul L.

Mezey, Mathy; Mitty, Ethel; Ramsey, Gloria. Assessment of decision-making capacity: nursing's role. *Journal of Gerontological Nursing.* 1997 Mar; 23(3): 28–35.
(INFORMED CONSENT)

Mezey, Mathy; Ramsey, Gloria C.; Mitty, Ethel. Making the PSDA work for the elderly. *Generations (American Society on Aging).* 1994 Winter; 18(4): 13–18.
(ADVANCE DIRECTIVES)

Micco, Guy P. see Wu, Albert W.

Micetich, Kenneth C. see Thomasma, David C.

Michael, Adam. Europe/Japan face up to legal hurdles to cloning. [News]. *Nature Biotechnology.* 1997 Jul; 15(7): 609–610.
(CLONING)

Michaels, Meredith W. Other mothers: toward an ethic of postmaternal practice. *Hypatia.* 1996 Spring; 11(2): 49–70.
(REPRODUCTIVE TECHNOLOGIES; SURROGATE MOTHERS)

Michalowski, Sabine. Medical confidentiality and medical privilege -- a comparison of French and German law. *European Journal of Health Law.* 1998 Jun; 5(2): 89–116.
(CONFIDENTIALITY/LEGAL ASPECTS)

Michel, Lee. Consent: Ohio appellate court affirms confidentiality claim. *Journal of Law, Medicine and Ethics.* 1998 Winter; 26(4): 355–356.
(CONFIDENTIALITY/LEGAL ASPECTS)

Michel, Vicki. Factoring ethnic and racial differences into bioethics decision making. *Generations (American Society on Aging).* 1994 Winter; 18(4): 23–26.
(PROFESSIONAL PATIENT RELATIONSHIP; TRUTH DISCLOSURE)

Michels, Robert. Are research ethics bad for our mental health? *New England Journal of Medicine.* 1999 May 6; 340(18): 1427–1430.
(HUMAN EXPERIMENTATION/REGULATION; HUMAN EXPERIMENTATION/SPECIAL POPULATIONS)

Michie, Helena; Cahn, Naomi R. Confinements: Fertility and Infertility in Contemporary Culture. New Brunswick, NJ: Rutgers University Press; 1997. 187 p.
(REPRODUCTION; REPRODUCTIVE TECHNOLOGIES)

Michie, Susan see Clarke, Angus

Michigan Catholic Conference. Living and dying according to the voice of faith. *Origins.* 1997 Oct 23; 27(19): 317, 319–322.
(SUICIDE; TERMINAL CARE)

Middleton, A.; Hewison, J.; Mueller, R.F. A pilot study of attitudes of deaf and hearing parents towards issues surrounding genetic testing for deafness. [Abstract]. *American Journal of Human Genetics.* 1997 Oct; 61(4): A190.
(ABORTION/ATTITUDES; GENETIC SCREENING; PRENATAL DIAGNOSIS)

Midwest Bioethics Center. Kansas City Area Ethics Committee Consortium. Considerations regarding withholding/withdrawing life-sustaining treatment. *Bioethics Forum.* 1998 Summer; 14(2): SS1–SS8.
(ALLOWING TO DIE)

Midwest Bioethics Center. Kansas City Area Ethics Committee Consortium. Honoring do-not-resuscitate (DNR) orders during invasive procedures. *Bioethics Forum.* 1998 Spring; 14(1): 23–26.
(RESUSCITATION ORDERS)

Mieth, Dietmar. Reflections on genetic testing in childhood. *In:* Clarke, Angus, ed. The Genetic Testing of Children. Washington, DC: BIOS Scientific Publishers; 1998: 37–45.
(GENETIC SCREENING)

Mieth, Dietmar see Hildt, Elisabeth

Mika, Karin; Hurst, Bonnie. One way to be born? Legislative inaction and the posthumous child. *Marquette Law Review.* 1996 Summer; 79(4): 993–1019.
(REPRODUCTION; REPRODUCTIVE TECHNOLOGIES)

Miles, Al see Awong, Linda

Miles, Jeremy see van der Valk, Jan

Miles, Stephen H. see Koepp, Robert

Miles, Steven. Death in a technological and pluralistic culture. *In:* Youngner, Stuart J.; Arnold, Robert M.; Schapiro, Renie, eds. The Definition of Death: Contemporary Controversies. Baltimore, MD: Johns Hopkins University Press; 1999: 311–318.
(DETERMINATION OF DEATH)

Miles, Steven. Managed care issues in genetic testing for Alzheimer disease. *In:* Post, Stephen G.; Whitehouse, Peter J., eds. Genetic Testing for Alzheimer Disease: Ethical and Clinical Issues. Baltimore, MD: Johns Hopkins University Press; 1998: 209–221.
(GENETIC SCREENING; HEALTH CARE/ECONOMICS)

Miles, Steven H. A challenge to licensing boards: the stigma of mental illness. *JAMA.* 1998 Sep 9; 280(10): 865.
(CONFIDENTIALITY/MENTAL HEALTH)

Miles, Steven H. Restraints: controlling a symptom or a symptom of control. *HEC (HealthCare Ethics Committee) Forum.* 1998 Sep–Dec; 10(3–4): 235–243.
(BEHAVIOR CONTROL; PATIENT CARE/AGED)

Milford, Edgar L. Organ transplantation -- barriers, outcomes, and evolving policies. [Editorial]. *JAMA.* 1998 Oct 7; 280(13): 1184–1185.
(ORGAN AND TISSUE TRANSPLANTATION; RESOURCE ALLOCATION/BIOMEDICAL TECHNOLOGIES; SELECTION FOR TREATMENT)

Millard, Dietra D. Toxicology testing in neonates: is it ethical, and what does it mean? *Clinics in Perinatology.*

1996 Sep; 23(3): 491–507.
(MASS SCREENING; PRENATAL INJURIES)

Miller, Bradley W. A time to kill: Ronald Dworkin and the ethics of euthanasia. *Res Publica.* 1996; 2(1): 31–61.
(EUTHANASIA; SUICIDE)

Miller, Deborah J. see O'Rourke, Kevin

Miller, Douglas P. see Stead, William W.

Miller, Elizabeth R. see Merz, Jon F.

Miller, Franklin G.; Rosenstein, Donald L. Protocol review within the context of a research program. *IRB: A Review of Human Subjects Research.* 1998 Jul–Aug; 20(4): 7–10.
(HUMAN EXPERIMENTATION/ETHICS COMMITTEES; HUMAN EXPERIMENTATION/RESEARCH DESIGN)

Miller, Franklin G.; Rosenstein, Donald L.; DeRenzo, Evan G. Professional integrity in clinical research. *JAMA.* 1998 Oct 28; 280(16): 1449–1454.
(HUMAN EXPERIMENTATION; PROFESSIONAL PATIENT RELATIONSHIP)

Miller, Franklin G. see Brody, Howard

Miller, Franklin G. see Fins, Joseph J.

Miller, Franklin G. see Stead, William W.

Miller, Henry see Barton, John

Miller, Henry I. Policy Controversy in Biotechnology: An Insider's View. Austin, TX: R.G. Landes; 1997. 221 p.
(GENETIC INTERVENTION; RECOMBINANT DNA RESEARCH/REGULATION)

Miller, Judith see Blumenthal, Ralph

Miller, Linda J.; Bloom, Floyd E. Publishing controversial research. [Editorial]. *Science.* 1998 Nov 6; 282(5391): 1045.
(BIOMEDICAL RESEARCH; EMBRYO AND FETAL RESEARCH)

Miller, Michelle D. The informed-consent policy of the International Conference on Harmonization of Technical Requirements for Registration of Pharmaceuticals for Human Use: knowledge is the best medicine. [Note]. *Cornell International Law Journal.* 1997; 30(1): 203–244.
(HUMAN EXPERIMENTATION/INFORMED CONSENT; HUMAN EXPERIMENTATION/REGULATION)

Miller, Norman M. see Graham, Peter E.

Miller, Robert D. The continuum of coercion: constitutional and clinical considerations in the treatment of mentally disordered persons. *Denver University Law Review.* 1997; 74(4): 1169–1214.
(PATIENT CARE/MENTALLY DISABLED)

Miller, Saul see Limentani, Alexander E.

Miller, Tracy E. Center stage on the patient protection agenda: grievance and appeal rights. *Journal of Law, Medicine and Ethics.* 1998 Summer; 26(2): 89–99.
(HEALTH CARE/ECONOMICS; PATIENTS' RIGHTS)

Miller, Tracy E.; Sage, William M. Disclosing physician financial incentives. *JAMA*. 1999 Apr 21; 281(15): 1424–1430.
(HEALTH CARE/ECONOMICS)

Milunsky, Aubrey. The "new" genetics: from research to reality. *Suffolk University Law Review*. 1993 Winter; 27(4): 1307–1325.
(GENETIC INTERVENTION; GENETIC SCREENING)

Milunsky, Aubrey see **Handelin, Barbara**

Minkoff, Howard see **Balano, Kirsten**

Minnesota Medical Association. Use and care of animals in research and teaching: MMA policy statement. *Minnesota Medicine*. 1997 Sep; 80(9): 28.
(ANIMAL EXPERIMENTATION)

Minnesota. Supreme Court. Women of the State of Minnesota v. Gomez. *North Western Reporter, 2d Series*. 1995 Dec 15 (date of decision). 542: 17–42.
(ABORTION/FINANCIAL SUPPORT; ABORTION/LEGAL ASPECTS)

Mirsky, Judith; Radlett, Marty, eds.; Panos Institute. Private Decisions, Public Debate: Women, Reproduction and Population. London: Panos Publications; 1994. 185 p.
(CONTRACEPTION; HEALTH)

Mishima, Shuuichi see **Kitamura, Fusako**

Mishkin, Douglas B. Proffering bioethicists as experts. *Judges' Journal*. 1997 Summer; 36(3): 50–51, 88–89.
(ETHICISTS AND ETHICS COMMITTEES)

Mitchell, C. Ben. Patenting life: an Evangelical response. *In:* Demy, Timothy J.; Stewart, Gary P., eds. Genetic Engineering: A Christian Response: Crucial Considerations in Shaping Life. Grand Rapids, MI: Kregel Publications; 1999: 88–102.
(PATENTING LIFE FORMS)

Mitchell, John J. Administering mercy: the ethics of pain management. *Cancer Investigation*. 1994; 12(3): 343–349.
(TERMINAL CARE)

Mitchell, John J. see **Hutcheon, R. Gordon**

Mitchell, Peter. Alleged unlicensed gene–therapy trial comes to light. [News]. *Lancet*. 1999 Jul 17; 354(9174): 225.
(GENE THERAPY; HUMAN EXPERIMENTATION/FOREIGN COUNTRIES)

Mitchell, Peter. Human xenotransplantation trials may be licensed in the UK. [News]. *Lancet*. 1998 Aug 8; 352(9126): 464.
(HUMAN EXPERIMENTATION/FOREIGN COUNTRIES; HUMAN EXPERIMENTATION/REGULATION; ORGAN AND TISSUE TRANSPLANTATION)

Mitka, Mike. Do-it-yourself report on patient privacy. [News]. *JAMA*. 1998 Dec 9; 280(22): 1897.
(CONFIDENTIALITY; HEALTH CARE/ECONOMICS)

Mittman, Ilana Suez; Secundy, Marion Gray. A national dialogue on genetics and minority issues. *Community Genetics*. 1998; 1(3): 190–200.
(GENETIC RESEARCH; GENETIC SERVICES)

Mitty, Ethel see **Mezey, Mathy**

Mlinek, Edward J.; Pierce, Jessica. Confidentiality and privacy breaches in a university hospital emergency department. *Academic Emergency Medicine*. 1997 Dec; 4(12): 1142–1146.
(CONFIDENTIALITY)

Mlot, C. Panel backs widening net of genetic test. [News]. *Science News*. 1997 Apr 26; 151(17): 253.
(GENETIC SCREENING)

Mobeireek, Abdullah. The do-not-resuscitate order: indications on the current practice in Riyadh. *Annals of Saudi Medicine*. 1995 Jan; 15(1): 6–9.
(RESUSCITATION ORDERS)

Moczynski, Nancy P. see **Holzer, Jacob C.**

Mohler, R. Albert see **Brown, Harold O.J.**

Möhr–Baumann, E. see **Müller, H.J.**

Mohr, M.; Kettler, D. Ethical aspects of prehospital CPR. *Acta Anaesthesiologica Scandinavica*. 1997; 41(Suppl. 111): 298–300.
(RESUSCITATION ORDERS)

Mokalla, Mani see **Lantos, John D.**

Mokalla, Mani see **Meadow, William**

Mold, James W.; Looney, Stephen W.; Viviani, Nancy J.; Quiggins, Patricia A. Predicting the health–related values and preferences of geriatric patients. *Journal of Family Practice*. 1994 Nov; 39(5): 461–467.
(ADVANCE DIRECTIVES; PATIENT CARE/AGED)

Moldow, D. Gay. VHA ethics rounds: [refusal to eat]. *NCCE News (Veterans Health Administration National Center for Clinical Ethics)*. 1994 Fall; 2(4): 4–5.
(TREATMENT REFUSAL/MENTALLY DISABLED)

Moldow, D. Gay see **Carlsen, Mary S.**

Molinari, Victor see **Workman, Richard H.**

Molnar, Beth E. Juveniles and psychiatric institutionalization: toward better due process and treatment review in the United States. *Health and Human Rights*. 1997; 2(2): 99–116.
(BEHAVIOR CONTROL; INVOLUNTARY COMMITMENT/MINORS)

Monafo, William see **Phipps, Etienne**

Monahan, Emmy S. An analysis of the mandatory notification procedure pertaining to termination of life in the Netherlands and recent developments. *Saint Louis University Public Law Review*. 1996; 15(2): 411–422.
(EUTHANASIA/LEGAL ASPECTS; SUICIDE)

Mondragon, Delfi see **Krainacker, David A.**

Montenegro, Hugo D. see **Daly, Barbara J.**

Montgomery, Jonathan. Confidentiality in the modernised NHS: the challenge of data protection. *Bulletin of Medical Ethics*. 1999 Mar; No. 146: 18–21.
(CONFIDENTIALITY/LEGAL ASPECTS)

Mook, Bertha see Bergsma, Jurrit

Mooney, Gavin; Jan, Stephen. Vertical equity: weighing outcomes? or establishing procedures? *Health Policy.* 1997 Jan; 39(1): 79–87.
(HEALTH CARE; RESOURCE ALLOCATION)

Moore, Andrew see Peart, Nicola

Moore, Andrew see Wilkinson, Martin

Moore, Brad see Rosenbaum, Sara

Moore, Donna E. see Brown, Janet

Moore, Kirsten; Randolph, Kate; Toubia, Nahid; Kirberger, Elizabeth. The synergistic relationship between health and human rights: a case study using female genital mutilation. *Health and Human Rights.* 1997; 2(2): 137–146.
(HEALTH)

Moore, Lorna Grindlay see West, Charles

Moore, Michael L. see MacKay, Charles

Moore, Michael R. see Kosseff, Andrew L.

Moore, R. Andrew see Tramèr, Martin R.

Mor, Vincent see Teno, Joan M.

Mor-Yosef, Shlomo. Cost effectiveness of *in vitro* fertilization. *Journal of Assisted Reproduction and Genetics.* 1995 Sep; 12(8): 524–530.
(IN VITRO FERTILIZATION)

Mora-Corrasco, Fernando see Egilman, David

Morabia, Alfredo see Dolian, Gayane

Moraczewski, Albert S. Cloning testimony. *Ethics and Medics.* 1997 May; 22(5): 3–4.
(CLONING)

Mordini, Emilio. Mandatory hospitalisation in mental health. *Bulletin of Medical Ethics.* 1997 Nov; No. 133: 18–21.
(INVOLUNTARY COMMITMENT)

Moreno, Jonathan; Caplan, Arthur L.; Wolpe, Paul Root; Project on Informed Consent, Human Research Ethics Group (University of Pennsylvania Health System, Center for Bioethics). Updating protections for human subjects involved in research. *JAMA.* 1998 Dec 9; 280(22): 1951–1958.
(HUMAN EXPERIMENTATION/REGULATION)

Moreno, Jonathan D. Bioethics is a naturalism. *In:* McGee, Glenn, ed. Pragmatic Bioethics. Nashville, TN: Vanderbilt University Press; 1999: 5–17, 257–258.
(BIOETHICS)

Moreno, Jonathan D. Ethics committees and ethics consultants. *In:* Kuhse, Helga; Singer, Peter, eds. A Companion to Bioethics. Malden, MA: Blackwell; 1998: 475–484.
(ETHICISTS AND ETHICS COMMITTEES)

Moreno, Jonathan D. IRBs under the microscope.

Kennedy Institute of Ethics Journal. 1998 Sep; 8(3): 329–337.
(HUMAN EXPERIMENTATION/ETHICS COMMITTEES; HUMAN EXPERIMENTATION/REGULATION)

Morgan, Frank. Babe the magnificent organ donor? The perils and promises surrounding xenotransplantation. [Comment]. *Journal of Contemporary Health Law and Policy.* 1997 Fall; 14(1): 127–160.
(HUMAN EXPERIMENTATION/REGULATION; ORGAN AND TISSUE TRANSPLANTATION)

Morgan, G.L. Is there a right to fetal tissue transplantation? *University of Tasmania Law Review.* 1991; 10(2): 129–156.
(FETUSES; HUMAN EXPERIMENTATION; ORGAN AND TISSUE TRANSPLANTATION)

Morgan, John, ed. An Easeful Death? Perspectives on Death, Dying and Euthanasia. Sydney, NSW, Australia: Federation Press; 1996. 218 p.
(EUTHANASIA; TERMINAL CARE)

Morgan, Lynn M. Fetal relationality in feminist philosophy: an anthropological critique. *Hypatia.* 1996 Summer; 11(3): 47–70.
(FETUSES; PERSONHOOD)

Morgenweck, Cynthiane J. see Kane, Richard S.

Mori, Maurizio. On the concept of pre-embryo: the basis for a new "Copernican revolution" in the current view about human reproduction. *In:* Harris, John; Holm, Søren, eds. The Future of Human Reproduction: Ethics, Choice, and Regulation. New York, NY: Oxford University Press; 1998: 38–54.
(FETUSES; PERSONHOOD)

Morin, Karine. The standard of disclosure in human subject experimentation. *Journal of Legal Medicine.* 1998 Jun; 19(2): 157–221.
(HUMAN EXPERIMENTATION/INFORMED CONSENT)

Morishita, Mayumi see Hamajima, Nobuyuki

Morita, Shigeho see Nakata, Yoshinori

Moritaka, Shigeko see Hamajima, Nobuyuki

Morlock, Laura L. see Weisman, Carol S.

Morray, Barbara H. The lottery of life: should organ transplants be used to even the odds? *Dimensions of Critical Care Nursing.* 1995 Sep–Oct; 14(5): 266–272.
(ORGAN AND TISSUE TRANSPLANTATION; SELECTION FOR TREATMENT)

Morreim, E. Haavi. Bioethics and the press. *Journal of Medicine and Philosophy.* 1999 Apr; 24(2): 103–107.
(BIOETHICS)

Morreim, E. Haavi. Managed care, ethics, and academic health centers: maximizing potential, minimizing drawbacks. *Academic Medicine.* 1997 May; 72(5): 332–340.
(HEALTH CARE/ECONOMICS)

Morreim, E. Haavi. To tell the truth: disclosing the incentives and limits of managed care. *American Journal Of Managed Care.* 1997 Jan; 3(1): 35–43.
(HEALTH CARE/ECONOMICS)

Morris, Alan see Truog, Robert D.

Morris, David B. Illness and Culture in the Postmodern Age. Berkeley, CA: University of California Press; 1998. 345 p.
(HEALTH)

Morris, John see **Teno, Joan M.**

Morris, Kelly. US military face punishment for refusing anthrax vaccine. [News]. *Lancet.* 1999 Jan 9; 353(9147): 130.
(IMMUNIZATION; WAR)

Morris, Kelly see **Watts, Jonathan**

Morris, Lynn; Martin, Desmond J.; Quinn, Thomas C.; Chaisson, Richard E. The importance of doing HIV research in developing countries. *Nature Medicine.* 1998 Nov; 4(11): 1228–1229.
(AIDS/HUMAN EXPERIMENTATION; BIOMEDICAL RESEARCH; HUMAN EXPERIMENTATION/FOREIGN COUNTRIES; RESOURCE ALLOCATION)

Morris, Monica B. see **Neuhaus, Richard John**

Morrison, Catherine J. see **Clouser, K. Danner**

Morrison, Mary F. Obstacles to doctor–patient communication at the end of life. *In:* Steinberg, Maurice D.; Youngner, Stuart J., eds. End–of–Life Decisions: A Psychosocial Perspective. Washington, DC: American Psychiatric Press; 1998: 109–136.
(ALLOWING TO DIE; PROFESSIONAL PATIENT RELATIONSHIP; TERMINAL CARE)

Morrison, P.J. Implications of genetic testing for insurance in the UK. *Lancet.* 1998 Nov 21; 352(9141): 1647–1648.
(GENETIC SCREENING)

Morrison, R. Sean; Meier, Diane E. Physician–assisted dying: fashioning public policy with an absence of data. *Generations (American Society on Aging).* 1994 Winter; 18(4): 48–53.
(EUTHANASIA; SUICIDE)

Morrison, R. Sean; Zayas, Luis H.; Mulvihill, Michael; Baskin, Shari A.; Meier, Diane E. Barriers to completion of health care proxies: an examination of ethnic differences. *Archives of Internal Medicine.* 1998 Dec 7–21; 158(22): 2493–2497.
(ADVANCE DIRECTIVES)

Morrison, R. Sean see **Preston, Thomas A.**

Morton, Newton E. Hippocratic or hypocritic: birth pangs of an ethical code. [Letter]. *Nature Genetics.* 1998 Jan; 18(1): 18.
(EUGENICS)

Moseley, Charles B. The impact of restraints on nursing home resident outcomes. *American Journal of Medical Quality.* 1997 Summer; 12(2): 94–102.
(PATIENT CARE/AGED)

Moser, H. see **Müller, H.J.**

Moses, Hamilton. Managing managed care. *Clinical Performance and Quality Health Care.* 1996 Oct–Dec; 4(4): 200–202.
(HEALTH CARE/ECONOMICS)

Mosier, Alicia see **Brown, Harold O.J.**

Moskowitz, Ellen H. see **Henderson, Shelley**

Moss, Alvin H. The application of the Task Force report in rural and frontier settings. *Journal of Clinical Ethics.* 1999 Spring; 10(1): 42–48.
(ETHICISTS AND ETHICS COMMITTEES)

Moss, Alvin H. see **Hines, Stephen C.**

Moss, Alvin H. see **MacKay, Karen**

Moss, Alvin H. see **McKenzie, John K.**

Moss, Sue; Cuckle, Howard. Trial of mammography in women under 50 is ethical. [Letter]. *BMJ (British Medical Journal).* 1998 Dec 5; 317(7172): 1589–1590.
(HUMAN EXPERIMENTATION/FOREIGN COUNTRIES; HUMAN EXPERIMENTATION/INFORMED CONSENT; MASS SCREENING)

Motluk, Alison. Insurers fight shy of gene tests. [News]. *New Scientist.* 1997 Feb 22; 153(2070): 7.
(GENETIC SCREENING)

Motluk, Alison. Young people question vivisection. [News]. *New Scientist.* 1998 Jun 6; 158(2137): 23.
(ANIMAL EXPERIMENTATION)

Moustarah, Fady. Organ procurement: let's presume consent. *Canadian Medical Association Journal.* 1998 Jan 27; 158(2): 231–234.
(ORGAN AND TISSUE DONATION)

Moyers, Peter. A Rawlsian case for physician–assisted suicide. *Princeton Journal of Bioethics.* 1998 Spring; 1(1): 23–31.
(SUICIDE)

Mozes, Tamar see **Mester, Roberto**

Msamanga, Gernard see **Desvarieux, Moïse**

Mudge, C. see **Weiss, A.H.**

Mudur, Ganapati. Indian Supreme Court rules that HIV positive people inform spouses. [News]. *BMJ (British Medical Journal).* 1998 Nov 28; 317(7171): 1474.
(AIDS/CONFIDENTIALITY)

Mudur, Ganapati. Indian surgeon challenges ban on xenotransplantation. [News]. *BMJ (British Medical Journal).* 1999 Jan 9; 318(7176): 79.
(ORGAN AND TISSUE TRANSPLANTATION)

Mudur, Ganapati. Indian women's groups question contraceptive vaccine research. [News]. *BMJ (British Medical Journal).* 1998 Nov 14; 317(7169): 1340.
(CONTRACEPTION; HUMAN EXPERIMENTATION/FOREIGN COUNTRIES; HUMAN EXPERIMENTATION/SPECIAL POPULATIONS)

Mueller, Mary–Rose. Science versus care: physicians, nurses, and the dilemma of clinical research. *In:* Elston, Mary Ann, ed. The Sociology of Medical Science and Technology. Malden, MA: Blackwell; 1997: 57–78.
(AIDS/HUMAN EXPERIMENTATION)

Mueller, R.F. see **Middleton, A.**

Mugerwa, Roy D. see **Desvarieux, Moïse**

Mulkay, Michael. Galileo and the embryos: religion and science in parliamentary debate over research on human embryos. *Social Studies of Science.* 1995 Aug; 25(3): 499–532.
(EMBRYO AND FETAL RESEARCH)

Mullens, Anne. 7:10 am, Nov. 8, 1994. *Canadian Medical Association Journal.* 1998 Feb 24; 158(4): 528–531.
(ABORTION)

Müller, H.J.; Deonna, Th.; Abbt, I.; Bachmann, C.; Bär, W.; Brückner, Ch.; Bühler, E.; Courvoisier, B.; Dayer, P.; Fuchs, E.; Gelzer, J.; Guillod, O.; Gutzwiller, F.; Heierli, C.; Hitzig, W.; Moser, H.; Möhr-Baumann, E.; Pescia, G.; Sitter-Liver, B.; Thévoz, J.M.; Waldboth, Y.; Weber, W.; Wicki, S. Medical-ethical guidelines for genetic investigations in humans. *Schweizerische Medizinische Wochenschrift.* 1994 Jun 4; 124(22): 974–979.
(GENETIC COUNSELING; GENETIC SCREENING; PRENATAL DIAGNOSIS)

Muller, Martien T. see **Onwuteaka-Philipsen, Bregje D.**

Mulley, G.P. see **Turner, N.J.**

Mulvihill, Michael see **Morrison, R. Sean**

Mulvihill, Michael see **Zelenik, Jomarie**

Muncie, Herbert L.; Magaziner, Jay; Hebel, J. Richard; Warren, John W. Proxies' decisions about clinical research participation for their charges. *Journal of the American Geriatrics Society.* 1997 Aug; 45(8): 929–933.
(HUMAN EXPERIMENTATION/INFORMED CONSENT; HUMAN EXPERIMENTATION/SPECIAL POPULATIONS)

Muncie, Herbert L. see **Lynn, Joanne**

Munn, Rita K. see **Andrykowski, Michael A.**

Munoz, Rodrigo see **Rosenheck, Robert**

Munro, Lyle. From vilification to accommodation: making a common cause movement. *Cambridge Quarterly of Healthcare Ethics.* 1999 Winter; 8(1): 46–57.
(ANIMAL EXPERIMENTATION)

Muramoto, Osamu. Bioethics of the refusal of blood by Jehovah's Witnesses: Part 1. Should bioethical deliberation consider dissidents' views? *Journal of Medical Ethics.* 1998 Aug; 24(4): 223–230.
(TREATMENT REFUSAL)

Muramoto, Osamu. Bioethics of the refusal of blood by Jehovah's Witnesses: Part 2. A novel approach based on rational non-interventional paternalism. *Journal of Medical Ethics.* 1998 Oct; 24(5): 295–301.
(TREATMENT REFUSAL)

Muramoto, Osamu. Jehovah's Witnesses and blood transfusions. [Letter]. *Lancet.* 1998 Sep 5; 352(9130): 824.
(TREATMENT REFUSAL)

Muraskas, Jonathan; Marshall, Patricia A.; Tomich, Paul; Myers, Thomas F.; Gianopoulos, John G.;

Thomasma, David C. Neonatal viability in the 1990s: held hostage by technology. *Cambridge Quarterly of Healthcare Ethics.* 1999 Spring; 8(2): 160–172.
(ALLOWING TO DIE/INFANTS; BIOMEDICAL TECHNOLOGIES; SELECTION FOR TREATMENT)

Murphy, Donald; Buchanan, Susan Fox. Community guidelines for end-of-life care: incremental change or significant reform? *Bioethics Forum.* 1998 Summer; 14(2): 19–24.
(ALLOWING TO DIE; TERMINAL CARE)

Murphy, Donald J.; Barbour, Elizabeth. GUIDe (Guidelines for the Use of Intensive Care in Denver): a community effort to define futile and inappropriate care. *New Horizons.* 1994 Aug; 2(3): 326–331.
(ALLOWING TO DIE; SELECTION FOR TREATMENT)

Murphy, Edmond A.; Butzow, James J.; Suarez-Murias, Edward L. Underpinnings of Medical Ethics. Baltimore, MD: Johns Hopkins University Press; 1997. 480 p.
(MEDICAL ETHICS)

Murphy, Julien S. Should lesbians count as infertile couples? Antilesbian discrimination in assisted reproduction. *In:* Donchin, Anne; Purdy, Laura M., eds. Embodying Bioethics: Recent Feminist Advances. Lanham, MD: Rowman and Littlefield; 1999: 103–120.
(ARTIFICIAL INSEMINATION; SELECTION FOR TREATMENT)

Murphy, Michael J.; DeBernardo, Caren R.; Shoemaker, Wendy E. Impact of managed care on independent practice and professional ethics: a survey of independent practitioners. *Professional Psychology: Research and Practice.* 1998 Feb; 29(1): 43–51.
(HEALTH CARE/ECONOMICS; PATIENT CARE/MENTALLY DISABLED)

Murphy, Patricia D. see **MacKay, Charles**

Murphy, Sheigla; Rosenbaum, Marsha. Pregnant Women on Drugs: Combating Stereotypes and Stigma. New Brunswick, NJ: Rutgers University Press; 1999. 204 p.
(PRENATAL INJURIES)

Murphy, Timothy F. Entitlement to cloning: response to "Cloning and infertilty" by Carson Strong (*CQ*, 1998 Summer; 7(3): 279–293). *Cambridge Quarterly of Healthcare Ethics.* 1999 Summer; 8(3): 364–368.
(CLONING; SELECTION FOR TREATMENT)

Murphy, Timothy F. Mapping the human genome. *In:* Kuhse, Helga; Singer, Peter, eds. A Companion to Bioethics. Malden, MA: Blackwell; 1998: 198–205.
(GENOME MAPPING)

Murphy, Timothy F. see **Merson, Michael H.**

Murray, Jeffrey C. see **Cutter, Mary Ann G.**

Murray, Joseph E. see **Bleich, J. David**

Murray, Robert. The ethics of predictive genetic screening: are the benefits worth the risks? *In:* Smith, Edward; Sapp, Walter, eds. Plain Talk about the Human Genome Project: A Tuskegee University Conference on Its Promise and Perils ... and Matters of Race. Tuskegee, AL: Tuskegee University Press; 1997:

139–150.
(GENETIC SCREENING)

Murray, Thomas. Genetic discrimination in health insurance and why it is wrong. *In:* Smith, Edward; Sapp, Walter, eds. Plain Talk about the Human Genome Project: A Tuskegee University Conference on Its Promise and Perils ... and Matters of Race. Tuskegee, AL: Tuskegee University Press; 1997: 159–168.
(GENETIC SCREENING)

Murray, Thomas see **Kodish, Eric**

Murray, Thomas H. Money-back guarantees for IVF: an ethical critique. *Journal of Law, Medicine and Ethics.* 1997 Winter; 25(4): 292–294.
(IN VITRO FERTILIZATION)

Murray, Thomas H. What do we mean by "narrative ethics"? *Medical Humanities Review.* 1997 Fall; 11(2): 44–57.
(BIOETHICS)

Murray, Thomas H. see **Binstock, Robert H.**

Murray, Thomas H. see **Klugman, Craig M.**

Murri, Rita see **Albert, Steven M.**

Muscari, Mary E. Rebels with a cause: when adolescents won't follow medical advice. *American Journal of Nursing.* 1998 Dec; 98(12): 26–31.
(PATIENT CARE/MINORS)

Mwinga, Alwyn see **Edi-Osagie, E.C.O.**

Myers, Ronald E. see **Lerman, Caryn**

Myers, Steven Lee. Airman discharged for refusal to take anthrax vaccine as rebellion grows. [News]. *New York Times.* 1999 Mar 11: A24.
(IMMUNIZATION; WAR)

Myers, Thomas F. see **Muraskas, Jonathan**

Myser, Catherine. How bioethics is being taught: a critical review. *In:* Kuhse, Helga; Singer, Peter, eds. A Companion to Bioethics. Malden, MA: Blackwell; 1998: 484–500.
(BIOETHICS/EDUCATION)

N

Nab, Jan see **van der Valk, Jan**

Nachmias, Solomon see **Jaworowski, Solomon**

Nachtigall, Robert D.; Tschann, Jeanne M.; Quiroga, Seline Szkupinski; Pitcher, Linda; Becker, Gay. Stigma, disclosure, and family functioning among parents of children conceived through donor insemination. *Fertility and Sterility.* 1997 Jul; 68(1): 83–89.
(ARTIFICIAL INSEMINATION)

Nadelson, Carol C. Ethics and empathy in a changing health care system. *Pharos.* 1996 Fall; 59(4): 29–32.
(HEALTH CARE/ECONOMICS; PROFESSIONAL PATIENT RELATIONSHIP)

Nader, Claire; Newman, Stuart A. Human cloning. [Letter]. *Science.* 1998 Dec 4; 282(5395): 1824–1825.

(CLONING)

Nadis, Steve. US concern grows over secrecy clauses. [News]. *Nature.* 1999 Apr 1; 398(6726): 359.
(BIOMEDICAL RESEARCH)

Naessens, Katrien. Egg donor, or seller? *Christian Science Monitor.* 1999 Apr 9: 11.
(REPRODUCTIVE TECHNOLOGIES)

Nagel, Denise see **Roberts, John**

Nagy, Anne-Marie; De Man, Xavier; Ruibal, Nike; Lints, Frédéric A. Scientific and ethical issues of preimplantation diagnosis. [Editorial]. *Annals of Medicine.* 1998 Feb; 30(1): 1–6.
(GENETIC SCREENING; PRENATAL DIAGNOSIS)

Nairn, Thomas A. Reclaiming our moral tradition: Catholic teaching calls us to accept the limits of medical technology. *Health Progress.* 1997 Nov–Dec; 78(6): 36–39, 42.
(ALLOWING TO DIE/RELIGIOUS ASPECTS)

Nakashima, Allyn K.; Horsley, Rosemarie; Frey, Robert L.; Sweeney, Patricia A.; Weber, J. Todd; Fleming, Patricia L. Effect of HIV reporting by name on use of HIV testing in publicly funded counseling and testing programs. *JAMA.* 1998 Oct 28; 280(16): 1421–1426.
(AIDS/CONFIDENTIALITY; AIDS/TESTING AND SCREENING)

Nakata, Yoshinori; Goto, Takahisa; Morita, Shigeho. Serving the emperor without asking: critical care ethics in Japan. *Journal of Medicine and Philosophy.* 1998 Dec; 23(6): 601–615.
(ALLOWING TO DIE; HEALTH CARE/FOREIGN COUNTRIES)

Nakazato, Paul Z. Controversial aspects of the current liver donor allocation system for liver transplantation. *Academic Radiology.* 1995 Mar; 2(3): 244–248.
(ORGAN AND TISSUE TRANSPLANTATION; RESOURCE ALLOCATION/BIOMEDICAL TECHNOLOGIES)

Nakchbandi, Inaam A. see **Wong, Jeffrey G.**

Nardi, Jason see **van der Valk, Jan**

Nasar, Sylvia. Princeton's new philosopher draws a stir. [News]. *New York Times.* 1999 Apr 10: 1, B11.
(ETHICISTS AND ETHICS COMMITTEES)

Nash, J. Madeleine. Cloning's Kevorkian. [News]. *Time.* 1998 Jan 19; 151(2): 58.
(CLONING)

Nash, J. Madeleine. The case for cloning. [News]. *Time.* 1998 Feb 9; 151(5): 81.
(CLONING)

Nash, Jean E. see **Schrock, Charles R.**

Nasto, Barbara. Xenotransplantation: proceed with caution. [News]. *Nature Biotechnology.* 1996 Apr; 14(4): 424, 426.
(ORGAN AND TISSUE TRANSPLANTATION)

Nathan, D.G.; Weatherall, D.J. Academia and industry: lessons from the unfortunate events in Toronto. *Lancet.* 1999 Mar 6; 353(9155): 771–772.

(BIOMEDICAL RESEARCH; HUMAN
EXPERIMENTATION/FOREIGN COUNTRIES)

Nathan, Richard see **Saegusa, Asako**

National Bioethics Advisory Commission. Cloning
Human Beings: Report and Recommendations of the
National Bioethics Advisory Commission. Executive
Summary. Rockville, MD: The Commission; 1997 Jun.
5 p.
(CLONING)

National Bioethics Advisory Commission. Cloning
Human Beings: Report and Recommendations of the
National Bioethics Advisory Commission. Volumme II:
Commission Papers. Rockville, MD: The Commission;
1997 Jun. 289 p.
(CLONING)

National Bioethics Advisory Commission. Research
Involving Persons with Mental Disorders That May
Affect Decisionmaking Capacity. Volume I: Report and
Recommendations of the National Bioethics Advisory
Commission. Rockville, MD: The Commission; 1998
Dec. 88 p.
(HUMAN EXPERIMENTATION/REGULATION; HUMAN
EXPERIMENTATION/SPECIAL POPULATIONS)

**National Bioethics Advisory Commission. Genetics
Subcommittee.** Transcript of the National Bioethics
Advisory Commission Genetics Subcommittee Meeting
held on 23 Nov 1997, in Bethesda, Maryland. Rockville,
MD: The Commission; 1997 Nov 23. 201 p.
(GENETIC RESEARCH; ORGAN AND TISSUE DONATION)

**National Committees on Scientific Dishonesty in the
Nordic Countries** see **Nylenna, Magne**

**National Council on Bioethics in Human Research
(Canada).** Facilitating ethical research: promoting
informed choice. *NCBHR Communique (National
Council on Bioethics in Human Research).* 1996 Dec; 7(2,
Suppl.): i–ii, 1–28.
(HUMAN EXPERIMENTATION/FOREIGN COUNTRIES;
HUMAN EXPERIMENTATION/INFORMED CONSENT)

**National Institute of Diabetes and Digestive and
Kidney Diseases. Liver Transplantation Database
Group** see **Showstack, Jonathan**

**National Research Council and Institute of Medicine.
Board on Children, Youth, and Families** see **Institute
of Medicine. Committee on Perinatal Transmission
of HIV**

Naughton, Michelle see **Hall, Mark A.**

Navarrete de Olivares, Victoria see
Hernández–Arriaga, Jorge

Nayfield, Susan G. Ethical and scientific considerations
for chemoprevention research in cohorts at genetic risk
for breast cancer. *Journal of Cellular Biochemistry.
Supplement.* 1996; 25: 123–130.
(GENETIC RESEARCH; GENETIC SCREENING; HUMAN
EXPERIMENTATION/RESEARCH DESIGN)

Naylor, A.R. see **Lloyd, A.J.**

Neal, Bernard W. Ethical aspects in the care of very low
birth weight infants. *Pediatrician.* 1990; 17(2): 92–99.

(RESOURCE ALLOCATION/BIOMEDICAL TECHNOLOGIES;
SELECTION FOR TREATMENT)

Nease, Donald E.; Doukas, David J. Research privacy
or freedom of information? [News]. *Hastings Center
Report.* 1999 May–Jun; 29(3): 47.
(CONFIDENTIALITY/LEGAL ASPECTS; HUMAN
EXPERIMENTATION/REGULATION)

**Neerhof, Mark G.; MacGregor, Scott N.; Kilner, John
F.** Congenital diaphragmatic hernia: in utero therapy
and ethical considerations. *Clinics in Perinatology.* 1996
Sep; 23(3): 465–472.
(FETUSES)

Neerhof, Mark G. see **Sprang, M. LeRoy**

Neiburger, Ellis J. see **Tessman, Irwin**

Neild, Patricia. Irreconcilable differences: a parent's right
to refuse to consent to the medical treatment of a child.
Family and Conciliation Courts Review. 1995 Jul; 33(3):
342–360.
(TREATMENT REFUSAL/MINORS)

Neilson, Jane. A patient's perspective on genetic
counseling and predictive testing for Alzheimer's disease.
Journal of Genetic Counseling. 1999 Feb; 8(1): 37–46.
(GENETIC COUNSELING; GENETIC SCREENING)

Nelkin, Dorothy. Publication and promotion: the
performance of science. *Lancet.* 1998 Sep 12; 352(9131):
893.
(BIOMEDICAL RESEARCH)

Nelkin, Dorothy; Andrews, Lori. Homo economicus:
commercialization of body tissue in the age of
biotechnology. *Hastings Center Report.* 1998 Sep–Oct;
28(5): 30–39.
(BIOMEDICAL RESEARCH; GENETIC RESEARCH; ORGAN
AND TISSUE DONATION)

Nelson, Beverly see **Constantino, Rose E.**

Nelson, Christine see **Cooper–Patrick, Lisa**

Nelson, Hilde Lindemann. *Feminist Approaches to
Bioethics: Theoretical Reflections and Practical
Applications*, by Rosemarie Tong. [Book review essay].
Hypatia. 1998 Fall; 13(4): 112–116.
(BIOETHICS)

Nelson, James Lindemann. Bioethics as several kinds of
writing. *Journal of Medicine and Philosophy.* 1999 Apr;
24(2): 148–163.
(BIOETHICS; ETHICISTS AND ETHICS COMMITTEES)

Nelson, Janet Cooper. Mistaking the periphery for the
center: a response to "Euthanasia" by Dan W. Brock.
Rhode Island Medicine. 1993 Dec; 76(12): 592–594.
(EUTHANASIA)

Nelson, Judith E. Saving lives and saving deaths. *Annals
of Internal Medicine.* 1999 May 4; 130(9): 776–777.
(PATIENT CARE; TERMINAL CARE)

Nelson, Robert M. Ethics in the intensive care unit:
creating an ethical environment. *Critical Care Clinics.*
1997 Jul; 13(3): 691–701.
(BIOMEDICAL TECHNOLOGIES; PATIENT CARE)

Nespoli, L. see **Burgio, G. Roberto**

Nessa, John; Malterud, Kirsti. Tell me what's wrong with me: a discourse analysis approach to the concept of patient autonomy. *Journal of Medical Ethics.* 1998 Dec; 24(6): 394–400.
(PROFESSIONAL PATIENT RELATIONSHIP)

Netherlands. Ministry of Health, Welfare and Sport. Documentation and Library Department see **Vlaardingerbroek, W.F.C.**

Neuberger, Julia; Tallis, Raymond. Do we need a new word for patients? [Article and commentary]. *BMJ (British Medical Journal).* 1999 Jun 26; 318(7200): 1756–1758.
(PROFESSIONAL PATIENT RELATIONSHIP)

Neuberger, Julia see **Limentani, Alexander E.**

Neuberger, Julia see **Selby, Mary**

Neufeld, Victor R. Physician as humanist: still an educational challenge. [Editorial]. *Canadian Medical Association Journal.* 1998 Oct 6; 159(7): 787–788.
(MEDICAL ETHICS/EDUCATION; PROFESSIONAL PATIENT RELATIONSHIP)

Neuhaus, Richard John; Morris, Monica B. Should surrogate motherhood be outlawed? *In:* Francoeur, Robert T., ed. Taking Sides: Clashing Views on Controversial Issues in Human Sexuality. Fifth Edition. Guilford, CT: Dushkin Publishing Group/Brown and Benchmark; 1996: 144–159.
(SURROGATE MOTHERS)

New England Regional Genetics Group. New England Regional Genetics Group (NERGG) policy statement on screening for cystic fibrosis. *Genetic Resource.* 1991; 6(1): 67–68.
(GENETIC SCREENING)

New York State Task Force on Life and the Law. When Death Is Sought: Assisted Suicide and Euthanasia in the Medical Context; Supplement to Report. New York, NY: The Task Force; 1997 Apr. 18 p.
(ALLOWING TO DIE/LEGAL ASPECTS; EUTHANASIA/LEGAL ASPECTS; SUICIDE)

New York. Supreme Court, Albany County. In re Finn. *New York Supplement, 2d Series.* 1995 Feb 21 (date of decision). 625: 809–814.
(RESUSCITATION ORDERS)

New York. Supreme Court, Appellate Division, Second Department. Kass v. Kass. *New York Supplement, 2d Series.* 1997 Sep 8 (date of decision). 663: 581–602.
(FETUSES; IN VITRO FERTILIZATION)

New York. Supreme Court, Queens County. In re Christopher. *New York Supplement, 2d Series.* 1998 May 21 (date of decision). 675: 807–810.
(ALLOWING TO DIE/LEGAL ASPECTS)

Newdick, Christopher. Resource allocation in the National Health Service. *American Journal of Law and Medicine.* 1997; 23(2–3): 291–318.
(HEALTH CARE/FOREIGN COUNTRIES; RESOURCE ALLOCATION)

Newell, Christopher. The ethics of narrative ethics: some teaching reflections. *Health Care Analysis.* 1998 Jun; 6(2): 171–174.
(BIOETHICS/EDUCATION)

Newell, Christopher. The social nature of disability, disease and genetics: a response to Gillam, Persson, Holtug, Draper and Chadwick. *Journal of Medical Ethics.* 1999 Apr; 25(2): 172–175.
(PRENATAL DIAGNOSIS)

Newell, Marie–Louise see **Graham, Wendy J.**

Newman, David H. A medical school honor code: what does it mean? *Pharos.* 1997 Spring; 60(2): 2–4.
(MEDICAL ETHICS/CODES OF ETHICS; MEDICAL ETHICS/EDUCATION)

Newman, Stuart A. Cloning our way to "the next level." *Nature Biotechnology.* 1997 Jun; 15(6): 488.
(CLONING)

Newman, Stuart A. Human cloning and the law. *Journal of Biolaw and Business.* 1998 Spring; 1(3): 59–62.
(CLONING)

Newman, Stuart A. see **Billings, Paul R.**

Newman, Stuart A. see **Nader, Claire**

Newson, Ainsley; Williamson, Robert. Should we undertake genetic research on intelligence? *Bioethics.* 1999 Jul; 13(3–4): 327–342.
(BEHAVIORAL GENETICS; GENETIC INTERVENTION; GENETIC RESEARCH)

Newton, Michael J. Precedent autonomy: life–sustaining intervention and the demented patient. *Cambridge Quarterly of Healthcare Ethics.* 1999 Spring; 8(2): 189–199.
(ADVANCE DIRECTIVES; ALLOWING TO DIE)

Ng, Valerie see **Balano, Kirsten**

Nicholas, Barbara. Strategies for effective transformation. *In:* Donchin, Anne; Purdy, Laura M., eds. Embodying Bioethics: Recent Feminist Advances. Lanham, MD: Rowman and Littlefield; 1999: 239–252.
(BIOETHICS; ETHICISTS AND ETHICS COMMITTEES)

Nicholas, Richard A. see **Margolis, Lewis H.**

Nicholls, Michael. Keyholders and flak jackets: consent to medical treatment for children. *Family Law.* 1994 Feb; 24: 81–85.
(INFORMED CONSENT/MINORS; TREATMENT REFUSAL/MINORS)

Nichols, David see **Gilhooly, Mary L.M.**

Nicholson, Michael L.; Bradley, J. Andrew. Renal transplantation from living donors. [Editorial]. *BMJ (British Medical Journal).* 1999 Feb 13; 318(7181): 409–410.
(ORGAN AND TISSUE DONATION; ORGAN AND TISSUE TRANSPLANTATION)

Nicholson, Richard see **Dickenson, Donna L.**

Nicholson, Richard H. "Don't die of ignorance." *Hastings Center Report.* 1999 May–Jun; 29(3): 6.
(MASS SCREENING)

Nicholson, Richard H. Power corrupts...? *Hastings Center Report.* 1998 Sep–Oct; 28(5): 6.
(PATENTING LIFE FORMS)

Nicholson, Richard H. Unity in diversity. *Hastings Center Report.* 1999 Jan–Feb; 29(1): 6.
(HUMAN EXPERIMENTATION/ETHICS COMMITTEES; HUMAN EXPERIMENTATION/FOREIGN COUNTRIES; HUMAN EXPERIMENTATION/REGULATION)

Nicolaides, K.H. see **Snijders, R.J.M.**

Nieland, M. see **Lui, S.C.**

Niermeyer, Susan see **West, Charles**

Nieuw, A.D. Informed consent. *Medicine and Law.* 1993; 12(1–2): 125–130.
(INFORMED CONSENT)

Nieves, Evelyn. Girl awaits father's 2d kidney, and decision by medical ethicists. [News]. *New York Times.* 1998 Dec 5: A1, A11.
(ORGAN AND TISSUE DONATION)

Nightingale, Stuart L. Categories of research eligible for expedited review by IRBs. [News]. *JAMA.* 1999 Jan 6; 281(1): 27.
(HUMAN EXPERIMENTATION/ETHICS COMMITTEES; HUMAN EXPERIMENTATION/REGULATION)

Nightingale, Stuart L.; Brown, Philip; Levin, Arthur Aaron; Inlander, Charles B.; Goldstein, Mark R.; Medawar, Charles. Advertising prescription-only drugs. [Letters]. *Lancet.* 1998 May 23; 351(9115): 1582–1584.
(PATIENT CARE/DRUGS)

Nilges, Richard G. see **Byrne, Paul A.**

Nilsson, Annika see **Rose, Joanna**

Nilstun, Tore; Ranstam, Jonas. Ethics in orthopedic research. [Editorial]. *Acta Orthopaedica Scandinavica.* 1997 Jun; 68(3): 205–206.
(HUMAN EXPERIMENTATION)

Nilstun, Tore see **Zwitter, Matjaz**

Nippert, I.; Horst, J.; Wolff, G.; Wertz, D. Ethical issues in genetic service provision: attitudes of human geneticists in Germany. [Abstract]. *American Journal of Human Genetics.* 1996 Oct; 59(4): A338.
(GENETIC COUNSELING; GENETIC SCREENING)

Nitschke, Philip see **Kissane, David W.**

Noble, Holcomb B. Of life, death and the rules of liver transplants. [News]. *New York Times.* 1999 Apr 6: F6.
(ORGAN AND TISSUE TRANSPLANTATION; SELECTION FOR TREATMENT)

Noble, P. see **Snijders, R.J.M.**

Noblin, Charles D. see **Richards, Karlotta A.**

Nolan, David. Abortion: should men have a say? *In:* Lee, Ellie, ed. Abortion Law and Politics Today. New York, NY: St. Martin's Press; 1998: 216–231.
(ABORTION/FOREIGN COUNTRIES; ABORTION/LEGAL ASPECTS)

Noll, Robert B. see **Kodish, Eric D.**

Norberg, Astrid see **Söderberg, Anna**

Nord, Erik see **Menzel, Paul**

Nordenfelt, Lennart. On medicine and other means of health enhancement: towards a conceptual framework. *In:* Hanson, Mark J.; Callahan, Daniel, eds. The Goals of Medicine: The Forgotten Issue in Health Care Reform. Washington, DC: Georgetown University Press; 1999: 69–87.
(HEALTH; HEALTH CARE)

Nordin, Ingemar. The limits of medical practice. *Theoretical Medicine and Bioethics.* 1999 Apr; 20(2): 105–123.
(HEALTH; HEALTH CARE; PUBLIC HEALTH)

Nordio, S. Beneficence, virtues and ethical committees in pediatrics: epistemology, bioethics and medical pedagogy in pediatrics. *In:* Burgio, G. Roberto; Lantos, John D., eds. *Primum Non Nocere* Today. Second Edition. New York, NY: Elsevier; 1998: 147–158.
(BIOETHICS; MEDICAL ETHICS/EDUCATION)

Normile, Dennis. Geneticists debate eugenics and China's infant health law. [News]. *Science.* 1998 Aug 21; 281(5380): 1118–1119.
(EUGENICS)

Norrie, Peter. Ethical decision-making in intensive care: are nurses suitable patient advocates? *Intensive and Critical Care Nursing.* 1997 Jun; 13(3): 167–169.
(PATIENT CARE)

Norris, John W. see **Alexandrov, Andrei V.**

Norris, Patrick. Sheep cloning: what next? *Health Care Ethics USA.* 1997 Spring; 5(2): 6–7.
(CLONING)

Norris, Peggy. Medical Ethics. Southport, Merseyside, England: Christian Theology Trust; 1992. 41 p.
(MEDICAL ETHICS)

North Carolina Medical Society. Bioethics Committee see **Sellers, Phil**

Northern Ireland. Supreme Court of Judicature, High Court of Justice, Family Division. Northern Health and Social Services Board v. F and G. *Northern Ireland Law Reports.* 1993 Oct 14 (date of decision). 1993: 268–278.
(ABORTION/FOREIGN COUNTRIES; ABORTION/MINORS)

Northridge, Mary. Annotation: new rules for authorship in the Journal: your contributions are recognized -- and published! [Editorial]. *American Journal of Public Health.* 1998 May; 88(5): 733–734.
(BIOMEDICAL RESEARCH)

Notarangelo, Luigi D. see **Candotti, Fabio**

Novack, Dennis H. see **Feldman, Debra S.**

Novaes, Simone Bateman; Salem, Tania. Embedding the embryo. *In:* Harris, John; Holm, Søren, eds. The Future of Human Reproduction: Ethics, Choice, and Regulation. New York, NY: Oxford University Press;

1998: 101–126.
(REPRODUCTION; REPRODUCTIVE TECHNOLOGIES)

Novick, Alvin. HIV surveillance: what's hot, what's not. *AIDS and Public Policy Journal.* 1998 Summer; 13(2): 51–55.
(AIDS)

Nowak, Rachel. Almost human. [News]. *New Scientist.* 1999 Feb 13; 161(2173): 20–21.
(ANIMAL EXPERIMENTATION)

Nuffield Council on Bioethics. Mental Disorders and Genetics: The Ethical Context. London: The Council; 1998 Sep. 117 p.
(GENETIC COUNSELING; GENETIC RESEARCH; GENETIC SCREENING)

Nussbaum, Martha C.; Sunstein, Cass R., eds. Clones and Clones: Facts and Fantasies about Human Cloning. New York, NY: Norton; 1998. 351 p.
(CLONING)

Nygaard, Richard Lowell. The ten commandments of behavioral genetic data and criminology. *Judges' Journal.* 1997 Summer; 36(3): 59–64, 94–96.
(BEHAVIORAL GENETICS)

Nylenna, Magne; Andersen, Daniel; Dahlquist, Gisela; Sarvas, Matti; Aakvaag, Asbjørn; National Committees on Scientific Dishonesty in the Nordic Countries. Handling of scientific dishonesty in the Nordic countries. *Lancet.* 1999 Jul 3; 354(9172): 57–61.
(BIOMEDICAL RESEARCH; FRAUD AND MISCONDUCT)

Nyman, Deborah J.; Eidelman, Leonid A.; Sprung, Charles L. Euthanasia. *Critical Care Clinics.* 1996 Jan; 12(1): 85–96.
(ALLOWING TO DIE; EUTHANASIA)

Nys, Herman. Therapeutic use of human organs and tissues under Belgian law. *Medicine and Law.* 1993; 12(1–2): 131–135.
(ORGAN AND TISSUE DONATION)

Nys, Herman see **Denekens, Joke P.M.**

O

Oakley, Justin. A virtue ethics approach. *In:* Kuhse, Helga; Singer, Peter, eds. A Companion to bioethics. Malden, MA: Blackwell; 1998: 86–97.
(BIOETHICS)

Oberfield, Sharon E. Growth hormone use in normal, short children -- a plea for reason. [Editorial]. *New England Journal of Medicine.* 1999 Feb 18; 340(7): 557–559.
(PATIENT CARE/MINORS; SELECTION FOR TREATMENT)

Oberlander, Jonathan see **Jacobs, Lawrence**

Oberman, Michelle. Real and perceived legal barriers to the inclusion of women in clinical trials. *In:* Dan, Alice J., ed. Reframing Women's Health: Multidisciplinary Research and Practice. Thousand Oaks, CA: Sage Publications; 1994: 266–276.
(HUMAN EXPERIMENTATION/SPECIAL POPULATIONS)

O'Brien, Daniel. Working for the common good: Catholic healthcare's opportunity to shape values–based managed care. *Health Progress.* 1997 Jan–Feb; 78(1): 40–42, 47.
(HEALTH CARE/ECONOMICS)

O'Brien, James G., ed. Ethical and Legal Issues in Care of the Elderly. Proceedings of a Conference at Michigan State University, 14 Jun 1985. Issued by the Dept. of Family Practice, Michigan State University, East Lansing, MI; 1988. 119 p.
(PATIENT CARE/AGED)

O'Brien, Louise see **West, Charles**

O'Connell, Laurence J. The role of religion in health–related decision making for elderly patients. *Generations (American Society on Aging).* 1994 Winter; 18(4): 27–30.
(PATIENT CARE/AGED)

O'Connor, Bonnie B. Culture and the use of patient restraints. *HEC (HealthCare Ethics Committee) Forum.* 1998 Sep–Dec; 10(3–4): 263–275.
(BEHAVIOR CONTROL; PATIENT CARE)

O'Conor, Rory see **Denley, Ian**

Odlind, Viveca. Induced abortion -- a global health problem. *Acta Obstetricia et Gynecologica Scandinavica.* 1997; 76(Suppl. 164): 43–45.
(ABORTION/FOREIGN COUNTRIES)

Oehmke, Thomas see **Brovins, Joan**

Office for Protection from Research Risks Review Panel. Report to the Advisory Committee to the Director, NIH. The Panel [online]. Downloaded from Internet Web site: http://www.nih.gov/grants/oprr/references/060399b.html on 7 Jun 1999; 1999 Jun 3. 16 p.
(ANIMAL EXPERIMENTATION; HUMAN EXPERIMENTATION/REGULATION)

Offit, Kenneth see **Garber, Judy E.**

Ogden, R.D. see **Starace, F.**

Ogden, Russel. AIDS, euthanasia and nursing. *Nursing Standard.* 1996 May 29; 10(36): 49–51.
(AIDS/HEALTH PERSONNEL; EUTHANASIA; SUICIDE)

Ogloff, James R.P. see **Achille, Marie A.**

O'Hare, Michael J. see **Mepham, T. Ben**

Okamura, Hitoshi; Uchitomi, Yosuke; Sasako, Mitsuru; Eguchi, Kenji; Kakizoe, Tadao. Guidelines for telling the truth to cancer patients. *Japanese Journal of Clinical Oncology.* 1998 Jan; 28(1): 1–4.
(TRUTH DISCLOSURE)

Okarma, Thomas B. Human primordial stem cells. [Symposium introduction]. *Hastings Center Report.* 1999 Mar–Apr; 29(2): 30.
(EMBRYO AND FETAL RESEARCH)

Okwo–Bele, J.M. see **Lee, J.W.**

Olaitan, Adeola see **Gbolade, Babatunde A.**

Oldenettel, Debra; Dye, Timothy D.; Artal, Raul. Prenatal HIV screening in pregnant women: a

medical–legal review. *Birth.* 1997 Sep; 24(3): 165–172.
(AIDS/TESTING AND SCREENING)

Olick, Robert S. Deciding for Incompetent Patients: The Nature and Limits of Prospective Autonomy and Advance Directives. Ann Arbor, MI: UMI Dissertation Services; 1996. 374 p. (2 v. in 1).
(ADVANCE DIRECTIVES; ALLOWING TO DIE; INFORMED CONSENT)

Oliver, Jo. Anorexia and the refusal of medical treatment. *Victoria University of Wellington Law Review.* 1997 Dec; 27(4): 621–647.
(FORCE FEEDING; TREATMENT REFUSAL)

Olopade, O.I. (Funmi) see **Garber, Judy E.**

Olsen, Douglas see **Tschudin, Verena**

Olsen, Douglas P. Ethical responsibility in health care reform dialogue. [Editorial]. *NursingConnections.* 1996 Summer; 9(2): 17–22.
(HEALTH CARE)

Olsen, Douglas P. Toward an ethical standard for coerced mental health treatment: least restrictive or most therapeutic? *Journal of Clinical Ethics.* 1998 Fall; 9(3): 235–246.
(PATIENT CARE/MENTALLY DISABLED)

Olson, Ellen. Treatment termination in long–term care: what about the physician? What about the family? *Journal of Long Term Home Health Care.* 1997 Winter; 16(1): 14–21.
(ALLOWING TO DIE)

Olsthoorn–Heim, Els T.M. HIV testing and private insurance. *Medicine and Law.* 1993; 12(1–2): 11–14.
(AIDS/TESTING AND SCREENING)

O'Mathúna, Dónal P. Applying justice to genetics. *In:* Demy, Timothy J.; Stewart, Gary P., eds. Genetic Engineering: A Christian Response: Crucial Considerations in Shaping Life. Grand Rapids, MI: Kregel Publications; 1999: 50–69.
(GENETIC INTERVENTION)

O'Mathúna, Dónal P. see **Stewart, Gary P.**

O'Neil, Mary see **Swartz, Richard D.**

O'Neill, J. A peaceful death. [Personal view]. *BMJ (British Medical Journal).* 1999 Jul 31; 319(7205): 327.
(TERMINAL CARE)

O'Neill, Kathryn see **Kerr, Susan M.**

O'Neill, Patrick. Negotiating Consent in Psychotherapy. New York, NY: New York University Press; 1998. 188 p.
(INFORMED CONSENT/MENTALLY DISABLED; PROFESSIONAL PATIENT RELATIONSHIP)

O'Neill, Terry. Biomedical Ethics. [Juvenile literature]. San Diego, CA: Greenhaven Press; 1999. 144 p.
(BIOETHICS)

Ono, Yumiko see **Peters, Malte**

Onorato, Ida see **Kirsch, Michael**

Onwuteaka–Philipsen, Bregje D.; Muller, Martien T.; van der Wal, Gerrit. Euthanatics: implementation of a protocol to standardise euthanatics among pharmacists and GPs. *Patient Education and Counseling.* 1997 Jun; 31(2): 131–137.
(EUTHANASIA; SUICIDE)

Onwuteaka–Philipsen, Bregje D. see **Haverkate, Ilinka**

Oppé, Thomas E. Ethical aspects of AIDS in childhood in England. *Pediatrician.* 1990; 17(2): 115–117.
(AIDS; PATIENT CARE/MINORS)

Oppenheim, Arieh see **Sprung, Charles L.**

Orentlicher, David. Paying physicians more to do less: financial incentives to limit care. *University of Richmond Law Review.* 1996 Jan; 30(1): 155–197.
(HEALTH CARE/ECONOMICS; RESOURCE ALLOCATION)

Orentlicher, David. The Supreme Court and terminal sedation: rejecting assisted suicide, embracing euthanasia. *Hastings Constitutional Law Quarterly.* 1997 Summer; 24(4): 947–968.
(ALLOWING TO DIE/LEGAL ASPECTS; EUTHANASIA/LEGAL ASPECTS; SUICIDE)

Orentlicher, David see **Tonelli, Mark R.**

Oreopoulos, D.G. see **Velasco, N.**

Orlans, F. Barbara. Ethical evaluation of animal research protocols: how it can be enhanced. *In:* van Zutphen, L.F.M.; Balls, M., eds. Animal Alternatives, Welfare and Ethics. New York, NY: Elsevier; 1997: 385–390.
(ANIMAL EXPERIMENTATION)

Orlans, F. Barbara. History and ethical regulation of animal experimentation: an international perspective. *In:* Kuhse, Helga; Singer, Peter, eds. A Companion to Bioethics. Malden, MA: Blackwell; 1998: 399–410.
(ANIMAL EXPERIMENTATION)

Ormel, Johan see **Sullivan, Mark**

O'Rourke, Dennis. Half Life: A Parable for the Nuclear Age. [Videorecording]. Available from Direct Cinema Ltd., P.O. Box 69799, Los Angeles, CA, 90069, (213)396-4774; 1986. Videocassette; 86 min.; sd., color; VHS.
(FRAUD AND MISCONDUCT; HUMAN EXPERIMENTATION/SPECIAL POPULATIONS; WAR)

O'Rourke, Kevin. Surrogate decision making: ethical issues. *Health Care Ethics USA.* 1998 Summer; 6(3): 2–3.
(ALLOWING TO DIE/ATTITUDES; INFORMED CONSENT)

O'Rourke, Kevin; Sulmasy, Daniel P.; Terry, Peter B.; Miller, Deborah J. Accuracy of substituted judgments in patients with terminal diagnoses. [Letter and response]. *Annals of Internal Medicine.* 1998 Dec 15; 129(12): 1082–1083.
(ALLOWING TO DIE; INFORMED CONSENT)

O'Rourke, Kevin see **Keenan, James F.**

O'Rourke, Kevin see **Rainey, R. Randall**

O'Rourke, Kevin D. Applying the Directives: The *Ethical and Religious Directives* concerning three medical situations require some elucidation. *Health Progress.* 1998

Jul–Aug; 79(4): 64–69.
(ABORTION/RELIGIOUS ASPECTS; ALLOWING TO
DIE/RELIGIOUS ASPECTS; CONTRACEPTION)

O'Rourke, Kevin D. Physician assisted suicide, a religious perspective. *Saint Louis University Public Law Review.* 1996; 15(2): 433–446.
(SUICIDE)

O'Rourke, Kevin D.; Boyle, Philip. Medical Ethics: Sources of Catholic Teachings. Third Edition. Washington, DC: Georgetown University Press; 1999. 442 p.
(BIOETHICS)

Orr, Robert D. The temptation of human cloning. *Today's Christian Doctor.* 1997 Fall; 28(3): 4–7.
(CLONING)

Orr, Robert D.; Genesen, Leigh B. Medicine, ethics and religion: rational or irrational? *Journal of Medical Ethics.* 1998 Dec; 24(6): 385–387.
(ALLOWING TO DIE/RELIGIOUS ASPECTS; PATIENT CARE)

Orr, Robert D. see **Kilner, John F.**

Orr, Robert D. see **Larimore, Walter L.**

Orr, William B. see **Barton, C. Dennis**

Orris, Peter see **Brodkin, C. Andrew**

Ortega, Rafael see **Dal–Ré, Rafael**

Ortona, Luigi see **Albert, Steven M.**

Osher, Trina W.; Telesford, Mary. Involving families to improve research. *In:* Hoagwood, Kimberly; Jensen, Peter S.; Fisher, Celia B., eds. Ethical Issues in Mental Health Research with Children and Adolescents. Mahwah, NJ: Lawrence Erlbaum Associates; 1996: 29–39.
(HUMAN EXPERIMENTATION/MINORS; HUMAN EXPERIMENTATION/SPECIAL POPULATIONS)

Osmond, Dennis see **Bindman, Andrew B.**

Osmond, Dennis see **Grumbach, Kevin**

Ost, Katherine see **Agarwal, Manoj R.**

Ostrer, Harry; Scheuermann, Richard H.; Picker, Louis J. Benefits and dangers of genetic tests. [Letters]. *Nature.* 1998 Mar 5; 392(6671): 14.
(GENETIC RESEARCH; GENETIC SCREENING; ORGAN AND TISSUE DONATION)

O'Sullivan, Helen see **Hill, Ruaraidh**

O'Sullivan, Mary Jo see **Balano, Kirsten**

Osuna, E. see **Pacheco, R.**

Oswald, Nigel see **Jones, Steve**

O'Toole, Brian. Four ways people approach ethics: a practical guide to reaching consensus on moral problems. *Health Progress.* 1998 Nov–Dec; 79(6): 38–41, 43.
(PROFESSIONAL ETHICS)

Otte, Kimberly K. see **Gervais, Karen G.**

Otten, Marc. Parents refuse to allow life–saving treatment for newborn: our moral obligation. *Princeton Journal of Bioethics.* 1998 Spring; 1(1): 61–64.
(ALLOWING TO DIE/INFANTS; TREATMENT REFUSAL/MINORS)

Overall, Stephen W. see **Sexson, William R.**

Oye, Robert see **Wenger, Neil**

P

Paauw, Douglas S. see **Margolis, Lewis H.**

Pace, Nicholas see **West, Charles**

Pacheco, R.; Osuna, E.; Gómez–Zapata, M.; Luna, A. Medicolegal problems associated with do not resuscitate orders. *Medicine and Law.* 1994; 13(5–6): 461–466.
(RESUSCITATION ORDERS)

Packer, Samuel. Capitated care is unethical. *Archives of Ophthalmology.* 1997 Sep; 115(9): 1195–1196.
(HEALTH CARE/ECONOMICS)

Paddock, John R. see **Loftus, Elizabeth F.**

Page, David C. see **Reilly, Philip R.**

Paine, Shirley J. see **Brown, Lowell C.**

Paintin, David, ed. Ante–Natal Screening and Abortion for Fetal Abnormality. London: Birth Control Trust; 1997. 96 p.
(ABORTION; PRENATAL DIAGNOSIS)

Palleschi, Massimo see **Zuccaro, Stefano Maria**

Pallis, Chris. On the brainstem criterion of death. *In:* Youngner, Stuart J.; Arnold, Robert M.; Schapiro, Renie, eds. The Definition of Death: Contemporary Controversies Baltimore, MD: Johns Hopkins University Press; 1999: 93–100.
(DETERMINATION OF DEATH/BRAIN DEATH)

Palmer, Eileen Alexa. Genetic Choice, Disability, and Regret. Ann Arbor, MI: UMI Dissertation Services; 1997. 159 p.
(EUGENICS; REPRODUCTION)

Palmer, Louis J. Organ Transplants from Executed Prisoners: An Argument for the Creation of Death Sentence Organ Removal Statutes. Jefferson, NC: McFarland; 1999. 156 p.
(CAPITAL PUNISHMENT; ORGAN AND TISSUE DONATION)

Palmer, Michael. Moral Problems in Medicine: A Practical Coursebook. Buffalo, NY: University of Toronto Press; 1999. 190 p.
(BIOETHICS)

Palmour, Roberta M. see **Glass, Kathleen Cranley**

Palmstierna, Tom see **Kjellin, Lars**

Palumbo, Michael G. see **Kopelman, Loretta M.**

Pan, Richard J.D. see **Simon, Steven R.**

Pandit, Jaideep J. Ethical commentaries must be based

on sound science. [Letter]. *BMJ (British Medical Journal)*. 1998 Dec 5; 317(7172): 1594–1595.
(HUMAN EXPERIMENTATION/MINORS)

Paneth, Nigel. Separating authorship responsibility and authorship credit: a proposal for biomedical journals. *American Journal of Public Health*. 1998 May; 88(5): 824–826.
(BIOMEDICAL RESEARCH)

Pang, Mei–che Samantha. Protective truthfulness: the Chinese way of safeguarding patients in informed treatment decisions. *Journal of Medical Ethics*. 1999 Jun; 25(3): 247–253.
(INFORMED CONSENT; MEDICAL ETHICS; PROFESSIONAL PATIENT RELATIONSHIP; TRUTH DISCLOSURE)

Panos Institute see **Mirsky, Judith**

Panossian, André A.; Panossian, Vahé; Doumanian, Nancy P. Criminalization of perinatal HIV transmission. *Journal of Legal Medicine*. 1998 Jun; 19(2): 223–255.
(AIDS; PRENATAL INJURIES)

Panossian, Vahé see **Panossian, André A.**

Panush, Richard S. Upon finding a Nazi anatomy atlas: the lessons of Nazi medicine. *Pharos*. 1996 Fall; 59(4): 18–22.
(FRAUD AND MISCONDUCT)

Parazzini, Fabio see **Gbolade, Babatunde A.**

Pardo, Antonio. Human cloning. *Dolentium Hominum: Church and Health in the World*. 1997; 36(12th Yr., No. 3): 28–31.
(CLONING)

Parens, Erik, ed. Enhancing Human Traits: Ethical and Social Implications. Washington, DC: Georgetown University Press; 1998. 258 p.
(BIOMEDICAL TECHNOLOGIES; HEALTH; HEALTH CARE)

Parens, Erik. Researchers close in on primordial stem cells. [News]. *Hastings Center Report*. 1999 Jan–Feb; 29(1): 51–52.
(EMBRYO AND FETAL RESEARCH)

Pargiter, Russell; Bloch, Sidney. The ethics committee of a psychiatric college: its procedures and themes. *Australian and New Zealand Journal of Psychiatry*. 1997 Feb; 31(1): 76–82.
(ETHICISTS AND ETHICS COMMITTEES; MEDICAL ETHICS)

Paris, John J. Hugh Finn's "right to die." *America*. 1998 Oct 31; 179(13): 13–15.
(ALLOWING TO DIE/RELIGIOUS ASPECTS)

Paris, John J.; Schreiber, Michael D. Parental discretion in refusal of treatment for newborns: a real but limited right. *Clinics in Perinatology*. 1996 Sep; 23(3): 573–581.
(ALLOWING TO DIE/INFANTS; TREATMENT REFUSAL/MINORS)

Paris, John J.; Schreiber, Michael D. Physicians' refusal to provide life–prolonging medical interventions. *Clinics in Perinatology*. 1996 Sep; 23(3): 563–571.
(ALLOWING TO DIE)

Park, Yon see **Tolle, Susan W.**

Parker, James see **Conn, P. Michael**

Parker, Kelly A. The bioethics committee: a consensus–recommendation model. *In:* McGee, Glenn, ed. Pragamatic Bioethics. Nashville, TN: Vanderbilt University Press; 1999: 60–70, 264–265.
(ETHICISTS AND ETHICS COMMITTEES)

Parker, Lisa S. Reproduction: *Who's Afraid of Human Cloning?* by Gregory E. Pence. [Book review essay]. *JAMA*. 1998 Nov 25; 280(20): 1798–1799.
(CLONING)

Parker, Michael see **Pattison, Stephen**

Parkins, K. see **West, Charles**

Parness, Jeffrey A. Arming the pregnancy police: more outlandish concoctions? *Louisiana Law Review*. 1992 Nov; 53(2): 427–448.
(PRENATAL INJURIES)

Parry, Richard D. Death, dignity and morality. *America*. 1998 Nov 14; 179(15): 20–21.
(TERMINAL CARE)

Parshad, Omkar see **Wray, Samuel R.**

Parsons, John see **Wincze, John P.**

Pascual, Julio; Liaño, Fernando; Madrid Acute Renal Failure Study Group. Causes and prognosis of acute renal failure in the very old. *Journal of the American Geriatrics Society*. 1998 Jun; 46(6): 721–725.
(PATIENT CARE/AGED; SELECTION FOR TREATMENT)

Pask, Eleanor G. see **Maher, John T.**

Passero, Mary Ann see **Lafayette, DeeDee**

Patenaude, Andrea Farkas. Cancer susceptibility testing: risks, benefits and personal beliefs. *In:* Clarke, Angus, ed. The Genetic Testing of Children. Washington, DC: BIOS Scientific Publishers; 1998: 145–156.
(GENETIC SCREENING)

Paterson, Ron. Rationing access to dialysis in New Zealand. *Ethics and Intellectual Disability*. 1999 Winter; 4(1): 5.
(RESOURCE ALLOCATION/BIOMEDICAL TECHNOLOGIES; SELECTION FOR TREATMENT)

Patrinos, Ari see **Collins, Francis S.**

Patterson, James R. see **Preston, Thomas A.**

Pattison, Stephen; Dickenson, Donna; Parker, Michael; Heller, Tom. Do case studies mislead about the nature of reality? *Journal of Medical Ethics*. 1999 Feb; 25(1): 42–46.
(BIOETHICS/EDUCATION)

Pauer–Studer, Herlinde. Peter Singer on euthanasia. *Monist*. 1993 Apr; 76(2): 135–157.
(ALLOWING TO DIE/INFANTS; EUTHANASIA; PERSONHOOD)

Pauker, S.P. see **Mecsas–Faxon, S.**

Paul, Diane B. The Politics of Heredity: Essays on

Eugenics, Biomedicine, and the Nature–Nurture Debate. Albany, NY: State University of New York Press; 1998. 219 p.
(EUGENICS)

Pauly, Mark V. see **Ramsey, Scott D.**

Payne, Doug. More British abortions for Irish women. [News]. *BMJ (British Medical Journal).* 1999 Jan 9; 318(7176): 77.
(ABORTION/FOREIGN COUNTRIES)

Payne, S. A.; Langley–Evans, A.; Hillier, R. Perceptions of a "good" death: a comparative study of the views of hospice staff and patients. *Palliative Medicine.* 1996 Oct; 10(4): 307–312.
(TERMINAL CARE)

Payne, William D. The rational development of liver allocation policy. *Liver Transplantation and Surgery.* 1995 Jan; 1(1): 58–61.
(ORGAN AND TISSUE TRANSPLANTATION; RESOURCE ALLOCATION/BIOMEDICAL TECHNOLOGIES)

Peabody, Joyce L.; Martin, Gilbert I. From how small is too small to how much is too much: ethical issues at the limits of neonatal viability. *Clinics in Perinatology.* 1996 Sep; 23(3): 473–489.
(ALLOWING TO DIE/INFANTS; SELECTION FOR TREATMENT)

Pear, Robert. F.D.A. will require companies to test drugs on children. [News]. *New York Times.* 1998 Nov 28: A1, A10.
(HUMAN EXPERIMENTATION/MINORS; HUMAN EXPERIMENTATION/REGULATION)

Pear, Robert. Future bleak for bill to keep health records confidential. [News]. *New York Times.* 1999 Jun 21: A12.
(CONFIDENTIALITY/LEGAL ASPECTS)

Pear, Robert. Inquiry criticizes A.M.A. backing of abortion procedure ban. [News]. *New York Times.* 1998 Dec 4: A27.
(ABORTION/LEGAL ASPECTS)

Pearlman, Theodore see **Bursztajn, Harold J.**

Pearlman, Theodore see **Weinstock, Robert**

Pearson, Graham S. How to make microbes safer. *Nature.* 1998 Jul 16; 394(6690): 217–218.
(GENETIC INTERVENTION; WAR)

Peart, Nicola; Moore, Andrew. Compensation for injuries suffered by participants in commercially sponsored clinical trials in New Zealand. *Medical Law Review.* 1997 Spring; 5(1): 1–21.
(HUMAN EXPERIMENTATION/FOREIGN COUNTRIES; HUMAN EXPERIMENTATION/REGULATION)

Peck, M. Scott. Denial of the Soul: Spiritual and Medical Perspectives on Euthanasia and Mortality. New York, NY: Harmony Books; 1997. 242 p.
(SUICIDE)

Pedersen, Jette see **Zwitter, Matjaz**

Peerenboom, Ellen. Germany funds two new bioethics programs. [News]. *Nature Medicine.* 1998 Mar; 4(3): 261.
(BIOETHICS)

Peerenboom, Ellen. Germany still pays donors. [News]. *Nature Medicine.* 1998 Feb; 4(2): 139.
(BLOOD DONATION)

Peiris, Vasum see **Bradley, Elizabeth H.**

Pelias, Mary Z. see **Baumiller, Robert C.**

Pelin, Serap Sahinoglu. The question of virginity testing in Turkey. *Bioethics.* 1999 Jul; 13(3–4): 256–261.
(BEHAVIOR CONTROL)

Pellegrino, Edmund see **Bowes, Watson**

Pellegrino, Edmund D. Clinical ethics consultations: some reflections on the report of the SHHV–SBC. *Journal of Clinical Ethics.* 1999 Spring; 10(1): 5–12.
(ETHICISTS AND ETHICS COMMITTEES)

Pellegrino, Edmund D. The goals and ends of medicine: how are they to be defined? *In:* Hanson, Mark J.; Callahan, Daniel, eds. The Goals of Medicine: The Forgotten Issue in Health Care Reform. Washington, DC: Georgetown University Press; 1999: 55–68.
(HEALTH CARE; MEDICAL ETHICS)

Pellegrino, Edmund D. The origins and evolution of bioethics: some personal reflections. *Kennedy Institute of Ethics Journal.* 1999 Mar; 9(1): 73–88.
(BIOETHICS)

Pellegrino, Edmund D. What the philosophy of medicine is. *Theoretical Medicine and Bioethics.* 1998 Aug; 19(4): 315–336.
(BIOETHICS)

Pellegrino, Edmund D. see **Sulmasy, Daniel P.**

Pellissier, James M.; Venta, Enrique R. Introducing patient values into the decision making process for breast cancer screening. *Women and Health.* 1996; 24(4): 47–67.
(MASS SCREENING; PROFESSIONAL PATIENT RELATIONSHIP)

Pels, Richard J. see **Branch, William T.**

Pence, Gregory E.; Smolkin, Mitchell T.; Effros, Richard M.; Gilbert, Scott F.; Annas, George J.; Robertson, John A. Human cloning. [Letters and responses]. *New England Journal of Medicine.* 1998 Nov 19; 339(21): 1558–1559.
(CLONING)

Peng, Rui–cong. The goals of medicine and public health. *In:* Hanson, Mark J.; Callahan, Daniel, eds. The Goals of Medicine: The Forgotten Issue in Health Care Reform. Washington, DC: Georgetown University Press; 1999: 174–180.
(PUBLIC HEALTH)

Pennings, Guido. Age and assisted reproduction. *International Journal of Medicine and Law.* 1995; 14(7/8): 531–541.
(REPRODUCTIVE TECHNOLOGIES; SELECTION FOR TREATMENT)

Pennings, Guido. The internal coherence of donor insemination practice: attracting the right type of donor without paying. *Human Reproduction.* 1997 Sep; 12(9): 1842–1844.
(ARTIFICIAL INSEMINATION)

Penticuff, Joy Hinson. Ethical dimensions in genetic screening: a look into the future. *Journal of Obstetric, Gynecologic and Neonatal Nursing.* 1996 Nov–Dec; 25(9): 785–789.
(GENETIC SCREENING)

Pentz, Rebecca D. Beyond case consultation: an expanded model for organizational ethics. *Journal of Clinical Ethics.* 1999 Spring; 10(1): 34–41.
(ETHICISTS AND ETHICS COMMITTEES; PROFESSIONAL ETHICS)

Pentz, Rebecca D. Genetic counseling: guidance for chilling choices. *In:* Demy, Timothy J.; Stewart, Gary P., eds. Genetic Engineering: A Christian Response: Crucial Considerations in Shaping Life. Grand Rapids, MI: Kregel Publications; 1999: 188–195.
(GENE THERAPY; GENETIC COUNSELING; GENETIC SCREENING)

Pentz, Rebecca D. see **Kodish, Eric D.**

Perentesis, Patricia see **Sugarman, Jeremy**

Pérez–Peña, Richard; Blair, Jayson. Albany plan widely expands sampling of criminals DNA. [News]. *New York Times.* 1999 Aug 7: A1, B4.
(DNA FINGERPRINTING)

Pergament, Eugene see **Fiddler, Morris**

Perkins, David V.; Hudson, Brenda L.; Gray, Diana M.; Stewart, Mary. Decisions and justifications by community mental health providers about hypothetical ethical dilemmas. *Psychiatric Services.* 1998 Oct; 49(10): 1317–1322.
(CONFIDENTIALITY/MENTAL HEALTH; PROFESSIONAL ETHICS; PROFESSIONAL PATIENT RELATIONSHIP)

Pernick, Martin S. Brain death in a cultural context: the reconstruction of death, 1967–1981. *In:* Youngner, Stuart J.; Arnold, Robert M.; Schapiro, Renie, eds. The Definition of Death: Contemporary Controversies. Baltimore, MD: Johns Hopkins University Press; 1999: 3–33.
(DETERMINATION OF DEATH/BRAIN DEATH)

Perone, Nicola; Chervenak, Frank A.; McCullough, Laurence B.; Chez, Ronald A. Physicians should not be allowed to enter into contractual agreements with managed care companies that do not meet basic ethical standards. [Letter and response]. *American Journal of Obstetrics and Gynecology.* 1997 Aug; 177(2): 481–482.
(HEALTH CARE/ECONOMICS)

Perrin, Kathleen Ouimet. Giving voice to the wishes of elders for end-of-life care. *Journal of Gerontological Nursing.* 1997 Mar; 23(3): 18–27.
(ADVANCE DIRECTIVES; TERMINAL CARE)

Perry, Clifton. Children's suits for suffering life. *Pediatrician.* 1990; 17(2): 79–86.
(WRONGFUL LIFE)

Perry, Clifton; Kuruc, Joan Wallman. Psychotherapists' sexual relationships with their patients. *Annals of Health Law.* 1993; 2: 35–54.
(FRAUD AND MISCONDUCT; PROFESSIONAL PATIENT RELATIONSHIP)

Perry, Erica; Swartz, Richard; Smith–Wheelock,

Linda; Westbrook, Joan; Buck, Catherine. Why is it difficult for staff to discuss advance directives with chronic dialysis patients? *Journal of the American Society of Nephrology.* 1996 Oct; 7(10): 2160–2168.
(ADVANCE DIRECTIVES)

Perry, Erica see **Swartz, Richard D.**

Perry, Michael A. see **Anderson, Warwick P.**

Persson, Ingmar. Equality and selection for existence. *Journal of Medical Ethics.* 1999 Apr; 25(2): 130–136.
(GENETIC SCREENING; PRENATAL DIAGNOSIS)

Persson, Ingmar. Harming the non–conscious. *Bioethics.* 1999 Jul; 13(3–4): 294–305.
(ABORTION; EMBRYO AND FETAL RESEARCH; FETUSES)

Peru. Supreme Decree No. 014–88–SA of 19 May 1988. (*Revista de Legislacifn y Jurisprudencia: Normas Legales,* May–Jun 1988, Vol. 152, p. 167–171). [Summary]. *International Digest of Health Legislation.* 1994. 45(1). 36–37.
(ORGAN AND TISSUE DONATION)

Pescia, G. see **Müller, H.J.**

Peshkin, Beth N.; Lerman, Caryn. Genetic counselling for hereditary breast cancer. *Lancet.* 1999 Jun 26; 353(9171): 2176–2177.
(GENETIC COUNSELING; GENETIC SCREENING)

Petchesky, Rosalind P.; Judd, Karen, eds.; International Reproductive Rights Research Action Group (IRRRAG). Negotiating Reproductive Rights: Women's Perspectives Across Countries and Cultures. New York, NY: Zed Books; 1998. 358 p.
(REPRODUCTION)

Peters, Antoinette S. see **Simon, Steven R.**

Peters, Ellen Ash. The care and treatment of the terminally ill: questions raised by *McConnell v. Beverly Enterprises–Connecticut, Inc.. Connecticut Law Review.* 1989 Spring; 21(3): 543–550.
(ALLOWING TO DIE/LEGAL ASPECTS)

Peters, Keith see **Sherwood, Thomas**

Peters, Malte; Ono, Yumiko; Shimizu, Koji; Hesse, Manfred. Selected bioethical issues in Japanese and German textbooks of biology for lower secondary schools. *Journal of Moral Education.* 1997 Dec; 26(4): 473–489.
(BIOETHICS/EDUCATION)

Peters, Philip G. When physicians balk at futile care: implications of the disability rights laws. *Northwestern University Law Review.* 1997 Spring; 91(3): 798–864.
(ALLOWING TO DIE/LEGAL ASPECTS)

Peters, Ted. Should we patent God's creation? *Dialog: A Journal of Theology.* 1996 Spring; 35(2): 117–132.
(GENETIC RESEARCH; PATENTING LIFE FORMS)

Peterson, Mark A. Managed care: ethics, trust, and accountability. [Editorial]. *Journal of Health Politics, Policy and Law.* 1998 Aug; 23(4): 611–615.
(HEALTH CARE/ECONOMICS)

Petrila, John. Ethics, money, and the problem of coercion in managed behavioral health care. *Saint Louis University Law Journal.* 1996 Spring; 40(2): 359–405.
(HEALTH CARE/ECONOMICS; PATIENT CARE/MENTALLY DISABLED)

Petrinovich, Lewis. Morality and animal research: research is...; setting research and educational policy. *In: his* Darwinian Dominion: Animal Welfare and Human Interests. Cambridge, MA: MIT Press; 1999: 239–337.
(ANIMAL EXPERIMENTATION)

Pfeffer, Naomi; Alderson, Priscilla; Campbell, Harry, et al. Informed consent. [Letters]. *BMJ (British Medical Journal).* 1997 Jul 26; 315(7102): 247–254.
(HUMAN EXPERIMENTATION/INFORMED CONSENT)

Pfettscher, Susan. Nephrology nurses, euthanasia, and assisted suicide. *ANNA Journal (American Nephrology Nurses' Association).* 1996 Oct; 23(5): 524–525.
(ALLOWING TO DIE; SUICIDE)

Pfettscher, Susan A. Making decisions about end–stage renal disease treatment: a review of theories and issues. *Advances in Renal Replacement Therapy.* 1997 Jan; 4(1): 81–88.
(PATIENT CARE; PROFESSIONAL PATIENT RELATIONSHIP)

Philipp, Robin see **Limentani, Alexander E.**

Phillips, Alan see **Redenbaugh, Russell**

Phillips, Ben; Reagan, James E. VHA ethics rounds: [truth–telling]. *NCCE News (Veterans Health Administration National Center for Clinical Ethics).* 1998 Winter; 6(1): 4–5.
(TRUTH DISCLOSURE)

Phillips, Benjamin. The Concept of Futility in Medical Care. Ann Arbor, MI: UMI Dissertation Services; 1996 Dec. 159 p.
(ALLOWING TO DIE)

Phillips, Charles D. see **Teno, Joan M.**

Phillips, Donald F. Erecting an ethical framework for managed care. [Meeting report]. *JAMA.* 1998 Dec 23–30; 280(24): 2060–2062.
(HEALTH CARE/ECONOMICS)

Phillips, Donald F. New report rejects accrediting of those who provide ethics consultation services. [News]. *JAMA.* 1999 Jun 2; 281(21): 1976.
(ETHICISTS AND ETHICS COMMITTEES)

Phillips, Russell S. see **Hamel, Mary Beth**

Phipps, Etienne; Shelton, Wayne; Monafo, William; Krizek, Thomas J. Forgoing medical treatment in severe facial trauma. *Journal of Trauma.* 1997 Dec; 43(6): 970–974.
(ALLOWING TO DIE)

Pianelli, James V. see **Angelides, Kimon**

Piattelli, Abramo Alberto. Health, illness, and healing in the great religions: III. Judaism. *Dolentium Hominum: Church and Health in the World.* 1998; No. 37 [yr. 13(1)]: 116–117.
(HEALTH)

Pichayangkura, Chart see **Achrekar, Abinash**

Pickar, David see **Pinals, Debra A.**

Picker, Louis J. see **Ostrer, Harry**

Pierce, Jessica; Kerby, Christina. The global ethics of latex gloves: reflections on natural resource use in healthcare. *Cambridge Quarterly of Healthcare Ethics.* 1999 Winter; 8(1): 98–107.
(BIOMEDICAL TECHNOLOGIES)

Pierce, Jessica see **Mlinek, Edward J.**

Pieters, Toine. Marketing medicines through randomised controlled trials: the case of interferon. *BMJ (British Medical Journal).* 1998 Oct 31; 317(7167): 1231–1233.
(HUMAN EXPERIMENTATION/RESEARCH DESIGN)

Pinals, Debra A.; Malhotra, Anil K.; Breier, Alan; Pickar, David. Informed consent in schizophrenia research. [Letter]. *Psychiatric Services.* 1998 Feb; 49(2): 244.
(HUMAN EXPERIMENTATION/INFORMED CONSENT; HUMAN EXPERIMENTATION/SPECIAL POPULATIONS)

Pinch, Trevor see **Collins, Harry**

Pincus, Harold Alan; Lieberman, Jeffrey A.; Ferris, Sandy, eds. Ethics in Psychiatric Research: A Resource Manual for Human Subjects Protection. Washington, DC: American Psychiatric Association; 1999. 341 p.
(HUMAN EXPERIMENTATION/SPECIAL POPULATIONS)

Pincus, Harold Alan see **Finestone, Albert J.**

Pincus, Theodore; Esther, Robert; DeWalt, Darren A.; Callahan, Leigh F. Social conditions and self–management are more powerful determinants of health than access to care. *Annals of Internal Medicine.* 1998 Sep 1; 129(5): 406–411.
(HEALTH; HEALTH CARE)

Pincus, Theodore see **Stein, C. Michael**

Pinkus, Rosa Lynn. Editorial comment on 'the ethicist's role.' *Clinical Transplantation.* 1993 Dec; 7(6): 565–566.
(ETHICISTS AND ETHICS COMMITTEES; ORGAN AND TISSUE TRANSPLANTATION)

Pinkus, Rosa Lynn B. see **Kuczewski, Mark G.**

Pinto–Prades, Jose–Louis see **Menzel, Paul**

Piot, Peter; Timberlake, Susan. HIV/AIDS and human rights: continued commitment in the second decade. *Health and Human Rights.* 1998; 3(1): 1–6.
(AIDS)

Piot, Peter see **Merson, Michael H.**

Pisetsky, David S. see **Knudsen, Nancy S.**

Pitcher, Linda see **Nachtigall, Robert D.**

Pitkofsky, Rob. Race and tuberculosis: coincidence or correlation? *Princeton Journal of Bioethics.* 1998 Spring; 1(1): 32–41.
(PUBLIC HEALTH)

Place, Michael D. How faith and public policy intersect. *Health Progress.* 1999 Jan–Feb; 80(1): 10–13.
(SUICIDE)

Plachta, Michael. The right to die in Canadian legislation, case law and legal doctrine. *Medicine and Law.* 1994; 13(7–8): 639–680.
(ALLOWING TO DIE/LEGAL ASPECTS)

Platt, Jeffrey L. see **Sachs, David H.**

Platt, M.P. Ward see **West, Charles**

Platzer, Hazel see **James, Trudi**

Pleming, Nigel see **Thomas, Sandy**

Plueckhahn, Vernon D. see **Breen, Kerry J.**

Plum, Fred. Clinical standards and technological confirmatory tests in diagnosing brain death. *In:* Youngner, Stuart J.; Arnold, Robert M.; Schapiro, Renie, eds. The Definition of Death: Contemporary Controversies. Baltimore, MD: Johns Hopkins University Press; 1999: 34–65.
(DETERMINATION OF DEATH/BRAIN DEATH)

Plutko, Lawrence A. Pursuing justice in an era of managed care: Seattle-based system makes room for the underserved and uninsured. *Health Progress.* 1997 Jan–Feb; 78(1): 37–39, 48.
(HEALTH CARE/ECONOMICS)

Pochard, Frédéric see **Letvak, Richard**

Pocock, Stuart; White, Ian. Trials stopped early: too good to be true? *Lancet.* 1999 Mar 20; 353(9157): 943–944.
(HUMAN EXPERIMENTATION/RESEARCH DESIGN)

Poenisch, Carol. Merian Frederick's story. *New England Journal of Medicine.* 1998 Oct 1; 339(14): 996–998.
(SUICIDE)

Poets, C. see **West, Charles**

Pokorski, Robert J. Insurance underwriting in the genetic era. *Cancer.* 1997 Aug; 80(3, Suppl.): 587–599.
(GENETIC SCREENING)

Pokorski, Robert J.; Sanderson, Patricia; Bennett, Nancy; Costanza, Mary; Dicke, Arnold A.; Eyre, Harmon; Hall, Phyllis H.; Hausman, Shawn; Lynch, Jane; Meyer, Roberta B.; Sener, Stephen; Wender, Richard; Zeitz, Kathleen. Insurance issues and genetic testing: challenges and recommendations: workshop no. 1. *Cancer.* 1997 Aug 1; 80(3, Suppl.): 627.
(GENETIC SCREENING)

Poland. Law of 30 Aug 1996 amending the law on family planning, protection of human fetuses, and the conditions under which pregnancy termination is permissable, and amending other laws. (*Dziennik Ustaw Rzeczypospolitej,* 4 Dec 1996, No. 139, Text No. 646, pp. 2885–2888). *International Digest of Health Legislation.* 1997; 48(2): 176–178.
(ABORTION/FOREIGN COUNTRIES; ABORTION/LEGAL ASPECTS)

Poland, Susan Cartier. Bioethics commissions: town meetings with a "blue, blue ribbon". [Bibliography]. *Kennedy Institute of Ethics Journal.* 1998 Mar; 8(1): 91–109.
(BIOETHICS; ETHICISTS AND ETHICS COMMITTEES)

Polin, Glenn see **Kerr, Susan M.**

Pollak, Michael. Doctors fighting backlash over vaccines. [News]. *New York Times.* 1999 Apr 27: F7.
(IMMUNIZATION)

Pollock, Donald. Healing dilemmas. *Anthropological Quarterly.* 1996 Jul; 69(3): 149–157.
(PATIENT CARE)

Pomeroy, Claire see **Carlsen, Mary S.**

Ponjaert-Kristoffersen, I. see **Baetens, P.**

Pontifical Academy for Life see **Vial Correa, Juan de Dios**

Pontificia Academia pro Vita see **Vial Correa, Juan de Dios**

Pörn, Ingmar. The meaning of 'rights' in the right to know debate. *In:* Chadwick, Ruth; Levitt, Mairi; Shickle, Darren, eds. The Right to Know and the Right Not to Know. Brookfield, VT: Ashgate; 1997: 37–42.
(GENETIC COUNSELING; GENETIC SCREENING)

Poroch, Davina see **McAlpine, Heather**

Port, Friedrich K. see **Leggat, John E.**

Porta, Miguel; Busquet, Xavier; Jariod, Manuel. Attitudes and views of physicians and nurses towards cancer patients dying at home. *Palliative Medicine.* 1997 Mar; 11(2): 116–126.
(TERMINAL CARE)

Porter, Elisabeth. Abortion ethics: rights and responsibilities. *Hypatia.* 1994 Summer; 9(3): 66–87.
(ABORTION)

Porter, Ian see **Baumiller, Robert C.**

Porter, Joan P. Regulatory considerations in research involving children and adolescents with mental disorders. *In:* Hoagwood, Kimberly; Jensen, Peter S.; Fisher, Celia B., eds. Ethical Issues in Mental Health Research with Children and Adolescents. Mahwah, NJ: Lawrence Erlbaum Associates; 1996: 15–28.
(HUMAN EXPERIMENTATION/MINORS; HUMAN EXPERIMENTATION/REGULATION; HUMAN EXPERIMENTATION/SPECIAL POPULATIONS)

Porter, John see **Edi-Osagie, E.C.O.**

Portmann, John. Cutting bodies to harvest organs. *Cambridge Quarterly of Healthcare Ethics.* 1999 Summer; 8(3): 288–298.
(ORGAN AND TISSUE DONATION)

Posner, Eric A.; Posner, Richard A. The demand for human cloning. *In:* Nussbaum, Martha C.; Sunstein, Cass R., eds. Clones and Clones: Facts and Fantasies About Human Cloning. New York, NY: Norton; 1998: 233–261.
(CLONING; REPRODUCTION)

Posner, Richard A. see Posner, Eric A.

Post, Linda Farber; Blustein, Jeffrey; Dubler, Nancy Neveloff. The doctor-proxy relationship: an untapped resource: introduction. *Journal of Law, Medicine and Ethics.* 1999 Spring; 27(1): 5-12.
(ADVANCE DIRECTIVES; INFORMED CONSENT)

Post, Linda Farber see Fleischman, Alan R.

Post, Linda Farber see Zelenik, Jomarie

Post, Stephen G.; Whitehouse, Peter J. Emerging antidementia drugs: a preliminary ethical view. *Journal of the American Geriatrics Society.* 1998 Jun; 46(6): 784-787.
(PATIENT CARE/DRUGS; PATIENT CARE/MENTALLY DISABLED)

Post, Stephen G.; Whitehouse, Peter J., eds. Genetic Testing for Alzheimer Disease: Ethical and Clinical Issues. Baltimore, MD: Johns Hopkins University Press; 1998. 284 p.
(GENETIC SCREENING)

Post, Stephen G. see Rakowski, Eric

Poste, George see Fears, Robin

Poteat, G. Michael see Wuensch, Karl L.

Potter, David see Brown, Janet

Potter, Robert; Emmott, Helen. Barney says "no." [Case study and study questions]. *Bioethics Forum.* 1998 Summer; 14(2): 29-30.
(ALLOWING TO DIE)

Potter, Robert Lyman. Treatment redirection: moving from curative to palliative care. *Bioethics Forum.* 1998 Summer; 14(2): 3-9.
(TERMINAL CARE)

Potter, Van Rensselaer. Bioethics, biology, *and* the biosphere: fragmented ethics and "bridge bioethics". *Hastings Center Report.* 1999 Jan-Feb; 29(1): 38-40.
(BIOETHICS)

Potts, John T.; Herdman, Roger C.; Beauchamp, Thomas L.; Robertson, John A. Commentary: clear thinking and open discussion guide IOM's report on organ donation. *Journal of Law, Medicine and Ethics.* 1998 Summer; 26(2): 166-168.
(DETERMINATION OF DEATH; ORGAN AND TISSUE DONATION)

Potts, John T. see Herdman, Roger

Poulakou-Rebelakou, Effie see Lascaratos, John

Pouloudi, Athanasia. Conflicting concerns over the privacy of electronic medical records in the NHSnet. *Business Ethics: A European Review.* 1997 Apr; 6(2): 94-101.
(CONFIDENTIALITY)

Powe, Neil R. see Cooper-Patrick, Lisa

Powe, Neil R. see Gross, Cary P.

Powell, Donald see Slovenko, Ralph

Powell, Donald see Sugarman, Jeremy

Powell, John. Abortion: The Silent Holocaust. Allen, TX: Tabor; 1981. 183 p.
(ABORTION/RELIGIOUS ASPECTS)

Powell, Marion G. Ensuring access to abortion in an era of cutbacks. [Editorial]. *Canadian Medical Association Journal.* 1997 Jun 1; 156(11): 1545-1547.
(ABORTION)

Powell, T. see Sloan, R.P.

Powell, Tia. Consultation-liaison psychiatry and clinical ethics: representative cases. *Psychosomatics.* 1997 Jul-Aug; 38(4): 321-326.
(ETHICISTS AND ETHICS COMMITTEES)

Powell, Tia. Extubating Mrs. K: psychological aspects of surrogate decision making. *Journal of Law, Medicine and Ethics.* 1999 Spring; 27(1): 81-86.
(ADVANCE DIRECTIVES; ALLOWING TO DIE; INFORMED CONSENT)

Pownall, Mark. Falsifying data is main problem in US research fraud review. [News]. *BMJ (British Medical Journal).* 1999 May 1; 318(7192): 1164.
(BIOMEDICAL RESEARCH; FRAUD AND MISCONDUCT)

Poythress, Norman G. see Cascardi, Michele

Prado, C.G.; Taylor, S.J. Assisted Suicide: Theory and Practice in Elective Death. Amherst, NY: Humanity Books; 1999. 223 p.
(SUICIDE; TERMINAL CARE)

Prechter, Gary C. see Kosseff, Andrew L.

Preece, Alan see Evans, Donald

Prentice, Ernest D.; Gordon, Bruce. IRB review of adverse events in investigational drug studies. *IRB: A Review of Human Subjects Research.* 1997 Nov-Dec; 19(6): 1-4.
(HUMAN EXPERIMENTATION/ETHICS COMMITTEES)

Prentice, Ross L. see Brown, Norman K.

Prescott, Nicholas see Merson, Michael H.

Press, Nancy see Markens, Susan

Preston, Thomas A. Physician involvement in life-ending practices. *Seattle University Law Review.* 1995 Spring; 18(3): 531-544.
(ALLOWING TO DIE; SUICIDE; TERMINAL CARE)

Preston, Thomas A.; Patterson, James R.; Hodges, Marian O.; Shorr, Andrew F.; Manfredi, Paolo L.; Morrison, R. Sean; Meier, Diane E.; Quill, Timothy E.; Dresser, Rebecca; Brock, Dan W. The rule of double effect. [Letters and response]. *New England Journal of Medicine.* 1998 May 7; 338(19): 1389-1390.
(TERMINAL CARE)

Preves, Sharon E. For the sake of the children: destigmatizing intersexuality. *Journal of Clinical Ethics.* 1998 Winter; 9(4): 411-420.

(PATIENT CARE/MINORS; TRUTH DISCLOSURE)

Price, David; Akveld, Hans. Living donor organ transplantation in Europe: re–evaluating its role. *European Journal of Health Law.* 1998 Mar; 5(1): 19–44.
(ORGAN AND TISSUE DONATION)

Price, David; Akveld, Hans. Rotterdam Symposium on living organ donation (Rotterdam, 6–7 Nov 1995). [Meeting report]. *International Digest of Health Legislation.* 1997; 48(1): 77–80.
(ORGAN AND TISSUE DONATION)

Price, David P.T. Assisted suicide and refusing medical treatment: linguistics, morals and legal contortions. *Medical Law Review.* 1996 Autumn; 4(3): 270–299.
(SUICIDE; TREATMENT REFUSAL)

Price, David P.T. Civil commitment of the mentally ill: compelling arguments for reform. *Medical Law Review.* 1994 Autumn; 2(3): 321–352.
(INVOLUNTARY COMMITMENT/FOREIGN COUNTRIES)

Priester, Reinhard see **Gervais, Karen G.**

Prilleltensky, Isaac. Values, assumptions, and practices: assessing the moral implications of psychological discourse and action. *American Psychologist.* 1997 May; 52(5): 517–535.
(PROFESSIONAL ETHICS)

Pritchard, Michael S. Conflicts of interest: conceptual and normative issues. *Academic Medicine.* 1996 Dec; 71(12): 1305–1313.
(BIOMEDICAL RESEARCH)

Pritchard, Robert S.; Fisher, Elliott S.; Teno, Joan M.; Sharp, Sandra M.; Reding, Douglas J.; Knaus, William A.; Wennberg, John E.; Lynn, Joanne. Influence of patient preferences and local health system characteristics on the place of death. [For the SUPPORT Investigators]. *Journal of the American Geriatrics Society.* 1998 Oct; 46(10): 1242–1250.
(TERMINAL CARE)

Proctor, Susan see **Baram, Michael**

Project on Informed Consent, Human Research Ethics Group (University of Pennsylvania Health System, Center for Bioethics) see **Moreno, Jonathan**

Proulx, Amy J. Should you call a code? When a patient's condition is terminal, how do you handle a code? *American Journal of Nursing.* 1998 Jun; 98(6): 41.
(NURSING ETHICS; RESUSCITATION ORDERS)

Pulimood, R. see **Rajagopalan, M.**

Pullicino, Patrick M. see **Alexandrov, Andrei V.**

Pullman, Daryl. Role conflict and conflict of interest: a professional practice dilemma. *Journal of the American Optometric Association.* 1996 Feb; 67(2): 98–108.
(PROFESSIONAL ETHICS; PROFESSIONAL PATIENT RELATIONSHIP)

Puplick, Chris. Washington's teeth: patients' rights and dentists' rights -- where are we heading? *Annals of the Royal Australasian College of Dental Surgeons.* 1996 Apr; 13: 221–236.
(AIDS/HEALTH PERSONNEL)

Purcell, Carol. Withdrawing treatment from a critically–ill child. *Intensive and Critical Care Nursing.* 1997 Apr; 13(2): 103–107.
(ALLOWING TO DIE)

Purdy, Laura M. Assisted reproduction. *In:* Kuhse, Helga; Singer, Peter, eds. A Companion to Bioethics. Malden, MA: Blackwell; 1998: 163–172.
(REPRODUCTIVE TECHNOLOGIES)

Purdy, Laura M. see **Donchin, Anne**

Purtell, Dennis J.; Brakman, Sarah–Vaughan. Autonomy and the mentally disabled. [Letter and response]. *Hastings Center Report.* 1999 Jul–Aug; 29(4): 5.
(INFORMED CONSENT/MENTALLY DISABLED; TREATMENT REFUSAL/MENTALLY DISABLED)

Purtilo, Ruth B. What kind of a good is a donor liver anyway, and why should we care? *Liver Transplantation and Surgery.* 1995 Jan; 1(1): 75–80.
(ORGAN AND TISSUE TRANSPLANTATION; RESOURCE ALLOCATION/BIOMEDICAL TECHNOLOGIES)

Putnam, Frank W.; Liss, Marsha B.; Landsverk, John. Ethical issues in maltreatment research with children and adolescents. *In:* Hoagwood, Kimberly; Jensen, Peter S.; Fisher, Celia B., eds. Ethical Issues in Mental Health Research with Children and Adolescents. Mahwah, NJ: Lawrence Erlbaum Associates; 1996: 113–132.
(BEHAVIORAL RESEARCH/MINORS; BEHAVIORAL RESEARCH/SPECIAL POPULATIONS)

Pyeritz, Reed E. see **Grody, Wayne W.**

Q

Qizilbash, Nawab see **Koepp, Robert**

Quaid, Kimberly A. Implications of genetic susceptibility testing with apolipoprotein E. *In:* Post, Stephen G.; Whitehouse, Peter J., eds. Genetic Testing for Alzheimer Disease: Ethical and Clinical Issues. Baltimore, MD: Johns Hopkins University Press; 1998: 118–139.
(GENETIC COUNSELING; GENETIC SCREENING)

Quaid, Kimberly A. see **Smith, David H.**

Quesenberry, Charles see **Grumbach, Kevin**

Quiggins, Patricia A. see **Mold, James W.**

Quigley, Maria see **Edi–Osagie, E.C.O.**

Quill, Timothy see **Karlawish, Jason H.T.**

Quill, Timothy see **Lo, Bernard**

Quill, Timothy E. see **Letvak, Richard**

Quill, Timothy E. see **Preston, Thomas A.**

Quill, Timothy E. see **Stead, William W.**

Quinn, M.W. see **Shah, V.S.**

Quinn, Thomas C. see **Morris, Lynn**

Quintero, Ruben A. see **Evans, Mark I.**

Quiroga, Seline Szkupinski see **Nachtigall, Robert D.**

Quist, Norman see **Shamoo, Adil E.**

Qureshi, Sarah N. Global ostracism of HIV–positive aliens: international restrictions barring HIV–positive aliens. *Maryland Journal of International Law and Trade.* 1995 Spring; 19(1): 81–120.
(AIDS)

R

Rabinovich, Regina see **Matz, Robert**

Rabinowitz, Jonathan. A method for preserving confidentiality when linking computerized registries. [Letter]. *American Journal of Public Health.* 1998 May; 88(5): 836.
(CONFIDENTIALITY)

Rabinowitz, Jonathan see **Bar El, Yair Carlos**

Rabinson, Jakob see **Hammerman, Cathy**

Rachels, James. Ethical theory and bioethics. *In:* Kuhse, Helga; Singer, Peter, eds. A Companion to Bioethics. Malden, MA: Blackwell; 1998: 15–23.
(BIOETHICS)

Radlett, Marty see **Mirsky, Judith**

Rae, Scott B. Ethical issues and concerns about human cloning. *In:* Demy, Timothy J.; Stewart, Gary P., eds. Genetic Engineering: A Christian Response: Crucial Considerations in Shaping Life. Grand Rapids, MI: Kregel Publications; 1999: 278–292.
(CLONING; EMBRYO AND FETAL RESEARCH)

Rae, Scott B.; Cox, Paul M. Bioethics: A Christian Approach in a Pluralistic Age. Grand Rapids, MI: W.B. Eerdmans; 1999. 326 p.
(BIOETHICS)

Raffensperger, J. A philosophical approach to conjoined twins. *Pediatric Surgery International.* 1997 Apr; 12(4): 249–255.
(ALLOWING TO DIE/INFANTS; PATIENT CARE/MINORS; SELECTION FOR TREATMENT)

Raffin, T.A. see **McConnell, L.M.**

Raffin, Thomas A. see **Gilligan, Timothy**

Raffin, Thomas A. see **Koenig, Barbara A.**

Ragas, Rasa see **Jain, Renu**

Rai, Arti K. Reflective choice in health care: using information technology to present allocation options. *American Journal of Law and Medicine.* 1999; 25(2–3): 387–402.
(HEALTH CARE/ECONOMICS; RESOURCE ALLOCATION)

Rainey, R. Randall; Magill, Gerard, eds. Abortion and Public Policy: An Interdisciplinary Investigation within the Catholic Tradition. Omaha, NE: Creighton University Press; 1996. 254 p.
(ABORTION/RELIGIOUS ASPECTS)

Rainey, R. Randall; Magill, Gerard; O'Rourke, Kevin. Introduction: abortion, the Catholic Church, and public policy. *In:* Rainey, R. Randall; Magill, Gerard, eds. Abortion and Public Policy: An Interdisciplinary Investigation within the Catholic Tradition. Omaha, NE: Creighton University Press; 1996: 1–46.
(ABORTION/RELIGIOUS ASPECTS)

Rajagopalan, M.; Pulimood, R. Attitudes of medical and nursing students towards blood donation. *National Medical Journal of India.* 1998 Jan–Feb; 11(1): 12–13.
(BLOOD DONATION)

Rakowski, Eric; Post, Stephen G. Should health care be rationed by age? Yes [and] No. *In:* Scharlach, Andrew E.; Kaye, Lenard W., eds. Controversial Issues in Aging. Boston, MA: Allyn and Bacon; 1997: 103–113.
(PATIENT CARE/AGED; RESOURCE ALLOCATION/BIOMEDICAL TECHNOLOGIES; SELECTION FOR TREATMENT)

Ralph, David see **Swinn, Michael**

Ramsay, Sarah. Call to strengthen UK ban on human clones. [News]. *Lancet.* 1998 Dec 12; 352(9144): 1917.
(CLONING)

Ramsay, Sarah. National body unites UK ethics committees. [News]. *Lancet.* 1999 Mar 20; 353(9157): 993.
(HUMAN EXPERIMENTATION/ETHICS COMMITTEES)

Ramsay, Sarah. UK "Bristol case" inquiry formally opened. [News]. *Lancet.* 1999 Mar 20; 353(9157): 987.
(FRAUD AND MISCONDUCT; PATIENT CARE/MINORS)

Ramsay, Sarah. UK psychiatrists refuse to treat the untreatable. [News]. *Lancet.* 1999 Feb 20; 353(9153): 647.
(INVOLUNTARY COMMITMENT/FOREIGN COUNTRIES)

Ramsey, Gloria see **Mezey, Mathy**

Ramsey, Gloria C. see **Mezey, Mathy**

Ramsey, Scott D.; Hillman, Alan L.; Pauly, Mark V. The effects of health insurance on access to new medical technologies. *International Journal of Technology Assessment in Health Care.* 1997 Spring; 13(2): 357–367.
(BIOMEDICAL TECHNOLOGIES; HEALTH CARE/ECONOMICS)

Rand, Justin. AIDS and HIV: Colorado court upholds privacy rights in disclosure of test results. *Journal of Law, Medicine and Ethics.* 1998 Winter; 26(4): 353–355.
(AIDS/CONFIDENTIALITY; AIDS/TESTING AND SCREENING; CONFIDENTIALITY/LEGAL ASPECTS)

Randall, Vernellia R. Slavery, segregation and racism: trusting the health care system ain't always easy! An African American perspective on bioethics. *Saint Louis University Public Law Review.* 1996; 15(2): 191–235.
(BIOETHICS; HEALTH CARE)

Randolph, Adrienne see **Truog, Robert D.**

Randolph, Kate see **Moore, Kirsten**

Ranjadayalan, Kulasegaram see **Barakat, Khalid**

Ranstam, Jonas see **Nilstun, Tore**

Raphaely, Den. Informed consent near death: myth and actuality. *Family Systems Medicine.* 1991 Winter; 9(4): 343–370.

(INFORMED CONSENT)

Rapkin, Bruce D. see **Costantini–Ferrando, Maria F.**

Rapp, Rayna. Refusing prenatal diagnosis: the meanings of bioscience in a multicultural world. *Science, Technology, and Human Values.* 1998 Winter; 23(1): 45–70.
(PRENATAL DIAGNOSIS)

Rappaport, Shabtai A. Genetic engineering: technology, creation, and interference. *Jewish Medical Ethics.* 1997 Jan; 3(1): 3–4.
(GENETIC INTERVENTION)

Ratanakul, Pinit. Buddhist health care ethics. *In:* Coward, Harold; Ratanakul, Pinit, eds. A Cross–Cultural Dialogue on Health Care Ethics. Waterloo, ON: Wilfrid Laurier University Press; 1999: 119–127.
(BIOETHICS)

Ratanakul, Pinit see **Burgess, Michael**

Ratanakul, Pinit see **Coward, Harold**

Rath, Satyajit see **Basu, Sandip K.**

Ravilly, Sophie see **Robinson, Walter M.**

Raymond, Janice see **Callum, Janet**

Raymond, Lawrence W. see **Merrill, William W.**

Rayner, John D. A matter of life and death. *In: his* Jewish Religious Law: A Progressive Perspective. New York, NY: Berghahn Books; 1998: 130–137.
(ALLOWING TO DIE/RELIGIOUS ASPECTS; DETERMINATION OF DEATH)

Rayner, John D. Euthanasia. *In: his* Jewish Religious Law: A Progressive Perspective. New York, NY: Berghahn Books; 1998: 138–143.
(ALLOWING TO DIE/RELIGIOUS ASPECTS; EUTHANASIA/RELIGIOUS ASPECTS)

Rayner, John D. Medical confidentiality. *In: his* Jewish Religious Law: A Progressive Perspective. New York, NY: Berghahn Books; 1998: 116–123.
(CONFIDENTIALITY)

Rayner, John D. Organ transplantation. *In: his* Jewish Religious Law: A Progressive Perspective. New York, NY: Berghahn Books; 1998: 124–129.
(ORGAN AND TISSUE DONATION; ORGAN AND TISSUE TRANSPLANTATION)

Reagan, James E. see **Phillips, Ben**

Reagan, Peter. Helen. *Lancet.* 1999 Apr 10; 353(9160): 1265–1267.
(SUICIDE)

Reatig, Natalie see **de Jong, Judith**

Reay, Trish. Allocating scarce resources in a publicly funded health system: ethical considerations of a Canadian managed care proposal. *Nursing Ethics.* 1999 May; 6(3): 240–249.
(HEALTH CARE/ECONOMICS; HEALTH CARE/FOREIGN COUNTRIES; RESOURCE ALLOCATION)

Redding, Barbara A. see **Selleck, Cynthia S.**

Redenbaugh, Russell; Phillips, Alan; Fisher, Barbara Loe; Allen, Arthur; Children's Defense Fund; U.S. Centers for Disease Control and Prevention. Are government vaccination programs beneficial? *In:* Dudley, William, ed. Epidemics: Opposing Viewpoints. San Diego, CA: Greenhaven Press; 1999: 86–134, 174.
(IMMUNIZATION)

Reding, Douglas J. see **Pritchard, Robert S.**

Regan, Priscilla M. Genetic testing and workplace surveillance: implications for privacy. *In:* Lyon, David; Zureik, Elia, eds. Computers, Surveillance, and Privacy. Minneapolis, MN: University of Minnesota Press; 1996: 21–46.
(CONFIDENTIALITY; GENETIC SCREENING)

Rehmann–Sutter, Christoph. Liberating gene therapy. [Book review essay]. *Hastings Center Report.* 1999 May–Jun; 29(3): 43.
(GENE THERAPY)

Reich, Theodore see **Chatterji, Somnath**

Reich, Warren Thomas. Experiential ethics as a foundation for dialogue between health communication and health–care ethics. *Journal of Applied Communication Research.* 1988 Spring; 16(1): 16–28.
(BIOETHICS)

Reich, Warren Thomas. The "wider view": André Hellegers's passionate, integrating intellect and the creation of bioethics. *Kennedy Institute of Ethics Journal.* 1999 Mar; 9(1): 25–51.
(BIOETHICS)

Reich, Warren Thomas see **McCullough, Laurence B.**

Reichhardt, Tony. Europe will fly animals on space station. [News]. *Nature.* 1999 Apr 22; 398(6729): 642.
(ANIMAL EXPERIMENTATION)

Reichhardt, Tony see **Butler, Declan**

Reiling, Jennifer, ed. *JAMA* 100 years ago: euphoria vs. euthanasia. [Reprint]. *JAMA.* 1999 Mar 24–31; 281(12): 1068f.
(EUTHANASIA)

Reiling, Jennifer, ed. *JAMA* 100 years ago: the right to die. [Reprint]. *JAMA.* 1999 Sep 22–29; 282(12): 1112*b*.
(EUTHANASIA/ATTITUDES; SUICIDE)

Reilly, Philip see **Handelin, Barbara**

Reilly, Philip R. Carrier screening for cystic fibrosis: a commentary on current legal and social policy issues. *Genetic Resource.* 1991; 6(1): 65–66.
(GENETIC SCREENING)

Reilly, Philip R. Public policy and legal issues raised by advances in genetic screening and testing. *Suffolk University Law Review.* 1993 Winter; 27(4): 1327–1357.
(CONFIDENTIALITY/LEGAL ASPECTS; GENETIC SCREENING)

Reilly, Philip R.; Page, David C. We're off to see the genome. *Nature Genetics.* 1998 Sep; 20(1): 15–17.
(GENETIC RESEARCH)

Reiman, Jeffrey. Abortion and the Ways We Value Human Life. Lanham, MD: Rowman and Littlefield; 1999. 127 p.
(ABORTION)

Reimshisel, Tyler see **Meadow, William**

Reinarz, James A. see **Chavey, William E.**

Reinders, Hans S. Euthanasia and justice: response to "Euthanasia and health reform in Canada" by Michael Stingl (*CQ* Vol. 7, No. 4). *Cambridge Quarterly of Healthcare Ethics.* 1999 Spring; 8(2): 238–240.
(EUTHANASIA; HEALTH CARE)

Reinecke, Robert D. see **Davidoff, Frank**

Reiner, William G. see **Wilson, Bruce E.**

Reingold, Arthur see **Bindman, Andrew B.**

Reinhardt, Christoph A. see **Mepham, T. Ben**

Reinhardt, Uwe E. see **Epstein, Richard A.**

Reiss, Michael J. see **Richardson, Michael K.**

Reiter–Theil, Stella. The voice of the patient: experiences with the patients' medical ethics forum. *Bulletin of Medical Ethics.* 1998 Feb; No. 135: 18–21.
(BIOETHICS/EDUCATION)

Reitman, James S.; Calhoun, Byron C.; Hoeldtke, Nathan J. Perinatal hospice: a response to early termination for severe congenital anomalies. *In:* Demy, Timothy J.; Stewart, Gary P., eds. Genetic Engineering: A Christian Response: Crucial Considerations in Shaping Life. Grand Rapids, MI: Kregel Publications; 1999: 196–211.
(ABORTION/RELIGIOUS ASPECTS; TERMINAL CARE/HOSPICES)

Renal Physicians Association; American Society of Nephrology. RPA/ASN position on quality of care at the end of life. [Position paper]. *Dialysis and Transplantation.* 1997 Nov; 26(11): 776, 778–780, 782–783.
(ALLOWING TO DIE; TERMINAL CARE)

Rennie, Drummond see **Davies, Huw T.O.**

Rennie, Drummond see **Greenfield, Barak**

Rennie, Drummond see **Yank, Veronica**

Resnik, David. Social epistemology and the ethics of research. *Studies in History and Philosophy of Science.* 1996 Dec; 27(4): 565–586.
(BIOMEDICAL RESEARCH; PROFESSIONAL ETHICS)

Resnik, David B. Replies to commentaries. *Bioethics.* 1998 Oct; 12(4): 331–333.
(AIDS/HUMAN EXPERIMENTATION; HUMAN EXPERIMENTATION/FOREIGN COUNTRIES; HUMAN EXPERIMENTATION/RESEARCH DESIGN)

Resnik, David B. The commodification of human reproductive materials. *Journal of Medical Ethics.* 1998 Dec; 24(6): 388–393.
(FETUSES; ORGAN AND TISSUE DONATION; REPRODUCTIVE TECHNOLOGIES)

Resnik, David B. The ethics of HIV research in developing nations. *Bioethics.* 1998 Oct; 12(4): 286–306.
(AIDS/HUMAN EXPERIMENTATION; HUMAN EXPERIMENTATION/FOREIGN COUNTRIES; HUMAN EXPERIMENTATION/RESEARCH DESIGN; HUMAN EXPERIMENTATION/SPECIAL POPULATIONS)

Resnik, David B. The Ethics of Science: An Introduction. New York, NY: Routledge; 1998. 221 p.
(BIOMEDICAL RESEARCH; FRAUD AND MISCONDUCT; PROFESSIONAL ETHICS)

Resnik, David B.; Steinkraus, Holly B.; Langer, Pamela J. Human Germline Gene Therapy: Scientific, Moral and Political Issues. Austin, TX: R.G. Landes; 1999. 189 p.
(GENE THERAPY; GENETIC INTERVENTION)

Resnik, Robert. Cancer during pregnancy. [Editorial]. *New England Journal of Medicine.* 1999 Jul 8; 341(2): 120–121.
(FETUSES; PATIENT CARE)

Reuben, David B. see **Maly, Rose C.**

Revicki, Dennis see **Albert, Steven M.**

Reynolds, D. John M. see **Tramèr, Martin R.**

Reynolds, Don F.; Garrett, Celia K. Avoiding resuscitation in non–hospital settings: *no consent* forms. *Bioethics Forum.* 1998 Spring; 14(1): 13–19.
(ADVANCE DIRECTIVES; RESUSCITATION ORDERS)

Reynolds, Susan see **Margolis, Lewis H.**

Rezabek, Pamela see **Workman, Richard H.**

Rhodes, Rosamond. Organ transplantation. *In:* Kuhse, Helga; Singer, Peter, eds. A Companion to Bioethics. Malden, MA: Blackwell; 1998: 329–340.
(ORGAN AND TISSUE DONATION; ORGAN AND TISSUE TRANSPLANTATION)

Rhodes, Rosamond see **Kuczewski, Mark G.**

Riccabona, U.M. see **Waibel, U.G.**

Ricci, Elena see **Gbolade, Babatunde A.**

Rich, Barbara A. see **Trull, Frankie L.**

Rich, Harlin see **Segal, Eran**

Richard–Hughes, Sharon. Attitudes and beliefs of Afro–Americans related to organ and tissue donation. *International Journal of Trauma Nursing.* 1997 Oct–Dec; 3(4): 119–123.
(ORGAN AND TISSUE DONATION)

Richards, Bill. How a corporate feud doomed human trials of promising therapy. [News]. *Wall Street Journal.* 1999 Aug 6: A1, A6.
(BIOMEDICAL TECHNOLOGIES; HUMAN EXPERIMENTATION; ORGAN AND TISSUE TRANSPLANTATION)

Richards, Cory L. see **Gold, Rachel Benson**

Richards, Edward P. HIV testing, screening, and confidentiality: an American perspective. *In:* Bennett, Rebecca; Erin, Charles A., eds. HIV and AIDS: Testing,

Screening, and Confidentiality. New York, NY: Oxford University Press; 1999: 75–90.
(AIDS/TESTING AND SCREENING)

Richards, Jeff see **Wincze, John P.**

Richards, Karlotta A.; Noblin, Charles D. Sanctions for ethics violations: does licensure of socioeconomic status matter? *Ethics and Behavior.* 1999; 9(2): 119–126.
(FRAUD AND MISCONDUCT; PROFESSIONAL PATIENT RELATIONSHIP)

Richards, Martin. The genetic testing of children: adult attitudes and children's understanding. *In:* Clarke, Angus, ed. The Genetic Testing of Children. Washington, DC: BIOS Scientific Publishers; 1998: 157–168.
(GENETIC SCREENING)

Richards, Martin see **Thomas, Sandy**

Richards, Tessa. Patients' priorities. [Editorial]. *BMJ (British Medical Journal).* 1999 Jan 30; 318(7179): 277.
(PATIENT CARE)

Richardson, Jeff see **Menzel, Paul**

Richardson, Lynda. AIDS groups stunned by vote for partner notification. [News]. *New York Times.* 1998 Jun 20: B2.
(AIDS/CONFIDENTIALITY)

Richardson, Lynda. New Jersey's H.I.V. list: valuable, and still secret. [News]. *New York Times.* 1998 May 29: A1, B8.
(AIDS/CONFIDENTIALITY)

Richardson, Lynda. Wave of laws aimed at people with H.I.V. [News]. *New York Times.* 1998 Sep 25: A1, B4.
(AIDS)

Richardson, Michael K.; Reiss, Michael J. What does the human embryo look like, and does it matter? *Lancet.* 1999 Jul 17; 354(9174): 246–248.
(FETUSES)

Richey, Warren. A vaccination war erupts in military. [News]. *Christian Science Monitor.* 1999 Jan 28: 2.
(IMMUNIZATION; WAR)

Richter, Gerd. Treatment of metastatic breast cancer -- economic and ethical considerations. *Cancer Investigation.* 1997; 15(4): 335–341.
(HUMAN EXPERIMENTATION; PATIENT CARE; RESOURCE ALLOCATION)

Richter, Gerd; Bacchetta, Matthew D. Interventions in the human genome: some moral and ethical considerations. *Journal of Medicine and Philosophy.* 1998 Jun; 23(3): 303–317.
(GENE THERAPY; GENETIC INTERVENTION)

Richter, Gerd see **Fletcher, John C.**

Richter, Jörg see **Eisemann, Martin**

Ricketts, Maura see **King, Susan M.**

Riddle, Mark see **Leonard, Henrietta**

Ridway, Derry. No-fault vaccine insurance: lessons from the National Vaccine Injury Compensation Program. *Journal of Health Politics, Policy and Law.* 1999 Feb; 24(1): 59–90.
(IMMUNIZATION)

Ridzon, Renée see **Kirsch, Michael**

Rieger, Dean see **Back, Anthony**

Rifkin, Jeremy. Who will decide between defect and perfect? *Washington Post.* 1998 Apr 19: C4.
(EUGENICS; GENETIC INTERVENTION)

Rigali, Justin; Law, Bernard; Mahony, Roger; Graff, Sylvester. Proposed sale of two Catholic hospitals to for-profit chain. *Origins.* 1997 Nov 6; 27(21): 362–364.
(HEALTH CARE)

Riggs, Garrett. What should we do about Eduard Pernkopf's atlas? *Academic Medicine.* 1998 Apr; 73(4): 380–386.
(FRAUD AND MISCONDUCT)

Rind, David M. see **Roberts, John**

Rischitelli, Gary see **Uzych, Leo**

Ristinen, Elaine; Mamtani, Ravinder. Ethics of transmission of hepatitis B virus by health-care workers. *Lancet.* 1998 Oct 24; 352(9137): 1381–1383.
(PATIENT CARE)

Ritchie, Janet; Sklar, Ron; Steiner, Warren. Advance directives in psychiatry: resolving issues of autonomy and competence. *International Journal of Law and Psychiatry.* 1998 Summer; 21(3): 245–260.
(ADVANCE DIRECTIVES)

Rix, Bo Andreassen. Brain death, ethics, and politics in Denmark. *In:* Youngner, Stuart J.; Arnold, Robert M.; Schapiro, Renie, eds. The Definition of Death: Contemporary Controversies. Baltimore, MD: Johns Hopkins University Press; 1999: 227–238.
(DETERMINATION OF DEATH/BRAIN DEATH)

Rix, Gary; Cutting, Keith. Clinical audit, the case for ethical scrutiny? *International Journal of Health Care Quality Assurance.* 1996; 9(6): 18–20.
(HEALTH CARE)

Rizzo, John A. see **Bradley, Elizabeth H.**

Roach, William H.; Aspen Health Law and Compliance Center. Access to medical record information. *In: their* Medical Records and the Law. Third Edition. Gaithersburg, MD: Aspen Publishers; 1998: 87–139.
(CONFIDENTIALITY/LEGAL ASPECTS; PATIENT ACCESS TO RECORDS)

Roach, William H.; Aspen Health Law and Compliance Center. Documenting consent to treatment. *In: their* Medical Records and the Law. Third Edition. Gaithersburg, MD: Aspen Publishers; 1998: 62–86.
(INFORMED CONSENT)

Roach, William H.; Aspen Health Law and Compliance Center. HIV/AIDS: mandatory reporting and confidentiality. *In: their* Medical Records and the Law. Third Edition. Gaithersburg, MD: Aspen Publishers; 1998: 213–239.
(AIDS/CONFIDENTIALITY; CONFIDENTIALITY/LEGAL

ASPECTS)

Robb, Carol S. Liberties, claims, entitlements, and trumps: reproductive rights and ecological responsibilities. *Journal of Religious Ethics.* 1998 Fall; 26(2): 283–294.
(POPULATION CONTROL; REPRODUCTION)

Robb, Nancy. The Morrison ruling: the case may be closed but the issues it raised are not. *Canadian Medical Association Journal.* 1998 Apr 21; 158(8): 1071–1072.
(EUTHANASIA/LEGAL ASPECTS)

Robb, Yvonne A. Ethical considerations relating to terminal weaning in intensive care. *Intensive and Critical Care Nursing.* 1997 Jun; 13(3): 156–162.
(ALLOWING TO DIE; TERMINAL CARE)

Robbins, Dennis. Integrating Managed Care and Ethics: Transforming Challenges into Positive Outcomes. New York, NY: McGraw-Hill; 1998. 327 p.
(HEALTH CARE/ECONOMICS)

Roberts, Dorothy E. The genetic tie. *University of Chicago Law Review.* 1995 Winter; 62(1): 209–273.
(REPRODUCTION; REPRODUCTIVE TECHNOLOGIES)

Roberts, E. Francine. Academic misconduct in schools of nursing. *NursingConnections.* 1997 Fall; 10(3): 28–36.
(FRAUD AND MISCONDUCT; NURSING ETHICS/EDUCATION)

Roberts, John; Decter, Sheila R.; Nagel, Denise; Rind, David M.; Szolovits, Peter; Kohane, Isaac S. Confidentiality and electronic medical records. [Letter and response]. *Annals of Internal Medicine.* 1998 Mar 15; 128(6): 510–511.
(CONFIDENTIALITY)

Roberts, Laura Weiss; Battaglia, John; Smithpeter, Margaret; Epstein, Richard S. An office on Main Street: health care dilemmas in small communities. *Hastings Center Report.* 1999 Jul–Aug; 29(4): 28–37.
(BIOETHICS; HEALTH CARE; PATIENT CARE)

Roberts, Melinda A. Child versus Childmaker: Future Persons and Present Duties in Ethics and the Law. Lanham, MD: Rowman and Littlefield; 1998. 235 p.
(CLONING; REPRODUCTION; WRONGFUL LIFE)

Roberts, Melinda A. Present duties and future persons: when are existence-inducing acts wrong? *Law and Philosophy.* 1995 Nov; 14(3–4): 297–327.
(REPRODUCTION; REPRODUCTIVE TECHNOLOGIES; WRONGFUL LIFE)

Robertson, Channing R. see **Hurt, Richard D.**

Robertson, Donald. The withdrawal of medical treatment from patients: fundamental legal issues. *Australian Law Journal.* 1996 Sep; 70(9): 723–746.
(ALLOWING TO DIE/LEGAL ASPECTS; EUTHANASIA/LEGAL ASPECTS)

Robertson, Gerald see **Caulfield, Timothy**

Robertson, John see **Forster, Heidi P.**

Robertson, John A. Abortion to obtain fetal tissue for transplant. *Suffolk University Law Review.* 1993 Winter; 27(4): 1359–1389.
(ABORTION/LEGAL ASPECTS; FETUSES; ORGAN AND TISSUE DONATION)

Robertson, John A. Ethics and policy in embryonic stem cell research. *Kennedy Institute of Ethics Journal.* 1999 June; 9(2): 109–136.
(EMBRYO AND FETAL RESEARCH)

Robertson, John A.; Schneyer, Theodore J. Professional self-regulation and shared-risk programs for in vitro fertilization. *Journal of Law, Medicine and Ethics.* 1997 Winter; 25(4): 283–291.
(IN VITRO FERTILIZATION)

Robertson, John A. see **Bleich, J. David**

Robertson, John A. see **Lizza, John B.**

Robertson, John A. see **Pence, Gregory E.**

Robertson, John A. see **Potts, John T.**

Robertson, Stephen. The ethics of human cloning. [Letter]. *Journal of Medical Ethics.* 1998 Aug; 24(4): 282.
(CLONING)

Robin, Eugene D.; McCauly, Robert F. A Hippocratic oath for our times. *Nurse Practitioner.* 1995 Jul; 20(7): 14–15.
(PROFESSIONAL ETHICS/CODES OF ETHICS)

Robinson, Bruce E. see **Schonwetter, Ronald S.**

Robinson, Carol see **Valdiserri, Ronald O.**

Robinson, J. see **Lui, S.C.**

Robinson, John H.; Berry, Roberta M.; McDonnell, Kevin, eds. Bioethics. *In: their* A Health Law Reader: An Interdisciplinary Approach. Durham, NC: Carolina Academic Press; 1999: 5–72.
(BIOETHICS)

Robinson, John H.; Berry, Roberta M.; McDonnell, Kevin, eds. Death and dying. *In: their* A Health Law Reader: An Interdisciplinary Approach. Durham, NC: Carolina Academic Press; 1999: 339–426.
(ADVANCE DIRECTIVES; ALLOWING TO DIE/LEGAL ASPECTS; EUTHANASIA/LEGAL ASPECTS; SUICIDE)

Robinson, John H.; Berry, Roberta M.; McDonnell, Kevin, eds. Issues in adult health care. *In: their* A Health Law Reader: An Interdisciplinary Approach. Durham, NC: Carolina Academic Press; 1999: 239–337.
(CONFIDENTIALITY/LEGAL ASPECTS; INFORMED CONSENT; ORGAN AND TISSUE DONATION; ORGAN AND TISSUE TRANSPLANTATION)

Robinson, John H.; Berry, Roberta M.; McDonnell, Kevin, eds. Neonates and children. *In: their* A Health Law Reader: An Interdisciplinary Approach. Durham, NC: Carolina Academic Press; 1999: 181–238.
(ALLOWING TO DIE/INFANTS; ALLOWING TO DIE/LEGAL ASPECTS; ORGAN AND TISSUE DONATION; TREATMENT REFUSAL/MINORS)

Robinson, John H.; Berry, Roberta M.; McDonnell, Kevin, eds. Reproduction. *In: their* A Health Law Reader: An Interdisciplinary Approach. Durham, NC: Carolina Academic Press; 1999: 73–180.
(ABORTION; GENETIC INTERVENTION; REPRODUCTION; REPRODUCTIVE TECHNOLOGIES)

Robinson, Paul. Prenatal screening, sex selection and

cloning. *In:* Kuhse, Helga; Singer, Peter, eds. A Companion to Bioethics. Malden, MA: Blackwell; 1998: 173–185.
(ABORTION; PRENATAL DIAGNOSIS)

Robinson, Walter see **Truog, Robert D.**

Robinson, Walter M.; Ravilly, Sophie; Berde, Charles; Wohl, Mary Ellen. End-of-life care in cystic fibrosis. *Pediatrics.* 1997 Aug; 100(2, Pt. 1): 205–209.
(TERMINAL CARE)

Roche, Patricia; Glantz, Leonard H.; Annas, George J. The Genetic Privacy Act: a proposal for national legislation. *In:* Smith, Edward; Sapp, Walter, eds. Plain Talk about the Human Genome Project: A Tuskegee University Conference on Its Promise and Perils ... and Matters of Race. Tuskegee, AL: Tuskegee University Press; 1997: 187–196.
(CONFIDENTIALITY/LEGAL ASPECTS; GENETIC SCREENING)

Roche, Patricia A.; Grodin, Michael A. Why single out pregnant women? Comments on ACOG's recommendations for involving pregnant women in research. *Women's Health Issues.* 1999 Jul–Aug; 9(4): 202–205.
(HUMAN EXPERIMENTATION/SPECIAL POPULATIONS)

Rodney, Patricia see **Blue, Arthur**

Rodney, Patricia see **Burgess, Michael**

Rodriguez, Daniel Torres see **Fusilier, Marcelline**

Rodriguez, Eduardo. Genetic discrimination and health care: ethical reflections. *Linacre Quarterly.* 1996 Nov; 63(4): 30–36.
(GENETIC SCREENING)

Rodriguez, Gonzalo Herranz. Contemporary ethical codes of professional conduct. *Dolentium Hominum: Church and Health in the World.* 1996; 31(11th Yr., No. 1): 33–36.
(MEDICAL ETHICS/CODES OF ETHICS; PATIENT CARE)

Roels, L.; Deschoolmeester, G.; Vanrenterghem, Y. A profile of people objecting to organ donation in a country with a presumed consent law: data from the Belgian National Registry. *Transplantation Proceedings.* 1997 Feb–Mar; 29(1–2): 1473–1475.
(ORGAN AND TISSUE DONATION)

Rogers, Joan see **DeSantis, Joe**

Rogers, Martha F. see **Merson, Michael H.**

Rogers, Wendy A. Menopause: is this a disease and should we treat it? *In:* Donchin, Anne; Purdy, Laura M., eds. Embodying Bioethics: Recent Feminist Advances. Lanham, MD: Rowman and Littlefield; 1999: 203–219.
(HEALTH; PATIENT CARE/DRUGS)

Rohde, David. Black parents prevail in embryo mix-up. [News]. *New York Times.* 1999 Jul 17: B3.
(IN VITRO FERTILIZATION)

Rohde, David. Quietly, DNA testing transforms sleuth's job -- but practice alarms civil libertarians. *New York Times.* 1999 Mar 9: B1, B5.
(DNA FINGERPRINTING)

Rohter, Larry. Brazil rights group hopes to bar doctors linked to torture. [News]. *New York Times.* 1999 Mar 11: A15.
(TORTURE)

Rojanksy, Nathan; Schenker, Joseph G. Ethical aspects of assisted reproduction in AIDS patients. *Journal of Assisted Reproduction and Genetics.* 1995 Sep; 12(8): 537–542.
(AIDS; REPRODUCTIVE TECHNOLOGIES)

Rollin, Bernard E. The moral status of animals and their use as experimental subjects. *In:* Kuhse, Helga; Singer, Peter, eds. A Companion to Bioethics. Malden, MA: Blackwell; 1998: 411–422.
(ANIMAL EXPERIMENTATION)

Rollin, Bernard E. The Unheeded Cry: Animal Consciousness, Animal Pain, and Science. Expanded Edition. Ames, IA: Iowa State University Press; 1998. 330 p.
(ANIMAL EXPERIMENTATION)

Root, Jane; Stableford, Sue. Easy-to-read consumer communications: a missing link in Medicaid managed care. *Journal of Health Politics, Policy and Law.* 1999 Feb; 24(1): 1–26.
(HEALTH CARE/ECONOMICS)

Roper Willson, Nancy see **Baumiller, Robert C.**

Rorty, Mary V. Feminism and elective fetal reduction. *In:* Donchin, Anne; Purdy, Laura M., eds. Embodying Bioethics: Recent Feminist Advances. Lanham, MD: Rowman and Littlefield; 1999: 159–175.
(ABORTION)

Roscam Abbing, Henriette D.C. New developments in international health law. *European Journal of Health Law.* 1998 Jun; 5(2): 155–169.
(CLONING; GENETIC RESEARCH; GENOME MAPPING; ORGAN AND TISSUE TRANSPLANTATION)

Rose, Joanna; Nilsson, Annika. Sweden considers more oversight of research. [News]. *Science.* 1999 Mar 19; 283(5409): 1829.
(HUMAN EXPERIMENTATION/FOREIGN COUNTRIES; HUMAN EXPERIMENTATION/REGULATION)

Rose, Margaret. Animal ethics committees: do we need to re-examine their purpose? *In:* van Zutphen, L.F.M.; Balls, M., eds. Animal Alternatives, Welfare and Ethics. New York, NY: Elsevier; 1997: 361–366.
(ANIMAL EXPERIMENTATION)

Rose, Mary R. see **Tulsky, James A.**

Rose, Steven P.R. Neurogenetic determinism and the new euphenics. *BMJ (British Medical Journal).* 1998 Dec 19–26; 317(7174): 1707–1708.
(BEHAVIOR CONTROL; BEHAVIORAL GENETICS; PATIENT CARE/DRUGS)

Rosen, Elisabeth. Bioethics committees as consensus shapers. *Bulletin of Medical Ethics.* 1999 Feb; No. 145: 13–18.
(BIOETHICS; ETHICISTS AND ETHICS COMMITTEES)

Rosenbaum, Marsha see **Murphy, Sheigla**

Rosenbaum, Peter L. see **Saigal, Saroj**

Rosenbaum, Sara; Frankford, David M.; Moore, Brad; Borzi, Phyllis. Who should determine when health care is medically necessary? *New England Journal of Medicine.* 1999 Jan 21; 340(3): 229–232.
(HEALTH CARE/ECONOMICS)

Rosenberg, James. The voice of God. *Rhode Island Medicine.* 1993 Dec; 76(12): 600.
(EUTHANASIA/RELIGIOUS ASPECTS)

Rosenblatt, Abram see **Attkisson, C. Clifford**

Rosenczweig, Carolyn. Should relatives witness resuscitation? Ethical issues and practical considerations. *Canadian Medical Association Journal.* 1998 Mar 10; 158(5): 617–620.
(PATIENT CARE)

Rosendale, John D. see **Lin, Hung-Mo**

Rosenfeld, Albert. The journalist's role in bioethics. *Journal of Medicine and Philosophy.* 1999 Apr; 24(2): 108–129.
(BIOETHICS)

Rosenfeld, Anne G. see **Tolle, Susan W.**

Rosenheck, Robert; Armstrong, Moe; Callahan, Daniel; Dea, Robin; Del Vecchio, Paolo; Flynn, Laurie; Fox, Renée C.; Goldman, Howard H.; Horvath, Thomas; Munoz, Rodrigo. Obligation to the least well off in setting mental health service priorities: a consensus statement. *Psychiatric Services.* 1998 Oct; 49(10): 1273–1274, 1290.
(HEALTH CARE/ECONOMICS; MENTAL HEALTH; RESOURCE ALLOCATION; SELECTION FOR TREATMENT)

Rosenstein, Donald L. see **Miller, Franklin G.**

Rosenthal, Elisabeth. Scientists debate China's law on sterilizing the carriers of genetic defects. [News]. *New York Times.* 1998 Aug 16: 14.
(EUGENICS; STERILIZATION)

Rosenthal, Elisabeth. West's medicine is raising bills for China's sick. [News]. *New York Times.* 1998 Nov 19: A1, A12.
(HEALTH CARE/ECONOMICS; HEALTH CARE/FOREIGN COUNTRIES; PATIENT CARE/DRUGS)

Rosner, Fred. The definition of death in Jewish law. *In:* Youngner, Stuart J.; Arnold, Robert M.; Schapiro, Renie, eds. The Definition of Death: Contemporary Controversies. Baltimore, MD: Johns Hopkins University Press; 1999: 210–221.
(DETERMINATION OF DEATH/BRAIN DEATH)

Rosner, Fred. The imperative to heal in traditional Judaism. *Mount Sinai Journal of Medicine.* 1997 Nov; 64(6): 413–416.
(AIDS/HEALTH PERSONNEL; PATIENT CARE)

Rosner, Fred see **Margolis, Lewis H.**

Rosner, Mary; Johnson, T.R. Telling stories: metaphors of the Human Genome Project. *Hypatia.* 1995 Fall; 10(4): 104–129.
(GENOME MAPPING)

Rosoff, Arnold J. Informed consent in the electronic age. *American Journal of Law and Medicine.* 1999; 25(2–3): 367–386.
(INFORMED CONSENT; PROFESSIONAL PATIENT RELATIONSHIP)

Ross, Judith Wilson. The Task Force report: comprehensible forest or unknown beetles? *Journal of Clinical Ethics.* 1999 Spring; 10(1): 26–33.
(ETHICISTS AND ETHICS COMMITTEES)

Ross, Lainie Friedman. Children, Families, and Health Care Decision Making. New York, NY: Clarendon Press; 1998. 197 p.
(HUMAN EXPERIMENTATION/MINORS; INFORMED CONSENT/MINORS; ORGAN AND TISSUE DONATION; PATIENT CARE/MINORS; TREATMENT REFUSAL/MINORS)

Ross, Saul; Malloy, David Cruise. Biomedical Ethics: Concepts and Cases for Health Care Professionals. Buffalo, NY: Thompson Educational Publishing; 1999. 192 p.
(BIOETHICS; MEDICAL ETHICS)

Rossel, Peter; Holm, Søren. How does the public perceive the motives of medical researchers for doing research? *Bulletin of Medical Ethics.* 1999 Mar; No. 146: 16–17.
(HUMAN EXPERIMENTATION/FOREIGN COUNTRIES)

Rossel, Peter see **Bjørn, Else**

Rossel, Peter see **Holm, Søren**

Rosser, Sue V. Gender bias in clinical research: the difference it makes. *In:* Dan, Alice J., ed. Reframing Women's Health: Multidisciplinary Research and Practice. Thousand Oaks, CA: Sage Publications; 1994: 253–265.
(HUMAN EXPERIMENTATION/SPECIAL POPULATIONS)

Rosser, Walter W. Application of evidence from randomised controlled trials to general practice. *Lancet.* 1999 Feb 20; 353(9153): 661–664.
(HUMAN EXPERIMENTATION/RESEARCH DESIGN; PATIENT CARE)

Rossignol, Michel see **Druzin, Paul**

Rossiter, Belinda see **Cutter, Mary Ann G.**

Rothenberg, Karen H. Gender matters: implications for clinical research and women's health care. *Houston Law Review.* 1996 Symposium; 32(5): 1201–1272.
(HUMAN EXPERIMENTATION/REGULATION; HUMAN EXPERIMENTATION/SPECIAL POPULATIONS)

Rothenberg, Karen H.; Rutkin, Amy B. Toward a framework of mutualism: the Jewish community in genetics research. *Community Genetics.* 1998; 1(3): 148–153.
(GENETIC RESEARCH)

Rothenberg, Karen H. see **Wilfond, Benjamin S.**

Rothman, David J. see **Lerner, Barron H.**

Rothman, David J. see **Wu, John**

Rothman, Harry see **Glasner, Peter**

Rothschild, Bruce M. see **Kirsch, Michael**

Rothstein, Julie A. see **Swenson, Sara L.**

Rothstein, Mark A. Preventing the discovery of plaintiff genetic profiles by defendants seeking to limit damages in personal injury litigation. *Indiana Law Journal.* 1996 Fall; 71(4): 877–910.
(CONFIDENTIALITY/LEGAL ASPECTS; GENETIC SCREENING)

Rouse, Dwight J. see **Stringer, Jeffrey S.A.**

Rovner, Julie. Politicians squabble over stem-cell research. [News]. *Lancet.* 1999 Jun 5; 353(9168): 1948.
(EMBRYO AND FETAL RESEARCH)

Rowan, Andrew N. Scientists and animal research: Dr. Jekyll or Mr. Hyde? *Social Research.* 1995 Fall; 62(3): 787–800.
(ANIMAL EXPERIMENTATION)

Rowan, Andrew N. The search for animal well-being. *In:* Hart, Lynette A., ed. Responsible Conduct with Animals in Research. New York, NY: Oxford University Press; 1998: 119–131.
(ANIMAL EXPERIMENTATION)

Rowan, Cathy. Court-ordered caesareans -- choice or control? *Nursing Ethics.* 1998 Nov; 5(6): 542–544.
(FETUSES; TREATMENT REFUSAL)

Rowell, Mary see **Koch, Tom**

Rowland, Lewis P. Assisted suicide and alternatives in amyotrophic lateral sclerosis. [Editorial]. *New England Journal of Medicine.* 1998 Oct 1; 339(14): 987–989.
(SUICIDE; TERMINAL CARE)

Roy, David J. The relief of pain and suffering: ethical principles and imperatives. [Editorial]. *Journal of Palliative Care.* 1998 Summer; 14(2): 3–5.
(PATIENT CARE/DRUGS; TERMINAL CARE)

Royal College of Nursing see **British Medical Association**

Royal College of Obstetricians and Gynaecologists. Ethics Committee. Sex Selection. London: Royal College of Obstetricians and Gynaecologists Press; 1993. 16 p.
(SEX DETERMINATION; SEX PRESELECTION)

Royal College of Physicians. Setting Priorities in the NHS: A Framework for Decision-Making. A Report of the Royal College of Physicians. London: Royal College of Physicians of London; 1995 Sep. 38 p.
(HEALTH CARE/ECONOMICS; HEALTH CARE/FOREIGN COUNTRIES; RESOURCE ALLOCATION)

Royal College of Psychiatrists. Consent of Non-Volitional Patients and *De Facto* Detention of Informal Patients. Issued by the Royal College of Psychiatrists, 17 Belgrave Sq., London SW1X 8PG, England; 1989 Oct. 23 p.
(BEHAVIOR CONTROL; INFORMED CONSENT/MENTALLY DISABLED)

Royal College of Psychiatrists. Guidelines to Good Practice in the Use of Behavioral Treatments. Issued by the Royal College of Psychiatrists, 17 Belgrave Sq., London SW1X 8PG, England; 1989 Oct. 26 p.
(BEHAVIOR CONTROL)

Royal College of Psychiatrists. Position Statement on Confidentiality. Issued by the Royal College of Psychiatrists, 17 Belgrave Sq., London SW1X 8PG, England; 1989 Oct. 21 p.
(CONFIDENTIALITY/LEGAL ASPECTS; CONFIDENTIALITY/MENTAL HEALTH)

Royal Dutch Medical Association see **Legemaate, Johan**

Royal Dutch Medical Association. Medical Ethics Committee. Making Choices Professionally. Issued by the Association: Koninklijke Nederlandsche Maatschappij tot bevordering der Geneeskunst, P.O. Box 20051, 3502 LB, Utrecht, The Netherlands; 1992 Aug. 30 p.
(HEALTH CARE/ECONOMICS; HEALTH CARE/FOREIGN COUNTRIES)

Rubenstein, Jeffrey S.; Unti, Sharon M.; Winter, Robert J. Pediatric resident attitudes about technologic support of vegetative patients and the effects of parental input -- a longitudinal study. *Pediatrics.* 1994 Jul; 94(1): 8–12.
(ALLOWING TO DIE/ATTITUDES)

Rubin, Herbert see **Menendez, Roger**

Rubin, Rita see **Waldman, Steven**

Rubinstein, Helena Gail. If I am only for myself, what am I? A communitarian look at the privacy stalemate. *American Journal of Law and Medicine.* 1999; 25(2–3): 203–231.
(CONFIDENTIALITY/LEGAL ASPECTS)

Ruccione, Kathy see **Kodish, Eric D.**

Ruch, Martine see **Lot, Florence**

Ruddick, William. Hope and deception. *Bioethics.* 1999 Jul; 13(3–4): 343–357.
(TRUTH DISCLOSURE)

Rudin, Edward. A critique from the siding: response to "Paradigms for clinical ethics consultation practice" by Mark D. Fox, Glenn McGee, and Arthur L. Caplan (*CQ,* 1998 Summer; 7(3): 308–314). *Cambridge Quarterly of Healthcare Ethics.* 1999 Summer; 8(3): 351–357.
(BIOETHICS; ETHICISTS AND ETHICS COMMITTEES)

Rudy, Ellen B. see **Daly, Barbara J.**

Ruibal, Nike see **Nagy, Anne-Marie**

Rule, James T.; Shamoo, Adil E. Ethical issues in research relationships between universities and industry. *Accountability in Research.* 1997; 5(4): 239–249.
(BIOMEDICAL RESEARCH)

Ruminjo, J.K. see **Marjan, R.S.R.**

Runkle, Anna. In Good Conscience: A Practical, Emotional, and Spiritual Guide to Deciding Whether to Have an Abortion. San Francisco, CA: Jossey-Bass; 1998. 165 p.
(ABORTION)

Runtenberg, Christa see **Boshammer, Susanne**

Rural Advancement Foundation International (RAFI). Endangered or endangering indigenous peoples? *Splice*

of Life. 1996 Dec; 3(3): 5–6.
(GENOME MAPPING)

Rusche, B. see **Johnson, N.E.**

Rushbrooke, Rupert. Knowing me isn't knowing you. *Splice of Life.* 1998 Mar–Apr; 4(4): 6–7.
(CLONING)

Rushton, Cindy Hylton see **Scanlon, Colleen**

Russell, Jeanie. "I'm the most hated physician in America." *Good Housekeeping.* 1998 May; 226(5): 108–111, 180.
(SEX DETERMINATION)

Russell, Paul S. Understanding resource use in liver transplantation. [Editorial]. *JAMA.* 1999 Apr 21; 281(15): 1431–1432.
(HEALTH CARE/ECONOMICS; ORGAN AND TISSUE TRANSPLANTATION; RESOURCE ALLOCATION/BIOMEDICAL TECHNOLOGIES; SELECTION FOR TREATMENT)

Russell, Paul S. see **Sachs, David H.**

Russian Federation. Principles of the legislation of the Russion Federation on the protection of the health of citizens. Dated 22 Jul 1993. (*Rossijskaja Gazeta,* 18 Aug 1993, p. 4–7). [Summary]. *International Digest of Health Legislation.* 1994. 45(1). 3–6.
(HEALTH CARE/FOREIGN COUNTRIES; HEALTH CARE/RIGHTS)

Rutherford, Joan see **White, D.M.D.**

Rutkin, Amy B. see **Rothenberg, Karen H.**

Ryan, Christopher James. Pulling up the runaway: the effect of new evidence on euthanasia's slippery slope. *Journal of Medical Ethics.* 1998 Oct; 24(5): 341–344.
(EUTHANASIA; SUICIDE)

Ryan, Lesley see **Grisso, Jeane Ann**

Ryan, Neal see **Leonard, Henrietta**

Ryan, W. see **Cappelli, M.**

Ryder, Richard D. Painism: some moral rules for the civilized experimenter. *Cambridge Quarterly of Healthcare Ethics.* 1999 Winter; 8(1): 35–42.
(ANIMAL EXPERIMENTATION)

Rylance, George. Privacy, dignity, and confidentiality: interview study with structured questionnaire. *BMJ (British Medical Journal).* 1999 Jan 30; 318(7179): 301.
(CONFIDENTIALITY; PATIENT CARE/MINORS)

Rymer, Janice see **Breimer, Lars**

Ryynänen, Markku see **Heikkilä, Annaleena**

S

Saarikoski, Seppo see **Heikkilä, Annaleena**

Saatkamp, Herman J. Genetics and pragmatism. *In:* McGee, Glenn, ed. Pragmatic Bioethics. Nashville, TN: Vanderbilt University Press; 1999: 152–167, 278–279.
(EUGENICS; GENETIC INTERVENTION)

Sabatino, Charles P. The legal and functional status of the medical proxy: suggestions for statutory reform. *Journal of Law, Medicine and Ethics.* 1999 Spring; 27(1): 52–68.
(ADVANCE DIRECTIVES; INFORMED CONSENT)

Sabin, James E. Fairness as a problem of love and the heart: a clinician's perspective on priority setting. *BMJ (British Medical Journal).* 1998 Oct 10; 317(7164): 1002–1004.
(HEALTH CARE; RESOURCE ALLOCATION)

Sachs, David H.; Colvin, Robert B.; Cosimi, A. Benedict; Russell, Paul S.; Sykes, Megan; McGregor, Christopher G.A.; Platt, Jeffrey L.; Bach, Fritz H.; Forrow, Lachlan; Daniels, Norman; Fineberg, Harvey V.; Fishman, Jay A. Xenotransplantation –– caution, but no moratorium. [Letter and response]. *Nature Medicine.* 1998 Apr; 4(4): 372–373.
(ORGAN AND TISSUE TRANSPLANTATION)

Sachs, Greg A. Dementia and the goals of care. [Editorial]. *Journal of the American Geriatrics Society.* 1998 Jun; 46(6): 782–783.
(PATIENT CARE/AGED; PATIENT CARE/MENTALLY DISABLED)

Sachs, Greg A. Improving care of the the dying. *Generations (American Society on Aging).* 1994 Winter; 18(4): 19–22.
(TERMINAL CARE)

Sachs, Susan. Man accused of assisting wife's suicide. [News]. *New York Times.* 1999 Aug 7: B1, B3.
(SUICIDE)

Sackett, David. The Doctor's (Ethical and Economic) Dilemma: A Description of the Dilemmas Faced by a Physician Who Tries to Serve Both Individual Patients and Society. Office of Health Economics [OHE] Annual Lecture 1996. London: Office of Health Economics; 1996 Aug. 20 p.
(HEALTH CARE/ECONOMICS; HEALTH CARE/FOREIGN COUNTRIES; RESOURCE ALLOCATION)

Sade, Robert M. Cadaveric organ donation: rethinking donor motivation. *Archives of Internal Medicine.* 1999 Mar 8; 159(5): 438–442.
(ORGAN AND TISSUE DONATION)

Sadick, Mary H. see **Byrne, Paul A.**

Sadowski, Alexis see **Daly, Barbara J.**

Saegusa, Asako. Are Japanese researchers exploiting Thai HIV patients? [News]. *Nature Medicine.* 1998 May; 4(5): 540.
(AIDS/HUMAN EXPERIMENTATION; HUMAN EXPERIMENTATION/FOREIGN COUNTRIES; IMMUNIZATION)

Saegusa, Asako. Japan to ban human cloning. [News]. *Nature Medicine.* 1998 Sep; 4(9): 993.
(CLONING)

Saegusa, Asako. Japanese university approves genetic tests on in vitro embryos. [News]. *Nature.* 1999 Feb 11; 397(6719): 461.
(GENETIC SCREENING; PRENATAL DIAGNOSIS)

Saegusa, Asako. Japan's transplant law 'is too stringent'. [News]. *Nature.* 1999 Mar 11; 398(6723): 95.
(ORGAN AND TISSUE DONATION)

Saegusa, Asako. Private deal puts Japanese researcher in hot water. [News]. *Nature.* 1998 Nov 19; 396(6708): 205.
(BIOMEDICAL RESEARCH; FRAUD AND MISCONDUCT)

Saegusa, Asako. South Korean researchers under fire for claims of human cloning. [News]. *Nature.* 1998 Dec 24–31; 396(6713): 713.
(CLONING)

Saegusa, Asako; Nathan, Richard. Japan renews gene therapy efforts ... and plans transgenic medicine guidelines. [News]. *Nature Medicine.* 1998 Nov; 4(11): 1213.
(GENE THERAPY; GENETIC INTERVENTION; HUMAN EXPERIMENTATION/FOREIGN COUNTRIES)

Sage, William M. Fraud and abuse law. [Editorial]. *JAMA.* 1999 Sep 22–29; 282(12): 1179–1181.
(FRAUD AND MISCONDUCT; HEALTH CARE/ECONOMICS)

Sage, William M.; Jõe, Linda; Emanuel, Ezekiel J.; Battin, Margaret P. Potential cost savings from legalizing physician–assisted suicide. [Letters and response]. *New England Journal of Medicine.* 1998 Dec 10; 339(24): 1789–1790.
(SUICIDE; TERMINAL CARE)

Sage, William M. see **Miller, Tracy E.**

Saha, Somnath; Komaromy, Miriam; Koepsell, Thomas D.; Bindman, Andrew B. Patient–physician racial concordance and the perceived quality and use of health care. *Archives of Internal Medicine.* 1999 May 10; 159(9): 997–1004.
(HEALTH CARE; PROFESSIONAL PATIENT RELATIONSHIP)

Sahai, Suman. Bogus debate on bioethics. *Economic and Political Weekly (Bombay).* 1996 Dec 14; 31(50): 3231–3232.
(GENETIC INTERVENTION; GENETIC RESEARCH)

Saigal, Saroj; Stoskopf, Barbara L.; Feeny, David; Furlong, William; Burrows, Elizabeth; Rosenbaum, Peter L.; Hoult, Lorraine. Differences in preferences for neonatal outcomes among health care professionals, parents, and adolescents. *JAMA.* 1999 Jun 2; 281(21): 1991–1997.
(ALLOWING TO DIE/INFANTS; HEALTH; PATIENT CARE/MINORS)

St. Clair, Thomas. Informed consent in pediatric dentistry: a comprehensive overview. *Pediatric Dentistry.* 1995 Mar–Apr; 17(2): 90–97.
(INFORMED CONSENT/MINORS)

St. George, Ian M. see **Briant, Robin H.**

St. Peter, Robert F. see **Cunningham, Peter J.**

Sakai, Akio. Consensus formation in bioethical decisionmaking in Japan: present contexts and future perspectives. *In:* ten Have, Henk A.M.J.; Sass, Hans-Martin, eds. Consensus Formation in Healthcare Ethics. Boston, MA: Kluwer Academic; 1998: 93–105.
(BIOETHICS; BIOMEDICAL TECHNOLOGIES; DETERMINATION OF DEATH/BRAIN DEATH)

Sakakibara, Noriko see **Hamajima, Nobuyuki**

Sakamoto, Hyakudai. Towards a new "global bioethics". *Bioethics.* 1999 Jul; 13(3–4): 191–197.
(BIOETHICS)

Salem, Tania. Physician–assisted suicide: promoting autonomy –– or medicalizing suicide? *Hastings Center Report.* 1999 May–Jun; 29(3): 30–36.
(SUICIDE)

Salem, Tania see **Novaes, Simone Bateman**

Salinas, Jean–Louis see **Flanders, Steven**

Salladay, Susan A. Nursing ethics: growing beyond rules of conduct. *Journal of Christian Nursing.* 1997 Spring; 14(2): 20–23.
(NURSING ETHICS)

Salokangas, Raimo K.R. see **Kaltiala-Heino, Riittakerttu**

Saltman, Richard B. Equity and distributive justice in European health care reform. *International Journal of Health Services.* 1997; 27(3): 443–453.
(HEALTH CARE/FOREIGN COUNTRIES)

Salvucci, Angelo A. see **Koenig, Kristi L.**

Sanders, Arthur B. Do we need a clinical decision rule for the discontinuation of cardiac arrest resuscitations? [Editorial]. *Archives of Internal Medicine.* 1999 Jan 25; 159(2): 119–121.
(ALLOWING TO DIE; RESUSCITATION ORDERS; SELECTION FOR TREATMENT)

Sanders, Arthur B. When are resuscitation attempts futile? [Editorial]. *Academic Emergency Medicine.* 1997 Sep; 4(9): 852–853.
(RESUSCITATION ORDERS)

Sanderson, Patricia see **Pokorski, Robert J.**

Sandquist, Michael A. Do not go gently. *Pharos.* 1996 Fall; 59(4): 14–17.
(HEALTH CARE/ECONOMICS)

Sankar, Pamela see **Merz, Jon F.**

Santiago Delpin, Eduardo A. see **Wu, John**

Santorum, Rick see **Garver, Kenneth L.**

Saperstein, David see **Vorspan, Albert**

Sapp, Walter see **Smith, Edward**

Sarvas, Matti see **Nylenna, Magne**

Sasako, Mitsuru see **Okamura, Hitoshi**

Sass, Hans–Martin. Action driven consensus formation. *In:* ten Have, Henk A.M.J.; Sass, Hans-Martin, eds. Consensus Formation in Healthcare Ethics. Boston, MA: Kluwer Academic; 1998: 159–173.
(BIOETHICS)

Sass, Hans–Martin. Ethics of the allocation of highly advanced medical technologies. *Artificial Organs.* 1998

Mar; 22(3): 263–268.
(ORGAN AND TISSUE DONATION; ORGAN AND TISSUE TRANSPLANTATION; RESOURCE ALLOCATION/BIOMEDICAL TECHNOLOGIES)

Sass, Hans–Martin. Genotyping in clinical trials: towards a principle of informed request. *Journal of Medicine and Philosophy.* 1998 Jun; 23(3): 288–296.
(GENETIC RESEARCH; HUMAN EXPERIMENTATION/INFORMED CONSENT)

Sass, Hans–Martin. Introduction: why protect the human genome? *Journal of Medicine and Philosophy.* 1998 Jun; 23(3): 227–233.
(GENETIC INTERVENTION; GENETIC RESEARCH)

Sass, Hans–Martin. Moral aspects of risk and innovation. *Artificial Organs.* 1997 Nov; 21(11): 1217–1221.
(BIOMEDICAL TECHNOLOGIES)

Sass, Hans–Martin see **ten Have, Henk A.M.J.**

Savulescu, Julian. On the commercial exploitation of participants of research. [Letter]. *Journal of Medical Ethics.* 1997 Dec; 23(6): 392.
(HUMAN EXPERIMENTATION)

Savulescu, Julian. Should doctors intentionally do less than the best? *Journal of Medical Ethics.* 1999 Apr; 25(2): 121–126.
(CLONING; PRENATAL DIAGNOSIS; REPRODUCTION; REPRODUCTIVE TECHNOLOGIES)

Savulescu, Julian. Should we clone human beings? Cloning as a source of tissue for transplantation. *Journal of Medical Ethics.* 1999 Apr; 25(2): 87–95.
(CLONING)

Savulescu, Julian. The cost of refusing treatment and equality of outcome. *Journal of Medical Ethics.* 1998 Aug; 24(4): 231–236.
(RESOURCE ALLOCATION/BIOMEDICAL TECHNOLOGIES; TREATMENT REFUSAL)

Savulescu, Julian. Two worlds apart: religion and ethics. *Journal of Medical Ethics.* 1998 Dec; 24(6): 382–384.
(ALLOWING TO DIE/RELIGIOUS ASPECTS; PATIENT CARE)

Savulescu, Julian see **West, Charles**

Sawyer, Douglas see **Caulfield, Timothy**

Scanlon, Colleen; Rushton, Cindy Hylton. Assisted suicide: clinical realities and ethical challenges. *American Journal of Critical Care.* 1996 Nov; 5(6): 397–405.
(SUICIDE)

Scarnecchia, Suellyn; Field, Julie Kunce. Judging girls: decision making in parental consent to abortion cases. *Michigan Journal of Gender and Law.* 1995; 3(41): 75–123.
(ABORTION/LEGAL ASPECTS; ABORTION/MINORS; INFORMED CONSENT/MINORS)

Schäfer, Dieter see **Kettner, Matthias**

Schaffner, Kenneth F. Coming home to Hume: a sociobiological foundation for a concept of 'health' and morality. *Journal of Medicine and Philosophy.* 1999 Aug; 24(4): 365–375.
(HEALTH)

Schaffner, Kenneth F. Ethical considerations in human

investigation involving paradigm shifts: organ transplantation in the 1990s. *IRB: A Review of Human Subjects Research.* 1997 Nov–Dec; 19(6): 5–10.
(HUMAN EXPERIMENTATION/RESEARCH DESIGN; ORGAN AND TISSUE TRANSPLANTATION)

Schapiro, Renie see **Youngner, Stuart J.**

Schatz, Gottfried. The Swiss vote on gene technology. *Science.* 1998 Sep 18; 281(5384): 1810–1811.
(GENETIC INTERVENTION; RECOMBINANT DNA RESEARCH)

Schatz, Ulrich. Patents and morality. *In:* Sterckx, Sigrid, ed. Biotechnology, Patents and Morality. Proceedings of an International Workshop, "Biotechnology, Patents and Morality: Towards a Consensus," held in Ghent, Belgium, 17–19 Jan 1996. Brookfield, VT: Ashgate; 1997: 159–170.
(GENETIC INTERVENTION; PATENTING LIFE FORMS)

Scheck, Barry see **Handelin, Barbara**

Scheinkestel, Carlos D. The evolution of the intensivist: from health care provider to economic rationalist and ethicist. *Medical Journal of Australia.* 1996 Mar 4; 164(5): 310–312.
(RESOURCE ALLOCATION/BIOMEDICAL TECHNOLOGIES; SELECTION FOR TREATMENT)

Schenk, Maryjean see **Brodkin, C. Andrew**

Schenker, J.G. see **Eisenberg, V.H.**

Schenker, Joseph G. Sperm, oocyte, and pre–embryo donation. *Journal of Assisted Reproduction and Genetics.* 1995 Sep; 12(8): 499–508.
(ORGAN AND TISSUE DONATION; REPRODUCTIVE TECHNOLOGIES)

Schenker, Joseph G. see **Eisenberg, Vered H.**

Schenker, Joseph G. see **Rojanksy, Nathan**

Schenker, Joseph J. see **Eisenberg, Vered H.**

Scher, Richard K. see **Daniel, C. Ralph**

Scherer, Jennifer M.; Simon, Rita J. Euthanasia and the Right to Die: A Comparative View. Lanham, MD: Rowman and Littlefield; 1999. 151 p.
(ALLOWING TO DIE/LEGAL ASPECTS; EUTHANASIA; EUTHANASIA/LEGAL ASPECTS; SUICIDE)

Scheu, Jennifer see **Freilicher, Liza**

Scheuermann, Richard H. see **Ostrer, Harry**

Schiavone, Michele. Ethics and psychiatry. *Dolentium Hominum: Church and Health in the World.* 1997; 34(12th Yr., No. 1): 202–204.
(PATIENT CARE/MENTALLY DISABLED)

Schick, Ida Critelli. Protecting patients' privacy. *Health Progress.* 1998 May–Jun; 79(3): 26–31.
(CONFIDENTIALITY)

Schickendantz, S. see **Borowski, A.**

Schiermeier, Quirin. Animal rights activists turn the screw. [News]. *Nature.* 1998 Dec 10; 396(6711): 505.

(ANIMAL EXPERIMENTATION)

Schiermeier, Quirin. Germans mix support and scepticism for genetic engineering. [News]. *Nature.* 1998 May 28; 393(6683): 299.
(GENETIC INTERVENTION; RECOMBINANT DNA RESEARCH)

Schiermeier, Quirin. Swiss reject curbs on genetic engineering. [News]. *Nature.* 1998 Jun 11; 393(6685): 507.
(GENETIC INTERVENTION; RECOMBINANT DNA RESEARCH/REGULATION)

Schiff, Daniel. Developing *halakhic* attitudes to sex preselection. *In:* Jacob, Walter; Zemer, Moshe, eds. The Fetus and Fertility in Jewish Law: Essays and Responsa. Pittsburgh, PA: Rodef Shalom Press; Freehof Institute of Progressive Halakhah; 1995: 91–117.
(SEX PRESELECTION)

Schimmel, Michael S. see **Hammerman, Cathy**

Schlager, A. see **Waibel, U.G.**

Schlaudraff, Udo. Xenotransplantation: benefits and risks to society. *Bulletin of Medical Ethics.* 1999 Mar; No. 146: 13–15.
(ORGAN AND TISSUE TRANSPLANTATION)

Schlomann, Pamela; Fister, Susan. Parental perspectives related to decision–making and neonatal death. *Pediatric Nursing.* 1995 May–Jun; 21(3): 243–247, 254.
(ALLOWING TO DIE/ATTITUDES; ALLOWING TO DIE/INFANTS)

Schmacke, Norbert. Overdramatization of the burdens on health and social services: a continuing debate in the history of German medicine. *International Journal of Health Services.* 1997; 27(3): 559–574.
(EUGENICS; HEALTH CARE/ECONOMICS; HEALTH CARE/FOREIGN COUNTRIES)

Schmerler, Susan see **Hutcheon, R. Gordon**

Schmidt, Kelli. "Who are you to say what my best interest is?" Minors' due process rights when admitted by parents for inpatient mental health treatment. [Comment]. *Washington Law Review.* 1996 Oct; 71(4): 1187–1217.
(INVOLUNTARY COMMITMENT/MINORS; TREATMENT REFUSAL/MINORS)

Schmidt, Terri A. see **Koenig, Kristi L.**

Schmidt, Volker H. The politics of justice and the paradox of justification. *Social Justice Research.* 1998 Mar; 11(1): 3–19.
(ORGAN AND TISSUE TRANSPLANTATION; RESOURCE ALLOCATION/BIOMEDICAL TECHNOLOGIES; SELECTION FOR TREATMENT)

Schmiedebach, Heinz–Peter. The mentally ill patient caught between the state's demands and the professional interests of psychiatrists. *In:* Berg, Manfred; Cocks, Geoffrey, eds. Medicine and Modernity: Public Health and Medical Care in Nineteenth– and Twentieth–Century Germany. New York, NY: Cambridge University Press; 1997: 99–119.
(HEALTH CARE/FOREIGN COUNTRIES; MENTAL HEALTH; PATIENT CARE/MENTALLY DISABLED)

Schmitt, Roland W. Conflict or synergy: university–industry research relations. *Accountability in Research.* 1997; 5(4): 251–254.

(BIOMEDICAL RESEARCH)

Schneck, Stuart A. "Doctoring" doctors and their families. *JAMA.* 1998 Dec 16; 280(23): 2039–2042.
(PATIENT CARE; PROFESSIONAL PATIENT RELATIONSHIP)

Schneider, Carl see **Swartz, Richard D.**

Schneider, Carl E. Justification by faith. *Hastings Center Report.* 1999 Jan–Feb; 29(1): 24–25.
(TREATMENT REFUSAL/MINORS)

Schneider, Carl E. Regulating doctors. *Hastings Center Report.* 1999 Jul–Aug; 29(4): 21–22.
(PATIENT CARE)

Schneider, Carl E. The Practice of Autonomy: Patients, Doctors, and Medical Decisions. New York, NY: Oxford University Press; 1998. 307 p.
(INFORMED CONSENT; PROFESSIONAL PATIENT RELATIONSHIP)

Schneider, Holm see **Billings, Paul R.**

Schneider, Lon see **Koepp, Robert**

Schneiderman, Lawrence J. Medical futility and aging: ethical implications. *Generations (American Society on Aging).* 1994 Winter; 18(4): 61–65.
(ALLOWING TO DIE)

Schneiderman, Lawrence J. The family physician and end–of–life care. *Journal of Family Practice.* 1997 Sep; 45(3): 259–262.
(ADVANCE DIRECTIVES; ALLOWING TO DIE; TERMINAL CARE)

Schneyer, Theodore J. see **Robertson, John A.**

Schober, Justine Marut. A surgeon's response to the intersex controversy. *Journal of Clinical Ethics.* 1998 Winter; 9(4): 393–397.
(PATIENT CARE/MINORS)

Schoen, Johanna. "A Great Thing for Poor Folks": Birth Control, Sterilization, and Abortion in Public Health and Welfare in the Twentieth Century. Ann Arbor, MI: UMI Dissertation Services; 1996. 267 p.
(ABORTION; CONTRACEPTION; STERILIZATION)

Schoenfeld, Charles N. see **Marco, Catherine A.**

Schoenholtz, Jack C.; Freedman, Alfred M.; Halpern, Abraham L. The "legal" abuse of physicians in deaths in the United States: the erosion of ethics and morality in medicine. *Wayne Law Review.* 1996 Spring; 42(3): 1505–1601.
(CAPITAL PUNISHMENT; SUICIDE)

Schoenholtz, Jack C. see **Halpern, Abraham L.**

Schofer, Joel Martin. Violations of informed consent during war. *JAMA.* 1999 May 5; 281(17): 1657.
(HUMAN EXPERIMENTATION/INFORMED CONSENT; HUMAN EXPERIMENTATION/SPECIAL POPULATIONS; IMMUNIZATION; WAR)

Scholl, Ann. Legally protecting fetuses: a study of the legal protections afforded organically united individuals. *Public Affairs Quarterly.* 1997 Apr; 11(2): 141–161.
(FETUSES; PERSONHOOD)

Schöne–Seifert, Bettina. Defining death in Germany: brain death and its discontents. *In:* Youngner, Stuart J.; Arnold, Robert M.; Schapiro, Renie eds. The Definition of Death: Contemporary Controversies. Baltimore, MD: Johns Hopkins University Press; 1999: 257–271.
(DETERMINATION OF DEATH/BRAIN DEATH)

Schonwetter, Ronald S.; Walker, Robert M.; Robinson, Bruce E. The lack of advance directives among hospice patients. *Hospice Journal.* 1995; 10(3): 1–11.
(ADVANCE DIRECTIVES)

Schoonmaker, M.; Bernhardt, B.; Holtzman, N.A. Coverage of new genetic technologies: what matters to insurers? [Abstract]. *American Journal of Human Genetics.* 1996 Oct; 59(4): A3.
(GENETIC SCREENING)

Schotsmans, Paul see **Gastmans, Chris**

Schreiber, Michael D. see **Paris, John J.**

Schrock, Charles R.; Botkin, Jeffrey R.; McMahon, William M.; Smith, Ken R.; Nash, Jean E. Permission and confidentiality in publishing pedigrees. [Letter and response]. *JAMA.* 1998 Dec 2; 280(21): 1826–1827.
(CONFIDENTIALITY; GENETIC RESEARCH; HUMAN EXPERIMENTATION/INFORMED CONSENT)

Schrooten, W. see **Colebunders, Robert**

Schubert–Lehnhardt, Viola. Issues in the study of medical ethics. *Medicine and Law.* 1993; 12(1–2): 33–39.
(MEDICAL ETHICS/EDUCATION)

Schubert–Lehnhardt, Viola. Selective abortion after prenatal diagnosis. *Medicine and Law.* 1996; 15(1): 75–81.
(ABORTION/FOREIGN COUNTRIES; PRENATAL DIAGNOSIS)

Schubiner, Howard see **Butler, Dennis J.**

Schüklenk, Udo. Access to Experimental Drugs in Terminal Illness: Ethical Issues. New York, NY: Pharmaceutical Products Press; 1998. 228 p.
(AIDS/HUMAN EXPERIMENTATION; HUMAN EXPERIMENTATION/SPECIAL POPULATIONS)

Schüklenk, Udo. AIDS: individual and 'public' interests. *In:* Kuhse, Helga; Singer, Peter, eds. A Companion to Bioethics. Malden, MA: Blackwell; 1998: 343–354.
(AIDS)

Schüklenk, Udo. India fears patent and ethics abuses. [News]. *Nature Biotechnology.* 1997 Jul; 15(7): 613.
(GENETIC RESEARCH; GENOME MAPPING)

Schüklenk, Udo. Unethical perinatal HIV transmission trials establish bad precedent. *Bioethics.* 1998 Oct; 12(4): 312–319.
(AIDS/HUMAN EXPERIMENTATION; HUMAN EXPERIMENTATION/FOREIGN COUNTRIES; HUMAN EXPERIMENTATION/RESEARCH DESIGN; HUMAN EXPERIMENTATION/SPECIAL POPULATIONS)

Schüklenk, Udo; Chokevivat, Vichai; Del Rio, Carlos; Gbadegesin, Segun; Magis, Carlos. AIDS: ethical issues in the developing world. *In:* Kuhse, Helga; Singer, Peter, eds. A Companion to Bioethics. Malden, MA: Blackwell; 1998: 355–365.
(AIDS)

Schulman, Kevin A.; Berlin, Jesse A.; Harless, William; Kerner, Jon F.; Sistrunk, Shyrl; Gersh, Bernard J.; Dubé, Ross; Taleghani, Christopher K.; Burke, Jennifer E.; Williams, Sankey; Eisenberg, John M.; Escarce, José J. The effect of race and sex on physicians' recommendations for cardiac catheterization. *New England Journal of Medicine.* 1999 Feb 25; 340(8): 618–626.
(SELECTION FOR TREATMENT)

Schulman, Kevin A. see **Malter, Alex**

Schultz, Elizabeth A. Informed consent: an overview. *CRNA: The Clinical Forum for Nurse Anesthetists.* 1998 Feb; 9(1): 2–9.
(INFORMED CONSENT)

Schulz, Joerg see **Chandna, Shahid M.**

Schwartz, Jack see **Khanna, Vikram**

Schwartz, John. For sale in Iceland: a nation's genetic code. [News]. *Washington Post.* 1999 Jan 12: A1, A4.
(GENETIC RESEARCH)

Schwartz, Robert see **Chalmers, Don**

Schwartz, William B. Life Without Disease: The Pursuit of Medical Utopia. Berkeley, CA: University of California Press; 1998. 178 p.
(GENETIC INTERVENTION; HEALTH CARE/ECONOMICS; RESOURCE ALLOCATION/BIOMEDICAL TECHNOLOGIES)

Schwindt, Richard; Vining, Aidan. Proposal for a mutual insurance pool for transplant organs. *Journal of Health Politics, Policy and Law.* 1998 Oct; 23(5): 725–741.
(ORGAN AND TISSUE DONATION)

Schyve, Paul. Critiques and new directions [bioethics services]. *SBC Newsletter (Society for Bioethics Consultation).* 1996 Spring: 4–8.
(ETHICISTS AND ETHICS COMMITTEES)

Scofield, Giles R. Exposing some myths about physician–assisted suicide. *Seattle University Law Review.* 1995 Spring; 18(3): 473–493.
(SUICIDE)

Scofield, Giles R. Medical futility: can we talk? *Generations (American Society on Aging).* 1994 Winter; 18(4): 66–70.
(ALLOWING TO DIE)

Scott, Hilary see **White, D.M.D.**

Scott, Jonathan see **White, D.M.D.**

Scott, P. Anne. Autonomy, power, and control in palliative care. *Cambridge Quarterly of Healthcare Ethics.* 1999 Spring; 8(2): 139–147.
(PROFESSIONAL PATIENT RELATIONSHIP; TERMINAL CARE/HOSPICES)

Scott, P. Anne. Professional ethics: are we on the wrong track? *Nursing Ethics.* 1998 Nov; 5(6): 477–485.
(FRAUD AND MISCONDUCT; NURSING ETHICS)

Scottish Action on Dementia. Rights and Legal Protection Sub–Committee see **Gilhooly, Mary L.M.**

Sebire, N. see **Snijders, R.J.M.**

Seckinger, Daniel L. see **Gans Epner, Janet E.**

Secundy, Marian Gray. Ethical literacy and cultural competence. *In:* McGee, Glenn, ed. Pragmatic Bioethics. Nashville, TN: Vanderbilt University Press; 1999: 246–253, 288.
(ETHICISTS AND ETHICS COMMITTEES)

Secundy, Marion Gray see **Mittman, Ilana Suez**

Seedhouse, David. Death's moral sting. [Editorial]. *Health Care Analysis.* 1998 Dec; 6(4): 273–276.
(HEALTH CARE/ECONOMICS; PROFESSIONAL PATIENT RELATIONSHIP)

Seedhouse, David. Ethics: The Heart of Health Care. Second Edition. New York, NY: Wiley; 1998. 232 p.
(HEALTH CARE; PROFESSIONAL ETHICS)

Seely, John F. see **Stead, William W.**

Segal, Eran; Halamish-Shani, Talia; Rich, Harlin; Greenfield, L. John; Fried, Terri R.; Wachtel, Tom J.; Ish, Christopher; Krause, Robert G.; Gazelle, Gail. The slow code. [Letters and response]. *New England Journal of Medicine.* 1998 Jun 25; 338(26): 1921–1923.
(RESUSCITATION ORDERS)

Séguier, Jean–Christophe see **Lot, Florence**

Sehgal, Ashwini R. see **Alexander, G. Caleb**

Seidel, Gill. Confidentiality and HIV status in Kwazulu–Natal, South Africa: implications, resistances and challenges. *Health Policy and Planning.* 1996 Dec; 11(4): 418–427.
(AIDS/CONFIDENTIALITY)

Seiden, Dena J. see **Eiser, Arnold R.**

Seiden, Dena J. see **Kuczewski, Mark G.**

Seifert, Josef. Is 'brain death' actually death? *Monist.* 1993 Apr; 76(2): 175–202.
(DETERMINATION OF DEATH/BRAIN DEATH)

Selby, Joe V. see **Grumbach, Kevin**

Selby, Mary; Neuberger, Julia; Easmon, Charles; Gough, Pippa. Ethical dilemma: dealing with racist patients. [Article and commentaries]. *BMJ (British Medical Journal).* 1999 Apr 24; 318(7191): 1129–1131.
(PROFESSIONAL PATIENT RELATIONSHIP)

Selby, P.J. see **Turner, N.J.**

Selden, Steven. Inheriting Shame: The Story of Eugenics and Racism in America. New York, NY: Teachers College Press; 1999. 177 p.
(EUGENICS)

Selicorni, Angelo see **Sereni, Fabio**

Seligman, Dan. Talking back to the ethicists. *Forbes.* 1997 May 5; 159(9): 198–199.
(ETHICISTS AND ETHICS COMMITTEES)

Selleck, Cynthia S.; Redding, Barbara A. Knowledge and attitudes of registered nurses toward perinatal substance abuse. *Journal of Obstetric, Gynecologic and Neonatal Nursing.* 1998 Jan–Feb; 27(1): 70–77.
(PRENATAL INJURIES)

Sellers, Phil; North Carolina Medical Society. Bioethics Committee. The role of the medical profession in a managed care environment. Statement of the Bioethics Committee of the North Carolina Medical Society. [Policy statement and commentaries]. *North Carolina Medical Journal.* 1998 Mar–Apr; 59(2): 96–100.
(HEALTH CARE/ECONOMICS)

Selwyn, Peter A.; Arnold, Robert. From fate to tragedy: the changing meanings of life, death, and AIDS. *Annals of Internal Medicine.* 1998 Dec 1; 129(11): 899–902.
(AIDS; PATIENT CARE; TERMINAL CARE)

Sen, Amartya. Fertility and coercion. *University of Chicago Law Review.* 1996 Summer; 63(3): 1035–1061.
(POPULATION CONTROL)

Senak, Mark S. see **Coburn, Tom**

Sener, Stephen see **Pokorski, Robert J.**

Seppa, Nathan. Cancer tests can heighten anxiety. [News]. *Science News.* 1998 Nov 14; 154(20): 316.
(GENETIC SCREENING)

Sereni, Fabio; Selicorni, Angelo. General remarks on the ethical problems of pediatric research. *In:* Burgio, G. Roberto; Lantos, John D., eds. Primum Non Nocere Today. Second Edition. New York, NY: Elsevier; 1998: 107–112.
(HUMAN EXPERIMENTATION/MINORS)

Serhal, Paul see **Swinn, Michael**

Serour, Gamal I. Reproductive choice: a Muslim perspective. *In:* Harris, John; Holm, Søren, eds. The Future of Human Reproduction: Ethics, Choice, and Regulation. New York, NY: Oxford University Press; 1998: 191–202.
(EMBRYO AND FETAL RESEARCH; REPRODUCTION; REPRODUCTIVE TECHNOLOGIES)

Serovich, Julianne M. see **Greene, Kathryn**

Serra–Prat, Mateu; Gallo, Pedro; Jovell, Albert J.; Aymerich, Marta; Estrada, M. Dolors. Trade–offs in prenatal detection of Down syndrome. *American Journal of Public Health.* 1998 Apr; 88(4): 551–557.
(MASS SCREENING; PRENATAL DIAGNOSIS)

Sessions, Kimberly see **Wilfert, Catherine M.**

Setka, J. Relationship of medicine and physician toward patient at the advent of the 3rd millennium. *Sbornik Lekarsky.* 1997; 98(1): 11–19.
(PROFESSIONAL PATIENT RELATIONSHIP)

Sever, M.S.; Ecder, T.; Aydin, A.E.; Türkman, A.; Kiliçaslan, I.; Uysal, V.; Eraksoy, H.; Calangu, S.; Carin, M.; Eldegez, U. Living unrelated (paid) kidney transplantation in Third–World countries: high risk of complications besides the ethical problem. *Nephrology, Dialysis, Transplantation.* 1994; 9(4): 350–354.
(ORGAN AND TISSUE DONATION; ORGAN AND TISSUE

TRANSPLANTATION)

Severin, Matthew J. Breast carcinoma litigation: medical questions, legal answers. *Cancer.* 1997 Aug 1; 80(3, Suppl.): 600–605.
(GENETIC SCREENING)

Seward, P. John. Restoring the ethical balance in health care. *Health Affairs.* 1997 May–Jun; 16(3): 195–197.
(HEALTH CARE)

Sewell, Dorita. Introduction [to a set of articles by T.F. McGovern, W.A. Leigh, E.J. Trickett, and J. de Jong and N. Reatig; and a report on the Annapolis Participant Protection Conference held by the Substance Abuse and Mental Health Services Administration (SAMHSA)]. *Ethics and Behavior.* 1998; 8(4): 285–291.
(BEHAVIORAL RESEARCH/REGULATION; BEHAVIORAL RESEARCH/SPECIAL POPULATIONS)

Sewell, Herb see **Kennedy, Ian**

Sexson, William R.; Overall, Stephen W. Ethical decision making in perinatal asphyxia. *Clinics in Perinatology.* 1996 Sep; 23(3): 509–518.
(ALLOWING TO DIE/INFANTS)

Sexson, William R.; Thigpen, Janet. Organization and function of a hospital ethics committee. *Clinics in Perinatology.* 1996 Sep; 23(3): 429–436.
(ETHICISTS AND ETHICS COMMITTEES)

Seydel, Frank see **Baumiller, Robert C.**

Sgreccia, Elio see **Vial Correa, Juan de Dios**

Shade, Starley P. see **Gordon, Nancy P.**

Shaffer, Nathan see **Achrekar, Abinash**

Shah, Monica. Modern reproductive technologies: legal issues concerning cryopreservation and posthumous conception. *Journal of Legal Medicine.* 1996 Dec; 17(4): 547–571.
(REPRODUCTION; REPRODUCTIVE TECHNOLOGIES)

Shah, Nisha; Warner, James; Blizard, Bob; King, Michael. National survey of UK psychiatrists' attitudes to euthanasia. [Letter]. *Lancet.* 1998 Oct 24; 352(9137): 1360.
(ALLOWING TO DIE/ATTITUDES; EUTHANASIA/ATTITUDES; SUICIDE)

Shah, V.S.; Al–Khannan, M.; Quinn, M.W.; Tripp, J.H. Is venepuncture in neonatal research ethical? *Archives of Disease in Childhood. Fetal and Neonatal Edition.* 1997 Sep; 77(2): F141–F142.
(HUMAN EXPERIMENTATION/MINORS)

Shalala, Donna E. A Patients' Bill of Rights: the medical student's role. *JAMA.* 1999 Mar 3; 281(9): 857.
(HEALTH CARE/ECONOMICS; PATIENTS' RIGHTS)

Shamoo, Adil E.; Quist, Norman; Howe, Edmund G. Attempts at suppressing data. [Article and responses]. *Professional Ethics Report.* 1997 Winter; 10(1): 3–6.
(FRAUD AND MISCONDUCT)

Shamoo, Adil E. see **Rule, James T.**

Shandera, Wayne X. see **Alkas, Peri H.**

Shanner, Laura. Abortion, Chernobyl, and unanswered genetic questions. *In:* Donchin, Anne; Purdy, Laura M., eds. Embodying Bioethics: Recent Feminist Advances. Lanham, MD: Rowman and Littlefield; 1999: 85–102.
(BIOMEDICAL RESEARCH; REPRODUCTION)

Shapira, Amos. 'Wrongful life' lawsuits for faulty genetic counselling: should the impaired newborn be entitled to sue? *Journal of Medical Ethics.* 1998 Dec; 24(6): 369–375.
(GENETIC COUNSELING; WRONGFUL LIFE)

Shapiro, Arthur K.; Shapiro, Elaine. The Powerful Placebo: From Ancient Priest to Modern Physician. Baltimore, MD: Johns Hopkins University Press; 1997. 280 p.
(HUMAN EXPERIMENTATION/RESEARCH DESIGN; PATIENT CARE/DRUGS)

Shapiro, Daniel. Why even egalitarians should favor market health insurance. *Social Philosophy and Policy.* 1998 Summer; 15(2): 84–132.
(HEALTH CARE/ECONOMICS)

Shapiro, David. Think before you squawk. *New Scientist.* 1997 Aug 2; 155(2093): 47.
(CLONING; ETHICISTS AND ETHICS COMMITTEES)

Shapiro, Elaine see **Shapiro, Arthur K.**

Shapiro, Kenneth Joel. Animal Models of Human Psychology: Critique of Science, Ethics, and Policy. Seattle, WA: Hogrefe and Huber; 1998. 328 p.
(ANIMAL EXPERIMENTATION; BEHAVIORAL RESEARCH)

Shapiro, Robyn S. In re Edna MF: case law confusion in surrogate decision making. *Theoretical Medicine and Bioethics.* 1999 Jan; 20(1): 45–54.
(ALLOWING TO DIE/LEGAL ASPECTS; INFORMED CONSENT/MENTALLY DISABLED)

Shapiro, Stanley H. see **Glass, Kathleen Cranley**

Sharfstein, Steven S. see **Boronow, John**

Sharif, Shahnaaz K. see **Merson, Michael H.**

Sharkey, Joe. Bedlam: Greed, Profiteering, and Fraud in a Mental Health System Gone Crazy. New York, NY: St. Martin's Press; 1994. 294 p.
(FRAUD AND MISCONDUCT; MENTAL HEALTH; PATIENT CARE/MENTALLY DISABLED)

Sharma, Dinesh C. Indian organ donation goes ahead without consent. [News]. *Lancet.* 1999 Mar 27; 353(9158): 1076.
(INFORMED CONSENT; ORGAN AND TISSUE DONATION)

Sharma, Dinesh C. Indian welfare minister orders compulsory HIV testing for children in care. [News]. *Lancet.* 1999 Jan 30; 353(9150): 390.
(AIDS/TESTING AND SCREENING)

Sharma, Dinesh C. Indian xenotransplantation surgeon seeks damages from government. [News]. *Lancet.* 1999 Jan 2; 353(9146): 48.
(ORGAN AND TISSUE TRANSPLANTATION)

Sharma, Ursula see **Budd, Susan**

Sharp, Richard R.; Barrett, J. Carl. The Environmental Genome Project and bioethics. *Kennedy Institute of*

Ethics Journal. 1999 Jun; 9(2): 175–188.
(GENETIC RESEARCH; GENOME MAPPING)

Sharp, Richard R. see **Wilcox, Allen J.**

Sharp, Sandra M. see **Pritchard, Robert S.**

Sharpe, Virginia A. Ethical considerations? A commentary on ACOG committee opinion 213: "Ethical considerations in research involving pregnant women." *Women's Health Issues.* 1999 Jul–Aug; 9(4): 199–201.
(HUMAN EXPERIMENTATION/SPECIAL POPULATIONS)

Sharpe, Virginia A. see **Weisman, Carol S.**

Shattuck, Roger. Knowledge exploding: science and technology. *In: his* Forbidden Knowledge: From Prometheus to Pornography. San Diego, CA: Harcourt Brace; 1996: 173–225.
(EUGENICS; GENETIC INTERVENTION; GENETIC RESEARCH; GENOME MAPPING)

Shaul, Randi Zlotnik; Mendelssohn, David C. Scarce resource allocation decisions: issues of physician conflict and liability. *Humane Health Care International.* 1997 Spring; 13(1): 25–28.
(HEALTH CARE/ECONOMICS; HEALTH CARE/FOREIGN COUNTRIES; RESOURCE ALLOCATION/BIOMEDICAL TECHNOLOGIES)

Shaul, Randi Zlotnik see **Singer, Peter A.**

Shavers-Hornaday, Vickie L.; Lynch, Charles F.; Burmeister, Leon F.; Torner, James C. Why are African Americans under-represented in medical research studies? Impediments to participation. *Ethnicity and Health.* 1997 Mar–Jun; 2(1–2): 31–45.
(HUMAN EXPERIMENTATION/SPECIAL POPULATIONS)

Shaw, Allen B. Age as a basis for healthcare rationing: support for agist policies. *Drugs and Aging.* 1996 Dec; 9(6): 403–405.
(HEALTH CARE; PATIENT CARE/AGED; RESOURCE ALLOCATION; SELECTION FOR TREATMENT)

Sheckard, Denise see **Webb, Cynthia M.**

Sheil, A.G. Ross see **Wu, John**

Sheiner, Eyal; Shoham-Vardi, Ilana; Weitzman, Dalia; Gohar, Josef; Carmi, Rivka. Decisions regarding pregnancy termination among Bedouin couples referred to third level ultrasound clinic. *European Journal of Obstetrics, Gynecology, and Reproductive Biology.* 1998 Feb; 76(2): 141–146.
(ABORTION/FOREIGN COUNTRIES; PRENATAL DIAGNOSIS)

Shelanski, Vivien B. see **Flanders, Steven**

Sheldon, Sally; Wilkinson, Stephen. Female genital mutilation and cosmetic surgery: regulating non-therapeutic body modification. *Bioethics.* 1998 Oct; 12(4): 263–285.
(HEALTH)

Sheldon, Tony. Dutch regulate sponorship of hospitals. [News]. *BMJ (British Medical Journal).* 1999 Jun 19; 318(7199): 1644.
(HEALTH CARE/ECONOMICS; HEALTH CARE/FOREIGN COUNTRIES)

Sheldon, Tony. Euthanasia endorsed in Dutch patient with dementia. [News]. *BMJ (British Medical Journal).* 1999 Jul 10; 319(7202): 75.
(SUICIDE)

Sheldon, Tony see **Beecham, Linda**

Shelly, Judith Allen see **Kilner, John F.**

Shelman, Keith see **Menendez, Roger**

Shelton, Wayne. A broader look at medical futility. *Theoretical Medicine and Bioethics.* 1998 Aug; 19(4): 383–400.
(ALLOWING TO DIE; PATIENT CARE)

Shelton, Wayne see **Phipps, Etienne**

Shen, Jerome T.Y. see **Byrne, Paul A.**

Shenfield, F. Current ethical dilemmas in assisted reproduction. *International Journal of Andrology.* 1997; 20 (Suppl. 3): 74–78.
(REPRODUCTIVE TECHNOLOGIES)

Shenfield, Françoise. Recruitment and counselling of sperm donors: ethical problems. *Human Reproduction.* 1998 May; 13(Suppl. 2): 70–75.
(ARTIFICIAL INSEMINATION; ORGAN AND TISSUE DONATION)

Shepherd, H.R. see **Coburn, Tom**

Sheppard, Julie see **Abraham, John**

Sher, Geoffrey; Davis, Virginia Marriage; Stoess, Jean. Ethical implications of fertility technology. *In: their* In Vitro Fertilization: The A.R.T. of Making Babies. Updated Edition. New York, NY: Facts on File; 1998: 168–181.
(REPRODUCTIVE TECHNOLOGIES)

Sherr, Lorraine. Counselling and HIV testing: ethical dilemmas. *In:* Bennett, Rebecca; Erin, Charles A., eds. HIV and AIDS: Testing, Screening, and Confidentiality. New York, NY: Oxford University Press; 1999: 39–60.
(AIDS/TESTING AND SCREENING)

Sherr, Lorraine see **Hudson, C.N.**

Sherwin, Susan. Foundations, frameworks, lenses: the role of theories in bioethics. *Bioethics.* 1999 Jul; 13(3–4): 198–205.
(BIOETHICS)

Sherwin, Susan see **Baylis, Françoise**

Sherwin, Susan see **Downie, Jocelyn**

Sherwin, Susan see **Stingl, Michael**

Sherwood, Thomas; Peters, Keith. Publication and promotion: the value of discrimination. *Lancet.* 1998 Sep 12; 352(9131): 896–897.
(BIOMEDICAL RESEARCH)

Shewmon, D. Alan. "Brainstem death," "brain death" and death: a critical re-evaluation of the purported equivalence. *Issues in Law and Medicine.* 1998 Fall; 14(2): 125–145.
(DETERMINATION OF DEATH/BRAIN DEATH)

Shewmon, D. Alan. Recovery from "brain death": a neurologist's apologia. *Linacre Quarterly.* 1997 Feb; 64(1): 30–96.
(DETERMINATION OF DEATH/BRAIN DEATH; PERSONHOOD)

Shickle, Darren. Do 'all men desire to know'? A right of society to choose not to know about the genetics of personality traits. *In:* Chadwick, Ruth; Levitt, Mairi; Shickle, Darren, eds. The Right to Know and the Right Not to Know. Brookfield, VT: Ashgate; 1997: 69–77.
(BEHAVIORAL GENETICS; GENETIC RESEARCH)

Shickle, Darren see **Chadwick, Ruth**

Shield, Charles F. see **Lin, Hung–Mo**

Shih, Anthony see **Dwyer, James**

Shikiar, Rich see **Albert, Steven M.**

Shimizu, Koji see **Peters, Malte**

Shiner, Keith. Medical futility: a futile concept? [Note]. *Washington and Lee Law Review.* 1996; 53(2): 803–848.
(ALLOWING TO DIE/LEGAL ASPECTS)

Shlafman, Michael see **Bar El, Yair Carlos**

Shoemaker, Wendy E. see **Murphy, Michael J.**

Shoham–Vardi, Ilana see **Sheiner, Eyal**

Shorr, Andrew F. see **Preston, Thomas A.**

Showstack, Jonathan; Katz, Patricia P.; Lake, John R.; Brown, Robert S.; Dudley, R. Adams; Belle, Steven; Wiesner, Russell H.; Zetterman, Rowen K.; Everhart, James; National Institute of Diabetes and Digestive and Kidney Diseases. Liver Transplantation Database Group. Resource utilization in liver transplantation: effects of patient characteristics and clinical practice. *JAMA.* 1999 Apr 21; 281(15): 1381–1386.
(HEALTH CARE/ECONOMICS; ORGAN AND TISSUE TRANSPLANTATION; RESOURCE ALLOCATION/BIOMEDICAL TECHNOLOGIES)

Shrier, Ian see **Druzin, Paul**

Shuchman, Miriam. Independent review adds to controversy at Sick Kids. *Canadian Medical Association Journal.* 1999 Feb 9; 160(3): 386–388.
(BIOMEDICAL RESEARCH; HUMAN EXPERIMENTATION/FOREIGN COUNTRIES)

Shuchman, Miriam see **Kern, David G.**

Shulkin, David J. see **Bernard, David B.**

Shuman, C. see **Malkin, D.**

Sibbald, Barbara. Blood recipients and CJD: to notify or not to notify, that is the question. *Canadian Medical Association Journal.* 1998 Oct 6; 159(7): 829–831.
(BLOOD DONATION; TRUTH DISCLOSURE)

Sibbald, Barbara. CMA says no to mandatory hepatitis B vaccination, screening for MDs. *Canadian Medical Association Journal.* 1998 Jul 14; 159(1): 64–65.
(IMMUNIZATION; MASS SCREENING)

Siddiqui, Ataullah. Ethics in Islam: key concepts and contemporary challenges. *Journal of Moral Education.* 1997 Dec; 26(4): 423–431.
(BIOETHICS)

Sidley, Pat. Doctors contributed to poor health of black South Africans. [News]. *BMJ (British Medical Journal).* 1998 Nov 7; 317(7168): 1269.
(FRAUD AND MISCONDUCT; HEALTH CARE/FOREIGN COUNTRIES)

Sidley, Pat. South African research into AIDS "cure" severely criticised. [News]. *BMJ (British Medical Journal).* 1997 Mar 15; 314(7083): 771.
(AIDS/HUMAN EXPERIMENTATION; FRAUD AND MISCONDUCT; HUMAN EXPERIMENTATION/FOREIGN COUNTRIES)

Sidney, Stephen see **Krieger, Nancy**

Siegal, Nina. Critics say inmates again are shackled in childbirth. [News]. *New York Times.* 1999 Apr 11: 33.
(PATIENT CARE)

Siegel–Itzkovich, Judy see **Beecham, Linda**

Siegel, Mark C. Lethal pity: the Oregon Death with Dignity Act, its implications for the disabled, and the struggle for equality in an able–bodied world. *Law and Inequality.* 1998 Winter; 16(1): 259–288.
(SUICIDE)

Siegler, Mark see **McKenzie, John K.**

Sierra, Silvia see **Flanders, Steven**

Silberner, Joanne. Federal science policy: changing battle lines, new fronts. *Hastings Center Report.* 1999 Jul–Aug; 29(4): 6.
(BIOMEDICAL RESEARCH)

Silberner, Joanne. Turning pages, if not heads. *Hastings Center Report.* 1999 Mar–Apr; 29(2): 6.
(EMBRYO AND FETAL RESEARCH; ETHICISTS AND ETHICS COMMITTEES)

Silva, Mary Cipriano. Ethics of consumer rights in managed care. *NursingConnections.* 1997 Summer; 10(2): 24–26.
(HEALTH CARE/ECONOMICS; PATIENTS' RIGHTS)

Silva, Mary Cipriano. New ANA [American Nurses Association] guidelines for ethics in nursing research. *NursingConnections.* 1996 Summer; 9(2): 28–33.
(HUMAN EXPERIMENTATION; NURSING ETHICS)

Silver, Lee M. see **Golden, Frederic**

Silver, Lee M. see **Wright, Robert**

Silverberg, Heather L. see **Koenig, Barbara A.**

Silverman, Henry see **Khanna, Vikram**

Silverman, Jerald. The use of animals in biomedical research and teaching: searching for a common goal. *Cambridge Quarterly of Healthcare Ethics.* 1999 Winter; 8(1): 64–72.
(ANIMAL EXPERIMENTATION)

Silverman, Marvin see **Ferris, Lorraine E.**

Silverman, Ralph. Informing the cancer patient. *Missouri Medicine.* 1997 Jul; 94(7): 317–318.
(TRUTH DISCLOSURE)

Silverman, William A. Where's the Evidence? Controversies in Modern Medicine. New York, NY: Oxford University Press; 1998. 259 p.
(BIOETHICS; HUMAN EXPERIMENTATION/MINORS; HUMAN EXPERIMENTATION/RESEARCH DESIGN; PATIENT CARE/MINORS)

Silvers, Anita. A fatal attraction to normalizing: treating disabilities as deviations from "species-typical" functioning. *In:* Parens, Erik, ed. Enhancing Human Traits: Ethical and Social Implications. Washington, DC: Georgetown University Press; 1998: 95–123.
(BIOMEDICAL TECHNOLOGIES; HEALTH; HEALTH CARE; RESOURCE ALLOCATION/BIOMEDICAL TECHNOLOGIES)

Silvers, Anita. On not iterating women's disability: a crossover perspective on genetic dilemmas. *In:* Donchin, Anne; Purdy, Laura M., eds. Embodying Bioethics: Recent Feminist Advances. Lanham, MD: Rowman and Littlefield; 1999: 177–202.
(BIOETHICS; GENETIC COUNSELING)

Silvers, Anita; Wasserman, David; Mahowald, Mary B. Disability, Difference, Discrimination: Perspectives on Justice in Bioethics and Public Policy. Lanham, MD: Rowman and Littlefield; 1998. 343 p.
(PATIENT CARE)

Silversides, Ann. Private sector becoming the key to research funding in Canada. *Canadian Medical Association Journal.* 1998 Aug 25; 159(4): 397–398.
(BIOMEDICAL RESEARCH)

Silversides, Ann. With HIV prevalence among women increasing, more provinces encourage prenatal testing. *Canadian Medical Association Journal.* 1998 Jun 2; 158(11): 1518–1519.
(AIDS/TESTING AND SCREENING)

Sim, Julius. Respect for autonomy: issues in neurological rehabilitation. *Clinical Rehabilitation.* 1998 Feb; 12(1): 3–10.
(PATIENT CARE)

Simini, Bruno. Italy moves on with in-vitro fertilisation legislation. [News]. *Lancet.* 1999 Jun 5; 353(9168): 1950.
(IN VITRO FERTILIZATION; REPRODUCTIVE TECHNOLOGIES)

Simini, Bruno. US human organ dealer arrested in Italy. [News]. *Lancet.* 1998 Oct 17; 352(9136): 1289.
(ORGAN AND TISSUE DONATION)

Siminoff, Laura A.; Arnold, Robert. Increasing organ donation in the African–American community: altruism in the face of an untrustworthy system. [Editorial]. *Annals of Internal Medicine.* 1999 Apr 6; 130(7): 607–609.
(ORGAN AND TISSUE DONATION)

Siminoff, Laura A.; Bloch, Alexia. American attitudes and beliefs about brain death: the empirical literature. *In:* Youngner, Stuart J.; Arnold, Robert M.; Schapiro, Renie, eds. The Definition of Death: Contemporary Controversies. Baltimore, MD: Johns Hopkins University Press; 1999: 183–193.
(DETERMINATION OF DEATH/BRAIN DEATH; ORGAN AND TISSUE DONATION)

Siminoff, Laura A. see **Arnold, Robert M.**

Simon, Alfred. Establishing clinical [healthcare] ethics committees in Germany. [Letter]. *HEC (HealthCare Ethics Committee) Forum.* 1998 Sep–Dec; 10(3–4): 359–360.
(ETHICISTS AND ETHICS COMMITTEES)

Simon, Frank G. see **Byrne, Paul A.**

Simon, Philippe see **Lot, Florence**

Simon, Rita J. see **Scherer, Jennifer M.**

Simon, Steven R.; Pan, Richard J.D.; Sullivan, Amy M.; Clark–Chiarelli, Nancy; Connelly, Maureen T.; Peters, Antoinette S.; Singer, Judith D.; Inui, Thomas S.; Block, Susan D. Views of managed care: a survey of students, residents, faculty, and deans at medical schools in the United States. *New England Journal of Medicine.* 1999 Mar 25; 340(12): 928–936.
(HEALTH CARE/ECONOMICS)

Simonds, R.J. see **Merson, Michael H.**

Simone, Charles B. see **Charlton, Rodger**

Simone, Charles B., II see **Charlton, Rodger**

Simone, Nicole L. see **Charlton, Rodger**

Simpson, Wendy M.; Johnstone, Frank D.; Goldberg, David J.; Gormley, Siobhan M.; Hart, Graham J. Antenatal HIV testing: assessment of a routine voluntary approach. *BMJ (British Medical Journal).* 1999 Jun 19; 318(7199): 1660–1661.
(AIDS/TESTING AND SCREENING)

Simpson, William G. A different kind of Holocaust: from euthanasia to tyranny. *Linacre Quarterly.* 1997 Aug; 64(3): 87–92.
(ABORTION; EUTHANASIA; SUICIDE)

Sims, Calvin. Using gifts as bait, Peru sterilizes poor women. [News]. *New York Times.* 1998 Feb 15: 1, 12.
(STERILIZATION)

Singer, Beth J. Mental illness: rights, competence, and communication. *In:* McGee, Glenn, ed. Pragmatic Bioethics. Nashville, TN: Vanderbilt University Press; 1999: 141–151, 275–278.
(TREATMENT REFUSAL/MENTALLY DISABLED)

Singer, Judith D. see **Simon, Steven R.**

Singer, Maxine see **Berg, Paul**

Singer, Peter. Ethics into Action: Henry Spira and the Animal Rights Movement. Lanham, MD: Rowman and Littlefield; 1998. 222 p.
(ANIMAL EXPERIMENTATION)

Singer, Peter. Henry Spira's search for common ground on animal testing. *Cambridge Quarterly of Healthcare Ethics.* 1999 Winter; 8(1): 9–22.
(ANIMAL EXPERIMENTATION)

Singer, Peter. Living and dying. [Interview]. *Psychology Today.* 1999 Jan-Feb; 32(1): 56–59, 78–79.
(ANIMAL EXPERIMENTATION; ETHICISTS AND ETHICS

COMMITTEES; EUTHANASIA)

Singer, Peter; Kuhse, Helga. More on euthanasia: a response to Pauer–Studer. *Monist.* 1993 Apr; 76(2): 158–174.
(ALLOWING TO DIE; ALLOWING TO DIE/INFANTS; EUTHANASIA)

Singer, Peter see **Kuhse, Helga**

Singer, Peter A. University of Toronto Centre for Bioethics living will. *Ontario Medical Review.* 1993 Jan: 35, 37, 39–41.
(ADVANCE DIRECTIVES)

Singer, Peter A.; MacDonald, Neil. Bioethics for clinicians: 15. Quality end–of–life care. *Canadian Medical Association Journal.* 1998 Jul 28; 159(2): 159–162.
(TERMINAL CARE)

Singer, Peter A.; Martin, Douglas K.; Kelner, Merrijoy. Quality end–of–life care: patients' perspectives. *JAMA.* 1999 Jan 13; 281(2): 163–168.
(TERMINAL CARE)

Singer, Peter A.; Shaul, Randi Zlotnik. Resource allocation in coronary revascularization. *Canadian Journal of Cardiology.* 1997 Dec; 13(Suppl. D): 64D–66D.
(HEALTH CARE/FOREIGN COUNTRIES; RESOURCE ALLOCATION/BIOMEDICAL TECHNOLOGIES)

Singer, Peter A. see **Aikman, Peter J.**

Singer, Peter A. see **Colebunders, Robert**

Singer, Peter A. see **Martin, Douglas K.**

Singer, Peter A. see **Weijer, Charles**

Singh, Meharban. Ethical considerations in pediatric intensive care unit: Indian perspective. [Editorial]. *Indian Pediatrics.* 1996 Apr; 33(4): 271–278.
(ALLOWING TO DIE; PATIENT CARE/MINORS)

Siriwasin, Wimol see **Achrekar, Abinash**

Sistrunk, Shyrl see **Schulman, Kevin A.**

Sitter–Liver, B. see **Müller, H.J.**

Skene, Loane. Patients' rights or family responsibilities? Two approaches to genetic testing. *Medical Law Review.* 1998 Spring; 6(1): 1–41.
(GENETIC SCREENING)

Skene, Loane; Charlesworth, Max. The new genetics: legal and ethical implications for medicine. [Editorial]. *Medical Journal of Australia.* 1996 Sep 16; 165(6): 301–302.
(GENETIC SCREENING)

Skinner, Andrew see **Breimer, Lars**

Sklar, Ron see **Ritchie, Janet**

Skolnick, Andrew A. Critics denounce staffing jails and prisons with physicians convicted of misconduct. [News]. *JAMA.* 1998 Oct 28; 280(16): 1391–1392.
(FRAUD AND MISCONDUCT; PATIENT CARE)

Skolnick, Andrew A. Drug firm suit fails to halt

publication of Canadian Health Technology Report. [News]. *JAMA.* 1998 Aug 26; 280(8): 683–684.
(BIOMEDICAL RESEARCH; BIOMEDICAL TECHNOLOGIES)

Skolnick, Andrew A. Prison deaths spotlight how boards handle impaired, disciplined physicians. [News]. *JAMA.* 1998 Oct 28; 280(16): 1387–1390.
(FRAUD AND MISCONDUCT; PATIENT CARE)

Slevin, Eamonn see **Long, Ann**

Sloan, R.P.; Bagiella, E.; Powell, T. Religion, spirituality, and medicine. *Lancet.* 1999 Feb 20; 353(9153): 664–667.
(HEALTH; PATIENT CARE)

Slomka, Jacquelyn; Agich, George J.; Stagno, Susan J.; Smith, Martin L. Physical restraint elimination in the acute care setting: ethical considerations. *HEC (HealthCare Ethics Committee) Forum.* 1998 Sep–Dec; 10(3–4): 244–262.
(BEHAVIOR CONTROL; PATIENT CARE/MENTALLY DISABLED)

Slomka, Jacquelyn see **Lawry, Kathleen**

Slovenko, Ralph. Informed consent: information about the physician. *Medicine and Law.* 1994; 13(5–6): 467–472.
(AIDS/HEALTH PERSONNEL; INFORMED CONSENT)

Slovenko, Ralph. Psychotherapy and Confidentiality: Testimonial Privileged Communication, Breach of Confidentiality, and Reporting Duties. Springfield, IL: Charles C. Thomas; 1998. 640 p.
(CONFIDENTIALITY/MENTAL HEALTH)

Slovenko, Ralph; Sugarman, Jeremy; McCrory, Douglas C.; Powell, Donald; Krasny, Alex; Adams, Betsy; Ball, Eric; Cassell, Cynthia. Why study informed consent? [Letter and response]. *Hastings Center Report.* 1999 Jul–Aug; 29(4): 4.
(INFORMED CONSENT)

Slovenko, Ralph see **Bursztajn, Harold J.**

Sly, R. Michael. Ethical scientific writing and responsible medical practice. *Annals of Allergy, Asthma, and Immunology.* 1997 Dec; 79(6): 489–494.
(BIOMEDICAL RESEARCH; FRAUD AND MISCONDUCT)

Sly, William S. When does human life begin? Does science provide the answer? *In:* Rainey, R. Randall; Magill, Gerard, eds. Abortion and Public Policy: An Interdisciplinary Investigation within the Catholic Tradition. Omaha, NE: Creighton University Press; 1996: 62–71.
(FETUSES; PERSONHOOD)

Smit, D. Van Zyl. Reconciling the irreconcilable? Recent developments in the German law on abortion. *Medical Law Review.* 1994 Autumn; 2(3): 302–320.
(ABORTION/FOREIGN COUNTRIES; ABORTION/LEGAL ASPECTS)

Smith, Alexander McCall. Beyond autonomy. *Journal of Contemporary Health Law and Policy.* 1997 Fall; 14(1): 23–39.
(BIOETHICS)

Smith, Alexander McCall see **Gilhooly, Mary L.M.**

Smith, Carol M. see Lin, Hung-Mo

Smith, David Barton. Addressing racial inequities in health care: civil rights monitoring and report cards. *Journal of Health Politics, Policy and Law.* 1998 Feb; 23(1): 75–105.
(HEALTH CARE)

Smith, David Gary see Wong, Jeffrey G.

Smith, David H. Communication as a reflection of, and a source for, values in health. *Journal of Applied Communication Research.* 1988 Spring; 16(1): 29–38.
(HEALTH CARE)

Smith, David H. Ethics in the doctor-patient relationship. *Critical Care Clinics.* 1996 Jan; 12(1): 179–197.
(PROFESSIONAL PATIENT RELATIONSHIP)

Smith, David H.; Quaid, Kimberly A.; Dworkin, Roger B.; Gramelspacher, Gregory P.; Granbois, Judith A.; Vance, Gail H. Early Warning: Cases and Ethical Guidance for Presymptomatic Testing in Genetic Disease. Bloomington, IN: Indiana University Press; 1998. 188 p.
(GENETIC COUNSELING; GENETIC SCREENING)

Smith, David M. see Lee, Melinda A.

Smith, Edward; Sapp, Walter, eds. Plain Talk about the Human Genome Project: A Tuskegee University Conference on Its Promise and Perils...and Matters of Race. Tuskegee, AL: Tuskegee University Press; 1997. 292 p.
(GENOME MAPPING)

Smith, G. Kenneth; Kettelberger, Denise M. Patents and the Human Genome Project. *AIPLA Quarterly Journal (American Intellectual Property Law Association).* 1994; 22(1): 27–64.
(GENOME MAPPING)

Smith, George P. Assisted reproductive technologies: artificial insemination, surrogation, and *in vitro* fertilization. *In: his* Family Values and the New Society: Dilemmas of the 21st Century. Westport, CT: Praeger; 1998: 95–140.
(REPRODUCTIVE TECHNOLOGIES)

Smith, George P. Bioethics and the Administration of Justice. Available from the author, Catholic University of America School of Law, 3600 John McCormack Rd., NE, Washington, DC 20064; 1998. 32 p.
(BIOETHICS)

Smith, George P. Death. *In: his* Family Values and the New Society: Dilemmas of the 21st Century. Westport, CT: Praeger; 1998: 217–246.
(ALLOWING TO DIE/LEGAL ASPECTS; EUTHANASIA/LEGAL ASPECTS; SUICIDE)

Smith, George P. Developing a Standard for Advancing Genetic Health and Scientific Investigation. Available from the author, 3600 John McCormack Rd., NE, Washington, DC 20064; 1997. 17 p.
(GENETIC INTERVENTION)

Smith, George P. Ethical imperatives in law and medicine. Available from the author, 3600 John McCormack Rd., NE, Washington, DC 20064; 1997. 25 p.
(ALLOWING TO DIE)

Smith, George P. Harnessing the human genome through legislative constraint. *European Journal of Health Law.* 1998 Mar; 5(1): 53–65.
(GENETIC SCREENING)

Smith, George P. Organ harvesting: salvaging a new beginning. *In: his* Family Values and the New Society: Dilemmas of the 21st Century. Westport, CT: Praeger; 1998: 247–267.
(ORGAN AND TISSUE DONATION)

Smith, George P. Our hearts were once young and gay: health care rationing and the elderly. *University of Florida Journal of Law and Public Policy.* 1996 Fall; 8(1): 1–23.
(PATIENT CARE/AGED; RESOURCE ALLOCATION)

Smith, George P. Pathways to immortality in the new millenium: human responsibility, theological direction, or legal mandate. *Saint Louis University Public Law Review.* 1996; 15(2): 447–469.
(BIOMEDICAL TECHNOLOGIES; GENETIC INTERVENTION)

Smith, George P. Procreative Liberty or Procreative Responsibility? Available from the author, Catholic University of America School of Law, 3600 John McCormack Rd., NE, Washington, DC 20064; 1998. 22 p.
(PRENATAL INJURIES)

Smith, George P. Terminal sedation as palliative care: revalidating a right to a good death. *Cambridge Quarterly of Healthcare Ethics.* 1998 Fall; 7(4): 382–387.
(PATIENT CARE/DRUGS; TERMINAL CARE)

Smith, George P. Testing the limits of procreational autonomy. *In: his* Family Values and the New Society: Dilemmas of the 21st Century. Westport, CT: Praeger; 1998: 69–92.
(REPRODUCTIVE TECHNOLOGIES)

Smith, I. see West, Charles

Smith, Janet E. Sterilizations reconsidered? *Christian Bioethics.* 1998 Apr; 4(1): 45–62.
(STERILIZATION)

Smith, Janet E. see Brown, Harold O.J.

Smith, Ken R. see Schrock, Charles R.

Smith, Martin see Swinn, Michael

Smith, Martin L. Ethical perspectives on Jehovah's Witnesses' refusal of blood. *Cleveland Clinic Journal of Medicine.* 1997 Oct; 64(9): 475–481.
(TREATMENT REFUSAL; TREATMENT REFUSAL/MINORS)

Smith, Martin L. see Slomka, Jacquelyn

Smith, Orla. Theatre: a gamete gambol. *Science.* 1999 Jul 2; 285(5424): 56.
(REPRODUCTIVE TECHNOLOGIES)

Smith, Richard. Viagra and rationing: let the sunlight in, let the people speak. [Editorial]. *BMJ (British Medical Journal).* 1998 Sep 19; 317(7161): 760–761.
(HEALTH CARE/FOREIGN COUNTRIES; PATIENT CARE/DRUGS; RESOURCE ALLOCATION/BIOMEDICAL TECHNOLOGIES)

Smith, Richard; Hiatt, Howard; Berwick, Donald. A

shared statement of ethical principles for those who shape and give health care: a working draft from the Tavistock Group. *Annals of Internal Medicine.* 1999 Jan 19; 130(2): 143–147.
(HEALTH CARE; PROFESSIONAL ETHICS/CODES OF ETHICS)

Smith, Richard; Hiatt, Howard; Berwick, Donald. Shared ethical principles for everybody in health care: a working draft from the Tavistock group. Introduction. *BMJ (British Medical Journal).* 1999 Jan 23; 318(7178): 248–249.
(HEALTH CARE; PROFESSIONAL ETHICS/CODES OF ETHICS)

Smith, Robert A. see **MacKay, Charles**

Smith, Shepherd see **Solomon, Liza**

Smith, Simon Weston see **Denley, Ian**

Smith, Stacey. Parents refuse to allow life–saving treatment for newborn: the right to choose. *Princeton Journal of Bioethics.* 1998 Spring; 1(1): 58–60.
(ALLOWING TO DIE/INFANTS; TREATMENT REFUSAL/MINORS)

Smith, Teresa Rust see **Hall, Mark A.**

Smith, Thomas J. see **Costantini-Ferrando, Maria F.**

Smith, Trevor. Ethics in Medical Research: A Handbook of Good Practice. New York, NY: Cambridge University Press; 1999. 403 p.
(HUMAN EXPERIMENTATION/ETHICS COMMITTEES; HUMAN EXPERIMENTATION/RESEARCH DESIGN; PROFESSIONAL ETHICS)

Smith, Wesley J. Assisted suicide comes to Oregon. *Human Life Review.* 1995 Spring; 21(2): 25–40.
(SUICIDE)

Smith, Wesley J. Forced Exit: The Slippery Slope from Assisted Suicide to Legalized Murder. New York, NY: Times Books; 1997. 291 p.
(EUTHANASIA; SUICIDE)

Smith–Wheelock, Linda see **Perry, Erica**

Smithpeter, Margaret see **Roberts, Laura Weiss**

Smolkin, Mitchell T. see **Pence, Gregory E.**

Smugar, Steve see **Kerr, Susan M.**

Snider, Dixie E. see **Kirsch, Michael**

Snijders, R.J.M.; Noble, P.; Sebire, N.; Souka, A.; Nicolaides, K.H. UK multicentre project on assessment of risk of trisomy 21 by maternal age and fetal nuchal–translucency thickness at 10–14 weeks of gestation. [For the Fetal Medicine Foundation First Trimester Screening Group (Great Britain)]. *Lancet.* 1998 Aug 1; 352(9125): 343–346.
(PRENATAL DIAGNOSIS)

Snyder, Lois see **Battin, Margaret Pabst**

Snyder, Lois see **Lo, Bernard**

Snyder, Maryhelen. Ethical Issues in Feminist Family

Therapy. New York, NY: Haworth Press; 1994. 83 p.
(PATIENT CARE/MENTALLY DISABLED)

Snyder, Rebecca S. Reproductive technology and stolen ova: who is the mother? [Note]. *Law and Inequality.* 1998 Winter; 16(1): 289–334.
(REPRODUCTIVE TECHNOLOGIES)

Sobol, H. see **Julian-Reyneir, C.**

Society for Academic Emergency Medicine. Ethics Committee see **Adams, James**

Society for Low Temperature Biology (Great Britain) see **Institute of Biology (Great Britain)**

Söderberg, Anna; Gilje, Fredricka; Norberg, Astrid. Dignity in situations of ethical difficulty in intensive care. *Intensive and Critical Care Nursing.* 1997 Jun; 13(3): 135–144.
(NURSING ETHICS; PATIENT CARE)

Solberg, Mary M. see **Gervais, Karen G.**

Solinger, Rickie, ed. Abortion Wars: A Half Century of Struggle, 1950–2000. Berkeley, CA: University of California Press; 1998. 413 p.
(ABORTION)

Soll, Roger. Consensus and controversy over resuscitation of the newborn infant. *Lancet.* 1999 Jul 3; 354(9172): 4–5.
(PATIENT CARE/MINORS; RESUSCITATION ORDERS)

Solomon, Liza; Benjamin, Georges; Fernando, M. Daniel; Coburn, Tom A.; Smith, Shepherd; Gostin, Lawrence O.; Ward, John W.; Baker, A. Cornelius. National HIV case reporting. [Letters and response]. *New England Journal of Medicine.* 1998 Feb 26; 338(9): 626–627.
(AIDS/TESTING AND SCREENING)

Solter, Davor. Dolly *is* a clone -- and no longer alone. [News]. *Nature.* 1998 Jul 23; 394(6691): 315–316.
(CLONING)

Somerville, Margaret A. Euthanasia in the media: jounalists' values, media ethics and "public square" messages. *Humane Health Care International.* 1997 Spring; 13(1): 17–20.
(EUTHANASIA; SUICIDE)

Somerville, Margaret A. Making health, not war -- musings on global disparities in health and human rights: a critical commentary by Solomon R. Benatar. *American Journal of Public Health.* 1998 Feb; 88(2): 301–303.
(HEALTH)

Sommer, Alfred see **Edi-Osagie, E.C.O.**

Sommerville, Ann; English, Veronica. Genetic privacy: orthodoxy or oxymoron? *Journal of Medical Ethics.* 1999 Apr; 25(2): 144–150.
(CONFIDENTIALITY; GENETIC SCREENING)

Sommerville, Ann see **Fisher, Fleur**

Song, Rhayun see **Daly, Barbara J.**

Sootak, Jaan; Kurm, Margus. A wish to have a baby

and the dignity of the child and embryo: about the law on artificial insemination and embryo protection of the Republic of Estonia. *European Journal of Health Law.* 1998 Jun; 5(2): 191–201.
(ARTIFICIAL INSEMINATION)

Soper, Charles see **Velasco, N.**

Sorell, Tom, ed. Health Care, Ethics and Insurance. New York, NY: Routledge; 1998. 240 p.
(HEALTH CARE/ECONOMICS)

Sorell, Tom; Draper, Heather. AIDS and insurance. *In:* Bennett, Rebecca; Erin, Charles A., eds. HIV and AIDS: Testing, Screening, and Confidentiality. New York, NY: Oxford University Press; 1999: 216–227.
(AIDS/TESTING AND SCREENING)

Sosna, Dennis. Advance directives for emergency medical service workers: the struggle continues. *Bioethics Forum.* 1998 Spring; 14(1): 33–36.
(ADVANCE DIRECTIVES; RESUSCITATION ORDERS)

Souka, A. see **Snijders, R.J.M.**

South Africa. An act (No. 92 of 1996) to determine the circumstances in which and conditions under which the pregnancy of a woman may be terminated; and to provide for matters connected therewith. Date of assent: 12 Nov 1996. (The Choice on Termination of Pregnancy Act, 1996). (*Government Gazette*, 22 Nov 1996, Vol 377, No. 17602, pp. 1–10). [Summary]. *International Digest of Health Legislation.* 1997; 48(2): 178–181.
(ABORTION/FOREIGN COUNTRIES; ABORTION/LEGAL ASPECTS)

South Africa. Supreme Court, Cape Provincial Division. Castell v. De Greef. *South Africa Law Reports.* 1994 Feb 17 (date of decision). 1994(4): 408–441.
(INFORMED CONSENT)

Southall, David see **West, Charles**

Spady, Donald W. Advance directives for severely mentally and physically handicapped adults who have never been competent. *Bioethics Bulletin.* 1996 Nov; 8(2): 10–11.
(ADVANCE DIRECTIVES)

Spann, Stephen J. see **Chavey, William E.**

Specter, Michael. Uganda AIDS vaccine test: urgency affects ethics rules. [News]. *New York Times.* 1998 Oct 1: A1, A6.
(AIDS/HUMAN EXPERIMENTATION; HUMAN EXPERIMENTATION/FOREIGN COUNTRIES; IMMUNIZATION)

Speece, Mark see **Butler, Dennis J.**

Spencer, Donald E. Practical implications for health care providers in a physician–assisted suicide environment. *Seattle University Law Review.* 1995 Spring; 18(3): 545–556.
(SUICIDE; TERMINAL CARE)

Spencer, Edward M. Ethical conundrums: "Are ethics programs obsolete?" *SBC Newsletter (Society for Bioethics Consultation).* 1996 Spring: 8–9.
(ETHICISTS AND ETHICS COMMITTEES)

Spicker, Stuart F. Introduction: bioethic(s): one or many? *Journal of Medicine and Philosophy.* 1998 Aug; 23(4): 347–355.
(BIOETHICS)

Spicker, Stuart F. The process of coherence formation in healthcare ethics committees: the consensus process, social authority and ethical judgments. *In:* ten Have, Henk A.M.J.; Sass, Hans–Martin, eds. Consensus Formation in Healthcare Ethics. Boston, MA: Kluwer Academic; 1998: 35–44.
(ETHICISTS AND ETHICS COMMITTEES)

Spiegel, David see **Whitney, Simon N.**

Spielberg, Alissa R. On call and online: sociohistorical, legal, and ethical implications of e-mail for the patient–physician relationship. *JAMA.* 1998 Oct 21; 280(15): 1353–1359.
(CONFIDENTIALITY/LEGAL ASPECTS; PROFESSIONAL PATIENT RELATIONSHIP)

Spielberg, Alissa R. Online without a net: physician–patient communication by electronic mail. *American Journal of Law and Medicine.* 1999; 25(2–3): 267–295.
(CONFIDENTIALITY/LEGAL ASPECTS; PROFESSIONAL PATIENT RELATIONSHIP)

Spike, Jeffrey. Brain death, pregnancy, and posthumous motherhood. [Case study]. *Journal of Clinical Ethics.* 1999 Spring; 10(1): 57–65.
(ALLOWING TO DIE; FETUSES; PATIENT CARE)

Spike, Jeffrey. Physicians' responsibilities in the care of suicidal patients: three case studies. *Journal of Clinical Ethics.* 1998 Fall; 9(3): 306–313.
(ALLOWING TO DIE; SUICIDE)

Spinks, Nelda see **Wells, Barron**

Spinsanti, Sandro. Obtaining consent from the family: a horizon for clinical ethics. *In:* ten Have, Henk A.M.J.; Sass, Hans–Martin, eds. Consensus Formation in Healthcare Ethics. Boston, MA: Kluwer Academic; 1998: 209–217.
(INFORMED CONSENT; TRUTH DISCLOSURE)

Spiro, Howard. The Power of Hope: A Doctor's Perspective. New Haven, CT: Yale University Press; 1998. 288 p.
(PATIENT CARE)

Spivak, Baruch see **Mester, Roberto**

Sponholz, Gerlinde; Baitsch, Helmut; Ahr, Willfried; Harr, Helmut; Hölzer, Michael; Keller, Frieder; Meier–Allmendinger, Diana; Straif, Kurt; Allert, Gebhard. Genetic medicine: a new Copernican turning point? *In:* Hanson, Mark J.; Callahan, Daniel, eds. The Goals of Medicine: The Forgotten Issue in Health Care Reform. Washington, DC: Georgetown University Press; 1999: 162–173.
(GENETIC RESEARCH)

Sponholz, Gerlinde see **Allert, Gebhard**

Sprague, Joey; Greer, Margaret. Standpoints and the discourse on abortion: the reproductive debate. *Women and Politics.* 1998; 19(3): 49–80.
(ABORTION)

Sprang, M. LeRoy; Neerhof, Mark G. Rationale for banning abortions late in pregnancy. *JAMA.* 1998 Aug 26; 280(8): 744–747.
(ABORTION)

Sprung, Charles L.; Oppenheim, Arieh. End-of-life decisions in critical care medicine -- where are we headed? [Editorial]. *Critical Care Medicine.* 1998 Feb; 26(2): 200–202.
(ALLOWING TO DIE; EUTHANASIA; SUICIDE)

Sprung, Charles L. see **Nyman, Deborah J.**

Spurgeon, David. Canadian case questions funding. [News]. *BMJ (British Medical Journal).* 1999 Jan 9; 318(7176): 77.
(BIOMEDICAL RESEARCH; HUMAN EXPERIMENTATION/FOREIGN COUNTRIES)

Spurgeon, David. Canadian research councils publish joint code on ethics. [News]. *Nature.* 1998 Oct 1; 395(6701): 420.
(BEHAVIORAL RESEARCH/FOREIGN COUNTRIES; BEHAVIORAL RESEARCH/REGULATION; HUMAN EXPERIMENTATION/FOREIGN COUNTRIES; HUMAN EXPERIMENTATION/REGULATION)

Spurgeon, David. Canadian whistleblower row prompts broader code of conduct. [News]. *Nature.* 1998 Dec 24–31; 396(6713): 715.
(BIOMEDICAL RESEARCH; HUMAN EXPERIMENTATION/FOREIGN COUNTRIES)

Square, David. Court verdict "splendid," ethics professor says. [News]. *Canadian Medical Association Journal.* 1998 Jan 27; 158(2): 159–160.
(RESUSCITATION ORDERS)

Stableford, Sue see **Root, Jane**

Stagno, Susan J. see **Slomka, Jacquelyn**

Staitman, Mark N. Withdrawing or withholding nutrition, hydration or oxygen from patients. *In:* Jacob, Walter; Zemer, Moshe, eds. Death and Euthanasia in Jewish Law: Essays and Responsa. Pittsburgh, PA: Freehof Institute of Progressive Halakhah: Rodef Shalom Press; 1995: 1–10.
(ALLOWING TO DIE/RELIGIOUS ASPECTS)

Stanberry, Ben. The legal and ethical aspects of telemedicine. 3: Telemedicine and malpractice. *Journal of Telemedicine and Telecare.* 1998; 4(2): 72–79.
(INFORMED CONSENT; PATIENT CARE)

Stanford Program in Genomics, Ethics and Society. Alzheimer Disease Working Group see **McConnell, L.M.**

Stanisstreet, Martin see **Hill, Ruaraidh**

Starace, F.; Ogden, R.D. Suicidal behaviours and euthanasia. *AIDS Care.* 1997 Feb; 9(1): 106–108.
(AIDS; EUTHANASIA; SUICIDE)

Starr, Douglas. Blood: An Epic History of Medicine and Commerce. New York, NY: Alfred A. Knopf; 1998. 441 p.
(BLOOD DONATION)

Starr, Joann; Zawacki, Bruce E. Voices from the silent world of doctor and patient. *Cambridge Quarterly of*

Healthcare Ethics. 1999 Spring; 8(2): 129–138.
(PATIENT CARE; PROFESSIONAL PATIENT RELATIONSHIP; TREATMENT REFUSAL)

Starr, Paul. Health and the right to privacy. *American Journal of Law and Medicine.* 1999; 25(2–3): 193–201.
(CONFIDENTIALITY/LEGAL ASPECTS)

Starzomski, Rosalie see **Blue, Arthur**

Stead, William W.; Miller, Douglas P.; Lewis, Gregory L.; Hoefler, James M.; Seely, John F.; Miller, Franklin G.; Meier, Diane E.; Quill, Timothy E.; Block, Susan D.; Billings, J. Andrew. Terminal dehydration as an alternative to physician–assisted suicide. [Letters and responses]. *Annals of Internal Medicine.* 1998 Dec 15; 129(12): 1080–1082.
(SUICIDE; TERMINAL CARE; TREATMENT REFUSAL)

Stebbens, Valerie see **West, Charles**

Stein, C. Michael; Pincus, Theodore. Placebo–controlled studies in rheumatoid arthritis: ethical issues. *Lancet.* 1999 Jan 30; 353(9150): 400–403.
(HUMAN EXPERIMENTATION/RESEARCH DESIGN)

Stein, Robert E. see **Coburn, Tom**

Steinberg, A. see **Elstein, D.**

Steinberg, Avraham. Medical–halachic decisions of Rabbi Shlomo Zalman Auerbach (1910–1995). *Jewish Medical Ethics.* 1997 Jan; 3(1): 30–43.
(BIOETHICS)

Steinberg, Avraham. The foundations and the development of modern medical ethics. *Journal of Assisted Reproduction and Genetics.* 1995 Sep; 12(8): 473–476.
(BIOETHICS)

Steinberg, Deborah Lynn see **Swinn, Michael**

Steinberg, Karen see **MacKay, Charles**

Steinberg, Maurice D. Psychiatry and bioethics: an exploration of the relationship. *Psychosomatics.* 1997 Jul–Aug; 38(4): 313–320.
(ETHICISTS AND ETHICS COMMITTEES)

Steinberg, Maurice D.; Youngner, Stuart J., eds. End–of–Life Decisions: A Psychosocial Perspective. Washington, DC: American Psychiatric Press; 1998. 322 p.
(ALLOWING TO DIE; SUICIDE)

Steinbock, Bonnie. A philosopher looks at assisted reproduction. *Journal of Assisted Reproduction and Genetics.* 1995 Sep; 12(8): 543–551.
(REPRODUCTION; REPRODUCTIVE TECHNOLOGIES)

Steinbock, Bonnie. Mother–fetus conflict. *In:* Kuhse, Helga; Singer, Peter, eds. A Companion to Bioethics. Malden, MA: Blackwell; 1998: 135–146.
(FETUSES; PRENATAL INJURIES; TREATMENT REFUSAL)

Steinbock, Bonnie. Prenatal genetic testing for Alzheimer disease. *In:* Post, Stephen G.; Whitehouse, Peter J., eds. Genetic Testing for Alzheimer Disease: Ethical and Clinical Issues. Baltimore, MD: Johns Hopkins University Press; 1998: 140–151.

Steinbock, Bonnie. Sperm as property. *In:* Harris, John; Holm, Søren, eds. The Future of Human Reproduction: Ethics, Choice, and Regulation. New York, NY: Oxford University Press; 1998: 150–161.
(ARTIFICIAL INSEMINATION; REPRODUCTION; REPRODUCTIVE TECHNOLOGIES)

Steinbrook, Robert. Caring for people with human immunodeficiency virus infection. [Editorial]. *New England Journal of Medicine.* 1998 Dec 24; 339(26): 1926–1928.
(AIDS; HEALTH CARE/ECONOMICS; PATIENT CARE/DRUGS)

Steiner, Warren see **Ritchie, Janet**

Steinfels, Peter. Beliefs: wide-ranging, tough questions have been provoked by the broadcast of Kevorkian's video. *New York Times.* 1998 Nov 28: B7.
(EUTHANASIA)

Steinfels, Peter; Callahan, Daniel. A longtime leader in biomedical ethics reflects on his field's explosive growth, the backlash against it and 'false hopes' in America's health care quest. [Interview]. *New York Times.* 1998 May 2: A11.
(BIOETHICS)

Steinkraus, Holly B. see **Resnik, David B.**

Stell, Lance K. Stopping treatment on grounds of futility: a role for institutional policy. *Saint Louis University Public Law Review.* 1992; 11(2): 481–497.
(ALLOWING TO DIE/LEGAL ASPECTS)

Stempsey, William E. Laying down one's life for oneself. *Christian Bioethics.* 1998 Aug; 4(2): 202–224.
(SUICIDE)

Stenger, Christine E. Taking Tarasoff where no one has gone before: looking at "duty to warn" under the AIDS crisis. [Comment]. *Saint Louis University Public Law Review.* 1996; 15(2): 471–504.
(AIDS/CONFIDENTIALITY; CONFIDENTIALITY/LEGAL ASPECTS)

Stepanuk, Natalie Anne. Genetic information and third party access to information: New Jersey's pioneering legislation as a model for federal privacy protection of genetic information. [Comment]. *Catholic University Law Review.* 1998 Spring; 47(3): 1105–1144.
(CONFIDENTIALITY/LEGAL ASPECTS; GENETIC SCREENING)

Stephany, Theresa. Assisted suicide for the terminally ill: why we must have the choice. *Home Care Provider.* 1997 Oct; 2(5): 212–213.
(SUICIDE)

Stephenson, Peter. Expanding notions of culture for cross-cultural ethics in health and medicine. *In:* Coward, Harold; Ratanakul, Pinit, eds. A Cross-Cultural Dialogue on Health Care Ethics. Waterloo, ON: Wilfrid Laurier University Press; 1999: 68–91.
(HEALTH; HEALTH CARE)

Stephenson, Peter see **Burgess, Michael**

Sterckx, Sigrid, ed. Biotechnology, Patents and Morality. Brookfield, VT: Ashgate; 1997. 324 p.

Stern, Kristina. Advance directives. *Medical Law Review.* 1994 Spring; 2(1): 57–76.
(ADVANCE DIRECTIVES)

Stetson, Dorothy McBride. Feminist perspectives on abortion and reproductive technologies. *In:* Githens, Marianne; Stetson, Dorothy McBride, eds. Abortion Politics: Public Policy in Cross-Cultural Perspective. New York, NY: Routledge; 1996: 211–223.
(ABORTION; REPRODUCTIVE TECHNOLOGIES)

Stetson, Dorothy McBride see **Githens, Marianne**

Stevens, Andrew J. see **Edwards, Sarah J.L.**

Stevens, Christine A.; Hassan, Riaz. Nurses and the management of death, dying and euthanasia. *Medicine and Law.* 1994; 13(5–6): 541–554.
(ALLOWING TO DIE/ATTITUDES; EUTHANASIA/ATTITUDES)

Stevenson, David K.; Goldworth, Amnon. Commentary: neonatal viability in the 1990s: held hostage by technology. *Cambridge Quarterly of Healthcare Ethics.* 1999 Spring; 8(2): 170–172.
(ALLOWING TO DIE/INFANTS; SELECTION FOR TREATMENT)

Stewart, Barbara. Grand jury refuses to indict in an assisted suicide. [News]. *New York Times.* 1999 Jul 17: B1, B4.
(SUICIDE)

Stewart, Gary P.; Cutrer, William R.; Demy, Timothy J.; O'Mathúna, Dónal P.; Cunningham, Paige C.; Kilner, John F.; Bevington, Linda K. Basic Questions on Sexuality and Reproductive Technology: When Is It Right to Intervene? Grand Rapids, MI: Kregel Publications; 1998. 77 p.
(REPRODUCTIVE TECHNOLOGIES)

Stewart, Gary P. see **Demy, Timothy J.**

Stewart, J.A.D. Best interests and persistent vegetative state. [Letter]. *Journal of Medical Ethics.* 1998 Oct; 24(5): 350.
(ALLOWING TO DIE/LEGAL ASPECTS)

Stewart, Kevin see **Bacon, Mike**

Stewart, Mary see **Perkins, David V.**

Stewart, Robert see **Brown, Janet**

Stiell, Ian G. see **van Walraven, Carl**

Stingl, Michael; Burgess, Michael M.; Hubert, John; Sherwin, Susan. Euthanasia and health reform in Canada. [Article and commentaries]. *Cambridge Quarterly of Healthcare Ethics.* 1998 Fall; 7(4): 348–370.
(EUTHANASIA; HEALTH CARE/FOREIGN COUNTRIES; TERMINAL CARE)

Stocking, Carol B. see **McKenzie, John K.**

Stoddard, Jim. A practical approach to DNR discussions. *Bioethics Forum.* 1998 Spring; 14(1): 27–32.
(RESUSCITATION ORDERS)

Stoddard, Joan C.; Billings, Paul R.; Astrue, Michael J.; Tennenbaum, David; Lynch, Eugene C. Health care providers, insurers, and individual patients; the right to treatment; economic and policy issues. [Proceedings of the International Symposium on Law and Science at the Crossroads: Biomedical Technology, Ethics, Public Policy, and the Law; panel discussion]. *Suffolk University Law Review.* 1993 Winter; 27(4): 1499–1523.
(HEALTH CARE/ECONOMICS; ORGAN AND TISSUE TRANSPLANTATION)

Stoess, Jean see Sher, Geoffrey

Stoff, David M. see Arnold, L. Eugene

Stoffell, Brian. Voluntary euthanasia, suicide and physician–assisted suicide. *In:* Kuhse, Helga; Singer, Peter, eds. A Companion to Bioethics. Malden, MA: Blackwell; 1998: 272–279.
(EUTHANASIA; SUICIDE)

Stokes, William S. see Hill, Richard N.

Stolberg, Sheryl Gay. Animals as organ donors? Not until they're germ-free. *New York Times.* 1998 Feb 3: F1, F6.
(ORGAN AND TISSUE DONATION; ORGAN AND TISSUE TRANSPLANTATION)

Stolberg, Sheryl Gay. As life ebbs, so does time to elect comforts of hospice. *New York Times.* 1998 Mar 4: A1, A18.
(TERMINAL CARE/HOSPICES)

Stolberg, Sheryl Gay. Assisted suicides are rare, survey of doctors finds. [News]. *New York Times.* 1998 Apr 23: A1, A21.
(EUTHANASIA/ATTITUDES; SUICIDE)

Stolberg, Sheryl Gay. Decisive moment on Parkinson's fetal–cell transplants. [News]. *New York Times.* 1999 Apr 20: F2.
(HUMAN EXPERIMENTATION/RESEARCH DESIGN; ORGAN AND TISSUE TRANSPLANTATION)

Stolberg, Sheryl Gay. Fight over organs shifts to states from Washington. [News]. *New York Times.* 1999 Mar 11: A1, A26.
(ORGAN AND TISSUE TRANSPLANTATION; RESOURCE ALLOCATION/BIOMEDICAL TECHNOLOGIES)

Stolberg, Sheryl Gay. Health identifier for all Americans runs into hurdles: privacy debate heats up. [News]. *New York Times.* 1998 Jul 20: A1, A11.
(CONFIDENTIALITY)

Stolberg, Sheryl Gay. Health secretary urges donor priority for sickest patients. [News]. *New York Times.* 1998 Feb 27: A16.
(ORGAN AND TISSUE TRANSPLANTATION; RESOURCE ALLOCATION/BIOMEDICAL TECHNOLOGIES; SELECTION FOR TREATMENT)

Stolberg, Sheryl Gay. In death, the goal is no questions asked. [News]. *New York Times.* 1998 Apr 26: WK 3.
(SUICIDE)

Stolberg, Sheryl Gay. Internet prescriptions boom in the "Wild West" of the Web: a special report. *New York Times.* 1999 Jun 27: 1, 14.
(PATIENT CARE/DRUGS)

Stolberg, Sheryl Gay. New rules will force doctors to disclose ties to drug industry. [News]. *New York Times.* 1998 Feb 3: A12.
(BIOMEDICAL RESEARCH; HEALTH CARE/ECONOMICS; HUMAN EXPERIMENTATION/REGULATION)

Stolberg, Sheryl Gay. Organ transplant panel urges a broad sharing of livers. [News]. *New York Times.* 1999 Jul 21: A14.
(ORGAN AND TISSUE TRANSPLANTATION; RESOURCE ALLOCATION/BIOMEDICAL TECHNOLOGIES)

Stolberg, Sheryl Gay. Pennsylvania set to break taboo on reward for organ donation. [News]. *New York Times.* 1999 May 6: A1, A30.
(ORGAN AND TISSUE DONATION)

Stolberg, Sheryl Gay. Placebo use is suspended in overseas AIDS trials. [News]. *New York Times.* 1998 Feb 19: A16.
(AIDS/HUMAN EXPERIMENTATION; HUMAN EXPERIMENTATION/FOREIGN COUNTRIES; HUMAN EXPERIMENTATION/RESEARCH DESIGN; HUMAN EXPERIMENTATION/SPECIAL POPULATIONS)

Stolberg, Sheryl Gay. Sham surgery returns as a research tool. [News]. *New York Times.* 1999 Apr 25: WK 3.
(HUMAN EXPERIMENTATION/RESEARCH DESIGN)

Stolberg, Sheryl Gay see Hilts, Philip J.

Stoline, Anne see Boronow, John

Stoller, David. Prenatal genetic screening: the enigma of selective abortion. *Journal of Law and Health.* 1997–98; 12(1): 121–140.
(ABORTION/LEGAL ASPECTS; GENETIC SCREENING; PRENATAL DIAGNOSIS)

Stoskopf, Barbara L. see Saigal, Saroj

Stoto, Michael A.; Almario, Donna A.; McCormick, Marie C., eds.; Institute of Medicine. Committee on Perinatal Transmission of HIV; National Research Council and Institute of Medicine. Board on Children, Youth, and Families. Reducing the Odds: Preventing Perinatal Transmission of HIV in the United States. Washington, DC: National Academy Press; 1999. 397 p.
(AIDS; AIDS/TESTING AND SCREENING)

Straif, Kurt see Sponholz, Gerlinde

Strasburger, Larry H. see Bursztajn, Harold J.

Straus, Joseph. Patenting human genes in Europe -- past developments and prospects for the future. *IIC: International Review of Industrial Property and Copyright Law.* 1995 Dec; 26(6): 920–950.
(GENOME MAPPING; PATENTING LIFE FORMS)

Street, Annette see Kissane, David W.

Stringer, Anthony Y. see Banja, John D.

Stringer, Jeffrey S.A.; Rouse, Dwight J.; Goldenberg, Robert L. Prophylactic cesarean delivery for the prevention of perinatal human immunodeficiency virus transmission: the case for restraint. *JAMA.* 1999 May 26; 281(20): 1946–1949.
(AIDS)

Strong, Carson. Is there no common morality? [Book review essay]. *Medical Humanities Review.* 1997 Spring; 11(1): 39–45.
(BIOETHICS)

Stubbs, Cassandra see Egilman, David

Studdert, David M. Direct contracts, data sharing and employee risk selection: new stakes for patient privacy in tomorrow's health insurance markets. *American Journal of Law and Medicine.* 1999; 25(2–3): 233–265.
(CONFIDENTIALITY/LEGAL ASPECTS; HEALTH CARE/ECONOMICS; OCCUPATIONAL HEALTH)

Studts, Jamie L. see Andrykowski, Michael A.

Stuer, Hugo see Denekens, Joke P.M.

Suarez–Murias, Edward L. see Murphy, Edmond A.

Sugarman, Jeremy; Burk, Larry. Physicians' ethical obligations regarding alternative medicine. *JAMA.* 1998 Nov 11; 280(18): 1623–1625.
(PATIENT CARE)

Sugarman, Jeremy; Kass, Nancy E.; Goodman, Steven N.; Perentesis, Patricia; Fernandes, Praveen; Faden, Ruth R. What patients say about medical research. *IRB: A Review of Human Subjects Research.* 1998 Jul–Aug; 20(4): 1–7.
(HUMAN EXPERIMENTATION)

Sugarman, Jeremy; McCrory, Douglas C.; Hubal, Robert C. Getting meaningful informed consent from older adults: a structured literature review of empirical research. *Journal of the American Geriatrics Society.* 1998 Apr; 46(4): 517–524.
(HUMAN EXPERIMENTATION/INFORMED CONSENT; HUMAN EXPERIMENTATION/SPECIAL POPULATIONS; INFORMED CONSENT; PATIENT CARE/AGED)

Sugarman, Jeremy; McCrory, Douglas C.; Powell, Donald; Krasny, Alex; Adams, Betsy; Ball, Eric; Cassell, Cynthia, comps. Empirical research on informed consent: an annotated bibliography. *Hastings Center Report.* 1999 Jan–Feb; 29(1): S1–S42.
(HUMAN EXPERIMENTATION/INFORMED CONSENT; INFORMED CONSENT)

Sugarman, Jeremy see Slovenko, Ralph

Sullivan, Amy M. see Simon, Steven R.

Sullivan, George M. see Virgo, Katherine S.

Sullivan, Kevin see Jordan, Mary

Sullivan, M. C. The changing order of things [resuscitation]. *Bioethics Forum.* 1998 Spring; 14(1): 37–40.
(RESUSCITATION ORDERS)

Sullivan, Mark; Ormel, Johan; Kempen, G.I.J.M.; Tymstra, Tj. Beliefs concerning death, dying, and hastening death among older, functionally impaired Dutch adults: a one-year longitudinal study. *Journal of the American Geriatrics Society.* 1998 Oct; 46(10): 1251–1257.
(ALLOWING TO DIE/ATTITUDES; EUTHANASIA/ATTITUDES; SUICIDE)

Sullivan, Mark see Back, Anthony

Sullivan, Mark D. see Werth, James L.

Sullivan, Michael see Lysaker, John T.

Sullivan, Patrick. Move to market gene pool angers Iceland's MDs. *Canadian Medical Association Journal.* 1999 Aug 10; 161(3): 305.
(GENETIC RESEARCH)

Sullivan, William M. What is left of professionalism after managed care? *Hastings Center Report.* 1999 Mar–Apr; 29(2): 7–13.
(HEALTH CARE/ECONOMICS)

Sulmasy, Daniel P. Cancer, managed care, and therapeutic research: an ethicist's view. *HMO Practice.* 1997 Jun; 11(2): 59–62.
(HEALTH CARE/ECONOMICS; HUMAN EXPERIMENTATION)

Sulmasy, Daniel P.; Pellegrino, Edmund D. The rule of double effect: clearing up the double talk. *Archives of Internal Medicine.* 1999 Mar 22; 159(6): 545–550.
(TERMINAL CARE)

Sulmasy, Daniel P. see Buss, Mary K.

Sulmasy, Daniel P. see Malter, Alex

Sulmasy, Daniel P. see O'Rourke, Kevin

Summer, David. Maryland court rules on embryo standing. [News]. *Journal of Law, Medicine and Ethics.* 1995 Spring; 23(1): 108.
(EMBRYO AND FETAL RESEARCH)

Sumner, Edward D. see Dickinson, George E.

Sunstein, Cass R. The Constitution and the clone. In: Nussbaum, Martha C.; Sunstein, Cass R., eds. Clones and Clones: Facts and Fantasies About Human Cloning. New York, NY: Norton; 1998: 207–220.
(CLONING)

Sunstein, Cass R. The right to die. *Yale Law Journal.* 1997 Jan; 106(4): 1123–1163.
(SUICIDE)

Sunstein, Cass R. see Nussbaum, Martha C.

Supanich, Barbara see Doukas, David J.

Surace, Matteo see Gbolade, Babatunde A.

Surh, L. see Cappelli, M.

Susser, Mervyn. The prevention of perinatal HIV transmission in the less-developed world. [Editorial]. *American Journal of Public Health.* 1998 Apr; 88(4): 547–548.
(AIDS/HUMAN EXPERIMENTATION; HUMAN EXPERIMENTATION/FOREIGN COUNTRIES; HUMAN EXPERIMENTATION/RESEARCH DESIGN; HUMAN EXPERIMENTATION/SPECIAL POPULATIONS)

Susser, Mervyn see Karim, Quarraisha Abdool

Sutcliffe, Alastair G.; Taylor, Brent; Grudzinskas, Gedis; Thornton, Simon; Lieberman, Brian; Bowen, Jennifer R. Children conceived by intracytoplasmic

sperm injection. [Letter and response]. *Lancet.* 1998 Aug 15; 352(9127): 578–579.
(REPRODUCTIVE TECHNOLOGIES)

Suwonnakote, Khannika see **Burgess, Michael**

Svatos, Michele. Biotechnology and the utilitarian argument for patents. *In:* Paul, Ellen Frankel; Miller, Fred D.; Paul, Jeffrey, eds. Scientific Innovation, Philosophy, and Public Policy. New York, NY: Cambridge University Press; 1996: 113–144.
(BIOMEDICAL RESEARCH; BIOMEDICAL TECHNOLOGIES)

Svatos, Michele. Patents and morality: a philosophical commentary on the conference 'Biotechnology, patents and morality.' *In:* Sterckx, Sigrid, ed. Biotechnology, Patents and Morality. Proceedings of an International Workshop, "Biotechnology, Patents and Morality: Towards a Consensus," held in Ghent, Belgium, 17–19 Jan 1996. Brookfield, VT: Ashgate; 1997: 291–306.
(GENETIC INTERVENTION; PATENTING LIFE FORMS)

Swartz, Richard see **Perry, Erica**

Swartz, Richard D.; Perry, Erica; Schneider, Carl; Burdette, Tom; Curtis, George; O'Neil, Mary. The option to withdraw from chronic dialysis treatment. *Advances in Renal Replacement Therapy.* 1994 Oct; 1(3): 264–273.
(ALLOWING TO DIE; TREATMENT REFUSAL)

Swartz, Richard D. see **Leggat, John E.**

Sweeney, Patricia A. see **Nakashima, Allyn K.**

Swenson, Sara L.; Rothstein, Julie A. Navigating the wards: teaching medical students to use their moral compasses. *Academic Medicine.* 1996 Jun; 71(6): 591–594.
(MEDICAL ETHICS/EDUCATION)

Swick, Herbert M.; Szenas, Philip; Danoff, Deborah; Whitcomb, Michael E. Teaching professionalism in undergraduate medical education. *JAMA.* 1999 Sep 1; 282(9): 830–832.
(MEDICAL ETHICS/EDUCATION)

Swigart, Valerie Anne. A Study of Family Decision–Making about Life Support Using the Grounded Theory Method. Ann Arbor, MI: UMI Dissertation Services; 1994. 220 p.
(ALLOWING TO DIE)

Swiglo, B.A.; Lebel, R.R. Re–contact to advise of testing available to detect high risk for carcinoma: response to letters sent to persons initially ascertained for other genetic reasons. [Abstract]. *American Journal of Human Genetics.* 1997 Oct; 61(4): A390.
(GENETIC COUNSELING)

Swinburn, J.M.A.; Ali, S.M.; Banerjee, D.J.; Khan, Z.P. Ethical dilemma: discontinuation of ventilation after brain stem death: to whom is our duty of care? *BMJ (British Medical Journal).* 1999 Jun 26; 318(7200): 1753–1754.
(ALLOWING TO DIE; DETERMINATION OF DEATH/BRAIN DEATH)

Swinn, Michael; Emberton, Mark; Ralph, David; Smith, Martin; Serhal, Paul; Bewley, Susan; Lichterman, Boleslav; Steinberg, Deborah Lynn. Retrieving semen from a dead patient: Utilitarianism in

the absence of definitive guidelines; The patient was assaulted; Some ethical concerns were ignored; [and] An ethic of ambivalence. *BMJ (British Medical Journal).* 1998 Dec 5; 317(7172): 1583–1585.
(ORGAN AND TISSUE DONATION; REPRODUCTIVE TECHNOLOGIES)

Swisher, Laura Lee; Krueger–Brophy, Carol. Legal and Ethical Issues in Physical Therapy. Boston, MA: Butterworth–Heinemann; 1998. 231 p.
(PROFESSIONAL ETHICS)

Sy, Peter A. see **de Castro, Leonardo D.**

Sy, Susanna Leong Huey see **Leng, Ter Kah**

Sykes, Megan see **Sachs, David H.**

Szasz, Thomas. Parity for mental illness, disparity for the mental patient. *Lancet.* 1998 Oct 10; 352(9135): 1213–1215.
(ADVANCE DIRECTIVES; TREATMENT REFUSAL/MENTALLY DISABLED)

Szasz, Thomas see **Joy, Mark**

Szawarski, Zbigniew. The stick, the eye, and ownership of the body. *In:* ten Have, Henk A.M.J.; Welie, Jos V.M., eds. Ownership of the Human Body: Philosophical Considerations on the Use of the Human Body and Its Parts in Healthcare. Boston, MA: Kluwer Academic; 1998: 81–96.
(ORGAN AND TISSUE DONATION)

Szebik, Imre. Altering the mitochondrial genome: is it just a technical issue? Response to "Germ line therapy to cure mitochondrial disease: protocol and ethics of in vitro ovum nuclear transplantation" by Donald S. Rubenstein, David C. Thomasma, Eric A. Schon, and Michael J. Zinaman (*CQ*, 1995 Summer; 4(3): 316–339). *Cambridge Quarterly of Healthcare Ethics.* 1999 Summer; 8(3): 369–374.
(GENE THERAPY)

Szenas, Philip see **Swick, Herbert M.**

Szmukler, George see **Thorns, Andrew**

Szmukler, George I.; Bloch, Sidney. Family involvement in the care of people with psychoses: an ethical argument. [Editorial]. *British Journal of Psychiatry.* 1997 Nov; 171: 401–405.
(PATIENT CARE/MENTALLY DISABLED)

Szolovits, Peter see **Roberts, John**

Szulc, R. Ethics and research. [Editorial]. *European Journal of Anaesthesiology.* 1996 Mar; 13(2): 93–94.
(HUMAN EXPERIMENTATION)

T

Tabak, Nili. Informed consent: the nurse's dilemma. *Medicine and Law.* 1996; 15(1): 7–16.
(INFORMED CONSENT)

Tabarrok, Alexander. Genetic testing: an economic and contractarian analysis. *Journal of Health Economics.* 1994 Mar; 13(1): 75–91.
(GENETIC SCREENING; HEALTH CARE/ECONOMICS)

Tackaberry, Eilleen; Ganz, Peter R. Xenotransplantation: assessing the unknowns. [Editorial]. *Canadian Medical Association Journal.* 1998 Jul 14; 159(1): 41–43.
(ORGAN AND TISSUE TRANSPLANTATION)

Tacket, Carol O. see **Matz, Robert**

Tafesse, Eskinder see **Merson, Michael H.**

Tagliaferro, Linda. Genetic Engineering: Progress or Peril? [Juvenile literature]. Minneapolis, MN: Lerner Publications; 1997. 128 p.
(GENETIC INTERVENTION)

Taimi, Kitty. A new challenge for IRBs: medical surveillance for former DOE workers. *Protecting Human Subjects.* 1997 Fall: 6–8.
(HUMAN EXPERIMENTATION; OCCUPATIONAL HEALTH)

Tajima, Kazuo see **Hamajima, Nobuyuki**

Takala, Tuija. The right to genetic ignorance confirmed. *Bioethics.* 1999 Jul; 13(3–4): 288–293.
(GENETIC SCREENING; TRUTH DISCLOSURE)

Taleghani, Christopher K. see **Schulman, Kevin A.**

Tallis, Raymond see **Neuberger, Julia**

Tan, K.H. see **Gbolade, Babatunde A.**

Tanaka, Makoto see **Kitamura, Fusako**

Tanaka, Yuki. Japanese biological warfare plans and experiments on POWs. *In: his* Hidden Horrors: Japanese War Crimes in World War II. Boulder, CO: Westview Press; 1996: 135–165, 238–242.
(FRAUD AND MISCONDUCT; HUMAN EXPERIMENTATION/FOREIGN COUNTRIES; HUMAN EXPERIMENTATION/SPECIAL POPULATIONS; WAR)

Tang, Julie. The United States' immigration laws: prospects for relief for foreign nationals seeking refuge from coercive sterilization or abortion practices in their homelands. *Saint Louis University Public Law Review.* 1996; 15(2): 371–401.
(ABORTION/FOREIGN COUNTRIES; POPULATION CONTROL; STERILIZATION)

Tangwa, Godfrey B. Globalisation or Westernisation? Ethical concerns in the whole bio–business. *Bioethics.* 1999 Jul; 13(3–4): 218–226.
(BIOETHICS)

Tanida, Noritoshi see **Charlton, Rodger**

Tantravahi, Umadevi see **Lafayette, DeeDee**

Tapper, Melbourne. In the Blood: Sickle Cell Anemia and the Politics of Race. Philadelphia, PA: University of Pennsylvania Press; 1999. 163 p.
(GENETIC SCREENING; HEALTH)

Tarantola, Daniel; Gruskin, Sofia. Children confronting HIV/AIDS: charting the confluence of rights and health. *Health and Human Rights.* 1998; 3(1): 60–86.
(AIDS)

Tarantola, Daniel see **Gruskin, Sofia**

Tarlos–Benka, Judy see **Burton, Laurel Arthur**

Tarnow, Eugene. When extra authors get in on the act. [Letter]. *Nature.* 1999 Apr 22; 398(6729): 657.
(BIOMEDICAL RESEARCH; FRAUD AND MISCONDUCT)

Tarnow–Mordi, W.O. see **Fowlie, P.W.**

Tataryn, Douglas see **Chochinov, Harvey Max**

Tattam, Amanda. Australia considers human cloning for therapeutic purposes. [News]. *Lancet.* 1999 Mar 27; 353(9158): 1076.
(CLONING)

Taube, Sheila E. see **Merz, Jon F.**

Tauber, Alfred I. Confessions of a Medicine Man: An Essay in Popular Philosophy. Cambridge, MA: MIT Press; 1999. 159 p.
(MEDICAL ETHICS; PROFESSIONAL PATIENT RELATIONSHIP)

Tauer, Carol see **Lebacqz, Karen**

Tauer, Carol A. Private ethics boards and public debate. [Symposium: human primordial stem cells]. *Hastings Center Report.* 1999 Mar–Apr; 29(2): 43–45.
(EMBRYO AND FETAL RESEARCH)

Tavistock Group see **Benatar, Solomon R.**

Taylor, Brent see **Sutcliffe, Alastair G.**

Taylor, Carol. Medical futility and nursing. *Image: The Journal of Nursing Scholarship.* 1995 Winter; 27(4): 301–306.
(ALLOWING TO DIE)

Taylor, Carol R. Reflections on "Nursing considered as moral practice." *Kennedy Institute of Ethics Journal.* 1998 Mar; 8(1): 71–82.
(NURSING ETHICS)

Taylor, Jack A. see **Wilcox, Allen J.**

Taylor, Pamela see **Thomas, Sandy**

Taylor, Robert. Superhumans. *New Scientist.* 1998 Oct 3; 160(2154): 24–29.
(GENE THERAPY; GENETIC INTERVENTION)

Taylor, S.J. see **Prado, C.G.**

Teicher, Stacy A. When minors refuse medical treatment. [News]. *Christian Science Monitor.* 1999 Feb 9: 3.
(TREATMENT REFUSAL/MINORS)

Teitelbaum, Alexander see **Bar El, Yair Carlos**

Telesford, Mary see **Osher, Trina W.**

Telling, Douglas Cushman. Science in Politics: Eugenics, Sterilization, and Genetic Screening. Ann Arbor, MI: UMI Dissertation Services; 1988. 264 p.
(EUGENICS; GENETIC SCREENING; STERILIZATION)

Temianka, Daniel see **Kosseff, Andrew L.**

ten Have, Henk. Living with the future: genetic

information and human existence. *In:* Chadwick, Ruth; Levitt, Mairi; Shickle, Darren, eds. The Right to Know and the Right Not to Know. Brookfield, VT: Ashgate; 1997: 87–95.
(GENETIC SCREENING)

ten Have, Henk see **Chadwick, Ruth**

ten Have, Henk see **Hoedemaekers, Rogeer**

ten Have, Henk A.M.J. Consensus formation and healthcare policy. *In:* ten Have, Henk A.M.J.; Sass, Hans–Martin, eds. Consensus Formation in Healthcare Ethics. Boston, MA: Kluwer Academic; 1998: 45–59.
(HEALTH CARE/FOREIGN COUNTRIES; RESOURCE ALLOCATION)

ten Have, Henk A.M.J.; Sass, Hans–Martin, eds. Consensus Formation in Healthcare Ethics. Boston, MA: Kluwer Academic; 1998. 256 p.
(BIOETHICS)

ten Have, Henk A.M.J.; Welie, Jos V.M. Euthanasia in the Netherlands. *Critical Care Clinics.* 1996 Jan; 12(1): 97–108.
(EUTHANASIA)

ten Have, Henk A.M.J.; Welie, Jos V.M., eds. Ownership of the Human Body: Philosophical Considerations on the Use of the Human Body and Its Parts in Healthcare. Boston, MA: Kluwer Academic; 1998. 235 p.
(BIOETHICS; ORGAN AND TISSUE DONATION)

ten Have, Henk A.M.J. see **Dekkers, Wim J.M.**

Tenery, Robert M. see **Margolis, Lewis H.**

Tennenbaum, David see **Stoddard, Joan C.**

Tennessee. Supreme Court, at Knoxville see **Hopkins, Patrick D.**

Teno, Joan see **Wasson, John H.**

Teno, Joan M.; Branco, Kenneth J.; Mor, Vincent; Phillips, Charles D.; Hawes, Catherine; Morris, John; Fries, Brant E. Changes in advance care planning in nursing homes before and after the Patient Self–Determination Act: report of a 10–state survey. *Journal of the American Geriatrics Society.* 1997 Aug; 45(8): 939–944.
(ADVANCE DIRECTIVES; RESUSCITATION ORDERS)

Teno, Joan M. see **Hamel, Mary Beth**

Teno, Joan M. see **Pritchard, Robert S.**

Teo, K.P. see **Gbolade, Babatunde A.**

Terry, Peter B. see **Korzick, Karen A.**

Terry, Peter B. see **O'Rourke, Kevin**

Terry, Sara. The ethics of selecting child's sex. *Christian Science Monitor.* 1998 Sep 17: 1, 4.
(SEX PRESELECTION)

Tessman, Irwin; Neiburger, Ellis J.; Greely, Henry T.; Annas, George J. Bragdon v. Abbott: the Americans

with Disabilities Act and HIV infection. [Letters and response]. *New England Journal of Medicine.* 1999 Apr 15; 340(15): 1212–1214.
(AIDS/HEALTH PERSONNEL)

Thévoz, J.M. see **Müller, H.J.**

Thiel, Elaine C. see **Aikman, Peter J.**

Thiel, Elaine C. see **Martin, Douglas K.**

Thigpen, Janet see **Sexson, William R.**

Thom, David H.; Campbell, Bruce. Patient–physician trust: an exploratory study. *Journal of Family Practice.* 1997 Feb; 44(2): 169–176.
(PROFESSIONAL PATIENT RELATIONSHIP)

Thomas, Claire D. see **Enbom, John A.**

Thomas, Joe. Ethical challenges of HIV clinical trials in developing countries. *Bioethics.* 1998 Oct; 12(4): 320–327.
(AIDS/HUMAN EXPERIMENTATION; HUMAN EXPERIMENTATION/FOREIGN COUNTRIES; HUMAN EXPERIMENTATION/RESEARCH DESIGN; HUMAN EXPERIMENTATION/SPECIAL POPULATIONS)

Thomas, Sandy; Caldicott, Fiona; Barchard, Chris; Bartlett, Rachel; Haldane, John; Hornby, Sonia; McGuffin, Peter; Pleming, Nigel; Richards, Martin; Taylor, Pamela; Wilkie, Andrew; Young, Sally. Restrict genetic susceptibility tests. [Letter]. *Nature.* 1998 Sep 24; 395(6700): 317.
(GENETIC RESEARCH; GENETIC SCREENING)

Thomasma, David C. Assessing the arguments for and against euthanasia and assisted suicide: part two. *Cambridge Quarterly of Healthcare Ethics.* 1998 Fall; 7(4): 388–401.
(EUTHANASIA; SUICIDE)

Thomasma, David C. Assisted death and martyrdom. *Christian Bioethics.* 1998 Aug; 4(2): 122–142.
(EUTHANASIA/RELIGIOUS ASPECTS; SUICIDE)

Thomasma, David C. Bioethics and international human rights. *Journal of Law, Medicine and Ethics.* 1997 Winter; 25(4): 295–306.
(BIOETHICS)

Thomasma, David C. Stewardship of the aged: meeting the ethical challenge of ageism. *Cambridge Quarterly of Healthcare Ethics.* 1999 Spring; 8(2): 148–159.
(MEDICAL ETHICS; PATIENT CARE/AGED; PROFESSIONAL PATIENT RELATIONSHIP)

Thomasma, David C. Toward a 21st century bioethic. *Alternative Therapies in Health and Medicine.* 1995 Mar; 1(1): 74–75.
(BIOETHICS; BIOMEDICAL TECHNOLOGIES)

Thomasma, David C.; Kimbrough–Kushner, Thomasine; Kimsma, Gerrit K.; Ciesielski–Carlucci, Chris, eds. Asking to Die: Inside the Dutch Debate About Euthanasia. Boston, MA: Kluwer Academic; 1998. 584 p.
(EUTHANASIA; SUICIDE)

Thomasma, David C.; Micetich, Kenneth C.; Brems, John; Van Theil, David. The ethics of competition in liver transplantation. *Cambridge Quarterly of*

Healthcare Ethics. 1999 Summer; 8(3): 321–329.
(FRAUD AND MISCONDUCT; ORGAN AND TISSUE TRANSPLANTATION; RESOURCE ALLOCATION/BIOMEDICAL TECHNOLOGIES; SELECTION FOR TREATMENT)

Thomasma, David C. see **Jain, Renu**

Thomasma, David C. see **Muraskas, Jonathan**

Thompson, Angela. International protection of women's rights: an analysis of *Open Door Counselling Ltd. and Dublin Well Woman Centre v. Ireland. Boston University International Law Journal.* 1994; 12: 371–406.
(ABORTION/FOREIGN COUNTRIES; ABORTION/LEGAL ASPECTS)

Thompson, Dennis F. The institutional turn in professional ethics. *Ethics and Behavior.* 1999; 9(2): 109–118.
(PROFESSIONAL ETHICS; SUICIDE)

Thompson, Dick see **Lemonick, Michael D.**

Thompson, Donovan J. see **Brown, Norman K.**

Thompson, M. see **Williams, L.**

Thompson, Nancy J. see **Clemency, Mary V.**

Thomson, B. Time for reassessment of use of all medical information by UK insurers. *Lancet.* 1998 Oct 10; 352(9135): 1216–1218.
(GENETIC SCREENING)

Thomson, Elizabeth. The Ethical, Legal, and Social Implications Program at the National Human Genome Research Institute, NIH. *In:* Smith, Edward; Sapp, Walter, eds. Plain Talk about the Human Genome Project: A Tuskegee University Conference on Its Promise and Perils ... and Matters of Race. Tuskegee, AL: Tuskegee University Press; 1997: 123–130.
(GENETIC RESEARCH; GENOME MAPPING)

Thomson, Elizabeth J. see **Wilfond, Benjamin S.**

Thomson, Mathew. Sterilization, segregation and community care: ideology and solutions to the problem of mental deficiency in inter-war Britain. *History of Psychiatry.* 1992 Dec; 3(12): 473–498.
(EUGENICS; STERILIZATION/MENTALLY DISABLED)

Thomson, Mathew. The Problem of Mental Deficiency: Eugenics, Democracy, and Social Policy in Britain c. 1870–1959. New York, NY: Oxford University Press; 1998. 351 p.
(EUGENICS; STERILIZATION/MENTALLY DISABLED)

Thomson, Michael. Reproducing Narrative: Gender, Reproduction and Law. Brookfield, VT: Ashgate; 1998. 228 p.
(ABORTION; REPRODUCTION)

Thorne, Emanuel D. When private parts are made public goods: the economics of market–inalienability. *Yale Journal on Regulation.* 1998 Winter; 15(1): 149–175.
(ORGAN AND TISSUE DONATION)

Thorns, Andrew; Lloyd, Geoffrey; Szmukler, George; Welsh, James. Certifying fitness for corporal punishment: ethical debate. [Case study, commentaries, and response]. *BMJ (British Medical Journal).* 1998 Oct

3; 317(7163): 939–941.
(FRAUD AND MISCONDUCT)

Thornton, Simon see **Sutcliffe, Alastair G.**

Tichtchenko, Pavel. New bioethics association is founded for the post-socialist countries. [News]. *Bulletin of Medical Ethics.* 1999 Apr; No. 147: 6.
(BIOETHICS; ETHICISTS AND ETHICS COMMITTEES)

Tiedje, Linda Beth. Ethical and legal issues in the care of substance–using women. *Journal of Obstetric, Gynecologic and Neonatal Nursing.* 1998 Jan–Feb; 27(1): 92–98.
(PATIENT CARE; PRENATAL INJURIES)

Tiefel, Hans O. Human cloning in ethical perspectives. *In:* Humber, James M.; Almeder, Robert F.,eds. Human Cloning. Totowa, NJ: Humana Press; 1998: 177–207.
(CLONING)

Tierney, William M. see **Gramelspacher, Gregory P.**

Til Occam Ltd. Medical Research Ethics Committee Directory: United Kingdom and Republic of Ireland. 1996 Version. [Looseleaf format]. Surrey Research Park, Guildford, England: Til Occam; 1996. 247 p.
(HUMAN EXPERIMENTATION/ETHICS COMMITTEES; HUMAN EXPERIMENTATION/FOREIGN COUNTRIES)

Tilden, Virginia P. see **Tolle, Susan W.**

Timberlake, Susan. UNAIDS: human rights, ethics, and law. *Health and Human Rights.* 1998; 3(1): 87–106.
(AIDS)

Timberlake, Susan see **Piot, Peter**

Timmis, Adam see **Barakat, Khalid**

Tishler, L. Carl; Gordon, Lisa B. Ethical parameters of challenge studies inducing psychosis with ketamine. *Ethics and Behavior.* 1999; 9(3): 211–217.
(HUMAN EXPERIMENTATION/RESEARCH DESIGN; HUMAN EXPERIMENTATION/SPECIAL POPULATIONS)

Tishler, S. see **Mecsas–Faxon, S.**

Tizzard, Juliet. Reproductive technology: new ethical dilemmas and old moral prejudices. *In:* Lee, Ellie, ed. Abortion Law and Politics Today. New York, NY: St. Martin's Press; 1998: 184–197.
(REPRODUCTIVE TECHNOLOGIES)

Tokuda, Yasuharu; Kadlec, Robert F.; Zelicoff, Alan P. Physicians and biological warfare agents. [Letter and response]. *JAMA.* 1998 Jan 28; 279(4): 273–274.
(WAR)

Tolle, Susan W.; Rosenfeld, Anne G.; Tilden, Virginia P.; Park, Yon. Oregon's low in–hospital death rates: what determines where people die and satisfaction with decisions on place of death? *Annals of Internal Medicine.* 1999 Apr 20; 130(8): 681–685.
(TERMINAL CARE)

Tolle, Susan W. see **Chiodo, Gary T.**

Tolle, Susan W. see **Ganzini, Linda**

Tollefsen, Christopher. Advance directives and voluntary

slavery: response to "Reassessing the reliability of advance directives," by Thomas May (*CQ* Vol. 6., No. 3). *Cambridge Quarterly of Healthcare Ethics.* 1998 Fall; 7(4): 405–413.
(ADVANCE DIRECTIVES; PERSONHOOD)

Tollefsen, Christopher. Donagan, abortion, and civil rebellion. *Public Affairs Quarterly.* 1997 Jul; 11(3): 303–312.
(ABORTION)

Tomich, Paul see **Muraskas, Jonathan**

Tomlin, P.J. A memorable incident: when a spade is not a spade. *BMJ (British Medical Journal).* 1999 Jan 23; 318(7178): 256.
(TREATMENT REFUSAL)

Tomlinson, Tom see **Andre, Judith**

Tomoda, Atsuko see **Kitamura, Fusako**

Tompkins, Catherine see **Hoffmann, Diane E.**

Tonelli, Mark R.; Lynn, Joanne; Orentlicher, David. Terminal sedation. [Letters and response]. *New England Journal of Medicine.* 1998 Apr 23; 338(17): 1230–1231.
(EUTHANASIA; TERMINAL CARE)

Tong, Rosemarie. Just caring about maternal–fetal relations: the case of cocaine–using pregnant women. *In:* Donchin, Anne; Purdy, Laura M., eds. Embodying Bioethics: Recent Feminist Advances. Lanham, MD: Rowman and Littlefield; 1999: 33–43.
(PRENATAL INJURIES)

Tong, Rosemarie. The way of feminist bioethics. [Book review essay]. *Medical Humanities Review.* 1997 Spring; 11(1): 72–75.
(BIOETHICS; REPRODUCTION)

Tooley, Michael. Personhood. *In:* Kuhse, Helga; Singer, Peter, eds. A Companion to Bioethics. Malden, MA: Blackwell; 1998: 117–126.
(PERSONHOOD)

Tooley, Michael. The moral status of the cloning of humans. *In:* Humber, James M.;Almeder, Robert F.,eds. Human Cloning. Totowa, NJ: Humana Press; 1998: 65–101.
(CLONING)

Topol, Eric J. Publication and promotion: drafter and draftees. *Lancet.* 1998 Sep 12; 352(9131): 897–898.
(BIOMEDICAL RESEARCH)

Torner, James C. see **Shavers–Hornaday, Vickie L.**

Torrance, Caroline J.; Das, Robert; Allison, Miles C. Use of chaperones in clinics for genitourinary medicine: survey of consultants. *BMJ (British Medical Journal).* 1999 Jul 17; 319(7203): 159–160.
(PATIENT CARE; PROFESSIONAL PATIENT RELATIONSHIP)

Toth, Ellen L.; Gill, Satvir; Godkin, Diane; Lee, Kwoc–Choy. Advance directives for insulin–using diabetic patients. [Letter]. *Canadian Medical Association Journal.* 1998 May 5; 158(9): 1130–1131.
(ADVANCE DIRECTIVES)

Toubia, Nahid see **Moore, Kirsten**

Townes, Emilie M. Breaking the Fine Rain of Death: African American Health Issues and a Womanist Ethic of Care. New York, NY: Continuum; 1998. 214 p.
(HEALTH CARE)

Tracy, David. Human cloning and the public realm: a defense of intuitions of the good. *In:* Nussbaum, Martha C.; Sunstein, Cass R., eds. Clones and Clones: Facts and Fantasies About Human Cloning. New York, NY: Norton; 1998: 190–203.
(CLONING)

Tracy, Mark J. see **Lerner, Barron H.**

Tramèr, Martin R.; Reynolds, D. John M.; Moore, R. Andrew; McQuay, Henry J. When placebo controlled trials are essential and equivalence trials are inadequate. *BMJ (British Medical Journal).* 1998 Sep 26; 317(7162): 875–880.
(HUMAN EXPERIMENTATION/RESEARCH DESIGN)

Treene, Eric W. see **Glendon, Mary Ann**

Treloar, Adrian see **Engelhart, Karlheinz**

Trevett, Kenneth P. see **Hsu, John**

Tribble, Jack L. Gene patents -- a pharmaceutical perspective. *Cambridge Quarterly of Healthcare Ethics.* 1998 Fall; 7(4): 429–432.
(GENOME MAPPING)

Tribe, Laurence. On not banning cloning for the wrong reasons. *In:* Nussbaum, Martha C.; Sunstein, Cass R., eds. Clones and Clones: Facts and Fantasies About Human Cloning. New York, NY: Norton; 1998: 221–232.
(CLONING)

Trickett, Edison J. Toward a framework for defining and resolving ethical issues in the protection of communities involved in primary prevention projects. *Ethics and Behavior.* 1998; 8(4): 321–337.
(BEHAVIORAL RESEARCH; MENTAL HEALTH; PUBLIC HEALTH)

Tripp, J.H. see **Shah, V.S.**

Trippitelli, Carol Lynn; Jamison, Kay R.; Folstein, Marshal F.; Bartko, John J.; DePaulo, J. Raymond. Pilot study on patients' and spouses' attitudes toward potential genetic testing for bipolar disorder. *American Journal of Psychiatry.* 1998 Jul; 155(7): 899–904.
(GENETIC SCREENING; PRENATAL DIAGNOSIS)

Trivedi, Sandhya see **Workman, Richard H.**

Trock, Bruce J. see **Lerman, Caryn**

Trotter, C. Griffin. The medical covenant: a Roycean perspective. *In:* McGee, Glenn, ed. Pragmatic Bioethics. Nashville, TN: Vanderbilt University Press; 1999: 84–96, 266–269.
(MEDICAL ETHICS; PROFESSIONAL PATIENT RELATIONSHIP)

Trotter, Griffin. Mandated choice for organ donation. *Health Care Ethics USA.* 1997 Spring; 5(2): 2–3.
(ORGAN AND TISSUE DONATION)

Troy, Edwin S. Flores. The Genetic Privacy Act: an

analysis of privacy and research concerns. *Journal of Law, Medicine and Ethics*. 1997 Winter; 25(4): 256–272.
(CONFIDENTIALITY/LEGAL ASPECTS; GENETIC SCREENING)

Trull, Frankie L.; Rich, Barbara A. More regulation of rodents. [Editorial]. *Science*. 1999 May 28; 284(5419): 1463.
(ANIMAL EXPERIMENTATION)

Truman, Alison see **Grumbach, Kevin**

Truog, Robert D.; Robinson, Walter; Randolph, Adrienne; Morris, Alan. Is informed consent always necessary for randomized, controlled trials? *New England Journal of Medicine*. 1999 Mar 11; 340(10): 804–807.
(HUMAN EXPERIMENTATION/INFORMED CONSENT)

Truog, Robert D. see **Lizza, John B.**

Tschann, Jeanne M. see **Nachtigall, Robert D.**

Tschudin, Verena; Hunt, Geoffrey; Olsen, Douglas, et al. International Centres for Nursing Ethics [ICNE]. [Editorial]. *Nursing Ethics*. 1999 May; 6(3): 187–188.
(NURSING ETHICS)

Tsuang, Ming T. see **Faraone, Stephen V.**

Tsuchin, Verena. Special issues facing nurses. *In:* Kuhse, Helga; Singer, Peter, eds. A Companion to Bioethics. Malden, MA: Blackwell; 1998: 463–471.
(NURSING ETHICS)

Tsuchiya, Takashi. Eugenic sterilizations in Japan and recent demands for an apology: a report. *Ethics and Intellectual Disability*. 1997 Fall; 3(1): 1–4.
(EUGENICS; STERILIZATION)

Tsukada, Kazumi see **Kitamura, Fusako**

Tucker, Bonnie see **Haimowitz, Stephan**

Tucker, Kathryn L.; Burman, David J. Physician aid in dying: a humane option, a constitutionally protected choice. *Seattle University Law Review*. 1995 Spring; 18(3): 495–508.
(SUICIDE)

Tuffs, Annette. German drug agency approves mifepristone. [News]. *BMJ (British Medical Journal)*. 1999 Jul 17; 319(7203): 141.
(ABORTION/FOREIGN COUNTRIES; ABORTION/LEGAL ASPECTS)

Tuffs, Annette. Max–Planck Society investigates misconduct. [News]. *BMJ (British Medical Journal)*. 1999 Jul 31; 319(7205): 274.
(BIOMEDICAL RESEARCH; FRAUD AND MISCONDUCT)

Tulsky, James see **Lo, Bernard**

Tulsky, James A.; Fischer, Gary S.; Rose, Mary R.; Arnold, Robert M. Opening the black box: how do physicians communicate about advance directives? *Annals of Internal Medicine*. 1998 Sep 15; 129(6): 441–449.
(ADVANCE DIRECTIVES)

Tunisia. Decree No. 93–1155 of 17 May 1993 promulgating the Code of Medical Ethics. (*Journal Official de la Republique Tunisienne*, 28 May and 1 Jun 1993, No. 40, p. 764–770). [Summary]. *International Digest of Health Legislation*. 1994. 45(1). 53–54.
(HUMAN EXPERIMENTATION/REGULATION)

Tuohey, John F. Covenant model of corporate compliance. *Health Progress*. 1998 Jul–Aug; 79(4): 70–75.
(HEALTH CARE)

Tuohey, John F. see **Cowdin, Daniel M.**

Tuppin, Phillippe see **Julvez, Jean**

Türkman, A. see **Sever, M.S.**

Turnbull, John see **Crelinsten, Gordon L.**

Turner, J.Z. I don't want to see the pictures: science writing and the visibility of animal experiments. *Public Understanding of Science*. 1998 Jan; 7(1): 27–40.
(ANIMAL EXPERIMENTATION)

Turner, Marie T. see **Desvarieux, Moïse**

Turner, N.J.; Haward, R.A.; Mulley, G.P.; Selby, P.J. Cancer in old age -- is it inadequately investigated and treated? *BMJ (British Medical Journal)*. 1999 Jul 31; 319(7205): 309–312.
(PATIENT CARE/AGED; SELECTION FOR TREATMENT)

Turner, Philip see **Brown, Harold O.J.**

Turney, Jon. Frankenstein's Footsteps: Science, Genetics and Popular Culture. New Haven, CT: Yale University Press; 1998. 276 p.
(GENETIC INTERVENTION; GENETIC RESEARCH; RECOMBINANT DNA RESEARCH)

Turone, Fabio see **Beecham, Linda**

Tuthill, Kathryn A. Human experimentation: protecting patient autonomy through informed consent. *Journal of Legal Medicine*. 1997 Jun; 18(2): 221–250.
(HUMAN EXPERIMENTATION/INFORMED CONSENT)

Tymstra, Tj. see **Sullivan, Mark**

Tzelepis, Angela see **Butler, Dennis J.**

U

U.S. Centers for Disease Control and Prevention. HIV Counseling, Testing, and Referral: Standards and Guidelines. Washington, DC: U.S. Government Printing Office; 1994 May. 15 p.
(AIDS/TESTING AND SCREENING)

U.S. Centers for Disease Control and Prevention see **Children's Defense Fund**

U.S. Congress. House. A bill to establish federal penalties for prohibited uses and disclosures of individually identifiable health information, to establish a right in an individual to inspect and copy their own health information, and for other purposes [Consumer Health and Research technology (CHART) Protection Act]. H.R. 3900, 105th Cong., 2d Sess. Introduced by Christopher Shays.; 1998 May 19. 48 p.
(CONFIDENTIALITY/LEGAL ASPECTS; PATIENT ACCESS TO RECORDS)

U.S. Congress. House. Committee on Commerce. Subcommittee on Health and Environment. Cloning: Legal, Medical, Ethical, and Social Issues. Hearing, 12 Feb 1998. Washington, DC: U.S. Government Printing Office; 1998. 141 p.
(CLONING)

U.S. Congress. House. Committee on Government Reform and Oversight. Subcommittee on Human Resources. Institutional Review Boards: A System in Jeopardy. Hearing, 11 Jun 1998. Washington, DC: U.S. Government Printing Office; 1999. 179 p.
(ETHICISTS AND ETHICS COMMITTEES; HUMAN EXPERIMENTATION/ETHICS COMMITTEES)

U.S. Congress. Senate. A bill to improve the access and choice of patients to quality, affordable health care [Patients' Bill of Rights Act of 1998]. S. 2330, 105th Cong., 2d Sess. Introduced by Trent Lott for Don Nickles, for himself, and others.; 1998 Jul 17 (first reading). 185 p.
(HEALTH CARE/ECONOMICS; PATIENTS' RIGHTS)

U.S. Congress. Senate. Committee on Appropriations. Subcommitte on Departments of Labor, Health and Human Services, and Education, and Related Agencies. Stem Cell Research. Special Hearings, 2 Dec 1998, 12 Jan 1999, 26 Jan 1999. Washington, DC: U.S. Government Printing Office; 1999. 148 p.
(EMBRYO AND FETAL RESEARCH)

U.S. Court of Appeals, Fifth Circuit. Hope Medical Group for Women v. Edwards. *Federal Reporter, 3d Series.* 1998 Sep 11 (date of decision). 63: 418–429.
(ABORTION/FINANCIAL SUPPORT; ABORTION/LEGAL ASPECTS)

U.S. Court of Appeals, Fourth Circuit. Planned Parenthood of the Blue Ridge v. Camblos. *Federal Reporter, 3d Series.* 1997 Jun 30 (date of decision). 116: 707–721.
(ABORTION/LEGAL ASPECTS; ABORTION/MINORS)

U.S. Court of Appeals, Ninth Circuit. Norman-Bloodsaw v. Lawrence Berkeley Laboratory. *Federal Reporter, 3d Series.* 1998 Feb 3 (date of decision). 135: 1260–1276.
(GENETIC SCREENING; MASS SCREENING)

U.S. Court of Appeals, Ninth Circuit. Wicklund v. Salvagni. *Federal Reporter, 3d Series.* 1996 Aug 16 (date of decision). 93: 567–572.
(ABORTION/LEGAL ASPECTS; ABORTION/MINORS)

U.S. Court of Appeals, Sixth Circuit. Women's Medical Professional Corporation v. Voinovich. *Federal Reporter, 3d Series.* 1997 Nov 18 (date of decision). 130: 187–219.
(ABORTION/LEGAL ASPECTS)

U.S. Court of Appeals, Tenth Circuit. Jane L. v. Bangerter. *Federal Reporter, 3d Series.* 1996 Dec 23 (date of decision). 102: 1112–1118.
(ABORTION/LEGAL ASPECTS)

U.S. Department of Health and Human Services. The Conduct of Clinical Trials of Maternal-Infant Transmission of HIV Supported by the United States Department of Health and Human Services in Developing Countries: A Summary of the Needs of Developing Countries, the Scientific Applications, and the Ethical Considerations Assessed by the National Institutes of Health and the Centers for Disease Control and Prevention, 1994–1997. Downloaded from Internet Web site: http://www.nih.gov/news/mathiv/mathiv.htm and http://www.nih.gov/news/mathiv/whodoc.htm (Appendix) on 6 Dec 1997; 1997 Jul. 10 p.
(AIDS/HUMAN EXPERIMENTATION; HUMAN EXPERIMENTATION/FOREIGN COUNTRIES; HUMAN EXPERIMENTATION/RESEARCH DESIGN; HUMAN EXPERIMENTATION/SPECIAL POPULATIONS)

U.S. Department of Health and Human Services. Secretary's Advisory Committee on Genetic Testing. A Public Consultation on Oversight of Genetic Tests, December 1, 1999 – January 31, 2000. Issued by the Committee, 6000 Executive Blvd., Suite 302, Bethesda, MD 20892, http://www4.od.nih.gov/oba/sacgt.htm; 1999 Dec. 39 p.
(GENETIC SCREENING)

U.S. Department of Health and Human Services. Secretary's Advisory Committee on Genetic Testing. A Public Consultation on Oversight of Genetic Tests, December 1, 1999 – January 31, 2000: Summary. Issued by the Committee, 6000 Executive Blvd., Suite 302, Bethesda, MD 20892, http://www4.od.nih.gov/oba/sacgt.htm; 1999 Dec. 8 p.
(GENETIC SCREENING)

U.S. District Court, D. Montana, Butte Division. Wicklund v. Lambert. *Federal Supplement.* 1997 Oct 9 (date of decision). 979: 1285–1290.
(ABORTION/LEGAL ASPECTS; ABORTION/MINORS)

U.S. District Court, D. Nebraska. Carhart v. Stenberg. *Federal Supplement.* 1997 Aug 14 (date of decision). 972: 507–531.
(ABORTION/LEGAL ASPECTS)

U.S. District Court, D. Nebraska. Orr v. Nelson. *Federal Supplement.* 1994 Nov 4 (date of decision). 902: 1019–1022.
(ABORTION/FINANCIAL SUPPORT; ABORTION/LEGAL ASPECTS)

U.S. District Court, D. Oregon. In the United States District Court for the District of Oregon: Lee v. State of Oregon, Order, Civil No. 94–6467-HO, 9 May 1996. *Issues in Law and Medicine.* 1996 Summer; 12(1): 79–92.
(SUICIDE)

U.S. District Court, D. Oregon. Lee v. State of Oregon. *Federal Supplement.* 1995 Aug 3 (date of decision). 891: 1429–1439.
(SUICIDE)

U.S. District Court, E.D. Louisiana. Okpalobi v. Foster. *Federal Supplement.* 1998 Jan 7 (date of decision). 981: 977–988.
(ABORTION/LEGAL ASPECTS)

U.S. District Court, E.D. Michigan, Southern Division. Evans v. Kelley. *Federal Supplement.* 1997 Jul 31 (date of decision). 977: 1283–1320.
(ABORTION/LEGAL ASPECTS)

U.S. District Court, W.D. Wisconsin. Karlin v. Foust. *Federal Supplement.* 1997 Oct 2 (date of decision). 975: 1177–1235.
(ABORTION/LEGAL ASPECTS)

U.S. District Court, W.D. Wisconsin. Planned Parenthood of Wisconsin v. Doyle. *Federal Supplement, 2d Series.* 1998 Jun 15 (date of decision). 9: 1033–1046.
(ABORTION/LEGAL ASPECTS)

U.S. Food and Drug Administration. Accessibility to new drugs for use in military and civilian exigencies when traditional human efficacy studies are not feasible; determination under the interim rule that informed consent is not feasible for military exigencies; request for comments. *Federal Register.* 1997 Jul 31; 62(147): 40996–41001.
(HUMAN EXPERIMENTATION/INFORMED CONSENT; HUMAN EXPERIMENTATION/SPECIAL POPULATIONS; WAR)

U.S. General Accounting Office. Department of Energy: Information on DOE's Human Tissue Analysis Work. Fact Sheet for Congressional Requesters. Washington, DC: U.S. General Accounting Office; 1995 May. 45 p.
(HUMAN EXPERIMENTATION)

U.S. General Accounting Office. Scientific Research: Continued Vigilance Critical to Protecting Human Subjects. Report to the Ranking Minority Member, Committee on Governmental Affairs, U.S. Senate. Washington, DC: U.S. General Accounting Office; 1996 Mar. 46 p.
(HUMAN EXPERIMENTATION/REGULATION)

U.S. General Accounting Office. Scientific Research: Continued Vigilance Critical to Protecting Human Subjects [Testimony: Statement of Sarah F. Jaggar before the Committee on Governmental Affairs, U.S. Senate]. Washington, DC: U.S. General Accounting Office; 1996 Mar 12. 9 p.
(HUMAN EXPERIMENTATION/REGULATION)

U.S. National Institutes of Health. Recombinant DNA research: actions under the guidelines; notice. *Federal Register.* 1995 Apr 27; 60(81): 20726–20737.
(GENE THERAPY; HUMAN EXPERIMENTATION/REGULATION; RECOMBINANT DNA RESEARCH/REGULATION)

U.S. National Institutes of Health. Cancer Genetics Studies Consortium see **Wilfond, Benjamin S.**

Ubel, Peter see **Menzel, Paul**

Ubel, Peter A.; Baron, Jonathan; Asch, David A. Social responsibility, personal responsibility, and prognosis in public judgments about transplant allocation. *Bioethics.* 1999 Jan; 13(1): 57–68.
(ORGAN AND TISSUE TRANSPLANTATION; RESOURCE ALLOCATION/BIOMEDICAL TECHNOLOGIES; SELECTION FOR TREATMENT)

Ubel, Peter A.; Caplan, Arthur L. Geographic favoritism in liver transplantation -- unfortunate or unfair? *New England Journal of Medicine.* 1998 Oct 29; 339(18): 1322–1325.
(ORGAN AND TISSUE TRANSPLANTATION; RESOURCE ALLOCATION/BIOMEDICAL TECHNOLOGIES; SELECTION FOR TREATMENT)

Uchitomi, Yosuke see **Okamura, Hitoshi**

Uddo, Basile J. The public law of abortion: a constitutional and statutory review of the present and future legal landscape. *In:* Rainey, R. Randall; Magill, Gerard, eds. Abortion and Public Policy: An Interdiscliplinary Investigation within the Catholic Tradition. Omaha, NE: Creighton University Press; 1996: 163–182.
(ABORTION/LEGAL ASPECTS)

Ugazio, Alberto G. see **Candotti, Fabio**

Ulrich, C.M.; Kristal, A.R.; Durfy, S.J.; Hunt, J.R.; White, E. Attitudes toward genetic testing for cancer risk among Washington State residents. [Abstract]. *American Journal of Human Genetics.* 1996 Oct; 59(4): A340.
(GENETIC SCREENING)

Underwood, James L. The Supreme Court's assisted suicide opinions in international perspective: avoiding a bureaucracy of death. *North Dakota Law Review.* 1997; 73(4): 641–684.
(EUTHANASIA/LEGAL ASPECTS; SUICIDE)

Unesco. Universal declaration on the human genome and human rights (revised draft). *Bulletin of Medical Ethics.* 1997 Mar; No. 126: 9–11.
(GENETIC RESEARCH; GENOME MAPPING)

Unesco. Universal Declaration on the Human Genome and Human Rights [UNESCO Document 27 V / 45, adopted by the Thirty-first General Assembly of UNESCO, Paris, 11 November 1997]. *Journal of Medicine and Philosophy.* 1998 Jun; 23(3): 334–341.
(GENETIC INTERVENTION; GENETIC RESEARCH; GENOME MAPPING)

Unesco. International Bioethics Committee. First Session. [Report of the first session of the International Bioethics Committee, Paris, 15–16 Sep 1993]. Paris: International Bioethics Committee; 1994 Feb 1. 10 p. plus annexes (90 p.).
(ETHICISTS AND ETHICS COMMITTEES)

Unesco. International Bioethics Committee. Proceedings of the Fourth Session, October 1996. Volume I. Paris: The Committee; 1998. 164 p.
(BIOETHICS; GENETIC INTERVENTION; GENETIC RESEARCH; GENOME MAPPING; HUMAN EXPERIMENTATION)

Unesco. International Bioethics Committee. Proceedings of the Fourth Session, October 1996. Volume II. Paris: The Committee; 1998. 94 p.
(BIOETHICS; GENETIC INTERVENTION; HUMAN EXPERIMENTATION)

United Nations. Economic and Social Council. Commission on Human Rights. Human Rights and Scientific and Technological Developments -- Human Rights and Bioethics. Report of the Secretary-General. New York, NY: United Nations; 1994 Nov 15. 34 p.
(BIOETHICS)

University of Manchester (U.K.). Centre for Social Ethics and Policy. AIDS: Ethics, Justice and European Policy: summary of conclusions and recommendations. *In:* Bennett, Rebecca; Erin, Charles A., eds. HIV and AIDS: Testing, Screening, and Confidentiality. New York, NY: Oxford University Press; 1999: 267–270.
(AIDS)

Unti, Sharon M. see **Rubenstein, Jeffrey S.**

Uratsu, Connie see **Grumbach, Kevin**

Urofsky, Melvin I. Leaving the door ajar: the Supreme

Court and assisted suicide. *University of Richmond Law Review.* 1998 Mar; 32(2): 313–405.
(SUICIDE)

Urowitz, Sara see **Kerr, Susan M.**

Uruguay. Decree No. 660/991 of 4 Dec 1991 updating Regulations No. 86/977, made for the implementation of Law No. 14005, for the purpose of determining the technical supervision of the National Organ and Tissue Bank. (*Diario Oficial de la Repdblic Oriental del Uruguay*, 10 Feb 1992, No. 23521, p. 194–A). [Summary]. *International Digest of Health Legislation.* 1994. 45(1). 38.
(ORGAN AND TISSUE DONATION)

Uysal, V. see **Sever, M.S.**

Uzych, Leo. Bioethics and NBAC. [Letter]. *Nature Biotechnology.* 1996 Sep; 14(9): 1057.
(ETHICISTS AND ETHICS COMMITTEES)

Uzych, Leo; Rischitelli, Gary. Genetic testing data. [Letter and response]. *Journal of Occupational and Environmental Medicine.* 1996 Jan; 38(1): 13–14.
(GENETIC SCREENING)

V

VACO [VA Central Office] Bioethics Committee. Allocation of expensive medications. Report. *NCCE News (Veterans Health Administration National Center for Clinical Ethics).* 1995 Spring; 3(2, Suppl.): S1–S9.
(PATIENT CARE/DRUGS; RESOURCE ALLOCATION/BIOMEDICAL TECHNOLOGIES)

Vafidis, Gilli see **Hingorani, Melanie**

Vaillant, George E. see **Lynn, David J.**

Valdiserri, Ronald O.; Robinson, Carol; Lin, Lillian S.; West, Gary R.; Holtgrave, David R. Determining allocations for HIV–prevention interventions: assessing a change in federal funding policy. *AIDS and Public Policy Journal.* 1997 Winter; 12(4): 138–148.
(AIDS; RESOURCE ALLOCATION)

Valentine–Adams, Nancy see **Freda, Margaret Comerford**

Valluzzi, Janet L. see **Brown, Sharan E.**

Valmana, Anton see **White, D.M.D.**

Valois, Pierre see **Blondeau, Danielle**

Van Allen, Margot I. see **Bernard, Lynn E.**

van Amerongen, Patrice see **Lot, Florence**

van Balen, Frank. Development of IVF children. *Developmental Review.* 1998 Mar; 18(1): 30–46.
(IN VITRO FERTILIZATION; REPRODUCTIVE TECHNOLOGIES)

Vance, Gail H. see **Smith, David H.**

van de Scheur, Ada; van der Arend, Arie. The role of nurses in euthanasia: a Dutch study. *Nursing Ethics.* 1998 Nov; 5(6): 497–508.
(EUTHANASIA)

van Delden, Johannes J.M. Slippery slopes in flat countries — a response. *Journal of Medical Ethics.* 1999 Feb; 25(1): 22–24.
(EUTHANASIA)

Van den Berghe, Herman see **Decruyenaere, Marleen**

Van den Berghe, Herman see **Welkenhuysen, Myriam**

van den Boom, Frans M. AIDS, euthanasia and grief. *AIDS Care.* 1995; 7(Suppl. 2): S175–S185.
(AIDS; EUTHANASIA)

Vandenbergh, John G. Animal welfare issues in animal behavior research. *In:* Hart, Lynette A., ed. Responsible Conduct with Animals in Research. New York, NY: Oxford University Press; 1998: 67–76.
(ANIMAL EXPERIMENTATION)

van der Arend, Arie see **van de Scheur, Ada**

van der Burg, Wibren. Law and bioethics. *In:* Kuhse, Helga; Singer, Peter, eds. A Companion to Bioethics. Malden, MA: Blackwell; 1998: 49–57.
(BIOETHICS)

Van der Feen, Julie R.; Jellinek, Michael S. Consultation to end–of–life treatment decisions in children. *In:* Steinberg, Maurice D.; Youngner, Stuart J., eds. End–of–Life Decisions: A Psychosocial Perspective. Washington, DC: American Psychiatric Press; 1998: 137–177.
(ALLOWING TO DIE)

van der Maas, Paul J. see **Cuperus–Bosma, Jacqueline M.**

van der Maas, Paul J. see **Haverkate, Ilinka**

van der Meer, Miriam see **Mepham, T. Ben**

van der Valk, Jan; Dewhurst, David; Hughes, Ian; Atkinson, Jeffrey; Balcombe, Jonathan; Braun, Hans; Gabrielson, Karin; Gruber, Franz; Miles, Jeremy; Nab, Jan; Nardi, Jason; van Wilgenburg, Henk; Zinko, Ursula; Zurlo, Joanne. Alternatives to the Use of Animals in Higher Education: The Report and Recommendations of ECVAM (European Centre for the Validation of Alternate Methods) Workshop 33. *ATLA: Alternatives to Laboratory Animals.* 1999 Jan–Feb; 27(1): 39–52.
(ANIMAL EXPERIMENTATION)

Vander Veer, Joseph B. Euthanasia and Law in the Netherlands, by John Griffiths, et al. [Book review essay]. *JAMA.* 1999 Feb 10; 281(6): 568–569.
(EUTHANASIA)

van der Wal, Gerrit see **Cuperus–Bosma, Jacqueline M.**

van der Wal, Gerrit see **Haverkate, Ilinka**

van der Wal, Gerrit see **Onwuteaka–Philipsen, Bregje D.**

van Es, Adriaan see **Welsh, James**

van Eyl, Diderico see **Baram, Michael**

Van Gerven, Veerle see **Welkenhuysen, Myriam**

Van Haeringen, Alison R.; Dadds, Mark; Armstrong, Kenneth L. The child abuse lottery -- will the doctor suspect and report? Physician attitudes towards and reporting of suspected child abuse and neglect. *Child Abuse and Neglect.* 1998 Mar; 22(3): 159–169.
(CONFIDENTIALITY; PATIENT CARE/MINORS)

van Hooft, Stan. Acting from the virtue of caring in nursing. *Nursing Ethics.* 1999 May; 6(3): 189–201.
(NURSING ETHICS)

van Hooft, Stan. The meanings of suffering. *Hastings Center Report.* 1998 Sep–Oct; 28(5): 13–19.
(BIOETHICS)

van Hooft, Stan; Gillam, Lynn; Byrnes, Margot. The logic of ethical thinking. *In: their* Facts and Values: An Introduction to Critical Thinking for Nurses. Philadelphia, PA: MacLennan and Petty; 1995: 185–270, 278.
(NURSING ETHICS)

Vanischseni, Suphak see **Des Jarlais, Don C.**

van Kreijl, Coen F. see **Mepham, T. Ben**

Van Overwalle, Geertrui. Biotechnology patents in Europe: from law to ethics. *In:* Sterckx, Sigrid, ed. Biotechnology, Patents and Morality. Proceedings of an International Workshop, "Biotechnology, Patents and Morality: Towards a Consensus," held in Ghent, Belgium, 17–19 Jan 1996. Brookfield, VT: Ashgate; 1997: 139–148.
(GENETIC INTERVENTION; PATENTING LIFE FORMS)

Vanrenterghem, Y. see **Roels, L.**

Van Steirteghem, A.C. see **Baetens, P.**

Van Theil, David see **Thomasma, David C.**

van Veenendaal, E. Child abuse: does disclosing the fact have implications for medical secrecy? *Medicine and Law.* 1993; 12(1–2): 25–28.
(CONFIDENTIALITY)

van Walraven, Carl; Forster, Alan J.; Stiell, Ian G. Derivation of a clinical decision rule for the discontinuation of in–hospital cardiac arrest resuscitations. *Archives of Internal Medicine.* 1999 Jan 25; 159(2): 129–134.
(ALLOWING TO DIE; RESUSCITATION ORDERS; SELECTION FOR TREATMENT)

van Wilgenburg, Henk see **van der Valk, Jan**

van Zeller, Anne–Marie see **Mepham, T. Ben**

van Zutphen, L.F.M.; Balls, M., eds. Animal Alternatives, Welfare and Ethics. New York, NY: Elsevier; 1997. 1,260 p.
(ANIMAL EXPERIMENTATION)

van Zutphen, L.F.M. see **Festing, M.F.W.**

Varekamp, Inge; Meiland, Franka J.M.; Hoos, Aloysia M.; Wendte, Johannes F.; de Haes, Johanna C.J.M.; Krol, Leendert J. The meaning of urgency in the allocation of scarce health care resources; a comparison between renal transplantation and psychogeriatric nursing home care. *Health Policy.* 1998 May; 44(2): 135–148.
(ORGAN AND TISSUE TRANSPLANTATION; PATIENT CARE/AGED; RESOURCE ALLOCATION; SELECTION FOR TREATMENT)

Varghese, Francis T. see **Kelly, Brian**

Varmus, Harold. Evaluating the burden of disease and spending the research dollars of the National Institutes of Health. [Editorial]. *New England Journal of Medicine.* 1999 Jun 17; 340(24): 1914–1915.
(BIOMEDICAL RESEARCH; RESOURCE ALLOCATION)

Vassilas, C.A.; Donaldson, J. Few GPs tell patients of their diagnosis of Alzheimer's disease. [Letter]. *BMJ (British Medical Journal).* 1999 Feb 20; 318(7182): 536.
(TRUTH DISCLOSURE)

Vaught, Wayne; Lamdan, Ruth M. An ethics committee explores restraint use and practices. *HEC (HealthCare Ethics Committee) Forum.* 1998 Sep–Dec; 10(3–4): 306–316.
(BEHAVIOR CONTROL; PATIENT CARE)

Vaux, Kenneth L.; Vaux, Sara A. Dying Well. Nashville, TN: Abingdon Press; 1996. 147 p.
(TERMINAL CARE)

Vaux, Sara A. see **Vaux, Kenneth L.**

Vawter, Dorothy E. see **Gervais, Karen G.**

Veatch, Robert M. Egalitarian and maximin theories of justice: directed donation of organs for transplant. *Journal of Medicine and Philosophy.* 1998 Oct; 23(5): 456–476.
(ORGAN AND TISSUE DONATION; ORGAN AND TISSUE TRANSPLANTATION; RESOURCE ALLOCATION/BIOMEDICAL TECHNOLOGIES; SELECTION FOR TREATMENT)

Veatch, Robert M. Ethical consensus formation in clinical cases. *In:* ten Have, Henk A.M.J.; Sass, Hans–Martin, eds. Consensus Formation in Healthcare Ethics. Boston, MA: Kluwer Academic; 1998: 17–34.
(BIOETHICS; ETHICISTS AND ETHICS COMMITTEES; PATIENT CARE)

Veatch, Robert M. The conscience clause: how much individual choice in defining death can our society tolerate? *In:* Youngner, Stuart J.; Arnold, Robert M.; Schapiro, Renie, eds. The Definition of Death: Contemporary Controversies. Baltimore, MD: Johns Hopkins University Press; 1999: 137–160.
(DETERMINATION OF DEATH; DETERMINATION OF DEATH/BRAIN DEATH)

Veatch, Robert M. The foundations of bioethics. *Bioethics.* 1999 Jul; 13(3–4): 206–217.
(BIOETHICS)

Veatch, Robert M.; Haddad, Amy. Case Studies in Pharmacy Ethics. New York, NY: Oxford University Press; 1999. 290 p.
(PATIENT CARE/DRUGS; PROFESSIONAL ETHICS)

Vedder, Anton. HIV/AIDS and the point and scope of medical confidentiality. *In:* Bennett, Rebecca; Erin, Charles A., eds. HIV and AIDS: Testing, Screening, and Confidentiality. New York, NY: Oxford University

Press; 1999: 140–148.
(AIDS/CONFIDENTIALITY)

Vehviläinen–Julkunen, Katri see **Kylmä, Jari**

Velasco, N.; Drukker, Alfred; Lyon, Sue; Oreopoulos, D.G.; Khan, Izhar H.; Soper, Charles. Organ donation and kidney sales. [Letters]. *Lancet.* 1998 Aug 8; 352(9126): 483–485.
(ORGAN AND TISSUE DONATION)

Venta, Enrique R. see **Pellissier, James M.**

Verdun–Jones, Simon; Weisstub, David N. The regulation of biomedical research experimentation in Canada: developing an effective apparatus for the implementation of ethical principles in a scientific milieu. *Ottawa Law Review.* 1996–1997; 28(2): 297–341.
(HUMAN EXPERIMENTATION/ETHICS COMMITTEES; HUMAN EXPERIMENTATION/FOREIGN COUNTRIES; HUMAN EXPERIMENTATION/REGULATION)

Verghese, Abraham. Showing doctors their biases. *New York Times.* 1999 Mar 1: A21.
(PROFESSIONAL PATIENT RELATIONSHIP)

Verhovek, Sam Howe. Legal suicide has killed 8, Oregeon says. [News]. *New York Times.* 1998 Aug 19: A16.
(SUICIDE)

Verhovek, Sam Howe. Oregon reporting 15 deaths in 1998 under suicide law. [News]. *New York Times.* 1999 Feb 18: A1, A17.
(SUICIDE)

Verkerk, Marian. A care perspective on coercion and autonomy. *Bioethics.* 1999 Jul; 13(3–4): 358–368.
(PROFESSIONAL PATIENT RELATIONSHIP)

Verma, S. see **Cappelli, M.**

Vermeersch, Etienne. Ethical aspects of genetic engineering. *In:* Sterckx, Sigrid, ed. Biotechnology, Patents and Morality. Proceedings of an International Workshop, "Biotechnology, Patents and Morality: Towards a Consensus," held in Ghent, Belgium, 17–19 Jan 1996. Brookfield, VT: Ashgate; 1997: 107–113.
(GENETIC INTERVENTION)

Vernon, Martin see **White, D.M.D.**

Verweij, Marcel. Medicalization as a moral problem for preventative medicine. *Bioethics.* 1999 Apr; 13(2): 89–113.
(HEALTH; HEALTH CARE; PUBLIC HEALTH)

Veterans Affairs National Headquarters. Bioethics Committee. Ethical Considerations in Equitable Allocation and Distribution of Limited Health Care Resources: Report. Issued by the VA National Center for Clinical Ethics, White River Junction, VT 05009; 1996 Jan. 15 p.
(HEALTH CARE; RESOURCE ALLOCATION)

Veterans Affairs National Headquarters. Bioethics Committee. Guidelines for the Allocation of Unproved Treatments: Report. Issued by the VA National Center for Clinical Ethics, White River Junction, VT 05009; 1996 Jan. 12 p.
(RESOURCE ALLOCATION/BIOMEDICAL TECHNOLOGIES)

Veterans Affairs National Headquarters. Bioethics Committee. Surrogate–Written Advance Directives: Report. Issued by the VA National Center for Clinical Ethics, White River Junction, VT 05009; 1996 Jan. 6 p.
(ADVANCE DIRECTIVES; ALLOWING TO DIE; INFORMED CONSENT)

Vial Correa, Juan de Dios; Sgreccia, Elio, eds.; Pontificia Academia pro Vita. Identity and Statute [Status] of [the] Human Embryo: Proceedings of [the] Third Assembly of the Pontifical Academy for Life (Vatican City, February 14–16, 1997). Vatican City: Libreria Editrice Vaticana; 1998. 458 p.
(FETUSES; PERSONHOOD)

Vial Correa, Juan de Dios; Sgreccia, Elio; Pontifical Academy for Life. Reflections on cloning. [English translation]. *Origins.* 1998 May 21; 28(1): 14–16.
(CLONING)

Vickers, M.R. see **Welton, A.J.**

Vikhanski, Luba. Israel introduces organ swap scheme. [News]. *Nature Medicine.* 1998 Apr; 4(4): 377.
(ORGAN AND TISSUE DONATION)

Villar, Armando J. Santini see **Fusilier, Marcelline**

Vineis, Paolo. Ethical issues in genetic screening for cancer. *Annals of Oncology.* 1997 Oct; 8(10): 945–949.
(GENETIC SCREENING)

Vining, Aidan see **Schwindt, Richard**

Virgo, John M. see **Virgo, Katherine S.**

Virgo, Katherine S.; Carr, T.R.; Hile, Allison; Virgo, John M.; Sullivan, George M.; Kaikati, Jack G. Medical versus surgical abortion: a survey of knowledge and attitudes among abortion clinic patients. *Women's Health Issues.* 1999 May–Jun; 9(3): 143–154.
(ABORTION/ATTITUDES)

Visser, A.A. Oranjemed -- Bloemfontein Protocols preamble. *Journal of the Dental Association of South Africa.* 1996 Nov; 51(11): 673–677.
(HEALTH CARE/ECONOMICS; HEALTH CARE/FOREIGN COUNTRIES)

Vithayasai, Vicharn see **Merson, Michael H.**

Vitiello, Benedetto see **Leonard, Henrietta**

Viviani, Nancy J. see **Mold, James W.**

Vlaardingerbroek, W.F.C., comp.; Netherlands. Ministry of Health, Welfare and Sport. Documentation and Library Department. Euthanasia and Physician–Assisted Suicide in the Netherlands: Bibliography 1984–1995. Rijswijk, Netherlands: Ministry of Health, Welfare and Sport; 1995 Feb. 20 p.
(EUTHANASIA; SUICIDE)

Vojir, Carol see **Anderson, Donna G.**

Volkenandt, Matthias. Supportive care and euthanasia -- an ethical dilemma? *Supportive Care in Cancer.* 1998 Mar; 6(2): 114–119.
(EUTHANASIA; PROFESSIONAL PATIENT RELATIONSHIP; SUICIDE; TERMINAL CARE)

Volpintesta, Edward see Finestone, Albert J.

Volpintesta, Edward J. see Kosseff, Andrew L.

Vorspan, Albert; Saperstein, David. Bioethics: thinking the unthinkable. *In: their* Jewish Dimensions of Social Justice: Tough Moral Choices of Our Time. New York, NY: UAHC Press; 1998: 47–73.
(BIOETHICS)

Vorspan, Albert; Saperstein, David. Life and death issues: policy on the edge. *In: their* Jewish Dimensions of Social Justice: Tough Moral Choices of Our Time. New York, NY: UAHC Press; 1998: 11–46.
(BIOETHICS)

Vranizan, Karen see Bindman, Andrew B.

Vranizan, Karen see Grumbach, Kevin

Vrbová, H.; Holmerová, I.; Hrubantová, L. Business ethics as a novel issue in health care economics. *Sbornik Lekarsky.* 1997; 98(3): 225–232.
(HEALTH CARE/ECONOMICS; HEALTH CARE/FOREIGN COUNTRIES; RESOURCE ALLOCATION)

Vu, Hong Thi see Cooper-Patrick, Lisa

W

Wachbroit, Robert. Rethinking medical confidentiality: the impact of genetics. *Suffolk University Law Review.* 1993 Winter; 27(4): 1391–1410.
(CONFIDENTIALITY; GENETIC COUNSELING)

Wachbroit, Robert see Handelin, Barbara

Wachtel, Tom J. see Segal, Eran

Wade, Nicholas. Advisory panel votes for use of embryonic cells in research. [News]. *New York Times.* 1999 Jun 29: A15.
(EMBRYO AND FETAL RESEARCH)

Wade, Nicholas. Clinton asks study of bid to form part-human, part-cow cells. [News]. *New York Times.* 1998 Nov 15: 31.
(EMBRYO AND FETAL RESEARCH; GENETIC INTERVENTION)

Wade, Nicholas. Embryo cell research: a clash of values. *New York Times.* 1999 Jul 2: A13.
(EMBRYO AND FETAL RESEARCH)

Wade, Nicholas. Ethics panel is guarded about hybrid of cow cells. [News]. *New York Times.* 1998 Nov 21: A9.
(GENETIC INTERVENTION)

Wade, Nicholas. Government says ban on human embryo research does not apply to cells. [News]. *New York Times.* 1999 Jan 20: A29.
(EMBRYO AND FETAL RESEARCH)

Wade, Nicholas. Human–cow hybrid cells are topic of ethics panel. [News]. *New York Times.* 1998 Nov 18: A27.
(GENETIC INTERVENTION)

Wade, Nicholas. No research on cloning of embryos, Geron says. [News]. *New York Times.* 1999 Jun 15: A21.
(EMBRYO AND FETAL RESEARCH)

Wade, Nicholas. Primordial cells fuel debate on ethics. [News]. *New York Times.* 1998 Nov 10: F1, F2.
(EMBRYO AND FETAL RESEARCH)

Wade, Nicholas. Recommendation is near on embryo cell research: ethics panel expected to urge end to ban. [News]. *New York Times.* 1999 May 24: A18.
(EMBRYO AND FETAL RESEARCH)

Wade, Nicholas. Researchers claim embryonic cell mix of human and cow. [News]. *New York Times.* 1998 Nov 12: A1, A26.
(EMBRYO AND FETAL RESEARCH; GENETIC INTERVENTION)

Wadeley, Alison. Ethics in Psychological Research and Practice. Leicester, England: British Psychological Association; 1991. 41 p.
(BEHAVIORAL RESEARCH; PROFESSIONAL ETHICS/EDUCATION)

Wadman, Meredith. Cloned mice fail to rekindle ethics debate. [News]. *Nature.* 1998 Jul 30; 394(6692): 408–409.
(CLONING)

Wadman, Meredith. Cloning without human clones. [News]. *Wall Street Journal.* 1998 Jan 20: A18.
(CLONING)

Wadman, Meredith. Congress may block stem-cell research. [News]. *Nature.* 1999 Feb 25; 397(6721): 639.
(EMBRYO AND FETAL RESEARCH)

Wadman, Meredith. Dilemma for journals over tobacco cash. [News]. *Nature.* 1998 Aug 13; 394(6694): 609.
(BIOMEDICAL RESEARCH; FRAUD AND MISCONDUCT)

Wadman, Meredith. DuPont opens up access to genetics tool. [News]. *Nature.* 1998 Aug 27; 394(6696): 819.
(GENETIC RESEARCH)

Wadman, Meredith. Embryonic stem-cell research exempt from ban, NIH is told. [News]. *Nature.* 1999 Jan 21; 397(6716): 185–186.
(EMBRYO AND FETAL RESEARCH)

Wadman, Meredith. Ethical protection for subjects 'could stifle psychiatric research.' [News]. *Nature.* 1998 Aug 20; 394(6695): 713.
(HUMAN EXPERIMENTATION/SPECIAL POPULATIONS)

Wadman, Meredith. Ethicists urge funding for extraction of embryo cells. [News]. *Nature.* 1999 May 27; 399(6734): 292.
(EMBRYO AND FETAL RESEARCH)

Wadman, Meredith. Financial doubts over future of chimp lab. [News]. *Nature.* 1999 Apr 22; 398(6729): 644.
(ANIMAL EXPERIMENTATION)

Wadman, Meredith. Gene therapy pushes on, despite doubts. [News]. *Nature.* 1999 Jan 14; 397(6715): 94.
(EMBRYO AND FETAL RESEARCH; GENE THERAPY)

Wadman, Meredith. Higher status for 'research risks' office? [News]. *Nature.* 1999 Feb 18; 397(6720): 550.
(HUMAN EXPERIMENTATION/REGULATION)

Wadman, Meredith. NIH ethics office clamps down on Duke...as basic scientists feel the pinch in LA. [News]. *Nature.* 1999 May 20; 399(6733): 190.

(FRAUD AND MISCONDUCT; HUMAN
EXPERIMENTATION/REGULATION)

Wadman, Meredith. NIH launches discussion of in utero gene therapy ... and seeks to repair 'flaw' in review process. [News]. *Nature.* 1998 Oct 1; 395(6701): 420.
(FETUSES; GENE THERAPY)

Wadman, Meredith. NIH 'should help sharing of research tools.' [News]. *Nature.* 1998 Jun 11; 393(6685): 505.
(BIOMEDICAL RESEARCH)

Wadman, Meredith. NIH stem–cell guidelines face stormy ride. [News]. *Nature.* 1999 Apr 15; 398(6728): 551.
(EMBRYO AND FETAL RESEARCH)

Wadman, Meredith. Pesticide tests on humans cause concern. [News]. *Nature.* 1998 Aug 6; 394(6693): 515.
(HUMAN EXPERIMENTATION)

Wadman, Meredith. US research safety system 'in jeopardy.' [News]. *Nature.* 1998 Jun 18; 393(6686): 610.
(HUMAN EXPERIMENTATION/ETHICS COMMITTEES)

Wagner, Bertil K.J.; Christian Pharmacists Fellowship International. Pharmacists should not participate in abortion or assisted suicide. [Position paper]. *Annals of Pharmacotherapy.* 1996 Oct; 30(10): 1192–1196.
(ABORTION/RELIGIOUS ASPECTS; SUICIDE)

Wagner, James T.; Higdon, Tami L. Spiritual issues and bioethics in the intensive care unit: the role of the chaplain. *Critical Care Clinics.* 1996 Jan; 12(1): 15–27.
(PATIENT CARE)

Waibel, U.G.; Huber, Ch.; Riccabona, U.M.; Schlager, A. Medicolegal aspects of patient information before regional anesthesia in Austria. *Acta Anaesthesiologica Scandinavica.* 1997; 111(Suppl.): 229–231.
(INFORMED CONSENT)

Waitzkin, Howard see **Asch, Steven**

Waldboth, Y. see **Müller, H.J.**

Waldholz, Michael. AZT price cut for Third World mothers–to–be. [News]. *Wall Street Journal.* 1998 Mar 5: B1, B12.
(AIDS; PATIENT CARE/DRUGS)

Waldman, Steven; Ackerman, Elise; Rubin, Rita. Abortions in America: so many women have them, so few talk about them. *U.S. News and World Report.* 1998 Jan 19; 124(2): 20–22, 24–31.
(ABORTION)

Waldron, Mary A. see **Gbolade, Babatunde A.**

Walker, Leslie; Blechner, Barbara; Gruman, Cynthia; Bradley, Elizabeth. Assessment of capacity to discuss advance care planning in nursing homes. [Letter]. *Journal of the American Geriatrics Society.* 1998 Aug; 46(8): 1055–1056.
(ADVANCE DIRECTIVES)

Walker, Paul see **Crelinsten, Gordon L.**

Walker, Robert M. see **Schonwetter, Ronald S.**

Wallace, Robert W. The Human Genome Diversity Project: medical benefits versus ethical concerns.

Molecular Medicine Today. 1998 Feb; 4(2): 59–62.
(GENETIC RESEARCH; GENOME MAPPING)

Wallace, Wes see **Egilman, David**

Wallenstein, Sylvan see **McGovern, Margaret M.**

Waller, Adele A.; Alcantara, Oscar L. Ownership of health information in the information age. *Journal of the American Health Information Management Association.* 1998 Mar; 69(3): 28–40.
(CONFIDENTIALITY/LEGAL ASPECTS; PATIENT ACCESS TO RECORDS)

Wallsten, Tuula see **Kjellin, Lars**

Walsh, Joseph T. see **Zweig, Franklin M.**

Walsh, Julia. Reproductive rights and the Human Genome Project. *Southern California Review of Law and Women's Studies.* 1994 Fall; 4(1): 145–181.
(GENETIC SCREENING; PRENATAL DIAGNOSIS)

Walsh, Marcia K. Difficult decisions in health care: one woman's journey. [Personal narrative]. *Bioethics Forum.* 1997 Summer; 13(2): 35–37.
(ADVANCE DIRECTIVES; ALLOWING TO DIE; TREATMENT REFUSAL)

Walsh, Marie E.; Graber, Glenn C.; Wolfe, Amy K. University–industry relationships in genetic research: potential opportunities and pitfalls. *Accountability in Research.* 1997; 5(4): 265–282.
(GENETIC RESEARCH)

Walsh, Pat see **Grubb, Andrew**

Walter, James J. Theological parameters: Catholic doctrine on abortion in a pluralist society. *In:* Rainey, R. Randall; Magill, Gerard, eds. Abortion and Public Policy: An Interdisciplinary Investigation within the Catholic Tradition. Omaha, NE: Creighton University Press; 1996: 91–130.
(ABORTION/RELIGIOUS ASPECTS)

Walters, D. Campbell. Just Take It Out! The Ethics and Economics of Cesarean Section and Hysterectomy. Mt. Vernon, IL: Topiary Publishing; 1998. 271 p.
(PATIENT CARE)

Walters, LeRoy; Kahn, Tamar Joy, eds. Bibliography of Bioethics, Volume 24. Washington, DC: Georgetown University, Kennedy Institute of Ethics; 1998. 766 p.
(BIOETHICS)

Walters, LeRoy; Kahn, Tamar Joy, eds. Bibliography of Bioethics, Volume 25. Washington, DC: Georgetown University, Kennedy Institute of Ethics; 1999. 752 p.
(BIOETHICS)

Walters, LeRoy see **Beauchamp, Tom L.**

Walters, LeRoy see **Collins, Francis S.**

Walters, LeRoy B. Testimony of LeRoy Walters [concerning written standards for human experimentation in the years 1945 to 1949]. *Accountability in Research.* 1998 Jan; 6(1–2): 149–166.
(HUMAN EXPERIMENTATION)

Wang, Justin. Scientific misconduct: Chinese journals

pledge crackdown. [News]. *Science.* 1999 Mar 5; 283(5407): 1427.
(FRAUD AND MISCONDUCT)

Wapner, Ronald see **Chervenak, Frank A.**

Ward, John W. see **Solomon, Liza**

Warden, John. Surrogate mothers should be paid expenses only. [News]. *BMJ (British Medical Journal).* 1998 Oct 24; 317(7166): 1104.
(SURROGATE MOTHERS)

Warner, James see **Shah, Nisha**

Warnock, Mary. Experimentation on human embryos and fetuses. *In:* Kuhse, Helga; Singer, Peter, eds. A Companion to Bioethics. Malden, MA: Blackwell; 1998: 390–396.
(EMBRYO AND FETAL RESEARCH)

Warren, Catherine see **Dunne, Cara**

Warren, John W. see **Lynn, Joanne**

Warren, John W. see **Muncie, Herbert L.**

Warren, Mary Anne. Abortion. *In:* Kuhse, Helga; Singer, Peter, eds. A Companion to Bioethics. Malden, MA: Blackwell; 1998: 127–134.
(ABORTION)

Warwick, Catherine see **Webb, John**

Washofsky, Mark. Abortion and the halakhic conversation: a liberal perspective. *In:* Jacob, Walter; Zemer, Moshe, eds. The Fetus and Fertility in Jewish Law: Essays and Responsa. Pittsburgh, PA: Rodef Shalom Press; Freehof Institute of Progressive Halakhah; 1995: 39–89.
(ABORTION/RELIGIOUS ASPECTS)

Wasserman, David see **Silvers, Anita**

Wasson, John H.; Bubolz, Thomas A.; Lynn, Joanne; Teno, Joan. Can we afford comprehensive, supportive care for the very old? *Journal of the American Geriatrics Society.* 1998 Jul; 46(7): 829–832.
(HEALTH CARE/ECONOMICS; PATIENT CARE/AGED; RESOURCE ALLOCATION)

Watanabe, Toru see **Aoki, Eiko**

Watkins, Elizabeth Siegel. On the Pill: A Social History of Oral Contraceptives, 1950–1970. Baltimore, MD: Johns Hopkins University Press; 1998. 183 p.
(CONTRACEPTION)

Watson, Heather see **King, Susan M.**

Watson, James D. All for the good: why genetic engineering must soldier on. *Time.* 1999 Jan 11; 153(1): 91.
(GENETIC INTERVENTION)

Watson, Sidney Dean. In search of the story: physicians and charity care. *Saint Louis University Public Law Review.* 1996; 15(2): 353–369.
(BIOETHICS; HEALTH CARE/ECONOMICS; PATIENT CARE)

Watt, Helen. Germ–line therapy for mitochondrial disease: some ethical objections. *Cambridge Quarterly of Healthcare Ethics.* 1999 Winter; 8(1): 88–96.
(GENE THERAPY)

Watts, Jonathan. Concept of brain death to be accepted in South Korea. [News]. *Lancet.* 1998 Dec 19–26; 352(9145): 1996.
(DETERMINATION OF DEATH/BRAIN DEATH; ORGAN AND TISSUE DONATION)

Watts, Jonathan. In-vitro fertilisation guidelines fall behind the times. [News]. *Lancet.* 1999 Jan 23; 353(9149): 303.
(IN VITRO FERTILIZATION; REPRODUCTIVE TECHNOLOGIES)

Watts, Jonathan. Japan dashes Seed's plans for clone clinic. [News]. *Lancet.* 1998 Dec 12; 352(9144): 1917.
(CLONING)

Watts, Jonathan. Japan does its first official heart and liver transplantations. [News]. *Lancet.* 1999 Mar 6; 353(9155): 821.
(DETERMINATION OF DEATH/BRAIN DEATH; ORGAN AND TISSUE TRANSPLANTATION)

Watts, Jonathan. Japan proposes ban on human cloning. [News]. *Lancet.* 1998 Aug 8; 352(9126): 465.
(CLONING)

Watts, Jonathan. Japanese victims of discrimination against lepers sue government. [News]. *Lancet.* 1998 Aug 22; 352(9128): 631.
(PATIENT CARE)

Watts, Jonathan. Patients not to be tied up in Japanese sanatoriums. [News]. *Lancet.* 1999 Jul 24; 354(9175): 316.
(BEHAVIOR CONTROL; PATIENT CARE/MENTALLY DISABLED)

Watts, Jonathan. When impotence leads contraception. [News]. *Lancet.* 1999 Mar 6; 353(9155): 819.
(CONTRACEPTION; PATIENT CARE/DRUGS)

Watts, Jonathan; Morris, Kelly. Human cloning trial met with outrage and scepticism. [News]. *Lancet.* 1999 Jan 2; 353(9146): 43.
(CLONING)

Watts, Sheldon. Epidemics and History: Disease, Power and Imperialism. New Haven, CT: Yale University Press; 1997. 400 p.
(PUBLIC HEALTH)

Way, Ruth L. Seriously ill, extremely low birthweight infants: ethical dilemmas of treatment. *New Zealand Medical Journal.* 1996 Oct 25; 109(1032): 391–393.
(ALLOWING TO DIE/INFANTS)

Weatherall, D.J. see **Nathan, D.G.**

Weaver, S.M. see **Lui, S.C.**

Webb, Cynthia M.; Sheckard, Denise; Wilder, Pauline; Marks, Beverly L.; Williams, Elizabeth; Keeth, Merrill Beth; Matzo, Marianne LaPorte. Over the past year, how many patients have asked you to inject drugs to intentionally end their lives? Have you ever injected drugs to intentionally end a patient's life? [Letters]. *Journal of Gerontological Nursing.* 1997 Mar;

23(3): 57–59.
(EUTHANASIA/ATTITUDES)

Webb, Gilbert W.; Huddleston, John F. Management of the pregnant woman who sustains severe brain damage. *Clinics in Perinatology.* 1996 Sep; 23(3): 453–464.
(ALLOWING TO DIE; FETUSES)

Webb, John; Warwick, Catherine. Getting it right: the teaching of philosophical health care ethics. *Nursing Ethics.* 1999 Mar; 6(2): 150–156.
(NURSING ETHICS/EDUCATION)

Webb, Marilyn. The Good Death: The New American Search to Reshape the End of Life. New York, NY: Bantam Books; 1997. 479 p.
(ALLOWING TO DIE; TERMINAL CARE)

Webber, David W. see **Gostin, Lawrence O.**

Weber, David O. Realignments, realpolitik, religion, and reproductive health. *Healthcare Forum Journal.* 1996 May–Jun; 39(3): 76–83.
(ABORTION/RELIGIOUS ASPECTS; CONTRACEPTION)

Weber, J. Todd see **Nakashima, Allyn K.**

Weber, James E. see **Larkin, Gregory Luke**

Weber, Leonard J. Taking on organizational ethics. *Health Progress.* 1997 May–Jun; 78(3): 20–23, 32.
(ETHICISTS AND ETHICS COMMITTEES)

Weber, W. see **Müller, H.J.**

Weed, Douglas L. Preventing scientific misconduct. *American Journal of Public Health.* 1998 Jan; 88(1): 125–129.
(BIOMEDICAL RESEARCH; FRAUD AND MISCONDUCT; PROFESSIONAL ETHICS)

Weeks, Jane C. see **Costantini–Ferrando, Maria F.**

Wehrwein, Peter. US physicians confused about end–of–life care. [News]. *Lancet.* 1998 Aug 15; 352(9127): 549.
(EUTHANASIA/ATTITUDES; SUICIDE)

Weijer, Charles. Cardiopulmonary resuscitation for patients in a persistent vegetative state: futile or acceptable? [Editorial]. *Canadian Medical Association Journal.* 1998 Feb 24; 158(4): 491–493.
(ALLOWING TO DIE; RESUSCITATION ORDERS)

Weijer, Charles. Duty and healing: the lifework of Benjamin Freedman. [Editorial]. *Canadian Medical Association Journal.* 1997 Jun 1; 156(11): 1553–1555.
(ETHICISTS AND ETHICS COMMITTEES)

Weijer, Charles. Selecting subjects for participation in clinical research: one sphere of justice. *Journal of Medical Ethics.* 1999 Feb; 25(1): 31–36.
(HUMAN EXPERIMENTATION/SPECIAL POPULATIONS)

Weijer, Charles. The IRB's role in assessing the generalizability of non–NIH–funded clinical trials. *IRB: A Review of Human Subjects Research.* 1998 Mar–Jun; 20(2–3): 1–5.
(HUMAN EXPERIMENTATION/ETHICS COMMITTEES; HUMAN EXPERIMENTATION/RESEARCH DESIGN; HUMAN EXPERIMENTATION/SPECIAL POPULATIONS)

Weijer, Charles; Singer, Peter A.; Dickens, Bernard M.; Workman, Stephen. Bioethics for clinicians: 16. Dealing with demands for inappropriate treatment. *Canadian Medical Association Journal.* 1998 Oct 6; 159(7): 817–821.
(ALLOWING TO DIE)

Weijer, Charles see **Crelinsten, Gordon L.**

Weijer, Charles see **Glass, Kathleen Cranley**

Weijer, Charles see **Lapierre, Yvon D.**

Weinberger, Yaakov see **Ilani, Zvi**

Weindling, Paul. Human experiments in Nazi Germany: reflections on Ernst Klee's book "Auschwitz, die NS–Medizin und ihre Opfer" (1997) and film "Ärzte ohne Gewissen" (1996). *Medizinhistorisches Journal.* 1998; 33(2): 161–178.
(FRAUD AND MISCONDUCT; HUMAN EXPERIMENTATION/FOREIGN COUNTRIES)

Weinstock, Robert; Pearlman, Theodore. Letters to the editor [responses to P.S. Appelbaum, "A theory of ethics for forensic psychiatry," *JAAPS* 1997; 25(3): 233–247]. *Journal of the American Academy of Psychiatry and the Law.* 1998; 26(1): 151–157.
(MEDICAL ETHICS)

Weisman, Carol S.; Khoury, Amal J.; Cassirer, Christopher; Sharpe, Virginia A.; Morlock, Laura L. The implications of affiliations between Catholic and non–Catholic health care organizations for availability of reproductive health services. *Women's Health Issues.* 1999 May–Jun; 9(3): 121–134.
(HEALTH CARE; REPRODUCTION)

Weiss, A.H.; Fortinsky, R.H.; Laughlin, J.; Lo, B.; Adler, N.E.; Mudge, C.; Dimand, R.J. Parental consent for pediatric cadaveric organ donation. *Transplantation Proceedings.* 1997 May; 29(3): 1896–1901.
(ORGAN AND TISSUE DONATION)

Weiss, J.O.; Kozma, C.; Lapham, E.V. Whom would you trust with your genetic information? [Abstract]. *American Journal of Human Genetics.* 1997 Oct; 61(4): A24.
(CONFIDENTIALITY; GENETIC SCREENING)

Weiss, J.O. see **Lapham, E.V.**

Weiss, Meira. For doctors' eyes only: medical records in two Israeli hospitals. *Culture, Medicine and Psychiatry.* 1997 Sep; 21(3): 283–302.
(PATIENT ACCESS TO RECORDS)

Weiss, Rick. Babies in limbo: law outpaced by fertility advances. [News]. *Washington Post.* 1998 Feb 8: A1, A16.
(REPRODUCTIVE TECHNOLOGIES)

Weiss, Rick. Federal embryo research is backed: ethicists see benefits overriding qualms. [News]. *Washington Post.* 1999 May 23: A1, A16.
(EMBRYO AND FETAL RESEARCH)

Weiss, Rick. Fertility innovation or exploitation? *Washington Post.* 1998 Feb 9: A1, A12.
(HUMAN EXPERIMENTATION/REGULATION; REPRODUCTIVE TECHNOLOGIES)

Weiss, Rick. What is patently offensive? [News]. *Washington Post.* 1998 May 11: A21.
(PATENTING LIFE FORMS)

Weiss, Robin A. Xenografts and retroviruses. *Science.* 1999 Aug 20; 285(5431): 1221–1222.
(ORGAN AND TISSUE TRANSPLANTATION)

Weiss, Robin A. Xenotransplantation. *BMJ (British Medical Journal).* 1998 Oct 3; 317(7163): 931–934.
(ORGAN AND TISSUE TRANSPLANTATION)

Weiss, Stefan C. Defining a "patients' bill of rights" for the next century. [Editorial]. *JAMA.* 1999 Mar 3; 281(9): 856.
(HEALTH CARE/ECONOMICS; PATIENTS' RIGHTS)

Weissman, David E.; Matson, Sandra. Pain assessment and management in the long–term care setting. *Theoretical Medicine and Bioethics.* 1999 Jan; 20(1): 31–43.
(PATIENT CARE/AGED; PATIENT CARE/DRUGS; PATIENT CARE/MENTALLY DISABLED)

Weisstub, David N.; Arboleda-Flórez, Julio. Ethical research with the developmentally disabled. *Canadian Journal of Psychiatry.* 1997 Jun; 42(5): 492–496.
(HUMAN EXPERIMENTATION/INFORMED CONSENT; HUMAN EXPERIMENTATION/SPECIAL POPULATIONS)

Weisstub, David N. see Arboleda-Flórez, Julio

Weisstub, David N. see McCubbin, Michael

Weisstub, David N. see Verdun-Jones, Simon

Weitzman, Dalia see Sheiner, Eyal

Weksberg, R. see Malkin, D.

Welch, H. Gilbert; Burke, Wylie. Uncertainties in genetic testing for chronic disease. *JAMA.* 1998 Nov 4; 280(17): 1525–1527.
(GENETIC SCREENING)

Welch, H. Gilbert see Fisher, Elliott S.

Welie, Jos V.M. In the Face of Suffering: The Philosophical-Anthropological Foundations of Clinical Ethics. Omaha, NE: Creighton University Press; 1998. 304 p.
(BIOETHICS; PROFESSIONAL PATIENT RELATIONSHIP)

Welie, Jos V.M. see ten Have, Henk A.M.J.

Welkenhuysen, Myriam; Evers-Kiebooms, Gerry; Decruyenaere, Marleen; Van den Berghe, Herman; Bande-Knops, Jacqueline; Van Gerven, Veerle. Adolescents' attitude towards carrier testing for cystic fibrosis and its relative stability over time. *European Journal of Human Genetics.* 1996; 4(1): 52–62.
(GENETIC SCREENING)

Wells, Barron; Spinks, Nelda. The context of ethics in the health care industry. *Health Manpower Management.* 1996; 22(1): 21–29.
(FRAUD AND MISCONDUCT; HEALTH CARE; PROFESSIONAL ETHICS)

Welsh, James. Truth and reconciliation ... and justice. *Lancet.* 1998 Dec 5; 352(9143): 1852–1853.
(FRAUD AND MISCONDUCT; TORTURE)

Welsh, James; van Es, Adriaan. Health and human rights: an international minefield. *Lancet.* 1998 Dec 19–26; 352 (Suppl. 4): 14.
(FRAUD AND MISCONDUCT; TORTURE)

Welsh, James see Thorns, Andrew

Welton, A.J.; Vickers, M.R.; Cooper, J.A.; Meade, T.W.; Marteau, T.M. Is recruitment more difficult with a placebo arm in randomised controlled trials? A quasirandomised, interview based study. *BMJ (British Medical Journal).* 1999 Apr 24; 318(7191): 1114–1117.
(HUMAN EXPERIMENTATION/RESEARCH DESIGN)

Wendell, Susan. Old women out of control: some thoughts on aging, ethics, and psychosomatic medicine. *In:* Walter, Margaret Urban, ed. Mother Time: Women, Aging, and Ethics. Lanham, MD: Rowman and Littlefield; 1999: 133–149.
(HEALTH; MENTAL HEALTH; PATIENT CARE)

Wender, Richard see Pokorski, Robert J.

Wendler, Dave. Understanding the 'conservative' view on abortion. *Bioethics.* 1999 Jan; 13(1): 32–56.
(ABORTION; FETUSES; PERSONHOOD)

Wendler, Dave. When should "riskier" subjects be excluded from research participation? *Kennedy Institute of Ethics Journal.* 1998 Sep; 8(3): 307–327.
(HUMAN EXPERIMENTATION/RESEARCH DESIGN; HUMAN EXPERIMENTATION/SPECIAL POPULATIONS)

Wendte, Johannes F. see Varekamp, Inge

Wenger, Neil; Kagawa-Singer, Marjorie; Bito, Seiji; Oye, Robert; Liu, Honghu; Kahn, Katherine. End of life decision making model of Japanese Americans. [Abstract]. *Abstract Book/Association for Health Services Research.* 1997; 14: 256.
(ALLOWING TO DIE/ATTITUDES)

Wenger, Neil see Hamel, Mary Beth

Wenger, Neil S.; Korenman, Stanley G.; Berk, Richard; Berry, Sandy. The ethics of scientific research: an analysis of focus groups of scientists and institutional representatives. *Journal of Investigative Medicine.* 1997 Aug; 45(6): 371–380.
(BIOMEDICAL RESEARCH; FRAUD AND MISCONDUCT; PROFESSIONAL ETHICS)

Wennberg, John E. see Pritchard, Robert S.

Werner, D. Leonard. Guest editorial: imperialism, research ethics and global health. [Letter]. *Journal of Medical Ethics.* 1999 Feb; 25(1): 62.
(BIOETHICS)

Werth, James L. Mental health professionals and assisted death: perceived ethical obligations and proposed guidelines for practice. *Ethics and Behavior.* 1999; 9(2): 159–183.
(SUICIDE)

Werth, James L. When is a mental health professional competent to assess a person's decision to hasten death? *Ethics and Behavior.* 1999; 9(2): 141–157.
(SUICIDE)

Werth, James L.; Gordon, Judith R.; Sullivan, Mark

D.; Ganzini, Linda; Youngner, Stuart J. Gatekeepers. [Letter and response]. *Hastings Center Report.* 1999 May–Jun; 29(3): 4.
(SUICIDE)

Wertz, D. see **Nippert, I.**

Wertz, D.C. Is there a "women's ethic" in genetics? A survey of ASHG and NSGC. [Abstract]. *American Journal of Human Genetics.* 1996 Oct; 59(4): A340.
(GENETIC COUNSELING; GENETIC SCREENING; PRENATAL DIAGNOSIS)

Wertz, D.C. see **Fletcher, J.C.**

Wertz, Dorothy. Genetics and eugenics. [Letter]. *New Scientist.* 1999 Feb 13; 161(2173): 55–56.
(GENETIC SCREENING)

Wertz, Dorothy C. Chinese genetics and ethics. [Letter]. *Nature Medicine.* 1999 Mar; 5(3): 247.
(GENETIC COUNSELING)

Wertz, Dorothy C. Guidelines point the way on genetics ethics. [Letter]. *Nature.* 1999 May 27; 399(6734): 297.
(GENETIC SERVICES)

Wertz, Dorothy C. International perspectives. *In:* Clarke, Angus, ed. The Genetic Testing of Children. Washington, DC: BIOS Scientific Publishers; 1998: 271–287.
(GENETIC SCREENING)

Wertz, Dorothy C. International perspectives on ethics and human genetics. *Suffolk University Law Review.* 1993 Winter; 27(4): 1411–1456.
(GENETIC COUNSELING; GENETIC SCREENING; PRENATAL DIAGNOSIS)

Wertz, Dorothy C. The difficulties of recruiting minorities to studies of ethics and values in genetics. *Community Genetics.* 1998; 1(3): 175–179.
(GENETIC COUNSELING; GENETIC SCREENING)

Wertz, Dorothy C.; Fletcher, John C.; Berg, Kåre; Boulyjenkov, Victor; World Health Organization. Hereditary Diseases Programme. Guidelines on Ethical Issues in Medical Genetics and the Provision of Genetics Services. Geneva: World Health Organization; 1995. 119 p.
(GENETIC COUNSELING; GENETIC SERVICES)

West, Charles; Pace, Nicholas; Niermeyer, Susan; Moore, Lorna Grindlay; Platt, M.P. Ward; Fleming, P.J.; Blair, P.S.; Leach, C.E.A.; Golding, J.; Smith, I.; Johnson, Paul; Savulescu, Julian; James, P.B.; Southall, David; Poets, C.; O'Brien, Louise; Stebbens, Valerie; Parkins, K. Hypoxic responses in infants. [Letters and response]. *BMJ (British Medical Journal).* 1998 Sep 5; 317(7159): 675–678.
(HUMAN EXPERIMENTATION/MINORS)

West, Doe. Radiation experiments on children at the Fernald and Wrentham schools: lessons for protocols in human subject research. *Accountability in Research.* 1998 Jan; 6(1–2): 103–125.
(FRAUD AND MISCONDUCT; HUMAN EXPERIMENTATION/MINORS; HUMAN EXPERIMENTATION/SPECIAL POPULATIONS)

West, Gary R. see **Valdiserri, Ronald O.**

Westbrook, Joan see **Perry, Erica**

Westergaard, Tine; Wohlfahrt, Jan; Aaby, Peter; Melbye, Mads. Population based study of rates of multiple pregnancies in Denmark, 1980–94. *BMJ (British Medical Journal).* 1997 Mar 15; 314(7083): 775–779.
(REPRODUCTIVE TECHNOLOGIES)

Westfall, John M. see **Margolis, Lewis H.**

Westrin, Claes–Göran see **Kjellin, Lars**

Wetanson, Suzanne see **Freilicher, Liza**

Wetle, Terrie see **Bradley, Elizabeth H.**

Wexler, Alice. Mapping Fate: A Memoir of Family, Risk, and Genetic Research. Berkeley, CA: University of California Press; 1995. 321 p.
(GENETIC RESEARCH)

Weyers, Heleen see **Griffiths, John**

Weyers, Wolfgang. Death of Medicine in Nazi Germany: Dermatology and Dermatopathology under the Swastika. Philadelphia, PA; Lanham, MD: Ardor Scribendi; Madison Books; 1998. 442 p.
(FRAUD AND MISCONDUCT)

Whalen, Christopher C. see **Desvarieux, Moïse**

Wharton, Robert H. Pedestrian vs. train. *Hastings Center Report.* 1999 May–Jun; 29(3): 28–29.
(PATIENT CARE; PROFESSIONAL PATIENT RELATIONSHIP)

Wharton, Robert H.; Levine, Karen R.; Buka, Stephen; Emanuel, Linda. Advance care planning for children with special health care needs: a survey of parental attitudes. *Pediatrics.* 1996 May; 97(5): 682–687.
(ADVANCE DIRECTIVES; PATIENT CARE/MINORS)

Wheale, Peter R. Moral and legal consequences for the fetus/unborn child of medical technologies derived from human genome research. *In:* Glasner, Peter; Rothman, Harry, eds. Genetic Imaginations: Ethical, Legal and Social Issues in Human Genome Research. Brookfield, VT: Ashgate; 1998: 83–96.
(ABORTION/FOREIGN COUNTRIES; ABORTION/LEGAL ASPECTS; EMBRYO AND FETAL RESEARCH; FETUSES; PERSONHOOD; WRONGFUL LIFE)

Whelan, Daniel. Human rights approaches to an expanded response to address women's vulnerability to HIV/AIDS. *Health and Human Rights.* 1998; 3(1): 20–36.
(AIDS)

Whelan, Robert, ed. Legal Abortion Examined: 21 Years of Abortion Statistics. London: SPUC Educational Research Trust; 1992. 32 p.
(ABORTION/FOREIGN COUNTRIES)

Whitcomb, Michael E. see **Swick, Herbert M.**

White, Becky Cox; Zimbelman, Joel. Abandoning informed consent: an idea whose time has not yet come. *Journal of Medicine and Philosophy.* 1998 Oct; 23(5): 477–499.
(INFORMED CONSENT)

White, Caroline. Banking on interest: "Test Tube Dads" (*Inside Story*, BBC1, 25 August 1998). [Medicine and

the media]. *BMJ (British Medical Journal)*. 1998 Aug 29; 317(7158): 607.
(ARTIFICIAL INSEMINATION)

White, D.M.D.; Hillam, Jonathan; Harper, Max; Vernon, Martin; Bennett, Gerry; Scott, Hilary; Valmana, Anton; Rutherford, Joan; Scott, Jonathan; Williams, Edwina R.L. Suspension of nurse who gave drug on consultant's instructions. [Letters]. *BMJ (British Medical Journal)*. 1997 Jan 25; 314(7076): 299–301.
(BEHAVIOR CONTROL; FRAUD AND MISCONDUCT)

White, E. see **Ulrich, C.M.**

White, Gillian see **Briant, Robin H.**

White, Gladys B. Foresight, insight, oversight. [Symposium: human primordial stem cells]. *Hastings Center Report*. 1999 Mar–Apr; 29(2): 41–42.
(EMBRYO AND FETAL RESEARCH)

White, Ian see **Pocock, Stuart**

White, Mary Terrell. Guidelines for IRB review of international collaborative medical research: a proposal. *Journal of Law, Medicine and Ethics*. 1999 Spring; 27(1): 87–94.
(HUMAN EXPERIMENTATION/ETHICS COMMITTEES; HUMAN EXPERIMENTATION/FOREIGN COUNTRIES)

White, Mary Terrell. Making responsible decisions: an interpretive ethic for genetic decisionmaking. *Hastings Center Report*. 1999 Jan–Feb; 29(1): 14–21.
(GENETIC COUNSELING)

White, T. Michael see **Menendez, Roger**

Whitehead, Anne see **Koepp, Robert**

Whitehouse, Peter see **Kodish, Eric**

Whitehouse, Peter J. Bioethics, biology, *and* the biosphere: the ecomedical disconnection syndrome. *Hastings Center Report*. 1999 Jan–Feb; 29(1): 41–44.
(BIOETHICS)

Whitehouse, Peter J. see **Martin, Richard J.**

Whitehouse, Peter J. see **Post, Stephen G.**

Whitlow, Barry see **McFadyen, Anne**

Whitney, Simon N.; Spiegel, David. The patient, the physician, and the truth. [Case study and commentaries]. *Hastings Center Report*. 1999 May–Jun; 29(3): 24–25.
(TRUTH DISCLOSURE)

Whittington, Richard M. see **Cheng, Leo H.H.**

Wicclair, Mark R. The continuing debate over risk–related standards of competence. *Bioethics*. 1999 Apr; 13(2): 149–153.
(INFORMED CONSENT; TREATMENT REFUSAL)

Wicki, S. see **Müller, H.J.**

Widdershoven, Guy A.M. Euthanasia in the Netherlands: some first experiences of evaluation committees. [News]. *Hastings Center Report*. 1999 Jul–Aug; 29(4): 47–48.
(EUTHANASIA)

Wiesing, Urban. Individual rights and genetics: the historical perspective. A comment on Ruth Chadwick's paper. *In:* Chadwick, Ruth; Levitt, Mairi; Shickle, Darren, eds. The Right to Know and the Right Not to Know. Brookfield, VT: Ashgate; 1997: 23–27.
(EUGENICS)

Wiesing, Urban see **Chadwick, Ruth**

Wiesner, Russell H. see **Showstack, Jonathan**

Wiggins, S.; Green, T.; Adam, S.; Hayden, M.R. A long term (ca 5 years) prospective assessment of psychological consequences of predictive testing for Huntington disease (HD). [For the Canadian Collaborative Study of Predictive Testing]. *American Journal of Human Genetics*. 1996 Oct; 59(4): A7.
(GENETIC SCREENING)

Wikler, Daniel. Can we learn from eugenics? *Journal of Medical Ethics*. 1999 Apr; 25(2): 183–194.
(EUGENICS)

Wikler, Daniel; Marchand, Sarah. Macro–allocation: dividing up the health care budget. *In:* Kuhse, Helga; Singer, Peter, eds. A Companion to Bioethics. Malden, MA: Blackwell; 1998: 306–315.
(HEALTH CARE; RESOURCE ALLOCATION)

Wikler, Daniel see **Marchand, Sarah**

Wilcox, Allen J.; Taylor, Jack A.; Sharp, Richard R.; London, Stephanie J. Genetic determinism and the overprotection of human subjects. [Letter]. *Nature Genetics*. 1999 Apr; 21(4): 362.
(GENETIC RESEARCH; HUMAN EXPERIMENTATION/INFORMED CONSENT)

Wilcox, Hervey see **Limentani, Alexander E.**

Wilcox, W. Bradford see **Coburn, Tom**

Wilder, Bruce L. Ethical issues related to the new reproductive technologies. *Current Opinion in Obstetrics and Gynecology*. 1995 Jun; 7(3): 199–202.
(REPRODUCTIVE TECHNOLOGIES)

Wilder, Pauline see **Webb, Cynthia M.**

Wildes, Kevin W. Libertarianism and ownership of the human body. *In:* ten Have, Henk A.M.J.; Welie, Jos V.M., eds. Ownership of the Human Body: Philosophical Considerations on the Use of the Human Body and Its Parts in Healthcare. Boston, MA: Kluwer Academic; 1998: 143–157.
(BIOETHICS)

Wildman, Martin. Quality and the invisible man. [Personal view]. *BMJ (British Medical Journal)*. 1998 Dec 12; 317(7173): 1667.
(HEALTH CARE/ECONOMICS)

Wilfert, Catherine M.; Ammann, Arthur; Bayer, Ronald; Curran, James W.; del Rio, Carlos; Faden, Ruth R.; Feinberg, Mark B.; Karlin, Patricia Devine; Levine, Robert J.; Luo, Chewe; Sessions, Kimberly. Science, ethics, and the future of research into maternal infant transmission of HIV–1: Consensus statement. [For the Perinatal HIV Intervention Research in Developing Countries Workshop Participants].

Lancet. 1999 Mar 6; 353(9155): 832–835.
(AIDS/HUMAN EXPERIMENTATION; HUMAN
EXPERIMENTATION/FOREIGN COUNTRIES; HUMAN
EXPERIMENTATION/RESEARCH DESIGN; HUMAN
EXPERIMENTATION/SPECIAL POPULATIONS)

Wilfond, Benjamin S.; Rothenberg, Karen H.; Thomson, Elizabeth J.; Lerman, Caryn; U.S. National Institutes of Health. Cancer Genetics Studies Consortium. Cancer genetic susceptibility testing: ethical and policy implications for future research and clinical practice. *Journal of Law, Medicine and Ethics.* 1997 Winter; 25(4): 243–251.
(GENETIC COUNSELING; GENETIC SCREENING)

Wilkie, Andrew see **Thomas, Sandy**

Wilkie, Patricia. Ethical issues in qualitative research in palliative care. *Palliative Medicine.* 1997 Jul; 11(4): 321–324.
(BEHAVIORAL RESEARCH)

Wilkie, Tom. Genetics and insurance in Britain: why more than just the Atlantic divides the English-speaking nations. *Nature Genetics.* 1998 Oct; 20(2): 119–121.
(CONFIDENTIALITY; GENETIC SCREENING)

Wilkie, Tom see **Low, Lawrence**

Wilkinson, Martin; Moore, Andrew. Inducements revisited. *Bioethics.* 1999 Apr; 13(2): 114–130.
(HUMAN EXPERIMENTATION)

Wilkinson, Paul see **Barakat, Khalid**

Wilkinson, Stephen see **Sheldon, Sally**

Wilks, Ian. Asymmetrical competence. *Bioethics.* 1999 Apr; 13(2): 154–159.
(INFORMED CONSENT; TREATMENT REFUSAL)

Williams, Alan. Intergenerational equity: an exploration of the 'fair innings' argument. *Health Economics.* 1997 Mar–Apr; 6(2): 117–132.
(HEALTH CARE; RESOURCE ALLOCATION)

Williams, Alan; Evans, J. Grimley. Rationing health care by age: the case for [and] The case against. *BMJ (British Medical Journal).* 1997 Mar 15; 314(7083): 820–825.
(HEALTH CARE/FOREIGN COUNTRIES; PATIENT CARE/AGED; RESOURCE ALLOCATION; SELECTION FOR TREATMENT)

Williams, Edwina R.L. see **White, D.M.D.**

Williams, Elizabeth see **Webb, Cynthia M.**

Williams, L.; Harris, A.; Thompson, M.; Brayshaw, A. Consent to treatment by minors attending accident and emergency departments: guidelines. *Journal of Accident and Emergency Medicine.* 1997 Sep; 14(5): 286–289.
(INFORMED CONSENT/MINORS; TREATMENT REFUSAL/MINORS)

Williams, S. see **Houghton, D.J.**

Williams, Sankey see **Schulman, Kevin A.**

Williams, Walter W. see **Gordon, Todd E.**

Williamson, Charlotte. The rise of doctor–patient working groups. *BMJ (British Medical Journal).* 1998 Nov 14; 317(7169): 1374–1377.
(PATIENT CARE; PROFESSIONAL PATIENT RELATIONSHIP)

Williamson, Robert. Human reproductive cloning is unethical because it undermines autonomy: commentary on Savulescu. *Journal of Medical Ethics.* 1999 Apr; 25(2): 96–97.
(CLONING)

Williamson, Robert. What's 'new' about 'genetics'? [Editorial]. *Journal of Medical Ethics.* 1999 Apr; 25(2): 75–76.
(GENETIC RESEARCH)

Williamson, Robert see **Allen, Katrina**

Williamson, Robert see **Dodson, Michael**

Williamson, Robert see **Newson, Ainsley**

Wilmut, Ian. Dolly's false legacy. *Time.* 1999 Jan 11; 153(1): 74, 76–77.
(CLONING)

Wilson, Bruce E.; Reiner, William G. Management of intersex: a shifting paradigm. *Journal of Clinical Ethics.* 1998 Winter; 9(4): 360–369.
(PATIENT CARE/MINORS; TRUTH DISCLOSURE)

Wilson, James Q. see **Kass, Leon R.**

Wilson, Kenneth C.M. see **Agarwal, Manoj R.**

Wilson, Petra. The Law Commission's report on mental incapacity: medically vulnerable adults or politically vulnerable law? *Medical Law Review.* 1996 Autumn; 4(3): 227–249.
(ADVANCE DIRECTIVES; INFORMED CONSENT/MENTALLY DISABLED)

Wincze, John P.; Richards, Jeff; Parsons, John; Bailey, Susan. A comparative survey of therapist sexual misconduct between an American state and an Australian state. *Professional Psychology: Research and Practice.* 1996 Jun; 27(3): 289–294.
(FRAUD AND MISCONDUCT; PROFESSIONAL PATIENT RELATIONSHIP)

Wineberg, Howard. Oregon's Death with Dignity Act: ten months later. [Letter]. *Annals of Internal Medicine.* 1999 Mar 16; 130(6): 538.
(SUICIDE)

Winerip, Michael. Bedlam on the streets. *New York Times Magazine.* 1999 May 23: 42–49, 56, 65–66, 70.
(HEALTH CARE/ECONOMICS; PATIENT CARE/MENTALLY DISABLED)

Winerup, Michael. Fighting for Jacob [experimental gene therapy for Canavan disease]. *New York Times Magazine.* 1998 Dec 6: 56–63, 78, 80, 82, 112.
(GENE THERAPY; HUMAN EXPERIMENTATION/MINORS)

Wingerson, Lois. Unnatural Selection: The Promise and Power of Human Gene Research. New York, NY: Bantam Books; 1998. 399 p.
(GENETIC RESEARCH; GENETIC SCREENING; PRENATAL DIAGNOSIS)

Winick, Bruce J. Advance directive instruments for those with mental illness. *University of Miami Law Review.* 1996 Oct; 51(1): 57–95.
(ADVANCE DIRECTIVES)

Winkler, Mary G. Devices and desires of our own hearts. *In:* Parens, Erik, ed. Enhancing Human Traits: Ethical and Social Implications. Washington, DC: Georgetown University Press; 1998: 238–250.
(BIOMEDICAL TECHNOLOGIES)

Winter, Bob; Cohen, Simon. ABC of intensive care: withdrawal of treatment. *BMJ (British Medical Journal).* 1999 Jul 31; 319(7205): 306–308.
(ALLOWING TO DIE)

Winter, Robert J. see **Rubenstein, Jeffrey S.**

Wisconsin. Court of Appeals. Schreiber v. Physicians Insurance Company. *North Western Reporter, 2d Series.* 1998 Feb 17 (date of decision). 579: 730–739.
(INFORMED CONSENT)

Wisconsin. Supreme Court. Schreiber v. Physicians Insurance Company. *North Western Reporter, 2d Series.* 1999 Jan 26 (date of decision). 588: 26–35.
(INFORMED CONSENT)

Wise, Jacqui. Aricept advertisement breached code. [News]. *BMJ (British Medical Journal).* 1998 Sep 19; 317(7161): 766.
(PATIENT CARE/DRUGS)

Wise, Jacqui. Australian euthanasia law throws up many difficulties. [News]. *BMJ (British Medical Journal).* 1998 Oct 10; 317(7164): 969.
(EUTHANASIA/LEGAL ASPECTS)

Witte, Kim. The manipulative nature of health communication research: ethical issues and guidelines. *American Behavioral Scientist.* 1994 Nov; 38(2): 285–293.
(BEHAVIOR CONTROL; HEALTH CARE; PUBLIC HEALTH)

Wodak, Alex. Health, HIV infection, human rights, and injecting drug use. *Health and Human Rights.* 1998; 2(4): 24–41.
(AIDS; PUBLIC HEALTH)

Wohl, Mary Ellen see **Robinson, Walter M.**

Wohlfahrt, Jan see **Westergaard, Tine**

Wolf, Don P. see **De Jonge, Christopher J.**

Wolf, Eckhard see **Mepham, T. Ben**

Wolf, Susan M. Bioethics and law symposium: deconstructing traditional paradigms in bioethics: race, gender, class, and culture. Foreword: bioethics -- from mirror to window. *Saint Louis University Public Law Review.* 1996; 15(2): 183–189.
(BIOETHICS)

Wolf, Susan M. Erasing difference: race, ethnicity, and gender in bioethics. *In:* Donchin, Anne; Purdy, Laura M., eds. Embodying Bioethics: Recent Feminist Advances. Lanham, MD: Rowman and Littlefield; 1999: 65–81.
(BIOETHICS)

Wolf, Susan M. Shifting paradigms in bioethics and health

law: the rise of a new pragmatism. *American Journal of Law and Medicine.* 1994; 20(4): 395–415.
(BIOETHICS)

Wolfe, Amy K. see **Walsh, Marie E.**

Wolfe, Sidney M. see **Edi-Osagie, E.C.O.**

Wolfe, Sidney M. see **Lurie, Peter**

Wolfe, Sidney M. see **Merson, Michael H.**

Wolff, G. see **Nippert, I.**

Wolpe, Paul Root. Reply to Barbara Pfeffer Billauer's "On Judaism and genes." *Kennedy Institute of Ethics Journal.* 1999 Jun; 9(2): 167–174.
(BEHAVIORAL GENETICS)

Wolpe, Paul Root. The freelance bioethicist, chapter one. [Irony]. *Cambridge Quarterly of Healthcare Ethics.* 1999 Winter; 8(1): 118–119.
(ETHICISTS AND ETHICS COMMITTEES)

Wolpe, Paul Root see **Moreno, Jonathan**

Wolpert, Lewis. Is science dangerous? *Nature.* 1999 Mar 25; 398(6725): 281–282.
(BIOMEDICAL RESEARCH; GENETIC INTERVENTION; GENETIC RESEARCH)

Wong, Jeffrey G.; Nakchbandi, Inaam A.; Longenecker, J. Craig; Smith, David Gary. HIV testing in pregnant women. [Letter and response]. *Annals of Internal Medicine.* 1998 Dec 15; 129(12): 1075.
(AIDS/TESTING AND SCREENING)

Wong, Jeremy see **Khamsi, Firouz**

Wong, Josephine see **Holland, Anthony J.**

Wong, K.K. see **Cheng, F.**

Wong, Kenman L. Medicine and the Marketplace: The Moral Dimensions of Managed Care. Notre Dame, IN: University of Notre Dame Press; 1998. 219 p.
(HEALTH CARE/ECONOMICS)

Wong, Tina see **Hingorani, Melanie**

Wood, Erica; Karp, Naomi. Mediation: reframing care conflicts in nursing homes. *Generations (American Society on Aging).* 1994 Winter; 18(4): 54–57.
(PATIENT CARE/AGED)

Wooddell, Victor; Kaplan, Kalman J. An expanded typology of suicide, assisted suicide, and euthanasia. *Omega: A Journal of Death and Dying.* 1997–1998; 36(3): 219–226.
(ALLOWING TO DIE; EUTHANASIA; SUICIDE)

Woodman, Richard. BMA calls for extra safeguards for life and death decisions. [News]. *BMJ (British Medical Journal).* 1999 Jun 26; 318(7200): 1717.
(ALLOWING TO DIE)

Woolfrey, Joan see **Campbell, Courtney S.**

Woolhandler, Steffie see **Himmelstein, David U.**

Working Group on Prioritisation in Health Care (Finland). From Values to Choices: Report. Helsinki, Finland: National Research and Development Centre for Welfare and Health (STAKES); 1995. 78 p.
(HEALTH CARE/FOREIGN COUNTRIES; RESOURCE ALLOCATION)

Workman, Richard H.; Molinari, Victor; Rezabek, Pamela; McCullough, Laurence B.; Khalsa, Devi Kirin; Trivedi, Sandhya; Kunik, Mark E. An ethical framework for understanding patients with antisocial personality disorder who develop dementia: diagnosing and managing disorders of autonomy. *Journal of Ethics, Law, and Aging.* 1997 Fall–Winter; 3(2): 79–90.
(PATIENT CARE/AGED; PATIENT CARE/MENTALLY DISABLED)

Workman, Stephen see **Weijer, Charles**

World Health Organization. Hereditary Diseases Programme see **Wertz, Dorothy C.**

World Health Organization. Human Genetics Programme. Proposed International Guidelines on Ethical Issues in Medical Genetics and Genetic Services: Report of a WHO Meeting on Ethical Issues in Medical Genetics, Geneva, 15–16 December 1997. Geneva: World Health Organization; 1998. 15 p.
(GENETIC SERVICES)

World Medical Association. Proposed revision of the Declaration of Helsinki. *Bulletin of Medical Ethics.* 1999 Apr; No. 147: 18–22.
(HUMAN EXPERIMENTATION)

Worsham, G. Fred see **MacKay, Charles**

Wray, Samuel R.; Parshad, Omkar; Young, Lauriann E. Ethics and law in the medical curriculum -- a University of the West Indies perspective. *Medicine and Law.* 1993; 12(1–2): 41–45.
(MEDICAL ETHICS/EDUCATION)

Wright, Clinton see **Arnold, L. Eugene**

Wright, David E. The federal research misconduct regulations as viewed from the research universities. *Centennial Review.* 1994 Spring; 38(2): 249–272.
(BIOMEDICAL RESEARCH; FRAUD AND MISCONDUCT)

Wright, Robert. Who gets the good genes? *Time.* 1999 Jan 11; 153(1): 67.
(EUGENICS; GENETIC INTERVENTION)

Wright, Robert; Gorney, Cynthia; Silver, Lee M.; Coles, Robert; Bartholet, Elizabeth; Arnold, Lori. Fertility for sale. *New York Times.* 1998 Mar 4: A21.
(REPRODUCTIVE TECHNOLOGIES)

Wright, Stephen G. The distribution of resources in health care. *Professional Nurse (London).* 1996 Jun; 11(9): 583–586.
(HEALTH CARE/FOREIGN COUNTRIES; RESOURCE ALLOCATION)

Wronska, Irena; Gozdek, Nina. Aims and ethics of palliative care: the views of a selected group of Polish nursing students. *Scandinavian Journal of Caring Sciences.* 1994; 8(1): 25–27.
(TERMINAL CARE)

Wu, Albert W.; Cavanaugh, Thomas A.; McPhee, Stephen J.; Lo, Bernard; Micco, Guy P. To tell the truth: ethical and practical issues in disclosing medical mistakes to patients. *Journal of General Internal Medicine.* 1997 Dec; 12(12): 770–775.
(PATIENT CARE; TRUTH DISCLOSURE)

Wu, John; Sheil, A.G. Ross; Guttmann, Ronald D.; Santiago Delpin, Eduardo A.; Rothman, David J. Spare parts. [Letters and response]. *Sciences.* 1998 May/Jun; 38(3): 5, 8.
(ORGAN AND TISSUE DONATION)

WuDunn, Sheryl. Death taboo weakening, Japan sees 1st transplant. [News]. *New York Times.* 1999 Mar 1: A8.
(DETERMINATION OF DEATH/BRAIN DEATH; ORGAN AND TISSUE DONATION; ORGAN AND TISSUE TRANSPLANTATION)

Wuensch, Karl L.; Poteat, G. Michael. Evaluating the morality of animal research: effects of ethical ideology, gender, and purpose. *Journal of Social Behavior and Personality.* 1998 Mar; 13(1): 139–150.
(ANIMAL EXPERIMENTATION)

Wulff, Henrik R. Contemporary trends in healthcare ethics. *In:* ten Have, Henk A.M.J.; Sass, Hans–Martin, eds. Consensus Formation in Healthcare Ethics. Boston, MA: Kluwer Academic; 1998: 63–72.
(BIOETHICS)

Y

Yacowar, Mayer see **Druzin, Paul**

Yakir, Avi; Glick, Shimon M. Medical students' attitudes to the physician's oath. *Medical Education.* 1998 Mar; 32(2): 133–137.
(MEDICAL ETHICS/CODES OF ETHICS; MEDICAL ETHICS/EDUCATION)

Yamamoto, Loren G. Application of informed consent principles in the emergency department evaluation of febrile children at risk for occult bacteremia. *Hawaii Medical Journal.* 1997 Nov; 56(11): 313–317, 320–322.
(INFORMED CONSENT/MINORS)

Yan, W.W. see **Cheng, F.**

Yank, Veronica; Rennie, Drummond. Disclosure of researcher contributions: a study of original research articles in *The Lancet. Annals of Internal Medicine.* 1999 Apr 20; 130(8): 661–670.
(BIOMEDICAL RESEARCH)

Yank, Veronica see **Greenfield, Barak**

Yankauer, Alfred. The neglected lesson of the Tuskegee study. [Letter]. *American Journal of Public Health.* 1998 Sep; 88(9): 1406.
(FRAUD AND MISCONDUCT; HUMAN EXPERIMENTATION/SPECIAL POPULATIONS)

Yardley, Jim. Health officials investigating to determine how woman got the embryo of another. [News]. *New York Times.* 1999 Mar 31: B3.
(REPRODUCTIVE TECHNOLOGIES)

Yates, Anne see **Hope, R.A.**

Yates, R. Animal ethics committees and the implementation of the Three Rs. *In:* van Zutphen,

L.F.M.; Balls, M., eds. Animal Alternatives, Welfare and Ethics. New York, NY: Elsevier; 1997: 367–371.
(ANIMAL EXPERIMENTATION)

Yoder, Scot D. Experts in ethics? The nature of ethical expertise. *Hastings Center Report.* 1998 Nov–Dec; 28(6): 11–19.
(ETHICISTS AND ETHICS COMMITTEES)

Young, Alexey. Natural death and the work of perfection. *Christian Bioethics.* 1998 Aug; 4(2): 168–182.
(SUICIDE)

Young, Frank E. Worldviews in conflict: human cloning and embryo manipulation. *In:* Demy, Timothy J.; Stewart, Gary P., eds. Genetic Engineering: A Christian Response: Crucial Considerations in Shaping Life. Grand Rapids, MI: Kregel Publications; 1999: 70–86.
(CLONING; EMBRYO AND FETAL RESEARCH)

Young, Lauriann E. see **Wray, Samuel R.**

Young, Melissa see **Dworkin, Mark**

Young, Robert. Informed consent and patient autonomy. *In:* Kuhse, Helga; Singer, Peter, eds. A Companion to Bioethics. Malden, MA: Blackwell; 1998: 441–451.
(INFORMED CONSENT)

Young, Sally see **Thomas, Sandy**

Younggren, Jeffrey N. see **Fisher, Celia B.**

Youngner, Stuart see **Bartels, Dianne**

Youngner, Stuart J. Competence to refuse life–sustaining treatment. *In:* Steinberg, Maurice D.; Youngner, Stuart J., eds. End–of–Life Decisions: A Psychosocial Perspective. Washington, DC: American Psychiatric Press; 1998: 19–54.
(ALLOWING TO DIE; TREATMENT REFUSAL)

Youngner, Stuart J. Consultation–liaison psychiatry and clinical ethics: historical parallels and diversions. *Psychosomatics.* 1997 Jul–Aug; 38(4): 309–312.
(ETHICISTS AND ETHICS COMMITTEES)

Youngner, Stuart J. Medical futility. *Critical Care Clinics.* 1996 Jan; 12(1): 165–178.
(ALLOWING TO DIE)

Youngner, Stuart J.; Arnold, Robert M.; Schapiro, Renie, eds. The Definition of Death: Contemporary Controversies. Baltimore, MD: Johns Hopkins University Press; 1999.
(DETERMINATION OF DEATH; DETERMINATION OF DEATH/BRAIN DEATH)

Youngner, Stuart J. see **Aulisio, Mark P.**

Youngner, Stuart J. see **Meisel, Alan**

Youngner, Stuart J. see **Steinberg, Maurice D.**

Youngner, Stuart J. see **Werth, James L.**

Yu, Victor Y.H. Ethical decision–making in newborn infants. *Acta Medica Portuguesa.* 1997 Feb–Mar; 10(2–3): 197–204.
(ALLOWING TO DIE/INFANTS)

Yuan, Zong F.; Baume, Peter. Attitudes of Sydney Chinese to voluntary euthanasia. [Letter]. *Australian and New Zealand Journal of Public Health.* 1997 Feb; 21(1): 106–107.
(EUTHANASIA/ATTITUDES)

Yutzy, Sean H. see **Dinwiddie, Stephen H.**

Z

Zabow, Aubrey see **Jaworowski, Solomon**

Zakotnik, Branko see **Zwitter, Matjaz**

Zalcberg, John R.; Buchanan, John D. Clinical issues in euthanasia. [Editorial]. *Medical Journal of Australia.* 1997 Feb 3; 166(3): 150–152.
(EUTHANASIA; TERMINAL CARE)

Zallen, Doris Teichler. Does It Run in the Family? A Consumer's Guide to DNA Testing for Genetic Disorders. New Brunswick, NJ: Rutgers University Press; 1997. 201 p.
(GENETIC SCREENING)

Zametkin, Alan see **Arnold, L. Eugene**

Zaner, Richard M. Surprise! You're just like me! Reflections on cloning, eugenics, and other utopias. *In:* Humber, James M.; Almeder, Robert F.,eds. Human Cloning. Totowa, NJ: Humana Press; 1998: 103–151.
(CLONING)

Zaner, Richard M. see **Finder, Stuart G.**

Zanobio, Bruno. The ethical dimension of Hippocratic medicine and its specific relationship to Christian morality. *Dolentium Hominum: Church and Health in the World.* 1996; 31(11th Yr., No. 1): 29–32.
(MEDICAL ETHICS)

Zarin, Deborah A. see **Finestone, Albert J.**

Zaslavsky, Alan M. see **Kao, Audiey C.**

Zawacki, Bruce E. International bioethics at the bedside. [Editorial]. *Burns.* 1997 May; 23(3): iii–iv.
(ALLOWING TO DIE; PROFESSIONAL PATIENT RELATIONSHIP)

Zawacki, Bruce E. see **Starr, Joann**

Zawadowski, Andrew see **Crelinsten, Gordon L.**

Zayas, Luis H. see **Morrison, R. Sean**

Zechnich, Andrew D. see **Koenig, Kristi L.**

Zeitz, Kathleen see **Pokorski, Robert J.**

Zelas, Karen. Sex and the doctor–patient relationship. *New Zealand Medical Journal.* 1997 Feb 28; 110(1038): 60–62.
(FRAUD AND MISCONDUCT; PROFESSIONAL PATIENT RELATIONSHIP)

Zelenik, Jomarie; Post, Linda Farber; Mulvihill, Michael; Jacobs, Laurie G.; Burton, William B.; Dubler, Nancy Neveloff. The doctor–proxy relationship: perception and communication. *Journal of Law, Medicine and Ethics.* 1999 Spring; 27(1): 13–19.
(ADVANCE DIRECTIVES; INFORMED CONSENT)

Zelicoff, Alan P. see Tokuda, Yasuharu

Zemer, Moshe. Determining death in Jewish law. *In:* Jacob, Walter; Zemer, Moshe, eds. Death and Euthanasia in Jewish Law: Essays and Responsa. Pittsburgh, PA: Freehof Institute of Progressive Halakhah; Rodef Shalom Press; 1995: 105–119.
(DETERMINATION OF DEATH)

Zemer, Moshe see Jacob, Walter

Zetterman, Rowen K. see Showstack, Jonathan

Zhou, Xiao-Hua see Gramelspacher, Gregory P.

Ziman, John M. Why must scientists become more ethically sensitive than they used to be? *Science.* 1998 Dec 4; 282(5395): 1813–1814.
(BIOMEDICAL RESEARCH; PROFESSIONAL ETHICS)

Zimbelman, Joel see White, Becky Cox

Zimmerman, Sheryl Itkin see Hoffmann, Diane E.

Zimmern, R.L. Genetic testing: a conceptual exploration. *Journal of Medical Ethics.* 1999 Apr; 25(2): 151–156.
(GENETIC SCREENING)

Zimran, A. see Elstein, D.

Zinko, Ursula see van der Valk, Jan

Zion, Deborah. Ethical considerations of clinical trials to prevent vertical transmission of HIV in developing countries. *Nature Medicine.* 1998 Jan; 4(1): 11–12.
(AIDS/HUMAN EXPERIMENTATION; HUMAN EXPERIMENTATION/FOREIGN COUNTRIES; HUMAN EXPERIMENTATION/RESEARCH DESIGN; HUMAN EXPERIMENTATION/SPECIAL POPULATIONS)

Zion, Deborah see Mann, Jonathan M.

Zlatnik, Gail P. see Beller, Fritz K.

Zola, John see Cutter, Mary Ann G.

Zook, Eric G. see Gordon, Todd E.

Zuccaro, Stefano Maria; Palleschi, Massimo; Italian Society of Hospital Geriatricians. Document on the rights of the sick elderly. *Dolentium Hominum: Church and Health in the World.* 1997; 36(12th Yr., No. 3): 32–35.
(HEALTH CARE/RIGHTS; PATIENT CARE/AGED; PATIENTS' RIGHTS)

Zuckerman, Connie. Clinical ethics in geriatric care settings. *Generations (American Society on Aging).* 1994 Winter; 18(4): 9–12.
(BIOETHICS; PATIENT CARE/AGED)

Zuckerman, Connie see Levine, Carol

Zuger, Abigail. Doctors' offices turn into salesrooms. [News]. *New York Times.* 1999 Mar 30: F1, F11.
(HEALTH CARE/ECONOMICS; PATIENT CARE/DRUGS)

Zungu, Busie Maya see Kunene, Sibusiso Sixtus

Zurlo, Joanne; Goldberg, Alan M. The role of an academic center in promoting common goals. *Cambridge Quarterly of Healthcare Ethics.* 1999 Winter; 8(1): 58–63.

(ANIMAL EXPERIMENTATION)

Zurlo, Joanne see van der Valk, Jan

Zusman, Jack. Restraint and Seclusion: Improving Practice and Conquering the JCAHO Standards. Marblehead, MA: Opus Communications; 1997. 198 p.
(PATIENT CARE)

Zwart, Hub. Moral deliberation and moral warfare: consensus formation in a pluralistic society. *In:* ten Have, Henk A.M.J.; Sass, Hans-Martin, eds. Consensus Formation in Healthcare Ethics. Boston, MA: Kluwer Academic; 1998: 73–91.
(BIOETHICS)

Zwart, Hub A.E. Why should remunerated blood donation be unethical? Ethical reflections on current blood donation policies and their philosophical origins. *In:* ten Have, Henk A.M.J.; Welie, Jos V.M., eds. Ownership of the Human Body: Philosophical Considerations on the Use of the Human Body and Its Parts in Healthcare. Boston, MA: Kluwer Academic; 1998: 39–48.
(BLOOD DONATION)

Zweig, Franklin M.; Walsh, Joseph T.; Freeman, Daniel M. Adjudicating neurogenetics at the crossroads: privacy, adoption, and the death sentence. *Judges' Journal.* 1997 Summer; 36(3): 52–55, 57–58, 90–93.
(BEHAVIORAL GENETICS; CONFIDENTIALITY/LEGAL ASPECTS; GENETIC SCREENING)

Zweig, Steven C. An alternate policy for CPR in nursing homes. *Bioethics Forum.* 1998 Spring; 14(1): 5–11.
(RESUSCITATION ORDERS)

Zweig, Steven C. Cardiopulmonary resuscitation and do-not-resuscitate orders in the nursing home. *Archives of Family Medicine.* 1997 Sep-Oct; 6(5): 424–429.
(RESUSCITATION ORDERS)

Zwelling-Aamot, Marcy L. see Menendez, Roger

Zwier, Paul J. Looking for a nonlegal process: physician-assisted suicide and the care perspective. *University of Richmond Law Review.* 1996 Jan; 30(1): 199–248.
(SUICIDE)

Zwitter, Matjaz; Nilstun, Tore; Knudsen, Lisbeth E.; Zakotnik, Branko; Klocker, Johann; Bremberg, Stefan; Frentz, Gerda; Klocker-Kaiser, Ursula; Pedersen, Jette. Professional and public attitudes towards unsolicited medical intervention. *BMJ (British Medical Journal).* 1999 Jan 23; 318(7178): 251–253.
(PATIENT CARE)

ANONYMOUS

A better death in Oregon. [Editorial]. *New York Times.* 1998 Mar 28: A14.
(SUICIDE)

A birth spurs debate on using sperm after death. [Editorial]. *New York Times.* 1999 Mar 27: All.
(INFORMED CONSENT; REPRODUCTION; REPRODUCTIVE TECHNOLOGIES)

A duty to publish. [Editorial]. *Nature Medicine.* 1998 Oct;

4(10): 1089.
(BIOMEDICAL RESEARCH)

A suicide tape on TV inflames the issue in Spain. [News]. *New York Times.* 1998 Mar 9: A9.
(SUICIDE)

A suitable case for treatment. [Editorial]. *Nature.* 1999 May 20; 399(6733): 183.
(FRAUD AND MISCONDUCT; HUMAN EXPERIMENTATION/REGULATION)

Adult cloning marches on. [Editorial]. *Nature.* 1998 Jul 23; 394(6691): 303.
(CLONING)

Advance directive; notification; negligence; life prolongation; damages -- Allore v. Flower Hospital. *Mental and Physical Disability Law Reporter.* 1997 Sep-Oct; 21(5): 597.
(ADVANCE DIRECTIVES; ALLOWING TO DIE/LEGAL ASPECTS)

Alberta to compensate victims of sterilization. [News]. *New York Times.* 1998 Jun 6: A6.
(STERILIZATION/MENTALLY DISABLED)

All too human. [News]. *Science.* 1999 Apr 2; 284(5411): 21.
(HUMAN EXPERIMENTATION/FOREIGN COUNTRIES)

An organ donation offer on death row is refused. [News]. *New York Times.* 1998 Sep 9: A23.
(CAPITAL PUNISHMENT; ORGAN AND TISSUE DONATION)

An uncalculated risk. [Editorial]. *New Scientist.* 1997 Oct 18; 156(2104): 3.
(ORGAN AND TISSUE TRANSPLANTATION)

Appendix 2: EUROSCREEN survey of attitudes to the genetic testing of children among members of the European Society of Human Genetics. *In:* Clarke, Angus, ed. The Genetic Testing of Children. Washington, DC: BIOS Scientific Publishers; 1998: 321-328.
(GENETIC SCREENING)

Assisted suicide, at state discretion. [Editorial]. *New York Times.* 1998 Jun 8: A20.
(SUICIDE)

Assisted suicide, in practice. [Editorial]. *New York Times.* 1999 Feb 27: A14.
(SUICIDE)

Australian call for repeal of restrictive cloning laws. [News]. *Nature.* 1999 Apr 15; 398(6728): 552.
(CLONING)

Banking Our Genes: DNA Data on the Information Highway. [Videorecording]. Boston, MA: Fanlight Productions; 1995. 1 videocassette; 33 min.; sd.; color; VHS.
(DNA FINGERPRINTING; GENETIC SCREENING)

Blood tests of workers restricted by court. [News]. *New York Times.* 1998 Feb 5: A19.
(GENETIC SCREENING; MASS SCREENING)

Can ELSI's principles inform consensus? [Editorial]. *Nature Biotechnology.* 1996 Jun; 14(6): 677.
(GENETIC RESEARCH; GENETIC SCREENING)

China's 'eugenics' law still disturbing despite relabelling.

[Editorial]. *Nature.* 1998 Aug 20; 394(6695): 707.
(EUGENICS)

Churches condemn plan to clone humans. [News]. *Christian Science Monitor.* 1998 Jan 13: 13.
(CLONING)

Clinic plans to destroy unclaimed embryos. [News]. *New York Times.* 1999 Jul 13: F14.
(FETUSES; IN VITRO FERTILIZATION)

Cloning a human cell. [Editorial]. *New York Times.* 1998 Dec 18: A34.
(CLONING)

Court rules that fetuses are not "persons" entitled to be counted in the census: John Desmond Slattery v. William J. Clinton and William M. Daley, et al. (U.S. District Court, Southern District of New York, 1997). [News]. *Reporter on Human Reproduction and the Law.* 1997 Nov-Dec; No. 11-12: 62-63.
(FETUSES; PERSONHOOD)

Court says mother has right to stop HIV drugs for son. *AIDS Policy and Law.* 1998 Oct 2; 13(18): 1, 4-5.
(AIDS; TREATMENT REFUSAL/MINORS)

Cultural reaction. [Editorial]. *New Scientist.* 1998 Oct 24; 160(2157): 3.
(EUGENICS)

Current European laws on gamete donation. *Human Reproduction.* 1998 May; 13(Suppl. 2): 105-134.
(ORGAN AND TISSUE DONATION; REPRODUCTIVE TECHNOLOGIES)

Declaration of Helsinki -- nothing to declare? [Editorial]. *Lancet.* 1999 Apr 17; 353(9161): 1285.
(HUMAN EXPERIMENTATION)

Detention of potentially dangerous people. [Editorial]. *Lancet.* 1998 Nov 21; 352(9141): 1641.
(INVOLUNTARY COMMITMENT/FOREIGN COUNTRIES)

DNA testing proposals. [Editorial]. *New York Times.* 1998 Dec 17: A32.
(DNA FINGERPRINTING)

Do-not-resuscitate order; public school -- ABC School and DEF School v. Mr. and Mrs. M. *Mental and Physical Disability Law Reporter.* 1997 Nov-Dec; 21(6): 735.
(RESUSCITATION ORDERS; TREATMENT REFUSAL/MINORS)

Does biomedical research need another moratorium? [Editorial]. *Nature Medicine.* 1998 Feb; 4(2): 131.
(ORGAN AND TISSUE TRANSPLANTATION)

Don't die of recklessness. [Editorial]. *New Scientist.* 1997 Oct 4; 156(2102): 3.
(HUMAN EXPERIMENTATION/SPECIAL POPULATIONS)

Dr. Kevorkian's luck runs out. [Editorial]. *New York Times.* 1999 Mar 27: A16.
(EUTHANASIA/LEGAL ASPECTS)

Duty to warn; negligence; AIDS/HIV; surgeon: Doe v. Noe. *Mental and Physical Disability Law Reporter.* 1998 Mar-Apr; 22(2): 250.
(AIDS/HEALTH PERSONNEL)

EC ethics group established. [News]. *Nature Biotechnology.* 1998 Feb; 16(2): 121.

(ETHICISTS AND ETHICS COMMITTEES; GENETIC INTERVENTION)

Educational resources: finding bioethics journal literature. *NCCE News (Veterans Health Administration National Center for Clinical Ethics)*. 1994 Fall; 2(4): 8.
(BIOETHICS)

Effort to increase child immunization is under attack in Idaho. [News]. *New York Times*. 1999 Mar 7: 25.
(IMMUNIZATION)

Employment entrance exam; genetic/medical tests; applicants' consent; statute of limitations: Norman–Bloodsaw v. Lawrence Berkeley Lab. *Mental and Physical Disability Law Reporter*. 1998 Mar–Apr; 22(2): 233.
(GENETIC SCREENING)

European Group on Ethics in Science and New Technologies. [News]. *Journal of Medical Ethics*. 1998 Aug; 24(4): 247.
(BIOETHICS; ETHICISTS AND ETHICS COMMITTEES)

Euthanasia study challenged. *American Nurses Association Center for Ethics and Human Rights Communique*. 1996 Spring; 5(1): 6.
(EUTHANASIA; SUICIDE)

Fasten your seatbelts. [Editorial]. *New Scientist*. 1997 Dec 6; 156(2111): 3.
(REPRODUCTIVE TECHNOLOGIES)

First principles in cloning. [Editorial]. *Lancet*. 1999 Jan 9; 353(9147): 81.
(CLONING)

Florida tries DNA sampling to protect children. [News]. *New York Times*. 1999 Jan 27: A14.
(DNA FINGERPRINTING)

French public say 'non' to modified organisms. [News]. *Nature*. 1998 Oct 22; 395(6704): 736.
(GENETIC INTERVENTION)

Gene therapy and the germline. [Editorial]. *Nature Medicine*. 1999 Mar; 5(3): 245.
(GENE THERAPY)

Genome Vikings. [Editorial]. *Nature Genetics*. 1998 Oct; 20(2): 99–101.
(GENETIC RESEARCH)

GM foods debate needs a recipe for restoring trust. [Editorial]. *Nature*. 1999 Apr 22; 398(6729): 639.
(GENETIC INTERVENTION)

Government sets up enquiry into adequacy of research controls in North Staffordshire. [News]. *Bulletin of Medical Ethics*. 1999 Feb; No. 145: 3–4.
(HUMAN EXPERIMENTATION/FOREIGN COUNTRIES; HUMAN EXPERIMENTATION/INFORMED CONSENT; HUMAN EXPERIMENTATION/MINORS)

Guidelines issued on assisted suicide. [News]. *New York Times*. 1998 Mar 4: A15.
(SUICIDE)

Health care in America: your money or your life. *Economist*. 1998 Mar 7–13; 346(8058): 23–24, 26.
(HEALTH CARE/ECONOMICS)

Hello, Dolly. [Editorial]. *Economist*. 1997 Mar 1: 17–18.

(CLONING)

Helsinki Declaration revising continues. [News]. *Bulletin of Medical Ethics*. 1999 Mar; No. 146: 3–5.
(HUMAN EXPERIMENTATION)

Hospital failed on human research policy. [News]. *Science*. 1998 Nov 6; 282(5391): 1035.
(HUMAN EXPERIMENTATION/ETHICS COMMITTEES; HUMAN EXPERIMENTATION/REGULATION)

Improving access to organs. [Editorial]. *New York Times*. 1999 Jul 26: A14.
(ORGAN AND TISSUE TRANSPLANTATION; RESOURCE ALLOCATION/BIOMEDICAL TECHNOLOGIES)

In your face: if the idea of a hand transplant seems hard to take, just wait.... [Editorial]. *New Scientist*. 1998 Oct 3; 160(2154): 3.
(ORGAN AND TISSUE TRANSPLANTATION)

Institutionalised racism in health care. [Editorial]. *Lancet*. 1999 Mar 6; 353(9155): 765.
(HEALTH CARE)

International Conference on Harmonisation of Technical Requirements for Registration of Pharmaceuticals for Human Use (ICH) adopts Consolidated Guideline on Good Clinical Practice in the Conduct of Clinical Trials on Medicinal Products for Human Use. [Introduction and Sections 2 and 3 of the Consolidated Guideline]. *International Digest of Health Legislation*. 1997; 48(2): 231–234.
(HUMAN EXPERIMENTATION/FOREIGN COUNTRIES; HUMAN EXPERIMENTATION/REGULATION)

Jail time for Dr. Kevorkian. [Editorial]. *New York Times*. 1999 Apr 15: A30.
(EUTHANASIA/LEGAL ASPECTS)

Japan bans human cloning. [News]. *Nature Biotechnology*. 1998 Sep; 16(9): 803.
(CLONING)

Judge orders divorcing couple's frozen embryos destroyed. [News]. *New York Times*. 1998 Sep 29: B6.
(FETUSES; IN VITRO FERTILIZATION)

Kevorkian offers organs in assisted–suicide case. [News]. *New York Times*. 1998 Jun 8: A18.
(ORGAN AND TISSUE DONATION; SUICIDE)

Legislative insurance against genetic discrimination is insurance for biotechnology. [Editorial]. *Nature Biotechnology*. 1996 May; 14(5): 547.
(GENETIC SCREENING)

Making Babies: A Frontline Television Program. [Videorecording]. Available from PBS Home Video, 1320 Braddock Pl., Alexandria, VA 22314; 1–800–328–PBS1; 1999. Videocassette; 58 min.; sd.; color; VHS.
(REPRODUCTIVE TECHNOLOGIES)

Misguided chauvinisim on organs. [Editorial]. *New York Times*. 1999 Mar 12: A22.
(ORGAN AND TISSUE TRANSPLANTATION; RESOURCE ALLOCATION/BIOMEDICAL TECHNOLOGIES)

Miss Evers' Boys. [Videorecording; "based on the true story of the infamous Tuskegee Experiment"]. New York, NY: HBO Home Video; 1997. 1 videocassette; 118 min.; sd.; color; VHS.
(FRAUD AND MISCONDUCT; HUMAN

EXPERIMENTATION/SPECIAL POPULATIONS)

NIH peer review: time for some changes. [Editorial]. *Nature Biotechnology.* 1998 May; 16(5): 395.
(BIOMEDICAL RESEARCH)

No ABA embryo policy. [News]. *Washington Post.* 1998 Feb 3: A5.
(FETUSES; IN VITRO FERTILIZATION)

Oregon lets state pay for suicides. [News]. *New York Times.* 1998 Feb 27: A10.
(SUICIDE)

Organisation of African Unity adopts resolution on bioethics. [Text of resolution]. *International Digest of Health Legislation.* 1997; 48(2): 239–240.
(BIOETHICS)

Partner notification for H.I.V. [Editorial]. *New York Times.* 1998 Jun 9: A20.
(AIDS/CONFIDENTIALITY)

Patients for hire, doctors for sale. [Editorial]. *New York Times.* 1999 May 22: A12.
(HUMAN EXPERIMENTATION; PATIENT CARE/DRUGS)

Patients or profits? *Economist.* 1998 Mar 7–13; (346)8058: 15.
(HEALTH CARE/ECONOMICS)

Paying for family planning. [Editorial]. *Lancet.* 1998 Sep 12; 352(9131): 831.
(CONTRACEPTION)

Physician–patient privilege; depression; alcoholism: McCormick v. England. *Mental and Physical Disability Law Reporter.* 1998 Mar–Apr; 22(2): 235–236.
(CONFIDENTIALITY/LEGAL ASPECTS)

Pig in the middle: a moratorium on clinical trials of animal transplantation is justified. [Editorial]. *Nature.* 1999 Jan 28; 397(6717): 279.
(HUMAN EXPERIMENTATION/REGULATION; ORGAN AND TISSUE TRANSPLANTATION)

Policy on papers' contributors. [Editorial]. *Nature.* 1999 Jun 3; 399(6735): 393.
(BIOMEDICAL RESEARCH; FRAUD AND MISCONDUCT)

Privacy matters. [Editorial]. *Nature Genetics.* 1998 Jul; 19(3): 207–208.
(CONFIDENTIALITY; GENETIC RESEARCH; HUMAN EXPERIMENTATION/INFORMED CONSENT)

Research guidelines issued for persons with mental disorders and impaired capacity to make decisions. [News]. *Psychiatric Services.* 1999 Jan; 50(1): 128–129.
(HUMAN EXPERIMENTATION/SPECIAL POPULATIONS)

Research involving human subjects: efforts to resolve current ethical controversies. [Introduction to a set of documents, p. S:279–S:348]. *In:* BioLaw: A Legal and Ethical Reporter of Medicine, Health Care, and Bioengineering. Special Sections 2(7–8). Frederick, MD: University Publications of America; 1998 Jul–Aug: S:241–S:277.
(HUMAN EXPERIMENTATION/ETHICS COMMITTEES; HUMAN EXPERIMENTATION/SPECIAL POPULATIONS)

Some demented patients are still able to execute advance directives. [News]. *Geriatrics.* 1996 Jul; 51(7): 23.
(ADVANCE DIRECTIVES)

Special section: organ transplantation: shaping policy and keeping public trust. [Bibliography]. *Cambridge Quarterly of Healthcare Ethics.* 1999 Summer; 8(3): 348–350.
(ORGAN AND TISSUE DONATION; ORGAN AND TISSUE TRANSPLANTATION)

State funding and data disclosure. [Editorial]. *Lancet.* 1999 Mar 27; 353(9158): 1027.
(BIOMEDICAL RESEARCH)

Surviving misconduct is one thing, accountability is another. [Editorial]. *Nature.* 1998 Oct 22; 395(6704): 727.
(BIOMEDICAL RESEARCH; FRAUD AND MISCONDUCT)

Sweden plans to pay sterilization victims. [News]. *New York Times.* 1999 Jan 27: A8.
(STERILIZATION)

Swimming or drowning? Can Iceland show the world how to commercialise a gene pool? [Editorial]. *New Scientist.* 1998 Dec 5; 160(2163): 3.
(GENETIC RESEARCH)

Taking stock of scientific fraud. [Editorial]. *Nature Biotechnology.* 1998 May; 16(5): 395.
(BIOMEDICAL RESEARCH; FRAUD AND MISCONDUCT)

Testing new drugs: joining a study can be rewarding -- but risky [and] How to find -- and survive -- a clinical trial. *Consumer Reports.* 1998 Dec; 63(12): 64–65.
(HUMAN EXPERIMENTATION)

The euthanasia war: last rights -- human beings do not start their own life; do they have the right to invite a doctor to end it? The pros and cons of doctor–assisted suicide. *Economist.* 1997 Jun 21; 343(8022): 21–24.
(EUTHANASIA; SUICIDE)

The Farmington Consensus. *Alcohol and Alcoholism.* 1998 Jan–Feb; 33(1): 6–8.
(BIOMEDICAL RESEARCH)

The great divide? [Editorial]. *New Scientist.* 1999 Feb 13; 161(2173): 3.
(ANIMAL EXPERIMENTATION)

The Lynchburg Story: Eugenic Sterilization in America. [Videorecording]. New York, NY: Filmakers Library; 1994. 1 videocassette; 55 min.; sd.; color; VHS.
(EUGENICS; STERILIZATION/MENTALLY DISABLED)

The need of the many ... when individuals suffer for the sake of society we must compensate them properly. [Editorial]. *New Scientist.* 1998 Mar 7; 157(2124): 3.
(IMMUNIZATION)

The perils of paediatric research. [Editorial]. *Lancet.* 1999 Feb 27; 353(9154): 685.
(FRAUD AND MISCONDUCT; HUMAN EXPERIMENTATION/FOREIGN COUNTRIES; HUMAN EXPERIMENTATION/INFORMED CONSENT; HUMAN EXPERIMENTATION/MINORS)

The right to choose to die. [Editorial]. *Economist.* 1997 Jun 21; 343(8022): 15–16.
(SUICIDE)

Time to lift embryo research ban. [Editorial]. *Nature.* 1998 Nov 12; 396(6707): 97.
(EMBRYO AND FETAL RESEARCH)

Too much of a good thing. [Editorial]. *New York Times.*

1998 Dec 23: A26.
(REPRODUCTIVE TECHNOLOGIES)

Towards the acceptance of embryo stem–cell therapies. [Editorial]. *Nature.* 1999 Jan 28; 397(6717): 279.
(EMBRYO AND FETAL RESEARCH)

Treatment; transsexualism; equal protection; deliberate indifference: Farmer v. Hawk. *Mental and Physical Disability Law Reporter.* 1998 Mar–Apr; 22(2): 174.
(HEALTH CARE/RIGHTS)

United Kingdom Government publishes response to House of Lords report on medical ethics. [Summary of *Government Response to the Report of the Select Committee on Medical Ethics*, presented to Parliament by command of Her Majesty, May 1994]. *International Digest of Health Legislation.* 1995; 46(4): 570–572.
(ALLOWING TO DIE; EUTHANASIA; SUICIDE; TERMINAL CARE)

Unneccessary Fuss. [Videorecording]. Available from People for the Ethical Treatment of Animals (PETA), P.O. Box 42516, Washington, DC 20015–0516, (202) 726–0156, (301) 770–7444.; 1985. Videocassette; 26 min.; sd.; color; VHS.
(ANIMAL EXPERIMENTATION; FRAUD AND MISCONDUCT)

What price perfection? [Editorial]. *New Scientist.* 1997 Feb 22; 153(2070): 3.
(EUGENICS; GENETIC SCREENING; PRENATAL DIAGNOSIS)

When mental patients are at risk. [Editorial]. *New York Times.* 1999 Mar 31: A24.
(FRAUD AND MISCONDUCT; HUMAN EXPERIMENTATION/REGULATION; HUMAN EXPERIMENTATION/SPECIAL POPULATIONS)

Where next on misconduct? [Editorial]. *Nature.* 1999 Mar 4; 398(6722): 1.
(BIOMEDICAL RESEARCH; FRAUD AND MISCONDUCT)

WHO steps closer to its responsibilities. [Editorial]. *Nature.* 1999 Mar 18; 398(6724): 175.
(BIOETHICS; BIOMEDICAL RESEARCH)

Wisconsin abortion law allowed to stand. [News]. *New York Times.* 1998 May 20: A15.
(ABORTION/LEGAL ASPECTS)

World Medical Association adopts statements, etc., on miscellaneous matters. [Texts of statements and declarations]. *International Digest of Health Legislation.* 1997; 48(1): 92–97.
(CONTRACEPTION; HUMAN EXPERIMENTATION; PATIENT CARE/DRUGS)

World Psychiatric Association approves Declaration of Madrid (25 Aug 1996). [Texts of the Declaration of Madrid and of related Guidelines Concerning Specific Situations]. *International Digest of Health Legislation.* 1997; 48(2): 240–242.
(MEDICAL ETHICS/CODES OF ETHICS)

Xenotransplant caution continues. [Editorial]. *Nature.* 1999 Apr 15; 398(6728): 543.
(ORGAN AND TISSUE TRANSPLANTATION)

Xenotransplantation and the "yuk" factor. [Editorial]. *Nature Biotechnology.* 1996 Apr; 14(4): 403–404.
(ORGAN AND TISSUE TRANSPLANTATION)

Xenotransplantation: International Policy Issues. Paris, France: Organisation for Economic Co–operation and Development; 1999. 114 p.
(ORGAN AND TISSUE TRANSPLANTATION)